CRITICAL CARE MEDICINE

PERIOPERATIVE MANAGEMENT

SECOND EDITION

CRITICAL CARE MEDICINE

PERIOPERATIVE MANAGEMENT

SECOND EDITION

Editors

MICHAEL J. MURRAY, M.D., Ph.D.
Dean, Mayo School of Health Sciences
Professor and Chair, Department of Anesthesiology
Mayo Clinic and Foundation
Jacksonville, Florida

DOUGLAS B. COURSIN, M.D.
Professor
Associate Director, Trauma and Life Support Center
Departments of Anesthesiology and Internal Medicine
University of Wisconsin School of Medicine
Madison, Wisconsin

RONALD G. PEARL, M.D., Ph.D.
Professor and Chairman
Department of Anesthesia
Stanford University School of Medicine
Stanford, California

DONALD S. PROUGH, M.D.
Professor and Chair
Department of Anesthesiology
The University of Texas Medical Branch
Galveston, Texas

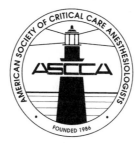

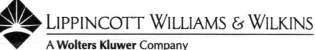

LIPPINCOTT WILLIAMS & WILKINS
A **Wolters Kluwer** Company

Philadelphia ▪ Baltimore ▪ New York ▪ London
Buenos Aires ▪ Hong Kong ▪ Sydney ▪ Tokyo

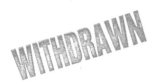

Acquisitions Editor: R. Craig Percy
Developmental Editor: Sonya L. Seigafuse
Production Editor: Robin E. Cook
Manufacturing Manager: Tim Reynolds
Cover Designer: Mark Lerner
Compositor: TechBooks
Printer: Maple Press

© 2002 by LIPPINCOTT WILLIAMS & WILKINS
530 Walnut Street
Philadelphia, PA 19106 USA
LWW.com

Printed in the USA.

Library of Congress Cataloging-in-Publication Data

Critical care medicine : perioperative management / editors, Michael J. Murray . . .
    [et al.]; American Society of Critical Anesthesiologists.—2nd ed.
        p. ; cm.
Includes bibliographical references and index.
ISBN 0-7817-2968-8
1. Critical care medicine.   I. Murray, Michael J. (Michael James), 1949–
II. American Society of Critical Care Anesthesiologists.
[DNLM: 1. Critical Care—methods. 2. Critical Illness. 3. Perioperative Care.
WX 218 C9361 2002]

RC86.7 .C743   2002
616′.028—dc21

                                        2001050525

                    10 9 8 7 6 5 4 3 2 1

To our families . . .

Drew, Marti, B and B, DRC and in memory of Robb W. Coursin—Douglas Coursin
Elise, Tess, Jennie, Karl, Greg, and Cate—Michael Murray
Mary C. Dunn, Jeremy and Nathan Pearl—Ronald Pearl
My wife Betty, my son Stephen, and my daughter Emily—Donald Prough

To our Patients and their Families, and to our colleagues who helped us care for them

CONTENTS

Contributing Authors xi
Preface xix
Acknowledgments xxi

SECTION I: PERIOPERATIVE ASSESSMENT AND ICU ORGANIZATION

1 Preoperative Assessment 1
Lee A. Fleisher and Stanley H. Rosenbaum

2 Intensive Care Unit Organization: Management, Staffing, and Ensuring Quality-of-Care 15
Neal H. Cohen

3 The Practice of Acute Care Medicine in Community Hospitals 29
Gerald A. Maccioli and Vincent L. Hoellerich

4 Ethical and End-of-Life Issues 45
Karen J. Schwenzer

SECTION II: PERIOPERATIVE INTERVENTIONS AND PATHOPHYSIOLOGY

5 Evidence-Based Medicine 55
Dan Connor, Jennifer Bayne, and William J. Sibbald

6 Genomics in Perioperative Critical Care 63
Kirk Hogan

7 Research in Critical Care Medicine 70
Anand Kumar, James E. Calvin, and Joseph E. Parrillo

8 Medical Informatics in the Intensive Care Unit 80
Keith Ruskin

9 Management of the Airway and Tracheal Intubation 89
Michael F. O'Connor and Andranik Ovassapian

10 Procedures in the Intensive Care Unit 102
Sylvia Y. Dolinski, Leanne Groban, and John Butterworth

11 Hemodynamic Assessment in the Critically Ill Patient 122
Jeffery S. Vender and Joseph W. Szokol

12 Fluid Management in Critically Ill Patients 137
Donald S. Prough and Mali Mathru

13 Sedative, Analgesic, and Neuromuscular Blocking Drugs 147
Christopher C. Young and Richard C. Prielipp

14 Surgical Considerations in the Intensive Care Unit 168
Michael S. Malian and Charles E. Lucas

15 Nutrition Support in the Critically Ill Patient 176
Michael J. Murray and Douglas W. Wilmore

16 Application of Pharmacokinetic and Pharmacodynamic Principles in Critically Ill Patients 186
Michael A. Duncan, Niamh McMahon, and Edmund G. Carton

17 Etiology and Pathophysiology of Shock 192
Robert M. Rodriguez and Myer H. Rosenthal

18 Diagnosis and Management of Acid–Base and Electrolyte Abnormalities 206
Donald S. Prough, Mali Mathru, and John D. Lang

SECTION III: NEUROLOGIC CRITICAL CARE

19 Principles of Cerebroprotection 225
Mark I. Rossberg, Anish Bhardwaj, Patricia D. Hurn, and Jeffrey R. Kirsch

20 Intensive Care Unit Management of Patients With Head and Spinal Cord Injury 236
Steven J. Allen

21 Diagnosis and Management of Comatose Patients in the Intensive Care Unit 244
Thomas P. Bleck

22 Postoperative Care of the Neurosurgical Patient 253
Patricia H. Petrozza

23 Subarachnoid Hemorrhage and Cerebrovascular Accident 264
Lauren C. Berkow, Marek Mirski, and Jeffrey R. Kirsch

24 The Diagnosis and Management of Brain-Dead and Nonheart-Beating Organ Donors 275
Jeffrey S. Plotkin, Megumi Nakamura, and Ake Grenvik

SECTION IV: CARDIOVASCULAR CRITICAL CARE

25 Cardiogenic Shock 287
Ashraf M. Ghobashy, Manuel Fontes, and Roberta L. Hines

26 Perioperative Myocardial Ischemia 303
James G. Ramsay and Gary Stolovitz

27 Acute Therapy in Patients with Cardiac Arrhythmias 320
Roger D. White

28 Care of the Hypertensive Patient in the Intensive Care Unit 333
Barry A. Harrison and Michael J. Murray

29 Perioperative Management of the Cardiac Surgical Patient 346
J. G. Reves, Steven E. Hill, Sam Thio Sum-Ping, John V. Booth, and Ian J. Welsby

30 Current Concepts in Cardiopulmonary Resuscitation 363
Charles W. Otto

SECTION V: PULMONARY CRITICAL CARE

31 Perioperative Evaluation of Pulmonary Diseases and Function 374
Peter J. Papadakos

32 Pneumonia 385
C. William Hanson, III

33 Perioperative Management of Obstructive and Restrictive Pulmonary Diseases 393
Stephen J. Ruoss

34 Acute Lung Injury and Acute Respiratory Distress Syndrome 408
Michael A. Matthay, Jeanine P. Wiener-Kronish, Ivan Cheng, and Michael A. Gropper

35 Perioperative Care of Thoracic Surgical Patients 417
Joanne Meyer and Brian P. Kavanagh

36 Respiratory Care 428
William T. Peruzzi and Barry A. Shapiro

37 Basic Principles and New Modes of Mechanical Ventilation 447
Neil R. MacIntyre

38 Weaning from Mechanical Ventilatory Support 460
E. Wesley Ely

SECTION VI: GASTROINTESTINAL CRITICAL CARE

39 Acute Abdominal Conditions in the Perioperative Intensive Care Patient 474
Bruce M. Potenza

40 Gastrointestinal Hemorrhage in the Critically Ill 485
Douglas B. Coursin and Kenneth E. Wood

41 Care of the Patient With Fulminant Hepatic Failure 495
Christopher J. Jankowski, Mark T. Keegan, and David J. Plevak

SECTION VII: RENAL CRITICAL CARE

42 Perioperative Renal Protection 503
H. T. Lee and Robert N. Sladen

43 Management of Acute Renal Failure in the Critically Ill Patient 521
Michelle A. Hladunewich and Richard A. Lafayette

SECTION VIII: HEMATOLOGIC CRITICAL CARE

44 An Approach to Venous Thromboembolism/ Pulmonary Embolism in the Critically Ill 533
Kenneth E. Wood

45 Perioperative Hemostasis and Coagulopathy 549
Carol A. Dion, Kathleen H. Chaimberg, Andrew Gettinger, and D. David Glass

46 Transfusion Medicine for the Intensivist 566
Eduardo N. Chini, Niki M. Dietz, and Ronald J. Faust

SECTION IX: INFECTION AND IMMUNOLOGY

47 Evaluation of Fever in the Intensive Care Unit 577
Kenneth E. Wood

48 Multiple-Organ Dysfunction Syndrome 588
Stephen O. Heard and Mitchell P. Fink

49 The Patient With Sepsis or the Systemic
Inflammatory Response Syndrome 601
*Sharon Orbach, Yoram G. Weiss, and
Clifford S. Deutschman*

50 Management of Life-Threatening Infection
in the Intensive Care Unit 616
Dennis G. Maki

51 Infections in the Immunocompromised 649
Anand Kumar and Bala Hota

52 The Use of Antimicrobials in the Intensive
Care Unit 672
Eugene Y. Cheng and Cynthia R. Hennen

SECTION X: TRANSPLANTATION

53 The Biology of Transplantation 690
L. Thomas Chin and Stuart J. Knechtle

54 Cardiopulmonary Transplantation 699
Byron P. Unger

55 Liver, Kidney, Pancreas Transplantation 724
Wolf H. Stapelfeldt

56 Hematopoietic Stem Cell Transplantation 740
Babak Kharrazi and Norman W. Rizk

SECTION XI: SPECIALIZED PERIOPERATIVE CARE

57 Care of the Patient With Endocrine Emergencies 752
Gary P. Zaloga

58 Care of Critically Ill Obstetric Patients 765
James W. Van Hook and Rakesh B. Vadhera

59 Pediatric Critical Care: Selected Aspects of
Perioperative Management of
Infants and Children 776
*Shekhar T. Venkataraman, Joseph A. Carcillo,
Mark W. Hall, Randall A. Ruppel,
and Patrick M. Kochanek*

60 Care of the Patient with Multiple Trauma 791
*Kimberly K. Nagy, Catherine Cagiannos,
and Kimberly T. Joseph*

61 Acute Care of Burns 801
R. E. Barrow and D. N. Herndon

62 Care of the Poisoned Patient 818
Brian S. Kaufman and Robert S. Hoffman

63 Advanced Imaging in the Intensive Care Unit 841
Janet E. Kuhlman

Subject Index 859

CONTRIBUTING AUTHORS

Steven J. Allen, M.D.
Professor, Department of Anesthesiology
The University of Texas-Houston Medical School
Department of Anesthesiology
Houston, Texas

R.E. Barrow, Ph.D.
Professor and Coordinator of Research
Department of General Surgery
The University of Texas Medical Branch
Shriner's Hospital for Children
Galveston, Texas

Jennifer Bayne, M.D.
The London Health Science Centre
Victoria Campus
London, Ontario
Canada

Lauren C. Berkow, M.D.
Assistant Professor
Department of Anesthesiology and Critical Care Medicine
Johns Hopkins University School of Medicine
Johns Hopkins Medical Institution
Baltimore, Maryland

Anish Bhardwaj, M.D.
Assistant Professor
The Johns Hopkins University School of Medicine
Department of Neurology
Baltimore, Maryland

Thomas P. Bleck, M.D.
The Louise Nerancy Eminent Scholar in Neurology and
Professor of Neurology, Neurological Surgery,
    and Internal Medicine
Director, Neuroscience Intensive Care Unit
The University of Virginia
Charlottesville Virginia

John V. Booth, F.R.C.A.
Assistant Professor
Department of Anesthesiology
Duke University Medical Center
Durham, North Carolina

John Butterworth, M.D.
Professor
Department of Anesthesiology
Wake Forest University School of Medicine
Medical Center Boulevard
Winston-Salem, North Carolina

Catherine Cagiannos, M.D., F.R.C.S.
Cook County Hospital
Department of Trauma
Chicago, Illinois

James E. Calvin, M.D.
Chairman, Division of Adult Cardiology
Cook County Hospital
Associate Professor of Medicine
Rush-Presbyterian-St. Luke's Medical Center
Chicago, Illinois

Joseph A. Carcillo, M.D.
Assistant Professor
Departments of Anesthesiology and Critical Care
    Medicine and Pediatrics
University of Pittsburgh School of Medicine
Associate Director
Pediatric Intensive Care Unit
Children's Hospital of Pittsburgh
Pittsburgh, Pennsylvania

Edmund G. Carton, M.D. F.F.A.R.C.S.I.
Consultant
Department of Intensive Care Medicine
Mater Misericordiae Hospital
Dublin, Ireland

Kathleen H. Chaimberg, M.D.
Assistant Professor of Anesthesiology
Department of Anesthesiology
Dartmouth-Hitchcock Medical Center
Lebanon, New Hampshire

Eugene Y. Cheng, M.D.
Professor of Anesthesiology and Medicine
Department of Anesthesiology
Medical College of Wisconsin
Associate Clinical Director of Anesthesiology and
    Critical Care
Department of Anesthesiology
Froedtert Memorial Lutheran Hospital
Milwaukee, Wisconsin

Ivan Cheng, M.D.
Fellow
Department of Pulmonary and
    Critical Care Medicine
University of California, San Francisco
San Francisco, California

L. Thomas Chin, M.D.
Assistant Professor
Department of Surgery
University of Wisconsin
Madison, Wisconsin

Eduardo N. Chini, M.D., Ph.D.
Assistant Professor
Department of Anesthesiology
Mayo Medical School
Senior Associate Consultant
Department of Anesthesiology
Mayo Clinic
Rochester, Minnesota

Neal H. Cohen, M.D., M.P.H., M.S.
Professor of Anesthesia and Medicine
Vice Dean for Academic Affairs
Director of Critical Care Medicine
University of California San Francisco
San Francisco, California

Dan Connor, M.B.B.S., F.A.N.Z.C.A.
Consultant, Anaesthesia and Intensive Care
Manning Base Hospital
Taree, New South Wales
Australia

Douglas B. Coursin, M.D.
Professor
Associate Director, Trauma and Life Support Center
Departments of Anesthesiology and
    Internal Medicine
University of Wisconsin School of Medicine
Madison, Wisconsin

Clifford S. Deutschman, M.D., F.C.C.M.
Professor, Department of Anesthesia
Hospital of the University of Pennsylvania
Philadelphia, Pennsylvania

Niki M. Dietz, M.D.
Associate Professor and Consultant
Department of Anesthesiology
Mayo Foundation
Mayo Clinic
Rochester, Minnesota

Carol A. Dion, M.D.
Staff Anesthesiologist and Intensivist
Department of Anesthesiology
Maine Medical Center
Portland, Maine

Sylvia Y. Dolinski, M.D.
Assistant Professor
Department of Anesthesiology
Wake Forest University School of Medicine
Medical Center Boulevard
Winston-Salem, North Carolina

Michael A. Duncan, F.F.A.R.C.S.I.
Registrar
Department of Intensive Care Medicine
Mater Miseriocordiae Hospital
Dublin, Ireland

E. Wesley Ely, M.D., M.P.H., F.C.C.P.
Assistant Professor of Medicine
Division on Allergy, Pulmonary and Critical Care Medicine
Center for Health Services Research
Vanderbilt University Medical Center
Nashville, Tennessee

Ronald J. Faust, M.D.
Professor
Department of Anesthesiology
Mayo Medical School
Rochester, Minnesota

Mitchell P. Fink, M.D.
Professor, Surgery, Anesthesiology and
    Critical Care Medicine
Chief, Critical Care Medicine
UPMC Health System
Pittsburgh, Pennsylvania

Lee A. Fleisher, M.D.
Associate Professor and Vice Chairman
    for Clinical Investigation
Department of Anesthesiology
Joint Appointments in Medicine and
    Health Policy and Management
Johns Hopkins University School of Medicine
Clinical Director of Operating Rooms
Department of Anesthesiology
Johns Hopkins Hospital
Baltimore, Maryland

Manuel Fontes, M.D.
Associate Professor
Department of Anesthesiology and
    Critical Care Medicine
Weill Medical College of Cornell University
Associate Clinical Professor
Cardiothoracic Department
New York Presbyterian Hospital
New York, New York

Andrew Gettinger, M.D.
Associate Professor
Department of Anesthesiology
Dartmouth Medical School
Associate Medical Director
Dartmouth-Hitchcock Medical Center
Lebanon, New Hampshire

Ashraf M. Ghobashy, M.D.
Assistant Professor
Department of Anesthesiology
Yale University School of Medicine
New Haven, Connecticut

D. David Glass, M.D.
Professor of Anesthesiology and Medicine
Dartmouth Medical School
Chairman, Department of Anesthesiology
Dartmouth-Hitchcock Medical Center
Lebanon, New Hampshire

Ake Grenvik, M.D., Ph.D.
Distinguished Service Professor of
    Critical Care Medicine
University of Pittsburgh School of Medicine
Pittsburgh, Pennsylvania

Leanne Groban, M.D.
Assistant Professor
Department of Anesthesiology
Wake Forest University School of Medicine
Winston-Salem, North Carolina

Michael A. Gropper, M.D.
Associate Professor
Departments of Anesthesiology and Physiology
University of California, San Francisco
Director, Department of Critical Care Medicine
Moffitt-Long Hospital
San Francisco, California

Mark W. Hall, M.D.
Instructor
Departments of Anesthesiology and
    Critical Care Medicine
University of Pittsburgh
Department of Pediatric Critical Care Medicine
Children's Hospital of Pittsburgh
Pittsburgh, Pennsylvania

C. William Hanson, III, M.D.
Professor of Anesthesia, Surgery, and Internal Medicine
Department of Anesthesia
University of Pennsylvania School of Medicine
Medical Director, Surgical Intensive Care Unit
Section Chief, Critical Care Medicine
Hospital of the University of Pennsylvania
Philadelphia, Pennsylvania

Barry A. Harrison, M.B.B.S.
Assistant Professor
Department of Anesthesia
Mayo Clinic Jacksonville
Jacksonville, Florida

Stephen O. Heard, M.D.
Professor and Executive Vice-Chair
Department of Anesthesiology
University of Massachusetts Medical School
Co-Director, Surgical Intensive Care Units
Department of Anesthesiology
Umass Memorial Medical Center
Worcester, Massachusetts

Cynthia R. Hennen, M.D.
Department of Pharmacy
Foredtert Memorial Lutheran Hospital
Milwaukee, Wisconsin

D. N. Herndon, M.D., F.A.C.S.
Chief of Staff & Director of Research
Shriners Burns Hospital-Galveston
Professor, Surgery and Pediatrics
Jesse H. Jones Distinguished Chair in Burn Surgery
Director of Burn Services
The University of Texas Medical Branch
Galveston, Texas

Steven E. Hill, M.D.
Assistant Professor
Department of Anesthesiology
Duke University Medical Center
Erwin Road
Durham, North Carolina

Roberta L. Hines, M.D.
Professor and Chairman
Department of Anesthesiology
Yale University School of Medicine
New Haven, Connecticut

Michelle A. Hladunewich, M.D.
Critical Care/Nephrology Fellow
Department of Medicine
Stanford University
Postdoctoral Fellow
Department of Medicine
Stanford Medical Center
Stanford, California

Vincent L. Hoellerich, M.D.
Vice-Chairman
Department of Anesthesiology & Critical Care Medicine
Rex Hospital
Raleigh, North Carolina

Robert S. Hoffman, M.D.
Assistant Professor
Departments of Surgery and Emergency Medicine
NYU School of Medicine
Director, Poison Control Center
New York, New York

Kirk Hogan, M.D.
Associate Professor
Department of Anesthesiology
University of Wisconsin
Madison, Wisconsin

Bala Hota, M.D.
Fellow
Section of Infectious Diseases
Rush-Presbyterian-St. Luke's Medical Center
Chicago, Illinois

Patricia D. Hurn, Ph.D.
Associate Professor
Department of Anesthesiology and Critical Care Medicine
Johns Hopkins School of Medicine
Baltimore Maryland

Christopher J. Jankowski, M.D.
Assistant Professor
Department of Anesthesiology
Mayo Medical School
Consultant
Department of Anesthesiology
Mayo Clinic
Rochester, Minnesota

Kimberly T. Joseph, M.D., C.N.S.P., F.A.C.S.
Associate Director
Department of Trauma
Cook Country Hospital
Chicago, Illinois

Brian S. Kaufman, M.D.
Associate Clinical Professor
Departments of Anesthesiology, Medicine, and Neurosurgery
New York University School of Medicine
Co-Director
Department of Critical Care
Tisch University Hospital
New York, New York

Brian P. Kavanagh, M.B., F.R.C.P.(C), M.R.C.P.(I)
Associate Director
Department of Critical Care
University of Toronto
Research Director
Department of Critical Care
Hospital for Sick Children
Toronto, Ontario
Canada

Mark T. Keegan, M.D.
Assistant Professor
Department of Anesthesiology
Mayo Medical School
Senior Associate Consultant
Department of Anesthesiology
Division of Clinical Care
Mayo Clinic
Rochester, Minnesota

Babak Kharrazi, M.D.
Stanford University Medical Center
Pulmonary and Critical Care Division
Stanford, California

Jeffrey R. Kirsch, M.D.
Professor
Department of Anesthesiology and
    Critical Care Medicine
Johns Hopkins University
Vice Chairman, Education and Training
Department of Anesthesiology and
    Critical Care Medicine
Johns Hopkins Hospital
Baltimore, Maryland

Stuart J. Knechtle, M.D.
Professor
Department of Surgery
University of Wisconsin
Staff Surgeon
Department of Surgery
University of Wisconsin Hospitals and Clinics
Madison, Wisconsin

Patrick M. Kochanek, M.D.
Associate Professor
Department of Anesthesiology/Critical Care Medicine
Safar Center for Resuscitation Research
University of Pittsburgh School of Medicine
Associate Director
Department of Pediatric Critical Care Medicine
Children's Hospital of Pittsburgh
Pittsburgh, Pennsylvania

Janet E. Kuhlman, M.D.
Professor of Radiology
Thoracic Imaging Division
University of Wisconsin Medical School
Madison, Wisconsin

Anand Kumar, M.D.
Assistant Professor
Section of Critical Care Medicine/
    Section of Infectious Diseases
Department of Medicine
Rush University
Attending Physician
Section of Critical Care Medicine
Rush-Presbyterian-St. Luke's Medical Center
Chicago, Illinois

Richard A. Lafayette, M.D.
Associate Professor
Associate Chief, Division of Nephrology
Department of Medicine
Stanford University
Clinical Director of Nephrology
Department of Medicine
Stanford University Medical Center
Stanford, California

John D. Lang, M.D.
Department of Anesthesiology
The University of Texas Medical Branch
Galveston, Texas

H. T. Lee, M.D., Ph.D.
Assistant Professor
Department of Anesthesiology
Columbia University College of Physicians and Surgeons
Assistant Attending
Department of Anesthesiology
New York Presbyterian Medical Center
New York, New York

Charles E. Lucas, M.D.
Professor, Department of Surgery
Wayne State University
Senior Attending
Department of Surgery
Detroit Receiving Hospital
Detroit, Michigan

Gerald A. Maccioli, M.D., F.C.C.M.
Assistant Consulting Professor of Anesthesiology
Duke University Medical Center
Director of Critical Care Medicine
Critical Health Systems, Inc.
Raleigh Practice Center
Raleigh, North Carolina

Dennis G. Maki, M.D.
Ovid O. Meyer Professor of Medicine
Head, Section of Infectious Diseases
University of Wisconsin Medical School
Attending Physician
Center for Trauma and Life Support
University of Wisconsin Hospital and Clinics
Madison, Wisconsin

Michael S. Malian, M.D.
Senior Associate Consultant in Surgery
Mayo Clinic
Rochester, Minnesota

Mali Mathru, M.D.
Department of Anesthesiology
The University of Texas Medical Branch
Galveston, Texas

Michael A. Matthay, M.D.
Professor
Department of Medicine and Anesthesia
Cardiovascular Research Institute
Associate Director, Intensive Care Unit
Department of Critical Care Medicine
University of California at San Francisco
San Francisco, California

Neil R. MacIntyre, M.D.
Professor
Department of Medicine
Duke University Medical Center
Associate Chief
Department of Pulmonary and Critical
    Care Medicine
Duke Hospital
Durham, North Carolina

Niamh McMahon
Pharmacist
Department of Intensive Care Medicine
Mater Misericordiae Hospital
Dublin, Ireland

Joanne Meyer, M.D. F.R.C.P.C.
Staff Intensivist
Toronto General Hospital
Toronto, Ontario Canada

Marek Mirski, M.D., Ph.D.
Associate Professor
Chief of Neuroanesthesiology
Director, Neuroscience Critical Care Unit
Departments of Anesthesia, Critical Care Medicine,
    Neurology, and Neurosurgery
Johns Hopkins University
Baltimore, Maryland

Michael J. Murray, M.D., Ph.D.
Dean, Mayo School of Health Sciences
Professor and Chair, Department of Anesthesiology
Mayo Clinic and Foundation
Jacksonville, Florida

Kimberly K. Nagy, M.D., F.A.C.S.
Associate Professor
Department of General Surgery
Rush Medical College
Director of Trauma Education
Department of Trauma
Cook County Hospital
Chicago, Illinois

Megumi Nakamura, M.D.
Department of Anesthesiology
Georgetown University Medical Center
Washington, D.C.

Michael F. O'Connor, M.D.
Associate Professor
Department of Anesthesia and Critical Care
University of Chicago
Chicago, Illinois

Sharon Orbach, M.D.
Department of Anesthesia and Critical Care Medicine
Hadassah Hebrew University Medical Center
Jerusalem, Israel

Charles W. Otto, M.D., F.C.C.M.
Professor
Department of Anesthesiology
University of Arizona College of Medicine
Tucson, Arizona

Andranik Ovassapian, M.D.
Professor
Director, Airway Study and Training Center
Department of Anesthesia and Critical Care
University of Chicago
Chicago, Illinois

Peter J. Papadakos, M.D., F.C.C.P., F.C.C.M.
Associate Professor
Director, Division of Critical Care Medicine
Departments of Anesthesiology and Surgery
University of Rochester
Rochester, New York

Joseph E. Parrillo, M.D.
James B. Herrick Professor of Medicine
Department of Internal Medicine
Rush Medical College
Chief, Division of Cardiovascular Diseases and
    Critical Care Medicine
Department of Internal Medicine
Rush-Presbyterian-St. Luke's Medical Center
Chicago, Illinois

William T. Peruzzi, M.D., F.C.C.M.
Associate Professor
Department of Anesthesiology
Northwestern University Medical School
Northwestern Memorial Hospital
Medical Director
Department of Respiratory Care
Chicago, Illinois

Patricia H. Petrozza, M.D.
Professor of Anesthesiology
Section Head, Neurosurgical Anesthesiology
Wake Forest University School of Medicine
Winston-Salem, North Carolina

David J. Plevak, M.D.
Professor
Department and Anesthesiology
Mayo Medical School
Head, Department of Liver Transplant Anesthesiology
Mayo Clinic
Rochester, Minnesota

Jeffrey S. Plotkin, M.D.
Associate Professor
Departments of Surgery and Anesthesiology
Georgetown University Medical Center
Director of Transplant Anesthesiology and Clinical Care
Georgetown Transplant Institute
Washington, D.C.

Bruce M. Potenza, M.D., F.A.C.S., F.A.C.P.
Assistant Professor of Clinical Surgery
Department of Surgery
University of California at San Diego
San Diego, California

Richard C. Prielipp, M.D., F.C.C.M.
Professor, Department of Cardiothoracic
Anesthesiology Section Head, Critical Care Medicine
Wake Forest University School of Medicine
Winston-Salem, North Carolina

Donald S. Prough, M.D.
Professor and Chair
Department of Anesthesiology
The University of Texas Medical Branch
Galveston, Texas

James G. Ramsay, M.D.
Professor and Service Chief
Department of Anesthesiology
Emory University School of Medicine
Emory University Hospital
Atlanta, Georgia

J. G. Reves
Vice President for Medical Affairs
Dean, College of Medicine
Medical University of South Carolina
Charleston, South Carolina

Norman W. Rizk, M.D., F.C.C.P.
Professor of Medicine
Senior Associate Chair for Clinical Affairs
Stanford University Medical Center
Pulmonary and Critical Care Division
Stanford, California

Robert M. Rodriguez, M.D.
Assistant Clinical Professor
Department of Emergency Medicine
University of California, San Francisco
San Francisco, California
Attending Physician
Alameda County Medical Center
Okland, California

Stanley H. Rosenbaum, M.D.
Professor of Anesthesiology, Medicine, and Surgery
Department of Anesthesiology
Yale University School of Medicine
Vice Chairman for Academic Affairs
Department of Anesthesiology
Yale-New Haven Hospital
New Haven, Connecticut

Myer H. Rosenthal, M.D.
Professor
Departments of Anesthesia, Medicine, and Surgery
Stanford University School of Medicine
Stanford, California

Mark I. Rossberg, M.D.
Assistant Professor
Anesthesiology/Critical Care Medicine
Johns Hopkins Medical Inst./ACCM
Baltimore, Maryland

Stephen J. Ruoss, M.D.
Associate Professor
Division of Pulmonary and Critical Care Medicine
Department of Medicine
Stanford University School of Medicine
Associate Director of Critical Care
Department of Medicine
Stanford University Medical Center
Stanford, California

Randall A. Ruppel, M.D.
Assistant Professor
Departments of Anesthesiology and Critical
    Care Medicine
University of Pittsburgh
Department of Pediatric Critical Care Medicine
Children's Hospital of Pittsburgh
Pittsburgh, Pennsylvania

Keith Ruskin, M.D.
Associate Professor
Department of Anesthesiology
Yale School of Medicine
New Haven, Connecticut

Karen J. Schwenzer, M.D.
Associate Professor
Department of Anesthesiology
University of Virginia Health System
Charlottesville, Virginia

Barry A. Shapiro, M.D.
Professor Emeritus
Department of Anesthesiology
Northwestern University Medical School
Chicago, Illinois

William J. Sibbald, M.D., F.R.C.P.C., F.C.C.H.S.E.
Physician-in-Chief
Department of Medicine
Sunnybrook & Women's College
    Health Sciences Centre
Toronto, Ontario
Canada

Robert N. Sladen, M.B. Ch.B., M.R.C.P.
Professor of and Vice-Chair
Department of Anesthesiology
College of Physicians and Surgeons of
    Columbia University
Director, Cardiothoracic and Surgical
    Intensive Care Units
New York Presbyterian Hospital—Columbia
    Medical Center
New York, New York

Wolf H. Stapelfeldt, M.D.
Chair, Division of Transplant Anesthesia
Vice Chair for Education
Department of Anesthesiology
Mayo Clinic Jacksonville
Jacksonville, Florida

Gary Stolovitz, M.D.
Staff Anesthesiologist
Piedmont Hospital
Atlanta, Georgia

Sam Thio Sum-Ping, M.B.Ch.B., F.R.C.A.
Associate Professor
Department of Anesthesiology
Duke University Medical Center
Medical Director, SICU
Department of Anesthesiology
Durham Veterans Affairs Medical Center
Durham, North Carolina

Joseph W. Szokol, M.D.
Assistant Professor
Northwestern University Medical School
Chicago, Illinois
Vice Chairman
Department of Anesthesiology
Evanstan Northwestern Healthcare
Evanston, Illinois

Byron P. Unger, M.D., F.R.C.P.C.
Clinical Assistant Professor
Department of Anesthesiology and Pain Medicine
University of Alberta Hospital
Edmonton, Alberta
Canada

Rakesh B. Vadhera, M.D., F.R.C.A., F.F.A.R.C.S.I.
Associate Professor
University of Texas Medical Branch
Department of Anesthesiology
Galveston, Texas

James W. Van Hook, M.D.
Assistant Professor
Department of Obstetrics and Gynecology
University of Texas Medical Branch
Director of Critical Care Obstetrics
Department of Obstetrics and Gynecology
John Sealy Hospital
Galveston, Texas

Jeffery S. Vender, M.D.
Professor
Northwestern University Medical School
Chicago, Illinois
Chairman, Department of Anesthesiology
Evanston Northwestern Healthcare
Evanston, Illinois

Shekhar T. Venkataraman, M.D.
Departments of Anesthesiology and
   Critical Care Medicine and Pediatrics
Children's Hospital of Pittsburgh
Safar Center for Resuscitation Research
Pittsburgh, Pennsylvania

Yoram G. Weiss, M.D.
Lecturer in Anesthesia
Department of Anesthesia and Critical
   Care Medicine
Hadassah Hebrew University Medical Center
Jerusalem, Israel

Ian J. Welsby, B.Sc., M.B.B.S., F.R.C.A.
Associate Professor
Department of Anesthesiology
Duke University Medical Center
Durham, North Carolina

Roger D. White, M.D.
Professor and Consultant
Department of Anesthesiology
Mayo Medical School
Mayo Clinic
Rochester, Minnesota

Jeanine P. Wiener-Kronish, M.D.
Associate Professor
Departments of Anesthesia and Medicine
University of California, San Francisco
San Francisco, California

Douglas W. Wilmore, M.D.
Frank Sawyer Professor of Surgery
Harvard Medical School
Brigham and Women's Hospital
Boston, Massachusetts

Kenneth E. Wood, D.O.
Associate Professor
Director of Critical Care Medicine
Section of Pulmonary and Critical Care Medicine
University of Wisconsin Hospital and Clinics
Madison, Wisconsin

Christopher C. Young, M.D.
Associate Professor of Anesthesiology
Chief, Critical Care Medicine
Duke University Medical Center
Duke Hospital
Durham, North Carolina

Gary P. Zaloga, M.D.
Professor of Medicine
Indiana University School of Medicine
Medical Cirector
Methodist Research Institute
Clarian Health Partners
Indianapolis, Indiana

PREFACE

The first edition of *Critical Care Medicine: Perioperative Management* was written to address a unique time frame in intensive care unit (ICU) management. The special needs of this commonly encountered patient population are frequently not a central point of comprehensive ICU texts or briefer subspecialty-directed critical care commentaries. Therefore, the first edition focused on preoperative evaluation and risk stratification, intraoperative issues that impact on morbidity, mortality and need for critical care, and postoperative acute care of patients ranging from obstetrics through children and adults.

The inaugural text was divided into ten sections: an overview of patient assessment and ICU organization followed by procedural and pathophysiologic commentaries, organ-specific discussions, and subspecialty critical care medicine reviews. Because it was published to critical acclaim from both reviewers and readers, the editors have maintained the basic organization of the text, and key words and key point summaries are again included in the chapters to highlight important topics and seminal themes in patient care.

The five years between editions of *Critical Care Medicine: Perioperative Management* have been filled with exciting technological and therapeutic developments, particularly in the areas of ventilatory management of the acute respiratory distress syndrome and in the modulation of the coagulation abnormalities associated with the sepsis syndrome. Each of these advances has helped critical care physicians improve the clinical outcome of relatively common, yet often devastating, pathologies. These major breakthroughs are discussed thoroughly in "Acute Lung Injury and Acute Respiratory Distress Syndrome" by Michael Matthay, Jeanine Wiener-Kronish, Ivan Cheng, and Michael Gropper and "Diagnosis and Treatment of Infection" by Dennis Maki.

The pivotal role of critical care physicians in improving survival of acutely ill patients with cost-effective therapies has been increasingly recognized since the first edition. As Neal Cohen comments in "ICU Organization," it is the charge and challenge of the intensivist to provide quality care, counterbalanced with the judicious use of advanced technology and other costly resources, and to achieve shortened length of stay and improve outcomes. To that end, the Leapfrog Group, a consortium of large companies providing health care to approximately 20 million employees and their families, underscores the value of critical care physicians. This group has made the "presence of dedicated intensive care practitioners" one of the top three criteria to become a qualified provider of efficient and optimal care within its network.

In order to enhance this second edition and keep pace with important advances, the editors and authors have completely revised previous chapters, eliminated or consolidated some topics, and added new information on timely subjects. This includes five new chapters, starting with "Medical Informatics in the Intensive Care Unit," by Keith Ruskin. Dr. Ruskin is the editor of GASNET, one of the largest web-based specialty resources. In addition to discussing the basics of information acquisition and management in his chapter, Dr. Ruskin also comments on artificial intelligence/learning and outlines the unique needs of physicians in his attempt to improve the interface between information specialists and practitioners. William Sibbald and colleagues succinctly review the need for evidence-based medicine in critical care and the appropriate application of this increasingly available technique. Kirk Hogan provides an exciting template for the role of human genomics in the ICU population. The clinical use of refined molecular biologic tools will continue to change the face of critical care diagnostics and therapies. Joseph

Parrillo, Anand Kumar, and James Calvin provide an insightful overview of the need for research in critical care medicine, combined with a guide to establishing a clinical research career. Finally, Janet Kuhlman skillfully fills a void in the first edition of this text with a detailed discussion on imaging in the ICU.

The editors have drawn from the collective experience of an expanded group of internationally recognized authors from multiple disciplines in this new edition. Leading experts in anesthesiology, internal medicine, pediatrics, neurology, radiology, and surgery have provided their insights and concise discussions in an attempt to cover the broad spectrum of patients seen in perioperative critical care settings.

It is our hope that this updated, expanded, and comprehensive approach to critical care medicine and perioperative patient management will provide you with the state-of-the art information needed to provide quality care to your most challenging patients.

—The Editors

ACKNOWLEDGMENTS

The editors thank the many contributors to this text as well as the editorial assistance of Joyce Kelly and Drew Coursin, and the administrative support from Robin Williams, Tehra Meyer, Jaclyn Schultz, and Gary Malchow. Thank you to Craig Percy and Sonya Seigafuse for their patience, perseverance, and editorial guidance, and the support personnel from our individual institutions as well as our colleagues and trainees.

PREOPERATIVE ASSESSMENT

LEE A. FLEISHER
STANLEY H. ROSENBAUM

> **KEY WORDS**
>
> - Risk index
> - APACHE Score
> - TRISS
> - Abbreviated Injury Scale
> - Complications, postoperative
> - Myocardial infarction
> - Coronary artery disease
> - Pulmonary complications
> - Emphysema
> - Chronic bronchitis
> - Asthma
> - Diabetes
> - Hypothyroidism
> - Hyperthyroidism
> - Adrenocortical suppression

INTRODUCTION

The assessment of a patient's overall medical and surgical condition and the reduction of the associated perioperative risks are broad undertakings. With the ever-increasing safety of modern surgical and anesthetic techniques there is a temptation to assume that a full assessment is not essential for every patient. But even for the relatively healthy patient having less stressful surgery, an overview is important.

The basic approach to the assessment of a preoperative patient can be separated into four parts (Table 1). First, the diagnoses of the patient's relevant medical problems must be entered into what can be a formal or informal database. There is, admittedly, an assumption here that this knowledge is helpful. While this might be difficult to prove, it is certain that ignorance cannot be advantageous. Next, where appropriate, diagnosed medical problems should be optimized. This principle derives from multiple arguments. Of these, most relevant is the implication of the informed consent that the planned procedure is being done with all the risks reasonably minimized. Optimization can be limited by resistant disease processes; but the worse the underlying conditions the more attention that should be directed at them. Of course, optimization must be done within the context of the risks of the planned surgery and the risks of the optimization itself. Some categories of optimization may themselves be either unacceptably risky (e.g., coronary artery stenting or bypass grafting in preparation for minor surgery), or may be unachievable because of patient choice (e.g.,

refusal to cease smoking or reduce severe obesity prior to elective surgery).

Third, an actual assessment of the risks of the planned procedure is needed. This also derives from our belief that a fully informed patient consent necessitates that the patients know what is likely to happen to them, as well as the more common or important risks that they may encounter. This risk assessment is also a critical part of the planning by internists, surgeons, and anesthesiologists as they make their own decisions regarding what surgery to recommend to patients, how to approach that procedure, and how to manage the patient during and afterward. Risk assessment is a difficult and subjective problem often approached by categorizing both patient status and surgical stress separately, occasionally via numerical (but poorly substantiated) scores. (These scores are discussed later in this chapter.) The often unmentioned factors of an individual surgeon's skill or an institution's overall experience are also certainly relevant, but only recently becoming available to patients and referring physicians (Fig. 1).

The last component of the preoperative assessment process is consideration of the actual plans for the perioperative period. This extends from the early preoperative time when chemotherapy, nutritional support, beta blockade, and other therapies might be initiated, through the immediate preoperative day when bowel preparation and antiasthma steroids might be started. For the postoperative period, early planning is helpful regarding hospitalization issues from the recommendation for same-day surgery up to requests for intensive care unit (ICU) beds, and beyond to scheduling posthospitalization skilled nursing care.

Much of the information necessary to define this database can be obtained from a good patient history with supplemental information from the primary care giver or specialist involved in the patient's care. From the anesthesiologist's and surgeon's perspectives, it is important to define the specific questions required from the primary care giver/specialist in order to complete the database. Similarly, these primary care givers should provide information on the stability of disease and any potential interventions that might be contemplated to improve care. It is then critical to define the need for additional diagnostic testing, such as basic studies including hemoglobin and electrolytes or sophisticated noninvasive or invasive cardiovascular modalities. In interpreting these tests, the definition of both normal and abnormal results depends upon the clinical picture (i.e., is a function of the prior probability of disease) (1). For example, a spot on

TABLE 1. COMPONENTS OF THE PREOPERATIVE EVALUATION

- Diagnosis
- Optimization
- Risk assessment
- Perioperative management plan

a chest radiograph may have very different interpretation in a young healthy individual than in an older chronic smoker. In an age of economic constraints, it is also important that testing be limited to cases in which it will influence perioperative care. Among the rationales for further diagnostic testing is the decision to utilize, or not utilize, postoperative intensive care.

CARDIAC DISEASE

As the population ages, an increasing number of older adults present for surgery. These patients often have coexisting diseases, such as atherosclerosis. Of the 23 million Americans anesthetized annually, approximately 7 to 8 million have known or risk factors for coronary artery disease (CAD) (2). Because data suggest that patients at high risk for cardiovascular complications have improved outcomes when managed in an ICU by a dedicated specialist (e.g., patients undergoing abdominal aortic aneurysm resection), the preoperative evaluation should identify patients who might benefit from increased perioperative resource utilization (3).

The identification of significant CAD has traditionally been approached from two perspectives: multifactorial risk indices and evaluation of new preoperative testing modalities in specific patient groups. The first area was popularized by the pioneering work of Dr. Dripps and the American Society of Anesthesiologists Physical Status Index and then Dr. Lee Goldman and colleagues (Cardiac Risk Index) (4,5). The second area involves the assessment of new noninvasive testing modalities, and has received extensive attention during the previous two decades. Specific testing modalities will be addressed later in the chapter.

Multifactorial indices are predicated on certain assumptions that are critical to understanding how best to utilize them. The first is that data are available on all of the potentially important variables. Second, eliminating variables from the model must be based upon biological significance, and not just statistical importance.

Noncardiac Risk Indices

In 1977, Goldman and colleagues published their landmark article studying 1,001 patients undergoing noncardiac surgical procedures, excluding transurethral resection of the prostate (TURP) (4). The authors excluded this surgery because of their impression of a low morbidity rate when performed under spinal anesthesia. They identified nine risk factors, and gave each factor a certain number of points (Goldman Cardiac Risk Index or CRI). A myocardial infarction and S3 gallop were identified as the most significant risk factors. By adding up the total number of points, patients were placed in one of four classes. The patient's class could then be compared to the rates of morbidity and mortality from the original cohort.

The CRI was subsequently validated in another cohort of patients; however, it has not been found to be predictive in patients undergoing major vascular surgery (6,7). Multiple studies have demonstrated that major vascular surgery is associated with a higher rate of morbidity and mortality compared to nonvascular surgery (4,8–10). In order to rectify this problem, Detsky

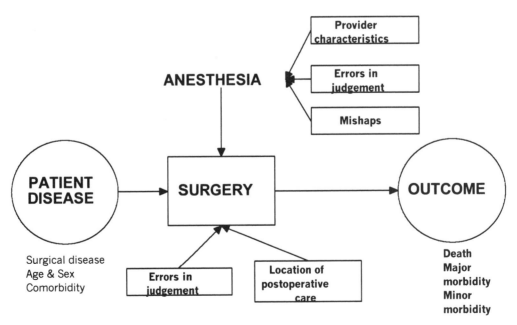

FIGURE 1. Multifactorial influences upon perioperative risk. (Adapted with permission from Fleither LA. Risk of anesthesia. In: Miller R, Miller ED, eds. *Anesthesia*, 5th ed. New York: Churchill-Livingstone, 2000:795–823.)

and colleagues proposed a modification of the CRI for vascular patients (11).

Although both of these indices were extremely useful when initially proposed, perioperative care has changed significantly in the intervening years. Goldman class III and IV continue to represent a high-risk cohort; however, recent mortality has been lower than originally reported (12). In addition, the presence of peripheral vascular disease is not a factor in the index and many vascular surgery patients would be classified as low risk, despite the high incidence of occult coronary artery disease (7). Important changes in the medical care of the patient with coronary artery disease has had profound impact on the perioperative period.

In an attempt to update the original index, Goldman and colleagues studied 4,315 patients, all 50 years of age, who were undergoing elective major noncardiac procedures in a tertiary-care teaching hospital (13). Six independent predictors of complications were identified and included in a Revised Cardiac Risk Index: high-risk type of surgery, history of ischemic heart disease, history of congestive heart failure, history of cerebrovascular disease, preoperative treatment with insulin, and preoperative serum creatinine greater than 2.0 mg per dL. Rates of major cardiac complication with none, one, two, or three of these factors were 0.5%, 1.3%, 4%, and 9%, respectively, in the derivation cohort and 0.4%, 0.9%, 7%, and 11%, respectively, among 1,422 patients in the validation cohort.

A primary issue with all of these indices is that a simple estimate of risk does not change perioperative management, but may provide information to assess the probability of risk. In contrast, the anesthesiologist is most concerned with defining the cardiovascular risk factors and symptoms or signs of unstable cardiac disease states such as myocardial ischemia, congestive heart failure, valvular heart disease, and significant cardiac arrhythmias. Therefore, risk indices are often helpful to nonanesthesiologists in estimating the probability of sustaining perioperative complications and may be used in risk/benefit assessment for the planned surgery. The anesthesiologist, however, will incorporate additional information such as specific details of the planned surgery and local management factors into their assessment of risk. In fact, the American Society of Anesthesiologists Physical Status Index provides almost as much information on the risk of perioperative complications as the more objective numerical indices (13). Providing a specific category of risk by the primary care giver should never substitute for details relating to the medical condition.

Cardiac Surgery Specific Risk Indices

Over the years there have been a number of risk indices developed to predict complications and resource utilization after cardiac surgery. Clinical and Angiographic Predictors of Operative Mortality were initially defined from the Collaborative Study in Coronary Artery Surgery (14). A total of 6,630 patients underwent isolated coronary artery bypass graft (CABG) between 1975 and 1978. Women had a significantly higher mortality than men, with mortality increasing with advancing age in men, but not significantly with women. Increasing severity of angina, manifestations of heart failure, and number and extent of coronary

artery stenoses all correlated with higher mortality, while ejection fraction was not a predictor. Urgency of surgery was a very strong predictor of outcome, with those patients requiring emergent surgery in the presence of a 90% left main coronary stenosis sustaining a 40% mortality.

O'Connor and associates used data collected from 3,055 patients undergoing isolated CABG at five clinical centers between 1987 and 1989 to develop a multivariate numerical score (15). A regression model was developed in a training set and subsequently validated in a test set. Independent predictors of mortality included age, body surface area, comorbidity score, prior CABG, ejection fraction, left ventricular end diastolic pressure, and priority of surgery.

One of the most commonly used scoring systems for CABG, developed by Parsonnet and colleagues (16), identified 14 risk factors following univariate regression analysis of 3,500 consecutive operations. An additive model was constructed and prospectively evaluated in 1,332 open heart procedures. Five categories of risk were associated with increasing mortality rates at the Newark Beth Israel Medical Center. The Parsonnet Index is often used as a benchmark for comparison between institutions.

Higgins developed a Clinical Severity Score for CABG at the Cleveland Clinic (17). A multivariate logistic regression model to predict perioperative risk was developed in 5,051 patients and subsequently validated in a cohort of 4,069 patients. Each independent predictor was assigned a weight or score, with increasing morbidity and mortality associated with an increasing total score.

Recently, Dupuis and colleagues have attempted to simplify the approach to risk of cardiac surgical procedures in a manner similar to the original American Society of Anesthesiologists (ASA) physical status classification (18). They developed a score that utilizes a simple continuous categorization using five classes plus an emergency status (Table 2). The Cardiac Anesthesia Risk Evaluation (CARE) Score demonstrates similar or superior predictive characteristics than the more complex indices.

Clinical Evaluation in Patients Undergoing Noncardiac Surgery

In patients with symptomatic coronary disease, the preoperative evaluation may disclose a change in the frequency or pattern of anginal symptoms. Symptoms of cardiovascular disease should be carefully determined, especially characteristics of chest pain, if present. Certain populations of patients, for example, older adults, women, or diabetics, may present with more atypical features. The presence of unstable angina has been associated with a high perioperative risk of myocardial infarction (MI) (19). The perioperative period is associated with a hypercoagulable state and surges in endogenous catecholamines, both of which may exacerbate the underlying process in unstable angina, and increase the risk of acute infarction (20). The preoperative evaluation can impact on both a patient's short- and long-term health by instituting treatment of unstable angina.

The patient with stable angina represents a continuum from mild angina with extreme exertion to dyspnea with angina after walking up a few stairs. The patient who only manifests angina after strenuous exercise does not demonstrate signs of left ventricular dysfunction and would not be a candidate for changes in

TABLE 2. CARDIAC ANESTHESIA RISK EVALUATION (CARE) SCORE

1	Patient with stable cardiac disease and no other medical problem. A noncomplex surgery is undertaken.
2	Patient with stable cardiac disease and one or more controlled medical problems.[a] A noncomplex surgery is undertaken.
3	Patient with any uncontrolled medical problem[b] or patient in whom a complex surgery is undertaken.[c]
4	Patient with any uncontrolled medical problem and in whom a complex surgery is undertaken.
5	Patient with chronic or advanced cardiac disease for whom cardiac surgery is undertaken as a last hope to save or improve life.
E	*Emergency*—surgery as soon as diagnosis is made and operating room is available.

[a] Examples: controlled hypertension, diabetes mellitus, peripheral vascular disease, chronic obstructive pulmonary disease, controlled systemic diseases, others as judged by clinicians.
[b] Examples: unstable angina treated with intravenous heparin or nitroglycerin, preoperative intraaortic balloon pump, heart failure with pulmonary or peripheral edema, uncontrolled hypertension, renal insufficiency (creatinine level >140 μmol/L), debilitating systemic diseases, others as judged by clinicians.
[c] Examples: reoperation, combined valve and coronary artery surgery, multiple valve surgery, left ventricular aneurysmectomy, repair of ventricular septal defect after myocardial infarction, coronary artery bypass of diffuse or heavily calcified vessels, others as judged by clinicians. (Reproduced with permission from Dupuis JY, et al. The Cardiac Anesthesia Risk Evaluation Score: a clinically useful predictor of mortality and morbidity after cardiac surgery. *Anesthesiology* 2001;94:194–204.)

management. In contrast, a patient with dyspnea on mild exertion would be at high risk for developing perioperative ventricular dysfunction, myocardial ischemia, and possible MI. These patients have an extremely high probability of having extensive coronary artery disease and additional monitoring or cardiovascular testing should be contemplated, depending upon the surgical procedure and institutional factors.

In virtually all studies, the presence of active congestive heart failure preoperatively has been associated with an increased incidence of perioperative cardiac morbidity (4,11). Stabilization of ventricular function and treatment for pulmonary congestion is prudent prior to elective surgery. Also, it is important to determine the etiology of the left heart failure. Congestive symptoms may be due to nonischemic cardiomyopathy or vascular disease. Since the type of perioperative monitoring and treatments would be different, clarifying the cause of cardiac congestion is important. There are numerous studies that have evaluated the impact of pulmonary artery catheter monitoring on outcome, including randomized clinical trials of patients undergoing abdominal aortic aneurysm resection (21–23). Using perioperative MI or cardiac death as an endpoint, none of the studies demonstrated any difference in outcome between those monitored with a pulmonary artery versus central venous catheter. Importantly, these studies selected patients at low cardiac risk (i.e., no symptoms or history or a negative noninvasive diagnostic test). No study directly addressed the issue of monitoring in a patient with congestive heart failure. In fact, patients with asymmetric hypertrophic subaortic stenosis are at low risk for perioperative MI or death but high risk of perioperative congestive heart failure (24).

Patients with a prior MI have coronary artery disease, although a small group of patients may sustain an MI from a nonatherosclerotic mechanism. Traditionally, risk assessment for noncardiac surgery was based upon the time interval between the MI and surgery. Multiple studies have demonstrated an increased incidence of reinfarction if the MI was within 6 months of surgery (25–27). With improvements in perioperative care, this difference has decreased (28). Therefore, the importance of the intervening time interval may no longer be valid in the current era of thrombolytics, angioplasty, and risk stratification after an acute MI. Although many patients with an MI may continue to have myocardium at risk for subsequent ischemia and infarction, other patients may have their critical coronary stenosis either totally occluded or widely patent. For example, the use of percutaneous transluminal coronary angioplasty, thrombolysis, medical therapy, and early coronary artery bypass grafting has changed the natural history of the disease (29–31). Therefore, patients should be evaluated for their risk for ongoing ischemia. The American Heart Association/American College of Cardiology Task Force on Perioperative Evaluation of the Cardiac Patient undergoing Noncardiac Surgery has defined three risk groups and advocates the use of an MI less than 30 days before noncardiac surgery as the group at highest risk, while after that period, a prior MI places the patient at intermediate risk (32) (Table 3).

TABLE 3. CLINICAL PREDICTORS OF INCREASED PERIOPERATIVE CARDIOVASCULAR RISK (MYOCARDIAL INFARCTION, CONGESTIVE HEART FAILURE, DEATH)

Major
Unstable coronary syndromes
    Recent myocardial infarction[a] with evidence of important ischemic risk by clinical symptoms or noninvasive study
    Unstable or severe[b] angina (Canadian class III or IV)[c]
Decompensated congestive heart failure
Significant arrhythmias
    High-grade atrioventricular block
    Symptomatic ventricular arrhythmias in the presence of underlying heart disease
    Supraventricular arrhythmias with uncontrolled ventricular rate
Severe valvular disease

Intermediate
Mild angina pectoris (Canadian class I or II)
Prior myocardial infarction by history or pathologic Q waves
Compensated or prior congestive heart failure
Diabetes mellitus

Minor
Advanced age
Abnormal ECG (left ventricular hypertrophy, left bundle branch block, ST-T abnormalities)
Rhythm other than sinus (e.g., atrial fibrillation)
Low functional capacity (e.g., inability to climb one flight of stairs with a bag of groceries)
History of stroke
Uncontrolled systemic hypertension

ECG, electrocardiogram.
[a] The American College of Cardiology National Database Library defines recent myocardial infarction as greater than 7 days but less than or equal to 1 month (30 days).
[b] May include "stable" angina in patients who are unusually sedentary.
[c] Campeau L. Grading of angina pectoris. *Circulation.* 1976;54:522–523.
(Reproduced with permission from Eagle K, et al. Guidelines for perioperative cardiovascular evaluation of the noncardiac surgery. A report of the American Heart Association/American College of Cardiology Task Force on Assessment of Diagnostic and Therapeutic Cardiovascular Procedures. *Circulation* 1996;93:1278–1317.)

Patients at Risk for Coronary Artery Disease (CAD)

For those patients without overt symptoms or history, the probability of CAD varies with the type and number of atherosclerotic risk factors present. Peripheral arterial disease has been associated with CAD in multiple studies. Hertzer and colleagues studied 1,000 consecutive patients scheduled for major vascular surgery and found that approximately 60% of patients had at least one coronary artery with a critical stenosis (33).

Diabetes mellitus is common in the older adult and represents a disease that impacts on multiple organ systems. Complications of diabetes mellitus are often the cause of urgent or emergent surgery, especially in older adults. Diabetes accelerates the progression of atherosclerosis, which can often be silent in nature. Diabetics have a higher probability of CAD than nondiabetics do. There is a high incidence of both silent MI and myocardial ischemia (34). Eagle and coworkers demonstrated that diabetes is an independent risk factor for perioperative cardiac morbidity (35). In attempting to determine the degree of this increased probability, the length of the disease and other associated end-organ dysfunction should be taken into account. Autonomic neuropathy has recently been found to be the best predictor of silent coronary artery disease (36). Since these patients are at very high risk for silent MI, the electrocardiogram (ECG) should be obtained to examine for the presence of Q waves.

Hypertension has also been associated with an increased incidence of silent myocardial ischemia and infarction (34). Those hypertensive patients with left ventricular hypertrophy who are undergoing noncardiac surgery are at a higher perioperative risk than nonhypertensive patients (37). Investigators have suggested that the presence of a strain pattern on ECG suggests a chronic ischemic state (38). Therefore, these patients should also be considered to have an increased probability of CAD and developing cardiovascular morbidity.

There is a great deal of debate regarding a trigger to delay or cancel a surgical procedure in a patient with poorly or untreated hypertension. Although Goldman and Caldera suggest that a case should be delayed if the diastolic pressure is greater than 110 mm Hg, they demonstrated no major morbidity in this small cohort of individuals in their study (39). In the absence of end-organ changes, such as renal insufficiency or left ventricular hypertrophy with strain, it would seem appropriate to proceed with surgery. In contrast, a patient with a markedly elevated blood pressure and the new onset of a headache should have surgery delayed for further treatment.

Several other risk factors suggest an increased probability of CAD. These include the atherosclerotic processes associated with tobacco use and hypercholesterolemia. Although these risk factors increase the probability of developing coronary artery disease, they have not been shown to increase perioperative risk. When attempting to determine the overall probability of disease, the number and severity of the risk factors are important.

Importance of Surgical Procedure

The surgical procedure influences the extent of the preoperative evaluation required by determining the potential range of changes in perioperative management. For example, a pulmonary artery catheter or transesophageal echocardiography may be appropriate for a patient undergoing major abdominal or vascular surgery, but would not be considered appropriate for ambulatory surgery. Similarly, coronary revascularization may be beneficial for procedures associated with a high incidence of morbidity and mortality, but not those associated with a low incidence, as described below. Few objective data define the surgery specific incidence of complications. It is known that peripheral procedures, such as those included in a study of ambulatory surgery completed at the Mayo Clinic, are associated with an extremely low incidence of morbidity and mortality (40). Similarly, major vascular procedures are associated with among the highest incidence of complications, with a similar incidence documented for infrainguinal and aortic surgery (41). Eagle and colleagues published data on the incidence of perioperative MI and mortality by procedure for patients enrolled in the coronary artery surgery study (CASS) (42). They determined the overall risk of perioperative morbidity in patients with known coronary artery disease on medical treatment, and the potential reduced rate of perioperative morbidity in those patients who had a prior coronary artery bypass grafting. High-risk procedures include major vascular, abdominal, thoracic, and orthopedic surgery. The American Heart Association/ American College of Cardiology Guidelines defined three tiers of surgical stress, which are shown in Table 4 (32).

Importance of Exercise Tolerance

Exercise tolerance is one of the most important determinants of perioperative risk and the need for invasive monitoring (43). An excellent exercise tolerance, even in patients with stable angina,

TABLE 4. CARDIAC RISK[a] STRATIFICATION FOR NONCARDIAC SURGICAL PROCEDURES

High	(Reported cardiac risk often >5%)
	Emergent major operations, particularly in older adults
	Aortic and other major vascular
	Peripheral vascular
	Anticipated prolonged surgical procedures associated with large fluid shifts and/or blood loss
Intermediate	(Reported cardiac risk generally <5%)
	Carotid endarterectomy
	Head and neck
	Intraperitoneal and intrathoracic
	Orthopedic
	Prostate
Low[b]	(Reported cardiac risk generally <1%)
	Endoscopic procedures
	Superficial procedure
	Cataract
	Breast

[a] Combined incidence of cardiac death and nonfatal myocardial infarction.
[b] Do not generally require further preoperative cardiac testing.
(Reproduced with permission from Eagle K, et al. Guidelines for perioperative cardiovascular evaluation of the noncardiac surgery. A report of the American Heart Association/American College of Cardiology Task Force on Assessment of Diagnostic and Therapeutic Cardiovascular Procedures. *Circulation* 1996;93:1278–1317.)

TABLE 5. ESTIMATED ENERGY REQUIREMENT FOR VARIOUS ACTIVITIES[a]

1 MET	Can you take care of yourself?	4 METs	Climb a flight of stairs or walk up a hill?
	Eat, dress, or use the toilet?		Walk on level ground at 4 mph or 6.4 km/h?
	Walk indoors around the house?		Run a short distance[2]?
	Walk a block or two on level		Do heavy work around the house like scrubbing
	ground at 2–3 mph or 3.2–4.8 km/h?		floors or lifting or moving heavy furniture?
	Do light work around the house like		Participate in moderate recreational activities like golf,
	dusting or washing dishes?		bowling, dancing, doubles tennis, or throwing a baseball or football?
		>10 METs	Participate in strenuous sports like swimming, singles tennis,
			football, basketball, or skiing?

MET, metabolic equivalent.
[a] Adapted from the Duke Activity Status Index and American Heart Association Exercise Standards.
(Reproduced with permission from Eagle K, et al. Guidelines for perioperative cardiovascular evaluation of the noncardiac surgery. A report of the American Heart Association/American College of Cardiology Task Force on Assessment of Diagnostic and Therapeutic Cardiovascular Procedures. *Circulation* 1996;93:1278–1317.)

suggests that the myocardium can be stressed without becoming dysfunctional. If a patient can walk a mile without becoming short of breath, then the probability of extensive coronary artery disease is small. Alternatively, if patients become dyspneic associated with chest pain during minimal exertion, then the probability of extensive coronary artery disease is high. A greater degree of coronary artery disease has been associated with a higher perioperative risk (44). Additionally, these patients are at risk for developing hypotension with ischemia, and therefore may benefit from more extensive monitoring or coronary revascularization. Exercise tolerance can be assessed with formal treadmill testing or with a questionnaire that assesses activities of daily living (Table 5) (32).

Reilly and colleagues have evaluated the predictive value of self-reported exercise tolerance for serious perioperative complications, and demonstrated that a poor exercise tolerance (could not walk four blocks and climb two flights of stairs) independently predicted a complication with an odds ratio of 1.94 (45). The likelihood of a serious adverse event was inversely related to the number of blocks that could be walked. Therefore, there is good evidence to suggest that minimal additional testing is necessary if the patient is able to relate a good exercise tolerance.

Approach to the Patient

Multiple algorithms have been proposed to determine who requires further testing. As described previously, the risk associated with the proposed surgical procedure influences the decision to perform further diagnostic testing and interventions, tempered by recent studies in which perioperative cardiac morbidity was greatly reduced by perioperative beta-adrenergic blockade administration (46,47). With the reduction in perioperative morbidity, it has been suggested that extensive cardiovascular testing is not necessary (13). However, further testing may be warranted.

The algorithm to determine the need for testing proposed by the American College of Cardiology/American Heart Association Task Force is based upon the available evidence and expert opinion and integrates clinical history, surgery specific risk, and exercise tolerance. (Fig. 2) (32). First, the clinician must evaluate the urgency of the surgery and the appropriateness of a formal preoperative assessment. Next, it must be determined if

the patient has undergone a previous revascularization procedure or coronary evaluation. Those patients with unstable coronary syndromes should be identified, and appropriate treatment instituted. Finally, the decision to undergo further testing depends upon the interaction of the clinical risk factors, surgery-specific risk, and functional capacity. For patients at intermediate clinical risk, both exercise tolerance and the extent of planned surgery are considered. Importantly, no preoperative cardiovascular testing should be performed if the results will not change perioperative management.

The American College of Physicians Guidelines attempts to apply the evidence-based approach (48). The initial decision point is the assessment of risk using the Detsky modification of the Cardiac Risk Index (11). If patients are class II or III, they are considered high risk. If they are class I, the presence of other clinical factors according to work by Eagle and colleagues or Vanzetto and colleagues is used to further stratify risk (32,49). Those with multiple markers for cardiovascular disease according to these risk indices and undergoing major vascular surgery are considered appropriate for further diagnostic testing by either dipyridamole imaging or dobutamine stress echocardiography. The Guidelines suggest that there is insufficient evidence to recommend diagnostic testing for nonvascular surgery patients.

There have been numerous diagnostic imaging modalities that have been advocated as means of assessing the extent of coronary artery disease. There are multiple noninvasive diagnostic tests that have been proposed to evaluate the extent of coronary artery disease before noncardiac surgery. The exercise ECG has been the traditional method of evaluating individuals for the presence of coronary artery disease, however, as outlined previously, patients with a good exercise tolerance will rarely benefit from further testing.

A significant number of high-risk patients are either unable to exercise or have contraindications to exercise. In surgical patients, this phenomenon is most evident in those patients with claudication or an abdominal aortic aneurysm undergoing vascular surgery, both of which have a high rate of perioperative cardiac morbidity. Therefore, pharmacologic stress testing has become popular, particularly as a preoperative test in vascular surgery patients.

Pharmacologic stress for the detection of CAD can be divided into two categories: (a) those that result in coronary artery

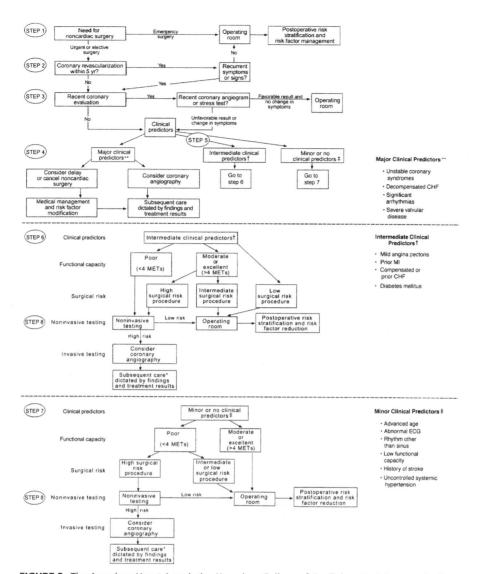

FIGURE 2. The American Heart Association/American College of Cardiology Task Force on Perioperative Evaluation of Cardiac Patients Undergoing Noncardiac Surgery has proposed an algorithm for decisions regarding the need for further evaluation. This represents one of multiple algorithms proposed in the literature. It is based upon expert opinion, and incorporates six steps. First, the clinician must evaluate the urgency of the surgery and the appropriateness of a formal preoperative assessment. Next, he or she must determine whether the patient has had a previous revascularization procedure or coronary evaluation. Those patients with unstable coronary syndromes should be identified, and appropriate treatment should be instituted. The decision to have further testing depends on the interaction of the clinical risk factors, surgery-specific risk, and functional capacity. (Adapted with permission from Eagle K, et al. Guidelines for perioperative cardiovascular evaluation of the noncardiac surgery. A report of the AHA/ACC task force on Assessment of Diagnostic and the Therapeutic Cardiovascular Procedures. *Circulation* 1996;93:1278–1317.)

vasodilation such as dipyridamole and (b) those that increase myocardial oxygen demand such as dobutamine. The coronary artery vasodilators work by producing differential flows in normal coronary arteries when compared to stenotic arteries. Several authors have shown that a redistribution defect on dipyridamole thallium imaging in patients undergoing peripheral vascular surgery is predictive of postoperative cardiac events (50–53). In order to increase the predictive value of the test, several strategies have been suggested. Lung uptake, left ventricular cavity dilation, and redistribution defect size have all been shown to be predictive of subsequent morbidity. Fleisher and associates demonstrated that

the delineation of "low" and "high" risk thallium scans markedly improved the test's predictive value (44). Only patients with "high" risk thallium scans were at increased risk for perioperative morbidity and long-term mortality.

Stress echocardiography has received attention as a preoperative test. The appearance of new or worsened regional wall motion abnormalities is considered a positive test. These findings represent areas at-risk for myocardial ischemia. Dobutamine echocardiography has also been studied and found to have among the best positive and negative predictive values for postoperative cardiac events (54). Poldermans and coworkers demonstrated that the group at greatest risk were those who had regional wall motion abnormalities at low heart rates (55).

Bartels and others prospectively studied a group of vascular surgery patients and performed preoperative testing solely based upon an algorithm similar to that proposed by the American Heart Association/American College of Cardiology (56). They demonstrated low rates of complications, supporting the approach taken in the Guidelines.

RESPIRATORY DISEASE

The preoperative assessment of the patient with pulmonary disease should focus on the demands made of the patient in the postoperative period. The patient needs not only to breathe adequately, but to breathe deeply enough to prevent atelectasis, and to be able to cough well enough to clear secretions. In this context, the classic division of pulmonary disease into "restrictive" and "obstructive" components, although a beginning, is not sufficient (Table 6).

The postoperative patient is limited by surgical pain, by the depressant effects of medication and illness, and by the weakness caused directly by the surgical incisions and indirectly by the stress of the surgery and anesthesia. Furthermore, atelectasis, pulmonary congestion, infection, and possible bronchospasm may all decrease pulmonary efficiency and increase respiratory effort.

For the patient with restrictive lung disease (e.g., obesity, chest wall or spinal abnormalities, or intrinsic lung processes) the respiratory pattern tends to be more rapid and shallow than normal. Such patients may, at their baseline, have trouble taking a deep breath, and may have very marginal reserve ability to maintain an adequate volume of ventilation. With the impairments brought on by surgery and illness there is the direct risk of respiratory failure. The indirect risk of atelectasis worsens pulmonary efficiency (causing respiratory failure), and also can increase risk of pulmonary infection in the regions of lung collapse.

Because chronic obstructive pulmonary disease (COPD) is generally the result of long-term cigarette smoking, it is often viewed as a single lung disease. However, for the perioperative patient COPD should be viewed as a combination of its three separate components: emphysema, chronic bronchitis, and bronchospasm.

The patient with emphysema, pathologically defined as dilation and destruction of the alveoli with impaired elastic recoil, has a relatively fixed process during the perioperative period. These patients may have very inefficient lungs, may even retain CO_2, and are often very sensitive to the pulmonary effects of fluid overload. Except for the fluid issues (which are often extremely important), surgery does not make this condition worse nor are there any specific therapeutic concerns. Preoperative pulmonary function studies and blood gas determinations are the best way to assess the severity of emphysema (57).

Chronic bronchitis is the most difficult respiratory disease to manage perioperatively. Severity is assessed from a history of cigarette smoking and chronic sputum production. The problem for surgical patients is to continue to cough sufficiently to clear their secretion given the impairments resulting from pain, sedation, and surgical incisions. Because pulmonary secretions are likely to be increased by infection or fluid overload, the vulnerable patient must deal with the problems both of excess secretions and impaired cough. Furthermore, as secretions accumulate, respiratory work increases and the patient weakens. Postoperative respiratory failure is a very real possibility for the patient with increased secretions. Hence, control of infection, careful fluid balance, and vigorous chest physical therapy (including tracheal suctioning) are all important therapies for these patients.

Bronchospasm is a process that can be easily triggered, going from absent to severe in moments. In the usual outpatient setting, bronchospasm is often initiated by an allergic or infectious process. In the perioperative setting, airway instrumentation, pulmonary secretion or infection, and fluid overload are most likely to cause bronchospasm. Except for the most severe cases, this is generally readily treated with bronchodilators. Because bronchospasm is so variable, it is difficult to assess severity preoperatively. When bronchospasm does develop, a careful search for the trigger factors (fluid, secretions, infection) is necessary; a default diagnosis of "asthma" is rarely sufficient.

Congestive heart failure (i.e., left ventricular overload leading to increased pulmonary fluid and atelectasis), is a problem that both exacerbates intrinsic pulmonary disorders and can be a problem in itself. The greater the fluid accumulation in tissue edema and other extravascular spaces, the greater the necessity for the patient to be mobilized postoperatively. For the patient

TABLE 6. EVALUATION OF THE PATIENT WITH PULMONARY DISEASE

Disease Type	Problems	Variability	Surgical Significance
Restrictive lung disease	Impaired breathing Atelectasis Weak cough	Slight	++
COPD—emphysema	Impaired breathing	None	+
COPD—asthma	Impaired breathing Atelectasis	Variable, usually treatable	++
COPD—chronic bronchitis	Retained secretions	Very variable depending on pain and strength	+++
CHF	Impaired breathing Atelectasis	Very variable	+++

COPD, chronic obstructive pulmonary disease; CHF, congestive heart failure.

with an impaired left ventricle, this can lead to pulmonary vascular congestion or even frank pulmonary edema. The heavy wet lung leads to worsened respiratory efficiency and may result in atelectasis, infection, or bronchospasm. Preoperative assessment of cardiac reserve, combined with a prediction of the fluid shifts during surgery can yield a prediction of the likelihood of pulmonary congestion postoperatively. Careful fluid balance, and diuretic or cardiac medication is a common part of postoperative care.

ENDOCRINE

Diabetes

Diabetes mellitus is a complex systemic illness with multiple potential end-organ pathologies that may add to the risks of the perioperative period. Of these complicating comorbidities, occult coronary artery disease is probably the most important, especially since it may appear in patients who are relatively young and may be asymptomatic until serious problems arise (34). It is therefore prudent to maintain a high degree of suspicion regarding the risks of cardiac ischemia in diabetic patients, especially those who have had the disease from an early age or for a long time.

Renal insufficiency is also unusually common in the diabetic population. Perioperative hypovolemia, especially if induced by intravenous contrast loads, may promote the progression of renal insufficiency to overt renal failure.

The classic hallmark of diabetes mellitus is hyperglycemia. Tight control of blood sugar (in the range of 100 to 150 mg per dL) is important for long-term management of diabetes because it minimizes many of the end-organ problems; in the perioperative period such precise glucose management is not necessary. The problems associated with hyperglycemia in the perioperative period are those of fluid balance, especially if there is a significant osmotic diuresis, and electrolyte imbalance (especially K^+). Severe hyperglycemia may precipitate hyperosmolarity and impairment of white cell function becomes a relevant risk. Blood sugar in the range of 200 to 300 mg per dL is acceptable for this time, although not ideal.

Perhaps most important is the avoidance of profound hypoglycemia (blood sugars below 50 mg per dL are a potential risk) that may lead to permanent brain damage. In an anesthetized or sedated patient the abnormal mentation of early hypoglycemia may not be recognized promptly. Hence, it is common to manage diabetes perioperatively with mild hyperglycemia so as to avoid hypoglycemia. It is good practice to control the amount of glucose given to an adult patient to the 5 to 10 g per hour range, both to prevent hypoglycemia and to avoid extreme hyperglycemia that is difficult (and certainly tedious) to manage.

The septic or traumatized diabetic patient, especially if illness has prevented usual insulin dosing, is at risk for the perioperative development of diabetic ketoacidosis. This is best managed, as in the usual medical intensive care setting, with careful (e.g., hourly flow sheet) separate monitoring of insulin, fluids, electrolytes (especially bicarbonate and potassium), and arterial blood gases. An awake patient with severe acidosis may have very marked hyperventilation with very low $PaCO_2$; care must be taken that a conversion to mechanical ventilation does not severely worsen the acid-base status.

Thyroid Disease

Hyperthyroidism in the perioperative period risks a concomitant hypermetabolic state leading to tachycardia, fever, cardiac dysrhythmias (especially atrial fibrillation), and agitation. Mild hyperthyroidism may be difficult to distinguish from other physiologic stress, and is managed similarly. If severe, the syndrome of thyroid storm may be elicited by either the underlying illness or the stress of surgery, with marked metabolic decompensation. In addition to symptomatic therapy (beta blockade, antipyretics, mild sedation, antiarrhythmics, and careful fluid balance) specific antithyroid therapy and supplemental corticosteroids may be necessary.

Mild hypothyroidism is difficult to appreciate in the perioperative patient and is not likely to cause major problems unless there is marked stress. Lethargy, bradycardia, hypothermia, and poor fluid balance are all potential risks if the hypothyroidism is more severe. There is also a significant risk with the rapid correction of hypothyroidism because the abrupt increase in metabolic rate is a potent stimulus to the development of cardiac ischemia in the vulnerable patient.

Adrenocortical Suppression

Adrenocortical suppression occurs perioperatively in a significant percentage of surgical patients. Multiple etiologies include primary tumors of the adrenal cortex, tumors of the pituitary gland, and most commonly from recent or prolonged steroid use. In patients with prolonged use of glucocorticoids, a Cushing syndrome can develop. The hallmark of this syndrome includes truncal obesity, moon facies, skin striations, easy bruisability, hypertension, and hypovolemia. Preoperative preparation includes correction of fluid and electrolyte abnormalities. In patients on long-term corticosteroids, perioperative steroid supplementation is indicated to cover the stress of anesthesia and surgery. In patients who have a short course of steroids within the 12 months prior to surgery, the use of supplemental steroids is somewhat controversial, although most clinicians would favor their use (Table 7) (58).

HEPATIC DISEASE

For patients with liver disease, the synthetic function may be decreased and the volume of distribution increased. Both of these factors may influence the effects of anesthetic and other perioperative drugs. Most of the coagulation factors are produced in the liver, and hepatic dysfunction is associated with coagulopathies perioperatively. For patients in whom poor synthetic function is suspected, prothrombin time is the best screening test.

RENAL DISEASE

The presence of renal disease has important implications for both the metabolism of drugs and fluid management. Preoperative

TABLE 7. PERIOPERATIVE CORTICOSTEROID COVERAGE

For minor surgery	The patient should take 1.5–2× his or her usual prednisone dose on the morning of surgery. The following day the patient should take his or her normal prednisone dose (or parenteral equivalent if gut cannot be used). The surgeon and anesthesiologist should be aware that the patient is glucocorticoid-dependent and they should be prepared to administer more "steroids" if the surgery becomes prolonged or more extensive.
For moderate surgery	The patient should be given 2× his or her usual glucocorticoid dose orally (if possible) on the morning of surgery and/or 25 mg hydrocortisone i.v. before surgery, then 75 mg hydrocortisone i.v. during surgery, 50 mg hydrocortisone i.v. after surgery, then the dose should be rapidly tapered over 48 h to the usual dose—if postoperative course is uncomplicated.
For major surgery	The patient should be given 2× his or her usual glucocorticoid dose orally (if possible) on the morning of surgery and/or 50 mg hydrocortisone i.v. before surgery, then 100 mg hydrocortisone i.v. during surgery. After surgery 100 mg i.v. q8h × 24 h should be administered and then rapidly tapered (over 48–72 h) to the patient's usual glucocorticoid dose—if the postoperative course is uncomplicated.

(Adapted from Brussel T, Chernow B. Perioperative management of endocrine problems: thyroid, adrenal cortex, pituitary. *Am Soc Anesthesiol* 1990;3:48, with permission.)

evaluation should determine the type of dialysis, the last dialysis, the serum potassium, and hematocrit. Patients with chronic renal failure, especially those on dialysis, are prone to congestive heart failure, hyperkalemia, and platelet dysfunction. After hemodialysis, patients may actually be hypovolemic, and require administration of fluid prior to induction of general anesthesia. Patients often exhibit chronic anemia, which is responsive to long-term erythropoietin treatment (59). These patients exhibit multiple mechanisms to compensate for the low hematocrit, which will allow them to tolerate a lower hematocrit perioperatively than other patients. However, these compensatory mechanisms must be balanced against the high incidence of coronary artery disease in selected renal patients.

HEMATOLOGIC AND INFECTIOUS ISSUES

The anesthesiologist must be concerned with the presence of infectious diseases. Part of the questioning should be directed at determining the presence of both hepatitis and human immunodeficiency virus (HIV) infection. Although universal precautions should be used in all patients, knowledge of disease state should increase safety.

There are multiple hematologic problems that can influence anesthetic management. Patients who demonstrated anemia (hematocrit less than 10g per dL) preoperatively should be evaluated for the cause, although anemia of chronic disease is often

the etiology. In patients with gastrointestinal bleeding or systemic diseases such as chronic renal failure, further evaluation is unnecessary. However, a low hematocrit may signify sickle cell disease or thalassemia.

An area of major concern and continued debate is the evaluation of coagulation disorders. Coagulation disorders can impact on the decision to perform regional anesthesia and direct perioperative utilization of blood products. The patient should be questioned regarding a history of a bleeding diathesis, such as easy bruising, epistaxis, or bleeding from the gums. The use of any medications that can influence platelet function (i.e., nonsteroidal antiinflammatory drug) should be determined. Platelet dysfunction is associated with bleeding of the mucocutaneous surfaces, such as petechiae, epistaxis, and hematuria. The anesthesiologist should also review any in-hospital medications to determine if low molecular weight heparins have been given.

NEUROLOGIC DISEASE

The extent of the neurologic history often depends upon the surgical procedure. Neurologic deficits can be divided into those primarily affecting the central versus peripheral nervous system. A history of a stroke identifies patients with an increased risk of a perioperative stroke. Evaluation of any residual neurologic defects as a baseline status should be performed in order to compare any changes postoperatively. In patients with a recent trauma, signs of increased intracranial pressure should be elicited. The presence of a change in mental status, lethargy, headache, or change in vision should alert the anesthesiologist to increased intracranial pressure and a risk for herniation. The Glasgow Coma Scale is often used to assess the level of consciousness (Table 8). Physical signs may include hypertension, bradycardia, arrhythmias, focal sensory or motor deficits, and slurred speech.

TABLE 8. GLASGOW COMA SCALE

Response	Score
Eye opening	
Spontaneous	4
To speech	3
To pain	2
Nil	1
Best motor response	
Obeys	6
Localizes	5
Withdraws (flexion)	4
Abnormal flexion	3
Extensor response	2
Nil	1
Verbal response	
Oriented	5
Confused conversation	4
Inappropriate words	3
Incomprehensible sounds	2
Nil	1

RISK INDICES FOR INTENSIVE CARE UNIT MORTALITY AND UTILIZATION

The majority of this chapter has focused on the preoperative evaluation of the patient presenting for elective surgery. As described previously, the goal is to diagnose and optimize the patient in order to develop a perioperative plan. Part of this plan includes allocation of scarce and expensive resources (i.e., the ICU). Several groups have attempted to develop severity of illness scores that predict ICU resource utilization in an acutely ill patient. Several different systems have been developed and even commercialized, and have been reviewed in greater detail elsewhere (60). The pediatric severity of illness scores represents a unique case and will not be dealt with in this chapter. The characteristics of the common scoring systems to predict surgical risk are shown in Table 9.

The most commonly used severity of illness scoring system is the Acute Physiology and Chronic Health Evaluation (APACHE) (61). The APACHE system sums the worst physiologic variables within the first 24 hours of ICU care for medical or surgical patients or measurements made in the emergency department for trauma victims and adds age and chronic health. The initial iteration was composed of 34 physiologic variables. The APACHE II has simplified the score by reducing it to 12 variables and adding age and chronic health (62). The APACHE II has also been used in a mortality prediction model, with variable results. It tends to underestimate death in high-risk patients and overestimate death in low-risk patients (63,64). The newest iteration, APACHE III, considers 18 physiologic variables and chronic health and has been used as an indicator of daily progress in the ICU (65). The Simplified Acute Physiology Score (SAPS) is another derivative of the APACHE score, using 14 of the original variables to predict death (66).

The Trauma Injury Severity Score (TRISS) and a severity characterization of trauma (ASCOT) are based upon the anatomic locale of the injury and selected physiologic parameters. The TRISS is derived from the Abbreviated Injury Scale for the three most severely injured body systems and respiratory rate, systolic blood pressure, and the Glasgow Coma Scale (67). TRISS is less accurate than the APACHE II in the severely injured (68).

The Physiological and Operative Severity Score for Enumeration of Mortality and Morbidity (POSSUM) has been developed specifically for prediction in surgical patients. It uses 12 physiologic and 6 operative variables to give a calculated risk of morbidity and death (69). Since it requires the inclusion of operative information, it can only be calculated postoperatively.

Value of Risk Indices

How are these risk indices utilized in clinical practice? The identification of important risk factors, via an index or simple research protocol, is critical in defining targets for intervention. One of the best examples of this approach has been the Framingham health study in which hypertension and other public health hazards were clearly identified and prompted changes in management of chronic diseases (70). Risk indices can also be used to compare groups at two different locations or with different provider characteristics of care.

TABLE 9. COMMON SCORING SYSTEMS AND THEIR COMPONENTS

	APACHE II	APACHE III	SAPS	POSSUM
Temperature	+	+	+	
Blood pressure	+	+	+	+
Pulse rate	+	+	+	+
Respiratory rate	+	+	+	
Pao$_2$	+	+		
pH	+	+		
Bicarbonate			+	
Hemoglobin				+
Hematocrit	+	+	+	
White blood count	+	+	+	+
Sodium	+	+	+	+
Potassium	+		+	+
Creatinine	+	+		
Albumin		+		
Bilirubin		+		
Glucose		+	+	
BUN/urea		+	+	+
Urine output		+	+	
Glasgow coma scale	+	+	+	+
ECG				+
Cardiac sign				+
Respiratory signs				+
Age	+		+	+
Chronic health	+	+		

APACHE, Acute Physiologic and Chronic Health Evaluation; SAPS, Simplified Acute Physiology Score; POSSUM, Physiological and Operative Severity Score for the Enumeration of Mortality and Morbidity; Pao$_2$, arterial partial pressure of oxygen; BUN, blood urea nitrogen; ECG, electrocardiogram.
(Adapted from Jones HJS, de Cossart L. Risk scoring in surgical patients. *Br J Surg* 1999;86:151, with permission.)

However, anesthesiologists effectively use subjective scores to assess risk. Physicians from other specialties may continue to use risk indices as means of determining baseline rates of complications in their decision if there is a threshold for action. Importantly, the ability to calculate a simple number (e.g., risk category) may detract from the dissemination of important clinical information since the risk category does not provide the anesthesiologist with the information he or she needs to modify care. Therefore, risk indices are most useful as a means of risk stratifying outcomes, comparing populations, and as a resource tool to identify areas that warrant targeted interventions, but have minimal impact on perioperative care.

SUMMARY

The preoperative evaluation of the surgical patient continues to be an important component of the anesthesiologist's role. It is critical that medical conditions be diagnosed, optimized, and risk-assessed, and a treatment plan developed. A thorough history and physical examination can be used to identify those medical conditions that might impact on perioperative management and direct further laboratory testing which impacts on perioperative management such as ICU utilization. Although risk indices may be useful in benchmarking local data to national standards or for comparing groups, they have less utility in defining care for the individual patient.

KEY POINTS

An estimate of perioperative risk provides nonanesthesiologists with information regarding the possibility of perioperative complications but anesthesiologists require additional information about the details of the planned surgical procedure and the severity and stability of preexisting disease in order to plan management.

The group of patients at highest risk of perioperative complications after previous myocardial infarction (MI) are those in whom the infarction occurred less than 30 days previously.

The algorithm recommended by the American College of Cardiology/American Heart Association Task Force for preoperative testing for cardiac disease incorporates three factors: clinical history, surgery-specific risk factors, and exercise tolerance.

Chronic obstructive pulmonary disease (COPD) increases perioperative risk, but the risk should be assessed as a function of the three components of COPD (i.e., emphysema, chronic bronchitis, and bronchospasm).

The perioperative management of the diabetic patient should emphasize avoidance of hypoglycemia and thus should tolerate mild hyperglycemia.

The Acute Physiologic and Chronic Health Evaluation (APACHE) combines physiologic variables from the first 24 hours of ICU care with age and chronic health assessment to predict the likelihood of mortality from critical illness.

REFERENCES

1. Shuman P. Bayes' theorem: a review. *Cardiol Clin* 1984;2:319–328.
2. Mangano DT. Perioperative cardiac morbidity. *Anesthesiology* 1990; 72:153–184.
3. Pronovost PJ, Jenckes MW, Dorman T, et al. Organizational characteristics of intensive care units related to outcomes of abdominal aortic surgery. *JAMA* 1999;281:1310–1317.
4. Goldman L, Caldera DL, Nussbaum SR, et al. Multifactorial index of cardiac risk in noncardiac surgical procedures. *N Engl J Med* 1977; 297:845–850.
5. Keats AS. The ASA classification of physical status—a recapitulation. *Anesthesiology* 1978;49:233.
6. Zeldin RA. Assessing cardiac risk in patients who undergo noncardiac surgical procedures. *Can J Surg* 1984;27:402.
7. McEnroe CS, O'Donnell TF, Yeager A, et al. Comparison of ejection fraction and Goldman risk factor analysis to dipyridamole-thallium imaging. 201 studies in the evaluation of cardiac morbidity after aortic aneurysm surgery. *J Vasc Surg* 1990;11:497–504.
8. Fleisher L, Rosenbaum S, Nelson A, et al. The predictive value of preoperative silent ischemia for postoperative ischemic cardiac events in vascular and nonvascular surgical patients. *Am Heart J* 1991;122:980–986.
9. Calvin JE, Kieser TM, Walley VM, et al. Cardiac mortality and morbidity after vascular surgery. *Can J Surg* 1986;29:93–97.
10. Mangano DT, Browner WS, Hollenberg M, et al. Association of perioperative myocardial ischemia with cardiac morbidity and mortality in men undergoing noncardiac surgery. *N Engl J Med* 1990;323:1781–1788.
11. Detsky A, Abrams H, McLaughlin J, et al. Predicting cardiac complications in patients undergoing non-cardiac surgery. *J Gen Intern Med* 1986;1:211–219.
12. Shah K, Kleinman B, Rao T, et al. Reduction in mortality from cardiac causes in Goldman class IV patients. *J Cardiothorac Anesth* 1988;2:789.
13. Lee TH, Marcantonio ER, Mangione CM, et al. Derivation and prospective validation of a simple index for prediction of cardiac risk of major noncardiac surgery. *Circulation* 1999;100:1043–1049.
14. Kennedy JW, Kaiser GC, Fisher LD, et al. Clinical and angiographic predictors of operative mortality from the Collaborative Study in Coronary Artery Surgery (CASS). *Circulation* 1981;63:793–802.
15. O'Connor G, Plume S, Olmstead E, et al. Multivariate prediction of in-hospital mortality associated with coronary artery by-pass graft surgery. *Circulation* 1992;85:2110–2118.
16. Parsonnet V, Dean D, Bernstein A. A method of uniform stratification of risk for evaluating the results of surgery in acquired adult heart disease. *Circulation* 1989;79:I3–I12.
17. Higgins T, Estafanous F, Loop F, et al. Stratification of morbidity and mortality outcome by preoperative risk factors in coronary artery bypass patients. *JAMA* 1992;267:2344–2348.
18. Dupuis JY, Wang F, Nathan H, et al. The Cardiac Anesthesia Risk Evaluation Score: a clinically useful predictor of mortality and morbidity after cardiac surgery. *Anesthesiology* 2001;94:194–204.
19. Shah KB, Kleinman BS, Rao T, et al. Angina and other risk factors in patients with cardiac diseases undergoing noncardiac operations. *Anesth Analg* 1990;70:240–247.
20. Tuman KJ, McCarthy RJ, March RJ, et al. Effects of epidural anesthesia and analgesia on coagulation and outcome after major vascular surgery. *Anesth Analg* 1991;73:696–704.
21. Isaacson IJ, Lowdon JD, Berry AJ, et al. The value of pulmonary artery

and central venous monitoring in patients undergoing abdominal aortic reconstructive surgery: a comparative study of two selected, randomized groups. *J Vasc Surg* 1990;12:754–760.

22. Bender J, Smith-Meek M, Jones C. Routine pulmonary artery catheterization does not reduce morbidity and mortality of elective vascular surgery: results of a prospective, randomized trial. *Ann Surg* 1997;226:229–236; discussion 236–237.

23. Valentine RJ, Duke ML, Inman MH, et al. Effectiveness of pulmonary artery catheters in aortic surgery: a randomized trial. *J Vasc Surg* 1998;27:203–211; discussion 211–212.

24. Haering JM, Comunale ME, Parker RA, et al. Cardiac risk of noncardiac surgery in patients with asymmetric septal hypertrophy. *Anesthesiology* 1996;85:254–259.

25. Tarhan S, Moffitt EA, Taylor WF, et al. Myocardial infarction after general anesthesia. *JAMA* 1972;220:1451–1454.

26. Rao TK, Jacobs KH, El-Etr AA. Reinfarction following anesthesia in patients with myocardial infarction. *Anesthesiology* 1983;59.

27. Shah KB, Kleinman BS, Sami H, et al. Reevaluation of perioperative myocardial infarction in patients with prior myocardial infarction undergoing noncardiac operations. *Anesth Analg* 1990;71. 231–235.

28. Rivers SP, Scher LA, Gupta SK, et al. Safety of peripheral vascular surgery after recent acute myocardial infarction. *J Vasc Surg* 1990;11:70–75.

29. Califf RM, Topol EJ, George BS, et al. One-year outcome after therapy with tissue plasminogen activator: report from the Thrombolysis and Angioplasty in Myocardial Infarction trial. *Am Heart J* 1990;119:777–785.

30. Merz CN, Rozanski A, Forrester JS. The secondary prevention of coronary artery disease. *Am J Med* 1997;102:572–581.

31. Ryan TJ, Antman EM, Brooks NH, et al. 1999 update: ACC/AHA Guidelines for the Management of Patients with Acute Myocardial Infarction: Executive Summary and Recommendations: A report of the American College of Cardiology/American Heart Association Task Force on Practice Guidelines (Committee on Management of Acute Myocardial Infarction). *Circulation* 1999;100:1016–1030.

32. Eagle K, Brundage B, Chaitman B, et al. Guidelines for perioperative cardiovascular evaluation of the noncardiac surgery. A report of the American Heart Association/American College of Cardiology Task Force on Assessment of Diagnostic and Therapeutic Cardiovascular Procedures. *Circulation* 1996;93:1278–1317.

33. Hertzer NR, Bevan EG, Young JR, et al. Coronary artery disease in peripheral vascular patients: a classification of 1,000 coronary angiograms and results of surgical management. *Ann Surg* 1984;199:223–233.

34. Kannel W, Abbott R. Incidence and prognosis of unrecognized myocardial infarction: an update on the Framingham Study. *N Engl J Med* 1984;311:1144–1147.

35. Eagle KA, Coley CM, Newell JB, et al. Combining clinical and thallium data optimizes preoperative assessment of cardiac risk before major vascular surgery. *Ann Intern Med* 1989;110:859–866.

36. Acharya DU, Shekhar YC, Aggarwal A, et al. Lack of pain during myocardial infarction in diabetics—is autonomic dysfunction responsible? *Am J Cardiol* 1991;68:793–796.

37. Hollenberg M, Mangano DT, Browner WS, et al. Predictors of postoperative myocardial ischemia in patients undergoing noncardiac surgery. The Study of Perioperative Ischemia Research. *JAMA* 1992;268:205–209.

38. Pringle SD, MacFarlane PW, McKillop JH, et al. Pathophysiologic assessment of left ventricular hypertrophy and strain in asymptomatic patients with essential hypertension. *J Am Coll Cardiol* 1989;13:1377–1381.

39. Goldman L, Caldera DL. Risks of general anesthesia and elective operation in the hypertensive patient. *Anesthesiology* 1979;50:285–292.

40. Warner MA, Shields SE, Chute CG. Major morbidity and mortality within 1 month of ambulatory surgery and anesthesia. *JAMA* 1993;270:1437–1441.

41. Krupski WC, Layug EL, Reilly LM, et al. Comparison of cardiac morbidity between aortic and infrainguinal operations. Study of Perioperative Ischemia (SPI) Research Group. *J Vasc Surg* 1992;15:354–363.

42. Eagle KA, Rihal CS, Mickel MC, et al. Cardiac risk of noncardiac surgery: influence of coronary disease and type of surgery in 3,368 operations. CASS Investigators and University of Michigan Heart Care Program. Coronary Artery Surgery Study. *Circulation* 1997;96:1882–1887.

43. McPhail N, Calvin JE, Shariatmadar A, et al. The use of preoperative exercise testing to predict cardiac complications after arterial reconstruction. *J Vasc Surg* 1988;7:60–68.

44. Fleisher LA, Rosenbaum SH, Nelson AH, et al. Preoperative dipyridamole thallium imaging and Holter monitoring as a predictor of perioperative cardiac events and long tem outcome. *Anesthesiology* 1995;83:906–917.

45. Reilly DF, McNeely MJ, Doerner D, et al. Self-reported exercise tolerance and the risk of serious perioperative complications. *Arch Intern Med* 1999;159:2185–2192.

46. Mangano DT, Layug EL, Wallace A, et al. Effect of atenolol on mortality and cardiovascular morbidity after noncardiac surgery. Multicenter Study of Perioperative Ischemia Research Group. *N Engl J Med* 1996;335:1713–1720.

47. Poldermans D, Boersma E, Bax JJ, et al. The effect of bisoprolol on perioperative mortality and myocardial infarction in high-risk patients undergoing vascular surgery. Dutch Echocardiographic Cardiac Risk Evaluation Applying Stress Echocardiography Study Group. *N Engl J Med* 1999;341:1789–1794.

48. Palda V, Detsky A. Guidelines for assessing and managing the perioperative risk from coronary artery disease associated with major noncardiac surgery. *Ann Intern Med* 1997;127:313–328.

49. Vanzetto G, Machecourt J, Blendea D, et al. Additive value of thallium single-photon emission computed tomography myocardial imaging for prediction of perioperative events in clinically selected high cardiac risk patients having abdominal aortic surgery. *Am J Cardiol* 1996;77:143–148.

50. Boucher CA, Brewster DC, Darling RC, et al. Determination of cardiac risk by dipyridamole-thallium imaging before peripheral vascular surgery. *N Engl J Med* 1985;312:389–394.

51. Eagle KA, Singer DE, Brewster DC, et al. Dipyridamole-thallium scanning in patients undergoing vascular surgery. Optimizing preoperative evaluation of cardiac risk. *JAMA* 1987;257:2185–2189.

52. Cutler BS, Leppo JA. Dipyridamole thallium 201 scintigraphy to detect coronary artery disease before abdominal aortic surgery. *J Vasc Surg* 1987;5:91–100.

53. Lette J, Waters D, Cerino M, et al. Preoperative coronary artery disease risk stratification based on dipyridamole imaging and a simple three-step, three-segment model for patients undergoing noncardiac vascular surgery or major general surgery. *Am J Cardiol* 1992;69:1553–1558.

54. Poldermans D, Fioretti PM, Forster T, et al. Dobutamine stress echocardiography for assessment of perioperative cardiac risk in patients undergoing major vascular surgery. *Circulation* 1993;87:1506–1512.

55. Poldermans D, Arnese M, Fioretti PM, et al. Improved cardiac risk stratification in major vascular surgery with dobutamine-atropine stress echocardiography. *J Am Coll Cardiol* 1995;26:648–653.

56. Bartels C, Bechtel J, Hossmann V, et al. Cardiac risk stratification for high-risk vascular surgery. *Circulation* 1997;95:2473–2475.

57. Smetana GW. Preoperative pulmonary evaluation. *N Engl J Med* 1999;340:937–944.

58. Salem M, Tainsh RE Jr, Bromberg J, et al. Perioperative glucocorticoid coverage. A reassessment 42 years after emergence of a problem. *Ann Surg* 1994;219:416–425.

59. Paganini EP, Miller T. Erythropoietin therapy in renal failure. *Adv Intern Med* 1993;38:223–243.

60. Jones HJ, de Cossart L. Risk scoring in surgical patients. *Br J Surg* 1999;86:149–157.

61. Knaus WA, Zimmerman JE, Wagner DP, et al. APACHE-acute physiology and chronic health evaluation: a physiologically based classification system. *Crit Care Med* 1981;9:591–597.

62. Knaus WA, Draper EA, Wagner DP, et al. APACHE II: a severity of disease classification system. *Crit Care Med* 1985;13:818–829.

63. Berger MM, Marazzi A, Freeman J, et al. Evaluation of the consistency of Acute Physiology and Chronic Health Evaluation (APACHE II) scoring in a surgical intensive care unit. *Crit Care Med* 1992;20:1681–1687.

64. Vassar MJ, Wilkerson CL, Duran PJ, et al. Comparison of APACHE II, TRISS, and a proposed 24-hour ICU point system for prediction of outcome in ICU trauma patients. *J Trauma* 1992;32:490–9; discussion 499–500.

65. Knaus WA, Wagner DP, Draper EA, et al. The APACHE III prognostic system. Risk prediction of hospital mortality for critically ill hospitalized adults. *Chest* 1991;100:1619–1636.

66. Le Gall JR, Loirat P, Alperovitch A, et al. A simplified acute physiology score for ICU patients. *Crit Care Med* 1984;12:975–977.

67. Boyd CR, Tolson MA, Copes WS. Evaluating trauma care: the TRISS method. Trauma Score and the Injury Severity Score. *J Trauma* 1987;27:370–378.

68. Demetriades D, Chan LS, Velmahos G, et al. TRISS methodology in trauma: the need for alternatives. *Br J Surg* 1998;85:379–384.

69. Copeland GP, Jones D, Walters M. POSSUM: a scoring system for surgical audit. *Br J Surg* 1991;78:355–360.

70. Kannel WB. Framingham study insights into hypertensive risk of cardiovascular disease. *Hypertens Res* 1995;18:181–196.

INTENSIVE CARE UNIT ORGANIZATION: MANAGEMENT, STAFFING, AND ENSURING QUALITY-OF-CARE

NEAL H. COHEN

KEY WORDS

- Acuity systems
- APACHE
- Clinical information systems
- HIPAA
- Outcomes
- Performance improvement
- Practice guidelines
- Privacy and security
- Quality improvement
- Scoring systems
- Standards of practice

INTRODUCTION

Intensive care units (ICUs) are assuming an ever-increasing role in hospital inpatient care. A greater number of inpatient beds are dedicated to the management of critically ill patients, in some cases within traditional ICU and in other cases in a variety of transitional or intermediate care settings. The primary reason for the increase in the percentage of beds devoted to specialized care is the complexity of inpatient needs. Only the sickest patients are now cared for within the acute care hospital; for many of these patients their needs can only be satisfactorily fulfilled within an intensively monitored environment staffed by dedicated intensive care providers. The increase in intensive care beds is also related to the improved clinical capabilities of ICUs and the improved quality of life and reduced overall costs that can be achieved in these specialized units because of the care provided (1–7). As a result, the management and staffing of the ICU requires special attention. The ICU must have an administrative structure that provides the framework for ensuring that care is optimized and resources are utilized effectively. It must have a medical director and nurse manager, who have the knowledge and skills necessary to ensure that the care delivery model is effective and the resources are available to optimize care. It must be staffed with an adequate number of providers, with the correct skill set, to provide care to the patient population. Finally, the ICU management team must develop a method to assess the quality-of-care and appropriateness of resource utilization and identify ways to modify or improve the delivery of care based on a critical evaluation of new approaches to clinical management.

INTENSIVE CARE UNIT MANAGEMENT

The approach to the clinical management of the ICU patient depends on a number of variables, including institutional capabilities, clinical needs, availability of physician services, and unit staffing patterns and resources. ICUs were originally developed to centralize nursing staff and high-cost monitoring equipment. Over the past two decades, the clinical needs and unit requirements have changed significantly. As a result, the definition of an ICU has become, in some respects, more focused and in some ways, more diffuse. A wide variety of ICUs now exist, often with very different purposes. The clinical capabilities within the ICU vary from one institution to another, and often within a single hospital (1–3,8–11). Because of the varying capabilities, a patient in one hospital might require care in an ICU, while a patient with the same clinical needs in another hospital will be cared for in a different setting. In some hospitals, specialty units have been created to focus care on subsets of patients with specific physiologic problems (cardiac disease, medical versus surgical ICUs) or based on surgical procedures (cardiac surgery, transplant, neurosurgery). In other cases, multidisciplinary units have been created. The approach to the patient will obviously differ depending on the skills of the staff, their familiarity with the clinical problems, and the administrative structure of the ICU.

Administrative Structure

To ensure that the ICU is capable of providing the care required for the patient population it serves, it must have a clearly defined administrative structure with a dedicated medical director and nurse manager. This team is responsible for defining the staffing needs, provider-to-patient ratios, and required staff skills; developing staffing models to optimize care; defining appropriate resource utilization; ensuring compliance with institutional and external regulatory requirements; and developing evaluation tools to monitor quality-of-care and define ways to improve it.

The most appropriate administrative model for an ICU is dependent on institutional needs, staffing capabilities, the physical environment, and the political climate within an institution. No single model can be defined and not one model is appropriate for all settings. Despite this reality, each ICU must fulfill specific requirements no matter what the patient population or the institutional needs. The definition of the ICU includes specific components, not the least of which is dedicated space and the availability of certain clinical capabilities.

No matter how the ICU is organized, each unit must have a medical director and nurse (patient care) manager (12–14). External regulatory agencies mandate that each of these individuals have clearly delineated roles and responsibilities. Although these mandates are important, more essential is the commitment of the physician and nurse leader to assume responsibility for oversight of clinical practices and day-to-day operation of the ICU as well as to participate more broadly as members of the overall hospital management team.

The specific duties of the ICU director are defined in part by the regulatory mandates and administrative needs of the ICU (12), but are also dependent on the clinical capabilities and management skills of the individual physician. Some general expectations are clear-cut. The clinical training of the medical director requires an overall understanding of critical illness. The physician must provide care to patients with a wide variety of clinical problems, must possess a broad fund of knowledge and experience in the management of multisystem problems, and must be able to define the most appropriate diagnostic and therapeutic options for each patient. The patient population cared for in the ICU and their clinical needs dictate the specific specialty training and skills required of the medical director. The medical director should have training appropriate to the clinical needs of the patient population in the ICU. The specific specialty training is not as important as the specific breadth and depth of critical care training relative to the patient population. The physician may be board certified in any medical specialty, including medicine, pulmonary medicine, cardiology, anesthesiology, or surgery, but should also have fulfilled special qualifications in critical care medicine (2,15–17).

The medical director of the ICU must work cooperatively in a dynamic and often politically sensitive environment. Although the medical director may or may not provide personal care for every patient in the unit, the director is responsible for maintaining standards of care for all patients, developing and implementing policies and procedures for the unit, and defining the standards of care. The medical director must know the current clinical status and needs of every patient in the ICU and must ensure that each patient receives the necessary and appropriate care. The director must also ensure that such care is effective, efficient, and carried out with respect for the dignity of the patient and patient's family. When unavailable, the medical director must identify a designee to assume these same responsibilities.

The ICU must also have a nurse (patient care) manager who is responsible for staffing by nurses and ancillary personnel (hospital assistants, other assistive personnel). The medical director and nurse manager have responsibility for developing unit policies and procedures and establishing a performance improvement program to ensure that patient care is delivered within accepted

standards and that standards of practice change as additional knowledge is acquired.

The medical director and nurse manager must work collaboratively to ensure not only that the unit is adequately staffed with appropriately skilled providers, but also that the supplies and equipment necessary for patient care are available. In many hospital settings the administrative leadership of the ICU participates in the selection and purchasing decisions about capital equipment, including monitors and electronic record-keeping systems, as well as supplies and materials. This level of participation ensures that the supplies and equipment will meet clinical needs, but also that the selection is based on both clinical and economic requirements, rather than one to the exclusion of the other. The medical director and nurse manager must also develop a budget for the unit, including personnel needs and supply and equipment requirements, and work closely with the hospital administrators to ensure that decisions are financially responsible but do not compromise clinical needs.

In addition to the ICU medical director and nurse manager, each ICU should have a management committee to assist the physician and nurse manager in procedural and clinical decision making. The committee should include all dedicated critical care physicians, the nursing leadership, including the nurse manager and assistant manager, clinical nurse specialist, nurse educator, and other unit-dedicated staff.

The ICU management team is critical to the effective functioning of the unit, but equally important is the availability of a well-integrated team of direct patient care providers with a wide variety of skills. Although each member of this team has specifically delineated responsibilities, the most effective ICU is one in which all providers work together to ensure the efficient and effective delivery of care, consistent with institutional resources, patient needs and expectations, and standards of practice.

An ICU must have written policies and procedures in place appropriate to the needs of the patient population. The policies should define lines of decision-making authority; specify admission and discharge criteria; outline triage procedures; and document clinical management protocols and the evidence upon which they are based. The policies should be developed and approved by the management committee under the direction of the medical director and nurse manager. Input into the policies and procedures should be obtained from the entire staff to ensure that they understand the basis for the policies and accept them. The other providers should understand how the policies and procedures can be modified, the method by which they can raise their concerns or recommendations, and the lines of authority for decision making.

Models of Care

A number of models for ICU management and care are used in both university and community hospitals. Some ICUs are "open" units and some are "closed" (18,19). In an "open" unit model, the primary (admitting) physician continues to participate in and coordinate the care of the patient after transfer to the ICU. The ICU physicians provide consultative care to the patient, similar to the care provided by other consultants. The extent to which the ICU physician has responsibility for any aspect of the patient's care varies. Because the critical care physician is physically present and therefore more readily available in most open ICUs, they provide emergency and resuscitative care and is responsible for airway management; many critical care physicians also assume responsibility for ventilatory support. The extent to which the ICU physician provides more comprehensive care is dependent on the skills and availability of the primary physician, the capabilities and availability of the ICU physician, and institutional politics. In each situation, if care is to be optimized, it must be carefully coordinated despite the fact that primary responsibility remains with the patient's primary care provider, surgeon, or perhaps a dedicated hospital-based physician (hospitalist) (8,11,18,20,21).

The "closed" ICU uses a different model of care. In this model, responsibility for all aspects of the patient's care is transferred to the ICU physician. In most such situations, whether in an academic or community hospital, a dedicated ICU physician is physically present or readily available to the ICU 24 hours a day, seven days a week. Although the care is transferred to the ICU physician, the need to coordinate care remains critical. The patient's primary physician may not be participating in the minute-to-minute care of the patient and, in more complex clinical situations, may not even understand some aspects of the patient's care needs. Nonetheless, the provider who often has a long-standing relationship with the patient and who will probably assume responsibility for the patient's care after discharge from the ICU, should be apprised of all changes in the patient's condition and should participate in discussions about patient care and post-ICU disposition.

Although both models of ICU management exist and either can be successful, the closed ICU has been demonstrated to improve patient outcome (3,19,22–26). Whichever model is used in an individual institution, however, the key criterion for providing optimal patient care is the participation of a critical care-trained physician. The ICU physician can help coordinate care from ICU admission to ICU discharge and ensure effective communication between all providers, including the admitting physician, consultants, other hospital-based physicians, and outpatient primary care provider. This communication will ensure that all patient and family needs are addressed, long-standing relationships with the patient are maintained, and the transition of care into and out of the ICU is accomplished without compromise to patient care.

Finally, from a management perspective, one of the greatest challenges is to ensure that the care is provided in a cost-effective and efficient manner (22,27–31). ICU care is resource-intensive, in terms of personnel costs, supplies, and equipment, and as a result, is expensive. The percentage of health care dollars devoted to ICU care (and end-of-life care) has increased. In many cases the costs do not relate to improved outcome or quality of life. As a result, as clinical capabilities have improved and critical care providers have gained new insights into the pathophysiology of critical illness and developed new monitoring techniques and therapeutic modalities, it has become incumbent on them to more effectively determine when critical care is appropriate and when it is not. ICU care, therefore, creates economic and ethical dilemmas that must be addressed each time a patient is admitted.

Intensive Care Unit Staffing

The ICU is a complex environment, requiring a diverse group of providers, including physicians, nurses, respiratory therapists, nutritionists, physical therapists, and other support staff, each of whom must have a wide variety of skills.

Physician Staffing

The ICU should be staffed with critical care-trained physicians. The participation of an intensive care specialist in the care of the critically ill patient has repeatedly been identified as a reason for reduced morbidity and mortality (3,4,18,22,23,26), decreased length of ICU and hospital stay (22,23,26), and lower costs (3,18,22). The ICU physician provides direct patient care, is responsible for ensuring that admission and discharge criteria are followed, and when appropriate, alternative sites for care are identified (8,22,26). They also often assume a triage function for the hospital as a whole, determining the most appropriate patient placement when ICU beds are in short supply (8,11,17,23). The value of the dedicated ICU physician is now acknowledged by the health care industry. The Leapfrog Group, an alliance of Fortune 500 companies and the Federal Employee Health Plan, now recommends that employers only contract with hospitals that have dedicated, specially trained ICU physicians (32,33).

Critical Care Nurses

The foundation of good clinical management for the ICU patient remains the dedicated care provided by the bedside ICU nurse (34). The care includes the traditional nursing functions, such as monitoring and recording of vital signs, completing a nursing assessment, and preventing complications associated with extended care. While these tasks are an essential component of good nursing care, the primary value of the specially trained ICU nurse is the judgment brought to the bedside that allows the nurse to anticipate potential clinical problems and respond to subtle changes in clinical condition to avoid complications.

Recent changes in reimbursement and the financial solvency of hospitals have created staffing challenges for the ICU. Since many of the specific functions fulfilled by the bedside nurse could be assumed by less skilled providers, there has been a tendency to consider alternative staffing patterns. In some settings, respiratory therapists have assumed some of the monitoring functions traditionally fulfilled by the registered nurse. In other cases, non-licensed personnel have been trained to obtain and record vital signs, monitor urine flow, and provide comfort measures. These changes have challenged the policies of institutions and the mandates of regulatory agencies for specific nurse-to-patient ratios and traditional staff skill mixes. The need to redefine the models of care delivery is also being required due to the shortage of skilled staff.

The current shortage of registered nurses and the aging of the nursing staff will put further pressures on us to develop new models of care (10,35–38). We will have to consider methods to cross-train a variety of providers to ensure that the basic care requirements are met, while at the same time developing better ways to utilize the extensive skills, experience, and judgment of the experienced nurse. Nurses will probably have to assume more of a coordinating role as care managers. They may be asked to coordinate the care provided by a team of staff and to direct the care of multiple patients, rather than providing all aspects of bedside care personally. Technology can facilitate this change in management by providing better ways to monitor patients using centralized systems that alert the nurse to a change in patient condition and direct the nurse to the patient who requires immediate attention.

As a result of the shortage of qualified nurses, the nurse manager, nurse educator, and physician staff must also develop recruitment strategies and creative ways to retain staff. Educational and career development opportunities will have to be provided to the nursing staff to improve their knowledge base and skills, improve their morale, and retain them within the unit.

Because of the complexity of clinical problems and the highly technical nature of critical care nursing, most ICUs also have critical care clinical nurse specialists or nurse educators to provide support and training of the bedside nursing staff. The knowledge and skills of the clinical nurse specialist and the other resources required to ensure that the standards of care are upheld depend on the patient population, the clinical capabilities of the staff, and the therapies that are available within the ICU. Particularly when highly technical treatments, such are extracorporeal circulatory support systems and continuous veno-venous hemofiltration and dialysis are required, the need for highly specialized and broadly trained educators becomes essential to provide educational and technical support to the nursing staff.

Respiratory Therapists

Because of the high patient acuity and the impact of respiratory disease on the need for ICU care, the respiratory therapist is an integral part of the ICU staff. The role of the respiratory therapist is being expanded, in part due to the complexity of ventilatory management and the pulmonary rehabilitative needs of the patients, and in part as a result of the changing ICU skill mix. Many of the respiratory care needs of patients within the ICU are being directed by the respiratory therapists using therapist-driven protocols developed jointly by the critical care physician staff and respiratory therapists. These protocols for management of mechanical ventilation, weaning, and airway management have resulted in improved clinical outcome, reduced ICU length of stay and lower costs of care (35,36,39–41).

In addition to the traditional clinical responsibilities of respiratory therapists, many hospitals are expanding the role of the therapist to include duties such as phlebotomy, recording electrocardiograms (ECGs), and measuring vital signs. Whether this expanded role will prove to be cost-effective or of clinical benefit remains unclear. Clearly if the assumption of these responsibilities distract the therapist from their primary role in optimizing pulmonary care, the economic benefit may be far outweighed by the clinical cost (35,40).

Pharmacists

Because of the complexity of pharmacologic interventions required to care for the patient with multisystem disease and the potential for adverse reactions or deleterious drug interactions, the role of the pharmacist in the ICU has expanded (42). The pharmacist has extensive knowledge of the pharmacokinetics and pharmacodynamics of the drugs commonly used in the ICU setting. The pharmacist can provide ongoing evaluation of potential drug incompatibilities and assessment of the impact of renal and hepatic dysfunction on drug metabolism and clearance. Because of the high risk of antibiotic resistance and nosocomial infection, pharmacists have served as "gatekeepers" for the use of some of the newer and more expensive antibiotics, to ensure that they are used appropriately and not indiscriminately (43–45). ICU pharmacists can also be helpful by providing a knowledgeable review of all drug orders, drug selection, and alternatives, and can assist with the drug administration during cardiopulmonary resuscitation (CPR). These efforts have proven to have significant economic benefit in addition to clinical value (46).

Nutritionist

As the outcome of ICU care has improved, the need to address nutritional needs has increased. The catabolic effects of critical illness can be overwhelming. For many patients who require an extended ICU stay, malnutrition often becomes a major factor influencing outcome and length of rehabilitation. Many studies have documented the value of early refeeding on ICU length of stay and outcome (47–50). As important has been the recent demonstration that many patients who previously received extended and expensive parenteral nutritional support actually benefit from enteral feedings, with reduced complications and improved nutritional status (51,52). For example, the traditional training that enteral feedings are contraindicated for the patient with pancreatitis has now been refuted by recent studies that encourage early institution of enteral feeding into the small bowel (48,49). In these situations, the nutritionist brings a level of knowledge, experience, and skill to the ICU setting and is an integral member of the ICU care team.

Social Worker

The complexity of the clinical and social issues that arise in the ICU setting requires that the social worker play an integral role in the patient's care. In some cases, the services provided to the patient and family are typical of the social work services provided in other inpatient and outpatient settings. In other cases, the social worker can serve as a filter for the providers, interpreting patient and family needs to facilitate communication about clinical care, expectations, and goals. During family discussions, the social worker can serve as a knowledgeable observer and can provide feedback to the physician about whether the family has been adequately informed. The role of the social worker has also expanded. Because of the complexity of health insurance coverage and some of the limitations placed on what services can be provided and in what settings, the social worker is an invaluable source of information about clinical alternatives, disposition options, and discharge planning needs.

Other Clinical Staff

A number of other health care personnel serve an essential role in the care of patients in the ICU. One of the recent additions to the ICU staff is the nurse practitioner, physician assistant, or physician extender (38,53). In part due to the shortage of nursing staff and in part to address the high costs of ICU care, some ICUs are utilizing nurse practitioners or physician assistants to perform physical examinations or to write routine orders in consultation with a supervising physician or under an approved protocol. In some settings, the nurse practitioner or physician assistant provides ongoing communication with the patient and family when the physician is unavailable. These staff also coordinate care with consultants and other providers. Depending on training and state licensure requirements, some nurse practitioners or physician assistants perform invasive procedures or institute cardiopulmonary resuscitation. In models where physician assistants are commonly used and adequate levels of training for the job expectations are ensured, the care has been demonstrated to be the same as physician-only care models (53).

ENSURING QUALITY-OF-CARE

Critical care units were originally created to centralize clinical services most needed by critically ill patients. The implicit, or in some cases explicit reason for the creation of specialized ICUs was to ensure that by consolidating services and resources, care would be optimized. As the economic environment changed, some of the focus of ICU care has been on the cost-effectiveness and efficiency, rather than quality-of-care. The challenge for the ICU providers is to fulfill the clinical expectations to provide the highest quality-of-care possible, while, at the same time, attempting to optimize resource utilization and reduce costs. We cannot take the quality-of-care for granted and must design ways to evaluate it, and when necessary, to change systems or approaches to care to improve it.

For critical care, evaluating and optimizing the quality-of-care is a significant challenge. Critical care medicine, by its very nature, is undergoing constant evolution. Standards of practice are not written in stone, but continue to change as our knowledge improves. Therapeutic interventions that are now used routinely were either not considered or were not available until recently. The standard of care also changes based on our ever-expanding understanding of critical illness (54–56). Perhaps more significantly, the assessment of quality-of-care is difficult. First, we are challenged to define quality in any clinical setting. Second, quality has so many different components that quantifying it can also be difficult. Assessing quality-of-care requires an understanding of the existing standards of care, a methodology for defining appropriate utilization of resources, and a method for evaluating the clinical and economic costs of care (57). Perhaps most important in the evaluation of quality-of-care is the assessment of outcome and whether it is consistent with the goals of therapy for both the patient and provider. Patient (and family) goals and expectations must also be addressed as part of the assessment of quality-of-care.

Quality assessment in the ICU is more complicated than in other settings for other reasons as well. ICU patients are sicker, require more resources and more interventions, and are cared for by a greater number of providers. As a result, the likelihood of a side effect or complication is greater.

The need to assess the quality-of-care is not only important to the individual patient who may suffer consequences of poor quality care, but also has major implications for the institution and providers (58). Accrediting agencies, such as the Joint Commission on Accreditation of Healthcare Organizations (JCAHO) (12,13) and state (14) and local governments, as well as government (59–61) and third party payors (32,33), mandate evaluation and documentation of the quality-of-care. Many payors prepare "report cards" to define outcomes of care and compare institutions. These comparisons often serve as the basis for a payor to contract for services in one institution rather than another. They have also served as a way of defining centers of excellence that become primary sites for delivery of specialized care. Quality assessment techniques also provide information about practitioner capabilities that are used for credentialing purposes and as monitors of individual clinical performance.

To properly assess the quality-of-care in the ICU requires that the critical care physician understands the principles of quality management and develops methods to assess quality of patient care (6,15,28). Effective evaluative techniques mandate an understanding of the standards for care in the specific environment, appropriate benchmarks to compare one unit or practice to another, and methods to identify systematic problems with care delivery within an institution that influence outcomes of care. A comprehensive quality management program will allow critical care providers to continue to improve care as our knowledge about the pathophysiology of critical illness evolves.

Quality-Management Techniques

Traditional Approaches to Assessing Quality

Intensive Care Unit Policies and Procedures as Quality-of-Care Tools

Each ICU should have written policies and procedures to ensure that the structure of the unit supports patient care and that the resources are provided to allow the delivery of high-quality clinical services. The policies should define the administrative structure for the unit, the staffing pattern, and how care is to be delivered and by whom. The specific policies and procedures must comply with the requirements of external regulatory agencies, including the JCAHO (12,13) and state (14) and local agencies. Some of the mandatory policies include a definition of admission and discharge criteria, triage procedures, disaster planning, and policies describing lines of authority and clinical areas of responsibility, particularly for multidisciplinary ICUs. The policies should describe who has the authority to accept a patient for ICU admission; when discharge criteria are met; and, perhaps most important, how disagreements are resolved. The policies and procedures are useful, not only to define for the medical and nursing staffs how the ICU is administered and how care is provided, but they also serve as the standard upon which the ICU is evaluated by accrediting agencies.

One of the most important reasons to have written policies and procedures is that they ensure defined standards for evaluating the quality-of-care, assess new clinical practices, and identify systematic problems that could potentially compromise care and how those problems will be addressed (8,18,41,58,62,63). The care should be evaluated on the basis of institutional measures of outcome and complication rates and by comparison of institutional outcomes to community standards. The specific community standard for comparison varies depending on the patient acuity, the nature of the patient population, and the practice environment. A community hospital ICU would be expected to have different practices and standards than would a unit in an academic medical center that cares for patients with multisystem failure. Multidisciplinary critical care units, such as medical–surgical units caring for a wide variety of patients with multisystem disease, will require more complex quality assessment techniques to address the needs of varying patient populations and to ensure that the staff maintains the skills necessary to care for these patients. The written policies and procedures should be specific to the ICU patient needs and staffing patterns.

Quality-Assurance Programs

The standard approach to evaluating the quality-of-care is through the departmental review of patient care activities and outcomes. In this type of review, a clinical problem is identified and an assessment of the causes for the problem completed. Based on the review, either educational efforts or changes in practice are implemented to reduce the likelihood of the problem recurring. The impact of the changes in practice can then be evaluated by completing a follow-up audit.

Most ICUs perform these traditional quality-assurance (QA) activities to evaluate clinical outcomes. For example, many ICUs monitor the frequency of accidental tracheal extubation or complications of central line insertion. The frequency of complications or bad outcome is measured and compared to a previously defined standard (57,64–68). While this approach does provide some useful information about areas on which to focus educational efforts, it is not a very effective method for improving overall care. It usually provides retrospective information about the performance of an individual provider or a set of circumstances that resulted in poor outcome. The reporting of clinical problems depends on the identification of the poor outcome and a subjective reporting system. In many cases the reporting is haphazard. For many of the problems, even when identified, a follow-up evaluation to determine if the proposed solution has been implemented and works is not performed unless the problem recurs. Finally, these focused QA activities do not identify trends across departments or units or do not allow comparison within an institution in such a way that systematic problems can be identified and corrected.

Morbidity and Mortality Review

Another very common way to evaluate the quality-of-care and educate providers about ways to improve it is through morbidity and mortality reviews. Morbidity and mortality reviews are typically conducted on a departmental basis, with discussion of an isolated adverse event. The goal of the review is to assess whether the care was appropriate and within the standard of care and to determine what, if anything, could or should have been done differently that might have altered the outcome. Although these reviews generally do not identify systematic ways to improve care, they provide an opportunity to evaluate specific problems and to educate providers about alternative ways of caring for patients. If this process is to be used and to have value to the providers and patients, the reviews should be conducted on a regular basis and include a systematic method to identify clinical problems.

The approach to morbidity and mortality review for patients cared for in the ICU is more comprehensive than is necessary for other services. Because critical care medicine requires a multidisciplinary approach, critical care mortality and morbidity review should include the participation of numerous departments involved in patient care. At the University of California, San Francisco, the monthly morbidity and mortality review includes participation of the ICU physicians (residents, attending physicians, and medical students), nurses, social workers, pharmacists, and representatives of the infection control staff. Other providers are encouraged to participate. Feedback is provided to other services involved in the care of the patient as needed. When necessary, formal feedback regarding the discussion and any concerns about patient care are reported to the program for further follow-up. The conference includes a discussion of all significant complications and a review of all patient deaths. The mortality review is performed to determine if any change in management might have altered the outcome. When patients die in the ICU, the death is classified according to a hospital-wide classification system. This system categorizes each death based on whether it was due to the underlying disease or a complication of patient management and whether the death was avoidable. As part of the review, the pathologists discuss autopsy findings and review specimens, when appropriate. The correlation between the clinical management and pathologic findings provides an opportunity for the critical care staff to discuss clinical management options and to determine if any unknown clinical conditions existed that might have altered clinical management. Minutes of the meetings and the discussions are an important component of the monthly program for the ICU.

Standards of Practice in Critical Care Medicine

Quality-of-care is, in large part, determined by the standards of practice for each environment. The definition of the standard of care in the critical care environment is difficult. First, the scope of critical care services continues to expand. New diagnostic and therapeutic interventions are continually being developed (35,38). The standards of care generally accepted today are very different from those of the recent past. As more knowledge and experience have been acquired in the most effective management of specific critical care patient populations, critical care providers have become better able to define those elements of care that are appropriate to provide and those that are ineffective. Second, standards of practice vary; not every provider would acknowledge the same standards, and the standards in one clinical environment are different from standards in another setting. Some generic standards do exist, most often defined within the local medical community, developed by specialty organizations, or mandated by accrediting agencies. Because these standards do apply to each critical care practice, it is essential that every critical care provider understand them.

Most standards of care evolve from clinical practice and experience. Although most clinically derived standards are applied in all clinical sites of care, some standards vary by clinical site, facility, or community. For example, the level of care and expectations for an ICU within an academic medical center is different than the standard of care for an ICU in a small community hospital. Patient acuity, diversity of the patient population, and clinical needs dictate the level and standards of care that are expected.

Despite this variability in the expected standard of care from one environment to another, some basic standards can be defined. A variety of methods are used to determine the standard of care in an ICU. Clinical experience is an important determinant of the standard of care to be expected in a given ICU. Clinicians also use medical knowledge obtained from peer-reviewed publications to maintain and refine clinical skills and judgment based on the current level of understanding of pathophysiology and clinical capabilities. Within the medical staff structure, peer-review methods are used to assess whether a provider is delivering the expected standard of care for each approved credential. This method of defining clinically acceptable quality is important, but also difficult to monitor.

Another mechanism designed to ensure minimum levels of competence is the certification process. Physicians and nurses must be licensed to provide care. The examination process to obtain licensure includes some assessment of knowledge and skills in clinical practice. Board certification in medical specialty and subspecialty training and certification in critical care medicine also imply a certain standard of care.

The ultimate definition of standard of care comes from the legal system. Traditional "standards of care" in medicine are based upon the judicial standard of the "reasonable person," a standard that is upheld when allegations of neglect are brought before a court of law. This "reasonable person" standard is determined by expert testimony that describes the community standard. Questions about malpractice are raised when care is believed to be below the community standard. Using the jury process, which evaluates the testimony of clinical experts, the court system ultimately assesses whether the quality-of-care delivered was within the accepted standard. This method for evaluating quality-of-care should only be used when peer-review mechanisms and standard clinical methods have failed.

MORE EFFECTIVE METHODS OF ASSESSING QUALITY

Performance Improvement

Over the past few years traditional QA activities have been replaced by performance improvement strategies specifically designed to optimize clinical management rather than to describe breaches in the standard of care (58). The JCAHO is emphasizing performance improvement methods and systematic evaluation of potential barriers to providing optimal patient care rather than the traditional QA methods (12,13). The JCAHO is particularly interested in identifying ways in which multidisciplinary teams can work together to solve systematic problems in care delivery. The JCAHO standards require that each department develops a performance improvement system that is multidisciplinary in nature and addresses all aspects of patient care, communication, patient rights, and safety. These areas have particular relevance to the ICU, since critical care medicine is multidisciplinary and requires demonstrated competence in a wide variety of procedures and aspects of care.

Performance improvement activities are focused on systems of care and are designed to evaluate how policies and procedures influence performance, and as a result, outcome of care. They are designed to continuously analyze data about the methods for care delivery so that policies and procedures can be consistently modified to meet the current state of knowledge. The JCAHO now defines standard methods for instituting performance improvement activities and requires that each institution establish a planned, systematic, and organization-wide approach to performance measurement, analysis, and improvement. Effective performance improvement programs result in identification of ineffective policies and procedures that prevent clinicians from providing appropriate care and implementation of new procedures that facilitate the delivery of improved care. They should demonstrate that the desired goals have been achieved and sustained, rather than be directed to solving an isolated clinical problem (57,68).

Evidence-Based Standards

The trend toward basing clinical management on data, as opposed to personal clinical experience, is also an effective way to assess and improve performance. Over the past few years, attempts have been made to evaluate practices based on evidence published in peer-reviewed journals. The goal of this approach is to ensure that experts in the field validate that the practices are appropriate and that care delivered to each patient is based on a sound scientific foundation. The publication of evidence-based guidelines provides a mechanism for leaders in a field to provide a scholarly review of the state of the practice and make recommendations for clinical management. Many critical care groups have developed practice guidelines for a variety of critical care services. By publishing guidelines or standards of care in specialty journals and texts, a number of health care and specialty organizations have attempted to define standards of care to ensure the quality-of-care provided to critically ill patients. Because critical care continues to evolve, the guidelines should provide some guidance to the provider, but should not be accepted as rigid principles of management (2,8,15,16,37).

Critical Care Clinical Practice Guidelines

A number of specialty societies have published clinical practice guidelines or advisories that can be helpful in defining the most effective therapeutic or diagnostic approaches to the ICU patient. The Society of Critical Care Medicine (SCCM), the American Society of Anesthesiologists (ASA), and other organizations have developed guidelines for management based on a consensus of experts who have reviewed the relevant literature. The SCCM has guidelines that define the qualifications for a critical care provider and provide a description of the requirements for granting privileges to physicians who perform procedures in critically ill patients (15,34,69). The SCCM also provides a recommendation that any physician practicing critical care medicine complete an approved training program in critical care medicine and/or obtain a certificate of special qualifications. The ASA and other organizations have published guidelines for the use of pulmonary artery catheters, the use of transesophageal echocardiography, and other clinical practices (34,70,71).

The American Association of Critical-Care Nurses (AACN) has also drafted standards for care of the critically ill patient (34). These standards describe the role of the critical care nurse in the care of the ICU patient. The standards acknowledge the dynamic interaction between the critical care nurse, the critically ill patient, and the ICU environment. AACN standards of practice require demonstration of a critical care nurse's clinical competence through a clinical preceptorship, continuing education, and ongoing peer review.

MANDATORY PRACTICE STANDARDS

Joint Commission on Accreditation of Healthcare Organizations

A number of regulatory agencies have responsibility for ensuring patient safety and the quality-of-care delivered in the ICU (13). The most notable oversight agency is the JCAHO. Most hospitals in the United States are accredited by the JCAHO; the accreditation is mandatory for any institution that wants to receive funding from the Medicare or Medicaid programs. The JCAHO accreditation methodology is designed to "ensure (and improve) the quality of health care." The JCAHO defines quality of patient care as the "degree to which health services for individuals and populations increase the likelihood of desired health outcomes and are consistent with current professional knowledge" (13). The JCAHO has recently changed its emphasis to organizational performance improvement, emphasizing the importance of the environment of care on clinical outcomes and a systems approach to care delivery. Because of the complexity of the ICU environment and the resources required to care for the critically ill patient, the ICU is a major focus of each JCAHO inpatient survey.

The JCAHO has also mandated that each institution establish a system that evaluates the safety of the clinical environment, identifies sentinel events, and develops a mechanism for analyzing their cause and preventing them (12). A sentinel event is any event that results in significant patient harm and is avoidable. The JCAHO allows each institution to develop their own sentinel event monitoring and reporting system, but mandates that there be a method for systematic review and development of prevention strategies. Some examples of sentinel events that warrant this kind of review include: (a) an event that has resulted in an unanticipated death or major permanent loss of function, not related to the natural course of a patient's disease or underlying condition; (b) hemolytic transfusion reaction; (c) surgery or an invasive procedure on the wrong patient or body part; (d) patient suicide while being cared for in a monitored environment; (e) infant abduction; (f) rape in a hospital setting; (g) patient death as a result of use of restraints or patient

seclusion; (h) patient elopement resulting in death or major loss of function; and (i) assault or other criminal act leading to death or permanent injury.

The identification of a sentinel event must initiate a formal process, known as a root cause analysis. A root cause analysis is a systematic review of all elements in the process of care that might have contributed to the event. To complete the investigation, a group of providers and administrators should be appointed by the hospital chief of staff to analyze the cause for the event. The group should interview all relevant parties to the event. Based on the investigation, an action plan should be designed to correct any systematic issues that might have contributed to the event and to define solutions to minimize the likelihood that a similar problem will occur in the future. Finally, the root cause analysis should create a monitoring mechanism to ensure that the corrective action has been implemented and to provide a method to monitor for compliance with any changes in practice implemented as a result of the review. The sentinel event procedures are particularly relevant to the ICU environment, since many of the patients in whom a sentinel event has occurred may be cared for in the ICU either at the time of the event or as a result of the event. The ICU medical director, nurse manager, and other staff often participate in the root cause analysis and are instrumental in identifying ways to minimize some of the events for which the complex ICU patient is at risk.

Three other areas being evaluated by the JACHO during its site visits warrant discussion (13). First, the JCAHO is assessing the use of and need for patient restraints. The JCAHO mandates that a physician on a regular basis must evaluate every patient who requires either physical or pharmacologic restraint, and that orders for the restraints be renewed if they are required on a daily basis. Second, pain assessment has been defined as the "fifth vital sign". Each ICU must have specific methods for evaluating pain, even for patients who cannot speak, or who, for clinical reasons, may be difficult to assess. A variety of pain management techniques must be available and the physician and nursing staff must work together to ensure that adequate analgesia is available to the patient and is administered based on objective criteria. The third area of concern relates to patients both within and outside of the ICU. The administration of sedatives and hypnotic agents to patients for procedures or to facilitate patient care must be provided by clinicians capable of managing any complications of the therapy. Although most ICU physicians and nurses have the skills required to administer moderate sedation, additional assessment skills must be assured. Since the sedation might compromise the patient's ability to protect the airway, the clinicians must be able to assess the patient continuously, to provide supplemental oxygen as needed, and to maintain an airway should the patient's level of consciousness deteriorate. Since many patients require sedation either during transport to or from the ICU or during procedures outside of the ICU, the skilled and knowledgeable ICU staff is often involved in the development of sedation protocols for the hospital. The protocols should ensure that the level of care provided to each patient is the same regardless of location; each provider administering moderate or deep sedation must be credentialed to do so; and the specific skills required to administer and monitor patients must be clearly delineated.

Government Agencies

Each state government also defines standards for health care facilities within the state. For example, in California, Title 22 of the California Administrative Code for licensing and certification of health facilities, defines what is required for a unit to be licensed as an ICU and defines the necessary policies and procedures, staffing and equipment needs, and space allocation (14). The code also mandates that a committee of the medical staff evaluates quality of patient care services. The Department of Health Services and the California Medical Association, through its Institute on Medical Quality, completes a site visit in conjunction with the JCAHO accreditation visit. Critical care providers should be familiar with the requirements of the JCAHO and their state agencies and should ensure that the requirements are fulfilled.

Payor-Mandated Assessment of Quality-of-Care

Most insurance companies and government funding agencies require a method for evaluating quality-of-care. In most cases, the requirements are consistent with those of the JCAHO and state agencies. The Health Care Financing Administration (HCFA), which oversees Medicare funding and the Medicaid program, requires accreditation by the JCAHO in order to receive federal funds. The Agency for Health Care Policy and Research and the Professional Standards Review Organization have also defined national practice standards and monitoring requirements.

All private insurers also require that hospitals have quality-of-care monitoring activities and that the quality-of-care is consistent with community standards. They also require utilization review of patient-care activities. Through the utilization review process, third-party payors will deny reimbursement if the level of care provided to the patient is inappropriate. The hospital and physicians will not be reimbursed for clinical services that are determined to be unnecessary or excessive. The utilization review process is particularly important for the critically ill patient, since the specific services for which the patient remains in an ICU may not be understood by the utilization review staff as requiring an ICU level of care. In these situations, it is essential that the critical care physician participate in the decision to either keep the patient in the ICU or transfer the patient based on specific clinical need, rather than bed availability. The documentation in the medical record often becomes the basis for approval or denial of a day in the ICU, so the physician note must clearly define the required clinical services and the need for continued ICU care.

Patient-Acuity Systems as Quality Assessment Tools

Patient-acuity systems can also serve as a QA tool, with respect to both evaluating the care provided in an ICU and as a method for benchmarking and comparing care from one unit to another. A number of patient-acuity systems have been developed that help define an ICU patient population, describe clinical and resource needs, and define the expected outcome of care. While most of the systems were originally developed to assist with staffing and estimating patient needs, the value of acuity systems has changed. As the patient population has gotten sicker and the clinical capabilities in the ICU have improved, the high cost of advanced medical technology places the utilization of critical care resources at the core of hospital cost-containment strategies. Apportionment of these critical care resources will have to include a more rational approach to the use of equipment, staff, and medications. Acuity systems or scoring systems that help clarify potential costs of care and predict outcome could be very useful guides to allocating resources.

A variety of scoring systems, including the Therapeutic Intervention Scoring System (TISS) (73), acute physiology assessment and chronic health evaluation (APACHE) (1,74), the mortality prediction model (30), and other systems have been developed as management tools for critical care units. Some systems are designed to document severity of illness and estimate resource needs; others are designed to assess prognosis to identify the patients most likely to benefit from ICU care. Those scoring systems that were designed to assess utilization of resources have concentrated on staffing needs, which account for the majority of costs in providing care in an ICU. Several other systems have been developed to evaluate staffing needs, many quantifying the hours or minutes required for each aspect of the care delivered. Although intended to define personnel needs, many of these systems allow predictions of resource use, providing quantitative assessments of care.

TISS is one of the earliest systems used to evaluate the relationship between severity of illness of ICU patients and resource use (73). It was the first quantitative measure of intensive care services and patient acuity. TISS assigns each therapeutic intervention a score. Based on the cumulative points assigned to the interventions, overall clinical needs can be determined for an individual patient. Resources required for one patient can be compared with those required to care for another patient, either in the same ICU or to compare across units. Although TISS was developed over 25 years ago, it remains a useful guide to nurse staffing needs. It has also been used to determine appropriate utilization of ICU facilities and to estimate costs of ICU care (9,30,63,75). As a measure of risk for complications or severity of illness, TISS has been used to stratify ICU patients (62,76).

Although TISS was designed to quantify services provided to ICU patients, it has been used for other purposes. Some investigators have tried to use TISS to measure severity of illness. For this application, it has significant limitations (27). TISS does not directly measure physiologic abnormalities and does not account for differences in clinical practice among providers. Comparison of TISS scores between institutions or between two ICUs in the same institution is difficult, since the range of services provided may differ considerably, even if the patient populations are similar. Despite these limitations, TISS can provide an assessment of resource utilization in an ICU and can be very useful as a management tool for the nurse and physician managers.

A number of physiologic scoring systems have also been developed to try to address some of the limitations of those systems that use resource allocation to estimate severity of illness. The APACHE scoring system is probably the most widely used of these systems (1,74). The APACHE system includes scores that account for both the acute changes of critical illness and any underlying abnormalities that might influence outcome. APACHE has two components, an acute physiology score and a chronic health evaluation status. The Acute Physiologic Score (APS) is derived from 34 distinct physiologic measures, usually obtained at the time of ICU admission. They include vital signs, hematocrit, electrolytes, urine output, liver function studies, and Glasgow Coma Scale. The chronic health evaluation is derived from the medical history and assessment of functional status to estimate a patient's underlying health status.

APACHE has undergone extensive evaluation and modification in order to better predict severity of illness and potentially predict outcomes of ICU care. The most recent version of APACHE, APACHE III, is a commercially available classification system (77–79).

Although the physiologic scoring system is a useful way to evaluate and compare clinical conditions from one patient to another, the specific value of either the APACHE system or any of the other physiologic scoring systems as a predictor of outcome has not been confirmed. While the APACHE system is able to classify patients according to likelihood of survival or death, it cannot be relied upon to guide management decisions for the individual patient. The primary value of the APACHE system is that it provides a consistent methodology for defining physiologic status of patients and allows comparisons of patient acuity from one ICU to another (80).

Clinical Information Systems as a Quality-Management Tool

Computerized clinical information systems have been successfully used as a quality-improvement tool in the ICU (81,82). Software programs allow for the collection and extraction of detailed information and trends from virtually every ICU chart on a continuous basis. Once collated from the computerized bedside record, data reflecting severity of illness can be integrated with other hospital databases to provide information about quality-of-care, morbidity and mortality, and resource utilization. This highly efficient method of data collection not only avoids the tedious traditional methods of chart review and manual data retrieval but, more significantly, serves as the foundation for continuous quality improvement.

Many ICUs now routinely utilize automated data collection methods to evaluate quality-of-care and monitor outcomes of care. In some ICUs, TISS and a physiologic scoring system are recorded routinely to allow correlation of severity of illness with resource use. For example, in one ICU the Simplified Acute Physiology Score (SAPS) is obtained for each ICU patient and is integrated with the TISS to produce a Computerized Intensity Intervention Score (CIIS). The CIIS has been shown to be a reliable predictor of ICU and in-hospital deaths for this ICU (83). As computerized charting systems become more prevalent in the intensive care setting, this type of automated quality-improvement program will become an integral part of critical care quality management. In order to manage the large quantity of data accumulated as part of the routine care for the ICU patient, every ICU will have to implement automated medical

record systems (84). The changing critical care environment and the complexity of patient care needs will mandate that clinical information be available to providers in remote locations. For example, digitized radiologic studies will be electronically transmitted to a radiologist who might be some distance from the ICU (or in another facility). An electronic record-keeping system will also be required to provide complete archiving of all clinical information.

Cost–Benefit Analysis

Quality management mandates that critical care providers demonstrate the value of the care provided. The changing health care environment requires that we assess the benefits to be gained by using high-cost approaches to care (29,31). This cost–benefit analysis has been lacking for most critical care services. For example. although the use of the pulmonary artery (PA) catheter has become a standard practice to evaluate cardiac function in critically ill patients, the benefits of this technique have rarely been documented. The value of the information provided by the PA catheter and its influence on patient outcome when used to monitor patients with sepsis, renal failure, or adult respiratory distress syndrome has never been confirmed (72). After years of experience with the PA catheter, we still cannot define those situations in which it is essential and those for which the information has clinical value. Multicenter studies are currently underway to determine if the value of the PA catheter is outweighed by its potential or real risks.

This example illustrates the importance of and need for better cost–benefit studies in critical care medicine. In order to determine what resources we need to care for the ICU patient and to ensure that they are available to us, we must develop better methods to determine the actual costs of the care we provide. As part of the cost accounting, we will also have to define the benefits of each of our interventions and determine which improve outcome sufficiently to warrant the expense. This analysis will be required of every ICU physician in order to justify the resources required to provide ICU care, and at the same time, ensure the financial viability of the hospital.

Calculating the costs of care, particularly those costs associated with the use of technology, is difficult. A number of elements of cost, such as acquisition costs, costs for associated supplies, labor costs, and additional costs incurred as a result of complications, must be included in the analysis. Professional fees must also be included in any cost analysis, at least from the point of view of the payors. The complexity inherent in technology cost analysis explains why meaningful objective data are so difficult to obtain.

Assessing the benefits of technology is equally difficult. Improved clinical care is the most obvious benefit, but it is difficult to quantify. Some benefits, such as reduced ICU length of stay or lower complication rates, are easy to quantify. Others, such as patient satisfaction or better quality of life, are much harder, although equally important, to assess. In fact, third-party payors and patients are putting premiums on increased satisfaction by providing bonuses to physicians who improve patient satisfaction. As part of a comprehensive quality-management program, assessing the cost and benefits of ICU care will take on increasing importance, particularly as critical care accounts for an ever-increasing proportion of inpatient care.

Other Regulatory Requirements Influencing Quality-of-Care

Medicare and the Health Care Financing Administration (HCFA) (59–61) mandate compliance with regulatory requirements for documentation of clinical services within the ICU and appropriate billing for those services. The risks associated with noncompliance are significant. First, if billing is not consistent with the level of service provided, HCFA will charge the provider with fraudulent billing practices. In the case of the ICU provider, the documentation for the extensive level of care often required can be onerous. The documentation in the medical record must support the level of evaluation and management services provided. Whether billing for a critical care service or a subsequent hospital visit, the note must include a thorough (interval) history, relevant review of systems, physical examination, and documentation of clinical decision making. Since most ICU patients require ongoing care over a 24-hour period, the specific services provided often vary throughout the day. HCFA does not compensate the physician for any discussions or follow-up by phone, or for time spent away from the patient's bedside. The critical care provider is responsible for understanding all billing and documentation requirements, including the 45,000 pages of regulations.

The compliance risk is significant. Although not specifically related to ICU care, HCFA has fined many health care organizations and physicians for compliance violations. They have also begun to educate seniors to discover Medicare billing problems and to report them. HCFA has allocated $7 million to fund a "fraud squad" to improve reporting of inappropriate billing.

In order to minimize the risk of Medicare fraud, each unit should develop clearly defined standards for documentation and billing. Standards of practice should be clearly defined and disseminated to all providers. Enforcement procedures should also be developed. Only services personally provided should be billed. Coding should be based on the level of service as documented in the medical record. If the individual provider is coding the level of service, the coding should be based on the documentation, not on a perception of the level of service provided. Use of an independent coder can minimize the risk of over- or undercoding. The compliance program should also define methods for voluntary disclosure of billing errors and a nonretaliatory reporting mechanism. The physicians should receive ongoing education about the coding requirements for each payor and any changes in billing and documentation procedures.

Patient Privacy and Security

The Health Insurance Portability and Accountability Act (HIPAA) of 1996 (85) was designed to ensure that patients had access to health insurance if they changed employers. The goal of the legislation was to "improve the efficiency and effectiveness of information transfers related to the provision, management, and financing of health care." The act included a number of other important changes that affect critical care services. HIPAA defined an administrative simplification procedure that mandates

standard billing policies and procedures. These administrative changes include the use of a national health identifier and common billing forms. Although the health insurance industry has opposed these changes and has tried to delay their implementation, the current administration has approved the implementation of these requirements in April 2001. The common billing forms should facilitate timely and consistent billing practices from one payor to another and might improve reimbursement for critical care services.

HIPAA has other and more important mandates that will significantly impact the delivery of critical care services. Patients must be assured of privacy and security with respect to the use and dissemination of medical information. Providers cannot disclose clinical information without patient consent. Although the information can be exchanged with other providers who have a "need to know" the information, the exact definition of "need to know" has not yet been defined. The legislation also requires that each institution identify a privacy officer to monitor compliance with the HIPAA requirements and provide patient safeguards. Since the legislation is new and the interpretation of the requirements still a matter of debate, critical care providers will have to use care in sharing health care information, while ensuring that important clinical information is available to the providers who need to have it. Confidential patient information should only be shared with those providers who have a clear-cut clinical need to know it, and it should, whenever possible, be disseminated only after obtaining patient consent. The other implication of the legislation that will affect patient management relates to the care that must be instituted in eliminating patient identifiers from patient census boards and cautious distribution of any aspect of the medical record. Unit specific laboratory reports or other administrative reports must not identify any patient by name or other identifying information. Patient identifiers must be used cautiously during morbidity and mortality reports and all such conferences must be managed within the medical staff structure with the inherent protections afforded it. Electronic medical records will make the requirements of the legislation easier to fulfill, as long as the electronic systems have appropriate security systems.

SUMMARY

The ICU is a complex and resource intensive clinical environment. In order to provide care to the wide variety of patients and fulfill the expectations of each patient, the ICU must have an administrative structure and staffing pattern appropriate to the patient population. Specific policies and procedures must be developed that define how patients will be cared for, by whom, and with what resources. Each ICU must develop a comprehensive quality-management program that evaluates all aspects of care and identifies ways to improve them. The program must define how new technologies will be evaluated and under what circumstances they will be introduced into clinical use. This last requirement is a particular challenge for the ICU, since critical care is a constantly evolving specialty. Technologic and therapeutic advances make the practice of critical care medicine exciting and the monitoring challenging.

KEY POINTS

As the number of hospital beds decreases, the number and percentage of acute and intensive care beds grows, and patient acuity increases, care of the critically ill consumes a greater amount of hospital-based resources. Appropriate institutional organization and allocation is crucial to optimize the efficient and cost-effective use of limited services such as critical care.

A well-organized intensive care unit (ICU) medical and nursing administration provides the foundation for proper utilization of personnel, risk management, peer review, quality assurance, benchmarking against accepted standards of care, and application of innovative therapies. Guidelines and external standards that are regularly revised and reviewed by government agencies and nongovernment organizations such as the Joint Commission on Accreditation of Healthcare Organizations (JCAHO) must be understood by the management team and systems put in place to assure compliance with them. Compliance with federal and state directives and private sector initiatives must also be documented and confirmed through institutional and ICU-specific review processes.

Various tools such as physiologic scoring systems can assist in the evaluation of the care of the critically ill patient, can serve as benchmarks upon which to monitor the efficacy of care in the ICU, and can identify the impact of changes in resource allocation or institution of new therapies.

Oversight of clinical practices has increased and the need to monitor ICU clinical care has become even more important. The documentation of patient care along with provision of patient confidentiality remain growing challenges to critical care providers. Fraudulent billing and inappropriate disclosure of confidential information must be identified, eliminated, or preferably avoided.

Proper ICU organization is crucial in maintaining the highest levels of patient care, meeting constantly changing reimbursement directives, and providing a mechanism to address "sentinel" events or shifting demands on precious resources such as critical care practitioners.

REFERENCES

1. Knaus WA, Wagner DP, Zimmerman JE, et al. Variations in mortality and length of stay in intensive care units. *Ann Intern Med* 1993;118:753–761.
2. Society of Critical Care Medicine. Guidelines for intensive care unit design. Guidelines/Practice Parameters Committee of the American College of Critical Care Medicine. *Crit Care Med* 1995;23:582–588.
3. Reynolds HN, Haupt MT, Thill-Baharozian MC, et al. Impact of critical care physician staffing on patients with septic shock in a university hospital medical intensive care unit. *JAMA* 1988;260:3446–3450.
4. Brown JJ, Sullivan G. Effect on ICU mortality of a full-time critical care specialist. *Chest* 1989;96(1):127–129.
5. Hanson CW, Deutschman CS, Anderson HL, et al. Effects of an organized critical care service on outcomes and resource utilization: a cohort study. *Crit Care Med* 1999;27:270–274.
6. Marini, JJ. Streamlining critical care: responsibilities and cost-effectiveness in intensive care unit organization. *Mayo Clin Proc* 1997;72:483–485.
7. Pronovost P, Jenckes M, Dorman T, et al. Organizational characteristics of intensive care units related to outcomes of abdominal aortic surgery. *JAMA* 1999;281:1310–1317.
8. American College of Critical Care Medicine, the Society of Critical Care Medicine, and Nasraway SA, Cohen IL, Dennis RC, et al. Guidelines on admission and discharge for adult intermediate care units. *Crit Care Med* 1998;26:607–610.
9. Gemke RJ, Bonsel GJ, McDonnell J, et al. Patient characteristics and resource utilisation in paediatric intensive care. *Arch Dis Child* 1994;71:291–296.
10. Lathrop JP. *Restructuring health care: the patient-focused paradigm.* San Francisco: Jossey-Bass Publishers, 1993.
11. Zimmerman JE, Wagner DP, Knaus WA, et al. The use of risk predictions to identify candidates for intermediate care units: implications for intensive care utilization and cost. *Chest* 1995;108:490–499.
12. Joint Commission on Accreditation of Healthcare Organizations. *Accreditation manual for hospitals,* vol 1: "Standards." Oakbrook Terrace, IL: JCAHO, 2000.
13. Joint Commission on Accreditation of Healthcare Organizations. Available at: http://www.jcaho.org. Accessed October 1, 2001.
14. Title 22. Social Security, division 5: licensure and certification of health facilities, home health agencies, clinics, and referral agencies. *The California code of regulations,* vol 30. South San Francisco: Barclays Law Publishers, 1990.
15. Society of Critical Care Medicine, Guidelines Committee. Guidelines for the definition of an intensivist and the practice of critical care medicine. *Crit Care Med* 1992;20:540–542.
16. American Society of Anesthesiologists. Guidelines for the practice of critical care medicine by anesthesiologists. Available at: http://www.asahq.org/Standards/31.html. Accessed October 1, 2001.
17. Strosberg MA. Intensive care units in the triage mode: an organizational perspective. *Crit Care Clin* 1993;9:415–424.
18. Carson SS, Stocking C, Podsadecki T, et al. Effects of organizational change in the medical intensive care unit of a teaching hospital: a comparison of "open" and "closed" formats. *JAMA* 1996;276:322–328.
19. Ghorra S, Reinert SE, Cioffi W, et al. Analysis of the effect of conversion from open to closed surgical intensive care unit. *Ann Surg* 1999;229:163–171.
20. Nelson JR, Winthrop FW. The hospitalist: how we've grown, where we're going. *Today's Internist* 1998;September/October:10–13.
21. Wachter RM, Goldman L. The emerging role of "hospitalists" in the American health care system. *N Engl J Med* 1996;335:514.
22. Li TC, Phillips MC, Shaw L, et al. On-site physician staffing in a community hospital intensive care unit: impact on test and procedure use and patient outcome. *JAMA* 1984;252:2023–2027.
23. Manthous CA, Amoateng-Adjepong Y, Al-Kharrat T, et al. Effects of a medical intensivist on patient care in a community teaching hospital. *Mayo Clin Proc* 1997;72:391–399.
24. Multz AS, Samson I, Scharf SM. A "closed" ICU is more efficient compared to an "open" ICU. *Crit Care Med* 1997;25[Suppl]:A106.
25. Multz AS, Chalfin DB, Samson IM, et al. A "closed" medical intensive care unit (MICU) improves resource utilization when compared with an "open" MICU. *Am J Resp Crit Care Med* 1998;157:1468–1473.
26. Pollack MM, Katz RW, Ruttiman UE, et al. Improving the outcome and efficiency of intensive care: the impact of an intensivist. *Crit Care Med* 1988;16:11.
27. Chen FG, Khoo ST. Critical care medicine–a review of the outcome prediction in critical care. *Ann Acad Med Singapore* 1993;22:360–364.

28. Esserman L, Belkora J, Lenert L. Potentially ineffective care: a new outcome to assess the limits of critical care. *JAMA* 1995;274:1544–1551.

29. Johnstone RE, Martinec CL. Cost of anesthesia. *Anesth Analg* 1993;76:840–848.

30. Rapoport J, Teres D, Lemeshow S, et al. Explaining variability of cost using a severity-of-illness measure for ICU patients. *Med Care* 1990;28:338–348.

31. Tuman KJ, Ivankovich AD. High cost, high tech medicine: are we getting our money's worth? *J Clin Anesth* 1993;5:168–177.

32. Birkmeyer JD, Birkmeyer CM, Wennberg DE, et al. *Leapfrog safety standards: potential benefits of universal adoption.* The Leapfrog Group: Washington, DC, 2000.

33. The Leapfrog Group for Patient Safety. Available at: http://www.leapfroggroup.org. Accessed.

34. Sanford SJ, Disch JM. *Standards for nursing care of the critically ill,* 2nd ed. Aliso Viejo, CA: American Association of Critical-Care Nurses, 1989.

35. Cohen IL. Establishing and justifying specialized teams in intensive care units for nutrition, ventilator management, and palliative care. *Crit Care Clin* 1993;9:511–520.

36. Cohen IL. Weaning from mechanical ventilation—the team approach and beyond. *Intensive Care Med* 1994;20:317–318.

37. Eddy DM. *Assessing health practices and designing practice policies.* Philadelphia: American College of Physicians, 1992.

38. Meyer C. Visions of tomorrow's ICU. *Am J Nurs* 1993;93:26–31.

39. Burton GG, Tietsort JA. *Therapist-driven respiratory care protocols (TDP): a practitioner's guide.* Los Angeles: Academy Medical Systems, Inc., 1993.

40. Wood G, MacLeod B, Moffatt S. Weaning from mechanical ventilation: physician-directed vs. a respiratory-therapist-directed protocol. *Respiratory Care* 1995;40:219–224.

41. Marelich GP. Protocol weaning of mechanical ventilation in medical and surgical patients by respiratory care practitioners and nurses: effect on weaning time and incidence of ventilator-associated pneumonia. *Chest* 2000;118(2):459–467.

42. Montazeri M, Cook DJ. Impact of a clinical pharmacist in a multidisciplinary intensive care unit. *Crit Care Med* 1994;2:1044–1048.

43. Burkiewicz JS, Kostiuk KA, Jacobs RA, et al. Impact of an intravenous fluconazole restriction policy on patient outcomes. *Ann Pharmacother* 2001;35:9–13.

44. Guglielmo BJ, Luber AD, Corelli RL, et al. Prevention of adverse events in hospitalized patients using an antimicrobial review program. *West J Med* 1999;171:159–162.

45. Luber AD, Corelli RL, Flaherty JF, et al. The evolution of an antimicrobial review system at a university hospital. *J Infect Dis Pharmacotherapy* 1996;2:65–84.

46. Dasta JF. Critical care pharmacy update. *Ann Pharmacother* 1992;26:823–825.

47. Hamaoui E, Lefkowitz R, Olender L, et al. Enteral nutrition in the early postoperative period: a new semi-elemental formula versus total parenteral nutrition. *J Parenteral Enteral Nutr* 1990;14:501–507.

48. Moore EE, Jones TN. Benefits of immediate jejunostomy feeding after major abdominal trauma—a prospective, randomized study. *J Trauma* 1986;26:874–881.

49. Alexander JW. Nutrition and translocation. *J Parenteral Enteral Nutr* 1990; 14:170S–174S.

50. Peterson VM, Moore EE, Jones TN, et al. Total enteral nutrition versus total parenteral nutrition after major torso injury: attenuation of hepatic protein reprioritization. *Surgery* 1988;104:199–207.

51. Lobo DN, Memon MA, Allison SP, et al. Evolution of nutritional support in acute pancreatitis. *Br J Surg* 2000; 87:695–707.

52. McClave SA, Greene LM, Snider HL, et al. Comparison of the safety of early enteral vs. parenteral nutrition in mild acute pancreatitis. *J Parenteral Enteral Nutr* 1997;21:14–20.

53. Dubaybo BA, Samson MK, Carlson RW. The role of physician-assistants in critical care units. *Chest* 1991;99:89–91.

54. Bernard GR, Vincent J-L, Laterre P-F, et al., for the Recombinant Human Activated Protein C Worldwide Evaluation in Severe Sepsis (PROWESS) Study Group. Efficacy and safety of recombinant human activated protein C for severe sepsis. *N Engl J Med* 2001;344:699–709.

55. Morris AH, Wallace CJ, Menlove RL, et al. Randomized clinical trial of pressure-controlled inverse ratio ventilation and extracorporeal CO_2 removal for acute respiratory distress syndrome. *Am J Respir Crit Care Med* 1994;149:295–305.

56. The Acute Respiratory Distress Syndrome Network. Ventilation with lower tidal volume as compared with traditional tidal volumes for acute lung injury and the acute respiratory distress syndrome. *N Engl J Med* 2000;342:1301–1308.

57. Couch NS, Dorgan NE. Vecuronium use in MICU: a quality improvement study. *Nurs Mgmt* 1993;24:96J–96P.

58. Davis ER. There's more to quality improvement than a name change. *J Healthcare Quality: Promoting Excellence in Healthcare* 1993;15:33–35.

59. Health Care Financing Administration. HCFA Compliance. Available at: http://www.hcfa.gov/facts/fsy2k.htm. Accessed October 1, 2001.

60. HCMS Board of Socioeconomics. Conomikes Medicine Hotline, July 1–Aug. 2000.

61. HCMS Board of Socioeconomics. HCFA compliance, part 1. Available at: http://www.hcms.org/hcfa/partone.html. Accessed.

62. Becker RB, Zimmerman JE, Knaus WA, et al. The use of APACHE III to evaluate ICU length of stay, resource use, and mortality after coronary artery by-pass surgery. *J Cardiovasc Surg* 1995;36:1–11.

63. Hjortso E, Buch T, Ryding J, et al. The nursing care recording system. A preliminary study of a system for assessment of nursing care demands in the ICU. *Acta Anaesthesiol Scand* 1992;36:610–614.

64. Grap MJ, Glass C, Lindamood MO. Factors related to unplanned extubation of endotracheal tubes. *Crit Care Nurse* 1995;15:57–65.

65. Taggart JA, Lind MA. Evaluating unplanned endotracheal extubations. *DCCN: Dimensions of Critical Care Nursing* 1994;13:114–122.

66. Agee KA, Balk RA. Central venous catheterization in the critically ill patient. *Crit Care Clin* 1992;8:677–686.

67. Puri VK, Carlson RW, Bander JJ, et al. Complications of vascular catheterization in the critically ill. A prospective study. *Crit Care Med* 1980;8:495–499.

68. Kollef MH, Legare EJ, Damiano M. Endotracheal tube misplacement: incidence, risk factors, and impact of a quality improvement program. *South Med J* 1994;87:248–254.

69. Society of Critical Care Medicine, Guidelines Committee. Guidelines for granting privileges for the performance of procedures in critically ill patients. *Crit Care Med* 1993;21:292–293.

70. American Society of Anesthesiologists. Practice guidelines for perioperative transesophageal echocardiography. *Anesthesiology* 1996;84:986–1006.

71. American Society of Anesthesiologists. Practice guidelines for pulmonary artery catheterization. *Anesthesiology* 1993;78:380–394.

72. Iberti TJ, Fischer EP, Leibowitz AB, et al. A multicenter study of physicians' knowledge of the pulmonary artery catheter. Pulmonary Artery Catheter Study Group. *JAMA* 1990;264:2928–2932.

73. Cullen DJ, Civetta JM, Briggs BA, et al. Therapeutic intervention scoring system: a method for quantitative comparison of patient care. *Crit Care Med* 1974;2:57–60.

74. Knaus WA, Zimmerman JE, Wagner DP, et al. APACHE—acute physiology and chronic health evaluation: a physiologically based classification system. *Crit Care Med* 1981;9:591–597.

75. Malstam J, Lind L. Therapeutic intervention scoring system (TISS)—a method for measuring workload and calculating costs in the ICU. *Acta Anaesthesiol Scand* 1992;36:758–763.

76. Bueno-Cavanillas A, Rodriguez-Contreras R, Lopez-Luque A, et al. Usefulness of severity indices in intensive care medicine as a predictor of nosocomial infection risk. *Intensive Care Med* 1991;17:336–339.

77. Wagner D, Draper E, Knaus W. Development of APACHE III. APACHE III study design: analytic plan for evaluation of severity and outcome. *Crit Care Med* 1989;17:S199–S203.

78. Knaus WA, Wagner DP, Draper EA, et al. The APACHE III prognostic system. Risk prediction of hospital mortality for critically ill hospitalized adults. *Chest* 1991;100:1619–1636.

79. Zimmerman JE, Wagner DP, Draper EA, et al. Evaluation of acute physiology and chronic health evaluation III predictions of hospital mortality in an independent database. *Crit Care Med* 1998;26:1317–1326.

80. Lemeshow S, LeGall J-R. Modeling the severity of illness of ICU patients: a systems update. *JAMA* 1994; 272:1049–1055.

81. Brimm JE. Computers and critical care. *Crit Care Q* 1987;9:53–63.

82. Gardner RM, Huff SM. Computers in the ICU: Why? What? And so what? *Int J Clin Monit Comput* 1992;9:199–205.

83. Shabot MM, Bjerke HS, LoBue M, et al. Quality assurance and utilization assessment: the major by-products of an ICU clinical information system. In: Proceedings of the Annual Symposium on Computer Applied Medical Care 1991;554–558.

84. Buchman TG. Computers in the intensive care unit: promises yet to be fulfilled. *J Intensive Care Med* 1995;10:234–240.

85. Health Care Financing Administration. Health Insurance Portability and Accountability Act. Available at: http://www.hcfa.gov/medlearn/hipaa.htm. Accessed.

3

THE PRACTICE OF ACUTE CARE
MEDICINE IN COMMUNITY HOSPITALS

GERALD A. MACCIOLI
VINCENT L. HOELLERICH

KEY WORDS

- Acute care medicine
- Clinical pathways
- Hospital organization
- Hospitalist
- Outcomes
- Perioperative medicine
- Preoperative assessment
- Intraoperative management
- Critical care medicine
- Pain management

INTRODUCTION

Anesthesiologists have provided critical care services for decades, with many anesthesiologists intimately involved in the development of intensive care units (ICUs) throughout the world (1). As the practice of anesthesiology has evolved, participation and interest in critical care medicine has waxed and waned, depending on the physician's personal interests and training and on the traditions of particular hospitals and anesthesiology departments. Although many academic departments have become "full-service" departments of anesthesiology and critical care medicine, few private or community hospitals have departments that function in such a capacity. However, many practicing anesthesiologists without specific critical care training are often involved with the perioperative care of ICU patients.

The community hospital practice of anesthesiology and critical care medicine varies from one institution to another and is likely to change in the future. Change is most likely to come from the pressure of third-party carriers' ongoing quest for absolute dollar savings. Anesthesiologists may provide one-on-one care of patients by primarily providing anesthesia in operating rooms (ORs) (i.e., the traditional approach to anesthetic practice). In other settings, anesthesiologists provide a much broader scope of services including comprehensive perioperative care of surgical patients. Furthermore, there are some anesthesiology groups that provide pain management and critical care, as well as other consultative services for general inpatient care and management (e.g., "hospitalist" care).

One way of viewing these full-service departments is to look at the anesthesiologist as the provider of acute care medicine: the perioperative care of surgical patients, the care of critically ill patients in the ICU, and the diagnosis and treatment of acutely ill patients elsewhere in the hospital (2,3). This chapter outlines the fundamental issues that anesthesiologists face when providing acute and critical care medicine services in private hospitals and examines various models of such practices.

PRACTICE FRAMEWORK

The primary function of an anesthesiology group is to provide OR anesthesia and comprehensive perioperative medicine services. Perioperative medicine in this model comprises a thorough preoperative assessment, intraoperative management, and postoperative care. Preoperative assessment in general occurs through a pretesting visit where every patient has an opportunity to meet an anesthesiologist. At this time, all preoperative tests are performed, a tour of the facility is offered, preoperative education is conducted, and an introduction for rehabilitation and recovery strategies is performed. Groups have the option of developing state-of-the-art guidelines for preoperative tests such as the cardiac evaluation for patients undergoing noncardiac surgery (Fig 1). Preoperative consultation is the area where the anesthesiologist/intensivist may have the greatest impact. The two most common areas of perioperative concern are prevention of postoperative pulmonary complications and perioperative cardiac events. Poldermans and colleagues recently published a study on the effect of beta-blocker therapy on perioperative mortality and myocardial infarction in "high-risk" patients undergoing vascular surgery (4). The efficacy of perioperative beta-blockade on the incidence of death from cardiac causes and nonfatal myocardial infarction within 30 days of major vascular surgery was evaluated. The authors concluded beta-blockade, bisoprolol in this study, reduces the perioperative incidence of death from cardiac causes and nonfatal myocardial infarction in high-risk patients undergoing vascular reconstruction. The anesthesiologist/intensivist in the community is most likely to be the physician who institutes beta-blocker therapy.

Likewise, several recent reviews comment on the role of anesthesiologists as perioperative physicians and the role they play in preoperative pulmonary evaluation and prevention of

CHS Guidelines for Pre-Op Cardiac Evaluations

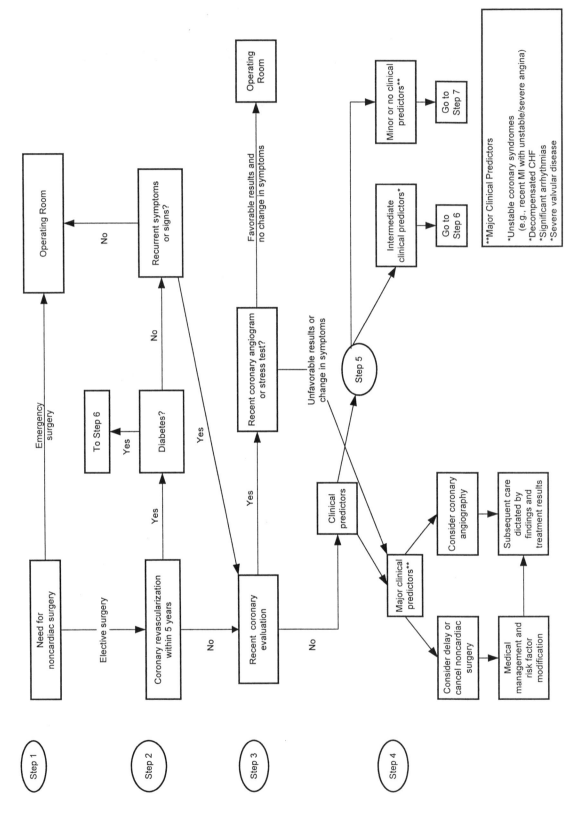

FIGURE 1. Perioperative cardiac evaluation decision analysis form. Modified from the guidelines for Perioperative Cardiovascular Evaluation for Non-Cardiac Surgery. *Circulation* 1996.

CHS Guidelines for Pre-Op Cardiac Evaluations

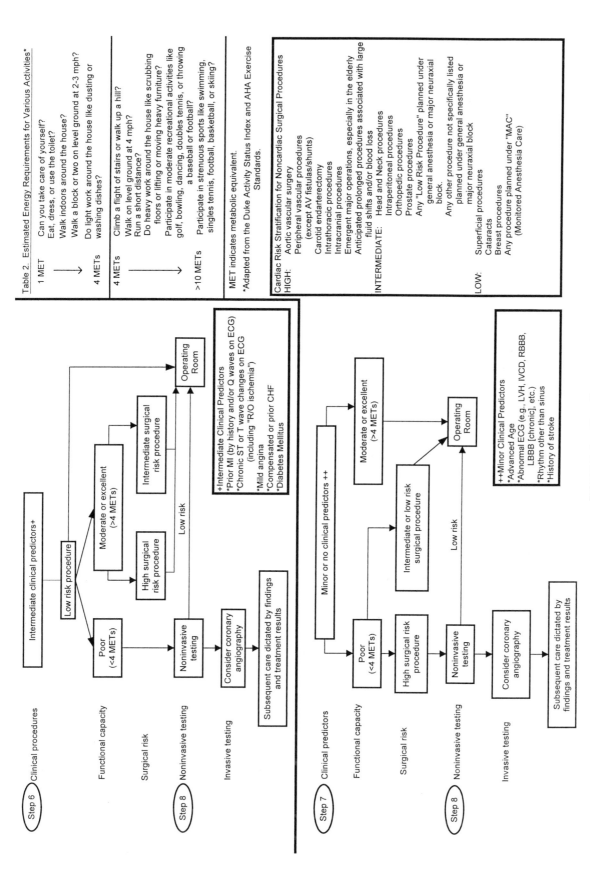

FIGURE 1. (*continued*)

Table 2. Estimated Energy Requirements for Various Activities*

1 MET	Can you take care of yourself?
	Eat, dress, or use the toilet?
	Walk indoors around the house?
	Walk a block or two on level ground at 2-3 mph?
↓	Do light work around the house like dusting or washing dishes?
4 METs	
4 METs	Climb a flight of stairs or walk up a hill?
	Walk on level ground at 4 mph?
	Run a short distance?
	Do heavy work around the house like scrubbing floors or lifting or moving heavy furniture?
	Participate in moderate recreational activities like golf, bowling, dancing, doubles tennis, or throwing a baseball or football?
>10 METs	Participate in strenuous sports like swimming, singles tennis, football, basketball, or skiing?

MET indicates metabolic equivalent.
*Adapted from the Duke Activity Status Index and AHA Exercise Standards.

Cardiac Risk Stratification for Noncardiac Surgical Procedures
HIGH: Aortic vascular surgery
           Peripheral vascular procedures (except AV fistulas/shunts)
           Carotid endarterectomy
           Intrathoracic procedures
           Intracranial procedures
           Emergent major operations, especially in the elderly
           Anticipated prolonged procedures associated with large fluid shifts and/or blood loss
INTERMEDIATE: Head and Neck procedures
           Intraperitoneal procedures
           Orthopedic procedures
           Prostate procedures
           Any "Low Risk Procedure" planned under general anesthesia or major neuraxial block.
           Any other procedure not specifically listed planned under general anesthesia or major neuraxial block
LOW: Superficial procedures
           Cataracts
           Breast procedures
           Any procedure planned under "MAC" (Monitored Anesthesia Care)

31

postoperative complications (5,6). Perioperative care, including risk-reduction strategies, is usually performed at the initiation of the anesthesiologist (6,7).

Given the current economic paradigm of cost-containment, optimal resource utilization, and an insufficient number of both anesthesia care providers and specialist intensivists, the anesthesia care team approach simultaneously facilitates quality care in the OR and ICU. Perioperative care of patients has become increasingly sophisticated and safe. Along with this improvement in safety, physicians continue to push the envelope of medicine by providing care to older and more severely ill patients while applying innovative techniques. One only has to compare current anesthetizing locations with their myriad monitoring equipment, standardized anesthetic delivery systems, and data management capabilities with those used only 10 to 20 years ago to appreciate the magnitude of these paradigm shifts. Applications of pulse oximetry and breath-to-breath capnography with end-tidal agent analysis, in particular, have dramatically increased the safety of anesthesiology. The benefits have been most pronounced during the intraoperative period. These positive developments must be continued and efforts focused on improving outcome through enhanced perioperative care, particularly in preoperative screening and postoperative management of pain and recovery from surgical intervention. Who supplies this care, how they provide care, how many are needed to provide perioperative care, and what skills are required to provide care are some of the crucial questions that the specialty must address (8,9).

Perioperative medicine will be defined in this chapter as the practice of medicine directly caring for patients in the perioperative period in an acute care facility (Table 1). It includes many aspects of what has previously been discussed, but is more comprehensive. The components of acute care medicine in a traditional hospital setting include the practices of anesthesi-

ology, perioperative medicine, pain management, critical care, general inpatient care and management, and the care of emergency department patients. Anesthesiologists are best positioned as hospital-based physicians specializing in acute intervention. The most important component of being part of a successful and efficient acute care team is to be able and willing to manage acutely ill patients anywhere in the hospital.

Preoperative Evaluation Clinic

A preoperative area should be adjacent to the main OR suite and patients should be seen by any anesthesiologist who regularly staffs the ORs. The hospital provides both the space and the staff for the clinic, and many clinicians believe that the optimization of day of surgery OR efficiency is worth the cost of the preoperative clinic. In other words, the preoperative clinic helps to avoid last minute cancellations due to inadequate workup or other problems and thereby assures an extremely low rate of surgical cancellations on any given day in the main OR.

The anesthesiologist who sees the patient during the preoperative evaluation is not necessarily the anesthesiologist who will help provide care on the day of surgery. However, all pertinent information related to the case including American Society of Anesthesiologists (ASA) status, medical diagnoses, medications, type of anesthesia discussed and planned, as well as additional concerns about difficult airway management, invasive monitoring, and postoperative issues are documented on a form that becomes part of the daily schedule on the day the surgery is actually performed. This model helps with early identification of those patients who will require postoperative intensive care, mechanical ventilation, nutritional support, or other interventions.

Compensation of anesthesiologists on a nonproductivity basis assures the preoperative obligation is simply an expected part of all of the anesthesiologist's duties on a given day. This requires the anesthesiologist to be self-motivated and understand that in addition to managing the ORs, overseeing aspects of patient care in the postanesthesia care unit and other related issues, their obligations involve routine rotations through the preoperative clinic. This can best be facilitated in hospitals in which the main OR suite, postanesthesia care unit, as well as the preoperative clinic are all located within close proximity to each other.

Standardizing the approach to preoperative testing and developing a set of guidelines by which any given patient would have appropriate tests ordered automatically, unless otherwise ordered by the anesthesiologist conducting the preoperative evaluation, improves efficiency and enhances uniformity of quality. Example preoperative orders as well as the guidelines are shown in Table 2 and Fig. 2. The orders facilitate the care of the patient on the day of surgery and the guidelines allow rapid assessment of what tests need to be performed based on the patient's medical history. Guidelines are developed after consultation with the entire group and review of all of the current literature related to preoperative testing. The guidelines are evaluated on a continual basis—a most recent change in the guidelines includes the elimination of the routine ordering of electrocardiograms (ECGs) on any patient undergoing cataract surgery under monitored anesthesia care (MAC). This change was made after evaluation of the

TABLE 1. ANESTHESIOLOGY AND PERIOPERATIVE MANAGEMENT[a]

Anesthesiology is the practice of medicine dealing with, but not limited to:
1. Assessment of, consultation for, and preparation of, patients for anesthesia.
2. Relief and prevention of pain during and following surgical, obstetric, therapeutic, and diagnostic procedures.
3. Monitoring and maintenance of normal physiology during the perioperative period.
4. Management of critically ill patients.
5. Diagnosis and treatment of acute, chronic, and cancer-related pain.
6. Clinical management and teaching of cardiac and pulmonary resuscitation.
7. Evaluation of respiratory function and application of respiratory therapy.
8. Conduct of clinical, translational, and basic science research.
9. Supervision, teaching, and evaluation of personnel, both medical and paramedical, involved in perioperative care.
10. Administrative involvement in health care facilities and organizations and medical schools necessary to implement these responsibilities.

[a] As defined, with permission, by the American Board of Anesthesiology.

TABLE 2. ANESTHESIA PREOPERATIVE PROTOCOL

1. i.v.: Start LR 1,000 mL at KVO rate on all patients having general, MAC, regional, or spinal anesthesia, except for the following:
   Patients diagnosed with diabetes
   Patients diagnosed with renal failure (NS 500 mL with micro-drip tubing)
   Patients under 16 years of age

2. Start 18-gauge i.v. on all patients receiving general, MAC, regional, or spinal anesthesia, except for the following:
   Patients under 16 years of age are evaluated by Anesthesia on an individual basis.
   Patients undergoing Cataract surgery may have an 18 or 20 gauge IV.

3. Blood sugars on Patient Care Unit:
   On-call on all insulin dependent diabetics. Call Anesthesia if glucose ≥ 250 or less than 100.
   On-call on all non-insulin dependent diabetics if BMP glucose > 250. Call Anesthesia if glucose ≥ 250.

4. Notify anesthesiologist and surgeon, if applicable, of any of the following abnormal labs, CXR, ECG results unless they represent chronic abnormalities:

Labs	hgb < 9.5	hct < 29	WBC < 2.5 or > 15	Platelets < 100	PT (INR) > 1.5	PTT > 50	Creatinine > 1.9	K⁺ < 3.0 or > 5.5	Glucose (nondiabetic patient) > 180
ECG	Infarct	Ischemia	ST depressions or elevations	Tachycardia > 120	Sinus bradycardia < 40	Undetermined rhythm	Abnormal changes from last ECG		
CXR	New onset CHF	Pneumonia	Infiltrates	Undiagnosed mass	Full lobe atelectasis				

5. Give preoperative medication to all SSU patients upon arrival to the unit or as soon as admission information is obtained. Do not wait for a medication call from the Operating Room.

BMP, basic metabolic panel; SSU, short stay unit.

---

true benefit of ECGs in this patient population, in an attempt to improve patient flow, and after review of the state of the art in the medical literature regarding the cost/benefit of preoperative testing in this patient population.

Intraoperative Care

In the OR, the anesthesiologist directs the provision of anesthesia services and coordinates the daily OR schedule in collaboration with OR nursing management. The physicians in the practice group can participate in the long-range planning for OR management and has extensive knowledge of the entire OR environment. In this role, the group essentially plays the role of the "OR physician" while being both a patient and OR staff advocate.

Postoperative Care

In the postoperative period, the anesthesiologist medically directs the postanesthesia care unit care for patients and can provide medical direction and care of patients in a combined medical–surgical ICU. Often the anesthesiologist continues the care of patients after they leave the ICU, especially those that have complex medical problems or require prolonged ventilatory support postoperatively. Postsurgical pain is another area where anesthesiologists are often involved. Moreover, because of their broad view of the perioperative period, anesthesiologists have provided guidance in development of surgical "clinical pathways".

Surgical Clinical Pathways

The departments of anesthesiology and critical care medicine should be involved in the development of surgical clinical pathways including pathways for coronary artery bypass graft, total joint replacement, and colon surgery. The influence of pathways on perioperative practice includes standardization of laboratory testing and postoperative analgesia in certain patient populations throughout the hospital stay. With a volunteer medical staff, the pathways have been most successful where single medical groups are caring for patients. A single group of cardiac or orthopedic surgeons has allowed compliance with the voluntary guidelines to be much higher than that of the colon pathway, where a number of different general surgical groups are involved. The effectiveness of the pathways is monitored both in terms of total hospital costs related to these specific diagnoses as well as patient outcomes as part of an overall performance improvement program.

Critical Care

Community hospitals usually have combined medical–surgical ICUs as opposed to a variety of subspecialty units found in the university or academic medical center. (10,11) Rounds should be made in the ICU by the anesthesiologist/intensivist each morning. Several days a week, multidisciplinary rounds are held with anesthesiologists leading those discussions. Generally, these units are operated in an open fashion, where consults for anesthesiology/critical care are voluntary. Medical direction for the ICU is actually provided by the anesthesiology department. Some aspects of this open arrangement may be difficult at times, but mandatory closed units by any single specialty are viewed as threatening the livelihood and independence of other medical staff members. Therefore, "closing" of units has not been rigorously pursued in the community setting considering the political realities of dealing with a community hospital and a voluntary medical staff.

Consults for the anesthesiology/critical care service are obtained and responsibilities are delineated in a standing order form (Fig. 3). On this form, comprehensive involvement can be requested as well as more limited involvement related to ventilator management, sedation and analgesia services, or other special issues where the in-house service can be best utilized.

ANESTHESIA PRE-OPERATIVE ORDERS

LABORATORY STUDIES:

1. For **ALL** patients – select the required data and [✔] to order diagnostic studies.
2. Do not repeat lab test if done within past 3 months; ECG within past 2 years. On the day of surgery, order BMP (STAT) on renal failure patients, order PT (STAT) for patients receiving Warfarin (Coumadin).

	CBC	PT	BMP	LFT	ECG *
[ ] Cardiovascular Disease – Specify:	[ ]		[ ]		[ ]
[ ] Hypertension			[ ] K+		[ ]
[ ] Diabetes	[ ]		[ ]		
[ ] Hepatic Disease – Specify:	[ ]	[ ]	[ ]	[ ]	
[ ] Renal Disease – Specify:	[ ]		[ ]		
[ ] Use of Diuretics – Specify Reason for Medication:			[ ] K+		
[ ] Use of Digoxin – Specify Reason for Medication:			[ ] K+		[ ]
[ ] Use of Steroids – Specify Reason for Medication:			[ ]		
[ ] Use of Coumadin – Specify Reason for Medication:	[ ]	[ ]			
[ ] Hematologic Disease – Specify:	[ ]				
[ ] Procedure Performed for Bleeding – Specify:	[ ]				
[ ] INPATIENT 50+ years and/or Diabetic	[ ]		[ ]		[ ]
[ ] SMAs 50+ years and/or Diabetic	[ ]		[ ]		[ ]
[ ] Procedure requires T&S or T&C (See Standard Surgical Blood Order Schedule-on unit).	[ ]				

* ECG not required for Cataract surgery scheduled under MAC

FIGURE 2. Anesthesiology guidelines for preoperative testing.

Development of protocols to standardize the approach to common patient care issues in the unit including magnesium replacement, insulin/glucose management, and potassium repletion, as well as a sedation protocol for those patients on ventilators (Tables 3 through 6; Figs. 4 and 5) greatly facilitates patient care. Furthermore, the departments of anesthesiology and critical care medicine are the logical choices to provide medical direction of the respiratory therapy department given their 24-hour, 7-day a week presence coupled with expertise in airway management and treatment of acute ventilatory failure. Again, development of a ventilator protocol to facilitate the care of patients who have more predictable courses of assisted ventilation (Table 7) enhances standardization of patient care (12). Community hospitals, in general, do not have house staff, and protocols allow the anesthesiology-based intensivist to optimize time and resource utilization.

We will focus on the ICU as an area where a group of perioperative anesthesiologists can demonstrate benefit to the internal customer base (i.e., the hospital administration). In a typical hospital, ICUs usually compromise 8% to 10% of inpatient beds and consume 33% of resources. This represents an area of great concern to administrators. How can a perioperative anesthesiology group address this concern?

Numerous studies have shown that appropriately trained intensivists have profound effects on patient care and resource utilization in the ICU. These effects include, but are not limited to, reduction in predicted mortality, ICU and possibly hospital length of stay, duration of mechanical ventilation, and resource utilization (13–19). Thus, a primary focus and concern of the internal customer base is addressed in a positive and proactive fashion. Furthermore, the reported reduction in iatrogenic complications, bacteremia, acute renal failure, blood product utilization, and Medicare charges is a positive for the internal and external customer base (e.g., the patients and referring physicians) (20–22).

A key component of a successful strategy is data collection to demonstrate the value the perioperative services bring to the institution and the referring physician base. A variety of options exist including the Society of Critical Care Medicine's (SCCM) Project Impact for data collection and analysis. Other specialties, notably nephrology, have demonstrated databases can be used to

ANESTHESIOLOGY/CRITICAL CARE MEDICINE ORDERS

[ ] 1. CONSULT Anesthesiology/Critical Care Service for COMPREHENSIVE patient management.

OR

[ ] 2. CONSULT Anesthesiology/Critical Care Service for the following:

    [ ] Respiratory and ventilator management.

    [ ] Pain management (including sedation).

    [ ] Hemodynamic management (including fluids and vasoactive drugs).

    [ ] Daily visits/consultation only. This service includes management and maintenance of vascular catheters, i.e., PA Catheters, CVPs, arterial lines, and 24 hour/day availability for bedside critical care interventions (if requested).

3. Please notify Dr. _____ for any of the following:

    a. Transfusion of blood products.

    b. _____

    c. _____

    d. _____

Signature: _____

        (Admitting/Attending Physician)   Date

FIGURE 3. Orders for requesting type of anesthesiology/critical care medicine intensive care unit consultation.

improve clinical outcomes (23). Data showing actual improvement in outcomes and decreased lengths of stay might justify a more aggressive approach to either "close" the units or at least to require appropriate anesthesia/critical care consultations in the future. An added benefit of full-time critical care is the increased patient capacity, which improved care and optimized outcomes facilitate. More patients can be cared for within the same number of beds and nursing staff by this approach to care (24).

PHILOSOPHICAL AND PRACTICAL APPROACH

Hospital Organization Involvement

Groups of anesthesiologists that provide a broad range of acute care medicine services should remain actively involved in hospital activities, especially those that impact patient care. Acute care medicine physicians participate in the care of patients not only in ORs, ICUs and, if applicable, obstetric units, but also throughout the hospital including the patient wards, emergency department, endoscopy, and radiology suites. Examples of hospital administrative activities in which anesthesiologists participate include the development of ad hoc committees to oversee all aspects of sedation for procedures, including the policies and procedures, as well as the credentialing of physicians. Another example includes the development of surgical services operations committees that can review the efficiency of ORs more carefully and review patient care issues during the perioperative period. Finally, the provision of an anesthesiologist as medical director for ICUs can facilitate coordination of activities in the medical and surgical ICUs. The director can assist in triage when necessary, provide quality

TABLE 3. MAGNESIUM REPLACEMENT PROTOCOL

A. Assessment
1. If the Magnesium Replacement Protocol is ordered but no baseline magnesium level has been obtained, order a magnesium level and initiate the protocol as necessary.
2. If serum magnesium level is ≤2 mg/dL and serum creatinine ≤2.0 mg/dL, utilize this protocol.
   If a patient has not had a creatinine level measured, order a BMP.[a]
3. Use oral route for replacement if:
   a. No nausea and/or vomiting
   b. Patient is not n.p.o.
4. *Do not* crush for NG tube administration.
5. Administer magnesium i.v. if unable to give orally or patient has an NG tube.

B. Intervention
1. If Mg^{++} level ≤2 mg/dL, replace magnesium according to the table below.
2. Write order on Physician Order sheet for the amount of magnesium needed for replacement.
3. Document medication administration in "One-Time" Orders section of Patient Medication Record.
4. Continue to follow Protocol as long as rechecked Mg^{++} ≤2 mg/dL *and* serum creatinine ≤2.0 mg/dL.
5. Discontinue Magnesium Replacement Protocol if TPN initiated. Magnesium replacement will be managed through physician orders and TPN orders.

	Oral	Intravenous	Labs
Mg^{++} 1.5–2.0 mg/dL	Magnesium oxide 400 mg p.o. b.i.d. × 24 h (13.9 mEq Mg^{++} = 7 mm)	Magnesium sulfate 2 g over 2 h in 100 mL (16.2 mEq Mg^{++} = 8 mm)	Recheck Mg^{++} in a.m. or 6 h after infusion complete (whichever is first)
Mg^{++} ≤1.5 mg/dL		Magnesium sulfate 4 g i.v. over 4 h (dilute in at least 200 mL) (32.4 mEq Mg^{++} = 16 mm)	Recheck Mg^{++} next a.m. or 6 h after infusion complete (whichever is first)
Mg^{++} <1.0 mg/dL		Magnesium sulfate 4 g i.v. over 4 h (dilute in at least 200 mL) (32.4 mEq mg^{++} = 16 mm)	Recheck Mg^{++} 6 h after dose complete (whichever is first)

[a]BMP, basic metabolic panel (Na, K, Cl, HCO_3, Glu, BUN, Ca); NG, nasogastric; TPN, total parenteral nutrition.

TABLE 4. INTENSIVE CARE UNIT CLINICAL PROTOCOL

Standard Sliding Scale Insulin Protocol

Goal: Maintain serum glucose between 80 and 140 mg/dL
Monitoring:
1. Check blood glucose q4h by glucometer (if glucometer unable to give reading, send sample to the laboratory) until stable (three values in the desired range). The checks can then be reduced to q6h if on continuous enteral feeding or qAC & HS[a] if on intermittent feeding.
2. All insulin used is Humulin insulin given *subcutaneous administration*, unless otherwise specified.
3. If potassium is <3.5 units, start Potassium Replacement Protocol.
If glucose remains outside 80–140 mg/dL, the RN will automatically advance one level up from initial physician order for sliding scale regimen. If blood glucose remains outside 80–140 mg/dL, notify physician for further orders.

Glucose Level (Fingerstick)	Low Dose Regimen	Medium Dose Regimen	High Dose Regimen	Very High Dose Regimen
<80	Call MD	Call MD	Call MD	Call MD
81–140	0	0	0	5 U
141–180	1 U	2 U	4 U	10 U
181–240	2 U	4 U	8 U	15 U
241–300	4 U	6 U	12 U	20 U
301–400	6 U	9 U	16 U	25 U
>400	8 U	12 U	20 U	30 U

[a]qAC & HS, before each meal.
HS, hour of sleep.

TABLE 5. REGULAR INSULIN INFUSION[a] PROTOCOL

Goal: To maintain serum glucose between 120 and 180 mg/dL.
Monitoring:
1. Check glucose q1h until result within desired range ×3, then q4h and p.r.n.
2. Check glucose q1h if <60 or >350 or if fluctuating rapidly.
3. Check K when insulin infusion initiated and p.r.n. during infusion.

Initiating Insulin Infusion: **Mixed in standard concentration of 1 U/mL of fluid**

Glucose	180–240 mg/dL	241–300 mg/dL	301–360 mg/dL	361–420 mg/dL	>420 mg/dL
	Give 3 U insulin i.v.p. and start infusion @ 2 U/h	Give 6 U insulin i.v.p. and start infusion @ 2 U/h	Give 8 U insulin i.v.p. and start infusion @ 2 U/h	Give 10 U insulin i.v.p. and start infusion @ 2 U/h	Call MD for orders

Titrating Insulin Infusion: **Glucose ≤120 mg/dL**

	Infusion Rate 1–3 U/h	Infusion Rate 4–6 U/h	Infusion Rate 7–9 U/h	Infusion Rate 10–12 U/h	Infusion Rate 13–16 U/h	Infusion Rate >16 U/h
<60 mg/dL	D/C infusion and give 50 mL D50 i.v.p.	D/C infusion and give 50 mL D50 i.v.p.	D/C infusion and give 50 mL D50 i.v.p.	D/C infusion and give 50 mL D50 i.v.p.	D/C infusion and give 50 mL D50 i.v.p.	D/C infusion and give 50 mL D50 i.v.p.
61–80 mg/dL	D/C infusion and give 25 mL D50 i.v.p.	D/C infusion and give 25 mL D50 i.v.p.	D/C infusion and give 25 mL D50 i.v.p.	D/C infusion and give 25 mL D50 i.v.p.	D/C infusion and give 25 mL D50 i.v.p.	D/C infusion and give 25 mL D50 i.v.p.
81–100 mg/dL	D/C infusion	D/C infusion rate by 50%	D/C infusion rate by 50%	D/C infusion rate by 50%	D/C infusion rate by 50%	D/C infusion rate by 50%
101–120 mg/dL	D/C infusion rate by 1 U/h	D/C infusion rate by 2 U/h	D/C infusion rate by 3 U/h	D/C infusion rate by 4 U/h	D/C infusion rate by 5 U/h	D/C infusion rate by 6 U/h

Glucose 121–180 mg/dL: No change

Glucose >180 mg/dL

	Infusion Rate 1–5 U/h	Infusion Rate 6–10 U/h	Infusion Rate 11–16 U/h	Infusion Rate >16 U/h
181–240 mg/dL	Give 3 U insulin i.v.p. and increase rate by 1 U/h	Give 3 U insulin i.v.p. and increase rate by 2 U/h	Give 3 U insulin i.v.p. and increase rate by 3 U/h	Call physician for new orders
241–300 mg/dL	Give 5 U insulin i.v.p. and increase rate by 1 U/h	Give 5 U insulin i.v.p. and increase rate by 2 U/h	Give 5 U insulin i.v.p. and increase rate by 3 U/h	Call physician for new orders
301–360 mg/dL	Give 8 U insulin i.v.p. and increase rate by 2 U/h	Give 8 U insulin i.v.p. and increase rate by 3 U/h	Give 8 U insulin i.v.p. and increase rate by 4 U/h	Call physician for new orders
361–420 mg/dL	Give 10 U insulin i.v.p. and increase rate by 2 U/h	Give 10 U insulin i.v.p. and increase rate by 3 U/h	Give 10 U insulin i.v.p. and increase rate by 4 U/h	Call physician for new orders
>420 mg/dL	Call physician for new order	Call physician for new order	Call physician for new order	Call physician for new orders

[a] Insulin adheres to i.v. tubing; coat the i.v. tubing by wasting at least 50 mL of solution during priming the first bag or whenever tubing is changed. Administer via i.v. pump.
D/C, discontinue; D50, ; i.v.p., intravenous push.

TABLE 6. POTASSIUM REPLACEMENT PROTOCOL

A. Assessment
1. Obtain physician's order before initiating this protocol. Order to include at what level replacement is to begin (i.e., K^+ <4.0 mMol/L or K^+ <3.5 mMol/L).
   If no level ordered, replace K^+ at <3.5 mMol/L level.
2. Initiate this protocol only if serum creatinine ≤2.0 mg/dL. If patient has not had a creatinine level measured, order a BMP.
   If serum creatinine >2.0 mg/dL, **do not use this protocol**, and notify physician.
3. If serum potassium <2.7 mMol/L or patient is on a diuretic, check serum magnesium, and follow Magnesium Replacement Protocol.
4. Administer potassium i.v. if unable to use NG/oral route, giving varied doses for peripheral vs. central line access.
   Potassium i.v. is preferably given via central access, and can be mixed at a concentration of 40 mEq KCl/100 mL i.v. fluid.
   K^+ infusions administered via peripheral access **should not exceed 20 mEq KCl/100 mL i.v. fluid.**
5. Never administer potassium as a direct i.v. push or in an undiluted form.
6. Patients must be on continuous ECG monitoring if receiving >20 mEq/h.

B. Intervention
1. Write order on Physician Order sheet for the amount of potassium needed for replacement.
2. Document medication administration in "One-Time" Orders section of Patient Medication Record.
3. Continue to follow Protocol as long as rechecked K^+ less than ordered value *and* creatinine ≤2.0 mg/dL.
4. May check K^+ p.r.n. for increased diuresis or if patient has cardiac monitor showing ectopy.
5. Only order K^+ level when rechecking potassium blood level.
6. D/C use of this protocol if TPN is initiated; K^+ replacement will be managed through physician orders and TPN orders.

	Nasogastric/Oral	Intravenous		Labs
	Potassium chloride liquid 20 mEq/15 mL	*Central* KCl 40 mEq/100 mL concentration concentration (pre-i.v.p.b.)	*Peripheral* KCl 20 mEq/100 mL mixed	
K^+ 2.7–3.4 mMol/L	Potassium chloride liquid 20 mEq NG/P.O. q4h × 3 doses *or→*	KCl 40 mEq/100 mL (infuse over 1 h[a]) × 1 100 mL	KCl 20 mEq i.v. diluted in q1h × 2 (infuse each over 1 h)	Recheck K^+ in a.m.
K^+ <2.7 mMol/L	Potassium chloride liquid 20 mEq NG/p.o. q2h × 4 doses	KCl 40 mEq/100 mL ×2 (infuse each dose in 100 mL over 1 h[a])	KCl 20 mEq i.v. diluted q1h × 4 (infuse each over 1 h)	Recheck K^+ 1 h after dose completed (if rechecked K^+ normal, repeat electrolytes in 4 h.) Check serum Mg^{++} and use Mg protocol if <2.1 mg/dL

[a] For patients not on cardiac monitor, infuse over 2 h.
D/C, discontinue; BMP, basic metabolic panel; NG, nasogastric; ECG, electrocardiogram; TPN, total parenteral nutrition; i.v.p.b., intravenous push bolus.

assurance, and perform improvement activities for the entire hospital. In addition, the director can be a representative to the medical staff and hospital leadership including the medical executive committee and the board of trustees.

Groups can undertake a variety of such administrative roles to expand their influence, secure and stabilize their position in the hospital, and ultimately improve patient care. Despite a rapidly changing health care environment, this level of involvement adds great stability to any group practice; it allows groups to help develop policies and procedures that ultimately affect the care of all patients in the facility. Furthermore, this level of involvement may allow the group to recruit the brightest new anesthesiology graduates who have strong interest in practicing as acute care physicians.

Recruiting and Training of Anesthesiologists

Groups of anesthesiologists that include acute care medicine in their practice are often successful in recruiting the best and most well-trained anesthesiologists in the United States. Anesthesiologists who serve the needs of such practices are those that envision themselves providing broad-based acute care and perioperative medicine services, and also view themselves as physicians, not only anesthesiologists, in such an environment. In some academic departments where perioperative medicine residencies or fellowships have been contemplated, anesthesiologists who would have completed such training would be very attractive to practices that are committed to acute care services, and it is likely that the philosophies of individuals with such training would complement that of such groups.

Because of the broad range of knowledge and technical skills required to provide acute care medicine services throughout the institution, groups should strongly mandate continuing education by all of their members. Special time on an annual basis should be afforded every anesthesiologist to participate in continuing education in general areas or in specific areas of interest. Sharing technical information and advanced medical knowledge with other members of the group should be encouraged. Presentations of clinical advancements and innovative technical procedures can be done at weekly or monthly practice meetings where information can be analyzed and evaluated, and decisions made regarding integrating new patient care strategies into the practice. In addition, sharing the current state of the art knowledge with other members of the medical staff is also strongly encouraged, either in a grand rounds setting or periodic presentations at other departmental meetings.

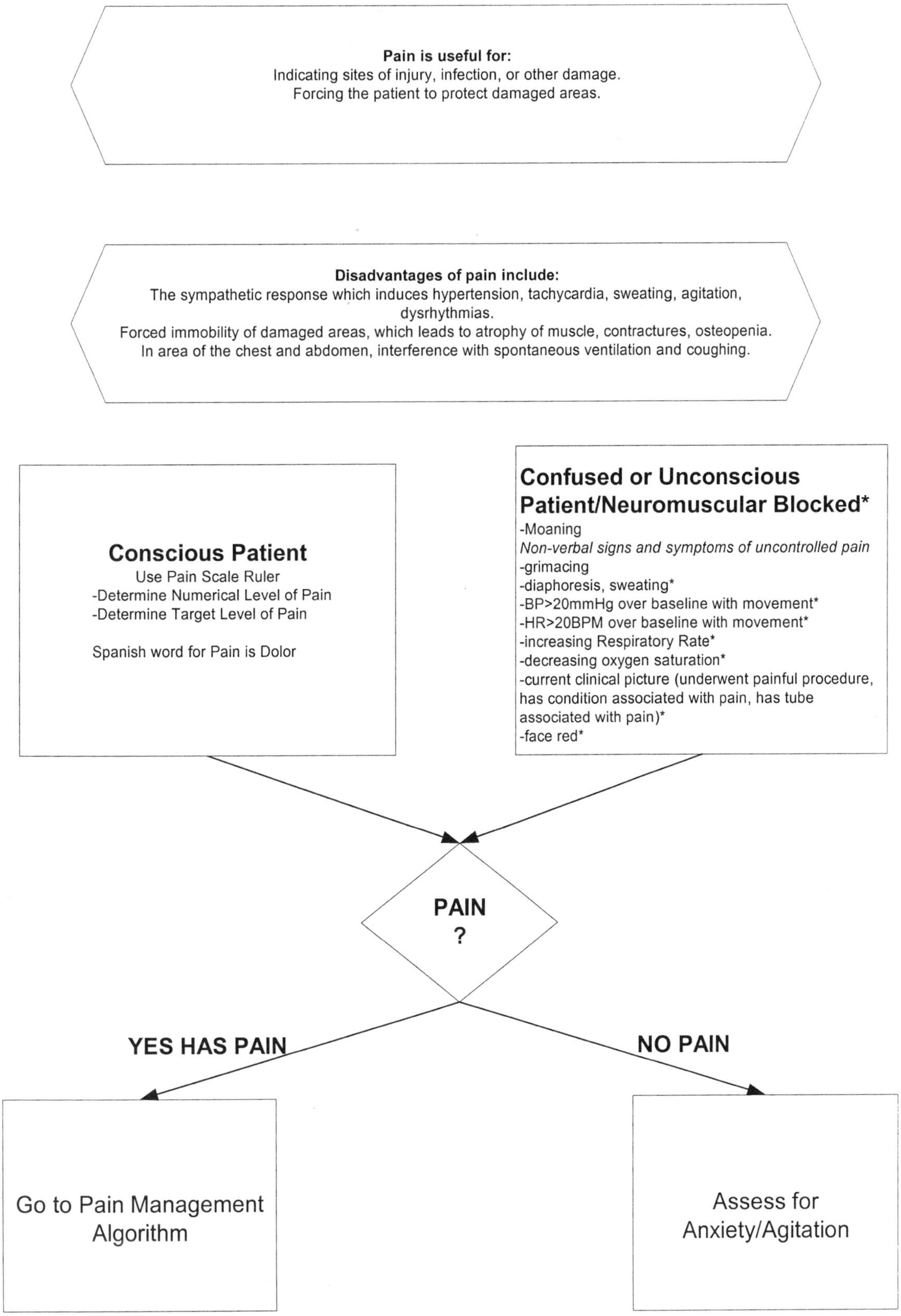

Pain is useful for:
Indicating sites of injury, infection, or other damage.
Forcing the patient to protect damaged areas.

Disadvantages of pain include:
The sympathetic response which induces hypertension, tachycardia, sweating, agitation, dysrhythmias.
Forced immobility of damaged areas, which leads to atrophy of muscle, contractures, osteopenia.
In area of the chest and abdomen, interference with spontaneous ventilation and coughing.

Conscious Patient
Use Pain Scale Ruler
-Determine Numerical Level of Pain
-Determine Target Level of Pain

Spanish word for Pain is Dolor

Confused or Unconscious Patient/Neuromuscular Blocked*
-Moaning
Non-verbal signs and symptoms of uncontrolled pain
-grimacing
-diaphoresis, sweating*
-BP>20mmHg over baseline with movement*
-HR>20BPM over baseline with movement*
-increasing Respiratory Rate*
-decreasing oxygen saturation*
-current clinical picture (underwent painful procedure, has condition associated with pain, has tube associated with pain)*
-face red*

PAIN ?

YES HAS PAIN

NO PAIN

Go to Pain Management Algorithm

Assess for Anxiety/Agitation

FIGURE 4. Pain assessment algorithm.

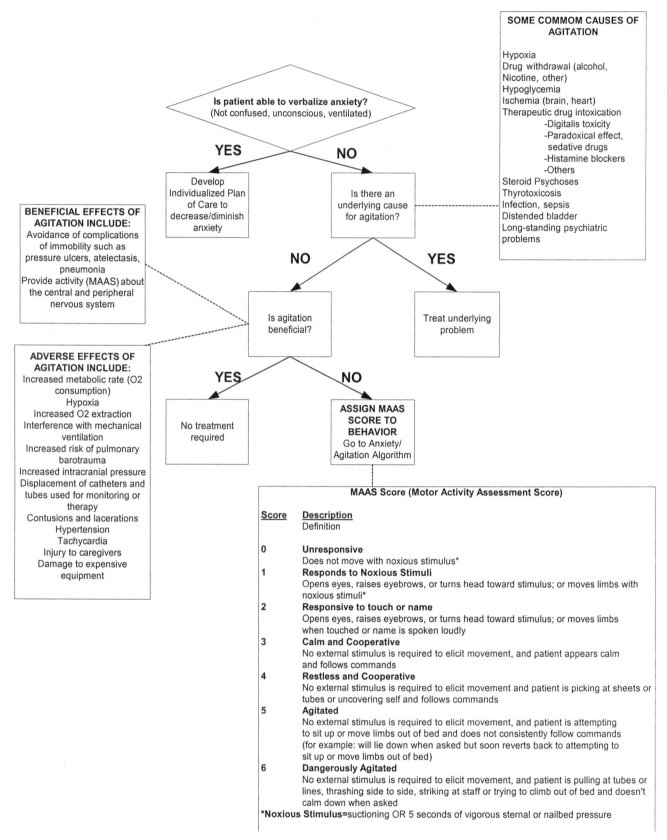

FIGURE 5. Anxiety/agitation assessment algorithm.

TABLE 7. MECHANICAL VENTILATION PROTOCOL FOR ROUTINE VENTILATOR MANAGEMENT (NOT FOR PATIENTS WITH ALI OR ARDS)

Procedure

A. General Guidelines
1. On day 2 of mechanical ventilation, the staff nurse and respiratory therapist in collaboration with the primary care physician, or physician managing the ventilator will assess if the patient meets "Mechanical Ventilator Management Protocol" criteria. The team will request implementation of the protocol if the patient meets criteria.
2. The RCP (Respiratory Care Provider) will be primarily responsible for all mechanical ventilator intervention under protocol guidelines.
3. Physician orders will supersede protocol directions.
4. RCPs will work closely and communicate effectively with appropriate nursing and medical staff in the management of ventilator patients.
5. Related Patient Care Service policies and procedures pertaining to ventilator care will be adhered to in the course of ventilator management.
6. Arterial blood gas (ABG) samples will be acquired within the initial hour of mechanical ventilation, and as needed to assure protocol compliance.
7. End tidal CO_2 (A-aDCO_2) and pulse oximetry (SpO_2) trending is mandatory to decrease ABG acquisition.
8. The Ventilator Team will evaluate the protocol as needed.
9. The RCP will assure that airway care and bronchodilation are optimized during mechanical ventilatory support and postextubation.
10. Indirect calorimetry measurements will be performed on day 3 of mechanical ventilation to assess nutritional support. The nutritional team will assess metabolic results and provide recommendations to the physician after rounds.
11. A chest radiograph will be performed immediately after endotracheal intubation and as clinically indicated.
12. Standard Protocol Goals:[a,b]
    a. Arterial pH to be between 7.30 and 7.45
    b. Arterial PaO_2 to be between 55 torr and 90 torr
    c. Pulse oximeter SpO_2 to be between 88% and 95%
    d. Inspiratory plateau pressure (Pplatt) to be below 35 cm H_2O

Protocols

B. Total Mechanical Ventilatory Support (Severe Respiratory Failure)
1. Clinical indications for total support:
    a. Inadequate alveolar ventilation (respiratory acidosis)
    b. Inadequate oxygenation not amenable to routine oxygen therapy (PaO_2/FiO_2 <200 or PEEP >10 or FiO_2 >0.60
    c. Intolerance to partial mechanical ventilatory support
    d. Apnea
2. Total support parameters:
    a. Initial mode will be volume ventilation.
    b. Tidal volume range will be 8 cc/kg–12 cc/kg to assist in producing the desired minute ventilation and plateau pressure.
    c. Ventilator rate shall be titrated as needed to meet Standard Protocol Goals. Rates above 20/min should be avoided.
    d. FiO_2 and PEEP should be adjusted to maintain protocol oxygen goals (as a general rule PEEP should not be >5 while FiO_2 <0.60. PEEP >12 will be assessed by the Ventilator Team).
    e. Inspiratory flow rates (volume) will be adjusted to maximize patient inspiratory demand while minimizing air trapping while utilizing waveform analysis.
    f. Pressure support may be provided up to the level of the patient's plateau pressure.
    g. I:E ratios will be 1:1 to 1:4. I:E ratios exceeding 1:1 will require a physician's order.
C. Partial Mechanical Ventilatory Support (patients assessed by the Ventilator Team to be capable of providing the majority of the work of breathing):
1. Clinical indications for partial support (*must have all*):
    a. PEEP <10, FiO_2 <0.60
    b. Reliable respiratory drive present
    c. Chest radiograph stable or improving
    d. Patients tolerate pressure support (see "Tolerance Criteria", Appendix 1 at the end of this table)
    e. Hemodynamic stability (dopamine <10 μg/kg/min or dobutamine <10 μg/kg/min, no other inotropes or pressors)
2. Patients meeting above criteria will receive daily weaning mechanics to assess spontaneous work of breathing after 5 minutes of CPAP. If NIF is <−25, and CPAP tolerated (see Appendix 1), continue on CPAP and PS 5 for 60 min and consider extubation (see Appendix 2 at the end of this table). Patients not meeting "Tolerance" or "Extubation"[c] criteria during CPAP and PS 5 may be placed on partial support weaning protocols below.
3. The choice of partial support weaning techniques is at the discretion of the Ventilator Team. In general, rapidly resolving processes should be done with T-Piece/CPAP, more slowly resolving processes (e.g., repeatedly failed T-piece/CPAP trials), should be done with pressure support. SIMV should only be considered if respiratory drive is questionable (e.g., anesthesia, heavy sedation).
D. Partial Mechanical Ventilatory Support Guidelines (may be amended by Ventilator Team)
1. *T-piece/CPAP Trial*
    a. Place patient on flow-by (15 LPM flow/3 LPM sensitivity) and ≤5 CPAP through the ventilator circuit.
    b. Monitor patient according to Appendices 1 and 2.
    c. Adjust duration of T-piece trials until 60-min duration is achieved (opportunity for extubation).
2. *Pressure Support (PS) Weaning*
    a. Begin weaning at a PS level delivering a tidal volume of 8 cc/kg.
    b. Wean PS by 2 cm H_2O, as tolerated (Appendix 1).
    c. Once patient tolerates (Appendix 1) a PS 5, assess for extubation (Appendix 2).
3. *SIMV Weaning*
    a. Initial SIMV rate to achieve partial support goals is decreased by two BPM (PS 5 may be added), as tolerated (Appendix 1), until a rate of two BPM is achieved.
    b. If patient is able to tolerate a rate of two BPM, assess for extubation (Appendix 2).[d]

Appendix 1: Tolerance Criteria

Patient will be considered intolerant if *any* of the following exists:
1. Development of rapid, shallow breathing. Respiratory rate (RR) ≥35 or increase of >10 BPM over previous RR.
2. Intolerable dyspnea, diaphoresis, excessive use of accessory muscles, or development of paradoxic respirations.
3. Heart rate (HR) >120 BPM or change in heart rate of 20 BPM over previous HR.
4. Diastolic blood pressure change of ≥20 mm Hg.
5. Development of cardiac arrhythmias, deterioration of mental status, or deterioration of arterial blood gases.

(continued)

TABLE 7. (continued)

Appendix 2: Extubation Criteria

Patients should be considered for extubation if they meet the following criteria:
1. NIFM >−25 cm H_2O
2. VC >12 mL/kg
3. RR >10 and <30 BPM
4. Tidal volume >5 mL/kg
5. $Pao_2/Fio_2 > 200 − (PEEP/CPAP < 6$ and $Fio_2 < 60\%)$
6. Mental status: awake, alert, appropriate
7. Neuromuscular status: head lift > 5 sec
8. Adequate airway protection and secretion control

[a] Appropriate physician will be notified if patient falls outside of "Standard Protocol Goals" or does not meet "Tolerance Criteria."
[b] Ventilator Team may adjust "Standard Protocol Goals" according to patient specificity.
[c] Extubation is only upon physician's order.
[d] Patients who do not meet "Tolerance Criteria" will be placed on previously tolerated ventilator settings and monitored.
ALI, acute lung injury; ARDS, adult respiratory distress syndorne; PEEP, positive end expiratory pressure; CPAP, continuous positive airway pressure; NIF, negative inspiratory force; PS 5, pressure support, level 5; SIMV, synchronized intermittent mandatory ventilation; LPM, licensed practical nurse; BPM, beats per minute; VC, vital capacity.

ACUTE CARE MEDICINE: ADDED VALUE FOR ANESTHESIOLOGY DEPARTMENTS

Anesthesiology groups that have been successful in aggressively pursuing perioperative and acute care medicine activities have grown to become more respected in their institutions than might otherwise have been the case if they had only provided OR anesthesia services and had not involved themselves in a variety of areas throughout the hospital. Such groups need to continue to evaluate additional opportunities in perioperative and acute care medicine as they become available. The group should pursue all of the activities outside the OR that can add to the value of the group, the medical staff, and the hospital itself, as well as translate into improved financial and job security.

Additional activities should not be evaluated solely on the basis of financial gain since many of the activities have secondary benefits that may be of greater overall benefit to the group even if the service itself does not generate significant income. Groups should evaluate current and future opportunities based on the possibility for increased visibility and exposure of the group outside of the OR, the potential for joint ventures with other medical groups or the hospital, and the likelihood of filling a void in a community or medical service. When evaluated against these ideals, decisions whether or not to continue to offer a service or to expand services become more clear.

The potential added value of integrating acute care medicine services into any anesthesiology department must be evaluated on a department-by-department basis. Each hospital environment remains so unique that the particular strategies involved in developing acute care services cannot be provided by a cookie-cutter approach. Each individual environment, hospital, and medical staff must be evaluated in a broad context to decide what additional opportunities exist for a group of anesthesiologists, and, more specifically, what type of strategies might succeed best in expanding the role of the anesthesiology group.

The Role of Hospitalist Teams in Acute Care Services

Over the next decade and beyond, the acuity of patients admitted to the hospital setting will increase and will demand special knowledge and skills by physicians caring for these patients.

Well-trained, motivated physicians who are available in the hospital 24 hours a day should play a key role in the provision of care for these acutely and critically ill patients. Of those physicians currently in hospital-based practices—namely the pathologists, radiologists, emergency medicine physicians, and anesthesiologists—who meets such qualifications? Perhaps a hospital medicine specialist is a better answer, and this concept has been suggested and developed by several hospitals nationwide in just the last few years. Physicians trained in hospital medicine who become hospital-based and no longer practice in office settings may be the type of physicians best trained and logistically positioned for this group of patients. The emerging role of the hospitalist in the United States health care system was first described in 1996 (25), and there has been a rapid growth of specialists in inpatient medicine since then who have become responsible for managing care of hospitalized patients. The "hospitalist trend" has become more visible both at teaching and community hospitals throughout the country.

Some anesthesiologists would look at a model where anesthesiologists provide only OR anesthesia services and hospitalists provide all other aspects of inpatient care as the obvious match of complementary services, and the extent to which anesthesiologists should be involved in acute care. However, the idea that the hospitalist team might better be organized as a multispecialty group has been identified: "a model in which a team of hospitalists, some trained as generalists, others as specialists, shares responsibility for the management of inpatient care" (25). Anesthesiology groups that have integrated acute care medicine into their practice believe that anesthesiologists, with expertise in critical care, perioperative care, and pain management as well as resuscitation medicine, complement the skills of general internists who may be providing hospital medicine services.

The complementary services of the perioperative or acute care medicine services and hospitalists are exemplified further in the perioperative care of surgical patients. Anesthesiologists, who are trained not only in anesthesiology but in other related areas including critical care and pain management, provide knowledge, expertise, and clinical skills, and truly understand many aspects of the care of the surgical patient. Hospitalists, who provide excellent inpatient care for general medical patients, are often internists who have not had broad exposure to the perioperative care of surgical patients. Anesthesiologists with an interest in

TABLE 8. TOP 10 ADMITTING DIAGNOSES

1986	1999
1. Obstetrics	1. Obstetrics
2. Postsurgery after care	2. Coronary artery disease
3. Maintenance chemotherapy	3. Pneumonia
4. Pneumonia	4. Congestive heart failure
5. Asthma	5. Chest pain
6. Kidney stones	6. Hypovolemia
7. Abdominal pain	7. Chronic obstructive pulmonary disease
8. Open hand wound	Hysterectomy
9. Otitis media	9. Cerebral artery occlusion
10. Congestive heart failure	Subendocardial myocardial infarction

acute care can provide outstanding perioperative management of surgical patients in these settings.

Currently, a much more acutely ill population is being admitted to the hospital than was the case 10 or 15 years ago. The top ten admitting diagnoses in 1986 and 1999 at Rex Hospital (Raleigh, NC) are shown in Table 8. Analysis of these two lists suggests that not only is the inpatient population much more acutely ill, but also that the disease processes of which anesthesiologists are often familiar with and manage daily in OR settings are included in most of the current top ten admitting diagnoses. In other words, the scope of care for these types of patients includes skills and knowledge that anesthesiologists already possess.

There are many examples around the United States where groups of internists work as hospitalists and coordinate patient care with an anesthesiology acute care medicine team to provide outstanding and comprehensive care to all hospitalized patients. Teams such as this provide quality, cost-efficient care in many areas, with anesthesiologists providing services in critical care, the postanesthesia care unit, preoperative and postoperative management, resuscitation, acute and chronic pain management, oversight for sedation for procedures, labor analgesia, and OR anesthesia. Such coordinated efforts with hospitalist teams may indeed be a model for the medical care of hospitalized patients.

SUMMARY

The advent of hospitalist teams and the opportunities for anesthesiologists to complement the services that hospitalist teams provide has also produced the possibility for the intense competition in caring for acutely ill patients in hospital settings. In a variety of institutions around the United States, inpatient care has been entirely coordinated through internal medicine–based hospitalist services, and has included specialists in pulmonary and critical care to provide care for critically ill patients in ICUs. In many of these instances, the anesthesiology departments have had little or no involvement at all in the development of such programs.

As discussed herein, there are many anesthesiologists who believe that inpatient care outside of the OR is not in the purview of anesthesiologists. The sentiment that anesthesiology can continue to survive as a viable medical specialty by solely providing OR anesthesia, labor analgesia, and office-based anesthesia may not be particularly well founded given today's competitive health care environment. Anesthesiologists remain under intense competition from nurse anesthetists who have expanded their role to include significant involvement in providing OR anesthesia as well as analgesia for labor and delivery. Furthermore, nurse anesthetists have become extensively involved in providing office-based anesthesia services and are now exploring expanded roles in pain management. For the next decade or more, the competition for providing pure anesthesia services will remain significant and the opportunities for anesthesiologists to practice as acute care physicians, although available now, may disappear as other physician specialists step in to fill these areas of need. The opportunities for anesthesiologists to expand the scope of services they now provide remain extensive today. However, it is only through attitude, interest, experience, education, technical proficiency, work ethic, and affability that a group of anesthesiologists can expand their role to include a broad range of acute care medicine services in a hospital setting.

The viability of anesthesiology as a specialty, especially when incorporating acute care medicine, remains bright, but the window of opportunity is of limited duration. The opportunity to establish anesthesiology and acute care medicine as a significant and permanent medical specialty that will remain essential to the health care systems of the twenty-first century is a significant challenge that can only be met by concerted and organized efforts at both the local and national level. Failure to meet such a challenge will leave anesthesiology as a specialty extremely narrow in scope, and threatened by intense competition on three fronts. These include nurse anesthetists in the OR, medicine- and surgical-based critical care physicians in the ICUs, and internists, neurologists, and nurse anesthetists in the management of acute and chronic pain. The most effective means of maintaining anesthesiology as a preeminent medical specialty is for anesthesiologists to begin practicing acute care medicine in community hospital settings (26).

KEY POINTS

The organization of acute and critical care services in the community hospital may differ from the "classic" academic approach to these disciplines. The practice paradigm varies from hospital-to-hospital depending on institutional needs and history, scope of community practice, availability of resources and personnel, and local politics. Acute care medicine, critical care, and perioperative medicine are not mutually exclusive.

With the growing hospitalist movement, the integration of hospital-based physicians is required to provide optimal care and avoid deficiencies in coverage or unnecessary redundancies. Anesthesiologists have a long and distinguished role of active participation and innovative development in the history of acute care and critical care. However, most recently, intraoperative management has been the premier focus of many anesthesia practitioners.

From an economy of scale perspective, anesthesiologists are well suited to provide hospital-based acute and critical care along with perioperative management of surgical patients. This approach frees up primary care and office-based physicians and allows emergency room physicians to focus on their department and hospitalists to care for hospital-based nonsurgical patients.

Appropriate training and commitment to a broad practice are suggested as a flexible model for the anesthesiologist, particularly within a group, to act as a perioperative physician. The anesthesiologist's responsibilities include preoperative assessment, intraoperative direction of the anesthesia health care team, postoperative pain management and critical care, and coverage for in-house urgencies and emergencies. Administrative skills should be honed to facilitate hospital-based committee efforts and hospital leadership roles such as perioperative director, acute care director, and medical director of a facility.

REFERENCES

1. Löfstrom JB. The polio epidemic in Copenhagen in 1952—and how the anaesthetist came out of the operating room. *Acta Anaesthesiol Scand* 1994;38:419.
2. Saidman LJ. The 33rd Rovenstine Lecture. What I have learned from 9 years and 9,000 papers. *Anesthesiology* 1995;83:191–197.
3. Rosenthal MH. Critical care medicine: at the crossroads. *Anesth Analg* 1995;81:439–440.
4. Poldermans D, Boersma E, Bax JJ, et al. The effect of bisoprolol on perioperative mortality and myocardial infarction in high-risk patients undergoing vascular surgery. *N Engl J Med* 1999;341:1789–1794.
5. Smetana GW. Preoperative pulmonary evaluation. *N Engl J Med* 1999;340:937–944.
6. Warner DO. Preventing postoperative pulmonary complications—the role of the anesthesiologist. *Anesthesiology* 2000;92:1467–1472.
7. Cuschieri RJ, Morran CG, Howie JC, et al. Postoperative pain and pulmonary complications: comparison of three analgesic regimens. *Br J Surg* 1985;72:495–498.
8. Longnecker DE. Planning the future of anesthesiology. *Anesthesiology* 1996; 84:495–497.
9. Abt Associates. *Estimation of the physician work force requirements in anesthesiology.* Prepared for the American Society of Anesthesiologists, Inc., Park Ridge, IL, 1994.
10. Groeger JS, Strosberg MA, Halpern NA, et al. Descriptive analysis of critical care units in the United States. *Crit Care Med* 1992;20:846–863.
11. Calvin JE, Habet K, Parrillo JE. Critical care in the United States. Who are we and how did we get here? *Crit Care Clin* 1997:13(2):363–376.
12. Marelich GP. Protocol weaning of mechanical ventilation in medical and surgical patients by respiratory care practitioners and nurses: effect on weaning time and incidence of ventilator-associated pneumonia. *Chest* 2000;118(2):459–467.
13. Li TC, Phillips MC, Shaw L, et al. On-site physician staffing in a community hospital intensive care unit: impact on test and procedure use and on patient outcome. *JAMA* 1984;252:2023–2027.
14. Brown JJ, Sullivan G. Effect on ICU mortality of a full-time critical care specialist. *Chest* 1989;96:127–129.
15. Reynolds HN, Haupt MT, Thill-Baharozian MC, et al. Impact of critical care physician staffing on patients with septic shock in a university hospital medical intensive care unit. *JAMA* 1988;260:3446–3450.
16. Pollack MM, Katz RW, Ruttimann UE, et al. Improving the outcome and efficiency of intensive care: the impact of an intensivist. *Crit Care Med* 1988;16:11–17.
17. Multz AS, Samson I, Scharf SM. A "closed" ICU is more efficient compared to an "open" ICU. *Crit Care Med* 1997;25[Suppl]:A106(abst).
18. Manthous CA, Amoateng-Adjepong Y, Al-Kharrat T, et al. Effects of a medical intensivist on patient care in a community teaching hospital. *Mayo Clinic Proc* 1997;72(5):391–399.
19. Multz AS, Chalfin DB, Samson IM, et al. A "closed" medical intensive care unit (MICU) improves resource utilization when compared with an "open" MICU. *Am J Resp Crit Care Med* 1998;157(5):1468–1473.
20. Hanson CW, Deutschman CS, Anderson HL, et al. The effect of an organized critical care service on outcomes and resource utilization: a prospective cohort study. *Crit Care Med* 1999;27:270–274.
21. Pronovost P, Jenckes M, Dorman T, et al. Organizational characteristics of intensive care units related to outcomes of abdominal aortic surgery. *JAMA* 1999;281(14):1310–1317.
22. Ghorra S, Reinert SE, Cioffi W, et al. Analysis of the effect of conversion from open to closed surgical intensive care unit. *Ann Surg* 1999;229(2):163–171.
23. Bednar B. The use of a database to improve clinical outcomes. *Nephrol New Issues* 1996;10(6):18–21.
24. Mascia MF, Koch M, Medicis JJ. Pharmacoeconomic impact of rational use guidelines on the provision of analgesia, sedation, and neuromuscular blockade in critical care. *Crit Care Med* 2000;28(7):2300–2306.
25. Wachter, RM, Goldman L. The emerging role of "hospitalists" in the American health care system. *N Engl J Med* 1996;335(7):514–517.
26. Lindahl SGE. Future anesthesiologists will be as much outside as inside operating theaters. *Acta Anesthesiol Scand* 2000:44:906–909.

ETHICAL AND END-OF-LIFE ISSUES

KAREN J. SCHWENZER

ETHICAL CONSIDERATIONS IN CARING FOR PATIENTS

Physicians caring for critically ill patients in the perioperative setting often encounter moral dilemmas. The concerns of clinical ethics include: issues of capacity and informed consent, a patient's refusal of medically indicated treatment, decisions to forgo life-sustaining treatments, physician-assisted suicide, and conflicts with managed health care organizations.

What is the difference between the words *ethical* and *moral*? Some people use the term ethical to refer to their individual character traits or professional behavior. The more appropriate term, moral, describes the widely shared beliefs about the norms of right and wrong conduct prevailing in a particular culture or subculture. Clinical ethics is the practice of understanding and examining this moral life, including the conduct of individual health care professionals, patients and their families, health care organizations, and societal practices (1). The professional fields that deal with clinical ethics include medicine, nursing, law, sociology, philosophy, and theology, though today medical ethics is also recognized as its own discipline.

A moral dilemma occurs when ethical obligations justify the physician's performance of an action and refraining from performance of an action. The most frequently recurring moral dilemmas faced by critical care physicians arise in cases that require, or seem to require, infringements upon the basic obligations of physicians to patients regarding choices about treatment at or near the end of life.

PHYSICIANS' BASIC OBLIGATIONS (1)

Beneficence or Nonmaleficence

The relationship between the physician and the patient lies at the center of clinical ethics. The physician has an obligation to use his or her medical knowledge to determine what treatments benefit or prevent harm to the patient. Beneficence, or nonmaleficence, is that quality that physicians must possess to meet this obligation. Physicians have an obligation to care for sick and injured patients. In doing so, they are obligated to preserve life, to cure when possible, to heal, to restore or maintain bodily functions and mental capacities, to prevent disease or injury, to minimize risks or harm, and to relieve suffering.

Autonomy

Respect for patient self-determination and autonomy is another fundamental obligation of physicians. Capable adult patients have the right to determine for themselves whether they accept or refuse treatment. The right of self-determination also means that no treatment can be imposed on capable patients without their consent.

Distributive Justice

Physicians are obligated to ensure fairness in the distribution of medical resources as well as bedside rationing. The principle of distributive justice, along with the principles of beneficence, nonmaleficence, and autonomy, is one of the four major principles governing physicians. Even when faced with societal and economic pressures, physicians remain patients' main advocates for access to medically indicated health care and entitlements to coverage under private and public insurance plans.

Professional Integrity

Though patients are free to refuse treatment, they are not necessarily entitled to receive whatever treatment they demand. In order for physicians to preserve their professional integrity, to ensure beneficence, and to uphold their obligation to ensure fairness in the distribution of medical resources, they have no moral obligation to offer or provide treatment that is not medically indicated. Controversy exists, however, as to what constitutes futile care. A physician may view a treatment as having no reasonable medical benefit and merely prolonging the patient's dying process. Others may believe that the patient's life is worth prolonging. Disputes that focus on the interpretation of what constitutes a good quality of life preclude the physician from acting unilaterally, especially when forgoing life-sustaining treatments. In such situations, ethics committee consultation may be indicated to help all parties clarify the goals of medial treatment.

Privacy and Confidentiality

The right to privacy is one of the most basic human rights. Privacy involves both negative and positive rights. The negative right comprises the right to be left alone. It is a basic prerequisite of autonomy or self-determination. As a positive right, privacy involves an individual's prerogative to control access to and the distribution of information about one's self.

Confidentiality is one of the mechanisms by which a person's right to privacy is recognized and honored. The physician's obligation to protect the patient's privacy dates back to the time of Hippocrates. Contemporary sources of authority come from the American Hospital Association's Patient's Bill of Rights, professional codes of ethics, state statutes, case law, and institutional policies.

The realities of the current health care environment often prevent the traditional interpretation of this doctrine. After one of his patients complained about a respiratory therapist reading his chart, Siegler conducted an informal survey and determined that over 75 clinicians and hospital personnel had legitimate access to the patient's medical record (2).

Disclosure and Informed Consent

Patient autonomy is entwined with the physician's obligation to communicate honestly about all aspects of the patient's diagnosis, the nature and purpose of proposed treatments, the risks of proposed treatments, any alternatives, and the risks and consequences of no treatment, as well as determining the patient's comprehension of this information transfer. The physician is additionally obligated to disclose uncertainty and therapeutic errors.

To carry out such goals, the physician must treat the patient as a partner in the process of making health care decisions. Shared decision making implies sharing power, and the physician is obligated to examine the differentials of power between persons and groups and to prevent unnecessary power struggles (3).

An ethically valid informed consent is obtained in a voluntary fashion from a capable adult patient. In most cases, the determination of a patient's capacity to make decisions is a common sense issue. If uncertainty exists, a second opinion from a physician colleague, formal testing, or a psychiatric evaluation may be useful. Critically ill patients are not inherently incapacitated, and efforts should be made to communicate with patients with impaired speech due to endotracheal tubes, neuromuscular disorders, or strokes. Steps to enhance a patient's decision-making capacity, such as the temporary withholding of sedatives and neuromuscular-blocking agents, should also be undertaken to help determine the patient's preferences for treatment.

When patients are admitted to an intensive care unit (ICU), they have not given implied consent for all aspects of critical care, such as the placement of a central venous pressure (CVP) catheter or the institution of mechanical ventilation. If time permits, the physician should obtain consent from the patient for all proposed treatments, recognizing that the signed form alone does not represent a legally or ethically valid consent, but is only the written record of the process of disclosure and discussion.

It is not necessary to obtain an ethically valid informed consent in times of a medical emergency, a situation in which obtaining explicit consent would endanger the life or health of the patient. In such situations, the preferred method is to treat the patient with their best interests in mind and obtain consent at the first opportunity.

Patient Refusal of Treatment

Patients' wishes should be respected, and capable patients have the right to refuse treatment, even medically indicated life-sustaining treatments such as surgery, cardioversion, chest compressions, and endotracheal intubation. The ability of patients to forgo treatment is equally extended to other forms of treatment, including those considered by the physician to be of the most banal nature, such as the use of antibiotic drugs, intravenous (i.v.) hydration, and enteral tube nutrition.

People sometimes refuse proven, effective treatments for themselves or their children on the grounds of religious or other personal objections to traditional medicine. The classic moral dilemma faced by physicians is the Jehovah's Witness patient who refuses a lifesaving blood transfusion. Now well grounded in legal and ethical cases, problems continue to surface when capable adults with dependents or viable fetuses refuse life-sustaining treatment, when surrogate decision makers refuse treatment for incapacitated adults or children, and in emergency situations.

Death and Dying

Physicians have an obligation to communicate with the patient and family regarding end-of-life issues, to conduct a benefit–burden analysis within the confines of medical uncertainty, to disclose futility, to obtain ethically and legally valid advance directives, and to provide emotional support to the dying patient and their family.

Decision Making for the Incapacitated Patient

Critically ill patients are often incapable of participating in medical treatment decisions when the need arises, especially regarding life-sustaining treatments. Physicians are obligated to outline an ethically valid decision-making process for incapacitated patients. This process most often involves identifying an appropriate surrogate decision maker, usually a family member, in a hierarchy determined by state law. The patient's designated surrogate (as defined in an advance directive to function as the patient's health care proxy) would take precedence over other family members, and a person legally appointed as the patient's surrogate decision maker for health affairs would take precedent over all other decision makers. Most surrogates are willing to assume this role, in a process of shared decision making with the physician.

Two methods for guiding surrogate decision making may be used in order to aid the surrogate and physician. One is used when evidence, either verbal or written, exists that the patient communicated relevant preferences or values before becoming incapacitated. In such situations, a medical treatment decision can be reached using a substituted judgment of what the patient would have wanted if he or she were able to participate in the decision at hand. This standard was first clarified in the Clare Conroy case in New Jersey (4) and played a role in the United States Supreme Court ruling in the Nancy Cruzan case (5). When knowledge of the patient's previously expressed wishes is not available, or when the patient never had the ability to participate in decision making (i.e., pediatric patients), the physician and surrogate decision maker must reach a decision that would be in the best interest of the patient.

ADVANCE DIRECTIVES

The United States Congress enacted the Patient Self-Determination Act (PSDA) in order to enhance a patient's control over medical treatment decisions by promoting the use of ethically and legally binding advance directives (6). Most states have three written documents that help ensure that even if patients cannot speak for themselves, they will get only the care they desire. These are: (a) a living will, (b) a health care proxy (also known as a durable power of attorney for health affairs), and (c) a do-not-resuscitate order. While the first two are legal documents that are administered according to a state's laws, the third is a medical directive that is entered into the patient's medical record.

A living will outlines the types of medical treatment the patient would like or would not like to receive in the event that they have been given a terminal diagnosis or are in a terminally unconscious state. Though the spirit of a living will is to allow a patient to forgo burdensome medical treatments when death is imminent, it is often open to interpretation by physicians. In addition, a living will usually specifies that only "artificial treatment" should be forgone, and provisions for a surrogate decision maker are often not indicated (7).

A more powerful advance directive is a health care proxy. In most states, a health care proxy permits the patient to designate a surrogate to make medical treatment decisions if the patient becomes incapacitated. This durable power of attorney is implemented at any time the patient is incapacitated, not just near the end of life, and is applicable for any medical treatment decision.

Unfortunately, the majority of patients have not designated a health care proxy. Though these numbers are increasing, the goals of the PSDA are not being entirely reached, and greater efforts are needed to enhance and reinforce discussions about advance directives. Attainment of the goals is dependent upon the extent to which hospitals advocate and devote resources for effective discussion of advance directives, as well as the desire of primary care physicians to initiate the discussions before a patient becomes critically ill.

Do-Not-Resuscitate Orders

A decision to withhold cardiopulmonary resuscitation (CPR) in the event of a cardiac or respiratory arrest is another form of a written advance directive. The original intent of do-not-resuscitate (DNR) orders was for the patient, in the process of dying from a terminal condition, to forgo CPR. When making this end-of-life decision, the patient, family, and physician agree that the goal of further treatment is to provide comfort and symptom relief.

The use of DNR in the twenty-first century is much more ambiguous. Not only is the interpretation of what resuscitation entails broad, but a general misinterpretation and misunderstanding exist of a patient's intent to limit medical treatment. This ambiguity is further compounded when the decision to limit treatment is poorly communicated and documented in a patient's medical record. Patients may agree to forgo CPR but should be offered and may choose other treatment options, including surgery or intensive care therapy. A not uncommon, though not necessarily inappropriate, circumstance in ICUs in the United States is to see patients designated as DNR. For instance, a patient with end-stage chronic obstructive pulmonary disease and acute pneumonia may benefit from a trial of endotracheal intubation, mechanical ventilation, and antibiotic therapy, but no foreseeable benefit may be deemed for the use of chest compressions and cardioversion in the event of a cardiac arrest.

Forgoing Treatment Policies

The limitation of DNR orders has reinforced the need for health care institutions to develop forgoing treatment policies. Forgoing treatment policies emphasize the importance of goal-oriented treatment planning. Ideally, they can facilitate accurate communication between members of the health care team, patients, and families; and improve documentation of these decisions (8). Forgoing treatment orders should be clear and explicit. A basis for the medical treatment decision should be documented in the medical record and there should be an understanding that the order does not affect other aspects of medical care. Unfortunately, actual practice often falls short of the ideal. Interpretation of forgoing treatment orders is variable, often poorly communicated, and misunderstood.

Guidelines for Forgoing Life-Sustaining Treatments

The most difficult cases of withholding and withdrawing life-sustaining treatment in ICUs have a mix of medical uncertainty dealing with the probability of death without treatment, poor quality of life even with treatment, and the use of costly resources. This scenario occurs in a setting where more and more of the patients are incapacitated and unable to participate in the medical treatment decisions that need to be made. On the surface, the technologically advanced ICU may appear to be the focus of this problem. One cannot, however, ignore the societal demands placed on the physician to use this technology to prolong life, often without the physician having a logical analysis of the quality of that life. These technologies cannot cure the underlying disease process in some patients but, instead, have the potential to prolong the process of dying, causing needless suffering or maintaining the patient in a vegetative or profoundly impaired existence (9).

Finally, this moral dilemma is compounded by the increasing number of incapacitated patients occupying ICUs. The United States population is aging, with the fastest growing group being over age 85, including a population of patients with diminished capacity for medical treatment decisions due to stroke, dementia, the long-term effects of alcohol and other substance abuse, and head trauma (10). Studies have shown that only a small percentage of critically ill patients are capable of participating in medical treatment decisions, though family members are readily available and willing to function as surrogate decision makers (11–13).

Most patients in ICUs recover and are discharged with a good quality of life. Only a small percentage decide whether or not to forgo (i. e., withhold or withdraw) medical treatment. Of these patients, most die in the ICU following withdrawal of life-sustaining treatment, and the remainder die soon after transferring to the hospital ward.

On the surface, withdrawing treatment should apparently be morally more difficult than withholding treatment. For instance, a physician may be more reluctant to switch a ventilator off than to have never turned it on. The President's Commission for the Study of Ethical Problems strongly challenged this belief. The commission stressed that withholding any treatment that has not yet been tried with the patient ought to be morally more difficult than withdrawing any treatment that has been tried and has failed to benefit the patient (14). If doubt exists that a given treatment may or may not benefit the patient, all parties involved in making the decision should outline specific goals of treatment, and then a therapeutic trial should be undertaken. Once evidence becomes apparent that the treatment is not benefiting the patient, no moral obligation necessitates continuing the treatment, as no moral distinction exists between withholding and withdrawing treatments. In fact, continuing aggressive treatment, such as endotracheal intubation and mechanical ventilation for hopelessly ill patients, may cause discomfort and be contrary to the physician's obligation to provide comfort and symptom relief.

DO NOT RESUSCITATE AND FORGOING TREATMENT ORDERS IN THE OPERATING ROOM

Though DNR and forgoing treatment orders have been implemented in other areas of the hospital, only recently have anesthesiologists addressed this issue in the operating room (OR). The use of these two types of orders in the OR is the focus of previous debate (15,16).

The concept of DNR orders for patients presenting to the OR was addressed by the President's Commission in 1983 (14). This commission indicated that the order to not resuscitate had no implications for other treatments, including surgical care. Surgical interventions may take the form of palliative procedures, such as the placement of central venous catheters for the administration of analgesics; potential curative operations, such as appendectomies for acute appendicitis; and elective operations that could improve the patient's quality of life but are unrelated

to the patient's underlying illness, such as cataract extraction in a patient with an incurable malignancy.

Anesthesiologists have had a tradition of unilaterally suspending the DNR order perioperatively. Many reasons support the perioperative suspension of DNR orders. First, a cardiopulmonary arrest that results from an intervention in the OR or during the performance of a procedure (i.e., endoscopy with conscious sedation) is usually associated with a clearly identifiable cause unrelated to the patient's primary disease process and more likely to be successfully treated. Second, anesthesiologists find it extremely difficult to differentiate routine anesthetic care from resuscitative efforts. Further arguments for automatic suspension of DNR orders in the OR include the anesthesiologist's fear that the possibility of causing a respiratory or cardiac arrest from analgesics and sedatives will constrain them from providing optimum care. Many anesthesiologists believe that they will be envisioned as the champions of patients seeking physician-assisted suicide. This notion is compounded by the belief that patients with DNR orders are often terminally ill and are more likely to require resuscitation in the OR.

Assumed perioperative suspension of DNR orders and policies that automatically suspend DNR orders or other advance directives that limit treatment are passive attempts to usurp the basic rights of patients. Anesthesiologists have an obligation to respect a patient's or surrogate's wish to limit medical treatment.

Attempts to resolve this dilemma by distinguishing routine anesthetic practices from the aggressive maneuvers of electric cardioversion and chest compressions are flawed, as they do not address what to do with patients who have orders to forgo other treatments. A better strategy, as outlined by the American Society of Anesthesiologists and others, is to develop a policy of mandatory reassessment of DNR and forgoing treatment orders (17).

WITHDRAWAL OF LIFE-SUSTAINING TREATMENT

A decision to withdraw life-sustaining treatment from a critically ill patient is a difficult but necessary part of care in the ICU. More often than not, the patient will be unable to participate in the medical treatment decision. Efforts should be made, however, to determine if the patient had verbal or written advance directives that would aid the physician and surrogate decision maker. Lacking advance directives, the physician should conduct a benefit–burden analysis with the best interests of the patient in mind. Time-limited therapeutic trials can be attempted.

Unanimity should be attained among the health care team and the surrogate regarding forgoing treatment. Problems may arise when members of the team or family feel excluded from the decision-making process. Once a medical treatment decision is reached, it should be documented in the progress notes, and a forgoing treatment or DNR order should be entered in the medical record.

Sedatives and analgesics should be administered during the process of withdrawing life-sustaining treatment. The goal of further treatment is to (a) relieve physical pain; (b) produce an unconscious state before the withdrawal of artificial life support;

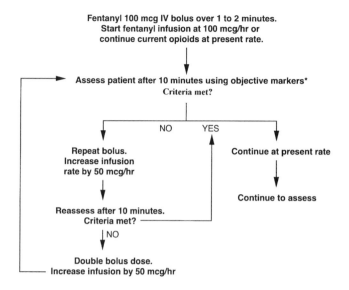

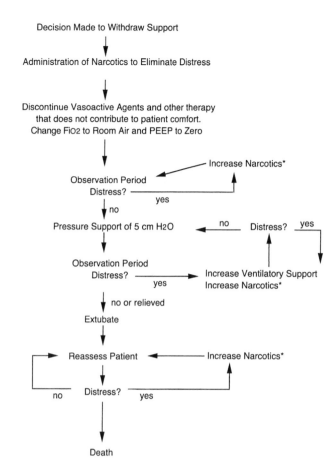

FIGURE 1. Suggested guidelines for pharmacologic intervention during the withdrawal of life-sustaining treatment using objective markers to ensure patient comfort. *RR*, respiratory rate; *HR*, heart rate; *MAP*, mean arterial pressure.

See figure one for guidelines to increase narcotics

FIGURE 2. Suggested algorithm for the withdrawal of mechanical ventilation. *F*IO₂, percentage of inspired oxygen; *PEEP*, positive end-expiratory pressure.

or (c) relieve nonphysical suffering (Fig. 1) (18). Standard drug dosages may be grossly inadequate to relieve a dying patient's suffering, and the physician should not hesitate to use high doses of analgesics, especially in patients who have developed tolerance to opioid medications. Emphasis on the intent of end-of-life treatment has led to the concept of double effect, which means that an act with both good and bad consequences could be carried out as long as certain conditions are met (19). The intent of administering opioids or sedatives is to relieve pain and suffering in a dying patient. The unintended consequence may be that these medications might cause either respiratory depression or excessive sedation, which might hasten a patient's death. The death is attributed to the disease or complications of the disease, combined in some circumstances with the withdrawal of life-sustaining treatments such as mechanical ventilation, vasoactive drugs, i.v. fluids, and nutrition.

Following an assessment of adequate relief of terminal symptoms, vasoactive agents and other therapies should be withdrawn (Fig. 2). The ventilator should be withdrawn next, with supplemental oxygen and positive end-expiratory pressure (PEEP) initially withdrawn and then any assist mode. If these actions do not result in the patient's death, the patient should then be extubated. Recognizing that pain is only one form of suffering,

the physician needs to make continual bedside assessments of the patient's level of comfort (Tables 1 and 2) (20).

WITHDRAWAL OF BASIC LIFE SUPPORT

Decisions to forgo basic life support, such as nutrition and hydration, are grounded in the same ethical principles as are those decisions to forgo other life-sustaining treatments (5,21). Nevertheless, withdrawing i.v. catheters or feeding tubes remains an emotionally charged issue and is a frequent impetus for ethics committee consultation. Closely monitoring the efficacy of symptom-relief measures will help to alleviate the surrogate's fear that the patient will suffer from hunger and thirst.

MEDIATING DISPUTES

When disputes arise with surrogate decision makers, the physician should continue to treat the patient until the dispute is resolved, except when treatment is harmful to the patient. This guideline is grounded in a premise that favors sustaining life. To

TABLE 1. SYMPTOMS OF SUFFERING

Pain
Dyspnea
Cough
Nausea and vomiting
Thirst
Hunger
Sleeplessness
Fatigue
Incontinence
Constipation
Itching
Perspiration
Hiccups
Excessive salivation
Decubitus ulcers
Mucosal ulcers

(From Humphry D. *Final exit*. Eugene, OR: The Hemlock Society, 1991:126–128, with permission.)

effect resolution of the dispute, all parties must assess the benefit and burden of each medical treatment. Any advance directives the patient may have made before becoming incapacitated should be considered. The physician should not hesitate to consult the hospital ethics committee or other mediators, such as social workers, patient representatives, psychiatrists, and clergy members. Resolution may not be simplistic or easy to accomplish.

In situations where the surrogate of an incapacitated patient demands that beneficial medical treatment be withheld from the patient and it is not clear if the patient may have wanted that treatment, the physician should not acquiesce to the surrogate's demand. Though the physician should attempt to resolve the dispute, they should put the patient's best interests above all other considerations. The burden of seeking legal action to stop treatment in this situation falls on the surrogate.

If the surrogate demands that futile medical treatment be started, the physician has an obligation to discuss the patient's poor prognosis with the surrogate and to express the opinion that a treatment is ineffective, unreasonable, or not in the patient's best interest. Recognize that some people may be suspicious and distrustful of the health care system. Poverty, lack of education, and low literacy levels may cause barriers in communicating effectively. The physician, after good faith efforts to resolve the dispute and with prior institutional approval and ethics committee consultation, should withhold the harmful treatment, even over

TABLE 2. OTHER FORMS OF SUFFERING

Changes in physical appearance associated with weight loss, tumor, or burn
Dependence on others
Loss of dignity associated with confusion, disorientation, forgetfulness
Other behavioral or intellectual changes
Leaving loved ones
Having unfulfilled dreams
Losing material possessions
Financial concerns
Anxiety that the suffering will become worse

(From Humphry D. *Final exit*. Eugene, OR: The Hemlock Society, 1991:126–128, with permission.)

the objections of the surrogate (22). The physician's ethical obligation of nonmaleficence takes precedence in these situations. A common conflict in the ICU arises when a surrogate demands that the physician "do everything," including medically inappropriate and burdensome CPR. Sound practice does not even offer CPR as an option for a patient who would not benefit from it, and the physician is obligated to discuss with the surrogate the medical reasons why CPR is inappropriate. If the dispute cannot be resolved, the physician should seek outside help, including making a good faith effort of transferring the patient to another physician. If this effort is also unsuccessful, the physician has no moral obligation to provide the treatment. Seeking legal relief ought to be an act of last resort in these disputes.

When the surrogate demands that harmful medical treatment be continued, the physician, after all attempts to mediate the dispute have failed, should strive to withdraw the treatment (22). In these cases, the physician should have prior institutional approval, and the institution should seek a court's approval for withdrawal of life-sustaining treatment or treatments. In cases where the dispute is largely about the patient's quality of life, respect for the surrogate's wishes and values is appropriate because the surrogate is considered to be in a better position to evaluate quality-of-life issues. The physician should recognize that spirituality and religious beliefs might significantly affect attitudes toward the dying process and the determination of what treatments the surrogate feels are appropriate. In such situations, taking unilateral action to withdraw treatment, such as turning off a ventilator, over a surrogate's objections runs contrary to a moral perspective that allows a surrogate to be the final interpreter of what "quality of life" means to that particular patient (14). If the case clearly involves harm to the patient, however, the physician's first loyalty is to the patient, and treatment should be withdrawn to prevent harm.

PEDIATRIC ISSUES

The ethical issues surrounding medical treatment decisions for children are not inherently different from those for adults. Truth telling, disclosure, informed consent, decisions to forgo life-sustaining treatment, and issues surrounding death and dying are all involved in caring for pediatric patients. Specific differences between pediatrics and other medical disciplines do, however, deserve special note.

Pediatric patients are not capable and never have been capable of making medical treatment decisions. The issue of surrogate decision making and the role of the parents are, therefore, of paramount importance and have evolved over the last 20 years. In 1982, the Department of Health and Human Services regulations surrounding the "Baby Doe" case sought to dictate rigid standards of care. On the other hand, pediatricians were criticized for their lack of respect for parental autonomy, especially when dealing with critically ill neonates. Compounding this moral dilemma is the increasing complexity of medical technology and the ability of children to make rapid and dramatic improvements in the face of tremendous medical uncertainty. Current guidelines now recognize that withholding or withdrawing life-sustaining treatment from critically ill, malformed, or handicapped neonates and critically ill older children is justifiable in some circumstances (23). Many of the moral dilemmas confronted by pediatric intensivists and neonatologists center upon this issue.

The legal system in the United States recognizes parents' autonomy in making medical treatment decisions for their child. Parents have a moral responsibility to care for their child, and as such, they should be in a position to determine what is best for their child. To function as surrogate decision makers, parents need full disclosure of their child's diagnosis, prognosis, and treatment options. Unfortunately, a variety of factors complicate this process. A family that is faced with their child's life-threatening problems is also faced with tremendous emotional issues. Feelings of denial, anger, depression, fear, and even disgust often overwhelm the parents. Most health care professionals believe that the parents' role is not unlimited in decisions regarding forgoing treatment. Circumstances exist in which the parents' decisions should be questioned; such as when a medical treatment decision is made that reflects not the child's best interests but others' interests, such as the burden foreseen by the parents in bringing up a physically or mentally handicapped child. In other situations, in attempting to adhere to their religious beliefs, parents may make medical treatment decisions for their child that are not in the child's best interests, such as the refusal of a Jehovah's Witness to authorize a lifesaving blood transfusion during their child's chemotherapy for a curable malignancy.

When disputes arise between the parent and the physician, the best approach is to use the model of shared decision making. The physician is obligated to communicate openly about diagnosis, prognosis, and treatment options, and should make recommendations to the parents. This disclosure provides the parents with insight into all of the issues involved with their child's care. The parents then bring their values, goals, and preferences to the discussion, and ideally, all can reach a morally acceptable medical treatment decision. Nevertheless, the physician has a responsibility to promote the child's best interests and to seek intervention if the moral dilemma cannot be satisfactorily resolved (1). The physician should not hesitate to involve the hospital ethics committee, clergy members, and social workers to help resolve the dispute in their advocacy for the child. In some situations, the physician may seek legal counsel in order to have the parents' medical treatment decision overridden by the courts.

Physicians should take into account an older child's opinion and values when sharing medical treatment decisions with the child's surrogates (i.e., parents). "Assent" is the term used to differentiate a child's agreement to receive treatment from an ethically and legally valid consent, which can only be obtained from the child's surrogate. Certain statutory exceptions exist for certain minors, however, that enable them to make medical treatment decisions for themselves. Emancipated minors, married minors or those who are parents, and minors in military service are all granted the same status as that of capable adult patients. Infrequently, mature minors may seek court orders granting them rights to participate in medical treatment decisions.

PHYSICIAN-ASSISTED SUICIDE (PAS) AND ACTIVE EUTHANASIA

Physicians are obligated to take steps to provide comfort and alleviate suffering. They also have an obligation to withdraw medical

TABLE 3. DEFINITIONS OF EUTHANASIA AND PHYSICIAN-ASSISTED SUICIDE

Term	Definition
Euthanasia	An action that of itself and by intention causes death, with the purpose of eliminating suffering
Voluntary active euthanasia	Administration of a lethal agent by a physician to a capable patient for the purpose of eliminating the patient's suffering
Involuntary active euthanasia	Euthanasia performed without the consent of a capable patient
Passive euthanasia	Forgoing life-sustaining treatment
Assisted suicide	Facilitation of a patient's death by provision of the necessary means to enable the patient to perform a life-ending act
Physician-assisted suicide	The physician provides the means to enable a patient to perform a life-ending act

treatment that is simply prolonging the life of a patient with an incurable illness (Table 3). Whether physicians have the moral obligation to help terminate the life of a patient who suffers from an incurable disease and wants to die remains an unresolved dilemma in the United States. What is clear is that individuals from broad segments of the population who are afflicted with terminal diseases or chronic diseases that impair their quality of life have requested physician assistance in dying.

In 1997 the Supreme Court unanimously upheld Washington and New York state laws banning PAS (24,25). The Court ruled that the United States Constitution does not guarantee citizens the right to end their lives with a physician's help, but left individual states the option of legalizing the practice. One such state that did this is Oregon. When Oregonians first endorsed the landmark Death with Dignity Act in 1994, they opened a Pandora's box of legal and ethical dilemmas. The law, which allows terminally ill adults to end their own lives, attracted national attention. Three years later, after surviving political challenges from everyone from district court judges to the United States Department of Justice, and in the face of sustained opposition, the world's first official, state-sponsored PAS law was back in the hands of Oregon voters, who approved the measure. Since the law went into effect in the winter of 1997, roughly 50 Oregonians have used the act to end their lives (26). Under the law, both an attending and consulting physician must first determine that a patient, who is required to be mentally capable and a resident of Oregon, is suffering from a terminal disease. A prescription for a lethal dose of drugs is written only after both patient and physician have followed a strict protocol. The patient makes two oral requests and one written request for medication over the course of 15 days; the prescription can be filled on the 15th day, which is also when the second oral request is presented. Physicians cannot administer the medication; a critical requirement of the Oregon law demands that patients be able to take the lethal dose themselves. If a physician suspects that a patient is depressed or otherwise mentally incapable of making an informed decision, they can refuse the prescription requests and refer the patient to a mental health professional.

Opponents of PAS object that physician participation in assisting people to die violates the basic moral obligations of physicians to do no harm. Issues centering on competency of those requesting death and to what degree physician involvement is

TABLE 4. GUIDELINES FOR JUSTIFIABLE PHYSICIAN-ASSISTED SUICIDE

1. A voluntary request by a capable adult patient
2. An ongoing patient–physician relationship
3. Mutual and informed decision making by patient and physician
4. A supportive yet critical and probing environment of decision making
5. A considered rejection of alternatives such as hospice care
6. Structured consultation with other parties in medicine
7. A persistent preference for death expressed by the patient
8. Unacceptable suffering by the patient
9. Use of a means that is as painless and comfortable as possible

(From Beauchamp RL, Childress JF. *Principles of biomedical ethics*, 4th ed. New York: Oxford University Press, 1994, with permission.)

necessary fuel the PAS debate. Observers of the European experience of voluntary euthanasia and PAS have seen abuses, such as the involuntary active euthanasia in the Netherlands of incapacitated patients and neonates. Opponents also fear that patients may be coerced into opting for death and that the traditional role of the physician as healer will be undermined by such practices.

Efforts to legalize PAS and voluntary euthanasia will likely continue. Advocates see no difference between these practices and forgoing life-sustaining treatment in patients with incurable illnesses. They contend that PAS will become one of a physician's moral obligations to their patients. Physicians remain polarized in their belief in and ability to participate in PAS (27–29). Restrictions and safeguards will be incorporated into any practice of legalized PAS (Table 4) and procedures for physicians who morally object to PAS and euthanasia must be present.

The fear of uncontrolled pain will lead many hopelessly ill patients to consider PAS as their only alternative. If nothing else, the PAS debate has improved the care of dying patients and comprehensive palliative care, which employ an interdisciplinary team of physicians, nurses, home health aides, ethicists, chaplains, and bereavement counselors, and is now an expected standard at the end of life. Unfortunately, many physicians are ill-equipped to abandon their traditional role of curing their patient and fighting for life in order to adopt a stance where the relief of their patient's suffering should supersede all other treatment goals. Medical schools and graduate medical education are addressing this need with end-of-life care as a regular part of the curriculum.

ALLOCATION OF MEDICAL RESOURCES

Rationing of health care has been defined as "the allocation of scarce health care resources among competing individuals"(30). Allocation of critical care services is not a new phenomenon. Recent examples of scarce resources are hemodialysis machines in the 1960s and the ongoing scarcity of organs for transplantation. More often, though, is the everyday occurrence in most ICUs of rationing of personnel, equipment, and space.

Physicians have a moral obligation to direct scarce, critical care resources to those patients most likely to benefit from those resources. A moral dilemma arises when physicians also are obligated to do all that they can for the benefit of an individual patient. In an attempt to resolve this conflict, physicians must consider the cost-effectiveness of particular treatments when

making medical treatment decisions. The Society of Critical Care Medicine's Consensus Statement on the Triage of Critically Ill Patients recommends that the physician in charge of triage decisions should make unilateral decisions regarding exclusion or discharge of patients from an ICU and outlines specific diagnostic categories of patients that should be excluded from admission to the unit. Beyond these diagnostic groups of patients, clear guidelines regarding the cost-effectiveness of expensive critical care are lacking. Limiting CPR is another strategy suggested to limit costs (31).

As more cost-effective studies are available, guidelines to limit care could be developed on a national, statewide, or even institutional basis to determine which treatments would be futile, disproportionate, or unreasonable. Patient autonomy and even physician autonomy would yield to organizational autonomy. The traditional balance between the four main ethical principles, currently weighted toward patient autonomy and beneficence, would swing toward the responsibility of the physician, as well as the patient, to society. The physician's obligation to their patient would no longer require an unlimited duty to advance the patient's interest regardless of the cost or the degree of the expected benefit.

HEALTH CARE SYSTEM REFORM

As a society we often talk about health care and health insurance as if it is a fundamental human right, similar to free speech or freedom of association. The reality is that about 15% of Americans (over 42 million individuals) have no health insurance, while everyone has a right to free speech. Hospitals and health systems are left to fill the gap between what is expected from health care— universal access—and what we as a society have been willing to pay for. What new sources of funding will be available to offset the cost of health care? How will hospitals support care given to the uninsured and underinsured? Many feel that the amount of money allocated to health care, approximately 13% of the U.S. gross national product, is already excessive and unfair, taking precedence over other expenditures such as education or national defense.

Since the 1990s increasing emphasis has been placed on minimizing costs in health care. One strategy to reduce expenditure is to revamp the health care delivery system. Many believe that tremendous cost savings can be realized if more money is spent on preventive health care services. Though spending on preventive medicine may increase the quality of life for many people, overall savings may not take place because patients will live longer and have greater health care needs later in life. Another major concern is that health care expenditures at or near the end of life have been targeted as areas for cost savings. Whether the increased use of advance directives, hospice care, and fewer technically aggressive interventions at or near the end of life can realize substantial cost savings is doubtful (32). Nevertheless, education of the public regarding their responsibilities as patients in medical treatment decisions and health care reform is necessary.

Areas targeted as more likely to generate cost savings include decreasing the size and cost of the medical bureaucracy surrounding health care financing and controlling pharmaceutical prices. Seen as politically correct by many people, these maneuvers should be viewed only as components of a more encompassing strategy of containing the rate of medical inflation (33). To control inflation and ensure long-lasting cost savings, the development of new technologies and treatments may need to be slowed, their use may need to be controlled, and they may even need to be rationed.

MANAGED CARE

Managed care refers to a cost-savings technique to conserve and equitably distribute scarce medical resources (34). In the old system, reimbursement policies rewarded the performance of technical procedures. In the managed care system, a variety of strategies are used to contain costs through competition. Managed care organizations use primary care physicians as "gatekeepers" and financial incentives to effect changes in physicians' behavior. Medical ethicists have examined the fairness of managed care schemes that are devised to lower costs through market competition (35) and many are concerned about the potential for conflict between the desire to hold down costs and the duties of health care providers to act as strong advocates for those in their care. The degree of conflict is directly related to the attitude of the organization. The ultimate motive of the organization should be quality of care. However, attempts by the health care organization to micromanage patient care can be seen as an intrusion by a third party into the physician–patient relationship and the clinical autonomy of physicians. Moral dilemmas regarding restrictions on patient autonomy of choice of physician, choice of treatment, and choice of treatment site do occur. The organization may deny or curtail treatment based on compliance by the patient or the physician with the organization's rules. The organization's attempts to contain costs by limiting care to the exclusion of out-of-network physicians may directly impact on the patient's ability to obtain quality critical care. Anesthesiologists are particularly affected if attempts to contain costs are accomplished by limiting the number and types of surgical procedures performed.

HOSPITAL ETHICS COMMITTEES

In the field of clinical ethics, controversy remains over the role of hospital ethics committees and clinical ethicists. In the United States, ethics committees differ widely in their composition and function. An ethics committee may function as an educational resource within an institution, providing valuable information to both health care professionals and the public. An ethics committee can also function to develop and comment upon explicit hospital policies. The most useful and salient task of an ethics committee is to provide consultation when a patient, family, and physician need help in reaching a difficult medical treatment decision. When providing consultation, an ethics committee should aid physicians with moral dilemmas by making recommendations that are within a range of ethically acceptable alternatives, rather than by dictating a particular medical treatment decision. Ethics consultants should not impose their opinion upon the patient, family, physician, or other health care professionals. Rather, the ability to mediate and counsel these participants is paramount

to providing effective ethics consultation. Regardless of the role an ethics committee chooses to play within an institution, some method should be in place to review the actions of the committee (36).

ETHICAL AND LEGAL PROBLEMS

Clinical ethics and health care law evolved together in a dynamic and interactive relationship. Though related, the two disciplines do not entirely overlap. Law seeks to educate and to regulate by establishing a minimal standard of conduct, and by instituting disincentives for ignoring the standard. Negative sanctions such as suspension of license to practice, fines, or even imprisonment are imposed by our society and are carried out by the government. The field of medical ethics also endorses basic norms of behavior that are required by law; however, ethics extends beyond the law to prescribe desirable conduct and virtues to which we should aspire. Sanctions are generated by the praise or blame of our colleagues and are generally noncoercive.

The judicial system can be seen as intrusive in medical treatment decisions. The courts, as a routine, are often cumbersome, adversarial, unfamiliar with patients' goals, and usually strongly dependent on the physician's viewpoint. However, seeking a court ruling may be justifiable in some cases.

SUMMARY

Clinical ethics is an important part of the perioperative physician's area of expertise. Issues of capacity and informed consent and decisions to forgo life-sustaining treatment are integral to the critical care physician's practice. A previous emphasis on patient autonomy is being challenged by the concepts of beneficence and distributive justice. Managed health care has been rapidly integrated into our society. A critical care physician's obligation to their patient is oftentimes in conflict with a managed health care organization's obligation to control the escalating costs of expensive, technologically advanced medical treatments.

Simultaneously, end-of-life issues are in the forefront of the public's consciousness. Patients are executing their rights to make advance directives for health care and many are in favor of legalizing PAS. When discussing end-of-life decisions, the critical care physician must maintain a balanced approach, with special attention on relieving pain and suffering, and must maintain respect for the patient's informed decisions.

EYE TO THE FUTURE

New genetic technologies promise to make medical ethics an even more central part of social decision making. The Human Genome Project, a 15-year, federally funded $3 billion effort to code the entire human genetic map, has already resulted in the discovery of a number of genes that may lead to particular diseases or traits. This project will also give individuals more information about their own genetic make-up. Medical ethicists are debating whether or not this genetic information is the exclusive property of patients, or is instead the concern of insurers, employers, and society.

The explosion in genetic diagnosis and therapy poses a variety of challenges to society. Many wonder if our abilities to collect information and undertake efforts at therapeutic intervention are racing ahead faster than law, ethics, and public policy can respond.

During this dynamic period, physicians with competence in clinical ethics will assume a vital role within health care organizations to ensure that ethical medical care is provided.

KEY POINTS

Truth telling, disclosure, informed consent, decisions to forgo life-sustaining treatment, and issues surrounding death and dying are involved in the care of critically ill patients. The physician must determine the ability of a critically ill patient to make an informed medical treatment decision, and if the patient is deemed incapacitated, the physician must identify an appropriate surrogate decision maker for the patient.

Physicians caring for incapacitated critically ill patients are often confronted with difficult decisions to forgo life-sustaining treatment due to the uncertainty of the patient's death if treatment is forgone, the possibility of a poor quality of life even with treatment, and the absence of an advance directive. Such medical treatment decisions are made by the physician and the patient's surrogate decision maker in a process of shared decision making, using a benefit–burden analysis, with the patient's best interests in mind.

Not all technologically possible means of prolonging life need be or should be used in every case. Though physicians are obligated to take steps to provide comfort and alleviate suffering, they may not be obligated to actively assist in a patient's death. In managed health care systems, conflicts arise when a physician's obligation to the patient and to the managed care organization's rules and cost-containment efforts conflict.

REFERENCES

1. Beauchamp TL, Childress JF. *Principles of biomedical ethics*, 4th ed. New York: Oxford University Press, 1994.
2. Siegler, M. Sounding boards. Confidentiality in medicine a decrepit concept. *N Engl J Med* 1982;307:1518–1521.
3. Brody H. *The healing power*. New Haven, CT: Yale University Press, 1992.
4. *Conroy*, 98 NJ 321, 486 A2d 1209, (N.J. Supreme Court 1985).
5. *Cruzan v Director, Missouri Department of Health*, 1990 US Lexis 3301, United States Supreme Court June 25, 1990.
6. Omnibus Budget Reconciliation Act of 1990. Title IV, Section 4206. Congressional Record, October 26, 1990;136:H2456.
7. Annas GJ. The health care proxy and the living will. *N Engl J Med* 1991;324:1210–1213.
8. O'Toole EE, Youngner SJ, Juknialis BW, et al. Evaluation of a treatment limitation policy with a specific treatment-limiting order page. *Arch Intern Med* 1994;154:425–432.
9. Fletcher JC. Decisions to forgo life-sustaining treatment when the patient is incapacitated. In: *Introduction to clinical ethics*. Frederick, MD: University Publishing Group, 1995.
10. U.S. Congress, Office of Technology Assessment. *Losing a million minds: confronting the tragedy of Alzheimer's disease and other dementias*. Washington, DC: U.S. Government Printing Office, 1987:15–22. Pub. no. OTA-BA-323.
11. Danis M, Southerlan LI, Garrett JM, et al. A prospective study of advance directives for life-sustaining care. *N Engl J Med* 1991;324:882–888.
12. Smedira NG, Evans BH, Grais LS, et al. Withholding and withdrawal of life support from the critically ill. *N Engl J Med* 1990;322:309–315.
13. Lee DK, Swinburne AJ, Fedullo AJ, et al. Withdrawing care. Experience in a medical intensive care unit. *JAMA* 1994;271:1358–1361.
14. President's Commission for the Study of Ethical Problems in Medicine and Biomedical Research. *Deciding to forego life-sustaining treatment*. Washington, DC: U.S. Government Printing Office, 1983.
15. Truog RD. "Do-not-resuscitate" orders during anesthesia and surgery. *Anesthesiology* 1991;74:606–608.
16. Cohen CB, Cohen PJ. Do-not-resuscitate orders in the operating room. *N Engl J Med* 1991;325:1879–1882.
17. American Society of Anesthesiologists. Standards, Guidelines, and Statements, October 1996. Ethical guidelines for the anesthesia care of patients with do-not-resuscitate orders or other directives that limit treatment. Park Ridge, IL: American Society of Anesthesiologists,1997.
18. Truog RD, Berde CB, Mitchell C, Grier HE. Barbiturates in the care of the terminally-ill. *New Engl J Med* 1992;327:1678.
19. Quill TE, Dresser R, Brock DW. The rule of double effect—a critique of its role in end-of-life decision making. *N Engl J Med* 1997;337:1768–1771.
20. Humphry D. *Final exit*. Eugene, OR: The Hemlock Society, 1991:126–128.
21. Ruark JE, Raffin TA. Initiating and withdrawing life support. Principles and practice in adult medicine. *N Engl J Med* 1988;318:25–30.
22. Luce JM. Physicians do not have a responsibility to provide futile or unreasonable care if a patient or family insists. *Crit Care Med* 1995;23:760–766.
23. Nelson LJ, Nelson RM. Ethics and the provision of futile, harmful, or burdensome treatment to children. *Crit Care Med* 1992;20:427–433.
24. *Washington v Glucksberg*, 117 S. Ct. 2258 (1997).
25. *Vacco v Quill*, 117 S. Ct. 2293 (1997).
26. Sullivan AJ, Hedberg K, Fleming DW. Legalized physician-assisted suicide in Oregon—the second year. *N Engl J Med* 2000;342:598–604.
27. Bachman JG, Alcser KH, Doukas DJ, et al. Attitudes of Michigan physicians and the public toward legalizing physician-assisted suicide and voluntary euthanasia. *N Engl J Med* 1996;334:303–309.
28. Lee MA, Nelson HD, Tilden VP, et al. Legalizing assisted suicide—views of physicians in Oregon. *N Engl J Med* 1996;334:310–315.
29. Cohen JS, Fihn SD, Boyko EJ, et al. Attitudes toward assisted suicide and euthanasia among physicians in Washington State. *N Engl J Med* 1994;331:89–94.
30. Kalb PE, Miller DH. Utilization strategies for intensive care units. *JAMA* 1989;261:2389–2395.
31. Murphy DJ, Finucane TE. New do-not-resuscitate policies. A first step in cost control. *Arch Intern Med* 1993;153:1641–1648.
32. Emanuel EJ, Emanuel LL. The economics of dying. The illusion of cost savings at the end of life. *N Engl J Med* 1994;330:540–544.
33. Massaro TA. Impact of new technologies on health care costs and on the nation's "health." *Clin Chem* 1990;36:1612–1616.
34. Igelhart JK. Physicians and the growth of managed care. *N Engl J Med* 1994;331:1167–1171.
35. Wolf SM. Health care reform and the future of physician ethics. *Hastings Center Report* 1994;24:28–41.
36. Auliso MP, Arnold RM, Younger SJ, et al. Health care ethics consultation: nature, goals, and competencies: a position paper from the Society for Health and Human Value–Society for Bioethics Consultation Task Force on Standards for Bioethics Consultation. *Ann Intern Med* 2000;133:59–69.

5

EVIDENCE-BASED MEDICINE

DAN CONNOR
JENNIFER BAYNE
WILLIAM J. SIBBALD

KEY WORDS

- Cochrane Library
- Evidence-based medicine
- Information systems
- Levels of evidence
- Medical subject headings (MeSH)
- Meta-analysis
- Outcomes research
- Randomized controlled trial
- Systematic review

INTRODUCTION

Adopting an evidence-based approach to the practice of medicine is not new for most physicians who have made continuing medical education an integral part of their work. What is new is how readily one can now access so many facets of the repository of medical knowledge. In the past, we were restricted to textbooks, journals, and collegial advice. Now we have access to huge electronic databases that contain not only journal archives but also other sources that collect, critically appraise, summarize, and reference thousands of studies. The challenge is to learn the most efficient ways to access and evaluate this "evidence." It is not practical to spend hours searching and reviewing the literature every time there is a challenging clinical question. The following section focuses on creating an efficient system to search and appraise relevant medical literature and to do so rapidly.

BACKGROUND AND NEED FOR EVIDENCE-BASED MEDICINE

Within the past 25 years, the number of published documents has doubled and technological advances such as the Internet have created a system where distribution of these data is occurring at an exponentially increasing rate. The combination of increased availability of information with improved channels of information distribution requires innovative methods to manage effectively the flow of information. Enhancing the clinician's ability to manage and evaluate research data can reduce the amount of information overload and reduce the delay in incorporating research findings into clinical practice, concepts that were drivers

for the development of the theoretical framework for evidence-based medicine (EBM). As originally described, EBM was a systematic process whereby a clinician would effectively find and implement the "best evidence" to answer specific clinical questions. Since its inception, the growth of the EBM paradigm has been extensive and has given birth to many journal-based and electronic "spinoffs" that attempt to integrate and deliver to the clinician the best available evidence to assist in improving patient outcomes and overall health system efficiencies. At the same time, the rapid growth of EBM has led to criticisms that EBM is no longer a pure science to be used at the patient's bedside but, rather, has become a "catch phrase" that has diluted its underlying premise. EBM has become more of an information management system compared with its initial construct as a method to formulate principles that enable clinicians to select preferentially the information most appropriate to a particular clinical situation. In contrast to seeking advice from local experts or a textbook (also called *authority-based medicine*), EBM promotes advances in regard to underlying methodologies used by health care practitioners to answer clinical questions.

The most frequently used definition of EBM is "the conscientious, explicit and judicious use of current best evidence in making decisions about the care of the individual patients" (1). Initially, clinicians convert their information needs into a structured question. Next they conduct an efficient search for relevant literature to address the question. This approach empowers the clinician independently to locate and critically appraise the evidence for validity and generalizability and then subsequently to integrate the best evidence into patient care. This method results in clinical decisions based on evidence from population, patient, and laboratory studies rather than from popular opinion alone.

SOME OF THE SKILL SETS REQUIRED

One of the key skill sets required by clinicians in using EBM is the *critical appraisal* process of individual data sets and manuscripts to determine what evidence is valid and relevant to one's patient. There are, however, large variations in both the quality and appropriateness of such data. Because of this variability, published studies initially are categorized into primary and secondary levels. *Primary* evidence indicates original articles, such as the randomized controlled trial (RCT) and meta-analysis, and *secondary* evidence is generated from other sources such as editorials, expert opinion, and practice guidelines. To judge the value of either primary or secondary evidence, the clinician must learn analytical skills or a practical and working knowledge related to the various research designs. Understanding the strengths and weaknesses of different research methodologies is essential if the clinician is to weigh adequately the overall clinical value of the available evidence.

The Evidence-Based Medicine Working Group published a series of articles over the past decade entitled *The Users' Guides to the Medical Literature*. Now including 36 publications, this series aims to provide a systematic approach to the appraisal of various types of published medical reports to determine their level of evidence and applicability to clinical practice. This series allows the clinician to appraise quickly a study based on peer-accepted evaluative criteria. The results of this series are widely referenced in the peer-reviewed literature and have been used as an evaluative framework by many investigators. Publications in this series are of value to the clinician requiring a structured approach to determining the "best available evidence."

The *levels of evidence* method is a hierarchic method proposed to evaluate the strength of research or evidence. In this process, a level is assigned to a publication based on the study methodology. There are at least three accepted methods of categorizing the level of evidence, and these methods differ only in the nomenclature used to distinguish levels. In all three methods, the RCT is awarded higher levels of evidence than that of opinion leaders in the field, and practitioner opinion receives the lowest level of evidence.

In this chapter, we use clinical scenarios to demonstrate how an evidence-based approach can help practitioners make decisions for individual patients. Of necessity, this chapter cannot detail all the strengths and weaknesses of an evidence-based approach to patient care. What we can do is provide a demonstration of how this approach can be used to benefit both the decision maker and the patient; so the reader is encouraged to read more. In using a clinical scenario method, we analyze approaches to addressing clinically relevance. Our focus is on using electronic databases such as Medline, Cochrane Library, and UpToDate to find quality answers quickly. A list of useful website addresses with a focus on EBM also is included.

SCENARIO 1

A 64-year-old woman has been admitted to the intensive care unit (ICU) following a total hip replacement. During the procedure, she developed significant but transient ST segment depression. She was hemodynamically stable throughout the procedure. Now in the ICU, her 12-lead electrocardiograph (ECG) shows new ST- and T-wave changes consistent with a non–Q-wave myocardial infarction (MI). Her cardiac enzyme profile confirms MI. She is treated with aspirin. Because of her history of beta-blocker–induced asthma, you are considering starting a calcium channel blocker such as diltiazem or verapamil as an alternative to the beta-blockers. You are unsure, however, whether they are recommended in this situation and decide to find out whether there is evidence to support your decision.

Search Strategy

Evidence-based medicine is arguably a combination, or even a tradeoff, between searching for all the best evidence and practical limits. So the first thing to do is to try to articulate clearly your needs in a particular situation. To be easily achievable and practical, the searching process first must take into account the following factors:

- How much time do you have to make a decision? Do you need to know the answer immediately, in a week, or in a month? For example, you may want to retrieve every clinical trial on diltiazem. If you need to make a decision within 10 minutes, that approach would be impractical and overwhelming.
- How quickly is the information available? Do you have access to full text, or do you need to order an article from elsewhere?
- How much information do you need and are able to absorb? Are two excellent trials enough, or do you need a broader selection?
- How current must the information be? Is last month's Medline file sufficient, or do you need everything back to 1966?
- What tangents are you prepared to accept or reject, at least in principle? Are you interested only in elderly patients in the ICU, or would literature on younger patients with the same or similar diagnosis be useful?

The medical subject headings (MeSH) browser of Medline provides a good definition for EBM as being "the process of systematically finding, appraising, and using contemporaneous research findings as the basis for clinical decisions. Evidence-based medicine asks questions, finds and appraises the relevant data, and harnesses that information for everyday clinical practice. EBM follows four steps: formulate a clear clinical question from a patient's problem; search the literature for relevant clinical articles; evaluate (critically appraise) the evidence for its validity and usefulness; and implement useful findings in clinical practice. The term "evidence-based medicine" was coined at McMaster Medical School in Canada in the 1980's to label this clinical strategy, which people at the school had been developing for over a decade (1).

This definition outlines four steps for a search strategy:

1. *Formulate* a clear clinical question from a patient's problem.
2. *Search* the literature for relevant clinical articles.
3. *Evaluate* (critically appraise) the evidence for its validity and usefulness.
4. *Implement* useful findings in clinical practice.

Formulate the Question

Because the searchable databases, such as Medline, Embase, and Cochrane Library, contain millions of words, hundreds of thousands of journal articles, and more than 30,000 terms and synonyms in their thesauri, it is necessary to choose search terms that will retrieve the most appropriate information. The most efficient way to do this is first to identify a clinical topic and then divide the topic into its constituent parts:

- The *type of patient*, subject group, or problem
- The *intervention* being considered

- A *comparison* or alternative intervention, if appropriate
- The desired *outcome*

This is known as the *base clinical set.*

One also must identify at this stage the language for the publication, the age group of the patients, and the types of studies. The goal is to retrieve the most methodologically sound articles for the current scenario; so the following filters will be used:

- Clinical trial
- Multicenter trial
- Controlled clinical trial
- Randomized controlled trial

Evidence-based medicine divides the research literature into four main areas: therapy, diagnosis, etiology, and prognosis. Specific types of studies are best suited to answer questions related to each of these areas of research and clinical work, and are outlined in Table 1. In anesthesia and critical care, most clinical questions relate to therapy. For prognosis, etiology, and diagnostic testing questions, the search process is similar, but the critical appraisal of the evidence follows a different path. The *JAMA* users' guides outline the approach for all types of clinical questions and can be accessed through the excellent Evidence-Based Medicine Tool Kit website at http://www.med.ualberta.ca/ebm/ebm.htm.

A good description of the classes of studies available, the advantages and disadvantages of each study type, and Table 1 can be found at the Duke University Medical Center Library website: http://www.mc.duke.edu/mclibrary/respub/guides/ebm.html#top.

Systematic reviews, meta-analyses, and practice guidelines are termed *synthesis articles* and can be used to find information for any type of question. As our clinical question relates to a treatment or therapy, it is best answered by a randomized controlled trial.

In our scenario, we now can construct the clinical question, Does the use of diltiazem, representing a prototypical calcium channel blocker, in patients with myocardial infarction improve survival or decrease morbidity compared with beta-blockers?

- The *type of patient*, subject group, or problem: myocardial infarction, human adult subjects
- The *intervention* being considered: diltiazem
- *Comparison* or alternative intervention: beta-blockers
- The desired *outcome*: improved survival, decreased morbidity

Search the Literature for Relevant Clinical Articles

We now have a clinical question as a framework for searching the literature. Next we must decide where to start the search. Numerous databases provide access to reviews that are critically

TABLE 1. TYPE OF STUDIES*^a* TO ANSWER A SPECIFIC TYPE OF QUESTION

Therapy	Randomized controlled trial, controlled clinical trial
Diagnostic testing	Prospective, blind comparison to gold standard
Etiology/harm	Cohort study > case–control > case series
Prognosis	Cohort study > case–control > case series

^a In order of usefulness.

appraised and well referenced. If the information we require can be found in these databases, use of these databases could save a significant amount of work and may provide a summary of the subject. The two best databases are the *Cochrane Library* at http://www.updateusa.com/cochrane/navbar.html and *UpToDate* at http://www.uptodate.com. Medline also could be included here because it is the preeminent biomedical database, but it is discussed later in this chapter.

We will start with the Cochrane Library to determine whether there are any systematic reviews in this area. The Cochrane Library is a quarterly updated electronic publication that specializes in the production of high-quality systematic reviews and information about the Cochrane Collaboration. The Collaboration was named after Archie Cochrane, a British epidemiologist who in 1972 first drew attention to the urgent need for clinicians to have ready access to current and reliable reviews of medical evidence (2). The Collaboration is an international collective of researchers, health care professionals, consumers, and others, divided into small, topic-based review groups and larger Cochrane Centres. Each review group collects and assesses all relevant studies pertaining to clinical subjects and then prepares and maintains a systematic review. The information is presented within the Cochrane Library in one of several databases:

1. *The Cochrane Database of Systematic Reviews (CDSR)*: Cochrane Reviews are full-text articles that review the effects of health care interventions. The reviews are highly structured and systematic, with evidence included or excluded on the basis of explicit quality criteria to minimize bias.
2. *The Database of Abstracts of Reviews of Effectiveness (DARE)*: DARE includes structured abstracts of systematic reviews from around the world that have been critically appraised by reviewers at the National Health Service (NHS) Centre for Reviews and Dissemination at the University of York, England.
3. *The Cochrane Controlled Trials Register (CCTR)*: CCTR is a bibliography of controlled trials identified by contributors to the Cochrane Collaboration and others as part of an international effort to hand search the world's journals and create an unbiased source of data for systematic reviews.

In the end, busy clinicians have easy access to databases of the best available systematic reviews and more recent RCTs. At present, there are 795 systematic reviews within CDSR, 1,634 reviews within DARE, and more than 263,000 references in CCTR. Access to the Cochrane Library can be by personal subscription or through a university, college, or hospital library institutional subscription. Searching the database is simple as long as a few rules are followed; these can be found in the Help Rules for Searches section of the Help Index of the Cochrane Library. Medline also now searches and identifies articles within the Cochrane Library.

We begin our search using the terms *diltiazem* and *MI* and find one reference (3) within CDSR and five references in DARE (4–8). Four of the references within DARE appear to be quite relevant, and the other (6) is still in the Cochrane Library assessment stage. The abstracts are available via Medline and the full text from the hospital library. Many libraries and some private organizations (9) offer full-text Internet download of journal articles for subscribers free or at reasonable costs, allowing nearly instant access to useful data.

Next we search *UpToDate*, an electronic clinical reference presented primarily for medicine subspecialists and internists. It is sold both as a compact disk (or CD, updated every 4 months) or online and provides access to abstracts from Medline, a drug database, and thousands of graphics. The information in UpToDate is a summary on specific topics, and although it does not have a set of explicit methodologic criteria for each article (like the Cochrane Library), it references only high-quality studies. Experts in each clinical field critically appraise articles from up to 150 journals to provide specific, well-referenced recommendations on diagnosis and therapy.

UpToDate searches with only one word or term and then matches that word or term with key words within the database. Each key word then is subdivided on a subsequent screen into *most relevant topics* and *related topics*. These topics provide an overview of each of the major trials in the associated clinical area and then a well-referenced summary by expert clinicians.

We begin our search with *calcium-channel blockers* and find three matching key words and the related topics. There are 15 *most relevant* topics and 128 *related topics*. Selecting the topic *calcium-channel blockers in myocardial infarction*, we find a succinct review of trials (4,10–18) using nifedipine, diltiazem, or verapamil for patients with MI. In the summary, there are already some answers to our clinical question.

Critically Appraise the Evidence

In the Cochrane Library, the review by Opie in *Cardiovascular Drugs and Therapy* (3) highlights the role of diltiazem for patients with a non–Q-wave infarction and equates the advantages of beta-blockers with calcium-channel blockers in these patients as long as there is no evidence of cardiac failure. In Persson's article in *Drugs* (18), the summary states, "A reliable theoretical background exists to support a secondary preventive effect of calcium antagonists after myocardial infarction. Recent studies also indicate that positive results can be achieved with diltiazem and, in particular, verapamil, provided that they are not given to patients suffering clinically manifest myocardial failure during the acute phase of the disease." The study by Held and Yusuf in *Coronary Artery Disease* (4) agrees with this assessment as they conclude, "Although nifedipine has not been conclusively proved to be harmful it seems unlikely to be beneficial. The effects of verapamil and diltiazem appear more promising. The interpretation of the possible subgroup effects is unclear, but it appears that a cautious approach should be taken to using a calcium antagonist in patients with signs and symptoms of left ventricular dysfunction."

The UpToDate summary states, "Verapamil or diltiazem were recommended as adjunctive therapy only in patients unable to take beta blockers in whom there is no congestive heart failure, left ventricular dysfunction, or atrioventricular block (class IIa recommendation). Diltiazem was recommended only in non-ST-elevation (i.e., non-Q wave) infarcts in patients without congestive heart failure or left ventricular dysfunction (class IIB recommendation). When used in this setting, diltiazem should be started after 24 hours and continued for one year."

The value of using the Cochrane Library or UpToDate to locate systematic reviews or topic summaries is that these are reviews mainly of RCTs, where evidence has been included or excluded on the basis of strict criteria to reduce or eliminate bias. Critical appraisal already has been completed on these reviews and summaries, and so we can look now to using this information in the clinical setting.

Implement Useful Findings in Clinical Practice

For scenario 1, it seems clear from the systematic reviews, trials, and summary that there is reasonable evidence, with caveats, to support the use of calcium-channel blockers, verapamil, or diltiazem in this situation. Based on this, you commence diltiazem and your patient makes an uneventful recovery.

In the next clinical scenario, we discuss critical appraisal of individual articles. A therapy type question is used again, but this time we use the question to explore Medline.

SCENARIO 2

A 45-year-old man who underwent radical cystectomy for bladder carcinoma 18 hours ago now has a hemoglobin level of 7.3 g per deciliter. The patient is hemodynamically stable and appears euvolemic. The surgeon questions whether the patient should receive a blood transfusion. You believe that blood transfusion is probably not necessary and search the literature for concrete evidence to support your decision.

As in our first scenario, we follow a search strategy and begin by formulating a question.

Formulate the Question

At what hemoglobin level is blood transfusion necessary in the critical care patient?

- The *type of patient*, subject group, or problem: critical care patients, hemoglobin concentration
- The *intervention* being considered: no blood transfusion
- *Comparison* or alternative intervention: blood transfusion
- The desired *outcome*: improved survival, decreased morbidity and transfusion requirements

Search the Literature for Relevant Clinical Articles

For this scenario, we assume that we do not have access to either the Cochrane Library or UpToDate. Our choice is to search in *Medline*, which is a bibliographic database created in 1966 by the National Library of Medicine (NLM) of the United States. This database covers the fields of medicine, nursing, dentistry, veterinary science, the health care system, and preclinical sciences. Of the approximately 14,000 health science serial publications in the world, Medline indexes the 4,000 it considers the most important. Some of the remaining 10,000 are indexed in other health sciences indexes, such as Embase, but most are not indexed at all. About 20% of the journals indexed by NLM in Medline are non–English-language journals.

Medline can be accessed in several ways. Grateful Med and PubMed (http://www.ncbi.nlm.nih.gov/PubMed/) are provided free by the NML and are available on the Internet. Ovid and SilverPlatter are two database products provided by health sciences libraries. We will access Medline using PubMed, a web-based database search software developed by the National Center for Biotechnology Information (NCBI) and licensed by the NLM for public searching of Medline. Searching the Medline database using the PubMed software is free, and there are no restrictions to its use.

The home page of Pubmed displays many different features and can be quite daunting to the uninitiated. Properly developing and implementing an appropriate search strategy from the start will result in improved search results. Rosenberg and colleagues (19) evaluated the effect on a group of medical students of attending a 3-hour training session on formulating questions and searching databases. They were able to show significant improvements in both search performance and quality of evidence retrieved. There are a number of journal articles, books, and websites (20–24) that offer tutorials or advice on searching strategies. Most hospital or university libraries have short tutorials for individuals or groups to give them an overview of PubMed and its inner workings. The PubMed site has a newly introduced tutorial feature providing PubMed online training available at the PubMed Homepage, http://www.ncbi.nlm.nih.gov/entrez/query.fcgi or by going directly to http://www.nlm.nih.gov/bsd/pubmed_tutorial /m1001.html. An excellent Ovid tutorial can be found on the Duke University Medical Center Library website at http://www .mc.duke.edu/mclibrary/respub/guides/ebm.html.

To begin a search in PubMed, enter search terms in the input query box, and then click the *Go* command button.

Unfortunately, simple textword searching of Medline may provide poor results or an overwhelming number of articles. A more focused search that uses a small number of searching techniques will be more efficient. The following are suggested techniques:

1. Selecting the best MeSH terms
2. Searching for each term separately
3. Combining the terms or sets
4. Limiting your retrieval to the most appropriate references

Selecting The Best MeSH (Medical Subject Headings) Terms

When words are entered in the query box, PubMed automatically performs the search in the MeSH fields as well as all other text word fields, such as the title or abstract. This does not guarantee that the text word is a topic of the article. It then combines significant words and terms together using the Boolean Operator AND.[1] What results is an extensive search for the word, not the subject. An alternative and more productive approach is to begin your search using MeSH terms.

The *Medical Subject Headings (MeSH)* comprise NLM's controlled vocabulary used for indexing articles, for cataloging books

and other holdings, and for searching MeSH-indexed databases, including Medline. NLM's reviewers read every article before adding it to the database, and they catalog it by assigning relevant MeSH terms. These MeSH terms provide a consistent way to retrieve information that may use different terminology for the same concepts.

The *MeSH Browser*, available on the PubMed's sidebar menu, can be used to find descriptors. This vocabulary look-up aid is designed to help quickly locate descriptors and to show the hierarchy in which they appear. The browser displays virtually complete MeSH records, including the scope notes, annotations, entry vocabulary, history notes, allowable qualifiers, and so on. It also provides links to relevant sections of the NLM Indexing Manual. MeSH organizes its descriptors in a hierarchical structure so that broad searches can include articles indexed more narrowly. This structure also provides an effective way for searchers to browse MeSH to find appropriate descriptors. Usually there are only one or two Major MeSH terms and up to ten additional MeSH terms applied to an article. In most circumstances, it is best not to limit the search to Major MeSH terms initially because to do so may narrow the search significantly.

PubMed also allows one to "explode" (or expand) a MeSH term. This feature provides retrieval of not only those articles that deal with the main subject but also all the associated subordinate subjects. During searching, it is important to be aware whether this feature is activated.

The MeSH vocabulary is updated continually by subject specialists in various areas. Each year, hundreds of new concepts are added and thousands of modifications are made. MeSH includes more than 19,000 *main headings*, 110,000 *supplementary concept records* (formerly *supplementary chemical records*), and an entry vocabulary of over 300,000 terms (25).

Searching for Each Term Separately

From our clinical question in scenario 2, we have a number of search terms: critically ill, human, adults, blood transfusion, survival, morbidity, RCT. When we enter *critically ill* into the MeSH Browser query box, we find that the associated MeSH term is *critical illness*. We can expand this MeSH term by accessing the *detailed display* and then include the subheadings, *mortality* and *therapy*. We add the MeSH term to our PubMed Query box via the *ADD* icon, and click on the *PubMed search* icon. We return to the MeSH Browser page once this search is completed and repeat this process with all our search terms (Table 2).

Note that entering the word *transfusion* into the MeSH Browser query box finds the terms *transfusion, blood* and *transfusion,* and

TABLE 2. MeSH SEARCH RESULTS

Clinical Search Term	MeSH Search Term	Search
Critically ill	Critical illness: mortality/ therapy	1
Transfusion	Erythrocyte transfusion	2
Hemoglobin levels	Hemoglobins	3

MeSH, medical subject headings.

---

[1]Boolean Operator relates to a combinatorial system devised by George Boole that combines propositions with the logical operators *AND* and *OR* and *NOT*.

erythrocyte. The hierarchical structure for these terms reveals that *transfusion, blood* is part of the MeSH "tree" for *transfusion, erythrocyte* and does not need to be searched separately.

Combining the Terms and Limiting Your Retrieval

The final search for *hemoglobins* ends in the results screen. Next we enter the *history* screen via the submenu below the query box. Here there is a summary of our three separate searches. This screen allows us to combine our searches using Boolean Operators and to preview these searches. We are also able to limit the searching to specific areas such as type of trial, age of patients, human subjects, and publication dates by activating the *limit submenu.*

Initially, we combine no.1 and no. 2, and our preview reveals five articles. Numbers 1 and 3 produce seven articles; and numbers 2 and 3 give us 128 articles. By using the limits *randomized controlled trial, all adult,* and *human,* the number of articles is reduced to 2, 3, and 19, respectively. Review of the abstracts results in the initial selection of five useful articles (26–30), but only two have direct relevance to critically ill patients, and one of these is the pilot study for the second study. We therefore select this paper (28) for critical appraisal.

Critically Appraise the Evidence

Until recently, critical appraisal of an article was performed primarily by the journal reviewers and editors. If a study appeared in a respected journal, it was assumed by most readers that the results had been interpreted correctly and the conclusions could be accepted without further critique. Unfortunately, many such published studies did not apply the necessary methods to allow results to be clinically significant, useful, or relevant. Since the early 1980s, there has been a worldwide movement driven by the EBM teams at McMasters and Oxford Universities to develop, disseminate, and then teach "critical appraisal" so that individuals without a background in research methodology can easily evaluate clinical articles. Numerous articles, books, and websites (see Table 3) are dedicated to this area of critical appraisal, but nearly all use the original series of *JAMA* users' guides (31–37) as a basis. A series of questions has been developed to help evaluate original articles on diagnosis, treatment, prognosis, and economic analysis as well as systematic reviews and meta-analyses. Many of the websites (Table 3) at the end of the chapter provide printable versions of worksheets with these questions. In our scenario on blood transfusion, the following questions are recommended to appraise an article on treatment.

Randomization

Was the assignment of patients to treatment randomized?

Patient Follow-up

Were all patients who entered the trial properly accounted for and attributed at its conclusion?

Analysis of patients

Were patients analyzed in the groups to which they were randomized?

Blinding

Were patients, health workers, and study personnel "blind" to treatment?

TABLE 3. OTHER SOURCES OF INFORMATION FOR THE EVIDENCE-BASED "EXPLORER"

American College of Physicians Journal Club
  http://www.acponline.org/journals/acpjc/jcmenu.htm
Bandolier: monthly journal of the NHS R & D Directorate
  http://www.jr2.ox.ac.uk:80/Bandolier/index.html
Centre for EBM, from Mt. Sinai Hospital
  http://www.library.utoronto.ca/medicine/ebm/
Critical Appraisal of Bio-medical Literature: Allan O'Rourke
  http://www.shef.ac.uk/uni/projects/wrp/ebpsem2.html
Duke University Medical Center Library
  http://www.mc.duke.edu/mclibrary/respub/guides/ebm.html#top
EBM–Evidence-Based Medicine: Ruth Lilly Medical Library/
  Indiana University School of Medicine
  http://www.medlib.iupui.edu/ebm/home.html
EBM Tool Kit
  http://www.med.ualberta.ca/ebm/ebm.htm
Evidence-based Surgery, from the Royal College of Surgeons
  of England
  http://www.rcseng.ac.uk/public/infores/reso_ir.htm
Netting the evidence
  http://www.shef.ac.uk/~scharr/ir/netting/
New York Academy of Medicine Library
  http://www.ebmny.org/thecentr2.html
Seeking the evidence
  http://www.shef.ac.uk/~scharr/ir/proto.html
SumSearch
  http://sumsearch.uthscsa.edu/searchform45.html
User's guide to the medical literature
  http://www.cche.net/principles/content_all.asp
The University of Texas Health Science Center at San Antonio
  http://clinical.uthscsa.edu/pubmed.htm
Wisdom Centre: NHS Informatics Program
  http://www.wisdom.org.uk/index.html

NHS, National Health Service; R & D, research and development; EBM, evidence-based medicine.

Baseline characteristics of patients
Were groups similar at the start of the trial?
Treatments
Aside from the experimental intervention, were the groups treated equally?
Results
What is the strength of the outcomes?
How large was the treatment effect?
How precise was the treatment effect?
Practical application
Are the results applicable to my patient?
Were all clinically important outcomes considered?
Are the benefits worth the potential harms and costs?

Implement Useful Findings in Clinical Practice

A critical appraisal of the transfusion study from the Canadian Critical Care Trials Group based on the preceding questions confirms that the study was valid and applicable, although we note that blinding was not achieved. Applied to our scenario, the results support a decision not to give transfusion to a patient younger than 55 years with no history of cardiac disease and an Acute Physiology and Chronic Health Evaluation (APACHE) score of less than 20 until the hemoglobin level is less than 7.0 g per deciliter.

SUMMARY

Evidence-based medicine is a strategy that involves a sequential process to identify a question and then find and appraise its answer. It is a process that challenges the clinician to accept that he or she does not know everything. The growth of medical knowledge is so rapid that clinicians need to increasingly become advocates for learning and appraising strategies proposed as meaningful to their patients' care. Application of EBM can help clinicians search for and appraise evidence that can benefit their patients.

KEY POINTS

Evidence-based medicine (EBM) is an approach designed to use existing best evidence to make individual patient care decisions.

EBM developed in response to the exponentially increasing rate of information available.

EBM begins with a search strategy to obtain relevant studies and reviews.

Critical appraisal of the evidence can be based on the users' guides published in *JAMA*.

The Cochrane Library and UpToDate are two databases that provide systematic reviews and summaries of many topics.

The utility of the Medline database can be improved by better search strategies.

EBM is part of a life-long commitment to learning.

REFERENCES

1. Sackett D. *How to practice and teach EBM*. New York: Churchill Livingstone, 1998.
2. Cochrane AL. *Effectiveness and efficiency: random reflections on health services*. London: Nuffield Provincial Hospitals Trusts, 1973.
3. Opie LH. Calcium channel antagonists. Part II: Use and comparative properties of the three prototypical calcium antagonists in ischemic heart disease, including recommendations based on an analysis of 41 trials. *Cardiovasc Drugs Ther* 1988;1:461–491.
4. Held PH, Yusuf S. Calcium antagonists in the treatment of ischemic heart disease: myocardial infarction. *Coron Artery Dis* 1994;5:21–26.
5. McAlister FA. Antiarrhythmic therapies for the prevention of sudden cardiac death. *Drugs* 1997;54:235–252.
6. Sakai H. An application of meta-analysis techniques in the evaluation of adverse experiences with antihypertensive agents. *Pharmacoepidemiology & Drug Safety* 1999;8:169–177.
7. Heidenreich PA. Meta-analysis of trials comparing B-blockers, calcium antagonists, and nitrates for stable angina. *JAMA* 1999;281:1927–1936.
8. Lievre M. Nifedipine and coronary heart disease: reasons for controversy. *Therapie* 1997;52:37–45,239–240.
9. Aries Systems Corporation. Knowledge Finder, 2001. http://www.kfinder.com/newweb/home.html. Accessed October 4, 2001.
10. The Multicenter Diltiazem Postinfarction Trial Research Group. The effect of diltiazem on mortality and reinfarction after myocardial infarction. *N Engl J Med* 1988;319:385–389.
11. Danish Verapamil Infarction Trial 2 Group. Effect of verapamil on mortality and major events after acute myocardial infarction. *Am J Cardiol* 1990;66:779–785.
12. Braunwald E. Mechanism of action of calcium-channel-blocking agents. *N Engl J Med* 1982;307:1618–1627.
13. Gibson RS, Boden WE, Theroux P, et al. Diltiazem and reinfarction in patients with non-Q-wave myocardial infarction: results of a double-blind, randomized, multicenter trial. *N Engl J Med* 1986;315:423–429.
14. Koenig W, Lowel H, Lewis M, et al. Long-term survival after myocardial infarction: relationship with thrombolysis and discharge medication. Results of the Augsburg Myocardial Infarction Follow-up Study 1985 to 1993. *Eur Heart J* 1996;17:1199–1206.
15. Rengo F, Carbonin P, Pahor M, et al. A controlled trial of verapamil in patients after acute myocardial infarction: results of the calcium antagonist reinfarction Italian study (CRIS) [see comments]. *Am J Cardiol* 1996;77:365–369.
16. Ryan TJ, Antman EM, Brooks NH, et al. 1999 update: ACC/AHA guidelines for the management of patients with acute myocardial infarction: executive summary and recommendations: a report of the American College of Cardiology/American Heart Association Task Force on Practice Guidelines (Committee on Management of Acute Myocardial Infarction) [In Process Citation]. *Circulation* 1999;100:1016–1030.
17. Theroux P, Gregoire J, Chin C, et al. Intravenous diltiazem in acute myocardial infarction. Diltiazem as adjunctive therapy to activase (DATA) trial. *J Am Coll Cardiol* 1998;32:620–628.
18. Persson S. Calcium antagonists in secondary prevention after myocardial infarction. *Drugs* 1991;42(Suppl) 2:54–60.
19. Rosenberg WM, Deeks J, Lusher A, et al. Improving searching skills and evidence retrieval. *JR Coll Physicians Lond* 1998;32:557–563.
20. Duke University Medical Center Library. Evidence-based medicine 1999. http://www.mc.duke.edu/mclibrary/respub/guides/ebm.html. Accessed October 4, 2001.
21. Greenhalgh T. How to read a paper. The Medline database. *BMJ* 1997;315:180–183.
22. Sackett D, Richardson WS, Rosenberg WM, et al. How to ask clinical questions you can answer. In: *Evidence based medicine, how to practice and teach EBM*. Anonymous. New York: Churchill Livingstone, 1997:21.
23. Sackett D, Richardson WS, Rosenberg WM, et al. Searching for the best evidence. In: *Evidence based medicine, how to practice and teach EBM*. Anonymous. New York: Churchill Livingstone, 1997:37.
24. University of Alberta Faculty of Medicine and Dentistry. Available from http://www.med.ualberta.ca/ebm/ebm.html. Accessed October 4, 2001.
25. PubMed Mesh Browser Help. http://www.ncbi.nlm.nih.gov:80/entrez/meshbrowser_help.html. Accessed October 4, 2001.
26. Bracey AW, Radovancevic R, Riggs SA, et al. Lowering the hemoglobin threshold for transfusion in coronary artery bypass procedures: effect on patient outcome. *Transfusion* 1999;39:1070–1077.
27. Hebert PC, Wells G, Marshall J, et al. Transfusion requirements in critical care: a pilot study. Canadian Critical Care Trials Group [published erratum appears in *JAMA* 1995;27;274:944]. *JAMA* 1995;273:1439–1444.
28. Hebert PC, Wells G, Blajchman MA, et al. A multicenter, randomized, controlled clinical trial of transfusion requirements in critical care. Transfusion Requirements in Critical Care Investigators, Canadian Critical Care Trials Group [see comments] [published erratum

appears in *N Engl J Med* 1999;340:1056]. *N Engl J Med* 1999;340:
409–417.

29. Carson JL, Terrin ML, Barton FB, et al. A pilot randomized trial comparing symptomatic vs. hemoglobin-level-driven red blood cell transfusions following hip fracture. *Transfusion* 1998;38:522–529.

30. Bush RL, Pevec WC, Holcroft JW. A prospective, randomized trial limiting perioperative red blood cell transfusions in vascular patients. *Am J Surg* 1997;174:143–148.

31. Oxman AD, Sackett DL, Guyatt GH. Users' guides to the medical literature. I. How to get started. The Evidence-Based Medicine Working Group. *JAMA* 1993;270:2093–2095.

32. Guyatt GH, Sackett DL, Cook DJ. Users' guides to the medical literature. II. How to use an article about therapy or prevention: A. Are the results of the study valid? Evidence-Based Medicine Working Group. *JAMA* 1993;270:2598–2601.

33. Guyatt GH, Sackett DL, Cook DJ. Users' guides to the medical literature. II. How to use an article about therapy or prevention: B. What were the results and will they help me in caring for my patients? Evidence-Based Medicine Working Group. *JAMA* 1994;271:59–63.

34. Jaeschke R, Guyatt G, Sackett DL. Users' guides to the medical literature. III. How to use an article about a diagnostic test: A. Are the results of the study valid? Evidence-Based Medicine Working Group. *JAMA* 1994;271: 389–391.

35. Jaeschke R, Guyatt GH, Sackett DL. Users' guides to the medical literature. III. How to use an article about a diagnostic test: B. What are the results and will they help me in caring for my patients? The Evidence-Based Medicine Working Group. *JAMA* 1994;271:703–707.

36. Levine M, Walter S, Lee H, et al. Users' guides to the medical literature: IV. How to use an article about harm. Evidence-Based Medicine Working Group. *JAMA* 1994;271:1615–1619.

37. Laupacis A, Wells G, Richardson WS, et al. Users' guides to the medical literature: V. How to use an article about prognosis. Evidence-Based Medicine Working Group. *JAMA* 1994;272:234–237.

GENOMICS IN PERIOPERATIVE CRITICAL CARE

KIRK HOGAN

KEY WORDS

- Pharmacogenetics
- Cloning
- DNA polymorphism
- Polymerase chain reaction
- Genotype
- Phenotype
- Linkage dysequilibrium
- Single nucleotide polymorphism
- Compound heterozygosity
- Genetic association
- Causal mutation
- Haplotype
- Genetic heterogeneity
- Candidate gene
- Mutation hot spot

INTRODUCTION

Acceleration of the Human Genome Project, coupled with technologies enabling rapid and precise detection of genetic variations, offers an unprecedented opportunity to tailor medical management in accord with each patient's singular genetic makeup. No other interventions represent a comparable degree of physiologic trespass as the trauma of surgery, the coma of anesthesia, and the pharmacologic and mechanical life support of critical care. It follows that nowhere else will interindividual differences in genetic constitution be more consequential to disparity in outcome. It is not my objective here to survey the foundations of molecular biology, a task better accomplished in allied treatises (1) and texts (2). Nor is the aim of this chapter to delve into the intricacies of frontier technologies or to catalog genes and mutations of potential interest to intensivists, although representative examples will be cited. Rather, I hope to assemble a framework within which to judge the value that knowledge of DNA sequence variation may render in the care of the critically ill.

Genomics, the science of nucleotide permutation between species, genders, ethnic groups, families, and individuals, is a term used in contradistinction to gene discovery, expression, or therapy. Its power in application resides in the strength of correlation between a patient's *genotype* (unique DNA sequence) and *phenotype* or characteristics that result from the interaction of a patient's genotype, environment, and life history. Different forms of a gene or DNA sequence inherited at a specific chromosomal site, or *locus*, are referred to as *alleles*. Alleles are *polymorphic* if two or more exist at significant frequencies in the population, that is, each occurs in one percent or greater of the population. Each individual inherits two alleles at a single site, one from each parent. By sorting an individual's polymorphic alleles, the aim of genomics is to segregate the majority of polymorphisms that fail to produce a phenotype from the minority that play a role in the genesis of a trait, that is, mutations causing disease. Early in the genetics revolution, data regarding human DNA sequence variation were rare and hard won, with phenotypic descriptors much more easily quantified. We now have passed an inflection point such that DNA sequence is almost absurdly easy to acquire, archive, and access, whereas the capacity to establish firm phenotypic correlations has become the rate-limiting step. As a consequence, the genomic playing field, which until the recent past slanted toward the laboratory bench, now tilts steeply to the bedside and clinic. In the years immediately ahead, physicians adept at identifying and corroborating novel genotype to phenotype associations will be responsible for fulfilling the promise of genomics, assuring more rapid and protracted recoveries for our patients.

CATEGORIES OF CRITICAL CARE GENOTYPES

Alleles for inclusion in patient genotyping are conveniently categorized in keeping with the purposes for which they are sought. Owing to their dramatic sequelae, pharmacogenetic syndromes involving drugs commonly used in perioperative settings, including nondepolarizing muscle relaxants and potent inhalational agents, were among the first to be recognized (3). Unanticipated responses to both classes of drugs reflecting pharmacokinetic (butyrylcholinesterase deficiency) and pharmacodynamic (malignant hyperthermia) genetic syndromes now have been fixed at the molecular level, either partially (4) or in full (5). Strong genomic predictors of drug interaction, toxicity, or failed response mediated by phase 1 hepatic oxidative (cytochrome P450) drug metabolism subsequently were established for a wide range of cardiovascular (6), analgesic, psychotropic, and sedative drugs (7). Because of the number of drugs administered, and primary or secondary dysfunction of the organs essential for metabolism and excretion, intensive care patients are particularly vulnerable

(8,9). Overlapping substrate specificities have precluded equivalent inferences for genes encoding phase 2 conjugative transferase enzymes to date (10). As underlying mechanisms are disclosed, panels of mutations in genes governing drug absorption, distribution, metabolism, excretion, and toxicology (i.e., *ADMET*) will enter routine use in the guidance of drug selection, dose, and regimen for all critically ill patients.

Although the detection of genomic differences underlying variability in drug response will help to ensure predictable efficacy, reducing adverse events and costs in the near future, genotyping critically ill patients for disease alleles may have greater impact over the long term. The differential diagnosis of outwardly identical disease phenotypes arising from distinct genetic mechanisms now can be elucidated at the molecular level for a rapidly expanding inventory of disorders, for example, hyperkalemic versus hypokalemic periodic paralysis (11). Furthermore, by triggering surveillance and specific interventions within the interval in which the greatest likelihood of benefit is preserved, genomic predispositions also may be solicited before signs and symptoms become apparent. Aberrant thrombosis accounts for up to 50% of deaths each year in North America (12), with deep venous thrombosis, pulmonary embolus, stroke, and myocardial infarction among the most feared complications of surgery and critical illness. Encumbering the procoagulant effects of pain, immobilization, and neuroendocrine responses attendant to trauma and organ failure are genetic polymorphisms that increase the incidence of thrombophilia in critically ill patients. Not only are patients with prevalent mutations in protein C (13), factor VII (14), factor V Leiden (15), and prothrombin II (16) most susceptible, but the alleles also may act in tandem to heighten susceptibility (17). Foreknowledge of these genomic liabilities enables scarce resources in monitoring to be targeted to those patients most likely to profit and confines risky regimens (e.g., aggressive anticoagulation) to those in greatest jeopardy.

Disorders that arise from perturbed tissue responses to inflammation also were traced to polymorphisms of genes encoding cytokine mediators. Patients with the tumor necrosis factor-alpha (TNF-α) promoter (-308) allele, and TNF-β intron ($+252$) allele, exhibit elevated TNF-α cytokine production and secretion, in correlation with higher risk for posttraumatic sepsis (18–20), postoperative susceptibility to septic shock (21), and elevated incidence of acute rejection (22,23) and infection (24) after solid-organ transplantation. In addition to confirming the risk of mortality intrinsic to the TNF-β_2 allele, Fang and colleagues found an increased frequency of the interleukin-1 receptor antagonist A2 (IL-1raA2) allele of the IL-1ra in patients with severe sepsis following surgery (25). Hence, alleles in distinct cytokine genes may be deleterious markers of sepsis risk, severity, or both, especially if present in aggregate. Identification of these alleles imparts improved estimates of patient prognosis to guide surgical decision making, but it also points to optimized immunosuppressive and antiinfectious therapies based on genetic idiosyncrasy in immune responsiveness.

A striking advantage of genomic profiling is that each patient's unique sequence remains invariant within all nonneoplastic, somatic cells over a lifespan. But this finite, albeit huge, compendium of singular DNA sequence does not fill the horizons of critical care relevance. Indeed, genomic analysis of host susceptibility and response (26), coupled with genetic identification of viral, bacterial, and fungal microbes, seems probable to represent the earliest broad-scale application of molecular technologies to critical care. Highly sensitive, rapid, and specific genetic methods for identification of many pathogens by direct assay of unique DNA or RNA sequences will soon be available for many clinical samples, for example, tracking of methicillin-resistant *Staphylococcus aureus* among intensive care unit (ICU) patients (27). Genomic techniques have been introduced to rapidly identify *Candida* from sputum, blood, and bronchoalveolar lavage (28) and to type *Mycobacterium tuberculosis*, allowing specific mutations conferring antibiotic resistance to be identified (29). Testing for the presence or absence of non–species-specific prokaryotic 16S ribosomal DNA in the plasma permits differentiation of a systemic inflammatory response with and without infection, thereby speeding initiation of appropriate therapy (30,31). Finally, the unique genomic signatures of picaresque viruses makes it possible to recount an infectious course from patient to health care worker and back, for example, hepatitis C (32).

In each category of patient-centered genomic testing, *heterozygosity* for a mutation (i.e., a single abnormal copy of the gene from either parent) may be sufficient to manifest a severe trait inherited as an *autosomal dominant*. For other alleles, a single abnormal copy may confer a disadvantage of lesser but still significant severity under the stressed circumstances of surgery or organ failure. In a growing number of disorders, *compound heterozygosity* (i.e, single mutant copies at two distinct loci within the same or different genes) may be as perilous as *homozygosity*, that is, *autosomal recessive* inheritance. Beyond a given trait's mechanism of inheritance, every application of genomic data to clinical subject matter must rest on three fundamental benchmarks. Knowledge of the genotype must be *analytically valid* (the chosen DNA-based method must detect the genotype accurately), *clinically valid* (the genotype must correctly predict the phenotype), and of clear-cut *clinical utility* (the genotype must specify an available step to improve patient safety). These criteria, which all tests must fulfill before adoption into clinical practice, will be considered in turn.

Analytical Validity

Inferences drawn from base pair by base pair inspection of a fragment of DNA sequence are grounded on the assumption that the reported linear string of nucleotide bases accurately reflects those to be found in the patient's cells. How good is this supposition? The first developments of human sequence characterization required replication of DNA segments in prokaryotic host cells to obtain sufficient amounts for analysis, that is, *cloning*. Variations then were detected either directly by sequencing or indirectly by digestion with enzymes that only cleave DNA at the site of a short recognition sequence of nucleotides, that is, *restriction fragment length polymorphism (RFLP)*. Both techniques remain in widespread use; however, interrogation by RFLP is slow, and results are often ambiguous as a result of partial digestion. Even sequencing is not fail-safe, with up to 30 errors for each million base pairs examined. With introduction of the *polymerase chain reaction (PCR)* in the late 1980s and its subsequent evolution, amplification, and analysis of DNA in the test tube became much more rapid and facile (32). Despite its suitability for research,

PCR is a labor-intensive, time-consuming, and expensive procedure, thereby inhibiting more widespread clinical use. Moreover, misincorporation and infidelities in replication occurring as often as 50 base pairs per million limit PCR-based techniques to applications able to tolerate an error rate of this magnitude.

The third major innovation in genomic technology grew out of the pharmaceutical industry's need to screen thousands of patients for many hundreds of thousands *of single nucleotide polymorphisms (SNPs)* in search of new drug targets. The great advantage bestowed by these methods for genotyping is tremendous compression of analysis time. Although novel high through-put detection assays, including *molecular beacons* (34), *oligonucleotide microarrays* ("gene chips") (35), and *mini-sequencing* (36), are capable of simultaneously scoring several thousands of genotypes on a single specimen, they remain dependent on preliminary target amplification steps such as PCR. In addition, they require expensive, dedicated equipment for precise detection, and they can miss heterozygotes. More recently, sensitive methods of mutation scoring based on signal rather than target amplification have been described (37,38). In all likelihood, the first incarnation of these innovative techniques to reach the bedside will incorporate the advantages of several detection schemes on miniaturized and automated platforms. The analytical method that is chosen must be flexible enough to discriminate a wide variety of genetic pathologies within a common assay format to include wild-type and mutant homozygotes and heterozygotes; single base pair substitutions in coding regions, introns and promoters; multiple alleles at a single locus; large and small insertions and deletions; detection within gene duplications and pseudogenes; and resolution of genetic heterogeneity underlying both monogenic and polygenic traits. Assays capable of distinguishing these changes with greater than 99% precision, at pennies per allele, in as short an interval as 1 to 2 hours, are soon to enter clinical practice. Because genetic analysis is identical in its essentials no matter the encoded gene product, genomic panels carry the potential to replace multiple laboratories required to directly assay functional proteins with equivalent breadth. Despite the science-fiction aura of these technologies, practitioners using test data must be versed in their practical as well as theoretical limitations, including the need for standardized protocols, details of specimen handling, and control over the onslaught of bioinformational data collected from each patient.

CLINICAL VALIDITY

Considered at large, the field of genomics remains entrenched within its discovery phase, with claims for associations between DNA sequence variations and traits proliferating at an explosive rate, followed by vague promises of emergent diagnostics and therapeutics. At the threshold of real world use of genomic data in the daily care of the severely ill or injured patient, these assertions require a much higher level of scrutiny than is acceptable for curiosity driven experimentation. Beyond its derivation from a specific tissue and organism and its translation into protein sequence based on an invariant code, what does DNA sequence mean? Simple inspection of a train of sequence yields few if any clues regarding its origin, its interpretation, or its implications

for clinical care. Here I wish to consider the sources of extrinsic knowledge, which must be compressed into DNA sequence variations to predict something of value about their corresponding phenotypes. The scope of evidence and the underlying principles are unlikely to change over coming decades, thereby enabling the practicing consumer of genotypic data to temper enthusiasm with requisite doubt before engaging in transfer of the technology to the bedside.

The primary distinction to be made falls between a DNA polymorphism, or random sequence variation that may have no functional role but may still be inherited, and a *causal mutation*, which either alone or in a major way contributes to the genesis of a phenotype. True neutral DNA polymorphisms, which give rise to neither harmful nor beneficial nor even detectable traits, nevertheless may be of extraordinary value in gene discovery because they are inherited together with the gene that does cause the trait. In most, if not all, clinical circumstances, however, awareness of the causal gene and its variations will be required when lives hang in the balance. Second, it is essential to recognize that a given sequence variation may become meaningful (i.e., causal) only if it is reported in the context of additional quantifiable genetic and environmental factors acting in concert. Finally, although ascending qualities of proof for discriminating a *genetic association* (i.e., by heredity alone) from a causal mutation are ordered here in parallel with their respective cost and difficulty, the original suggestion of causality may in fact appear at any point of entry.

Statistical Evidence For Genomic Causation

Population-based Genomic Association Studies: Identity by Phenotype

If a statistically significant association between a DNA polymorphism (e.g., TNF-α (−308)) and a phenotypic trait (e.g., the severity of postoperative sepsis) is declared on comparison of unrelated affected and unaffected individuals in a population, there are four possible explanations:

1. The DNA variation causes the trait.
2. The DNA variation is in *linkage dysequilibrium* with the trait. The basic principle behind linkage dysequilibrium mapping is that alleles at loci nearest a particular disease-influencing locus will show strong statistical associations with the disease, whereas alleles at distant loci will not. Thus, the presence of the tested allele predicts the presence of an untested causal mutation in unrelated patients, but it does not itself cause the trait of interest (i.e., the most likely explanation for the TNF-α (−308) polymorphism, sepsis association).
3. There has been uneven sampling of cases or controls in a subgroup of a heterogeneous population (i.e., confounding by population stratification).
4. The association occurs by chance alone.

A significance level of positive association by chance at less than 1 per 1,000 is generally adopted for research purposes, but for management decisions resting solely on population-based data, probabilities of erroneous association of fewer than 1 per 100,000 or 1 per 1,000,000 may be preferred. The advantages of case-control population studies for inference of a causal association between a genotypic risk factor and a phenotype include simplicity of data acquisition and ready generation of hypotheses. Challenges in matching cases to controls, the presence of known and unknown confounding variables—especially prevalent in patients with multiple organ failure—and the relative ease of statistical "data-chopping" unite to beget erroneous reports of significant results. These shortcomings may be addressed in part by brute force. Causation is supported if, in large numbers of patients, everyone with the genotype exhibits the identical trait, everyone without the genotype lacks the trait, and everyone without the trait lacks the genotype. In reality, population-based association studies rarely achieve this level of parsimony and often are tainted by inappropriate controls, inadequate statistical or sampling methods, and a bias for reporting positive associations.

Family-based Segregation Analysis: Identity by Descent

Cosegregation, or *coinheritance*, of a DNA sequence variation and a trait between family members is a more stringent test of causation because of shared genetic and environmental influences. In particular, if a group of genetic markers, or *haplotype*, surrounds the putative causal mutation and is inherited together as a block, arguments for causality are strengthened. Additional convincing factors for family-based studies of causation include the occurrence of the association in more than one family, its presence in more than two generations within a single family, and preservation of the association in all obligate carriers who pass the genotype from their parents to their offspring. Despite positive evidence for these factors, it remains possible to draw erroneous conclusions, even within the more narrowly restricted investigation of familial associations. Different traits commonly arise from the identical genotype (*variable expressivity*), and the identical trait may arise from other differences in the same or distinct genes (*allelic and locus genetic heterogeneity*) or from nongenetic causes (*phenocopies*). Even though a specific DNA sequence variation meets all the criteria for linkage in multiple families with a chance for error at less than 1 in 1,000, its association with the trait still may be mistaken for causality simply by virtue of its close proximity to a truly causal but still undiscovered gene. A serious limitation of family-based association studies aimed at characterizing alleles of interest to intensivists is that few pedigrees will be ascertained with a large enough proportion of members sharing a critical care course in multiple generations.

CIRCUMSTANTIAL EVIDENCE FOR GENOMIC CAUSATION

Among the first manipulations an investigator performs with novel DNA sequences, or a new variation of an old sequence, is to decipher its amino acid and protein composition by computer analysis and to test for causality in the context of collateral databases constructed from prior observations. This permits the amino acid constituents of a peptide to be queried for sequences of structural or functional significance that may be shared between proteins of the same class or between composite classes of proteins. DNA mutations generating alterations in these elements thereby become plausible candidates for causation without the investigator having to leave her desk. Nucleotide substitutions in genetic regulatory elements and in untranslated regions are more likely to cause a trait in question than those appearing in introns. Missense or nonsynonymous mutations in coding regions that alter amino acid translation are more likely still to underlie a faction of disease variation. The causality of a given mutation is bolstered if it appears in a region of a gene that is phylogenetically conserved between species, at a locus that is the site of previously identified causal mutations (i.e., a mutation "hot spot"), and if it predicts a change in a physical property of the protein (e.g., the amount, shape, or electrostatic charge). Finally, a cause-and-effect relationship is supported if the mutation is found in a component of a critical physiologic pathway with well-understood biochemical participants and interactions consistent with the trait, (i.e., the mutation appears in a credible candidate gene).

The value of circumstantial evidence for causation is constrained by the failure of protein alterations derived from DNA sequence to predict consistently the corresponding divergence in structure or other attributes. Moreover, expression of the mutation in the whole organism may not be observable because of compensatory homeostatic mechanisms or redundancy of physiologic functional reserves. Contributory mutations at a second-order or higher-order loci may be required to manifest the phenotype (i.e., polygenic and multifactorial inheritance of hypertension and diabetes), and compound or mixed heterozygotes are likely to be commonplace as traits in outbred human populations are resolved at the genetic level. None of these associations will be reliably detected in the absence of well-conceived and conducted bench experimentation.

EXPERIMENTAL EVIDENCE FOR BIOLOGIC CAUSATION

So firmly rooted is adherence to molecular biology's *central dogma* (i.e., the flow of sequence information from DNA to RNA to protein to trait by an invariant code) that a protein itself may only be directly sequenced as a cross-check in the event of anomalies in subsequent experiments. Assuming the accuracy of the gene's derived protein product, the causal consequences of DNA sequence variation can be tested according to the principles of scientific proof. Documentation of *in vivo* changes in protein shape clear a higher bar for causation than those detected *in vitro* (e.g., x-ray crystallography) but remains beyond the grasp of most contemporary technologies. Similarly, functional changes measured *in vitro* (e.g., enzyme kinetics) are less persuasive than *in vivo* alterations, particularly if more nearly physiologic conditions (e.g., temperature, pH) abolish differences between normal and mutant polypeptides. If confirmatory, functional validation using technologies such as differential gene expression, *in situ* hybridization, and immunohistochemistry may be invaluable in defining the temporal and spatial roles of plausible gene products.

Causation becomes much more certain if cellular function is altered in lines from an affected individual, by transfection of the mutant allele into a wild-type cell line with generation of an apposite phenotype, or by mutagenesis of cells to recreate the patient's genotype. In each case, isolation of the mutant protein may be followed by *in vitro* assays designed to compare closely whole-cell data with that collected from purified preparations. In exceptional circumstances it is possible to investigate the biologic repercussions of a genomic alteration in an animal model by spontaneous experiments of nature, for example, malignant hyperthermia caused by calcium release channel mutations in humans (4), swine (39), and dogs (40). Controlled breeding and selection experiments then allow quantification of genotype–phenotype correlations at all levels, including gene, protein, cell, tissue, and whole organism. Creation of the phenotype in a species that does not otherwise exhibit the trait is nearly irrefutable evidence for causation, but one that few human disorders will achieve because of the time and expense required for transgenic manipulation and selection.

PHENOTYPE ISSUES IN GENOMIC CAUSATION

Although insufficient attention has been given formally to assumptions of clinical validity implicit to the genotypic arm of causation, premises upholding the corresponding phenotypic arm typically are overlooked or concealed. Suspect disease classifications and spurious patient-to-patient distinctions doom DNA mapping studies to fallacious results from the outset. *A priori* segregation of population samples and subgroups may be wrong even if assured by the consensus of expert panels. Taken together, these two sources of error predispose to "definition drift" in follow-up investigations tending to tighten mistaken positive associations. Even so fundamental an issue as designation of a trait as *neutral, harmful,* or *beneficial* is semantic and culturally conditioned, reaching the level of paradox in debate over which the allele of a given gene is truly wild type (i.e., normal) and which is mutant. Moreover, recognition of a detrimental trait may simply be a function of the intensity of an investigator's motives. Is the phenotype apparent to unaided observation, that is, by history and physical examination? Or is technical assistance necessary? If so, what is the resolving power of the tools used, and what is their cost if many patients must undergo phenotyping? Explicit answers to these questions are needed to determine properties so fundamental as the mechanism of inheritance of a trait. As an example, until methods for phenotyping are improved, heterozygotes may be undetectable from wild-type homozygotes, not because of an inherent property of the mutation or its genetic background but rather due to limitations in the capacity to diagnose.

Often, disorders traditionally classified as *discrete diseases*, in fact, represent syndromes with many distinct contributing pathogenic mechanisms and outwardly unrelated environmental triggers. Quantitative DNA sequence variation is deceptively easy to acquire, computerize, and disseminate. Conversely, traits and diseases may be difficult to differentiate from background and from one another, qualitatively hard to measure, and yet harder to compare. Skepticism is urged when researchers choose from an expansive menu of euphemisms for causation to imply more than data warrants, intimating that a polymorphism "influences," "explains," "accounts for," "controls," or "is responsible for" a trait (the careful reader may spot several others in the preceding text). These considerations are frequently glossed over in human genomic research at the risk of recapitulating a contemporary phrenology, with DNA sequence variations standing in for cranial contours, but the exigencies of clinical decision making based on genomic data mandate a higher standard of phenotypic clarity. Headlines proclaiming an association between DNA polymorphisms and disease states must be viewed with great caution and subjected to standards of rigorous analysis identical to those that would be demanded for nongenomic risk factors, including large unambiguous effects in sufficient patient numbers, replication of observations by independent groups of investigators, and stringent control of confounding variables.

CLINICAL UTILITY

Genomic screening of the critically ill patient will become widespread only when the capacity to detect susceptibility is matched by the ability to modulate risk. Unless explicitly enrolled in research protocols, patients must not be tested for alleles in the absence of alternative interventions of documented benefit. Conversely, even if the list of all conceivable genotypes underlying a specific trait is partial, and even if the causality arguments for each genotype are incompletely settled, the positive presence of an at-risk genotype may be lifesaving if a meaningful alternative intervention is at hand. Lack of an at-risk genotype in a tested patient does not mean there is no risk, nor will genotyping ever substitute for vigilance and clinical judgment. By virtue of testing, however, net risk will be reduced to a measurable degree. Genomic testing of the critically ill patient thus may help to unravel complex clinical syndromes and raise warning signs of trouble ahead, but it does not guarantee complications or promise safety in the absence of intelligent experienced caregivers. Only by learning how patients subtly differ, one from the other, will we be able to avoid genetic problems *en bloc*, with less reliance on downstream detection and aptitude for rescue when warnings are issued.

ETHICAL, LEGAL, AND SOCIAL ISSUES

Perhaps the greatest barriers to widespread implementation of critical care genomics will be ethical, legal, and social constraints. Centering debates in terms of patient safety and perioperative risks pertinent to all, however, will shift the balance in favor of testing, especially if there is no coercion to be tested and firewalls against identifiability, breaches of confidentiality, and discrimination are assured. Genomic screening can be accomplished on a strict need-to-know basis. It is not necessary to collect data from family members or to investigate genetic loci unassociated with responses to anesthesia, surgery, or stress in the critically ill patient. Unlike screening patients for familial diseases, cancer, or progressive neurologic decline, genotyping the critically ill patient need not require costly genetic counseling to yield its maximal value to patients and caregivers alike. Samples and data can be shielded at the patient's request and recollected as needed in the future. Use of genomic data in the intensive care setting thus protects and enhances patient autonomy, calling attention to unique differences within vulnerable groups, including the very young, the very old, and the very sick.

SHORTCOMINGS OF GENOMICS IN PERIOPERATIVE CRITICAL CARE

As a practical matter, no contemporary or foreseeable genotyping methodology will be sensitive to all mechanisms of heredity (e.g., multifactorial inheritance, alternative splicing, posttranslational modification), and new predictive alleles will continue to be identified for many years hence (41). In turn, phenotypic tests will not be superseded in many circumstances; for example, genotyping for ABO blood groups (42) in all likelihood will remain confirmatory of serologic testing, with the latter's greater capacity to detect all significant host–donor interactions. For years to come, genotyping in real time may not be available for true emergencies. Nevertheless, technical advances reducing turnover times by the use of microfluidics, electrostatic addressing, microbead arrays, and laser detection are on the near horizon; nor have data arriving to the operating room or ICU after the patient necessarily shed their import. In this regard, genomic results are no different from other widely used and highly valued tests, for example, toxicology screens and tests for bacterial antibiotic sensitivity.

How revolutionary genomic knowledge will nest in existing practice patterns and habits of thought is of greater concern. Few busy intensivists, surgeons, or anesthesiologists are well informed about molecular biology, and they will not be able to learn readily on the job for lack of time and formal training. As genomic data exponentially accumulate, clinicians and their patients often will find themselves in a cross-fire of conflicting risks. Close balancing and clinical judgment always have been essential but now will be required at the genetic level. Though daunting, the advantages genomic information affords in safeguarding patients will outweigh these concerns for most current and all future practitioners in acquiring needed sophistication. A still larger issue is the requisite turnabout in attitudes now in vogue toward perioperative and postadmission screening in general. Standing orders for testing have recently been questioned and often abandoned because, in many cases, the data are of little or no predictive value (43). Decisions frequently are confronted over the proper response to unanticipated results, and patients have been harmed during what might, in retrospect, have been needless workups. For purposes of perioperative critical care, knowledge of a genotype is to be sought only if it is analytically valid, clinically valid, and of clear clinical utility. Either the prevalence of the allele must be high, or the trait must be severe if the allele is rare. Each allele must exhibit close genotype–phenotype correlation, and direct evidence for causality is strongly to be preferred. The overriding criterion is the availability of safe alternative interventions for patients carrying the targeted alleles, for example, intensified surveillance, focused prophylaxis, surrogate drugs, regimens, and procedures. Lastly, the risk of the substituted management must not outweigh the possibility of false-positive genomic results. In the ideal circumstance, false-positive genomic data would entail no added inconvenience, cost, or intrinsic risk.

SUMMARY

The role of genomics in perioperative critical care is not to screen populations based on the presence of preexisting markers or because of membership in at-risk pedigrees, but rather to screen individual patients exposed to potent medications and invasive procedures necessary to sustain life. Because risks from a large variety and number of predisposing genetic conditions can be effectively stratified using a shared technology, genomic profiling in life support is feasible and of immediate benefit, representing an ideal opportunity to introduce genomics into broad clinical practice. Scientific and technical barriers have been surmounted, and legal precedent favors testing through expeditious adoption of safety steps as they are proven to be of value. As comprehensive panels of alleles evolve, it will be possible to customize profiles for specific risk groups and procedures that clear thresholds for accuracy, cost, efficiency, and safety of the test itself, in assuring that genomic profiling will become a daily component of critical care.

KEY POINTS

In the interval from the first edition of this volume to the present, practice at the highest standards of intensive care medicine has been within the reach of those with virtually no knowledge of molecular biology. From this edition to the next, it will no longer be so. As the gestational period of the genetics revolution ends and its active labor begins, physicians embracing the new technology will be rewarded by strides in patient care without antecedent or bound. Because the enterprise pivots on how well DNA sequence variation predicts a trait of interest, criteria for performing this appraisal have been set forth here.

REFERENCES

1. Hogan K. Principles and techniques of molecular biology. In: Hopkins P, Hemmings HC, eds. *Basic and applied science for anesthesia*. New York: Mosby-Wolfe, 2000:37–54.
2. Strachan T, Read AP. *Human molecular genetics*, 2nd ed. New York: Bios Scientific Publishers Limited, 1999.
3. Kalow W, Grant DM. Pharmacogenetics. In: Scriver CR, Beaudet AL, Sly WS, et al., eds. *The metabolic and molecular basis of inherited disease*, 8th ed. New York: McGraw-Hill, 2001:225–255.
4. Jurkat-Rott KT, McCarthy T, Lehmann-Horn F. Genetics and pathogenesis of malignant hyperthermia. *Muscle Nerve* 2000;23:4–17.
5. La Du BN, Bartels CF, Nogueira CP, et al. Phenotypic and molecular biological analysis of human butyrylcholinesterase variants. *Clin Biochem* 1990;23:423–431.
6. Nakagawa K, Ishizaki T. Therapeutic relevance of pharmacogenetic factors in cardiovascular medicine. *Pharmacol Ther* 2000;86:1–28.
7. van der Weide J, Stejins LSW. Cytochrome P450 enzyme system: genetic polymorphisms and impact on clinical pharmacology. *Ann Clin Biochem* 1999;36:722–729.

8. Tanaka E. Update: Genetic polymorphism of drug metabolizing enzymes in humans. *J Clin Pharm and Ther* 1999;24:323–329.

9. Dale O, Olkkola KT. Cytochrome P450, molecular biology and anaesthesia. *Acta Anesthesiol Scand* 1998;42:1025–1027.

10. de Wildt SN, Kearns GL, Leeder JS, et al. Glucuronidation in humans: pharmacogenetic and developmental aspects. *Clin Pharmacokinet* 1999;36:429–452.

11. Fouad G, Dalakas M. Servidei S, et al. Genotype-phenotype correlations of DHP receptor α1 subunit gene mutations causing hypokalemic periodic paralysis. *Neuromuscl Disord* 1997;7:33–38.

12. Bick R. Preface. *Semin Thromb Hemost* 1999;25:251–253.

13. Ireland H, Thompson E, Lane DA. Gene mutations in 21 unrelated cases of phenotypic heterozygous protein C deficiency and thrombosis: Protein C Study Group. *Thromb Haemost* 1996;76:867–873.

14. Iacoviello L, Di Castelnuovo A, De Knijff P, et al. Polymorphisms in the coagulation factor VII gene and the risk of myocardial infarction. *N Engl J Med* 1998;338:79–85.

15. Simoni P, Prandoni P, Lensing AWA, et al. The risk of recurrent venous thromboembolism in patients with an Arg506Gln mutation in the gene for factor V (factor V Leiden). *N Engl J Med* 1997;336:399–403.

16. Nguyen A. Prothrombin G20210A polymorphism and thrombophilia. *Mayo Clin Proc* 2000;75:595–604.

17. DeStefano V, Martinelli I, Mannucci PM, et al. The risk of recurrent deep venous thrombosis among heterozygous carriers of both factor V Leiden and the G20210A prothrombin mutation. *N Engl Med* 1999;341:801–806.

18. Majetschak M, Flohe S, Obertacke U, et al. Relation of a TNF gene polymorphism to severe sepsis in trauma patients. *Ann Surg* 1999;230:207–214.

19. Stuber F, Petersen M, Bokelmann F, et al. A genomic polymorphism within the tumor necrosis locus influences plasma tumor necrosis factor-alpha concentrations and outcome of patients with severe sepsis. *Crit Care Med* 1996;24:381–386.

20. Flach R, Majetschak M, Heukamp T, et al. Relation of *ex vivo* stimulated blood cytokine synthesis to post-traumatic sepsis. *Cytokine* 1999;11:173–178.

21. Mira JP, Cariou A, Grall F, et al. Association of TNF2, a TNF-α promoter polymorphism with septic shock susceptibility and mortality: a multicenter study. *JAMA* 1999;282:561–568.

22. Pelleiter R, Pravica V, Perrey C, et al. Evidence for a genetic predisposition towards acute rejection after kidney and simultaneous kidney-pancreas transplantation. *Transplantation* 2000;70:674–680.

23. Suthanthiran M. The importance of genetic polymorphisms in renal transplantation. *Current Opinion in Urology* 2000;10:71–75.

24. Freeman RB, Tran CL, Mattoli J, et al. Tumor necrosis factor genetic polymorphisms correlate with infections after liver transplantation. *Transplantation* 1999;67:1005–1010.

25. Fang XM, Schroder S, Hoeft A, et al. Comparison of two polymorphisms of the interleukin-1 gene family: interleukin-1 receptor antagonist polymorphism contributes to susceptibility to severe sepsis. *Crit Care Med* 1999;27:1330–1334.

26. McNicholl JM, Cuenco KT. Host genes and infectious diseases: HIV, other pathogens, and a public health perspective. *Am J Prev Med* 1999;16:141–154.

27. Tambic A, Power EG, Talasnia H, et al. Analysis of an out-break of non-phage-typeable methicillin-resistant *Staphylococcus aureus* by using a randomly amplified polymorphic DNA assay. *J Clin Microbiol* 1997;35:3092–3097.

28. Einsele H, Hebart H, Roller G, et al. Detection and identification of fungal pathogens in blood using molecular probes. *J Clin Microbiol* 1997;35:1353–1360.

29. Goyal M, Shaw R, Benerjee DK, et al. Rapid detection of multi-drug resistant tuberculosis. *Eur Respir J* 1997;10:1120–1124.

30. Cursons RTM, Jeyerajah E, Sleigh JW, et al. The use of polymerase chain reaction to detect septicemia in critically ill patients. *Crit Care Med* 1999;27:937–940.

31. Teba L. Polymerase chain reaction: a new chapter in critical care diagnosis. *Crit Care Med* 1999;27:860–861.

32. Ross RS, Viazov S, Gross T, et al. Transmission of hepatitis C from a patient to an anesthesiology assistant to five patients. *N Engl J Med* 2001;343:1851–1853.

33. Fanning S, Gibbs RA. PCR in genome analysis. In: Birren B, Green ED, Klapholz S, et al., eds. *Genome analysis: a laboratory manual.* Plainview, NY: Cold Spring Harbor Laboratory Press, 1997:249–299.

34. Marras SA, Kramer FR, Tyagi S. Multiplex detection of single-nucleotide variations using molecular beacons. *Genet Anal* 1999;14:151–156.

35. Phimister B, ed. The chipping forecast. *Nat Genet* 1999;21(Suppl):1–60.

36. Fan JB, Chen X, Halushka MK, et al. Parallel genotyping of human SNPs using generic high-density oligonucleotide Tag arrays. *Genome Res* 2000;10: 853–860.

37. Isaksson A, Landegren U. Accessing genomic information: alternatives to PCR. *Curr Opin Biotechnol* 1999;10:11–15.

38. Kwiatkowski RW, Lyamichev V, de Arruda M, et al. Clinical, genetic and pharmacogenetic applications of the Invader assay. *Molecular Diagnosis* 1999;4:353–364.

39. Fujii J, Otsu K, Zorzato F, et al. Identification of a mutation in porcine ryanodine receptor associated with malignant hyperthermia. *Science* 1991;253:448–451.

40. Roberts MC, Mickelson JR, Patterson EE, et al. Autosomal dominant canine malignant hyperthermia is caused by a mutation in the gene encoding the skeletal muscle calcium release channel. *Anesthesiology* 2001;95:716–725.

41. Schork NJ. Genetics of complex disease: approaches, problems, and solutions. *Am J Respir Crit Care Med* 1997;156:S103–S109.

42. Rozman P, Dovc T, Gassner C. Differentiation of autologous ABO, RHD, RHCE, KEL, JK, and FY blood group genotypes by analysis of peripheral blood samples of patients who have recently received multiple transfusions. *Transfusion* 2000;40:936–942.

43. Roizen MF. Perioperative testing. In: Sweitzer B, ed. *Handbook of preoperative assessment and management.* Philadelphia: Lippincott Williams & Wilkins, 2000:16–38.

7

RESEARCH IN CRITICAL CARE MEDICINE

ANAND KUMAR
JAMES E. CALVIN
JOSEPH E. PARRILLO

KEY WORDS

- Acute respiratory distress syndrome
- Clinical trial: blinded, nonrandomized, prospective, randomized, retrospective, unblinded, uncontrolled
- Conflict of interest
- Consent types
- Cost analysis
- Inclusion/exclusion criteria

- Ethics
- Institutional Review Board
- Outcomes analysis
- Patient confidentiality
- Principal investigator
- Research
- Research subjects
- Resource utilization
- Sponsor
- Standards of care
- Study coordinator

INTRODUCTION

Critical care medicine (CCM) involves the care of patients with critical organ dysfunction. In 1983, the National Institutes of Health (NIH) Consensus Development Conference on CCM was held, involving scientists, physicians, and other health care professionals. The conference members defined CCM as "a multidisciplinary and multi-professional medical-nursing field concerned with patients who have sustained or are at risk of sustaining acute life-threatening single or multiple organ system failure because of disease or injury" (1). Since critical organ dysfunction can derive from several forms of injury and may require support from physicians of several disciplines, the field of CCM is, as noted, intrinsically multidisciplinary in nature. Within the intensive care unit (ICU) environment where CCM is practiced, CCM specialists from internal medicine, pediatrics, anesthesiology, and surgery deliver care. In addition, modern ICUs have evolved to encompass the contributions and involvement of dedicated teams of nurses, pharmacists, nutritionists, respiratory therapists, and social workers.

The origins of CCM and ICUs may be found in the postoperative recovery rooms following World War II and later the "iron lung" wards for polio sufferers in the 1950s. From there came the dedicated coronary care units of the 1960s that laid the foundations for the multiple specialized ICUs (neonatal, pediatric, medical, general surgical, neurosurgical, cardiovascular) found in modern institutions. Along with this profusion of ICUs has come a corresponding increase in total costs. Data from the early 1990s demonstrated that ICUs account for 20% to 30% of total hospital costs while using just 7% of hospital beds (2). About 1% of the gross national product (GNP) of the United States is spent annually on care of patients in critical care units (2).

If for no other reason than the tremendous expense of intensive care and relatively high morbidity and mortality of critically ill patients, all sectors in the society have a vested interest in finding better strategies for patient evaluation and treatment for the critically ill. Such efforts must span the breadth of health care research encompassing biological sciences, epidemiology of the critically ill, utilization of new technologies, and consumption of health care resources.

Over the years, CCM research has evolved with the problems of critically ill patients. During World War II, traumatic and hemorrhagic shock and their immediate complications were the major focus of critical care research (3,4). The Korean War fueled the research that demonstrated the relationship of acute tubular necrosis (ATN) and acute renal failure (ARF) to circulatory shock (3,4). In addition, studies of battlefield casualties showed the relationship between early resuscitation and survival (3,4). Subsequently, the polio epidemic stimulated interest in the management of respiratory failure. During the Vietnam conflict, with the widespread use of mechanical ventilators, the dominant research interest became postshock infection and "shock lung" [acute respiratory distress syndrome (ARDS)]. More recently, sepsis and shock-related multiple organ dysfunction syndrome (MODS) have come to the foreground (4).

The modern day ICU holds outstanding potential as a site for clinical research efforts. The many clinically indicated invasive monitoring devices routinely used in ICUs (e.g., pulmonary artery catheters for estimation of ventricular filling pressures and cardiac output, arterial catheters for measurement of blood pressure and arterial blood gases, and mechanical ventilators with advanced monitoring technology) offer an opportunity for clinical research and for insights into disease processes that can be gained nowhere else.

EVOLUTION OF CRITICAL CARE RESEARCH

During the 1983 NIH Conference on CCM, four important areas of CCM research were emphasized (1). Subsequently, in 1991, a special article by the Research Division of the Society of Critical Care Medicine (SCCM) revisited those four designated research areas, highlighting progress to date and providing guidance for key future studies (5). The following are the four key areas of research:

1. Natural history, risk, and outcomes analysis
2. ICU technology and therapy
3. Optimal ICU personnel and resource utilization
4. Pathophysiology of disease

Natural History, Risk, and Outcomes Analysis

This area of research involves the development of accurate criteria for diagnosis of illness/disease, acuity scoring, and the analysis of outcomes based on diagnosis and severity of illness (6–9). The development of these methodologies supports not only quality assurance but also allows better patient prognostication and aid in clinical research design. Although these tools predict patient population outcomes well, they have not yet been proven to be helpful in managing individual patients.

Intensive Care Unit Technology and Therapy

The goal of this area is to assess the cost benefit and cost effectiveness of sophisticated technologies and treatments available to critically ill patients. Many of these are expensive, and their value is largely unproved. Much of this technological and treatment assessment has been retrospective, uncontrolled, unblinded, and nonrandomized. Unfortunately, much cost and little benefit have been the results. The goals of technology assessment have been summarized previously and include (a) the technology's feasibility, (b) its efficacy, (c) its effectiveness, and (d) its economic impact (10).

Understanding all the necessary components of technology assessment highlights the importance of avoiding ineffective "in-house" studies that do not answer the important question of cost effectiveness of a given technology but rather serve to enhance diffusion of an unproved one.

Guyatt and colleagues (11) described a multistep process for the scientific assessment of diagnostic technologies to be undertaken before one does an economic (cost-benefit) evaluation including the following:

1. The demonstration of technological capability
2. The potential range of uses
3. The accuracy of the technology in comparison to a "gold standard"
4. The effect on the health care provider in terms of the importance, uniqueness, and timeliness of the information provided
5. The potential impact of the technology in changing therapy
6. The potential impact of the technology in improving outcome

In general, most technologies found in ICUs have been evaluated through the first three steps (10). Rarely have technologies been evaluated through steps 4 through 6 (12,13). In part, the failure to complete higher levels of evaluation is related to expense. Furthermore, outcome assessments for certain technologies, such as hemodynamic monitoring, are difficult to evaluate because they only provide information, and their efficacy depends on how the information is used and interpreted and the effectiveness of the treatment strategy (14,15). One potential example of this problem is the use of pulmonary artery catheters, an established diagnostic technology that has been associated with increased mortality (16,17).

Subsequent economic evaluations include cost–benefit analysis, cost-effectiveness analysis, and cost–utility analysis. Cost–benefit analysis is used to measure in dollar amounts the difference between costs and benefits resulting from an activity. Cost-effectiveness analysis compares strategies with similar outcomes. To determine the most efficient method of achieving a particular healthcare objective, cost–utility analysis examines the cost of a program compared to quality adjusted life years gained.

Optimal Personnel and Resources Utilization

Any lack of access to beneficial therapy undermines the effectiveness of a therapy as a health care advance. Necessary infrastructure must be developed and resources allocated to ensure adequate access and availability of effective treatments. Human resource studies are needed to develop adequate staffing models, not only within hospitals but also within cities, states, and regions. Data on optimal training in and evaluation of practice guidelines are also necessary. Examples of research in this area include studies that demonstrate improved outcome and decreased resource utilization with the introduction of intensivists to community or academic ICUs (18–20). Studies that show decreased incidence of catheter-related sepsis with dedicated catheter insertion and care teams also fit into this category (21–23).

Pathophysiology of Diseases

The goal of this research is a better understanding of the pathophysiology of diseases commonly seen in the ICU. In the last 25 years, an improved understanding of the physiologic derangement of organ failure has been integrated into the treatment of a variety of disorders. The use of vasodilators to reduce left ventricular afterload has resulted in improved mortality in patients with chronic congestive heart failure (24). The use of thrombolytic agents in acute myocardial infarction was based on the knowledge that acute coronary occlusion with thrombus was the basis of this clinical entity (25). Along with aspirin and β-blocker therapy, thrombolytic agents have reduced mortality in acute myocardial infarction (26). Even when studies have not resulted in new therapies, disease-oriented research can yield fruitful new areas for investigation. A series of studies demonstrated a role for nitric oxide in septic cardiovascular dysfunction (27–31). These investigations indirectly led to ongoing clinical trials of the efficacy of nitric oxide inhibitors in septic shock (32,33)

Further Advances in Critical Care Research

In 1993, a decade after the original NIH Conference on CCM, the National Heart, Lung and Blood Institute (NHLBI) of the NIH, at the request of U.S. House of Representatives Committee on Appropriations, convened the Task Force on Research in Cardiopulmonary Dysfunction in Critical Care Medicine (1,2). The task force comprised national experts in basic science, clinical, and epidemiologic research in CCM and further delineated priority areas for research in CCM. Three major research areas were recommended for support.

The highest priority was given to clinical research in the belief that advances in basic science had surpassed clinical application of those advances to that point. Recommended areas of clinical research included the following:

1. The development and validation of consensus definitions of ARDS, sepsis, MODS, and related terms
2. Investigation of mechanisms of disease such as inflammatory mediators, physical stresses, nutrition/nutritional supplements, oxygen transport/consumption, and their impact on outcome measures
3. Evaluation of standard (e.g., vasopressors, ionotropes, fluids and nutritional support) and experimental (e.g., artificial surfactant, tissue repair enhancers) pharmacologic therapies
4. Utility of standard and experimental ventilatory modes (including noninvasive ventilatory modes) and supportive related therapies (e.g., respiratory muscle training, biofeedback)
5. Utility of standard (pulmonary artery catheterization, echocardiography, other cardiac imaging techniques) and experimental (multiple-lead electrocardiograms, continuous electroencephalograms, assessment of drug levels and effects) techniques for patient monitoring

Epidemiologic research was recommended to be equal in priority to clinical research. The task force recommended two important areas for attention:

1. Outcome studies including quality of life; functional status; cost-effectiveness; and survival in relation to race, ethnicity, sex, age, socioeconomic status; other patient characteristics; comorbid conditions; admission diagnosis; and ICU complications for identification of potential inequalities in ICU use and outcome.
2. Risk stratification systems based on demographic characteristics and premorbid/comorbid conditions for identification of patient populations for which ICU care is most efficacious.

Although the task force recommended that clinical and epidemiologic research should carry a higher priority than basic research, the report of the task force made it clear that basic research efforts should not be compromised. The two areas of highest priority within the realm of basic research were the following:

1. Development of improved *in vitro* techniques and animal models for the study of cell–cell interactions, acute tissue injury, cellular response to inflammation, and cellular repair mechanisms as related to critical illness including trauma, sepsis, and organ failure.
2. Cellular and molecular studies to advance the understanding of the endogenous activity and regulation of cytokines,

adhesion molecules, oxygen metabolites, and antioxidant defenses. In addition, studies to examine mechanisms of microvascular response to alterations in concentration of oxygen, adenosine, endothelin, nitric oxide, and other endogenous mediators were recommended as was research into cellular energy metabolism during hypoxemia and sepsis.

In the future, a better understanding of the pathophysiology of disorders at the cellular and molecular level holds promise to reduce further morbidity and mortality in critical illness. For example, the demonstration that apoptosis is involved in human sepsis (34) yielded studies showing that apoptosis inhibitors (e.g., caspase inhibitors) can improve outcome in animal models of septic shock (35). Similarly, it is hoped that the demonstration of activation of transcription factors in cells exposed to human septic serum may result in therapies involving transcription factor inhibitors (36). The continued interaction of basic scientists and clinical researchers will be necessary for research to succeed in developing new advances in CCM.

Integrative Research in the ICU

Integrative research is particularly suited to the physician/scientist. *Integrative research* has been defined as molecular biologic investigation into the molecular/biologic processes that regulate the physiologic function of cells, tissues, organs, and intact organisms (37). The field requires integration of clinical and laboratory research efforts and the study of a particular research question at multiple levels ranging from molecular, cell biology, and physiology through to clinical studies. This field may be particularly attractive to intensivist/scientists because the ICU, in many ways, represents a human physiology laboratory. It is the only place where humans are routinely invasively monitored for cardiovascular, respiratory, and renal function. In the last decade, many clinical observations made in the ICU have been translated into bench or experimental animal research with the hope that experimental data then could be used to derive therapies that can be applied at the bedside. These studies include the initial confirmation of the existence of septic myocardial depression leading to identification of a circulating myocardial depressant substance (38–40). Demonstration of apoptosis in tissues of humans succumbing to septic shock, leading to studies showing increased survival in a murine septic shock model with an apoptosis inhibitor, is another example (34,35). Older examples of integrative research contributions to CCM practice include the development of stress ulcer prophylaxis in the critically ill (41,42) and the association of ventilator-associated pneumonia with the migration of gut organisms into the upper airway (43,44).

To perform integrative research effectively in an ICU setting, several prerequisites are needed. Overall, an appropriate organizational environment, physical plant and resources, and personnel are key. First and foremost, a secure and reliable patient population must be available. Research questions must be geared to the problems seen in the ICU population. It is intrinsically difficult to study wound trauma in a medical ICU or end-stage chronic obstructive pulmonary disease (COPD) in a surgical ICU. It is also helpful to have a sufficient degree of education in the subject population to facilitate patient recruitment. On the other hand, some problems tend to occur in populations with modest educational achievement and with less inclination to participate in clinical research efforts. Those populations also must be served. A second requirement is for a sufficient pool of research expertise. To perform correlative biochemistry, cell biology, molecular biology, and animal studies, a cadre of supporting researchers is needed. A third requirement for effective integrative research is state-of-the-art laboratory and clinical research facilities. This may include dedicated clinical study areas as well as laboratory equipment. A strong animal facility is the fourth prerequisite for successful integrative research. This animal facility should include assistance and expertise in the development and use of appropriate animal models of disease. The final two required elements are a supportive administrative structure, including an institutional commitment, and secure funding whether from internal funds or from established extramural sources.

The practicing intensivist scientist can contribute to research in many areas, although some may require specialized supplemental training in translational research. All intensivists, however, potentially can contribute in the clinical research arena. Relatively little material exists on the conduct of clinical trials in the ICU context. For this reason, and because the 1993 NHLBI Task Force on Cardiopulmonary Dysfunction in CCM recommended it as a priority item (2), the remainder of this chapter focuses on the history and conduct of clinical trials in the ICU.

CLINICAL TRIALS

History of Clinical Research

Clinical research as a fundamental component of medical practice is a relatively new concept in North America. Despite a centuries-long history of integration of clinical and research functions in European medical schools, it was not until the development of full-time faculty in university clinical departments in the early part of this century that North American physicians found a substantial research role (45–47). Until that time, North American physicians were almost uniformly considered to be clinicians rather than scientists.

The Flexner report by the New York Carnegie Foundation for the Advancement of Teaching in 1910 set the tone for future developments by stimulating the establishment of an increased number of full-time professorships in the clinical departments of medical schools (48). Subsequently, in 1917, the Committee on Medical Research of the Association of Medical Colleges recommended an expansion of clinical research responsibilities for all medical school faculty members (49). The result of these efforts was the growth of clinical research centers in dedicated clinical research laboratories and institutes at academic medical centers throughout the country.

Eventually, in 1930, the U.S. Congress, in recognizing that "scientific research is the most important function of the Federal Government as it relates to public health" established the NIH, an agency that since has become the principal federal sponsor for support of medical research (45,50). Following the success of federally sponsored research programs during and immediately following World War II (antibiotic development, trauma resuscitation), funding for the NIH expanded almost continu-

ously. Despite the support of 74 general clinical research centers at medical schools throughout the United States, a trend favoring basic science research and basic scientists in recent decades may have existed. In recent years, however, this trend has been recognized and partially reversed with rededication to support of clinical research efforts by physicians and scientists (51).

The Clinical Trial

The clinical trial (52), defined as a prospective study in human subjects examining the effect and value of an intervention compared to a control, is the most powerful and robust study design available. More than any other study design, a clinical trial has the ability to determine whether a given intervention has the postulated effect. A sound knowledge of experimental design, statistical techniques, and demonstration of organizational skills is mandatory to run an effective and valid trial.

To understand the organizational design of research activities within ICUs, a brief review of study design is necessary. In addition to using a control group (53), the other important characteristics of a clinical trial are (a) that it is prospective, (b) that there is a clearly defined intervention and clear endpoint to be tested, (c) that the treatment is randomized, and (d) that both patient and caregivers are blinded to what therapy the patient is receiving when possible (54).

It is important to review some other important elements of a clinical trial:

1. Prospective studies require "a priori" definition of the inclusion and exclusion criteria and follow-up of patients longitudinally forward from the initiation of the intervention.
2. The intervention, which may be a drug, device, test, or strategy, must be applied in a standard fashion.
3. The control group is an integral part of the trial and should be comparable in all important aspects to the test groups.
4. Randomization is processed so that all subjects have an equal chance of being assigned to the treatment or control group. This procedure protects against bias in the allocation of subject to one group or another and ensures comparable groups and the validity of the statistical methods.
5. The process of blinding is to guard insofar as possible against bias by patient or investigator.
6. There is a clearly defined endpoint that determines the success of the trial.

These elements make it apparent that a clearly written protocol is a necessary prerequisite of the clinical trial serving as an agreement between investigator, subject, scientific community, and funding source. The protocol must contain the background, the objectives, hypothesis to be tested, and the design and organization of the trial. It must be developed prior to the beginning of the trial and is a major portion of grant applications and requests for approval by institutional review boards (IRBs) (55).

The protocol also must contain the inclusion and exclusion criteria of the study population, sample-size estimates, the process of enrolling subjects (including informed consent, baseline examinations, and group allocation), description and schedule of intervention, follow-up schedule, ascertainment of response variables, and study organization.

This overall organization has particular relevance when determining whether a center should initiate a single center trial or participate in a multicenter trial. Description of inclusion and exclusion criteria and calculation of sample size help to determine the feasibility of being able to recruit a sufficient number of patients in a specific unit of time. A center with special expertise may be able to participate by providing specialized diagnostic or analytical services for all centers. A center providing such a core laboratory usually does not participate in patient recruitment.

The issue of patient recruitment is probably the most important question to be addressed when considering participation. One must ask whether it is realistic to recruit enough patients based on the best estimate from medical records and available databases. At this point, expanding the trial to other centers may be necessary to accomplish this task. It is obvious that considerable organizational assistance is necessary not only to gather the necessary data for recruitment estimates but also to screen potential test centers.

Patients who are possible subjects can be identified by standard screening techniques. Considerable care must be extended to keeping accurate and complete records. To accomplish this, staff must often be available during off-hours or during vacation periods. Quality checks must be performed periodically. Missing data often are used as an indicator of the quality of the research and must be minimized.

Other Forms of Clinical Studies

In addition to randomized clinical trials, other forms of clinical investigation are possible (56). Nonrandomized concurrent control studies can be used, but their major criticism is that the groups may be dissimilar and bias toward treatment allocation may exist (selection bias). Historical series have been used as a control and permit all new subjects to receive a new therapy. Again, groups may be dissimilar, there is vulnerability to bias, and outcomes may be secondary to confounded variables. Crossover designs are popular because smaller sample sizes can be used, but one cannot use this design to test treatments where the effects of the first treatment period may carry over to the second treatment.

Databases (57) often are used to assess an experience with a treatment technology. These reviews are usually retrospective, however, and often are lacking in necessary information because of the lack of *a priori* planning.

Organization of the Study

Little has been written about the organizational structure of research enterprises within the hospital, let alone the ICU. A great deal has been written, however, about the organizational structure of multicenter clinical trials (58–62). This offers a starting point for a discussion about the organization of critical care research within an institution.

Table 1 lists the composition of the management staff for a large multicenter clinical trial (62). The number of people involved in this endeavor can be enormous, although a few specific roles are common to all trials. In particular, the principal inves-

TABLE 1. COMPOSITION OF MANAGEMENT STAFF FOR A LARGE MULTICENTER TRIAL

Principal investigator(s)
Coinvestigators and assistant investigators
Members of Institutional Review Board
Professional consultants
Regulatory agency reviewers
Trial coordinators
Trial monitors
Monitoring committees
Project champions
Project managers
Supervisors of data processors
Statistical reviewers
Executives of sponsoring institutions
Data analysis committee members
Independent auditors of diagnoses, laboratory data, trial conduct
Independent review committee of trial results and interpretation

Adapted from Management styles, staff and systems. In: Spilker B, ed. New York: Raven Press, 1991:953–960, with permission.

tigator (PI) provides the leadership necessary to organize a sufficiently large and skilled enterprise to answer the major hypothesis tested. In concert with the study statistician and coinvestigators, the PI coordinates prestudy organizational meetings that select the hypothesis to be tested, determines the inclusion and exclusion criteria, and estimates the sample size and power calculations. An administrative or executive committee can be formed at this point; the first job of this committee is to determine which test centers will be involved. Other staff listed in Table 1 may be specific to the sponsoring agency or the study center or may be part of organizational committees or core laboratories.

Quality assurance of data collected by multicenter trials involves ensuring standardization of patient eligibility criteria, diagnostic classification, and assessment of the effects of treatment. To perform this function, an independent group or committee is formed that is not directly involved with actual patient recruitment or study execution. Such a committee also can act as a safety monitoring committee with preset rules for stopping the trial if there is evidence of harm occurring to either treatment or control groups.

The interpretation of specialized tests also should be performed by individuals who are not directly involved with patient recruitment, and these persons should remain blind to patient treatment. By organizing such persons as a central committee, variability can be assessed and reduced.

Other administrative committees are often necessary including executive, data and safety monitoring, data analysis, writing, and external advisory committees. A representative outline of such an organizational structure is depicted in Fig. 1.

ORGANIZATIONAL STRUCTURE WITHIN THE INSTITUTION

The organizational structure of research with an individual center recognizes the accountability to the funding agency that must exist. Accountability within the institution needs clarification, however.

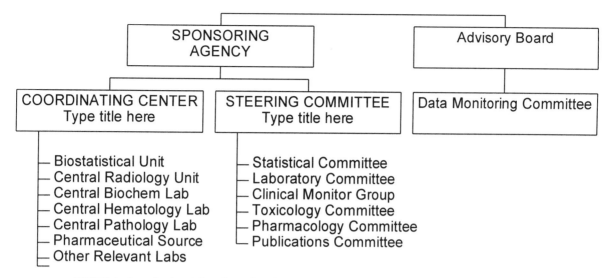

FIGURE 1. Organizational chart for a clinical trial. This is a representative model with coordinating and steering committees answering to the sponsoring agency. This model includes an Advisory Board and a Data Monitoring Committee. Other committees and core laboratories are established to handle various facets of the trial. In general, core laboratories answer to the coordinating center and organizational committees answer to the steering committee.

In the simplest scenario, the PI of a single study is accountable to either the funding agency or executive committee of a multicenter trial. Staff members who are fully dedicated to the project are responsible to the PI. The PI is also responsible to his section director or department head as representative of the institution. This implied matrix is necessary to protect interests of the study, the patient, and the institution.

In a more complex model of institutional research, several small projects are ongoing at the same time. The workload of each project may not be sufficient to justify a need for full-time personnel. In this scenario, research associates may work on more than one project and are not accountable to a single investigator. Because of the complexities of these arrangements, it is often useful to have an internal administrative committee oversee priorities and interact with either the funding agency or coordinating committee on financial matters. The PI is still responsible for the actual execution of the trial and providing necessary periodical reports to the institutional review body, funding agency, or a multicenter trial administrative committee.

In between these two models, various organizational structures may exist. Research staff may be largely responsible for a single project but provide coverage for vacation time and after-hours coverage for other studies. Advisory or administrative committees may have varying degrees of strictness over control of priorities and resources, depending on the experience and style of the institution. In single-center studies, in-house statistical consultation and data analysis are necessary.

Role of the Principal Investigator

The PI has the primary responsibility for the conduct of the trial. The PI is responsible not only for obtaining initial approval but also for filing periodic reports, advising the IRB of any change in the protocol, and advising of any serious adverse reactions. Form 1572 of the U.S. Food and Drug Administration (FDA) reviews the specific commitments of the investigator. These obligations include a commitment (a) personally to conduct or supervise the investigation in accordance with the relevant, current protocol; (b) to make changes to the protocol only after notifying the sponsor and IRB, except when necessary to protect the safety, rights, or welfare of research subjects; (c) to ensure that any research patients or persons used as controls are aware that study drugs that are being used for investigational purposes; (d) to ensure that requirements related to obtaining informed consent and IRB approval are appropriately met; (e) to report to the sponsor adverse experiences that occur in the course of the investigation; (f) to read and understand the information in the investigator's brochure including potential risks and side effects of the study intervention; (g) to ensure that all colleagues, associates and employees assisting in the conduct of the study are informed about their obligations with respect to these commitments; (h) to maintain adequate and accurate records and to make these records available for inspection as required by regulatory authorities; and (i) to ensure initial and ongoing review by an authorized IRB.

Role of the Study Coordinator

The study or trial coordinator handles most administrative tasks on a day-to-day basis. The coordinator's responsibilities range from patient scheduling, ensuring accurate and complete data recording, conducting the protocol, and acting as a major contact person. The coordinator plays the most important role of ensuring the most efficient conduct of the trial.

Role of the Institutional Review Board

Institutional approval for a research project or clinical trial is now mandated by the federal government for federally funded projects to ensure (a) that the conduct of a clinical trial is ethical and will do no harm; (b) that informed consent is obtained; (c) that potential conflicts of interest are eliminated; (d) that patient confidentiality is maintained; and (e) that confidentiality of the data is maintained.

An IRB must have at least five members, one of whom is not affiliated with the institution. It may not be composed entirely of men or women or from a single profession. Each IRB must include at least one member whose primary concerns are in scientific areas and at least one whose primary concerns are in nonscientific areas. No IRB may have a member participate in initial or continuing review of any project in which the member has a conflicting interest except to provide information as requested by the board.

In addition to providing initial and continuing review of clinical trials involving human subjects, the IRB is also responsible for overview of research involving stored clinical data and human tissue banks (63). In general, research investigations involving medical chart or database review or studies of human tissue specimens collected by others fall under federal regulations regarding informed consent (64). One major exception is made for situations in which all tissue donors are deceased (in which case the Office of Research Administration must verify that access to the tissue specimens complies with the requirements of the Uniform Anatomical Gift Act). The other major exception pertains to patient data (in databases or charts) that are accessed and used without any identifiers (coded or otherwise) in the extracted data such that identification of specific patients is impossible.

In the absence of such exclusion criteria, clinical tissue specimens and clinical data may be obtained from an IRB-supervised "repository" according to regulations of the Department of Health and Human Services (63). This "repository" model requires that informed consent be documented for specimens or data deposited into the repository. In addition, an IRB-approved protocol is required for study of data or tissues within the repository. Finally, a repository manager who has no conflict of interest and can ensure confidentiality for donors is essential. It is of note that clinical databases that could serve dual functions of clinical care and research should be designated as clinical data repositories requiring IRB supervision.

Funding Sources

Funding for both clinical and basic research can be acquired by contracting with third parties or by grant application to public funding agencies such as the NIH, private endowments, and foundations (65). Pharmaceutical-based contracts are a very common source of funding for some kinds of studies and present specific issues (see Conflict of Interest section) that are troublesome.

Various types of foundations exist, including special-interest foundations, corporate foundations, and family or community foundations. In general, funding from public agencies, endowments, and foundations are competitive and subject to peer review.

Estimating Costs of Research

The budget represents a major portion of a grant application. All costs must be identified (65). In general, these costs can be categorized as follows:

1. Personnel
2. Consultant fees
3. Equipment costs and maintenance
4. Supplies and reagents
5. Travel to either organizational meeting or to present the data
6. Patient care costs
7. Alteration or renovation to physical plant
8. Contractural costs
9. Miscellaneous costs

Granting agencies permit many of these costs, although certain equipment items or physical plant renovations often are borne by the institution. The budget requires careful scrutiny and integrity. Many funding agencies require multiple quotations on major equipment items and detailed explanations of why the equipment is necessary.

CONFLICT OF INTEREST IN CRITICAL CARE RESEARCH

There is a special need for the organization of research affairs within an institution to protect investigators against conflicts of interest (66). Such conflicts may be most immediate and intense in the clinical research arena but can exist in all forms of investigation. The potential for conflict of interest is most obvious in the relationship between investigators and pharmaceutical manufacturers, especially where the latter act as the funding agency. To emphasize the implication of potential conflicts of interest, one study found a correlation between the outcome of a study and its funding (67).

Another ethical issue that arises when investigators receive reimbursement for drug testing is *informed consent*. This issue arises because patients are rarely told that their physician will be paid for doing the study and that this financial incentive may influence the type of therapy the patient receives. Recent court decisions affirmed that a higher standard of disclosure is necessary for such research studies. In this context, it may be advisable that patients be informed about the source of funding and the investigator's potential conflict of interest in receiving renumeration for enrolling patients.

A few simple measures may help to alleviate concerns about potential conflict of interest in addition to the patient being told the source and mechanism of funding. This identifies to the patient the investigator's potential sources of bias. The direct financial incentive to investigators can be diminished if not eliminated by the institution taking control of the money through a process that pays direct costs of the project first, indirect costs of the institution second, and remaining funds allocated throughout the institution to investigators or projects on the basis of need and merit. Patients should be informed of the arrangement. This represents a mechanism analogous to the external peer-reviewed funding agency.

PROBLEMS OF CONDUCTING RESEARCH IN THE INTENSIVE CARE UNIT

Critically ill patients face the irony that, although they can benefit significantly from research activities, the ICU remains a complex and difficult arena for the conduct of research. The reasons for this complexity are numerous.

First, ICU patients often have MODS, which complicates the patients' response to therapy. Patients generally are receiving many drugs and often are undergoing multiple procedures. There are often compelling reasons for these multiple therapies, but they provide many confounding variables, making it a challenge for investigators to isolate the effects of a given investigational intervention.

Second, in view of the discomfort many patients may be experiencing and frequently poor prognosis, any evaluation of therapy often is debated in ethical terms. Other health care providers and families alike need to be reassured that the trial is in the patient's best interest (or at a minimum, not harmful) and that the study is important. Investigators must go out of their way to communicate the necessity of the study and address concerns regarding safety, patient distress, and importance. These concerns are justified and require careful and detailed discussions.

Third, it is important that staff performing the research are familiar with caring for such critically ill patients so that ongoing care is not compromised and other patient care issues are not neglected. This is often facilitated by having research staff members who are experienced in caring for the critically ill.

Fourth, the timing of study protocols must be worked into the patient's schedule for other treatments and tests. This requires excellent communication and significant effort, but it carries the highest priority.

Fifth, research on ICU patients necessarily involves patients who may be near the end of their lives. In recent years, a broader acceptance of termination or withdrawal of life-sustaining care (e.g., ventilation, vasopressors) in appropriate circumstances has evolved. This acceptance has resulted in the need for the design of ICU trials to accommodate unanticipated withdrawal of life support without engendering an inadvertent bias for or against an experimental treatment modality. Often this can be done through either *a priori* eligibility criteria that mandate aggressive life support or through defined criteria for withdrawal of life support.

Sixth, the issue of obtaining informed consent is a major handicap. Many IRBs have refused permission for research on acute-care patients because of the difficulty satisfying the patient's legal capacity to give voluntarily consent. Alternatives to informed consent have been explored, such as using surrogates (68,69), deferring consent (70), and using established waivers for informed consent (71) (so long as the IRB oversees these waivers in a stringent and ethical manner) (72). Federal regulations allow the use of surrogate consent for research when the subject is unable to participate in the decision-making process (64). State laws,

however, may supersede these regulations, resulting in a patchwork of approaches nationwide. In addition, FDA regulations (73) specifically allow an exception from informed consent requirements in emergency situations when there is a threat to life, when available treatments are unproved or unsatisfactory, when collection of valid scientific evidence to determine the safety and effectiveness of a particular intervention is needed, when participation in the research holds the prospect of direct benefit to the patient, when the clinical investigation could not be practically carried out without the waiver, and when obtaining informed consent is not feasible (e.g., in cardiopulmonary resuscitation research). An interesting requirement of this exception is that it applies only to research involving FDA-regulated products and requires community notification and consultation. Other alternatives to traditional informed consent in situations in which the subject is unable to provide consent continue to be discussed widely, but until consensus emerges, this issue will continue to present problems.

Finally, because of the severity of illness and the intensity of emotions experienced by patients, their families, and caregivers, it can be difficult to engender the support of crucial clinical staff members (e.g., nurses, physicians) whose cooperation is vital for the successful implementation of any research protocol. For this reason, it is crucial for the investigator to provide feedback to the clinical as well as research staff on trial results. Clinical research activities may be pointless unless they improve patient care in some way (including economics of care). Future staff support is fostered both by demonstrating evidence of improved patient care and recognizing the contribution of all patient care givers.

SUMMARY

Research in CCM remains in its infancy. NIH-sponsored consensus conferences over the last 20 years have delineated priority research areas in the field. These include clinical research of ICU technology and therapies, epidemiology of ICU disorders, and disease entity investigation involving basic research. Intensivists/scientists are particularly well positioned to make contributions in integrative research efforts that combine elements of clinical, animal, and bench investigations.

More emphasis needs to be placed on CCM research if we are to achieve the goals of improving the prognosis of the critically ill and making this care more cost efficient. The areas of necessary research activity have been identified, and the types of research studies reviewed; special attention was given to the clinical trial. Organization of clinical trials is discussed with emphasis on the interrelationships that exist.

KEY POINTS

Critical care consumes a large percentage of health care resources and allows patients to receive innovative but potentially harmful therapies and procedures. Clinicians and patients benefit from well-established, funded, organized programs that provide basic, applied, and translational research advances.

The prime areas of investigation for intensivists initially focused on the natural history, risk, and outcomes analysis of critically ill patients; application and development of ICU technology and therapy; the optimal use of ICU personnel and resource utilization; and the pathophysiology and natural course of various diseases, such as ARDS and MODS. A recent expert task force on critical care research emphasized the need for increased clinical efforts to provide consensus on terminology; identify cellular and molecular mechanisms of disease; evaluate standard and experimental pharmacologic therapies; determine the utility of standard and experimental ventilatory modes, hemodynamic techniques, and supportive related therapies. Additional priorities should be placed on epidemiologic research, with attention on clinical research outcome studies and risk stratification of critically ill patients in this era of cost consciousness and the need for careful resource allocation. Finally, the task force advocated continued strong support of basic research directed at the development

of improved *in vitro* techniques, animal models of disease, and cellular and molecular technologies.

Successful research requires proper training, sufficient personnel, and judicious allocation and application of resources. When possible, clinical studies should be prospective, randomized, controlled, and blinded. Well-organized multicenter trials may be required to provide sufficient breadth of patients and pathologies and to generate robust, readily accessible databases. Investigators must be familiar with various research regulations and ethical standards so that the confidentially, care, and rights of subjects are not compromised and conflicts of interest do not develop.

REFERENCES

1. Critical Care Medicine. *NIH Consensus Statement* 1983;Mar 7–9;4:1–26.
2. Lefant C. Task force on research in cardiopulmonary dysfunction in critical care medicine. *Circulation* 1995;91:1–7.
3. Anonymous. *Battle casualties in Korea: surgical research team in Korea.* Vol 1. Washington, DC: Army Medical Graduate School, Walter Reed Medical Center, 1954.
4. Kumar A, Parrillo JE. Shock: pathophysiology, classification and approach to management. In: Bone R, Parrillo JE, eds. *Textbook of critical care medicine,* 1st ed. Mosby, 1995.
5. Parrillo JE. Research in critical care medicine: Present status of critical care investigation. *Crit Care Med* 1991;19:569.
6. Knaus WA, Zimmerman JE, Wagner DP. APACHE-Acute physiology and chronic health evaluation: A physiologically based classification system. *Crit Care Med* 1981;9:591–597.
7. Knaus WA, Draper EA. APACHE II: a severity of disease classification system. *Crit Care Med* 1985;13:818–829.
8. Teskey RJ, Calvin JE, McPhail I. Disease severity in the coronary care unit. *Chest* 1991;100:1637–1642.
9. Bone RC, Balk R, Cerra FB, et al. ACCP/SCCM Consensus Conference: definitions for sepsis and organ failure and guidelines for use of innovative therapies in sepsis. *Chest* 1992;101:1644–1655.
10. Sibbald WJ, Escaf M, Calvin JE. How can new technology be introduced, evaluated, and financed in critical care? *Clin Chem* 1990;8(B):1604.
11. Guyatt G, Drummond M, Feeny D. Guidelines for the clinical and economic evaluation of health care technologies. *Soc Sci Med* 1986;22:393.
12. Bone RC, Slotman GJ, Maunder R, et al. Randomized double blind multi-centre study of prostaglandin E1 in patients with adult respiratory distress syndrome. Prostaglandin E1 study group. *Chest* 1989;96:114.
13. Holcroft JW, Vossar MJ, Weber CJ. Prostaglandin E1 and survival in patients with adult distress syndrome. *Ann Surg* 1986;203:371.
14. Calvin JE. Hemodynamic monitoring: a technology assessment. *Can Med Assoc J* 1991;145:114.
15. Zehender M, Kasper W, Kauder E, et al. Right ventricular infarction as an independent predictor of prognosis after acute inferior myocardial infarction. *N Engl J Med* 1993;328:981–988.
16. Naylor CD, Sibbald WJ, Sprung CL, et al. Pulmonary artery catheterization: can there be an integrated strategy for guideline development and research promotion? *JAMA* 1993;269:2407–2411.
17. Connors AF Jr, Speroff T, Dawson NV, et al. The effectiveness of right heart catheterization in the initial care of critically ill patients. *JAMA* 1996;276:889–897.
18. Reynolds HN, Haupt MT, Thill-Baharozian MC, et al. Impact of critical care physician staffing on patients with septic shock in a university hospital medical intensive care unit. *JAMA* 1988;260:3446–3450.
19. Pronovost PJ, Jenckes MW, Dorman T, et al. Organizational characteristics of intensive care units related to outcomes of abdominal aortic surgery. *JAMA* 1999;281:1310–1317.
20. Carson SS, Stocking C, Podsadecki T, et al. Effects of organizational change in the medical intensive care unit of a teaching hospital: a comparison of 'open' and 'closed' formats. *JAMA* 1996;276:322–328.
21. Faubion WC, Wesley JR, Khalidi N, et al. Total parenteral nutrition catheter sepsis: impact of the team approach. *J Parenter Enter Nutr* 1986;10:642–645.
22. Nelson DB, Kien CL, Mohr B. Dressing changes by specialized personnel reduced infection rates in patients receiving central venous parenteral nutrition. *J Parenter Enter Nutr* 1986;10:220–222.
23. Tomford JW, Hershey CO, McLaren CE. Intravenous therapy team and peripheral venous catheter-associated complications: a prospective controlled study. *Arch Intern Med* 1984;144:1191–1194.
24. Pfeffer MA, Braunwald E, Moye LA. Effect of captopril on mortality and morbidity in patients with left ventricular dysfunction after myocardial infarction. Results of the survival and ventricular enlargement trial. *N Engl J Med* 1992;327:669.
25. Gruppo Italiano per lo Studio della Streptochi-nasi nell'Infarto Miocardico (GISSI). Long-term effects of intravenous thrombolysis in acute myocardial infarction: Final report of the GISSI study. *Lancet* 1987;2:871–874.
26. Lau J, Antman EM, Jimenez-Silva J. Cumulative meta-analysis of therapeutic trials for myocardial infarction. *N Engl J Med* 1992;327:248.
27. Barthlen W, Stadler J, Lehn NL, et al. Serum levels of end products of nitric oxide synthesis correlate positively with tumor necrosis factor alpha and negatively with body temperature in patients with postoperative abdominal sepsis. *Shock* 1994;2:398–401.
28. Gomez-Jimenez J, Salgado A, Mourelle M, et al. L-arginine: nitric oxide pathway in endotoxemia and human septic shock. *Crit Care Med* 1995;23:253–258.
29. Hollenberg SM, Cunnion RE, Zimmerberg J. Nitric oxide synthase inhibition reverses arteriolar hyporesponsiveness to catecholamines in septic rats. *Am J Physiol* 1993;33:H660–H663.
30. Kumar A, Brar R, Wang P, et al. The role of nitric oxide and cyclic GMP in human septic serum-induced depression of cardiac myocyte contractility. *Am J Physiol* 1999;276:R265–R276.
31. Kumar A, Krieger A, Symeoneides S, et al. Myocardial dysfunction in septic shock. Part 2: role of cytokines and nitric oxide. *J Cardiovasc Thorac Anesth* 2001 (*in press*).
32. Grover R, Lopez A, Lorente J, et al. Multicenter, randomized, placebo-controlled, double-blind study of the nitric oxide inhibitor, 546C88: effect on survival in patients with septic shock. *Crit Care Med* 1999;27:A33(abst).
33. Grover R, Zaccardelli D, Colice G, et al. An open-label dose escalation study of the nitric oxide synthase inhibitor NG-methyl-L-arginine hydrochloride (546C88), in patients with septic shock. *Crit Care Med* 1999;27:913–922.
34. Hotchkiss RS, Swanson PE, Freeman BD, et al. Apoptotic cell death in patients with sepsis, shock, and multiple organ dysfunction. *Crit Care Med* 1999;27:1230–1251.
35. Hotchkiss RS, Tinsley KW, Swanson PE, et al. Prevention of lymphocyte

cell death in sepsis improves survival in mice. *Proc Natl Acad Sci* 1999;27:14541–14546.

36. Kumar A, Symeoneides S, Skorupa G, et al. Characterization of intracellular signalling components involved in sepsis. *Crit Care Med* 1999;27:A58(abst).

37. Minutes and Consensus of NHLBI Special Emphasis Panel on Integrative Research. April 19, 1996. http://www.nhlbi.nih.gov/meetings/workshops/intphys.txt. Accessed October 6, 2001.

38. Parrillo JE, Burch C, Shelhamer JH, et al. A circulating myocardial depressant substance in humans with septic shock. Septic shock patients with a reduced ejection fraction have a circulating factor that depresses *in vitro* myocardial cell performance. *J Clin Invest* 1985;76:1539–1553.

39. Parker MM, Shelhamer JH, Bacharach SL, et al. Profound but reversible myocardial depression in patients with septic shock. *Ann Intern Med* 1984;100:483–490.

40. Kumar A, Thota V, Dee L, et al. Tumor necrosis factor-alpha and interleukin-1 beta are responsible for depression of *in vitro* myocardial cell contractility induced by serum from humans with septic shock. *J Exp Med* 1996;183:949–958.

41. Hastings PR, Skillman JJ, Bushnell LS, et al. Antacid titration in the prevention of acute gastrointestinal bleeding: a controlled, randomized trial in 100 critically ill patients. *N Engl J Med* 1978;298:1041–1045.

42. Cook DJ, Reeve BK, Guyatt GH, et al. Stress ulcer prophylaxis in critically ill patients. Resolving discordant meta-analyses. *JAMA* 1996;275:308–314.

43. Dixon RE. Nosocomial respiratory infections. *Infect Control Hosp Epidemiol* 1983;4:376–381.

44. Bonten MJ, Gaillard CA, de Leeuw PW, et al. Role of colonization of the upper intestinal tract in the pathogenesis of ventilator-associated pneumonia. *Clin Infect Dis* 1997;24:309–319.

45. Pruitt BA Jr. The integration of clinical care and laboratory research: a model for medical progress. *Arch Surg* 1995;130:461–471.

46. Harvey AM. *Science at the bedside: clinical research in American medicine, 1905–1945.* Baltimore: John Hopkins University Press, 1981.

47. Sewall H. The beginnings of physiological research in America. *Science* 1923;58:187–195.

48. Flexner A. *Medical education in the United States and Canada.* New York: Carnegie Foundation for the Advancement of Teaching. Bulletin 4, 1910.

49. Lee FS, Cannon WB. Medical research in its relation to medical schools. *Proc Assoc Am Med Coll* 1917;27:19–31.

50. Fye WB. The origin of the full-time faculty system: implications for clinical research. *JAMA* 1991;265:1555–1562.

51. Zemlo TR, Garrison HH, Partridge NC, et al. The physician-scientist: career issues and challenges at the year 2000. *FASEB J* 2000;14:221–230.

52. Pocock SJ. *Clinical trials: a practical approach.* Toronto, Canada: John Wiley & Sons, 1983:28–49.

53. Spilker B. Controls used in clinical studies. In: *Guide to clinical studies and developing protocols.* New York: Raven Press, 1984:18–20.

54. Spilker B. Types of blinds. In: *Guide to clinical studies and developing protocols.* New York: Raven Press, 1984:14–17.

55. Spilker B. Standardized information across protocols (polishing the boilerplate). In: *Guide to clinical studies and developing protocols.* New York: Raven Press, 1984:154–184.

56. Wissow L, Pascoe J. Types of research models and methods. In: DeAngelis C, ed. *An introduction to clinical research.* Oxford: Oxford University Press, 1990:154–184.

57. McCormick M, Wasserman RC. Data collection management and analysis. In: DeAngelis C, ed. *An introduction to clinical research.* Oxford: Oxford University Press, 1990:75–110.

58. Spilker B. Comments on multicenter studies. In: *Guide to clinical studies and developing protocols.* New York: Raven Press, 1984:208–211.

59. Spilker B. Interview and selection of investigators. In: *Guide to clinical studies and developing protocols.* New York: Raven Press, 1984:217–225.

60. Spilker B. Monitoring and troubleshooting a study. In: *Guide to clinical studies and developing protocols.* New York: Raven Press, 1984:241–245.

61. Inmann KJ, Martin CM, Sibbald WJ. Design and conduct of clinical trials in critical care. *J Crit Care* 1992;7:118.

62. Spilker B. Management styles, staff and systems. In: *Guide to clinical trials.* New York: Raven Press, 1991:953–960.

63. Department of Health and Human Services, National Institutes of Health Office for Protection from Research Risks. Issues to consider in research use of stored data or tissues. Nov 7, 1997. http://ohrp.osophs.dhhs.gov/humansubjects/guidance/reposit.htm. Accessed October 6, 2001.

64. Department of Health and Human Services. *Federal policy for the protection of human services.* Code of Federal Regulations. Title 45. Public Welfare Part 46: Protection of Human Subjects, Subpart A: Section 46.116d. Basic DHHS Policy for Protection of Human Research Subjects. Revised June 18, 1991.

65. Duggan AK. Pragmatics. In: DeAngelis C, ed. *An introduction to clinical research.* Oxford: Oxford University Press, 1990:111–132.

66. Shimm DS. Industry reimbursement for entering patients into clinical trials: legal and ethical issues. *Ann Intern Med* 1991;115:148.

67. Davidson RA. Source of funding and outcome of clinical trials. *J Gen Intern Med* 1986;1:155.

68. Buchanan AE. *The ethics of surrogate decision making.* New York: Cambridge University Press, 1989.

69. Fost NC. A surrogate system for informed consent. *JAMA* 1975;233:800.

70. Miller BL. Philosophical, ethical, and legal aspects of resuscitation medicine. 1. Deferred consent and justification of resuscitation research. *Crit Care Med* 1988;16:1059.

71. National Commission for the Protection of Human Subjects of Biomedical and Behavioral Research. *The Belmont report*, OPPR. US Government Printing Office, 1983.

72. Iserson KV, Mahowald MB. Acute care research: is it ethical? *Crit Care Med* 1992;20:1032.

73. Code of Federal Regulations. Title 21 Food and Drugs, Part 50: Protection of Human Subjects, Subpart B: Informed Consent of Human Subjects, Section 24, Exception from informed consent requirements for emergency research. Revision date: April 1, 2000 (21CFR50.24).

MEDICAL INFORMATICS IN THE INTENSIVE CARE UNIT

KEITH RUSKIN

> ### KEY WORDS
>
> - Electronic medical record
> - Decision support systems; decision support methods, decision support technology, cost reduction
> - Clinical management databases; data mining, benchmarking
> - Internet, electronic mail, teleconferencing
> - Wireless technology
> - Security; encryption
> - Information-seeking behavior

INTRODUCTION

Critical care physicians can use computers for nearly all aspects of patient care, including medical record keeping, clinical databases, and decision support systems. Electronic medical records can help health care providers manage patient information while storing data in clinical databases that can be used to find subtle patterns in large volumes of data. In turn, this information can be used to create decision support systems that offer advice and treatment guidelines. The Internet provides universal access to resources and allows sharing of information by clinicians and researchers.

The Integrated Advanced Information Management Systems (IAIMS) model suggests that effective information management can improve patient care and reduce costs (1). Although the need for an information technology infrastructure seems obvious, the cost of implementing an information system in the intensive care unit (ICU) can be significant. A basic understanding of information technology is therefore essential in deciding when to invest in technology and when to pursue alternative strategies. The goal of medical informatics research is to improve patient care and decrease costs by integrating information technology into the work processes of health care professionals. This chapter explores practical applications of medical informatics in the ICU.

ELECTRONIC MEDICAL RECORD

The patient record is an integral part of the health care system that provides critical patient information to physicians, nurses, and ancillary staff at the point of care. Despite advances in nearly every other health care technology, the patient record in many institutions consists of pages clipped into a notebook, and information within it is frequently missing or inaccurate. Electronic medical records (EMRs) can solve many of the problems inherent to paper records. The Institute of Medicine defines the EMR as an "electronic patient record that resides in a system specifically designed to support users by providing accessibility to complete and accurate data, alerts, reminders, clinical decision support systems, links to medical knowledge, and other aids" (2).

Much research has focused on the development of an EMR, and systems that offer increasing levels of functionality have become commercially available. Although numerous attempts have been made to create an EMR system that stores all patient information, few systems completely eliminate the need for paper. Relatively few ICUs have adopted a completely paperless system, but implementing systems such as electronic order entry and laboratory results reporting can improve the efficiency of patient care.

Advantages

The chief advantage of EMRs is that they provide immediate access to critical information at the point of care. They are available 24 hours per day and do not need to be requested from the medical records department. Providers in different locations within the same institution or at other facilities can access the same records at the same time over secure networks.

Paper records are frequently incomplete and rarely present information in context to the task being performed. In one early study, between 5% and 20% of the information contained in patients' charts was missing, most of which were missing radiology reports or laboratory results. The same study found that as many as 30% of patients were seen without any medical records (3). Missing or incomplete information can delay or prevent clinical decision making, possibly resulting in increased length of stay. Missing information also may necessitate repeat studies, which increase the cost of patient care and may themselves cause complications.

Even if needed information is in the chart, handwritten notes and orders can be difficult or impossible to read. The Institute of Medicine has focused on illegible and misread orders and prescriptions as a factor that can significantly affect patient safety (4).

Typically, EMRs require that healthcare providers select treatment orders from a menu or drop-down box, practically eliminating illegible handwriting and spelling errors. The Leapfrog Group, which is composed of the health care buyers for several Fortune 500 companies, has recognized the potential for electronic order entry and prescriptions to improve patient safety and requests this capability during contract negotiations with health care providers.

By presenting information and reference materials in context to the task currently being performed, EMRs can decrease errors and improve the decision making process. For example, an EMR system can immediately alert physicians to new information, such as Food and Drug Administration (FDA) drug alerts. An EMR system can make a physician ordering an antibiotic aware of allergy information contained in another section of the chart. A physician ordering a drug that relies on renal excretion can be alerted to renal function studies that may have just become available. In one study on clinical alerts, Rind and colleagues showed that providing reminders to check renal function in hospitalized patients taking nephrotoxic drugs resulted in lower serum creatinine levels (5).

In addition, EMRs can improve billing accuracy and speed of payment. Most third-party payors now either prefer or require electronic submission. By automatically tracking hospital days and services rendered, EMRs can help hospitals and practitioners to avoid overbilling. They can provide billing personnel with a complete list of services and secondary diagnoses that otherwise might not have been reimbursed. One study by Hsia and colleagues reviewed bills submitted for reimbursement under Medicare and revealed an error rate of 20.8% in diagnosis related group (DRG) coding. Although older studies found that errors occurred randomly (i.e., half benefited the hospital financially and half penalized the hospital), Hsia and co-workers found that 61.7% of coding errors favored the hospital and concluded that "creep" resulting in overpayment occurs during coding of DRGs (6,7). Such billing errors are now being aggressively pursued by the U.S. federal government and by private payors and may result in substantial fines and possibly criminal charges.

Although the potential benefits of EMRs seem to be readily understandable, most of the evidence supporting their use is anecdotal. EMRs may decrease the time that health care professionals spend on charting, although this remains a subject of controversy. Implementation of a computerized record in a coronary care unit and medical ICU decreased the time nurses spent on charting from 17.4% to 10% and the time that they spent on data gathering from 7% to 4% (8). Several other studies suggest that EMRs increase productivity (9,10). In another study, however, physicians reported doubling the time that they spent on charting after introduction of an EMR system (11). Even if time is saved, the benefit is ambiguous. The study by Pierpont and Thilgen,

in which charting time was decreased, revealed that time spent for other tasks remained unchanged after implementation of the record (8).

Perhaps the simplest way to gauge user acceptance is to survey user satisfaction. Gardner and Lundsgaarde asked 360 physicians and 90 nurses about their EMR. They were asked to rank the importance of accessibility of various kinds of information on a scale from 1 (least important) to 5 (most important). The response rate was 68% for physicians and 90% for nurses. Physicians thought laboratory results, blood gas data, and demographic information are the most important pieces of information, whereas nurses considered laboratory results, blood gas data, and electrocardiographic (ECG) data with interpretation most important. Both physicians and nurses thought alerts for critical values and drug monitoring are helpful. Interestingly, nurses were less likely than physicians to believe that the EMR directly aided patient care (12). Tierney and colleagues surveyed medical students and house officers who used computer workstations for order entry and found that the opinions of the most junior students were most positive, whereas more senior house officers expressed increasing levels of dissatisfaction. This study concludes that widespread adoption of computing requires basic changes in medical education (13).

It is difficult to demonstrate the benefits of implementing an EMR using randomized controlled trials (1,14). At least one study showed that introduction of an EMR into a coronary and medical ICU did not result in an increase in patient care or the reduction of a full-time equivalent (FTE) resident (8). There are probably several factors that play a part in this phenomenon. One proposed explanation is that few EMRs are completely integrated into the ICU workflow, and manual charting is still required for some tasks. This can result in a duplication of effort and wasted time. An alternative explanation is that time saved by EMRs can be used for other tasks that are not reported by physicians.

The results of these studies suggest that it is important to determine which outcomes are of interest. Most studies involving EMRs use time-series techniques, in which workflow is analyzed before and after implementation of the EMR system. Most studies look at cost-effectiveness, clinical outcomes, and workflow studies (1). One recent workflow study described the implementation of an ICU EMR that had been designed to capture every mouse click and keystroke of every user over the course of one year. After analyzing this information, the researchers found that the majority of mistakes were made when first learning to use the system, and were able to modify their training programs to minimize errors. They also analyzed the workflow, and were able to maximize efficiency in the ICU by determining when physicians entered orders and when nurses subsequently implemented them.

Data Collection

Intensive care unit EMRs can include some or all of the data generated during an inpatient admission. Typically stored information includes vital signs, hemodynamic information, mechanical ventilation parameters, and laboratory data. Nursing or physician notes, medication lists, care plans, clinical pathways, and orders also may be stored. Bradshaw and colleagues found that laboratory information such as blood chemistry and blood gas results constituted the highest proportion of information that physicians used to make clinical decisions (42%). Drugs and fluid input and output were next at 22%, followed by physiologic monitoring data, which was used in only 13% of decisions (15). EMRs that store this information frequently offer trending or plotting features that make information easier to understand (e.g., charts or graphs of blood gas data or plots of cardiac output versus pulmonary capillary wedge pressure).

Data acquisition in clinical settings has been the topic of considerable research and debate. The Institute of Electric and Electronic Engineering (IEEE) has developed a standard for a medical information bus (MIB), referred to as the IEEE 1073 Standard for Medical Device Communications. The MIB is a system that allows the rapid exchange of data between up to 255 devices and provides clinicians with a relatively straightforward way to link bedside medical devices to a patient monitoring device or a computer network. This permits comprehensive data capture from devices such as infusion pumps, ventilators, and patient monitors connected to acutely ill patients. Several major pharmaceutical and medical equipment manufacturers currently support the MIB standard.

The MIB standard currently defines only the specific hardware that is used to connect devices (i.e., signal levels and connector pin designators). Languages such as HL-7 and DICOM have been developed in an effort to standardize communication between medical devices, but incompatibilities still exist. The IEEE Medical Device Communications Industry Group has developed tools to help medical device manufacturers develop standardized messaging systems. It has also developed infusion pump software that uses the IEEE 1073 standards. Despite these limitations, however, nurses in one study preferred using an MIB-controlled intravenous infusion device to a stand-alone pump or gravity-fed intravenous line (16).

Widespread adoption of the MIB standard will improve the accuracy of information stored within the medical record. Several studies have shown that information entered by health care professionals does not match information simultaneously acquired through the MIB. In one study, respiratory therapists recorded levels of inspired oxygen that were significantly lower than ventilators were set to deliver. Nurses in the same study frequently recorded a saturation that was much lower than that reported by the MIB (17). Several other studies suggest that differing kinds of information have different acceptance rates. For example, nurses in one study accepted reported values for heart rate, temperature, airway pressure, and noninvasive blood pressure more than 90% of the time, whereas respiratory rate, pulse oximetry, invasive blood pressure, and central venous blood pressure had only 75% to 90% acceptance rates (18).

Adopting An Electronic Medical Record System

The decision to implement an EMR system requires the commitment of significant levels of time and resources. It is therefore critical that the people who will use the EMR play a role in choosing and configuring the system. The most fundamental decisions

that must be made include determination of what information to acquire and store, how often to acquire it, and what checks are made as to its validity. The busy ICU environment demands a system that is intuitive and requires minimal training. The user interface is therefore of critical importance.

Comprehensive EMR systems for the ICU have been commercially available for several years and are steadily improving in quality, ease of use, and flexibility. Most systems are distributed by medical equipment manufacturers and are designed to work primarily with their equipment; nearly all of them can be adapted to work with competing manufacturers' equipment. Most systems consist of one or more dedicated servers that are connected to workstations used by clinicians for documentation and accessing the record and also are connected to physiologic monitors and medical devices. Although some systems use proprietary architecture, most commercial systems in current production use standard protocols and open systems, such as the Open Database Connectivity standard, that allow the information to be accessed by other software.

The Clinicomp International Clinical Information System (CIS) is an EMR that is designed for ambulatory, outpatient, and inpatient use. The CIS integrates current patient information and displays it at the point-of-care, at central stations, and from remote locations. It supports patient care functions, including charting, managing order entry, and analyzing data as part of a real-time clinical decision support system. The point-of-care module will work with nearly all standard bedside instruments, and it exchanges information via the HL-7 language, meaning that it can be integrated into an existing hospital information system. This system also contains a "clinical pathway administrator," which offers clinical pathways for patients with specific diagnoses. With this system, standard pathways can be designed based on the care model at a given facility. Once the system is in place, any deviations from a pathway are entered into the system as a variance linked to patient documentation. Variances are automatically tracked and reported either concurrently or retrospectively using the query capability of a data warehouse.

The Picis CareSuite is a suite of applications, including an EMR, an order entry system, a decision support tool, and a reporting system. The Chart+program is an EMR application that automatically collects, manages, integrates, and stores vital patient information required to evaluate the patient condition, to give care, and to generate the medical legal record. The system can be connected to a variety of medical devices, laboratory systems, and hospital information systems. The system also allows manual entry of vital signs, text entry, and calculation of derived parameters. The system addresses the transition from manual charting by using the Microsoft Windows interface, and working like other Windows programs. The CareSuite also offers a decision support tool called VisualCare. This system provides automatic order entry and care planning that is based on patient condition and hospital care standards. Each care standard can be customized by the hospital through a use configuration program. After an order has been entered, the VisualCare system gives the clinician the estimated cost of care prior to initiation, which the company claims can help to decrease cost.

DECISION SUPPORT SYSTEMS

As the amount of information that health care providers must assimilate and use has grown, computers have been increasingly used to aid the clinical decision-making process. In its report on patient safety, the Institute of Medicine has proposed the use of decision support systems that monitor drug allergies and interactions in an effort to decrease the likelihood of an adverse drug reaction (4). Information stored in an EMR or clinical database can be used to enhance the ability of health care providers to make decisions at the point of care. Such systems are referred to as clinical decision support systems and can offer guidelines, alerts, treatment recommendations, or access to pertinent reference materials. Decision support systems that provide timely, patient-specific information have been shown to be highly effective. A study looking at the efficacy of a computerized decision support system for mechanical ventilation demonstrated that instructions were followed 94% of the time and that patient morbidity significantly was decreased (19).

A substantial amount of information in the literature describes the design and implementation of decision support systems (20–22). Although these systems can offer various features, nearly every successful implementation has several things in common. Successful decision support systems ultimately save time while offering improved compliance with regulations and decreasing cost. The implementation of managed health care has resulted in increased patient volumes, greater demand for documentation, and fewer ancillary personnel. Any system that makes it easier for health care providers to comply with new regulations and documentation requirements while improving patient care will be well accepted.

Successful decision support systems are integrated into the existing workflow of the ICU and give patient-specific recommendations. Simply displaying guidelines that are already published in the literature will not change physician behavior (23). Systems that make information easier to understand or that offer automatic order entry dictated by clinical pathways, however, will save time, increase compliance, and may reduce costs. For example, a patient admitted to the hospital for a myocardial infarction might have most admitting orders, tests, and initial therapy generated according to specific guidelines.

Decision Support Methods

Computers can aid the decision-making process simply by presenting information in a way that makes it more usable (e.g., by creating flow sheets). The value of flow sheets in the management of chronic illness was established in a study by Whiting-O'Keefe and colleagues (24). Graphic displays of laboratory information can help physicians to place laboratory information in context and to spot trends (25). Health care providers readily accept these systems because they do not require any additional interaction, provide valuable information, and save time.

Clinical decision support systems that make treatment recommendations or offer guidelines rely on models that interpret available information about the patient (26). Some systems place reminders or suggestions into patient notes or "pop-up windows" that appear when relevant information is retrieved. Such

reminders usually consist of a short message that suggests an action, along with the clinical basis for the reminder. For example, a system might remind a physician to enter an NPO (nothing by mouth) order in a patient for whom a surgical procedure is being scheduled. They also can be integrated into order pathways (e.g., guidelines for preoperative laboratories appear when a blood test is selected as part of a preoperative order). The decision support system then can use rule-based management to decide whether the clinician needs to be notified about the critical event.

Decision support systems that provide current patient information in context to the task being performed can reduce the cost of a hospital stay by eliminating unnecessary interventions. Systems that provide this information also can reduce medication errors by warning about drug allergies, monitoring dosage limits, or alerting physicians to a drug that does not treat the patient's problem (27). One such system alerts physicians when the results of a culture and sensitivity test reveal an infection not treated by the patient's current antibiotic regimen (28). A study at the University of Indiana was able to decrease the number of tests ordered by 13% if the results of the previous test were displayed next to the current order (29).

One study demonstrated that "corollary" orders, or orders that should be considered when another one is placed, are much more likely to be ordered when presented at the time of order entry (30). Such systems typically use specific events as triggers. Decision support systems also can alert health care providers to new information that they might be otherwise unaware of, such as a "panic" laboratory value or a decision to move the patient to a higher level of care. In addition to adding alerts to the patient's chart, such systems also might send an alphanumeric page or electronic mail message.

Decision Support Technology

Decision support systems that offer recommendations for diagnosis or treatment typically use knowledge-based expert systems (31). *Expert systems* are collections of rules in the form of "if . . . then . . . else" statements and work well when a problem is easily broken down into a limited number of variables with simple interactions (32). For example, a rule regarding the dosing of phenytoin might be as follows: "If the serum level of phenytoin is less than 10, then advise the clinician to increase the dose."

More complex systems that require analysis of multiple interacting variables are not amenable to analysis by expert systems. Neural networks are an alternative method of extracting useful information from medical data. Neural networks consist of a computer program that simulates neuronal connections; neural networks are useful for pattern recognition, generalization, and trend prediction. They are fast, tolerant of imperfect data, and do not need formulas or rules. Neural networks learn by "experience"; they are trained by repeatedly presenting examples to the network. Each example includes both inputs (information that is used to make a decision) and outputs (the resulting decision, prediction, or response). The internal connections that are formed as a result of the training are poorly understood. When the results given by the neural network have reached the desired consistency with the input data, the training is complete (33).

Westenskow and colleagues used networks to analyze alarms from physiologic monitors during anesthesia and showed that they can reduce response time (34). These systems also have been used to predict patient outcome and for experimental decision support systems (35,36). Kovalerchuk and co-workers used a neural network to evaluate radiographic images of breast tumors (32). Although the software was 100% accurate on the training data, its accuracy fell to 66% when given test data.

Cost Reduction

Several studies document the ability of decision support systems to reduce costs associated with patient care (37). Gardner and colleagues analyzed the effect of an electronic pharmacy system that monitored drug reactions, laboratory studies, and allergies. In this study, only 0.7% of drug orders generated alerts, but these alerts generated a savings of $253,000 over 2 years (38). According to Bates and associates, adverse drug events increased the length of stay by 4.6 days in an ICU, and the estimated cost of these events was $4,685 (39). In another study on the effects of a decision support system on antibiotic use, Evans and colleagues developed a computer-assisted antimicrobial management system for use in the critical care unit. This system tracked patient allergies, pathogens, local patterns of antibiotic resistance, laboratory studies, and culture results. Manually assembling this information would have taken clinicians approximately 25 minutes per patient. The study showed that patients whose physicians used this system received fewer doses of antibiotic, were given fewer orders for drugs to which the patient was allergic, and had shorter lengths of stay with lower costs (40).

CLINICAL MANAGEMENT DATABASES

A clinical management database can provide systematic documentation of ICU resource utilization and performance and offers objective information about quality of care (23). Clinical management databases contain information that has been either automatically gathered by an EMR or is manually entered by data entry personnel. This information can be used for research, benchmarking, or development of decision support systems.

The ideal system would allow real-time collection of all clinical information, including physiologic, laboratory, and radiographic data, and key components of such a system are currently in development. Data dictionaries, which provide standard terms for describing medical events, terms, and conditions, will play an important role in allowing information from these databases to be shared and interpreted (41). Standard Nomenclature of Medicine (SNOMED), developed by the American College of Pathologists, is one such dictionary. Databases can be used to evaluate quality of care by recording adverse events such as readmission, hospital-acquired infections, and inadvertent extubation.

Data Mining

The widespread adoption of medical information systems offers new opportunities for extracting useful information from large observational data sets, such as information collected as part of an EMR. As computer systems have become more advanced, research in the area of knowledge discovery in databases, or data mining, has exploded. Specialized software examines this information for subtle relationships or patterns that can provide new knowledge (42,43). Specific techniques that can be used include predictive modeling, dependency modeling, and deviation detection (44).

The process of data mining is a complex process that involves many steps. The first step in the process is to define clearly the goals of the knowledge discovery process. After the goals of the process are identified, a target data set is created. The next steps involve validating the data, removing noise, developing strategies for handling missing data, selecting a hypothesis, and performing exploratory analyses. The purpose of these steps is to evaluate the selected model and mining technique and may result in modification of the original specifications. After these steps are completed, the data are mined for the variables identified in the previous steps. Specialized software then analyzes the data for patterns or relationships between the variables that have been selected, and any patterns are interpreted (45).

Data mining techniques have been used in one ICU to find shifts in patterns of infection and resistance to antimicrobial agents (46) and to study disease progression in patients with the human immunodeficiency virus (HIV) (45). Information gained from data mining techniques may lead to new scientific studies or simply to changes in the practice in a single ICU.

Benchmarking

Benchmarking, or using the data to compare outcomes of different providers, can be done by tracking sentinel events, comparing one provider to another, or comparing each provider to a predefined standard for a high-quality practice (47). This information can be used to improve the practice of individual physicians or of the entire group. One study done at Duke University found that simply alerting anesthesiologists to the cost of their techniques compared with that of their colleagues significantly decreased the use of costly medications (48). Benchmarking techniques are subject to errors introduced by differences in patient populations and by detection bias (unequal performance of measures that detect the occurrence of an outcome in two groups of patients) (23).

THE INTERNET

The Internet is a global network that connects millions of computers. Easy-to-use programs have made this technology available to nearly anyone with access to a modern computer and a modem. Many new computers come with preloaded Internet access software; when the computer is initially powered on, the user is offered the option of establishing a connection. Internet resources are accessed using a variety of computer programs referred to collectively as *Internet services*.

Electronic Mail

Electronic mail (e-mail) is a rapid, efficient method of communication, and it remains the most frequently used Internet service.

Individuals use e-mail to send messages across the Internet to a single person or to an entire group. Although e-mail originally was designed to transmit short messages containing only plain text, new e-mail systems can exchange items such as pictures and sounds and documents created by word processors or spreadsheets (49). Some e-mail servers impose limits on the size of messages that they deliver, which means that users who wish to exchange very large files (e.g., high resolution images or large databases) must use another type of Internet service such as the File Transfer Protocol.

Audio, Video, and Teleconferencing

Faster Internet connections and improved data compression techniques, combined with inexpensive hardware such as sound cards and video cameras, make it possible to send audio and video using only a desktop computer. Inexpensive teleconferencing programs allow two physicians to communicate or allow a single person to communicate with a large group. It is possible to add "streaming video" to World Wide Web (WWW) sites with software that is available for little or no cost. Internet broadcasting makes it possible to receive educational information such as lectures or make "virtual" visits to operating rooms. Physicians now use inexpensive software to hold "virtual meetings," and the use of Internet teleconferencing has been proposed to perform consultations on patients in remote locations (50,51).

WIRELESS TECHNOLOGY

Bluetooth is a short-range wireless network that has been designed to allow personal devices to communicate. An industrial consortium consisting of Ericsson, IBM, Nokia, Intel, and Toshiba developed this protocol (52). It operates in the internationally allocated Industrial, Scientific, and Medical band and offers high-speed communication within a range of approximately 10 m. The protocol is designed to work despite high levels of radiofrequency interference and uses multiple technologies to ensure data integrity, including rapid acknowledgment and forward error correction. The protocol is also designed to offer authentication and encryption at the physical layer. Bluetooth allows any device that has been added to the network to find printers or other peripherals or, for example, to allow a handheld computer to synchronize an address book with desktop computer. Medical applications of this technology may include linking monitors, infusion pumps, and computers.

For its continued widespread adoption, wireless technology must clear several hurdles. Dense coverage in the United States still is limited to major metropolitan areas, and service is limited in large buildings. Confidentiality is also a concern, because data are being transmitted over the public cellular telephone network. For this reason, most wireless data are encrypted between the device and the cellular tower. Many physicians worry about interference with physiologic monitors, infusion pumps, implantable cardioverter-defibrillators (ICDs), and cardiac pacemakers. Several studies found that, although mobile telephones may interfere with telemetry monitoring of ICDs, there are no false arrhythmia detections and that arrhythmia recognition takes place during induced ventricular fibrillation (53,54). Another study suggests that the amount of energy radiated by mobile telephones at 1 m is not sufficient to interfere with typical hospital monitoring equipment (55).

SECURITY

Every computer user should be concerned about the security of his or her computer and of information transmitted on the Internet. Fortunately, computer "hackers" represent only a small proportion of Internet users and are a small threat to most Internet users. A few simple precautions, combined with common sense, can minimize the risk of information theft or damage. Network access to personal computers should be allowed only when necessary, and computers should be protected by a carefully chosen password. A password ideally should consist of a series of letters, numerals, and punctuation marks that can be easily remembered by the owner of the computer but difficult to guess by anyone else. Passwords should be given only to persons well known to the owner of the computer and never should be sent by e-mail or posted on a WWW page.

A virus is a program that, when executed, "infects" one or more computer programs. These programs, when run, then infect other programs. Viruses can travel as part of an executable program or as part of a word processor, spreadsheet, or database file. Several new viruses are capable of attaching themselves to outgoing e-mail and infect new computers when the recipient opens and runs the attached program. Commercially available antivirus programs automatically scan information and files entering the computer for the presence of a virus and remove any virus that is found. It is advisable to use software provided by well-known sources and to open e-mail attachments only if the sender is well known to the recipient. All files should be scanned with an antivirus program before opening or using them. It is critically important to keep antivirus software updated because new viruses appear daily.

Encryption

The Internet is a "public network," meaning that it is possible for unauthorized personnel to view or even modify information as it is exchanged. It is therefore necessary to take steps to ensure the privacy (information is seen only by those intended) and authenticity (information arrives intact) of information used for critical applications such as clinical and research. Most of the time, the sheer volume of information traversing the network makes it unlikely that a specific message will be read. There are, however, tools, such as packet sniffers, that selectively filter information that is of interest to someone. Moreover, system administrators can read e-mail, and files can be viewed by other users of the same computer. For this reason, it is advisable to encrypt sensitive information or to avoid sending it over the Internet altogether.

Encryption software is relatively easy to use and is inexpensive or free. Software that uses Pretty Good Privacy (PGP) encryption technology is available free to individuals for noncommercial use and allows users to both sign and encrypt documents. It allows users to encrypt e-mail messages, data files, or even an entire hard disk using public key encryption (PKE) (56). PKE (PGP) uses two keys to encrypt and decrypt information: a private key, which is known only to its holder, and a public key, which is widely known. Information that has been encrypted with one key can be decrypted only with the other.

Users can use PGP to sign a document. When a document is signed, the encryption software does a mathematical operation on it. The results of this operation, along with information about the signer, are encrypted using the signer's private key. When the recipient feeds the signed message into his or her encryption software, the information is decrypted with the original signer's public key. This proves the authorship of the document. Next, the mathematical operation is performed on the document, and the results are compared with those in the signature. If they match, the document has arrived at its destination exactly as it was sent. In the United States, cryptographically signed documents are being accepted as legally binding.

INFORMATION-SEEKING BEHAVIOR (57–62)

Information systems in clinical settings allow researchers to explore information-seeking behavior of physicians. Physicians may not recognize all their information needs. Although educational researchers have developed electronic information systems that attempt to solve this problem, few ever progress beyond the demonstration phase. One possible reason for this is that physicians use information differently than many other groups. Because they must convert theoretic information into a series of tasks, simply presenting a list of facts may not be helpful. Moreover, nonphysicians, who may not understand how a physician approaches a given problem, often design these systems. For this reason, accurate models of how physicians use information are necessary to ensure continued use of information systems.

The information collected by information resources can help teachers to develop better educational materials because Internet users frequently "browse" for information when they recognize a need but cannot precisely identify it. By analyzing log files of a medical Internet resource, for example, it may be possible to determine the information needs of its users. This allows the developer of the resource to add more information on popular topics or to move important information to a location where it can be more easily accessed. It might ultimately be possible to infer the processes that physicians use to find information by examining how they follow hyperlinks or phrase queries to a search engine. Internet medical resources may help to improve all forms of medical education by giving teachers a better understanding of the information needs of physicians.

Information that is used by physicians may be classified into several types: *Unrecognized* needs refer to information that the physician is unaware that he does not know and that must be inferred by measurement of knowledge or finding errors in patient care. The clinician articulates recognized needs. *Pursued* needs refer to knowledge for which information-seeking behavior is observed. Unfortunately, little is known about how physicians choose to pursue a given area of knowledge. *Satisfied* needs refer to information for which pursuit has been successful.

Information systems in the ICU allow collection of information and possible understanding of how physicians use information. Information can be collected by analyzing log files or by direct observation. It is possible that use of hyperlinks or specific search phrases may represent thought processes, which ultimately might allow researchers to determine the information needs of entire groups or specific physicians.

SUMMARY

The science of medical informatics is becoming increasingly important in clinical practice as well as medical education and research. Electronic medical records and decision support systems can provide the information necessary for health care professionals to make decisions in critically ill patients. Information technology also offers educators new ways of determining what information physicians really need. It is clear that medical informatics will continue to play an important role in the critical care environment.

KEY POINTS

Information technology continues to explode. This rapid expansion limits our ability to maintain up-to-date material in a fixed reference such as a textbook. This chapter provides a framework that reviews the basics of the electronic medical record (EMR), with its advantages and applications to the practice of critical care. The EMR facilitates access to enhanced record keeping and tracking. This tool can be used securely by multiple individuals simultaneously from various access portals. It is also useful for data collection, correlation, and application for quality improvement and investigation purposed.

The use of decision-making techniques and algorithms will continue to grow. It is crucial for clinicians to be involved in development and review of these electronic pathways. Feed-back and refinement will enhance the utility of these systems. In addition, information can be shared locally or over long distances using the Internet and innovations in audio, video, and teleconferencing.

Information systems increasingly will come into play as a means to readily provide physician pertinent data to practitioners. This will allow us to know what we know, know what we need to know, alert us to important, potentially unrecognized information, and gain these insights in a timely and secure fashion.

Information technology is here to stay, is rapidly expanding, and will continue to impact on the quality of care for intensivists and our patients.

REFERENCES

1. Tierney WM, Overhage JM, McDonald C. Demonstrating the effects of an IAIMS on health care quality and cost. *J Am Med Inform Assoc* 1997;S41–S46.

2. Institute of Medicine, Committee on Improving the Medical Record. *The computer-based patient record: an essential technology for health care.* Washington, DC: National Academy Press, 1991.

3. Tufo HM, Speidel JJ. Problems with medical records. *Med Care* 1971;9:509–517.

4. Kohn LT, Corrigan JM, Donaldson MS, eds. Committee on Quality of Health Care in America, Institute of Medicine. *To err is human: building a safer health system.* Washington, DC: National Academy Press, 1999: 312 pp.

5. Rind DM, Safran C, Phillips RS, et al. Effect of computer-based alerts on the treatment and outcomes of hospitalized patients. *Arch Intern Med* 1994;154:1511–1517.

6. Hsia DC. Accuracy of Medicare reimbursement for cardiac arrest. *JAMA* 1990;264:59–62.

7. Hsia DC, Ahern CA, Ritchie BP, et al. Medicare reimbursement accuracy under the prospective payment system, 1985 to 1988. *JAMA* 1992;268:896–899.

8. Pierpont GL, Thilgen D. Effect of computerized charting on nursing activity in intensive care. *Crit Care Med* 1995;23:1067–1073.

9. Allen D, Davis M. A computerized CIS enhances bedside intensive care. *Nurs Manage* 1992;23:112I–112J,112N,112P.

10. Andrews RD, Gardner RM, Metcalf SM, et al. Computer charting: an evaluation of a respiratory care computer system. *Respir Care* 1985;30:695–707.

11. Birch and Davis Associates, Inc. Clinical information system benefits assessment study final report for the Composite Health Care System II benefits assessment study for the clinical information system Phase II. DOD Contract no. DASW01-95-D-0026, Washington, DC, 1998.

12. Gardner RM, Lundsgaarde HP. Evaluation of user acceptance of a clinical expert system. *J Am Med Inform Assoc* 1994;1:428–438.

13. Tierney WM, Overhage JM, McDonald CJ, et al. Medical students' and housestaff's opinions of computerized order-writing. *Acad Med* 1994;69:386–389.

14. McDonald CJ, Overhage JM, Tierney WM, et al. The Regenstrief Medical Record System: a quarter century experience. *Int J Med Inform* 1999;54:225–253.

15. Bradshaw KE, Gardner RM, Clemmer TP, et al. Physician decision-making—evaluation of data used in a computerized ICU. *Int J Clin Monit Comput* 1984;1:81–91.

16. Dalto JD, Johnson KV, Gardner RM, et al. Medical Information Bus usage for automated IV pump data acquisition: evaluation of usage patterns. *Int J Clin Monit Comput* 1997;14:151–154.

17. Gardner RM, Hawley WL, East TD, et al. Real time data acquisition: recommendations for the Medical Information Bus (MIB). *Int J Clin Monit Comput* 1991–1992;8:251–258.

18. Friesdorf W, Konichezky S, Gross-Alltag F, et al. Data quality of bedside monitoring in an intensive care unit. *Int J Clin Monit Comput* 1994;11:123–128.

19. East TD, Heermann LK, Bradshaw RL, et al. Efficacy of computerized decision support for mechanical ventilation: results of a prospective multi-center randomized trial. *Proc AMIA Symp* 1999; 251–255.

20. Callan K. Preparing for a decision support system. *Top Health Inf Manage* 2000;21:84–90.

21. Rivers JA, Rivers PA. The ABCs for deciding on a decision support system in the health care industry. *J Health Hum Serv Adm* 2000;22:346–353.

22. Heermann LK, Thompson CB, East TD. Clinical informatics case study: computerized protocols for ventilator management in ARDS patients: case study. *Comput Nurs* 1999;17:247–250.

23. Cowen JS. The Clinical Management Database. *Crit Care Clin* 1999;15:481–497.

24. Whiting-O'Keefe QE, Simborg DW, Epstein WV, et al. A computerized summary medical record system can provide more information than the standard medical record. *JAMA* 1985;254:1185–1192.

25. Powsner SM, Tufte ER. Graphical summary of patient status. *Lancet* 1994;344:386–389.

26. Shiffman RN. Representation of clinical practice guidelines in conventional and augmented decision tables. *J Am Med Inform Assoc* 1997;4:382–393.

27. Payne TH, Savarino J, Marshall R, Hoey CT. Use of a clinical event monitor to prevent and detect medication errors. *Proc AMIA Annu Symp* 2000;20(Suppl):640–644.

28. Payne TH. Computer decision support systems. *Chest* 2000;118: 47S–52S.

29. Tierney WM, McDonald CJ, Hui SL, et al. Computer predictions of abnormal test results: effects on outpatient testing. *JAMA* 1988;259:1194–1198.

30. Overhage JM, Tierney WM, Zhou XH, et al. A randomized trial of "corollary orders" to prevent errors of omission. *J Am Med Inform Assoc* 1997;4:364–375.

31. Sado AS. Electronic medical record in the intensive care unit. *Crit Care Clin* 1999;15:499–522.

32. Kovalerchuk B, Vityaev E, Ruiz JF. Consistent knowledge discovery in medical diagnosis. *IEEE Eng Med Biol Mag* 2000;19:26–37.

33. Lawrence J. *Introduction to neural networks,* 5 ed. Nevada City, CA: California Scientific Software, 1998.

34. Westenskow DR, Orr JA, Simon FH, et al. Intelligent alarms reduce anesthesiologist's response time to critical faults. *Anesthesiology* 1992;77:1074–1079.

35. Dombi GW, Nandi P, Saxe JM, et al. Prediction of rib fracture injury outcome by an artificial neural network. *J Trauma* 1995;39:915–921.

36. Frye KE, Izenberg SD, Williams MD. Simulated biologic intelligence used to predict length of stay and survival of burns. *J Burn Care Rehabil* 1996;17(6 Pt 1):540–546.

37. Bates DW, Teich JM, Lee J, et al. The impact of computerized physician order entry on medication error prevention. *J Am Med Inform Assoc* 1999;6:313–321.

38. Gardner RM, Hulse RK, Larsen KG. Assessing the effectiveness of a computerized pharmacy system. In: *Proc Annu Symp Comput Appl Med Care.* Washington, DC, 1990.

39. Bates DW, Spell N, Cullen DJ, et al. The costs of adverse drug events in hospitalized patients. Adverse Drug Events Prevention Study Group. *JAMA* 1997;277:307–311.

40. Evans RS, Larsen RA, Burke JP, et al. Computer surveillance of hospital-acquired infections and antibiotic use. *JAMA* 1986;256:1007–1011.

41. Linnarsson R, Wigertz O. The data dictionary—a controlled vocabulary for integrating clinical databases and medical knowledge bases. *Methods Inf Med* 1989;28:78–85.

42. Babic A. Knowledge discovery for advanced clinical data management and analysis. *Stud Health Technol Inform* 1999;68:409–413.

43. Prather JC, Lobach DF, Goodwin LK, et al. Medical data mining: knowledge discovery in a clinical data warehouse. *Proc AMIA Annu Fall Symp* 1997:101–105.

44. Lavrac N. Selected techniques for data mining in medicine. *Artif Intell Med* 1999;16:3–23.

45. Ramirez JC, Cook DJ, Peterson LL, et al. Temporal pattern discovery in course-of-disease data. *IEEE Eng Med Biol Mag* 2000;19:63–71.

46. Moser SA, Jones WT, Brossette SE. Application of data mining to intensive care unit microbiologic data. *Emerg Infect Dis* 1999;5:454–457.

47. Higgins MS. Data management for a perioperative medicine practice. *Anesthesiol Clin North Am* 2000;18:647–661.

48. Lubarsky DA, Sanderson IC, Gilbert WC, et al. Using an anesthesia information management system as a cost containment tool: description and validation. *Anesthesiology* 1997;86:1161–1169.

49. Levine JR, Baroudi C, Young M. *The Internet for dummies,* 6th ed. Foster City, California: IDG Books Worldwide, 1999.

50. Ruskin KJ, Palmer TEA, Hagenouw RRPM, et al. Internet teleconferencing as a clinical tool for anesthesiologists. *J Clin Monit Comput* 1998;14:183–189.

51. Palmer TEA, Cumpston PHV, Ruskin KJ, et al. WCALive: broadcasting a major medical conference on the Internet. *Int J Clin Mon Comput* 1997;14:209–216.

52. Bluetooth Special Interest Group. http://www.bluetooth.com. Accessed October 10, 2001.

53. Occhetta E, Plebani L, Bortnik M, et al. Implantable cardioverter defibrillators and cellular telephones: is there any interference? *Pacing Clin Electrophysiol* 1999;22:983–989.

54. Fetter JG, Ivans V, Benditt DG, Collins J. Digital cellular telephone interaction with implantable cardioverter-defibrillators. *J Am Coll Cardiol* 1998;31:623–628.

55. Robinson MP, Flintoft ID, Marvin AC. Interference to medical equipment from mobile phones. *J Med Eng Technol* 1997;21:141–146.

56. Pretty Good Privacy. http://www.pgp.com. Accessed October 10, 2001.

57. Barnett GO. Information technology and medical education. *J Am Med Inform Assoc* 1995;2:285–291.

58. D'Alessandro MP, Nguyen BC, D'Alessandro DM. Information needs and information seeking behaviors of on-call radiology residents. *Acad Radiol* 1999;6:16–21.

59. Haug JD. Physicians' preferences for information sources: a meta-analytic study. *Bull Med Libr Assoc* 1997;85:223–232.

60. Hernandez-Borges. Assessing the relative quality of anesthesiology and critical care medicine Internet mailing lists. *Anesth Analg* 1999;89:520–525.

61. Impicciatore P, Pandolfini C, Casella N, et al. Reliability of health information for the public on the world wide web: systematic survey of advice on managing fever in children at home. *BMJ* 1997;314:1875–1878.

62. Rotman BL, Sullivan AN, McDonald TW et al. A randomized controlled trial of a computer-based physician workstation in an outpatient setting: Implementation barriers to outcome evaluation. *JAMA* 1996;3:340–348.

MANAGEMENT OF THE AIRWAY AND TRACHEAL INTUBATION

MICHAEL F. O'CONNOR
ANDRANIK OVASSAPIAN

KEY WORDS

- Intubation
- Difficult airway
- Fiberoptic intubation
- Complications
- Laryngeal mask airway
- Extubation
- Reintubation
- ASA difficult airway algorithm
- Pharmacologic preparation
- Airway management
- Equipment list
- Indications for intubation

INTRODUCTION

Tracheal intubation is one of the most common lifesaving procedures performed in the intensive care unit (ICU). It is imperative that ICU physicians have a clear understanding of the indications for tracheal intubation, the issues surrounding the assessment of the patient, the tools and techniques used, and the consequences and complications of tracheal intubation. Although airway management is taught as a part of advanced cardiac life support (ACLS), certain considerations apply to its conduct in the ICU that differ from ACLS rescue situations. Similarly, although anesthesia personnel are taught airway management in the operating room (OR), some important issues are commonly encountered in critically ill patients but not in the OR.

INDICATIONS FOR INTUBATION

The decision to intubate the patient is no longer a simple, straightforward decision because noninvasive ventilation has been used in almost every type of respiratory failure and has been documented to improve outcome. Studies have been reported that support the use of noninvasive ventilation for every major cause of respiratory failure, including acute respiratory distress syndrome (ARDS), pneumonia, congestive heart failure (CHF), chronic obstructive pulmonary disease (COPD), and asthma (1–7). Intubation increasingly represents the conversion of a patient's airway and does not constitute the beginning of artificial or mechanical ventilation. Patients who fail noninvasive ventilation are likely to be more hypoxic, more hypercarbic, more hypotensive, and have a higher risk of mortality from both their underlying disease and interventional airway management. Hence, the decision to intubate a patient now depends more than ever on the judgment of the physicians assessing the patient (Table 1). Most experienced clinicians are able to synthesize the clinical and laboratory information and make a reasonable decision regarding the necessity for intubation.

In the setting of unfavorable airway anatomy of any cause, two decisions need to be made when the patient is evaluated: (a) Does this patient require an artificial airway? and (b) Does this patient require endotracheal intubation or tracheostomy? It may be difficult or impossible to succeed in translaryngeal intubation in patients with facial trauma, unstable cervical spines, small mandibles, airway tumors, severe edema, or hematomas. Preparation for tracheostomy should commence simultaneously with preparation for translaryngeal intubation in patients judged to be difficult and at high risk for failed intubation.

ASSESSING THE PATIENT BEFORE INTUBATION

All patients being evaluated for tracheal intubation should be treated with the highest fraction of inspired oxygen (FIO_2) obtainable in a closely monitored setting. Monitoring should include pulse oximetry, electrocardiogram (ECG), and frequent assessment of both blood pressure and respiratory effort. Blood gas analysis should be performed as indicated.

Patients who require urgent intubation also require rapid assessment of their underlying medical conditions and airway anatomy (Tables 2 and 3). Of the coexisting medical conditions, the possible presence of increased intracranial pressure or increased risk of intracranial bleeding is the most important to ascertain. Equal attention should be given to airway management and avoiding severe hypotension and increases in intracranial pressure. Whereas most airway manipulation in the ICU may be done safely with the patient awake, patients with elevated intracranial pressure and increased risk for intracranial hemorrhage may be best managed with intravenous general anesthesia.

TABLE 1. INDICATIONS FOR TRACHEAL INTUBATION

Airway support
  Diminished mental status/decreased ability to maintain airway and
    clear secretions (e.g., new quadriplegic, hepatic encephalopathy)
  Compromised airway anatomy (e.g., edema)
  Diminished airway reflexes, full stomach, and fluctuating
    consciousness (general anesthesia, drug overdose)
  Requirement for sedation in circumstances where airway control
    may not be easy to establish (e.g., CT, MRI)
  Pharyngeal instability (e.g., facial fractures)

Pulmonary disease
  Acute hypoxic respiratory failure (high and low pressure edema)
  Hypoventilation (including CNS causes and weakness)
  Lung disease with a work of breathing which exceeds the patient's
    ability to breathe (e.g., severe obstruction or restriction of any
    cause)

Circulatory
  Cardiopulmonary arrest
  Refractory or unresuscitated shock
  Sepsis

Other
  Elevated ICP requiring treatment
  Transportation of a patient at risk for deterioration

CT, computerized tomogram; MRI, magnetic resonance image; CNS, central
nervous system; ICP, intracranial pressure.

Laryngoscopy and tracheal intubation frequently provoke myocardial ischemia in at risk patients. Adequate topical or intravenous anesthesia can attenuate or obliterate the usual out-
pouring of catecholamines in response to laryngoscopy and the
myocardial ischemia associated with it. Inadequate anesthesia
can result in ischemia and arrhythmias. The use of intravenous
agents in this setting is fraught with hazard and high-risk tradeoffs. Insufficient intravenous agent can be associated with an

TABLE 2. MEDICAL EVALUATION FOR INTUBATION

Neurologic
  Elevated ICP
  Presence of intracranial bleed, AVM, or aneurysm
  Cervical spine pathology

Cardiovascular
  Ischemia, hypovolemia, history of MI, CHF, dysrhythmias
  Drug allergies

Pulmonary
  Severity of hypoxia, obstruction

Aspiration risk
  NPO status
  Morbid obesity
  Impaired gastric emptying/gastroparesis
  Pregnancy

Coagulation
  Thrombocytopenia, anticoagulant therapy, coagulopathy
  Recent or anticipated therapy with thrombolytics

Contraindications to succinylcholine
  Extensive burns, crush injuries, spinal cord injuries, malignant
    hyperthermia

ICP, intracranial pressure; AVM, arteriovenous malfunction; MI, myocardial
infarction; CHF, congestive heart failure.

TABLE 3. ANATOMIC CONDITIONS ASSOCIATED WITH DIFFICULT RIGID LARYNGOSCOPY

Poor mouth opening
Temporomandibular dysfunction
Receding mandible
Short thyromental distance
Mallampati class III and IV
Limited extension of the head at the base of the skull
Cervical instability
Supraglottic cyst
Obesity
Short, thick neck
Tumor and infections
Trauma
Pregnancy

increase in catecholamine release and myocardial ischemia. Excessive medication can result in hypotension, ischemia, vital organ hypoperfusion, and decreased rate of redistribution of the
offending agent. The use of intravenous agents is especially precarious in patients with decreased systolic function or valve
dysfunction.

Patients with severe respiratory failure may become hypoxic
very quickly during airway manipulation or when their respiratory efforts diminish or are ineffective. The more severe the
pulmonary pathology, the less likely ventilation with an Ambu
bag and mask is to be successful in maintaining adequate oxygenation. Typically, the use of a face mask and Ambu bag cannot
generate the level of pressures necessary to ventilate patients with
pulmonary edema or severe bronchospasm.

Aspiration is a major complication of airway manipulation
in the ICU. Critically ill patients typically have full stomachs.
The actual contents of the stomach differ but may include blood
(upper gastrointestinal hemorrhage), acid (stress gastritis), or bacteria (patients on histamine [H_2] blockers or proton pump inhibitors). Diabetic gastroparesis, pregnancy, and morbid obesity
all impair gastric emptying and increase the potential for aspiration. Cricoid pressure (the Sellick maneuver) should be performed whenever possible on patients undergoing airway manipulation in the ICU.

Coagulopathy is a relative contraindication to nasal intubation
and techniques associated with a risk of bleeding, such as transtracheal injection of anesthesia, superior laryngeal nerve blocks, and
retrograde intubation techniques. Nasal intubation is also contraindicated for immunosuppressed patients (e.g., on high-dose
steroids or immunosuppressants or with marked leukopenia), for
patients with complex facial injuries (e.g., basilar skull or crib-
riform plate fracture), and for any patient with a cerebral spinal
fluid leak.

Various anatomic conditions are well known to make laryngoscopy and intubation more difficult (Table 3). The American
Society of Anesthesiologists (ASA) recently incorporated into its
difficult airway algorithm a concise but thorough plan for airway assessment that many practitioners will find useful; however,
a thorough evaluation will fail to identify all the patients who
will be difficult to intubate (7a). Furthermore, details of some
of the bedside assessments in these patients are controversial. Patients with a supraglottic cyst or lingual tonsil hyperplasia will be

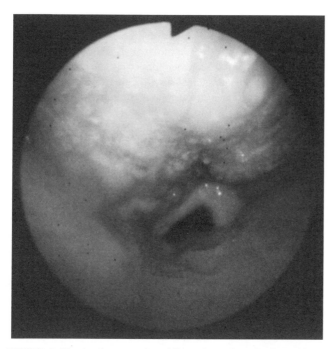

FIGURE 1. Massive hypertrophy of lingual tonsil at the base of the tongue has pushed the epiglottis posteriorly against the posterior pharyngeal wall. This interfered with the rigid laryngoscopic exposure of the glottis and caused failure of tracheal intubation. Face mask ventilation in this patient was satisfactory, but in some it could also be associated with impossible face mask ventilation.

TABLE 4. EQUIPMENT LIST FOR AIRWAY MANAGEMENT

Emergency ventilation
  Ventilation with Ambu bag
    or Jackson Reese set with
    face mask
  Oral and nasal airways
  Laryngeal mask airway
  Combitube
  Transtracheal jet ventilation

Emergency intubation
  Rigid laryngoscope (various sizes
    of curved and straight blades)
  Flexible fiberoptic bronchoscope
  Intubating laryngeal mask
  Blind nasal tube
  Light wand
  Retrograde intubation

Monitors
  Pulse oximeter
  Blood pressure
  Electrocardiography
  A means to measure
    end-tidal carbon dioxide

Drugs
  Resuscitation medications
  Topical anesthetics
    Lidocaine cream
    Lidocaine spray
  Muscle relaxants
  Antisialagogue

Other supplies and equipment
  Endotracheal tubes of
    different sizes
  Stylet
  Magill forceps
  Tape
  Suction with Yankauer tip
  Syringes
  Stethoscope
  Fiberoptic intubating airway
  Bronchoscopy swivel adapter
  O_2 delivery nasal cannula

difficult to intubate despite apparently normal airway assessment results (Fig. 1). History of difficulty with previous intubations is vital information but usually is not available in urgent circumstances. The possibility of a difficult airway makes asleep techniques for securing the airway more dangerous and makes awake, sedated, spontaneously breathing techniques more desirable. It also increases the attractiveness of techniques such as blind nasal and fiberoptic intubation. Tracheostomy may be the airway technique of choice in the patient with major airway or facial trauma, advanced airway tumors, or infections.

EQUIPMENT

Most airway manipulations can be accomplished using a very small subset of the available equipment listed in Table 4. Boxes or bags with such equipment can be stored throughout the hospital or ICU to be readily accessible to physicians or others tasked with managing an airway under urgent circumstances. A cart that is fully stocked with all the equipment required to manage a difficult airway should be available for airway management in the ICU. It is important that the box or bag is stocked and the equipment checked by the person who is to use it. It may be necessary in some institutions to place equipment and supplies under lock and key to prevent misuse or loss of vital equipment. Equipment should be checked regularly and restocked after every use. This practice allows the airway manager to devote attention to the patient during airway manipulation and not be distracted by equipment checks or preparation.

There is increasing evidence that the microaspiration of secretions around the cuff of the endotracheal tube may be a major cause of ventilator-associated pneumonia (VAP) and that the suctioning of subglottic secretions can significantly reduce the incidence of VAP or delay its onset (3–7, 8–11). Endotracheal tubes designed to facilitate this, such as the EVAC tube, are increasingly used for patients who are likely to require intubation for several days or longer. Endotracheal tubes of this or similar design are likely to become the standard of care for patients who require extended mechanical ventilation. Adequate cuff inflation is also increasingly recognized as an important factor in preventing VAP (10). Devices are being tested that ensure cuff inflation to pressures sufficient to prevent aspiration (12). Finally, there is evidence that the endotracheal tube itself may be a reservoir of bacteria (13). Endotracheal tubes with antimicrobial coatings may be developed to limit this problem. The era when patients in the ICU and emergency department (ED) were intubated with the same kinds of endotracheal tubes as those in the OR may be passing.

PREPARATION OF PATIENT

Experienced operators can manage most airways in the ICU with topical or local anesthesia alone. Pharmacologic preparation is used to allow safe and effective laryngoscopy and attenuate the discomfort associated with airway manipulation and its attendant hemodynamic and endocrine consequences. Many operators induce intravenous general anesthesia to facilitate establishment of the airway. This practice is safe in the setting of straightforward airway anatomy but is hazardous as conditions become less favorable.

A combination of drying agents and local anesthetic can be used to prepare the airway. Glycopyrrolate 0.2 to 0.4 mg is commonly used to dry the mouth to facilitate direct laryngoscopy.

Local anesthetic spray, including benzocaine 20% and lidocaine 4%, can be used to provide topical anesthesia of the airway. Lidocaine cream (5%) also can be smeared over the base of the tongue to accomplish oropharyngeal anesthesia. Because lidocaine is readily absorbed by the mucous membranes, care should be taken to avoid excessive doses (i.e., >6 mg/kg). As a consequence of co-oximeter incorporation in blood gas machines, benzocaine is increasingly recognized as a cause of methemoglobinemia when used to facilitate airway management. Techniques such as the superior laryngeal nerve block are not generally necessary in most ICU patients.

The use of sedatives will not significantly increase the success rate of relatively inexperienced or undertrained practitioners. A recent study demonstrated that the use of midazolam did not increase the success rate of paramedics intubating the trachea (14). Sivilotti and Ducharme performed a retrospective review of their experience using intravenous agents to facilitate airway management in the ED and found that thiopental was associated with hypotension, midazolam was associated with a delay in securing the airway, and fentanyl was associated with greater cardiovascular stability (15). Recent literature also suggests that some benefit may be gained by using etomidate to facilitate tracheal intubation in these circumstances, although no controlled trials have compared it with any of its alternatives (16).

The use of intravenous agents to facilitate tracheal intubation in the ICU is fraught with hazard. Hypovolemia, myocardial dysfunction, and shock are frequently present at the time of intubation, and doses of intravenous agents that are well tolerated by healthy patients can precipitate circulatory collapse, converting a serious situation into a desperate one. General anesthesia can be induced with as little as 50 mg of thiopental or 100 mg of lidocaine in patients with shock. Intravenous agents such as midazolam, fentanyl, thiopental, etomidate, propofol, and ketamine should be used only by experienced practitioners who can estimate what the appropriate dose may be.

NEUROMUSCULAR BLOCKING AGENTS

The neuromuscular blocking agent (NMBA) of choice for airway management outside the OR remains succinylcholine. This preference is reflected in the literature, which describes its widespread use in both the ICU and the ED (17–22). A single study suggests that the use of nondepolarizing agents may be associated with an increased risk of difficulty in obtaining an airway compared with succinylcholine, and hence their use should be avoided if possible (22). Some might advocate rapacuronium as the agent of choice in settings outside the OR, but hypotension associated with its use may make it undesirable in patients with coronary artery disease or hypotension from other causes (23).

Well-trained practitioners report success rates in the range of 94% to 99% when they use succinylcholine to facilitate tracheal intubation outside the OR (18–22). This range represents a failure rate of 1% to 6%, which is much higher than would be acceptable in the more elective setting of the OR. It is not clear what role NMBAs play in producing either success or failure in these reports. There are no prospective, randomized, or controlled studies that address this issue; hence, the question remains unanswered. A variety of useful benchmarks can be derived from these series. Approximately 70% of intubations will be done by rapid sequence induction, and 8% to 10% of intubations will be classified as difficult. More than 25% of patients will require more than one attempt at laryngoscopy; the success rate will be in the range of 94% to 99%, and 1% of patients will require cricothyroidotomy or a tracheostomy (17–21).

The use of paralytics to facilitate airway management outside the OR remains controversial. Once these agents are administered, it is imperative that a definitive airway be obtained within minutes. Attempts at ventilating most patients with respiratory failure with an Ambu bag and mask are difficult and frequently futile because the underlying decreased compliance of the lung or increased airway resistance makes it difficult or impossible to maintain adequate oxygenation. The impulse of inexperienced operators to attempt to use intravenous agents, including paralytics, to compensate for lack of confidence and skill should be strongly discouraged.

PROCEDURES FOR INTUBATION

Face-mask ventilation is commonly applied to improve oxygenation before intubation in the ICU, but it requires an advanced degree of understanding to realize its potential in this setting. Proper fit of the mask to the face is crucial to success; hence, masks of several different sizes should be available to airway managers. One of the most common mistakes is to push the mask into the mandible, which causes displacement of the tongue posteriorly, which in turn usually occludes the airway. Although an oral airway can be used to compensate for this, most experienced practitioners prefer to position the head in the sniffing position (head extended at the occiput) and pull the mandible into the mask, displacing the tongue anteriorly and opening up the hypopharyngeal airway. Ventilation with high pressures (>20 cm H_2O) usually opens the esophagus and result in gastric insufflation. This is undesirable because it both diverts ventilation from the lungs and increases the risk of aspiration. An oral airway may facilitate mask ventilation in edentulous patients by elongating the cheeks and increasing their tension and rigidity, which, in turn, improves the fit of the mask. When face-mask ventilation is difficult or impossible, other techniques for ventilation, such as classic laryngeal mask airway (LMA), Combitube, or jet ventilation, should be considered if tracheal intubation has failed (Figs. 2 and 3; Table 4).

Critically ill patients tend to desaturate quickly for a variety of reasons: lung pathology, decreased functional residual capacity (FRC), and increased metabolic rate, to name a few. Nonetheless, these patients do benefit from preoxygenation and mask ventilation, and all patients should be preoxygenated as time and circumstance allow.

Patients in cardiopulmonary arrest require no drug therapy to facilitate intubation, and intubation is relatively straightforward in these patients because they are typically unconscious and relatively flaccid. Direct laryngoscopy should be attempted immediately, and the appropriate size endotracheal tube should be

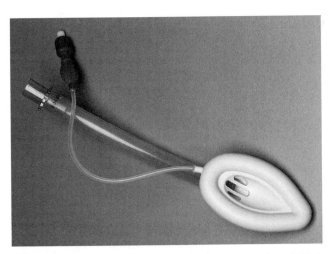

FIGURE 2. Laryngeal mask airway (LMA). The classic LMA is available in six different sizes that can be used. They range from neonates to large adults. It has gained wide recognition in airway management. Its role in difficult or impossible face mask ventilation is well established and has multiple applications in the American Society of Anesthesiologists' Difficult Airway Guideline algorithm published in 1993.

inserted into the trachea. Many patients will have large amounts of oral secretions or aspirated or gastric contents prior to or after their cardiopulmonary arrest and therefore will require suctioning of secretions to clear the airway and obtain adequate visualization of the glottis. Patients receiving cardiopulmonary resuscitation (CPR) typically do not deliver much carbon dioxide to their lungs. Hence, attempts to confirm tracheal intubation with CO_2 monitors are frequently futile. Cervical instability is one coexisting condition that might delay securing the airway of a patient receiving CPR and may mandate immediate tracheostomy.

Several studies published over the past several years have added substance to the controversy over oral versus nasal intubation route. Nasally intubated patients have a lower risk of self-extubation compared with orally intubated patients (24,25). The incidence of VAP is lower for patients who are orally intubated, as is the incidence of sinusitis (26,27). The incidence of both sinusitis and VAP appears to be reduced by aggressively diagnosing and treating maxillary sinusitis in nasally intubated patients (27).

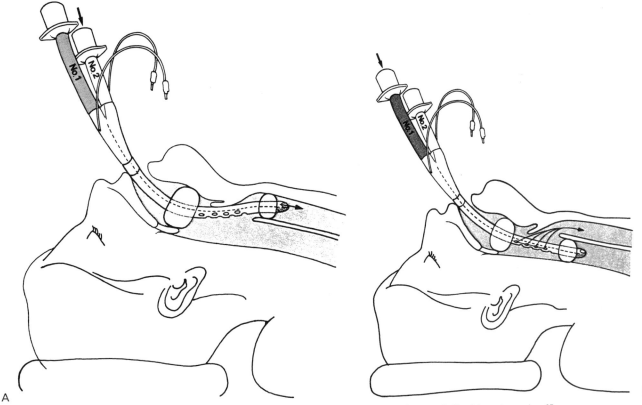

FIGURE 3. A: Combitube in esophagus. This double lumen tube with a small distal (esophageal cuff) and a large proximal (pharyngeal) cuff is designed for blind placement in the esophagus to ventilate the lungs when other techniques of establishing ventilation have failed. Inflation of the distal small cuff blocks the esophagus and prevents air entry into the stomach. Inflation of the pharyngeal cuff prevents air leak from the mouth and nose. Ventilation is provided through several side perforations of tube no. 1 positioned in the pharynx. **B:** Combitube positioned in the trachea. In this position, the distal cuff of tube no. 2 seals the trachea like an endotracheal tube. Ventilation is provided through tube no. 2 positioned inside the trachea. Inflation of the pharyngeal cuff makes the tube more stable and accidental dislodgment less likely. Combitube in either esophageal or tracheal position can be used for artificial ventilation, eliminating the need for further attempts at intubation. (Reprinted by permission from ref. 32a.)

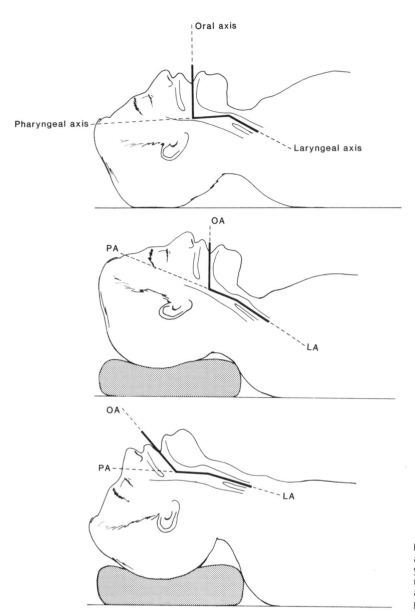

FIGURE 4. Position of the head during rigid laryngoscopy and intubation of trachea. The three axes of trachea, pharynx and oral cavity are brought more nearly into alignment using the sniffing position (flexion of cervical spine and extension of the atlantooccipital joint). (Reprinted by permission from ref. 27a.)

Orotracheal Intubation with a Rigid Laryngoscope

Most tracheal intubations in the ICU are accomplished via the oral route using a rigid laryngoscope. Its popularity is a consequence of both the comfort most operators have with it and the relative ease with which it is accomplished in many patients (27a) (Fig. 4). It can be accomplished using topical anesthesia alone or after induction of general anesthesia. Disadvantages of oral intubation include the stimulation of the gag reflex with laryngoscopy during awake intubation, risk of dental and cervical trauma, difficulty in securing the tube, limitations in maintaining oral hygiene, and problems with patients biting and occluding the tube.

For intubation with the patient under topical anesthesia, the oropharynx can be prepared with drying agents and topical anesthetics. The importance of the oral airway as a way to deliver lidocaine jelly and topical anesthetic spray to the retropharynx is emphasized because it is the quality of the hypopharyngeal anesthesia that allows direct awake laryngoscopy to be performed. Once the patient has been intubated, it is imperative to hold the tube firmly in place until it has been secured. Oral endotracheal tubes must be secured with at least tape and may be wired to secure teeth in circumstances where the use of tape is undesirable or impossible. Patients who are biting the endotracheal tube and cannot be adequately sedated may benefit from the placement of a bite block. This may be associated with substantial dental damage, however, if vigorous biting attempts continue.

Nasotracheal Intubation

Nasal intubation can be accomplished with the patient's head in a neutral position or traction and with the patient sitting bolt-upright in bed. Blind nasal and fiberoptic nasal intubations are readily accomplished in patients with air hunger. Blind nasal intubation is less likely to be successful in the patient making minimal or no respiratory efforts. Nasal endotracheal tubes are easy to secure, allow free access to the mouth, and cannot be occluded by biting. Disadvantages to nasal intubation include increased length of the endotracheal tube; trauma to the nasal mucosa, septum, and turbinates; and risk of purulent or serous otitis and sinusitis (27–29). Coagulopathy [including thrombocytopenia, platelet dysfunction, disseminated intravascular coagulopathy (DIC), and anticoagulation as indicated by the prothrombin time (PT) and partial thromboplastin time (PTT)], immunocompromise, and suspected or known base of skull trauma are all relative contraindications to nasal intubation. Nasal intubation can be performed blindly with direct laryngoscopy or fiberoptically with a bronchoscope. Whenever possible, an 8.0-mm endotracheal tube should be used for nasal intubation because it has low resistance and is large enough to allow bronchoscopy to be performed (30). Tubes designed specifically for blind nasal intubation, such as the Endotrol tube, are preferable to regular tubes in most patients.

Nasal intubation can be successfully performed with topical anesthesia alone in most patients. In most settings, cocaine or a combination of phenylephrine and lidocaine mixture is used for topical anesthesia (31). A nasal trumpet lubricated with lidocaine jelly can be used to provide topical anesthesia to the nose and to direct a local anesthetic spray at the vocal cords. Once the nose has been prepared, an appropriately sized tube, lubricated with lidocaine jelly, is introduced into the nasal passage and advanced with inspiration. Attempts to advance the tube in the face of substantial resistance are associated with mucosal lacerations, polypectomies, turbinectomies, crushed nasal septum, and tunneling of the endotracheal tube underneath the mucosa, all of which can be associated with spectacular bleeding. Trauma associated with failed attempts may increase the risk of subsequent infection (32). Nasotracheal intubation guided by laryngoscopy is undertaken in some patients (more commonly in the OR than the ICU). Magill intubating forceps are used to direct the tube through the glottis under direct visualization. During blind nasal intubation, the sensation of the tube popping through the cords, followed by efforts at a cough by the patient, suggests successful introduction of the tube into the trachea. Tape is used to secure the nasal tubes; in rare circumstances (facial burns, severe allergy to adhesive tape), suture may be used instead.

Fiberoptic Intubation

Most operators skilled in the use of the bronchoscope can perform the technique of fiberoptic intubation (32a) (Fig. 5). Because copious amounts of either blood or secretions can make fiberoptic intubation difficult or impossible, it is imperative that operators who might resort to using this technique take all possible measures to dry the airway and avoid airway trauma. It is easier to perform fiberoptic intubation in awake patients because their muscle tone maintains the airway in a way that favors the success of this technique. Preparation of the oropharynx or nasopharynx proceeds as described previously. An appropriately sized endotracheal tube is warmed to soften it and then threaded over a lubricated bronchoscope.

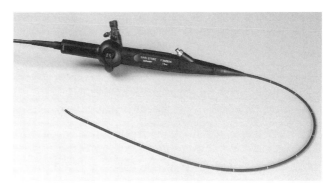

FIGURE 5. Storz flexible intubation fiberscope. (Karl Storz Endoscopy-America, Inc. Culver City, CA, U.S.A.)

An Ovassapian airway is very useful when attempting oral fiberoptic intubation, as it guides the tube to the midline, displaces the tongue, and prevents biting on the fiberscope (Fig. 6). The airway is inserted, the pharynx is suctioned, and an assistant delivers anterior thrust of the mandible. Alternatively, when the airway is not used, the assistant can pull on the tongue, displacing it anteriorly. The fiberoptic bronchoscope then is passed through the vocal cords, down the trachea, and next to the carina. The endotracheal tube is threaded over the bronchoscope with a smooth, twisting motion into the trachea. Tracheal intubation is confirmed with use of the bronchoscope as it is withdrawn from the trachea. The distance from the carina to the tip of the tube can be measured by observing how far the bronchoscope must be withdrawn from the carina before the tube becomes visible. Difficulty advancing the tube is usually a consequence of the endotracheal tube catching laryngeal structures and can be corrected by pulling the endotracheal tube back and readvancing it with a twisting motion. Rarely, the tube may be too large for the glottic opening, requiring the bronchoscope to be withdrawn and a smaller tube to be placed.

The nasal technique is similar in most regards to the oral technique. Some operators will insert the endotracheal tube through the nose and into the retropharynx, using it as a guide for the

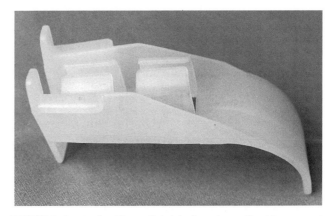

FIGURE 6. Ovassapian fiberoptic intubating airway. Provides open-air space in pharynx, protects fiberscope from patient's bite, and is removed from the mouth without disconnecting the endotracheal tube adapter.

bronchoscope. If the patient is asleep or unconscious, an assistant will be required to perform either a mandibular thrust or a tongue tug to facilitate the procedure. This technique is quite easy but can become a problem if the patient develops epistaxis associated with insertion of the tube. This is why other operators will perform the technique in the same manner as described for the oral route, waiting until the last possible moment to advance the tube into contact with the patient's tissues.

Intubating Laryngeal Mask Airway (Fastrack)

Since its recent introduction into clinical practice, the intubating LMA has become an important component in the management of the difficult airway in the OR (Fig. 7) (32b). Given this, it seems only reasonable to anticipate that it will play an increasing role in the management of airways in the ICU. Practitioners with lower levels of training and experience, however, have a high failure rate when using the intubating LMA (33,34). Additionally, the application of cricoid pressure reduces the chances of successfully intubating the trachea with the intubating LMA by 30% (35). This is a significant drawback to the technique of the intubating LMA as it is presently practiced and is likely to limit its utility for airway management in the ICU. Because the intubating LMA does not protect against aspiration, and because higher inspiratory pressures are undesirable, the utility of the intubating LMA in the patient with the difficult airway may not be as great in the ICU as it has been in the OR. Nonetheless, in the presence of upper airway bleeding, large amounts of secretions and failed rigid intubation, the Fastrack offers several advantages. It can help to restore oxygenation and prevent blood and secretions from reaching the larynx. Blind or fiberoptic-guided intubation using the intubating LMA is close to 100% successful in patients with difficult or failed rigid laryngoscopic intubations in the OR.

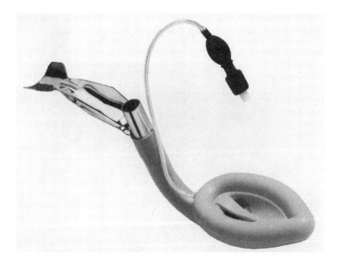

FIGURE 7. Intubating laryngeal mask airway (LMA; Fastrack). Is available in three adult sizes (3, 4, and 5). The Fastrack has a short, curved, stainless steel shaft covered with silicone, and a metal handle. The two bars of the classic LMA are replaced with a single epiglottic elevator bar. These new features have made blind tracheal intubation through the LMA easier, which results in a higher success rate. Endotracheal tubes up to 8 mm in diameter can be used with this device.

THE DIFFICULT AIRWAY

The difficult airway is encountered far more commonly in the ICU and ED than in the OR. Multiple attempts at laryngoscopy are common (25%), and 1 in 200 patients cannot be intubated (17–21). Copious secretions combined with obesity, an anterior larynx, small mandible, large tongue, short neck, prominent maxillary teeth, and inadequate positioning are common explanations for the increased rate of difficulty observed in the ICU. Delay in obtaining an airway in critically ill patients frequently is associated with the rapid onset of hypoxia, especially if deep sedation, intravenous general anesthesia, or paralytics have been administered. The ASA's Difficult Airway Algorithm was devised to outline the options available to practitioners faced with a challenging airway (Fig. 8). Choices in this circumstance include ventilate with the bag and mask, summon help in the form of another operator, reposition, attempt laryngoscopy with a different blade, and apply other techniques as appropriate. Attempts to ventilate the patient with an Ambu bag should occur concurrently as the operator prepares for the next attempt to secure the airway. If the patient can be adequately oxygenated with mask ventilation, the options available for airway management are substantially greater. Changing operators or blades sometimes allows successful laryngoscopy where previous attempts have failed. A straight blade, such as the Miller blade, can be especially useful in patients with prominent maxillary teeth, micrognathia, an anterior larynx, a floppy epiglottis, or trismus. The LMA can be useful as a bridge to oxygenate a patient who cannot be intubated, but it cannot be counted upon to do so in the presence of abnormal lung mechanics or anatomy (36). If it is inserted improperly or malpositioned, the LMA may insufflate the esophagus and increase the risk of aspiration. Even when the LMA is properly inserted, inflation pressures over 20 cm H_2O pressure with the LMA can cause both leaks and esophageal and gastric insufflation. The Combitube can be used to provide a stable airway in this situation as well and is commonly used for transport in the field. The choice between tracheostomy and cricothyroidotomy is based on institutional, operator, and patient factors. Emergency surgical airways such as tracheostomy have a complication rate of 30% (37). If trained personnel and suitable equipment are available in a timely fashion to establish a surgical airway, tracheostomy is generally preferable to cricothyroidotomy. Successful tracheostomy provides a cuffed, large-bore airway that both protects against aspiration and can be used for mechanical ventilation. Commercially available kits for tracheostomy and cricothyroidotomy contain all the necessary equipment, are sterile, and are relatively straightforward in their use. If the possibility of using such kits as part of airway management algorithm/practice is anticipated, the contents should be reviewed and the user should become familiar with the intended sequence of their use. Needle cricothyroidotomy is best viewed as a bridge either to further attempts at gaining airway control from above the glottis or tracheostomy, not as a definitive or acceptable airway by itself. If needle cricothyroidotomy is performed successfully, adequate oxygenation of patients with even mildly abnormal lung mechanics may require jet ventilation. Needle cricothyroidotomy and jet ventilation are increasingly accepted as the most likely to succeed approach when attempts to secure an airway via laryngoscopy fail (38). After a large catheter has been

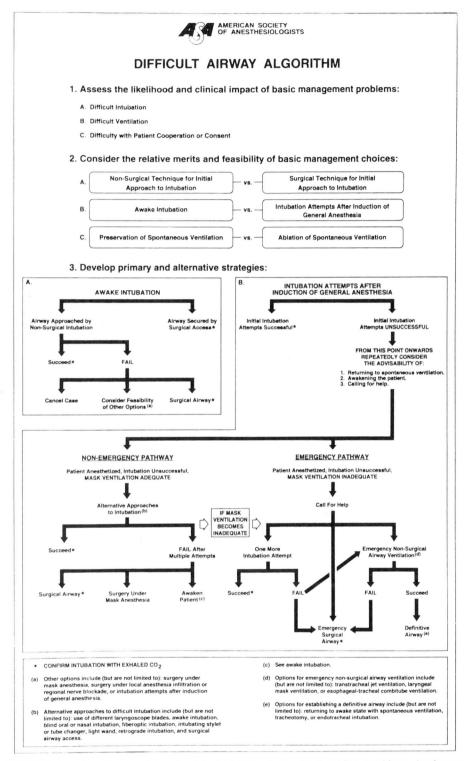

FIGURE 8. American Society of Anesthesiologists' Difficult Airway Algorithm provides a simple general guideline for management of an anticipated and unanticipated difficult airway. (Reprinted with permission from ref. 7a.)

passed through the cricothyroid membrane and air has been freely aspirated from it, the patient is ventilated with a specially designed device. Effective ventilation occurs with inspiratory pressures of 20 to 25 psi but still requires a patent airway to allow the patient to exhale.

CHANGING THE ENDOTRACHEAL TUBE

The most common indications for changing an existing endotracheal tube (ETT) are cuff leak, occlusion of the tube with inspissated secretions or clot, requirement for a tube different from the one originally inserted (one of a larger diameter or different type, such as double- to single-lumen) and sinusitis associated with nasal intubation. It is imperative that practitioners realize that changing the endotracheal tube of a critically ill patient may be one of the most hazardous undertakings in medicine. Complete occlusion of the endotracheal tube or cuff rupture constitute true emergencies; most other ETT changes are not and afford practitioners some time to prepare and assemble the necessary equipment and personnel.

The ease or difficulty of obtaining an airway has been documented at least once for the vast majority of intubated patients. If laryngoscopy was easily accomplished previously and the patient's airway anatomy has not changed appreciably (as a result of edema or trauma), most practitioners will perform endotracheal tube changes with direct laryngoscopy under sedation or anesthesia, and paralysis. Some experts recommend that tube changes be performed with the patient spontaneously breathing, if possible, because respiratory efforts by the patient will delay the onset of hypoxia in the event of difficulty in obtaining an airway.

Semirigid catheters, such as the Eschman stylet, can be very useful for changing the tube in difficult circumstances when the route of intubation remains the same but should not be relied on exclusively for endotracheal tube changes. Tube changers can kink or coil, preventing the tube from being threaded over them. They also can become dislodged during intubation. Finally, for a variety of reasons, it may be impossible to thread the new tube over them into the trachea. Some tube changers (such as the Cook Critical Care catheter) are designed to oxygenate patients through a lumen in the catheter in the event that a definitive airway cannot be established. Several assistants may be required for especially challenging patients, such as patients with massive facial edema or severe burns.

When the route of intubation is to be changed from oral to nasal or nose to mouth, rigid laryngoscopes or fiberoptic bronchoscopes can be used to change endotracheal tubes. When the bronchoscope is used in this role, it is introduced alongside the existing tube into the trachea, and the existing tube is withdrawn simultaneously with the new tube being advanced into the trachea. Additional safety can be obtained by withdrawing the old tube over a tube changer catheter. Given adequate preparation time and minimal trauma from previous manipulations of the airway, fiberoptic techniques are likely to be successful.

EXTUBATING PATIENTS IN THE INTENSIVE CARE UNIT

Many patients are transported to the ICU intubated postoperatively and are extubated after what is deemed a suitable period of observation. The accepted criteria for this have included adequate oxygenation on an F_{IO_2} below 60% and positive end-expiratory pressure (PEEP) below 5 cm H_2O pressure; respiratory rate below 30 to 40 per minute; stable pattern of respiration with a reasonable arterial CO_2; and the ability to sustain a 5-second head lift (which demonstrates satisfactory recovery from paralytic agents). Although this practice is widespread and commonly regarded as safe, there is growing literature that suggests some additional measures may improve outcome.

Trace doses of neuromuscular blockers depress the hypoxic drive to breathe in ways that are poorly understood (39,40) but occur independently from the effects of other anesthetic agents. This observation further supports the common practice of monitoring patients with pulse oximetry in the perioperative period and in the ICU. There is also growing evidence that previously accepted levels of recovery from paralytics may be associated with an increased risk of aspiration (41,42). The present standard, a train-of-four (TOF) ratio of 0.70, has been associated with an increased risk of aspiration in human volunteers not under the influence of any other drugs. Higher levels of recovery (TOF ratio ≥0.85) appear to be associated with a decreased risk of aspiration (41,42). Finally, a recent study suggested that residual paralysis is more common than previously documented in patients whose paralysis has been pharmacologically reversed, and residual paralysis is a strong risk factor for developing radiographically apparent infiltrates in the perioperative period (43). The risk of developing infiltrates was further increased in patients who underwent abdominal procedures (43).

Any strategy developed to reduce perioperative pulmonary complications in patients who undergo even short courses of mechanical ventilation in the ICU is going to have to reduce risk factors on several fronts. Patients whose recovery is scheduled to include a longer period of ventilation in the ICU may benefit from being intubated with an EVAC tube. The suction port on the tube probably should be attached to low intermittent suction from the commencement of anesthesia until the patient is extubated. Second, all paralytics should be reversed to very high levels of recovery prior to extubation. In practical terms, this means that long-acting paralytics should be forsaken in favor of shorter-acting or intermediate duration drugs and that they should be reversed regardless of what the clinical impression of the patient's degree of recovery may be. Finally, short-acting or ultra–short-acting sedative or analgesic drugs should be used to sedate or treat pain in these patients in the perioperative period prior to their extubation. The extubation of the patient with a known difficult airway requires complete preparation to manage the airway and the presence of experienced airway managers. Inadequate preparation, poor timing of extubation, and insufficiently experienced airway managers all can increase the damage of this inherently hazardous undertaking.

Reintubating Patients for Whom Extubation Fails

Patients for whom trials of extubation have failed have a high morbidity and mortality. The overall mortality for these patients is approximately 40% (44), and this is likely to increase over time. Patients fail a trial of extubation for many reasons, most of which can be associated with either an increased work of breathing or a decreased ability to sustain that work. Almost all cases of respiratory failure increase the work of breathing. Many patients who have been intubated for a long period will have respiratory muscle deconditioning and impaired airway reflexes. Myocardial ischemia frequently complicates efforts to liberate patients from the ventilator and is especially an issue in elderly patients with known coronary artery disease. Aspiration, either during intubation, prior to reintubation, or at the time of reintubation is common in these patients (45) and increases the likelihood they will become hypoxic around the time their airway is manipulated. The propensity of these patients to aspirate repeatedly is well recognized, and it is unlikely that the usual efforts at aggressive pulmonary toilet are effective. Practitioners reintubating these patients should assess them for the presence of ischemia and adapt their airway management plan as they deem appropriate. All feasible measures to prevent aspiration are also warranted in these patients.

Complications

Airway management in critically ill patients is an intrinsically hazardous undertaking. Death, hemodynamic instability, arrhythmias, hypoxia, airway trauma, aspiration, and failed intubation can all happen even when everything is performed properly.

Tracheal intubation and the institution of mechanical ventilation can be associated with a variety of physiologic responses. Endotracheal tubes increase the resistance to breathing as their lumen narrows. An 8.0-mm endotracheal tube causes a fixed increase in the airway resistance of 20% (46). The resistance increases exponentially with smaller tube diameters (30). As the lumen of the tube narrows from the accumulation of secretions, the resistance to flow will increase as a consequence of both narrowed diameter and increased turbulent flow. Using the largest possible tube will minimize the increase in resistance associated with intubation but may be associated with a greater rate of laryngeal trauma-related complications. Laryngoscopy and tracheal intubation also can trigger bronchospasm in susceptible individuals.

Hypertension, tachycardia, and variety of arrhythmias frequently accompany laryngoscopy and tracheal intubation and can be associated in turn with myocardial ischemia. Subsequent hypotension can have many causes (47). Myocardial ischemia can be precipitated by stress or hypoxia associated with the need for intubation. The hypertension and tachycardia that also can occur around the time of airway manipulation can exacerbate this ischemia. Severe myocardial ischemia can precipitate cardiac dysfunction, which in turn can cause hypotension. A variety of arrhythmias also may be triggered by the stress of airway management, including ventricular premature beats, ventricular tachycardia, ventricular fibrillation, and the full range of supraventricular tachycardias, including atrial fibrillation. Young patients may develop bradycardia as a manifestation of vagal outflow in response to airway manipulation.

Death occurs around the time of tracheal intubation in 0.5% to 3.0% of critically ill patients (17,20). Difficulty obtaining or maintaining an airway may play a role in some of these deaths. Mechanical ventilation replaces mean negative intrathoracic pressures with mean positive intrathoracic pressures, which can cause a decline in venous return and cardiac output. Catecholamine levels can plummet as hypoxia, hypercarbia, and dyspnea resolve. High-frequency ventilation with an Ambu bag or a ventilator can precipitate life-threatening levels of auto-PEEP and hypotension in susceptible patients, such as those with asthma, emphysema, and chronic bronchitis (48,49). High levels of PEEP or auto-PEEP can increase pulmonary vascular resistance (PVR) with an associated shift of the interventricular septum into the left ventricle (50,51). This septal shift, in turn, causes inadequate left ventricular filling, which results in decreased cardiac output. Initial ventilation strategies which use the least PEEP to ensure adequate oxygenation and which avoid creating high levels of auto-PEEP may be associated with a decreased risk of hypotension following intubation.

Right mainstem intubation commonly occurs when the practitioner advances the tube as far as possible prior to securing it. Right mainstem intubation could be averted in many cases by using the average tooth-to-carina distance, which is 28 cm in the average man and 24 cm in the average woman, and by taping tubes at 23 cm at the lip in men and 21 cm at the lip in women of average stature (52). Tooth-to-carina distance increases with height; a tube taped at 24 cm at the lip might be in perfect position for the average 180 cm man but might not even be in the trachea of a tall basketball player. Tube position can be confirmed using a bronchoscope by assessing its position relative to the carina. Chest radiographs should be obtained to confirm appropriate placement of the endotracheal tube because clinical assessment may be unreliable (53,54).

Esophageal intubation remains an inevitable complication of airway management. In theory, it should be recognized immediately and the malpositioned tube removed expeditiously. In practice, it occurs in circumstances where auscultation of the breath sounds is difficult or impossible and where tracheal intubation cannot be confirmed with capnography, such as neonates, patients with severe bronchospasm, and adults in full cardiopulmonary arrest (55).

Aspiration of gastric contents occurs in approximately 4% of ICU intubations (17) and in up to 30% of trauma patients who require intubation (56). Manipulation of the airway while the patient is awake with at least some intact airway reflexes and the application of cricoid pressure whenever possible during airway management are preventive measures.

Soft-tissue and dental injuries are well-described complications of rigid laryngoscopy in the ICU (57–61). There is a greater risk of laryngeal injuries in patients who are uncooperative, seizing, or have difficult airways (61). Modern dentistry can provide cosmetically and functionally effective treatments for dental damage, but at substantial expense. Domino and colleagues reported a series of cases of mediastinitis and retropharyngeal abscesses that were associated with tracheal and esophageal lacerations sustained during airway manipulation (32). Dysphagia is a well-described complication in critically ill patients and may be, in part, a consequence of soft-tissue injury associated with intubation (62).

SUMMARY

Airway management in the ICU is significantly different from that in the OR. Most patients in the ICU are intubated urgently or emergently, allowing little time for airway assessment or preparation for managing the airway. Those who manage the airway in the ICU typically do so with a subset of the equipment available in the OR and with significantly less skilled assistance. Paths of retreat such as mask ventilation or LMA ventilation are less effective in critically ill patients. Complications of intubation, including dental trauma, aspiration, hypertension, hypotension, arrhythmias, hypoxia, death, and failed intubation, are all more common in critically ill patients than in the OR.

KEY POINTS

Critically ill patients are frequently more susceptible to hypoxia during airway management than are those under other scenarios such as the operating room. Hypoxia or inadequate gas exchange may be exacerbated because of the frequent inefficiency of ventilation with an Ambu bag and mask or LMA in patients with respiratory failure because of their restrictive or obstructive lung mechanics. Critically ill patients also are at increased risk of having a full stomach or delayed gastric emptying, and the associated risk of aspiration is therefore increased in critically ill patients.

The use of intravenous agents and paralytics to facilitate airway management in the critically ill is a potentially hazardous practice, which entails a tradeoff between improved conditions for managing the airway and respiratory or circulatory depression for the patients. Therefore, awake intubation with topical anesthesia is preferable whenever possible.

Nasal intubation is associated with a lower risk of self-extubation but a higher risk of sinusitis and perhaps ventilator associated pneumonia. Coagulopathy and immunosuppression are relative contraindications to nasal intubation, whereas significant anatomic compromise of the nasal bones, basilar skull fracture, or cerebrospinal leak are absolute contraindications. Fiberoptic-guided intubation can be safely accomplished in most critically ill patients but requires adequate preparation and favorable operating conditions. Bleeding and trauma from failed intubations may make subsequent attempts with the fiberoptic bronchoscope difficult or impossible.

In critically ill patients, endotracheal tubes designed to suction subglottic secretions may be preferable to tubes of conventional design. Patients who require reintubation may have a variety of causes of their respiratory failure, including aspiration, myocardial ischemia, bronchospasm, and respiratory muscle deconditioning. Patients who require reintubation have a high mortality.

REFERENCES

1. Confalonieri M, Potena A, Carbone G, et al. Acute respiratory failure in patients with severe community-acquired pneumonia: a prospective randomized evaluation of non-invasive ventilation. *Am J Respir Crit Care Med* 1999;160:1585–1591.
2. Antonelli M, Conti G, Bufi M, et al. Noninvasive ventilation for treatment of acute respiratory failure in patients undergoing solid organ transplantation: a randomized trial. *JAMA* 2000;283:235–241.
3. Nourdine K, Combes P, Carton MJ et al. Does non-invasive ventilation reduce the ICU nosocomial infection risk? A prospective clinical survey. *Intensive Care Med* 1999;25:567–73.
4. Pang D, Keenan SP, Cook DJ, et al. The effect of positive pressure airway support on mortality and the need for endotracheal intubation in cardiogenic pulmonary edema: a systematic review. *Chest* 1998;114:1185–1192.
5. Rocker GM, Mackenzie MG, Williams B, et al. Noninvasive positive pressure ventilation: successful outcome in patients with acute lung injury/ARDS. *Chest* 1999;115:173–177.
6. Meduri GU, Turner RE, Abou-Shala N, et al. Noninvasive positive pressure ventilation via face mask: first line intervention in patients with acute hypercapnic and hypoxemic respiratory failure. *Chest* 1996;109:179–193.
7. Keenan SP, Kernerman PD, Cook DJ, et al. Effect of noninvasive positive pressure ventilation on mortality in patients admitted with respiratory failure: a meta-analysis. *Crit Care Med* 1997;25:1685–92.
7a. American Society of Anesthesiologists Task Force on Management of the Difficult Airway. Practice guidelines for management of the difficult airway. *Anesthesiology* 1993;78:597–602.
8. Kollef MH, Skubas NJ, Sundt TM. A randomized clinical trial of continuous aspiration of subglottic secretions in cardiac surgery patients. *Chest* 1999;116:1339–1346.
9. Mahul P, Auboyer C, Jospe R, et al. Prevention of nosocomial pneumonia in intubated patients: respective role of mechanical subglottic secretions drainage and stress ulcer prophylaxis. *Intensive Care Med* 1992;18:20–25.
10. Rello J, Sonora R, Jubert P, et al. Pneumonia in intubated patients: role of respiratory airway care. *Am J Respir Crit Care Med* 1996;154:111–115.
11. Valles J, Artigas A, Rello J, et al. Continuous aspiration of subglottic secretions in preventing ventilator associated pneumonia. *Ann Intern Med* 1995;122:179–86.
12. Young PJ, Basson C, Hamilton D, et al. Prevention of tracheal aspiration using the pressure-limited tracheal tube cuff. *Anaesthesia* 1999;54:559–563.
13. Adair CG, Gorman SP, Feron BM, et al. Implications of endotracheal biofilm for ventilator associated pneumonia. *Intensive Care Med* 1999;25:1072–1076.
14. Wang HE, O'Connor RE, Megargel RE, et al. The utilization of midazolam as a pharmacologic adjunct to endotracheal intubation by paramedics. *Prehosp Emerg Care* 2000;4:14–18.
15. Sivilotti ML, Ducharme J. Randomized, double-blind study on sedatives and hemodynamics during rapid sequence intubation in the emergency department: the SHRED study. *Ann Emerg Med* 1998;31:313–324.
16. Smith DC, Bergen JM, Smithline H, et al. A trial of etomidate for rapid sequence intubation in the emergency department. *J Emerg Med* 2000;18:13–16.
17. Schwartz DE, Matthay MA, Cohen NH. Death and other complications of emergency airway management in critically ill adults. *Anesthesiology* 1995;82:367–376.
18. Wayne MA, Friedland E. Prehospital use of succinylcholine: a 20 year review. *Prehosp Emerg Care* 1999;3:107–109.
19. Tayal VS, Riggs RW, Marx JA, et al. Rapid sequence intubation at an emergency medicine residency: success rate and adverse events during a two-year period. *Acad Emerg Med* 1999;6:31–37.
20. Sakles JC, Laurin EG, Rantapaa AA, et al. Airway management in the emergency department: a one year study of 620 tracheal intubations. *Ann Emerg Med* 1998;31:325–32.
21. Adnet F, Jouriles NJ, Le Toumelin P, et al. Survey of out-of-hospital emergency intubations in the French prehospital medical system: a multi-center study. *Ann Emerg Med* 1998;32:454–460.
22. Vijaykumar E, Bosscher H, Renzi FP, et al. The use of neuromuscular blocking agents in the emergency department to facilitate tracheal intubation in the trauma patient: help or hindrance? *J Crit Care* 1998;13:1–6.
23. McCourt KC, Elliott P, Mirakhur RK, et al. Haemodynamic effects of rapacuronium in adults with coronary artery or valvular disease. *Br J Anaesth* 1999;83:721–726.

24. Tindol GA, Jr, DiBenedetto RJ, Kosciuk L. Unplanned extubations. *Chest* 1994;105:1804–1807.

25. Chevron V, Menard J, Richard J, et al. Unplanned extubation: risk factors for the development and predictive criteria for reintubation. *Crit Care Med* 1998;26:1049–1053.

26. Holzapfel L, Chevret S, Madinier G, et al. Influence of long-term oro- or naso-tracheal intubation on nosocomial maxillary sinutsitis and pneumonia: results of a prospective, randomized clinical trial. *Crit Care Med* 1993;21:1132–1138.

27. Holzapfel L, Chastang C, Demingeon G, et al. A randomized study assessing the systematic search for maxillary sinusitis in nasotracheally mechanically ventilated patients. Influence of nosocomial maxillary sinusitis on the occurrence of ventilator-associated pneumonia. *Am J Resp Crit Care Med* 1999;159:695–701.

27a. Ovassapian A, Meyer RM, Airway management. In: Longnecker JE, Murphy FL, eds. *Dripps/Eckenhoff/Vandam: Introduction to Anesthesia*, 9th ed. Philadelphia: WB Saunders, 1997.

28. Rouby JJ, Laurent P, Gosnach M, et al. Risk factors and clinical relevance of nosocomial maxillary sinusitis in the clinically ill. *Am J Respir Crit Care Med* 1994;150:776–83.

29. Heffner JE. Nosocomial sinusitis: den of multiresistant thieves? *Am J Respir Crit Care Med* 1994;150:608–609.

30. Habib MP. Physiologic implications of artificial airways. *Chest* 1989;96:180–184.

31. Sessler CN, Vitaliti JC, Cooper KR, et al. Comparison of 4% lidocaine/0.5% phenylephrine with 5% cocaine: which dilates the nasal passages better? *Anesthesiology* 1986;64:274–277.

32. Domino KB, Posner KL, Caplan RA, et al. Airway injury during anesthesia: a closed claims analysis. *Anesthesiology* 1999;91:1703–1711.

32a. Ovassapian A. *Fiberoptic endoscopy and the difficult airway.* 2nd ed. Philadelphia: Lippincott-Raven, 1996.

32b. Brain AIJ, Verghese C, Addy EV, et al. The intubating laryngeal mask. II. A preliminary report of a new means of intubating the trachea. *Br J Anaesth* 1997;79:704–709.

33. Levitan RM, Ochroch EA, Stuart S, et al. Use of the intubating laryngeal mask airway by medical and non-medical personnel. *Am J Emerg Med* 2000;18:12–16.

34. Avidan MS, Harvey A, Chitkara N, et al. The intubating laryngeal mask airway compared with direct laryngoscopy. *Br J Anaesth* 1999;83:615–617.

35. Harry RM, Nolan JP. The use of cricoid pressure with the intubating laryngeal mask. *Anaesthesia* 1999;54:656–659.

36. Martin SE, Ochsner MG, Jarman RH, et al. Use of the laryngeal mask airway in air transport when intubation fails. *J Trauma* 1999;47:352–357.

37. Gillespie MB, Eisle DW. Outcomes of emergency surgical airway procedures in a hospital wide setting. *Laryngoscope* 1999;109:1766–1769.

38. Patel RG. Percutaneous transtracheal jet ventilation: a safe, quick, and temporary way to provide oxygenation and ventilation when conventional methods are unsuccessful. *Chest* 1999;116:1689–1694.

39. Eriksson L. Reduced hypoxic chemosensitivity in partially paralyzed man: a new property of muscle relaxants. *Acta Anasthesiol Scand* 1996;40:520–523.

40. Eriksson LI, Lennmarken C, Wyon N, et al. Attenuated ventilatory response to hypoxaemia with vecuronium-induced partial neuromuscular block. *Acta Anesthesiol Scand* 1992;36:710–715.

41. Kopman AF, Yee PS, Neuman GG. Relationship of the train-of-four fade ratio to clinical signs and symptoms of residual paralysis in awake volunteers. *Anesthesiology* 1997;86:765–761.

42. Eriksson LI, Sundman E, Olsso R, et al. Functional assessment of the pharynx at rest and during swallowing in partially paralyzed humans. *Anesthesiology* 1997; 87:1035–1043.

43. Berg H, Viby-Mogensen J, Roed J, et al. Residual neuromuscular block is a risk factor for postoperative pulmonary complications. *Acta Aneaesthesiol Scand* 1997;41:1095–1103.

44. Epstein SK, Ciubotaru RL. Independent effects of etiology of failure and time to reintubation on outcome for patients failing extubation. *Am J Respir Crit Care Med* 1998;158:489–493.

45. Torres A, Gatell JM, Aznar E, et al. Re-intubation increases the risk of nosocomial pneumonia in patients needing mechanical ventilation. *Am J Respir Crit Care Med* 1995;152:137–141.

46. Gal TJ. Pulmonary mechanics in normal subjects following endotracheal intubation. *Anesthesiology* 1980;52:27–35.

47. Franklin C, Samuel J, Hu T-C. Life-threatening hypotension associated with emergency intubation and the initiation of mechanical ventilation. *Am J Emerg Med* 1994;12:425–428.

48. Pepe PE, Marini JJ. Occult positive end-expiratory pressure in mechanically ventilated patients with airflow obstruction: the auto-PEEP effect. *Am Rev Respir Dis* 1982;126:166–170.

49. Rogers PL, Schlichtig R, Miro A, et al. Auto-PEEP during CPR: an "occult" cause of electromechanical dissociation? *Chest* 1991;99:492–493.

50. Jardin F, Farcot J-C, Boisante L, et al. Influence of positive end-expiratory pressure on left ventricular performance. *N Engl J Med* 1981;304:387–392.

51. Baigorri F, de Monte A, Blanch L, et al. Hemodynamic responses to external counterbalancing of auto-positive end-expiratory pressure in mechanically ventilated patients with chronic obstructive pulmonary disease. *Crit Care Med* 1994;22:1782–1791.

52. Owen RL, Cheney F. Endobronchial intubation: a preventable complication. *Anesthesiology* 1987;67:255–257.

53. Schwartz DE, Lieberman JA, Cohen NH. Women are at greater risk than men for malpositioning of the endotracheal tube after emergent intubation. *Crit Care Med* 1994;22:1127–1131.

54. Brunel W, Coleman DL, Schwartz DE, et al. Assessment of routine chest roentgenograms and the physical examination to confirm endotracheal tube position. *Chest* 1989;96:1043–1045.

55. Bagshaw O, Gillis J, Schell D. Delayed recognition of esophageal intubation in a neonate: role of radiologic diagnosis. *Crit Care Med* 1994;22:2020–2023.

56. Lockey DJ, Coats T, Parr MJ. Aspiration in severe trauma: a prospective study. *Anaesthesia* 1999;54:1097–1098.

57. Whited RE. Posterior commissure stenosis post long-term intubation. *Laryngoscope* 1983;93:1314–1318.

58. Belson TP. Cuff induced tracheal injury in dogs following prolonged intubation. *Laryngoscope* 1983;93:549–555.

59. Rashkin MC, Davis T. Acute complications of endotracheal intubation: relationship to reintubation, route, urgency, and duration. *Chest* 1986;89:165–167.

60. Kastanos N, Miró RE, Perez AM, et al. Laryngotracheal injury due to endotracheal intubation: incidence, evolution, and predisposing factors. a prospective long-term study. *Crit Care Med* 1983;11:362–67.

61. Thomas R, Kumar EV, Kameswaran M, et al. Post intubation laryngeal sequelae in an intensive care unit. *J Laryngol Otol* 1995;109:313–316.

62. de Larminat V, Montravers P, Dureuil B, et al. Alteration in swallowing reflex after extubation in intensive care unit patients. *Crit Care Med* 1995;23:486–490.

PROCEDURES IN THE INTENSIVE CARE UNIT

SYLVIA Y. DOLINSKI
LEANNE GROBAN
JOHN BUTTERWORTH

INTRODUCTION

With advances in technology, an increasing variety of invasive procedures are commonly performed in the intensive care unit (ICU). Large monographs have been written on the subject, so this chapter will highlight only a few topics: placement of arterial, central venous, and pulmonary arterial catheters; transesophageal echocardiography; and percutaneous tracheostomy. The authors chose to discuss the aforementioned procedures because we wanted to highlight basic and some of the newest procedures in the ICU. We recognize that there are numerous other important procedures and refer the reader to a procedures manual (1).

HEMODYNAMIC MONITORING

Arterial, central venous, and pulmonary artery catheters permit continuous assessment of critically ill patients during circulatory instability. Underlying medical conditions, fluid therapies, and vasoactive drugs may all result in major circulatory changes. Central venous or pulmonary artery catheters permit monitoring of right heart or left heart filling pressures. At times, peripheral venous access can be difficult or nearly impossible in burned, obese, or severely vasoconstricted patients. Noninvasive blood pressure monitoring can sometimes be impossible. Finally, indwelling arterial and central venous catheters simplify blood sampling, for good and for bad, avoiding repeated painful arterial or venous punctures, but making phlebotomy-induced anemia a common occurrence.

ARTERIAL CANNULATION

There are several peripheral arteries that are accessible for percutaneous cannulation, including the radial, ulnar, brachial, axillary, dorsalis pedis, posterior tibial, and femoral arteries. The site selected often depends on the operator's ability to detect the pulse, the absence of nearby infections, the adequacy of collateral blood flow, and the potential for complications. In general, more distal sites are selected before more proximal ones.

The most common arterial cannulation site remains the radial artery. Its companion vessel, the ulnar artery, tends to be the dominant arterial supply to the hand. The ulnar artery usually connects distally with the radial artery to form the superficial and deep palmar arches. The Allen test is often performed to assess the adequacy of collateral flow, although there is little evidence that an abnormal Allen test increases the risk of radial artery cannulation, or that a normal result predicts increased safety.

Technique of Radial Artery Cannulation

The wrist is dorsiflexed over a rolled towel and secured with adhesive tape to an armboard. The radial artery is palpated proximal to the distal wrist crease on the lateral aspect of the wrist. The skin is cleansed with an antiseptic solution (alcohol or povidone) and may be draped with sterile towels. A small skin wheal of 1% lidocaine is injected prior to skin puncture (Fig. 1).

Direct Cannulation

A 20-gauge angiocatheter, held like a dart, is advanced through the skin and underlying tissue at a 30- to 40-degree angle to the wrist in line with the radial pulse (Fig. 2). Upon visualization of a flash of blood, the catheter is lowered (Fig. 3, step A), and the angiocatheter needle assembly is advanced 1 mm further to ensure that the catheter itself has entered the artery, and not just the needle tip (Fig. 3, step B). The catheter is advanced over the needle into the artery, the needle is removed, and the catheter is

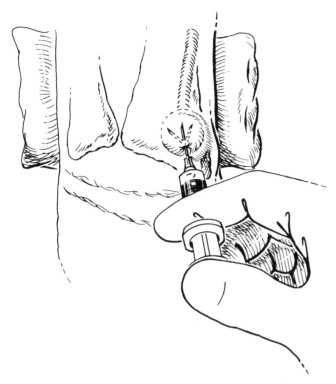

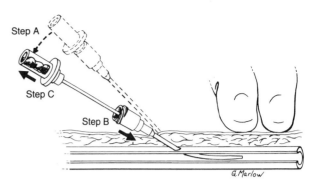

FIGURE 3. Direct arterial cannulation. **A:** Blood flushes into the hub of the needle and cannula, and the angiocatheter is lowered. **B:** Catheter and needle are advanced 1 mm. **C:** Cannula is advanced over the needle into the artery. (Reproduced with permission from Butterworth JF IV. *Atlas of procedures in anesthesia and critical care.* Philadelphia: WB Saunders, 1992.)

connected to a heparinized saline-filled transducer tubing (Fig. 4). If the artery is not entered during the first pass, then the next pass should usually be directed more mediad. Care should be taken to clear the tubing of air bubbles to avoid embolization during catheter flushes. The transducer should be zeroed at the level of the heart.

Transfixation Cannulation Technique

In an alternative method for arterial cannulation, the angiocatheter is passed through the anterior and posterior walls of the

FIGURE 1. Injection of 1% lidocaine in the shin at the intended puncture site with the wrist dorsiflexed. (Reproduced with permission from Butterworth JF IV. *Atlas of procedures in anesthesia and critical care.* Philadelphia: WB Saunders, 1992.)

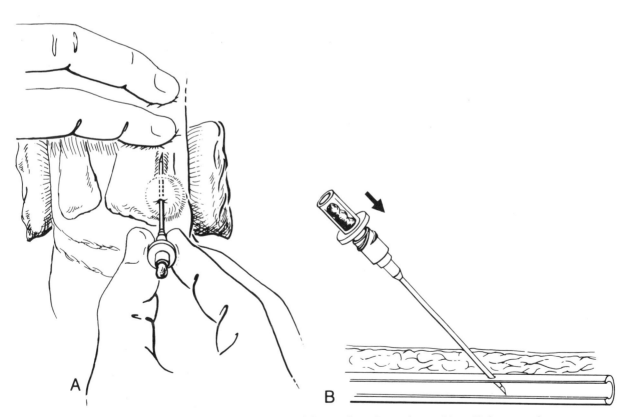

FIGURE 2. Diagram illustrating advancement of the needle and cannula at a 30- to 40-degree angle until the artery is entered. (Reproduced with permission from Butterworth JF IV. *Atlas of procedures in anesthesia and critical care.* Philadelphia: WB Saunders, 1992.)

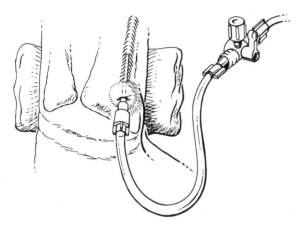

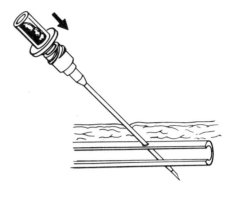

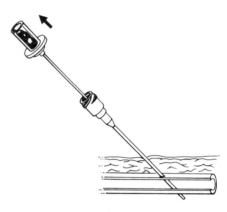

FIGURE 4. Radial arterial catheter connected to saline-filled transducer tubing. (Reproduced with permission from Butterworth JF IV. *Atlas of procedures in anesthesia and critical care.* Philadelphia: WB Saunders, 1992.)

artery, transfixing the artery (Fig. 5). After the needle is removed, the catheter is slowly withdrawn until blood returns through the catheter hub. The catheter can then be pushed directly or passed over a small sterile (0.018-inch) guidewire into the arterial lumen (Fig. 6). Radial artery cannulation kits with built-in guidewires are widely used. Once removed, the needle should not be reintroduced, because its sharp tip can shear off fragments of catheter that can embolize distally. The catheter is secured to skin with suture or tape. A sterile, dry dressing should cover the catheter insertion site.

The technique of arterial cannulation is identical at all sites except that a guidewire technique is nearly always used and longer catheters are necessary for femoral or axillary cannulations. The *femoral artery,* the second most common site of cannulation, is often chosen when arterial pulses are not palpable at other sites. The midpoint of a line drawn from the anterior superior iliac spine and symphysis pubis is a useful guide for locating the femoral artery. Using the sterile technique previously described for radial artery cannulation, a 6- to 7-cm long, 18- to 20-gauge thin-walled arteriotomy needle attached to a syringe is used to locate the femoral artery. The artery has been entered when arterial blood can be aspirated. The syringe is removed and a guidewire (preferably with a flexible "J" tip) is advanced through the needle into the artery. The needle is removed. A skin nick is made with a scalpel, permitting an 18-gauge (16-cm) catheter to be passed over the guidewire without encountering skin resistance.

The *axillary artery* is located within a sheath that also surrounds the axillary vein and brachial plexus. With the arm abducted at 90 degrees and externally rotated, the axillary pulse can be palpated dorsad to the biceps muscle. Using a Seldinger technique similar to that described for femoral artery cannulation, a needle and guidewire are placed in the artery, the needle is removed, and the catheter is slid over the wire.

The *dorsalis pedis* artery is located superficially and laterally to the extensor hallucis longus tendon, and cannulated at the level of the metatarsals. The *posterior tibial* artery lies posterior to the medial malleolus at the ankle, and is sometimes used for arterial pressure monitoring in children. The *brachial artery* is uncommonly cannulated for fear of thrombosis and limb loss from lack of collateral blood flow. Nevertheless, numerous studies

FIGURE 5. Transfixation cannulation technique. The angiocatheter needle is advanced farther after blood flushes back **(top diagram)**. The needle is removed **(middle diagram)**, and the catheter is slowly removed until blood returns in a pulsating fashion **(bottom diagram)**. (Reproduced with permission from Butterworth JF IV. *Atlas of procedures in anesthesia and critical care.* Philadelphia: WB Saunders, 1992.)

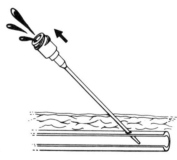

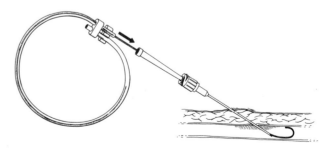

FIGURE 6. Diagram of the passage of a guidewire into the vessel lumen over which the catheter can be threaded. (Reproduced with permission from Butterworth JF IV. *Atlas of procedures in anesthesia and critical care.* Philadelphia: WB Saunders, 1992.)

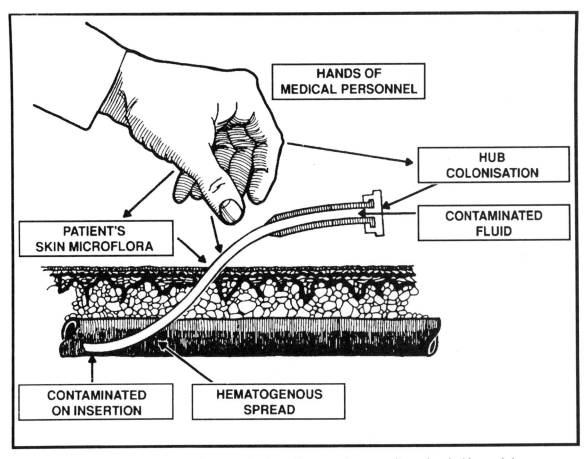

FIGURE 7. Potential sources for contamination of intravascular access. (Reproduced with permission from Pearson ML; the Hospital Infection Control Practices Advisory Committee: Guideline for Prevention of Intravascular Device-Related Infections. Division of Healthcare Quality Promotion, Centers for Disease Control and Prevention. Available at: http://www.cdc.gov/ncidod/hip/IV/Iv.htm. Accessed October 1, 2001.)

have documented that it can be used safely for periods of 1 to 2 days during and after cardiac surgery. It can be palpated and cannulated medial to the biceps tendon in the antecubital fossa.

Complications of Arterial Cannulation

Arterial catheters are sometimes maintained *in situ* long after hemodynamic stability has been achieved solely for convenient blood sampling. If a patient is undergoing only one withdrawal of blood per day, the arterial catheter should be removed. The mere presence of an arterial catheter increases both costs and iatrogenic blood loss (1a). Arterial catheterization sites are often located near

TABLE 1. COMPLICATIONS OF ARTERIAL LINE PLACEMENT

Iatrogenic blood loss
Peripheral nerve damage
Hemorrhage
Hematoma
Infection
Heparin-associated antibody
Thrombosis
Embolization
Accidental medication injection

nerves (ulnar nerve for ulnar catheters, brachial plexus for axillary catheters, median nerve for brachial catheters, and femoral nerve for femoral catheters), and nerve damage has been reported following arterial cannulation. Bleeding and hematomas secondary to arterial cannulation can also cause compression of neighboring nerves. As a consequence of transducer lines being flushed with heparin solutions, patients can develop a heparin antibody. Our institution has switched to heparin-free, saline-flushed catheters. Arterial catheter sites should be inspected daily for signs of infection. As the data in Fig. 7 indicate, there are several potential sources for contamination. Finally, arterial tubing and stopcocks can be confused with peripheral intravenous tubing and accidentally be injected with a vesicant medication. These several complications are summarized in Table 1.

CENTRAL VENOUS CATHETERIZATION

The indications and complications of central venous cannulation are listed in Tables 2 and 3. Fluid resuscitation per se is not an indication for central venous catheter placement. In fact, two short (3.0-cm) 18-gauge intravenous catheters allow greater fluid flow than a single 20-cm long, 16-gauge central venous cannula (2). The choice of the puncture site is usually based on physician preference and convenience, but sometimes patient factors

TABLE 2. INDICATIONS FOR CENTRAL VENOUS ACCESS

Secure venous access in patients lacking good peripheral sites
Monitoring of right-heart filling pressure (central venous pressure)
Conduit for pulmonary artery catheter placement
Site for dialysis
Administration of total parenteral nutrition
Administration of inotropic and vasoactive drugs

supersede. For example, if there are concerns about unstable cranial fractures, a recent carotid endarterectomy, or in the rare event that long-term parenteral nutrition will be required, a subclavian venous approach may be preferred to either internal or external jugular venous approaches. If hemodialysis catheters are to be placed, the internal jugular site is preferred to eliminate the potential for iatrogenic subclavian stenosis, which could limit future hemodialysis fistula sites. In patients with a coagulopathy, the internal or external jugular vein sites are preferred over the subclavian vein site, since direct pressure cannot be readily applied to bleeding punctured vessels.

TECHNIQUES OF INTERNAL JUGULAR VEIN CATHETERIZATION

The patient is placed supine with the head turned away from the puncture site. The patient's bed is placed in Trendelenburg position to distend the vein, facilitating venipuncture. It is sometimes helpful to place a rolled towel behind the scapulae to extend the neck. The area overlying the site of puncture should be cleansed with an antiseptic solution and allowed to dry. The operator should wear a mask and bonnet, don sterile gloves and gown, and the puncture site should be draped as a sterile field. The central venous catheter kit should be opened using aseptic technique, and its contents inspected and syringes prepared.

The internal jugular vein is located anterior and lateral to the carotid artery. Of the many approaches to the internal jugular vein, we will describe three: (a) the *anterior approach* whereby the medial border of the sternocleidomastoid (SCM) muscle serves as a landmark to find the internal jugular vein just lateral to the carotid pulse at the level of the thyroid cartilage; (b) the *central approach* whereby the internal jugular is located between the two

TABLE 3. SITE-SPECIFIC COMPLICATIONS ASSOCIATED WITH CENTRAL VENOUS ACCESS ACQUISITION

Catheter-related infections (all) (IJ > SC)
Arterial puncture (IJ > SC)
Severe arrhythmias (all) *rare*
Venous air embolism (all) *common*
Intravascular thrombosis (all)
Nerve injury (SC, IJ, F) *rare*
Pericardial tamponade (all) *rare*
Noncompressible bleeding in a patient with
  bleeding diathesis or coagulopathy (SC)
Cerebral spinal fluid tap (IJ) *rare*
Hemo-, pneumo- (SC > LIJ, RIJ), chylothorax (LIJ) *common*
Retroperitoneal bleeding (F) *rare*

IJ = internal jugular, (L) left, (R) right; SC = subclavian; F = femoral.

heads of the SCM muscle; and (c) the *posterior approach* whereby the lateral border of the SCM muscle as it is crossed by the external jugular vein serves as a landmark. Individual preference guides the selection of the approach; however, studies using sonography indicate that needles are less frequently directed toward the carotid artery during the anterior and central approaches than during the posterior approach.

The carotid pulse, dorsal and medial to the sternal head of the SCM muscle, should be located to avoid atrial puncture. The more craniad that the vein is punctured, the less likely the pleura of the lung (or on the left side, the thoracic duct) will be traumatized. Avoiding rotation of the head beyond 40 degrees from midline reduces the risk of carotid puncture. As the head is rotated, ultrasonography demonstrates that the internal jugular vein flattens and rotates over the carotid artery increasing the likelihood of carotid puncture (3).

In unsedated patients, the skin is infiltrated with 1% lidocaine and then the vein is located at the apex of the two muscle heads of the SCM (using the central approach) by aspirating venous blood through a 22-gauge, 4-cm "finder" needle attached to a syringe with the needle aimed toward the ipsilateral nipple at a 30- to 45-degree angle to the skin. It is helpful to use an empty syringe for aspiration, since local anesthetic solutions can alter the color of the aspirate, making it difficult to differentiate venous from arterial blood. The internal jugular vein can be located most often within 1.5 cm from skin penetration (4). Next, either an 18-gauge, thin-walled arteriotomy needle or 18-gauge angiocatheter attached to a syringe is inserted through the skin following the path identified by the finder needle. When venous blood is aspirated by the angiocatheter, the angiocatheter assembly is advanced an additional 1 to 2 mm to ensure the tip of the catheter is fully within the vein; the catheter is then advanced off the needle. On the other hand, the 18-gauge, thin-walled needle is not advanced once blood is freely aspirated. It is important to keep in mind the angle and depth at which the internal jugular vein was located by the finder needle, and avoid probing any deeper with the arteriotomy needle or angiocatheter. After an apparently unsuccessful pass with the needle, it is common to aspirate blood as the needle is withdrawn, because the jugular vein may be compressed by an advancing needle (4).

The venous placement of the catheter or needle can be verified by comparing the color of the blood aspirated from the cannula or syringe with a simultaneously drawn arterial sample. If the color of the two samples is similar, then the angiocatheter or needle is likely in the carotid and the procedure should not be continued. When an arterial blood sample is not available or if a color difference is questionable, the cannula or syringe is transduced with an electric transducer or a catheter manometer while maintaining aseptic technique. The appearance of central venous waveforms and pressure exclude the cannulation of the carotid artery. A venous manometer is readily obtained by attaching a sterile intravenous extension tubing to the cannula. After passively filling the tubing with blood, the tubing is held upright while attached to the cannula or needle. The height of the blood column establishes the central venous pressure. If the catheter or needle is in the carotid artery, pulsatile blood will overfill the tubing. In patients with pulmonary hypertension or others with high central venous pressures (e.g., tricuspid regurgitation) the column also will not fall despite venous cannulation. Ultrasonic imaging can also be used to locate the vein. Denys and Uretsky showed that in only 92% of 200 patients, the internal jugular vein was found in its expected anterolateral location in relation to the carotid artery (5). In another study, the internal jugular vein was located medially or anteromedially to the carotid artery as often as 5.5% of the time (6). It can also reduce the risk of arterial puncture. Ultrasound-guided cannulation of the internal jugular vein can also reduce the risk of arterial puncture. In two studies, the use of ultrasound decreased the risk of carotid atrial puncture from 8% to 2% (7,8).

When arterial puncture has been ruled out, the guidewire is inserted through the catheter or needle into the vein leaving about half of the guidewire outside of the patient. The average distance from all access sites to the superior vena cava–atrial junction is 18 cm; thus, the guidewire never need be introduced further than 18 cm (9). Next the catheter or needle is removed over the wire. Premature beats are common during wire insertion, especially when the wire has been advanced further than necessary and contacts the endocardial wall. A small skin incision is made at the puncture site and a plastic dilator is passed over the wire, then removed. After passage of the central venous catheter, the guidewire is withdrawn, and a gloved finger or syringe occludes the catheter hub to avoid air entrainment and embolism until it can be attached to an intravenous or transducer line. The catheter is secured to the skin with a nonabsorbable suture. A sterile dressing is placed with either sterile dry gauze or a transparent dressing. Antibiotic ointment is not recommended, because it has been found to allow *Candida* species to colonize the catheter site (10). We agree with the recommendations of the Food and Drug Administration that the catheter tip should not be maintained in the right atrium (11). To aid depth of central line insertion determination, two studies offer the following formulae for insertion depth (in cm; where H = patient height in cm): Centimeters of catheter inserted at the right jugular vein = H/10, whereas at the right subclavian vein: H/10 − 2, at the left internal jugular vein: H/10 + 4 and at the left subclavian vein: H/10 + 2 (12,13).

Since central venous catheters can migrate up to 3 cm further toward and into the heart, the catheter tip should be 2 to 3 cm above the cava–atrial junction on the postprocedure chest radiograph. This position will ensure that the catheter will be in the superior vena cava (SVC), but not within the pericardium. Approximately 3 cm of the SVC lie within the pericardium. When the catheter tip is located within the pericardium, erosion through a vessel may result in delayed cardiac tamponade. The pericardial sac ends below the level of the carina on the chest radiograph, making it a helpful landmark for correct placement (14,15). The catheter tip should not be allowed to abut a vein at 90 degrees (a possibility when catheters inserted from the left side are positioned using the carina as a landmark), as this appears to increase the risk of puncture and hemorrhage. Thus, catheters inserted from the patient's left side may need to be advanced within 3 cm of the cava–atrial junction in order to avoid leaving the catheter tip at a dangerous angle (16,17). An alternative safe location for the catheter tip introduced from the left access site would be in the left innominate vein before it enters the SVC (18).

The anterior and posterior approaches to the internal jugular vein have different sites of venipuncture. With the anterior approach, at the level of the cricoid, the carotid is palpable medial

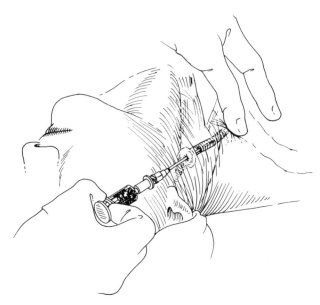

FIGURE 8. Illustration of external jugular vein cannulation. (Reproduced with permission from Butterworth JF IV. *Atlas of procedures in anesthesia and critical care*. Philadelphia: WB Saunders, 1992.)

to the medial border of the SCM muscle. Here the finder needle is inserted 0.5 to 1.0 cm lateral to the pulse. The landmark for the posterior approach is the point where the external jugular vein crosses the lateral border of the SCM. The needle is pointed caudad toward the suprasternal notch. Once the vein is identified, the technique used is identical to that described for the central approach.

TECHNIQUE OF EXTERNAL JUGULAR VENOUS CANNULATION

The external jugular vein traverses superficially the lateral border of the SCM muscle at the level of the cricothyroid membrane and provides a central access site. With the patient in the head down position, the vein becomes readily visible except in the dehydrated patient. The left index finger helps distend and stabilize the vein (Fig. 8). The external jugular is best entered with an angiocatheter (as compared to a thin wall arteriotomy needle), because it anchors the guidewire better through its winding path. A central venous catheter is then exchanged for the angiocatheter over the guidewire. Abduction of the ipsilateral arm 90 degrees or maintenance at the side while an assistant applies caudad traction before attempting to pass the guidewire facilitates passage of the guidewire underneath the clavicle.

PERIPHERALLY INSERTED CENTRAL VENOUS CATHETERS (PICC LINES)

In patients with limited peripheral venous sites or need for prolonged access, PICC lines are useful. They are usually inserted by radiologists from the antecubital fossa or the basilic or cephalic veins. The natural course of the basilic vein turns into the axillary vein; whereas the cephalic vein less reliably enters the axillary vein and does so at a more acute angle. The limitations of these lines are that they are typically long, small lumen intravenous catheters with slow infusion rates. A proximal tourniquet is applied to distend the basilic vein and while the patient's arm is kept at the side, the antecubital fossa is prepared aseptically and draped. Proximal to the antecubital crease, a commercially prepared catheter-though-a-needle assembly is advanced into the vein at a 45-degree angle. The tourniquet is released and the catheter is threaded through the needle until the distance traversed equals the distance from the insertion site to the sternomanubrial junction. The stiff inner wire is removed and attached to an infusion line. A chest radiograph confirms the position. If the catheter does not readily advance, another vein is tried. The success of placement is improved by fluoroscopy.

TECHNIQUE OF SUBCLAVIAN VENOUS CATHETERIZATION

With the patient in the Trendelenburg position with both arms at the side, a rolled towel is placed along the thoracic spine between the scapulae to extend the shoulders. The patient's upper chest and neck are prepared and draped as a sterile field and the physician dons sterile attire as previously described. We normally do not use either a finder needle or an angiocatheter because the depth of the subclavian vein is greater than the length of the finder needle and the angiocatheter is easily kinked.

An 18-gauge, thin-walled arteriotomy needle, inserted 1 to 2 cm inferior to the junction between the lateral and middle third of the clavicle, is directed underneath the clavicle and advanced toward the suprasternal notch until the subclavian vein is entered and blood can be aspirated. Some believe (we do not) that by orienting the bevel of the needle caudally, the guidewire will be directed toward the SVC. After an unsuccessful insertion, if the vein is not located after slow withdrawal of the needle, then another pass is made with the needle. Once the vein has been entered, guidewire placement and catheterization proceeds as described for the internal jugular method.

TECHNIQUE OF FEMORAL VENOUS CATHETERIZATION

The femoral vein presents an alternative puncture site for central venous cannulation when sites located craniad to the diaphragm are ruled out by bleeding diatheses, coagulopathy, or a tracheostomy. It is a particularly useful site in children. The midpoint of a line drawn from the anterior superior iliac spine and symphysis pubis is a useful landmark to locate the femoral artery. The femoral vein is located 1 to 1.5 cm medially to the femoral artery. The patient is prepared and draped and the physician dons sterile attire as previously described. Similar to the cannulation technique described for the internal jugular approach, the guidewire is placed via a needle or catheter next to the arterial pulsation 2 to 3 cm below the inguinal ligament (to reduce the risk of a retroperitoneal hematoma). Despite long-standing prejudice

against femoral venous catheters, recent reports demonstrate no higher rates of catheter sepsis at this site than at others (19).

COMPLICATIONS OF CENTRAL VENOUS CATHETERIZATION

Contamination and colonization of invasive vascular devices by microorganisms can contribute to nosocomial infection, increasing length of hospital stay, costs, and morbidity. In some circumstances, catheter-related infections carry a mortality rate of 10% to 25% (10). We believe that avoiding catheter-related infections is dependent on aseptic technique, including hand washing, sterile gloves, head covering, masks and gowns, and full-bed sterile drapes (20). Some studies show that skin preparation with chlorhexidine rather than povidone-iodine reduces the incidence of catheter-related sepsis (21). Daily site inspection with frequent aseptic dressing and intravenous tubing changes should be part of standard nursing operating procedures. Luer® locks and stop cocks should be accessed aseptically and replaced with a new sterile cap, since 22% of these caps become contaminated after three manipulations (22). Perhaps most important, the need for invasive monitors should be reassessed daily and the catheters removed as soon as possible, since the risk of infectious colonization is dramatically increased after 4 days (23). Catheters placed during emergency resuscitations before arrival in the ICU should be suspected of contamination. These catheters should be changed (24).

Whenever a catheter is suspected of being infected, it should be removed or replaced over a guidewire. The catheter tip should be sent for quantitative bacterial cultures; if there is no bacterial growth, the "new" catheter can be left in place. If the cultures confirm a catheter-related infection, then the "new" catheter should be removed and replaced aseptically at a different site. We do not recommend that central venous catheters be routinely replaced every 3 to 4 days over a guidewire (as was often the case in the past), since this practice does not reduce the rate of catheter infections (25,26).

In recent years, antimicrobial-coated and antiseptic-coated catheters have been developed that reduce colonization and bloodstream infections. When minocycline-rifampin–coated catheters were compared to chlorhexidine-silver-sulfadiazine–coated catheters, the minocycline-rifampin catheters were 3 times less likely to be colonized and 12 times less likely to be associated with a catheter-related bacteremia. Minocycline-rifampin–coated catheters retained their antimicrobial activity for 2 weeks (27). Because antimicrobial-coated catheters could, in theory, lead to antimicrobial resistance, these catheters are reserved for situations where infection rates are high. However, the antibiotics cannot be detected in blood, making the development of resistance by organisms residing at distant sites unlikely. Resistance infrequently occurs with multidrug therapy, and the decreased risk of catheter-related bloodstream infections might decrease the use of empiric antibiotics in critically ill patients, reducing the overall use of antibiotics (27). These potential advantages have not been assessed in clinical trials.

Other catheter-related complications can be reduced by anticipation and avoidance of common adverse events, and prompt treatment should they occur. Complications of invasive monitoring catheters can be described as either *immediate* (during catheter placement) or *delayed*. During attempted internal jugular or femoral venous catheter placement, the most common immediate complication is arterial puncture. Excessive hemorrhage can result in a hemothorax after the carotid subclavian vessels or SVC are punctured. If the carotid is cannulated accidentally, the catheter should be removed and direct pressure applied for 10 minutes. The airway is monitored for development of stridor or tracheal deviation. Another common immediate complication of attempted subclavian vein catheterization is pneumothorax, the incidence of which is estimated to be 1% to 2%. Should a pneumothorax occur in a patient who is mechanically ventilated, a thoracostomy tube should be placed to evacuate the pleural air. Spontaneously breathing patients with pneumothorax are evaluated on an individual basis for the need for air evacuation and thoracostomy tube placement. As previously noted, arrhythmias are common during placement of central venous catheters. Air embolism should be suspected when sudden hypoxemia or cardiovascular collapse develops during cannulation attempts.

As previously noted, an indwelling catheter that is abutting a vein at 90 degrees can erode through the vessel, leading to hemorrhage. Generally, this erosion occurs several days after catheter insertion. Cardiac tamponade can also occur when a guidewire or catheter perforates the intrapericardial SVC, the right atrium, right ventricle, or pulmonary artery (PA). Catheter-related thrombosis can occur. Misplaced catheters can result in interpleural administration of fluid, drugs, or nutritional support. Brachial plexopathy has been described after subclavian vein catheterization.

PULMONARY ARTERY CATHETERIZATION

Pulmonary artery catheters (PACs) are used to assess cardiac output (CO) and intravascular volume status and their response to therapy. Bedside estimation of cardiac preload is one of the more difficult tasks demanded of the intensivist. Blood pressure, urine output, neck vein distension, and skin turgor become unreliable predictors of adequate CO in the patient with critical illness. In a study of 103 PA catheterizations, physicians correctly predicted pulmonary arterial occlusion pressure (PAOP), CO, and right arterial pressure (RAP) 30%, 51%, and 55% of the time, respectively (28). Serial PAC measurements of cardiac performance using preload, CO, and afterload, although likely overused, nevertheless aid in the clinical management of unstable patients. Information obtainable from a PAC includes continuous monitoring of central venous and pulmonary artery pressure along with intermittent PAOP. CO measurements can be made by the thermodilution technique, either manually or nearly continuously with specially designed catheters. Mixed venous blood saturation, either continuously measured using a fiberoptic technique or intermittently with analysis of blood sample, can aid in assessing the adequacy of oxygen delivery relative to oxygen consumption. Right ventricular end-diastolic volume and ejection fraction can also be estimated using certain PACs. Some catheters have the capacity for right ventricular pacing, and in some cases, right atrial pacing.

The basic adult PA catheter is a 7.0F to 7.5F, polyvinyl chloride, radiopaque, multilumen catheter. It is 110-cm long and contains three lumens and a latex balloon at the tip. The PAC is marked every 10 cm from the tip with a black ring. The PA pressure is transduced and mixed venous blood samples are obtained from the distal lumen. The right ventricular lumen, 20 cm from the tip, is used for fluid and drug administration and in specialized catheters can serve as a port for a pacing electrode. The proximal lumen, located 30 cm from the tip, provides a portal for central venous pressure measurement, fluid and drug administration, and for thermodilution CO injectate. A thermistor at the tip connects to the CO monitor and measures the PA temperature. CO is calculated using the integral of PA temperature changes over time and the Stewart-Hamilton equation.

The PAC can be inserted at the bedside through an introducer sheath in any central vein, but most easily via the right internal jugular or left subclavian vein. As outlined in Table 4, the patient should be adequately monitored, prepared, and draped using aseptic techniques. The insertion method is identical to that described for central venous catheters, except that an introducer sheath is substituted for the venous catheter, and the dilator is inserted through the sheath before the entire unit is advanced over the guidewire into the vein. The wire and dilator are then pulled out together to keep a closed system and avoid air embolization. The introducer has a hemostasis valve through which the PAC will be inserted (Fig. 9).

Prior to insertion, a transparent sterility sheath is usually placed over the PAC. All lumens should be flushed with saline and the PA lumen connected to a pressure transducer. Function of the transducer(s) can be verified by "wiggling" the catheter and observing waveforms on the bedside monitor display. The PAC is advanced through the introducer sheath to the 20-cm mark at which point the balloon is inflated with 1.5 cc of air. As the PAC is gently advanced, the inflated balloon and blood flow guide the catheter from the vena cava, through the right atrium and ventricle, into the PA. Characteristic pressure waveforms are seen as the catheter advances through the heart chambers out into the PA and "wedges" in a PA segment (Fig. 10). Usually, the tip enters the right ventricle at 30 to 35 cm, the PA at approximately 40 to 45 cm, and the PA "wedge" position at 45 to 52 cm.

TABLE 4. EQUIPMENT NEEDED FOR CENTRAL VENOUS CATHETERIZATION

Mask, gown, head covering, eye protection, bed drape
Sterile gloves
Antiseptic solution
Intravenous infusion set or syringes with flush solution
Electrocardiography, pulse oximetry, noninvasive (or intraarterial) blood pressure
Resuscitation drugs
Central venous catheter tray/pulmonary artery catheter

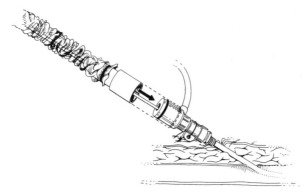

FIGURE 9. Illustration of placement of the pulmonary artery catheter through a sterility sheath into the introducer. The sheath is then advanced over the catheter and attached to the introducer. (Reproduced with permission from Butterworth JF IV. *Atlas of procedures in anesthesia and critical care.* Philadelphia: WB Saunders, 1992.)

Once the catheter enters a PA segment smaller in diameter than the inflated balloon, a PA occlusion pressure (PAOP, or "wedge") waveform will appear on the display. Once in the "wedge" position, the balloon is deflated and the pressure waveform should revert back to a PA pressure waveform. If it does not, then the catheter is withdrawn with the balloon deflated until a PA tracing returns.

When the catheter is well positioned, the PAOP and PA pressures can be obtained by a single, sequential inflation and deflation of the balloon. If the catheter has been advanced too far distally into the pulmonary vasculature, it may "wedge" continuously, increasing the risk of PA infarction or rupture. When the catheter tip is too proximally located in the PA, it may "whip" in and out of the right ventricle leading to a misdiagnosis of low PA diastolic pressures and increasing the risk of ventricular arrhythmias. Once the catheter is in proper position, the sterile sheath is advanced over the catheter and attached to the introducer assembly.

TABLE 5. ALTERATIONS OF NORMAL INTRACARDIAC PRESSURE–VOLUME RELATIONSHIP (PVR)

PAD > PAOP	PAOP > LVEDP	PAOP < LVEDP
Increased PVR	Positive pressure	Aortic insufficiency
Heart rate > 120	ventilation	
	PEEP	
	Mitral valve disease	

PAD, pulmonary artery diastolic pressure; PAOP, pulmonary arterial occlusion pressure; LVEDP, left-ventricular end-diastolic pressure; PEEP, positive end-expiratory pressure.

There is widespread agreement that clinicians who insert and manage PACs must be able to interpret the PAC data and initiate appropriate therapeutic actions based on these data. Unfortunately, multiple studies have identified deficits in clinicians' knowledge as far as indications, insertion technique, and interpretation of PAC data are concerned. In two studies only 53% and 77%, respectively, of physicians were able to determine PAOP correctly when given an original wave tracing (29,30).

To properly interpret the data obtained from the PAC, one must understand the relationship between PAOP and left ventricular pressure and volume. Ideally, when PAOP is obtained, the PAC resides in a region of the lung where PA pressure exceeds pulmonary venous and alveolar pressures. In this position, it is assumed that a static column of fluid exists between the tip of the PAC and the left ventricle. In the absence of valvular heart disease, excessive positive airway pressure, or major alterations of ventricular compliance, PAOP will approximate LAP, which in turn approximates the left ventricular end-diastolic pressure (LVEDP). The LVEDP relates to the left ventricular end-diastolic volume. Thus, the PAOP estimates left ventricular preload. However, the pressure–volume relationship is altered under many circumstances (Table 5). PAOP always should be measured at end-expiration. Both spontaneous and mechanical ventilation can confound the interpretation of the PAOP waveform (Fig. 11).

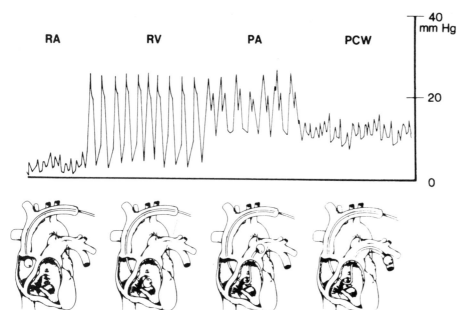

FIGURE 10. Pulmonary artery catheter pressure waveforms as the catheter passes through the right atrium (*RA*), right ventricle (*RV*), and pulmonary artery (*PA*), until it wedges (*PCW*). (Reproduced with permission from Rorie DK. Monitoring during cardiovascular surgery. In: Tarhan S, ed. *Cardiovascular anesthesia and postoperative care.* Chicago: Year Book Medical Publishers, Inc., 1982.)

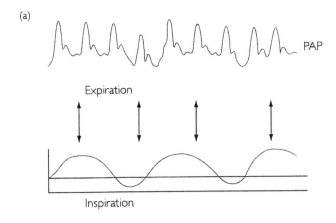

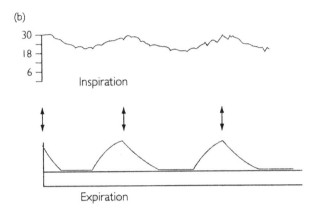

FIGURE 11. A: During normal respiration, the pulmonary artery (PA) waveforms on inspiration will be negative due to a decrease in intrathoracic pressure. On expiration, the intrathoracic pressure will result in positive deflections in the PA waveforms. The values recorded should be obtained at end-expiration when the intrathoracic pressure influence is minimal. **B:** When a patient is mechanically ventilated, the intrathoracic pressure during inspiration is at a positive level with ventilated breaths. On expiration, the values are negative due to the relative negative intrathoracic pressure. PAP are to be read to end-expiration.

Newer Pulmonary Artery Catheter Variants: Continuous Cardiac Output, Mixed Venous Oximetry Monitoring, and Right Ventricular Ejection Fraction Pulmonary Artery Catheters

Continuous cardiac output (CCO) monitoring uses thermodilution to estimate blood flow. Heat is released in pulses from a filament in the right ventricular portion of the catheter. The average CO over the past 3 to 6 minutes is displayed; thus the CCO is a continually updated average rather than a true, real-time continuous value. CCO is reliable and accurate compared to intermittent thermodilution CO measurements. Since CCO is averaged over several minutes, it is recorded throughout the respiratory cycle and may provide a more accurate estimate in patients who are mechanically ventilated. Currently the acquisition cost of this catheter is roughly twice that of a standard thermodilution PAC (31).

Continuous mixed-venous oximetry PA catheters use fiberoptics to determine the venous hemoglobin saturation using similar technology to that of a pulse oximeter. Mixed-venous oximetry

assesses the adequacy of the CO by measuring oxygen consumption by the body. This catheter is roughly four times as expensive as a conventional thermodilution catheter, and there are no studies showing improved patient outcome with its use (31).

When patients are subjected to increasing levels of positive end-expiratory pressure (PEEP), interpretation of increased PAOP or central venous pressure measurements become increasingly difficult. The right ventricular ejection fraction (RVEF) catheter was designed particularly for such patients. During fluid resuscitation from hypovolemia, the right ventricular end-diastolic volume index correlates well with the cardiac index. A right ventricular end-diastolic volume index of less than 140 mL/m^2 predicts improvement in cardiac index following a fluid challenge; conversely an index greater than 140 mL/m^2 predicts no improvement in cardiac index following a fluid challenge (32). We have found this catheter to be useful for resuscitation of critically ill trauma patients; however, there are no clinical trials demonstrating improved patient outcome with use of the RVEF catheter. This PAC also is considerably more expensive than the standard PAC.

TRANSPULMONARY THERMODILUTION

An alternative method of determining CO that is less invasive than a PAC is the pulse contour cardiac output monitor (PiCCO). It requires a simple central venous catheter and a specialized 4F femoral arterial catheter with an integrated thermistor (Pulsiocath, Pulsion Medical Systems) that is advanced into the abdominal aorta. It is considered less invasive, since a PAC is not needed and most critically ill patients have both a central and arterial line in place. In addition, there are small catheters available for use in small children. This technique should perhaps not be used in patients with abdominal aortic atherosclerosis or aneurysms. Transpulmonary thermodilution is a technique whereby cold fluid is injected into a central line port to measure CO. The cold indicator solution passes through the right side of the heart, the lungs, and through the left side of the heart until temperature is measured in the lower abdominal aorta. The transpulmonary CO measurement correlates well with PA thermodilution CO (33–35) (Fig. 12). The CO is slightly overestimated (by 3% to 5%), which is thought to be due to the dissipation of heat by the time the cold injectate reaches the thermistor located in the abdominal aorta. The femoral catheter also allows for the arterial pressure monitoring and withdrawal of blood samples.

TRANSESOPHAGEAL ECHOCARDIOGRAPHY

Transesophageal echocardiography (TEE) is increasingly utilized to evaluate critically ill patients. It can be performed rapidly and safely and the information obtained can be utilized to diagnose and manage acute hemodynamic decompensation. Even though PAC monitoring is typically used in this situation, methodologic limitations associated with its use (36) have resulted in controversy concerning its utility (37). For example, high amounts

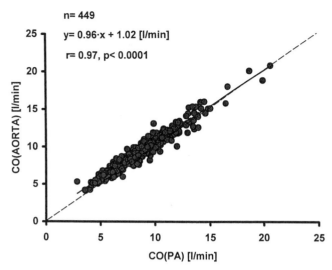

n= 449

y= 0.96·x + 1.02 [l/min]

r= 0.97, p< 0.0001

FIGURE 12. Linear regression analysis of transpulmonary cardiac output measurement, CO(AORTA), compared to traditional pulmonary artery, CO(PA), cardiac output measurement. (Reproduced with permission from Sakka SG, Reinhart K, Meier-Hellmann A. Comparison of pulmonary artery and arterial thermodilution cardiac output in critically ill patients. *Intensive Care Med* 1999;25:843–846.)

of PEEP and high PA pressures can provide misleading data in the presence of severe lung injury. Likewise, transthoracic echocardiography may have limited value because of interference from mechanical ventilation, surgical wound dressings, chest tubes, obesity, profound obstructive lung disease, and the inability to turn the patient laterally (38). TEE overcomes many of these technical limitations in that an ultrasound probe is placed into the esophagus which lies in close proximity to the heart and great vessels, and with its high frequency transducer (5 MHz), provides excellent image resolution. For the intensivist who is neither a cardiologist nor a cardiac anesthesiologist, a basic TEE examination can aid in the diagnosis of hemodynamic instability through rapid assessment of preload, ventricular performance, and extracardiac fluid. Interrogation of valvular pathology and aortic integrity requires more advanced TEE skills. Indications for TEE in the intensive care setting are listed in Table 6 (39).

Most critically ill patients in whom the intensivist desires to perform TEE are mechanically ventilated. Those who are not, can often wait for a cardiologist's examination. However, if an unintubated patient's respiratory status is severely compromised, it is recommended that the airway be secured with an endotracheal tube before placing the TEE probe. Correspondingly, gastric contents should be evacuated via an oral gastric or nasogastric tube as delayed gastric emptying is commonly seen in the critically ill patient. Nasal feeding and gastric tubes should, in turn, be removed prior to probe insertion in order to ensure good contact with the esophagus, essential for clear images. When performing the bedside TEE procedure, continuous electrocardiogram (ECG), blood pressure, and pulse oximetry should be monitored and resuscitative equipment should be available. Depending upon the mental and hemodynamic status of the patient, sedation may be warranted. TEE is contraindicated in

TABLE 6. INDICATIONS FOR TRANSESOPHAGEAL ECHOCARDIOGRAPHY IN THE INTENSIVE CARE UNIT[a]

1. Aorta
   Dissection
   Transection
2. **Hemodynamic instability**
   Unexplained shock
   Unexplained unstable hemodynamics
3. Cardiac contusion
   Clinical evidence and unstable hemodynamics
4. Evaluation of function of potential donor heart
5. **Extracardiac fluid**
   Tamponade
   Localized effusion
6. **Complication or diagnosis of myocardial infarction**
   Ventricular septal defect
   Valve dysfunction
7. Source of embolism (thrombus, air, tumor)
8. Endocarditis

[a]Headings in bold are addressed in the text.

those patients with severe esophageal or gastric pathology, including esophageal diverticula, stricture, perforation, varices, tumors, or recent esophageal or antral surgery (38). Performance of a TEE examination is also avoided in the patient with an unstable cervical spine. Although rare (1% to 3%), complications from performing TEE in the ICU include airway obstruction, right mainstem advancement of an endotracheal tube, tracheal extubation, vascular compromise, esophageal trauma and bleeding, and arrhythmias (38,40).

Basic Two-Dimensional Examination

(The views presented in Fig. 13 are taken from reference 41.)

With the patient in the supine position, the lubricated and unlocked probe is placed into the esophagus (35 to 40 cm) and gently advanced into the stomach. Anteflexing the probe at this level with the transducer at 0 degrees provides an excellent image for assessment of left ventricular filling. This is the *transgastric mid-short axis (TG-SAX)* view (Fig. 13D). At 90 degrees, the transgastric two-chamber view (TG-2 chamber) allows for interrogation of the anterior and inferior walls of the left ventricle (LV) and the mitral valve apparatus (Fig. 13E). At 120 degrees and with clockwise torque of the probe, the right atrium, right ventricle (RV), and tricuspid valve come into view; this is referred to as the transgastric right ventricular inflow view (TG RV inflow) (Fig. 13N) Then, after returning to 0 degrees, the probe is withdrawn into the *middle of the esophagus (30 cm)* where the four-chamber view is best seen (ME 4-chamber) (Fig.13A). To "drop" the LV down so that it is not foreshortened, the large wheel of the multiplane probe is turned counterclockwise and withdrawn a few centimeters so that the RA, RV, LA, LV, IAS, MV, and TV are visualized. At 30 degrees, the probe is withdrawn and turned slightly clockwise until all three leaflets of the aortic valve (AV) are seen (ME SAX AV); this is often termed the "Mercedes-Benz sign" (Fig. 13H). At 45 to 60 degrees, the right ventricular inflow-outflow tract can be interrogated (Fig. 13M) as well as the IAS, LA, LAA, and LUPV. At 90 degrees, several other structures

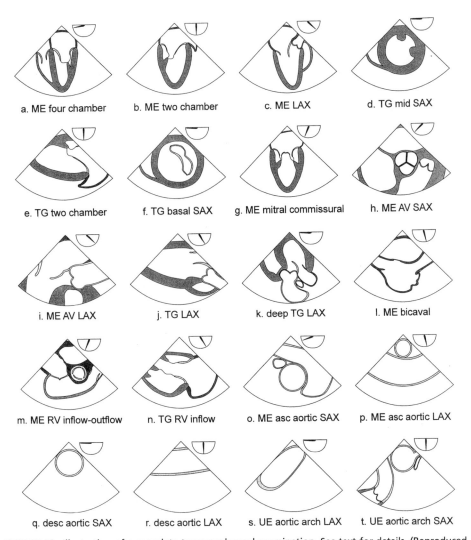

a. ME four chamber   b. ME two chamber   c. ME LAX   d. TG mid SAX

e. TG two chamber   f. TG basal SAX   g. ME mitral commissural   h. ME AV SAX

i. ME AV LAX   j. TG LAX   k. deep TG LAX   l. ME bicaval

m. ME RV inflow-outflow   n. TG RV inflow   o. ME asc aortic SAX   p. ME asc aortic LAX

q. desc aortic SAX   r. desc aortic LAX   s. UE aortic arch LAX   t. UE aortic arch SAX

FIGURE 13. Illustration of a complete transesophageal examination. See text for details. (Reproduced with permission from Shanewise JS, Cheung AT, Aronson S, et al. ASE/SCA guidelines for performing a comprehensive intraoperative multiplane transesophageal echocardiography examination: recommendations of the American Society of Echocardiography Council for Intraoperative Echocardiography and the Society of Cardiovascular Anesthesiologists Task Force for Certification in Perioperative Transesophageal Echocardiography. *Anesth Analg* 1999;89:870–884.)

can be evaluated by simply rotating the probe clockwise and counterclockwise. A hard counterclockwise torque will provide the two-chamber view: LA, LV, MV, and sometimes the LAA (Fig. 13B). A hard clockwise turn of the probe will bring in the inferior vena cava (IVC), RA, and SVC or bicaval view (Fig.13L). Between 110 and 130 degrees, and a slight clockwise rotation of the probe will layout the AV and ascending aorta into long-axis view (ME AV LAX) (Fig. 13I). Withdrawing the probe and turning the larger wheel clockwise will provide an even better view of the ascending aorta. The descending aorta is imaged after returning to the ME four-chamber view. The probe is rotated clockwise or counterclockwise until the aorta is seen in cross-section (Fig. 13Q). The probe is then advanced to the level of the diaphragm and then slowly withdrawn to the aortic arch, signified by an elongated image of the aorta (Fig. 13S). At this point, the angle of the transducer is turned to 60 degrees and the probe and large wheel are torqued clockwise to allow for visualization of the left subclavian artery. This view is of particular interest if there is concern of aortic dissection since traumatic rupture or transection usually occurs a couple of centimeters below the takeoff of the left subclavian artery at the aortic isthmus.

Left Ventricular Filling or Volume Status

The initial assessment of left ventricular filling is usually performed in the transgastric short axis view at the level of the papillary muscles. If the patient's volume status is jeopardized then "kissing" papillary muscles or cavitary obliteration of the left ventricle is seen during systole. In addition, left ventricular end-diastolic dimensions are reduced (42,43). Normal cross-sectional dimensions in this view range between 3.5 to 6.1 cm for

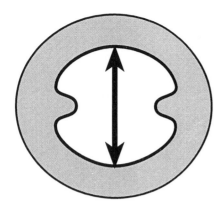

Diastole   3.5 – 6.1 cm
Systole   2.3 – 4.1 cm

FIGURE 14. Schematic of normal cross-sectional dimensions in transgastric short-axis view.

a body surface area of 1.4 to 2.0 m². Fig. 14 shows site of measurement (44). This can further lead to a turbulent flow pattern in the left ventricular outflow tract visualized by color Doppler. Certainly, whenever left ventricular filling is assessed, the underlying function of the ventricle must be taken into consideration. For example, in the case of cardiomyopathy, the echocardiographic indices of hypovolemia may be very subtle whereas in the case of a hyperdynamic myocardium (i.e., sepsis, liver failure), systolic cavitary obliteration may be the norm (38). In such circumstances, additional data from the PAC may be useful.

Left Ventricular Performance

Echocardiographic images of the left ventricle provide reliable quantitative and qualitative estimates of global left ventricular function. Quantitative assessment of systolic function is customarily performed using the transgastric short-axis view at the mid-papillary level. Fractional area change (FAC) of the left ventricle can be obtained by first freezing the left ventricular image at end-diastole (corresponding to the peak of the R wave on the ECG) and the operator can trace the cavity, or endocardial border, by hand manipulating the trackball. The computer will then calculate the end-diastolic area (EDA). Similarly, the end-systolic area (ESA) can be obtained by tracing the frozen echocardiographic image when the left ventricle is the smallest (usually

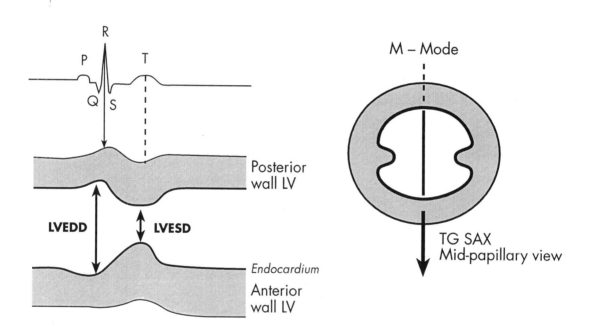

Fractional shortening: EDD – ESD/EDD x 100%

LVEDD = Left ventricular end diastolic dimension
LVESD = Left ventricular end systolic dimension
TG   = Transgastric
SAX   = Short axis

FIGURE 15. Schematic of M-mode transesophageal echocardiography of the left ventricle obtained from the transgastric short-axis view. Fractional shortening, an index of systolic function, is calculated using linear dimensions from M-mode measurements. Fractional shortening (%) of the left ventricle is the left ventricle end-diastolic dimension (LVEDD) minus left ventricle end-systolic dimension (LVESD) divided by the LVEDD.

corresponding to the peak of the T wave on the ECG). The FAC can then be derived by the formula:

$$(EDA - ESA)/EDA$$

This is analogous to ejection fraction. Fractional shortening (FS) is another measure of global systolic function. Assuming no regional wall motion abnormalities, two times FS is a good one-dimensional estimate of ejection fraction. It is usually calculated automatically from online software using M-mode left ventricular dimensions in diastole (LVDD) and left ventricular dimensions in systole (LVSD) at the transgastric short-axis midpapillary level (Fig. 15). Normal adult ranges for FS (%) are 28 to 44. One important limitation however to these indices of systolic function is that they are load-dependent: changes in preload and afterload can cause marked changes in FAC without changing the intrinsic properties of ventricular function.

Qualitative assessment of left ventricular performance requires no special formula, but does require an experienced echocardiographer. In the hypotensive, critically ill patient, a qualitative assessment of left ventricular filling and function may serve as a practical guide to administration of fluid, inotropes, and vasopressors (45). Table 7 summarizes the echocardiographic findings associated with the more common causes of hypotension in the critical care setting.

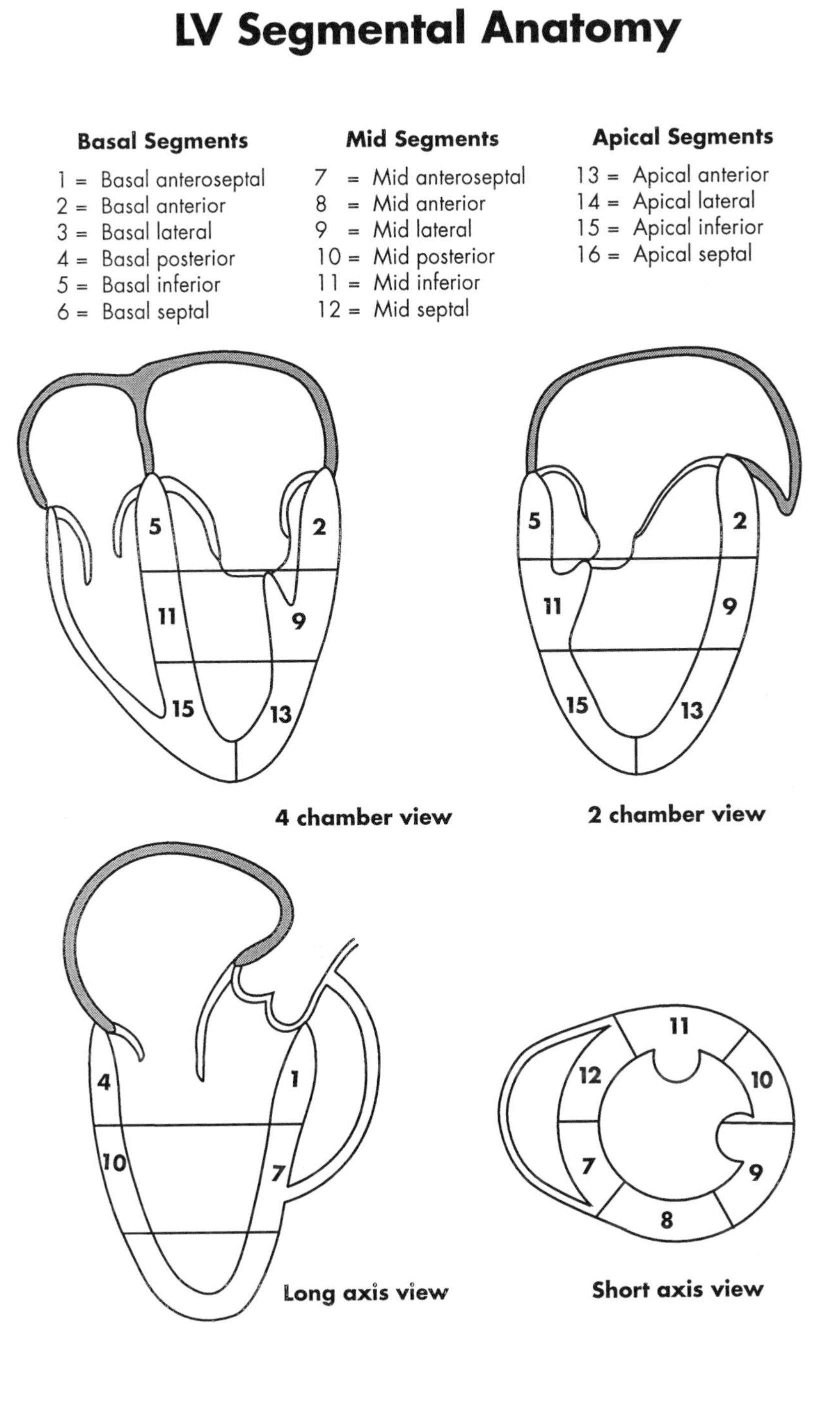

LV Segmental Anatomy

Basal Segments	**Mid Segments**	**Apical Segments**
1 = Basal anteroseptal	7 = Mid anteroseptal	13 = Apical anterior
2 = Basal anterior	8 = Mid anterior	14 = Apical lateral
3 = Basal lateral	9 = Mid lateral	15 = Apical inferior
4 = Basal posterior	10 = Mid posterior	16 = Apical septal
5 = Basal inferior	11 = Mid inferior	
6 = Basal septal	12 = Mid septal	

4 chamber view

2 chamber view

Long axis view

Short axis view

FIGURE 16. Four left ventricular views to identify 16 wall segments for assessment of ischemia.

TABLE 7. ETIOLOGY OF ACUTE HYPOTENSION USING ECHOCARDIOGRAPHIC ESTIMATES OF END-DIASTOLIC AREA (EDA) AND EJECTION FRACTION (EF)

EDA	EF (Estimated)	Etiology	Treatment
⇓⇓	⇑⇑ > 80%	Hypovolemia	Fluid or blood
⇑⇑	⇓⇓ < 20%	LV failure	Inotropes
Normal	⇑⇑ > 80%	SVR (r/o severe MR or AR, or VSD)	Vasopressors

EDA, end-diastolic area; EF, ejection fraction; LV, left ventricular; SVR, systemic vascular resistance; MR, mitral regurgitation; AR, atrial regurgitation; VSD, ventricular septal defect.

Transesophageal echocardiography aids in the early detection of myocardial ischemia through assessment of regional wall motion abnormalities (RWMA). Four views of the left ventricle are routinely used to identify the 16 wall segments recommended by the American Society of Echocardiography for evaluation of ischemia (Fig. 16). These segments are supplied by the three coronary arteries (Fig. 17). Wall motion is based on inward excursion toward the center of the left ventricular cavity and segmental thickening during systole. Both assessments are necessary because infarcted tissue, for example, may appear to be moving inward as it is "tethered" to adjacent normal segments. The absence of systolic wall thickening, however, helps delineate the damaged wall segment. The qualitative grading system used to assess RWMA is:

1 = normal (marked thickening and greater than 30% systolic reduction in radius)

2 = mildly hypokinetic (moderate thickening and 10% to 30% systolic reduction in radius)

3 = severely hypokinetic (minimal thickening and 0% to 10% systolic reduction in radius)

4 = akinetic (no thickening and no change in radius)

5 = dyskinetic (thinning and paradoxic, outward movement during systole) (45)

TEE is also useful in identifying the presence of extracardiac fluid that may be responsible for acute hemodynamic decompensation in the critically ill patient. Specifically, TEE can aid in the rapid and early diagnosis of cardiac tamponade or loculated pericardial effusions that might otherwise be delayed or missed by conventional hemodynamic monitoring techniques. The two-dimensional echocardiographic findings of tamponade include right atrial inversion, right ventricular diastolic collapse, and a decrease in dimensions of both ventricles during systole and diastole. Using Doppler, exaggerated transmitral and tricuspid flow velocities can also be observed. If the critically ill patient has an increased right ventricular afterload due to acute lung injury then these echocardiographic signs of tamponade may be delayed. On the other hand, if the patient has preexisting left ventricular dysfunction then the echocardiographic findings of excessive extracardiac fluid will appear earlier (38). Nevertheless, it remains essential that multiple echocardiographic views are employed in order to identify evidence of regional tamponade or a loculated effusion that may be responsible for hemodynamic decompensation.

In those patients who are not intubated or who possess the aforementioned contraindications to TEE, transthoracic echocardiography (TTE) can be performed easily at the bedside using a 2.5 to 3.5 MHz-phased array transducer to aid in the differential diagnosis of hypotension and the suspicion of pericardial tamponade. Although the optimal position of the patient for examination is often in the left lateral decubitus position, the critically ill patient may be uncooperative necessitating the supine position. The various locations for placement of the transthoracic transducer for the two-dimensional examination of the heart are shown in Fig. 18. The four basic transducer positions include the parasternal (left of the sternum), suprasternal (in the suprasternal notch), apical (apex of the heart), and subcostal positions. The relationship of the TTE and TEE examinations is displayed in Fig. 19. The sector apex in the short-axis and long-axis views is displayed downward reflecting the transthoracic image while the TEE approach views the heart from the opposite direction.

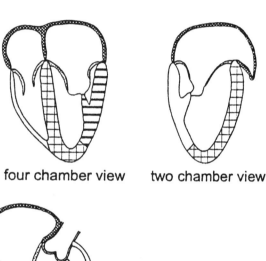

four chamber view   **two chamber view**

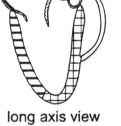

long axis view

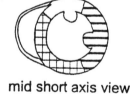

mid short axis view

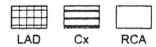

LAD   Cx   RCA

FIGURE 17. Illustration of coronary artery blood supply to various wall segments. (Reproduced with permission from Shanewise JS, Cheung AT, Aronson S, et al. ASE/SCA guidelines for performing a comprehensive intraoperative multiplane transesophageal echocardiography examination: recommendations of the American Society of Echocardiography Council for Intraoperative Echocardiography and the Society of Cardiovascular Anesthesiologists Task Force for Certification in Perioperative Transesophageal Echocardiography. *Anesth Analg* 1999;89:870–884.)

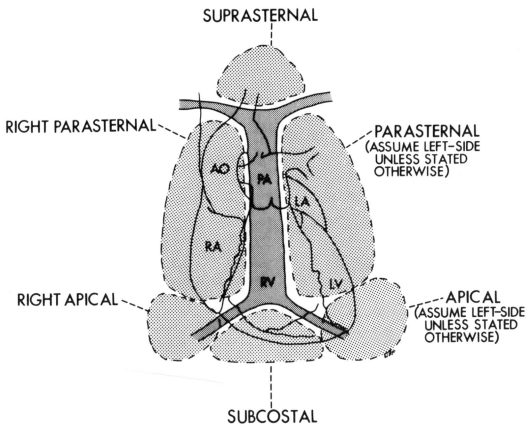

FIGURE 18. Diagram showing the locations for the placement of the transthoracic transducer for the two-dimensional examination of the heart. (Reproduced from Henry WL, DeMaria A, Gramiak R, et al. Report of the American Society of Echocardiography Committee on Nomenclature and Standards in Two-Dimensional Echocardiography. *Circulation* 1980;62:212–215, with permission from the American Heart Association, Inc.)

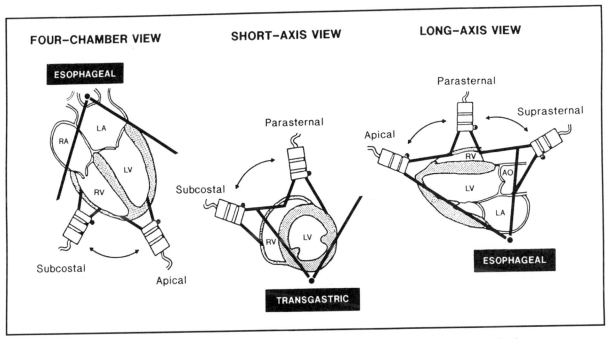

FIGURE 19. Diagram showing the relationship of the transthoracic and transesophageal examinations. (Reproduced with permission from Seward JB, Khandheria BK, Edwards WD, et al. Biplanar transesophageal echocardiography: anatomic correlations, image orientation, and clinical applications. *Mayo Clin Proc* 1990;65:1193–1194.)

PERCUTANEOUS DILATIONAL TRACHEOSTOMY

Percutaneous dilational tracheostomy (PcT), the bedside insertion of a cannula into the trachea, is increasingly popular relative to conventional open tracheostomy, as it avoids unnecessary transfers of critically ill patients to and from the operating room, providing more convenient scheduling (since tracheostomy procedures are often "added on" to the regular surgery schedule), and reducing exposure of healthy surgical patients to sick ICU patients bearing drug-resistant organisms (46). There may also be fewer short- and long-term complications. The bedside technique requires one or two persons to perform the procedure and a nurse to monitor the patient. The cost has been estimated at one-half to one-third that of standard operative tracheostomies (46,47). However, it is difficult to compare PcT to surgical tracheostomy because there have been four different PcT techniques, and multiple surgical tracheostomy techniques described. The Rapitrach kit is no longer performed due to increased complication rates. The three remaining techniques include: the single dilator technique of Toy and Weinstein (48), the Griggs technique (49), and the PDT kit of Ciaglia (50,51). The first two techniques use a needle and a guidewire to enter the trachea, and a dilator forceps to spread open the trachea. Use of the dilator forceps increases the risk of tracheal injury, bleeding, and loss of airway. At present the most popular PcT technique is the PDT kit of Ciaglia. This technique has been reported to have a low incidence of perioperative complications comparable to those associated with open tracheostomy.

The timing of tracheostomy remains controversial and has been reviewed elsewhere (52–54). Hemodynamically unstable patients, patients requiring high amounts of PEEP or FIO_2, or patients with bleeding diatheses should have the procedure postponed to avoid potentially life-threatening hypoxemia, death, or bleeding. Inability to extend the neck due to confirmed or potential cervical fracture also precludes the placement of a tracheostomy, since the neck must be extended during the procedure. A short, fat neck often makes placement difficult. Although recent median sternotomy is often considered a contraindication to tracheostomy due to proximity of the healing surgical wound to tracheal secretions, early studies of PcT in cardiac surgical patients show no increased risk of sternal wound infection even when performed within 2 weeks of surgery (55,56).

PcT should only be performed by a person skilled at this procedure. The necessary equipment to perform a PcT is outlined in Table 8. Experience with open tracheostomy helps the operator to better appreciate the anatomy, and facilitates a switch to an open technique should that be required. Using the Ciaglia Percutaneous Introducer Set (Cook, Inc.), the patient is placed on a hard board in the ICU bed with a rolled towel placed along the thoracic spine between the scapulae to extend the shoulders. After donning sterile apparel, the operator prepares the neck with aseptic solution and drapes it. The existing endotracheal tube is withdrawn until its tip lies just caudad to the glottic opening. After appropriate sedation, local anesthetic is injected for a 2-cm skin incision made 1 cm below the cricoid cartilage. The trachea is palpated and entered between the first and third tracheal rings with an 18-gauge, thin-walled arteriotomy needle or an

TABLE 8. COMPLICATIONS OF PERCUTANEOUS TRACHEOSTOMY

	Incidence (%)	Refs
Initial complications:		
Hemorrhage	0–6	46, 51, 55, 58
Posterior mucosal wall laceration	<2	59, 60
Paratracheal malpositioning	<1	55, 60
Subcutaneous emphysema	<5	51, 55
Pneumothorax	<1	51, 60
Infection	<2	46, 55
Delayed complications:		
Tracheoinnominate artery fistula	<1	46
Tracheoesophageal fistula	<1	46, 55
Tracheal stenosis (symptomatic)	<2	46, 51, 58

appropriate size intravenous needle–cannula assembly directed caudad (Fig. 20). Tracheal entrance is confirmed by aspiration of air. The orotracheal tube is twisted to ensure it has not been speared by the needle. A guidewire is passed through the needle (or cannula) and the needle (or cannula) removed. Dilators of increasing size (from 12F to 36F) are passed over the guidewire complex (Fig. 21). The tracheostomy tube is mounted over the largest dilator, and with firm pressure is advanced with a twisting motion into the trachea (Fig. 22). Difficulty can be encountered at this point from "buckling" of the anterior tracheal wall. (The Sims Per-Fit percutaneous dilational tracheostomy kit [Sims, Inc.] has a tracheostomy tube specifically designed to fit the dilator/introducer.) The trachea is suctioned (to remove secretions and blood) and the cuff of the cannula is inflated. Correct position is confirmed by auscultation of lung sounds and detection of carbon dioxide in end-tidal gas. Finally, the indwelling transoral endotracheal tube is removed and the tracheostomy tube is secured with sutures and tracheostomy tape. Bronchoscopy through the indwelling endotracheal tube can be helpful by allowing direct vision of needle puncture into the trachea and confirming that the existing endotracheal tube has not been punctured, and that the wire has not passed outside the trachea.

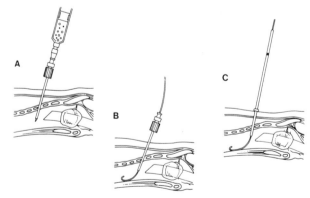

FIGURE 20. Illustration of percutaneous tracheostomy placement. **A:** Air aspiration confirms tracheal entrance of catheter. **B:** A guidewire is placed through the catheter. **C:** A dilator is exchanged over the guidewire for the catheter. (Reproduced with permission from Powell DM, Price PD, Forrest LA. Review of percutaneous tracheostomy. *Laryngoscope* 1998;108:170–177.)

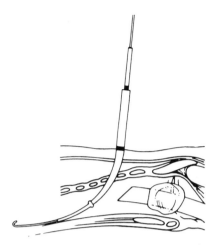

FIGURE 21. Illustration of dilator placement. (Reproduced with permission from Powell DM, Price PD, Forrest LA. Review of percutaneous tracheostomy. *Laryngoscope* 1998;108:170–177.)

Complications of Percutaneous Dilational Tracheostomy

The morbidity of tracheostomy comes acutely from airway loss, airway obstruction, hemorrhage, pneumothorax, or subcutaneous emphysema (46,47,57). A freshly placed cannula can be dislodged from the trachea while remaining in the patient, indicated by high ventilatory pressure alarms or the inability to pass a suction catheter through the cannula. When this occurs, it is best to intubate the patient orally, since the tracheostomy canal is not stable and may collapse when the cannula is removed. If the cannula is electively exchanged, an airway exchange device

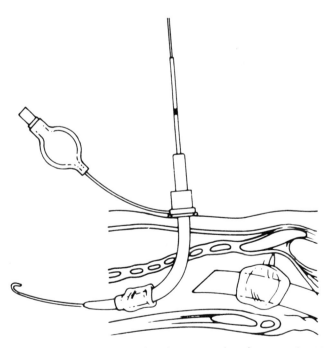

FIGURE 22. Demonstration of tracheostomy tube advancement over the largest dilator. (Reproduced with permission from Powell DM, Price PD, Forrest LA. Review of percutaneous tracheostomy. *Laryngoscope* 1998;108:170–177.)

TABLE 9. EQUIPMENT FOR PERCUTANEOUS TRACHEOSTOMY

Usual monitoring—electrocardiography, pulse oximetry, noninvasive blood pressure
Resuscitation drugs
Suction apparatus
Antiseptic solution
Sterile gloves, apparel, cap, mask
Standard intubation equipment
Percutaneous tracheostomy tray
Fiberoptic bronchoscopy (optional)
Tracheostomy tapes
Chest tube tray at bedside

should be used. Infection at the cannulation site is uncommon and usually responds to antibiotic therapy. It may become necessary to convert to an open tracheostomy if one is unable to pass the cannula over a dilator or if excessive bleeding occurs. Bleeding usually can be stopped by applying direct pressure. Acute and delayed complications with PcT are summarized in Table 9.

Rare delayed complications include: (a) a tracheoinnominate artery fistula, (b) a tracheoesophageal fistula, (c) voice changes, and (d) tracheal stenosis. Symptomatic tracheal stenosis is reported to occur in less than 2% of patients, while subclinical stenosis defined as 10% stenosis is reported after about 40% of PcT. In contrast, subclinical stenosis is reported after 60% to 75% of traditional surgical tracheostomies (58). Overall, PcT is a simple technique that can usually be performed in less than 15 minutes (47,57–59). Complications can be reduced by selecting appropriate patients and by excluding those with short, fat necks whose tracheal rings cannot be palpated.

SUMMARY

Multiple procedures are routinely used in the care of critically ill patients. Attention to detail in performing invasive techniques is important in limiting morbidity. Arterial cannulation, a basic technique for monitoring blood pressure in unstable patients and for obtaining frequent blood samples, can be performed at several accessible sites, including the radial, dorsalis pedis, femoral, brachial, and axillary arteries. The order of the preceding list is the usual order of preference. Although infectious complications of arterial catheterization are infrequent, infectious complications of central venous catheterization (including pulmonary arterial catheterization) are common. Therefore, central venous catheterization should be performed using scrupulous sterile technique including mask, cap, gown, and gloves. Central venous catheters suspected of infection, but without evidence of local skin purulence, can be replaced over a wire and the new catheter can be left in place if quantitative tip cultures are negative for bacterial growth. Pulmonary arterial catheters provide valuable hemodynamic information in many patients, but at the expense of occasional life-threatening complications. Pulmonary arterial catheters should be positioned so that they "wedge" with the appropriate balloon volume and are neither continuously wedged nor located so that they whip in and out of the right ventricle. TEE offers a less invasive technique for assessing hemodynamic status. Basic skills in TEE include the ability to assess ventricular preload, ventricular performance, and extracardiac fluid; advanced skills include the ability to assess valvular pathology and aortic integrity. Although the general topic of airway management is beyond the scope of this chapter, one technique for long-term management of ventilated patients merits discussion. PcT avoids unnecessary transfers of critically ill patients to and from the operating room, avoids use of expensive time in the operating room, and reduces movement of potentially drug-resistant organisms around the hospital.

KEY POINTS

Arterial cannulation can be performed at several accessible sites, including the radial, brachial, axillary, dorsalis pedis, and femoral arteries. In general, more distal sites are selected first.

Central venous catheterization should be performed using scrupulous sterile technique including mask, cap, gown, and gloves.

Central venous catheters suspected of infection, but without evidence of local skin purulence, can be replaced over a wire and the new catheter can be left in place if quantitative tip cultures are negative for bacterial growth.

Pulmonary arterial catheters should be positioned so that they "wedge" with the appropriate balloon volume and are neither continuously wedged nor located so that they whip in and out of the right ventricle.

Basic skills in transesophageal echocardiography include the ability to assess ventricular preload, ventricular performance, and extracardiac fluid; advanced skills include the ability to assess valvular pathology and aortic integrity.

Percutaneous dilational tracheostomy avoids unnecessary transfers of critically ill patients to and from the operating room, avoids use of expensive time in the operating room, and reduces movement of potentially drug-resistant organisms around the hospital.

REFERENCES

1. Rippe RM, ed. *Procedures and techniques in intensive care medicine.* Boston: Little, Brown, 1995.
1a. Low LL, Harrington GR, Stoltzfus DP. The effect of arterial lines on blood-drawing practices and costs in intensive care units. *Chest* 1995;108:216–219.
2. Graber D, Dailey RH. Catheter flow rates updated. *JACEP* 1977;6:518.
3. Sulek CA, Gravenstein N, Blackshear RH, et al. Head rotation during internal jugular vein cannulation and the risk of carotid artery puncture. *Anesth Analg* 1996;82:125–128.
4. Maruyama K, Nakajima Y, Hayashi Y, et al. A guide to preventing deep insertion of the cannulation needle during catheterization of the internal jugular vein. *J Cardiothorac Vasc Anesth* 1997;11:192–194.
5. Denys BG, Uretsky BF. Anatomical variations of internal jugular vein location: impact on central venous access. *Crit Care Med* 1991;19:1516–1519.
6. Gordon AC, Saliken JC, Johns D, et al. US-guided puncture of the internal jugular vein: complications and anatomic considerations. *J Vasc Interv Radiol* 1998;9:333–338.
7. Denys BG, Uretsky BF, Reddy PS. Ultrasound-assisted cannulation of the internal jugular vein. A prospective comparison to the external landmark-guided technique. *Circulation* 1993;87:1557–1562.
8. Troianos CA, Jobes DR, Ellison N. Ultrasound-guided cannulation of the internal jugular vein. A prospective, randomized study. *Anesth Analg* 1991;72:823–826.
9. Andrews RT, Bova DA, Venbrux AC. How much guidewire is too much? Direct measurement of the distance from subclavian and internal jugular vein access sites to the superior vena cava-atrial junction during central venous catheter placement. *Crit Care Med* 2000;28:138–142.
10. Mermel LA. Prevention of intravascular catheter-related infections. *Ann Intern Med* 2000;132:391–402.
11. FDA Task Force. Precautions necessary with central venous catheters. *FDA Drug Bulletin* 1989;19(2):15–16.
12. Peres PW. Positioning central venous catheters—a prospective survey. *Anaesth Intensive Care* 1990;18:536–539.
13. Czepizak CA, O'Callaghan JM, Venus B. Evaluation of formulas for optimal positioning of central venous catheters. *Chest* 1995;107:1662–1664.
14. Shuster M, Nave H, Piepenbrock S, et al. The carina as a landmark in central venous catheter placement. *Br J Anaesth* 2000;85:192–194.
15. Chalkiadis GA, Goucke CR. Depth of central venous catheter insertion in adults: an audit and assessment of a technique to improve tip position. *Anaesth Intensive Care* 1998;26:61–66.
16. Tocino IM, Watanabe A. Impending catheter perforation of superior vena cava: radiographic recognition. *AJR Am J Roentgenol* 1986;146:487–490.
17. Duntley P, Siever J, Korwes ML, et al. Vascular erosion by central venous catheters. *Chest* 1992;101:1633–1638.
18. Fletcher SJ, Bodenham AR. Safe placement of central venous catheters: where should the tip of the catheter lie? *Br J Anaesth* 2000;85:188–191.
19. Kruse JA, Carlson RW. Infectious complications of femoral vs internal jugular and subclavian vein central venous catheterization. *Crit Care Med* 1991;19:S84.
20. Sherertz RJ, Ely EW, Westbrook DM, et al. Education of physicians-in-training can decrease the risk for vascular catheter infection. *Ann Intern Med* 2000;132:641–648.
21. Maki DG, Ringer M, Alvarado CJ. Prospective randomised trial of povidone-iodine, alcohol, and chlorhexidine for the prevention of infection associated with central venous and arterial catheters. *Lancet* 1991;338:339–343.
22. Tebbs SE, Ghose A, Elliott TS. Microbial contamination of intravenous and arterial catheters. *Intensive Care Med* 1996;22:272–273.
23. Samsoondar W, Freeman JB, Coultish I, et al. Colonization of intravascular catheters in the intensive care unit. *Am J Surg* 1985;149:730–732.
24. Norwood S, Ruby A, Civetta J, et al. Catheter-related infections and associated septicemia. *Chest* 1991;99:968–975.
25. Cobb DK, High KP, Sawyer RG, et al. A controlled trial of scheduled replacement of central venous and pulmonary artery catheters. *N Engl J Med* 1992;327:1062–1068.
26. Cook D, Randolph A, Kernerman P, et al. Central venous catheter replacement strategies: a systematic review of the literature. *Crit Care Med* 1997;25:1417–1424.
27. Darouiche RO, Raad II, Heard SO, et al. A comparison of two antimicrobial-impregnated central venous catheters. *N Engl J Med* 1999;340:1–8.
28. Eisenberg PR, Jaffe AS, Schuster DP. Clinical evaluation compared to pulmonary artery catheterization in the hemodynamic assessment of critically ill patients. *Crit Care Med* 1984;12:549–553.

29. Iberti TJ, Fischer EP, Leibowitz AB, et al. A multicenter study of physicians' knowledge of the pulmonary artery catheter. Pulmonary artery catheter study group. *JAMA* 1991;264:2928–2932.

30. Trottier SJ, Taylor RW. Physicians' attitudes toward and knowledge of the pulmonary artery catheter. Society of Critical Care Medicine membership survey. *New Horiz* 1997;5:201–205.

31. Nelson LD. The new pulmonary artery catheters: continuous venous oximetry, right ventricular ejection fraction, and continuous cardiac output. *New Horiz* 1997;5:251–258.

32. Diebel LN, Wilson RF, Tagett MG, et al. End-diastolic volume: a better indicator of preload in the critically ill. *Arch Surg* 1992;127:817–822.

33. Sakka SG, Reinhart K, Meier-Hellmann A. Comparison of pulmonary artery and arterial thermodilution cardiac output in critically ill patients. *Intensive Care Med* 1999;25:843–846.

34. Goedje O, Peyerl M, Seebauer T, et al. Reproducibility of double indicator dilution measurements of intrathoracic blood volume compartments, extravascular lung water, and liver function. *Chest* 1998;113:1070–1077.

35. Goedje O, Hoeke K, Lichtwarck-Aschoff M, et al. Continuous cardiac output by femoral arterial thermodilution calibrated pulse contour analysis: comparison with pulmonary arterial thermodilution. *Crit Care Med* 1999;27:2407–2412.

36. Van Aken H, Vandermeersch E. Reliability of PCWP as an index for left ventricular preload. *Br J Anaesth* 1988;60:85S–89S.

37. Conners AF Jr, Speroff T, Dawson NV, et al. The effectiveness of right heart catheterization in the initial care of critically ill patients. *JAMA* 1996;276:889–897.

38. Porembka DT, Hanson CW III. New technologies for the perioperative physician. *Anesthesiol Clin North Am* 1997;15:833–877.

39. Kerut EK, McIlwain EF, Plotnick GD. Critical care. In: *Handbook of echo-Doppler interpretation*. Armonk, NY: Futura Publishing Co, Inc., 1996.

40. Pearson AC, Castello R, Labovitz AJ. Safety and utility of transesophageal echocardiography in the critically ill patient. *Am Heart J* 1990;119:1083.

41. Shanewise JS, Cheung AT, Aronson S, et al. ASE/SCA guidelines for performing a comprehensive intraoperative multiplane transesophageal echocardiography examination: recommendations of the American Society of Echocardiography Council for Intraoperative Echocardiography and the Society of Cardiovascular Anesthesiologists Task Force for Certification in Perioperative Transesophageal Echocardiography. *Anesth Analg* 1999;89:870–884.

42. Cheung AT, Savino JS, Weiss SJ, et al. Echocardiographic and hemodynamic indexes of left ventricular preload in patients with normal and abnormal ventricular function. *Anesthesiology* 1994;81:376.

43. Leung JM, Levine EH. Left ventricular end-systolic cavity obliteration as an estimate of intraoperative hypovolemia. *Anesthesiology* 1994;81:1102.

44. Rimington H, Chambers J. *Echocardiography: a practical guide for reporting.* Pearl River, NY: Parthenon Publishing Group Ltd., 1998.

45. Cahalan M. Ventricular systolic function: regional and global LV and RV function. Paper presented at: 3rd Annual Comprehensive Review of Intraoperative Echo; February 2000; San Diego.

46. Powell DM, Price PD, Forrest LA. Review of percutaneous tracheostomy. *Laryngoscope* 1998;108:170–177.

47. Hill BB, Zweng TN, Maley RH, et al. Percutaneous dilational tracheostomy: report of 356 cases. *J Trauma* 1996;41:238–244.

48. Toy FJ, Weinstein JD. A percutaneous tracheostomy device. *Surgery* 1969;65:384–389.

49. Griggs WM, Worthley LI, Gilligan JE, et al. A simple percutaneous tracheostomy technique. *Surg Gynecol Obstet* 1990;170:543–555.

50. Ciaglia P, Firsching R, Syniec C. Elective percutaneous dilational tracheostomy. A new simple bedside procedure: preliminary report. *Chest* 1985;87:715–719.

51. Ciaglia P, Graniero KD. Percutaneous dilational tracheostomy. Results and long-term follow-up. *Chest* 1992;101:464–467.

52. Heffner JE, Miller KS, Sahn SA. Tracheostomy in the intensive care unit. Part 2: complications. *Chest* 1986;90:430–436.

53. Heffner JE, Miller KS, Sahn SA. Tracheostomy in the intensive care unit. Part 1: indications, technique, management. *Chest* 1986;90:269–274.

54. Plummer AL, Gracey DR. Consensus conference on artificial airways in patients receiving mechanical ventilation. *Chest* 1989;96:178–180.

55. Hubner N, Rees W, Seufert K, et al. Percutaneous dilational tracheostomy done early after cardiac surgery: outcome and incidence of mediastinitis. *Thorac Cardiovasc Surg* 1998;46:89–92.

56. Byhahn C, Rinne T, Halbig S, et al. Frühelektive perkutane tracheotomie nach medianer sternotomie. *Z Herz-Thorax-Gefäß chir* 1999;13:221–227.

57. Leonard RC, Lewis RH, Singh B, et al. Late outcome from percutaneous tracheostomy using the Portex kit. *Chest* 1999;115:1070–1075.

58. Walz MK, Peitgen K, Thurauf N, et al. Percutaneous dilatational tracheostomy—early results and long-term outcome of 326 critically ill patients. *Intensive Care Med* 1998;24:685–690.

59. Petros S, Engelmann L. Percutaneous dilatational tracheostomy in a medical ICU. *Intensive Care Med* 1997;23:630–634.

60. Berrouschot J, Oaken J, Steineger L, et al. Perioperative complications of percutaneous dilational tracheostomy. *Laryngoscope* 1997; 107:1538–1544.

HEMODYNAMIC ASSESSMENT IN THE CRITICALLY ILL PATIENT

JEFFERY S. VENDER
JOSEPH W. SZOKOL

KEY WORDS

- Intravascular monitoring
- Oxygen delivery
- Pulmonary artery catheter
- Pulmonary artery occlusion pressure
- Right ventricular ejection fraction
- Thermodilution cardiac output
- Transesophageal echocardiography
- Transthoracic echocardiography

INTRODUCTION

The growth in the field of intensive care medicine has paralleled advances in biotechnology. A primary advance in biotechnology that has had a dramatic impact on intensive care medicine was the development of monitors that allow continuous measuring and recording of physiologic variables. Anesthesiologists, who had considerable experience monitoring the hemodynamic status of patients in the operating room, extended their expertise to the critical care arena.

Clinical monitoring, which began with simple systemic blood pressure monitoring, changed dramatically with the development of continuous indwelling catheters and hardware support for cardiovascular assessment. These developments increased the scope of clinical monitoring to include intravascular (central venous and pulmonary artery pressure) monitoring. Technological advances in monitoring should continue to occur as severity of illness and expectation for improved outcome occur.

This chapter will discuss monitoring of the cardiovascular system, with primary emphasis on the pulmonary artery catheter (PAC). The focus will include: (a) the accuracy and interpretation of data obtained from pulmonary artery (PA) pressure monitoring; (b) physical complications of PA monitoring; (c) thermodilution cardiac output measurement; (d) mixed venous-oxygen saturation (Svo_2) monitoring; (e) new technologic advances in PACs (right ventricular ejection fraction [RVEF]); continuous cardiac output (CCO); newer, noninvasive modalities to mea-

sure cardiac output; and (f) clinical use of PACs. The second part of the chapter will review the recent and growing application of transesophageal echocardiography in the management of critically ill patients.

PULMONARY ARTERY CATHETER

Because clinical observation is often subjective or inadequate (1,2) and medical therapy based on clinical observation alone may be harmful, the quantitative assessment of hemodynamic function is essential for the management of critically ill patients. Measurement of right heart pressures provides an unreliable determinant of left ventricular (LV)-filling pressure (3). The central venous pressure monitoring in older adult surgical patients or patients with cardiopulmonary disease may vary inversely with the pulmonary artery occlusion pressure (PAOP) (4). Therefore, flow-directed, balloon-flotation PACs have proven to be a major advance in hemodynamic monitoring.

The clinical advantages of using PACs include the ability to measure intracardiac pressures, determine cardiac output (through thermodilution), and obtain intracardiac and mixed-venous blood samples. The resulting information can be used to assess volume status and ventricular performance, calculate the derived hemodynamic and respiratory indexes, evaluate total tissue-oxygen balance, determine the etiology of clinical dilemmas, and monitor pathophysiologic progression and responses to therapy. Optimal PAC use depends upon the critical care provider understanding the complications associated with the use of PACs and what factors alter the validity of the measurements, appropriately applying the data, and appreciating the use and benefits of recent PAC modifications.

The recent article by Connors and colleagues rekindles a decade-old debate regarding the indications and clinical benefit of PAC monitoring (5,6). When PACs were initially developed, they were not critically evaluated under strict protocols; however, they quickly became a standard of care. These concerns have led to the development of guidelines for the use of PACs by several organizations including the American Society of Anesthesiologists (7).

Though PACs have been in use for more than two decades, several studies have demonstrated an inadequate and nonuniform knowledge of PAC monitoring (8–11). These studies analyzed the knowledge base among various medical specialties and critical care nurses in several countries including the United States, Canada, and Europe. Before a clinical benefit can be demonstrated, it is imperative that clinicians (and other caregivers) understand the physiologic principles and limitations of the monitoring employed and apply the data appropriately.

DATA MEASUREMENT AND INTERPRETATION

The primary function of PAC monitoring includes the monitoring of cardiac function (i.e., cardiac output) and intracardiac pressures (i.e., PAOP). The accuracy and validity of the data depend on proper functioning of the monitoring equipment, an understanding of the various factors that alter the relationship between PAOP and other cardiac pressures and volumes, and obtaining the most accurate reflection of the PAOP from the tracing. Technical errors due to pressure-monitoring equipment commonly occur. The equipment necessary for PAC monitoring includes the catheter, pressure transducer, tubing, flush system, connectors, and oscilloscope.

Catheter "fling" and "dampened" tracings, which result from "under" and "over" dampening of the recording system, may affect both systolic- and diastolic-pressure values. Fling refers to catheter motion produced by cardiac contraction in an underdampened system. A dampened tracing results from air bubbles or a blood clot in the tubing system as well as from the following: loose, damaged fittings; long, wide-bore, compliant, or kinked tubing; too many stopcocks; apposition of the catheter tip against the vessel wall; or inadequate flushing following aspiration of blood from the PA. To achieve an accurate tracing, the clinician must first ascertain that the system is appropriately calibrated and must then rapidly flush the line and assess the system response. A detailed discussion of the dynamic response characteristics (i.e., natural resonant frequency and dampening coefficient) of pressure-monitoring systems is beyond the scope of this chapter and is reviewed elsewhere (12).

HEMODYNAMIC PRESSURE MONITORING

The hemodynamic monitoring of critically ill patients requires an understanding of the various physiologic determinants of cardiac output, arterial pressure, and oxygen delivery (DO_2) (Fig. 1). Preload, defined as the ventricular fiber length at end diastole, has direct effects on cardiac performance. Preload is determined clinically by the ventricular end-diastolic volume, but end-diastolic volume is difficult to measure routinely at the bedside. Changes in LV end-diastolic volume (LVEDV) alter LV end-diastolic pressure (LVEDP), and the relationship of LVEDV to LVEDP is dependent on ventricular compliance (discussed later in the chapter). PAC monitoring is used to measure PAOP as a reflection of LVEDP. Figure 2 depicts the relationship between PA diastolic pressure (PADP), PAOP (often interchangeably called the PA wedge pressure or pulmonary capillary pressure [PCP]), pulmonary venous pressure, left atrial (LA) pressure, and LVEDP. In

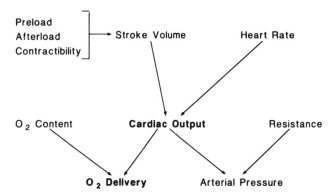

FIGURE 1. The primary determinants of cardiac output and oxygen delivery. (Reproduced from Vender JS. Pulmonary artery catheter monitoring. In: Barash PG, ed. *Cardiac monitoring*. Philadelphia: WB Saunders 1988:743–767, with permission.)

the past, estimates of each of these pressures have been used as a guide to determine the LVEDV. The accuracy of these pressure estimates is directly related to the measurement site's proximity to the left ventricle.

When the PAC balloon is inflated, blood ceases to flow forward in the "wedged" or "occluded" PA segment; at end-diastole, a static fluid column exists between the left ventricle and the PAC tip. Without a pressure gradient, the PAOP will equilibrate with the LVEDP. In healthy individuals, all proximal end-diastolic pressures (i.e., PADP, PAOP, pulmonary venous pressure, and LA pressure) reflect the LVEDP. As with any static fluid column, however, alterations in internal and external forces will diminish the catheter's ability to reflect the true LVEDP.

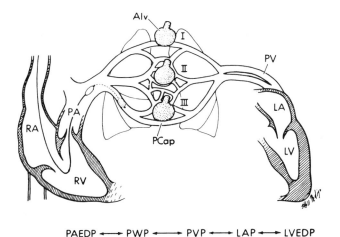

FIGURE 2. The anatomic position of a pulmonary artery catheter in the pulmonary artery. The *shaded areas* position the inflated balloon in the "wedged" position. The *bottom line* shows the progressive correlation of vascular pressures. *RA*, right atrium; *RV*, right ventricle; *PA*, pulmonary artery; *Alv*, alveolus; *PCap*, pulmonary capillary; *PV*, pulmonary vein; *LA*, left atrium; *LV*, left ventricle; *I, II*, and *III* characterize the relationship of alveolar pressure, arterial pressure, and venous pressure as described by West et al. (see ref. 15); *PADP*, pulmonary artery end-diastolic pressure; *PWP*, pulmonary capillary wedge pressure; *PVP*, pulmonary venous pressure; *LAP*, left atrial pressure; *LVEDP*, left ventricular end-diastolic pressure. (Reproduced from Vender JS. Pulmonary artery catheter monitoring. In: Barash PG, ed. *Cardiac monitoring*. Philadelphia: WB Saunders, 1988:743–767, with permission.)

HEMODYNAMIC ASSESSMENT

In clinical practice, balloon occlusion of the PAC represents the PAOP. Although numerous publications refer to this pressure as the PCP or pulmonary capillary wedge pressure (PCWP), the PAOP reflects the pulmonary venous pressure, LA pressure, and LVEDP, but is not the true PCP. For forward flow to occur, the PCP must exceed the PAOP. Under normal physiologic conditions, the PAOP and PCP are quite close, but an increase in pulmonary vascular resistance (PVR) causes the PCP to further exceed the PAOP. The PCP can be estimated from the PAOP profile (13).

Certain factors alter the clinician's ability to obtain accurate and meaningful data from PACs. Under normal conditions, pulmonary capillary resistance is low, impedance to flow is limited, and the PADP is dependent on all distal pressures (e.g., pulmonary venous pressure, LA pressure, and LVEDP). Vasoactive drug use, pulmonary emboli, alveolar hypoxia, acidosis, hypoxemia, and acute or chronic parenchymal pulmonary disease can increase PVR. An elevated PVR alters the direct relationship of PADP to PAOP. Tachycardia above 120 beats per minute reduces cardiac diastolic time, thereby reducing the amount of time for distal runoff to occur and altering the relationship between PADP and PAOP. When PVR is increased, or when significant tachycardia exists, the PADP cannot be an assumed surrogate for the measured PAOP or any distal end-diastolic pressure.

Other factors that influence the PAOP measurement and interpretation are well described (14). PAC tip location, a change in positive end-expiratory pressure (PEEP) levels, and hypovolemia can alter the correlation between PAOP and pulmonary venous pressure. West and associates describe a gravity-dependent difference between ventilation and perfusion in the lung (15). These authors categorize the differences into three zones based on the relationship between local PA pressure, PA alveolar pressure (P_{ALV}), and pulmonary venous pressure (Fig. 2). In zone I, P_{ALV} is greater than the PA and pulmonary venous pressure. In zone II, P_{ALV} is greater than pulmonary venous pressure, but is less than PA pressure. In zone III, PA and pulmonary venous pressures are greater than P_{ALV}. In zone III, uninterrupted blood flow allows the PAC tip to communicate continuously with the distal vascular pressures during diastole. Pressures recorded from a catheter in zones I and II can reflect alveolar rather than vascular pressure. With increasing alveolar pressure (e.g., increasing levels of PEEP), change in position, or decreased intravascular volume, zone III areas can revert to zone II or zone I. The PAC tip must be in zone III for reliable PAOP monitoring to occur. Because the catheters are flow directed, they tend to migrate or advance to areas of higher, continuous blood flow. This migration usually occurs spontaneously to dependent areas of the lung (zone III). Changes in a patient's position (e.g., supine to head up) postinsertion can alter the zone in which the PAC tip resides.

The following characteristics suggest that the catheter tip may be outside zone III: (a) the PAOP tracing is smooth; (b) the PADP is less than the PAOP; (c) the PAOP increases by more than an attendant 50% change in P_{ALV}; and (d) the PAOP decreases by more than a 50% reduction in PEEP (15). When the PAC is located in zone III, the clinician should be able to easily aspirate blood from the distal tip of the catheter, and when the catheter is in the "wedge" position, the blood should be a capillary and not PA or mixed-venous sample. A lateral chest radiograph can help confirm the catheter tip location relative to the left atrium. Increasing intravascular volume or decreasing P_{ALV} can convert zones I or II to zone III. Alternatively, the catheter or patient can be repositioned so that the catheter tip is in a dependent position (zone III). The impact of airway pressure is reduced in the patient with pulmonary parenchymal injury. Many critically ill patients have noncompliant lungs, a condition that reduces the transmission of alveolar pressure to the pulmonary vasculature (16).

PERIOPERATIVE INTERVENTIONS AND PATHOPHYSIOLOGY

A pressure gradient does not often develop between the pulmonary veins (pulmonary venous pressure) and the left atrium, but occlusion of the pulmonary veins (as can occur with tumors, fibrosis, or vasculitis) can cause the pulmonary venous pressure to exceed the LA pressure (15). Furthermore, pulmonary venoconstriction can occur in patients with endotoxemia and sepsis (17).

Normally, the mean LA pressure approximates the LVEDP; however, valvular heart disease and alterations in ventricular compliance can alter this relationship. In patients with mitral stenosis, the LA pressure exceeds the LVEDP. In patients with mitral insufficiency, ventricular systole causes retrograde ejection so that the LA pressure can exceed the LVEDP. This change appears on the PAOP tracing as a large "v" wave, which can cause the clinician to misinterpret the tracing as a nonoccluded PA tracing. Aortic regurgitation and premature closure of the mitral valve can cause continual retrograde ventricular filling from the aorta, resulting in a reverse pressure gradient (in which the LVEDP is greater than the LA pressure).

A decrease in LV compliance can cause a disparity between the LA pressure and the LVEDP. The A wave of the PAOP tracing best reflects the LVEDP in patients with decreased ventricular compliance (18). In a patient with normal PVR and right bundle-branch block, the block can delay right ventricular (RV) systole, causing the PAOP to be lower than the mean LA pressure (19).

An accurate PAOP tracing does not ensure that a linear relationship exists between the LVEDP (PAOP) and the LVEDV; normally, there is a curvilinear relationship between LVEDP (PAOP) and LVEDV. As mentioned earlier, LVEDV determines fiber length and preload is the length of the myocardial fiber at end-diastole. Therefore, the relationship between LVEDP and LVEDV is dependent on ventricular compliance (Fig. 3). With increasing compliance, LVEDV will increase with only small changes in LVEDP (PAOP). The reverse occurs with decreased compliance; LVEDP (PAOP) increases with minimal change in LVEDV. A decrease in ventricular compliance always results in an increase in LVEDP, an occurrence that explains the development of hydrostatic pulmonary edema in some patients with normal LVEDV (e.g., myocardial ischemia). Ventricular compliance is dynamic and can change abruptly with physiologic or therapeutic alterations. The nonlinear nature of the compliance curve mandates that compliance cannot be thought of as a single

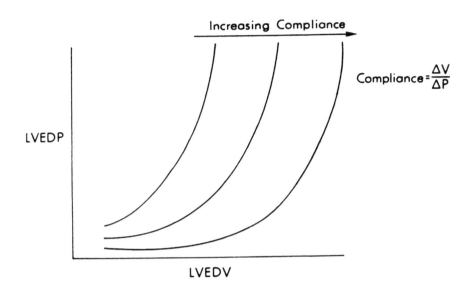

Increasing Compliance

$$Compliance = \frac{\Delta V}{\Delta P}$$

LVEDP

LVEDV

FIGURE 3. Typical series of left ventricular compliance curves. *LVEDP*, left ventricular end-diastolic pressure; *LVEDV*, left ventricular end-diastolic volume. (Reproduced from Vender JS. Pulmonary artery catheter monitoring. In: Barash PG, ed. *Cardiac monitoring.* Philadelphia: WB Saunders 1988:743–767, with permission.)

number. Table 1 lists some of the factors that decrease LV compliance (12).

The LVEDV correlates better with the transmural pressure of the ventricle, defined as the net distending pressure, than with the LVEDP (PAOP), an intravascular pressure. Transmural pressure is calculated by subtracting the juxtacardiac pressure from the intracavitary pressure (LVEDP). Juxtacardiac pressure, the pressure surrounding the heart, is approximated by measuring the intrathoracic (intrapleural) pressure (20). During spontaneous ventilation, the intrapleural pressure approaches zero at end-expiration. When this occurs, the transmural pressure approximates the LVEDP.

The effects of PEEP on transmural ventricular pressure can affect the relationship of LVEDP (PAOP) to LVEDV. In addition to the effects of PEEP on zone-I or zone-II lung, PEEP can also alter ventricular distensibility by increasing juxtacardiac pressure and decreasing venous return. The reduced distensibility causes a decrease in transmural pressure and a disproportionate increase in LVEDP (PAOP) relative to LVEDV (i.e., it decreases compliance). The effects of PEEP on transmural pressure can be assessed by measuring pleural pressure. In clinical practice, pleural pressure is reflected by the midesophageal pressure obtained with the patient in the lateral decubitus position (20). During PEEP therapy, pulmonary compliance and a reduction in venous return limit the increase in LVEDP (PAOP) and effects on trans-

mural pressure. As the lung becomes noncompliant, the effect on pleural pressure is reduced, and the LVEDP (PAOP) correlates better with the transmural pressure. Auto-PEEP is a phenomenon in which airflow obstruction during expiration and residual air trapping causes the P_{ALV} in mechanically ventilated patients to progressively increase (21). The effects of auto-PEEP on transmural and intrapleural pressures are similar to the effects that occur with the use of PEEP. PEEP levels of less than 10 cm H_2O have a limited clinical effect on intrapleural pressure, making the LVEDP (PAOP) in this circumstance a close reflection of the transmural pressure.

The pressure-volume relationship of the left ventricle is also dependent on the end-diastolic volume of the right ventricle. This ventricular interdependence can be caused by displacement of the interventricular septum in the presence of an intact pericardium that constrains the two ventricles. Factors that actually increase RV preload (i.e., increases in RVEDV or RV afterload) can result in a leftward shift of the interventricular septum, causing the septum to encroach upon the left ventricle. This encroachment produces a decrease in LV compliance, which causes an increase in the LVEDP (PAOP) despite a simultaneous decrease in the LVEDV. Acute changes in pulmonary pressures (e.g., embolism) or reduced RVEF can produce this phenomenon.

Alterations in ventilatory patterns can cause fluctuations in intrapleural pressure. Large swings in intrapleural pressure occur with positive-pressure ventilation or when the patient experiences labored respiratory efforts, performs the Valsalva maneuver, or coughs. These fluctuations can cause the clinician to overestimate or underestimate the LVEDP (PAOP).

The best representation of PAOP requires the following steps. Whenever possible, measurements should be derived from a scaled strip-chart recorder or oscilloscope. Digital displays are often inaccurate because they are time-based electrical samplings averaged over a predetermined interval. Measurements should be made at end-expiration because end-expiration minimizes the influence of intrapleural pressure swings and is usually identifiable on the oscilloscope.

TABLE 1. FACTORS THAT DECREASE LEFT VENTRICULAR COMPLIANCE

Myocardial ischemia
Restrictive cardiomyopathy
Right-to-left interventricular septal shift
Aortic stenosis
Cardiac tamponade and effusion
Myocardial fibrosis
Inotropic-drug use
Hypertension

The effects of PEEP on PAOP can also be determined by measuring intrapleural pressure or, alternatively, the PAOP value can be adjusted according to the patient's pulmonary compliance (22). An approximation of PAOP can be made by subtracting a portion of the amount of PEEP from the PAOP; for simplicity, in patients with compliant lungs, this amount is one-half the PEEP level, and in patients with noncompliant lungs, the amount is one-fourth the PEEP level.

Though several investigators recommend discontinuing the patient's mechanical ventilation and PEEP while the PAOP is being measured (14), problems can occur with this technique. Changes in venous return when PEEP is discontinued can cause an "autotransfusion effect" and potential cardiopulmonary decompensation. Abrupt discontinuation of high PEEP can alter respiratory mechanics and gas exchange. More important, because the LVEDP (PAOP)-to-LVEDV ratio is nonlinear and dependent on the state of ventricular compliance, assessing changes and trends in the PAOP relative to medical therapy (e.g., volume, inotrope or vasodilator use, diuresis, airway-pressure change) is more significant than knowing an absolute number.

In addition to PEEP, other modes of mechanical ventilatory support may impair the measurement and assessment of hemodynamic indexes (e.g., PAOP or transmural pressures). Inverse-ratio ventilation can produce an overestimation of the true PAOP by shortening expiratory time and increasing end-expiratory lung volume (23). Airway-pressure–release ventilation, in contrast to conventional modes, typically results in lower mean-airway and pleural pressures. With airway-pressure–release ventilation, large transpulmonary gradients are necessary for ventilation. The PAOP should be measured, therefore, at the end of the positive-pressure plateau.

PHYSICAL COMPLICATIONS OF PULMONARY ARTERY CATHETER MONITORING

PAC use is associated with complications (7) attributed to central venous cannulation (insertion), catheter passage (advancement), or catheter presence (maintenance) (see Chapter 10). The reports and review articles describe varying complication rates (Table 2), and depending on its potential for increasing morbidity or mortality, the complication is often classified as minor or major. A prospective study that reviewed 6,245 PAC insertions reported a relatively low incidence of morbidity associated with this procedure (24). The simplicity and safety of PAC insertion has created a cavalier attitude among many professionals. The authors of this study concluded that experience of the person inserting the catheter, supervision of trainees, and attention to detail were of primary importance in minimizing the incidence of complications.

CENTRAL VENOUS CANNULATION

Complications of venous cannulation are identical for central venous access and for PAC insertion. Arterial puncture is a common complication of venous cannulation. Hemorrhage, hematoma formation with airway compromise (associated with internal

TABLE 2. REPORTED INCIDENCE OF COMPLICATIONS ASSOCIATED WITH PULMONARY ARTERY MONITORING

Complications	Incidence (%)
Of vascular access:	
Arterial puncture	1.1–1.3
Bleeding at cutdown site	5.3
Postoperative neuropathy	0.3–1.1
Pneumothorax	0.3–4.5
Air embolism	0.5
Of placement:	
Minor dysrhythmias	4.7–68.9
Severe dysrhythmias	0.3–62.7
Right bundle-branch block	0.1–4.3
Complete heart block	0–8.5
Of catheter residence:	
PA rupture	0.1–1.5
Positive culture of PA tip	1.4–34.8
Catheter-related sepsis	0.7–11.4
Thrombophlebitis	6.5
Venous thrombosis	0.5–66.7
Pulmonary infarction	0.1–5.6
mural thrombus	
Valvular/endocardial vegetations or documented endocarditis	2.2–100
Deaths attributed to PA catheter	0.02–1.5

PA, pulmonary artery. (Reprinted from A report from the American Society of Anesthesiologists Task Force on Pulmonary Artery Catheterization. Practice guidelines for pulmonary artery catheterization. *Anesthesiology* 1993;78:380–394, with permission.)

jugular cannulation), and embolization of atherosclerotic plaques are uncommon but occasionally reported sequelae of unintentional arterial puncture. Persistent bleeding, hematoma, and hemothorax are possible complications of venous cannulation. When a patient is scheduled to undergo a surgical procedure that requires systemic heparinization (e.g., cardiopulmonary bypass or a major vascular operation), accidental arterial puncture with a large-bore cannula is a relative indication for postponing surgery.

Pneumothorax, another well-known complication of venous cannulation, occurs less often with cannulation of the internal jugular vein than with cannulation of the subclavian vein. Injury can also occur to other structures adjacent to the intended vascular route. Horner syndrome, brachial-plexus injury, thoracic duct trauma with a subsequent chylothorax, and transient phrenic nerve injury (25) are all reported complications. Misplacement of the catheter into the mediastinum or pleural space can result in the infusion of large volumes of fluid into nonvascular spaces (e.g., cardiac tamponade or hydrothorax). Air embolization is an uncommon but potentially lethal complication of PAC insertion. Catheter placement with the patient in Trendelenburg position or when the patient performs a Valsalva maneuver limits the potential for air embolism.

CATHETER PASSAGE

Placement of the PAC is discussed in Chapter 10. Several of the complications associated with passage of the PAC can also occur with the catheter in place. Arrhythmias are a frequent complication of PAC insertion and removal. Premature ventricular contractions are often noted with balloon passage through the right ventricle, and ventricular tachycardia can occur. In addition, other arrhythmias (e.g., premature atrial contraction and atrial fibrillation), various conduction disturbances (right bundle-branch block), and complete heart block can occur. If there is potential for complete heart block to develop (e.g., in a patient with preexisting left bundle-branch block), placement of a catheter with pacing capabilities should be considered, or an external pacemaker should be available.

Coiling, looping, or knotting of the catheter can occur during insertion of PACs. These complications occur more often in patients with a low-flow state, in patients with large intracardiac cavities, with the use of small-gauge PACs, or when an excessive length of catheter is inserted without obtaining the anticipated pressure tracing or verifying the catheter position. Ventricular enlargement, low-output states, congenital cardiac defects, tricuspid insufficiency, and venospasm (of peripheral veins) can increase the difficulty of passage. When the clinician encounters difficulty in passing the catheter, having the patient change positions (e.g., head up, left side down) or take a deep breath may be useful. Fluoroscopic guidance may be necessary.

CATHETER PRESENCE IN THE PULMONARY ARTERY

Patients with PACs have an increased risk of associated morbidity and even mortality. A common, but usually asymptomatic, problem is venous thrombosis at the site of PAC insertion; however, the incidence of this complication is reportedly reduced by the use of heparin-bonded catheters (26). Embolization can also result from distal migration of the PAC tip or from prolonged balloon inflation that occludes distal blood flow in the PA. A pulmonary infarction can be a serious sequela, especially in patients with low-flow states in which collateral blood flow is reduced. The incidence of this complication can be decreased by continuous monitoring of the PA tracing, avoiding prolonged balloon inflation, placing the catheter proximally, and using continuous high-pressure, heparin-flush devices.

Catheter-related infections, sepsis, and endocarditis cause morbidity. Bacterial or fungal colonization of the catheter is common. Factors that increase the incidence of catheter-induced infections include: catheterization for longer than 72 hours; multiple catheter manipulations; nonaseptic insertion and maintenance; system (i.e., infusion-set or cardiac output–syringe) contamination; and skin puncture site infections. Surgical cutdowns have higher infection rates than percutaneous insertions. The benefits of protective catheter sheaths have not been conclusively determined. Recently published data suggest that catheter changes should be done using a guidewire and should reuse the old catheter site, unless the catheter or the insertion site is infected. The risk-to-benefit ratio of when and how to change catheters remains controversial (27).

The most dramatic and acutely catastrophic complication of PAC insertion or maintenance is PA perforation and hemorrhage. Barash and colleagues have delineated several mechanisms for this complication (28). Factors that increase the risk of PA perfora-

tion include catheter insertion in patients with advanced age, pulmonary hypertension, or hypothermia, and when the clinician deviates from standard insertion techniques. Patients who have received anticoagulant medications or who have coagulopathies may have a higher mortality rate secondary to perforation. Suggested ways to avoid this complication include: carefully selecting patients; using the PADP (when the reading is consistent with the PAOP) to minimize the frequency of balloon inflations; continuously monitoring the PA tracing; inflating the 1.5-mL balloon during catheter insertion to ensure proximal catheter tip location in the PA; gradually inflating the balloon during occlusion-pressure recordings; and determining the concentricity of the balloon before inserting it. Overwedging usually indicates distal catheter placement or balloon herniation over the tip and causes a falsely elevated PA pressure. When overwedging occurs, the balloon should be deflated immediately, the catheter should be withdrawn 1 to 2 cm, and the balloon should be slowly reinflated. Supportive care is usually adequate to manage most PA perforations, but if massive bleeding occurs, surgical intervention may be needed.

PRINCIPLES OF THERMODILUTION CARDIAC OUTPUT MEASUREMENT

Deriving accurate hemodynamic indexes and selecting appropriate therapies in critically ill patients requires accurate measurement of cardiac output. Thermodilution cardiac output has become an acceptable substitute for use of the Fick method or dye-dilution technique to measure cardiac output (29).

The Stewart-Hamilton equation links cardiac output to temperature changes.

$$Q = \frac{V(TB - T1) K1 \times K2}{f \Delta TB(t)dt}$$

where $\sim Q$ = cardiac output, V = volume injected,

TB = blood temperature,

TI = injectate temperature,

K1 and K2 = computational constants, and

TB(t) = blood temperature as a function of time.

The thermodilution technique is similar to the dye-dilution technique, but rather than using an injectate of dye, thermodilution uses an injectate of "cold" saline. A cardiac output computer integrates the temperature information derived from a thermistor at the tip of the catheter to provide a cardiac output curve. The area under the curve is inversely proportional to the cardiac output.

The clinician must understand several technical considerations to minimize errors with the thermodilution method. The catheter thermistor must be positioned freely in the lumen of the PA. Falsely elevated cardiac output readings will occur if the thermistor impinges on the vessel wall, insulating it from the "cool" thermal indicator. Irregular cardiac output curves can produce inaccurate cardiac output results. These irregular curves can be caused by an inadequate mixture of the injectate and the blood, contact between the thermistor and the vessel wall, changes in heart rate or blood pressure, and abnormal respiratory patterns.

Injectate volume and temperature also affect thermodilution cardiac output measurements. Typically, 10 mL of a 5% dextrose or saline solution is used, but when volume overload is a concern (e.g., in children), smaller volumes (2.5 to 5 mL) can be used without significantly affecting the results. Injectate temperature can range from 0° to 24°C. When patients are hypothermic (25°C), as occurs during cardiopulmonary bypass (CPB), using cold injectate (0° to 4°C) may be necessary to increase the signal-to-noise ratio. Falsely elevated and decreased cardiac output measurements can result when the volume or temperature of the injectate is incorrectly programmed into the computer (e.g., if the computer is programmed for 10 cc and 8 cc is injected, it will produce falsely elevated cardiac output). The speed of the injection appears to be of minimal consequence if the 10-mL injectate is delivered in less than 4 seconds.

Timing the injection with the respiratory cycle can improve the reproducibility of cardiac output measurements. Because the temperature of PA blood can vary with phases of the respiratory cycle, cardiac output measurements should be done at end-expiration. When patients are receiving positive-pressure ventilation, the readings of the thermodilution cardiac output correlate with cyclic variations in RV cardiac output. Because it may be difficult to synchronize the injection with end-expiration, multiple determinations of the cardiac output should be made. An average of three evenly spaced determinations represents an accurate estimate of cardiac output. Modern computers help compensate for respiratory-cycle–related temperature shifts by averaging the blood temperature for a short time before the injection.

Certain conditions prevent appropriate mixing or directional flow of the indicator solution. Intracardiac shunts, tricuspid regurgitation, and cardiac arrhythmias—which affect beat-to-beat cardiac ejection—can all affect the accuracy of thermodilution cardiac output measurements.

Cardiac output measurements are commonly used in clinical care. As a singular parameter, the clinical application of cardiac output has limitations. Indeed, cardiac output (or index) can be a misleading gauge of myocardial function. Tachycardia can compensate for decreased stroke volume. The cardiac output must be evaluated in combination with other indexes, such as SvO_2 or urine output, to better assess the adequacy of tissue perfusion. A normal cardiac index suggests adequate myocardial function when tissue perfusion could, in fact, be luxuriant, adequate, or suboptimal, depending on arterial oxygen content and the metabolic needs of the tissue (see SvO_2 discussion).

SPECIAL PURPOSE PULMONARY ARTERY CATHETERS

PACs, by virtue of their traversing of the right atrium and outflow tract of the right ventricle, have been adapted for special functions. Each modification offers additional diagnostic and therapeutic capabilities. SvO_2 modifications are commonly used in clinical practice. The ability to provide cardiac pacing via a PAC can be therapeutically beneficial. Newer PACs have the capability of measuring the RVEF and cardiac output continuously (CCO).

MIXED-VENOUS OXYGEN-SATURATION CATHETERS

Routine measurements of cardiac-filling pressure and cardiac output do not assure adequacy of perfusion. In assessing a patient's pulmonary status, physicians are seldom concerned with the minute ventilation alone, but instead are concerned about the $PaCO_2$, which is determined by the adequacy of minute ventilation in relation to the patient's metabolic rate. In contrast, cardiac output is often the focal point in the diagnostic and therapeutic assessment of the high-risk surgical patient. As can be seen in Fig. 4, cardiac output is positioned parallel to minute ventilation. Cardiac output is the product of stroke volume times heart rate. What is needed is a parameter comparable to $PaCO_2$ that would help determine adequacy of perfusion. In this regard, SvO_2 has been suggested as a measure that can help reflect the balance of total tissue oxygen supply-and-demand dynamics.

PACs provide access for the intermittent sampling of mixed-venous blood from the PA. Advances in fiberoptic technology have led to the development of catheters that continuously measure SvO_2.

The use of SvO_2 to assess total tissue-oxygen balance requires an understanding of oxygen delivery (DO_2), oxygen demand, and oxygen consumption. Oxygen delivery equals arterial oxygen content times the cardiac output. The following formula ignores dissolved oxygen content, which is usually insignificant.

$$DO_2 = (Hgb \times 13.9)\, SaO_2 \times cardiac\ output$$
$$= 800 - 1000\ mL/min$$

The 13.9 constant is a product of the 1.39 mL of oxygen per gram of hemoglobin (Hgb) times a factor of 10 to convert the units for Hgb to grams per liter. DO_2, therefore, is determined by cardiac output, Hgb level, and SaO_2. The saturation of Hgb is determined by arterial oxygen partial pressure and the oxyhemoglobin dissociation curve. DO_2 must be sufficient to supply the oxygen needed for cellular metabolism of the various organ systems (O_2 demand). Oxygen consumption ($V \times O_2$) is the amount of oxygen used by the tissues. $V \times O_2$ is determined by the amount of arterial oxygen delivered minus the mixed venous O_2 returned. Ignoring dissolved oxygen content,

$$V \times O_2(mLO_2) = [(Hgb \times 13.9)SaO_2 \times cardiac\ output]$$
$$- [(Hgb \times 13.9)SvO_2 \times cardiac\ output]$$

A further derivation of this equation shows the relationship of SvO_2 to the other indexes:

$$SvO_2 = SaO_2 - \frac{V \times O_2}{Hgb \times 13.9 \times cardiac\ output}$$

Minute Ventilation	Cardiac Output
[Tidal Volume × Respiratory Rate]	[Stroke Volume × Heart Rate]
↓	↓
PaCO₂	?SvO₂?

FIGURE 4. Similarities between minute ventilation and cardiac output. (Reproduced from Vender JS. Pulmonary artery catheter monitoring. In: Barash PG, ed. *Cardiac monitoring.* Philadelphia: WB Saunders, 1988:743–767, with permission.)

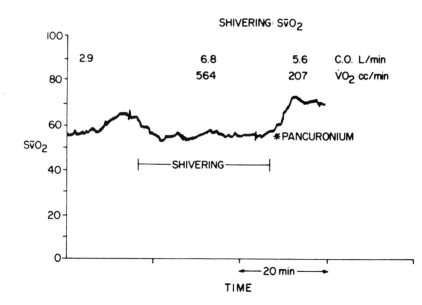

FIGURE 5. This Sv_{O_2} recording in a patient after a coronary artery bypass operation demonstrates the effects and treatment of shivering and the relationship between Sv_{O_2}, cardiac output (CO), and metabolic rate ($V \times O_2$). (Reproduced from Vender JS. Pulmonary artery catheter monitoring. In: Barash PG, ed. *Cardiac monitoring.* Philadelphia: WB Saunders, 1988:743–767, with permission.)

Sv_{O_2} varies directly with cardiac output, Hgb, and Sa_{O_2} and inversely with metabolic rate. Normal Sv_{O_2} is approximately 75% ($Pv_{O_2} = 40$ mm Hg), which indicates that normal metabolic needs are met by extraction of 25% of delivered oxygen. An acute increase in cardiac output or oxygen extraction initially compensates for an increase in oxygen demand or a decrease in arterial oxygen content. Critically ill patients can have limited cardiac reserves so that if oxygen demand increases, the Sv_{O_2} decreases further. At a critical level of DO_2, extraction of oxygen is maximal, the Sv_{O_2} reaches a plateau, and $V \times O_2$ becomes delivery-dependent. When the Sv_{O_2} is 50% or less, the tissue–oxygen balance is compromised and the potential for anaerobic metabolism and lactic acidosis increases (30).

Figure 5 shows an Sv_{O_2} recording from a patient who has undergone a coronary artery bypass operation. Despite having a seemingly acceptable cardiac output value, the patient has a significant decrease in Sv_{O_2}, which suggests an imbalance in the tissues' supply of and demand for oxygen. The metabolic rate has significantly increased with the onset of shivering. The changes in the Sv_{O_2} clearly track the patient's inability to adequately compensate for the increased oxygen demand, despite having an increased cardiac output. Variables that alter oxygen supply or demand and that must be evaluated when the Sv_{O_2} decreases include: cardiac output, Hgb, Sa_{O_2}, and metabolic rate. When arterial oxygen content and the $V \times O_2$ are stable, the Sv_{O_2} will correlate directly with fluctuations in cardiac output.

Abnormal increases in Sv_{O_2} are more difficult to interpret. Sepsis, arteriovenous fistulas, cirrhosis, left-to-right cardiac shunts, peripheral shunts, cyanide poisoning, hypothermia, unintentional PAC wedging, and rapid withdrawal of arterial blood from the PAC can cause an increase in the Sv_{O_2} (4). Valid Sv_{O_2} monitoring requires a true mixed-venous sample; inadequate mixing of blood from the superior vena cava, inferior vena cava, and coronary sinus makes venous measurements from the right atrium less reliable. The presence of a left-to-right intracardiac shunt makes the determination of an accurate Sv_{O_2} sample from the PA impossible.

Sv_{O_2} can be used in critically ill patients as a diagnostic tool (e.g., acute ventricular septal defect) and to monitor therapeutic interventions. Combining a pulse oximeter with an Sv_{O_2} oximeter (dual oximetry) provides a way to monitor the cardiopulmonary effects of PEEP in the management of acute respiratory failure. Sv_{O_2} measured via PACs does not detect inadequate regional perfusion and, therefore, should be regarded solely as an index of total tissue–oxygen balance.

RIGHT VENTRICULAR EJECTION FRACTION CATHETER

RVEF catheters are a technological advance in PAC monitoring that have enabled the measurement of RVEF and RV volumes from the exponential decay of the thermodilution curve (31). The principal modification in the catheter is the use of a rapid response (50 msec) thermistor to measure beat-to-beat end-diastolic temperature variation using the R wave signal from the ECG. From this data, the "mean residual fraction" (RF mean) is determined. The RVEF (normal = 40%) is calculated by the equation: $EF = 1 - RF$ mean. Using the EF, RV end-diastolic is computed by dividing stroke volume (cardiac output/heart rate [HR]) by the EF. RV end-systolic volume is derived by subtracting the RV stroke volume from the RV end-diastolic volume.

$$EF = 1 - RF \text{ mean}$$
$$\text{Stroke volume} = \text{cardiac output/HR}$$
$$RVED = RV \text{ stroke volume/RVEF}$$
$$RVES = RVED - RV \text{ stroke volume}$$

RVEF has been clinically validated against *in vivo* radionuclear and echocardiographic techniques in animal and human studies (32). Accuracy of the measurement necessitates a regular R-R interval, the injectate port in the right atrium just proximal to the tricuspid valve, and instantaneous mixing in the RV.

The existence of cardiac dysrhythmias (e.g., atrial fibrillation) or tricuspid insufficiency can impact the RVEF measurement. Averaging the thermal curves over several beats reduces the problems caused by a nonsinus rhythm.

The clinical utilization of RVEF catheters could be justified in situations where acute changes in RVEF may occur: pulmonary hypertension (acute lung injury), right coronary artery disease with RV ischemia/infarction, and following a heart transplant.

CONTINUOUS CARDIAC OUTPUT CATHETER

Numerous efforts have been made to develop a method for automated continuous (near continuous) cardiac output (CCO) monitoring (31). Various methodologies have been investigated for PAC-CCO including Doppler, thermodeprivation, cyclic cooling, and pulse thermodilution (33).

The clinically available methodology employs a PAC modified with a 10-cm thermal filament coiled around a portion of the PAC that lies in the RA and RV (34). The thermal filament generates a low-power heat, cycled intermittently in a pseudorandom sequence, which is sensed at a distal thermistor. Using a proprietary signal processing system (Stochastic), the downstream temperature is cross-correlated with the input sequence to produce a thermodilution washout curve. The pseudorandom sequence and signal processing enhance the signal identification and reduce the impact of extraneous thermal noise. The resultant cardiac output typically represents an averaging of the previous several minutes and is updated approximately every 30 seconds.

The application of this technology has been validated against bolus thermodilution in both animals and humans over a wide range of cardiac outputs and clinical settings (35). Reportedly, accuracy decreases at higher cardiac outputs and response time delays are greater with acute hemodynamic changes. Various algorithms offer a trend versus stat mode (36). PAC-CCO is also available in combination with continuous SvO_2 monitoring.

OTHER MEANS TO DETERMINE CARDIAC OUTPUT

Doppler Ultrasonography

Doppler ultrasonography measures the frequency shift of reflected sound waves to determine the velocity of blood within the thoracic aorta or the pulmonary artery. For velocities measured in the aorta, cardiac output can be determined by utilization of a probe placed either on the distal portion of an endotracheal tube or a stand-alone device located within the esophagus and directed toward the aorta. The following equation is then used to determine cardiac output:

$$\Pi(D/2)^2 = CSA$$
$$SV = CSA \times VTI$$
$$CO = SV \times HR$$

D = diameter; CSA = cross-sectional area; SV = stroke volume; VTI = velocity-time integral; CO = cardiac output.

The diameter of the aorta is determined either from a nomogram based on weight, height, age, and gender, or may be measured directly. The angle between the probe and the structure to be interrogated should be less than 20% or the alignment of the blood velocity and the probe will no longer be in parallel and the precision of the measurement will be sacrificed. The advantage that Doppler ultrasonography possesses over cardiac output determination by traditional thermodilution methods is that Doppler ultrasonography is noninvasive and may avoid the need to place a PAC with its attendant risks. Doppler ultrasonography may be used in lieu of a PAC to allow optimization of fluid status in patients undergoing surgery. This optimization may lead to significantly faster postoperative recovery and a reduction in hospital stay (37).

Thoracic Impedance Cardiography

The thorax is viewed as a homogeneous electrical conductor occupied by blood. Thoracic impedance cardiography (TIC) involves placing up to ten electrodes on the thorax and measuring changes in electrical conductance between the current transmitting electrodes and the sensing electrodes. The synchronous changes in impedance come from volume changes in the cardiovascular system. Sources of error include incorrect electrode placement, intrathoracic fluid shifts, and changes in hematocrit. In a metaanalysis of 154 studies, the overall r^2 value was 0.67, but the r^2 for single measurements was only 0.53. The conclusion to be drawn is that TIC is useful for trend analysis but at this date is unreliable for single, isolated measurements (38).

Lithium Dilution

Cardiac output may be measured by a bolus injection of lithium chloride into the circulation through a central venous catheter with the arterial plasma lithium concentration measured via a peripheral arterial catheter and then determining cardiac output from the lithium dilution curve. This method might avoid the need for a PAC and may be more accurate than traditional thermodilution methods (39).

Arterial Pressure Wave

The measurement of the waveform of the arterial pulse through a peripheral arterial catheter may permit the determination of cardiac output. This allows beat-to-beat measurement of cardiac output and may be a reliable and accurate indicator of cardiac output (40).

Partial CO$_2$ Rebreathing

Pulmonary capillary blood flow can be measured using a noninvasive method employing CO_2 rebreathing. Cardiac output can be determined in mechanically ventilated patients by applying a 30- to 60-second period of partial rebreathing using additional dead space. The ratio of change in end-tidal CO_2 and CO_2 excretion can then be employed to yield the cardiac output using a differential Fick equation (41). Validation studies have demonstrated that this method may be a clinically useful means of determining cardiac output in ventilated patients (42). Limitations to this technology have been discussed, with future studies necessary to determine its clinical use.

CLINICAL APPLICATION OF PULMONARY ARTERY MONITORING

PACs are often used for monitoring patients with specific disease entities (e.g., congestive heart failure, pulmonary edema, valvular dysfunction, acute respiratory distress syndrome, or sepsis). Use should be based on the physiologic information obtained from the catheter for diagnosing and managing the underlying pathology. A brief discussion of some of the uses of PACs follows, but this discussion does not include all applications.

Volume assessment and fluid management are the most common uses of PACs. Support of tissue perfusion is the primary goal of fluid therapy (see Chapter 12). Because monitoring PAOP is an indirect reflection of LVEDV, following changes over time in PAOP, cardiac output, and tissue perfusion in response to rapid fluid administration is more important than is a single measurement.

When the patient has inadequate tissue perfusion, the response of PAOP to a fluid challenge can be used to assess and guide therapy (43). In this situation, fluid is rapidly administered (over approximately a 10-minute period) in predetermined increments (50 to 200 mL), and the change in PAOP is monitored. The magnitude of change in PAOP is determined by the patient's individual ventricular compliance curve. A large increase from baseline PAOP (greater than 7 mmHg) or the development of pulmonary edema suggests an excessive increase in LVEDP (preload) and a position on the steep portion of the curve (Fig. 3). Further volume administration increases the LVEDP and increases myocardial $V \times O_2$ without improving cardiac output. If the PAOP does not increase at least 3 mm Hg and perfusion remains inadequate, administration of additional fluid boluses are necessary until systemic perfusion returns. If the patient's intravascular volume is at an optimal level and tissue perfusion remains inadequate, further intervention is required. Inotropic support, afterload reduction, and chronotropic modification may adequately enhance the cardiac output.

PACs can be used for early diagnosis and monitoring of myocardial ischemia. Ischemia produces an acute decrease in ventricular compliance; the LVEDP (PAOP) rises disproportionately to the LVEDV. Additionally, an acute alteration in ventricular compliance can produce "a" waves on the PAOP tracing. Papillary muscle dysfunction due to subendocardial ischemia can produce mitral insufficiency and prominent large "v" waves. The presence of normal ventricular function in patients with significant coronary artery disease does not obviate the use of PACs for the monitoring of myocardial ischemia (35). It is recognized that changes in ventricular compliance and wall-motion abnormalities are more reliably detected with echocardiography than with PACs (discussed later in the chapter).

Measurement of PAOP can help distinguish cardiogenic from noncardiogenic pulmonary edema. Lung water is directly related to PCP. This relationship is magnified in conditions of leaky alveolar capillary membranes. In patients with acute lung injury, pulmonary edema can occur with normal PCP; cardiogenic pulmonary edema is associated with elevated PCP. An optimal ventricular-filling pressure is produced by an LVEDV that is adequate for tissue perfusion (cardiac output) but does not result in pulmonary edema.

Other diagnostic uses of PACs include differentiation of a ventricular septal defect from mitral insufficiency and detection of cardiac tamponade. A new systolic murmur that occurs after a myocardial infraction (MI) can be due to a ventricular septal defect or acquired mitral insufficiency. With a ventricular septal defect, blood drawn from the various cardiac chambers shows a step-up in oxygen saturation between the right atrium and the RV due to left-to-right shunting of highly oxygenated LV blood across the ventricular septum. Cardiac output may be falsely elevated when measured by thermodilution in patients with left-to-right shunting. If the murmur is due to acute mitral insufficiency, no step-up occurs in oxygen saturation and a large "v" wave can be seen on the PAOP tracing (Fig. 6). Though cardiac tamponade is definitively diagnosed by echocardiography, the equalization of all diastolic pressures (right atrium, right ventricle, PAOP) is highly suggestive of a constrictive cardiac process.

PAC monitoring has been used to classify hemodynamic function after a patient has an MI. Defining subsets of patients with MIs and correlating PAOP and cardiac index can aid in selecting therapy and determining prognosis. Del Guercio and

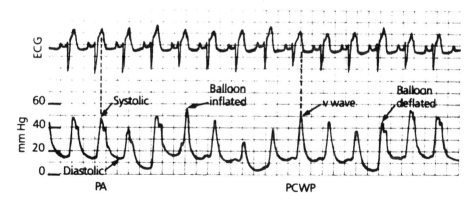

FIGURE 6. Pulmonary artery (PA) and pulmonary capillary wedge pressure (PCWP) tracings in a patient with acute mitral regurgitation. Note the large waves in the PCWP with balloon inflation. (Reproduced from Amin DK, Shah PK, Swan HJC. The Swan-Ganz catheter: indications for insertion. Diagnostic, therapeutic, and prognostic applications. *J Crit Illness* 1986;1:54–61, with permission.)

Cohn demonstrated the benefit of preoperative PAC monitoring hemodynamic for assessing hemodynamic function, evaluating therapeutic interventions, and classifying prognosis for older adult surgical patients (44).

EFFICACY OF THE PULMONARY ARTERY CATHETER

Since the introduction of PAC monitoring in 1970, the indications for its use have broadened dramatically. PACs are used to obtain hemodynamic data for the assessment, monitoring, and therapeutic management of critically ill, high-risk surgical patients.

Because of potential complications associated with PAC monitoring, numerous editorials and articles have questioned the procedure's risk-to-benefit ratio (5,6). These articles address the inadequacy of outcome data and suggest that PA monitoring does not confer a benefit to patients. Subgroups of patients have been identified, however, in whom PAC monitoring data have altered the clinicians' assessments and subsequent patients' care (1,2,45). Rao and associates (46) report that PAC monitoring is associated with a decreased mortality rate in surgical patients with recent MIs.

Many studies and metaanalyses have had disparate results regarding the benefit of PAC monitoring. Several studies have shown a positive outcome difference in patients managed with PAC data and optimization of cardiac function. In a prospective study, Shoemaker and associates evaluated the impact of PAC monitoring on mortality, with an emphasis on how information from the PAC was used (47). Several studies have assessed the impact of supranormal oxygen delivery results (48–50). Mimoz and colleagues report improved outcome in septic patients managed with PACs (51).

Unfortunately, deficiencies exist in most studies published due to sample size, concomitant therapy and disease, study design, blinding, equivalence of caregiver competency, and so forth. Practical difficulties have limited our ability to design and implement a large multicenter randomized controlled trial (RCT) on PAC monitoring and outcome in critically ill patients (52). Ivanov and coworkers performed a metaanalysis showing a nonsignificant trend toward reduced mortality in patients managed with a PAC (53). A more recent metaanalysis of RCTs has suggested a statistically significant difference on major morbidity with PAC monitoring (54).

The clinical value of PAC monitoring necessitates a thorough understanding of the technology, indications, limitations, and risks. An inadequate and nonuniform knowledge among various medical specialties and critical care nurses in the United States, Canada, and Europe has been demonstrated (8–11). The Ontario Intensive Care Study Group articulated the ethical difficulties in doing RCT outcome studies (52). Clinical misinterpretation and misapplication of PAC data are immediate impediments to improved patient outcome or the ability to demonstrate a clinical benefit to PAC monitoring.

Several medical organizations have published practice guidelines in an effort to address appropriate indications for PAC use (7,55,56). More recently, a joint effort has been undertaken to produce a comprehensive clinical education program for PAC monitoring. Until the educational process and knowledge base has assured an acceptable level of competency by "all" those who utilize PAC monitoring (data) for the care of critically ill patients, we cannot appropriately assess the clinical efficacy and subsequent cost-effectiveness of PAC monitoring.

TRANSESOPHAGEAL ECHOCARDIOGRAPHY

The primary indications for transesophageal echocardiography (TEE) include: evaluation of preload, cardiac output (57,58); myocardial performance and ischemia; pericardial effusions or tamponade; valvular disease; ruptured papillary muscles or chordae tendinae; aortic dissections or aneurysms (59–61); intracardiac masses (62,63) or valvular vegetations; intracardiac shunts (ventricular septal or atrial septal defects); pulmonary emboli; and the function of prosthetic heart valves. Table 3 lists hemodynamic parameters obtainable with TEE.

Echocardiography uses the principle of ultrasound and the ultrasound waves generated by piezoelectric crystals to evaluate the structure, function, and hemodynamic state of the heart and great vessels. The ultrasound transducer sends out sound waves of high frequency that are used to interrogate the structures in question. This mechanical information is then translated into an electric signal that is ultimately converted into an image on the monitor. The most common modes used in echocardiography are the M-mode, two-dimensional-mode, and color flow Doppler. The frequency range of most ultrasound probes is from 2.5 to 7.5 megahertz. Frequency is inversely proportional to the wavelength. The image resolution obtained is improved with higher frequencies, but the strength of the ultrasound beam is reduced as it is attenuated by structures that the beam must cross. Doppler is used to examine the direction and velocity of blood flow by comparing the ultrasound frequency sent out to the returning ultrasound waves obtained by the transducer.

The advantage that TEE possesses relative to transthoracic echocardiography (TTE) is that the ultrasound probe is placed

TABLE 3. HEMODYNAMIC INFORMATION THAT CAN BE ACQUIRED WITH ECHOCARDIOGRAPHY

Valve area
  Stenotic valve area
  Transvalvular pressure gradients
Volume measurements
  Stroke volume
  Cardiac output
  Regurgitant valve volume
  Shunt values (Qp/Qs)
Pressure measurements
  Right ventricle systolic pressure
  Pulmonary artery systolic pressure
  Mean pulmonary artery pressure
  Pulmonary artery end-diastolic pressure
  Left atrial pressure
  Left ventricle end-diastolic pressure

(Adapted from Oh JK, Seward JB, Tajik AJ. *The echo manual*, 2nd ed. Philadelphia: Lippincott-Raven, 1999.)

in the esophagus and positioned directly behind the heart. This permits the use of higher frequencies since the ultrasound beam has a shorter distance to travel. This higher frequency allows a better resolution of images. Transthoracic ultrasound might employ lower frequencies since the ultrasound beam must use a longer wavelength to travel farther distances, leading to a reduction in resolution. This is especially true for those patients that may have chronic obstructive pulmonary disease, obesity, or surgical wounds and dressings on their thorax. Similarly, TEE may have an advantage over TTE in evaluating bacterial endocarditis, the functioning of prosthetic heart valves, and severe mitral regurgitation caused by ruptured chordae tendinae.

TEE is a generally safe procedure but might lead to dental injuries, pharyngeal or laryngeal trauma, esophageal trauma, arrhythmias, hemodynamic compromise, respiratory embarrassment (especially in the small pediatric population), or dysphagia. The use of intraoperative TEE may be associated with an increased risk of postprocedure dysphagia (64,65), but a multicenter study concluded that TEE studies are associated with an acceptable low risk when performed by an experienced operator (66). The introduction of the esophageal probe into the mouth and then into the stomach should never be forced. If difficulty is encountered inserting the probe, either use a different technique or have someone with greater experience perform this procedure. Probably the most severe complication is operator inexperience resulting in the presentation of incorrect information and subsequent treatment based on erroneous conclusions. Absolute contraindications to TEE include esophageal strictures, tumor, and recent surgery of the esophagus and stomach. There exists a relative contraindication to placement of the TEE probe in patients with esophageal varices, but this risk must be weighed against the potential benefit of obtaining accurate information concerning the patient's underlying hemodynamic state. The American Society of Echocardiography (ASE) and the Society of Cardiovascular Anesthesiologists (SCA) published guidelines for performing a comprehensive intraoperative TEE examination (67). This publication was the outcome of an effort by both anesthesiologists and cardiologists to establish consistent acquisition and description of intraoperative echocardiographic data, and is also to be used as a tool for quality improvement. This examination in qualified hands can be done in fewer than 10 minutes. These guidelines established a set of anatomically directed cross-sectional views of the heart and can be used by the echocardiographer as a starting point in the examination of the heart.

Recent publication of practice guidelines (68) on "Perioperative TEE" by the American Society of Anesthesiologists and the SCA established three categories documenting the utility of TEE during the perioperative period. Category I included indications that were supported by strong evidence or expert opinion. TEE is often useful in improving clinical outcomes in the settings described. Category II indications were supported by weaker evidence and expert consensus. TEE may be useful in improving clinical outcomes in these circumstances, but suitable indications are less certain than in category I; category III indications lack scientific support.

Table 4 lists the category I and II indications. The use of the TEE is justified as a category I indication in the intensive care setting if there are unexplained hemodynamic disturbances,

TABLE 4. PRACTICE GUIDELINES FOR PERIOPERATIVE TRANSESOPHAGEAL ECHOCARDIOGRAPHY (TEE)

Category I indications: Supported by the strongest evidence or opinion; TEE is often useful in improving clinical outcomes in these settings and is often indicated, depending on individual circumstances.

- Intraoperative evaluation of acute, persistent, and life-threatening hemodynamic disturbances in which ventricular function and its determinants are uncertain and have not responded to treatment
- Intraoperative use in valve repair
- Intraoperative use in congenital heart surgery for most lesions requiring cardiopulmonary bypass
- Intraoperative use in repair of hypertrophic obstructive cardiomyopathy
- Intraoperative use for endocarditis when preoperative testing is inadequate or extension of infection to perivalvular tissue is suspected
- Preoperative use in unstable patients with suspected thoracic aortic aneurysms, dissection, or disruption who need to be evaluated quickly
- Intraoperative assessment of aortic valve function in repair of aortic dissections with possible aortic valve involvement
- Intraoperative evaluation of pericardial window procedures
- Use in the intensive care unit for unstable patients with unexplained hemodynamic disturbances, suspected valve disease, or thromboembolic problems (if other tests or monitoring have not confirmed the diagnosis or patients are too unstable to undergo other tests)*a*

Category II indications: Supported by weaker evidence and expert consensus; TEE may be useful in improving clinical outcomes in these settings, depending on individual circumstances, but appropriate indications are less certain.

- Perioperative use in patients with increased risk of myocardial ischemia or infarction
- Perioperative use in patients with increased risk of hemodynamic disturbances
- Intraoperative assessment of valve replacement
- Intraoperative assessment of repair of cardiac aneurysms
- Intraoperative evaluation of removal of cardiac tumors
- Intraoperative detection of foreign bodies
- Intraoperative detection of air emboli during cardiotomy, heart transplant operations, and upright neurosurgical procedures
- Intraoperative use during intracardiac thrombectomy
- Intraoperative use during pulmonary embolectomy
- Intraoperative use for suspected cardiac trauma
- Preoperative assessment of patients with suspected thoracic aortic dissections, aneurysms, or disruption
- Intraoperative use during repair of thoracic aortic dissections without suspected aortic valve involvement
- Intraoperative detection of aortic atheromatous disease or other sources of aortic emboli
- Intraoperative evaluation of pericardiectomy, pericardial effusions, or evaluation of pericardial surgery
- Intraoperative evaluation of anastomotic sites during heart and/or lung transplantation
- Monitoring placement and function of assist devices

(Reprinted from Practice Guidelines for Perioperative Transesophageal Echocardiography: A Report by the American Society of Anesthesiologists and the Society of Cardiovascular Anesthesiologists Task Force on Transesophageal Echocardiography. *Anesthesiology* 1996;84:986–1006, with permission.)
*a*Emphasis added.

suspected valvular disease, or thromboembolic complications in unstable intensive care unit (ICU) patients. Further, TEE is a category I indicated test if other tests or monitoring techniques have been unable to confirm or establish a diagnosis and the patient is too unstable to transport for other tests. The exact length and training necessary for an intensivist to undergo in order to competently perform a comprehensive TEE examination is uncertain, but an intensivist can be trained in a relatively short period of time to perform a goal-directed, limited-scope TEE evaluation of LV function. One study (69) examined five surgical intensivists with no previous familiarity with echocardiography under the supervision of a cardiologist. This study involved 100 patients. Forty-eight of the patients had a TEE study performed by an intensivist in conjunction with a cardiologist. Fifty-two examinations were done without supervision but were reviewed later. The endpoints were the determination of cardiac volume, LV wall thickness, and global LV function and regional wall motion. The intensivists' analysis was deemed correct in 93% of cases for LV wall thickness, 87% for intracardiac volume status, and 81% for regional wall motion abnormalities. The TEE data disagreed with the PAC determination of volume status in 55% of the 100 pts. and in 39% of the 100 pts. regarding myocardial function. This study demonstrated that limited TEE acquisition skills can be accomplished in a relatively short time span, and that the data obtained would yield useful information in addition to knowledge gained from a PAC. TEE has proven its capability in the operating room, but it also is an important tool in evaluating the postsurgical patient. This is especially true in the hypotensive patient after cardiac surgery. A study from the Netherlands (70) looked at 60 patients who were hypotensive after cardiac surgery. The TEE determined that 14 of the patients were hypotensive secondary to hypovolemia, 6 had cardiac tamponade, and 16 had evidence of LV failure. Eleven patients demonstrated RV failure, and 8 patients demonstrated biventricular failure. Two of the patients with tamponade and 6 patients with hypovolemia were undiagnosed with standard hemodynamic data. Reoperation was avoided in 5 patients.

TEE is also a valuable tool in the noncardiac surgery ICU patient. Poelaert and coworkers (71) performed a retrospective analysis of 108 consecutive TEE videos in a combined medical and surgical ICU. The results of this study found that TEE provided additional information to that gathered by a PAC. Of the 64% of patients with a PAC, 44% underwent therapy changes after TEE interrogation of the heart. Forty-one percent of patients without a PAC had changes in their therapy based on TEE findings. Another prospective study assessed unexplained hypotension (for a period of 60 minutes or longer) in critically ill patients (72). This study of 61 adult patients utilized both TEE and TTE. Twenty-nine (64%) of 45 of the surface studies were deemed inadequate compared to only 2 (3%) of the 61 TEE examinations. TEE contributed clinically new diagnoses in 17 patients, leading to surgery in 20% of these patients. TEE is a technology that can be readily used to obtain quick and accurate information regarding a critically ill patient's underlying hemodynamic performance. TEE may also provide information faster than that obtained with a PAC. Kaul and colleagues (73) looked in a prospective manner at 49 consecutive critically ill patients with hypotension, pulmonary edema, or both, and determined

if the cause was cardiac or noncardiac. The TEE and PAC agreed in 86% of cases as to whether the causes of hypotension or pulmonary edema were due to cardiac or noncardiac causes. But the TEE information was obtained in 19 + 7 minutes versus the 63 + 45 minutes it took to place the PAC.

TEE has the ability to detect linear changes in LV end-diastolic area with a blood loss of as little as 2.5% of estimated blood volume (74). These changes were reflected by corresponding changes in cardiac output, stroke volume, and PAOP. These changes were noted even in those patients with LV wall motion abnormalities. TEE may be a better indicator of myocardial ischemia than PAOP. Van Daele and associates (75) studied 98 anesthetized patients for coronary artery bypass surgery and found that at the onset of wall motion changes determined by TEE, these patients had a mean increase of PAOP of 3.5 + 4.8 mm Hg. This translated into a 25% PAOP sensitivity detecting ischemia and a positive predictive value of 16%. Ten of the 14 patients who had ischemia demonstrated by TEE had concomitant ST segment depression of a minimum of 1 mm on at least one lead of a 12-lead electrocardiogram (ECG). Only one patient had ST segment depression that was not diagnosed by TEE. Changes in LV myocardial function detectable by TEE typically precede either changes in the ECG or PAC hemodynamic parameters (76). Clements and colleagues (77) compared radionuclide angiography (RNA) with two-dimensional TEE to estimate LV volume and ejection fraction. They determined that TEE and RNA had a strong correlation, whereas the numbers that were derived from the PAOP had a poor correlation to those volume measurements obtained from RNA and TEE.

The role of TEE in critical care is growing as cardiology and intraoperative experiences have demonstrated its clinical utility. The minimal invasiveness in conjunction with the accuracy of the information makes TEE a valuable diagnostic tool in the armamentarium of the critical care practitioner. Because of the learning curve and cost, it is improbable that TEE will replace (near term) the role of PAC as a routine monitor for the care and management of critically ill patients in the ICU setting.

SUMMARY

Hemodynamic assessment remains an important clinical tool in evaluating and managing critically ill patients. The proper choice and application of current techniques such as the PAC and bedside echocardiography continue to evolve.

Appropriate application of modern technology combined with proper interpretation of information is crucial to optimizing the efficacy and safety of such devices. The lack of prospective, randomized, and controlled trials evaluating the proper use of the PAC, as well as identification of the lack of knowledge in interpreting and troubleshooting monitoring systems, must be considered when guidelines are created on the proper use of hemodynamic assessment.

Miniaturization of transesophageal probes and improved biocompatibility of invasive materials, which may limit infectious and thrombotic risk, along with refinement of noninvasive techniques, may further simplify and enhance hemodynamic evaluation in the ICU.

REFERENCES

1. Steingrub JS, Celoria G, Vickers-Lahti M, et al. Therapeutic impact of pulmonary artery catheterization in a medical/surgical ICU. *Chest* 1991;99:1451–1455.
2. Eisenberg PR, Jaffe AS, Schuster DP. Clinical evaluation compared to pulmonary artery catheterization in the hemodynamic assessment of critically ill patients. *Crit Care Med* 1984;12:549–553.
3. Swan HJC. Central venous pressure monitoring is an outmoded procedure of limited practical value. In: Ingelfinger FJ, Ebert RV, Finland M, et al, eds. *Controversies in internal medicine.* Philadelphia: WB Saunders, 1974:185.
4. Forrester JS, Diamond G, McHugh TJ, et al. Filling pressures in right and left sides of the heart in acute myocardial infarction. A reappraisal of central-venous-pressure monitoring. *N Engl J Med* 1971;285:190–193.
5. Connors AF, Speroff T, Dawson NV, et al. The effectiveness of right heart catheterization in the initial care of critically ill patients. *JAMA,* 1996;276:889–897.
6. Dale JE, Bone RC. Is it time to pull the pulmonary artery catheter? *JAMA,* 1996;276:916–918.
7. Anonymous. A Report from the American Society of Anesthesiologists Task Force on Pulmonary Artery Catheterization. Practice guidelines for pulmonary artery catheterization. *Anesthesiology* 1993;78:380–394.
8. Iberti TJ, Fischer EP, Leibowitz AB, et al. A multicenter study of physicians' knowledge of the pulmonary artery catheter. Pulmonary Artery Catheter Study Group. *JAMA* 1990;264:2928–2932.
9. Gnaegi A, Feihl F, Perret C. Intensive care physician's insufficient knowledge of right-heart catheterization at bedside: Time to act? *Crit Care Med* 1997;25:213–220.
10. Iberti TJ, Dailey EK, Leibowitz AB, et al. Assessment of critical care nurses' knowledge of pulmonary artery catheter. *Crit Care Med* 1994;22: 1674–1678.
11. Trottier SJ, Taylor RW. Society of Critical Care Medicine: Pulmonary artery catheter membership survey. *New Horiz* 197;5:201–206.
12. Gardner RM. Direct blood pressure measurement-dynamic response requirements. *Anesthesiology* 1981;54:227–236.
13. Cope DK, Allison RC, Permentier JL, et al. Measurement of effective pulmonary capillary pressure using the pressure profile after artery occlusion. *Crit Care Med* 1986;14:16–22.
14. Marini JJ. Obtaining meaningful data from the Swan-Ganz catheter. *Respiratory Care* 1985;30:572–585.
15. West JB, Dollery CT, Naimark A. Distribution of blood flow in isolated lung; relation to vascular and alveolar pressures. *J Appl Physiol* 1964;19:713.
16. Berryhill RE, Benumof JL. PEEP-induced discrepancy between pulmonary arterial wedge pressure and left atrial pressure: the effects of controlled vs. spontaneous ventilation and compliant vs. noncompliant lungs in the dog. *Anesthesiology* 1979;51:303–308.
17. Marini JJ. Acute lung injury. Hemodynamic monitoring with the pulmonary artery catheter. *Crit Care Clin* 1986;2:551–572.
18. Donovan KD. Invasive monitoring and support of the circulation. *Clin Anesthes* 1985;3:909–953.
19. Herbert WH. Pulmonary artery and left heart end-diastolic pressure relations. *Br Heart J* 1970;32:774–778.
20. Marini JJ, O'Quin R, Culver BH, et al. Estimation of transmural cardiac pressures during ventilation with PEEP. *J Appl Physiol* 1982;53:384–391.
21. Pepe PE, Marini JJ. Occult positive end-expiratory pressure in mechanically ventilated patients with airflow obstruction: the auto-PEEP effect. *Am Rev Respir Dis* 1982;126:166–170.
22. Jardin F, Farcot JC, Boisante L, et al. Influence of positive end-expiratory pressure on left ventricular performance. *N Engl J Med* 1981;304:387–392.
23. Gurevitch MJ, Van Dyke J, Young ES, et al. Improved oxygenation and lower peak airway pressure in severe adult respiratory distress syndrome. Treatment with inverse ratio ventilation. *Chest* 1986;89:211–213.
24. Shah KB, Rao TK, Laughlin S, et al. A review of pulmonary artery catheterization in 6,245 patients. *Anesthesiology* 1984;61:271–275.
25. Obel IW. Transient phrenic-nerve paralysis following subclavian venipuncture. *Anesthesiology* 1970;33:369–370.
26. Hoar PF, Wilson RM, Mangano DT, et al. Heparin bonding reduces thrombogenicity of pulmonary-artery catheters. *N Engl J Med* 1981;305:993–995.
27. Cobb DK, High KP, Sawyer RG, et al. A controlled trial of scheduled replacement of central venous and pulmonary-artery catheters. *N Engl J Med* 1992;327:1062–1068.
28. Barash PG, Nardi D, Hammond G, et al. Catheter-induced pulmonary artery perforation. Mechanisms, management, and modifications. *J Thorac Cardiovasc Surg* 1981;82:5–12.
29. Ganz W, Donoso R, Marcus HS, et al. A new technique for measurement of cardiac output by thermodilution in man. *Am J Cardiol* 1971;27:392–396.
30. Mohsenifar Z, Goldbach P, Tashkin DP, et al. Relationship between O2 delivery and O2 consumption in the adult respiratory distress syndrome. *Chest* 1983;84:267–271.
31. Nelson LD. The new pulmonary arterial catheters. Right ventricle ejections fraction and continuous cardiac output. *Crit Care Clin* 1996;52:795–818.
32. Spinale FG, Smith AC, Carabello BA, et al. Right ventricular function computed by thermodilution and ventriculography. A comparison of methods. *J Thorac Cardiovasc Surg* 1990;99:141–152.
33. Jansen JR, Johnson RW, Yan JY, et al. Near continuous cardiac output thermodilution. *J Clin Monit* 1997;13:233–299.
34. Yelderman ML, Ramsay MA, Quinn MD, et al. Continuous thermodilution cardiac output measurement in intensive care unit patients. *J Cardiothorac Vasc Anesth* 1992;6:270–274.
35. Mangano DT. Monitoring pulmonary arterial pressure in coronary-artery disease. *Anesthesiology* 1980;53:364–370.
36. Lazor MA, Pierce ET, Stanley GD, et al. Evaluation of the accuracy and response time of STAT-mode continuous cardiac output. *J Cardiothorac Vasc Anesth* 1997;11:432–466.
37. Sinclair S, James S, Singer M. Intraoperative intravascular volume optimisation and length of hospital stay after repair of proximal femoral fracture: randomized controlled trial. *Br Med J* 1997;315:909–912.
38. Raaijmakers E, Faes TJ, Scholten RJ, et al. A meta-analysis of three decades of validating thoracic impedance cardiography. *Crit Care Med* 1999; 27:1203–1213.
39. Linton RA, Band DM, Haire KM. A new method of measuring cardiac output in man using lithium dilution. *Br J Anaesth* 1993;71:262–266.

40. Zollner C, Haller M, Weiss M, et al. Beat-to-beat measurement of cardiac output by intravascular pulse contour analysis: a prospective criterion standard study in patients after cardiac surgery. *J Cardiothorac Vasc Anesth* 2000;14:125–129.

41. Capek JM, Roy RJ. Noninvasive measurement of cardiac output using partial CO_2 rebreathing. *IEEE Trans Biomed Eng* 1988;35:653–661.

42. Watt RC, Loeb RG, Orr JA. Comparison of a new non-invasive cardiac output technique with invasive bolus and continuous thermodilution. *Anesthesiology* 1998, 89(3A):A543.

43. Wil MH, Henning RJ. New concepts in diagnosis and fluid treatment in circulatory shock. *Anesth Analg* 1979;58:124–132.

44. Del Guercio LR, Cohn JD. Monitoring operative risk in the elderly. *JAMA* 1980;243:1350–1355.

45. Tuchschmidt J, Sharma OP. Impact of hemodynamic monitoring in a medical intensive care unit. *Crit Care Med* 1987;15:840–843.

46. Rao TLK, Jacobs KH, El-Etr AA. Reinfarction following anesthesia in patients with myocardial infarction. *Anesthesiology* 1983;59:499–505.

47. Shoemaker WC, Appel PL, Kram HB, et al. Prospective trial of supranormal values of survivors as therapeutic goals in high-risk surgical patients. *Chest* 1988;94:1176–1186.

48. Bishop MH, Shoemaker WC, Appel PL, et al. Prospective, randomized trial of survivor values of cardiac index, oxygen delivery, and oxygen consumption as resuscitation endpoints in severe trauma. *J Trauma* 1995;38:780–787.

49. Gattinoni L, Brazzi L, Pelosi P, et al. A trial of goal-oriented hemodynamic therapy in critically ill patients. SvO_2 Collaborative Group. *N Engl J Med* 1995;333:1025–1032.

50. Boyd O, Ground RM, Bennett ED. A randomized clinical trial of the effects of deliberate perioperative increase of oxygen delivery on mortality in high-risk surgical patients. *JAMA* 1993;270:2699–2707.

51. Mimoz O, Rauss A, Rekik N, et al. Pulmonary artery catheterization in critically ill patients: a prospective analysis of outcome changes associated with catheter-prompted changes in therapy. *Crit Care Med* 1994;27:573–579.

52. Ontario Intensive Care Group. A randomized controlled trial of right heart catheterization in critically ill patients. *J Intensive Care Med* 1991;6:91–95.

53. Ivanov R, Allen J, Sandham D, et al. Pulmonary artery catheterization: a narrative systematic critique of randomized controlled trials and recommendations for the future. *New Horiz* 1997;5:268–276.

54. Ivanov R, Allen J, Calvin JE. The incidence of major morbidity in critically ill patients managed with pulmonary artery catheter. A meta-analysis. *Crit Care Med* 2000;28:615–619.

55. American College of Physicians/American College of Cardiology/American Heart Association Task Force on critical privileges in cardiology clinical competence in hemodynamics monitoring. *J Am Coll Cardiol* 1990;15:1460–1464.

56. Chernow B. Pulmonary artery flotation catheters: a statement by the American College of Chest Physicians and the American Thoracic Society. *Chest* 1997;111:261.

57. Perrino AC, Harris SN, Luther MA. Intraoperative determination of cardiac output using multiplane transesophageal echocardiography: A comparison to thermodilution. *Anesthesiology* 1998;89:350–357.

58. Hozumi T, Shakudo M, Applegate R, et al. Accuracy of cardiac output estimation with biplane transesophageal echocardiography. *J Am Soc Echocardiogr* 1993;6:62–68.

59. Buckmaster MJ, Kearney PA, Johnson SB, et al. Further experience with transesophageal echocardiography in the evaluation of thoracic aortic injury. *J Trauma* 1994;37:989–995.

60. Nienaber CA, von Kodolitsch Y, Nicolas V, et al. The diagnosis of thoracic aortic dissection by noninvasive imaging procedures. *N Eng J Med* 1993;328:1–9.

61. Banning AP, Masani ND, Fraser AG, et al. Transesophageal echocardiography as the sole diagnostic investigation in patients with suspected thoracic aortic dissection. *Br Heart J* 1994;72:461–465.

62. Reeder GS, Khandheria BK, Seward JB, et al. Transesophageal echocardiography and cardiac masses. *Mayo Clin Proc* 1991;66:1101–1109.

63. Mugge A, Daniel WG, Haverich A, et al. Diagnosis of noninfective cardiac mass lesions by two-dimensional echocardiography. Comparison of the transthoracic and transesophageal approaches. *Circulation* 1991;83:70–78.

64. Rousou JA, Tighe DA, Garb JL, et al. Risk of dysphagia after transesophageal echocardiography during cardiac operations. *Ann Thorac Surg* 2000;69:486–490.

65. Hogue CW, Lappas GD, Creswell LL, et al. Swallowing dysfunction after cardiac operations. Associated adverse outcomes and risk factors including intraoperative transesophageal echocardiography. *J Thorac Cardiovasc Surg* 1995;110:517–522.

66. Daniel WG, Erbel R, Kasper W, et al. Safety of transesophageal echocardiography. A multicenter survey of 10,419 examinations. *Circulation* 1991;83:817–821.

67. Shanewise JS, Cheung AT, Aronson S, et al. ASE/SCA guidelines for performing a comprehensive intraoperative multiplane echocardiography examination: recommendation of the American Society of Echocardiography Council for Intraoperative Echocardiography and the Society of Cardiovascular Anesthesiologists Task Force for Certification in Perioperative Transesophageal Echocardiography. *Anesth Analg* 1999;89:870–884.

68. Thys DM, Abel M, Bollen BA, et al. Practice guidelines for perioperative transesophageal echocardiography: a report by the American Society of Anesthesiologists and the Society of Cardiovascular Anesthesiologists Task Force on Transesophageal Echocardiography. *Anesthesiology* 1996;84:986–1006.

69. Benjamin E, Griffin K, Leibowitz AB, et al. Goal-directed transesophageal echocardiography performed by intensivists to assess left ventricular function: comparison with pulmonary artery catheterization. *J Cardiothorac Vasc Anesth* 1998;12:10–15.

70. Reichert CL, Visser CA, Koolen JJ, et al. Transesophageal echocardiography in hypotensive patients after cardiac operations. Comparison with hemodynamic parameters. *J Thorac Cardiovasc Surg* 1992;104:321–326.

71. Poelaert JI, Trouerbach J, De Buyzere M, et al. Evaluation of transesophageal echocardiography as a diagnostic and therapeutic aid in a critical care setting. *Chest* 1995;107:774–779.

72. Heidenreich PA, Stainback RF, Redberg RF, et al. Transesophageal echocardiography predicts mortality in critically ill patients with unexplained hypotension. *J Am Coll Cardiol* 1995;26:152–158.

73. Kaul S, Stratienko AA, Pollock SG, et al. Value of two-dimensional echocardiography for determining the basis of hemodynamic compromise in critically ill patients: a prospective study. *J Am Soc Echocardiogr* 1994;7:598–606.

74. Cheung AT, Savino JS, Weiss SJ, et al. Echocardiographic and hemodynamic indexes of left ventricular preload in patients with normal and abnormal ventricular function. *Anesthesiology* 1994;81:376–387.

75. Van Daele ME, Sutherland GR, Mitchell MM, et al. Do changes in pulmonary capillary wedge pressure adequately reflect myocardial ischemia during anesthesia? A correlative preoperative hemodynamic, electrocardiographic, and transesophageal echocardiographic study. *Circulation* 1990;81:865–871.

76. Smith JS, Cahalan MK, Benefiel DJ, et al. Intraoperative detection of myocardial ischemia in high-risk patients: electrocardiography versus two-dimensional transesophageal echocardiography. *Circulation* 1985;72:1015–1021.

77. Clements FM, Harpole DH, Quill T, et al. Estimation of left ventricular volume and ejection fraction by two-dimensional transoesophageal echocardiography: comparison of short axis imaging and simultaneous radionuclide angiography. *Br J Anaesth* 1990;64:31–336.

FLUID MANAGEMENT IN CRITICALLY ILL PATIENTS

DONALD S. PROUGH
MALI MATHRU

KEY WORDS

- Colloid fluids
- Crystalloid fluids
- Dextrose
- Extracellular volume
- Fluid kinetics
- Hypertonic fluids
- Interstitial fluid
- Intracellular
- Intracranial pressure
- Osmolality
- Oxygen delivery
- Plasma volume
- Starling equation
- Total body water

INTRODUCTION

Trauma, surgery, and critical illness alter the volumes and composition of the intracellular and extracellular spaces and the kinetics of fluid distribution and excretion. Therapeutic infusion of fluids further alters compartmental volumes and composition and the kinetics of fluid redistribution and excretion. Recognition of the multiple influences on perioperative fluid therapy and management of fluids to limit adverse consequences may limit surgical morbidity and mortality.

PHYSIOLOGIC PRINCIPLES OF VOLUME HOMEOSTASIS

Body Fluid Compartments

Accurate replacement of fluid deficits requires an understanding of the distribution spaces of water, sodium, and colloid (Fig. 1). Total body water (TBW), which approximates 60% of total body weight, includes intracellular volume (ICV; 40% of total body weight) and extracellular volume (ECV; 20% of body weight). ECV serves as the distribution volume for sodium. Plasma volume (PV) equals about one-fifth of ECV, the remainder of which is interstitial fluid (IF). Red cell volume, approximately 2 L, is part of ECV.

Sodium concentration [Na^+] is equal in PV and IF (approximately 140 mEq per L). The predominant intracellular cation, potassium, has an intracellular concentration approximating 150 mEq per L. Albumin is unequally distributed in PV ($\sim$4 g per dL) and IF ($\sim$1 g per dL). ECV is the distribution volume for colloid, although the concentrations in PV and IF are unequal.

Distribution of Infused Fluids

Conventional prediction of PV expansion after fluid infusion assumes static fluid spaces and ignores fluid excretion. For example, assume that a 70-kg patient requires replacement of an acute blood loss of 1,000 mL. The formula describing the effects on PV of infusion of any fluid is as follows:

$$PV\ increment = (Volume\ infused \times normal\ PV)/distribution\ volume$$

To replace 1.0 L of blood loss using 5% dextrose in water (D5W):

$$1.0\,L = 14\,L \times 3.0\,L/42\,L$$

where 1.0 L is the desired PV increment, 3.0 L is the normal estimated PV in a 70-kg person, and 42 L is the TBW (the distribution volume of sodium-free water).

To replace 1.0 L of blood loss using lactated Ringer solution (which has a distribution volume approximately similar to ECV):

$$1.0\,L = 4.7\,L \times 3.0\,L/14\,L$$

where 14 L is the ECV in a 70-kg person.

If 5% albumin, which exerts colloid osmotic pressure similar to plasma and has a distribution volume similar to PV, were infused, the infused volume initially would remain in the PV. Twenty-five percent human serum albumin, a concentrated colloid, would expand PV by approximately 400 mL for each 100 mL infused (i.e., 1.0 L of blood loss could be replaced temporarily by 250 mL of 25% albumin).

Prediction of Plasma Volume Expansion Using Kinetic Analysis

Kinetic analysis of the responses of PV to fluid infusion serves the same purposes as pharmacokinetic analysis of drug concentrations (i.e., estimating peak volume expansion and rates of

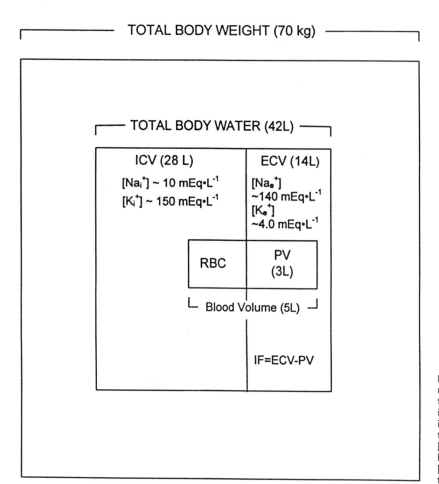

FIGURE 1. The distribution volume of water, approximately 60% of total body weight, includes both the extracellular (ECV) and intracellular volume (ICV). Sodium is distributed primarily in the ECV. If capillary integrity is preserved, the concentration of colloid is higher in the plasma volume (PV) than in interstitial fluid (IF). $[Na_i^+]$ and $[Na_e^+]$ indicate intracellular and extracellular concentrations of sodium, respectively; $[K_i^+]$ and $[K_e^+]$ represent intracellular and extracellular concentrations of potassium.

clearance of infused fluid from PV). As an alternative to the drug concentrations that are analyzed in pharmacokinetic analysis, fluid kinetics usually analyze changes in hemoglobin concentration (1). In normovolemic volunteers, rapid infusion of crystalloid solutions results in minimal expansion of PV; most of the infused fluid is rapidly excreted (2). In contrast, in mildly hypovolemic volunteers, a larger fraction is retained in PV (3) and in moderately hypovolemic volunteers, nearly all is retained in the short term (4). Preliminary data suggest that sepsis (5) and hypoproteinemia (6) exert surprisingly small influences on fluid kinetics. During administration of isoflurane in conscious sheep, the fraction of fluid remaining in PV is small and similar to that remaining intravascularly in conscious animals, but the fluid is not excreted; rather, fluid accumulates in the interstitial fluid volume (7).

Regulation of Extracellular Fluid Volume

Changes in retention and excretion of infused fluid are regulated by the kidneys and the sympathetic nervous system. Renal adaptation to hypovolemia (and decreased cardiac output) occurs through three primary mechanisms: a reduction in renal blood flow (RBF), a reduction in the glomerular filtration rate (GFR), and increased tubular reabsorption of sodium and water (1). Initially, RBF is maintained (i.e., autoregulated) as perfusion pressure decreases by decreases in renal afferent arteriolar resis-

tance. Further decreases in cardiac output redistribute blood flow from the kidneys and other less essential tissues to the heart and brain.

Renal perfusion during hypovolemia is determined by the balance between renal vasoconstrictive factors (the renal sympathetic nerves, angiotensin II, and catecholamines) and vasodilatory mechanisms (intrinsic renal autoregulation and the renal vasodilatory effects of prostaglandins). Autoregulation may be impaired or lost during severe, acute hypovolemia and may be lost in the inner medulla with even less reduction in perfusion pressure (3). Renal sympathetic stimulation, resulting in secretion of α-adrenergic catecholamines and angiotensin II, increases renal vascular resistance.

To preserve PV, reabsorption of filtered water and sodium is enhanced by antidiuretic hormone (ADH) and aldosterone and by reduced secretion of atrial natriuretic peptide (ANP). A 10% to 20% decrease in blood volume is necessary before ADH secretion from the posterior pituitary increases (8). ADH acts primarily on the medullary collecting ducts to increase water reabsorption, thereby causing excretion of smaller volumes of more highly concentrated urine. Sodium conservation results from both decreased filtration and increased distal tubular reabsorption of sodium, mediated by aldosterone. Hypoperfusion stimulates the granular cells of the renal juxtaglomerular apparatus to release renin, which catalyzes the conversion of angiotensinogen to angiotensin I. Angiotensin-converting enzyme converts angiotensin I to angiotensin II, which stimulates the adrenal cortex to synthesize and release aldosterone. ANP, which exerts vasodilatory effects and increases the renal excretion of sodium and water (9), is released from the cardiac atria in smaller quantities in hypovolemia.

The kidney also synthesizes vasodilator prostaglandins that play a crucial role in protecting the kidney from vasoconstrictor hormones and in maintaining RBF during hypovolemia. The protective effect of endogenous renal prostaglandins may be antagonized by nonsteroidal antiinflammatory drugs (10).

FLUID MANAGEMENT

Colloids, Crystalloids, and Hypertonic Solutions

Physiology and Pharmacology

Osmotically active particles attract water across semipermeable membranes until equilibrium is attained. Osmolality, a measurement of the number of osmotically active particles per kilogram of solvent, can be estimated as follows:

$$\text{Osmolality} = ([Na^+] \times 2.0) + (\text{Glucose}/18) + (\text{BUN}/2.3)$$

where osmolality is expressed in mmol per kg, $[Na^+]$ is expressed in mEq per L, serum glucose is expressed in mg per dL, and BUN is blood urea nitrogen expressed in mg per dL. Sugars, alcohols, and radiographic dyes increase measured osmolality.

A hyperosmolar state occurs whenever the concentration of osmotically active particles is high. Both uremia (increased BUN) and hypernatremia (increased serum $[Na^+]$) increase serum osmolality. Because sodium is largely restricted to the ECV, hypernatremia causes hypertonicity (i.e., osmotically mediated redistribution of water from ICV to ECV). However, because urea distributes throughout TBW, an increase in BUN does not cause hypertonicity.

The small proportion of osmotically active particles consisting of plasma proteins is essential in determining the equilibrium of fluid between IF and PV. The reflection coefficient (σ) describes the permeability of capillary membranes to individual solutes, with 0 representing free permeability and 1.0 representing complete impermeability. The σ for albumin ranges from 0.6 to nearly 1.0 in various capillary beds. Because capillary protein concentrations exceed interstitial concentrations, the osmotic pressure exerted by plasma proteins (termed colloid osmotic pressure or oncotic pressure and symbolized by π) is higher than interstitial oncotic pressure (π_i) and tends to preserve PV. The filtration rate of fluid from the capillaries into the interstitial space is the net result of the gradient from capillary π (π_c) to π_i and the gradient between intravascular and interstitial hydrostatic pressures, as expressed in the Starling equation:

$$Q = kA \left[(P_c - P_i) + \sigma(\pi_i - \pi_c) \right]$$

where Q is the fluid filtration, k is the capillary filtration coefficient (conductivity of water), A is the area of the capillary membrane, P_c is the capillary hydrostatic pressure, and P_i is the interstitial hydrostatic pressure.

P_c, the most powerful factor promoting fluid filtration, is determined by capillary flow, arterial resistance, venous resistance, and venous pressure. If capillary filtration increases, the rate of water and sodium filtration usually exceeds protein filtration, resulting in preservation of π_c, dilution of π_i, and an increase in the colloid osmotic pressure gradient. When coupled with increased lymphatic drainage, an increase in the oncotic pressure gradient limits the accumulation of IF. If P_c increases at a time when lymphatic drainage is maximal, then IF accumulates, forming edema. In chronically edematous states, IF pressure is reduced by enhanced lymphatic drainage through dilated lymphatic vessels. Increased fluid filtration also dilutes the proteoglycan matrix in the IF, increasing capillary permeability; dehydration of the interstitium reduces vascular permeability (11).

Clinical Implications of Choices Between Crystalloid and Colloid

If membrane permeability is intact, colloids such as albumin or hydroxyethyl starch preferentially expand PV rather than IF. Concentrated colloid-containing solutions (i.e., 25% albumin) may translocate IF into the PV. PV expansion unaccompanied by IF expansion offers apparent advantages: lower fluid requirements, less peripheral and pulmonary edema accumulation, and reduced concern about later fluid mobilization.

Exhaustive research however has failed to establish the superiority of either colloid-containing or crystalloid-containing fluids (Table 1). In fact, systematic reviews of randomized trials comparing colloid and crystalloid solutions (12) or specifically comparing albumin and crystalloid solutions (13) have suggested that colloid solutions are associated with increased mortality. These systematic reviews have been extensively criticized, but at the very least prompt careful examination of perioperative fluid strategies.

Much of the crystalloid-colloid debate has centered on the relative risk of pulmonary edema associated with the two types of fluids. Crystalloid solutions are associated with pulmonary

TABLE 1. ADVANTAGES AND DISADVANTAGES OF COLLOID VS. CRYSTALLOID INTRAVENOUS FLUIDS

Solution	Advantages	Disadvantages
Colloid	Smaller infused volume	Greater cost
	Prolonged increase in plasma volume	Coagulopathy (dextran > HES)
	Greater peripheral edema	Pulmonary edema (capillary leak states)
		Decreased GFR
		Osmotic diuresis (low-molecular-weight dextran)
Crystalloid	Lower cost	Transient hemodynamic improvement
	Greater urinary flow	Peripheral edema (protein dilution)
	Replaces interstitial fluid	Pulmonary edema (protein dilution plus high PAOP)

HES, hydroxyethyl starch; GFR, glomerular filtration rate; PAOP, pulmonary artery occlusion pressure.

edema, usually as a result of increased P_c, perhaps in combination with a reduction in π_c. Colloid may also produce increases, often of greater duration, in P_c. Moreover, in disease states associated with increased pulmonary capillary permeability (i.e., sepsis or the *acute* respiratory distress syndrome), infusion of colloid may aggravate pulmonary edema. Increased microvascular permeability decreases the gradient between π_c and π_i so that the term "$\sigma(\pi_i - \pi_c)$" in the previous equation approaches zero. In the absence of an oncotic pressure gradient, small increases in the hydrostatic gradient can result in clinically important pulmonary edema.

Hypoproteinemia in critically ill patients has been associated with the development of pulmonary edema and with increased mortality. However, either crystalloid or colloid administration, if sufficient to substantially increase pulmonary microvascular pressure, may precipitate pulmonary edema in patients who have valvular heart disease, decreased left ventricular compliance, or decreased left ventricular contractility (i.e., heart failure). After experimentally increasing microvascular permeability, Pearl and colleagues (14) found no differences between increases in extravascular lung water induced by colloid or crystalloid.

In surgical patients at risk for the development of pulmonary edema, pulmonary arterial catheterization and measurement of pulmonary arterial occlusion pressure (PAOP) may facilitate management and should be maintained at the lowest level compatible with adequate systemic perfusion. Theoretically, maintenance of a relatively low PAOP, coupled with fluid therapy with colloid (to preserve π_c) should minimize edema formation. However, little data support that approach. Rather, most clinical experience suggests that a more practical approach is to scrupulously avoid infusion of fluid in excess of that necessary to support cardiac output.

Hydroxyethyl starch, the most commonly used synthetic colloid, is less expensive than albumin. Although large doses of some formulations of hydroxyethyl starch produce laboratory evidence of coagulopathy, 6.0% hydroxyethyl starch, used in recommended volumes (10 to 15 mL per kg), has not been associated with clinically important coagulopathy in patients undergoing abdominal aortic aneurysm surgery (15). More recently, changes in the mixture of sizes of hydroxyethyl starch molecules and changes in the composition of the carrier fluids have produced fluids that have potentially desirable characteristics (16,17). Hydroxyethyl starch, derived from amylopectin, is a mixture of molecules of different sizes. Hydroxyethyl groups can be substituted at any or all of three carbons, C_2, C_3, and C_6. The size, extent of substitution, and the C_2/C_6 ratio determine the rates of degradation and excretion and the magnitude of effects on coagulation.

Consequently, mixtures of these molecules are defined in terms of their mean molecular weight, their degree of substitution, and their C_2/C_6 ratio. Hetastarch, the most commonly used hydroxyethyl starch formulation in the United States, has a mean molecular weight of 450,000 daltons and a hydroxyethyl group is substituted at seven-tenths of the potential sites; therefore, hetastarch can be described as 450,000/0.7. Pentastarch, used in Europe for fluid replacement but used in the United States only as replacement for plasmapheresis is designated 200,000/0.5. Other formulations are undergoing clinical trials, such as the low-molecular-weight, low-substitution product, 130,000/0.4,

which appears to minimally influence coagulation and to be more rapidly excreted (18). Further clinical trials will be necessary to define the most appropriate composition of hydroxyethyl starch fluids.

Part of the difficulty in comparing individual crystalloid or colloid fluids is directly attributable to the difficulty of defining comparable endpoints in clinically relevant experimental models (19). More recently developed models replicate clinical situations, permitting more accurate comparison of crystalloid and colloid solutions. In animals infused with *Escherichia coli*, lipopolysaccharide, which mimics some aspects of clinical sepsis, lactated Ringer solution, or 6% hydroxyethyl starch, produced comparable effects on the critical endpoint of systemic oxygen delivery ($\dot{D}O_2$) while producing the expected differences in extravascular fluid accumulation (20). In a more complex porcine model, consisting of temporary exteriorization of the small intestine accompanied by incremental hemorrhage and replacement, colloid solutions produced superior restoration of cardiac output, $\dot{D}O_2$, and oxygen consumption (21).

Implications of Crystalloid and Colloid Infusions on Intracranial Pressure

Because the cerebral capillary membrane, the blood–brain barrier, is highly impermeable to protein, clinicians have assumed that administration of colloid-containing solutions should increase intracranial pressure (ICP) less than crystalloid solutions would. In anesthetized rabbits, plasmapheresis to reduce plasma osmolality by 13 mOsm per kg (baseline value = 295 mOsm per kg) increased cortical water content and ICP; reducing colloid osmotic pressure from 20 to 7.0 mm Hg produced no significant change in either variable (22). Similar independence of brain water and ICP from colloid osmotic pressure has been demonstrated in animals after forebrain ischemia (23) and focal cryogenic injury (24). However, after experimental traumatic brain injury, Drummond and coworkers (25) demonstrated that colloid osmotic pressure also could influence brain water accumulation, perhaps because of dysfunction of the blood–brain barrier.

FLUID REPLACEMENT THERAPY

Maintenance Requirements for Water, Sodium, and Potassium

Two simple formulas are used interchangeably to estimate maintenance water requirements. The first provides 4.0 mL per kg per hour for each of the first 10 kg of body weight, 2.0 mL per kg per hour for each of the next 10 kg, and 1.0 mL per kg per hour for any kg greater than 20. The second formula provides 100 mL per kg per day for each of the first 10 kg of body weight, 50 mL per kg per day for each of the next 10 kg, and 20 mL per kg per day for any kg greater than 20. In healthy adults, sufficient water is required to balance gastrointestinal losses of 100 to 200 mL per day, insensible losses of 500 to 1,000 mL per day (one-half of which is respiratory and one-half cutaneous), and urinary losses of 1,000 mL per day. Urinary losses exceeding 1,000 mL per day may represent an inability to conserve salt or water or an appropriate physiologic response to ECV expansion.

TABLE 2. PREDICTED VS. REPORTED CHANGES IN SERUM BICARBONATE [HCO$_3^-$] AFTER SALINE INFUSION IN HUMANS

	Infusion		Postinfusion		
First Author	Volume (mL/kg)	[HCO$_3^-$] (mEq/L)	Estimated ECV (L)	Predicted [HCO$_3^-$] (mEq/L)	Actual [HCO$_3^-$] (mEq/L)
Waters and Bernstein (29)	14.9	0	15.8	25.1	25.0
Rehm, et al. (30)	23.7	0	13.1[a]	21.0	21.6
Liskaser, et al. (31)	19.7	0	16.7[a]	22.9	20.4
McFarlane and Lee (27)	53.4	0	14.2[a]	20.4	21.0
Scheingraber, et al. (28)[b]	71	0	17.1[a]	18.6	18.4

[a] Estimated as baseline extracellular volume (ECV) minus plasma volume removed plus colloid infused.
[b] Data at 120 min of surgery.
(Reprinted from Prough DS. Acidosis associated with perioperative saline administration: dilution or delusion? *Anesthesiology* 2000;93:1167–1169, with permission.)

Sodium balance is maintained by renal mechanisms despite wide variation in sodium intake. Sodium excretion can decrease to less than 10 mEq per day or greatly exceed normal daily requirements (~75 mEq). Because renal conservation and excretion of potassium is less efficient, requirements slightly exceed 40 mEq.

Fluid Management

Combining the predicted daily maintenance requirements for water, sodium, and potassium in healthy, 70-kg adults results in an estimated 2,500 mL per day of a solution containing a [Na$^+$] of 30 mEq per L and a [K$^+$] of 15 to 20 mEq per L. Intraoperatively, fluids containing sodium-free water (i.e., [Na$^+$] less than 130 mEq per L) are rarely employed in adults because most surgical losses (blood loss and accumulation of tissue edema) are isotonic. Postoperatively, lactated Ringer solution or 0.9% saline is commonly used until patients are hemodynamically stable. Subsequently, if cardiac and renal functions are satisfactory, patients tolerate fluids containing more free water (i.e., 0.45% saline) but still containing [Na$^+$] in excess of maintenance requirements.

Dextrose

Traditionally, physicians have infused glucose-containing intravenous fluids perioperatively in an effort to prevent hypoglycemia and limit protein catabolism. However, due to the hyperglycemic response associated with surgical stress, only infants and patients receiving insulin or drugs that interfere with glucose synthesis or patients with severe liver disease and limited glycogen stores are at risk for hypoglycemia. Iatrogenic hyperglycemia can induce an osmotic diuresis and may aggravate ischemic and traumatic brain injury (26).

Surgical Fluid Requirements

Surgical patients require replacement of PV and ECV losses secondary to wound or burn edema, ascites, and gastrointestinal secretions. Wound and burn edema and ascitic fluid are protein rich and contain electrolytes in concentrations similar to those found in plasma. If ECV is adequate and renal and cardiovascular function are normal, all gastrointestinal secretions, including high-chloride gastric secretions and high-bicarbonate intestinal secretions, can be replaced using lactated Ringer solution or 0.9% ("normal") saline; if renal or cardiovascular function is compromised, more precise replacement is necessary. Substantial loss of gastrointestinal fluids requires replacement of other electrolytes (e.g., potassium, magnesium, phosphate). Chronic gastric losses may produce hypochloremic metabolic alkalosis that can be corrected with 0.9% saline; chronic diarrhea may produce hyperchloremic metabolic acidosis that may be prevented or corrected by infusion of fluid containing bicarbonate or bicarbonate substrate (i.e., lactate or acetate).

Infusion of large volumes of fluids also may substantially alter acid-base balance. For example, clinicians have long recognized that the lactate present in lactated Ringer solution, once metabolized to bicarbonate, may result in hyperbicarbonatremia in proportion to the volume of fluid infused. More recently, several studies have demonstrated that infusion of 0.9% saline, or colloids suspended in 0.9% saline, will produce a dose-dependent, hyperchloremic metabolic acidosis (Table 2) (27–32). There is little evidence that mild hyperchloremic acidosis is physiologically harmful; however, diagnostic confusion between this predictable effect of saline infusion on bicarbonate concentration and the more threatening occurrence of lactic acidosis after trauma or surgery may prompt inappropriate treatment (33). Calculation of the anion gap (which should be normal in hyperchloremic acidosis and increased in lactic acidosis) or measurement of serum lactate concentration can clarify the clinical situation.

Although hyperchloremic acidosis could be avoided by using a balanced salt solution that has a lower chloride concentration than 0.9% saline, experimental data suggest that there may be adverse effects of other constituents of intravenous infusions. For example, in rats that are resuscitated from hemorrhage shock using lactated Ringer solution, apoptosis was increased in the gastrointestinal tract and liver in comparison to rats resuscitated with a lactate-free fluid (34). Also in rats, lactate resuscitation was associated with infusion rate-dependent immune suppression (35). In contrast, in rats with massive hemorrhage, lactated Ringer solution improved survival in comparison to saline (36).

Replacement of intraoperative fluid losses must compensate for the acute reduction of functional IF that accompanies trauma, hemorrhage, and tissue manipulation. For example, otherwise healthy subjects who received no intraoperative sodium while undergoing gastric or gallbladder surgery demonstrated a decline

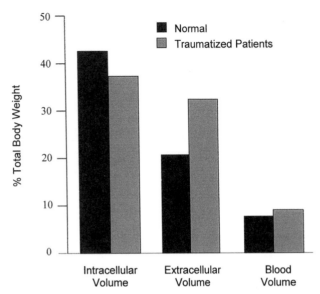

FIGURE 2. In comparison with normal individuals, patients recently subjected to severe trauma (fluid and blood requirements exceeding an average of 21 L on the day of admission) have a slight decrease in intracellular volume (as percentage of body weight) and a substantial increase in extracellular volume. (Data redrawn from Böck JC, Barker BC, Clinton AG, et al. Post-traumatic changes in, and effect of colloid osmotic pressure on the distribution of body water. *Ann Surg* 1989;210:395–405, with permission.)

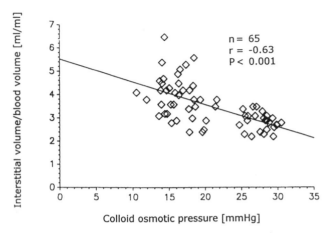

FIGURE 3. Correlation between plasma colloid osmotic pressure and the ratio of interstitial volume to blood volume in patients after severe trauma and resuscitation. Note that the ratio of interstitial volume to plasma volume would be higher. For instance, if the ratio of interstitial volume to blood volume is 4:1 and hematocrit is 30, the ratio of interstitial volume to plasma volume would be 5.7:1. (Reproduced from Böck JC, Barker BC, Clinton AG, et al. Post-traumatic changes in, and effect of colloid osmotic pressure on the distribution of body water. *Ann Surg* 1989;210:395–405, with permission.)

in ECV of nearly 2.0 L and a 13% decline in GFR (37). In contrast, patients who received lactated Ringer solution maintained ECV and increased GFR by 10%. No data describe changes in PV, IF, and ICV during acute, unresuscitated shock in humans. During prolonged experimental hemorrhagic shock, both sodium and water accumulate intracellularly (38) but appear to return to normal once systemic hemodynamic stability is restored. Patients studied during the first 10 days after resuscitation from massive trauma demonstrated a 55% increase in IF volume (Fig. 2) and, in association with a reduction in colloid osmotic pressure, an increased ratio of IF to blood volume (Fig. 3) (39).

Based on the previous considerations, guidelines have been developed for replacement of fluid shifts during surgical procedures. The simplest formula provides, in addition to maintenance fluids and replacement of estimated blood loss, $4\ mL \times kg^{-1} \times h^{-1}$ of lactated Ringer solution or 0.9% saline for procedures involving minimal trauma, $6\ mL \times kg^{-1} \times h^{-1}$ for those involving moderate trauma, and $8\ mL \times kg^{-1} \times h^{-1}$ for those involving extreme trauma. Guidelines for fluid administration, however, must be applied with care. Clinical data suggest that many patients undergoing surgery develop pulmonary edema, often without antecedent cardiac compromise, and that many of these patients may die as a consequence of this complication of fluid therapy (40).

An important corollary of the inevitable IF expansion that accompanies intraoperative fluid resuscitation is the mobilization and return of accumulated fluid to the ECV and the PV, colloquially termed "deresuscitation." In most patients, mobilization occurs on approximately the third postoperative day. If the cardiovascular system and kidneys can effectively transport and excrete mobilized fluid, no important physiologic consequences follow. If not, hypervolemia and pulmonary edema may occur.

Clinical Implications of Hypertonic Fluid Administration

An ideal alternative to conventional crystalloid and colloid fluids would be inexpensive, produce minimal peripheral or pulmonary edema, generate sustained hemodynamic effects, and be effective even if administered in small volumes. Hypertonic, hypernatremic solutions combined with colloid appear to fulfill some of these criteria (Table 3). Small volumes (6.0 mL per kg) of 7.5% hypertonic saline restored blood pressure and cardiac output and increased mesenteric blood flow to greater than control values in hemorrhaged dogs; all animals survived (41). Although posttreatment serum osmolality exceeded 330 mOsm per kg, no animal showed adverse effects.

Hypertonic solutions also may improve microvascular perfusion. *In vivo* experimental evidence suggests that resuscitation with 7.2% NaCl + 10% hydroxyethyl starch facilitates the passage of leukocytes through the microvascular network (42). In experimental animals, the acute effects of hypertonic infusions also include favorable alterations in neutrophil cytotoxicity, pulmonary sequestration of neutrophils, priming of neutrophils, and endotoxin-induced increases in vascular permeability.

Hypertonic solutions exert favorable effects on cerebral hemodynamics, in part because the impermeability to sodium of the blood–brain barrier in uninjured brain causes the brain to shrink in response to acute increases in serum [Na$^+$]. In dogs with intracranial mass lesions, intracranial pressure increased during resuscitation from hemorrhagic shock with 0.8% saline but remained unchanged if 7.2% saline was infused in a sufficient volume to comparably improve systemic hemodynamics (43). Hypertonic solutions restored regional cerebral blood flow better than did slightly hypotonic solutions (43). In hemorrhaged rats subjected to mechanical brain injury, brain water content was lower in uninjured brain (but similar in injured brain) after resuscitation with a hyperosmotic solution (44). However, when

TABLE 3. HYPERTONIC RESUSCITATION FLUIDS: ADVANTAGES AND DISADVANTAGES

Solution	Advantages	Disadvantages
Hypertonic crystalloid	Inexpensive Promotes urinary flow Small initial volume Improved myocardial contractility? Arteriolar dilation Reduced peripheral edema Lower intracranial pressure Sustained hemodynamic response	Hypertonicity Subdural hemorrhage Transient effect Added expense

Hypertonic crystalloid
  plus colloid (in comparison to
  hypertonic crystalloid alone)
	Reduced subsequent volume requirements	Coagulopathy (dextran > HES)
		Osmotic diuresis
		Impaired crossmatch (dextran)
		Hypertonicity

HES, hydroxyethyl starch.
(Reprinted from Prough DS, Johnston WE. Fluid resuscitation in septic shock: no solution yet. *Anesth Analg* 1989;69:699–704, with permission.)

considering maintenance fluid therapy, differences between fluids of varying tonicity become negligible (45).

Clinical Experience with Hypertonic Fluid Management

Unfortunately, after initial improvement, both cardiac output and blood pressure rapidly decline after single-dose resuscitation with hypertonic saline. Strategies to prolong the therapeutic effects beyond 30 to 60 minutes include continued infusion of hypertonic saline, subsequent infusion of blood or conventional fluids, or addition of colloid to hypertonic resuscitation. In a recent randomized study, Vassar and colleagues (46) evaluated the effects of 250 mL of 7.5% sodium chloride with and without 6% and 12% dextran 70 for the prehospital resuscitation of hypotensive trauma patients. Addition of dextran did not improve the blood pressure changes associated with administration of hypertonic saline alone. A small subgroup of patients with Glasgow Coma Scale scores of less than 8, but without severe anatomic injury, seemed to benefit most from hypertonic resuscitation (46). Mattox and associates (47) also reported improved survival in traumatized patients initially resuscitated with 7.5% saline and requiring surgery. In humans resuscitated with hypertonic saline, acute increases in serum [Na^+] to 155 to 160 mEq per L produced no apparent harm (46,47). Central pontine myelinolysis, which follows rapid correction of severe, chronic hyponatremia, has not been observed in clinical trials of hypertonic resuscitation.

Hypertonic solutions have also been evaluated for management of intracranial hypertension in patients requiring intensive care for neurologic and neurosurgical critical illness. In general, clinical experience has been favorable, with hypertonic therapy well tolerated and with good control of intracranial hypertension in comparison to conventional management (48–50). However, available evidence is not yet sufficient to support the use of hypertonic solutions for routine neurointensive care.

The clinical efficacy of hypertonic resuscitation in comparison to conventional fluids remains unclear because many preclinical studies have compared the effects of single boluses of experimental and control fluids. In contrast, clinical fluid resuscitation continues until no additional fluid is required. Comparison of two or more resuscitation regimens that alter more than one hemodynamic variable may generate misleading conclusions. For example, because hypertonic fluids reduce systemic vascular resistance, ventricular ejection may improve, leading to decreased PAOP; theoretically, more fluid would therefore be necessary to restore a filling pressure similar to that produced by a colloid solution.

Will clinicians routinely use hypertonic or combination hypertonic/hyperoncotic fluids for resuscitation in the future? Pending further preclinical work, the theoretical advantages of such fluids appear most attractive in the acute resuscitation of hypovolemic patients with head-injuries.

FLUID STATUS: ASSESSMENT AND MONITORING

Assessment of Hypovolemia and Tissue Hypoperfusion

Two contrasting methods are used to assess the adequacy of intravascular volume. The first, conventional clinical assessment, is appropriate for most patients; the second, goal-directed hemodynamic management, may be superior for high-risk surgical patients.

Clinical quantification of blood volume and ECV is difficult, beginning with recognition of settings in which deficits are likely, such as bowel obstruction, chronic diuretic use, sepsis, burns, pancreatitis, and trauma. Although the physical signs of hypovolemia are insensitive and nonspecific, suggestive evidence includes oliguria, supine hypotension, and a positive "tilt test." Oliguria implies hypovolemia, although hypovolemic patients may be nonoliguric and normovolemic patients may be oliguric because of renal failure or stress-induced endocrine responses. Supine hypotension implies a blood volume deficit exceeding 30%. However, arterial blood pressure within the normal range could represent relative hypotension in an elderly or chronically hypertensive patient. Substantial depletion of blood volume and organ hypoperfusion may occur, despite an apparently normal blood pressure and heart rate. The value of the tilt test is limited by a high incidence of false-positive and false-negative findings. Young, healthy subjects can withstand acute loss of 20% of blood volume while exhibiting only postural tachycardia and variable postural hypotension. In contrast, 20% to 30% of older adult patients may demonstrate orthostatic changes in blood pressure, despite normal blood volume (51).

Laboratory evidence that is compatible with the diagnoses of hypovolemia or ECV depletion includes hemoconcentration, azotemia, low urinary [Na^+], metabolic alkalosis, and metabolic acidosis. Hematocrit, a poor indicator of intravascular volume, is virtually unchanged by acute hemorrhage; later, hemodilution occurs as fluids are administered or as fluid shifts from the interstitial to the intravascular space. If intravascular volume has been restored, hematocrit more accurately reflects red cell mass. BUN, normally 8 to 20 mg per dL, is increased by hypovolemia, high protein intake, gastrointestinal bleeding, or accelerated catabolism and decreased by severe hepatic dysfunction. Serum creatinine (SCr), a product of muscle catabolism, may be misleadingly low in older adults, in females, and in debilitated or malnourished patients. In contrast, in muscular or acutely catabolic patients, SCr may exceed the normal range (0.5 to 1.5 mg per dL) because of greater turnover of muscle protein. A ratio of BUN:SCr exceeding the normal range (10 to 20) suggests dehydration or other factors that alter the serum concentrations. In prerenal oliguria, enhanced sodium reabsorption should reduce urinary [Na^+] to less than 20 mEq per L and enhanced water reabsorption should increase urinary concentration (i.e., urinary osmolality greater than 400; urine/plasma creatinine ratio greater than 40:1). However, the sensitivity and specificity of measurements of urinary [Na^+], osmolality, and creatinine ratios may be misleading in acute situations. ECV depletion is a potent stimulus for the maintenance of metabolic alkalosis. Severe hypovolemia may result in systemic hypoperfusion and lactic acidosis.

The adequacy of perioperative fluid resuscitation must be ascertained by evaluating multiple clinical variables, including heart rate, arterial blood pressure, urinary output, and arterial blood gases. Tachycardia is a nonspecific indicator of hypovolemia. Preservation of blood pressure, accompanied by a central venous pressure of 6 to 12 mm Hg, suggests adequate replacement. During profound hypovolemia, indirect measurements of blood pressure may inaccurately reflect intraarterial pressure.

Urinary output usually decreases precipitously during moderate to severe hypovolemia. Therefore, in the absence of glycosuria or diuretic administration, a urinary output of 0.5 to 1.0 mL $\times$ kg^{-1} $\times$ h^{-1} suggests adequate renal perfusion. Serum bicarbonate and arterial pH may decrease only when tissue hypoperfusion becomes severe. Cardiac output can be normal despite severely reduced regional blood flow. Mixed venous hemoglobin desaturation, a specific indicator of poor systemic perfusion, reflects average perfusion in multiple organs and cannot supplant regional monitors such as urinary output.

No intraoperative monitor is sufficiently sensitive or specific to detect hypoperfusion in all patients. Moreover, acute renal failure, hepatic failure, and sepsis may result from unrecognized, subclinical tissue hypoperfusion. One key variable that has been associated with survival is a $\dot{D}O_2 \geq 600$ mL $O_2 \times$ min$^{-1} \times$ m^{-2}. A theoretically attractive goal for resuscitation, $\dot{D}O_2$ combines in a single-term cardiac index (CI) and arterial oxygen content (CaO$_2$) according to the equation:

$$\dot{D}O_2 = CI \times CaO_2 \times 10$$

where the factor 10 corrects CaO$_2$, measured in mL O$_2$ per dL, to mL per L.

Because fluid resuscitation using crystalloid, colloid, or hypertonic solutions both increases cardiac output and decreases hemoglobin concentration, the use of $\dot{D}O_2$ as a goal may be preferable. The concept underlying the use of $\dot{D}O_2$ as a goal for resuscitation is that critically ill patients are at risk for subclinical tissue hypoperfusion (i.e., tissue hypoperfusion at a regional or global level that is not evident from any monitored variable). Theoretically, regional or global oxygen consumption would increase if tissue perfusion increased; therefore, increasing $\dot{D}O_2$ could eliminate subclinical tissue hypoperfusion. Such an improvement could be reflected in increased oxygen consumption, although clinical data do not strongly support the utility of oxygen consumption as an endpoint for resuscitation.

A number of caveats however pertain to the use of an arbitrary targeted level of $\dot{D}O_2$ as an endpoint for resuscitation. First, red cell transfusion increases hemoglobin concentration but may not increase $\dot{D}O_2$ because of a reciprocal decrease in CI. Second, the use of catecholamines to increase $\dot{D}O_2$ may produce a misleading increase in oxygen consumption because of the calorigenic effects of β-agonists. Third, various catecholamines may exert unequal effects. Fourth, patients who attain the targeted $\dot{D}O_2$, either spontaneously or as a result of hemodynamic support, may be inherently more robust and more likely to survive than those who fail to attain the targeted $\dot{D}O_2$. Finally, the use of specific monitors to define resolution of tissue hypoperfusion in specific organ systems (e.g., gastrointestinal intramucosal pH) should be superior to using a global target such as $\dot{D}O_2$.

Several recent studies have examined the utility of this endpoint but have reached inconsistent conclusions. Boyd and coworkers (52) randomized high-risk surgical patients to conventional treatment or $\dot{D}O_2 \geq 600$ mL O$_2 \times$ min$^{-1} \times$ m^{-2} and demonstrated a decrease in mortality and in the number of complications in the patients managed at the higher level of $\dot{D}O_2$. In contrast, Hayes and colleagues (53) randomized a broader range of critically ill patients to conventional treatment or $\dot{D}O_2 \geq$ 600 mL O$_2 \times$ min$^{-1} \times$ m^{-2} using a combination of volume and dobutamine. They demonstrated increased mortality in the group maintained at the higher levels and speculated that aggressive elevations in $\dot{D}O_2$ actually may have been harmful. Wilson and others (54) performed a randomized clinical trial of preoperative optimization of $\dot{D}O_2$ for major elective surgery in 138 patients scheduled to undergo surgery of at least 2 hours' duration and involving aortic, upper gastrointestinal, or other extensive procedures. Patients were randomized to three groups: routine care; hemodynamic monitoring accompanied by fluid plus *dopexamine*

TABLE 4. OUTCOME OF TRAUMA PATIENTS RANDOMIZED TO ENHANCEMENT OF OXYGEN DELIVERY OR ROUTINE PERIOPERATIVE CARE

Outcome Measure	Optimal Group ($n = 40$)	Control Group ($n = 35$)	P Value
Death	15% (6)	11% (4)	0.74
Organ failure	38% (15)	57% (20)	0.11
Sepsis	40% (16)	51% (18)	0.36
All complications	62% (24)	71% (25)	0.47
ICU days	15 ± 23	15 ± 12	0.91
Hospital days	25 ± 24	27 ± 21	0.72

(Reprinted from Velmahos GC, et al. Endpoints of resuscitation of critically injured patients: normal or supranormal? A prospective randomized trial. *Ann Surg* 2000;232:409–418, with permission.)

to attain the target $\dot{D}O_2$; or monitoring accompanied by fluid plus *epinephrine* to attain the target $\dot{D}O_2$. Mortality was significantly higher in the routine care group (17%) versus 4% in the dopamine group and 2% in the epinephrine group. However, complications were lower in the dopamine group (30%) than in the routine care group (61%) or epinephrine group (52%). In contrast, Takala and colleagues (55) compared routine administration of either of two doses of dopamine (0.5 mg per kg per minute or 2.0 mg per kg per minute) to placebo in a multicenter placebo-controlled, randomized clinical trial or patients after

major abdominal surgery and found no significant difference in outcome between the groups. Bishop and associates (56) performed a single-institution prospective randomized controlled trial comparing $\dot{D}O_2$ greater than 670 mL per minute per m^2 versus conventional endpoints in 115 severely traumatized patients. Both mortality (18% versus 37%) and the number of organ failures (0.74 ± 0.28 versus 1.62 ± 0.28) per patient were significantly fewer in the protocol group. However, in a follow-up study in the same hospital, Velmahos and coworkers (57) were unable to confirm those results (Table 4).

Taken together, these data suggest that aggressive, goal-directed hemodynamic support in certain high-risk surgical patients may limit the mortality and morbidity that result from clinically inapparent hypoperfusion but that further clinical trials are necessary to define the appropriate populations and the proper interventions.

SUMMARY

Careful fluid management is essential in limiting morbidity and mortality in critically ill surgical patients. Maintenance of systemic perfusion is a critical strategy in avoiding shock and the late consequences of the multiple system organ failure syndrome.

KEY POINTS

Total body water approximates 60% of total body weight; intracellular volume constitutes 40% of total body weight; and extracellular volume constitutes 20% of body weight. Plasma volume equals about one-fifth of extracellular volume, the remainder of which is interstitial fluid volume.

Osmotically active particles attract water across semipermeable membranes until equilibrium is attained. Osmolality, a measurement of the number of osmotically active particles per kilogram, is largely attributable to sodium ions.

The osmotic pressure contributed by plasma proteins is less than 1% of total osmotic pressure, but is essential in determining the distribution of fluid between the plasma volume

and interstitial fluid volume. Colloid osmotic pressure is also termed oncotic pressure.

Routine use of dextrose-containing solutions for resuscitation is discouraged because of the risk of aggravating neurologic injury; however, dextrose-containing solutions should be used in patients at risk for hypoglycemia.

Hypertonic saline solutions reduce intracranial pressure while transiently increasing cardiac output.

Oxygen delivery, the product of cardiac output and arterial oxygen content, has been used as a target for resuscitation; however, the data at this time are inconsistent regarding the utility of that target.

REFERENCES

1. Prough DS, Brauer KI. Application of kinetic principles to intravenous fluid therapy. *Prob Anesth* 1999;11:419–433.
2. Svensén C, Hahn RG. Volume kinetics of Ringer solution, dextran 70, and hypertonic saline in male volunteers. *Anesthesiology* 1997;87:204–212.
3. Drobin D, Hahn RG. Volume kinetics of Ringer's solution in hypovolemic volunteers. *Anesthesiology* 1999;90:81–91.
4. Riddez L, Johnson L, Hahn RG. Central and regional hemodynamics during crystalloid fluid therapy after uncontrolled intra-abdominal bleeding. *J Trauma* 1998;44:433–439.
5. Brauer KI, Prough DS, Clifton JB, et al. Sepsis does not alter plasma volume expansion (PVE) in response to 0.9% saline infusion in sheep. *Crit Care Med* 1999;27:A49.

6. Brauer KI, Prough DS, Traber LD, et al. Hypoproteinemia does not alter plasma volume expansion (PVE) in response to 0.9% saline infusion in sheep. *Crit Care Med* 1999;27:A60.
7. Brauer KI, Svensén C, Hahn RG, et al. Volume kinetic analysis of the distribution of 0.9% saline in conscious versus isoflurane-anesthetized sheep. *Anesthesiology* 2001 *(in press)*.
8. Robinson AG, Verbalis JG. Diabetes insipidus. *Curr Ther Endocrinol Metab* 1997;6:1–7.
9. Needleman P, Greenwald JE. Atriopeptin: a cardiac hormone intimately involved in fluid, electrolyte, and blood-pressure homeostasis. *N Engl J Med* 1986;314:828–834.
10. Murray MD, Brater DC. Adverse effect of nonsteroidal anti-inflammatory drugs on renal function. *Ann Intern Med* 1990;112:559–560.
11. Demling RH. Shock and fluids. In: Chernow B, Shoemaker WC, eds. *Critical care: state of the art.* Fullerton, CA: Society of Critical Care Medicine, 1986:301–351.

12. Schierhout G, Roberts I. Fluid resuscitation with colloid or crystalloid solutions in critically ill patients: a systematic review of randomised trials. *Br Med J* 1998;316:961–964.

13. Cochrane Injuries Group Albumin Reviewers. Human albumin administration in critically ill patients: systematic review of randomised controlled trials. *Br Med J* 1998;317:235–240.

14. Pearl RG, Halperin BD, Mihm FG, et al. Pulmonary effects of crystalloid and colloid resuscitation from hemorrhagic shock in the presence of oleic acid-induced pulmonary capillary injury in the dog. *Anesthesiology* 1988;68:12–20.

15. Gold MS, Russo J, Tissot M, et al. Comparison of hetastarch to albumin for perioperative bleeding in patients undergoing abdominal aortic aneurysm surgery: a prospective, randomized study. *Ann Surg* 1990;211:482–485.

16. Entholzner EK, Mielke LL, Calatzis AN, et al. Coagulation effects of a recently developed hydroxyethyl starch (HES 130/0.4) compared to hydroxyethyl starches with higher molecular weight. *Acta Anaesthesiol Scand* 2000;44:1116–1121.

17. Gan TJ, Bennett-Guerrero E, Phillips-Bute B, et al. Hextend, a physiologically balanced plasma expander for large volume use in major surgery: a randomized phase III clinical trial. *Anesth Analg* 1999;88:992–998.

18. Haisch G, Boldt J, Krebs C, et al. The influence of intravascular volume therapy with a new hydroxyethyl starch preparation (6% HES 130/0.4) on coagulation in patients undergoing major abdominal surgery. *Anesth Analg* 2001;92:565–571.

19. Prough DS, Johnston WE. Fluid resuscitation in septic shock: no solution yet. *Anesth Analg* 1989;69:699–704.

20. Baum TD, Wang H, Rothschild HR, et al. Mesenteric oxygen metabolism, ileal mucosal hydrogen ion concentration, and tissue edema after crystalloid of colloid resuscitation in porcine endotoxic shock: comparison of Ringer's lactate and 6% hetastarch. *Circ Shock* 1990;30:385–397.

21. Linko K, Makelainen A. Cardiorespiratory function after replacement of blood loss with hydroxyethyl starch 120, dextran-70, and Ringer's acetate in pigs. *Crit Care Med* 1989;17:1031–1035.

22. Zornow MH, Todd MM, Moore SS. The acute cerebral effects of changes in plasma osmolality and oncotic pressure. *Anesthesiology* 1987;67:936–941.

23. Warner DS, Boehland LA. Effects of iso-osmolal intravenous fluid therapy on post-ischemic brain water content in the rat. *Anesthesiology* 1988;68:86–91.

24. Zornow MH, Scheller MS, Todd MM, et al. Acute cerebral effects of isotonic crystalloid and colloid solutions following cryogenic brain injury in the rabbit. *Anesthesiology* 1988;69:180–184.

25. Drummond JC, Patel PM, Cole DJ, et al. The effect of the reduction of colloid oncotic pressure, with and without reduction of osmolality, on post-traumatic cerebral edema. *Anesthesiology* 1998;88:993–1002.

26. Lam AM, Winn HR, Cullen BF, et al. Hyperglycemia and neurological outcome in patients with head injury. *J Neurosurg* 1991;75:545–551.

27. McFarlane C, Lee A. A comparison of plasmalyte 148 and 0.9% saline for intra-operative fluid replacement. *Anaesthesia* 1994;49:779–781.

28. Scheingraber S, Rehm M, Sehmisch C, et al. Rapid saline infusion produces hyperchloremic acidosis in patients undergoing gynecologic surgery. *Anesthesiology* 1999;90:1265–1270.

29. Waters JH, Bernstein CA. Dilutional acidosis following hetastarch or albumin in healthy volunteers. *Anesthesiology* 2000;93:1184–1187.

30. Rehm M, Orth V, Scheingraber S, et al. Acid-base changes caused by 5% albumin versus 6% hydroxyethyl starch solution in patients undergoing acute normovolemic hemodilution: a randomized prospective study. *Anesthesiology* 2000;93:1174–1183.

31. Liskaser FJ, Bellomo R, Hayhoe M, et al. The role of pump prime in the etiology and pathogenesis of cardiopulmonary bypass associated acidosis. *Anesthesiology* 2000;93:1170–1173.

32. Prough DS. Acidosis associated with perioperative saline administration: dilution or delusion? *Anesthesiology* 2000;93:1167–1169.

33. Prough DS, Bidani A. Hyperchloremic metabolic acidosis is a predictable consequence of intraoperative infusion of 0.9% saline. *Anesthesiology* 1999;90:1247–1249.

34. Deb S, Martin B, Sun L, et al. Resuscitation with lactated Ringer's solution in rats with hemorrhagic shock induces immediate apoptosis. *J Trauma* 1999;46:582–589.

35. Knoferl MW, Angele MK, Ayala A, et al. Do different rates of fluid resuscitation adversely or beneficially influence immune responses after trauma-hemorrhage? *J Trauma* 1999;46:23–33.

36. Healey MA, Davis RE, Liu FC, et al. Lactated Ringer's is superior to normal saline in a model of massive hemorrhage and resuscitation. *J Trauma* 1998;45:894–899.

37. Roberts JP, Roberts JD Jr, Skinner C, et al. Extracellular fluid deficit following operation and its correction with Ringer's lactate: a reassessment. *Ann Surg* 1985;202:1–8.

38. Chiao JJC, Minei JP, Shires GT III, et al. In vivo myocyte sodium activity and concentration during hemorrhagic shock. *Am J Physiol* 1990;258:R684–R689.

39. Böck JC, Barker BC, Clinton AG, et al. Post-traumatic changes in, and effect of colloid osmotic pressure on the distribution of body water. *Ann Surg* 1989;210:395–405.

40. Arieff AI. Fatal postoperative pulmonary edema. Pathogenesis and literature review. *Chest* 1999;115:1371–1377.

41. Velasco IT, Pontieri V, Rocha e Silva M Jr, et al. Hyperosmotic NaCl and severe hemorrhagic shock. *Am J Physiol* 1980;239:H664–H673.

42. Vollmar B, Lang G, Menger MD, et al. Hypertonic hydroxyethyl starch restores hepatic microvascular perfusion in hemorrhagic shock. *Am J Physiol (Heart Circ Physiol)* 1994;266:H1927–H1934.

43. Prough DS, Whitley JM, Taylor CL, et al. Regional cerebral blood flow following resuscitation from hemorrhagic shock with hypertonic saline: influence of a subdural mass. *Anesthesiology* 1991;75:319–327.

44. Wisner DH, Schuster L, Quinn C. Hypertonic saline resuscitation of head injury: effects on cerebral water content. *J Trauma* 1990;30:75–78.

45. Whitley JM, Prough DS, Taylor CL, et al. Cerebrovascular effects of small volume resuscitation from hemorrhagic shock: comparison of hypertonic saline and concentrated hydroxyethyl starch in dogs. *J Neurosurg Anesthesiol* 1991;3:47–55.

46. Vassar MJ, Fischer RP, O'Brien PE, et al. A multicenter trial for resuscitation of injured patients with 7.5% sodium chloride: the effect of added dextran 70. *Arch Surg* 1993;128:1003–1013.

47. Mattox KL, Maningas PA, Moore EE, et al. Prehospital hypertonic saline/dextran infusion for post-traumatic hypotension. The U.S.A. Multicenter Trial. *Ann Surg* 1991;213:482–491.

48. Simma B, Burger R, Falk M, et al. A prospective, randomized, and controlled study of fluid management in children with severe head injury: lactated Ringer's solution versus hypertonic saline. *Crit Care Med* 1998;26:1265–1270.

49. Khanna S, Davis D, Peterson B, et al. Use of hypertonic saline in the treatment of severe refractory posttraumatic intracranial hypertension in pediatric traumatic brain injury. *Crit Care Med* 2000;28:1144–1151.

50. Qureshi AI, Suarez JI, Castro A, et al. Use of hypertonic saline/acetate infusion in treatment of cerebral edema in patients with head trauma: experience at a single center. *J Trauma* 1999;47:659–665.

51. Lipsitz LA. Orthostatic hypotension in the elderly. *N Engl J Med* 1989;321:952–957.

52. Boyd O, Grounds RM, Bennett ED. A randomized clinical trial of the effect of deliberate perioperative increase of oxygen delivery on mortality in high-risk surgical patients. *JAMA* 1993;270:2699–2707.

53. Hayes MA, Timmins AC, Yau EHS, et al. Elevation of systemic oxygen delivery in the treatment of critically ill patients. *N Engl J Med* 1994;330:1717–1722.

54. Wilson J, Woods I, Fawcett J, et al. Reducing the risk of major elective surgery: randomised controlled trial of preoperative optimisation of oxygen delivery. *Br Med J* 1999;318:1099–1103.

55. Takala J, Meier-Hellmann A, Eddleston J, et al. Effect of dopexamine on outcome after major abdominal surgery: a prospective, randomized, controlled multicenter study. *Crit Care Med* 2000;28:3417–3423.

56. Bishop MH, Shoemaker WC, Appel PL, et al. Prospective, randomized trial of survivor values of cardiac index, oxygen delivery, and oxygen consumption as resuscitation endpoints in severe trauma. *J Trauma* 1995;38:780–787.

57. Velmahos GC, Demetriades D, Shoemaker WC, et al. Endpoints of resuscitation of critically injured patients: normal or supranormal? A prospective randomized trial. *Ann Surg* 2000;232:409–418.

13

SEDATIVE, ANALGESIC, AND NEUROMUSCULAR BLOCKING DRUGS

CHRISTOPHER C. YOUNG
RICHARD C. PRIELIPP

KEY WORDS

- Sedatives; α2-agonists
- Analgesics; opioids
- Neuromuscular blocking agents
- Neuromuscular junction
- Transcutaneous nerve stimulation
- Pharmacology

SEDATIVE AND ANALGESIC DRUGS IN INTENSIVE CARE UNIT PATIENTS

Intensivists must ensure adequate analgesia (for pain relief) and sedation (for anxiolytic, hypnotic, and amnestic needs) of the intensive care unit (ICU) patient (1). Anxiolysis is the reduction of the emotional and physical responses to real or perceived danger the patient experiences in the ICU. Hypnosis refers to a state of minimal motor activity and appears physically similar to sleep. Amnesia is impairment or cessation of memory due to alteration in attention, arousal, or mood and is generally considered desirable for patients in the ICU. While sedative drugs produce multiple effects within the spectrum of anxiolysis, hypnosis, and amnesia, most are devoid of analgesic activity.

Failure to meet appropriate sedation goals may have deleterious physical and emotional effects on the critically ill patient. Sedative drugs are therefore prescribed in the ICU to decrease patient anxiety and diminish recall of noxious events. Inadequate administration of sedatives can lead to patient anxiety and agitation and add to the stress response, a complex set of neurohumoral and endocrine responses to illness or injury that may compromise patient outcome. The stress response to critical illness may be reduced when sedatives are dosed appropriately (2). Overdosage of sedative agents, however, can have detrimental effects as well. Overly sedated patients are at risk for venous stasis, thromboembolic events, pressure ulceration, and aspiration pneumonia. In addition, recent evidence suggests that when ICU patients are oversedated, it delays weaning of mechanical ventilation and increases the duration and cost of the ICU stay (3,4).

Sedative Drugs

Sedative needs of individual ICU patients constantly change depending on the nature and course of their disease, interaction with other therapies (e.g., analgesic agents), time of day, and response to the external environment. The ideal level of sedation varies from patient to patient and in different situations, but in general, most intensivists seek to maintain a patient who is tranquil and sleepy, but easily aroused (5). Deeper sedation should be reserved for select patients, such as those receiving neuromuscular blocking (NMB) drugs or those with inadequate ventilation and oxygen delivery (6).

A standard scoring system for sedation of ICU patients has been difficult to develop and implement (7). The Ramsay score, a numeric scale of motor responsiveness graduated according to increased depth of sedation, was developed to assess drug-induced sedation (Table 1) (8). While the Ramsay score fails to adequately account for the agitated or oversedated patient, it has been the standard measure of sedation in most comparative studies. The Riker Sedation-Agitation Scale (Table 2) was designed to overcome some of the shortcomings of the Ramsay scoring system (9). With the Riker scale, a seven-point scale is used to better describe patients at the extremes of agitation or oversedation. Sedation scales are generally useful for targeting a level of sedation consistent between multiple medical providers, as well as for comparative studies, but other factors, such as a patient's acute disease process and use of analgesic or neuromuscular blocking agents, can influence the appropriate level of sedation and its assessment.

The Benzodiazepines: Diazepam, Lorazepam, and Midazolam

Benzodiazepines, in particular diazepam, lorazepam, and midazolam are commonly used to provide sedation and amnesia in the ICU. Although dose-related degrees of respiratory depression and hypotension can be seen following benzodiazepine administration, complications from this class of drug are rare. The benzodiazepines exert their anxiolytic, anticonvulsant, and muscle-relaxing effects through interaction of specific binding sites on the γ-aminobutyric acid (GABA) receptor. Receptor binding results in increased chloride conductance and hyperpolarization

TABLE 1. RAMSAY SEDATION SCORE (8)

Awake Levels	1	Patient anxious and agitated, or restless, or both
	2	Patient cooperative, oriented, and tranquil
	3	Patient responds to verbal commands
Asleep Levels	4	Brisk response to a light glabellar tap or loud auditory stimulus
	5	Sluggish response to a light glabellar tap or loud auditory stimulus
	6	No response to a light glabellar tap or loud auditory stimulus

of the neuronal cell. Chronic administration of benzodiazepines can lead to receptor downregulation and drug tolerance. Acute tolerance appears to be a common finding in ICU patients receiving benzodiazepines or other sedative agents for more than 24 hours (10). Withdrawal syndromes have been reported with cessation of both midazolam and propofol infusions. Risk factors for acute withdrawal include high infusion rates, prolonged duration, and abrupt cessation. For these reasons, gradual tapering of sedative infusions and substitution with longer-acting agents (e.g., diazepam) are suggested to reduce the chance of withdrawal reactions.

Diazepam is the oldest benzodiazepine commonly used in the ICU. The original propylene glycol intravenous formulation can produce thrombophlebitis, thrombosis, and even metabolic acidosis. These problems are reduced by a new diazepam formulation in sterile fat emulsion. The half-life of diazepam is increased in older adults, neonates, and patients with liver disease. Diazepam is metabolized to active compounds such as desmethyldiazepam, which has a very long half-life (200 hours) and is dependent upon the kidneys for elimination. Prolonged elimination of diazepam and its metabolites limits its usefulness in the ICU environment.

Lorazepam is the least lipid soluble of the three benzodiazepines and traverses the blood–brain barrier most slowly, resulting in delayed onset and prolonged duration of effect (11). Lorazepam can be administered by both intermittent injections and by continuous infusion. It is metabolized to inactive products by hepatic glucuronidation. This unique metabolic pathway among benzodiazepines renders lorazepam resistant to drug interactions

involving oxidative hepatic drug elimination. For this reason, the pharmacokinetics of lorazepam do not change significantly in the older adult or critically ill populations. Lorazepam is manufactured with propylene glycol and polyethylene glycol, a drug vehicle associated with lactic acidosis, hyperosmolar coma, and nephrotoxicity after high doses or prolonged infusion (12). The overall favorable pharmacokinetics of lorazepam and its lower cost relative to other agents favor its use if rapid and predictable arousal is not essential or when long-term sedation is desired.

Midazolam has gained popularity both in the operating room and in the ICU. Midazolam is a water-soluble compound *ex vivo* that becomes highly lipid-soluble at physiologic pH, and therefore, relatively rapid in onset of action. Midazolam is highly protein-bound and metabolized via hepatic microsomal oxidation. The oxidative pathway is susceptible to many factors including hepatic disease, advanced age, and drug inhibition. A number of drugs, including cimetidine, erythromycin, propofol, and diltiazem have been reported to delay midazolam metabolism and therefore increase its duration of effect. Midazolam may exert an increased effect in patients with renal failure owing to an increase in the active, unbound portion of the drug. However, in ICU patients with minimal end-organ disease, drug clearance is unchanged.

Midazolam is biotransformed to an active metabolite, alpha-hydroxymidazolam. Although this metabolite is pharmacologically active, it is less potent and much shorter lasting than the parent compound (13). The recent introduction of generic formulations of midazolam has led to decreased drug acquisition cost. Because midazolam has the shortest half-life of the benzodiazepines, lacks active metabolites, is water-soluble, and is well suited for continuous infusion, it is often preferred to other benzodiazepines in the ICU (14).

Propofol

Propofol has been used to sedate ICU patients since the late 1980s, even though Food and Drug Administration (FDA) approval for ICU sedation did not occur until 1993. Propofol activates the GABA receptor to produce CNS depression, similar to benzodiazepines. Because of its rapid onset and the hypotensive response observed after bolus doses, propofol is generally administered as a continuous infusion (without loading dose) in the ICU (15). Propofol infusions are associated with dose-related decreases in blood pressure, heart rate, tidal volume, and minute ventilation. Early pharmacokinetic studies involving bolus injections or short-term infusions of propofol demonstrated very rapid elimination from the central compartment. In addition, propofol elimination and pharmacodynamics are unchanged in patients with renal or hepatic disease, but elimination is delayed in older adult patients. Hepatic enzyme induction by drugs such as barbiturates, carbamazepine, phenytoin, and rifampin, enhance propofol clearance and shorten the duration of effect. However, the terminal elimination half-life of propofol is long despite its brief clinical effect because of drug pooled in highly lipophilic and poorly perfused tissue compartments (i.e., adipose). Nonetheless, propofol is cleared three to five times faster than midazolam despite its larger apparent volume of distribution. Propofol is typically characterized by a rapid recovery from its sedative

TABLE 2. RIKER SEDATION-AGITATION SCALE (SAS) (9)

Score	Description	Example
7	Dangerous agitation	Pulling at endotracheal tube, trying to remove catheters, striking at staff
6	Very agitated	Does not calm to voice, requires physical restraints
5	Agitated	Anxious or mildly agitated, verbal instruction calms patient
4	Calm and cooperative	Calm, awakens easily, follows commands
3	Sedated	Difficult to arouse; awakens to verbal stimuli or gentle shaking
2	Very sedated	Arouses to physical stimuli, does not follow commands
1	Unarousable	Minimal or no response to noxious stimuli

and electroencephalogram (EEG) effects, particularly when dosed to deeper levels of sedation. Thus, there is an association between use of propofol (compared to other ICU sedatives) and shorter time to extubation and reduced costs (14). The ability of patients to rapidly awaken from deep levels of sedation has led to the adoption of propofol algorithms for many fast-track postoperative cardiac surgical patients and for patients with brain injury requiring frequent neurologic examinations. However, after very long infusions, plasma concentrations steadily increase unless the infusion rate is decreased. Thus, intensivists question the rapidity of recovery following infusions longer than 12 hours (16).

Because of the high lipophilicity of propofol, it requires a phospholipid emulsion carrier (10% Intralipid). The nutritional value of this lipid carrier, which provides 1.1 kcal per mL, must be considered in patients receiving moderate- to high-dose propofol infusions. Potential infectious complications relating to propofol are also a consequence of the lipid component of the drug vehicle. The recent addition of EDTA or sodium metabisulfite to the lipid formulations decreases the incidence of bacterial contamination, but special handling precautions of this product are still indicated (17). Long-term or high-dose infusions can result in hypertriglyceridemia, which may be associated with elevated pancreatic enzymes, and on occasion, pancreatitis. Propofol is contraindicated in patients sensitive to soybean oil, egg lecithin, or glycerol, and is not recommended for ICU administration in children.

Dexmedetomidine

Dexmedetomidine is a new, highly selective alpha-2 adrenoreceptor agonist approved by the FDA in 2000 for sedation of "initially intubated and mechanically ventilated ICU patients." Dexmedetomidine produces anxiolysis, analgesia, hypnosis, and reduction in the stress response associated with surgery and critical illness. Dexmedetomidine is seven to eight times more selective for the alpha-2 receptor than clonidine. Alpha-2 receptors are found in the spinal cord, CNS, peripheral nerves, autonomic ganglia, and in the postsynaptic region of vascular smooth muscle. Activation of presynaptic alpha-2 receptors inhibits the release of the neurotransmitter norepinephrine. Activation of postsynaptic alpha-2 receptors in the CNS inhibits sympathetic activity (decreasing blood pressure and heart rate) and produces dose-dependent anxiolysis. Activation of alpha-2 receptors in the spinal cord produces the analgesic effect of dexmedetomidine. Following loading-dose infusion of dexmedetomidine (over 10 to 20 minutes), a transient increase in blood pressure and resulting bradycardia may be noted, a direct effect of activation of alpha-2 receptors in vascular smooth muscle. For this reason, bolus administration of dexmedetomidine is contraindicated, and loading-dose administration should be carefully monitored in those patients with low resting heart rate or conduction block. The package insert for dexmedetomidine notes that drug administration should not exceed 24 hours. Published information characterizing longer infusions are sparse, although a clinical trial is in progress that specifically addresses these issues. So far, dexmedetomidine does not appear to be cumulative or to be associated with rebound when it is discontinued. While long-term infusions (1 week) diminish the cortisol response to corticotropin (ACTH)

by 40% in *animal* studies (18), minimal information is available regarding this response in humans.

Patients receiving dexmedetomidine infusions appear asleep but are easily arousable. The quality of sedation achieved with dexmedetomidine is unlike that seen with other agents. Patients wake rapidly to verbal stimuli or light touch and are able to interact with caregivers and family members. When left unstimulated, patients receiving dexmedetomidine return rapidly to a hypnotic state. It achieves these clinical endpoints without producing respiratory depression (19). For this reason, dexmedetomidine infusion can be continued through the process of weaning of mechanical ventilation, including extubation. Its analgesic effect results in a reduction of opioid needs by approximately 50% (20). One caveat is that a significant number of patients receiving dexmedetomidine in clinical trials (20,21) reported recall of ICU events. Therefore, at currently recommended doses, it is probably an inadequate sole sedative choice for patients receiving NMB drugs.

Dexmedetomidine is highly protein bound, but nonetheless, is extensively distributed to tissues within 5 minutes of administration. It undergoes extensive hepatic metabolism to methyl and glucuronide conjugates. These end products are dependent on renal function for their elimination. Dexmedetomidine pharmacokinetics are markedly affected by hepatic insufficiency, and decreased requirements are to be anticipated in patients with hepatic insufficiency. Dexmedetomidine appears to have little effect on the cytochrome P450 hepatic enzyme system, and thus far, there are few noteworthy interactions with other drugs.

Other Sedatives

Other agents are used occasionally to provide sedation in the ICU. Ketamine is an anesthetic induction agent that is structurally related to phencyclidine (PCP) and other hallucinogenic drugs. It may be useful in patients with severe hypotension or respiratory depression requiring sedation because of its cardiovascular and neurologic excitatory effects. It will also reduce opioid requirements because of its potent analgesic effect.

Etomidate is a short-acting agent used for the induction of anesthesia in patients with hemodynamic instability. It provides amnesia and hypnosis with minimal cardiovascular effect. It is useful for inducing anesthesia in the critically ill because of the stable hemodynamics. However, it is not recommended for prolonged sedation as etomidate-induced suppression of adrenal steroid synthesis has been associated with increased mortality when given by continuous infusion for sedation in the ICU (22).

Barbiturates are sometimes used in the ICU as an adjunct to sedation, for cerebral protection, and to treat seizures. All these agents possess long elimination half-lives and thus are generally unsuitable for routine sedation. Phenothiazine and butyrophenone derivatives are sometimes used to provide sedation, particularly when an element of psychosis is contributing to agitation. They may also be an adjunct when benzodiazepines are believed to be contributing to patient confusion or agitation. The butyrophenones produce mild hypotension due to their alpha-blocking properties. Other side effects include prolonged QT interval, extrapyramidal effects, and precipitation of neuroleptic malignant syndrome. Fortunately, these side effects are rarely seen

TABLE 3. COMPARISON OF COMMON INTENSIVE CARE UNIT SEDATIVE DRUGS

Property	Lorazepam	Midazolam	Propofol	Dexmedetomidine
Rapid onset	−	+	+	±
Short duration	−	±	+	−
Minimal cardiovascular/ respiratory depression	+	±	−	+ +
Inactive metabolites	+	−	+	+
Elimination minimally dependent on hepatic function	−	−	+	−
Elimination minimally dependent on renal function	−	−	+	+
Few adverse side effects	+	+	±	+
No associated tolerance or withdrawal	−	−	−	?
Inexpensive	+	±	−	−

−, drug is devoid of, or displays minimal activity; +, prominent drug action; ±, drug is intermediate in responsiveness.

in the ICU, perhaps due to frequent concomitant benzodiazepine administration (23).

Inhaled anesthetic drugs are rarely used to provide sedation in the ICU for a variety of reasons. They require sophisticated delivery systems, additional monitoring modalities, and exhaled gases must be scavenged to prevent workplace environmental contamination. Although the newer agents (isoflurane, sevoflurane) undergo significantly less metabolism than the older ones (halothane, enflurane), excessive fluoride concentrations may result from prolonged isoflurane sedation (24). The levels of fluoride generated may be greater than the concentration thought to be nephrotoxic (greater than 50 μM). In addition, the cost of some agents delivered through high-flow ventilator circuits is prohibitive (25).

Summary

Ideally, the choice of drug should be based on pharmacokinetic and pharmacodynamic characteristics that allow safe, efficacious, and titratable use in the ICU. Costs of therapy must also be considered. These include the cost of the drug itself and its delivery apparatus, as well as the expense associated with treating side effects. All of the currently available intravenous sedative agents fall short of being "ideal" (Table 3). Pharmacokinetic variables for diazepam, lorazepam, midazolam, propofol, and dexmedetomidine are listed in Table 4. The rate constants for the commonly used sedatives are obtained in healthy volunteers and may be significantly altered in the critically ill. As critically ill patients present with significant organ system dysfunction and hemodynamic instability, there is significant interindividual variation in the response to sedative agents and their metabolism. Because there are few studies of the disposition of these drugs in ICU patients, most data are extrapolated from studies in other patient populations.

Analgesic Drugs

Untreated or undertreated pain results in physiologic responses (hypercoagulability, immunosuppression, and persistent catabolism) that are associated with poor outcomes (26). Pain increases levels of sympathetic nervous system activity and catecholamine release, which places additional demands on the cardiovascular system in critically ill patients. The hypermetabolic state following injury is exacerbated by pain, and this can lead to diminished immune function and impaired wound healing (27). Prolonged pain can result in the development of severe anxiety and even delirium (28). Therefore, adequate analgesia is of primary importance in managing these patients.

The degree of pain is most often assessed by the use of a visual analog scale (VAS), a numeric (0 to 10) scale that allows the patient to indicate a level of pain. However, VAS is often impractical in critically ill patients owing to concurrent sedative agents, restraints, endotracheal intubation, or other impediments to communication. In these cases, observation of somatic (grimacing, wincing, tearing) or autonomic (hypertension, tachycardia) responses must suffice. These signs are less precise, particularly in those patients receiving NMB drugs or vasoactive infusions. Up to 25% of patients may not demonstrate increased sympathetic activity, yet still have inadequate analgesia (29).

Nonsteroidal Antiinflammatory Drugs

Aspirin, acetaminophen, and nonsteroidal antiinflammatory drugs (NSAIDs) are recommended as first-line drugs in the treatment of acute pain syndromes (30). With increasing doses, acetaminophen, aspirin, and the other NSAIDs all reach a ceiling for their maximum analgesic effect. For aspirin and acetaminophen, the maximum analgesic effect usually occurs with single oral doses between 650 and 1,300 mg. The ceiling effect for some NSAIDs is relatively higher and the duration of analgesia effect may be longer than with aspirin or acetaminophen. Use of these agents, however, is limited in the ICU for a number of reasons. Aspirin can produce bleeding by irreversibly inhibiting platelet function for the 8- to 10-day life span of the platelet. It is also associated with gastric ulceration and can precipitate asthma in aspirin-sensitive patients. Acetaminophen is similar in analgesic effect to aspirin with fewer adverse effects. However, overdosage can cause serious or fatal hepatic injury, and even lower doses may be hepatotoxic to some ICU patients (alcoholics, patients who are fasting, and those taking cytochrome P450 enzyme-inducing drugs). Aspirin and acetaminophen are only available as enteral preparations, limiting their usefulness as analgesics in the ICU.

TABLE 4. PHARMACOKINETIC VARIABLES OF COMMON INTENSIVE CARE UNIT SEDATIVE DRUGS

	Diazepam	Lorazepam	Midazolam	Propofol	Dexmedetomidine
Vd (L/kg)	0.7–1.7	1.1–1.3	1.1–1.7	5.4–7.8	1.3
Clearance (mL/kg/min)	0.2–0.5	1.5–1.1	6.4–11.1	26–29	8.3
Alpha $t_{1/2}$ (min)	30–66	3–20	6–15	2–3	6
Beta $t_{1/2}$ (h)	24–57	14	1.7–2.6	0.5–1.0	2–3
Route of elimination	Hepatic hydroxylation and conjugation	Hepatic glucuronidation	Hepatic glucuronidation and oxidation	Hepatic glucuronidation	Hepatic glucuronidation and conjugation

Most NSAIDs are more effective analgesics than aspirin or acetaminophen, and some can equal or exceed the analgesic effects of injected opioids. Ketorolac is the only injectable NSAID available in the United States. Ketorolac, 30 mg intravenous (i.v.) or intramuscular (i.m.), has analgesic efficacy comparable to moderate doses of morphine or meperidine, with a somewhat slower onset but longer duration of action (31). The dose of ketorolac should be reduced in patients over 65 years of age or with renal dysfunction. NSAIDs are associated with an increased risk of gastrointestinal bleeding, ulceration, and perforation. Ketorolac use should be limited to 5 days and is contraindicated before and during surgery and whenever bleeding could be a problem (e.g., after neurosurgery) because NSAIDs cause reversible inhibition of platelet aggregation. Normal platelet function resumes when most of the drug has been eliminated. Lastly, NSAIDs decrease synthesis of renal vasodilator prostaglandins, decrease renal blood flow, cause fluid retention, and may cause renal failure, particularly in older adults and those with congestive heart failure, renal insufficiency, ascites, volume depletion, and diuretic usage (32).

Opioids

Opioids are classified as full agonists, partial agonists, and mixed agonist-antagonists based on their interactions with specific opiate receptors. Agonists interact with the mu receptor to produce analgesia, respiratory depression, and bradycardia. The kappa receptor mediates some analgesia and sedation, while the sigma receptor mediates dysphoric effects. Opioids are considered the drugs of choice for severe acute pain, even though in some circumstances NSAIDs may be as effective (33). Morphine sulfate and fentanyl citrate are the most commonly used opioids in ICUs in the United States. In addition to potent analgesic effects, these full agonists provide synergy with sedative agents, thereby decreasing overall dosage required for adequate sedation. However, opioids are devoid of intrinsic amnestic properties despite their demonstrated synergy with sedative agents. The i.v. route of administration, often by the use of patient-controlled analgesia (PCA) devices, is preferred to i.m. or subcutaneous dosing due to more reliable absorption. Occasionally, transdermal delivery of fentanyl can be utilized, but skin blood flow and drug absorption by this route can also be unpredictable in the critically ill patient.

Morphine, fentanyl, and other full agonists have no ceiling for their analgesic effectiveness except that imposed by adverse effects. The adverse effects of most concern are respiratory depression and impaired gastrointestinal motility. Respiratory depression with an increase in blood CO_2 tension is thought to be the primary means of intracranial pressure (ICP) elevation associated with the opioids. Myoclonus and muscle rigidity are more commonly seen with the high-potency opioids and may further impair ventilation. Morphine can stimulate histamine release from mast cells, resulting in bronchospasm and hypotension. Alternate routes of administration (intrathecal, epidural, patient-controlled analgesia) and combination therapies (local anesthetics, alpha-2 agonists, antidepressants, anticonvulsants) can be used to limit the adverse effects associated with systemic administration (Table 5). The mixed agonists-antagonists, such as pentazocine, butorphanol, nalbuphine, and buprenorphine, exhibit fewer side effects, but are more likely to produce acute psychomimetic responses and acute opioid withdrawal in opioid-dependent patients. In addition, these drugs demonstrate a ceiling effect, making them of limited usefulness in the ICU.

Morphine sulfate is a prototypical opioid analgesic with a half-life of 2 to 3 hours in healthy volunteers, but the half-life is significantly increased (more than 24 hours) in patients with severe

TABLE 5. ALTERNATE DRUGS AND ROUTES OF ADMINISTRATION OF INTENSIVE CARE UNIT ANALGESIA

Drug	Routes of Administration
Opioids	Intravenous Patient controlled analgesia Oral Transdermal Intrathecal Epidural
Local anesthetics	Intrathecal Epidural Epidural patient-controlled analgesia Regional block (e.g., brachial plexus) Intrapleural Intercostal/paravertebral Local infiltration
Anticonvulsants	Intravenous Oral
Antidepressants	Intravenous Oral
Alpha-2 agonists	Intravenous (dexmedetomidine) Epidural (clonidine) Transdermal (clonidine) Oral (clonidine)

cirrhosis or burns. Septic shock and renal impairment decrease the clearance of morphine and its active glucuronide metabolites, so caution must be exercised when repeat boluses or continuous infusions of morphine are used (34). Hydromorphone has a half-life of 2 to 3 hours, but clearance of the drug is susceptible to changes in hepatic blood flow and protein binding, Its primary metabolite, hydromorphone-3-glucuronide, can accumulate in the setting of renal failure and cause neuroexcitation and cognitive impairment.

Fentanyl is a short-acting, high-potency, synthetic opioid commonly administered by continuous infusion. Its metabolism is not significantly affected by renal disease, but clearance is dependent on hepatic blood flow. It is highly protein bound, so increased effect can be anticipated in the setting of renal failure. Long duration infusion can result in prolonged drug effect because of accumulation of drug outside the central compartment. Alfentanil is another short-acting, high-potency, synthetic opioid. It may have some advantage in the ICU since renal insufficiency does not alter its pharmacokinetic profile. Sufentanil, another high-potency synthetic opioid, has more variable elimination in ICU patients compared to healthy individuals (35). The expense associated with alfentanil and sufentanil compared to fentanyl may outweigh their advantages however, and they are rarely used for analgesia in the ICU. Remifentanil is extremely short acting and has a unique route of metabolism. It is degraded by nonspecific blood and tissue esterases. Its pharmacokinetic profile is unchanged in the presence liver or renal impairment. It has been successfully applied in fast-track postoperative cardiac surgical protocols as a means of providing potent, but rapidly terminated analgesia (36).

Meperidine is generally not recommended for analgesia in the ICU. It is shorter acting than morphine and far less potent than fentanyl. Repeated doses of the drug lead to accumulation of normeperidine, a toxic metabolite with a 15- to 20-hour half-life that can cause dysphoria, irritability, tremors, myoclonus, and seizures. In patients taking a monoamine oxidase inhibitor, meperidine can cause severe encephalopathy and death.

The sedative and analgesic agents are essential elements in the care of the critically ill. Initial assessment of analgesic and sedative needs and subsequent assessment of response to therapy is required to maximize efficacy of sedation while avoiding untoward effects. Knowledge of the pharmacology of the commonly used sedative and analgesic agents is essential for appropriate and cost-effective use of these drugs in the ICU environment.

NEUROMUSCULAR BLOCKING DRUGS IN THE INTENSIVE CARE UNIT

Administration of NMB drugs in ICU patients peaked in the 1980s, but is currently declining because of: (a) aggressive use of sedative and analgesic agents such as propofol, dexmedetomidine, and fentanyl, which decrease or eliminate the need for NMB drugs, and (b) increased recognition of the morbidity and costs of untoward NMB drug side effects such as accumulation of toxic metabolites, prolonged motor weakness, and myopathy (37,38). Nonetheless, there will always be a small cadre of ICU patients for whom these drugs optimize care (39). Potential

problems associated with these drugs may be diminished by improved understanding of NMB drug selection and administration, identification of drug–drug interactions, optimization of drug delivery, monitoring depth of neuromuscular blockade, and recognition of risk factors associated with NMB-induced neuromuscular injury.

Physiology of the Neuromuscular Junction

The neuromuscular junction is the triad of a motor nerve terminus, the neurotransmitter acetylcholine (ACh), and the postsynaptic muscle endplate that controls voluntary muscle contraction. An action potential reaching the motor nerve terminus causes release of ACh from synaptic vesicles, each one containing about 10,000 molecules of the neurotransmitter. This concentrated release of ACh rapidly diffuses across the 10- to 20-nm gap to the postsynaptic endplate (Fig. 1). The motor endplate contains specialized ligand-gated, nicotinic ACh receptors (nAChRs), which convert the chemical signal (i.e., binding of two ACh molecules) into electric signals (i.e., a transient permeability change and depolarization in the postsynaptic membrane of striated muscle) (40). Voluntary muscle contraction follows.

Nicotinic-AChRs are clustered at the muscle endplate, concentrated on the crests of the postjunctional membrane folds. Each nAChR is a pentameric glycoprotein complex composed of five subunits, alpha, beta, delta, and epsilon in a ratio of 2:1:1:1 (40). Each of the two alpha subunits act as an ACh-binding site

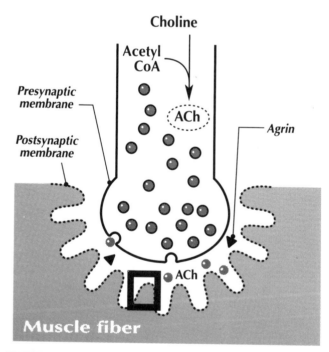

FIGURE 1. Diagram of the neuromuscular junction, site of 1 to 10 million nicotinic acetylcholine receptors (nAChRs) concentrated in the junctional folds of the muscle endplate. The neurotransmitter acetylcholine is released from axonal vesicles in response to neuronal action potentials. (Reprinted with permission from Wall MH, Prielipp RC. Monitoring the neuromuscular junction. In: Lake CL, Hines RL, Blitt CD, eds. *Clinical monitoring: practical applications for anesthesia and critical care.* Philadelphia: WB Saunders, 2001:120.)

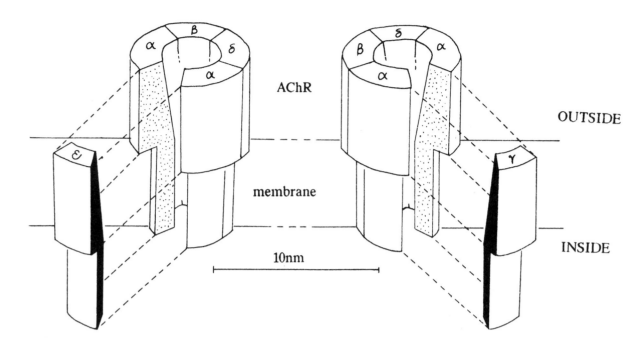

AChR

OUTSIDE

membrane

INSIDE

10nm

mature/innervated

fetal/denervated

FIGURE 2. The mature nicotinic acetylcholine receptor (nAChR) **(left)** with its glycoprotein subunits arranged around the central cation core. Two molecules of acetylcholine bind simultaneously to the two alpha-subunits to convert the channel to an open state. The immature, or fetal-variant receptor with a single subunit substitution **(right)** follows major stress (e.g., burns or denervation). These immature receptors are characterized by tenfold greater ionic activity, rapid metabolic turnover, and extrajunctional proliferation. Use of a depolarizing muscle relaxant (succinylcholine) in patients with proliferating, immature nAChR will lead to severe, acute hyperkalemia. (Reprinted with permission from Martyn JAJ, White DA, Gronert GA, et al. Up-and-down regulation of skeletal muscle acetylcholine receptors. *Anesthesiology* 1992;76:825).

(Fig. 2). When stimulated, the channel undergoes conformational change and opens for one millisecond, allowing nonselective passage of small positively charged ions, mainly sodium (Na^+, peak rate of $\geq 30,000$ ions per channel per millisecond), potassium, and calcium. This Na^+ influx depolarizes the nearby muscle membrane, triggering local voltage-gated Na^+-channels, and thereby creates a self-propagating depolarization (i.e., a muscle action potential). Excitation-contraction coupling results in voluntary muscle contraction. Under most circumstances, a "safety margin" for neuromuscular transmission exists whereby excess ACh is released to ensure effective signal transduction. The action of ACh is terminated by dissociation and passive diffusion away from the endplate, along with enzymatic degradation by acetylcholinesterase. Subsequently, the nAChR channel transitions rapidly through desensitized and closed states to ready itself for another nerve impulse.

Adult skeletal muscle retains an ability to synthesize both the mature, adult AChR, as well as an immature nAChR variant (Fig. 2), in which a gamma subunit is substituted for the normal epsilon subunit (40). In diseases and injuries such as Guillain-Barré, stroke, polio, spinal cord injury, burns, severe muscle trauma, enforced immobilization, or other conditions producing loss of nerve function, synthesis of immature (fetal) receptors may be triggered. These immature nAChRs are distinguished by three features. First, immature receptors are not localized to the muscle endplate, but migrate across the entire membrane surface (40). Second, the immature receptors are metabolically short-lived (less than 24 hours) and more ionically active, having a two- to tenfold longer channel "open time." Lastly, these immature receptors are more sensitive to the depolarizing effects of drugs such as succinylcholine, and more resistant to the effects of competitive antagonists such as d-tubocurarine. The clinical consequences of upregulation of these abnormal receptors are profound and problematic (40). For example, in acute spinal cord injury and burn patients, denervation-induced proliferation of immature (gamma-subunit) nAChR may explain the observed sensitivity and potentially lethal hyperkalemic response to depolarizing agonists like succinylcholine. In addition, this same phenomenon explains NMB drug resistance and tachyphylaxis to nondepolarizing NMB drugs such as d-tubocurarine, vecuronium, and atracurium in these same ICU patients.

One of the striking features of the neuromuscular junction is the concentration of nAChR on the postsynaptic membrane. Normal neural activity and stimulation of the motor endplate regulates the translation and membrane integration of the nAChR. Before synapse formation, AChRs are evenly distributed across the muscle membrane, but within hours after interaction with the nerve, receptor density increases 1,000-fold to a concentration of $\geq 10,000$ receptors per μ^2. Figure 3 shows a schematic model of the organization and structure of this postsynaptic

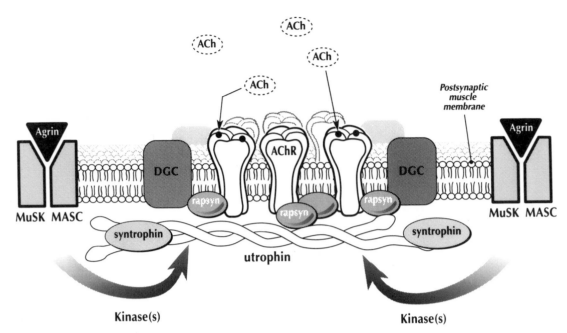

FIGURE 3. Schematic drawing of the molecular organization of the nicotinic acetylcholine receptors (nAChRs) in the postsynaptic muscle membrane. Agrin is the *nerve-derived* ~ K-D protein that triggers clustering of receptor proteins during synapse formation, as well as concentrating other synaptic proteins such as acetylcholinesterase, rapsyn, and utrophin. Evidence suggests that MuSK (muscle-specific kinase), along with a cofactor MASC (myotube-associated specificity component) activates certain kinase activity which initiates clustering of synaptic proteins. Receptor aggregation occurs in distinct steps however, initiated with nAChR localization by rapsyn. Meanwhile, ∂-dystroglycan (not shown), the extracellular component of dystrophin-associated glycoprotein complex (DGC), may also function as an agrin receptor, and promotes further nAChR clustering. The final process utilizes the structural organization of additional proteins like utrophin, which stabilize the mature, immobile domains by interaction with the underlying cytoskeleton (F-actin). When completed, this process concentrates nAChR density 1,000-fold compared to unmodified muscle membrane. The agrin signaling mechanism must remain active throughout the life of the synapse in order to maintain stability. (Reprinted with permission from Wall MH, Prielipp RC. Monitoring the neuromuscular junction. In: Lake CL, Hines RL, Blitt CD, eds. *Clinical monitoring: practical applications for anesthesia and critical care*. Philadelphia: WB Saunders, 2001:121.)

region. Agrin is the nerve-derived extracellular protein that is instrumental in triggering receptor clustering during synapse formation (41). However, receptor aggregation appears to occur in distinct steps, with small clusters followed by formation of larger ones. Utrophin bridges the maturing clusters to underlying strands of F-actin in the internal muscle cytoskeleton, thus forming immobile, mature, functional receptor domains.

Neuromuscular Blocking Drugs

Indications and Interactions of Neuromuscular Blocking Drugs in the Intensive Care Unit

Because NMB drugs are totally devoid of sedative and analgesic activity, they should be accompanied by coadministration of amnestic drugs, opioids, or sedatives (see earlier sections in this chapter). Indeed, many ICU patients may be adequately ventilated and managed without NMB drugs if appropriate quantities of analgesics and sedatives are administered. The common and generally recognized uses of NMB drugs in the ICU are summarized in Table 6. Optimization of mechanical ventilation is the most frequent indication, especially in patients with acute lung injury requiring newer, more sophisticated modes of ventilation. Pharmacokinetic and pharmacodynamic properties of

NMB drugs are summarized in Table 13.7, while adverse effects are outlined in Table 8. Lastly, the interactions of NMB agents with other drugs are summarized in Table 9.

TABLE 6. USES OF NEUROMUSCULAR BLOCKING DRUGS IN INTENSIVE CARE UNIT PATIENTS

Common indications:
  Facilitate synchrony, or decrease airway pressure, in mechanically ventilated patients (e.g., status asthmaticus)
  Facilitate endotracheal intubation
  Attenuate increases in intracranial hypertension
  Eliminate shivering
  Decrease O_2 consumption
  Optimize conditions for imaging or diagnostic studies
  Ensure patient immobility during invasive procedures, or patient transport
  Establish control of agitated or combative (intubated) patient
Less frequent indications:
  Supportive therapy of tetanus or status epilepticus (with EEG monitoring)
  Selected patients with severe cardiovascular instability or support devices (e.g., left ventricular assist devices; ECMO)

EEG, electroencephalogram; ECMO, extracorporeal membrane oxygenation.

TABLE 7. NEUROMUSCULAR BLOCKING DRUGS FOR INTENSIVE CARE UNIT (ICU) USE

Selected Benzylisoquinolinium Drugs/Generic (Trade Name)	Tubocurarine (Curare)	Cisatracurium (Nimbex)	Atracurium (Tracrium)	Doxacurium (Nuromax)	Mivacurium (Mivacron)
Introduced (yr)	1942	1995	1983	1991	1992
ED$_{95}$ dose (mg/kg)	0.51	0.05	0.25	0.025–0.030	0.075
Initial dose (mg/kg)	0.2–0.3	0.20	0.4–0.5	up to 0.1	0.15–0.25
Duration (min)	80	45–60	25–35	120–150	10–20
Infusion described	rare	yes	yes	yes	yes
Infusion dose (μg/kg/min)	—	2.5–3.0	4–12	0.3–0.5	9–10
Recovery (min)	80–180	90	40–60	120–180	10–20
% Renal excretion	40–45	Hofmann elimination	5–10 (uses Hofmann elimination)	70	inactive metabolites
Renal failure	increased effect	no change	no change	increased effect	increased duration
% Biliary excretion	10–40	Hofmann elimination	minimal (uses Hofmann elimination)	unclear	—
Hepatic failure	minimal change to mild increased effect	minimal to no change	minimal to no change	?	increased duration
Active metabolites	no	no	no, but can accumulate laudanosine	?	no
Histamine release hypotension	marked	no	minimal but dose-dependent	none	minimal but dose-dependent
Vagal block tachycardia	minimal	no	no	no	no
Ganglionic blockade hypotension	marked	no	minimal to none	no	no
Prolonged ICU block	?	rare	rare	rare	?
Estimated U.S. ICU use	rare	increasing	minimal	infrequent	rare; N.R.
Cost ($) (24-h estimate)	N.R.	decreasing	decreasing	intermediate	very costly

Selected Aminosteroids/ Generic (Trade Name)	Pancuronium (Pavulon)	Vecuronium (Norcuron)	Pipecuronium (Arduan)	Rocuronium (Zemuron)	Rapacuronium (Raplon)
Introduced (yr)	1972	1984	1991	1994	1999
ED$_{95}$ dose (mg/kg)	0.07	0.05	0.05	0.3	1.5
Initial dose (mg/kg)	0.1	0.1	0.085–0.1	0.6–1.0	1.5–2.0
Duration (min)	90–100	35–45	90–100	30	15–20
Infusion described	yes	yes	no	yes	N.R.
Infusion dose (μg/kg/min)	1–2	1–2	0.5–2.0	10–12	N.R.
Recovery (min)	120–180	45–60	55–160	20–30	30
% Renal excretion	45–70	50	50+	33	significant
Renal failure	increased effect	increased effect, especially metabolites	increased duration	minimal	accumulation of Org 9488 (active, potent metabolite)
% Biliary excretion	10–15	35–50	minimal	≅75%	?
Hepatic failure	mild increased effect	variable, mild	minimal	moderate	?
Active metabolites	yes: 3-OH and 17-OH-pancuronium	yes: 3-desacetyl-vecuronium	not reported	no	yes: 3-OH-rapacuronium
Histamine release hypotension	none	none	none	none	yes: 2%–3% incidence bronchospasm
Vagal block tachycardia	modest to marked	no	no	some at higher doses	mild tachycardia
Ganglionic blockade hypotension	no	no	no	no	mild hypotension
Prolonged ICU block	yes	yes	no reports	no reports	N.R.
Estimated U.S. ICU use	variable	decreasing	uncommon	variable	N.R.
Cost (24-h estimate)	inexpensive	decreasing	rarely used	more costly	N.R.

N.R., not recommended
(Modified with permission from Prielipp RC, Coursin DB. *New Horz* 1994;2:34.)

Structure-Activity Relationship

All nondepolarizing NMB drugs competitively antagonize post-junctional ACh receptors. The neurotransmitter, ACh, has a positively charged quaternary ammonium ($[N-C_4]^+$) group which binds with the negatively charged alpha-subunit of the cholinergic receptor. The remarkable specificity of NMB drugs relates to the molecular structure of the ACh molecule being functionally duplicated within the structure of NMB drugs like pancuronium (Fig. 4).

Drug Action

Succinylcholine, composed of two ACh molecules attached end to end via acetate groups, is a depolarizing NMB drug that produces sustained activation of nAChRs, resulting in muscle

TABLE 8. POTENTIAL ADVERSE EFFECTS OF NEUROMUSCULAR BLOCKING DRUGS IN THE INTENSIVE CARE UNIT

Anxiety, stress, potential unpleasant recall in the awake, but paralyzed patient
Risk of ventilator disconnect or airway mishap
Autonomic and cardiovascular interactions
   Tachycardia or bradycardia
   Hypotension or hypertension
Accumulation of parent drug or drug metabolites (e.g., laudanosine; 3-desacetyl-vecuronium)
Decreased lymphatic flow, respiratory clearance
Risk of skeletal muscle deconditioning, skin breakdown, peripheral nerve injury
Risk of prolonged muscle weakness and "postparalytic syndrome" (myopathy)
Central nervous system toxicity with prolonged administration
Interactions with leukocytes (i.e., immune suppression)
Drug cost

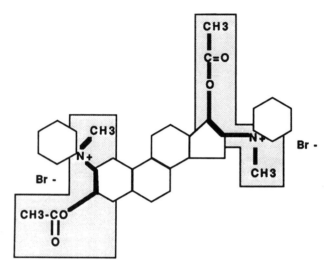

FIGURE 4. Receptor specificity is imparted by the incorporation of the basic acetylcholine molecule **(highlighted, bold)** within the basic structure of the aminosteroid neuromuscular blocking (NMB) drugs like pancuronium. NMB drug binding occurs at the alpha-subunit of the nicotinic acetylcholine receptor (nAChR). The presence of the bulky, steroid backbone of the NMB drug (pancuronium) assists in effectively blocking the cation channel. (Reprinted with permission from Prielipp RC, Coursin DB. Applied pharmacology of common neuromuscular blocking agents in critical care. *New Horiz* 1994;2:37.)

endplate depolarization (fasciculations) followed by receptor desensitization and flaccid paralysis. On the other hand, nondepolarizing NMB drugs competitively bind to the nAChR, preventing ACh activation of receptors. These compounds are large, bulky structures that are chemically categorized in two classes: the benzylisoquinolinium (42) and the aminosteroid compounds (43), and can be further categorized by their duration of action.

Depolarizing Neuromuscular Block

Succinylcholine is the only depolarizing NMB agent in common use today. The administration of 1.0 mg per kg of succinylcholine

TABLE 9. DRUG INTERACTIONS WITH NEUROMUSCULAR BLOCKING (NMB) DRUGS

Drugs that potentiate the actions of nondepolarizing NMB drugs
  Halogenated anesthetics
  Local anesthetics
  Lidocaine
  Antibiotics
    Aminoglycosides (gentamicin, tobramycin, amikacin)
    Polypeptides (polymyxin B)
    Other antibiotics (clindamycin, tetracycline)
  Antiarrhythmics
    Procainamide
    Quinidine
  Magnesium
  Calcium-channel blockers
  ß-adrenergic blockers
  Chemotherapeutic agents
    Cyclophosphamide
  Dantrolene
  Diuretics
    Furosemide (biphasic response)
    Thiazides
  Lithium carbonate
  Cyclosporine
Drugs that antagonize the actions of nondepolarizing NMB drugs
  Phenytoin
  Carbamazepine
  Theophylline
  Sympathomimetic agents
  Chronic exposure to nondepolarizing NMB drugs

i.v. ($2 \times$ the ED_{95}) causes fasciculations, followed by flaccid paralysis within 30 to 60 seconds. This flaccid paralysis lasts 7 to 12 minutes as the succinylcholine diffuses away from the neuromuscular junction and is metabolized to choline and succinylmonocholine by plasma cholinesterase (also known as pseudo- or butyryoholinesterase).

Cardiac arrhythmias, myalgias and myoglobinuria, increases in intragastric pressure and ICP, malignant hyperthermia, and (lethal) hyperkalemia are all potential adverse effects of succinylcholine. Classic risk factors for hyperkalemia are major burns, spinal cord injury or other denervation, significant trauma with crushed muscle, and certain muscular dystrophies (i.e., myotonia congenita or dystrophica). Of particular note for ICU considerations is the association of *prolonged immobilization* and the upregulation of nAChR, which also renders (some) ICU patients susceptible to succinylcholine-induced hyperkalemia.

Nondepolarizing (Competitive) Neuromuscular Block

The benzylisoquinolinium drugs tend to be potent (and therefore slower in onset) NMB drugs that are eliminated by the kidneys or Hofmann elimination, and may trigger histamine release. Conversely, the aminosteroid compounds are less potent, have a faster onset of action, are eliminated by the liver with active metabolites, and generally lack significant histamine release or autonomic interactions.

Short-Acting Neuromuscular Blocking Drugs

Mivacurium is currently the shortest-acting, nondepolarizing (benzylisoquinolinium) NMB drug (42). It may be associated with histamine release and has a duration of action of 15 to

25 minutes when administered as a bolus. Mivacurium is metabolized by plasma cholinesterase, the same enzyme that degrades succinylcholine. Therefore, prolonged neuromuscular blockade can occur in the same clinical situations described with succinylcholine. The short duration of action requires that this drug be administered as a continuous infusion in the ICU; however, the cost of such an infusion is prohibitive. Thus, mivacurium may be used for intubation in the ICU patient in whom succinylcholine is contraindicated. Major metabolites of mivacurium are renally excreted.

Intermediate-Acting Drugs

Atracurium is an intermediate-acting, benzylisoquinolinium NMB drug marketed as a racemic mixture of 10 stereoisomers (42). Neuromuscular block occurs over 3 to 4 minutes after injection of 0.3 to 0.6 mg per kg. Rapid administration may trigger histamine release with secondary hypotension. The most unique aspect of atracurium is its degradation via the Hofmann reaction, a nonenzymatic, spontaneous breakdown that occurs at normal body temperature and pH, which is independent of renal or hepatic function (42,44,45). However, accumulation of one major metabolite, laudanosine, may produce excitatory CNS toxicity, perhaps even seizures. The threshold for laudanosine CNS stimulation in humans remains unknown, but because laudanosine is renally excreted, it may accumulate to a greater degree when prolonged infusions are used in critically ill patients with renal failure.

Cisatracurium is the R, *cis*-R′, *cis*-isomer that constitutes about 15% of the commercial NMB drug mixture marketed as atracurium. Attributes of cisatracurium are threefold greater potency, lack of histamine release, minimal interaction with autonomic ganglia, and decreased generation of the metabolite, laudanosine. Similar to atracurium, it undergoes Hofmann elimination, so that drug elimination occurs independent of end-organ function. Intravenous doses of 0.2 mg per kg ($4 \times ED_{95}$) provide good conditions for endotracheal intubation in 90 to 120 seconds, and last 60 to 80 minutes. Infusions may be titrated from 2.5 to 3.0 μg per kg per minute in ICU patients (46).

Vecuronium is an aminosteroid that differs in structure from pancuronium by the deletion of a methyl group at the 2 N-piperdino position of the steroid molecule (43). This substitution eliminates the vagolytic effects such as tachycardia and hypertension associated with pancuronium. Vecuronium is administered in the ICU as an intermittent bolus or continuous infusion (46). It undergoes hepatic hydrolysis to three different desacetyl metabolites: 3-desacetyl-, 17-desacetyl-, and 3,17-desacetyl-vecuronium, which vary in NMB activity. The 3-desacetyl metabolite is estimated to be 80% as potent as the parent compound, while the others are far less potent (37). Metabolites such as 3-desacetyl-vecuronium accumulate in renal failure, especially when complicated by uremia, have a longer elimination half-life, and may cause prolonged weakness in this group of patients (37,47). These metabolites are not removed by hemodialysis.

Rocuronium, introduced in 1994, is also an aminosteroid NMB drug chemically related to vecuronium. Intravenous doses of 0.6 to 1.2 mg per kg produce good to excellent intubating conditions within 60 seconds, rivaling succinylcholine for speed of onset. Rocuronium has an intermediate duration of action

(30 to 45 minutes), no cardiovascular side effects, and is eliminated primarily via the hepatobiliary system (but with minimal liver metabolism). Either intermittent bolus (doses of 15 to 70 mg per hour) or continuous infusion (30 to 50 mg per hour) may be utilized in adult and pediatric ICU patients (48). However, the $T_{1/2}\beta$ (terminal half-life) at least triples in ICU patients when the drug is given for prolonged periods because the volume of distribution increases threefold (48).

Long-Acting Neuromuscular Blocking Drugs

D-tubocurarine (curare) is the prototypical, benzylisoquinolinium NMB drug (42). Although the first NMB used in the ICU (for the treatment of tetanus), it is rarely used now because of associated histamine release and ganglionic blockade producing hypotension. It undergoes predominantly renal elimination with some minor biliary excretion. The $T_{1/2}\beta$ of curare is markedly prolonged in patients with renal and hepatic dysfunction.

Metocurine is a trimethylated derivative of d-tubocurarine. It is twice as potent as the parent compound and associated with far less histamine release and less ganglionic blockade (42). It is minimally metabolized, undergoes predominantly renal excretion, and has an extended half-life in patients with renal failure since it does not undergo hepatic or biliary elimination.

Pancuronium is a synthetic, bisquaternary aminosteroid NMB drug (43), which is vagolytic and sympathomimetic. These changes in autonomic tone may result in tachycardia, hypertension, and increased cardiac output (49), and are likely to occur despite the timing and method of drug delivery in ICU patients. Pancuronium is metabolized to hydroxylated derivatives such as 3-OH-pancuronium, which is 50% as potent as the parent drug (43). Thus, the NMB effects of pancuronium accumulate with repeated dosing. Because pancuronium and its metabolites are mainly excreted by the kidney, the duration of action may be prolonged in patients with either hepatic or renal insufficiency. The long duration of action permits administration in the ICU as either intermittent boluses or continuous infusion (49).

Pipercuronium is also a long-acting aminosteroid NMB drug, facilitating its ICU administration via intermittent boluses. It is longer acting than pancuronium, but is not associated with cardiovascular side effects or autonomic interactions. It is metabolized by the liver to 3-desacetyl pipercuronium, and then renally excreted.

Doxacurium chloride, a benzylisoquinolinium NMB drug introduced in 1991, is noted for its potency ($ED_{95} = 0.025$ mg per kg) and lack of hemodynamic or autonomic interactions (42,50). Repeated doxacurium dosing in operating room patients and ICU patients (49) has not been associated with tachycardia or accumulation. The drug is primarily excreted unchanged by the kidneys, and minimally metabolized. There may be modest prolongation of doxacurium blockade in patients with renal or hepatic insufficiency.

Monitoring Neuromuscular Blocking Drug Blockade: Theory of Nerve Stimulators

Neuromuscular twitch monitoring facilitates assessment of the degree of neuromuscular blockade independent of confounding

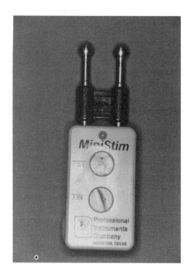
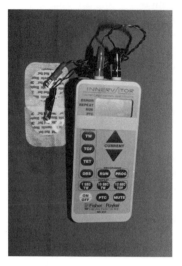
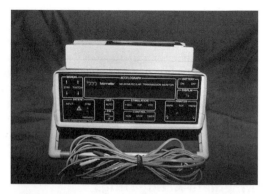
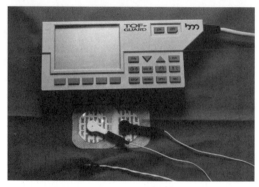

FIGURE 5. Four models of commercially available peripheral nerve stimulators are pictured. All units deliver variable voltage, constant current nerve stimulation for monitoring the depth of neuromuscular block. The more complex (and expensive) models provide improved accuracy, greater operator control of current selection, and a wider array of available stimulation patterns. From left to right are the MiniStim (Professional Instruments Co.); the Innervator Model NS 252 (Fisher & Paykel Healthcare); the Accelograph Model US 1 (Biometer International AS) (top); and the TOF-Guard (Biometer Turnhout) (bottom). The first two stimulators rely on visual or tactile response of the adductor pollicis brevis muscle to ulnar nerve stimulation. The latter two stimulators use an acceleration transducer attached to the thumb to automatically record the muscle twitch response to stimulation. Skeletal muscle acceleration is linearly related to traditional force-displacement measurements usually recorded in scientific or research studies. (Reprinted with permission from Wall MH, Prielipp RC. Monitoring the neuromuscular junction. In: Lake CL, Hines RL, Blitt CD, eds. *Clinical monitoring: practical applications for anesthesia and critical care.* Philadelphia: WB Saunders, 2001:124.)

variables such as sedation, alterations in mental status, or patient cooperation. We recommend routine use of a hand-held peripheral nerve stimulator in the ICU to titrate the depth of neuromuscular blockade, which should prevent significant and unnecessary NMB drug overdose.

Peripheral nerve stimulators are the simplest, most reliable means to assess neuromuscular function (Fig. 5). Traditionally, the ulnar nerve at the wrist is stimulated while evaluating the motor response of the adductor pollicis brevis muscle of the thumb. Other peripheral nerve sites (such as facial nerve stimulation while grading the orbicularis oculi muscle, or stimulating the peroneal nerve of the upper leg and grading foot dorsiflexion) are also available, but exhibit slightly different neuromuscular blockade profiles. Patients with strokes, paraplegia, or dense peripheral neuropathies should be monitored on *unaffected limbs,* since affected extremities will exhibit resistance to neuromuscular blockade.

Nerve stimulators pass an electric current across peripheral nerves to generate an action potential, leading to mechanical skeletal muscle contraction (51,52). Because peripheral nerves are made up of a large number of axons of different sizes and depolarizing thresholds, not all nerves will depolarize at equal

currents. The lowest current needed to generate muscular activity is the initial threshold for stimulation (ITS) current. The supramaximal current will usually be 2.75 to 3 times the ITS.

Surface electrodes using pregelled sodium/sodium chloride (Na/NaCl), silver/silver chloride, or conductive rubber are commonly used. If possible, the negative (black or stimulating) electrode should be placed distally over the nerve, while the positive (red) electrode should be placed more proximally (not over any other nerves). This electrode orientation minimizes the stimulation threshold.

Patterns of Stimulation

Nondepolarizing neuromuscular block is characterized by decreased single-twitch height, as well as fade with tetanus, train-of-four (TOF) and double burst stimulation, and posttetanic facilitation (Fig. 6).

Single Twitch

A supramaximal stimulus current is applied at intervals of 1 per 10 seconds and the twitch height is compared to a pre-NMB

Nondepolarizing drug

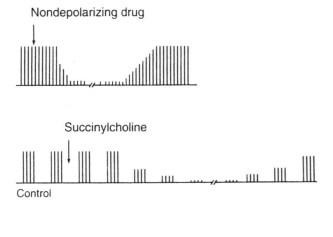

Succinylcholine

Control

Nondepolarizing drug   Neostigmine

Control

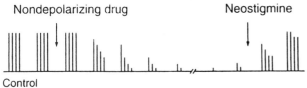

FIGURE 6. Top panel shows the effect of a nondepolarizing neuromuscular blocking (NMB) drug (e.g., pancuronium) on the single twitch response at 1 Hz. The middle panel shows the effect of succinylcholine (a depolarizing NMB drug) on the train-of-four (TOF) response applied at 2 Hz after a baseline period is established. Note that all four twitches are depressed equally, and that there is no fade of the response during either onset or recovery from this type of neuromuscular block. The bottom panel shows the more common effect of a nondepolarizing NMB drug producing a decrement in the TOF response ("fade"). The TOF response can be advantageous in that no baseline period is required for effective monitoring. In this case, recovery was hastened by use of the anticholinesterase drug, neostigmine. (Reprinted with permission from Hunter JM. Neuromuscular blocking drugs. *N Engl J Med* 1995;332:1691.)

drug baseline. The need for a predrug baseline is one of the major limitations of this simple modality.

Tetanus

Tetanus at 50 Hz for 5 seconds is a useful modality because there is no need for a baseline measurement. Absence of fade usually correlates with the ability to protect the airway after tracheal extubation. The main disadvantage of tetanus stimulation is that it is painful in awake patients.

Train-of-Four

The TOF response delivers four supramaximal stimuli (40 to 80 mA current) at 2 Hz (one stimulus every 0.5 sec), while the motor twitch response of the fourth twitch (T4) is compared to the twitch response of the first stimulus (T1). Visual or tactile evaluation of the TOF response is adequate for most clinical applications. The advantage of TOF stimulation is there is no need for a baseline and its semiquantitative endpoints (Table 10).

Double Burst Stimulation

This is a new pattern of nerve stimulation (two train-of-three stimulations, 0.2 msec duration at 50 Hz, separated by 750 msec)

designed to detect residual neuromuscular blockade in awake patients without causing excessive discomfort. Fade after double burst stimulation (DBS) is easier to detect by tactile examination than is fade associated with the T4/T1 ratio.

Recording Responses of Neuromuscular Junction

Visual and Tactile

The simplest, least expensive, and by far the most common method for neuromuscular monitoring is to look or feel for a muscle contraction response. However, multiple studies have shown that TOF fade or tetanic fade is often not perceived accurately by practitioners at the bedside, even when the T4/T1 ratio is as low as 0.3.

Accelerography

Accelerography measures the acceleration of muscle contraction (rather than force of contraction) by a piezoelectric transducer. The responses of force translation and accelerography have similar T4/T1 ratios.

Monitoring Limitations

One significant shortcoming of peripheral nerve stimulation is that global skeletal muscle function is inferred from the response of a single peripheral muscle group (53). For instance, the diaphragm and laryngeal muscles are more resistant to neuromuscular blockade than the adductor pollicis brevis muscle and also recover more quickly after cessation of NMB drugs (Fig. 7). In some patients, a TOF count of 0 at the adductor pollicis muscle may not correlate with a level of neuromuscular block sufficient to adequately manage clinical endpoints such as elimination of coughing during suctioning, elimination of peripheral motor movements, or dyssynchrony ("triggering") of the ventilator. Thus, a TOF count of 0 does not necessarily represent a failure of monitoring or drug titration, but reflects both the difficulty of administering NMB drugs in the ICU and the need for clinical endpoints discrepant with the monitored twitch response at the adductor pollicis. It is important therefore to use a combination of both peripheral nerve stimulation and clinical assessment to evaluate neuromuscular function and needed degree of neuromuscular blockade.

SIDE EFFECTS AND COMPLICATIONS OF NEUROMUSCULAR BLOCKING DRUGS IN THE INTENSIVE CARE UNIT

Use of NMB drugs in the ICU may be associated with numerous potential adverse effects (Table 8). Precautions to limit these effects include a secured, patent, mechanical airway, adequate ventilation, appropriate inspired oxygen concentration, concurrent sedation and analgesia, precautions with pressure points on the eyes or skin, prophylaxis for deep venous thrombosis, and intermittent neurologic assessment.

TABLE 10. RELATIONSHIP OF RECEPTOR OCCUPANCY/NEUROMUSCULAR MONITORING/CLINICAL SIGNS AT ADDUCTOR POLLICIS MUSCLE WITH NONDEPOLARIZING NEUROMUSCULAR BLOCKADE

% NMJ Receptors Blocked	T1 Twitch % Baseline	T4 Twitch % Baseline	TOFr	TOFc	Tetanus	Comments[a]
100	0	0	0	0		
95	5	0	0	0		
90	10	0	0	1	fade at 30 Hz	PTC ≈10
	20	0	0	2		
80	25	0	0	3		
80	80–90	55–65	0.6–0.7	4		Vc = 15 cc/kg, MIP = −22, V_T = 8 cc/kg,
	95	65–70	0.7–0.75	4		sustained eye opening, hand grip
75	100	75–100	0.75–1	4	sustained at 50 Hz	diplopia common, 5 sec leg lift, 5 sec
	100	90–100	0.8–1	4		head lift, MIP = −42, effective swallowing,
			0.9–1	4		masseter strength normal, normal UES
						tone, pharangeal function
50	100	100	1.0	4	fade at 100 Hz	
35	100	100	1.0	4	onset fade at 200 Hz	

[a]Clinical signs: tests do not always correlate with TOFr and TOFc and do not always ensure normal NMJ function, adequacy of ventilatory function, or the ability to protect the airway.
NMJ,neuromuscular junction; T1, first twitch; T4, fourth twitch; TOFr, train-of-four ratio (T4/T1); TOFc, train-of-four count; PTC, posttetanic count; Vc, vital capacity; MIP, maximum inspired pressure (cm H_2O); V_T, tidal volume; UES, upper esophageal sphincter.
(Modified from *Silverman DG, Brull SJ. Patterns of stimulation: In: Silverman DG, ed. Neuromuscular block in perioperative and intensive care.* Philadelphia: JB Lippincott Co., 1994:37–50.)

In addition to the issues noted above, case reports and other evidence document prolonged weakness and even myopathy (Table 11) after use of NMB drugs in the ICU. The incidence of prolonged weakness or myopathy remains unknown, but evidence suggests the problems may afflict up to 5% (39) to 10% (54) of patients. The actual incidence is likely dependent on numerous factors, including the administration of various antibiotics (aminoglycosides), corticosteroids, anticonvulsants, magnesium, calcium-channel blocking drugs, and other medications that interact with NMB drugs. The incidence of true *myopathy* may be related to the inappropriate or excessive duration of NMB blockade, excessive depth of neuromuscular blockade, the specific drug administered, and particularly NMB drug interactions with corticosteroids (54) (Table 9). Unresolved issues

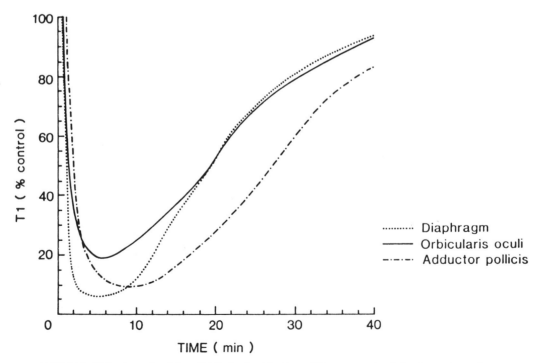

FIGURE 7. T1 in the train-of-four (TOF) obtained in three different muscles following a dose of vecuronium (0.04 mg per kg) showing onset and recovery of the diaphragm occurs before the adductor pollicis. (Reprinted with permission from Donati F, Meistelman C, Plaud B. Vecuronium neuromuscular blockade at the diaphragm, the orbicularis oculi, and adductor pollicis muscles. *Anesthesiology* 1990;73:873.)

TABLE 11. DIAGNOSTIC CHARACTERISTICS IN INTENSIVE CARE UNIT PATIENTS WITH PROLONGED WEAKNESS AND "FAILURE-TO-WEAN"

		Onset and Duration of Relaxants			
Diagnosis	History	Physical Examination and Labs	Muscle Bx/Nerve Bx	EMG/NCS	Course
Acute quadriplegic myopathy	NMB use, especially with concurrent steroids	Diffuse weakness Sparing of sensory function Potential for elevation in CK	Early change: selective thick filament degeneration in EM or local loss of ATPase activity on LM Late change: muscle fiber necrosis	Small CMAP NL SNAP NL or near NL NCV Myopathic change (only in patients with steroids and NMBs) NMB alone see type II atrophy (disuse)	Favorable for the most part, but patient may have prolonged recovery period
Critical illness polyneuropathy	Commonly occurs with sepsis More frequent in older adults, severely ill patients	Sensory and motor involvement Flaccid limbs Failure to wean Usually normal CK	Predominantly axonal degeneration Denervation atrophy No inflammation	Consistent with distal axonal sensorimotor polyneuropathy Abnormal MAP Abnormal SNAP	May have protracted process with unfavorable outcome Outcome mainly related to underlying pathology
Steroid-induced myopathy	Acute or chronic process Occurs more commonly in proximal muscles	Systemic sequelae of steroid use (skin changes, diabetes, body habitus, hypertension)	Type II muscle fiber atrophy	NL or if severe–mild myopathic change	Tends to be favorable
Deconditioning syndrome	Occurs with immobile, highly catabolic patients in the ICU May be exacerbated by deafferentation associated with dense neuromuscular blockade	Diffuse weakness and loss of muscle mass and skin Muscle wasting CK = normal	Muscle Bx not indicated, but if done shows type II fiber atrophy	Essentially NL	Dependent on underlying pathology
Guillain-Barré	Associated with underlying viral infection and ascending polyneuropathy	Diffuse motor weakness Potential involvement of cranial nerves Possible autonomic lability	Not indicated	Compatible with demyelinating sensorimotor polyneuropathy	Favorable, appears to improve with immunoglobulin or plasmapheresis
Myasthenia gravis	Variable but often progressive fatigue and bulbar signs	Muscle fatigability	Not indicated	Decremental response on repetitive stimulation at 2 Hz MUP variability on EMG	Dependent on aggressiveness of disease, favorable with cholinesterase inhibitors, steroids, and thymectomy as needed
Acute rhabdomyolysis	Associated with crush injuries, drug overdose, or toxic ingestions	Increased CK Check HPO_4^- Urine myoglobin	Diffuse muscle fiber necrosis	Spontaneous activity with myopathic changes	Favorable, depends on associated pathology and injury
Central pontine myelinolysis	Rapid electrolyte alterations	Locked-in syndrome	Not indicated	NL	Poor

Bx, biopsy; EMG, electromyogram; NCS, nerve conduction study; NMB, neuromuscular blocking; CMAP, compound muscle action potentials; EM, electron microscopy; ATPase, adenosine triphosphatase; LM, light microscopy; NL, normal; SNAP, sensory nerve action potential; NCV, nerve conduction velocity; CK, creative kinase; MAP, muscle action potential; MUP, motor unit potential; (Modified from Prielipp RC, et al. Complications associated with sedative and neuromuscular blocking drugs in critically ill patients. *Crit Care Clin* 1995;11(4):983–1003.)

include the protection inferred by routine monitoring of neuromuscular blockade, the effects of prolonged immobility, and the severity of systemic illness with associated neuromuscular pathology. It is helpful to characterize these adverse effects into *pharmacologic, physiologic,* and *toxic* mechanisms. "Prolonged weakness" will be defined as neuromuscular recovery that requires significantly longer than expected (e.g., greater than 120 minutes after discontinuation of intermediate-acting NMB drugs such as

cisatracurium or vecuronium) based on usual pharmacokinetic parameters recognized for these NMB drugs.

Pharmacologic

The steroid-based NMB drugs, pancuronium and vecuronium, are still commonly used in the ICU. (An informal, 1999 Internet survey of intensivists found these two NMB drugs were the preferred agents in 60% of institutions.) Not surprisingly, therefore, most case reports of ICU patients with prolonged weakness and myopathy are of patients who received steroid-based NMB drugs. But it is unclear if there is a unique, specific risk inferred by steroid-based, compared to benzylisoquinolinium-based, NMB drugs. Any comparison must examine the complex milieu of ICU patients receiving multiple drugs manifesting altered drug metabolism. For instance, vecuronium undergoes extensive hepatic hydrolysis, with the 3-desacetyl metabolite estimated to be 80% as potent as the parent compound. The 3-desacetyl-vecuronium metabolite accumulates in patients in renal failure, and is poorly dialyzed and minimally ultrafiltrated. In addition, the hepatic elimination of 3-desacetyl-vecuronium is decreased in patients uremic for at least 36 hours. Thus, accumulation of both 3-desacetyl-vecuronium and vecuronium in patients with renal failure contributes to prolonged weakness in this subset of ICU patients. Similarly, pancuronium is a bisquaternary NMB drug which is desacetylated at the C_3-position of the steroid nucleus to 3-desacetyl-pancuronium. The 3-OH metabolite is lipophilic, 90% bound to plasma proteins, approximately 50% as active as the parent pancuronium, and accumulates in patients with renal insufficiency. The combination of decreased clearance, increased volume of distribution, and accumulation of active 3-OH-metabolites is a likely pharmacologic explanation for prolonged weakness in ICU patients with renal insufficiency.

There are also a wide range of drugs with complex interactions with NMB drugs. These drug–drug interactions commonly potentiate the density of NMB motor block. For instance, aminoglycosides, cyclosporin, and other drugs (Table 9) may have a potent "curare-like" action, simulating a pharmacologic denervation.

Physiologic

Pathophysiologic changes occur at the nerve, neuromuscular junction, and muscle in critically ill patients. In ICU patients receiving long-term infusions of NMB drugs, the basement membrane of the neuromuscular junction may act as a reservoir of active drug, maintaining NMB drug at the nAChRs long after the drug has disappeared from the plasma. Other physiologic changes are enhanced in patients immobilized for long periods, in those suffering spinal cord injury and denervation, and patients receiving prolonged NMB drug-induced paralysis. The nAChR may be triggered to revert to a fetal variant structure, characterized by an increase in total number, greater ionic activity, rapid metabolic turnover, frequent extrajunctional proliferation, and "resistance" to nondepolarizing NMB drugs (Fig. 2). This may account for the observations of some ICU patients developing tachyphylaxis to NMB drugs, often resulting in a tripling or quadrupling of the starting NMB drug dose (55). The proliferation and distribution of these altered receptors across the myomembrane simultaneously sensitizes patients to depolarizing drugs such as succinylcholine. Succinylcholine stimulation of the immature, fetal receptors manifests as life-threatening hyperkalemia and cardiac arrest.

Toxic

Skeletal muscle injury in ICU patients is designated by a confusing and oftentimes overlapping list of names and syndromes including acute quadriplegic myopathy syndrome (AQMS), floppy-man syndrome, critical illness polyneuropathy (CIP), acute myopathy of intensive care, rapidly evolving myopathy, acute myopathy with selective lysis of myosin filaments, acute steroid myopathy, and neurogenic weakness (56–64). Prolonged weakness, also called prolonged recovery, is primarily a phenomenon of accumulating NMB drug, or drug metabolites, as described earlier. By comparison, a true myopathy in ICU patients is the clinical triad of acute clinical paresis, myonecrosis with increased creatine phosphokinase (CK) concentrations, and abnormal electromyography (EMG) and nerve conduction studies. The neurophysiologic abnormalities seen in these patients are characterized in three basic groups:

1. Pure sensory axonal neuropathy
2. Pure motor syndrome with weakness of both the upper and lower limbs
3. A mixed motor and sensory disturbance (57,58,60).

When the clinical paresis syndromes are examined early, they exhibit features most consistent with neuronal dysfunction, whereas later examination (meaning days to weeks) is typified by signs consistent with skeletal muscle atrophy and necrosis (58,59). Regardless, the patients with clinical paresis manifest severely reduced compound muscle action potentials (CMAP), indicating an abnormality of the distal motor neuron and/or the neuromuscular junction. Common causes and characteristics of skeletal muscle weakness in ICU patients are summarized in Table 11 and are discussed below.

TOXIC NEUROMYOPATHIES IN INTENSIVE CARE UNIT PATIENTS

Dysfunction of peripheral nerves, the neuromuscular junction, and disruption of skeletal muscle cytoarchitecture is increasingly recognized during severe illness in ICU patients. AQMS, also referred to as postparalytic quadriparesis and other names, is an infrequent, but major complication in ICU patients after administration of NMB drugs (56–64). Again, this entity must be differentiated from other neuromuscular pathologies (Tables 11 and 12), and requires extensive testing (and often muscle biopsy) for diagnosis. Of special note, reports of AQMS in patients receiving NMB drugs *alone* are quite limited. Indeed, no experimental (animal) model has been able to produce the histopathology of this myopathy by the administration of just NMB drugs. Afflicted patients demonstrate diffuse weakness that persists long after the NMB drug administration is discontinued (and the elimination of any active drug metabolites). Neurologic examination reveals a global motor deficit with decreased motor reflexes, and afflicts proximal and distal muscles in both the upper and lower extremities. However, extraocular muscle function is usually preserved. This myopathy is characterized by low amplitude CMAPs and muscle fibrillations, but normal (or near normal) sensory nerve conduction studies (59,62). Muscle biopsy shows prominent vacuolization of muscle fibers without inflammatory infiltrate, patchy type 2 muscle fiber atrophy, or sporadic myofiber necrosis, but usually does *not* show loss of thick, myosin filaments (contrast this with biopsy findings noted below in patients receiving

TABLE 12. DIFFERENTIAL DIAGNOSIS IN PATIENTS WITH PROLONGED WEAKNESS AFTER NEUROMUSCULAR BLOCKING (NMB) DRUGS

Residual NMB drug effect—secondary to parent drug, drug metabolite, or drug–drug interaction
Myasthenia gravis
Eaton-Lambert syndrome
Muscular dystrophies
Guillain-Barré
Central nervous system injury or lesion
Spinal cord injury
Steroid myopathy
Critical illness polyneuropathy (CIP)
Disuse atrophy
Severe electrolyte toxicity (e.g., magnesium)
Severe electrolyte deficiency (e.g., hypophosphatemia)

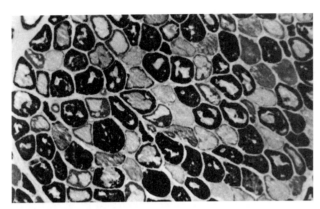

FIGURE 8. A 20-year-old woman developed flaccid quadriplegia and areflexia after 10 days of treatment for status asthmaticus that included bronchodilators, aminoglycoside antibiotics, corticosteroids (methylprednisolone 500 mg per day), and vecuronium to facilitate mechanical ventilation. This photomicrograph is the muscle biopsy of histochemical type 1 and type 2 muscle fibers demonstrating extensive central pallor, reflecting the unusual and selective loss of thick myofilaments (myosin). Also common in some cells is the accumulation of fat droplets. (Reprinted with permission from Danon MJ, Carpenter S. Myopathy with thick filament (myosin) loss following prolonged paralysis with vecuronium during steroid treatment. *Muscle Nerve* 1991;14:1133.)

corticosteroids and NMB drugs). Modest CK increases (zero to 15-fold above normal range) are noted in about half the patients, largely dependent on appropriate timing of enzyme determinations and the initiation of the myopathic process. Thus, there may be some justification in routinely screening high risk patients with serial CK determinations during the infusion of NMB drugs, particularly if the patients are concurrently treated with corticosteroids (see below). Other factors that may contribute include nutritional deprivation, concurrent drug administration with aminoglycosides or cyclosporin, hyperglycemia, renal and hepatic dysfunction, fever, and severe metabolic or electrolyte disorders.

Evidence supports, but occasionally refutes (62) the association of concurrent administration of NMB drugs plus exogenous corticosteroids and ICU neuromyopathy. The incidence of myopathy may be as high as 30% in patients with status asthmaticus who are treated with combinations of corticosteroids and NMB drugs (54). While no period of paralysis is risk free, NMB administration beyond 1 to 2 days clearly increases the risk of myopathy in this setting (54,57). Similarly, there is an inconsistent correlation with the dose of corticosteroids and myopathy, but probably total doses in excess of 1,000 mg of methylprednisolone (or equivalent) increase the risk. Afflicted patients manifest an acute, diffuse, flaccid weakness and an inability to wean from mechanical ventilation. Sensory function is generally preserved. Muscle biopsy shows extensive type 2 fiber atrophy, myonecrosis, disarray of sarcomere architecture, and an *extensive, selective loss of myosin* (Fig. 8) (65). Supporting this hypothesis is experimental evidence that denervation for more than 24 hours in animals induces profound negative nitrogen balance and increases expression of steroid receptors in muscle (66). This denervation sensitizes muscle to even normal corticosteroid concentrations, and evidence suggests the combination of denervation and high-dose dexamethasone precipitates myosinolysis.

Acute myopathy in ICU patients is also reported after ICU administration of the benzylisoquinolinium NMB drugs (i.e., doxacurium, atracurium, cisatracurium) (63). Common to all these reports is the coadministration of benzylisoquinolinium NMB drugs and large doses of corticosteroids, aminoglycosides, or other drugs that affect neuromuscular transmission. The syndrome is identical to that described earlier with acute myopathy mani-

festing as failure to wean and clinical quadriparesis, increased CK concentrations, and abnormal EMG studies, with normal or minimally disrupted sensory function.

Other disorders of nerve and muscle have been recognized in the last decade in ICU patients. For instance, CIP is a sensory and motor polyneuropathy identified in older adult, septic patients or those with multiorgan failure (64,67,68). The diagnosis is often overlooked, however, until patients fail to wean from mechanical ventilation, and the appropriate differential diagnosis is considered (Table 12). CIP reflects a profound, diffuse sensorimotor deficit producing a clinical quadriplegia with marked muscle atrophy, sometimes even affecting facial muscles and cranial nerves, and decreased or absent deep tendon reflexes. Blood CK levels are usually normal. EMG testing reveals decreased CMAP, fibrillation potentials, and positive sharp waves. CIP is primarily an axonopathy, and may be related to microvascular ischemia of the nerve during the systemic inflammatory response syndrome, but is not directly related to use of NMB drugs. The course of the neuropathy parallels that of the systemic illness. Thus, recovery requires a protracted period (weeks to months) of hospitalization and supportive care.

The diagnosis of the patient with prolonged weakness, paresis, and possible myopathy after discontinuation of NMB drugs requires a systematic approach. First, potential residual neuromuscular blockade should be investigated with a peripheral nerve stimulator. In addition, early neurologic consultation with appropriate diagnostic examination including EMG/NCV (nerve conduction velocity) studies, CK analysis, and muscle biopsy may be considered. Prognosis is guarded, as the myopathy may require weeks or months of additional ICU care. One economic analysis of ten patients who developed ICU myopathy found the median additional hospital charges were $66,000 per patient (excluding rehabilitation), but could reach $200,000 in some cases (69).

Recommendations to Avoid Prolonged Weakness During Use of Neuromuscular Blocking Drugs in the Intensive Care Unit

The following are recommendations to avoid prolonged weakness during use of NMB drugs in the ICU.

1. Routine use of nerve stimulators to titrate NMB administration.
2. Prolonged weakness is more likely in patients with concurrent renal insufficiency. Thus, the use of atracurium or cisatracurium in patients with renal failure is recommended to avoid accumulation of active NMB drug metabolites.
3. The risk of AQMS is *markedly* increased if patients receive concurrent NMB drugs and corticosteroids. Thus, we recommend administration of NMB drugs be limited to 24 hours, whenever possible.

Selected, Prospective Studies Using Neuromuscular Blocking Drugs in the Intensive Care Unit

Rocuronium

Bolus administration of rocuronium in ICU patients requires 0.34 mg per kg per hour, with a median recovery time of 100 minutes. Dosing for a continuous infusion is $\cong$ 0.5 mg per kg per hour, with recovery occurring in 60 minutes (48). Rocuronium requirements decrease during the first 6 to 9 hours, because the $T^{1/2\beta}$ (terminal half-life) and the volume of distribution at steady state increase.

Doxacurium and Pancuronium

Bolus doses of pancuronium and doxacurium were compared in a trial of ICU patients paralyzed for 2 to 3 days (49). Only pancuronium significantly increased heart rate (by 11 beats per minute). Neuromuscular recovery was more variable and prolonged (279 $\pm$ 229 minutes) after pancuronium (especially for patients with renal insufficiency), compared to recovery following doxacurium (138 $\pm$ 46 minutes).

Doxacurium was used as a continuous infusion in ICU patients with head injuries paralyzed for 66 $\pm$ 12 hours (50). The doxacurium infusion rate was similar at the beginning (1.0 $\pm$ 0.1 mg per hour) and end of the study (1.3 $\pm$ 0.4 mg per hour). Doxacurium bolus had no effect on heart rate, mean arterial pressure, or ICP. After discontinuation of doxacurium infusion, neuromuscular recovery required 2 hours.

Cisatracurium and Vecuronium

The dose-response and recovery pharmacodynamics of either cisatracurium or vecuronium were compared in a prospective, randomized, double-blind, multicenter study in 58 critically ill adults (46). Patients received cisatracurium for an average of 80 hours at 2.6 $\pm$ 0.2 μg $\times$ kg^{-1} $\times$ min^{-1}, followed by recovery in only 63 $\pm$ 12 minutes. Vecuronium infusion averaged 0.9 $\pm$ 0.1 μg $\times$ kg^{-1} $\times$ min^{-1} for a mean duration of 66 $\pm$ 12 hours.

However, recovery required significantly longer time (387 $\pm$ 163 minutes).

Cisatracurium and Atracurium

Twelve mechanically ventilated ICU patients were paralyzed for 1 to 2 days with either cisatracurium or atracurium. Neuromuscular recovery required one hour with either drug. Cisatracurium was 2.5 times more potent than atracurium, which translated into significantly lower plasma laudanosine concentrations after cisatracurium (peak value = 1.3 μg per mL) compared to atracurium (maximum concentration = 4.4 μg per mL) (70).

Other Considerations with Neuromuscular Blocking Drugs in the Intensive Care Unit

Head Trauma

While patients with severe head injury often manifest increased ICP, the use of NMB drugs is changing in this population. Paralysis was once routinely used to prevent or blunt sympathetic reflexes to tracheal suctioning, and facilitate the use of controlled hyperventilation. However, the administration of NMB drugs as part of a *routine* protocol in these patients may *worsen* outcome with significantly longer ICU stay, more frequent pneumonia, and a trend toward a higher rate of sepsis (71).

Central Nervous System Effects of Neuromuscular Blocking Drugs

Curare (d-tubocurarine) causes marked CNS excitation in animals when applied directly to the cerebral cortex. It is unknown what drug concentration develops in the cerebrospinal fluid of patients receiving prolonged administration of NMB drugs in the ICU, particularly if head trauma has disrupted the blood–brain barrier. Some suggest that the mechanism of CNS toxicity may be due to accumulation of intracellular calcium secondary to sustained activation of ACh receptors.

Reversal of Neuromuscular Blockade

Anticholinesterase drugs such as neostigmine or edrophonium may be administered to accelerate reversal of NMB drug blockade. In the operating room, this issue is controversial because the use of short- or intermediate-acting NMB drugs often allows sufficient time for complete, spontaneous recovery to occur. Thus, the necessity of administering anticholinesterase drugs in this situation is debated, especially considering the side effects of neostigmine such as increased nausea and vomiting, cardiac arrhythmias, bronchospasm, and so forth. Nonetheless, intensivists should recognize that in the acute perioperative period, residual neuromuscular block is often documented in patients in the recovery room and ICU after anesthesia using NMB drugs. The incidence is especially common in patients paralyzed with long-acting NMB drugs (e.g., 40% of patients paralyzed with pancuronium have a TOF ratio less than 0.70 in the PACU). This residual block may modify the respiratory response to hypoxia, result in uncoordinated swallowing, and predispose patients to gastric aspiration. Retrospective evidence suggests this partial, residual neuromuscular block increases the incidence of postoperative pneumonia, especially in older adult patients. In general, if ICU patients have recently arrived from the operating room and are part of an accelerated clinical pathway ("fast-track protocol"), the clinician should consider administering a combination of neostigmine and an anticholinergic drug to ensure full recovery of neuromuscular function prior to extubation. While recovery is more rapid after the administration of edrophonium rather than neostigmine, recovery is more reliable using neostigmine. Also, the more intense the residual block, the longer it will take to achieve acceptable standards of neuromuscular recovery. Lastly, pharmacologic reversal occurs rapidly in infants and children, but much more slowly in older adult patients.

Myositis Ossificans (Heterotopic Ossification)

The term myositis ossificans is misleading because the process involves connective tissue (not muscle), and because inflammation is not characteristic of the ailment. The name originates from the ossification that occurs within the connective tissue of muscle,

but may also be seen in ligaments, tendons, fascia, aponeuroses, and joint capsules. The basic defect is the inappropriate differentiation of fibroblasts into osteoblasts, and is usually triggered by trauma and muscle injury, paraplegia or quadriplegia, tetanus, and burns. Recently, several case reports have appeared documenting the process in patients paralyzed with NMB drugs (curare, vecuronium, and pancuronium) as well. Treatment is active range of motion around the affected joint, and surgery when necessary.

SUMMARY

NMB drugs are administered in large doses over prolonged periods to severely ill patients with one or more organ failures in the ICU. Major concerns focus on appropriate drug selection and delivery, monitoring, and neuromuscular recovery of patients who receive NMB drugs ≥ 24 hours. The myopathy and paresis reported in patients after prolonged use of NMB drugs in ICU patients needs further investigation to identify those at risk, and outline mechanisms to prevent or limit the injury. Pathophysiologic changes in the nerve, muscle, or neuromuscular junction may also play a role in the development of some cases of prolonged weakness or myopathy.

KEY POINTS

- Adequate analgesia and sedative administration prevents deleterious physical and emotional sequelae in intensive care unit (ICU) patients.
- Benzodiazepine drugs interact on the γ-aminobutyric acid receptor providing potent amnesia and sedation.
- Propofol is noteworthy for its titratability (rapid onset and offset), but should not be used for sedation in the pediatric ICU population.
- Dexmedetomidine is a new α-agonist with unique sedative properties, largely devoid of respiratory depression.
- Inadequately treated pain results in hypercoagulability, immunosuppression, a catabolic state, and poorer outcomes.
- Neuromuscular blocking (NMB) drugs are totally devoid of

sedative, analgesic, or amnestic properties, and may be classified as aminosteroid or benzylisoquinolinium compounds.
- Peripheral nerve stimulators facilitate proper NMB dosing, and diminish the likelihood of significant drug overdose.
- Among patients receiving NMB drugs, prolonged recovery of neuromuscular function is more likely in those with renal insufficiency.
- NMB use in ICU patients may be associated with severe muscle dysfunction, termed acute quadriplegic myopathy syndrome (AQMS).
- Patients receiving NMB drugs and concurrent corticosteroids are at greatest risk for AQMS.

REFERENCES

1. Shapiro B, Warren J, Egol A, et al. Practice parameters for intravenous analgesia and sedation for adult patients in the intensive care unit: an executive summary. *Crit Care Med* 1995;23:1596–1600.
2. Cohen D, Horiuchi K, Kemper M, Weissman C. Modulating effects of propofol on metabolic and cardiopulmonary responses to stressful intensive care unit procedures. *Crit Care Med* 1996;24: 612–617.
3. Kress JP, Pohlman AS, O'Connor MF, et al. Daily interruption of sedative infusions in critically ill patients undergoing mechanical ventilation. *N Engl J Med* 2000;342: 1471–1477.
4. Kollef MH, Levy NT, Ahrens TS, et al. The use of continuous IV sedation is associated with prolongation of mechanical ventilation. *Chest* 1998;114: 541–548.
5. Bion JF, Ledingham IM. Sedation in intensive care—a postal survey. *Intensive Care Med* 1987;13: 215–216.

6. Burns AM, Shelly MP, Park GR. The use of sedative agents in critically ill patients. *Drugs* 1992;43: 507–515.
7. Marx C, Smith P, Lowrie L, et al. Optimal sedation of mechanically ventilated pediatric critical care patients. *Crit Care Med* 1994;22:163–170.
8. Ramsay M, Savege T, Simpson B, et al. Controlled sedation with alphaxalon–alphadolone. *BMJ* 1974;2:656–659.
9. Riker RR, Picard JT, Fraser GL. Prospective evaluation of the Sedation-Agitation Scale for adult critically ill patients. *Crit Care Med* 1999;27:1325–1329.
10. Shafer A. Complications of sedation with midazolam in the intensive care unit and a comparison with other sedative regimens. *Crit Care Med* 1998;26:947–956.
11. McNulty S, Gratch D, Costello D, et al. The effect of midazolam and lorazepam on post-operative recovery after cardiac surgery. *Anesth Analg* 1995;81:404–407.
12. Laine GA, Hossain SM, Solis RT, et al. Polyethylene glycol

nephrotoxicity secondary to prolonged high-dose intravenous lo-razepam. *Ann Pharmacother* 1995;29:1110–1114.

13. Driessen JJ, Vree TB, Guelen PJ. The effects of acute changes in re-nal function on the pharmacokinetics of midazolam during long-term infusion in ICU patients. *Acta Anaesthesiol Belg* 1991;42:149–155.

14. Young C, Knudsen N, Hilton A, Reves JG. Sedation in the intensive care unit. *Crit Care Med* 2000;28:854–866.

15. Wagner BKJ, O'Hara DA. Pharmacokinetics and pharmacodynamics of sedatives and analgesics in the treatment of agitated critically ill patients. *Clin Pharmacokinet* 1997;33:426–453.

16. Bailie GR, Cockshott ID, Douglas EJ, et al. Pharmacokinetics of propo-fol during and after long-term continuous infusion for maintenance of sedation in ICU patients. *Br J Anaesth* 1992;68:486–491.

17. Bennett S, McNeil M, Bland L, et al. Postoperative infections traced to contamination of an intravenous anesthetic, propofol. *N Engl J Med* 1995;333:147–154.

18. Maze M, Virtanen R, Daunt D, et al. Effects of dexmedetomidine, a novel imidazole sedative-anesthetic agent, on adrenal steroidogenesis: *in vivo* and *in vitro* studies. *Anesth Analg* 1991;73:204–208.

19. Belleville JP, Ward DS, Bloor BC, et al. Effects of intravenous dexmedeto-midine in humans. I. Sedation, ventilation, and metabolic rate. *Anesthe-siology* 1992;77:1125–1133.

20. Venn RM, Bradshaw CJ, Spencer R, et al. Preliminary UK experience of dexmedetomidine, a novel agent for postoperative sedation in the intensive care unit. *Anaesthesia* 1999;54:1136–1142.

21. Hall JE, Uhrich TD, Barney JA, et al. Sedative, amnestic, and anal-gesic properties of small-dose dexmedetomidine infusions. *Anesth Analg* 2000;90:699–705.

22. Wagner RL, White PF, Kan PB, et al. Inhibition of adrenal steroido-genesis by the anesthetic etomidate. *N Engl J Med* 1984;310:1415–1421.

23. Aubree JC, Lader MH. High and very high dosage antipsychotics: a critical review. *J Clin Psychiatry* 1980;41:341–350.

24. Spencer EM, Willatts SM, Prys-Roberts C. Plasma inorganic fluoride concentrations during and after prolonged (>24 h) isoflurane sedation: effect on renal function. *Anesth Analg* 1991;73:731–737.

25. Armstrong DK, Crisp CB. Pharmacoeconomic issues of sedation, analgesia, and neuromuscular blockade in critical care. *New Horiz* 1994;2:85–93.

26. Lewis K, Whipple J, Michael K, et al. Effect of analgesic treatment on the physiological consequences of acute pain. *Am J Hosp Pharm* 1994;51:1539–1554.

27. Cuthbertson DP. Alterations in metabolism following injury: part I. *Injury* 1980;11:175–179.

28. Bond MR. Psychological and psychiatric aspects of pain. *Anaesthesia* 1978;33:355–361.

29. Murray MJ, Plevak DJ. Analgesia in the critically ill patient. *New Horiz* 1994;2:56–63.

30. Agency for Healthcare Policy and Research. *Acute pain management: op-erative or medical procedure and trauma.* Rockville, MD: US Department of Health and Human Services, 1992.

31. Gillis JC, Brogden RN. Ketorolac. A reappraisal of its pharmacodynamic and pharmacokinetic properties and therapeutic use in pain manage-ment. *Drugs* 1997;53:139–188.

32. DeBroe ME, Elseviers MM. Analgesic nephropathy. *N Engl J Med* 1998;338:446–452.

33. Levy MH. Pharmacologic treatment of cancer pain. *N Engl J Med* 1996;335:1124–1132.

34. Macnab MSP, Macrae DJ, Guy E, et al. Profound reduction in mor-phine clearance and liver blood flow in shock. *Intensive Care Med* 1986;12:366–369.

35. Alazia M, Albanese J, Martin C, et al. Pharmacokinetics of long term sufentanil infusion (72 hours) used for sedation in patients in the ICU. *Anesthesiology* 1992;77:A364.

36. Servin F. Remifentanil: when and how to use it. *Eur J Anaesth* 1997;15:41–44.

37. Segredo V, Caldwell JE, Matthay MA, et al. Persistent paralysis in criti-cally ill patients after long-term administration of vecuronium. *N Engl J Med* 1992;327:524–528.

38. Watling SM, Dasta JF. Prolonged paralysis in intensive care unit patients after the use of neuromuscular blocking agents: a review of the literature. *Crit Care Med* 1994;22:884–893.

39. Murray MJ, Strickland RA, Weiler C. The use of neuromuscular block-ing drugs in the intensive care unit: a US perspective. *Intensive Care Med* 1993;19[Suppl 2]:S40–S44.

40. Martyn JA, White DA, Gronert GA, et al. Up-and-down regulation of skeletal muscle acetylcholine receptors. Effects on neuromuscular block-ers. *Anesthesiology* 1992;76:822–843.

41. Apel ED, Merlie JP. Assembly of the postsynaptic apparatus. *Curr Opin Neurobiol* 1995;5:62–67.

42. Belmont MR, Maehr RB, Wastila WB, et al. Pharmacodynamics and pharmacokinetics of benzylisoquinolinium (curare-like) neuromuscular blocking drugs. *Anesthesiol Clin North Am* 1993;11(2):251–281.

43. Ducharme J, Donati F. Pharmacokinetics and pharmacodynamics of steroidal muscle relaxants. *Anesthesiol Clin North Am* 1993;11(2):283–307.

44. Prielipp RC, Coursin DB. Applied pharmacology of common neuro-muscular blocking agents in critical care. *New Horiz* 1994;2:34–47.

45. Prielipp RC, Jackson MJ, Coursin DB. Comparison of the neuromus-cular recovery after paralysis with atracurium versus vecuronium in an ICU patient with renal insufficiency. *Anesth Analg* 1994;78:775–778.

46. Prielipp RC, Coursin DB, Scuderi PE, et al. Comparison of the infusion requirements and recovery profiles of vecuronium and cisatracurium 51W89 in intensive care unit patients. *Anesth Analg* 1995;81:3–12.

47. Rudis MI, Guslits BJ, Peterson EL, et al. Economic impact of prolonged motor weakness complicating neuromuscular blockade in the intensive care unit. *Crit Care Med* 1996;24:1749–1756.

48. Sparr HJ, Wierda JM, Proost JH, et al. Pharmacodynamics and phar-macokinetics of rocuronium in intensive care patients. *Br J Anaesth* 1997;78:267–273.

49. Murray MJ, Coursin DB, Scuderi PE, et al. Double-blind, randomized, multicenter study of doxacurium vs. pancuronium in intensive care unit patients who require neuromuscular-blocking agents. *Crit Care Med* 1995;23:450–458.

50. Prielipp RC, Robinson JC, Wilson JA, et al. Dose response, recovery, and cost of doxacurium as a continuous infusion in neurosurgical intensive care unit patients. *Crit Care Med* 1997;25:1236–1241.

51. Hudes E, Lee KC. Clinical use of peripheral nerve stimulators in anaes-thesia. *Can J Anaesth* 1987;34:525–534.

52. Brull SJ. An update on monitoring of neuromuscular function. *Curr Opin Anaesthesiol* 1992;5:577–583.

53. Donati F, Bejan DR. Not all muscles are the same. *Br J Anaesth* 1992;68:235–236.

54. Behbehani NA, Al-Mane F, D'yachkova Y, et al. Myopathy following mechanical ventilation for acute severe asthma. The role of muscle re-laxants and corticosteroids. *Chest* 1999;115:1627–1631.

55. Coursin DB, Meyer DA, Prielipp RC. Doxacurium infusion in criti-cally ill patients with atracurium tachyphylaxis. *Am J Health Syst Pharm* 1995;52:635–639.

56. Lacomis D, Giuliani MJ, Van Cott A, et al. Acute myopathy of intensive care: clinical, electromyographic, and pathological aspects. *Ann Neurol* 1996;40:645–654.

57. Leatherman JW, Fluegel WL, David WS, et al. Muscle weakness in mechanically ventilated patients with severe asthma. *Am J Respir Crit Care Med* 1996;153:1686–1690.

58. David WS, Roehr CL, Leatherman JW. EMG findings in acute myopa-thy with status asthmaticus, steroids and paralytics. Clinical and elec-trophysiologic correlation. *Electromyogr Clin Neurophysiol* 1998;38:371–376.

59. Barohn RJ, Jackson CE, Rogers SJ, et al. Prolonged paralysis due to non-depolarizing neuromuscular blocking agents and corticosteroids. *Muscle Nerve* 1994;17:647–654.

60. Faragher MW, Day BJ, Dennett X. Critical care myopathy: an electro-physiological and histological study. *Muscle Nerve* 1996;19:516–518.

61. Latronico N, Fenzi F, Recupero D, et al. Critical illness myopathy and neuropathy. *Lancet* 1996;347:1579–1582.

62. Zochodne DW, Ramsay DA, Saly V, et al. Acute necrotizing myopathy of intensive care: electrophysiologic studies. *Muscle Nerve* 1994;17:285–292.

63. Meyer KC, Prielipp RC, Grossman JE, et al. Prolonged weakness after

infusion of atracurium in two intensive care unit patients. *Anesth Analg* 1994;78:772–774.

64. Hund EF, Fogel W, Krieger D, et al. Critical illness polyneuropathy: clinical findings and outcomes of a frequent cause of neuromuscular weaning failure. *Crit Care Med* 1996;24:1328–1333.
65. Danon MJ, Carpenter S. Myopathy with thick filament (myosin) loss following prolonged paralysis with vecuronium during steroid treatment. *Muscle Nerve* 1991;14:1131–1139.
66. Shin Y-S, Fink H, Khiroya R, et al. Prednisolone-induced muscle dysfunction is caused more by atrophy than by altered acetylcholine receptor expression. *Anesth Analg* 2000;91:322–328.
67. Bolton CF. Muscle weakness and difficulty in weaning from the ventilator in the critical care unit. *Chest* 1994;106:1–2.
68. Witt NJ, Zochodne DW, Bolton CF, et al. Peripheral nerve function in sepsis and multiple organ failure. *Chest* 1991;99:176–184.
69. Watling SM, Dasta JF. Prolonged paralysis in intensive care unit patients after the use of neuromuscular blocking agents: a review of the literature. *Crit Care Med* 1994;22:884–893.
70. Boyd AH, Eastwood NB, Parker CJ, et al. Comparison of the pharmacodynamics and pharmacokinetics of an infusion of cis-atracurium (51W89) or atracurium in critically ill patients undergoing mechanical ventilation in an intensive therapy unit. *Br J Anaesth* 1996;76:382–388.
71. Hsiang JK, Chestnut RM, Crisp CB, et al. Early, routine paralysis for intracranial pressure control in severe head injury: is it necessary? *Crit Care Med* 1994;22:1471–1476.

14

SURGICAL CONSIDERATIONS IN THE INTENSIVE CARE UNIT

MICHAEL S. MALIAN
CHARLES E. LUCAS

KEY WORDS

- Shock
- Systemic inflammatory response syndrome
- Sepsis
- Fascial dehiscence
- Peritonitis
- Stomas
- Intraabdominal hypertension
- Abdominal compartment syndrome
- Open abdomen
- Temporary abdominal closure
- Gastrostomy
- Duodenostomy
- Jejunostomy
- Ileostomy
- Colostomy
- Cecostomy
- Enterocutaneous fistula
- Cholecystitis
- Cholecystostomy
- Necrotizing pancreatitis

INTRODUCTION

The postoperative surgical patient often requires intensive care management for a variety of reasons. Most of the common challenges to patient care following an operation are expected and therefore anticipated. Patients often require hemodynamic monitoring following extensive major elective procedures or when significant comorbidities exist following lesser procedures. Many of these comorbid conditions relate to underlying medical problems, including cardiac, pulmonary, or renal insufficiency. Both intraoperative hemorrhage and perioperative infection may lead to instability and attendant need for ongoing resuscitation. The likelihood is that this will be much more common after emergency surgical procedures. Less commonly, patients without major comorbidity or significant operative insult are transferred to the floor and suddenly decompensate requiring admission to the intensive care unit (ICU).

Severe blunt or penetrating trauma also leads to hemodynamic instability and often an immediate inflammatory response brought about by severe bone and soft tissue injury. The severity of insult as represented by the duration of hypovolemic shock and the number of transfusions required to correct the deficit correlate directly with patients' physiologic changes necessitating

critical care. Blunt thoracic injury compromises cardiopulmonary function through a multitude of mechanisms, including myocardial contusion, pulmonary contusion, rib-cage disruption, and flail chest. An even greater total-body insult is created in patients who have nontrauma emergencies related to perforated viscus or necrotic bowel. Each insult leads to a systemic inflammatory response, which may progress to multiple-organ failure if appropriate intervention is not provided. Collectively, these surgical patients represent a large number of admissions to the ICU. They also share many of the physiologic responses and complications that should be familiar to all intensivists. The goal of this treatise is to identify common problems and their solutions for this type of surgical patient.

PHYSIOLOGIC RESPONSE TO SURGICAL INSULT

All surgical procedures are associated with fluid and electrolyte shifts. The extent of these shifts is directly related to the underlying physiologic insult. Surgical dissection, tissue trauma, and hemorrhage result in extravascular fluid and electrolyte relocation and redistribution. These changes are much more significant when hemorrhagic shock accompanies the preceding insults. Patients receiving 10 U or more of blood to correct hemorrhagic shock typically have marked expansion of the interstitial fluid compartment with at least 5 L of sequestrated fluid. This obligatory expansion of the interstitial fluid space occurs at the expense of the plasma volume. Adequate resuscitation therefore requires reexpansion of not only hemoglobin levels and plasma volume but also accommodation to the rapidly expanding interstitial fluid space. These physiologic responses to hemorrhagic shock present as three sequential but distinct phases. The initial phase is the period of active hemorrhage that ends when hemostasis has been achieved during operation. The second phase is characterized by the obligatory uptake or sequestration of balanced electrolyte solution that is sequestrated primarily in the interstitial fluid space and, to a lesser extent, in the intracellular space. This obligatory sequestration phase generally lasts 24 to 48 hours. The duration and extent of this second phase vary with the extent of the insult as reflected by the degree of hypotension and the number of units of blood needed to restore circulatory volume. The third phase is characterized by the mobilization of fluid from the interstitial fluid space into the plasma, where it is excreted by the kidneys. Whereas aggressive fluid replacement is required to maintain plasma volume and organ perfusion during the fluid uptake phase, fluid restriction—sometimes diuresis—is essential during this mobilization phase to prevent hypervolemia and its detrimental effects on cardiac and pulmonary function (1).

The postoperative septic patient also exhibits an obligatory extravascular fluid sequestration phase. The pathophysiologic responses, however, are more complex than those seen with pure hypovolemic shock from hemorrhage. The duration and extent of the interstitial fluid expansion vary according to the primary insult. Following early operation and closure of a perforated duodenal ulcer, the fluid uptake will be short lived, less than 12 hours, and the extent of fluid sequestration typically will be less than 2 L. In contrast, a patient with a perforated sigmoid diverticulitis with a large spill of colonic material will likely sequester more than 10 L of fluid within the interstitial space. As seen in patients with hemorrhagic shock, this relocation into the interstitial space is obligatory, with the result that fluid restriction will lead to hypovolemia, poor organ perfusion, and multiple organ failure. Concomitantly, the septic patient often exhibits a reduction in total peripheral vascular resistance and an increase in cardiac index, which aggravates the hemodynamic instability associated with the extravascular relocation of balanced electrolyte. The combination of extravascular fluid relocation plus intravascular vasodilation requires balanced electrolyte and fluid resuscitation to maintain a plasma volume sufficient to perfuse all critical organs. The release of various cellular factors contributes to this syndrome, which in the absence of a bacterial source is known as the systemic inflammatory response syndrome (SIRS). The hypotension sometimes associated with acute vasodilation may require the temporary use of a vasopressor agent to maintain an adequate mean arterial pressure. These treatment interventions, however, should not replace adequate volume replacement. During the ensuing resuscitation, the patient may appear overloaded with evidence of fluid retention and even may exhibit an unappealing countenance with diffuse body and facial swelling. This picture of anasarca should not discourage the appropriate use of fluid therapy as judged by effective plasma volume, cardiac efficacy, and urine output (2). Invasive hemodynamic monitoring aids in the appropriate administration of fluids and inotropic agents in this setting. The premature use of diuretics to reduce forcibly this physiologic bloating and anasarca is futile and even dangerous. In contrast, when the subsequent fluid mobilization begins in the septic patient or the patient with SIRS, there may be a rapid increase in plasma volume resulting from autoinfusion from the interstitial fluid space. This may lead rapidly to hypervolemia and may be associated with cardiopulmonary compromise requiring fluid restriction and concomitant diuresis.

Sustained Systemic Inflammatory Response

Siegel and co-workers identified four categories of pathophysiologic derangement secondary to SIRS. The first stage represents the normal response to surgical stress, injury, or illness with modest reduction in systemic vascular resistance (SVR) and mild

increase in cardiac output (CO). There is also a modest increase in oxygen consumption secondary to this mild hypermetabolic state. The second stage is an extension of the first phase with a more significant reduction in SVR. Large preload volume requirements are needed to prevent hypotension. The lactate level may be elevated, and there may be an increased venous oxygen saturation resulting from compromise of peripheral oxygen utilization. Evidence for multiple organ failure, especially renal, respiratory, and hepatic dysfunction or failure, may unfold. The third stage of SIRS is manifested by cardiopulmonary decompensation with a profound decrease in SVR and hypotension. Large volumes of fluid replacement plus organ support are necessary to prevent total cardiovascular collapse. Central monitoring is essential. The fourth stage is generally a preterminal period when hypodynamic circulation, increased SVR, and cardiac failure evolve. This fourth stage of SIRS generally occurs when death is imminent (3).

The goals, then, of the intensivist are to optimize the patient that arrives with signs of sepsis or SIRS with aggressive fluid resuscitation within the first 24 hours. Organ dysfunction and failure appear to arise in the wake of inadequate or delayed resuscitation. Optimally, resuscitation is best guided by the use of invasive hemodynamic monitoring, including the pulmonary artery catheter. Whereas the use of the pulmonary artery catheter remains controversial, it has been demonstrated to improve mortality when treatment changes occur in response to catheter-guided therapy (4).

Numerous studies have investigated hyperdynamic resuscitation with a goal of achieving supraphysiologic cardiac and oxygen delivery indices to improve survival in these critically ill patients. This approach was introduced as a result of a prospective trial in high-risk surgical patients (5). The results of these studies have been conflicting. Mixing a heterogenous population of patients with different endpoints of resuscitation has marred the studies. No study has conclusively demonstrated an improved outcome. One study actually reported increased mortality rate for patients driven to a hyperdynamic state (6). Nevertheless, the goal of optimizing resuscitation of the critically ill patient remains paramount to the intensivist.

A new generation of catheters is available with the ability to provide continuous mixed venous oximetry, continuous CO, and right ventricular function. Optimization of oxygen delivery is dependent on an adequate ventricular preload, which is a measure of the volume of the heart. The standard pulmonary artery catheter measures filling pressures and hence pulmonary artery occlusion pressures (PAOP) have been criticized for not accurately reflecting the true preload. Several studies have reported end diastolic volume as a better measure of preload status in the critically ill surgical patient (7,8). Nevertheless, it remains to be determined what the optimal goal for resuscitation should be.

Postoperative Fever

The etiology of fever following operative intervention for most disease is similar for patients in the ICU setting in the surgical ward. Fever beginning during the first 24 hours is typically due to pulmonary dysfunction, beginning with atelectasis and progressing to pneumonia. Patients with a greater severity of insult related to hemorrhagic shock or infection are at greater risk of developing worsening pulmonary functions. Fever within the first 48 hours often is related to urinary tract infections, especially in patients with indwelling Foley catheters, which, of course, are routinely used in critically ill patients for a number of days. One of the most common and, at the same time, preventable complication relates to phlebitis from both peripheral and central venous lines. These complications are much more likely to occur in the ICU setting because of the multiple indwelling catheters that are being used and the tendency to use lines beyond 72 hours because of the long-term need for intravenous therapy. When intravenous lines become infected, the responsible bacteria are filtered in the lungs, thus increasing the likelihood of pulmonary infection or injury and then are available to the systemic circulation thus increasing the likelihood for bacteremia. When this occurs, organ function is threatened. Consequently, one must place great emphasis on sterile technique and frequent culturing of such lines to identify when line changes are necessary.

A major factor with postoperative fever in the surgical patient relates to wound complications. The threat of postoperative wound infection led to the routine administration of perioperative antibiotic therapy, placing great emphasis on having a proper antibiotic level within the wound during the operative procedure. Despite these precautions, patients may develop superficial or deep wound infections that are more likely to occur as the magnitude of the operation increases and the amount of soilage increases. Early signs of wound infection, such as erythema, edema, induration, and tenderness, often do not present themselves until the fourth postoperative day. Although evidence of cellulitis around the wound without underlying fluid transudation or exudation may respond to the reinstitution of antibiotic therapy, careful observation and examination are mandatory to look for wound drainage. When purulent discharge occurs, it is essential to open the wound down to the fascia, thereby allowing the underlying tissues to be exposed to the atmosphere. When more extensive cellulitis, such as erysipelas, is present, wound debridement and high-dose antibiotic therapy may be lifesaving.

Generally, antibiotics are required. Discharge through the sutures or staples requires open evacuation of the wound followed by frequent dressing changes. More extensive cellulitis, sometimes referred to as *erysipelas*, may be life threatening. Beta-hemolytic streptococci, if unchecked, may progress rapidly and cause systemic toxicity because of bacteria exotoxinemia. Treatment consists of high-dose penicillin and debridement of infected tissue.

Most necrotizing infections of the skin are polymicrobial and often involve anaerobic gram-positive cocci and gram-negative bacilli. Necrotizing cellulitis that is monomicrobial usually results from groups A beta-hemolytic streptococcus. The infection spares the subcutaneous tissues and debridement is limited to the skin. Necrotizing fasciitis is often a mixed aerobic–anaerobic gas producing infection that involves primarily the subcutaneous tissues usually as an extension of a skin lesion. Systemic toxicity is common, and extensive debridement is necessary.

Myonecrosis or clostridial gas gangrene is caused by *C. perfringens.* The massive production of toxin has devastating effects, with rapid spread of necrosis along fascial tissue planes. Even with prompt antibiotic therapy and radical surgical debridement, mortality remains high. Antibiotic therapy should include penicillin to cover clostridia, enterococci, and peptostreptococcus. Clindamycin is used for anaerobic coverage of *B. fragilis.* Finally, an aminoglycoside or third generation cephalosporin is employed for coverage of *Enterobacteriaceae* and other gram-negative organisms (9).

Fascial Disruption

Wound disruption has many etiologies and its presentations varies according to the extent of dehiscence. The presence of serosanguinous drainage from a wound between postoperative days three and seven typically is the first sign of a loss of fascial integrity. Dehiscence or separation of the fascial margin is the likely cause. Although the initial presentation may follow coughing or straining, the underlying cause relates to either the technique of wound closure or superimposed wound infection. Once suspected in a stable patient, the wound is opened to inspect the fascia, and fascial separation is confirmed; then the fascia is closed. When a patient will not tolerate operative reexploration, the wound is not widely opened, whereas an ostomy appliance bag can be fitted at the site of drainage to prevent soilage. In the event of an anastomotic leak at the time of reexploration with obvious peritonitis and soilage, a full exploration is needed. Such patients often need to have a stoma constructed. If the fascial integrity is in question and a great deal of tension is encountered, a primary closure should be deferred. The interim placement of mesh, preferably absorbable, may provide this temporary closure.

Stomas

Stomas are a common problem in postoperative patients undergoing emergency general surgery. Stomas may be constructed because intraabdominal contamination does not permit safe construction of a primary closure or anastomosis. Stomas should be inspected periodically for viability. Aggressive resuscitation, obesity, intraabdominal hypertension, steroid dependence, and profound malnutrition may lead to stomal problems. Complications include simple skin irritation, necrosis, and stomal retraction with intraperitoneal leakage, stenosis, and bleeding (10). Skin irritation usually is due to improper location or construction of the stoma, leading to difficulty in maintaining a good seal around the stoma. Postoperative fluid resuscitation may contribute to distortion of the stoma with retraction and subsequent necrosis if the stoma is exteriorized with tension. A normal stoma will sit at least 2 to 3 cm above the skin and be pink. A change in color is an ominous sign. If the stoma darkens and remains dusky, ischemia of the stoma is likely. A black stoma signifies necrosis. Inspection of the mucosa through a glass tube or scope will determine whether the ischemia or necrosis extends below the skin line. Extension beyond the external wound warrants reexploration and revision of the ostomy to prevent peritonitis. Stomal retraction or stenosis may require revision if parastomal infection is evident or if a localized fistula develops. Bleeding from a stoma is usually arising from the stomal mesentery or the surrounding abdominal wall. Bleeding from the stomal itself may be due to local trauma to the mucosa. Persistent bleeding not evident from the local mucosa will require endoscopic evaluation. Control of bleeding usually can be achieved by electrocoagulation or suture ligature.

The construction of an ileostomy may result in metabolic complications resulting from high-volume fluid losses and electrolyte disturbances. This is more likely when the distal four inches of ileum are resected.

Peritonitis

The prevailing condition in the postoperative patient that is most likely to drive the SIRS is peritonitis. Failure to recognize and treat peritonitis allows proliferation of SIRS and leads to multiorgan dysfunction syndrome (MODS).

Peritonitis can be subdivided into three types. *Primary* peritonitis is generally a nonsurgical condition whereby a pathogen is introduced into the peritoneal cavity by lymphatic or hematogenous spread. Primary peritonitis typically is monomicrobial and is most commonly found in the patient with ascites brought on by hepatic or cardiac failure. Treatment is with antimicrobials alone (11).

Secondary peritonitis is seen more commonly in the surgical patient as a result of enteric or biliary disease contamination. Gastrointestinal tract perforation and necrosis are common causes. Gastroduodenal perforation results in a chemical peritonitis with few microorganisms resulting from the high acidity of the upper gastrointestinal tract. Lower gastrointestinal perforation has a higher density of microorganisms. Microbial dissemination ensues, leading to an intense inflammatory response. Dead tissue and blood products (i.e., hemoglobin and fibrin) act as adjuvants potentiating the response (12).

The normal physiologic response to diffuse microbial contamination is to sweep pathogens superiorly to the diaphragm, where they enter the lymphatic system (13). If the microbial burden is overwhelming, the peritoneal cavity responds by attempting to wall off the pathogens, leading to the formation of a phlegmon or an abscess. Abscesses form in the dependent areas or quadrants or within potential spaces between loops of bowel (14). Prompt percutaneous or open drainage of abscesses is often lifesaving.

Postoperative confirmation of ongoing peritonitis is sometimes difficult. Fever and leukocytosis may or may not be present. A computerized tomographic scan may demonstrate localized intraabdominal fluid, which may be accessible by the percutaneous route. Refractory peritonitis after surgery with evolution of MODS signifies an intraabdominal catastrophe warranting reexploration.

Massive peritoneal contamination may lead to a chronic state of peritonitis with an open abdomen and an intense inflammatory fibrinopurulent reaction described as tertiary peritonitis. These patients require aggressive local wound care as well as antibiotics. Special care must be exercised not to injure exposed bowel that might cause formation of a fistula, which ultimately may become a fatal complication.

Abdominal Compartment Syndrome

Intraabdominal hypertension is a common feature of the postoperative abdomen. The abdominal compartment syndrome (ACS) is a manifestation of severe intraabdominal hypertension and is characterized by massive abdominal distension with attendant cardiovascular, respiratory, and renal insufficiency (15). ACS

TABLE 1. CAUSES OF INTRAABDOMINAL HYPERTENSION

Severe adynamic ileus
Bowel obstruction
Retroperitoneal hematoma
Necrotizing pancreatitis
Massive fluid resuscitation for sepsis or trauma
Hemoperitoneum
Hepatic ascites
Abdominal closure under tension

often arises in the wake of aggressive fluid resuscitation of the unstable patient with shock or sepsis. Several entities may cause intraabdominal hypertension, leading to the ACS (Table 1).

The clinical features of ACS are a tense, distended abdomen, hemodynamic instability, oliguria, and diminished pulmonary compliance (Table 2). Frequently, the first sign of ACS is compromised ventilation. Diaphragmatic excursion is impaired, resulting in increased airway pressures and decreased pulmonary compliance (16).

The consequences of this intraabdominal hypertension on the cardiovascular system are devastating. CO is profoundly diminished because of a decreased preload, a decrease in ventricular compliance, and an increase in afterload (17).

When intraabdominal pressure exceeds 20 mm Hg, renal blood flow and glomerular filtration rate decrease such that oliguria occurs as a result of diminished filtration. As the intraabdominal pressure approaches 40 mm Hg, oliguria progresses to anuria (18). Splanchnic hypoperfusion, intestinal mucosal acidosis, and failure of mucosal barrier function also have been demonstrated. Hepatic and portal blood flow is reduced (19). Measurement of intraabdominal pressure is helpful in deciding the severity of the condition and the need for decompression. Measurement is most easily accomplished through transvesical pressure measurements (20) (Table 3).

The clinical course begins with abdominal distension, increased peak airway pressure, and an increased $PaCO_2$. The mean arterial pressure generally remains stable unless the patient is also hypovolemic. The cardiac index begins to fall and the SVR rises. Urine output diminishes and remains unresponsive to fluid challenges and inotropic agents. The use of diuretics is discouraged. The lower extremities may become cool compared with the upper extremities, and pulses may be diminished.

When abdominal pressures in excess of 25 mm Hg attend these clinical features, decompressive laparotomy is advised (21). Decompression usually results in prompt restoration of ventilation as inspiratory pressures fall. Urine output and hemodynamics normalize. If the patient is too unstable, the procedure may be

TABLE 2. CLINICAL MANIFESTATIONS OF ABDOMINAL COMPARTMENT SYNDROME

Distended, tense abdomen
Inability to ventilate with increased airway pressures due to decreased pulmonary compliance, hypercarbia, and hypoxemia
Renal insufficiency with oliguria leading to anuria
Diminished cardiac output with high filling pressures and increased systemic vascular resistance

TABLE 3. TRANSVESICAL MEASUREMENT OF INTRAABDOMINAL PRESSURE

Bladder catheter is connected to transducer
Patient is supine
Instill 100 mL of saline
Measure during expiration
Zero at pubic symphysis

performed at the bedside unless it is suspected that hemoperitoneum from an intraperitoneal bleeding is the cause. One must maintain adequate intravascular volume when ACS is suspected. In particular, it is important to achieve a relative hypervolemia, particularly at decompression. Otherwise, there may be profound cardiovascular collapse. Delayed decompression in cases of severe ACS may result in massive bowel infarction, hepatic infarction, and early death.

As a result of the increased recognition of this problem, prevention has become a mainstay of therapy. Prophylaxis entails the use of a tension-free abdominal closure using nonabsorbable mesh rather than primary closure in patients at high risk (22). If recovery occurs rapidly within a 2-week period, the mesh subsequently may be removed and secondary fascial closure performed. Often a sustained inflammatory response delays recovery and does not permit secondary closure. Meticulous wound care leads to the formation of granulation tissue above the intestines. It is important to exercise good wound care to avoid the formation of enterocutaneous fistula.

MANAGEMENT OF THE OPEN ABDOMEN

The management of severe trauma or severe abdominal sepsis has increasingly resulted in the use of an open abdominal technique. The most common examples of this are necrotizing pancreatitis requiring frequent return to the operating room for pancreatic debridement. Reexploration of patients with abdominal sepsis from bowel infarction or peritonitis from bowel perforation is another common reason for leaving the abdomen open. Patients at risk for ACS are also candidates for open abdominal care. Temporary closure is performed using a variety of materials, including intravenous bags, Silastic, or mesh sutured or stapled to the skin or fascia. Visceral packing with a combination of rayon cloth, gauze packs, and retention sutures also has been described (23).

If recovery occurs within a period of 1 to 14 days with concomitant fluid mobilization and diuresis, primary fascial closure once again may be attempted. More often than not, however, an absorbable mesh is sutured to the fascia to facilitate granulation and healing. This, then, is followed by skin grafting after a well-formed layer of granulation tissue has been laid. The patients then are often discharged and returned months later for primary closure facilitated often by tissue expansion or advancement flap techniques to repair this planned ventral hernia.

Tubes and Drains

Patients return from complicated abdominal procedures often with several tubes or drains in place. The nasogastric tube is the most commonly placed tube intraoperatively to maintain gastric decompression. These tubes must be kept patent to prevent accumulation of gastric juices and intestinal gas. Otherwise, the patient may be at risk for chemical aspiration of regurgitated fluids and subsequent pulmonary decompensation.

The largest sump nasogastric tube no. 18 French is most desirable for postoperative decompression. The sump is a double-lumen tube with the larger lumen connected to wall suction and the smaller lumen open to help maintain air circulation. Gastrostomy tubes sometimes are placed intraoperatively for suctioning and aspiration to replace or avoid the need for a nasogastric tube. They may also be placed for subsequent use for enteral nutrition when gastrointestinal function returns. They require periodic irrigation to maintain patency.

Tubes may be placed in the duodenum after gastric resection when intestinal continuity is restored by a gastrojejunostomy because of difficulty with duodenal stump closure. This permits controlled evacuation of the duodenal contents, but the patient may still eat. The drainage through the duodenostomy tube decreases as bowel function is restored. Once the drainage has ceased, the tube can be removed.

Jejunostomy tubes generally are placed for enteral nutrition, particularly when gastric ileus or atony is a major problem or when gastroesophageal reflux is more likely due to impaired lower esophageal sphincter function. Unlike gastrostomy feedings, which are given in bolus fashion to assimilate normal physiology, jejunostomy feedings are continuous. These tubes are generally placed approximately 20 cm distal to the ligament of Treitz.

Tubes are infrequently placed in the cecum for decompression of massive colonic ileus. These are generally undesirable and are placed when colonoscopy and decompression transrectally cannot be accomplished.

In addition to tubes, drains often are placed intraoperatively to control local intraperitoneal fluid collections, thus avoiding abscess formation. Drains most often are placed in the pelvis, in the pericolic gutters, in the subhepatic space, in the bed of the pancreas, as well as above the liver or in either subdiaphragmatic space. Most drains placed nowadays are attached to a closed drainage system to prevent bacterial migration through the drains into the abdomen. These drains are placed strategically as described in the previously listed locations and remain in place as long as there is a significant volume of fluid collected. A change in color, quality, or consistency may signal the formation of a fistula. Radiographs taken using water-soluble contrast through these drains determine the size and extent of an abscess cavity and whether it is shrinking or whether a fistula exists or has developed with a hollow viscous.

Enterocutaneous Fistulas

Fistulas are abnormal communications between two epithelial surfaces. The most significant fistulas are those that form postoperatively that communicate with the skin. The fistulas arise as a result of spontaneous intestinal perforation, as an anastomotic leakage or breakdown, or as a weakening of a serosa surface as a result of injury intraoperatively.

Leakage of intestinal contents results in abscess formation. If this abscess finds its way to the abdominal wall via a surgical wound, a fistula develops. The level at which the fistula occurs determines the volume of output through the fistula. Fistulas require attentive, organized management. Volume losses may be extremely high and also can lead to electrolyte disturbances, depending on the level of the fistula. Appropriate volume restoration and electrolyte repletion are imperative. If patients develop a septic response with hemodynamic instability, invasive hemodynamic monitoring is necessary. Fistulas emanating from high in the gastrointestinal tract may exude a very high volume of fluid. In particular, pancreatic and duodenal fistulas may have high bicarbonate losses, leading to metabolic acidosis. Severe electrolyte imbalance may warrant chemical evaluation of the fistula effluent to guide appropriate electrolyte therapy. The pancreatic enzymes (trypsin and chymotrypsin) can digest the skin surrounding the fistula. This problem will not occur when the pancreatic juices have not been activated by contact with enteric juices. Barrier devices, pastes, and zinc oxide may protect and allow for healing of excoriated skin, which is in contact with activated pancreatic enzymes.

Patients with fistulas typically are hypercatabolic and nutritionally depleted. Oral or enteral nutrition often must be withheld until the fistula is healed. Central hyperalimentation is necessary to maintain adequate caloric intake. After stabilization, the anatomy of the fistula should be defined. Drainage of an associated abscess via percutaneous radiologic drainage may at least control the fistula until definitive surgical management can be accomplished. If percutaneous drainage is not feasible, early reoperation may be necessary and invariably entails damage control, with the goals of surgery being drainage and fistula control to prevent ongoing sepsis.

Biliary Sepsis

Acute cholecystitis may develop in the critically ill postoperative patient at any time in patients with or without cholelithiasis. The clinical features of cholecystitis include fever, leukocytosis, right upper-quadrant tenderness, and elevated liver enzymes, including bilirubin. The pathogenesis of acute cholecystitis in this setting is complex and not completely understood. Bile stasis resulting from postoperative fasting may be a contributing factor. Subsequent feeding may result in impaction of stones or viscous bile in the cystic duct. Prolonged mechanical ventilation in association with elevated positive end expiratory pressure diminishes portal perfusion and increases hepatic venous pressure, possibly leading to ischemia (24). Total parenteral nutrition has been associated with the increased incidence of gallbladder sludge, which may lead to obstruction of the cystic duct. The administration of cholecystokinin results in contraction of the gallbladder and diminished formation of sludge. It has not been demonstrated to reduce the incidence of cholecystitis. It appears that the etiology of cholecystitis is multifactorial, with gallbladder ischemia, increased intraluminal gallbladder pressure resulting from inspissated viscous bile, and stasis collectively contributing to the root cause. The diagnosis is made by ultrasound or by computed tomography (CT) scan. Diagnostic radiologic criteria include (a) gallbladder wall thickness greater than 3.5 mm, (b) pericholecystic fluid or subserosal edema without ascites, (c) intramural gas, (d) sloughed mucosal membrane, (e) gallbladder distension, and (f) the presence of biliary sludge. These findings in association with clinical signs warrant immediate attention. Percutaneous cholecystostomy offers safe diagnosis and therapy in the critically ill patient by avoiding the risks of surgical intervention. Rapid resolution of symptoms usually follows. Persistent symptoms and worsening sepsis manifested by increased leukocytosis or fever suggest gangrenous or emphysematous cholecystitis that does require surgical intervention. Mortality is high under these circumstances. Nevertheless, ongoing fever and signs of sepsis without other sources should herald a consideration of occult biliary tract disease.

Necrotizing Pancreatitis

Necrotizing pancreatitis remains an ominous surgical condition associated with a high mortality rate. An intense inflammatory response, often with the development of multiorgan system dysfunction, is characteristic. This entity may present as a manifestation of complicated bilary tract disease, alcohol abuse, or from idiopathic causes. These patients often require massive fluid resuscitation, because of the sequestration of a large volume of fluid both interstitially and intraperitoneally with resultant visceral edema. Necrosis is identified on CT scan by nonenhancement of pancreatic tissue. If necrosis is suspected to be superinfected, fine-needle aspiration can confirm the diagnosis. These patients require surgical intervention with pancreatic debridement and appropriate drain placement. Peritoneal lavage may be helpful. Hemorrhage, persistent sepsis, and enterocutaneous and pancreatic fistulas are common, often fatal complications (25). Ischemic necrosis of the transverse colon requires colectomy with proximal ostomy. These patients often require open abdominal management because of the intense fluid sequestration and visceral edema, and they may require frequent returns to the operating room for further pancreatic debridement. The open wound often is protected by temporary abdominal closure by open intravenous bag and Silastic or a mesh placement. Necrotizing pancreatitis remains a formidable intensive care challenge.

SUMMARY

The postoperative surgical patient is often difficult to evaluate. Postoperative fluid and electrolyte management is necessary to achieve adequate resuscitation. The desired endpoint of adequate resuscitation is often difficult to identify. Therefore, invasive monitoring is an important adjunct during this critical postoperative period. A marked SIRS may affect hemodynamic stability. The rational use of fluids, blood products, and inotropic agents is augmented with invasive monitoring.

Attention to wounds, stomas, drains, and other tubes may identify underlying problems. Ongoing peritonitis, abscess formation, recurrent obstruction, and fistula formation may further complicate care by driving the SIRS.

Surgeons are recognizing a growing need to treat complex intraabdominal pathology and peritonitis with an open abdomen. Recurrent trips to the operating room help to avoid a situation of tertiary peritonitis with resultant development of sustained SIRS and the evolution of irreversible organ dysfunction. Nevertheless, occasionally an abdomen is closed without tension, but postoperative conditions can lead to a severe intraabdominal hypertension and subsequent abdominal compartment syndrome. The intensivist should be cognizant of this problem and should be able to evaluate the severity of intraabdominal hypertension by serial transvesical intraabdominal pressure measurements. Maintaining an adequate preload in the face of abdominal compartment syndrome is essential in optimizing the patient for successful abdominal decompression.

Biliary sepsis is not an infrequent complication seen in the ICU patient. If cholecystitis is demonstrated on ultrasound and the patient is too unstable for surgical intervention, radiologic percutaneous drainage generally can be accomplished. Failure to respond manifesting by a worsening clinical picture may warrant definitive surgical intervention because the gallbladder is often gangrenous in patients with acute cholecystitis.

Necrotizing pancreatitis remains a formidable problem in the ICU setting. Patients often develop multiorgan dysfunction and need frequent return trips to the operating room for additional debridement. Open abdominal management is becoming more and more common in these critically ill patients.

KEY POINTS

The postoperative surgical patient may require aggressive resuscitation, which is aided by invasive hemodynamic monitoring. The goals of resuscitation are to maintain or restore intravascular volume and optimize oxygen delivery.

Emergent surgery for perforated viscus often reveals severe peritonitis, which leads to a sustained inflammatory response requiring large volume resuscitation. This phase may last for days, with fluid being sequestered in the interstitial spaces. Recovery is heralded by a spontaneous diuresis.

Patients often return from the operating room with a variety of tubes and drains. The intensivist should be aware of the purpose of these retained foreign bodies.

Postoperative wound infection ranges from simple cellulitis to full-blown necrotizing fasciitis. It is import to inspect wounds frequently. Necrotizing infection requires prompt surgical debridement.

Infected wounds in the immunocompromised patient may lead to fascial dehiscence or outright evisceration. Both require prompt surgical attention.

Fascial dehiscence often heralds a more severe intraabdominal process.

Ostomies need to be inspected daily for viability and other problems. Bleeding, local infection, retraction, and frank necrosis are all potential problems. Revision is occasionally necessary.

Intraabdominal hypertension is of serious concern in the critically ill postoperative patient. Sustained intraabdominal hypertension with signs of multiple organ dysfunction defines the abdominal compartment syndrome. Decompression leads to return of organ function.

Patients with severe intraabdominal infection are being cared for increasingly by open abdominal management, which leads to planned ventral hernias left for definitive repair at a later date.

Biliary sepsis is an important cause of hepatobiliary dysfunction in the critically ill postoperative patient. Cholecystostomy drainage is an acceptable means of gallbladder decompression in most cases.

Necrotizing pancreatitis poses a formidable challenge for the intensivist. The decision to operate on these patients is predicated on the evidence for infected necrosis. Surgical care entails frequent returns to the operating room for debridement with temporary abdominal closure.

REFERENCES

1. Lucas CE. The water of life: a century of confusion. *J Am Coll Surg* 2001;192:86–93.
2. Lucas CE, Ledgerwood AM. The fluid problem in the critically ill. *Surg Clin North Am* 1983;63:439–454.
3. Siegel JH, Cerra FB, Coleman B, et al. Physiologic and metabolic correlates in human sepsis. *Surgery* 1979;86:163–193.
4. Mimoz O, Rauss A, Rekik N, et al. Pulmonary artery catheterization in critically ill patients: a prospective analysis of outcome changes associated with catheter prompted changes in therapy. *Crit Care Med* 1994;22:573–579.
5. Shoemaker WC, Kran KB, Appel PL, et al. Prospective trial of the effect of deliberate perioperative increase in oxygen delivery on mortality in high-risk surgical patients. *Chest* 1988;94:1176–1186.
6. Hayes MA, Timmins AC, Yau EHE, et al. Elevation of systemic oxygen delivery in critically ill patients. *N Engl J Med* 1994;330:1717–1722.
7. Diebel LN, Wilson RF, Tagett MG, et al. End diastolic volume: a better indicator of preload in the critically ill. *Arch Surg* 1992;127:817–822.
8. Cheatham ML, Nelson LD, Chang MC, et al. Right ventricular ends diastolic volume index as a predictor of preload status in patients on positive end expiratory pressure. *Crit Care Med* 1998;26:1801–1806.
9. Patino JF, Castro D. Necrotizing lesions of soft tissues: a review. *World J Surg* 1991;15:235–239.
10. Pearl RK, Prasad ML, Orsay CP, et al. Early local complications for intestinal stomas. *Arch Surg* 1985;120:1145–1147.
11. Hoefs JC, Runyon BA. Spontaneous bacterial peritonitis. *Dis Mon* 1985;31:1–48.
12. Pruett TL, Rotstein OD, Fiegel VD, et al. Mechanisms of the adjuvant effect of hemoglobin in experimental peritonitis: VII. A leukotoxin is produced by *E. coli* metabolism in hemoglobin. *Surgery* 1984;96:375–383.
13. Tsibilary EC, Wissig SL. Absorption from the peritoneal cavity: SEM study of the mesothelium covering the peritoneal surface of the muscular portion of the diaphragm. *Am J Anat* 1977;149:127–132.
14. Fry DE, Garrison RN, Heitsch RC, et al. Determinants of death in patients with intraabdominal abscess. *Surgery* 1980;89:517–523.
15. Ivatury RR, Diebel LN, Porter JM, et al. Intraabdominal hypertension and the abdominal compartment syndrome. *Surg Clin North Am* 1997;77:783–812.
16. Ridings PC, Loomfield GL, Blochs CR, et al. Cardiopulmonary effects of raised intraabdominal pressure before and after intravascular volume expansion. *J Trauma* 1995;39:1071–1075.

17. Schein M, Wittmann DH, Aprahamian CC, et al. The abdominal compartment syndrome: the physiological and clinical consequences of elevated intraabdominal pressure. J Am *Coll Surg* 1995;180:745–753.

18. Diebel LN, Dulchavsky SA, Wilson RF. Effects of increased abdominal pressure on mesenteric and intestinal mucosal blood flow. *J Trauma* 1992;33:45–49.

19. Obeid F, Saba A, Fath J, et al. Increases in intraabdominal pressure affect pulmonary compliance. *Arch Surg* 1995;130:544–548.

20. Kron IL, Harmon PK, Nolan SP. Measurement of intraabdominal pressure as a criterion for abdominal re-exploration. *Ann Surg* 1984;199:28–30.

21. Meldrum DR, More FA, Moore EE, et al. Prospective characterization and selective management of the abdominal compartment syndrome. *Am J Surg* 1997;174:667–673.

22. Mayberry JC, Mullins RJ, Crass RA, et al. Prevention of abdominal compartment syndrome by absorbable mesh prosthesis closure. *ArchSurg* 1997;132:957–962.

23. Bender JS, Bailey CE, Saxe JM, et al. The technique of visceral packing: recommended management of difficult fascial closure in trauma patients. *J Trauma* 1994;36:182–185.

24. Melin MM, Sarr MG, Bender CE, et al. Percutaneous cholecystostomy: a valuable technique in high-risk surgical patients with presumed acute cholecystitis. *Br J Surg* 1995;82:1274–1277.

25. Berger HG, Isenmann R. Management of necrotizing pancreatitis. *Surg Clin North Am* 1995;79:783–800.

15

NUTRITION SUPPORT IN THE CRITICALLY ILL PATIENT

MICHAEL J. MURRAY
DOUGLAS W. WILMORE

KEY WORDS

- Anabolic phases
- Assessment of nutrition status
- Calorimetry
- Catabolic phase
- Carbohydrates
- Enteral tube feeding
- Lipids
- Metabolic response to surgery
- Minerals
- Nitrogen balance
- Nutrition requirements
- Protein
- Trace elements
- Total parenteral nutrition
- Vitamins

INTRODUCTION

Nutrition is essential for survival because cellular function and structure disintegrate in the absence of adequate nutrients. Appropriate nutrition support may hasten a patient's recovery from an operation or critical illness and may decrease associated complications. Select nutrients are available that may alter cellular response to stress, which may favorably influence the disease process.

To implement a nutrition support plan for a patient, one must first assess the patient's nutrition status and then formulate a plan that takes into account the patient's metabolic response to injury. Most patients tolerate brief periods of "starvation"; however, clinicians should consider providing nutrition therapy within 5 to 10 days for previously well-nourished patients or within 0 to 7 days for malnourished patients (1).

METABOLIC RESPONSE TO INJURY

When a stress such as trauma, an operation, or a critical illness occurs, a catabolic phase ensues, followed by an early anabolic phase, and then a late anabolic phase, described as a slow convalescence stage (2). The boundaries of the three phases are ill defined, and the first phase may be and often is prolonged by ongoing disease processes, such as an infection or a cardiac event (Fig. 1).

The catabolic phase is characterized by an obligatory increase in energy expenditure and protein wasting. During this catabolic phase, serum concentrations of catecholamines, glucocorticoids, and glucagon are increased and insulin levels are decreased, all of which favor protein breakdown, lipolysis, and gluconeogenesis. Following a major stress, carbohydrate stores, primarily in the form of liver and muscle glycogen, provide the basal caloric requirement for less than a day. Metabolism of skeletal proteins supplies substrate for gluconeogenesis and energy production. The obligatory nitrogen loss associated with protein catabolism may reach 10 to 15 g per day or higher, much of which is excreted in urine and is proportional to the magnitude of the injury or illness. If starvation is absolute and prolonged, the body will catabolize both fat and protein as major sources of energy (3). With time, ketones produced by the liver gradually displace glucose as the major fuel used by the brain.

A wide variety of cytokines, including interleukin-1, interleukin-6, and tumor necrosis factor, are present in the circulation during this catabolic phase. The sequelae of the release of these cytokines may include anorexia, fever, leukocytosis, redistribution of plasma trace elements and minerals, hypoalbuminemia, and production of acute-phase proteins. The extent and duration of the catabolic response to stress are modified by endogenous and exogenous factors: resuscitation, infection control, and specific therapies. Volatile anesthetics and anesthetic doses of opioids suppress adrenocortical hormone and catecholamine surges during the perioperative period, probably through the inhibition of hypothalamic function (4,5). By interrupting afferent neurogenic stimuli, regional anesthetic techniques also attenuate the hormonal response to stress (6,7).

The early anabolic phase begins 2 to 3 days following an uncomplicated elective operation. Its onset is characterized by diuresis of retained free water and normalization of glucocorticoid levels. Nitrogen excretion declines, and lean body mass gradually increases. The early anabolic phase may last from a few weeks to a few months. The late anabolic phase overlaps with the early anabolic phase and lasts for several weeks to several months following a major illness. The late anabolic phase is characterized by gradual restoration of adipose and protein stores.

ASSESSMENT OF NUTRITION STATUS

The ideal management of any intensive care unit (ICU) patient includes a nutrition assessment that should identify and stratify

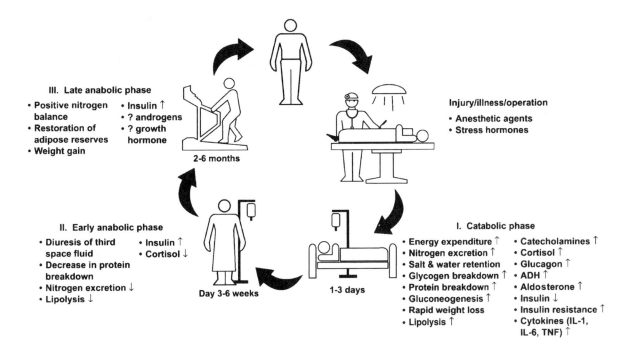

FIGURE 1. Stages of metabolic response following injury.

any preexisting malnutrition and identify factors that may allow the clinician to customize the nutrition regimen according to the patient's illness and needs. Up to 50% of hospitalized patients show evidence of preexisting protein–calorie malnutrition (8,9), which is often overlooked in developing nutrition support plans. Chronic caloric deficiency leads to *marasmus*, a syndrome characterized by growth failure in children, loss of adipose tissue, and generalized wasting of lean body mass without edema in adults. In contrast, chronic protein deficiency manifests as *kwashiorkor*, a syndrome characterized by growth failure in children, hypoalbuminemia, anasarca, fatty liver, and preservation of adipose tissue. A mixed form of protein–calorie malnutrition (kwashiorkor-marasmus) is seen most often. Unplanned weight loss of more than 10% of body weight over 6 months or body weight of less than 80% of the ideal without hypoalbuminemia is sometimes referred to as *adult marasmus*, and hypoalbuminemia alone is termed *adult kwashiorkor*. The clinician must differentiate such individuals from healthy individuals (e.g., athletes) who have low ideal body weight but whose nutrition status does not place them at increased risk (Table 1).

HISTORY

The first step in assessing a patient's nutrition status is to obtain a thorough nutrition history. By determining the nature and duration of any underlying illness, eating habits, and medication and alcohol use and the presence of weight loss or gain, it should be possible to identify conditions that may accompany malnutrition or predispose a patient to developing malnutrition. A history

of weight loss of greater than 10% during the preceding 3 to 6 months is an important indicator of increased risk for morbidity and mortality. Such persons should receive further evaluation and need to be considered for early nutrition support.

EXAMINATION

Physical examination of a patient in an ICU, trying to assess whether a patient is malnourished, is not usually helpful unless the patient is obviously cachetic. There are no specific markers for carbohydrate or lipid deficiencies unless the patient is receiving lipid-free parenteral nutrition, in which case he or she may have manifestations of essential fatty acid deficiency, that is, exfoliating skin lesions. With respect to protein deficiency, the patient may have evidence of hypoproteinemia manifested by peripheral edema or ascites.

One might also look for evidence of vitamin deficiency (i.e., scurvy, vitamin C; rickets, vitamin D; neuropathy, vitamin E; anemia, B_{12} or folate), but these are not necessarily associated with critical illness per se and are usually manifestations of chronic inadequate intake or malabsorption.

SUBJECTIVE GLOBAL ASSESSMENT

Jeejeebhoy and colleagues found that a history and physical examination with a clinical assessment based on the history and examination were as effective as a more intensive nutritional assessment. In their original study, they found that two examiners,

TABLE 1. NUTRITIONAL ASSESSMENTS USED IN DETERMINING DEGREE OF MALNUTRITION

Assessment Technique	Parameter Assessed	Mild Malnutrition	Moderate Malnutrition	Severe Malnutrition
History				
Weight loss over 6 mo	Fat reserve, total protein	<10%	10%–19%	>20%
Physical examination[a]				
Kwashiorkor	Protein deficiency	−	−/+	+
Marasmus	Caloric deficiency	−	−/+	+
Vitamin deficiencies	Vitamins	−	−/+	+
Element deficiencies	Trace elements	−	−/+	+
Anthropometric measurements				
Weight as percent ideal (%)	Fat reserve, total protein	80th–90th	79th–70th	<70th
Triceps skinfold thickness (percentile)	Fat reserve	40th–50th	30th–39th	<30th
Arm-muscle circumference (percentile)	Somatic protein	40th–50th	30th–39th	<30th
Biochemical parameters				
Serum albumin (g/dL)	Hepatic secretory protein	2.8–3.4	2.1–2.7	<2.1
Serum transferrin (mg/dL)	Hepatic secretory protein	150–300	100–149	<100
Serum prealbumin (ng/dL)	Hepatic secretory protein	10–15	5–9	<5
Immune competence				
Skin antigen tests	Cell-mediated immunity	Reactive	Reactive	Anergic
Total lymphocyte count	Cell-mediated immunity	1,200–2,000	800–1,199	<800

[a]+ One or more physical signs of deficiency; − Signs not related to nutritional status; −/+ Probable malnutrition in combination with other factors.
(Modified from World Health Organization (WHO). WHO Expert Committee on Medical Assessment of Nutritional Status. World Health Organization; Geneva: 1963; WHO Technical Report Series no. 258, with permission.)

based on using their clinical acumen, were able to classify patients as well nourished versus mild or severely malnourished with concordance between the two examiners approximately 90% of the time (10).

The recommendation is that patients in an ICU require an assessment of their nutritional status as part of their initial examination. The focus should be on determining whether the patient is previously malnourished, the degree of current stress, what route the patient might tolerate if he or she should be fed, and whether there are particular nutrient deficiencies that should be replaced. This is done using a subjective global assessment and incorporating laboratory measurements as appropriate.

LABORATORY EVALUATION

Biochemical Parameters

The levels of several plasma proteins, including serum albumin, transferrin, prealbumin, and retinol-binding proteins, in part reflect hepatic synthetic capacity. During both stress and starvation, these proteins are decreased. The low levels of plasma proteins may be the result of decreased synthesis, increased catabolism, or sequestration into the extravascular space. No matter what the cause, albumin concentration is the single most predictive factor of surgical risk as demonstrated by patients studied prospectively in the Veterans Administration hospital system. Serial measurement of plasma proteins can reflect the adequacy of nutrition intervention. Because prealbumin (half-life 2 days) and transferrin (half-life 8 days) have shorter half-lives than albumin (half-life 20 days), prealbumin and transferrin are often considered better markers than is albumin for evaluating acute changes in nutrition deprivation and repletion. Also, patients' serum albumin levels may remain depressed, independent of the patients' nutrition status. The serum albumin level may reflect, instead,

a nonspecific cytokine-mediated response to stress and, as such, is a better marker of the severity of stress than it is of nutrition status. Despite these limitations and independent of its cause, a strong correlation exists between the degree of hypoalbuminemia and the mortality rate in hospitalized patients (11).

Other laboratory tests that may be part of a nutrition assessment are measurements of serum glucose, creatinine, blood urea nitrogen (BUN), and electrolytes (sodium, potassium, magnesium, calcium, and phosphorus). Some patients have vitamin or trace-element deficiencies because of either the underlying disease process or inadequate intake or absorption. These situations must be assessed individually. By being alert to the possibility of patients having vitamin deficits, clinicians can identify patients whose vitamin and trace element levels should be measured.

Immunologic Tests

Although the loss of reactivity to commonly used skin tests (e.g., mumps, *Candida*, *Trichophyton*) correlates with malnutrition, the results from these tests correlate no better with outcome than do plasma protein markers. An important reason for the decline in the use of these tests has been recognition that many nonnutrition elements can influence the reactivity rate. Skin-antigen testing is therefore not recommended for routine nutrition assessment.

Nitrogen Balance

A fundamental goal of nutritional support is to increase protein synthesis to equal or exceed the rate of the patients' protein catabolism. Nitrogen-balance studies are an integral part of nutrition assessment and can be used to calculate the degree of protein breakdown, estimate the magnitude of the stress response as reflected in the catabolic rate, and assess the efficiency of nutrition interventions.

The balance measurement, determined by measuring the patient's daily protein intake and nitrogen loss, defines whether a patient is in positive or negative balance. Because dietary protein has an average nitrogen content of 16%, the patient's protein intake divided by 6.25 equals the nitrogen intake. The next step in the equation is to determine the patient's nitrogen loss.

The body loses nitrogen via the skin and feces and in urine as urea, creatinine, and ammonia. Typically, a 24-hour urine specimen is collected, and the total amount of nitrogen in the urine (*Kjeldahl method*) or in urea (the *major source*) is measured. The small amount lost in the gastrointestinal tract or skin is assumed to be about 2 g per day. If only urine urea is measured, an additional 2 g per day as nonurea nitrogen is assumed to be lost. Therefore:

$$N_2 \text{ balance} = N_2 \text{ in} - N_2 \text{ out}$$
$$N_2 \text{ out} = \text{urine urea } N_2 + 2\,g \text{ (nonurea) } N_2$$
$$+ 2\,g \text{ (fecal and skin) } N_2$$

or

$$N_2 \text{ out} = \text{Total urine } N_2 + 2\,g \text{ (fecal and skin) } N_2$$

The major problem with this determination is ensuring an adequate 24-hour urine collection. Total urine creatinine should be measured and generally can be used as a measure of adequacy of collection.

The *catabolic index* (CI) is a measure of stress in which total urea excretion is divided into that amount arising from exogenous protein administration and that arising from gluconeogenesis (glucose–alanine cycle) (12). The CI is equal to the difference between the measured and predicted urine urea nitrogen:

$$CI = 24\text{-hour urine } N_2 - (0.53\,N_2 \text{ intake} + 3\,g)$$

A CI of less than 0 indicates minimal stress, 0 to 5 indicates moderate stress, and greater than 5 indicates severe stress.

Some authorities believe that nitrogen-balance studies should be performed at baseline and after 3 to 7 days of nutrition support, adjusting protein intake to try to match protein loss. Unfortunately, an increase in nitrogen intake, although it may increase protein synthesis, may cause an equal degree of protein catabolism (13).

Energy Balance

Patients with a positive or slightly negative energy balance have a better outcome than do those patients with a more negative balance. Caloric intake is easier to measure than is caloric expenditure, but the latter must be known to calculate energy balance. Direct calorimeters that measure heat production exist mainly in research laboratories. The preferred clinical technique for measuring energy expenditure is by indirect calorimetry, which measures oxygen consumption and carbon-dioxide production. The small amount of protein metabolized by nonoxidative processes can be taken into account in calculating energy expenditure, but this is rarely done because the amount constitutes less than 2% of daily energy expenditure.

All the commercially available indirect calorimeters have limitations. They must be run by experienced personnel and must be carefully calibrated. In addition, they are difficult to use for certain groups of patients, such as endotracheally intubated patients who require mechanical ventilation with an inspired oxygen concentration of greater than 0.5. Furthermore, the sicker the patient, the less accurate the measurements.

Given some clinicians' proclivity to overfeed ICU patients, indirect calorimetry may have a role in establishing a reasonable level of caloric support. Certain admonitions, however, must be kept in mind. In stressed patients, one measures resting metabolic rate (RMR) and documents that rate for a brief period (10–30 minutes). The true metabolic rate of an ICU patient over a 24-hour period is 10% to 30% higher than the RMR. Trying to calculate 24-hour energy expenditure from a single measurement can be difficult. Some mechanical ventilators have continuous built-in indirect calorimeters, giving a measurement of energy expenditure over the entire course of the day, which theoretically should better measure 24-hour energy expenditure. In some institutions, indirect calorimetry is performed only at baseline and periodically thereafter; in others, caloric needs are estimated, alimentation is begun, and the initial measurement is performed 48 to 72 hours later.

Several nomograms can be used to estimate patients' energy requirements. The Harris–Benedict equation is widely used to estimate daily energy requirements:

For men,

$$RMR = 66.4 + 13.8\,W + 5\,H - 6.8\,A$$

For women,

$$RMR = 66.5 + 9.6\,W + 1.8\,H - 4.7\,A$$

Where W = weight (kg),
H = height (cm), and
A = age (yr)

Alternatively, most patients require about 25 to 30 kcal per kilogram of body weight daily. Burn or trauma patients and those with severe sepsis are the exception to this rule; because of their hypermetabolism, they have increased energy demands.

Laboratory-based Nutritional Assessment

Assessment begins with a brief history and examination, including a plasma protein marker, if appropriate, with an assessment of the patient's energy balance. If the patient is moderately or severely malnourished (as documented by a weight loss of greater than 12%–15%) or is in a negative energy balance and is expected to remain so for at least 5 to 7 days, further steps should be taken. A nitrogen-balance study can be started, and indirect calorimetry can be performed.

For example, a 37-year-old man with Crohn disease is brought to the ICU with sepsis after having undergone a small-bowel resection. He has lost 16 pounds (15%) over the previous 6 months. His adipose stores are depleted, and his serum albumin level is 2.9 g per deciliter. This patient is malnourished and stressed. Nitrogen-balance and indirect-calorimetry studies may further help guide nutrition intervention, but the gradual initiation of nutrition support can be initiated without the studies.

WHEN TO FEED

Many clinicians believe a patient should be fed enterally or parenterally within 24 hours of their admission to an ICU if the patient is unable to take an adequate amount of nutrients orally. Evidence to support this recommendation, however, is lacking. One study of patients who underwent nutrition support in the early postoperative period with hypocaloric parenteral nutrition demonstrated that patients tolerated these infusions well and the support was sufficient to ameliorate some, but not all, of the catabolic response (14).

Another study of patients who had sustained severe closed-head injury assessed the effects of early versus delayed parenteral nutrition on immune function. T-lymphocyte expression of CD-4 and CD-8 cell surface antigens and interleukin-6 were measured as endpoints. The study demonstrated that early nutrition support increased CD-4 cells, the CD4:CD8 ratio, and T-lymphocyte responsiveness to a known stimulant (15).

Both studies assessed early parenteral nutrition support. A recent meta-analysis of these and many other studies of TPN in surgical patients demonstrated no influence on outcome; a decrease in morbidity was seen in some studies, but many of these studies had flaws that make interpretation difficult (16). This is not to argue against early nutrition support, but no one has yet convincingly demonstrated in ICU patients that early nutrition support is better than nutrition support started later during the ICU stay, perhaps 5 to 10 days after admission to the ICU. Early nutrition support may lead to more frequent adverse events such as aspiration pneumonia (enteral feeding) or infectious complications (TPN).

HOW TO FEED

Enteral Nutrition

Once a decision is made that a patient should be fed, the next question to be addressed is how the patient should be fed. There is an increasing body of evidence that patients fed enterally, compared with parenterally, do better. The evidence for this, however, is not well established either. From one meta-analysis of 12 studies reporting on whether enteral feeding had a lower incidence of complications compared to parenteral feeding, the authors found that total parenteral nutrition (TPN) compared with enteral feeding had a higher rate of sepsis. Many of the studies had type II errors or were deficient in other ways (17). Despite these limitations, however, when nutrition support is indicated, enteral nutrition should be used preferentially over parenteral nutrition (18). The reasons for this recommendation include the safety associated with this approach, the greater variety of nutrients that can be administered, the presumed advantages enteral nutrition offers to the bowel mucosa, and the reduced cost.

Enteral feedings most commonly are administered through a nasal–enteral feeding tube commonly placed so that the tip is through the pylorus; nasogastric feedings are associated with a higher complication rate (19). For patients undergoing a laparotomy, there has been interest in placing catheters at the time of a surgical procedure using either a standard or a needle catheter jejunostomy. Such catheters, however, have a high incidence

TABLE 2. TUBE FEEDING PROBLEMS AND THEIR CAUSES

Problem	Cause
Vomiting	Improper tube placement
	Rate of feeding too fast
	Residual volume too great
	Osmolality of feeding too high
	Medications given with feeding
	Critical illness
	Gastric atony
Diarrhea	Rate of feeding too high
	Osmolality of feeding too high
	Intolerance to formula ingredients
	Medications (e.g., antibiotics)
	Severe protein–calorie malnutrition
	Malabsorption
	Bacterial overgrowth
Constipation	Lack of bulk in diet
	Inadequate fluid
	Lack of activity/opioids
Dyspnea	↓Functional residual capacity due to gastric/intestinal distention
Decreased activity	Feeding tube in trachea
	Abdominal distention

Modified from Murray MJ. Nutritional support in the critically ill. In: Hoyt JW, Tonnesen AS, Allen SJ, (eds). *Critical care practice.* Philadelphia: WB Saunders, 1991: 477–495, with permission.

of complications. In one retrospective survey of 122 patients, 22 were noted to have short-term complications, including infectious complications (one abscess, two abdominal wall infections, one local soft-tissue infection), mechanical problems (nine dislodgments, three blockages, three leaks), and one had an enterocutaneous fistula. In a subgroup of 50 patients who were contacted by telephone, 19 had long-term complications, two of which required reoperation (20). If a catheter is placed surgically or at the time of a laparostomy, a standard gastrotomy or jejunostomy probably should be performed (21).

For patients fed enterally, there is concern about complications related to bacterial overgrowth within the gastrointestinal tract (Table 2). Nasogastric tube feedings increase gastric pH, which has been associated with growth of microbes in an otherwise sterile environment. Bacterial overgrowth in the gastrointestinal tract is associated with an increased incidence of tracheal colonization and pneumonitis, especially ventilator-associated pneumonitis. Antacid prophylaxis with sucralfate does not appear to decrease the incidence of gastric colonization (22). In an attempt to decrease the incidence of bacterial overgrowth and lower the gastric pH, one study compared continuous enteral feedings versus intermittent feedings. Similarly, no differences in the incidence of bacterial overgrowth were found between the two approaches (23).

The benefits of enteral feeding are thought to occur because the approach is more physiologic; feeding nutrients enterally will provide a trophic stimulus to the gastrointestinal tract, which may be important in maintaining the integrity of the gastrointestinal barrier to the translocation of bacteria and endotoxin. Because glutamine is an important nutrient for the enterocytes lining the lumen of the gastrointestinal tract, it has been advocated for alimenting ICU patients. Unfortunately, glutamine added to tube feedings in doses less than 20 g per day, in hopes of raising plasma glutamine levels, does not appear to increase plasma glutamine levels (24). Glutamine in tube feedings, however, can increase glutamine levels in cells lining the gastrointestinal tract if coadministered with growth hormone (25).

TECHNIQUES FOR TUBE PLACEMENT

If patients are to be fed enterally, successful placement of the feeding tube is imperative. One study of pediatric patients showed that a technique using pH monitoring of the feeding tube aspirate facilitated placement of enteral feeding tubes in the postpyloric position. The technique was further associated with decreased costs and an increased success rate of placement. A pH greater than 5.6 accurately predicted transpyloric placement in 33 of 34 individuals (26). Another study demonstrated the safety of early feeding after percutaneous endoscopic gastrotomy (PEG), early feeding defined as feeding started within 3 hours after placement of the PEG (27).

Other techniques for placement of postpyloric feeding tubes include magnetic (28), sonographic (29), fluoroscopic, and endoscopic (30) techniques. The preferred technique is one that can be performed blind at the bedside (31). Insufflation of air or cold saline through a small-bore feeding tube with the patient in the right lateral position is often tried, along with the use of a procontractility agent (metoclopramide) to facilitate transpyloric tube placement. Whatever technique is used, the feeding tube position must be documented prior to its use because there are numerous reports of tubes placed in a mainstem bronchus in intubated, sedated patients with disastrous consequences if feedings had been started.

TOTAL PARENTERAL NUTRITION

Patients who cannot be fed enterally for whatever reason and for whom a decision to feed has been made should be fed parenterally. Concerns about increased infectious complications associated with TPN are valid but should not deter initiation of nutrition support in a patient who requires such support. Sedman and colleagues confirmed previous studies when they demonstrated that TPN was not associated with mucosal atrophy or bacterial translocation in humans (32). Although this is a problem in animals, no clinical study has demonstrated TPN-associated mucosal atrophy in humans. In patients who sustained abdominal trauma, TPN has been associated with positive nitrogen balance and an increase in serum albumin, prealbumin, fibronectin, and transferrin levels (33).

When using TPN in patients in whom there is no alternative, line-related infection continues to be a major problem. Controlling hyperglycemia (glucose level <180 mg/dL) may play an important role in decreasing the incidence of infectious complications (34). In a prospective survey of 92 peripherally inserted central catheters (PICCs), the incidence of venous thrombosis was significantly decreased if the tip of the catheter was within the superior vena cava (16%) compared with the incidence of 61% when the catheter was proximal to the superior vena cava (35).

SPECIFIC NUTRIENTS

Protein

Nitrogen-balance studies have been used to recommend the administration of large amounts of protein (>2.0 g of protein/kg daily). Feeding more than 1.4 g of protein per kilogram daily, although it does increase protein synthesis, also increases protein catabolism so that there is no net protein gain to the patient (13). Patients should be given 1.0 to 1.4 g of protein/kg daily (36). This quantity is decreased as indicated in patients with renal insufficiency or severe liver dysfunction and may be increased to 2 g per kilogram daily in patients with severe burns (37).

The recommendation is to give 1.0 to 1.5 g of protein per kilogram daily to critically ill patients who require supplementation. Patients with liver failure should receive lesser amounts and, if encephalopathic, may benefit from formulas that contained increased amounts of branched chain amino acids and decreased aromatic amino acids. If there is no improvement in the encephalopathy after 2 to 3 days on such formulas, there is no reason to continue them. Patients with renal failure, especially if on continuous renal replacement therapy (CRRT), should be alimented as any other critically ill patient would be (38).

Glucose and Fat

Most patients' energy needs should come from glucose and lipids. If a patient is febrile, hypermetabolic, and has a high metabolic rate, it would seem that one should administer more glucose. Inhibition of the metabolic process involved in the oxidation of glucose, however, is such that the most severely stressed patients cannot oxidize more than about 6 g of glucose per kilogram of body weight daily (4 mg/kg/min), or about 400 g of glucose per daily in a 70-kg patient (39). Glucose administered in excess of this level may lead to the development of a fatty liver and drive the production of lactate in hypoperfused areas of the body.

Originally, parenteral lipids were developed to be administered to avoid the sequelae of the essential fatty acid deficiency in patients with short bowel syndromes. It is now recognized that because of the insulin resistance associated with glucose administration, lipids are a logical source of calories in critically ill patients; however, there is similar inhibition of the enzymatic processes involved in the metabolism of lipids at the mitochondrial level. In patients who are most severely ill, their cells cannot metabolize greater than 1.0 to 1.5 g of fat per kilogram daily (40).

The recommendation is that, in establishing nutritional support, the energy requirement be calculated and about 1.5 g of protein per kilogram daily be administered. Then the calories contained in this protein are subtracted from the patient's total requirement and the remaining caloric support provided from glucose (approximately 60%) and lipids (approximately 40%).

OTHER CONSIDERATIONS

The preceding determinations should be made independent of whether the patient is fed enterally or parenterally. Although there is less leeway when feeding enterally for making adjustments to the carbohydrates, lipids, and protein contained in enteral products, there are ways to optimize enteral formulas to meet these recommendations.

Electrolytes

Many ICU patients develop hyponatremia, hypokalemia, and other electrolyte abnormalities. Therefore, sodium, potassium, magnesium, and calcium need to be monitored on a regular basis and deficiencies corrected. If the patient is fed enterally, electrolytes are commonly given parenterally. If the patient is fed parenterally, between one-third and two-thirds of the daily electrolyte requirements, especially for potassium, are added to the TPN, and the remainder is given orally or through a separate intravenous infusion, depending on the circumstance.

Hypophosphatemia was a frequently noted complication of parenteral nutrition in the 1970s, leading to muscle weakness and ventilator dependency. Patients are still at risk for developing hypophosphatemia, and so this complication needs to be recognized, appropriate monitoring standards established, and abnormalities treated.

Chloride and acetate must be administered to maintain the electroneutrality of any administered cations, and so chloride and bicarbonate levels should also be monitored. For the patient who has a metabolic alkalosis, exogenous chloride administration should be maximized. For patients who have a metabolic acidosis, exogenous acetate should be supplied. Along with electrolytes, trace elements should be administered (Table 3). These electrolyte and trace elements must be monitored on a periodic basis, usually by institutional or ICU protocol.

Fluids

Nutrients and electrolytes should be administered in a minimal amount of fluid. Patients who receive excess fluid during the perioperative and ICU stay, adjusting for severity of illness, have worse outcomes (41,42).

Vitamins

Vitamins should be administered on a daily basis, with vitamin K administered when necessary because most multivitamin supplements do not contain vitamin K; thiamine must be supplemented in alcoholics; and fat-soluble vitamins must be given in excess to patients with short bowel syndromes who have vitamin deficiencies. Studies are in progress to evaluate supranormal doses of antioxidant vitamins (A, C, E) and minerals (Zn and Se), but recommendations cannot be made regarding this approach at this time.

Immune-enhancing Diets

In addition to supporting the patient during the acute hypermetabolic phase, some authorities believe that nutrients can be used to manipulate endogenous mediators and the immune response; hence, these formulas (mostly enteral) are referred to as immune-enhancing formulae. Although many animal studies are promising, clinical information is limited but is increasing and improving. For example, there has been enthusiasm for using growth hormone or insulin-like growth factor (iLGF) to promote anabolism in critically ill patients (43), but prospective controlled studies have shown benefit only to the use of growth hormone in thermally injured children (44). Likewise, although glutamine is an important amino acid used preferentially for energy by intestinal mucosal cells and as a precursor for gluconeogenesis in the liver (45), only small studies have demonstrated that supplemented glutamine leads to improved outcome. Unfortunately, giving exogenous glutamine does not necessarily increase intracellular levels of glutamine because of altered transport and metabolism.

Arginine is another amino acid that has received a great deal of attention (46). It is the substrate from which nitric oxide is released; nitric oxide has been demonstrated to play an important role in a large number of physiologic events. Unfortunately, the administration or deletion of arginine in the diet has not been demonstrated to have any effect on endogenous nitric oxide levels.

Animal studies have demonstrated that omega-3 fatty acids modify the arachidonic acid cascade and the immune response. Several studies have claimed benefit (decreased ICU and hospital length of stay) to enteral diets supplemented with omega-3 fatty acids and other nutrients (47,48). Presumably, the patients' immune response was enhanced or the release of endogenous mediators attenuated. Some of these diets contain other nutrients, including ribonucleic acids and arginine, that may play a role in improving outcome. Although several studies have demonstrated a decrease in morbidity, no study has demonstrated decreased mortality that may explain why there has not been widespread adoption of these diets for use in critically ill patients (49,50). Moreover, one meta-analysis demonstrated increased mortality associated with the risk of these diets; so caution is advised (51).

A recent consensus conference found that immune-enhancing therapy may be of benefit in patients with blunt or penetrating

TABLE 3. DAILY REQUIREMENTS OF TRACE ELEMENTS IN TOTAL PARENTERAL NUTRITION

Trace Element	Recommended Intake	Effects of Deficiency
Zinc	3–12 mg	Dermatitis, alopecia, impaired wound healing, gonadal atrophy, impaired immune function, psychologic disturbances
Copper	300–500 μg	Anemia, demineralization of bone, vascular aneurysms
Iron	1–2 μg	Anemia
Selenium	50–100 μg	Cardiomyopathy, myositis, arthritis, hair and nail changes
Chromium	10–15 μg	Glucose intolerance, peripheral neuropathy, hyperlipidemia
Manganese	2–5 mg	Bleeding disorders, impaired wound healing
Molybdenum	10–50 μg	Amino-acid intolerance
Magnesium[a]	120–240 mg	Neuromuscular irritability, tetany, dysrhythmias
Phosphorus[a]	400–900 mg	Muscle weakness, red-blood-cell rigidity, reduced oxygen release from hemoglobin

[a]These are not trace elements but are included here for completeness.

torso trauma, but insufficient evidence and data are available to make more definitive recommendations of other groups of critically ill patients (52).

SPECIFIC DISEASE STATES

Renal Failure

Patients in renal failure, whether undergoing dialysis or not, commonly require alteration in their nutrition support. Patients who cannot excrete a normal volume of urine should receive as little free water in their diets as possible. Frequently, the amount of protein in the diet must be decreased. Most patients with chronic renal failure do well with a diet restricted in protein to less than 0.4 g of protein per kilogram of body weight daily. Critically ill patients with renal failure, however, may require protein up to 1 g of protein per kilogram of body weight daily, and patients undergoing dialysis may benefit from protein given up to 1.4 g of protein per kilogram of body weight daily (38). Decisions regarding protein doses should be further guided by assessing the importance of positive nitrogen balance and its influence on wound healing, strength, and cellular integrity; the need for and frequency of dialysis; and blood urea and creatinine levels. Although these patients once were thought to require alteration in the type of protein they receive, most outcome studies have not shown any benefit with diets that contain only essential amino acids.

Tubular defects, along with the defect in clearance of free water, also may lead to electrolyte abnormalities, especially hyperkalemia and metabolic acidosis. Although these patients must be assessed individually, treatment commonly includes a decrease in the amount of administered potassium, phosphorus, and magnesium and an increase in the amount of acetate to combat the metabolic acidosis.

Respiratory Failure

Nutrition status can affect the pulmonary system in a number of ways. Protein malnutrition can lead to emphysematous changes in the lung, loss of diaphragmatic mass and strength, and increased susceptibility to infection as a result of altered immune status. Nutrition replenishment has several potentially adverse side effects. Too many calories will increase oxygen consumption and carbon-dioxide production, and large amounts of intravenously administered amino acids increase the respiratory drive, none of which may be tolerated in patients with marginal respiratory reserves. Large amounts of intravenously administered fat emulsions may alter thromboxane and prostaglandin ratios, impairing lung perfusion, ventilation, and possibly immune function.

The goal in treating patients with respiratory failure is to supply adequate, but not excessive, amounts of protein (1–1.4 g/kg of protein daily) and calories (90%–120% of the RMR). The caloric composition is controversial. Some authorities believe that patients with respiratory failure should receive a large proportion (30%–70%) of their calories from dietary lipids. Oxidation of lipid decreases carbon-dioxide production, which may benefit patients in respiratory failure. Apart from lowering carbon-dioxide production, lipid diets rich in ω-3 polyunsaturated fatty acids

(ω-3 PUFAs) possess modest antiinflammatory properties. Omega-3 PUFAs, through their role in reducing dienoic eicosanoids (prostaglandin$_2$, prostaglandin I$_2$, thromboxane B$_2$ production, attenuate pulmonary dysfunction, and enhance the immune response during sepsis. No clinical study has demonstrated improvement in outcome using such an approach (48).

Hepatic Failure

Patients with preexisting liver disease require adequate carbohydrate calories and restriction of protein, salt, and water. A wide variety of factors (including elevated levels of antidiuretic hormone and aldosterone, hypoalbuminemia, renal impairment, and portal hypertension) can cause salt and water retention. Fluid retention can range from mild pitting edema to frank ascites. In patients with ascites, restrictions of sodium (200 mg daily) and water intake (1,000 mL daily) may help in the medical management of fluid retention. Because glycogen stores are diminished in liver disease, provision of adequate calories avoids the occurrence of hypoglycemia and also diminishes muscle breakdown for gluconeogenesis. Most patients with stable cirrhosis and intercurrent illness require protein at 0.8 to 1.2 g per kilogram of protein daily. With the onset of hepatic encephalopathy, protein intake should be restricted to 0.5 kg daily and should be completely stopped if coma ensues. The clinical impression is that such patients tolerate intravenous protein better than enteral protein. This is because encephalopathy is thought to be caused by ammonia and other nitrogenous metabolites that are generated within the gut and absorbed but not detoxified by the liver. Enteral administration of lactulose, a nonabsorbable disaccharide, diminishes the production and absorption of ammonia. Oral administration of neomycin sulfate also decreases the bacterial breakdown of protein. Even with the onset of coma, protein should be withheld only on a short-term basis. After a few days, protein should be reintroduced carefully in small increments to prevent negative nitrogen balance. Hepatic encephalopathy is associated with elevated levels of aromatic amino acids and decreased amounts of branched-chain amino acids. Specially formulated nutrition products with elevated levels of branched-chain amino acids and decreased levels of aromatic amino acids may benefit some encephalopathic patients to a modest extent. Because hepatic encephalopathy has a number of causes, however, not all patients benefit from such regimens.

SUMMARY

Prolonged starvation must be avoided in patients during the postoperative period. Provision of adequate calories and protein may limit the effects of obligatory catabolic phase that follows surgery. Overfeeding, however, should be avoided. Based on an objective evaluation of the patients' nutrition needs and the severity of stress, only the required amount of nutrients should be provided to the critically ill patient. Patients with functioning guts should be fed by the enteral route because this route is economical, safe, and physiologically appropriate. Specialized dietary formulations with altered amino acid composition or lipid contents may be of benefit in specific disease states.

KEY POINTS

Nutritional assessment of critically ill patients can be readily achieved using clinical acumen and a few readily available laboratory tests.

Nutrition support is recommended for any patient who does not have adequate oral intake. Knowing when to administer alimentation to such a patient is not firmly established, but many experts recommend feeding a patient enterally on the day of ICU admission. Others reserve such an aggressive approach for only those patients who are moderately to severely malnourished and unable to be fed orally.

Patients fed enterally should be fed with a postpyloric feeding tube if they are at risk for developing pulmonary aspiration.

Patients fed parenterally should be fed less than 6 g of glucose per kilogram of body weight daily and 1.0 to 1.5 g of fat per kilogram daily.

Patients should be fed at approximately 90% to 120% of their calculated or measured resting energy expenditure. Critically ill patients should not be overfed.

Protein should be administered at 1.0 to 1.4 g per kilogram of protein daily.

Monitoring of glucose, electrolytes, trace elements, and vitamins should be individualized and initiated whenever parenteral or enteral alimentation is instituted. Deficits should be corrected.

Nutrients, especially if given parenterally, should be administered in a concentrated volume and overhydration should be avoided.

Immune-enhancing diets are safe, appear to be well tolerated, and may be of benefit in select patient populations.

REFERENCES

1. Buzby GP. Overview of randomized clinical trials of total parenteral nutrition for malnourished surgical patients. *World J Surg* 1993;17:173–177.
2. Lowry SF. Host metabolic response to injury. In: Shires GT, Davis JM, eds. *Host defenses advance in trauma and surgery*. New York: JB Lippincott, 1986.
3. Bovill JG, Sebel PS, Fiolet JWT, et al. The influence of sufentanil on endocrine and metabolic responses to cardiac surgery. *Anesth Analg* 1983;62:391–397.
4. Roizen MF, Horrigan RW, Frazer BM. Anesthetic doses blocking adrenergic (stress) and cardiovascular responses to incision—MAC BAR. *Anesthesiology* 1981;54:390–398.
5. Bonnet F, Harari A, Thibonnier M, et al. Suppression of antidiuretic hormone hypersecretion during surgery by extradural anesthesia. *Br J Anaesth* 1982;54:29–36.
6. Engquist A, Brandt MR, Fernandes A, et al. The blocking effect of epidural analgesia on the adrenocortical and hyperglycemic responses to surgery. *Acta Anaesthesiol Scand* 1977;21:330–335.
7. Pflug AE, Halter JB. Effect of spinal anesthesia on adrenergic tone and the neuroendocrine responses to surgical stress in humans. *Anesthesiology* 1981;55:120–126.
8. Bistrian BR, Blackburn GL, Vitale J, et al. Prevalence of malnutrition in general medical patients. *JAMA* 1976;235:1567–1570.
9. Bistrian BR, Blackburn GL, Hallowell E, et al. Protein status of general surgical patients. *JAMA* 1974;230:858–860.
10. Hirsch S, de Obaldia N, Petermann M, et al. Subjective global assessment of nutritional status: further validation. *Nutrition* 1991;7:35–38.
11. Reinhardt GF, Myscofski JW, Wilkens DB, et al. Incidence and mortality of hypoalbuminemic patients in hospitalized veterans. *JPEN J Parenter Enter Nutr* 1980;4:357–359.
12. Bistrian BR. A simple technique to estimate severity of stress. *Surg Gynecol Obstet* 1979;148:675–678.
13. Wolfe RR, Goodenough RD, Burke JF, et al. Response of protein and urea kinetics in burn patients to different levels of protein intake. *Ann Surg* 1983;197:163–171.
14. Jauch KW, Kroner G, Hermann A, et al. Postoperative infusion therapy: electrolyte solution in comparison with hypocaloric glucose and carbohydrate exchange-amino acid solutions. *Zentralbl Chir* 1995;120:682–688.
15. Sacks GS, Brown RO, Teague D, et al. Early nutrition support modifies immune function in patients sustaining severe head injury. *JPEN J Parenter Enteral Nutr* 1995;19:387–392.

16. Heyland DK, MacDonald S, Keefe L, et al. Total parenteral nutrition in the critically ill patient: a meta-analysis. *JAMA* 1998;280:2013–2019.
17. Petit J, Kaeffer N, Dechelotte P, et al. Respective indications of enteral or parenteral nutrition during pre- and post-operative periods. *Ann Fr Anesth Reanim* 1995;14:127–136.
18. Heyland DK. Parenteral nutrition in the critically-ill patient: more harm than good? *Proc Nutr Soc* 2000;59:457–466.
19. Smith GH, Orlando R III. Enteral nutrition: should we feed the stomach? *Crit Care Med* 1999;27:1652–1653.
20. Eddy VA, Snell JE, Morris JA Jr. Analysis of complications and long-term outcome of trauma patients with needle catheter jejunostomy. *Am Surg* 1996;62:40–44.
21. Fox KA, Mularski RA, Sarfati MR, et al. Aspiration pneumonia following surgically placed feeding tubes. *Am J Surg* 1995;170:564–567.
22. Bonten MJ, Gaillard CA, van der Geest S, et al. The role of intragastric acidity and stress ulcer prophylaxis on colonization and infection in mechanically ventilated ICU patients: a stratified, randomized, double-blind study of sucralfate versus antacids. *Am J Respir Crit Care Med* 1995;152:1825–1834.
23. Spilker CA, Hinthorn DR, Pingleton SK. Intermittent enteral feeding in mechanically ventilated patients: the effect on gastric pH and gastric cultures. *Chest* 1996;110:243–248.
24. Long CL, Borghesi L, Stahl R, et al. Impact of enteral feeding of a glutamine-supplemented formula on the hypoaminoacidemic response in trauma patients. *J Trauma* 1996;40:97–102.
25. Mjaaland M, Unneberg K, Jenssen TG, et al. Experimental study to show that growth hormone treatment before trauma increases glutamine uptake in the intestinal tract. *Br J Surg* 1995;2:1076–1079.
26. Krafte-Jacobs B, Persinger M, Carver J, et al. Rapid placement of transpyloric feeding tubes: a comparison of pH-assisted and standard insertion techniques in children. *Pediatrics* 1996;98:242–248.
27. Brown DN, Miedema BW, King PD, et al. Safety of early feeding after percutaneous endoscopic gastrostomy. *J Clin Gastroenterol* 1995;21:330–331.
28. Gabriel SA, Ackermann RJ, Castresana MR. A new technique for placement of nasoenteral feeding tubes using external magnetic guidance. *Crit Care Med* 1997;25:641–645.
29. Hernandez-Socorro CR, Marin J, Ruiz-Santana S, et al. Bedside sonographic-guided versus blind nasoenteric feeding tube placement in critically ill patients. *Crit Care Med* 1996;24:1690–1694.
30. Grathwohl KW, Gibbons RV, Dillard TA, et al. Bedside videoscopic placement of feeding tubes: development of fiberoptics through the tube. *Crit Care Med* 1997;25:629–634.
31. Zaloga GP, Roberts PR. Bedside placement of enteral feeding tubes in the intensive care unit. *Crit Care Med* 1998;26:987–988.

32. Sedman PC, MacFie J, Palmer MD, et al. Preoperative total parenteral nutrition is not associated with mucosal atrophy or bacterial translocation in humans. *Br J Surg* 1995;82:1663–1667.

33. Shu Z, Li J. Total parenteral nutrition support for patients with major abdominal trauma. *Chung Hua Wai Ko Tsa Chih* 1995;33:279–281.

34. Murray MJ. Total parenteral nutrition: can we decrease infectious complications? *Crit Care Med* 2000;28:3756–3757.

35. Kearns PJ, Coleman S, Wehner JH. Complications of long arm-catheters: a randomized trial of central vs peripheral tip location. *JPEN J Parenter Enteral Nutr* 1996;20:20–24.

36. Jolliet P, Pichard C, Biolo G, et al. Enteral nutrition in intensive care patients: a practical approach. *Intensive Care Med* 1998;24:848–859.

37. Cerra FB, Benitez MR, Blackburn GL, et al. Applied nutrition in ICU patients: a consensus statement of the American College of Chest Physicians. *Chest* 1997;111:769–778.

38. National Kidney Foundation. Clinical practice guidelines for nutrition in chronic renal failure. *Am J Kidney Dis* 2000;35:S1–S140.

39. Burke JF, Wolfe RR, Mullany CJ, et al. Glucose requirements following burn injury: parameters of optimal glucose infusion and possible hepatic and respiratory abnormalities following excessive glucose intake. *Ann Surg* 1979;190:274–285.

40. Goodenough RD, Wolfe RR. Effect of total parenteral nutrition on free fatty acid metabolism in burned patients. *JPEN J Parenter Enteral Nutr* 1984;8:357–360.

41. Lowell JA, Schifferdecker C, Driscoll DF, et al. Postoperative fluid overload: not a benign problem. *Crit Care Med* 1990;18:728–733.

42. Schuller D, Mitchell JP, Calandrino FS, et al. Fluid balance during pulmonary edema. Is fluid gain a marker or a cause of poor outcome? *Chest* 1991;100:1068–1075.

43. Kupfer SR, Underwood LE, Baxter RC, et al. Enhancement of the anabolic effects of growth hormone and insulin-like growth factor I by use of both agents simultaneously. *J Clin Invest* 1993;91:391–396.

44. Ramirez RJ, Wolf SE, Barrow RE, et al. Growth hormone treatment in pediatric burns: a safe therapeutic approach. *Ann Surg* 1998;228:439–448.

45. Souba WW. Intestinal glutamine metabolism and nutrition. *J Nutr Biochem* 1993;4:2–9.

46. Brittenden J, Heys SD, Ross J, et al. Nutritional pharmacology: effects of L-arginine on host defenses, response to trauma and tumour growth. *Clin Sci* 1994;86:123–132.

47. Bower RH, Cerra FB, Bershadsky B, et al. Early enteral administration of a formula (Impact®) supplemented with arginine, nucleotides, and fish oil in intensive care unit patients: results of a multicenter, prospective, randomized, clinical trial. *Crit Care Med* 1995;23:436–449.

48. Gadek JE, DeMichele SJ, Karlstad MD, et al. Effect of enteral feeding with eicosapentaenoic acid, gamma-linolenic acid, and antioxidants in patients with acute respiratory distress syndrome. Enteral Nutrition in ARDS Study Group. *Crit Care Med* 1999;27:1409–1420.

49. Jurkovich GJ. Outcome studies using immune-enhancing diets: blunt and penetrating torso trauma patients. *JPEN J Parenter Enteral Nutr* 2001;25:S14–S17.

50. Van Way CW III. Perioperative nutritional support: an old controversy in nutritional care. *Nutr Clin Pract* 2001;16:67–68.

51. Heyland DK, Novak F. Immunonutrition in the critically ill patient: more harm than good? *JPEN J Parenter Enteral Nutr* 2001;25:S51–S55.

52. Anonymous. Consensus recommendations from the U.S. summit on immune-enhancing enteral therapy. *Can J Surg* 2001;44:102–111.

APPLICATION OF PHARMACOKINETIC AND PHARMACODYNAMIC PRINCIPLES IN CRITICALLY ILL PATIENTS

MICHAEL A. DUNCAN
NIAMH McMAHON
EDMUND G. CARTON

KEY WORDS

- Pharmacokinetics
- Pharmacodynamics
- Renal failure
- Hepatic failure
- Heart failure
- Plasma drug monitoring

INTRODUCTION

The basis of all drug therapy involves the administration of an appropriate amount of drug to achieve a useful clinical effect with minimal drug toxicity. Physicians involved in perioperative care are familiar with the concept of titrating drug dosage to achieve desired therapeutic effects. When the therapeutic endpoint is an easily quantified parameter, such as blood pressure or heart rate, small increments of drug dose can be titrated to provide optimal clinical effect.

For many drugs used in critically ill patients, the therapeutic index (the ratio between toxic and therapeutic drug concentration) is low; so toxic effects may occur at drug concentrations that are close to those associated with therapeutic effect. In these cases, application of pharmacokinetic and pharmacodynamic principles may help to guide therapy and predict both drug toxicity and undesirable drug interaction.

Pharmacokinetic and pharmacodynamic concepts have been developed to quantify the complex relationships between drug administration and clinical response (1). *Pharmacokinetic* principles define drug disposition within the body and predict how rapidly and for how long a given drug concentration will be achieved at a site of action. *Pharmacodynamic* principles describe a patient's intrinsic responsiveness to a given drug concentration.

DRUG DISPOSITION AFTER SINGLE INTRAVENOUS DOSE

Many drugs are administered intravenously to critically ill patients as a single bolus dose. The change in plasma drug concentration after bolus intravenous administration is most commonly described by a two-phase decline in the semilogarithmic plot of plasma drug concentration against time (Fig. 1).

Immediately after administration, essentially all the drug is confined to the intravascular space. The initially high plasma concentration declines rapidly during the distribution phase as the drug is transported to extravascular sites. When the rate of drug movement out of the plasma is matched by the return of the drug to the intravascular space, the concentration of drug in the plasma and tissue declines at the same rate; this is referred to as the *equilibrium* or *elimination* phase.

FIRST-ORDER AND DOSE-DEPENDENT KINETICS

The pattern of decline in plasma drug concentration during the equilibrium phase forms the basis of an important classification of drug disposition. Most commonly used drugs are eliminated by a *first-order process*, which implies that there is a linear relationship between the plasma concentration and time during the equilibrium phase (Fig. 1). This straight-line relationship is quantified by the half-life ($t_{1/2}$), the time required for the plasma concentration to decrease by 50%.

The constant rate of decline regardless of the starting point is a defining property of first-order processes. A characteristic of all first-order processes (both drug accumulation and elimination) is that they almost reach completion after four to five half-lives. Therefore, for drugs with a known half-life and that obey first-order kinetics, the time for almost complete drug elimination after a single bolus dose can be reliably predicted.

A relatively small but important group of drugs (e.g., phenytoin) do not follow first-order principles. With these drugs, the rate of decline of plasma concentration is not predictable and varies with the dose administered (*dose-dependent kinetics*).

Volume of Distribution and Clearance

After a single-bolus dose, the extent of extravascular drug distribution (volume of distribution) and the rate of drug elimination

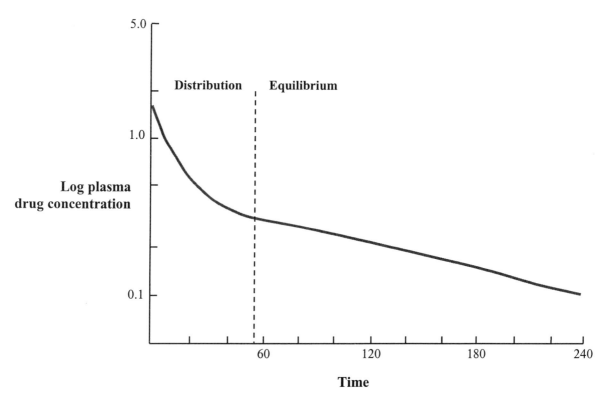

FIGURE 1. Plasma drug concentration versus time after bolus intravenous administration.

(clearance) are the two processes that determine the plasma concentration at any given time. The volume of distribution (V_d) is the theoretical volume available for drug distribution and is defined as the relationship between the total amount of drug in the body relative to the plasma concentration during the equilibrium phase:

$$V_d = \frac{\text{total amount in body}}{\text{plasma concentration}}$$

The volume of distribution also gives some indication of the proportion of the drug in the plasma and therefore available to the liver and kidney for elimination. When the volume of distribution is large, only a small proportion of the drug is in the vascular compartment, whereas when the volume of distribution approaches the plasma volume, most of the drug remains in the plasma.

Clearance (Cl) is defined as the volume of plasma that is completely cleared of drug per unit time. It is a measure of the efficiency of drug elimination and takes account of drug clearance by all the organs of elimination. Only drugs in the vascular compartment can be cleared by passage through the organs of elimination; thus, clearance is closely related to volume of distribution.

The rate of elimination of all first-order kinetic drugs is proportional to the declining amount of drug in the body. Drug half-life is shortened when drug clearance is increased with hepatic enzyme induction, whereas half-life is prolonged when drug clearance is decreased as a result of renal impairment.

$$t_{1/2} = \frac{0.693\,V_d}{Cl}$$

Binding of drugs to plasma proteins also can influence drug clearance if the elimination process is restricted to the unbound

drug only. For many drugs, however, the renal and hepatic clearance is such that both bound and unbound drugs are eliminated.

Drug Accumulation and Loading Dose

Drugs are rarely given as an isolated single-bolus dose. To sustain the clinical effect, repeated doses are administered. If drug elimination is incomplete when subsequent doses are administered, both the plasma concentration and pharmacologic effect will increase until a steady state has been reached. Similarly, when a drug is administered as a constant infusion, there will be a predictable rise to a steady state plasma concentration and clinical effect. With all first-order drugs, drug accumulation (as with drug elimination) will be almost complete after four or five half-lives. In addition, when drug dose is altered, drug accumulation to a new steady-state plasma concentration will take a similar time. In patients with normal renal function, the half-life of digoxin is 36 to 48 hours; therefore, after daily administration, drug accumulation to steady state will take about 6 to 8 days. At steady-state conditions, drug clearance is equal to the rate of drug administration. The steady-state plasma drug concentration (Cpss) and thus the intensity of the clinical response can be altered by changing drug dose, dosing interval, or drug clearance.

$$\text{Cpss} = \text{dose/interval} \times \text{Cl}$$

Clinicians should anticipate an increase in steady-state plasma drug concentration and clinical effect when there is a reduction in drug clearance. In the presence of decreased Cl, Cpss and clinical effect can be returned to normal by a reduction in dose with the same dosage interval or by maintaining the same drug dose and increasing the dosage interval. In most cases, decreasing the dose while maintaining the dosage interval is chosen so that prolonged periods of subtherapeutic plasma concentrations can be avoided.

If the time required to achieve steady state is prolonged and a more immediate clinical effect is required, a loading dose is administered to achieve rapidly an effective steady-state plasma concentration. The loading dose (LD) is calculated by multiplying the desired therapeutic plasma concentration by the volume of distribution.

$$LD = Vd \times Cpss$$

Because the elimination of the loading dose is essentially complete after four to five half-lives, the steady-state plasma concentration is independent of the loading dose after this interval. When the therapeutic index is low, fractionating the loading dose will avoid high plasma concentrations and associated drug toxicity (e.g., digoxin).

NON–FIRST-ORDER DRUG KINETICS

The rate of elimination of drugs with dose-dependent kinetics varies with the amount of drug in the body. Unlike first-order drugs, the time for the plasma drug concentration to decrease by 50% is not constant. At very high plasma concentration, the rate of elimination can be disproportionally prolonged, and the clearance increases as the concentration falls. Important dose dependent drugs include phenytoin and salicylate. Saturation of a rate-limiting step or feedback inhibition may explain these dose-dependent processes.

EFFECT OF RENAL FAILURE ON DRUG DISPOSITION

Urinary excretion is a major route of drug elimination and in the presence of renal impairment potentially nephrotoxic drugs should be avoided or the dose decreased to minimize toxicity. Impaired elimination of both parent drug and potentially active metabolites should be anticipated (e.g., meperidine, allopurinol, sodium nitroprusside). The decrease in creatinine clearance in patients with chronic stable renal failure will be mirrored by a decrease in renal drug clearance, and there should be a proportional reduction in drug dose to achieve the same average plasma concentration as in patients with normal renal function (2). Dosage adjustment in patients with unstable acute renal deterioration is more difficult to predict, and frequent measurement of drug plasma levels is essential to avoid both toxicity and inadequate therapy.

There is no need to change the loading dose in patients with renal impairment. The loading dose may need to be altered, however, when the extracellular volume is expanded (*edema*) or contracted (*cachexia*).

As drug elimination is decreased in renal failure, the time required (i.e., four to five half-lives) to achieve steady-state concentrations will be prolonged. Therefore, in patients with chronic stable renal failure, there may be an increase in the number of drugs in which consideration should be given to using a loading dose to attain steady-state conditions more rapidly.

The serum drug concentration of nephrotoxic antibiotics (e.g., gentamicin) should be monitored daily in patients with renal im-

pairment. The bactericidal activity of aminoglycoside antibiotics is concentration dependent; therefore, large, infrequent doses may be more effective (3). Serial random drug levels will identify when satisfactory trough levels have been achieved and repeat administration is required. Decreased renal tubular function is associated with decreased penicillin clearance because tubular secretion is an important means of renal excretion of these drugs.

Active or toxic metabolites may accumulate in renal failure. Delayed excretion of polar metabolites of morphine may prolong narcosis. In renal failure, accumulation of normeperidine, a meperidine metabolite, is associated with seizure activity. The potential of retained metabolites to cause undesirable effects is not reflected in the plasma concentration of the parent drug.

The clearance of drugs by renal replacement therapy is related to the molecular weight of the drug, its solubility, and the degree of protein binding. It will be influenced also by the properties of the dialysis system itself and the amount of drug in the plasma and hence to the volume of distribution of the drug (4). After intermittent hemodialysis, a supplementary dose of piperacillin/azobactam may be required to avoid subtherapeutic drug concentrations. The reduced dose of meropenem used in renal failure may need to be increased in the presence of continuous renal replacement.

EFFECT OF LIVER FAILURE ON DRUG DISPOSITION

With progressive hepatic dysfunction, there may be a variable and frequently unpredictable reduction in effective hepatic blood flow, hepatic drug metabolizing capacity, and plasma protein binding (5). The result may be an increased, decreased, or unchanged hepatic drug clearance. Conjugative biotransformation reactions seem to be less impaired than oxidative reactions by chronic hepatic dysfunction. Drugs excreted unchanged in the bile (e.g., fucidic acid, rifampicin) may accumulate in obstructive jaundice. The effect of changes in plasma protein binding on drug disposition in patients with liver disease remains uncertain. Moreover, alterations in drug disposition do not correlate with standard indices of hepatic function. In liver failure, drug administration must be adjusted according to careful clinical assessment of drug effects and through judicious use of plasma drug levels. Toxic effects may be seen at lower drug doses (e.g., valproate) in patients with hepatic impairment. In patients with portocaval shunts, there is a decrease in effective hepatic blood flow. Hepatic clearance of highly extracted drugs will be decreased and bioavailability after an oral dose may be increased.

Patients with Child's class A hepatic dysfunction require minimal manipulation of their medication, although there may be altered pharmacodynamic responses. Patients with Child's class C dysfunction require significant alteration in medication, especially if there is accompanying renal impairment.

EFFECT OF HEART FAILURE ON DRUG DISPOSITION

The decrease in tissue perfusion associated with heart failure from any cause is associated with preferential perfusion of the highly perfused organs. The consequent reduction in volume of distribution leads to higher plasma drug concentrations and increased risk of toxicity if the same loading dose is used (6). Heart failure also may be associated with decreased renal and hepatic clearance, resulting in an increase in plasma level and prolongation of the half-life (e.g., theophylline). If clearance and volume of distribution are decreased by a similar extent, there may be little change in half-life, but the steady-state plasma level and clinical effect will be increased secondary to the change in clearance. There are no reliable predictors of these changes in patients with heart failure, and drug dosage is guided by careful observation for signs of toxicity and repeated measurement of drug plasma concentration.

EFFECT OF CHANGES IN PLASMA PROTEIN BINDING ON DRUG DISPOSITION

Although most plasma drug assays measure total drug (both bound and unbound), there is increasing evidence that the concentration of unbound drug may be more closely associated with clinical effect (therapeutic or toxic) than total drug plasma concentration. For some drugs, distribution and elimination are restricted to the unbound drug. Passage of lidocaine across the blood–brain barrier is influenced by the plasma concentration of unbound lidocaine (7). Even small changes in the concentration of carrier protein will have a significant effect on the plasma concentration of the unbound drug, particularly for drugs that are highly bound. These drugs include midazolam, thiopentone, fentanyl, lidocaine, bupivicaine, warfarin, digoxin, and cephalosporin antibiotics.

Weak bases (e.g., propranolol, lidocaine) bind to α-1-acid glycoprotein (AAG), an acute phase reactant, whereas acidic drugs (e.g., warfarin, phenytoin, salicylate) bind to albumin. An abrupt increase in AAG after trauma or surgery may be associated with increased drug binding, a decrease in volume of distribution, and a decrease in free drug concentration. This may explain an ineffective therapeutic result despite normal total drug plasma concentration.

The decrease in albumin concentration in the perioperative period is due predominantly to transfer of albumin from the intravascular to the extravascular space. This transfer may lead to an increase in volume of distribution and a decrease in bound drug concentration in plasma. The effect on plasma-free drug concentration is more difficult to predict, but it may increase due to relative lack of binding sites. There may be an increased risk of drug toxicity in patients with low albumin concentration, despite normal total drug plasma concentration (e.g., phenytoin). The increase in free drug also may lead to increased clearance, which, in conjunction with the increase in volume of distribution, would tend to keep the half-life relatively unchanged.

In all these cases, adjustment of dosage should be based on careful clinical assessment of the therapeutic effect and, where available, measurement of plasma unbound drug concentration. The effect of exogenously administered colloid solutions on anionic drug disposition is not known, particularly in patients with increased capillary endothelium permeability.

DRUG DISPOSITION IN ELDERLY PATIENTS

It is not uncommon to prescribe multiple medications for elderly patients. In addition to the age-related changes in body composition and organ function, there is an increased prevalence of cardiac, renal, and neurologic disease processes in this population. There may be impaired cardiovascular responses that predispose to arterial hypotension. The decreased functional reserve of the organs of elimination is associated with reduced clearance with or without an increased volume of distribution. These changes can lead to prolonged elimination half-life and drug dose and frequency should be adjusted accordingly. Even allowing for these pharmacokinetic changes, there may be increased sensitivity to many medications (sedatives, narcotic analgesics) in elderly patients.

DRUG INTERACTIONS

The possibility of adverse drug interactions should be considered in all patients in whom multiple concomitant medications are being administered. These interactions may be pharmacokinetic and may alter the concentration of the drug at its site of action; or they may be pharmacodynamic interactions, leading to altered sensitivity to a given drug concentration.

Decreased plasma drug concentration may be associated with increased clearance secondary to hepatic enzyme induction following coadministration of drugs such as phenobarbitone. Increased plasma drug concentration may be associated with hepatic enzyme inhibition by coadministration of drugs such as cimetidine (Table 1). There may be considerable interpatient variability in the extent to which important drug interactions occur. Displacement of a highly protein-bound drug by the administration of a second highly bound drug may lead to an increase in the plasma concentration of free drug and an exaggerated clinical response (e.g., phenytoin) on administration in a patient who is receiving warfarin therapy.

PRACTICAL USE OF PLASMA DRUG CONCENTRATION

Variations in clinical response to a given drug dose may be due to a wide range of factors. Genetic differences in metabolizing capacity, concomitant drug administration, and age- or disease-related changes in organs of elimination all may contribute to

TABLE 1. HEPATIC ENZYME INDUCERS/INHIBITORS

Inducers	Inhibitors
Phenobarbitone	Cimetidine
Rimfampicin	Erythromycin
Phenytoin	Ketoconazole
Carbamazepine	Amiodarone

Note: Increased hepatic clearance of drugs is associated with coadministration of hepatic enzyme inducers. Decreased clearance is associated with coadministration of hepatic enzyme inhibitors.

First-order kinetics

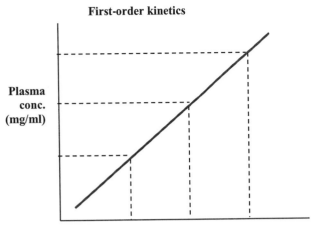

A

Drug dose (mg)

Zero-order kinetics

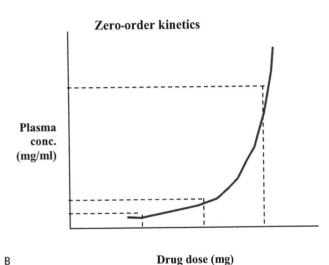

B   **Drug dose (mg)**

FIGURE 2. A: An increase in dose of drugs with first-order kinetics leads to a proportional increase in plasma concentration at steady state conditions. **B:** A similar increase in dose of drugs with zero-order kinetics leads to a disproportionate increase in plasma concentration at steady state.

unpredictable clinical response. When the therapeutic index is low, careful clinical assessment for signs of toxicity may be usefully supplemented by repeated measurement of plasma drug concentration.

If the plasma concentration reflects the concentration at the site of action (e.g., lidocaine), both the therapeutic and toxic effects will be most apparent during the distribution phase. For drugs that are distributed to their site of action more slowly (e.g., digoxin), the plasma concentration will reflect the drug concentration at the site of action only at the end of the distribution phase. Plasma concentrations of digoxin taken before the distribution phase is complete may be misleading. When high concentrations of a drug are not associated with toxicity, supranormal doses may be administered to prolong the clinical effect of rapidly eliminated drugs (e.g., penicillin).

For drugs with first-order kinetics, doubling the dose leads to a doubling of the plasma concentration after steady-state conditions have been achieved. For dose-dependent drugs, an alteration in drug dose may be associated with a wide range of plasma concentrations, and repeated determination of plasma drug concentration will guide therapy, particularly when there are ongoing changes in cardiac and renal function (Fig. 2). In critically ill patients, the dose of drugs such as digoxin, theophylline, lidocaine, aminoglycoside antibiotics, and anticonvulsants should be adjusted with reference to plasma concentration.

SUMMARY

Pharmacokinetic variables may change rapidly in critically ill patients, and pathologic states may be associated with atypical pharmacodynamic responses or may predispose patients to drug toxicity. In addition, interindividual pharmacokinetic and pharmacodynamic variability is common. Factors such as age, sex, diet, presence of inflammatory mediators, and the use of multiple concurrent medications may profoundly affect the already complex relationship between drug administration and drug effect. An understanding of basic pharmacokinetic and pharmacodynamic principles will guide drug therapy under these dynamic conditions to minimize unwanted effects and maximize therapeutic benefit.

KEY POINTS

Most commonly used drugs in the ICU are eliminated by a first-order process, which implies that there is a linear relationship between the plasma concentration and time during this elimination or equilibrium phase.

A relatively small but very important group of drugs (phenytoin, salicylate, and theophylline) do not follow first-order principles. The rate of decline of plasma concentration is unpredictable and varies with the dose administered.

Volume of distribution (V_d) is the theoretical volume available for drug distribution defined as the relationship between the total amount of drug in the body relative to the plasma concentration during the equilibrium phase.

When the rate of drug movement out of the plasma is matched by the return of the drug to the intravascular space, the concentration of drug in plasma and tissue declines at the same rate during this elimination (equilibrium) phase.

Clearance is defined as the volume of plasma that is completely cleared of drug per unit time.

With first-order drugs, drug accumulation will be almost complete after three to four doses.

REFERENCES

1. Park GR. Pharmacokinetics and pharmacodynamics in the critically ill patient. *Xenobiotica* 1993;23:1195–1230.
2. Bennett W, et al. *Drug prescribing in renal failure—dosing guidelines.* Philadelphia: American College of Physicians, 1999.
3. Parker SE, Davey PG. Once-daily aminoglycoside dosing. *Lancet* 1993;341:346–347.
4. Bressolle F, Kinowski JM, de la Coussaye JE, et al. Clinical pharmacoki-netics during continuous haemofiltration. *Clin Pharmacokinet* 1994;26:457–471.
5. Williams RL. Drug administration in hepatic disease. *N Engl J Med* 1983;309:1616–1622.
6. Williams RL, Bennet LZ. Drug pharmacokinetics in cardiac and hepatic disease. *Annu Rev Pharmacol Toxicol* 1980;20:389–413.
7. Marathe PH, Shen DD, Arttu AA, et al. Effect of serum protein binding on the entry of lidnocaine into brain and CSF in dogs. *Anesthesiology* 1991;75:804–812.

ETIOLOGY AND PATHOPHYSIOLOGY
OF SHOCK

ROBERT M. RODRIGUEZ
MYER H. ROSENTHAL

KEY WORDS

- Cardiogenic shock
- Classification of shock
- Cytokines
- Hyperdynamic shock
- Hypovolemic shock
- Lactate
- Obstructive mechanisms of shock
- Oxygen delivery
- Pathophysiology of shock
- Septic shock
- Vasopressor agents
- Approach to the patient with shock

INTRODUCTION

Shock is one of the most common causes of death in the United States today and, together with respiratory failure, accounts for most emergent intensive care unit (ICU) admissions. The Centers for Disease Control and Prevention (CDC) statistics for 1998 show that "septicemia" alone was the eleventh leading cause of death (1). "Accidents and adverse effects" was the fifth leading cause of death, with 40% of deaths in this category related to hemorrhage and hemorrhagic shock (1,2). Likewise, many patients included in the number one cause of death, "diseases of the heart," died of cardiogenic shock.

The magnitude of the problem of shock is illustrated not only by absolute numbers of deaths but also in the high mortality percentages seen with various types of shock. Septic shock is generally considered to have a mortality rate between 40% and 60%, and cardiogenic shock has an even higher mortality rate (3,4). For these reasons, shock has, and will continue to be, a major focus of research in critical care medicine.

Many diverse etiologies produce shock, and although physicians generally focus on singular pathophysiologic mechanisms in individual patients, it is clear that the shock state in many, if not most, patients arises from complex interactions of several mechanisms. Splanchnic hypoperfusion, regardless of etiology, impairs both intestinal-barrier and hepatic-reticuloendothelial functions, leading to bacterial translocation and increased levels of circulating endotoxin and cytokines. Consequently, hypovolemic and cardiogenic shock may be complicated by the low vascular resistance that is characteristic of hyperdynamic or septic shock. Likewise, widespread vasodilation and altered capillary permeability lead to both relative and absolute hypovolemia in patients with septic shock. Finally, depressed cardiac function, secondary to coronary hypoperfusion and negative inotropic effects of myocardial depressant factor or factors, commonly exacerbates septic shock. Figure 1 demonstrates the interrelationships of these three shock states.

Despite this physiologic complexity and the myriad etiologic mechanisms, the diversity of shock converges at the tissue and cellular levels. Central to any definition of shock is the concept of inadequate systemic perfusion to tissues and cells. This inadequacy of perfusion causes cellular hypoxia, which inhibits oxidative phosphorylation, the process by which 95% of the body's energy is generated. Under these anaerobic conditions, the physiologic energy source is the inefficient glycolytic cycle, which produces two adenosine triphosphate (ATP) molecules, four hydrogen ions, and two pyruvate molecules from each glucose molecule. Accumulation of pyruvate and hydrogen ions, according to the law of mass action, would prevent further glycolysis. In the presence of the nicotinamide adenine dinucleotide (NAD^+) co-factor, however, pyruvate and hydrogen combine to form lactic acid, a critical metabolite that is discussed later in this chapter.

Also critical to the understanding of shock is the concept that shock is an end-stage of a continuum of progressive physiologic derangement. Examining sepsis and the progression from the systemic inflammatory response syndrome (SIRS) to septic shock in a large cohort of patients, Rangel-Frausto and colleagues found that 71% of patients with culture-proven septic shock had been previously identified in the milder categories of SIRS, sepsis, or severe sepsis (5). Yet only 4% of patients with SIRS progressed to full septic shock. Patients suffering from hemorrhagic shock also exhibit a physiologic continuum from tachycardia and narrowed pulse pressure to marked hypotension as shock progresses. It is imperative, therefore, that clinicians recognize the early stages of shock at a time when it will be more responsive to treatment. The early signs that are common to nearly all types of shock are tachycardia, tachypnea, decreased urine output, and altered mental status. Skin signs of decreased perfusion, such as mottling, are also common early features of shock; however, patients with early septic or distributive shock may have inappropriately dilated

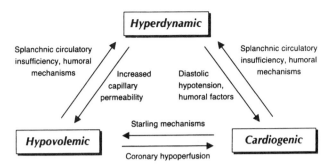

FIGURE 1. The interrelationships of the three principal shock states and the pathophysiologic mechanisms influencing these relationships.

and warm skin. Hypotension is deliberately excluded from this list of early signs because once it occurs, the shock state is usually obvious and may be quite advanced. The physician must not wait for the patient to exhibit hypotension before diagnosing shock.

Another important concept is that most patients do not die from the hypotensive shock state itself, but rather they ultimately die as a result of the sequelae of shock, namely, organ dysfunction and failure. While the brain, cardiovascular system, and kidneys show the most obvious signs of failure, essentially all organs are affected by cellular hypoxia and by inflammatory response–mediated microvascular injury. Anaerobic metabolism leads to lactic acidosis. The worsening of hypoxemia, diffuse pulmonary infiltrates, and decreased lung compliance herald progression from acute lung injury to acute respiratory distress syndrome (ARDS), which develops in approximately 64% of patients with septic shock (6). Likewise, hyperbilirubinemia and transaminase elevations mark the onset of hepatic dysfunction, and decreased bowel motility and gastrointestinal hemorrhage indicate intestinal ischemia. Together, these and other organ-system abnormalities constitute the multiple-organ dysfunction syndrome (MODS), a high-mortality condition that is discussed more fully in Chapter 18. The clinician's challenges are thus to recognize promptly the various shock states and to treat both the pathophysiologic hemodynamic alterations and their etiologies to prevent deterioration to MODS.

CLASSIFICATION OF SHOCK

Because patients and their physiologies do not often fall into clearly defined categories, many worthwhile shock classification schemes have been proposed. The most frequently cited categorization divides shock into three types: *septic* (hyperdynamic), *cardiogenic*, and *hypovolemic* (hemorrhagic). As discussed earlier in this chapter, shock states evolve, and several mechanisms of hypoperfusion interact in each patient. A patient with septic shock initially may present in a classic compensated high cardiac output (CO), low systemic vascular resistance (SVR) state. If this same septic patient's mechanisms of compensation fail, CO may decrease, SVR may increase, and the patient will no longer exhibit the classic picture of sepsis. With this in mind, a modification of the previous categorization is proposed in this chapter (Table 1). Several obstructive causes of shock should be diagnosed and treated rapidly before the physician considers other causes of

shock. Cardiac output and intravascular volume status are used to construct this classification. Examining three major physiologic categories of shock, the findings of the physical examination and invasive hemodynamic monitoring for patients in each category are presented. Specific disease entities are discussed in the most relevant categories.

Obstructive Mechanisms of Shock

Three principal reasons exist for the decision to discuss the obstructive mechanisms of shock as a separate consideration. First, these obstructive mechanisms share the common sign of distended neck veins or elevated central venous pressure, which in most patients would point to volume overload. The true physiologic state, however, is one of decreased left ventricular preload with associated low CO secondary to obstruction of filling of the left and sometimes right ventricle. Treatment of these disorders includes fluid resuscitation rather than the withholding of fluids as the clinical sign of venous distention might direct. Second, these causes of shock have specific therapies, such as pericardiocentesis for cardiac tamponade, that may quickly relieve the obstruction and reverse the shock. Third, and most important, shock resulting from obstructive mechanisms may progress rapidly to pulseless cardiac electrical activity, a state with a very poor prognosis. It is critical, therefore, that the physician faced with a patient who is developing shock rapidly consider these causes before moving on to the more common causes.

The first obstructive mechanism to consider is tension pneumothorax, in which a one-way valve defect of the lung or chest wall causes progressive accumulation of air in the thoracic cavity, producing lung collapse, mediastinal shift, and obstruction of venous return to the right side of the heart. Risk factors include trauma to the neck, back, or torso; insertion of jugular or subclavian central venous catheters; bronchoscopy; thoracoscopy; and mechanical ventilation with high tidal volumes and high airway pressures. In addition to hypotension, tachycardia, and distended neck veins, a major sign of tension pneumothorax is absent or markedly decreased breath sounds on one side of the chest with unilateral tympany to percussion. Bilateral absent breath sounds with shock may indicate the unusual case of bilateral tension pneumothorax. Deviated trachea and cyanosis are inconsistent and late signs. Treatment of tension pneumothorax consists of immediate decompression with a 14-gauge catheter placed in the second intercostal space at the midclavicular line, usually followed by chest-tube placement. In the presence of hemodynamic instability, treatment should not be delayed for radiographic confirmation of the pneumothorax.

Accumulation of fluid in the pericardial space may result in cardiac tamponade, a second obstructive cause of shock. Using a canine model of tamponade, Ditchey et al. demonstrated that right ventricular (RV) failure precedes left ventricular (LV) failure, indicating that shock from tamponade results primarily from compression and decreased filling of the right side of the heart (7). Because the signs of tamponade are both insensitive and nonspecific, the physician must maintain a high index of suspicion. Wilson and Bassett found that the full Beck's triad of hypotension, distended neck veins, and muffled heart signs was present in only 41% of patients with acute traumatic tamponade (8).

TABLE 1. CLASSIFICATION OF SHOCK

Type of shock	Signs	Hemodynamics	Disorders in which shock state is found
Obstructive	Narrow pulse pressure	CVP↑	Tension pneumothorax
	Distended neck veins	PAOP↓↑	Pericardial tamponade
	Poor skin or extremity perfusion	CO↓	Massive PE
	Absence of rales or signs of left-sided heart failure	SVR↑	RV infarction
			PEEP or auto-PEEP
Hyperdynamic	Wide pulse pressure	CVP↔↓↑	Sepsis
	Hyperdynamic precordium	PAOP↔↓↑	Anaphylaxis
	Warm skin and extremities	CO↑	Acute liver failure
		SVR↓	Severe anemia without hypovolemia
Hypervolemic cardiogenic	Distended neck veins	CVP↑	Large MI
	Rales	PAOP↑	Valvular heart disease (mitral or aortic regurgiation)
	S_3, S_4 on cardiac auscultation	CO↓	
	Laterally displaced precordial impulse	SVR↑	Dysrhythmias
	Poor skin or extremity perfusion		Cardiomyopathies
Hypovolemic	Weak pulse	↓CVP	Hemorrhage
	Narrow pulse pressure	↓PAOP	Gastrointestinal fluid loss
	Poor peripheral perfusion	↓CO	Diuresis
		↑SVR	Increased capillary permeability

CVP, central venous pressure; PAOP, pulmonary artery occlusion pressure; PE, pulmonary embolism; SVR, systemic vascular resistance; RV, right ventricular; PEEP, positive end-expiratory pressure; MI, myocardial infarction.

Other suggestive clues include pulsus paradoxus [a marked decrease in pulse or blood pressure (BP) during inspiration] and Kussmaul sign (distention of neck veins on spontaneous inspiration). The classic finding in patients who have pulmonary artery (PA) catheters is equalization of pressures, in which right atrial (RA) diastolic, PA diastolic, and pulmonary artery occlusion pressure (PAOP) are nearly equal. Echocardiography provides confirmatory evidence. In the profoundly hypotensive patient, initial treatment with fluid boluses and removal of fluid by subxiphoid pericardiocentesis should not be delayed.

Another obstructive cause of low CO shock is massive pulmonary embolism (PE), which produces obstruction to RV outflow. In patients whose hypotension is due to PE, signs of acute right-sided heart failure, such as RV heave and distended neck veins, may be present. Hypoxemia and increased arterial–alveolar tension gradient are inconsistent signs in patients presenting with PE (9), but persons with massive hemodynamically significant PE are more likely to have these findings. Data from the large Urokinase Pulmonary Embolism Trial revealed that electrocardiographic findings include nonspecific T-wave abnormalities in 40% of patients with angiographic evidence of PE, whereas RV-strain patterns, such as the often-cited S1Q3T3, occurred in only 25% (10,11). Patients with massive PE and shock were more likely to have signs of acute right heart strain on electrocardiography (ECG). Ventilation-perfusion (V/Q) lung scanning, pulmonary angiography, or rapid computed tomography (CT) scanning confirms the diagnosis; but, as with the other obstructive mechanisms, the patient may not tolerate treatment delays. Portable echocardiography to demonstrate elevated PA pressures and RV failure is an alternative rapid diagnostic modality. Unless contraindicated, thrombolysis has replaced surgical intervention as the initial therapy of choice for massive PE with hemodynamic compromise.

A fourth major "obstructive" mechanism of low CO shock is RV infarction, which occurs in association with almost half

of all inferior myocardial infarctions (MI) and may present with physical findings of right-sided heart failure that are identical to those seen with massive PE (12). In this case, obstruction is caused by a functional blockage of RV inflow and outflow with decreased compliance, poor filling, and poor contraction of the right ventricle. History and a normal alveolar–arterial oxygen gradient help to distinguish this diagnosis from massive PE. The RV infarct electrocardiographic pattern is best seen with right-sided chest leads, especially lead V4R. Serial cardiac enzyme studies and echocardiography may further aid in diagnosis. Volume loading, inotropic support, thrombolysis, and angioplasty are the mainstays of therapy.

High levels of positive end-expiratory pressure (PEEP), whether intrinsic (auto-PEEP) or administered, cause elevations in pleural and intrathoracic pressures that obstruct venous return to the heart and may lead to shock, especially in hypovolemic patients. In addition to their obstruction to cardiac inflow, increased intrapulmonary pressures are transmitted from the pulmonary alveoli to the pulmonary vasculature and increase pulmonary vascular resistance and RV afterload, with resultant decreased RV outflow. Conversely, increased pleural and intrathoracic pressure may decrease transmyocardial pressure and ventricular wall tension, producing a reduction in afterload-induced myocardial ischemia. The presence of auto-PEEP should be considered for patients with obstructive pulmonary disease, specifically those with bronchospasm and air trapping, and also for patients with high minute ventilation. On physical examination, the patient with auto-PEEP has signs of hyperinflation of the chest and prolonged expiratory time. Momentary occlusion of the expiratory outflow of some ventilators at the end of expiration allows measurement of auto-PEEP. Improvement in CO and BP with temporary disconnection from the ventilator, often with an associated rush of air from the endotracheal tube, confirms PEEP (intrinsic, extrinsic, or both) as the cause of circulatory shock. Volume loading, reduction of PEEP and auto-PEEP, and longer expiratory times are the treatments for shock associated with these mechanisms.

Hyperdynamic Shock

Once the mechanisms of obstructive shock have been considered, the clinician should investigate the other more common pathophysiologic mechanisms of shock: hyperdynamic, cardiogenic, and hypovolemic (13). To understand more fully the physiologic complexities of the various types of shock as they relate to stroke volume (SV) and CO, the physician should use the concepts developed by Starling and colleagues between 1895 and 1916 (14,15). The Starling concept describes the influence of preload on ventricular SV in the normal heart; as preload or cardiac filling increases, SV also increases. Figure 2 demonstrates this relationship in the normal physiologic state and further describes alterations expected with changes in myocardial contractility.

An alternative physiologic approach to the examination of hemodynamic dysfunction was initiated by the description of pressure–volume loops by Otto Frank in 1895 (16). Using a theoretical description of ventricular function in the frog heart, Frank provided a diagrammatic depiction of cardiac function that allows for the independent effects of preload, contractility, and afterload. Application of Starling concepts usually take end-diastolic pressure as a measure of preload. This practice fails to recognize the impact of diastolic dysfunction where decreases in ventricular compliance alter the pressure-volume relationship so that elevated ventricular end-diastolic pressure (VEDP) occurs despite decreases in ventricular end-diastolic volume (VEDV). Figure 3 shows the pressure–volume loop diagram. The end-diastolic pressure volume relationship (EDPVR) demonstrates the impact of changes in ventricular compliance; the end-systolic pressure volume relationship (ESPVR) represents contractility; and the effective arterial elastance (EAE) is a function of vascular resistance (17). The effects of the various shock pathophysiologies on the pressure–volume loop are described for each shock syndrome.

The physical findings of widened pulse pressure with a decreased diastolic BP, bounding precordial impulses, and warm skin and extremities can assist the physician in distinguishing hyperdynamic shock from the other types of shock. Central venous pressure (CVP) and PAOP generally are normal or decreased in hyperdynamic shock. Sepsis is the leading cause of

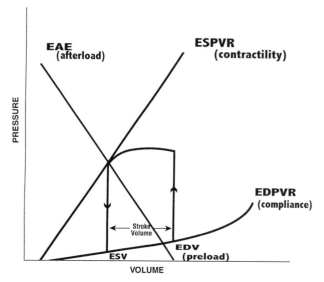

FIGURE 3. The pressure-volume loop where the end-diastolic pressure volume relationship (EDPVR) represents ventricular compliance (the relationship of end-diastolic volume (EDV) to end-diastolic pressure); the end-systolic pressure volume relationship (ESPVR) represents contractility; the effective arterial elastance (EAE) represents vascular resistance which is the major determinant of afterload. ESV, end-systolic pressure.

hyperdynamic shock; yet, as discussed earlier, not all hyperdynamic shock is a result of sepsis. The mechanisms, diagnosis, and treatments of septic shock are complex, and our understanding of these mechanisms is continuously evolving. Prevailing theory invokes exotoxin or endotoxin release as the central inciting event leading to sepsis. These toxins activate immunologic effector cells and the vascular endothelium, causing the amplified release of cytokines, arachidonic acid metabolites, and other mediators that interact to produce the various phenomena seen in sepsis. Perhaps most well-known of these effects is widespread vasodilation, but vasoconstriction and microvascular occlusion with platelets and leukocytes also occur. These vascular abnormalities precipitate metabolic mismatch and cellular and tissue hypoperfusion, with resultant ischemia and lactic acidosis. Essentially any microorganisms—i.e., bacteria, viruses, fungi—may initiate this cascade of humoral factors, leading to sepsis and hyperdynamic shock.

The cardiac and hemodynamic profile of sepsis may evolve to include elements of all three of the nonobstructive types of shock. Systemic vasodilation and increased capillary permeability initially cause hypovolemia, which, if not treated with fluid resuscitation, may progress to low CO hypovolemic shock. When fluids are given, the expected hyperdynamic picture follows. Despite the hyperdynamic state, a significant component of cardiac dysfunction occurs in septic shock. The production of myocardial depressant factor(s) (MDF) causes a decrease in myocardial contractility, resulting in increased ventricular volumes and decreased ejection fraction (18). Additionally, diastolic hypotension may precipitate myocardial ischemia in patients with coronary artery disease. Thus, the hemodynamic sequelae of sepsis depend on prior resuscitation measures (fluids and pressors) and on the progression of the underlying disorder.

The pressure–volume loop shown in Figure 4 represents one possible state of hyperdynamic shock. The slope of the EAE is

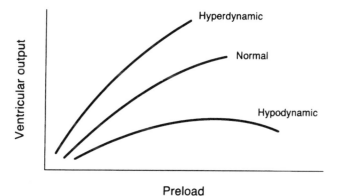

FIGURE 2. Starling ventricular function curves demonstrating the effect of changes in contractility.

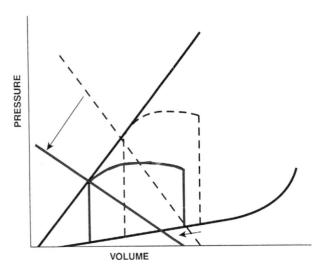

FIGURE 4. The pressure–volume loop demonstrating the changes to be expected in hyperdynamic/septic shock with unchanged myocardial contractility. Note the decreased slope of the effective arterial elastance (EAE) indicating vasodilation and the decrease in end-diastolic volume and pressure. (Refer to Fig. 3.)

decreased, representing the decrease in SVR; the slope of the ESPVR is unchanged, representing unchanged contractility, and the VEDV (preload) is decreased. Examination of Figure 4 reveals that, with a decreased slope of the ESPVR line (representing a reduction in contractility), stroke volume would remain elevated above normal, particularly if VEDV were returned to normal with fluid administration. The inability of the Starling relationship to describe this physiology arose from both dependence on the isolated heart preparation and the belief that vascular resistance had no effect on cardiac function (19).

Among the many potential manifestations of anaphylaxis is hyperdynamic shock. A complete discussion of the various mechanisms of anaphylaxis is beyond the scope of this chapter, but common to all of these mechanisms is a release of histamine, prostaglandins, leukotrienes, and other mediators from mast cells and basophils. Beyond the more common urticarial, pruritic, bronchospastic, and angioedema reactions, these mediators can cause severe systemic vasodilation and increased capillary permeability with resultant cardiovascular collapse. Prompt identification of this syndrome is paramount because treatment with epinephrine, steroids, and antihistamines can rapidly reverse the shock, bronchospasm, and other sequelae. Historical information and the presence of urticaria or wheezing are key to differentiating anaphylaxis from sepsis. In a patient who lacks these findings and has had a prolonged ICU course with risks for both sepsis and drug reactions, the distinction may be difficult to make. Antibiotic and contrast-media reactions account for the great majority of anaphylactic deaths in the United States (20), whereas histamine-releasing neuromuscular-blocking agents and opioids are implicated in many of the anaphylactic reactions that occur during anesthesia (21).

Severe anemia without hypovolemia causes a hyperdynamic shock state without the hypermetabolic signs of warm skin and extremities. The body initially compensates for the lack of oxygen-carrying capacity by increasing CO and systemic oxygen extrac-

tion (22). As this mechanism fails, however, anaerobic metabolism, acidosis, and organ failure ensue.

Cardiogenic Shock

In low CO shock, findings include a narrow pulse pressure, a hypodynamic precordium, and poor skin and extremity perfusion, including slow capillary refill and mottling. On physical examination, cardiogenic shock is characterized further by signs of heart failure, such as distended neck veins, rales, a laterally and inferiorly displaced precordial impulse, and a summation cardiac gallop. PA catheter assessment reveals low CO, high SVR, and high CVP and PAOP.

The most common cause of cardiogenic shock is LV infarction. Studies published in the early 1970s found that a loss of 40% or more of LV myocardium often resulted in shock (23,24). Among patients with MI, risk factors for shock include anterior MI, older age, diabetes mellitus, prior MI, and prior congestive heart failure (CHF) (3). Diagnosis of this cause of shock is made by taking the patient's history and according to the ECG and echocardiography findings. Details of its pathophysiology and treatment are presented in Chapter 27. Valvular heart disease, most commonly mitral and aortic regurgitation, alone or in combination with other heart disease, may cause cardiogenic shock. In addition to signs of left-sided heart failure, characteristic murmurs are the best clues to these diagnoses. PAOP tracings may show large V waves in the patient with mitral regurgitation. Echocardiography is the diagnostic modality of choice for nearly all valvular lesions. Medical treatment for the patient with severe left-sided heart failure and valvular–regurgitant pathology consists of a combination of inotropes, diuretics, and afterload reduction.

Cardiac output is the product of heart rate (HR) and SV. Tachydysrhythmias precipitate shock by significantly reducing SV. Limitation of adequate diastolic filling time of the ventricles, loss of coordinated atrioventricular synchrony, and induction of myocardial ischemia are the primary mechanisms leading to this decreased SV. Because nearly all types of shock are accompanied by tachycardia, confusion may arise as to whether a patient's tachycardia is a beneficial physiologic response to another cause of shock or a detrimental true precipitant of shock. Rhythm identification and clinical history are the keys to resolving this dilemma. Generally, sinus tachycardia should be considered a physiologic response to shock, whereas ventricular tachycardia is clearly deleterious. Rapid atrial fibrillation in a patient with septic shock and long-standing atrial fibrillation presents a complex problem; the hypotension may be due to several mechanisms, and the physician must decide how much to slow the ventricular response to the fibrillating atria. Treatment of tachydysrhythmias and bradydysrhythmias are discussed in Chapter 29.

Multiple other causes of cardiogenic shock exist, and many of these are included in the general category of cardiomyopathy. Space limitations preclude their discussion here. One etiology that deserves brief mention is hypotension occurring after cardiopulmonary bypass (CPB). LV dysfunction, anesthetic–drug effects, postoperative dysrhythmias, and the vasodilation associated with rewarming all may contribute to post-CPB shock, which often lasts up to 48 hours. Additionally, a circulating polypeptide similar to MDF has been identified as a cause of decreased

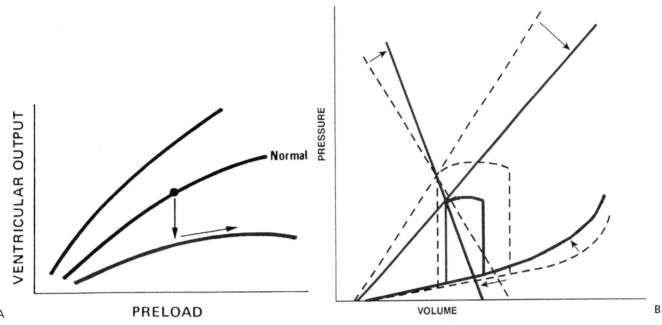

FIGURE 5. A: The Starling ventricular function curve demonstrating changes of cardiogenic shock with decreased contractility and increased preload as often measured by indices of ventricular end-diastolic pressure. **B:** The pressure–volume loop representing changes as observed in cardiogenic shock. The decrease in contractility (ESPVR) is accompanied by a decrease in compliance of the ventricle (EDPVR). The result is a decrease in true preload (end-diastolic volume, EDV) with unchanged end-diastolic pressure. Compensatory vasoconstriction is evident by the increased slope of the effective arterial elastance (EAE). The stroke volume is decreased. Envision the effect of a further reduction in compliance leading to increased EDP and decreased EDV. (Refer to Fig. 3.)

cardiac contractility following CPB (25). Treatment includes optimizing ventricular-filling pressures, inotropic support, afterload reduction, and control of dysrhythmias (Chapter 31).

Figure 5 shows the comparative physiologic descriptions of cardiogenic shock using Starling and pressure–volume diagrams. Note that in Figure 5B, a decrease in diastolic compliance often existing in cardiogenic shock allows for the demonstration of the perceived increase in preload that would be observed if pressure were used in the Starling curve (Fig. 5A). The pressure–volume loop accurately represents the potential for a reduction in VEDV in cardiogenic shock with the elevation in the EDPVR, which occurs with reduced ventricular compliance. Care must be exercised with volume administration because the accompanying increase in VEDP may result in increased pulmonary capillary hydrostatic pressure and pulmonary edema unless ventricular compliance is improved.

Hypovolemic Shock

Hypovolemic shock is defined on physical examination by signs of poor perfusion accompanied by the lack of signs of heart failure (flat neck veins, no rales, a precordial impulse that is not displaced or is not palpable, and absence of an S3 cardiac gallop). If the hypovolemia is of significant duration (>several hours), signs of dehydration such as poor skin turgor and dry mucous membranes may be present. If available, PA catheter findings show low CO, high SVR, and low CVP and PAOP.

Acute hemorrhage is a frequent cause of hypovolemic shock. Otherwise healthy patients with acute blood loss of 15% to 30% of blood volume develop tachycardia, tachypnea, and narrowed pulse pressure (26). Increased levels of endogenous circulating catecholamines account for these findings and produce the patient's appearance of apprehension and anxiety. So efficient are the physiologic compensatory mechanisms that a blood loss of 30% of a patient's blood volume (approximately 1,500 mL in an adult) is necessary to produce a decrease in mean systemic BP (26). Hemorrhagic shock is discussed more fully in Chapter 26.

Postoperative "third spacing" of fluids is another common cause of hypovolemic shock. Major abdominal and retroperitoneal operations, such as repair of abdominal aortic aneurysms, commonly lead to massive transudative fluid loss into the peritoneum, bowel wall, and planes of tissue injury. This sequestered fluid temporarily becomes part of a "nonfunctional" compartment. Recognition of patients at risk is essential for diagnosis because the fluid losses may not be obvious and the only physical signs may be distention of the abdomen or other tissues.

Extensive burns cause shock through several mechanisms. In the first 24 to 36 hours, the major mechanism is increased capillary permeability with resultant fluid extravasation into the interstitium. Without adequate volume resuscitation, hypovolemic shock occurs. After this initial fluid loss, a hyperdynamic hypermetabolic state follows. Inflammatory mediators similar to those active in sepsis may cause systemic vasodilation and hypotension. Loss of the skin's protective barrier, changes in cellular immunity, and instrumentation also may lead to infection and sepsis. Finally, burn patients, with or without sepsis, may produce MDF, which causes depressed cardiac contractility throughout these various stages (27).

Spinal-cord injury may produce a shock syndrome that physiologically resembles both hypovolemic and hyperdynamic shock. Often referred to as *neurogenic shock*, this syndrome occurs most frequently with cervical-cord lesions and has several well-defined pathogenic mechanisms. The primary cause appears to be a loss of peripheral sympathetic tone that results in inappropriate systemic vasodilation, which produces the hyperdynamic features of warm skin and extremities. Yet this vasodilation, combined with paralytic-induced loss of venous return, also causes a significant decrease in ventricular preload, producing functional hypovolemia. Loss of cardiac sympathetic tone may prevent inotropic and chronotropic augmentation of CO, further limiting the patient's response to hypoperfusion.

Figure 6 compares the descriptions of hypovolemic shock as demonstrated by the Starling curve and the pressure–volume loop. Both are able to describe the reductions in preload and stroke volume that exist in this shock state; the pressure–volume loop in Figure 6 also demonstrates the compensatory increase in vascular resistance (increased slope of the EAE), attempting to maintain perfusion pressure.

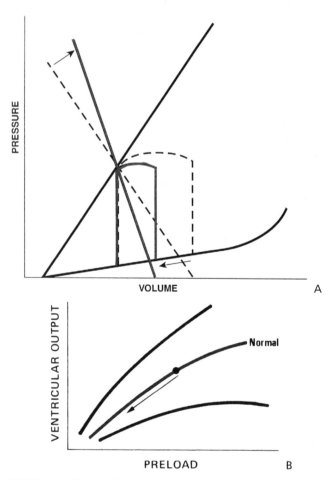

FIGURE 6. A: The Starling ventricular function curve demonstrating changes expected in hypovolemic shock with decreased preload and ventricular output. **B:** The pressure–volume loop representing the changes observed in hypovolemic shock with a reduction in preload (end-diastolic volume and end-diastolic pressure, or EDV and EDP) and compensatory vasoconstriction as the slope of the effective arterial elastance (EAE) is increased. (Refer to Fig. 3.)

MONITORING AND THERAPY

Before addressing the major treatment modalities of shock, one must first define therapeutic goals and techniques used to evaluate progress toward those goals. Specific therapies, such as choice of antibiotics or inhibitors of endogenous mediators of sepsis, are discussed later (see Chapters 52, 53, and 55). We will therefore focus primarily on initial stabilization and on hemodynamic support of patients with shock. *Shock* was defined earlier as a failure of tissue and cellular perfusion; the prime goal, therefore, is to reverse this perfusion failure. A monitored physiologic approach to therapy provides the best opportunity for successful outcome and avoidance of organ dysfunction. How the physician monitors success toward this goal depends on the type and severity of the shock state. The initial resuscitative technique may not be as important as is continuous evaluation of the patient's condition. Critical to the strategy of the treatment of shock is diligent serial therapeutic testing to find out whether the chosen therapy is improving hemodynamics and perfusion.

Following the standard variables of HR, BP, pulse pressure, and urine output may be all that is necessary in the monitoring of the patient with pure hypovolemic shock. The physician must be aware, however, of other influences on these variables; β-adrenergic blockers will blunt the tachycardic response, pain and anxiety will increase HR, and diuretics may produce a physiologically inappropriate high urine output. Additional useful information in the monitoring of hypovolemic shock may be obtained from CVP measurements.

Information derived from use of the flow-directed PA catheter may be used to monitor response to treatment in hyperdynamic septic and cardiogenic shock. Standard measurements of CVP and PAOP are used as indicators of filling volumes of the ventricles. The clinician must recognize, however, that decreased ventricular compliance will alter the ability of these pressure measurements to describe correctly the adequacy of intravascular volume. It is just such reliance on pressure correlates of preload in cardiogenic shock that might lead to aggravation of hypoperfusion with diuretic therapy. The use of echocardiographic estimates of VEDV can be helpful in accurately assessing preload in the presence of altered ventricular compliance.

Serial determinations of CO, oxygen delivery (DO_2), and SVR are the main benefits gained from the PA catheter. By measuring CO, DO_2, and SVR before and after institution of a vasopressor, the physician may discern whether the pressor is truly augmenting perfusion and DO_2 or merely raising BP by increasing vascular tone. Selection of initial therapy and evaluation of its effectiveness are best accomplished by first approximating the existing shock physiology using concepts described in the Starling ventricular-function family of curves (Fig. 7). Following initiation of the selected therapy, results must be rapidly examined to determine the success of treatment and to consider alternative pathophysiology (Fig. 8). The Starling curves still provide the easiest and most readily available description of hemodynamic pathophysiology. The flow-directed pulmonary artery catheter, which provides assessment of CVP, PAOP, and CO and the calculation of SVR and pulmonary vascular resistance (PVR), may thus be a valuable tool in shock management. Limitations in describing the pathophysiology of septic shock with cardiac

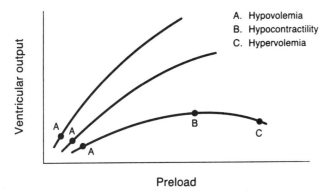

FIGURE 7. Using the Starling ventricular-function family of curves to estimate existing pathophysiology of cardiac function in patients with hemodynamic instability.

insufficiency and the altered relationships of VEDV and VEDP with decreased ventricular compliance must be recognized. The concepts described by the pressure–volume loop thus greatly assist in evaluating existing pathophysiology and response to therapy.

The concept that trauma and septic patients have a pathologic relationship between oxygen supply and oxygen demand remains controversial. Those supporting such a concept contend that augmenting DO_2 to "supranormal" levels increases oxygen consumption and, thereby, decreases organ failure and mortality (28–30). This delivery-dependent oxygen demand was first described in critically ill surgical patients who exhibited a critical DO_2, below which oxygen consumption (VO_2) decreased and above which VO_2 was constant (29,30). Guidelines for achieving this level of DO_2 were proposed and later applied to other groups of critically ill patients. More recent investigation has cast considerable doubt on this therapeutic approach of augmentation of DO_2 (31–35). These studies have indicated that a pathologic DO_2/VO_2 relationship does not exist but, rather, that elevations in VO_2 reflect a phenomenon of mathematic coupling intrinsic to prior study methods (35,36). Using a more valid, indirect calorimetry method of determining VO_2 has demonstrated no dependence of VO_2 to DO_2 in septic patients (32,33), and recent trials failed to demonstrate improved mortality with elevation of DO_2 (33,34). It is clear that hypotensive septic patients generally require fluid challenges, initially followed often by inotropic sup-

port, but the question remains unanswered as to whether "supranormal" DO_2 should be used as a universal goal of therapy. For the present, increasing CO above normal to maintain perfusion pressure in the presence of decreased SVR may be preferable to pharmacologic vasoconstriction. The optimal levels of CO and DO2 in the normotensive patient and the ideal timing of vasoconstrictor agents in the treatment of hypotension require further investigation.

Indicators of oxygen debt and tissue hypoperfusion are indispensable tools to the physician caring for the patient with shock. As described earlier, cells produce lactate during anaerobic metabolism in response to cellular hypoxia. Measurement of serum lactate, therefore, is an important marker of inadequacy of perfusion. Lactate is rapidly metabolized in the liver and kidney; therefore, for patients with satisfactory hepatic and renal function, it is an excellent index of response to therapy. For many years, studies have shown that elevated lactate levels are associated with increased mortality and that persistence of elevated lactate levels after therapy correlates with poor outcome. In 1965, Blair and co-workers reported that lactate levels above 3 mmol per liter were associated with high mortality in patients with septic shock (37). Bakker and colleagues demonstrated that patients with septic shock who, after therapy, continue to show high lactate levels have significantly greater mortality than those whose lactate levels decrease (38). Perret and Enrico demonstrated that the prognostic utility of lactate levels is not limited to septic shock (39). Examining patients with cardiogenic shock, they found that survivors had lower levels of lactate than did nonsurvivors. In patients with hemorrhagic shock, these investigators demonstrated a nonsignificant trend toward survival with lower lactate levels. With the advent of rapid, easily performed lactate measurements, a greater role for its use in the monitoring of shock treatment is likely. Aduen and colleagues reported accurate measurements of lactate on small blood samples within 2 minutes using a portable instrument (40).

Another modality of monitoring the severity of shock and adequacy of resuscitation is gastric tonometry, which measures gastric intramucosal pH, a marker of gastrointestinal tract ischemia. Maynard and co-workers proposed that other measures of tissue oxygenation (lactate levels, DO_2, and others) examine only global perfusion and do not identify important areas of regional hypoperfusion, specifically the splanchnic circulation (41). In a prospective study of 83 patients with shock, they found that gastric mucosal pH had a higher sensitivity (88%) for predicting mortality than did any of the conventional measures studied. Gutierrez and associates reported that therapy designed to maintain a normal gastric mucosal pH improved outcome in critically ill patients (42). Based on failure to improve outcomes in other studies, however, more recent investigators questioned the utility of gastric tonometry as a guide to therapy (43).

Oxygenation and Acid–Base Balance

To prevent deterioration and complications from shock, the physician must aggressively diagnose and treat the underlying cause, whether it be splenic rupture producing hypovolemic shock, urinary tract infection producing hyperdynamic septic shock, or MI causing cardiogenic shock. A critical first step in

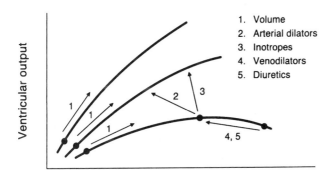

FIGURE 8. Expected hemodynamic responses to therapeutic options using the Starling curves from Fig. 7.

the treatment of shock is to ensure adequate alveolar ventilation and oxygenation. The patient's mental status and the patency of the airway must be assessed immediately to determine the need for intubation of the trachea. Even if the patient is able to maintain an adequate airway, he or she may require intubation. The patient may need higher levels of inspired oxygen and PEEP than can be achieved with mask delivery systems, or the patient may not be able to independently sustain the work of breathing. Finally, the patient may not be able to clear secretions and avoid atelectasis. It must be recognized that if ventilatory support is initiated in a hypovolemic patient, positive-pressure ventilation and PEEP may decrease venous return to the heart and produce further hemodynamic compromise.

The previous standard practice of administering bicarbonate to patients with acidosis has been revised. For many years, clinicians aggressively treated patients with shock and lactic acidosis with bicarbonate, often using calculations based on bicarbonate levels and base excess. Acidosis was believed to decrease the response to endogenous and exogenous catecholamines. It was further assumed that maintenance of a normal serum pH was essential for optimal microcirculatory integrity, cardiac function, central nervous system (CNS) function, and metabolism. More recent evidence, however, demonstrated that metabolic acidosis of the plasma may in fact be protective in shock states and that bicarbonate administration may transiently decrease intracellular and cerebrospinal fluid pH (44). The mechanism for this phenomenon is production of CO_2 as a product of the bicarbonate buffering of hydrogen ion and the rapid diffusion of this nonionized CO_2 across cellular membranes. This paradoxical intracellular acidosis has been shown to hinder brain and cardiac function (45,46). Consequently, a less aggressive approach with respect to the use of bicarbonate in patients with mild metabolic acidosis (pH > 7.25) is recommended.

Fluids

Common to all etiologies of hemodynamic instability and shock is the need to provide optimal intravascular volume to ensure adequacy of preload. Because the major types of shock often require increased levels of preload as initial therapy to improve ventricular output, it is appropriate to begin fluid administration in all shock patients who lack signs of pulmonary edema and LV overload. A normal lung examination may be deceiving, however, in patients with long-standing CHF. Stevenson and Perloff found rales in only 11% of patients whose subsequently measured PAOP was greater than or equal to 35 mm Hg (47).

Few issues in resuscitation have ignited as much controversy as that involving the use of colloid versus crystalloid solutions for resuscitation. In hemorrhagic shock, the use of blood for volume resuscitation is essential (see Chapter 26). Several meta-analyses determined that there is no benefit and even perhaps mild increased morbidity associated with the use of colloids instead of crystalloids for fluid resuscitation (48,49). What is most important when either type of fluid is used is to determine responses to these fluid challenges. Bolus instead of continuous-infusion therapy is therefore preferable to allow evaluation of response.

In isolated hypovolemic shock, changes in HR, pulse pressure, and urine output are usually sufficient to assess response to fluids, but patients with hyperdynamic and cardiogenic shock may need invasive monitoring to guide therapy. Optimal therapy generally means administering the quantity of fluid that maximizes DO_2 while avoiding LV overload and pulmonary edema. Because DO_2 is affected by many variables and because HR is a major determinant of CO, augmentation of SV is probably the most specific single indicator of a beneficial response to fluids in shock. Using the PAOP as an indirect indicator of left ventricular end-diastolic volume, the clinician may administer fluids while monitoring SV versus PAOP curve. The dynamic nature of shock prohibits the identification of a precise optimal PAOP for all patients or even a constant optimal PAOP for a single patient. Of prime importance is the provision of sufficient preload before or during institution of pharmacologic therapy for hypoperfusion. Use of a vasoconstrictor in a hypovolemic patient may worsen perfusion. Likewise, afterload reduction in the hypovolemic patient with cardiogenic shock may produce catastrophic hypotension. A PAOP of 12 to 15 mm Hg prior to and during the use of pharmacologic support is sufficient for most patients with shock, but some will need higher cardiac-filling pressures for optimal SV and CO, particularly if decreased ventricular compliance uncouples VEDP/VEDV relationships.

Vasopressor Agents

The pharmacologic approach to treating patients in shock involves initial patient assessment, choice and institution of an agent, and reassessment (Figs. 7 and 8). Because every agent can produce deleterious effects, it is essential that the physician recognize the pharmacologic spectrum of each vasopressor. Another important consideration is that of variability of patients' responses. Charts and tables listing manufacturer-suggested dose ranges are widely available, but the clinician must understand that these are only general guides. Altered pharmacokinetics and pharmacodynamics are to be expected in shock patients, and pressor therapy must therefore be individually adjusted to achieve specific goals. For example, β-receptors are typically less responsive in patients with septic shock, leading to lesser inotropic results with standard doses (50). Dopamine dosage ranges serve as an excellent illustration of this concept of variability of patient response. Physicians and textbooks typically categorize doses of dopamine in this manner: dopaminergic effects (1–3 μg/kg per minute), predominantly more β than α effects (3–10 μg/kg per minute), predominantly α effects (over 10 μg/kg per minute). Yet the lines of demarcation of these groupings of effects are not distinct. Tachycardia and other β effects are commonly seen in patients at low doses of dopamine, and α effects may predominate at doses lower than 10 μg per kilogram of body weight per minute.

In a discussion of the various drugs used to treat the hemodynamics of shock and hypotension, the term *pressor*, which refers to any substance that raises BP, is nonspecific and gives no insight as to mechanism of action. We will divide vasopressor agents into (a) inotropes/chronotropes (i.e., drugs that increase CO by increasing cardiac contractility and HR); (b) vasoconstrictors (i.e., agents that raise BP by increasing systemic vascular resistance); and (c) mixed pressor agents (i.e., drugs that act through both mechanisms) (Table 2).

TABLE 2. VASOPRESSOR AGENTS

	Receptors	Primary uses
Inotrope/ chronotropes		
Dobutamine	β_1, β_2	First-line cardiogenic shock Septic shock
Amrinone/ milrinone	Phosphodiesterase inhibitors	Adjunct for cardiogenic shock
Dopexamine	β_2, Dopaminergic$_1$, β_1	CHF
Isoproterenol	β_1, β_2	Essentially only for refractory hypotensive bradycardia until pacing available
Digitalis	Na–K ATPase inhibition	Chronic CHF failure
Vasoconstrictor		
Phenylephrine	α	Hypotension in septic shock not responding to epinephrine or norepinephrine Neurogenic shock
Mixed agents		
Dopamine	Low dose, dopaminergic$_1$ Intermediate dose, $\beta > \alpha$ High-dose, $\alpha > \beta$	Diuretic and possible renal protective at low dose Septic shock
Epinephrine	α, β	Septic shock
Norepinephrine	α, β Has more α effect than epinephrine	Septic shock

CHF, congestive heart failure.

Inotropic or Chronotropic Agents

Dobutamine hydrochloride, a synthetic β_1, β_2 receptor agonist, is often chosen for inotropic support in cardiogenic shock. Its pharmacologic properties, which are ideally suited to treatment of the failing heart, include increased myocardial contractility and CO, afterload reduction through peripheral vasodilation, and decreased left ventricular filling pressure with resultant improved diastolic coronary blood flow. Improvements in collateral blood flow and in balance between oxygen supply and demand prevent dobutamine from increasing infarct size in patients with acute MI (51,52). Tachycardia may be observed with higher infusion rates, but it is less likely at doses less than 15 μg per kilogram of body weight per minute. Because of β_2-mediated vasodilation, caution must be observed if dobutamine is administered to hypotensive patients, especially patients who have coexistent hypovolemia. Dobutamine also has been advocated for augmentation of DO$_2$ to supranormal levels in septic and other critically ill patients (28,30). Hayes et al., however, demonstrated increased mortality in patients treated with dobutamine for this purpose (33).

Milrinone lactate, a selective phosphodiesterase III inhibitor, increases inotropy and decreases SVR by preventing the degradation of cyclic adenosine monophosphate (cAMP). The hemodynamic effects are similar to those of dobutamine. Amrinone, another phosphodiesterase III inhibitor, is rarely used because of excessive vasodilation and thrombocytopenia following long-

term use. Milrinone may be useful for synergy in patients already taking β-agonists and for patients receiving β-blocking agents.

Dopexamine, a synthetic catecholamine, augments cardiac performance through both beta-2 mediated afterload reduction and baroreceptor-reflex-mediated inotropy. A further benefit is its dopaminergic-mediated increase in renal blood flow. Most studies of this new agent have involved patients with acute CHF or post–cardiac surgery ventricular failure (53), but trials of its use in combination with other drugs for the treatment of septic shock have demonstrated potential benefit (54).

The essentially pure β-receptor agonist, isoproterenol hydrochloride, produces CO augmentation by increasing both HR and contractility. Attendant marked increases in myocardial oxygen requirement and dysrhythmogenicity greatly limit the utility of isoproterenol.

The previously discussed agents produce their inotropy by cAMP-mediated increases in intracellular ionized calcium. Digitalis also produces increases in intracellular calcium by blocking the sodium-potassium pump, thereby opening calcium channels. Older studies indicated some benefit in the management of gram-negative bacteremic-induced myocardial hypocontractility (55). Because of slow onset of action and low potency, digitalis preparations have limited use in treating acute states of hypoperfusion. They may have some role for use synergistically with other agents in the treatment of acute heart failure.

Vasoconstrictor Agents

The primary vasoconstrictor agents are norepinephrine bitartrate, phenylephrine hydrochloride, and vasopressin. Phenylephrine produces selective postsynaptic α-receptor-mediated vasoconstriction, thereby increasing BP, generally decreasing CO, and often causing a reflex slowing of the HR. Phenylephrine can be used effectively as a first-line agent in the patient with neurogenic shock. It is used to augment the pathologically lowered SVR and BP. It also can be useful in patients who, despite maximal fluid and inotropic support, remain hypotensive with evidence of vital-organ hypoperfusion, such as the patient with septic shock whose widespread vasodilation and hypotension have not responded sufficiently to inotropic and mixed-pressor agents. The physician must recognize that pure vasoconstrictors may compromise flow and perfusion, especially in patients whose hypotension and low SVR are due to shunting, such as patients with end-stage liver disease, pregnancy, or arteriovenous fistulae. Thus, when using phenylephrine, attention to renal function, acid–base balance, serum lactate, and DO$_2$ is imperative. In addition to its vasoconstrictive effects, norepinephrine also has significant β_1 adrenergic activity and therefore is discussed in the following section describing mixed agents.

Vasopressin, an endogenous vasoconstrictor, is released by a baroreflex response. Vasopressin acts by the direct stimulation of endothelin, the principal mediator of vasoconstriction whose activity, coupled to that of endothelium-derived relaxant factor (nitric oxide), maintains normal vascular tone. The identification of α-receptor hyporesponsiveness and the demonstration of reduction in endogenous vasopressin production in 85% of patients in septic shock provided the option to use vasopressin as an alternative therapy for vasodilator shock, particularly in situations where α-stimulation does not produce a satisfactory vasoconstrictor response (56,57). Vasopressin is a direct coronary vasoconstrictor and may produce detrimental myocardial ischemia. Doses of vasopressin for treating systemic vasodilation have not been clearly defined, but most studies have used doses between 0.01 and 0.1 U per minute (58,59).

Mixed Pressor Agents

Pharmacologic agents that exhibit combined α- and β-sympathomimetic effects often are used for the management of hypoperfusion states. The principal agents in this group—dopamine, norepinephrine, and epinephrine—are all endogenous catecholamines that arise from the metabolism of tyrosine (Fig. 9).

Dopamine, a precursor of norepinephrine, is commonly used as an initial pressor agent, acting at several receptors in a dose-related manner. These varied actions of dopamine allow the physician to titrate this single agent toward achieving different aims of therapy: dopaminergic effects (e.g., vasodilation of renal and splanchnic vascular beds), β effects (e.g., augmentation of cardiac contractility and HR), and α effects (e.g., vasoconstriction). Much overlap exists at the various ranges of therapy. Dopaminergic-1 afferent renal arteriolar dilatation with resultant increase in ultrafiltration and urine output has been well described in animals. Debate continues, however, as to whether dopamine truly improves renal function or merely increases urine output through diuretic effects. Trials comparing the diuretic and creatinine clearance effects of dopamine versus dobutamine have yielded contrasting results; some have shown that dopamine is more effective, whereas others have favored dobutamine (60–62). Other investigators have shown that low-dose dopamine may reverse some of the deleterious effects of norepinephrine infusions on renal hemodynamics and function (61). The lack of convincing clinical evidence for any improvement in renal function or outcome with the use of dopamine for dopaminergic stimulation led to decreasing enthusiasm for its routine use to protect the kidneys from hypoperfusion insults or as a means to promote urine output in posthypoperfusion oliguria (63). Studies suggesting reversal of vasoconstrictor-induced increases in renal vascular resistance (61–64) indicate consideration for the use of dopamine at 2-3 mcg per kilogram of body weight per minute during vasoconstrictor infusion.

Recognizing the low inotropic potency of dopamine in patients with septic shock, many clinicians instead use the more potent endogenous catecholamines epinephrine and norepinephrine to treat hypotension and hypoperfusion in these patients. In a randomized, double-blind prospective trial, Martin and colleagues found that norepinephrine was more effective than dopamine at treating the hemodynamics of septic shock; norepinephrine also produced greater urine output and lower lactate levels than did dopamine (65). Likewise, Marik and Mohedin demonstrated that both norepinephrine and dopamine produce increases in mean arterial pressure, global oxygen delivery, and oxygen consumption in patients with septic shock (66). Dopamine, however, produced significant decreases in gastric mucosal pHi, whereas norepinephrine increased pHi. These researchers concluded that norepinephrine may improve splanchnic oxygen dynamics in sepsis, whereas dopamine may precipitate a splanchnic oxygen debt.

Epinephrine may be a preferable inotrope over the less potent dopamine in the presence of sepsis-induced decreases in β-receptor responsiveness and decreased dopamine β-hydroxylase activity (50,67). Given its mast cell stabilization effects, epinephrine is the preferred pressor for the treatment of anaphylactic shock. As with the use of all agents with vasoconstrictor properties, surveillance for organ ischemia is essential.

Studies indicating preferential effects of a combination of dobutamine and norepinephrine compared with epinephrine on splanchnic oxygenation must be scrutinized as to the doses of epinephrine used. In these studies, doses far exceeded those demonstrated to be optimal for inotropic therapy in septic shock (<170 ng/kg per minute) (68–70). Once such a dose is attained for inotropic support, further increases would be expected to result in reduction in cardiac output and oxygen delivery with an increase in SVR as α stimulation begins to predominate. At this point, with the need for further inotropic support one should consider the addition of agents with alternate mechanisms of action such as milrinone (71).

It should be recognized that all currently used vasopressor agents (α- or β-receptor agonists, cAMP phosphodiesterase inhibitors, or the sodium-potassium ATPase inhibitor digoxin) ultimately produce their effects by increasing intracellular ionized calcium concentration. Normal ionized calcium concentrations should be maintained in any patient who is dependent on vasopressor support.

Vasodilator Agents

Vasodilator agents to reduce afterload and improve CO are mainstays in the management of acute and chronic ventricular failure. Shock may exist in the normotensive or even hypertensive patient when BP is maintained by excessive vasoconstriction. Such patients are suitable candidates for acute afterload reduction to improve forward flow, CO, and perfusion. In the selection of the most appropriate vasodilator agent, the physician must

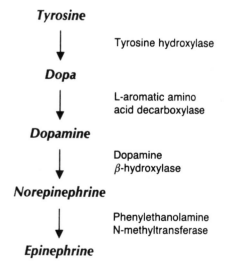

FIGURE 9. *In vivo* metabolic pathway for catecholamine production, identifying the presence of dopamine and the role of the enzyme, dopamine β-hydroxylase.

consider the patient's pathophysiologic state and the properties of the various agents. For acute venodilation and preload reduction, nitroglycerin is the agent of choice; for afterload reduction, sodium nitroprusside, angiotensin-converting-enzyme inhibitors (ACE-I), hydralazine hydrochloride, and fenoldopam are preferable. Finally, patients with right-sided heart failure, as determined on the basis of pulmonary hypertension, may benefit from the pulmonary vasodilators prostacyclin, prostaglandin E1, and inhaled nitric oxide. To avoid serious hypotension, caution in maintaining satisfactory preload must accompany the administration of vasodilators. Other specific drug-related toxicities, such as nitroprusside-induced thiocyanate and cyanide toxicity and ACEI-mediated renal insufficiency, also must be considered.

Steroids

Steroid administration as an adjunct to therapy in hyperdynamic/septic shock was nearly the standard of care 30 years ago. Supraphysiologic doses of methylprednisolone (30 mg/kg) were used (72). Subsequent prospective, double-blind, randomized, multicenter studies later demonstrated no benefit, and the practice of routine administration of high-dose steroids was abandoned (73,74). More recently, data emerged to suggest a decrease in the endogenous production of stress steroids in sepsis, resulting in vasopressor dependence and failure to respond to therapy (75,76). These studies indicated the potential benefit of administration of hydrocortisone at doses of 100 mg every 8 hours. In these recent studies, these physiologic stress doses have been shown to reduce the duration of vasopressor dependence and quicken the reversal of shock. The mechanism for benefit may be reversal of catecholamine receptor downregulation or prevention of inflammatory-mediated induction of nitric oxide synthase. Consideration should be given to administration of the preceding recommended doses to patients with septic shock who require increasing doses of vasopressor or do not respond within 24 hours of therapy.

THE FUTURE

Much of future research on shock will be centered on investigation of several major areas. The question of whether oxygen-delivery augmentation truly improves patient outcome will continue to be addressed. It is possible that certain populations, specifically young trauma or postoperative patients, may benefit from this approach. Current data, however, do not support the routine use of supranormal hemodynamic goals in critically ill patients.

The search for ideal monitors of CO and perfusion will continue. Despite recent controversy over its cost-effectiveness and its effects on morbidity and mortality rates, the PA catheter will likely persist as the primary CO and volume status monitor. The use of less invasive CO monitors, however, such as esophageal Doppler, impedance modalities, and echocardiography, will increase. These techniques provide measurement of both CO and intravascular volume status. Investigation of tissue perfusion markers will continue. Continuous CO monitors and gastric mucosal pH monitors are already in use.

The release of proinflammatory cytokines is one of the pathways to MODS in shock (77). The use of receptor and enzymatic blockers as well as immunotherapy to minimize the effects of these agents have generally shown little promise (78). Antibodies to endotoxin, platelet activating factor, and tumor necrosis factor, receptor blockers to interleukin 1, administration of the antiinflammatory cytokine interleukin 10, and inhibition of nitric oxide synthase have not been effective in randomized studies of patients with SIRS (79–83). Studies of activated protein C (APC) have supported its role as an endogenous antiinflammatory compound that also blocks thrombin-induced microcoagulation (84). APC levels are decreased in 85% of patients with sepsis and SIRS. A recent randomized, controlled clinical trial demonstrated that the administration of human recombinant activated protein C (drotrecogin α-activated) to patients demonstrating evidence of infection complicated by SIRS and at least single-organ dysfunction reduces mortality from 30.8% to 24.7% (84). The economic implication of APC therapy cannot be ignored: The recommendation is for the early (within 24 hours of diagnosis) administration of this agent to all patients with three of four indices of SIRS, known or suspected infection, and single-organ dysfunction that, among others, includes a mean arterial pressure below 70 mm Hg. The results of this study, with its reduction in 28-day mortality rate, indicated a need to treat 16 patients to prevent one death.

SUMMARY

Produced by multiple interacting mechanisms, shock is a complex, dynamic disorder of tissue and cellular hypoperfusion that may lead to MODS and death. Successful treatment of patients with shock requires prompt recognition of the shock state and a thorough understanding of the pathophysiology of the various types of shock. Fluids and pharmacologic agents are the mainstays in the treatment of shock. Response to therapy is monitored by following indicators of both total systemic and individual organ perfusion.

KEY POINTS

Shock, a state of tissue hypoperfusion that results in anaerobic metabolism, arises from complex interactions of multiple pathophysiologic mechanisms.

Although shock states are generally classified into one of three major categories (cardiogenic, septic, hypovolemic), delineation in individual patients is not completely distinct.

Shock states evolve, and patients often exhibit elements of all three types of shock.

Hypotension and malperfusion incite cytokine responses and produce organ dysfunction, such as renal failure and ARDS, which in turn lead to mortality from shock.

When caring for the patient with shock, it is critical to diagnose and treat the obstructive mechanisms of shock: tension pneumothorax, pericardial tamponade, massive PE, RV infarction, and high PEEP.

In addition to treating the underlying cause of shock, the major goal of therapy is to correct cellular hypoxia and tissue malperfusion.

Serial monitoring of perfusion indices is essential in the management of shock. In mild hypovolemic shock, one only need follow urine output and vital signs, whereas in severe septic or cardiogenic shock, one must examine other parameters such as CO, DO_2, lactate levels, and gastric mucosal pH.

Fluids and vasopressors, chosen according to the patient's physiologic state, are the mainstays in the treatment of the hemodynamics of shock.

REFERENCES

1. Murphy SL. Deaths: final data for 1998. *National Vital Statistics Reports* 2000;48(11):1–105.
2. Deitch EA. Shock resuscitation: is the glass half-empty or half full? *Crit Care Med* 2000;28:2665–2666.
3. Rackow EC, Astiz ME. Pathophysiology and treatment of septic shock. *JAMA* 1991;266:548–554.
4. Califf RM, Bengston JR. Cardiogenic shock. *N Engl J Med* 1994;330:1724–1730.
5. Rangel-Frausto MS, Pittet D, Costigan M, et al. The natural history of the systemic inflammatory response syndrome. *JAMA* 1995;273:117–123.
6. Fein AM, Lippmann M, Holtzman H, et al. The risk factors, incidence and prognosis of ARDS following septicemia. *Chest* 1983;83:40–42.
7. Ditchey R, Engler R, LeWinter M, et al. The role of the right heart in acute cardiac tamponade in dogs. *Circ Res* 1981;48:701–710.
8. Wilson RF, Bassett JS. Penetrating wounds of the pericardium or its contents. *JAMA* 1966;195:513–518.
9. Stein PD, Goldhaber SZ, Henry JW, et al. Arterial blood gas analysis in the assessment of suspected acute pulmonary embolism. *Chest* 1996;109:78–81.
10. Koerner S. Diagnosis and treatment of pulmonary embolism. *Cardiol Clin* 1991;9:761–772.
11. Urokinase pulmonary embolism trial. Phase 1 results: a cooperative study. *JAMA* 1974;214:2163–2168.
12. Kinch JW, Ryan TJ. Right ventricular infarction. *N Engl J Med* 1994;330:1211–1217.
13. Mouchawar A, Rosenthal M. A pathophysiological approach to the patient in shock. *Int Anesthesiol Clin* 1993;31:1–20.
14. Starling EH. The Linacre lecture on the law of the heart. In: Chapman CB, Mitchell JH, eds. *Starling on the heart*. London: Dawsons of Pall Mall, 1965:119–147.
15. Patterson SW, Starling EH. On the mechanical factors which determine the output of the ventricles. *J Physiol (Lond)* 1914;48:357–359.
16. Frank O. Zur Dynamik des Herzuskels. *Z Biol* 1895;32:370–447.
17. Sagawa K, Maughan L, Suga H, et al. *Cardiac contraction and the pressure–volume relationship*. New York: Oxford University Press, 1988.
18. Parrillo JE. Pathogenetic mechanisms of septic shock. *N Engl J Med* 1993;328:1471–1477.
19. Patterson SW, Piper H, Starling EH. The regulation of the heart beat.1914;48:465–513.
20. Atkinson TP, Kaliner MA. Anaphylaxis. *Med Clin North Am* 1992;76:841–855.
21. Fisher M, Baldo BA. Anaphylaxis during anaesthesia: current aspects of diagnosis and prevention. *Eur J Anaesthesiol* 1994;11:263–284.
22. Weiskopf RB, Viele MK, Feiner J, et al. Human cardiovascular and metabolic response to acute severe isovolemic anemia. *JAMA* 1998;279:217–221.
23. Harnarayan C, Bennett MA, Pentecost BL, et al. Quantitative study of infarcted myocardium in cardiogenic shock. *Br Heart J* 1970;32:728–732.
24. Alonso DR, Scheidt S, Post M, et al. Pathophysiology of cardiogenic shock: quantification of myocardial necrosis, clinical, pathologic and electrocardiographic correlations. *Circulation* 1973;48:588–596.
25. Coraim FI, Laufer G, Ilias W, et al. Release of myocardial depressant factor (MDF) during cardiopulmonary bypass (CPB): influence of corticosteroids (methylprednisolone) and protease inhibitor (aprotinin). *Prog Clin Biol Res* 1987;236A:611–620.
26. American College of Surgeons. *Advanced trauma life support student manual*. Chicago: American College of Surgeons, 1997.
27. Petroff P, Pruitt BA. Pulmonary disease in the burn patient. In: Artz C, Moncrief W, Pruitt B, eds. *Burns, a team approach*. Philadelphia: WB Saunders Co, 1979:95–160.
28. Wolf YG, Cotev S, Perel A, et al. Dependence of oxygen consumption on cardiac output in sepsis. *Crit Care Med* 1987;15:198–203.
29. Shoemaker WC, Kram HB, Appel PL. Therapy of shock based on pathophysiology, monitoring, and outcome prediction. *Crit Care Med* 1990;18:S19–S25.
30. Boyd O, Grounds RM, Bennett ED. A randomized clinical trial of the effect of deliberate perioperative increase of oxygen delivery on mortality in high-risk surgical patients. *JAMA* 1993;270:2699–2707.
31. Ronco JJ, Fenwick JC, Tweeddale MG, et al. Identification of the critical oxygen delivery for anaerobic metabolism in critically ill septic and nonseptic humans. *JAMA* 1993;270:1724–1730.
32. Mira JP, Fabre JE, Baigorri F, et al. Lack of oxygen supply dependency in patients with severe sepsis: a study of oxygen delivery increased by military antishock trouser and dobutamine. *Chest* 1994;106:1524–1531.
33. Hayes MA, Timmins AC, Yau EHS, et al. Elevation of systemic oxygen delivery in the treatment of critically ill patients. *N Engl J Med* 1994; 330:1717–1722.
34. Gattinoni L, Brazzi L, Pelosi P, et al. A trial of goal-oriented hemodynamic therapy in critically ill patients. Svo2 Collaborative Group. *N Engl J Med* 1995;333:1025–1032.
35. Wysocki M, Besbes M, Roupie E, et al. Modification of oxygen extraction ratio by change in oxygen transport in septic shock. *Chest* 1992;102:221–226.
36. Archie JP Jr. Mathematical coupling of data: a common source of error. *Ann Surg* 1981;193:296–303.
37. Blair E, Cowley A, Tait MK. Refractory septic shock in man. *Am Surg* 1965;31:537–540.
38. Bakker J, Vincent JL, Gris P, et al. Veno-arterial carbon dioxide gradient in human septic shock. *Chest* 1992;101:509–515.
39. Perret C, Enrico JF. Lactate in acute circulatory failure. In: Bossart H, Perret C, eds. *Lactate in acute conditions*. NewYork: S Karger, 1979:69–82.
40. Aduen J, Bernstein WK, Khastgir T, et al. The use and clinical importance of a substrate-specific electrode for rapid determination of blood lactate concentrations. *JAMA* 1994;272:1678–1685.
41. Maynard N, Bihari D, Beale R, et al. Assessment of splanchnic oxygenation by gastric tonometry in patients with acute circulatory failure. *JAMA* 1993;270:1203–1210.
42. Gutierrez G, Palizas F, Doglio G, et al. Gastric intramucosal pH as a therapeutic index of tissue oxygenation in critically ill patients. *Lancet* 1992;339:195–199.
43. Gomersall CD, Joynt GM, Freebairn RC, et al. Resuscitation of critically

ill patients based on the results of gastric tonometry: a prospective, randomized, controlled trial. *Crit Care Med* 2000;28:607–614.

44. Arieff AI. Efficacy of buffers in the management of cardiac arrest. *Crit Care Med* 1998;26:1311–1313.

45. Bersin RM, Chatterjee K, Arieff AI. Metabolic and hemodynamic consequences of sodium bicarbonate administration in patients with heart disease. *Am J Med* 1989;87:7–14.

46. Hope PL, Cady EB, Delpy DT, et al. Brain metabolism and intracellular pH during ischemia: effects of systemic glucose and bicarbonate administration studied by 31P and 1H nuclear magnetic resonance spectroscopy *in vivo* in the lamb. *J Neurochem* 1988;50:1394–1402.

47. Stevenson LW, Perloff JK. The limited reliability of physical signs for estimating hemodynamics in chronic heart failure. *JAMA* 1989;261:884–888.

48. Schierhout G, Roberts I. Fluid resuscitation with colloid or crystalloid solutions in critically ill patients: a systematic review of randomised trials. *BMJ* 1998;316:961–964.

49. Choi PTL, Yip G, Qinonez LG, et al. Crystalloids vs. colloids in fluid resuscitation: a systematic review. *Crit Care Med* 1999;27:200–210.

50. Silverman HJ, Penaranda R, Orens JB, et al. Impaired b-adrenergic receptor stimulation of cyclic adenosine monophosphate in human septic shock: association with myocardial hyporesponsiveness to catecholamines. *Crit Care Med* 1993;21:31–39.

51. Gillespie TA, Ambos HD, Sobel BE, et al. Effects of dobutamine in patients with acute myocardial infarction. *Am J Cardiol* 1977;39:588–594.

52. Leier CV. Acute inotropic support. In: Leier CV, ed. *Cardiotonic drugs: a clinical survey.* New York: Marcel Dekker, 1986.

53. Fitton A, Benfield P. Dopexamine hydrochloride: a review of its pharmacodynamic and pharmacokinetic properties and therapeutic potential in acute cardiac insufficiency. *Drugs* 1990;39:308–330.

54. Task Force of American College of Critical Care Medicine, Society of Critical Care Medicine. Practice parameters for hemodynamic support of sepsis in adult patients in sepsis. *Crit Care Med* 1999;27:639–660.

55. Hinshaw L. Role of the heart in the pathogenesis of endotoxin shock: a review of the clinical findings and observations on animal species. *J Surg Res* 1974;17:134–145.

56. Rozenfeld V, Cheng JW. The role of vasopressin in the treatment of vasodilation in shock states. *Ann Pharmacother* 2000;34:250–254.

57. Landry DW, Levin HR, Gallant EM, et al. Vasopressin deficiency contributes to the vasodilation of septic shock. *Circulation* 1997;95:1122–1125.

58. Argenziano M, Choudhri AF, Oz MC, et al. A prospective randomized trial of arginine vasopressin in the treatment of vasodilatory shock after left ventricular assist device placement. *Circulation* 1997;96:286–290.

59. Malay MB, Ashton RC, Landry DW, et al. Low-dose vasopressin in the treatment of vasodilatory shock. *J Trauma* 1999;47:699–703.

60. Ichai C, Soubielle J, Carles M, et al. Comparison of the renal effects of low to high doses of dopamine and dobutamine in critically ill patients: a single-blind randomized study. *Crit Care Med* 2000;28:921–928.

61. Hoogenberg K, Smit AJ, Girbes ARJ. Effects of low-dose dopamine on renal and systemic hemodynamics during incremental norepinephrine infusion in healthy volunteers. *Crit Care Med* 1998;26:260–265.

62. Duke GJ, Briedis JH, Weaver RA. Renal support in critically ill patients: low-dose dopamine or low-dose dobutamine? *Crit Care Med* 1994;22:1919–1925.

63. Bellomo R, Chapman M, Finfer S, et al. Low-dose dopamine in patients with early renal dysfunction: a placebo-controlled randomised trial: Australian and New Zealand Intensive Care Society (ANZICS) Clinical Trials Group. *Lancet* 2000;356:2139–2143.

64. Schaer GL, Fink MP, Parillo JE. Norepinephrine alone versus nor-

65. Martin C, Papazian L, Perrin G, et al. Norepinephrine or dopamine for the treatment of hyperdynamic septic shock? *Chest* 1993;103:1826–1831.

66. Marik PE, Mohedin M. The contrasting effects of dopamine and norepinephrine on systemic and splanchnic oxygen utilization in hyperdynamic sepsis. *JAMA* 1994;272:1354–1357.

67. Harari A, Martin E. Decreased dopamine beta hydroxylase activity in septic shock. *Anesthesiology* 1979;51:S155.

68. Moran JL, O'Fathartaigh MS, Peisach AR, et al. Epinephrine as an inotropic agent in septic shock: a dose-profile ananlysis. *Crit Care Med* 1993;21:70–77.

69. Levy B, Bollaert PE, Charpentier C, et al. Comparison of norepinephrine and dobutamine to epinephrine for hemodynamics, lactate metabolism and gastric tonometric variables in septic shock: a prospective randomized study. *Intensive Care Med* 1997;23:282–287.

70. Meier-Hellamn A, Reinhart K, Bredle DL. Epinephrine impairs splanchnic perfusion in septic shock. *Crit Care Med* 1997;25:399–404.

71. Gilbert EM, Hershberger RE, Weichmann RJ, et al. Pharmacologic and hemodynamic effects of combined beta-agonist stimulation and phosphodiesterase inhibition in the failing heart. *Chest* 1995;108:1524–1532.

72. Schumer W. Steroids in the treatment of clinical septic shock. *Ann Surg* 1976;184:333–339.

73. Bone RC, Fisher CJ, Clemmer TP, et al. A controlled clinical trial of high-dose methylprednisolone in the treatment of severe sepsis and septic shock. *N Engl J Med* 1987;317:653–658.

74. The Veterans Administration Systemic Sepsis Cooperative Study Group. Effect of high-dose glucocorticoid therapy on mortality in patients with clinical signs of systemic sepsis. *N Engl J Med* 1987;317:659–665.

75. Bollaert PE, Charpentier C, Levy B, et al. Reversal of late septic shock with supraphysiologic doses of hydrocortisone. *Crit Care Med* 1998;26:645–650.

76. Briegel J, Forst H, Hummel T, et al. Stress doses of hydrocortisone reverse hyperdynamic septic shock: a prospective, randomized, double-blind, single-center study. *Crit Care Med* 1999;27:723–732.

77. Bone RC. Toward a theory regarding the pathogenesis of systemic inflammatory response syndrome: what we do and do not know about cytokine regulation. *Crit Care Med* 1996;24:163–172.

78. Zeni F, Freeman B, Natanson C. Anti-inflammatory therapies to treat sepsis and septic shock: a reassessment. *Crit Care Med* 1997;25:1095–1100.

79. Angus DC, Birmingham MC, Balk RA, at el. E5 murine monoclonal antiendotoxin antibody in gram-negative sepsis: a randomized controlled trial. *JAMA* 2000;283:1723–1730.

80. Cohen J, Carlet J. INTERSEPT: an international, multicenter, placebo-controlled trial of monoclonal antibody to human tumor necrosis factor-alpha in patients with sepsis. International Sepsis Trial Study Group. *Crit Care Med* 1996;24:1431–1440.

81. Opal SM, Fisher CJ, Dhainaut JFA. Confirmatory interleukin-1 receptor antagonist trial in severe sepsis: a phase III, randomized, double-blind, placebo-controlled, multicenter trial. *Crit Care Med* 1997;25:1115–1124.

82. Remick DG, Garg SJ, Newcomb DE, et al. Exogenous interleukin-10 fails to decrease the mortality and morbidity of sepsis. *Crit Care Med* 1998;26:895–904.

83. Avontaur JAM, Nothenius RPT, Bujik SLCE, et al. Effect of L-NAME, an inhibitor of nitric oxide synthesis, on cardiopulmonary function in human septic shock. *Chest* 1998;113:1640–1646.

84. Bernard GR, Vincent JL, Laterre PF, et al. Efficacy and safety of recombinant human activated protein C for severe sepsis. *N Engl J Med* 2001;344:699–709.

18

DIAGNOSIS AND MANAGEMENT OF ACID–BASE AND ELECTROLYTE ABNORMALITIES

DONALD S. PROUGH
MALI MATHRU
JOHN D. LANG

KEY WORDS

- Acidemia
- Alkalemia
- Metabolic acidosis and alkalosis
- Metabolic compensation
- Respiratory acidosis and alkalosis
- Respiratory compensation
- Sodium bicarbonate
- Central pontine myelinosis
- Effective osmolality

- Hyperkalemia
- Hypernatremia
- Hypermagnesemia
- Hyperphosphatemia
- Hypocalcemia
- Hypokalemia
- Hyponatremia
- Hypomagnesemia
- Hypophosphatemia
- Syndrome of inappropriate antidiuretic hormone secretion (SIADH)

INTRODUCTION

Disorders of the composition of extracellular fluid occur commonly in critically ill surgical patients. Prompt diagnosis and appropriate treatment of acid–base disturbances and abnormalities in the concentrations of sodium, potassium, magnesium, and phosphate are particularly important. This chapter reviews the diagnosis, physiologic implications, and treatment of these disorders.

OVERVIEW OF ACID–BASE EQUILIBRIUM

The conventional approach to describing acid–base equilibrium uses the Henderson–Hasselbalch equation:

$$pH = 6.1 + \log[HCO_3^-]/0.032 \times Pa_{CO_2}$$

where pH is the negative logarithm of the hydrogen ion concentration ($[H^+]$), 6.1 is the pK_a of carbonic acid, $[HCO_3^-]$ is the bicarbonate concentration, and 0.032 is the solubility coefficient of carbon dioxide (CO_2) in blood.

Conventionally, acid–base interpretation defines disorders in terms of metabolic disturbances (i.e., those in which $[HCO_3^-]$ is primarily increased or decreased) and respiratory disturbances (i.e., those in which Pa_{CO_2} is primarily increased or decreased).

An alternative to the Henderson–Hasselbalch equation, the simpler Henderson equation, is useful in quickly determining if an arterial blood gas (ABG) has been mistranscribed and therefore does not balance:

$$[H^+] = 24 \times Pa_{CO_2}/[HCO_3^-]$$

Conversion of pH to $[H^+]$ can be accomplished by knowing four rules: (a) $[H^+]$ is 40 nmol per liter at a pH of 7.4; (b) each increase in pH of 0.10 pH units reduces $[H^+]$ to 0.8 × the starting $[H^+]$ concentration; (c) each decrease in pH of 0.10 pH units increases $[H^+]$ by a factor of 1.25; and (d) small changes (i.e., ≤0.05 pH units) produce approximately a 1.0 nmol per liter increase in $[H^+]$ for each 0.01 decrease in pH or a decrease in $[H^+]$ of 1 nmol per liter per 0.01 increase in pH.

An alternate approach to acid–base interpretation, proposed by Stewart and reviewed by Eicker, distinguishes between the independent variables and dependent variables that define pH [1,2]. The only independent variables are Pa_{CO_2}, the strong (i.e., highly dissociated) ion difference (SID), and the concentration of proteins, which usually are not strong ions. The strong ions, important because they are present in large concentrations, include sodium (Na^+), potassium (K^+), chloride (Cl^-), and lactate. The SID, calculated as ($Na^+ + K^+ - Cl^-$), normally is approximately 42 mEq per liter. By using a series of equations, the acid–base status can be accurately described using the Stewart approach. In addition, clinical data suggest that calculation of unmeasured anions using equations derived from the Stewart approach may predict mortality better than calculation of the anion gap or measurement of serum lactate [3]. However, there is little evidence that the clinical interpretation or treatment of acid–base disturbances is handicapped by the simpler constructs of the conventional approach.

TABLE 1. RULES OF THUMB FOR RESPIRATORY COMPENSATION FOR METABOLIC ALKALOSIS AND METABOLIC ACIDOSIS

Metabolic alkalosis
  Pa_{CO_2} increases approximately 0.5 to 0.6 mm Hg for each 1.0 mEq/L increase in $[HCO_3^-]$
  The last two digits of the pH should equal $[HCO_3^-] + 15$

Metabolic acidosis
  $Pa_{CO_2} = [HCO_3^-] \times 1.5 + 8$
  The last two digits of the pH should equal $[HCO_3^-] + 15$

METABOLIC ALKALOSIS

Metabolic alkalosis usually is characterized by an alkalemic pH (>7.45) and hyperbicarbonatemia (>27.0 mEq/L). The pathophysiology of metabolic alkalosis has been divided into generating and maintenance factors. Generating factors include, among others, nasogastric suction and diuretic administration. The maintenance of metabolic alkalosis is dependent on a continued stimulus, such as hypovolemia or hypokalemia, for the reabsorption of $[HCO_3^-]$ from the distal renal tubules. Metabolic alkalosis produces multiple physiologic effects, including hypokalemia and ionized hypocalcemia. Hypokalemia and alkalemia may precipitate ventricular arrhythmias, potentiate the toxicity of digoxin, and generate compensatory hypoventilation (hypercarbia) (Table 1). As Pa_{CO_2} increases, Pa_{O_2} will decrease, although hypoxemia due to hypoventilation is easily corrected by supplemental oxygen administration.

Serum electrolytes, even in the absence of ABGs, can suggest metabolic alkalosis. Because most carbon dioxide carried in the blood is in the form of $[HCO_3^-]$ (Fig.1) (4), the measurement of total CO_2 included in the electrolytes should be about 1.0 mEq per liter greater than $[HCO_3^-]$ calculated on simultaneously obtained ABGs (25 versus 24 mEq/L). If either measurement exceeds normal by 4.0 mEq per liter or more, the patient either has a primary metabolic alkalosis or has renally compensated for chronic hypercapnia by conserving $[HCO_3^-]$. Table 2 illustrates typical ABGs and electrolytes in metabolic alkalosis and the effects of superimposition of iatrogenic respiratory alkalosis. The expected effects of acutely decreasing Pa_{CO_2} on pH and $[HCO_3^-]$ are described in Table 3.

In general, treatment of metabolic alkalosis can be divided into etiologic (e.g., volume expansion or potassium repletion) and nonetiologic therapy. For a patient with metabolic alkalosis, 0.9% saline might be preferable to lactated Ringer solution for perioperative fluid resuscitation because lactate provides additional substrate for generation of $[HCO_3^-]$. Nonetiologic therapy includes the provision of hydrogen ions (in the form of ammonium chloride, arginine hydrochloride, or 0.1 N hydrochloric acid), the administration of acetazolamide (a carbonic anhydrase inhibitor that causes renal $[HCO_3^-]$ wasting), or dialysis against an acid bath (5).

METABOLIC ACIDOSIS

Metabolic acidosis, usually characterized by an acidemic pH (<7.35) and hypobicarbonatemia (<21 mEq/L), occurs as a con-

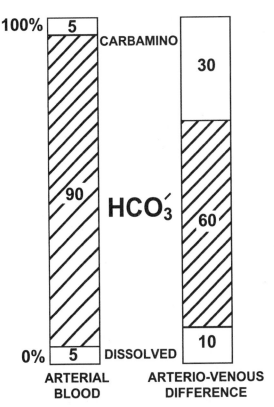

FIGURE 1. The left-hand stacked bar illustrates the components that comprise total CO_2 concentration in arterial blood. The second stacked bar shows the proportions that constitute the arterial–venous CO_2 difference. (Reprinted from West JB. *Respiratory physiology*, 4th ed. Baltimore: Williams & Wilkins, 1990:76, with permission.)

sequence of the buffering by $[HCO_3^-]$ of endogenous or exogenous acid loads or as a consequence of abnormal external loss of $[HCO_3^-]$. Two types of metabolic acidosis may be distinguished, based on whether the calculated anion gap is normal or increased (Table 4) (6). The "anion gap" $= [Na^+] - ([Cl^-] + [HCO_3^-])$. The anion gap is normal (9.0–13 mEq/L) in hyperchloremic metabolic acidosis, which is associated with situations, such as diarrhea, biliary drainage, and renal tubular acidosis, in which $[HCO_3^-]$ is lost externally or in situations in which extracellular volume is rapidly expanded with solutions containing high concentrations of chloride. Maintenance of a normal $[HCO_3^-]$ requires reabsorption of 4,500 mEq of filtered bicarbonate per day; reabsorption occurs in the proximal tubule (85%), in the thick ascending limb of Henle (10%), and by proton secretion in the collecting duct (7). Renal tubular acidosis, which produces hyperchloremic metabolic acidosis, can occur as a genetic defect or as an acquired disorder, as with loss of 70% to 80% of functioning nephron mass (7).

Metabolic acidosis associated with a high anion gap (>13 mEq/L) occurs as a result of excess production of lactic acid or ketoacids, increased retention of waste products (such as sulfate and phosphate), and ingestion of toxic quantities of substances such as aspirin, ethylene glycol, and methanol. The anion gap is increased because $[HCO_3^-]$, consumed in buffering hydrogen ions from metabolic acids, is displaced by the associated acid anion (for example, see Table 5).

TABLE 2. SUPERIMPOSITION OF RESPIRATORY ALKALOSIS ON PREVIOUSLY COMPENSATED METABOLIC ALKALOSIS

Blood gases	pH	7.40		7.47	Mechanical	7.62
	$Paco_2$ (mm Hg)	40	Chronic diuretic	45	hyperventilation	30
	$[HCO_3^-]$ (mEq/L)	24	→→→→→→	32	→→→→→→	29
Electrolytes	"CO_2" (mEq/L)	25		33		30
	Cl^- (mEq/L)	105		97		97
	Na^+ (mEq/L)	140		140		140
	K^+ (mEq/L)	4.0		2.8		2.4

Metabolic alkalosis, diagnosed by hyperbicarbonatemia and alkalemia, is suggested by the increased "CO_2" on the serum electrolytes. The increase in $Paco_2$ partially compensates for the increase in $[HCO_3^-]$.

The perioperative implications of metabolic acidosis are related to the severity of the underlying processes. If pH is sufficiently reduced, myocardial contractility may decrease, pulmonary vascular resistance may increase, and the response of the cardiovascular system to endogenous or exogenous catecholamines may be impaired (8). Although a patient with hyperchloremic metabolic acidosis may be relatively healthy, those with lactic acidosis, ketoacidosis, uremia, or toxic ingestions will be chronically or acutely ill. Assessment of the patient should focus on hypovolemia or hypoperfusion, abnormal renal function, and pulmonary pathology interfering with gas exchange. If shock is the cause, direct arterial pressure monitoring and, occasionally, pulmonary arterial catheterization may be indicated. Hypotensive responses to drugs and positive pressure ventilation may be exaggerated. When mechanically ventilating patients with metabolic acidosis, a level of ventilatory compensation comparable to usual physiologic compensation (Table 1) should be maintained until the primary process can be corrected (Table 5). The treatment of metabolic acidosis consists of the treatment of the primary pathophysiologic process, that is, correction of hypoperfusion or hypoxia, and, perhaps, if pH is severely decreased, administration of $NaHCO_3$. A commonly used calculation of an initial dose of $NaHCO_3$ is

$$NaHCO_3 (mEq) = Wt\ (kg) \times 0.3 \times (24\ mEq/L - Actual\ [HCO_3^-]/2)$$

where 0.3 is the assumed $[HCO_3^-]$ distribution space, 24 mEq per liter is the normal value for $[HCO_3^-]$ on ABG determination, and division by 2 is empirical. The calculation markedly underestimates dosage required to increase pH in severe metabolic acidosis.

In infants and children, an appropriate initial dose is 1.0 to 2.0 mEq per kilogram of body weight. If $[HCO_3^-]$ is infused, ABGs should be measured again after approximately 5 minutes. Hyperventilation, although an important compensatory response to metabolic acidosis, is not definitive therapy for metabolic acidosis.

Few data support the use of $NaHCO_3$ to treat lactic acidosis. In experimental animals, administration of $NaHCO_3$ transiently increases mean arterial blood pressure while increasing pH; however, intracellular pH does not improve (9). In animals with hypoxic acidosis, carbicarb (a combination of sodium bicarbonate and sodium carbonate) improved pH and cardiac index more than did $NaHCO_3$; $NaHCO_3$ increased $Paco_2$ because the buffering of $[H^+]$ by $[HCO_3^-]$ produced H_2CO_3, which dissociated to H_2O and CO_2 (10). In critically ill patients with lactic acidosis, there were no important differences between the hemodynamic effects of equimolar solutions of $NaHCO_3$ and sodium chloride (11), despite increases in pH, $[HCO_3^-]$, and $Paco_2$ after receiving sodium bicarbonate. It is important to note that $NaHCO_3$ did not improve the cardiovascular response to catecholamines but decreased plasma-ionized calcium (11). Although bicarbonate therapy appears to be safe in critically ill patients and in perioperative patients (12,13), no study has demonstrated that outcome is improved by treatment of pH with bicarbonate, carbicarb (13) or dichloroacetate (14). Although some clinicians continue to administer $NaHCO_3$ to patients with persistent lactic acidosis and ongoing deterioration (15), the efficacy of this treatment has been harshly criticized (16). The therapeutic value of bicarbonate administration also has been questioned in adult and pediatric patients with diabetic ketoacidosis in whom pH is between 6.9 and 7.1 (17,18).

TABLE 3. RULES OF THUMB FOR $[HCO_3^-]$ AND PH CHANGES IN RESPONSE TO ACUTE AND CHRONIC CHANGES IN $Paco_2$

Decreased $Paco_2$
  pH increases 0.10 for every decrease in $Paco_2$ of 10 mm Hg
  $[HCO_3^-]$ decreases 2 mEq/L for every decrease in $Paco_2$ of 10 mm Hg
  pH will nearly normalize if hypocarbia is sustained
  $[HCO_3^-]$ decreases 5 to 6 mEq/L for every chronic decrease in $Paco_2$ of 10 mm Hg[a]

Increased $Paco_2$
  pH decreases 0.05 for every increase in $PaCO_2$ of 10 mm Hg
  $[HCO_3^-]$ increases 1.0 mEq/L for every increase in $Paco_2$ of 10 mm Hg
  pH will return toward normal if hypercarbia is sustained
  $[HCO_3^-]$ increases 4 mEq/L for each chronic increase in $Paco_2$ of 10 mm Hg

[a] Hospitalized patients rarely develop compensation for hypocarbia because of sustained stimuli to reabsorb $[HCO_3^-]$.

TABLE 4. DIFFERENTIAL DIAGNOSIS OF METABOLIC ACIDOSIS

Elevated anion gap	Normal anion gap
Diseases	Renal tubular acidosis
Uremia	Diarrhea
Ketoacidosis	Carbonic anhydrase inhibition
Lactic acidosis	Ureteral diversions
Toxins	Early renal failure
Methanol	Hydronephrosis
Ethylene glycol	HCl administration
Salicylates	Rapid 0.9% or hypertonic saline administration
Paraldehyde	

TABLE 5. INCREASED ANION GAP METABOLIC ACIDOSIS COMPLICATED BY FAILURE TO MAINTAIN VENTILATORY COMPENSATION

Blood gases	pH	7.40		7.29		7.19
	Pa_{CO_2} (mm Hg)	40		29		49
	[HCO_3^-] (mEq/L)	24		14		16
Serum	Na^+ (mEq/L)	140	Lactic acidosis	140	Mechanical	140
electrolytes	Cl^- (mEq/L)	105	(hypoperfusion)	105	ventilation	105
	"CO_2" (mEq/L)	25	$\to\to\to\to\to\to$	15	$\to\to\to\to\to\to$	17
	Anion gap	10		20		20
	(mEq/L)	1.5		20		20
	Lactate (mEq/L)					10

As [HCO_3^-] is consumed in the buffering of hydrogen ions from lactic acid, lactate accumulates in the serum, increasing the anion gap. Appropriate respiratory compensation (hyperventilation) has developed. In the presence of metabolic acidosis, an otherwise innocuous increase in Pa_{CO_2} due to hypoventilation may create a dangerous decrease in pH.

RESPIRATORY ALKALOSIS

Respiratory alkalosis, usually characterized by an alkalemic pH (>7.45) and always characterized by hypocarbia ($Pa_{CO_2} \leq$ 35 mm Hg), results when minute ventilation exceeds the level required to excrete metabolic CO_2 production ($\dot{V}CO_2$). Patients may increase ventilation because of pain, anxiety, in response to hypoxemia or central nervous system disease, or as an early sign of systemic sepsis. Respiratory alkalosis, like metabolic alkalosis, may produce hypokalemia, hypocalcemia, cardiac dysrhythmias, bronchoconstriction, and hypotension and may potentiate the toxicity of digoxin. In addition, acute changes in Pa_{CO_2} alter cerebral blood flow. If minute ventilation is halved, Pa_{CO_2} and cerebral blood flow will double; conversely, doubling minute ventilation decreases Pa_{CO_2} to 20 mm Hg and halves cerebral blood flow. If minute ventilation and Pa_{CO_2} are maintained at abnormally high or low levels for 8 to 24 hours, cerebral blood flow will return toward previous levels as pH in cerebrospinal fluid returns toward normal (19). Subsequent changes in Pa_{CO_2}, after accommodation of the cerebrospinal fluid [HCO_3^-] and pH levels to chronic hypocapnia or hypercapnia, again will acutely change cerebral blood flow. For example, Table 6 illustrates a patient with closed head trauma, who, after 48 hours of therapeutic hyperventilation, was abruptly returned to normocapnia. Rules of thumb describing acute and chronic changes in pH and [HCO_3^-] in response to acute and chronic decreases in Pa_{CO_2} are described in Table 3.

RESPIRATORY ACIDOSIS

Respiratory acidosis, usually characterized by a low pH (<7.35) and always characterized by hypercarbia ($Pa_{CO_2} \geq$ 45 mm Hg), occurs when minute ventilation is insufficient to eliminate CO_2

production. Respiratory acidosis may be either acute, without compensation by renal [HCO_3^-] retention, or chronic, with [HCO_3^-] retention offsetting the decrease in pH (Table 3). Respiratory acidosis occurs because of a decrease in minute alveolar ventilation ($\dot{V}_A$), an increase in $\dot{V}CO_2$, or both, from the following equation:

$$Pa_{CO_2} = K/\dot{V}_A$$

where K = constant. A reduction in $\dot{V}_A$ may be due to an overall decrease in minute ventilation ($\dot{V}_E$) or to an increase in the amount of dead space ventilation ($\dot{V}_D$), according to the following equation:

$$\dot{V}_A = \dot{V}_E - \dot{V}_D$$

Decreases in $\dot{V}_E$ may occur because of central ventilatory depression by drugs or central nervous system injury, because of increased work of breathing, or because of airway obstruction or neuromuscular dysfunction. Increases in $\dot{V}_D$ occur with chronic obstructive pulmonary disease, pulmonary embolism, and most acute forms of respiratory failure. $\dot{V}CO_2$ may be increased by sepsis, high-glucose parenteral feeding, or fever.

In patients who are chronically unable to excrete CO_2 at a normal Pa_{CO_2}, the ventilatory decrease imposed by upper abdominal or thoracic surgery may be a particular risk. Administration of narcotics and sedatives, even in small doses, may cause hazardous ventilatory depression. Mechanical ventilation of patients with chronic hypercapnia should allow maintenance of a normal pH. An abrupt increase in minute ventilation to decrease Pa_{CO_2} to 40 mm Hg could result in profound alkalemia because the chronic elevation in [HCO_3^-] will persist. Postoperatively, ventilatory support may be required for selected patients with chronic hypercarbia. Epidural narcotic administration may provide adequate postoperative analgesia with less risk than parenteral narcotics of depressing ventilatory drive.

TABLE 6. HYPERVENTILATION ABRUPTLY TERMINATED AFTER 48 HOURS

Blood gases	pH	7.40	Acute hyperventilation	7.55	Hyperventilation for 48 h	7.55	Abrupt return to normoventilation	7.40
	Pa_{CO_2} (mm Hg)	40		25		25		40
	[HCO_3^-] (mEq/L)	24	$\to\to\to\to\to\to$	21	$\to\to\to\to\to\to$	21		21
CBF	(mL·100 g^{-1}·min^{-1})	50		30		50		80
ICP	(mm Hg)	30		8		18		40

CBF, cerebral blood flow; ICP, intracranial pressure.

The treatment of respiratory acidosis depends on the urgency of the clinical situation. Acute respiratory acidosis may require mechanical ventilation unless a simple etiologic factor (e.g., narcotic overdosage or residual muscular blockade) can be corrected rapidly. Bicarbonate administration is rarely indicated unless severe metabolic acidosis is also present or unless mechanical ventilation is ineffective in reducing acute hypercarbia. In contrast, chronic respiratory acidosis is rarely managed with mechanical ventilation. Rather, efforts are made to improve pulmonary function to permit more effective elimination of CO_2.

PRACTICAL APPROACH TO ACID–BASE INTERPRETATION

Rapid interpretation of acid–base status involves the integration of three sets of data: ABGs, electrolytes, and clinical presentation. The following stepwise approach facilitates interpretation (Table 7). Similar approaches have been described (20,21). More detailed descriptions of management of life-threatening acid–base disorders have been published (22,23).

Most acid–base problems can be assessed before therapy is initiated; however, some situations require immediate attention. Respiratory acidosis with a pH below 7.1 indicates the need for intubation and ventilatory support. Metabolic acidosis with a similar pH suggests the need for appropriate etiologic intervention and, perhaps, alkalinizing therapy.

The next step is to define the primary acid–base disturbance. The pH usually indicates the primary process; that is, acidosis produces acidemia (pH < 7.35). Alkalosis produces alkalemia (pH > 7.35). Note that the suffix "-osis" indicates a primary process that, if unopposed, will produce the corresponding pH change. The suffix "-emia" refers to the pH. More than one primary process may be present.

Step three addresses whether or not the entire ABG picture is consistent with (although not necessarily diagnostic of) a simple acute respiratory alkalosis or acidosis (Table 3). If the magnitude of the pH and $[HCO_3^-]$ changes are not consistent with a simple acute respiratory disturbance, a chronic respiratory acidosis or alkalosis ($\geq$24 h; Table 3) or a primary metabolic disturbance should be considered. The history often provides clues about whether the respiratory changes are acute or chronic. If neither an acute respiratory change nor a chronic compensatory change

can describe the entire ABG picture, then one must assume that a primary metabolic disturbance is also present.

Table 1 lists the rules for compensation that should occur in response to metabolic disturbances. Note that respiratory compensation occurs rapidly. Several general rules describe the compensation. First, overcompensation is rare. Second, inadequate or excessive compensation suggests an additional primary disturbance. Third, hypobicarbonatemia associated with an increased anion gap is never compensatory. Finally, the rules of thumb only approximate the logarithmic relationship between pH and $[H^+]$. The more the pH deviates from 7.40, the less accurate the rules become.

The sixth step, often inappropriately deleted, determines whether an increased anion gap is present. The electrolytes and anion gap should be assessed even if the ABGs appear straightforward. The simultaneous occurrence of metabolic alkalosis and metabolic acidosis (caused by an etiology associated with an increased anion gap) may result in an unremarkable pH and $[HCO_3^-]$; such a combined abnormality may be evident only by examining the anion gap (24). Failure to consider the presence or absence of an increased anion gap may result in an erroneous diagnosis and failure to initiate appropriate treatment.

The final question to ask is whether the clinical data are consistent with the ABG data. Failure to consider the clinical status of patients may lead to serious errors in acid–base interpretation.

Examples

The foregoing summarized an approach that simplifies interpretation. The following two hypothetical cases will be approached using the algorithm and previously discussed rules.

Example 1

A 65-year-old woman has undergone a 12-hour bilateral radical neck dissection and flap construction. To replace an estimated blood loss of 2,000 mL, she has received 3 U of packed red blood cells and 9 L of 0.9% saline. Her blood pressure and heart rate have remained stable on 0.5% to 1.0% isoflurane in 70:30 nitrous oxide and oxygen. Urinary output is about 60 mL per hour. ABGs and serum electrolytes are shown in Table 8.

The step-by-step interpretation is as follows:

1. The pH is not life threatening.
2. The pH is less than 7.40 but is not frankly acidemic.

TABLE 7. SEQUENTIAL APPROACH TO ACID–BASE INTERPRETATION

Is the pH life-threatening, requiring immediate intervention?
Is the pH acidemic or alkalemic?
Could the entire arterial blood-gas picture represent only an acute increase or decrease in Pa_{CO_2}?
If the answer to the preceding question is "no," is there evidence of a chronic respiratory disturbance or of an acute metabolic disturbance?
Are appropriate compensatory changes present?
Is the anion gap increased?
Do the clinical data fit the acid-base picture?

TABLE 8. HYPOBICARBONATEMIA AND SERUM ELECTROLYTES AFTER PROLONGED SURGERY

Blood gases	pH	7.38
	Pa_{CO_2}	32 mm Hg
	$[HCO_3^-]$	17 mEq/L
Serum electrolytes	Na^+	140 mEq/L
	Cl^-	112 mEq/L
	CO_2	18 mEq/L
	Anion gap	10 mEq/L

3. The ABGs cannot be adequately explained by acute hypocarbia. The predicted pH would be 7.48 and the predicted $[HCO_3^-]$ would be 22 mEq per liter (Table 3).
4. A metabolic acidosis appears to be present.
5. The question of respiratory compensation is not really relevant during general anesthesia, given that $PaCO_2$ is established by mechanical ventilation. This $PaCO_2$ would represent slight overcompensation for the calculated $[HCO_3^-]$ (Table 1) and thus suggests primary respiratory alkalosis.
6. Serum electrolytes (Table 8) demonstrate a normal anion gap, indicating that the metabolic acidosis is probably the result of dilution of the extracellular volume with high-chloride fluid (25,26). This benign condition requires no treatment; however, a misdiagnosis of lactic acidosis could have inappropriately prompted additional fluid therapy or other attempts to improve perfusion (27).
7. The clinical picture is consistent with the laboratory data.

Example 2

A 55-year-old man, an alcoholic, who was disoriented and complaining of recurrent vomiting and hematemesis, is scheduled for an emergency laparotomy. ABGs and electrolytes are summarized in Table 9.

1. The pH is not life threatening.
2. The patient has only a mild alkalemia.
3. Acute hypocarbia to 34 mm Hg should produce a pH of 7.45 and an $[HCO_3^-]$ of 23 mEq per L.
4. No other disorder is suggested by the ABGs alone.
5. No apparent compensation is present.
6. The electrolytes, however, show an anion gap of 26 mEq per liter, indicating a metabolic acidosis. Serum ketone levels are positive, providing the key to the diagnosis.
7. The patient has had several days of vomiting and thus has generated a substantial metabolic alkalosis (which normally would have increased $[HCO_3^-]$); however, because of inadequate fluid and carbohydrate intake, the patient also has developed an alcoholic ketoacidosis superimposed on an underlying metabolic alkalosis. Alcoholic ketoacidosis has reduced the $[HCO_3^-]$ from 37 mEq to 23 mEq per liter. In other words, the increase in the anion gap of 14 mEq has decreased serum $[HCO_3^-]$ by a similar amount. Thus, what superficially appears to be a simple mild respiratory alkalosis is, in fact, a triple acid–base disturbance that includes a primary metabolic alkalosis, a primary metabolic acidosis, and a primary respiratory alkalosis. Failure to calculate the anion gap would lead to an incorrect interpretation of the patient's acid–base status.

TABLE 9. DISORIENTATION AND HEMATEMESIS

Blood gases	pH	7.45
	$PaCO_2$	34 mm Hg
	$[HCO_3^-]$	23 mEq/L
Serum electrolytes	Na^+	135 mEq/L
	K^+	4.0 mEq/L
	Cl^-	85 mEq/L
	CO_2	24 mEq/L

SODIUM

Increases or decreases in total body sodium, the principal extracellular cation, and solute tend to increase or decrease extracellular volume and plasma volume. Disorders of sodium concentration ($[Na^+]$), that is, hyponatremia and hypernatremia, usually result from relative excesses or deficits, respectively, of water.

Hyponatremia

The signs and symptoms of hyponatremia ($[Na^+] < 130$ mEq/L) depend on both the rapidity and severity of the decrease in plasma $[Na^+]$. Symptoms that usually accompany $[Na^+] \leq 120$ mEq per liter include neurologic changes (altered consciousness, coma, seizures, and cerebral edema); loss of appetite; nausea; vomiting; cramps; and weakness (28). Because the blood–brain barrier is poorly permeable to sodium but freely permeable to water, a decrease in plasma $[Na^+]$ promptly increases both extracellular and intracellular brain water. The symptoms of cerebral overhydration are more severe in acute than in chronic hyponatremia. Compensatory responses to cerebral edema include bulk movement of interstitial fluid into the cerebrospinal fluid and loss of intracellular solutes, including potassium and organic osmolytes (previously termed *idiogenic osmoles*) such as taurine, phosphocreatine, myoinositol, glutamine, and glutamate (29). The symptoms of chronic hyponatremia probably relate to depletion of brain electrolytes. Once brain volume has compensated for hyponatremia, rapid correction may lead to abrupt brain dehydration.

Pseudohyponatremia occurs when hyperproteinemia (protein concentrations twice normal) or hyperlipidemia (severe enough to cause plasma lactescence) displaces water from plasma, thereby producing an apparently low plasma $[Na^+]$. Such patients, in whom true serum osmolality is normal, require no treatment.

True hyponatremia (Fig. 2) may be associated with normal, high, or low serum osmolality (30). Hypoosmolality may be associated with a high, low, or normal total body sodium and plasma volume. Hyponatremia with a normal or high serum osmolality results from the presence of a nonsodium solute, such as glucose or mannitol, which does not diffuse freely across cell membranes. A common cause of postoperative hyponatremia associated with a normal osmolality is the absorption of large volumes of isotonic, sodium-free irrigating solutions containing mannitol, glycine, or sorbitol during transurethral resection of the prostate. Osmolality can be estimated from the following equation:

$$Osmolality = [Na^+] + glucose/18 + BUN/2.8$$

where BUN is blood urea nitrogen. A discrepancy exceeding 10 mOsm per kilogram of body weight between the measured and calculated osmolality suggests either pseudohyponatremia or the presence of a nonsodium solute. Hypotonicity, which implies intracellular movement of water, may occur despite a normal or elevated serum osmolality in renal insufficiency because BUN, included in the calculation of total osmolality, distributes throughout both extracellular volume and intracellular volume.

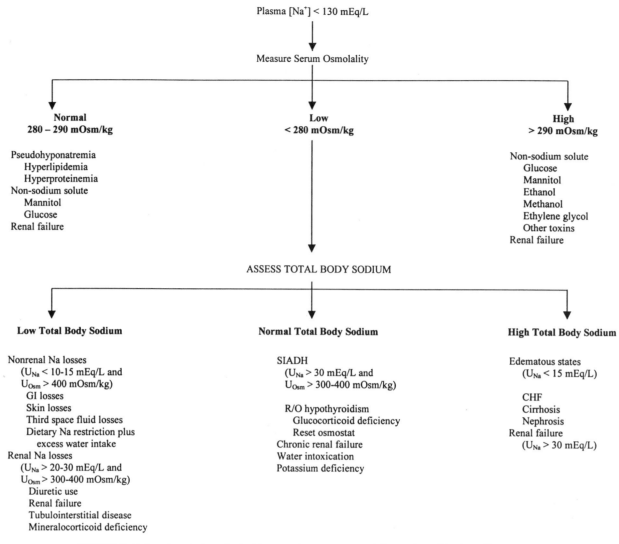

FIGURE 2. Hyponatremia is evaluated by assessing serum osmolality and total body sodium. SIADH, syndrome of inappropriate antidiuretic hormone secretion. (Reproduced from Prough DS, Mathru M. Acid–base, fluids and electrolytes. In: Barash PG, Cullen BF, Stoeltin RK, eds. *Clinical anesthesia*, 4th ed. Philadelphia: JB Lippincott, 2001:165–200, with permission.)

Effective osmolality is calculated as follows:

$$\text{Effective osmolality} = 2[\text{Na}^+] + \text{glucose}/18$$

Hyponatremia with hypoosmolality is evaluated by assessing total body sodium content, BUN, serum creatinine (SCr), urinary osmolality, and urinary [Na⁺]. Hyponatremia with increased total body sodium is characteristic of edematous states, for example, congestive heart failure and cirrhosis. In patients with renal insufficiency, reduced urinary diluting capacity coupled with excess free water intake can lead to hyponatremia. In hyponatremia with low total body sodium content (*hypovolemia*), volume-responsive antidiuretic hormone (ADH) secretion sacrifices tonicity but preserves intravascular volume. In euvolemic hyponatremia, total body sodium and extracellular volume are normal and edema is rarely evident. Almost invariably, this is due to the syndrome of inappropriate ADH secretion (SIADH). In postoperative patients, the diagnosis of SIADH may be applied incorrectly because postoperative patients frequently are functionally hypovolemic, in which case ADH secretion is appropriate (31).

The occasional postoperative occurrence of hyponatremia, mental status changes, and seizures has been attributed to intravenous administration of hypotonic fluids and SIADH. At least 4% of postoperative patients develop plasma [Na⁺] below 130 mEq per liter (32). Although neurologic manifestations are relatively uncommon, signs of hypervolemia are occasionally present (32). In extreme cases, administration of hypotonic fluids to healthy, young, female surgical patients has resulted in severe neurologic symptoms and death secondary to transtentorial herniation (33). Such problems may be more common in women because estrogen and progesterone inhibit the function of brain Na⁺/K⁺ adenosine triphosphatase (ATPase) activity, which is important in regulation of brain volume (34). Careful postoperative attention to fluid and electrolyte balance may minimize the occurrence of symptomatic hyponatremia.

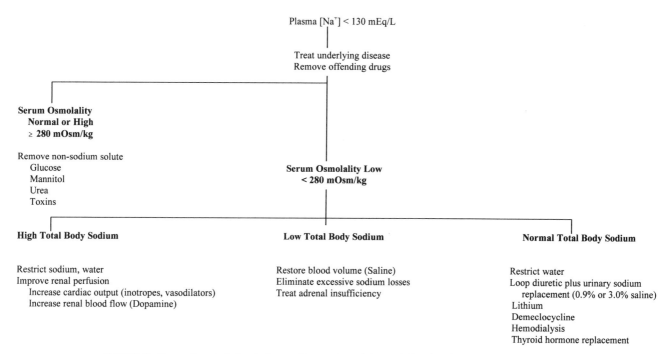

FIGURE 3. Hyponatremia is treated according to the etiology of the disturbance, the level of serum osmolality, and a clinical estimation of total body sodium. (Reproduced from Prough DS, Mathru M. Acid–base, fluids and electrolytes. In: Barash PG, Cullen BF, Stoelting RK, eds. *Clinical anesthesia*, 4th ed. Philadelphia: JB Lippincott, 2001:165–200, with permission.)

Treatment of hyponatremia (Fig. 3) associated with a normal or high serum osmolality requires reduction of the elevated concentrations of the responsible solute (30). Uremic patients are treated by restriction of free water or dialysis. Treatment of edematous (hypervolemic) patients necessitates restriction or removal of both sodium and water. Therapy is directed toward improving cardiac output and renal perfusion and using diuretics to inhibit sodium reabsorption. In hypovolemic, hyponatremic patients, blood volume must be restored, usually by infusion of 0.9% saline. The cornerstone of SIADH management is restriction of free water and elimination of precipitating causes. Water restriction sufficient to decrease total body water by 0.5 to 1.0 L daily, decreases extracellular volume, even if excessive ADH secretion continues. Free-water excretion can be increased by administering furosemide, which will induce greater urinary water losses than sodium losses, resulting in an increase in plasma [Na$^+$] and reducing the risk of excessive extracellular volume expansion secondary to concurrent administration of saline. In the future, antagonists of aquaporins, the recently discovered membrane water receptors that regulate water absorption in the renal collecting ducts, may permit a novel strategy for the treatment of hyponatremia (35,36).

Profound hyponatremia ([Na$^+$] < 115–120 mEq/L or neurologic symptoms) requires more aggressive therapy. Hypertonic (3%) saline is indicated in patients who have seizures or who acutely develop symptoms of water intoxication secondary to intravenous fluid administration. In such cases, 3% saline is administered at a rate of 1 to 2 mL $\cdot$ kg^{-1} $\cdot$ h^{-1} to increase plasma [Na$^+$] by 1 to 2 mEq $\cdot$ L^{-1} $\cdot$ h^{-1}; however, this treatment should not continue for more than a few hours. In extreme cases of

symptomatic hyponatremia, even 29.2% sodium chloride has been used safely in a dose of 50 mL (37).

The expected change in plasma [Na$^+$] resulting from infusion of one liter of infusate can be estimated from the equation (38):

$$\Delta[\text{Na}^+]_s = ([\text{Na}^+]_{\text{inf}} - [\text{Na}^+]_s)/(\text{TBW} + 1)$$

Where $\Delta[\text{Na}^+]_s$ is the change in the patient's serum sodium, $[\text{Na}^+]_{\text{inf}}$ is the sodium concentration of the infusate, $[\text{Na}^+]_s$ is the patient's serum sodium concentration, TBW is the patient's total body water in liters, and 1 is a factor added to take into account the volume of infusate.

Treatment of less severe hyponatremia remains controversial. Although severe hyponatremia may result in neurologic injury, excessively rapid correction can produce central pontine myelinolysis, cerebral hemorrhage, or congestive heart failure. The symptoms of central pontine myelinolysis vary from mild (transient behavioral disturbances or seizures) to severe (including pseudobulbar palsy and quadriparesis). The magnitude and chronicity of hyponatremia and the rate of correction appear to be the principal determinants of the likelihood of demyelinating lesions (39).

Predicting the rate at which plasma [Na$^+$] will increase is difficult because increases are determined not only by the composition of the infused fluid but also, to a major degree, by the rate of renal free-water excretion (40). Defining a safe rate of correction may be impossible, although more rapid correction is clearly more hazardous (41). Initially, plasma [Na$^+$] may be increased by 1 to 2 mEq $\cdot$ L^{-1} $\cdot$ h^{-1}; however, plasma [Na$^+$] should not increase more than 12 mEq per liter in 24 hours or 25 mEq per liter in

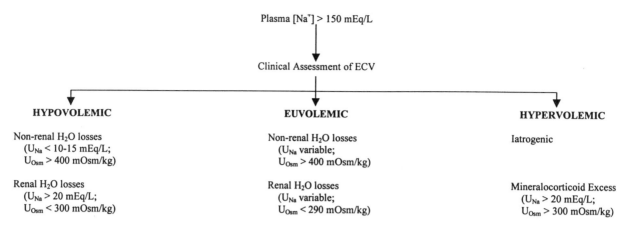

FIGURE 4. Severe hypernatremia is evaluated by first assessing extracellular volume (ECV) to separate patients into hypovolemic, euvolemic, and hypervolemic groups. Next, potential causes are diagnostically assessed. (Reproduced from Prough DS, Mathru M. Acid–base, fluids and electrolytes. In: Barash PG, Cullen BF, Stoelting RK, eds. *Clinical anesthesia*, 4th ed. Philadelphia: JB Lippincott, 2001:165–200, with permission.)

48 hours (42). Hypernatremia should be avoided. Once the plasma [Na$^+$] exceeds 120 to 125 mEq per liter, water restriction alone is usually sufficient to normalize [Na$^+$]. An alternative approach is to increase [Na$^+$] promptly by about 10 mmol and then to proceed more slowly, based on the rationale that cerebral water is increased by approximately 10% in chronic hyponatremia (43). As acute hyponatremia is corrected, central nervous system signs and symptoms usually improve within 24 to 96 hours. Once hyponatremia has improved, careful fluid restriction is necessary to avoid recurrence of hyponatremia.

Demeclocycline and lithium, although potentially toxic, have been used effectively to reverse SIADH in patients in whom the primary disease process is irreversible. Although better tolerated than lithium, demeclocycline may induce nephrotoxicity, a particular concern in patients with renal dysfunction. Hemodialysis is occasionally necessary in severely hyponatremic patients who cannot be adequately managed with drugs or hypertonic saline.

Hypernatremia

Hypernatremia ([Na$^+$] greater than 150 mEq/L) may produce neurologic symptoms (including stupor, coma, and seizures), hypovolemia, renal insufficiency (occasionally progressing to renal failure) and decreased urinary concentrating ability (44,45). Postoperative neurosurgical patients who have undergone pituitary surgery are at particular risk of developing transient or prolonged diabetes insipidus. The clinical consequences of hypernatremia are most serious at the extremes of age and when hypernatremia develops abruptly. Brain shrinkage may damage delicate cerebral vessels, leading to subdural hematoma, subcortical parenchymal hemorrhage, subarachnoid hemorrhage, and venous thrombosis. Polyuria may cause bladder distention, hydronephrosis, and permanent renal damage.

Hypernatremia indicates an absolute or relative water deficit and always is associated with hypertonicity. Signs of hypoperfusion also may be present. Before hypernatremia develops, an increased volume of hypotonic urine may suggest an abnormality

in water balance (46). The total body water (TBW) deficit can be estimated from the plasma [Na$^+$] using the following equation:

$$\text{TBW deficit (liters)} = \text{TBW} \times (1 - [140/\text{serum sodium}])$$

where TBW is 0.6 × current body weight. This formula, which underestimates the deficit in patients with hypotonic fluid losses (47), is useful primarily as a means of approximating anticipated therapy. Otherwise, the sometimes large quantities of fluid required may not be appreciated.

To determine therapy, hypernatremic patients must be separated into three groups, based on clinical assessment of extracellular volume (Fig. 4) (30). Treatment of hypernatremia resulting from water loss consists of repletion of water as well as associated deficits in total body sodium and other electrolytes (Table 10). Hypovolemia should be corrected promptly with 0.9% saline. Once hypovolemia is corrected, water can be replaced orally or intravenously using hypotonic fluids. Hypernatremia must be corrected slowly because of the risk of neurologic sequelae, such as seizures or cerebral edema (47,48). At the cellular level,

TABLE 10. HYPERNATREMIA: ACUTE TREATMENT

Sodium depletion (hypovolemia)
  Hypovolemia correction (0.9% saline)
  Hypernatremia correction (hypotonic fluids)
Sodium overload (hypervolemia)
  Enhance sodium removal (loop diuretics, dialysis)
  Replace water deficit (hypotonic fluids)
Normal total body sodium (euvolemia)
  Replace water deficit (hypotonic fluids)
  Control diabetes insipidus
    Central diabetes insipidus:
      DDAVP, 10–20 μg intranasally; 2.0–4.0 μg s.c.
      Aqueous vasopressin, 5.0 U q 2.0–4.0 h i.m. or s.c.
    Nephrogenic diabetes insipidus:
      Restrict sodium, water intake
      Thiazide diuretics

DDAVP, deamino-8-D-arginine vasopressin; s.c., subcutaneously; i.m., intramuscularly.

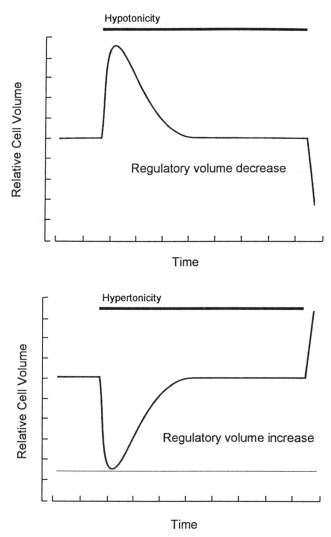

FIGURE 5. Activation of mechanisms regulating cell volume in response to acute osmotic stress. Regulatory volume decrease and regulatory volume increase refer to compensatory losses and gains of solutes. Although the course of these regulatory volume decreases and increases varies with the type of cell and experimental conditions, typically the responses occur over a period of minutes. Returning volume-regulated cells to normotonic conditions causes shrinkage or swelling. (Reproduced from McManus ML, Churchwill KB, Strange K. Regulation of cell volume in health and disease. *N Engl J Med* 1995;333:1260, with permission.)

restoration of cell volume occurs remarkably quickly after tonicity is altered (Fig. 5) (49). The plasma [Na$^+$] should not decrease by more than 1.0 to 2.0 mEq $\cdot$ L^{-1} $\cdot$ h^{-1}. Reversible underlying causes should be treated. In the occasional sodium-overloaded patient, sodium excretion can be accelerated using loop diuretics or dialysis.

The management of hypernatremia secondary to diabetes insipidus varies according to whether the etiology is central or nephrogenic (Table 10). The two most suitable agents for correcting central diabetes insipidus (an ADH deficiency syndrome) are desmopressin (DDAVP) and aqueous vasopressin. DDAVP, given subcutaneously in a dose of 1.0 to 4.0 μg or intranasally in a dose of 5.0 to 20 μg every 12 to 24 hours, is effective in most patients. DDAVP lacks the vasoconstrictor effects of vaso-

pressin and is less likely to produce abdominal cramping (50,51). In patients with incomplete ADH deficits (partial diabetes insipidus), the combination of chlorpropamide (100–250 mg/day) and clofibrate or a thiazide diuretic may be effective in patients who respond inadequately to either drug alone. In nephrogenic diabetes insipidus, urinary water losses can be decreased by using salt and water restriction or thiazide diuretics to induce extracellular volume contraction and enhance fluid reabsorption in the proximal tubules.

POTASSIUM

The intracellular concentration of potassium, the predominant intracellular cation, is normally 150 mEq per liter; the normal extracellular potassium concentration ([K$^+$]) is only 3.5 to 5.0 mEq per liter. Total body potassium in a 70-kg adult is approximately 4,256 mEq, of which 4,200 mEq is intracellular; of 56 mEq in the extracellular volume, only 12 mEq is located in the plasma volume. Potassium plays an important role in maintaining resting membrane potentials and in generating action potentials in the central nervous system and heart.

Total body potassium and [K$^+$] are regulated primarily by aldosterone, epinephrine, and insulin and by intrinsic renal mechanisms that regulate renal potassium excretion. Aldosterone increases renal reabsorption of sodium and excretion of potassium. Secretion of either epinephrine or insulin shifts potassium intracellularly and provides an important short-term response to hyperkalemia. Usually, only 40 to 120 mEq of potassium is lost daily in urine. Dietary potassium intake, unless greater than normal, can be excreted as long as the glomerular filtration rate (GFR) exceeds 8.0 mL per minute. In the proximal renal tubule, 50% to 70% of filtered potassium is passively reabsorbed. Potassium secretion into the distal convoluted tubules and cortical collecting ducts is increased by aldosterone, hyperkalemia, high urinary flow rates, and the presence in luminal fluid of nonreabsorbable anions, such as carbenicillin, phosphates, and sulfates. Additional potassium is reabsorbed from the medullary collecting ducts as part of a recycling loop. Within the distal nephron, a magnesium-dependent sodium/potassium ATPase enzyme plays a critical role in potassium reabsorption. Magnesium depletion impairs the activity of the enzyme, leading to renal potassium wasting.

Hypokalemia

Hypokalemia ([K$^+$] < 3.0 mEq/L) causes muscle weakness and, when severe, may even cause paralysis. Acute hypokalemia causes hyperpolarization of cardiac cells and may lead to ventricular escape activity, reentrant phenomena, ectopic tachycardias, and delayed conduction, but did not, in a prospective study, increase the incidence of intraoperative dysrhythmias (52). Potassium depletion reduces renal concentrating ability, resulting in polyuria and a decreased GFR. Potassium replacement improves GFR; however, the concentrating deficit may not improve for several months after treatment of hypokalemia. If hypokalemia is sufficiently prolonged, chronic renal interstitial damage may occur.

The plasma $[K^+]$ poorly reflects total body potassium; hypokalemia may occur with normal, low, or high total body potassium stores. As a general rule, a chronic decrement of 1.0 mEq per liter in the plasma $[K^+]$ corresponds to a total body deficit of approximately 200 to 300 mEq. In uncomplicated hypokalemia, the potassium deficit exceeds 300 mEq if plasma $[K^+]$ is less than 3.0 mEq per liter and 700 mEq if plasma $[K^+]$ is less than 2.0 mEq per liter.

Hypokalemia may result from acute redistribution of potassium from the extracellular to the intracellular space or from chronic depletion of total body potassium. Redistribution of potassium into cells occurs when the activity of the sodium-potassium ATPase pump is acutely increased by extracellular hyperkalemia or increased intracellular concentrations of sodium as well as by insulin, carbohydrate loading (which stimulates release of endogenous insulin), β_2 agonists, and aldosterone. Both metabolic and respiratory alkalosis lead to decreases in plasma $[K^+]$ (53). Respiratory acidosis tends to increase plasma $[K^+]$; however, organic acidoses (i.e., lactic acidosis, ketoacidosis) have little effect on $[K^+]$, whereas mineral acids cause significant cellular shifts.

Causes of chronic hypokalemia include those associated with renal potassium conservation (low urinary $[K^+]$) and those associated with renal potassium wasting (high urinary $[K^+]$). A low urinary $[K^+]$ suggests inadequate dietary intake or extrarenal depletion (in the absence of recent diuretic use). Diuretic-induced urinary potassium losses are frequently associated with hypokalemia, secondary to increased aldosterone secretion, alkalemia, and increased renal tubular flow. Aldosterone does not cause renal potassium wasting unless sodium ions are present; that is, aldosterone primarily controls sodium reabsorption, not potassium excretion. Renal tubular damage due to nephrotoxins such as aminoglycosides or amphotericin B also can cause renal potassium wasting.

Initial evaluation of hypokalemia includes a medical history (e.g., vomiting or diuretic use), physical examination (e.g., edema), and measurement of serum electrolytes (e.g., magnesium) and arterial pH. Measurement of 24-hour urinary excretion of sodium and potassium may distinguish extrarenal from renal causes. Plasma renin and aldosterone levels may be helpful in the differential diagnosis.

The treatment of hypokalemia consists of potassium repletion, correction of alkalemia, and removal of offending drugs. Hypokalemia secondary only to acute redistribution requires no treatment. If total body potassium is decreased, oral potassium supplementation is preferable to intravenous replacement. Potassium is usually replaced as the chloride salt because coexisting chloride deficiency may limit the ability of the kidney to conserve potassium. Potassium replacement may not be necessary in patients with asymptomatic, mild to moderate hypokalemia (3.0–3.5 mEq/L).

Potassium repletion must be performed cautiously, usually at a rate of less than or equal to 10 to 20 mEq per hour. The plasma $[K^+]$ and the electrocardiogram (ECG) must be monitored during rapid repletion (>20 mEq/h) to avoid hyperkalemic complications. Particular care should be taken in patients who have concurrent acidemia, type IV renal tubular acidosis, diabetes mellitus, or in those patients receiving nonsteroidal antiinflammatory agents, ACE inhibitors, or β-blockers, all of which delay movement of extracellular potassium into cells.

Hypokalemia associated with hyperaldosteronemia (e.g., primary aldosteronism, Cushing syndrome) usually responds favorably to reduced sodium intake and increased potassium intake. Intercurrent hypomagnesemia also should be treated. In patients who are both acidemic and hypokalemic, such as those who have diabetic ketoacidosis, potassium administration should precede correction of acidosis to avoid a precipitous decrease in plasma $[K^+]$ as pH increases.

Hyperkalemia

The most lethal manifestations of hyperkalemia ($[K^+]$ > 5.0 mEq/L) involve the cardiac conducting system and include dysrhythmias, conduction abnormalities, and cardiac arrest. If plasma $[K^+]$ is below 6.0 mEq per L, cardiac effects are negligible. As $[K^+]$ progressively increases, the ECG first shows tall, peaked T waves, especially in the precordial leads; then the P-R interval becomes prolonged, followed by a decrease in the amplitude of the P wave. Finally, the QRS complex widens as a prelude to cardiac standstill (Fig. 6) (54). Hyperkalemic cardiotoxicity is enhanced by hyponatremia, hypocalcemia, or acidosis. Progression to fatal cardiotoxicity is unpredictable and often swift. Ascending muscle weakness appears when plasma $[K^+]$ approaches 7.0 mEq per liter and may progress to flaccid paralysis, inability to phonate, and even respiratory arrest.

Hyperkalemia may occur with normal, high, or low total body potassium stores. A deficiency of aldosterone, a major regulator of potassium excretion, will lead to hyperkalemia. Because the kidneys excrete potassium, severe renal insufficiency commonly causes hyperkalemia. Patients with chronic renal insufficiency can maintain normal plasma $[K^+]$ by using tubular secretion until GFR falls below 8.0 mL per minute. Drugs that limit potassium excretion, including nonsteroidal antiinflammatory drugs, ACE inhibitors, cyclosporine, and potassium-sparing diuretics (e.g., triamterene), are now the most common cause of hyperkalemia (55). Drug effects most commonly occur in patients with other factors (e.g., advanced age) that predispose them to hyperkalemia (56). In patients who have normal total body potassium, hyperkalemia may accompany a sudden shift of potassium from the intracellular volume to the extracellular volume because of acidemia, increased catabolism, or rhabdomyolysis.

The treatment of hyperkalemia is aimed at eliminating the cause, reversing membrane hyperexcitability, and removing potassium from the body (Table 11). Mineralocorticoid deficiency can be treated with 9-alpha-fludrocortisone (0.1–0.2 mg/day). Hyperkalemia secondary to digitalis intoxication may be resistant to therapy because attempts to shift potassium from the extracellular volume to the intracellular volume are often ineffective. In this situation, use of digoxin-specific antibodies has been successful.

Membrane hyperexcitability can be antagonized by translocating potassium from the extracellular volume to the intracellular volume, removing excess potassium, or (transiently) by infusing calcium chloride ($CaCl_2$) to depress the membrane threshold potential. Acute alkalinization using sodium bicarbonate (50–100 mEq over 5–10 minutes in a 70-kg adult) transiently translocates potassium to the intracellular volume. Insulin, which increases the activity of the sodium/potassium ATPase pump, increases cellular uptake of potassium best when high insulin levels

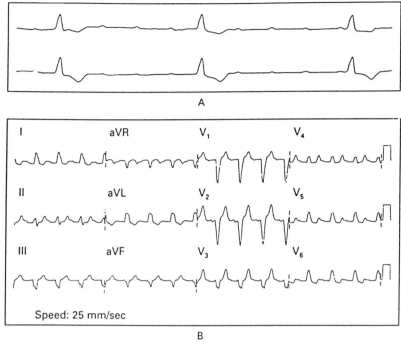

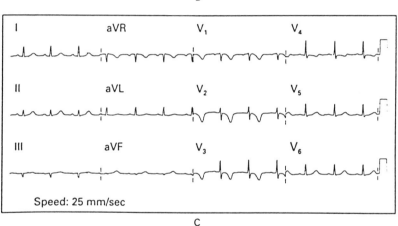

FIGURE 6. Electrocardiographic changes caused by hyperkalemia occurring in a 42-year-old woman undergoing placement of an arteriovenous fistula for permanent hemodialysis access to treat end-stage renal disease. During dissection of the brachial artery under local anesthesia, her cardiac rhythm converted from normal sinus rhythm to complete heart block with ventricular escape (approximately 25 beats per minute) (**A**). Two ampules of calcium gluconate (9.2 mEq) were administered intravenously. An electrocardiogram revealed sinus tachycardia with profound prolongation of the QRS interval (left-bundle-branch morphology), first-degree atrioventricular block, and "peaked" T waves (**B**). The serum potassium concentration was 8.6 mmol per liter. After reduction of the serum potassium concentration, the electrocardiogram showed sinus rhythm with normalization of the PR and QRS intervals. Anteroseptal ST wave and T wave changes were noted on subsequent electrocardiograms (**C**). A cardiac exercise imaging study did not show ischemia. (From Kuvin JT. Electrocardiographic changes of hyperkalemia. *N Engl J Med* 1998;338:662, with permission.)

are achieved by intravenous injection of 5 to 10 U of regular insulin accompanied by 50 mL of 50% glucose. Salbutamol, a selective β_2 agonist, decreases serum potassium acutely when

TABLE 11. SEVERE[a] HYPERKALEMIA: GOAL OF TREATMENT

Reverse membrane effects
   Calcium (10 mL of 10% calcium chloride i.v. over 2.0–5.0 min)
Transfer extracellular [K+] into cells
   Glucose and insulin (D10W + 5.0–10 U regular insulin per 25–50 g glucose)
   Sodium bicarbonate (50–100 mEq over 5.0–10 min)
   β_2 Agonists
Remove potassium from body
   Diuretics, proximal or loop
   Potassium-exchange resins (sodium polystyrene sulfonate)
   Hemodialysis
Monitor ECG and serum [K+] level

i.v., intravenous.
[a] Potassium concentration ([K+]) > 7.0 mEq/L or electrocardiographic (ECG) changes.

given by inhalation or intravenously. In 15 pediatric patients with mean baseline serum [K+] of 6.6 mEq per liter, a single infusion of salbutamol (5.0 μg/kg over 15 minutes) reduced serum [K+] to 5.7 mEq per liter after 30 minutes and 4.9 mEq per liter after 120 minutes (57). In adult patients with end-stage renal disease, addition of salbutamol (0.5 mg administered intravenously or 10 mg nebulized) to insulin and glucose may be effective (58). Insulin, which increases the activity of the Na+/K+ ATPase pump, increases cellular uptake of potassium best when high insulin levels are achieved by intravenous injection of 5.0 to 10 U of regular insulin, accompanied by 50 mL of 50% glucose. Pending definitive treatment, rapid infusion of CaCl₂ (i.e., 1 g over 3 minutes) may stabilize cardiac rhythm. Calcium should be given cautiously if digitalis intoxication is likely. Potassium may be removed from the body by the kidneys (using loop diuretics) or the gastrointestinal tract. Sodium polystyrene sulfonate resin (Kayexalate), which exchanges sodium for potassium, can be given orally (30 g) or as a retention enema (50 g in 200 mL of 20% sorbitol). Emergency hemodialysis, rarely necessary, may remove 25 to 50 mEq per hour.

CALCIUM

Because Chapter 57 discusses calcium metabolism, hypocalcemia, and hypercalcemia in detail, those topics will not be addressed in detail in this chapter.

Calcium is a divalent cation found primarily in the extracellular fluid. Calcium is regulated by multiple factors, including a calcium receptor (59) and several hormones, the most important of which are parathyroid hormone (PTH) and calcitriol (60). Calcitriol and PTH mobilize calcium from bone, increase reabsorption of calcium from the renal tubule, and enhance intestinal absorption of calcium. The free calcium $[Ca^{2+}]$ in extracellular volume is approximately 1 mM, whereas the free $[Ca^{2+}]$ in the intracellular volume approximates 100 nM. Circulating calcium includes protein-bound (40%), chelated (10%), and ionized fractions (50%); only the ionized fraction is physiologically active. Because mathematical formulae that "correct" total calcium measurements for albumin concentration are inaccurate in critically ill patients, ionized calcium should be measured directly. Acute acidemia increases and acute alkalemia decreases ionized calcium.

Calcium is essential for excitation–contraction coupling, muscle function, ciliary movement, mitosis, neurotransmitter release, enzyme secretion, hormonal secretion, and cellular metabolism. Important both for generation of the cardiac pacemaker activity and for generation of the cardiac action potential, calcium is the primary ion responsible for the plateau phase of the action potential.

Hypocalcemia

The hallmark of hypocalcemia is increased neuronal membrane irritability and tetany. In frank tetany, tonic contraction of respiratory muscles may lead to laryngospasm, bronchospasm, or respiratory arrest. Smooth-muscle spasm can result in abdominal cramping and urinary frequency. Mental status alterations include irritability, depression, psychosis, and dementia. Hypocalcemia has been associated with heart failure, hypotension, dysrhythmias, insensitivity to digitalis, and impaired β-adrenergic action. Reduced total serum calcium occurs in as many as 80% of critically ill and postsurgical patients. Fewer patients, however, develop ionized hypocalcemia, including 15% to 20% of critically ill patients, 20% of patients after cardiopulmonary bypass, and 30% to 40% after multiple trauma. In these situations, ionized hypocalcemia is clinically mild (ionized serum calcium concentrations 0.8 mM).

Hypocalcemia (ionized $[Ca^{2+}] < 4.0$ mg/dL or 1 mM) occurs as a result of failure of PTH or calcitriol action or because of calcium chelation or precipitation, not because of calcium deficiency alone. The differential diagnosis of hypocalcemia can be approached by addressing four issues: age of the patient, serum phosphate concentration, general clinical status, and duration of hypocalcemia (61). PTH deficiency can result from parathyroid suppression or surgical damage or removal. Parathyroid gland suppression may occur during severe hypomagnesemia or hypermagnesemia, burns, sepsis, or pancreatitis. Vitamin D deficiency may result from dietary lack or malabsorption in patients who lack sunlight exposure. High phosphate concentrations suggest renal failure or hypoparathyroidism. In renal insufficiency, reduced phosphorus excretion results in hyperphosphatemia, which downregulates the 1α-hydroxylase responsible for the renal conversion of calcidiol to calcitriol. This, in combination with decreased production of calcitriol secondary to reduced renal mass, causes reduced intestinal absorption of calcium and hypocalcemia (60). Hyperphosphatemia-induced hypocalcemia also may occur as a consequence of phosphate therapy, rhabdomyolysis, or cell lysis secondary to chemotherapy. Ionized calcium decreases approximately 0.019 mM for each 1.0-mM increase in phosphate concentration (62). In massive transfusion, citrate may produce transient, hemodynamically benign hypocalcemia by chelating calcium. A healthy, normothermic adult who has intact hepatic and renal function can metabolize the citrate present in 20 U of blood per hour without becoming hypocalcemic (63). When, however, citrate clearance is decreased (e.g., by hepatic or renal disease or hypothermia) and when blood transfusion rates are rapid (e.g., $0.5–2$ mL $\cdot$ kg^{-1} $\cdot$ min^{-1}), hypocalcemia and cardiovascular compromise may occur.

In treating hypocalcemia, unnecessary offending drugs should be discontinued. Hypocalcemia resulting from hypomagnesemia or hyperphosphatemia is treated by repletion or removal of magnesium or phosphate, respectively. Hyperkalemia and hypomagnesemia potentiate hypocalcemia-induced cardiac and neuromuscular irritability. In contrast, hypokalemia protects against hypocalcemic tetany; therefore, correction of hypokalemia without correction of hypocalcemia may provoke tetany. Mild, ionized hypocalcemia should not be overtreated. Calcium administration also has been questioned in the setting of mild hypocalcemia in patients suffering from sepsis and septic shock because of the possibility of interference with intracellular protective mechanisms (64).

The cornerstone of therapy for symptomatic, ionized hypocalcemia ($[Ca^{2+}] < 0.7$ mM) is calcium administration. In patients who have severe hypocalcemia or hypocalcemic symptoms, calcium should be administered intravenously. In emergency situations, in an average-sized adult, the "rule of tens" stipulates infusion of 10 mL of 10% calcium gluconate (93 mg elemental calcium) over 10 minutes. This infusion is followed by continuous infusion of elemental calcium, 0.3 to 2 mg $\cdot$ kg^{-1} $\cdot$ h^{-1} (i.e., 3–16 mL per hour of 10% calcium gluconate for a 70-kg adult). Calcium salts should be diluted in 50 to 100 mL of 5% dextrose in water (to limit venous irritation and thrombosis), should not be mixed with bicarbonate (to prevent precipitation), and must be given cautiously to patients receiving digoxin because calcium increases the toxicity of digoxin. Continuous ECG monitoring during initial therapy will detect cardiotoxicity (i.e., heart block, ventricular fibrillation). During calcium replacement, the clinician should monitor serum calcium, magnesium, phosphate, potassium, and SCr. Once the ionized $[Ca^{2+}]$ is stable in the range of 4 to 5 mg per deciliter (1.0–1.25 mM), oral calcium supplements can substitute for parenteral therapy. Urinary calcium should be monitored in an attempt to avoid hypercalciuria (>5.0 mg/kg per 24 hours) and urinary tract stone formation. Treatment of patients with both tetany and hyperphosphatemia requires coordination of therapy to avoid the consequences of metastatic soft-tissue calcification (Table 12) (65).

TABLE 12. TREATMENT OF CONCOMITANT HYPOCALCEMIA AND HYPERPHOSPHATEMIA

Treatment of Hyperphosphatemia	Treatment of Hypocalcemia
Increased renal excretion	Urgently required if symptomatic
Diuresis	
Dopamine	Calcium i.v. to increase $[Ca^{2+}]$
Redistribution	to low-normal
Dextrose/insulin	Immediate measures
Correct acidosis	to normalize $[PO_4]$
Deposition into bone	
Administer calcium	
Decreased absorption	
Oral phosphate binders	
Direct removal	
Hemodialysis	

i.v., intravenous; $[Ca^{2+}]$, ionized calcium concentration; $[PO_4]$, plasma phosphate concentration.
Reproduced from Sutters M, Gaboury CL, Bennett WM. Severe hyperphosphatemia and hypocalcemia: a dilemma in patient management. *J Am Soc Nephrol* 1996;7:2055, with permission.

Hypercalcemia

Although ionized $[Ca^{2+}]$ most accurately demonstrates hypercalcemia (ionized $[Ca^{2+}]$ >1.3 mM), *hypercalcemia* is defined conventionally as total serum calcium levels greater than 10.5 mg per deciliter. Patients in whom total serum calcium is below 11.5 mg per deciliter are usually asymptomatic. Patients with moderate hypercalcemia (total serum calcium 11.5–13 mg/dL) may have lethargy, anorexia, nausea, and polyuria. Severe hypercalcemia (total serum calcium >13 mg/dL) is associated with more severe symptoms, including muscle weakness, depression, impaired memory, emotional lability, lethargy, stupor, and coma. The cardiovascular effects of hypercalcemia include hypertension, arrhythmias, heart block, cardiac arrest, and digitalis sensitivity.

Hypercalcemia impairs urinary concentrating ability and renal excretion of calcium by irreversibly precipitating calcium salts within the renal parenchyma and by reducing renal blood flow and GFR. In response to hypovolemia, enhanced renal tubular reabsorption of sodium increases renal calcium reabsorption. Effective treatment of severe hypercalcemia is necessary to prevent progressive dehydration and renal failure leading to further increases in total serum calcium. Prolonged hypercalcemia may result in skeletal disease secondary to direct osteolysis or humoral bone resorption.

Hypercalcemia occurs when calcium enters the extracellular volume more rapidly than the kidneys can excrete the excess. Clinically, hypercalcemia most commonly results from an excess of bone resorption over bone formation, usually secondary to malignant disease, hyperparathyroidism, thyrotoxicosis, granulomatous diseases, or immobilization (66). Factors that promote hypercalcemia may be offset by coexisting disorders, such as pancreatitis, sepsis, or hyperphosphatemia, that reduce serum calcium.

Although definitive treatment of hypercalcemia requires correction of underlying causes, temporizing therapy may be necessary to avoid complications and to relieve symptoms. Total serum calcium exceeding 14 mg per deciliter represents a medical emergency. General supportive treatment includes hydration, correction of associated electrolyte abnormalities, removal of offending drugs, dietary calcium restriction, and increased physical activity. Because anorexia and antagonism by calcium of ADH action invariably lead to sodium and water depletion, infusion of 0.9% saline will dilute serum calcium, promote renal excretion, and can reduce total serum calcium by 1.5 to 3 mg per deciliter. Urinary output should be maintained at 200 to 300 mL per hour. As GFR increases, the sodium ion increases calcium excretion by competing with the calcium ion for reabsorption in the proximal renal tubules and loop of Henle. Furosemide further enhances calcium excretion by increasing tubular sodium. During saline infusion and forced diuresis, careful monitoring of cardiopulmonary status and electrolytes, especially magnesium and potassium, is required. Intensive diuresis and saline administration can achieve net calcium excretion rates of 2,000 to 4,000 mg per 24 hours, a rate eight times greater than saline alone, but still somewhat less than the rate of removal achieved by hemodialysis (i.e, 6,000 mg every 8 hours). Patients treated with phosphates should be well hydrated.

Bone resorption, the primary cause of hypercalcemia, can be minimized by mobilization and drug therapy. Specific drug therapy is based on the cause of the hypercalcemia and the pharmacodynamics and side effects of individual agents (67). Calcitonin is most effective in hypercalcemic states resulting from increased bone resorption (e.g., Paget disease, malignant disease, and immobilization). Calcitonin begins to reduce serum calcium within 1 to 2 hours after drug administration, with the maximal effect evident at 6 to 10 hours. Usually, calcitonin reduces total serum calcium by only 1 to 2 mg per deciliter. Mithramycin, a cytotoxic agent, lowers serum calcium primarily by inhibiting bone resorption, probably because of toxicity to osteoclasts. The hypocalcemic effect, usually seen within 12 to 24 hours after a single intravenous dose of 25 μg per kilogram of body weight, peaks at 48 to 72 hours, and persists for 5 to 7 days. Diphosphonate inhibits both bone resorption and mineralization. Pamidronate, an aminobisphosphonate 100 times more potent than etidronate, normalized serum calcium levels in 70% of patients with malignancy-associated hypercalcemia (68). Hydrocortisone is effective in treating hypercalcemic patients with lymphatic malignancies, vitamin D or A intoxication, and diseases associated with production of 1,25(OH)-D or osteoclast-activating factor by tumors or granulomas but rarely improves hypercalcemia secondary to malignancy or hyperparathyroidism.

Phosphates lower serum calcium by causing deposition of calcium in bone and soft tissue. Because the risk of extraskeletal calcification of organs such as the kidneys and myocardium is less if phosphates are given orally, the intravenous route should be reserved for patients with life-threatening hypercalcemia or patients in whom other measures have failed. The initial dose of intravenous phosphates should not exceed 50 mM within 8 hours.

MAGNESIUM

Magnesium is a multifunctional, divalent cation located primarily intracellularly. Approximately 50% of total body magnesium is located in bone, 25% in muscle, and less than 1% in serum. The normal serum concentration is 1.5 to 1.9 mEq per liter (0.75–0.95 mmol/L or 1.7-2.2 mg/dL) (69). Only ionized magnesium (55% of the serum concentration) is active. As a primary regulator or cofactor in many enzyme systems, magnesium is important for the regulation of the sodium–potassium pump, Ca^{2+}-ATPase enzymes, adenyl cyclase, proton pumps, and slow calcium channels. Magnesium has been called an endogenous calcium antagonist because regulation of slow calcium channels contributes to maintenance of normal vascular tone, prevention of vasospasm, and perhaps to prevention of calcium overload in many tissues. Because magnesium partially regulates PTH secretion and is important for the maintenance of end-organ sensitivity to both PTH and vitamin D, abnormalities in ionized magnesium concentration ($[Mg^{2+}]$) may result in abnormal calcium metabolism. Magnesium functions in potassium metabolism primarily through regulating sodium-potassium ATPase, an enzyme that controls potassium entry into cells, especially in potassium-depleted states, and controls reabsorption of potassium by the renal tubules. In addition, magnesium functions as a regulator of membrane excitability and serves as a structural component in both cell membranes and the skeleton.

Because magnesium stabilizes axonal membranes, reduction of magnesium concentration decreases the threshold of axonal stimulation and increases nerve-conduction velocity. Magnesium also influences the release of neurotransmitters at the neuromuscular junction by competitively inhibiting the entry of calcium into the presynaptic nerve terminals. The concentration of calcium required to trigger calcium release and the rate at which calcium is released from the sarcoplasmic reticulum are inversely related to the ambient magnesium concentration.

Serum $[Mg^{2+}]$ is regulated primarily by intrinsic renal mechanisms, although PTH and vitamin D exert minor influences. Whereas both magnesium and phosphate are regulated primarily by intrinsic renal mechanisms, PTH exerts a greater effect on renal loss of phosphate.

Hypomagnesemia

Magnesium deficiency has been identified in approximately 10% of hospitalized patients and as many as 40% of patients with other electrolyte disturbances (70). Of alcoholic patients admitted to the hospital, 30% are hypomagnesemic (71). The clinical features of hypomagnesemia ($[Mg^{2+}]$ <1.7 mg/dL), like those of hypocalcemia, are characterized by increased neuronal irritability and tetany (72). Although hypomagnesemia is common in critically ill patients, serum $[Mg^{2+}]$ may not reflect intracellular magnesium content (73). Symptoms are rare when the serum $[Mg^{2+}]$ is above 1.5 to 1.7 mg per deciliter; most symptomatic patients have serum $[Mg^{2+}]$ less than 1.0 mg per deciliter. Patients frequently complain of weakness, lethargy, muscle spasms, paresthesias, and depression. When severe, hypomagnesemia may induce seizures, confusion, and coma. Cardiovascular abnormalities include coronary artery spasm, cardiac failure, dysrhythmias, and hypotension.

Hypomagnesemia rarely results from inadequate dietary intake. The most common causes are inadequate gastrointestinal absorption, excessive magnesium losses, or failure of renal magnesium conservation (70). Excessive magnesium loss is associated with gastrointestinal disease, prolonged nasogastric suctioning, gastrointestinal or biliary fistulas, intestinal drains, and polyuria. Inability of the renal tubules to conserve magnesium complicates a variety of systemic and renal diseases, although advanced renal disease with a decreased GFR may lead to magnesium retention. Various drugs and toxins, including aminoglycosides, cis-platinum, cardiac glycosides, and diuretics, enhance urinary magnesium excretion. Intracellular shifts of magnesium as a result of thyroid hormone or insulin administration may also decrease serum $[Mg^{2+}]$.

Measurement of 24-hour urinary magnesium excretion is useful in separating renal from nonrenal causes of hypomagnesemia. Normal kidneys can reduce magnesium excretion to less than 1.0 to 2.0 mEq per day in response to magnesium depletion. Hypomagnesemia accompanied by high urinary excretion of magnesium (>3.0–4.0 mEq/day) suggests excessive renal losses. Parenteral magnesium tolerance testing is useful in confirming magnesium deficiency in the presence of normal renal function. In the magnesium-loading test, urinary $[Mg^{2+}]$ excretion is measured for 24 hours after an intravenous magnesium load (74).

Magnesium deficiency is treated by the administration of magnesium supplements (Table 13) (75). One gram of magnesium sulfate provides approximately 4 mmol (8.0 mEq, or 98 mg) of elemental magnesium. Symptomatic or severe hypomagnesemia ($[Mg^{2+}]$ <1.0 mg/dL) should be treated with parenteral magnesium: 1.0 to 2.0 g (8.0–16 mEq) of magnesium sulfate as an intravenous bolus over the first hour, followed by a continuous infusion of 0.5 to 1.0 g per hour (4.0–8.0 mEq/h). Therapy should be guided subsequently by the serum magnesium level. The rate of infusion should not exceed 1.0 mEq per minute, even in emergency situations, and the patient should receive continuous cardiac monitoring to detect cardiotoxicity. Because magnesium antagonizes calcium, blood pressure and cardiac function should be monitored, although clinical effects on myocardial contractility and blood pressure appear to be modest.

Magnesium has been used to help manage an impressive array of clinical problems, including cardiac dysrhythmias (76). Magnesium administration may decrease dysrhythmias by direct effects on myocardial membranes, altering cellular potassium and sodium concentrations, inhibiting cellular calcium entry, improving myocardial oxygen supply and demand, prolonging the effective refractory period, depressing conduction, antagonizing catecholamine action on the conducting system, and preventing vasospasm. Treatment of hypomagnesemia, which frequently occurs after cardiopulmonary bypass, decreases the incidence of ventricular dysrhythmias after heart surgery from 63% to 22% (77). In addition, magnesium may be useful as treatment for torsade de pointes, even in normomagnesemic patients. In such cases, the dose is 2.0 g over 10 to 15 minutes and can be repeated once if necessary (70). In patients with myocardial ischemia, magnesium can prevent the ischemic increase in action potential duration and membrane depolarization (78).

Because the sodium–potassium pump is magnesium dependent, hypomagnesemia increases myocardial sensitivity to digitalis preparations and may cause hypokalemia as a result of renal potassium wasting. Attempts to correct potassium deficits with potassium replacement therapy alone may not be successful

TABLE 13. THERAPY OF MAGNESIUM DEPLETION

| Form of Therapy | Indications | Total dose MgSO$_4$·7H$_2$O (g) | Elemental magnesium | | | Remarks |
			mg	mmol	mEq	
Emergency	Ventricular arrhythmias: neuromuscular hyperexcitability	2.0–4.0	200–400	8.0–16	16–32	Administer i.v. in 5% dextrose over 15–30 min
Urgent	Hyperreflexia; serum Mg^{2+} <1.0 mEq/L	6.0	600	25	50	Administer i.v. in 1.0 L 5% dextrose over 3 to 6 h
Non-urgent	Minimal to no symptoms; serum Mg^{2+} 1.0–1.5 mEq/L	6.0–8.0	600–800	25–33	50–66	Administer i.v. over 24 h
Maintenance	Prolonged i.v. sustenance; serum Mg^{2+} > 1.5 mEq/L	3.0–4.0	300–400	12.5–16.5	25–33	Add to daily infusions

i.v., intravenously.
Reproduced from Faber MD, Kupin WL, Heilig CW, et al. Common fluid-electrolyte and acid-base problems in the intensive care unit: selected issues. *Semin Nephrol* 1994;14:8–22, with permission.

without simultaneous magnesium therapy. The interrelationships of magnesium and potassium in cardiac tissue have probably the greatest clinical relevance in terms of arrhythmias, digoxin toxicity, and myocardial infarction. Both severe hypomagnesemia and hypermagnesemia suppress PTH secretion and can cause hypocalcemia. Severe hypomagnesemia also can impair end-organ responses to PTH.

During repletion, the patellar reflexes should be monitored frequently and magnesium withheld if they become suppressed. Patients who have renal insufficiency require careful monitoring during therapy. Repletion of systemic magnesium stores usually requires 5 to 7 days of therapy, after which daily maintenance doses of magnesium should be provided. Magnesium can be given orally, usually in a dose of 60 to 90 mEq per day of magnesium oxide. Hypocalcemic, hypomagnesemic patients should receive magnesium as the chloride salt because the sulfate ion can chelate calcium and further reduce the serum [Ca^{2+}].

Hypermagnesemia

Most cases of hypermagnesemia ([Mg^{2+}] > 2.5 mg/dL) are iatrogenic, resulting from the administration of magnesium in antacids, enemas, or parenteral nutrition, especially to patients with impaired renal function. Because magnesium antagonizes the release and effect of acetylcholine at the neuromuscular junction, hypermagnesemia depresses skeletal muscle function and may induce neuromuscular blockade. Magnesium potentiates the action of nondepolarizing muscle relaxants.

Therapeutic hypermagnesemia is used to treat patients with premature labor, preeclampsia, and eclampsia. Because magnesium blocks the release of catecholamines from adrenergic nerve terminals and the adrenal glands, magnesium has been used to reduce the hypertensive response to tracheal intubation and to reduce the effects of catecholamine excess in patients with tetanus and pheochromocytoma (79).

The neuromuscular and cardiac toxicity of hypermagnesemia can be acutely, but transiently, antagonized by giving intravenous calcium (5.0–10 mEq) to buy time while more definitive therapy is instituted (80). All magnesium-containing preparations must be stopped. Urinary excretion of magnesium can be increased by expanding extracellular volume and inducing diuresis with a combination of saline and furosemide. In emergency situations and in patients with renal failure, magnesium may be removed by dialysis.

PHOSPHATE

Phosphorus, in the form of phosphate, is distributed in similar concentrations throughout intracellular and extracellular fluid. Eighty-five percent of phosphate is osseous, and 15% is nonosseous. Phosphate circulates as free ions (55%), complexed ions (33%), and in a protein-bound form (12%). The normal total serum phosphate level ranges from 2.7 to 4.5 mg per deciliter in adults. Phosphates provide the primary energy bond in ATP and creatine phosphate. Therefore, severe phosphate depletion results in cellular energy depletion. Phosphorus is an essential element of second-messenger systems, including cAMP and phosphoinositides, and a major component of nucleic acids, phospholipids, and cell membranes. As part of 2,3-diphosphoglycerate, phosphate is important for off-loading oxygen from the hemoglobin molecule. Phosphorus also functions in protein phosphorylation and acts as a urinary buffer.

Hypophosphatemia

Hypophosphatemia is characterized by low levels of phosphate-containing cellular components, including ATP, 2,3-diphosphoglycerate, and membrane phospholipids. Serious life-threatening organ dysfunction may occur when the serum phosphate concentration ([PO$_4$]) falls below 1 mg per deciliter. Neurologic manifestations of hypophosphatemia include paresthesias, myopathy, encephalopathy, delirium, seizures, and coma (81). Hematologic abnormalities include dysfunction of erythrocytes, platelets, and leukocytes. Muscle weakness and malaise are common. In perioperative patients, respiratory muscle weakness and myocardial dysfunction are problems of particular concern.

Common in postoperative and traumatized patients (82), hypophosphatemia ([PO$_4$] <2.5 mg/dL) is caused by three primary abnormalities in [PO$_4$] homeostasis: an intracellular shift of

[PO$_4$], an increase in renal losses, and a decrease in gastrointestinal absorption. Carbohydrate-induced hypophosphatemia, mediated by insulin-induced cellular [PO$_4$] uptake, is the type most commonly encountered in hospitalized patients. Hypophosphatemia also may occur as catabolic patients become anabolic and during medical management of diabetic ketoacidosis. Acute alkalemia, which may reduce serum [PO$_4$] to 1.0 to 2.0 mg per deciliter, increases intracellular consumption of [PO$_4$] by increasing the rate of glycolysis. Respiratory alkalosis probably explains the hypophosphatemia associated with gram-negative bacteremia and salicylate poisoning. Excessive renal loss of [PO$_4$] explains the hypophosphatemia associated with hyperparathyroidism, hypomagnesemia, hypothermia, diuretic therapy, and renal tubular defects in [PO$_4$] absorption. Excess gastrointestinal loss of [PO$_4$] is most commonly secondary to the use of [PO$_4$]-binding antacids or to malabsorption syndromes.

Measurement of urinary [PO$_4$] aids in the differentiation of hypophosphatemia resulting from renal losses versus that caused by excessive gastrointestinal losses or redistribution of [PO$_4$] into cells. Extrarenal causes of hypophosphatemia cause avid renal tubular [PO$_4$] reabsorption, reducing urinary excretion to less than 100 mg daily.

Patients who have severe (<1.0 mg/dL) or symptomatic hypophosphatemia require intravenous phosphate administration (81). In chronically hypophosphatemic patients, 0.2 to 0.68 mmol per kilogram (5–16 mg/kg elemental phosphorus) should be infused over 12 hours. For moderately hypophosphatemic adult patients suffering from critical illness, the use of 15 mmol boluses (465 mg) mixed with 100 mL of 0.9% sodium chloride and given over a 2-hour period can replete phosphate safely (83). The dosage then is adjusted as indicated by the serum [PO$_4$] level because the cumulative deficit cannot be predicted accurately. In critically ill patients suffering from severe hypophosphatemia, larger doses (0.64 mmol/kg) of phosphate have been administered over 8 to 12 hours (84). Oral therapy can be substituted for parenteral [PO$_4$] once the serum [PO$_4$] level exceeds 2.0 mg per deciliter. Continued therapy with [PO$_4$] supplements is required for 5 to 10 days to replenish body stores.

Phosphate should be administered cautiously to hypocalcemic patients because of the risk of precipitating more severe hypocalcemia. In hypercalcemic patients, [PO$_4$] may cause soft-tissue calcification. Phosphorus must be given cautiously to patients with renal insufficiency because of impaired excretory ability. During treatment, close monitoring of serum [PO$_4$], calcium, magnesium, and potassium is essential to avoid complications.

Hyperphosphatemia

The clinical features of hyperphosphatemia ([PO$_4$] >5.0 mg/dL) relate primarily to the development of hypocalcemia and ectopic calcification.

Hyperphosphatemia is caused by three basic mechanisms: inadequate renal excretion, increased movement of [PO$_4$] out of cells, and increased [PO$_4$] or vitamin D intake. Renal excretion of [PO$_4$] remains adequate until the GFR falls below 20 to 25 mL per minute. Rapid cell lysis from chemotherapy, rhabdomyolysis, and sepsis can cause hyperphosphatemia, especially when renal function is impaired.

Measurements of BUN, SCr, GFR, and urinary [PO$_4$] are helpful in the differential diagnosis of hyperphosphatemia. Normal renal function accompanied by high [PO$_4$] excretion (>1,500 mg/day) indicates an oversupply of [PO$_4$]. An elevated BUN, elevated SCr, and low GFR suggest impaired renal excretion of [PO$_4$]. Normal renal function and [PO4] excretion less than 1,500 mg per day suggest increased [PO$_4$] reabsorption (i.e., hypoparathyroidism).

Hyperphosphatemia is corrected by eliminating the cause of the [PO$_4$] elevation and correcting the associated hypocalcemia. The serum concentration is reduced by restricting intake, increasing urinary excretion with saline and acetazolamide (500 mg every 6 hours), and increasing gastrointestinal losses by enteric administration of aluminum hydroxide (30–45 mL every 6 hours). Aluminum hydroxide absorbs [PO$_4$] secreted into the bowel lumen and increases [PO$_4$] loss even if none is ingested. Hemodialysis and peritoneal dialysis are effective in removing [PO$_4$] in patients who have renal failure.

SUMMARY

The appropriate identification of acid–base problems is of primary importance if complications of acid–base disturbances are to be avoided. The simple rules outlined here facilitate accurate diagnosis of most acid–base disturbances, thereby allowing appropriate management. The stepwise approach avoids inaccurate conclusions. Finally, the integration of clinical information into interpretation of the acid–base data must always be considered.

Commonly occurring in critically ill surgical patients, electrolyte disturbances cause dysfunction in multiple organ systems. Recognition and prompt therapy of disorders of concentrations of sodium, potassium, calcium, magnesium, and phosphate may limit morbidity and mortality.

KEY POINTS

The Henderson–Hasselbalch equation describes the relationship between pH, Pa$_{CO_2}$, and serum bicarbonate. The Henderson equation defines the previous relationship but substitutes hydrogen concentration for pH.

The pathophysiology of metabolic alkalosis is divided into generating and maintenance factors. A particularly important maintenance factor is renal hypoperfusion, which is often due to hypovolemia.

The addition of iatrogenic respiratory alkalosis to metabolic alkalosis can produce severe alkalemia.

Metabolic acidosis occurs as a consequence of the use of bicarbonate to buffer endogenous organic acids or as a consequence of external bicarbonate loss. The former causes an increase in the anion gap ($Na^+ - ([Cl^-] + [HCO_3^-])$).

When initiating mechanical ventilation in a patient with severe metabolic acidosis, it is important to maintain an appropriate level of ventilatory compensation, pending effective treatment of the primary cause for the metabolic acidosis.

Sodium bicarbonate, never proved to alter outcome in patients with lactic acidosis, should be reserved for those patients with severe acidemia.

Homeostatic mechanisms are usually adequate for the maintenance of electrolyte balance; however, critical illnesses and their treatment strategies can cause significant perturbations in electrolyte status, possibly leading to worsened patient outcome.

Disorders of the concentration of sodium, the principal extracellular cation, are dependent on the total body water concentration and can lead to neurologic dysfunction.

Disorders of potassium, the principal intracellular cation, are influenced primarily by insults that result in increased total body losses of potassium or changes in distribution.

Calcium, phosphorus, and magnesium are all essential for maintenance and function of the cardiovascular system. In addition, they also provide the milieu that ensures neuromuscular transmission. Disorders affecting any one of these electrolytes may lead to significant dysfunction and possibly result in cardiopulmonary arrest.

Whereas most imbalances encountered are only mild to moderate, proper diagnosis and treatment are essential to avoid the consequences associated with severe disorders.

REFERENCES

1. Stewart PA. Independent and dependent variables of acid-base control. *Respir Physiol* 1978;33:9–26.
2. Eicker SW. An introduction to strong ion difference. *Vet Clin North Am Food Anim Pract* 1990;8:45–49.
3. Balasubramanyan N, Havens PL, Hoffman GM. Unmeasured anions identified by the Fencl–Stewart method predict mortality better than base excess, anion gap, and lactate in patients in the pediatric intensive care unit. *Crit Care Med* 1999;27:1577–1581.
4. West JB. *Respiratory physiology.* Baltimore: Williams & Wilkins, 1990.
5. Ponce P, Santana A, Vinhas J. Treatment of severe metabolic alkalosis by "acid dialysis." *Crit Care Med* 1991;19:583–585.
6. Badrick T, Hickman PE. The anion gap: a reappraisal. *Am J Clin Pathol* 1992;98:249–252.
7. Gluck SL. Acid–base. *Lancet* 1998;352:474–479.
8. Stokke DB, Andersen PK, Brinklov MM, et al. Acid–base interactions with noradrenaline-induced contractile response of the rabbit isolated aorta. *Anesthesiology* 1984;60:400–404.
9. Beech JS, Nolan KM, Iles RA, et al. The effects of sodium bicarbonate and a mixture of sodium bicarbonate ("carbicarb") on skeletal muscle pH and hemodynamic status in rats with hypovolemic shock. *Metabolism* 1994;43:518–522.
10. Rhee KH, Toro LO, McDonald GG, et al. Carbicarb, sodium bicarbonate, and sodium chloride in hypoxic lactic acidosis: effect on arterial blood bases, lactate concentrations, hemodynamic variables, and myocardial intracellular pH. *Chest* 1993;104:913–918.
11. Cooper DJ, Walley KR, Wiggs BR, et al. Bicarbonate does not improve hemodynamics in critically ill patients who have lactic acidosis: a prospective, controlled clinical study. *Ann Intern Med* 1990;112:492–498.
12. Mark NH, Leung JM, Arieff AI, et al. Safety of low-dose intraoperative bicarbonate therapy: a prospective, double-blind, randomized study. *Crit Care Med* 1993;21:659–665.
13. Leung JM, Landow L, Franks M, et al. Safety and efficacy of intravenous carbicarb in patients undergoing surgery: comparison with sodium bicarbonate in the treatment of mild metabolic acidosis. *Crit Care Med* 1994;22:1540–1549.
14. Stacpoole PW, Wright EC, Baumgartner TG, et al. A controlled clinical trial of dichloroacetate for treatment of lactic acidosis in adults. *N Engl J Med* 1992;327:1564–1569.
15. Kaehny WD, Anderson RJ. Bicarbonate therapy of metabolic acidosis. *Crit Care Med* 1994;22:1525–1527.
16. Forsythe SM, Schmidt GA. Sodium bicarbonate for the treatment of lactic acidosis. *Chest* 2000;117:260–267.
17. Viallon A, Zeni F, Lafond P, et al. Does bicarbonate therapy improve the management of severe diabetic ketoacidosis? *Crit Care Med* 1999;27:2690–2693.
18. Green SM, Rothrock SG, Ho JD, et al. Failure of adjunctive bicarbonate to improve outcome in severe pediatric diabetic ketoacidosis. *Ann Emerg Med* 1998;31:41–48.
19. Christensen MS. Acid-base changes in cerebrospinal fluid and blood, and blood volumes changes following prolonged hyperventilation in man. *Br J Anaesth* 1974;46:348–357.
20. Fall PJ. A stepwise approach to acid-base disorders: practical patient evaluation for metabolic acidosis and other conditions. *Postgrad Med* 2000;107:249–257.
21. Williams AJ. ABC of oxygen: assessing and interpreting arterial blood gases and acid-base balance. *BMJ* 1998;317:1213–1216.
22. Adrogué HJ, Madias NE. Management of life-threatening acid-base disorders: first of two parts. *N Engl J Med* 1998;338:26–34.
23. Adrogué HJ, Madias NE. Management of life-threatening acid-base disorders: second of two parts. *N Engl J Med* 1998;338:107–111.
24. Elisaf MS, Tsatsoulis AA, Katopodis KP, et al. Acid-base and electrolyte disturbances in patients with diabetic ketoacidosis. *Diabetes Res Clin Pract* 1996;34:23–27.
25. McFarlane C, Lee A. A comparison of plasmalyte 148 and 0.9% saline for intra-operative fluid replacement. *Anaesthesia* 1994;49:779–781.
26. Scheingraber S, Rehm M, Sehmisch C, et al. Rapid saline infusion produces hyperchloremic acidosis in patients undergoing gynecologic surgery. *Anesthesiology* 1999;90:1265–1270.
27. Prough DS, Bidani A. Hyperchloremic metabolic acidosis is a predictable consequence of intraoperative infusion of 0.9% saline. *Anesthesiology* 1999;90:1247–1249.
28. Adrogué HJ, Madias NE. Hyponatremia. *N Engl J Med* 2000;342:1581–1589.
29. Lien YH, Shapiro JI, Chan L. Effects of hypernatremia on organic brain osmoles. *J Clin Invest* 1990;85:1427–1435.
30. Prough DS, Mathru M. Acid-base, fluids, and electrolytes. In: Barash PG, Cullen BF, Stoelting RK, eds. *Clinical anesthesia.* Philadelphia: Lippincott Williams & Wilkins, 2001:165–200.
31. Arieff AI. Postoperative hyponatraemic encephalopathy following elective surgery in children. *Paediatric Anesth* 1998;8:1–4.
32. Chung H, Kluge R, Schrier RW, et al. Postoperative hyponatremia: a prospective study. *Arch Intern Med* 1986;146:333–336.
33. Fraser CL, Arieff AI. Fatal central diabetes mellitus and insipidus resulting from untreated hyponatremia: a new syndrome. *Ann Intern Med* 1990;112:113–119.
34. Ayus JC, Arieff AI. Brain damage and postoperative hyponatremia: the role of gender. *Neurology* 1996;46:323–328.
35. Jamison RL. Hyponatremia: a re-examination. *Curr Opin Nephrol Hypertens* 1997;6:363–366.
36. Kitiyakara C, Wilcox CS. Vasopressin V2-receptor antagonists: panaceas for hyponatremia? *Curr Opin Nephrol Hypertens* 1997;6:461–467.
37. Soupart A, Decaux G. Therapeutic recommendations for management of severe hyponatremia: current concepts on pathogenesis and

prevention of neurologic complications. *Clin Nephrol* 1996;46:149–169.

38. Adrogué HJ, Madias NE. Aiding fluid prescription for the dysnatremias. *Intensive Care Med* 1997;23:309–316.

39. Laureno R, Karp BI. Myelinolysis after correction of hyponatremia. *Ann Intern Med* 1997;126:57–62.

40. Karmel KS, Bear RA. Treatment of hyponatremia: a quantitative analysis. *Am J Kidney Dis* 1994;21:439–443.

41. Pradhan S, Jha R, Singh MN, et al. Central pontine myelinolysis following 'slow' correction of hyponatremia. *Clin Neurol Neurosurg* 1995;97:340–343.

42. Berl T. Treating hyponatremia: what is all the controversy about? *Ann Intern Med* 1990;113:417–419.

43. Kumar S, Beri T. Sodium. *Lancet* 1998;352:220–228.

44. Hall J, Robertson G. Diabetes insipidus. *Probl Crit Care* 1990;4:342–354.

45. Ober KP. Endocrine crises: diabetes insipidus. *Crit Care Clin* 1991;7:109–125.

46. Robertson GL. Differential diagnosis of polyuria. *Annu Rev Med* 1988;39:425–442.

47. Adrogué HJ, Madias NE. Hypernatremia. *N Engl J Med* 2000;342:1493–1499.

48. Griffin KA, Bidani AK. How to manage disorders of sodium and water balance: five-step approach to evaluating appropriateness of renal response. *J Crit Illn* 1990;5:1054–1070.

49. McManus ML, Churchwill KB, Strange K. Regulation of cell volume in health and disease. *N Engl J Med* 1995;333:1260–1266.

50. Cobb WE, Spare S, Reichlin S. Neurogenic diabetes insipidus: management with dDAVP (1-desamino-8-D arginine vasopressin). *Ann Intern Med* 1978;88:183–188.

51. Chanson P, Jedynak CP, Dabrowski G, et al. Ultralow doses of vasopressin in the management of diabetes insipidus. *Crit Care Med* 1987;15:44–46.

52. Vitez TS, Soper LE, Wong KC, et al. Chronic hypokalemia and intraoperative dysrhythmias. *Anesthesiology* 1985;63:130–133.

53. Adrogué HJ, Madias NE. Changes in plasma potassium concentration during acute acid-base disturbances. *Am J Med* 1981;71:456–467.

54. Kuvin JT. Electrocardiographic changes of hyperkalemia. *N Engl J Med* 1998;338:662.

55. Rimmer JM, Horn JF, Gennari FJ. Hyperkalemia as a complication of drug therapy. *Arch Intern Med* 1987;147:867–869.

56. Perazella MA, Mahnensmith RL. Hyperkalemia in the elderly: drugs exacerbate impaired potassium homeostasis. *J Gen Intern Med* 1997;12:646–656.

57. Kemper MJ, Harps E, Müller-Wiefel DE. Hyperkalemia: therapeutic options in acute and chronic renal failure. *Clin Nephrol* 1996;46:67–69.

58. Liou HH, Chiang SS, Wu SC, et al. Hypokalemic effects of intravenous infusion or nebulization of salbutamol in patients with chronic renal failure: comparative study. *Am J Kidney Dis* 1994;23:266–271.

59. Brown EM, Pollak M, Seidman CE, et al. Calcium-ion-sensing cell-surface receptors. *N Engl J Med* 1995;333:234–240.

60. Bushinsky DA, Monk RD. Calcium. *Lancet* 1998;352:306–311.

61. Guise TA, Mundy GR. Evaluation of hypocalcemia in children and adults. *J Clin Endocrinol Metab* 1995;80:1473–1478.

62. Adler AJ, Ferran N, Berlyne GM. Effect of inorganic phosphate on serum ionized calcium concentration *in vitro*: a reassessment of the "trade-off hypothesis." *Kidney Int* 1985;28:932–935.

63. Rutledge R, Sheldon GF, Collins ML. Massive transfusion. *Crit Care Clin* 1986;2:791–805.

64. Vincent JL, Jankowski S. Why should ionized calcium be determined in acutely ill patients? *Acta Anaesthesiol Scand Suppl* 1995;107:281–286.

65. Sutters M, Gaboury CL, Bennett WM. Severe hyperphosphatemia and hypocalcemia: a dilemma in patient management. *J Am Soc Nephrol* 1996;7:2055–2061.

66. Davis KD, Attie MF. Management of severe hypercalcemia. *Crit Care Clin* 1991;7:175–190.

67. Jan de Beur SM, Levine MA. Hypercalcemia. *Curr Ther Endocrinol Metab* 1997;6:551–556.

68. Gucalp R, Ritch P, Wiernik PH, et al. Comparative study of pamidronate disodium and etidronate disodium in the treatment of cancer-related hypercalcemia. *J Clin Oncol* 1992;10:134–142.

69. Weisinger JR, Bellorin-Font E. Magnesium and phosphorus. *Lancet* 1998;352:391–396.

70. Fawcett WJ, Haxby EJ, Male DA. Magnesium: physiology and pharmacology. *Br J Anaesth* 1999;83:302–320.

71. Elisaf M, Merkouropoulos M, Tsianos EV, et al. Pathogenetic mechanisms of hypomagnesemia in alcoholic patients. *J Trace Elem Med Biol* 1995;9:210–214.

72. Salem M, Munoz R, Chernow B. Hypomagnesemia in critical illness: a common and clinically important problem. *Crit Care Clin* 1991;7:225–252.

73. Chernow B, Bamberger S, Stoiko M, et al. Hypomagnesemia in patients in postoperative intensive care. *Chest* 1989;95:391–397.

74. Hebert P, Mehta N, Wang J, et al. Functional magnesium deficiency in critically ill patients identified using a magnesium-loading test. *Crit Care Med* 1997;25:749–755.

75. Faber MD, Kupin WL, Heilig CW, et al. Common fluid-electrolyte and acid-base problems in the intensive care unit: selected issues. *Semin Nephrol* 1994;14:8–22.

76. McLean RM. Magnesium and its therapeutic uses: a review. *Am J Med* 1994;96:63–76.

77. Harris MNE, Crowther A, Jupp RA, et al. Magnesium and coronary revascularization. *Br J Anaesth* 1988;60:779–783.

78. Redwood SR, Taggart PI, Sutton PM, et al. Effect of magnesium on the monophasic action potential during early ischemia in the *in vivo* human heart. *J Am Coll Cardiol* 1996;28:1765–1769.

79. James MFM, Beer RE, Esser JD. Intravenous magnesium sulfate inhibits catecholamine release associated with tracheal intubation. *Anesth Analg* 1989;68:772–776.

80. van Hook JW. Hypermagnesemia. *Crit Care Clin* 1991;7:215–223.

81. Peppers MP, Geheb M, Desai T. Hypophosphatemia and hyperphosphatemia. *Crit Care Clin* 1991;7:201.

82. Zazzo JF, Troche G, Ruel P, et al. High incidence of hypophosphatemia in surgical intensive care patients: efficacy of phosphorus therapy on myocardial function. *Intensive Care Med* 1995;21:826–831.

83. Rosen GH, Boullata JI, O'Rangers EA, et al. Intravenous phosphate repletion regimen for critically ill patients with moderate hypophosphatemia. *Crit Care Med* 1995;23:1204–1210.

84. Clark CL, Sacks GS, Dickerson RN, et al. Treatment of hypophosphatemia in patients receiving specialized nutrition support using a graduated dosing scheme: results from a prospective clinical trial. *Crit Care Med* 1995;23:1504–1511.

19

PRINCIPLES OF CEREBROPROTECTION

MARK I. ROSSBERG
ANISH BHARDWAJ
PATRICIA D. HURN
JEFFREY R. KIRSCH

KEY WORDS

- Anesthetics
- Autoregulation
- Cerebral blood flow
- Cerebral ischemia
- Excitotoxicity
- Head trauma
- Injury mechanisms
- Neuroprotection
- Nitric oxide

INTRODUCTION

The high incidence and significant morbidity of neurologic dysfunction as encountered in the perioperative critical care setting provide a tremendous incentive to identify effective cerebroprotective strategies. These strategies must protect the brain from hemodynamic stressors, such as cardiopulmonary bypass or prolonged hypotension, and minimize ischemic damage from stroke, cardiac arrest, and head trauma. The overall goals of cerebroprotection are to optimally match cerebral blood flow (CBF) and metabolic demand, and to abort the complex pathophysiologic cascade of cellular and molecular events leading to the death of neurons, supportive glia, and vascular tissue. This chapter reviews the normal regulation of CBF and intracranial pressure (ICP), the mechanisms of injury inherent in cerebral ischemia and head injury, and current clinical and experimental therapeutic modalities with potential neuroprotective impact.

REGULATION OF CEREBROVASCULAR FUNCTION

Under physiologic conditions, CBF is tightly regulated and locally varies to meet regional tissue metabolic needs [for review, see (1)]. The major controllers of CBF are cerebral perfusion pressure (CPP), arterial oxygen tension, arterial CO_2 tension, and cerebral metabolic demand. In the brain, CPP is equal to mean arterial pressure (MAP) minus the cerebral outflow pressure. The latter is either mean ICP or cerebral venous pressure, whichever is greater. For most purposes, CPP = MAP − ICP. Because CBF is difficult to measure in the clinical setting, CPP is often used to assess the adequacy of cerebral perfusion. Normal human values for CPP are 70 to 100 mm Hg, while CBF averages approximately 50 mL per min^{-1} per 100 g^{-1} of brain tissue.

The influence of CPP on CBF is a function of the autoregulatory capacity of the cerebral vascular bed. In healthy, autoregulating brain, arteriolar diameter increases or decreases in response to decreasing or increasing CPP to maintain constant CBF over a range of approximately 60 to 160 mm Hg (Fig. 1). Because cerebral vasoconstriction occurs as CPP increases, cerebral blood volume actually decreases slightly. Below the autoregulatory range, a decrease in CPP results in decreased CBF and cerebral blood volume. As the "upper limit" of pressure autoregulation is exceeded, an increase in CPP results in increased CBF and cerebral blood volume. Persons with chronically low blood pressures (e.g., the young) demonstrate a leftward shift of the autoregulation curve, while chronic hypertension is associated with a rightward shift (Fig. 2). It is important to note that pressure autoregulation may be abnormal or lacking in the injured brain, with deleterious consequences.

Factors that influence ICP can influence CBF by altering CPP. The cranium is a closed space with a fixed volume. ICP, normally less than 15 mm Hg, reflects the volume of three compartments: brain parenchyma, cerebrospinal fluid (CSF), and intravascular blood. Because the intracranial vault is fixed in volume, increases in the size of one component of the intracranial contents require compensatory removal of an equivalent amount of another component if increases in ICP are to be avoided. Normally, small increases in any one intracranial component are tolerated without accompanying significant increases in pressure. Once a critical volume is reached, however, even small increments in the volume of the intracranial contents will result in large increases in ICP (Fig. 3). The point at which significant ICP elevation occurs is dependent on brain elastance and potential displacement of intracranial contents (e.g., CSF displacement). Intracranial blood volume is determined by two factors, CBF and capacitance vessel diameter (i.e., small veins and venules). Although CBF often changes in the same direction as cerebral blood volume, these variables are inversely related under some normal situations (e.g., autoregulation) or in pathologic situations. Furthermore, blood volume is not equally distributed throughout the brain; blood volume per unit weight is greater in gray than in white matter,

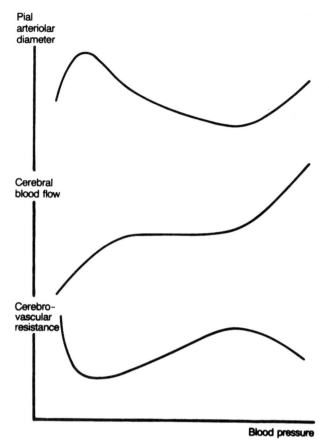

FIGURE 1. Relationship between brain arteriolar diameter, cerebral blood flow, and cerebrovascular resistance with blood pressure. Note that arteriolar diameter reaches maximum diameter below the lower limit of autoregulation. (From Paulson OB, Strandgaard S, Edvinsson L. Cerebral autoregulation. *Cerebrovasc Brain Metab Rev* 1990;2:161–192, with permission. Data from MacKenzie ET, Farrar JK, Fitch W, et al. Effects of hemorrhagic hypotension on the cerebral circulation. *Stroke* 1979;10:711–718, and MacKenzie ET, Strandgaard S, Graham DI, et al. Effect of acutely induced hypertension in cats on pial arteriolar caliber, local cerebral blood flow and the blood–brain barrier. *Circ Res* 1976;39:33–41.)

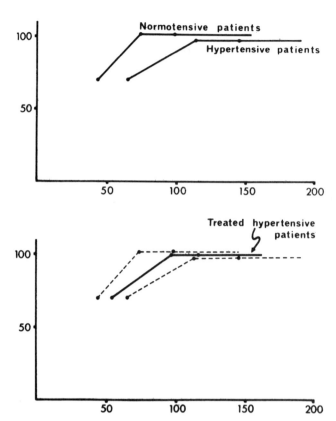

FIGURE 2. **Top:** Autoregulatory curves obtained in normotensive and severely hypertensive human subjects. Each curve is defined by the mean values of resting blood pressure, the lower limit of cerebral blood flow autoregulation and the lowest tolerated blood pressure. The curve from the hypertensive patients is shifted to the right. **Bottom:** Autoregulatory curves in patients with effective antihypertensive treatment. The curve falls between the two curves in the top panel, which are shown as *dotted lines*. (From Strandgaard S. Cerebral blood flow and hypertension. *Circulation* 1976;53:720–727, with permission.)

with further variation among the various nuclei. Pathology that affects either CBF or cerebral venous capacitance may modulate cerebral blood volume with subsequent effects on ICP. In the setting of reduced intracranial compliance, for example, either a decrease in CPP within the autoregulatory range, or an increase in CPP to above the autoregulatory range results in increased cerebral blood volume, which may result in an increase in ICP.

A second major determining factor of CBF is the arterial oxygen content (CaO_2). The brain responds to decreased CaO_2 by a compensatory rise in blood flow that acts to maintain adequate oxygen transport (i.e., oxygen transport = $CaO_2 \times CBF$) (Fig. 4). Thus, a 50% decrease in CaO_2 ordinarily results in a doubling of CBF. If CaO_2 is further reduced, increases in CBF cannot compensate, and the result is a decrease in the cerebral metabolic rate for oxygen ($CMRO_2$) and depression of electrical activity. The mechanism of the increase in CBF accompanying decreased CaO_2 remains controversial. Neurogenic mechanisms have been proposed to be involved in the cerebral vasodilator response to hypoxia; however, cerebral vasodilation is not affected by denervation of the carotid or aortic baroreceptors. Increased brain

adenosine is likely an important mechanism of cerebral hypoxic vasodilation. Increases in adenosine concentration are present in brain within seconds of hypoxia. Furthermore, adenosine antagonists, such as theophylline, caffeine, or phenyltheophylline, attenuate the vasodilation. Endothelium-dependent mechanisms have been implicated in the mechanism of cerebral vasodilation during anoxia (2). Regardless of mechanism, hypoxia can cause marked generalized cerebral vasodilation, an increase in cerebral blood volume, and a marked increase in ICP in patients with preexisting increased intracranial volume. If the increase in ICP impedes the normal increase in CBF and if CaO_2 is sufficiently low, extraction of oxygen from the blood may become maximal. In the injured brain, blood flow to damaged areas may actually decrease during hypoxia if there is less vasodilatory reserve in the injured region than in normal regions of the brain (intracerebral steal).

Changes in arterial CO_2 tension ($PaCO_2$) consistently alter CBF in the normal brain (Fig. 4), most likely mediated by changes in extracellular hydrogen ion concentration. However, arterioles in injured brain may be less responsive to $PaCO_2$; in this case, an increase in $PaCO_2$ may cause more of an increase in blood flow

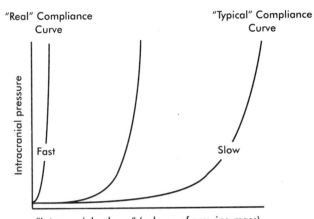

FIGURE 3. Intracranial pressure "compliance curves." If intracranial contents were noncompressible and the skull truly rigid, then the injection of any extra volume into the system would produce a very rapid increase in pressure (**left curve**, labeled "*real*"). However, this is not the pattern typically seen with a slowly growing mass lesion, which is shown on the **right curve** (labeled "*typical*"). Note that the x axis is the volume of growing mass. As a mass grows, total volume remains almost constant owing to compensatory mechanisms. Only when these mechanisms are exhausted does the pressure rise precipitously. Note also that the faster volume is added, the more quickly compensatory mechanisms are exhausted. (From Todd MM, Warner DS. Neuroanesthesia: a critical review. In: Rogers MC, Tinker, JH, Covino BG, et al., eds. *Principles and practice of anesthesiology*. St. Louis: Mosby Year Book, 1993:1599–1648, with permission.)

to normal tissue, "stealing" blood flow from damaged tissue. Increases in $PaCO_2$ may so dramatically increase cerebral blood volume that ICP also increases. In the setting of a preexisting elevated ICP, high or even normal $PaCO_2$ can cause excessive cerebral vasodilation, increase ICP, and reciprocally decrease CBF to already damaged brain. Clinicians often use hyperventilation, in the range of $PaCO_2$ of 25 to 30 mm Hg, as a means of decreasing cerebral blood volume and ICP. However, as discussed later in the chapter, this treatment can result in such marked cerebral vasoconstriction as to compromise CBF to previously normal brain. CBF is closely linked or "coupled" to cerebral metabolism.

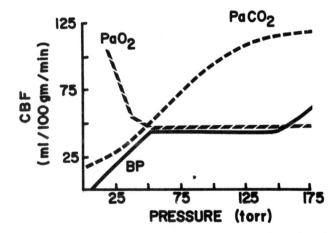

FIGURE 4. Changes in cerebral blood flow caused by independent alterations in arterial CO_2, O_2, and cerebral perfusion pressure. (From Drummond JC, Shapiro HM. Cerebral physiology. In: Miller R, ed. *Anesthesia*, 3rd ed. New York: Churchill Livingstone, 1990:621–628, with permission.)

TABLE 1. CEREBRAL OXYGEN SUPPLY AND UTILIZATION

Variable	Normal Value
Cerebral blood flow (CBF)	50 mL·100g^{-1}·min^{-1}
$CMRO_2 = CBF \times C(a\text{-}J_V)O_2$	3.5 mL·100g^{-1}·min^{-1}
$C(a\text{-}J_V)O_2$	7.0 mL·100g^{-1}
CaO_2	20 mL·100g^{-1}
$C_{JV}O_2$	13 mL·100g^{-1}
$S_{JV}O_2$	65%
$P_{JV}O_2$	35 mm Hg
$CDO_2 = CBF \times CaO_2$	10 mL·100g^{-1}

$CMRO_2$, cerebral metabolic rate for oxygen; CaO_2, arterial oxygen content; $C_{JV}O_2$, jugular bulb oxygen content; $C(a\text{-}J_V)O_2$, cerebral arteriovenous oxygen content difference; $S_{JV}O_2$, jugular bulb oxygen saturation; CDO_2, cerebral oxygen delivery; $P_{JV}O_2$.
(Reprinted from Prough DS, Dewitt DS. Cerebral protection. In: Chernow B, ed. *The pharmacologic approach to the critically ill patient,* 2nd ed. Baltimore: Williams and Wilkins, 1994;247–252, with permission.)

Central nervous system tissue uses predominantly glucose as substrate and has a high $CMRO_2$. Normal values for cerebral oxygen supply and utilization are listed in Table 1. Local metabolic needs (observed as changes in $CMRO_2$) are coupled with the required local CBF responses through metabolic autoregulation. The precise mechanisms behind this coupling remain elusive. Factors that increase $CMRO_2$ also increase CBF under physiologic conditions. Brain temperature is a notable example: $CMRO_2$ increases by approximately 6% with every 1°C increase in temperature. Conversely, hypothermia proportionately reduces $CMRO_2$. Although a decrease in metabolism does not usually result in dangerously low CBF, brain injury may occur if increased $CMRO_2$ exceeds the brain's vasodilatory capacity. In the setting of increased ICP, therapies that decrease $CMRO_2$ (e.g., hypothermia) may be useful in decreasing cerebral blood volume and thereby decreasing ICP.

CEREBRAL BLOOD FLOW THRESHOLDS

With graded reductions in CPP, a series of CBF thresholds has been observed experimentally. These thresholds are approximate and vary to some extent with species, metabolic rate, and anesthetic agents. In normal brain, reducing CPP to 50 mm Hg only modestly reduces CBF because of active vasodilation. With further reduction of CPP, CBF falls and oxygen extraction increases. With CPP below approximately 30 mm Hg, the increase in oxygen extraction generally is no longer adequate to maintain oxidative metabolism (3). Increases in brain lactate levels and decreases in brain pH and phosphocreatine become evident. When CBF is reduced below 20 mL min^{-1} 100 g^{-1}, corresponding to approximately a 60% reduction, significant abnormalities in the electroencephalogram (EEG) and somatosensory evoked potentials occur and surges in extracellular levels of neurotransmitters, such as glutamate, are detected. However, only modest decreases in cortical adenosine triphosphate (ATP) occur at this intermediate level of CBF, as the decrease in spontaneous electrical activity acts to conserve energy demand. Decreased high-energy phosphates in subcortical white matter precede decreases in high-energy phosphates in gray matter and may limit conduction of somatosensory evoked potentials. Impaired generation of somatosensory evoked potentials in brainstem and thalamus requires lower blood flow. The brainstem blood flow threshold for loss of brainstem auditory evoked responses is lower than the corresponding cortical blood flow threshold for loss of somatosensory evoked potentials, indicating a greater resistance to partial ischemia in the brainstem.

In the cortex, ATP progressively decreases when CBF is reduced below 10 to 12 mL min^{-1} 100 g^{-1} (4). With marked decreases in ATP, depolarization occurs, accompanied by a large potassium efflux and sodium and calcium influx. Thus, lower blood flow is required for depolarization than for loss of neurotransmission. Finally, with zero CBF (complete ischemia), depolarization and complete loss of ATP occur within 2 to 4 minutes. This series of CBF thresholds suggests a cascade of pathophysiologic mechanisms. As the severity and duration of ischemia increase, mechanisms of injury become multifactorial and pharmacologic strategies of cerebroprotection become increasingly complex.

PATHOPHYSIOLOGY OF CEREBRAL INJURY

Cerebral Ischemia/Reperfusion

Broadly defined, cerebral ischemia occurs when there is inadequate delivery of oxygen and substrate to brain tissue relative to its needs. A variety of experimental studies and clinical observations indicate that the brain is considerably vulnerable to short periods of ischemia, although some neuronal populations can survive 30 minutes or more of ischemia. The precise mechanism by which ischemia and reperfusion cause cell death remains to be elucidated and is generally assumed to be multifactorial. It is critical to consider the severity, duration, and distribution of CBF reduction when evaluating mechanisms of injury and the likely response to therapeutic interventions. The severity of ischemia refers to whether ischemia is complete (e.g., cardiac arrest) or incomplete (e.g., prolonged shock or intracranial hypertension); however, it can be difficult to evaluate severity when CBF is not measured or accurately inferred. The distribution of ischemia is commonly categorized as global (e.g., cardiac arrest, ventricular fibrillation) or focal (e.g., stroke) in which there is a spatial flow reduction gradient from the lesion core to surrounding salvageable tissue known as the penumbra. Much of what is known about ischemic mechanisms has been derived from experimental animal models of reversible global or focal ischemia.

The central and critically damaging event in ischemia is energy depletion [for reviews see (5,6)]. All cellular work is directly or indirectly accomplished using ATP produced by oxidative phosphorylation in the mitochondria or, less importantly, by glycolysis within the cytoplasm. When ischemia is severe (CBF, 10 mL min^{-1} 100^{-1} tissue) and ATP levels are compromised, an entire cascade of events has been hypothesized and experimentally demonstrated: rapid titration of brain high-energy phosphate sources (e.g., phosphocreatine via the creatine kinase reaction); loss of mitochondrial electron transport; accumulation of reduced compounds; and an increase in the NADH/NAD$^+$ ratio; loss of mitochondrial dehydrogenase activity, with accumulation of pyruvate; and a shift in the lactate dehydrogenase reaction toward pyruvate reduction and lactate formation. If effective circulation is restored, then extensive cell and tissue

recovery is possible, even after prolonged ischemia. If energy failure progresses, a cascade of injury mechanisms is called into play, many of which operate in parallel rather than in series.

Traumatic Brain Injury (TBI)

The essential factors that govern outcome in the head-injured patient are the primary damage sustained from the traumatic insult and any secondary injury due to hypoxia or ischemia related to hypotension or mass lesions. The traumatically injured brain is particularly sensitive to hypoxia and hypotension that would ordinarily be tolerated in the normal brain. Accordingly, one of the key goals in the critical care setting is to avoid these secondary insults.

Clinically significant TBI produces a depression of CMRo$_2$ and CBF (CBF may be reduced to a lesser degree or remain coupled to CMRo$_2$), a varying loss of autoregulation and responsivity to CO$_2$, and loss of blood–brain barrier integrity. For example, compensatory CBF responses to hemorrhagic hypotension (7) and hemodilution (8) are depressed in head-injured animals. One of the most established experimental models of TBI is the fluid-percussion model originally developed in cats (9) and adapted for use in rats [for review, see (10)]. The primary injury, thought to mimic human closed head injury electrophysiologically and hemodynamically, causes transient increases in CBF that rapidly return toward baseline values. Further, fluid-percussion injury reproducibly produces reflex suppression and motor deficits, possibly mediated by cholinergic mechanisms, as well as cognitive deficits and memory impairment. The normally tightly controlled coupling between CBF and metabolism may be impaired after TBI, with consequent derangement of regional energy metabolism. Alternative head injury models include the weight drop model and the most widely used model in small rodents, the controlled cortical impact (CCI) model. Both models simulate concussive brain injury and can be varied in injury severity from mild to severe damage (for review, see (11)]. The CCI method, which uses a rigid indenter to impact the brain at a controlled depth and velocity, has been well characterized in terms of histology, physiology, and cognitive outcomes. Mechanisms of injury, as with ischemia and reperfusion, are multifactorial and involve similar injury cascades as described below.

Cellular and Molecular Mechanisms

Brain injury cascades evolve over time and involve surprisingly large spaces, including tissue not directly involved in the initial insult. As an organizational tool, these mechanisms can be broadly divided into: (a) excitotoxicity, (b) inflammation, and (c) programmed cell death. The relative importance of each of these broad mechanisms, and abundance of cells injured by a specific molecular actor, depends on injury severity/duration and on available endogenous neuroprotection. A new and evolving concept in brain injury is that the brain has unique protective (and repair) mechanisms simulating developmental programming (12).

Excitotoxicity arises once neurons depolarize, releasing large loads of toxic neurotransmitters into the extracellular space. This early event is compounded by the loss of energy-dependent presynaptic neurotransmitter reuptake. The net effect is accumulation of excitatory amino acids such as glutamate, over-activation of postsynaptic glutamate receptors, and calcium overload within postsynaptic cells. Consequences of calcium overload on cell signaling are enormous, since calcium is a universal second messenger. Channels for monovalent ions also open, allowing Na^+, Cl^-, and water entry and cytotoxic cerebral edema. Inflammation begins within hours in injured tissue and persists over days. Many inflammatory mechanisms are linked to calcium activation of proteolytic enzymes which degrade cytoskeletal proteins (e.g., actin and spectrin) and extracellular matrix proteins (e.g., laminin), as well as key cell signaling enzymes. Activation of phospholipases and cyclooxygenase enzymes can generate oxygen radical species with consequent lipid peroxidation and further membrane damage. Mitochondria, an important source of and target for radicals, undergo radical-mediated disruption of the inner mitochondrial membrane and oxidation of electron transport proteins. Mitochondrial leakiness, partly due to the formation of a permeability transition pore, promotes swelling, renewed energy failure and loss of cytochrome C, likely triggering programmed cell death (6).

Neurons and glia that are compromised by excitotoxicity, calcium overload, radical injury, and DNA damage can die by necrosis or apoptosis (the pathology that is the hallmark of programmed cell death). Both endpoints are present in ischemic and TBI. Necrosis predominates in acute, severe injury, while milder insults allow the unmasking of a complex genetic death program, a so-called "cell suicide". Each of these events offers an opportunity for mechanistically or molecularly oriented treatments. The goal is to salvage peri-injury brain, direct inflammation toward repair and synaptic restructuring, and amplify endogenous neuroprotective resources.

Excitotoxicity

Ischemia, hypoxia, hypoglycemia, and head trauma cause accumulation of excitatory amino acids (e.g., glutamate, aspartate) in brain extracellular fluid [for reviews see (13–15)]. Clearance of glutamate can be slow, as evidenced by elevated glutamate levels in severely head-injured patients for up to 3 days after injury. Excitatory amino acids activate receptor-operated channels postsynaptically and allow influx of calcium ions and initiation of Ca^{2+}-dependent signaling and enzymatic function. There are three known types of glutamate receptors: those activated by N-methyl-d-aspartate (NMDA), and those activated by the non-NMDA agonists kainate and quisqualate/AMPA (a-amino-3-hydroxy-5-methyl-4-isoxazolepropionate). These receptors activate one of two types of agonist-operated channels; one gated by kainate or AMPA and one gated by NMDA. The former permits fast monovalent cation influx, such as Na^+ and K^+, whereas the latter permits predominantly Ca^{2+} influx. AMPA also binds to metabotropic receptors that stimulate phosphoinositide hydrolysis.

The discovery that NMDA and AMPA receptor inhibition provides some protection in animals against experimental ischemia, hypoglycemia, and TBI helped to solidify the concept of glutamate toxicity. Certain areas of the brain (e.g., hippocampus, neocortex) are selectively vulnerable to excitotoxic damage, perhaps related to greater excitatory amino acid concentrations, differences in receptors, or an imbalance of excitatory (more)

and inhibitory (less) neurotransmitters released by depolarization. The time frame for effective NMDA receptor antagonism is fairly short (1 to 2 hours) in most animal models and is somewhat longer for AMPA receptor blockade (16). Sodium influx through AMPA receptors also induces Ca^{2+} influx indirectly through depolarization of resting membrane potential and alleviating the physiologic Mg^{2+} block for NMDA receptor activation. Glutamate receptor activation should be considered as the gateway to excitotoxicity, but it must be recalled that glutamate is the primary excitatory neurotransmitter in normal neural conduction. Although blocking receptor function could alleviate excitotoxicity, serious adverse effects result such as pseudopsychosis and respiratory and cardiovascular dysfunction (17). Accordingly, interventions designed to act at critical downstream mechanisms have been studied (e.g., blocking Ca^{2+}-dependent nitric oxide synthase activation).

Nitric Oxide Toxicity and Oxidant Injury

Nitric oxide (NO) plays a complex multifaceted role in the brain as a regulator of CBF, a neurotransmitter, and a free radical, and thereby exerts a significant role in modulating ischemic brain injury [for reviews see (2,18)]. Pharmacologic and genetic approaches have enhanced our understanding of the actions of NO (19). Neuronal nitric oxide synthase (nNOS or type 1 NOS) is constitutively expressed in a small population of neurons in the brain. Glutamate and NMDA neurotoxicity are mediated largely via excess formation of NO from this source. Both direct and cooperative mechanisms by which NO produces cell death have been proposed (20). The prevailing hypothesis is that NO kills neighboring cells as a result of its reaction with superoxide to form peroxynitrite. Among other actions, peroxynitrite modifies and breaks DNA strands, activating DNA repair enzymes such as poly (ADP ribose) polymerase (PARP). Because PARP activation is energy-dependent, it contributes to neuronal injury and increases damage in experimental stroke (21). Endothelial NOS (eNOS, or type II) is constitutively expressed mostly in endothelial cells and its product serves as a prominent mediator of cerebrovascular hemodynamics by causing vasorelaxation. Thus, eNOS serves an important neuroprotective role in cerebral ischemia by maintaining regional CBF. Transgenic mice that lack eNOS had worse outcomes following focal cerebral ischemia. The inducible isoform of NOS, (iNOS or type III), is calcium-independent and expressed under pathologic conditions by neurons, microglia, and endothelial cells. This isoform also exacerbates glutamate excitotoxicity leading to delayed cell death.

Although NO participates in prooxidant injury, other types of radicals have historically been implicated in ischemic and traumatic brain injuries (22). A free radical's reactivity results from its unpaired electron, which rapidly strips an electron from neighboring molecules. Reactive oxygen species have been most intensely studied: superoxide anion; its protonated form, perhydroxyl radical; hydroxyl radical; and the nonradical, hydrogen peroxide. Radical-mediated brain injury involves many cell types: cells that generate radicals may be directly damaged or may indirectly damage neighboring cells through microcirculatory failure and edema formation, with consequent impaired oxygen and substrate supply to cell neighbors. For example, oxygen radicals impair capillary endothelial cell transport and alter membrane fluidity in the brain. Lipids are also an important target for radical mediated injury, specifically via lipid peroxidation. Once peroxidative reactions are initiated, they propagate as a chain in the presence of sufficient oxygen. Accumulation of conjugated dienes and thiobarbiturate reactive material (indirect measures of lipid peroxidation) has been reported in animal models of ischemia/reperfusion. Furthermore, a delayed increase in lipid peroxides occurs in selectively vulnerable regions during reperfusion, but not in permanently ischemic, infarcted tissue. Brain lipid peroxidation depends on the presence of oxygen radicals and iron at the site where radicals are produced. During reperfusion, whereas iron is elevated only transiently, lipid peroxidation progresses for many hours. Lipid peroxidation can be enhanced *in vitro* by lactic acidosis; however, it is not clear whether this effect is important *in vivo*. Lactic acidosis presumably increases the production of oxygen radicals because of its ability to dissociate protein-bound iron, making iron more available for production of hydroxyl radicals (23).

Inflammation

Calcium-activated second messenger systems, oxygen radical generation, and numerous injured cell constituents induce synthesis of important gene transcription factors, such as NFKB and hypoxia-inducible factor, which increase expression of proinflammatory gene products (e.g., tumor necrosis factor, TNFα, and interleukin IL-1β. The gene products, when displayed in appropriate subcellular localization in injured parenchymal cells, mediate the induction of endothelial cell surface adhesion molecules, including intercellular adhesion molecule 1 (ICAM-1) and the selectins (24). Adhesion molecules attract neutrophils that cross the vascular wall and enter brain parenchyma. Within 4 to 7 days of injury, large numbers of neutrophils, macrophages, and monocytes cross over and cluster in injured regions, joining with resident microglia in a profound inflammatory response. Chemokines are elaborated by injured brain and guide the migration of these cells toward the target. In addition to microvascular obstruction and vascular injury, inflammatory cells contribute to postischemic damage in many ways once localized within the brain. Inflammation results in production of inducible NOS; neuronal production of cyclooxygenase (COX$_2$), an enzyme that generates superoxide and prostanoids; cytokine production; and direct radical generation. Positive consequences for injured brain include inflammatory cell participation in tissue remodeling and repair. Consequently, treatments designed to modulate inflammation are promising. Recent evidence also suggests that inflammatory mediators are important in inducing programmed cell death.

Programmed Cell Death (PCD)

Brain injury is now known to trigger neuronal loss days after the original insult (coining the term, "delayed programmed cell death"). In general, cell death of this form is most readily seen in less densely injured brain regions, where it is not masked by overt necrosis. Cells with apoptotic morphology [oligonucleosomal DNA laddering, presence of apoptotic bodies, and positive TUNEL stain (terminal-deoxynucleotidyl-transferase–mediated

dUTP nick end-labeling) have been described widely in experimental stroke and TBI, and in human TBI (25,26). A family of protein-cleaving enzymes, caspases, or aspartate-specific cysteine proteases, and the Bcl2 gene family are likely key actors in this mechanism. Increased expression of Bcl2 suppresses cell death, while another family member, Bax, augments PCD. The genes for caspases are expressed at significant levels in ischemia and TBI, and early evidence suggests that caspase inhibitors produce resistance to ischemic damage

NONPHARMACOLOGIC CEREBROPROTECTIVE INTERVENTIONS

Promotion of Blood Flow and Oxygen Delivery

During reperfusion after ischemia, there is a variable period of hyperemia followed by "delayed hypoperfusion" associated with an elevated vascular resistance, vasoconstriction, and cerebral edema. Directly related to the severity and duration of the preceding ischemia, the mechanism for the depression of CBF remains elusive. Appropriate hemodynamic management and intravenous fluid administration are warranted to avoid hypotension and optimize CPP. After brain injury, parenteral administration of hypotonic solutions is likely to increase brain water and ICP. Glucose-containing solutions are usually avoided because of their potential to cause hyperglycemia, enhance tissue acidosis, and worsen neurologic outcomes in head-injured and stroke patients. In many patients, significant ICP elevation is observed.

Lower ICP is associated with better neurologic outcome after head injury. Therefore, most clinicians believe that elevated ICP must be treated to increase CPP, preserve CBF, and minimize secondary injury to abnormal and normal tissue. If there is significant tissue swelling, fluid restriction and diuretics may be of value. Chronic fluid restriction does not effectively reduce brain tissue volume. Osmotic diuretics (e.g., mannitol) and hypertonic saline rapidly cause tissue fluid loss by dehydrating normal brain, but may acutely increase ICP by increasing cerebral blood volume. Pretreatment with loop diuretics and hyperventilation can reduce this unwanted effect. Cerebrospinal fluid volume can be reduced mechanically by withdrawal through an intraventricular catheter that may be placed in patients with intraventricular hemorrhage, and in some situations, with intracranial hypertension.

Hyperventilation

Airway control protects against aspiration in the setting of decreased level of consciousness, assures adequate oxygenation, and allows early institution of therapeutic hyperventilation. Hypoxia must be strictly avoided, particularly to avoid cerebral vasodilation, increased blood volume, and increased ICP. Hyperventilation decreases blood volume by vasoconstricting normal arterioles. Therapeutic hyperventilation acutely decreases ICP by lowering blood flow to normal brain and may promote blood flow to regions of abnormal, vasoparalyzed brain. However, there is a risk of excessive vasoconstriction during acute hyperventilation, particularly in head-injured patients with depressed CBF. Moreover, it is important to realize that hyperventilation is only a temporary mode of therapy. Within hours of instituting the therapy, CBF returns toward prehyperventilation levels as a result of reduced extracellular bicarbonate concentration and normalization of extracellular pH. Any subsequent increase in $PaCO_2$ tension above the hyperventilated $PaCO_2$ results in increased CBF. Therefore, "normalizing" $PaCO_2$ after prolonged hyperventilation causes an increase in CBF and may be associated with increased ICP.

Hypothermia

Experimentally, preischemic hypothermia ameliorates "no-flow" lesions, delays intraischemic efflux of potassium, decreases accumulation of excitatory amino acids, lessens gross and histopathologic lesions, improves metabolic recovery, as measured by intracellular pH and high-energy phosphates, and improves neurologic recovery. The mechanism of hypothermic brain protection has been hypothesized to involve reduced excitatory amino acid accumulation and reduced prostanoid and oxygen radical production. Postischemic initiation of hypothermia has been less extensively studied. Hypothermia is associated with protection from brain injury when it is initiated after TBI in animals and humans. A phase II clinical study of moderate hypothermia (32° to 33°C) administered within 6 hours of nonpenetrating head injury, demonstrated minimal cardiovascular toxicity, a decreased incidence of seizures, and a small improvement in neurologic outcome 3 months after injury (27). However, a phase II trial reported no therapeutic efficacy of hypothermia after TBI (27a). Mild hypothermia (e.g., 34°C) provides neuronal protection, but data with prolonged application of mild hypothermia are lacking. Mild hyperthermia, in contrast, worsens neurologic injury after both global and focal cerebral ischemia.

PHARMACOLOGIC NEUROPROTECTANTS

Pathophysiologic investigations of ischemia and TBI have generated many experimental and clinical evaluations of potentially therapeutic compounds. Preischemic drug administration is often used to clarify mechanisms of injury, while clinical use requires efficacy after injury. Injury models evaluate the efficacy of therapeutic agents directly and indirectly by studying postischemic hyperemia and hypoperfusion, recovery of somatosensory evoked potentials, infarct volumes, recovery of high-energy phosphates, and functional neurologic recovery. Clinical efficacy must be established in terms of neurologic recovery. In general, effective therapeutic agents must gain access to the desired site at the appropriate time, perhaps as a sequential or parallel therapy, to be effective in the multimechanistic milieu of cerebral injury. Therefore, an efficacious agent should readily penetrate vascular endothelium and the blood–brain barrier (i.e., it should have a low molecular weight and not be ionized). Interestingly, large molecules with poor access to brain tissue produce positive outcomes in some studies, suggesting an important role of vascular endothelium in ischemic injury.

Osmotherapy

Cerebral edema and elevated ICP are often encountered in relationship to TBI, neurosurgery, subarachnoid and intracerebral hemorrhage, and large hemispheric infarctions. The key goals in the management of cerebral edema and elevated ICP are to maintain adequate cerebral perfusion with prevention of secondary neuronal ischemic injury and to prevent lethal compartmental shifts that may lead to compression of vital brain structures. Osmotherapy remains the cornerstone of pharmacologic intervention for brain resuscitation in acute brain injury. Historically, commonly used osmotic agents include mannitol, sorbitol, glycerol, urea, and various concentrations of hypertonic saline. These osmotic agents create and sustain a hyperosmolar state by drawing water from the interstitial, extracellular, and possibly intracellular spaces into the intravascular compartment, thereby reducing brain edema. An ideal osmotic agent should be nontoxic and be effectively excluded from the intact blood–brain barrier. However, rebound cerebral edema may occur due to the passage of osmotic agent into brain regions with disrupted blood–brain-barrier. To date, mannitol remains the osmotic agent of choice. In addition to its osmotic action, mannitol enhances CBF by reducing blood viscosity, acts as a free radical scavenger, and improves intracranial compliance by decreasing CSF production and reabsorption. However, mannitol often causes adverse side effects including hyperkalemia, dehydration, renal insufficiency, and rebound cerebral edema and intracranial hypertension. Recently, hypertonic saline has received attention because it may be excluded more effectively by the blood–brain-barrier and produces fewer side effects (28). Based on experimental studies and some small case series, hypertonic saline when given as an intravenous bolus rapidly and effectively decreases ICP without compromising cerebral perfusion. The efficacy of osmotherapy when given as a continuous intravenous infusion is less clear. Anecdotal case reports and small clinical case series suggest that continuous hypertonic saline infusion ameliorates cerebral edema and decreases ICP secondary to TBI and postoperative brain injury. This favorable result cannot necessarily be extended to cerebral ischemia and intracerebral hemorrhage. With experimental stroke, continuous hypertonic saline markedly worsens infarct volume (29). Accordingly, available data support the use of osmotherapy in the setting of brain resuscitation only. Caution is advised in the use of osmotic agents as continuous infusion therapy in cerebral ischemia until definitive data are forthcoming.

Calcium Channel Antagonists

Ischemia results in activation of sodium and calcium channels with translocation of extracellular calcium into the cell. Mitochondrial ATP production is disrupted, and free radicals are produced. Calcium-related enzymes are activated, including NOS, phospholipases, and proteases, and neuronal death ensues. However, calcium channel antagonists have provided little therapeutic benefit in the setting of hypoxic-ischemic injury or in focal or global ischemia (i.e., cardiac arrest). In animal models, pretreatment with these agents improves survival but does not improve neurologic function when given during recirculation. Clinical trials of nimodipine and lidoflazine after cardiac arrest have demonstrated no improvement in overall outcome.

Intravenous administration of L-type calcium channel blockers before experimental focal ischemia results in amelioration of blood flow reduction. Further, the extent of cellular damage with penumbral regions of the infarct is reduced. However, in large multicenter studies of nimodipine after stroke, overall mortality and neurologic outcome were not improved. Nimodipine is the single calcium channel blocker that has been demonstrated to improve outcome in aneurysmal subarachnoid hemorrhage. Additionally, both nimodipine and nicardipine have been evaluated in clinical trials of head-injured patients with no clinical benefit demonstrated. Newer mixed sodium/calcium antagonists are under investigation.

Excitatory Amino Acid Receptor Antagonists

Excitatory amino acid receptor antagonists have been tested for therapeutic efficacy in focal and global ischemia and in TBI, and an increasing number of these agents are currently in development and testing (30,31). There are numerous recognition sites for inhibition within the NMDA receptor-channel complex, hence a variety of therapeutic targets. However, because glutamate neurotransmission is essential to normal brain function, many NMDA receptor antagonists produce undesirable side effects that limit therapeutic potential. The NMDA receptor antagonist, dizocilpine (MK-801), ameliorates injury when administered before or up to 2 hours after permanent focal ischemia. Damage is also reduced when NMDA antagonists are administered before the onset of transient focal ischemia. When dizocilpine is administered in combination with nimodipine, neuroprotection is enhanced during transient focal ischemia. Pretreatment with NMDA receptor antagonists appears to improve recovery of neurologic function in transient global ischemia in a dose-dependent manner. NMDA receptor blockade has also been demonstrated to improve neurologic recovery after TBI and spinal cord injury. Remacemide hydrochloride is an NMDA antagonist with an active desglycinyl metabolite. Similar to dizocilpine (MK-801), it confers neuroprotection in animal focal ischemia models. In humans, it offers the advantages of oral and intravenous dosing, good oral bioavailability, and a lack of undesirable hemodynamic alterations. In the brain, concentrations of remacemide and its metabolites may be rapidly achieved within 1 hour of dosing, which may be advantageous given the narrow therapeutic window inherent in human stroke.

Nitric Oxide Synthase Inhibitors

Numerous studies have demonstrated that nNOS inhibition by concentrations of nonselective NOS inhibitors that do not alter eNOS activity, or by selective nNOS inhibitors such as 7-nitroindazole and ARL 17477, attenuates infarct volume as compared to controls. Transgenic mice lacking nNOS have reduced infarct volumes as compared to wild-type controls following focal cerebral ischemia. Treatment with the relatively selective iNOS inhibitor, aminoguanidine, results in attenuation of infarct volume as compared with vehicle-treated controls. Furthermore, iNOS null mice have significantly reduced stroke volume as compared with wild-type controls. Selective inhibition of nNOS and iNOS reduces delayed neuronal damage following global cerebral ischemia (32) and improves functional score and contusion volume in the fluid-percussion model of TBI (33). These experimental results strongly suggest the need for developing highly selective nNOS and iNOS inhibitors for ischemic neuroprotection, while maintaining eNOS function for adequate cerebral perfusion. Recently, PARP has been implicated as an injury mechanism in focal stroke (21), therefore therapies targeted toward pharmacologic inhibition of PARP can potentially provide significant neuroprotection.

Radical Scavengers

A variety of compounds that scavenge oxygen radicals have been investigated in animal or *in vitro* models of cerebral ischemia and head injury, including superoxide dismutase (with or without conjugation to polyethylene glycol), catalase, allopurinol, deferoxamine, dimethyl sulfoxide, and mannitol (22). Each of these agents is efficacious only in specific experimental conditions. The 21-aminosteroid compounds inhibit lipid peroxidation, scavenge lipid peroxyl radicals and oxygen radicals, and have α-tocopherol-sparing effects and membrane stabilizing action. Neuroprotective effects with this group of agents are inconsistent. Alpha-phenyl-n-tert-butyl-nitrone (PBN) and N-tert-butyl-(2-sulfophenyl)-nitrone (S-PBN) are free radical scavengers currently under investigation. PBN has been demonstrated to be effective in both global and focal ischemia models. Recently, S-PBN has also been shown to reduce cerebral infarct volume as effectively as does PBN in a rat focal ischemia model (34). Lastly, a promising new approach to drug design has yielded a bifunctional agent, BN80933, which scavenges radical species and inhibits nNOS (35). Future development of compounds that attack two or more prooxidant mechanisms may prove useful in stroke and neurotrauma.

Hormonal Neuroprotection

Recent studies underscore the importance of sex steroids (estrogen, progesterone, and testosterone) to outcome from ischemic and TBI [for reviews see (36,37)]. The most abundant evidence centers on estrogen as a neuroprotectant in a variety of global and focal ischemic animal models. In focal cerebral ischemia, 17β-estradiol treatment reduces histologic damage in male, ovariectomized female, and reproductively senescent female rats. Novel forms of estrogen have also been tested. LY353381.HCl, or 2-(4-methoxyphenyl)-3-[4-[2-(1-piperidinyl)ethoxy[phenoxy]benzo[b]thiophene-6-ol hydrochloride, is a selective estrogen receptor modulator (SERM) with a structure and *in vivo* activity profile similar to that of raloxifene. LY353381.HCl has central nervous system penetrability, and it confers neuroprotection via flow independent mechanisms in the rat (38). Clinical trials of postmenopausal estrogen replacement therapy and stroke risk and outcome are in progress.

Anesthetic Agents

The current concept that anesthesia could lessen brain injury arose from early clinical observations that patients under general anesthesia were more tolerant to cerebral ischemia than unanesthetized patients. An understanding of anesthesia-associated ischemic tolerance is important in forming an anesthetic plan for patients at high risk of cerebral ischemia (e.g., carotid endarterectomy, open-heart procedures) and as part of neuroprotective strategies in patients who have sustained cardiac arrest or a focal ischemic insult. It must be emphasized that all anesthetics

TABLE 2. ANESTHETIC EFFECTS AS THERAPEUTIC AGENTS DURING COMPLETE GLOBAL AND FOCAL/INCOMPLETE ISCHEMIA

Anesthetic	Complete Global Ischemia	Focal Incomplete Ischemia	Potential Mechanism of Protection
Barbiturates	No effect	Effective	1. Decreased $CMRO_2$ 2. Inhibition of agonist-induced cerebral vasoconstrictor response 3. Inhibition of protein kinase C 4. Decreased production of free fatty acids during ischemia 5. Inhibition of excitatory amino acid receptors
Inhalation agents	Not adequately evaluated	Effective	1. Decreased $CMRO_2$ 2. Increased CBF 3. Increased production of prostanoids 4. Inhibition of excitatory amino acid receptors 5. Attenuation of central dopamine release 6. Reduced excitatory amino acid-mediated calcium flux
Ketamine	Not adequately evaluated	Effective	1. NMDA-receptor antagonist 2. Attenuates systemic catecholamine response
Etomidate	Not adequately evaluated	Effective	1. Decreased $CMRO_2$ 2. Attenuates ischemia-induced dopamine release
Opiates	Not adequately evaluated	κ-receptor agonists are effective	1. κ-receptor agonists attenuate presynaptic excitotoxic mechanisms
Propofol	Not adequately evaluated	Effective	1. Decreased $CMRO_2$ 2. Decreased extracellular glycine accumulation
Alpha-2 agonists	Not adequately evaluated	Effective	1. Attenuated ischemia-induced catecholamine release within brain 2. Imidazole receptor ligand
Benzodiazepines	Not adequately evaluated	Limited effectiveness	1. Antiseizure 2. Decreased $CMRO_2$ 3. Increased affinity of GABA-receptor binding affinity

$CMRO_2$, cerebral metabolic rate for oxygen; CBF, cerebral blood flow; NMDA, N-methyl-d-aspartate; GABA, γ-aminobutyric acid.

exert some influence over CBF and neurologic function. Therefore, assessment of therapeutic potential for any selected anesthetic in animals or intraoperative subjects is often complicated by the presence of another baseline anesthetic agent. The baseline anesthetic may mask the therapeutic potential of the candidate drug if both agents share a neuroprotective mechanism. This fact has complicated our ability to uncover and understand important properties of anesthetics in cerebroprotection.

Although there are now numerous studies that evaluate anesthetic effects on cerebral hemodynamics and neurochemistry, only agents currently used in perioperative critical care are reviewed in this section. Table 2 summarizes these anesthetics and their beneficial or detrimental potential in brain injury. Efficacy in focal versus global insults should be considered in evaluating these agents. For example, barbiturates have been widely used preemptively for neuroprotection in cardiovascular and cerebrovascular surgery, in part because these agents decrease $CMRO_2$. Clinical investigators have been disappointed by the lack of therapeutic benefit when barbiturates are given after isolated cerebral ischemia, near-drowning, or resuscitation from cardiac arrest. However, barbiturates are still considered as potentially viable therapeutic agents in focal ischemia. To be effective in experimental focal ischemia, barbiturates must be given as a pretreatment or within approximately 1 hour of vascular occlusion. In addition, dosages that are therapeutic in experimental stroke may cause hemodynamic and respiratory depression in humans.

The neuroprotective efficacy of inhalational anesthetics has been well studied. Although most studies demonstrate similar neuroprotection efficacy of halothane, isoflurane, and barbiturates, more recent work suggests a small protective advantage for using isoflurane. Isoflurane produces superior metabolic suppression, although the duration of protection may be quite limited. Although mechanisms of neuroprotection vary among agents (Table 2), a key action is the ability to reduce metabolic needs of the brain, improve blood flow to penumbra, inhibit excitatory amino acid binding, attenuate dopamine release from corpus striatum, and reduce L-glutamate and NMDA-mediated calcium fluxes. Unlike the potent inhalational anesthetics, NO is likely detrimental to neurologic outcome following ischemia. Further, NO may decrease the neuroprotective activity of isoflurane by a mechanism related to increased cerebral metabolism. Because NO does not provide adequate surgical anesthesia when administered alone, its use is associated with high levels of systemic catecholamines. Accordingly, nitrous oxide would be expected to result in worsening of neurologic outcome following cerebral ischemia.

Nonvolatile anesthetics can be cerebroprotective as well. Although ketamine is not commonly used in clinical practice, it is of interest in that it acts as a noncompetitive NMDA receptor antagonist. In animals, high doses can provide cerebral protection following incomplete forebrain ischemia and improve outcome from focal ischemia to a similar degree as observed with halothane. Somewhat less is known about the neuroprotective efficacy of etomidate (1-(1-phenylethyl)-1H-imidazole-5-carboxylic acid ethyl ester). This agent provides EEG depression without hemodynamic instability, and pretreatment decreases brain injury following focal and global ischemia in animals. In humans, etomidate appears to have less efficacy in focal ischemia as compared to the inhalational anesthetics. Studies that evaluate the role of opiates in cerebral ischemia have concentrated predominately on K receptor agonists (e.g., nalbuphine) which produce analgesia and sedation. There is mounting evidence that K-receptor agonists, particularly the K-1 subtype, may be of benefit in brain injury even when administered hours after the onset of focal ischemia.

In healthy subjects, propofol (2,6-di-isopropyl phenol) reduces CBF, $CMRo_2$, and cerebral electrical activity. In animal models of transient focal ischemia, propofol clearly acts to protect the brain from subsequent injury. However, clinical use of high-dose propofol treatment has not been successful to date, (e.g., as a neuroprotective adjunct in open-heart surgery). Alpha-2 agonists and antagonists have also been evaluated, but current data are conflicting. For example, immediate postischemic administration of idazoxan, an $\alpha2$-receptor antagonist, ameliorates brain injury after forebrain ischemia in rats. Yet the $\alpha2$-adrenergic agonist and sedative, dexmedetomidine, also improves neurologic outcome from transient incomplete and focal ischemia. Further work is needed to clarify mechanisms by which this class of agents can reduce damage *in vivo*. Lastly, benzodiazepines have similar efficacy as barbiturates in the setting of transient incomplete global cerebral ischemia. These agents decrease electrical activity, cerebral metabolism, and CBF. Diazepam administration may be particularly effective in ameliorating forebrain injury when postischemic seizures are present. In contrast, midazolam has been less effective in experimental embolic stroke.

SUMMARY

Cerebral ischemia causes neurologic injury in diverse conditions such as stroke, cardiac arrest, and potentially during cardiopulmonary bypass, neurosurgical, and cerebrovascular procedures. Secondary deterioration after neurotrauma may also be related to ischemic processes. Pharmacologic treatment to prevent secondary injury is dependent on the presence of sufficient blood flow to injured brain for drug delivery. Similarly, therapies must address the fact that brain injury evolves over time and space and includes broad mechanisms such as excitotoxicity, inflammation, and programmed cell death. Effective concepts that guide postischemic therapy must reflect the possibility of synergism and competition among multiple injury mechanisms. Similarly, further study of innovative combination or sequential treatments is needed if we are to observe substantial, and functional, neuroprotection in patients.

Acknowledgments. Supported by National Institutes of Health grants NR03521, NS33668, and NS20020.

KEY POINTS

The injured brain is critically sensitive to hypoxia and hypotension that would likely be tolerated in the normal brain. Primary regulatory mechanisms of cerebral blood flow may be altered or abolished after cerebral ischemia or traumatic brain injury.

Brain injury cascades evolve over time and involve surprisingly large spaces, including tissue not directly involved in the initial insult. Injury mechanisms can be broadly divided into: (a) excitotoxicity, (b) inflammation, and (c) programmed cell death. The relative importance of each of these broad mechanisms, and abundance of cells injured by a specific molecular actor, depends on injury severity/duration and on available endogenous neuroprotection.

Nitric oxide is an important endogenous intracellular signaling agent that has been consistently implicated in neurotoxicity. One hypothesis is that nitric oxide reacts with other radical species (e.g., superoxide anion) to form lethal radical forms (e.g., peroxynitrite leading to DNA, membrane protein, and lipid damage).

Nonpharmacologic treatments (e.g., moderate hypothermia) and pharmacologic agents, such as subunit-specific glutamate receptor antagonists, neuronal NOS inhibitors, bifunctional antioxidant therapies, and hormones are promising neuroprotective measures at present.

REFERENCES

1. Paulson OB, Strandgaard S, Edvinsson L. Cerebral autoregulation. *Cerebrovasc Brain Metab Rev* 1990;2:161–192.
2. Iadecola C, Pelligrino DA, Moskowitz MA, et al. Nitric oxide synthase inhibition and cerebrovascular regulation. *J Cereb Blood Flow Metab* 1994;14:175–192.
3. Koehler RC, Backofen JE, McPherson RW, et al. Cerebral blood flow and evoked potentials during Cushing response in sheep. *Am J Physiol* 1989;256:HH779–HH788.
4. Hurn PD, Koehler RC, Norris SE, et al. Dependence of cerebral energy phosphate and evoked potential recovery on end-ischemic pH. *Am J Physiol* 1991;260:H532–H541.
5. Siesjö BK, Kristian T, Katsura KI. Overview of bioenergetic failure and metabolic cascades in brain ischemia. In: Ginsberg MD, Bogousslavsky J, eds. *Cerebrovascular disease: pathophysiology, diagnosis and management.* Oxford: Blackwell Science, 1998:3–13.
6. Fiskum G, Murphy AN, Beal MF. Mitochondria in neurodegeneration: acute ischemia and chronic neurodegenerative diseases. *J Cereb Blood Flow Metab* 1999;19:351–369.
7. DeWitt DS, Prough DS, Taylor CL, et al. Regional cerebrovascular responses to progressive hypotension after traumatic brain injury in cats. *Am J Physiol* 1993;32:H1276–H1284.
8. DeWitt DS, Prough DS, Deal DD, et al. Hypertonic saline does not improve cerebral oxygen delivery after head injury and mild hemorrhage in cats. *Crit Care Med* 1996;24:109–117.

9. Wei EP, Dietrich WD, Povlishock JT, et al. Functional, morphological and metabolic abnormalities of the cerebral microcirculation after concussive brain injury in cats. *Circ Res* 1980;46:37–47.

10. Povlishock JT, Hayes RL, Michel ME, et al. Workshop on animal models of traumatic brain injury. *J Neurotrauma* 1994;11:723–732.

11. Ohnishi ST, Ohnishi T, eds. *Central nervous system trauma: research techniques.* Boca Raton, FL: CRC Press, 1995.

12. Cramer SC, Chopp M. Recovery recapitulates ontogeny. *Trends Neurosci* 2000;23:265–271.

13. Diemer NH, Valente E, Bruhn T, et al. Glutamate receptor transmission and ischemic nerve cell damage: evidence for involvement of excitotoxic mechanisms. In: Kogure K, Hossmann KA, Siesjo BK, eds. *Progress in brain research,* vol 96. Amsterdam: Elsevier, 1993:105–124.

14. Lipton P. Ischemic cell death in brain neurons. *Physiol Rev* 1999; 79:1431–1568.

15. Nicotera P, Lipton SA. Excitotoxins in neuronal apoptosis and necrosis. *J Cereb Blood Flow Metab* 1999;19:583–591.

16. Turski L, Huth A, Sheardown M, et al. ZK200775: a phosphonate quinoxalinedione AMPA antagonist for neuroprotection in stroke and trauma. *Proc Natl Acad Sci* 1998;95:10960–10965.

17. Helfaer MA, Ichord R, Martin LJ, et al. Treatment with the competitive NMDA antagonist does not improve outcome after cardiac arrest in dogs. *Stroke* 1998;29:824–829.

18. Kirsch JR, Hurn PD, Traystman RJ. Nitric oxide and cerebral ischemia. In: Ignarro LJ, ed. *Nitric oxide: biology and pathobiology.* San Diego: Academic Press, 2000:439–451.

19. Samdani AF, Dawson TM, Dawson VL. Nitric oxide synthase in models of focal ischemia. *Stroke* 1997;28:1283–1288.

20. Dawson VL, Dawson TM. Nitric oxide in neurodegeneration. *Prog Brain Res* 1998;118:215–229.

21. Eliason MJL, Sampei K, Mandir AS, et al. Poly (ADP-ribose) polymerase gene disruption renders mice resistant to cerebral ischemia. *Nature Med* 1997;3:1089–1095.

22. Traystman RJ, Kirsch JR, Koehler RC. Oxygen radical mechanisms of brain injury following ischemia and reperfusion. *J Appl Physiol* 1991;71:1185–1195.

23. Hurn PD, Traystman RJ. pH-Mediated brain injury in cerebral ischemia and circulatory arrest. *J Intensive Care Med* 1996;11:205–218.

24. Del Zoppo G, Ginis I, Hallenbeck JM, et al. Inflammation and stroke: putative role for cytokines, adhesion molecules and iNOS in brain response to ischemia. *Brain Pathol* 2000;10:95–112.

25. Schulz JB, Weller M, Moskowitz MA. Caspases as treatment targets in stroke and neurodegenerative diseases. *Ann Neurol* 1999;45: 421–429.

26. Clark RS, Kochanek PM, Chen M, et al. Increases in Bcl-2 and cleavage of caspase-1 and caspase-3 in human brain after head injury. *FASEB J* 1999;13:813–821.

27. Clifton GL, Allen A, Barrodate P, et al. A phase II study of moderate hypothermia in severe brain injury. *J Neurotrauma* 1993;10:263–271.

27a. Clifton GL, Miller ER, Choi SC, et al. Lack of effect of induction of hypothermia after acute brain injury. *N Engl J Med* 2001;344:556–563.

28. Bhardwaj A, Ulatowski JA. Cerebral edema: hypertonic saline solutions. *Curr Treatment Options Neurol* 1999;1:179–187.

29. Bhardwaj A, Harukuni I, Murphy SJ, et al. Hypertonic saline worsens infarct volume after transient focal ischemia in rats. *Stroke* 2000;31:1694–1701.

30. Dyker AG, Lees KR. Remacemide hydrochloride: a double-blind, placebo-controlled, safety and tolerability study in patients with acute ischemic stroke. *Stroke* 1999;30:1796–1801.

31. Arrowsmith JE, Harrison MJ, Newman SP, et al. Neuroprotection of the brain during cardiopulmonary bypass: a randomized trial of remacemide during coronary artery bypass in 171 patients. *Stroke* 1998;29:2357–2362.

32. Nanri K, Montecot C, Springhetti V, et al. The selective inhibitor of neuronal nitric oxide synthase, 7-nitroindazole, reduces the delayed neuronal damage due to forebrain ischemia in rats. *Stroke* 1998;29:1248–1253.

33. Wada K, Chatzipanteli K, Kraydieh S, et al. Inducible nitric oxide synthase expression after traumatic brain injury and neuroprotection with aminoguanidine treatment in rats. *Neurosurgery* 1998;43:1427–1436.

34. Yang Y, Li Q, Shuaib A. Neuroprotection by 2-h postischemia administration of two free radical scavengers, alpha-phenyl-n-tert-butyl-nitrone (PBN) and N-tert-butyl-(2-sulfophenyl)-nitrone (S-PBN), in rats subjected to focal embolic cerebral ischemia. *Exp Neurol* 2000;163(1):39–45.

35. Chabrier PE, Auguet M, Spinnewyn B, et al. BN80933, A dual inhibitor of neuronal nitric oxide synthase and lipid peroxidation: a promising neuroprotective strategy. *PNAS* 1999;96:10824–10829.

36. Hurn PD, Macrae IM. Estrogen as neuroprotectant in stroke. *J Cereb Blood Flow Metab* 2000;20:631–652.

37. Roof RL, Hall ED. Gender differences in acute CNS trauma and stroke: neuroprotective effects of estrogen and progesterone. *J Neurotrauma* 2000;17:367–388.

38. Rossberg MI, Murphy SJ, Traystman RJ, et al. LY353381, A selective estrogen receptor modulator (SERM) and experimental stroke. *Stroke* 2000;31:3041–3046.

INTENSIVE CARE UNIT MANAGEMENT OF PATIENTS WITH HEAD AND SPINAL CORD INJURY

STEVEN J. ALLEN

TRAUMATIC BRAIN INJURY

Principles of Neurosurgical Critical Care and Initial Resuscitation

The principles behind the practice of neurosurgical critical care have much in common with the rest of intensive care medicine. By comprehensive monitoring of important physiologic variables and titrating specific therapy to those variables, we hope to give the patient's injured tissue the best chance of repairing itself. This process requires adequate delivery of appropriate substrates, such as oxygen and glucose, and the avoidance of deleterious factors such as infection. It is imperative to preserve residual viable nervous tissue because neurons cannot replicate or hypertrophy. Patients with neurologic injuries require the greatest attention to basic cardiopulmonary support.

Initial resuscitation is aimed at the rapid restoration of suitable arterial oxygen content and blood pressure because, compared to normal tissue, injured central nervous system (CNS) tissue tolerates hypoxemia and hypotension less well than uninjured nervous tissue. Hypoxemia, to which patients with acute brain trauma seem predisposed, results in deprivation of necessary substrate while increasing cerebral blood flow (CBF), thereby contributing to intracranial hypertension (1). The mechanism of hypoxemia associated with early head injury has not been elucidated. In roughly one-half of patients with severe brain injury, autoregulation to blood pressure is impaired (2). Thus, decreases in arterial blood pressure may cause detrimental decreases in CBF. Although the normal values for CBF and cerebral oxygen consumption (CMR_{O_2}) are 50 mL per minute^{-1} per 100 g^{-1} brain

and 3.3 mL O_2 per min^{-1} per 100 g^{-1} brain, respectively, in awake subjects, patients with impaired consciousness have different requirements. Decreases in the level of consciousness decrease CMR_{O_2} because the comatose brain consumes less oxygen and may not need the same CBF. Therefore, some monitoring of cerebral oxygen delivery adequacy, such as jugular bulb oxygen saturation, is desirable (see below).

Blood pressure should be rapidly restored to normal but not to hypertensive values with appropriate interventions. Hypotension resulting from brain injury alone is rare in patients who survive transport to the hospital. The differential diagnosis of hypotension in these patients should include concurrent spinal cord injury and hypovolemia.

The Glasgow Coma Scale (GCS) was developed to provide an objective means of describing a patient's level of consciousness (Table 1). Before the introduction of the GCS, clinicians used subjective terms, such as stuporous or semicomatose. By using a patient's specific verbal, motor, and eye opening response to stimuli, a score can be generated that is descriptive and reproducible from one examiner to the next. Coma is now defined as a GCS score of less than 8. This score generally describes patients who do not spontaneously open their eyes or follow commands. The GCS is typically reported at 6 hours after injury to minimize the potentially confounding effects of initial hypotension and hypoxemia.

Intracranial Hypertension

Pathophysiology and Treatment Rationale

Normal intracranial pressure (ICP) is less than 10 mm Hg with intracranial hypertension defined as ICP greater than 20 mm Hg. Intracranial hypertension in an awake patient is not necessarily associated with neurologic sequelae. For example, patients with pseudotumor cerebri may have intracranial hypertension for weeks without any evidence of neurologic deficits. However, patients with acute brain trauma appear to tolerate intracranial hypertension poorly. In these patients, increases in ICP are thought to result progressively in hypoperfusion, ischemia, and brain swelling, causing further increases in ICP. Because of the

TABLE 1. GLASGOW COMA SCALE

Eye Opening	Score	Motor	Score	Verbal	Score
Spontaneous	4	Follows command	6	Oriented	5
Voice	3	Localizes	5	Confused	4
Pain	2	Flexion/withdrawal	4	Words	3
None	1	Flexion	3	Moans	2
		Extensor	2	None	1
		Flaccid	1		
Range 3–15					

Severe head injury is commonly described as a Glasgow Coma Scale score ≤ 8.

association between poor outcome and intracranial hypertension, aggressive treatment of ICP has become an integral part of the management of severe acute traumatic brain injury. This has been reinforced by a consensus paper which reiterated the recommendation that ICP monitoring be instituted in the presence of GCS less than 8 and an abnormal CT scan (3).

One way to understand why intracranial hypertension may lead to hypoperfusion is to consider the concept of cerebral perfusion pressure (CPP). CPP is the difference between mean arterial blood pressure (MAP) and ICP (or cerebral pressure, whichever is higher). The lower the CPP, the less the pressure difference to drive blood flow across the brain. Evidence suggests that CPP

less than 70 mm Hg is associated with less favorable cerebral hemodynamics after brain injury (4).

Intracranial Compliance

The calvarium composes an essentially closed space. Compensatory mechanisms allow some increase in intracranial volume with little increase in ICP (Fig. 1). These compensatory mechanisms include shunting of cerebrospinal fluid (CSF) into the spinal subarachnoid space and compression of the dural venous sinuses. Once these events have occurred, even small increases in intracranial volume cause dramatic increases in ICP.

Cranial Vault Contents

The calvarium is composed of three fluid compartments: cerebral blood volume (CBV), CSF, and cerebral parenchyma. If intracranial hypertension develops and mass-occupying lesions such as hematomas or abscesses have been treated, then one of the three compartments must have increased in volume. Increases in CSF are by definition due to hydrocephalus. Hydrocephalus in acute brain trauma may be either communicating (no anatomic restriction to CSF outflow) or noncommunicating. Increases in the cerebral parenchymal compartment are due to edema. Edema in acute brain trauma may be due to either ischemia (cytotoxic) or impaired blood–brain barrier (BBB) function (vasogenic). Increases in CBV may be due to a number of factors, such as ischemia, acidosis, hypercapnia, increased venous pressure, and hyperthermia.

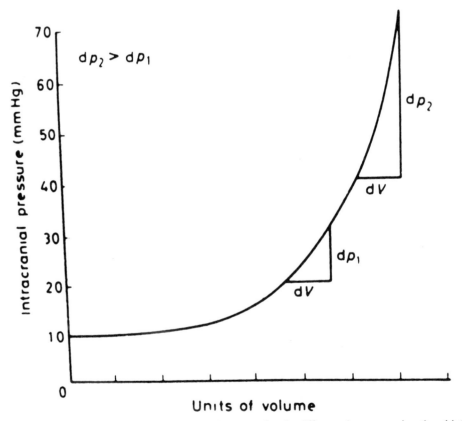

FIGURE 1. Intracranial pressure-volume curve demonstrating the difference in pressure elevations (*dp1*, *dp2*) for the same volume change (*dV*) at two separate locations. (Redrawn from data presented in Fig. 1 of Langfitt TW, Weinstein JD, Kassell NF. Cerebral vasomolor paralysis produced by intracranial hypertension. *Neurology* 1965;15:622–641, with permission.)

Intracranial Pressure Measurement

Intracranial hypertension cannot be intelligently treated without measuring ICP. The treatment for raised ICP is not benign; overzealous application of some therapies, such as hyperventilation, may exacerbate the injury. The gold standard for ICP measurement is ventriculostomy, which typically consists of placing a catheter into the frontal horn of one of the lateral ventricles through a burr hole. Advantages include excellent fidelity of waveform and ability to drain CSF. Contraindications include significant shift of brain structures and coagulopathy. Another technique, the subarachnoid bolt, is not contraindicated by shift or coagulopathy but does not allow CSF drainage and may lose accuracy as ICP increases. The most common method of ICP monitoring in the United States uses a transducer-tipped, fiberoptic catheter. The catheter is inserted a few centimeters into the parenchyma via a twist-drill burr hole and offers excellent waveform fidelity; however, CSF drainage is not possible. All ICP monitors carry a risk of infection that ranges up to 10% depending on the duration of monitoring. It is not clear that prophylactic antibiotics or routine changes of monitoring site reduce the infection risk.

ICP measurement is not a replacement for the neurologic examination. Catastrophic events may occur, especially in the posterior fossa, without an immediate change in ICP. ICP monitors can malfunction owing to a variety of causes. Thus, these patients should be examined in a conscientious manner on a regular basis or when any significant hemodynamic event occurs.

Management

Intracranial hypertension is not a disease, but a symptom of the underlying process. ICP can be elevated from a number of different causes and an attempt should be made to find the etiology and therapy directed accordingly.

Cerebral Blood Volume Reduction

CBV may be increased by increases in jugular venous pressure. Venous pressure may be elevated by head rotation, mechanical occlusion of the neck veins, posturing, and increased intrathoracic pressure. Maneuvers to decrease venous pressure include slight head elevation and midline position, sedation and muscle relaxation, and decreasing airway pressure.

Hyperventilation

Hyperventilation, a component of routine intracranial hypertension therapy for about 30 years, is based on the observation that CBF is linearly related to Pa_{CO_2}. CBF decreases approximately 3% for each mm Hg fall in Pa_{CO_2}. Thus, reducing a patient's Pa_{CO_2} from 40 to 25 mm Hg decreases CBF approximately 35% to 40% and decreases CBV and ICP. However, hypocapnia also decreases oxygen delivery to the brain and may aggravate neuronal injury. Studies have failed to demonstrate a benefit of routine hyperventilation and there are suggestions that it may be detrimental (5). A more rational way to employ hyperventilation is to titrate it to some physiologic endpoint such as jugular bulb oxygen saturation. As Pa_{CO_2} decreases, cerebral oxygen delivery decreases and the brain extracts a greater percentage of the oxygen delivered, resulting in a lower jugular venous oxygen saturation.

Maintenance of the jugular venous oxygen saturation above 50% is associated with improved outcome (6).

Normally, CBF is independent of MAP between the extremes of 50 and 150 mm Hg, a phenomenon known as autoregulation. About one-half of patients with severe brain trauma demonstrate altered autoregulation to blood pressure (2). Thus, relatively small decreases in MAP may result in critical reductions in CBF and cerebral oxygen delivery, while similar MAP increases may result in hyperemia and worsening intracranial hypertension. Accordingly, MAP should be kept as near normal as possible. Hypotension should be treated with attention to the cause such as hypovolemia or left ventricular dysfunction. Hypertension may be treated with a variety of agents, but drugs with direct vasodilatory effects, such as sodium nitroprusside, should be used with caution as they may worsen intracranial compliance and cause ICP to increase. Trimethaphan has not been reported to result in worsening intracranial hypertension, but the dilated pupils that arise from the ganglionic blockade may complicate evaluation. Beta-adrenergic blockers are most commonly used as first-line treatment if contraindications, such as cardiac failure or bronchospastic disease, do not exist. Nicardipine may also be considered as it is titratable and does not appear to be associated with increases in ICP.

Cerebrospinal Fluid Drainage

Decreasing the CSF space by drainage may decrease ICP. CSF is generated at a rate of 0.3 mL per kg^{-1} per $hour^{-1}$ or approximately 500 mL per day in an adult. However, only approximately 200 mL per day is accessible to the ventricular drain. Communicating and noncommunicating hydrocephalus can develop in head-injured patients but it rarely occurs in the first 2 to 3 days after injury. The treatment for hydrocephalus is CSF drainage, usually with a ventriculostomy, with shunt placement seldom necessary. Hydrocephalus should be considered in a patient in whom ICP has been under control for several days but subsequently develops intracranial hypertension. The diagnosis of hydrocephalus requires computed tomography (CT) or magnetic resonance imaging (MRI), as does the diagnosis of most neurosurgical lesions in these patients.

Brain Parenchyma Reduction

Hypertonic solutions have been advocated since the turn of the twentieth century for treatment of cerebral swelling. Mannitol is the solute of choice because of its inertness and slow half-life (approximately 2.3 hours) of equilibration across the BBB. The mechanism by which mannitol decreases ICP is controversial but any fluid removed probably comes from normal, and not edematous, tissue. Mannitol is unique in that it acts to increase CBF while decreasing ICP. This characteristic is advantageous when hyperventilation has been maximized and intracranial hypertension persists (7). As mannitol induces net free water excretion, serum sodium and osmolality should be monitored. We recommend not giving mannitol if serum osmolality is greater than 315 mOsm per L because there is evidence that at values greater than 330 mOsm per L, renal dysfunction occurs and the BBB begins to fail.

Steroids have been advocated to reduce edema associated with acute brain trauma, based on the often dramatic clinical effect of corticosteroids on peritumoral edema. However, a metaanalysis of 13 trials failed to show any beneficial effect (8).

Fluid Therapy

The goal of fluid therapy in brain trauma is to restore intravascular volume while minimizing cerebral edema. At one time, concern about cerebral edema led some clinicians to limit crystalloid fluid in head-injured patients. A few physicians even advocated hypovolemia as prevention or treatment of cerebral edema. This approach was based on an inaccurate concept of fluid balance in the CNS and was subsequently discredited when the deleterious effects of hypoperfusion were recognized. CNS fluid exchange occurs at the BBB. The BBB is formed by the tight junctions of the cerebral capillary endothelial cells and is the most impermeable microvascular exchange barrier of the vital organs. This low permeability is characterized by restricted passage of even small ions. In other organs, in which the capillary membranes are too permeable to allow sodium gradients to develop, plasma proteins are the main determinants of osmotic pressures. However, due to the relative impermeability of the BBB, sodium gradients can generate osmotic pressures severalfold greater than those produced by plasma proteins. For example, a normal protein concentration of 6 g per 100 mL generates a colloid osmotic pressure of about 20 mm Hg. In contrast, each milliosmole (0.5 mEq) of sodium can generate an osmotic pressure of 19.3 mm Hg. Studies have failed to show an impact of low protein solutions on ICP if the osmolality is normal. In contrast, normooncotic but hypoosmotic fluids increase cerebral water content. The clinical implication for fluid therapy in head-injured patients is that hypotonic fluid should be avoided. Even lactated Ringer solution is slightly hypoosmolar (273 mOsm per L) compared to plasma.

Heroics

As acute brain trauma tends to occur in young patients, heroic therapies are chosen sometimes when conventional management fails. These therapies are used for intractable intracranial hypertension, as defined by ICP greater than 25 mm Hg for 30 minutes, greater than 30 mm Hg for 15 minutes, or greater than 40 mm Hg for 5 minutes, despite maximal therapy and no evidence of a surgically correctable lesion on CT. As the success of these interventions is low and the risks are high, decisions should include input from family members.

Barbiturate Coma

Because hypoperfusion is a major concern in severe brain trauma, reduction of cerebral oxygen demand is an attractive intervention. Barbiturates can reduce cerebral oxygen demand without inducing cellular toxicity by causing electrical activity to cease. Titrating barbiturate administration to produce a 30- to 60-second burst suppression pattern on the electroencephalogram (EEG) is associated with maximum metabolic suppression. Barbiturate coma will decrease ICP in most patients, including those who are unresponsive to maximal conventional therapy. However, cardiovascular depression is a significant risk. Despite the ability to reduce ICP, it is not clear to what extent, if any, barbiturate

coma improves outcome in patients with intractable intracranial hypertension (9).

Hypothermia

Hypothermia also reduces cerebral oxygen demand and decreases ICP. Isoelectricity can be induced and the metabolic depression is probably greater than with barbiturate coma. However, no studies demonstrate whether iatrogenic hypothermia is of any benefit after intractable intracranial hypertension has developed. There is evidence that institution of hypothermia within 6 hours of injury does improve outcome (10,11). However, a multiinstitutional, randomized study involving 392 patients failed to show a decrease in the percentage of patients with bad outcomes (12). Nonetheless, the study suggests that there may be subpopulations that would benefit.

SPINAL CORD INJURIES

Pathophysiology

Spinal cord injuries occur with an incidence of approximately 50 cases per million population per year. Most cases in the United States are due to motor vehicle accidents but work- and sports-related injuries contribute about 10% each to the total. Autopsy studies demonstrate that even complete cord lesions are rarely associated with physical transection of the cord. Experimental studies show that spinal cord insult is associated with initiation of an injury response that results in neuronal destruction. This observation is the driving force behind the effort to develop pharmacologic interventions to modify this injury response and improve neurologic outcome.

Initial Resuscitation

As with any critically ill patient, timely resuscitation is the first priority in managing patients with spinal cord injury. In addition to addressing the pulmonary and cardiovascular effects associated with spinal cord injury mentioned below, immobilization of the neck should be ensured until cervical spine stabilization has occurred. Due to impaired sensation, other injuries may not produce symptoms and thus increase the risk that diagnosis of significant intraabdominal injury may be delayed.

Neurologic Examination

Early and sequential neurologic examinations are important to the management of patients with spinal cord injury, as they may guide timing of surgical intervention. In general, a patient with signs of neurologic deterioration may be a candidate for early surgery, while a patient who is improving will usually be managed more conservatively. The neurologic examination should assess motor and sensory function in enough detail to determine the level of the spinal cord lesion. Motor score can be effectively reported by using a 5-grade scale: 5 represents full strength, 4 is weak, 3 is ability to overcome gravity only, 2 is movement but not sufficient to overcome gravity, and 1 is flaccid. Table 2 shows the nerve root innervation of various muscles. Sensory function should include testing both pain and position in a

TABLE 2. SPINAL NERVE INNERVATION

Muscle	Spinal Roots
Trapezius	C4
Shoulder external rotators	C5
Shoulder internal rotators	C5
Shoulder abductors	C5
Biceps	C5, 6
Triceps	C7
Wrist extensors	C6, 7
Wrist flexors	C7, 8
Finger extensors	C8
Grasp	C8, T1
Hip flexors	L1, 2
Hip extensors	L5, S1
Knee flexors	S1
Knee extensors	L3, 4
Dorsiflexion	L4
Plantar flexion	S1, 2

fashion that determines the sensory level of the lesion (Fig. 2). Note that the lower cervical segments and upper thoracic segments often are not represented on the trunk and a complete sensory examination requires mapping the sensory level on the upper extremities.

Cord Injury Syndromes

Complete Cord Lesion

Patients present with complete loss of motor, sensory, and reflex activity below the injury level.

Central Cord Syndrome

This condition derives its name from the observation that the central part of the cord appears to be less injured than the other parts. This disparity results in greater strength in the legs than the arms. It probably results from an injury to the anterior spinal artery and generally improves with time.

Posterior Cord Syndrome

After a hyperflexion injury, the intervertebral disc may herniate straight back, compressing the spinal cord. A rare presentation is that of a spinal cord lesion in which only the posterior columns are spared. Thus, only position and vibratory sensation may be intact. Early surgery is sometimes indicated.

Brown-Séquard Syndrome

This presentation results from an injury to a lateral one-half of the spinal cord. Distal to the lesion, motor function and position and vibratory sensation are impaired ipsilaterally, while perception of pain and temperature is impaired contralaterally. This phenomenon occurs because the fibers of the spinothalamic tract (pain and temperature) cross in the cord about two to four levels above where they enter the cord while the motor fibers do not cross until they reach the brainstem. Therefore, there may be a

band just below the lesion where ipsilateral pain and temperature are impaired.

Spinal Shock

Spinal shock, a term sometimes confused with neurogenic shock, is used to describe the lack of neurologic function in the period from immediately after to approximately 4 weeks after trauma. Around 4 to 6 weeks, pathologic reflexes begin to develop due to disinhibition, and the cord is said to be out of shock. However, it is this transition that results in the patient becoming more susceptible to autonomic hyperreflexia (see below).

Systemic Effects

Although spinal cord injury affects all organ systems to some degree, it is the respiratory and cardiovascular effects that often result in admission to a critical care unit.

Respiratory

The degree of respiratory compromise associated with spinal cord injury is directly related to the level of the spinal cord lesion. Injury to the cord at or below the lower thoracic segments rarely poses pulmonary problems of clinical significance. Lesions above the thoracic levels result in loss of the intercostal muscles so that inspiration is mainly provided by the diaphragm, which is innervated by the phrenic nerve. Besides loss of the intercostal contribution to ventilation, the patient has essentially no active expiratory function, a deficit that interferes with secretion clearance. The phrenic nerves arise from C3-5, and injuries at these levels may result in the need for intubation and mechanical ventilation. In one study, only 2 of 11 patients with C5-6 injuries required intubation, while all of the patients with C4 injuries required intubation (13). Patients with spinal cord injuries above C3 may die of ventilatory failure before arrival of life support but some may be able to survive using accessory muscles. These patients are at great risk for developing apnea.

To understand how spinal cord injury at various levels results in the observed respiratory problems, a review of ventilatory mechanics is required. Normal tidal ventilation consists of maneuvers that maximize the efficiency of respiratory effort. The diaphragm contracts more effectively if it is stretched before onset of inspiration. This stretching is usually accomplished by contraction of the abdominal recti, which use the intraabdominal contents to stint the diaphragm to prevent it from descending. The intraabdominal contents could also be viewed as a fulcrum for the diaphragm. Loss of innervation to the lower thoracic segments may result in the diaphragm starting inspiration in a lower and less stretched (and, therefore, less efficient) position.

The intercostal muscles act in several ways to improve the efficiency of ventilation. Most obviously, they contract to expand the diameter of the rib cage, thereby lowering pleural pressure. Less well recognized is the role of the intercostal muscles in stabilizing the chest wall so that the negative pleural pressure does not result in paradoxic chest wall movement. Thus, cervical cord injury is associated with less efficient tidal breathing due to suboptimal diaphragm contraction and paradoxic chest wall movement. Cervical cord injury also weakens cough efforts by denervating the

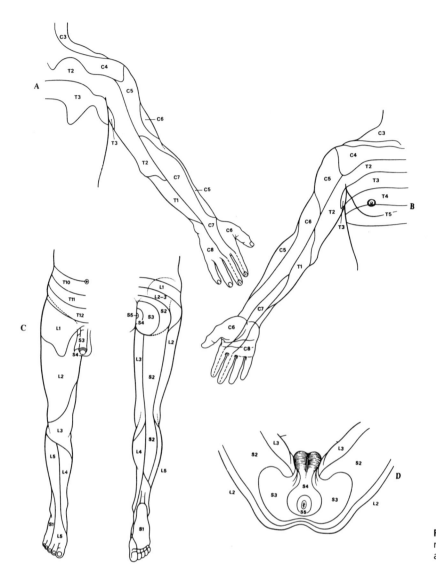

FIGURE 2. Distribution of sensory innervation of posterior (**A**) and anterior (**B**) trunk, neck, and upper extremity, and lower extremity (**C**) and perineal region (**D**).

primary muscles (intercostals and abdominal recti) used in active expiration.

Management of the respiratory effects of spinal cord injury consists of assistance with secretion clearance, maintenance of lung volumes, and timing of endotracheal intubation. Secretion mobilization is enhanced by position and chest physiotherapy, and by assisted cough maneuvers such as diaphragm thrust. However, these efforts may not be enough to prevent respiratory compromise and the need for intubation. We monitor tidal volume and maximum inspiratory pressure every 8 hours for the first 5 days after the acute injury. If the tidal volume decreases below 15 mL per kg or the maximum inspiratory pressure is not more negative than 25 cm H_2O, the patient is evaluated for intubation. In view of the potential for difficult airway visualization, we prefer to intubate these patients electively while gas exchange may be adequate but their pulmonary mechanics are decreasing, rather than to wait until respiratory distress ensues.

Although the major cause of death in the acutely quadriplegic patient is respiratory failure, respiratory mechanics tend to improve with time. Probably because of spasticity in the inter-

costal muscles, quadriplegic patients have better vital capacities 3 months after injury and pulmonary problems are more manageable. In addition, they can develop significant active expiratory efforts by learning to contract the clavicular portion of the pectoralis major.

Patients with cervical spinal cord injuries are also at risk for other respiratory complications, including direct rib cage injury, pulmonary embolism, gastric aspiration, and neurogenic pulmonary edema.

Cardiovascular

Cardiovascular problems after spinal cord injury are almost solely related to interruption of sympathetic pathways. Sympathetic fibers exit the spinal cord between the spinal roots T1-L2. Spinal cord lesions in the lower thoracic segments are not generally associated with clinically significant hemodynamic changes. However, cervical cord lesions are associated with hypotension and bradycardia as parasympathetic tone is unopposed. Bradycardia may be symptomatic and is usually associated with a stimulus such as turning or suctioning even if hypoxemia is avoided.

Pretreatment with vagolytics is sufficient for most patients who develop symptomatic bradycardia, which usually resolves within 2 months. It is the rare spinal cord injury patient who requires cardiac pacemaker insertion. Hypotension generally responds to mild intravascular volume enhancement and low doses of vasopressors unless a cardiac injury has occurred. Occasionally, a pulmonary arterial catheter may be needed to guide fluid therapy.

Autonomic Hyperreflexia

Loss of central inhibition leads to hyperreactive sympathetic reflex responses in the cord below the level of the lesion. As a result, stimuli such as bladder or bowel distension can result in severe hypertension, arrhythmias, and headache, with compensatory vasodilation above the lesion level. In addition to removing the stimulus, the hemodynamic effects may be treated with a mixed adrenergic blocker such as labetalol. Life-threatening hypertension in some patients may require a direct vasodilator such as sodium nitroprusside.

Metabolic Effects

Patients with spinal cord injury often develop adynamic ileus that usually resolves within 3 to 5 days, but may last 2 weeks. Because of their immobility, quadriplegic patients will remain in a negative nitrogen balance for several weeks and adequacy of nutritional support must be guided by other nutritional assessments. Patients with spinal cord injury may also develop hypercalcemia due to bone reabsorption and occasionally require long-term calcium therapy.

Neuroresuscitative Agents

With the recognition that the spinal cord is not physically transected in most of these patients, there has been intense interest in finding agents that may improve functional outcome. Many agents have been tested in animal and clinical trials. However, the only pharmacologic intervention that has been shown to improve neurologic outcome after spinal cord injury is high-dose steroids. The second National Acute Spinal Cord Injury Study randomized acute spinal injury patients to receive either placebo, naloxone, or methylprednisolone (14). Methylprednisolone was given as a 30 mg per kg bolus immediately, followed by 5.4 mg per kg^{-1} per hour for the next 23 hours. The steroid group had a statistically significant improvement of approximately one level, compared to the other groups (14). This treatment has become standard initial therapy for essentially all patients with suspected spinal cord injury, but appears to be effective only if given in the first 8 hours after injury. Geisler and colleagues report some modest improvements in neurologic function in patients receiving GM-1 ganglioside after spinal cord injury; however, differences between the placebo and treatment groups at baseline confound interpretation of those data (15).

SUMMARY

Head and spinal cord injuries remain serious problems in intensive care units. In both types of injury, careful attention to the principles of intensive care may limit the ultimate extent of injury and result in less disability in these often young patients.

KEY POINTS

Key points made in this chapter are:

- The assurance of adequate respiration and circulation is the most important part of the resuscitation of the neurologically injured patient.
- If intracranial hypertension is to be treated, intracranial pressure should be monitored.
- Intracranial hypertension is a symptom and not a disease process. It requires a differential diagnosis and directed therapy.
- Hyperventilation decreases oxygen delivery to the injured brain. It should be used cautiously and with some physiologic guidance.
- Resuscitation fluids should be iso- or hyperosmolar to prevent worsening of cerebral edema.
- The spinal cord is rarely physically transected in spinal cord injury.
- Loss of intercostal and rectus muscle function in cervical spinal cord injury results in inefficient inspiration and absence of active expiration.
- Respiratory complications are responsible for death in the first few months after spinal cord injury, while renal failure is more likely to cause death later.

- The use of corticosteroids in the first 8 hours following spinal cord injury provides a marginal improvement in function at 1 year.
- To date, no pharmacologic treatment can substantially reverse the consequences of either type of injury.

Similar to other progressive organ dysfunction seen in critically ill patients, the pathophysiology of acute brain trauma and spinal cord injury is related to the action of endogenous mediators. Animal studies and limited clinical experience suggest that modulation of mediator and cytokine action can significantly improve outcome in these conditions. Other compounds that modify the cytokine and opioid injury response will also be tested in clinical trials for neurologic injury.

The primitive state of central nervous system monitoring has led to the largely empiric manner in which neurologically injured patients are treated. There is a need for bedside monitors of cellular metabolism to guide therapy. These monitors would need to assess the adequacy of cerebral oxygen delivery (which obviates the need to follow cerebral perfusion pressure) in specific regions to guide therapy.

REFERENCES

1. Cooper KR, Boswell PA. Reduced functional residual capacity and abnormal oxygenation of patients with severe head injury. *Chest* 1983;84:29–35.
2. Bouma GJ, Muizelaar JP, Bandoh K, et al. Blood pressure and intracranial pressure-volume dynamics in severe head injury: relationship with cerebral blood flow. *J Neurosurg* 1992;77:15–19.
3. Bullock R, Chesnut RM, Clifton GL. Guidelines for the management of severe head injury. *J Neurotrauma* 2000;17:451–549.
4. Chan KH, Miller JD, Dearden NM, et al. The effect of changes in cerebral perfusion pressure upon middle cerebral artery blood flow velocity and jugular bulb venous oxygen saturation after severe brain injury. *J Neurosurg* 1992;77:55–61.
5. Muizelaar JP, Marmarou A, Ward JD, et al. Adverse effects of prolonged hyperventilation in patients with severe head injury: a randomized clinical trial. *J Neurosurg* 1991;75:731–739.
6. Sheinberg M, Kanter MJ, Robertson CS, et al. Continuous monitoring of jugular venous oxygen saturation in head-injured patients. *J Neurosurg* 1992;76:212–217.
7. Cruz J, Miner ME, Allen SJ, et al. Continuous monitoring of cerebral oxygenation in acute brain injury: injection of mannitol during hyperventilation. *J Neurosurg* 1990;73:725–730.
8. Alderson P, Roberts I. Corticosteroids in acute traumatic brain injury: systematic review of randomised controlled trials. *BMJ* 1997;314:1855–1859.
9. Eisenberg HM, Frankowski RF, Contant CF, et al. High-dose barbiturate control of elevated intracranial pressure in patients with severe head injury. *J Neurosurg* 1988;69:15–23.
10. Clifton GL, Allen SJ, Barrodale P, et al. A phase II study of moderate hypothermia in severe brain injury. *J Neurotrauma* 1993;10:263–271.
11. Marion DW, Obrist WD, Carlier PM, et al. The use of moderate therapeutic hypothermia for patients with severe head injuries: a preliminary report. *J Neurosurg* 1993;79:354–362.
12. Clifton GL, Miller ER, Choi SC, et al. Lack of effect of hypothermia in acute brain injury. *N Engl J Med* 2001;344:556–563.
13. Ledsome JR, Sharp JM. Pulmonary function in acute cervical cord injury. *Am Rev Respir Dis* 1981;124:41–44.
14. Bracken MB, Shepard JM, Collins WF, et al. A randomized, controlled trial of methylprednisolone or naloxone in the treatment of acute spinal cord injury: results of the second National Acute Spinal Cord Injury Study. *N Engl J Med* 1990;322:1405–1411.
15. Geisler FH, Dorsey FC, Coleman WP. Recovery of motor function after spinal-cord injury–a randomized, placebo-controlled trial with GM-1 ganglioside. *N Engl J Med* 1991;324:1829–1838.

DIAGNOSIS AND MANAGEMENT OF COMATOSE PATIENTS IN THE INTENSIVE CARE UNIT

THOMAS P. BLECK

KEY WORDS

- Brain death
- Coma
- Confusion
- Delirium
- Decerebrate
- Decorticate
- Extension posture; abnormal
- Flexion posture; abnormal

- Glasgow Coma Scale
- Herniation
- Locked-in syndrome
- Persistent vegetative state
- Psychogenic unresponsiveness
- Reticular formation
- Stupor

INTRODUCTION

In critical care practice, coma may seize the patient abruptly or may evolve so insidiously that the physician is not certain that the patient is changing in any important way. After general anesthesia, the patient may simply be someone slower than average to awaken, or may have suffered an intraoperative catastrophe. It is the task of the critical care staff to determine whether the patient's unresponsive state is expected or unusual, to assess the likely causes of abnormally altered consciousness with skill and speed, to reverse a set of immediately reversible causes of coma with deliberate speed, to determine which patients need emergent imaging or neurophysiologic studies, to institute emergent therapy for the potentially treatable etiologies, to assess prognosis, and to counsel the patient's loved ones. While intensivists will often call upon neurologic and neurosurgical colleagues for assistance, the initial steps of this process must be undertaken with such alacrity and frequency in the critical care setting that we must be able to institute analysis and management before others can arrive.

As one of the prototypic disorders of critical care, diagnostic studies and initial management procedures must proceed simultaneously. Within a few minutes of being called to the bedside, the intensivists should have completed the preliminary survey of neurologic function and excluded or treated hypotension, hypox-

emia, hypoglycemia, and thiamine deficiency. At this point one can decide what steps are next to be taken.

Comprehensive understanding of this topic requires a brief overview of the anatomy, physiology, and neurochemistry of consciousness. To discuss the concepts at all, however, we require a common set of definitions. In this regard one must acknowledge a debt to the work of a number of investigators whose œuvre form the basis for the masterful work of Plum and Posner (1).

DEFINITIONS

Consciousness is difficult to define but straightforward to recognize. Its major components are *arousal* and *content*. Arousal depends upon the midbrain reticular formation (RF) and its interaction with the thalamus and the cerebral cortex (2); if the midbrain RF fails, the cortex may be capable of normal function but will not be driven to consider either external stimuli or internal needs. If the RF arousal mechanisms are intact but the cortex cannot function, the patient may display spontaneous eye opening and sleep-wake cycling, but there is no awareness of the environment (cf. *akinetic mutism* below). In order for the brain to make the content of consciousness known to the outside world, it must have control of the motor neurons of the brainstem and spinal cord, and through them the muscles they innervate. The relatively rare *locked-in syndrome* denotes the presence of consciousness in a person who has lost most of the repertoire of motor function (3).

Many terms have evolved to describe the spectrum of abnormalities of consciousness; here we will not consider thought or mood disorders, in which the content of consciousness is disturbed, or focal abnormalities of brain function (except in differential diagnosis), but rather alterations of awareness in which (a) the cerebral cortex is globally affected or (b) the midbrain RF or its rostral connections are dysfunctional. Hence, one may view them as abnormalities of arousal (either of the arousal mechanism itself or of its end-organ, the cerebral cortex). We will also concentrate on a small vocabulary of definable terms.

Coma is a state in which the patient *usually* lies motionless, eyes closed, and does not make any understandable responses either to external stimuli or internal need. Under circumstances discussed below, the patient may have certain stereotypic movements (e.g., extensor posturing) and may have rhythmic eye opening (particularly in postanoxic states), but the remainder of the definition is never violated: a patient who makes understandable responses is by definition not comatose. While coma may superficially resemble normal sleep, it neither has the neurophysiologic correlates of normal sleep nor performs sleep's restorative function. General anesthesia is an induced and controlled form of coma.

To describe states in which the patient's level of awareness lies between normal and coma, we will use the terms *stupor, obtundation,* and *delirium.* Stuporous patients lie with their eyes closed unless stimulated; they then awaken and are able to follow some commands, although they are not usually normally responsive, and return to their unresponsive state when the stimulation ceases. Obtunded patients exhibit more spontaneous movement and interaction with the environment, but appear to spend excessive amounts of time asleep. Delirious patients are at the other end of the spectrum; they are excessively active, tend to sleep little if at all, and may hallucinate, especially visually. Although the *Diagnostic and Statistical Manual of Mental Disorders, Fourth Edition (DSM-IV)* downplays the importance of increased activity and agitation in its definition of delirium (4), confining the use of the term to patients with these manifestations increases its descriptive utility.

An alternative approach is simply to describe the patient's spontaneous behavior and response to external stimuli. This has the advantage of conveying the patient's state clearly to the next examiner. Various rating scales are also used, depending on the circumstances. Alteration in consciousness as a consequence of disease is traditionally rated via the Glasgow Coma Scale (GCS) scores (Table 1) (5). For convenience, a composite score (the sum of the eye, verbal, and motor components) is often employed, but changes in the individual component scores, especially the motor score, are important as well. Scoring the verbal response in intubated patients is problematic; while some impute a score, we prefer to rate only the eye and motor score. Adaptations of the GCS for small children are available (6).

For pharmacologically sedated patients, the Ramsay scale is commonly employed to describe the degree of responsiveness (Table 2) (7).

TABLE 1. GLASGOW COMA SCALE

Item	Response	Score
Verbal response	Oriented	5
	Confused	4
	Inappropriate words	3
	Incomprehensible	2
	None	1
Eye opening	Spontaneous	4
	To speech	3
	To pain	2
	None	1
Motor	Obeys commands	6
	Localizes pain	5
	Withdraws	4
	Abnormal flexion	3
	Abnormal extension	2
	Flaccid	1

TABLE 2. RAMSAY SEDATION SCALE

Level	Patient's State
1	Awake, anxious, and agitated, or restless, or both
2	Awake, cooperative, oriented, and tranquil
3	Awake but responds to commands only
4	Appears asleep (this is not true sleep), but responds briskly to a light glabellar tap or a loud auditory stimulus
5	Appears asleep, responds only sluggishly to a light glabellar tap or a loud auditory stimulus
6	Appears asleep, no response to stimuli

ANATOMY OF CONSCIOUSNESS

Arousal requires the interplay of the reticular formation with the cerebral hemispheres. The reticular components necessary for arousal reside in the midbrain and diencephalon; the pontine reticular formation is not necessary for consciousness. The midbrain functions as a driving center for the higher structures; loss of the midbrain reticular formation produces a state in which the cortex appears to be waiting for the command, or the ability, to function. This is manifested electroencephalographically as "alpha coma," in which the resting electrical activity of the cortex appears relatively normal but cannot be altered by external or internal stimuli (8).

The mechanism of diencephalic involvement is uncertain. Information from the midbrain reticular formation passes to the thalamus, through which signals must pass in order to allow the cortex to function. Disorders that distort the normal anatomic relationships of the midbrain, diencephalon, and cortex appear to impair arousal by interrupting flow from midbrain to cortex. It appears likely that the diencephalon plays a more active role in the control of arousal than that of a simple conduit. For example, in the prion disorder known as fatal familial insomnia, dysfunction of neurons in the anterior and ventral thalamic nuclei interfere with normal sleep-wake cycling to diminish or even completely prevent sleep (9).

Although older discussions of this material have stressed the role of downward shift of the midbrain in the production of coma, our concepts of pathologic anatomy have been revised by the availability of computed tomography (CT) and magnetic resonance imaging (MRI) (Figs. 1 through 5). It is now clear that in patients with lateralized masses the horizontal displacement of the diencephalon is more closely correlated with the degree of altered awareness than the vertical displacement (10). In patients with diffuse brain swelling caudal vertical displacement of the diencephalon is important, but the actual mechanism of coma may relate more to elevated intracranial pressure, which compromises cerebral perfusion more than the actual movement. Terminally, both lateral masses and diffuse supratentorial brain swelling displace the brainstem caudally, separating it from the basilar artery (which remains fixed to the clivus).

Loss of function of both cerebral hemispheres interferes with normal arousal mechanisms. However, over days to weeks following a severe global cortical injury (e.g., hypoxia), the central nervous system appears to reestablish some degree of arousal. This is clinically apparent in the vegetative state, in which the

Standard model

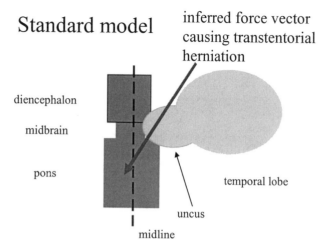

inferred force vector causing transtentorial herniation

diencephalon

midbrain

pons

temporal lobe

uncus

midline

FIGURE 1. Coronal view. The standard model of herniation inferred that coma was a consequence of downward movement of the brainstem because of force exerted by a supratentorial mass.

patient manifests sleep-wake cycling (11). This condition appears to represent arousal without awareness, and is histopathologically characterized by loss of the cortex with preservation of brainstem and diencephalic reticular structures.

EXAMINATION OF PATIENTS WITH ALTERED CONSCIOUSNESS

The examination of the patient with altered consciousness begins by ensuring that the patient's vital signs and basic biochemistry are adequate to support brain function. It should be ensured that blood pressure, respiration, and oxygen saturation are adequate, and that the patient is not hypoglycemic or thiamine-deficient, before proceeding with the examination. In many situations (e.g., emergency departments), naloxone is also administered at this

Current model

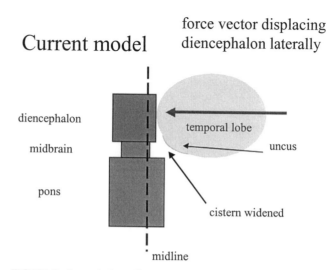

force vector displacing diencephalon laterally

diencephalon

midbrain

pons

temporal lobe

uncus

cistern widened

midline

FIGURE 3. Coronal view. The current model stresses shift of the diencephalon as the major cause of altered consciousness and signs of herniation. Note that the cistern is expected to be widened rather than obliterated (see also Fig. 5).

point to reverse the effects of opiates. The routine use of flumazenil to antagonize potential benzodiazepine intoxication is controversial because of the risk of provoking seizures or status epilepticus, especially in patients with mixed benzodiazepine and cyclic antidepressant overdoses (12).

The goals of the examination of the patient with altered consciousness are first to determine whether the patient is conscious; and then, in patients with altered awareness, to determine whether the reticular system is functional. Since altered awareness requires either reticular system dysfunction or bilateral hemispheric dysfunction, testing the structures immediately adjacent to the reticular system provides the major clues regarding the etiology of altered consciousness, and thereby determines the direction of subsequent investigations (13). The major findings on examination and their expected anatomic correlates are presented in Table 3. The types of respiratory abnormality are summarized in Table 4. Note that these correlations are with the level of

Standard model

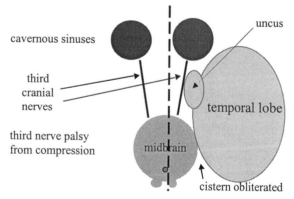

cavernous sinuses

uncus

third cranial nerves

temporal lobe

third nerve palsy from compression

midbrain

cistern obliterated

FIGURE 2. Horizontal view. In the standard model, the third nerve was thought to be compromised via direct compression by the uncus. The ipsilateral cistern would be obliterated by the medial movement of the temporal lobe. It is now apparent that this is an uncommon situation at the time physical findings (e.g., a third cranial nerve palsy) develop. In the rare cases where this does occur early, it usually reflects a lesion in the medial temporal region.

Current model

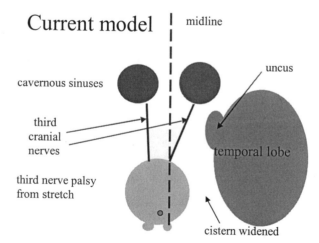

midline

uncus

cavernous sinuses

third cranial nerves

temporal lobe

third nerve palsy from stretch

cistern widened

FIGURE 4. Horizontal view. In the current model, the brainstem is pulled laterally by the diencephalon. The temporal lobe does not compress either the third nerve or the brainstem early in herniation.

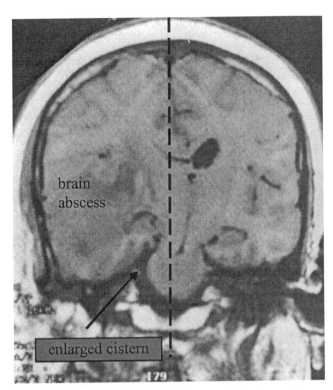

FIGURE 5. Coronal T1-weighted magnetic resonance image of a patient with a brain abscess. Note the shift of the diencephalic structures away from the midline (indicated by the *dotted line*) and the enlargement, rather than obliteration, of the ipsilateral cistern. (From Bleck TP, Greenlee JE. Approach to the patient with central nervous system infection. In: Mandell GM, Bennett JE, Dolin R, eds. *Principles and practice of infectious diseases*, 5th ed. New York: Churchill Livingstone, 2000:950–959.)

dysfunction, which may involve a substantially larger portion of the nervous system than the degree of actual *damage*.

The findings on these examinations are often summarized by use of the GCS (Table 1). This procedure is of value in indicating the severity of head injury, where a total score of 3 to 8 indicates severe trauma, 9 to 13 moderate trauma, and 14 to 15 mild trauma. However, the real purpose of the score is to provide a simple way of detecting changes in the examination over time, with good inter-rater reliability, in circumstances of global cerebral dysfunction (e.g., trauma, intoxication). The score has limited use in patients with focal neurologic dysfunction.

At all times in the examination of the patient with suspected impaired awareness, remain aware that the patient may in fact be capable of sensing and remembering. While noxious stimuli may be required for an adequate examination, the minimum necessary stimulation should be employed, and the examiner should always be cognizant of the need for explanation of procedures, especially potentially painful ones. This caveat should carry over from the first encounter with the patient throughout the course of treatment.

Attempts to communicate the level of sedation in patients are particularly problematic. For patients who are intoxicated or therapeutically sedated, the scale proposed by Ramsay and coworkers is commonly used (Table 2) (7).

The level of neurologic dysfunction is often best defined by the motor examination. If a patient responds to noxious stimuli by any defensive maneuver, such as withdrawal from the stimu-

lus, that patient is not truly comatose. Such a response may be seen in patients whose examinations otherwise suggest no cortical function, presumably because a noxious stimulus powerfully evokes an arousal response. Stereotyped posturing (spontaneous or induced) indicates that the cerebral cortices are no longer in command of the motor system. The physiologic levels of dysfunction are summarized in the motor component of the GCS.

Experiments in animals led to the concepts of *decorticate* and *decerebrate* rigidity. These terms have produced endless confusion, and these states are perhaps better called by the labels used in the GCS: decorticate rigidity is abnormal flexion, and decerebrate rigidity is abnormal extension. Physiologically, these states reflect loss of higher motor control functions, leaving either the rubrospinal system in command (in flexor posturing), or ceding control to the vestibulospinal and reticulospinal systems (in extensor posturing). These postures do not mean that the higher control centers have been destroyed, but indicate that they are not functioning. Patients with lateral mass lesions may demonstrate flexor posturing on one side of the body, and extensor posturing on the other (usually the side contralateral to the mass).

HERNIATION SYNDROMES

Herniation occurs when the brain is subjected to pressure gradients that cause portions of it to flow from one intracranial compartment to another (14). While the brain has substantial elasticity, the arteries and veins responsible for its blood supply are relatively fixed in space, producing a risk that brain shifts will cause the portions moving to lose their blood supply. In the case of lateral herniation, the hernia itself may compress or distort vessels, similarly disrupting blood flow. Herniation also appears to produce dysfunction in important white matter pathways, such as those connecting the midbrain reticular formation to the thalamus, probably via geometric distortion of the pathways themselves. Extracerebral structures, particularly the third cranial nerve, are also susceptible to distortion when the brain shifts.

These classic syndromes are well established in the clinical neurosciences; recent advances in imaging have changed some of our understanding of their pathologic anatomy, but their clinical semiology remains important.

Central

Central herniation occurs when diffuse brain swelling (e.g., after trauma) or a centrally located mass causes the diencephalon to move caudally through the tentorial notch. Dysfunction of the reticular formation and cerebral hypoperfusion due to intracranial pressure elevation are the leading hypotheses explaining alteration of consciousness in this setting. Diencephalic dysfunction initially produces small reactive pupils, due to loss of sympathetic output from the hypothalamus. At this stage, decorticate (flexor) posturing may be present spontaneously, or is often elicited by noxious stimuli. As the midbrain begins to fail, the pupils enlarge to midposition, and posturing becomes decerebrate (extensor). Attempts to elicit horizontal eye movements may reveal failure of adduction with either cervicoocular reflex (COR) or vestibuloocular reflex (VOR) testing; however, this is often only present

TABLE 3. CLINICAL FINDINGS WITH DIFFERENT LEVELS OF CENTRAL NERVOUS SYSTEM DYSFUNCTION

Dysfunction of	Response to Noxious Stimuli	Pupils	Eye Movements	Breathing
Both cortices	Withdrawal	Small, reactive	Spontaneous conjugate horizontal movements; if none, cervicoocular or vestibuloocular reflexes can be elicited	Posthyperventilation apnea or Cheyne-Stokes respiration
Thalamus	Decorticate posturing	Same as above, unless the optic tracts are also damaged	Same as above	Cheyne-Stokes respiration
Midbrain	Decorticate or decerebrate posturing	Midposition, fixed to light	Loss of ability to adduct	Usually same as above; potential for central reflex hyperpnea
Pons	Decerebrate posturing	Usually small; may exhibit bilateral pinpoint pupils (especially with midline pontine hemorrhage); Horner syndrome with lateral lesions	Loss of conjugate horizontal movements with retained vertical movements and accommodation	May exhibit central reflex hyperpnea, cluster (Biot) breathing, or apneustic breathing
Medulla	Weak leg flexion (or none)	Usually small; Horner syndrome with lateral lesions	Usually no effect on spontaneous eye movements; may interfere with reflex responses; rarely, nystagmus	Rarely, ataxic respiration; apnea if respiratory centers involved

Adapted from Bleck TP. Levels of consciousness and attention. In: Goetz CG, Pappert EJ, eds. *Textbook of clinical neurology.* Philadelphia: WB Saunders, 1998: 2–29.

briefly. Eventually, if the patient is breathing spontaneously, tidal volume decreases and the respiratory rhythm becomes irregular.

The initial cardiovascular response to diminished brainstem perfusion, regardless of etiology, is hypertension. Bradycardia, which in this setting is a reflex response to systemic hypertension, is commonly seen in children but less commonly in adults. There may be a tendency for bradycardia to occur more commonly in patients with posterior fossa masses, but this observation is confounded by the higher incidence of posterior fossa tumors in children. Respiratory disturbances, the third component of "Cushing triad," reflect the anatomic considerations discussed above and are not part of the same reflex system as the cardiovascular responses. In some clinical settings, such as head injury with diffuse brain swelling, spontaneous hyperventilation is commonly noted but its etiology remains obscure.

Lateral Mass Herniation (Uncal or Hippocampal Herniation)

As discussed above, concepts of herniation due to an expanding lateral cerebral mass have changed in the past decade. This has not led to new observations about the sequence in which physical findings develop. The initial signs are usually those related to the mass itself (e.g., contralateral hemiparesis); as the diencephalon begins to shift away from the mass, consciousness begins to diminish, and an ipsilateral third cranial nerve palsy develops in about 85% of patients. The remaining patients develop either simultaneous bilateral third nerve palsies, or on occasion an isolated nerve palsy. These findings presumably follow from the distortion of third nerve anatomy described above, although the bilateral disturbance may also relate to midbrain ischemia

as the brainstem begins to move away from the basilar artery. Imaging studies (CT or MRI) performed early in this process do not show transtentorial movement of the temporal lobe; this occurs later in the process, accounting for its implication as the cause of third nerve dysfunction in autopsy studies. Early in this process, the most common finding on imaging studies is an *enlargement* of the perimesencephalic cistern ipsilateral to the mass.

As lateral displacement of the midbrain continues, the contralateral corticospinal tract (in the cerebral peduncle) is compressed against the edge of the tentorium. This produces an *ipsilateral* hemiplegia, called the *Kernohan notch* phenomenon. If the herniation process continues, the diencephalon and the ipsilateral temporal lobe may actually herniate downward through the tentorial notch. Since the uncus (containing the amygdala) and the hippocampus are the most medial portions of the temporal lobe, they are the first structures to cross the tentorial edge; this accounts for the older terms of *uncal* or *hippocampal* herniation. Movement of the more posterior aspects of the medial temporal lobe may compress the posterior cerebral artery (or arteries), producing ischemia in the medial temporal lobe and sometimes in the occipital lobe(s).

Bilateral third nerve dysfunction usually implies rotation of the midbrain (15).

Subfalcine

Herniation of the medial frontal structures (e.g., the cingulate gyrus) beneath the falx is commonly observed in patients with frontal lobe masses. Most of these patients present with signs related either to the mass itself, or to the global increase in

TABLE 4. CENTRAL RESPIRATORY ABNORMALITIES

Pattern	Description	Localization	Comments
Posthyperventilation apnea	Apnea for more than 10 sec after five deep breaths	Bilateral hemispheric dysfunction	Normally, the cerebral cortex triggers another breath within 10 sec regardless of the $PaCO_2$
Cheyne-Stokes respiration	Rhythmic waxing and waning of respiratory amplitude	Bilateral hemispheric dysfunction	1. Periods of "apnea" are actually times when the respiratory amplitude is too low to measure, but the respiratory rhythm is unchanged 2. Congestive heart failure prolongs the reflex arc (blood leaving the lungs takes longer to reach the brainstem than is normal) and may produce this finding without any neurologic dysfunction
Central reflex hyperpnea (CRH) (formerly called central neurogenic hyperventilation)		Bilateral hemispheric (e.g., trauma), lower midbrain, upper pons, possibly medulla	When present in patients with brainstem lesions or subarachnoid hemorrhage, CRH is most commonly due to the hypoxia that accompanies neurogenic pulmonary edema. True central neurogenic hyperventilation is rare.
Apneustic respiration	Prolonged inspiratory time ("inspiratory cramp")	Pons	Does not support adequate ventilation (true for all following patterns as well). Isolated lesions at these levels do not produce coma.
Cluster (Biot) breathing	Clusters of breaths punctuated by apnea	Lower pons	
Ataxic respiration	infrequent, irregular breaths	Lower pons or upper medulla	
"Ondine's curse"	Failure of involuntary respiration with retained voluntary respiration	Medulla	
Apnea	No respiration	Medulla down to C4; peripheral nerve (e.g., acute inflammatory polyneuropathy), neuromuscular junction (e.g., myasthenia gravis), muscle	

Adapted from Bleck TP. Levels of consciousness and attention. In: Goetz CG, Pappert EJ, eds. *Textbook of clinical neurology.* Philadelphia: WB Saunders, 1998: 2–29.

intracranial pressure that accompanies it. Rarely, this subfalcine herniation causes ischemia in the distribution of the anterior cerebral arteries.

Cerebellar Tonsillar

Posterior fossa masses produce most of their findings by compression of the brainstem and cranial nerves, and by obstructive hydrocephalus. As the pressure gradient across the foramen magnum increases, however, the cerebellar tonsils may be pushed into, and eventually through, the foramen. This compresses the medulla, and may produce apnea by inducing dysfunction in the medullary respiratory centers. Before losing consciousness, patients with cerebellar tonsillar herniation may complain of a stiff neck.

Upward Transtentorial

Expanding posterior fossa masses usually herniate caudally because the obstructive hydrocephalus they produce prevents a pressure gradient across the tentorial opening. If these patients undergo ventriculostomy for relief of hydrocephalus, however, the

possibility of upward herniation of posterior fossa contents into the diencephalic region exists. Many neurosurgeons will prepare a patient for an emergent posterior fossa decompression just before performing the ventriculostomy in such cases.

PERSISTENT VEGETATIVE STATE

Following a severe brain insult, usually traumatic or anoxic, the comatose patient with a relatively intact brainstem usually begins to show the signs of the vegetative state discussed above. The prognosis for further recovery, to at least the level of ability to understand and follow commands, varies with the mechanism of injury and with the age of the patient. In general, patients who remain in a vegetative state 3 months after an anoxic injury are expected to persist in that state indefinitely. Patients in a vegetative state at the time of hospital discharge after head trauma have an almost 50% likelihood of further recovery over the next 12 months, and a small number will regain consciousness between 12 and 36 months. However, the prognosis for functional recovery (e.g., returning to work or to school) is worse. About one-third of trauma patients under the age of 30 who awaken after a prolonged vegetative state meet this criterion for functional recovery; only a few percent of those older than 30 do so.

DEATH BY BRAIN CRITERIA

The ability to successfully transplant organs led to the need for criteria for "brain death." In recent years, this state is more commonly referred to as "death by brain criteria," to underscore the recognition that this form of death should not be considered any less permanent than death by cardiorespiratory criteria. Many now argue that our current definitions are too restrictive, and that patients who can be defined as having no chance of regaining consciousness should be considered as potential organ donors. If this change is to occur, a substantial shift in societal thinking about life and death may need to precede it. In North America, death by brain criteria is still considered to be irreversible loss of brain (including brainstem) function. The single exception to this appears to be in the area of osmolar control; diabetes insipidus is not required for this diagnosis (16).

Currently, most jurisdictions recognize the existence of death by brain criteria, but its precise definition varies with local practice. In general, the first stage in pronouncing death by brain criteria is a *permissive diagnosis*; that is, there must be a diagnosis adequate to explain death of the brain, including the brainstem. This need not be an etiologic diagnosis; for example, a massive intracerebral hemorrhage qualifies as a permissive diagnosis, even if the etiology of the hemorrhage is unknown. This requirement helps to exclude cases of hypnosedative overdose, in which the patient may appear dead but still recover. This does not require demonstration of an anatomic lesion; a history of prolonged anoxia would suffice. One then proceeds to demonstrate that there is no detectable function above the level of the foramen magnum. Any sign of brainstem-mediated function, such as decerebrate posturing, eye movements, pupillary response to light, or coughing, negates the possibility of the diagnosis of death by brain criteria at that time. Brainstem testing includes apnea testing.

Apnea testing involves observing the brainstem response to hypercapnia without producing hypoxemia. In order to prevent hypoxemia, a period (e.g., 20 minutes) of ventilation with 100% oxygen is required before starting the test. Although acidosis, rather than hypercapnia, is the real afferent trigger for ventilation, a $PaCO_2$ of 60 torr (50 torr in the United Kingdom) is usually the endpoint for this test. In order to reach this endpoint before hypoxemia supervenes, it is advisable to regulate ventilation during the period of preapneic oxygenation so that the $PaCO_2$ reaches 40 to 45 torr before apnea begins. This period should also be used to ensure that the patient's core temperature is adequate (e.g., above 32°C), and that the results of assays for hypnosedative agents, if indicated, show that intoxication is not the cause of the patient's apparent lack of reflex responses.

Even though the patient has been adequately preoxygenated, some method of supplemental oxygen delivery is still necessary. This may be accomplished either by placing a suction catheter near the carina with a 10 L per minute oxygen flow, or by using a continuous positive airway pressure (CPAP) circuit with 10 cm H_2O pressure. A CPAP circuit does not provide ventilation, so it does not interfere with observation for spontaneous respirations.

Even with one of these methods employed, some patients with cardiorespiratory dysfunction may not tolerate the approximately 10 minutes of apnea necessary to raise the $PaCO_2$ to 60 torr without becoming hypoxemic and hypotensive. In this circumstance, a confirmatory test may be necessary.

Apnea is then allowed under observation until the $PaCO_2$ reaches 60 torr by arterial blood gas analysis. While it may be possible to predict this point by following the trend in end-tidal CO_2 ($PetCO_2$) measurements, there is enough discrepancy between arterial blood $PaCO_2$ and $PetCO_2$ to indicate use of the arterial measurement. Visual observation is the standard method for detecting respiratory movement; this may be supplemented by airway pressure monitoring. Any respiratory movement negates the diagnosis of apnea. However, if the patient remains apneic despite a $PaCO_2$ of 60 torr, the diagnosis of apnea is confirmed, and the patient, having met the other conditions cited as prerequisites, is declared dead by brain criteria.

If the patient is unable to tolerate the apnea test, or if some portion of the examination cannot be performed (e.g., trauma has rendered the face too swollen to examine the eyes), then a confirmatory test is necessary if the patient is to be diagnosed as dead. This is usually indicated only for potential organ donors, since there is no requirement that death be diagnosed in order to withdraw supportive measures, but may at times be helpful for the patient's family. Tests of cerebral perfusion (e.g., radionuclide angiography or conventional contrast angiography) are usually used to show that blood does not flow intracranially above the foramen magnum. Some clinicians consider transcranial Doppler blood flow velocity measurements adequate for this purpose. Electrophysiologic studies, such as electroencephalography (EEG), have been used for this purpose, but are prone to both false-positive (e.g., artifacts that cannot be distinguished from cerebral activity with certainty) and false-negative (due to hypothermia or hypnosedative drug intoxication) results.

PSYCHOGENIC UNRESPONSIVENESS

This category includes patients who have a diagnosable psychiatric condition such as catatonia or conversion disorder, and those who are malingering. The differential diagnosis of these conditions is beyond the scope of this chapter, but a few diagnostic points are important in order to raise the physician's suspicion of a psychogenic disorder. These conditions share two characteristics not seen in patients with neurologic reasons for coma: first, they have the COR and VOR responses characteristic of awake patients, and second, their EEGs are not indicative of coma.

EVALUATION GUIDELINES

The use of neurodiagnostic studies in patients with altered consciousness with specific syndromes is outlined in Table 5.

Neuroimaging studies should be selected based upon the history and the initial examination. If a structural lesion is suspected, an emergent CT scan should be obtained to guide therapy. Patients with bilateral hemispheric dysfunction do not usually benefit from emergent CT scanning. While MRI is almost always

TABLE 5. TESTS THAT HELP TO INTEGRATE CLINICAL SYNDROMES WITH VARIOUS ETIOLOGIES OF ALTERED LEVEL OF CONSCIOUSNESS

Location of Dysfunction	Neuroimaging	Electrophysiology	Fluid and Tissue Analysis
Bilateral cortical dysfunction: confusion and delirium	Usually normal; may show atrophy; rarely bilateral chronic subdural hematomata or evidence of herpes simplex encephalitis; dural enhancement in meningitis, especially neoplastic meningitides	Diffuse slowing; often, frontally predominant intermittent rhythmic delta activity (FIRDA); in herpes simplex encephalitis, periodic lateralized epileptiform activity (PLEDS)	Blood or urine analyses may reveal etiology; CSF may show evidence of infection or neoplastic cells
Diencephalic dysfunction	Lesion(s) in or displacement of diencephalon; also displays mass displacing the diencephalon	Usually diffuse slowing; rarely FIRDA; in displacement syndromes, effect of the mass producing displacement (e.g., focal delta activity, loss of faster rhythms)	Usually not helpful
Midbrain dysfunction	Lesion(s) in the midbrain or displacing it	Usually diffuse slowing; "alpha coma"; evoked response testing may demonstrate failure of conduction above the lesion	Rarely platelet or coagulation abnormalities
Pontine dysfunction	Lesion(s) producing syndrome; thrombosis of basilar artery	EEG usually normal; evoked responses usually normal	Rarely platelet or coagulation abnormalities
Medullary dysfunction	Lesion(s) producing dysfunction	EEG normal; brainstem auditory and somatosensory evoked responses may show conduction abnormalities	Rarely platelet or coagulation abnormalities
Herniation syndromes	Lesion(s) producing herniation; appearance of perimesencephalic cistern	Findings related to etiology	Findings related to etiology
Locked-in syndrome	Infarction of basis pontis	EEG and evoked potential studies normal	Findings related to etiology
Death by brain criteria	Absence of intracranial blood flow above the foramen magnum	EEG shows electrocerebral silence; evoked potential studies may show peripheral components (e.g., wave I of brainstem auditory evoked response) but no central conduction	Absence of hypnosedative drugs
Psychogenic unresponsiveness	Normal	Normal	Normal

CSF, cerebrospinal fluid; EEG, electroencephalogram.

superior in quality to CT, the pulse sequences currently employed may not detect all cases of acute intracranial bleeding. CT scanning is usually faster and more readily available in emergent circumstances.

An EEG is indicated in most patients with altered consciousness at some point in their evaluation. This is usually after a structural lesion has been excluded because the history and examination are inadequate to detect many cases of nonconvulsive status epilepticus. Patients, in whom supratentorial structural lesions are present but are not adequate to explain the patient's state based on their location and size, should also have an EEG performed.

Some EEG findings in patients with encephalopathy are characteristic; for example, frontally predominant rhythmic delta activity (FIRDA) and triphasic waves are common in metabolic disorders (17). An "alpha coma" pattern indicates either a midbrain lesion, anoxia, or hypnosedative drug overdose. In the latter setting, the patient has a good prognosis for recovery. An unexpectedly normal EEG, with alpha blocking on passive eye opening and normal sleep-wake cycling, should alert the physician to the likelihood of psychogenic unresponsiveness.

The EEG may also provide clues to otherwise unexpected diagnoses, such as subacute spongiform encephalopathy, which may come to medical attention in the guise of an acute encephalopathy.

Evoked response studies are of limited value in these patients. Although abnormalities may be present, as outlined in Table 5, these studies seldom contribute diagnostically or therapeutically useful data in this population.

Cerebrospinal fluid analysis is crucial in some conditions altering consciousness (e.g., suspected meningitis) and irrelevant in others. The decision to perform a lumbar puncture is thus based on the entire clinical picture. If bacterial meningitis is suspected, and the physician feels that an imaging study should precede the lumbar puncture in this patient, then appropriate antibiotic therapy should be started before the patient is sent for the imaging study. Pneumococcal and meningococcal meningitides may be so rapidly fatal that even a brief delay in instituting antibiotic treatment should not occur.

Although the concept of "routine" tests has fallen from favor in laboratory medicine circles due to pressure from third-party payors, the patient with unexplained bilateral hemispheric dysfunction should indeed have a battery of screening tests to allow the physician to rapidly detect treatable etiologies. At a minimum, these should include a complete blood count with differential, platelet estimate or count, prothrombin time, partial thromboplastin time, serum osmolality, and serum and urinary screening for drugs of abuse.

If oral drug ingestion is considered a possibility, gastric aspiration for analysis of the contents and removal of remaining unabsorbed drug is indicated. If the patient's airway protective reflexes are compromised, endotracheal intubation should first be performed. Induction of vomiting is no longer recommended in the emergency department since it may interfere with the use of activated charcoal to bind drugs. This substance may be used routinely unless acetaminophen ingestion is suspected, since it will interfere with the absorption of acetylcysteine as well.

SUMMARY

Since patients with alterations in consciousness are encountered regularly in the intensive care unit, intensivists must be prepared to provide rapid supportive care and acute intervention prior to interaction with neurologic, neuroradiologic, and neurosurgical consultants. When patients with an altered state progress to coma, it may be gradual or precipitous. A familiarity with the anatomy, physiology, and neurochemistry of consciousness aids the intensivist in rapidly assessing patients, initiating empiric therapy to arrest or reverse it, and applying various diagnostic modalities to establish the diagnosis and monitor therapy.

KEY POINTS

Progressive alteration in level of consciousness develops gradually or abruptly in critically ill patients. This deterioration may result in coma, defined as a state in which the patient lies motionless with eyes closed, not making an understandable response either to external stimuli or internal need. The intensivist must rapidly determine the severity, likely cause, and course of diminishing level of consciousness; initiate appropriate intervention to limit sequelae; obtain neurologic/neurosurgical guidance as warranted; and eliminate ongoing central nervous system insults.

Evaluation of the comatose patient requires immediate review of the history; performance of a focused physical examination to identify external trauma, hypothermia, fever, cerebral hypoperfusion secondary to abnormal cardiac rate, rhythm, or blood pressure (significant hypotension or hypertensive crisis), adequacy and pattern of ventilation; and measurement of the Glasgow Coma Scale to determine the best motor, verbal, and eye response combined with identification of focal neurologic findings. Complete blood count with differential, coagulation parameters, serum electrolytes and osmolarity, and blood glucose should be obtained emergently. Glucose and thiamine should be empirically administered. Antidotes such as flumazenil and naloxone should be administered judiciously in patients where there is a high suspicion of narcotic or benzodiazepine excess. Brain imaging, encephalographic assessment, and cerebral spinal fluid analysis should be acquired as warranted on a case-by-case basis.

REFERENCES

1. Plum F, Posner JB. *The diagnosis of stupor and coma*, ed 3. Philadelphia: FA Davis, 1980.
2. Moruzzi G, Magoun HW. Brain stem reticular formation and activation of the EEG. *Electroencephalog Clin Neurophysiol* 1949;1:455–473.
3. Hawkes CH. "Locked-in" syndrome: report of seven cases. *Br Med J* 1974;4:379–382.
4. American Psychiatric Association. *Diagnostic and statistical manual of mental disorders*, ed 4. Washington DC: American Psychiatric Association, 1994:124.
5. Teasdale G, Jennett B. Assessment of coma and impaired consciousness. A practical scale. *Lancet* 1974;2(872):81–84.
6. Durham SR, Clancy RR, Leuthardt E, et al. CHOP Infant Coma Scale ("Infant Face Scale"): a novel coma scale for children less than two years of age. *J Neurotrauma* 2000;17:729–737.
7. Ramsay MA, Savege TM, Simpson BR, et al. Controlled sedation with alphaxalone-alphadolone. *Br Med J* 1974;2(920):656–659.
8. Young GB. The EEG in coma. *J Clin Neurophysiol* 2000;17:473–485.
9. Wanschitz J, Kloppel S, Jarius C, et al. Alteration of the serotonergic nervous system in fatal familial insomnia. *Ann Neurol* 2000;48:788–791.
10. Ropper AH. A preliminary MRI study of the geometry of brain displacement and level of consciousness with acute intracranial masses. *Neurology* 1989;39:622–627.
11. Bleck TP. Vegetative state after closed-head injury. *Neurol Chron* 1992;1:10–11.
12. Gueye PN, Hoffman JR, Taboulet P, et al. Empiric use of flumazenil in comatose patients: limited applicability of criteria to define low risk. *Ann Emerg Med* 1996;27:730–735.
13. Bleck TP. Levels of consciousness and attention. In: Goetz CG, Pappert EJ, eds. *Textbook of clinical neurology*. Philadelphia: WB Saunders, 1998:2–29.
14. Bleck TP, Webb AR. The unconscious patient—causes and diagnosis. In: Webb AR, Shapiro MJ, Singer M, et al., eds. *The Oxford textbook of critical care*. Oxford: Oxford University Press, 1999:440–444.
15. Ropper AH. The opposite pupil in herniation. *Neurology* 1990; 40:1707–1709.
16. Wijdicks EF. The diagnosis of brain death. *N Engl J Med* 2001;344: 1215–1221.
17. Bleck TP. Metabolic encephalopathy. In: Weiner WJ, Shulman LM, eds. *Emergent and urgent neurology*, 2nd ed. Philadelphia: JB Lippincott Co, 1999:223–253.

POSTOPERATIVE CARE OF THE NEUROSURGICAL PATIENT

PATRICIA H. PETROZZA

KEY WORDS

- Carotid endarterectomy
- Craniotomy
- Intracranial pressure
- Intracranial aneurysm
- Vasospasm
- Arteriovenous malformation
- Decreased level of consciousness
- Cerebral ischemia
- Stroke
- Acute intracranial hypertension
- Acute intracranial hemorrhage

INTRODUCTION

Care of the neurosurgical patient can be especially challenging in the postoperative period. Good patient outcome often depends on prompt recognition and treatment of both frequent and infrequent complications. This chapter will focus on multiple complex conditions.

CAROTID ENDARTERECTOMY

After carotid endarterectomy, the overall incidence of serious postoperative complications is low, and the cost-effectiveness of direct intensive care unit (ICU) admission has been questioned. Some authors recommend a 2- to 4-hour period in the postanesthesia care unit (PACU) to identify those patients who will require additional intensive care (1). Careful monitoring is necessary to detect the occurrence of new neurologic deficits and to manage hemorrhage, hypertension, hypotension, and the hyperperfusion syndrome.

New neurologic deficits most often result from occlusion of the operated carotid artery or perioperative embolic events. Recognition of a new deficit should prompt immediate diagnostic evaluation. In the case of an arterial thrombus, Doppler ultrasound may demonstrate cessation of flow; angiography will confirm vascular occlusion. If carotid occlusion is diagnosed, reexploration may be necessary, occasionally without diagnostic confirmation. A computed tomography (CT) scan to rule out the presence of an intracranial hemorrhage is helpful if directed thrombolytic therapy distal to the carotid occlusion is an option.

Cranial nerve injuries during dissection are common, and subtle difficulties with phonation and swallowing may cause insidious patient morbidity. Loss of carotid body function in patients who have undergone bilateral carotid endarterectomy prevents circulatory or respiratory responses to hypoxia.

While soft tissue edema near the operative site is very common (2), hemorrhage after carotid endarterectomy may represent a challenge both to surgeons and intensivists. If hemorrhage is sufficiently severe to produce a large cervical hematoma, subsequent intubation may be difficult. Anticipation of a difficult intubation may necessitate the maintenance of spontaneous ventilation until the larynx can be visualized and the airway secured.

Since the most common cause of perioperative mortality in carotid endarterectomy patients is myocardial infarction, perioperative β-adrenergic blockade in high-risk patients may be appropriate. Hypertension and hypotension both occur frequently after carotid endarterectomy. Hypertension appears to be more common after general anesthesia, while hypotension is more common after regional anesthesia (3). The requirement for intravenous medication to control postoperative hypertension is often cited as the most compelling factor in instances of postoperative ICU admission (4). The etiology of blood pressure abnormalities is unclear, with hypertension attributed to circulating catecholamines and hypotension attributed to an abrupt increase in the perfusion pressure of the carotid sinus. Management of hypertension usually consists of administration of short-acting agents, such as sodium nitroprusside (SNP) or intravenous nitroglycerin; hypertension typically resolves within a few days except in patients who had uncontrolled hypertension preoperatively. Management of hypotension can be accomplished with volume administration or the infusion of phenylephrine. The use of an α-agonist is appropriate because the incidence of coronary artery disease is very high in patients with carotid artery lesions and β-agonists may increase myocardial oxygen demands. When hypotension is refractory, concern about a perioperative myocardial infarction is warranted.

The cerebral hyperperfusion syndrome is more likely in a patient with a preexisting cerebral infarct and is associated with postoperative hypertension, neurologic deficits, and increased cerebral blood flow (CBF) (5). The pathogenesis appears to be sudden restoration of perfusion pressure in a vascular bed that has been chronically perfused at low pressure. Preoperative transcranial Doppler (TCD) ultrasonography may identify patients at risk for this complication (5). Symptoms and signs include headache and occasional seizures typically arising 6 to 24 hours following the endarterectomy. Management consists of control of hypertension and treatment of associated complications such as seizures or intracerebral hemorrhage.

CRANIOTOMY

A craniotomy is performed for tumor resection, hematoma drainage, aneurysm clipping, or other intracranial procedures. Multiple challenges that can arise during postoperative intensive care are related to hemodynamic control, ventilatory support, hematoma detection and treatment, pain management, and fluid therapy.

After resection of a supratentorial tumor, most patients who follow commands can be safely extubated in the operating room. However, patients who preoperatively had compromised airway protection should remain intubated postoperatively. After posterior fossa surgery and skull base tumor resections, cranial nerve defects are common; therefore it is important to assess ability to handle secretions, as insidious aspiration is a common cause of postoperative morbidity (6). Elective tracheostomy and gastrostomy should be considered if deficits persist.

Postoperatively, most patients are positioned in a semirecumbent position with the head elevated 30 degrees to maximize cerebral venous drainage. Patients who should be maintained in the supine rather than the head-up position include those who have undergone drainage of a chronic subdural hematoma or repair of a cerebrospinal fluid leak. After transsphenoidal surgery, patients have extensive nasal packing and must breathe through their mouths. Significant elevation of the head and humidification of inspired gases improves postoperative comfort.

Ventilation should be assessed often in the immediate postoperative interval. Impaired swallowing ability may be related to residual neuromuscular blockade and not to cranial nerve dysfunction. A high percentage of patients newly admitted to the PACU demonstrate residual neuromuscular blockade (7). In addition to ventilatory mechanics, attention should be paid to ventilatory rhythm. Unusual or irregular breathing patterns such as Cheyne-Stokes respiration may signal brainstem compression by edema or hematoma.

In individual patients, the need to maintain communication and repeatedly assess level of consciousness must be weighed against the need to relieve discomfort from pain or nausea. The severity of pain following craniotomy has traditionally been underestimated. Carefully titrated doses of morphine (1 mg i.v.) can be administered without causing excessive sedation.

Postoperative nausea and vomiting in neurosurgical patients should be alleviated promptly, as these conditions may increase blood pressure and intracranial pressure (ICP). Refractory nausea should prompt consideration of the development of acute hydrocephalus or increased ICP secondary to brain edema or hematoma. Droperidol 0.625 to 2.5 mg i.v. and promethazine 12.5 to 25 mg i.v. or i.m., both commonly employed to treat nausea and vomiting, are dopamine antagonists and may

cause dystonic reactions or exacerbations of Parkinson disease. Ondansetron, administered 4 mg i.v., a selective blocking agent of the 5-HT$_3$ receptor type, is an effective, if expensive, antiemetic.

After craniotomy, patients may be relatively hypovolemic secondary to intraoperative diuresis or acute blood loss. As a first-line guide to the adequacy of blood volume, urinary output should be maintained at 0.5 mL per kg per hour through infusions of isotonic, nonglucose-containing solutions. Electrolytes should be measured early in the postoperative period to monitor changes in serum sodium and potassium, particularly if both mannitol and furosemide have been administered. If a suprasellar mass has been resected or the patient has suffered severe head injury, polyuria may signal the onset of diabetes insipidus; hyperglycemia or profound hypothermia are part of the differential diagnosis of polyuria. Urinary output often exceeds 200 to 400 mL per hour in diabetes insipidus and specific gravity is less than 1.005. Because mild hypothermia may protect the brain from ischemic injury, neurosurgical patients may be permitted to become somewhat hypothermic in the operating room and may arrive in the ICU in that state. Mild hypothermia, which can prolong emergence from anesthesia and increase oxygen consumption, can be corrected with warming lights, a circulating warm air mattress, and warmed fluids.

Prevention of seizures in the postoperative period is critical. Seizures may precipitate serious complications, including secondary intracranial bleeding, hypoxia, and aspiration. If seizures occur despite perioperative administration of anticonvulsants, control should be obtained with small doses of benzodiazepines while assuring an adequate airway. A recurrent intracranial mass should be suspected if a patient is not arousable within a short interval after termination of a seizure; cranial computed tomography (CT) is then indicated. Protracted complex partial seizures may cause a confusing and fluctuating level of consciousness from wakefulness to coma. An electroencephalographic investigation provides the diagnosis.

In neurosurgical patients, hypertension in the perioperative and postoperative period may be a sign of an evolving intracranial hematoma. Other causes of postoperative hypertension, including hypercarbia, pain, shivering, and bladder distention, also should be investigated. If there is no apparent primary cause of hypertension, aggressive efforts at control are warranted because of the risk that hypertension will precipitate intracranial hemorrhage or worsen cerebral edema. After supratentorial craniotomy for tumor, appropriate initial treatment consists of the administration of labetalol (5 to 10 mg increments i.v.) or small doses of esmolol. If hypertension persists and intracranial hypertension is unlikely, hydralazine administered at 10 to 20 mg i.v., nifedipine given at 10 to 20 mg sublingually, or, in rare cases, a continuous infusion of SNP may be required.

While a variety of focal neurologic deficits may be present, a depressed level of consciousness was the most consistent clinical presentation of postoperative intracranial hematomas (8), 35% of which presented within 12 hours of surgery. Coagulopathy and hypertension are precipitating factors for hematomas after brain tumor surgery. In a survey of approximately 5,000 intracranial procedures, most postoperative hematomas occurred in the operative site while 17% occurred at remote sites (8). In some patients who have suffered traumatic brain injury, ICP fails to rise despite clinical deterioration, and detection of a postcranial hematoma may be delayed if the clinical examination is discounted (9).

Even in the absence of intracranial hematomas, ICP commonly increases after elective intracranial surgery due to brain edema, with maximal pressure readings recorded approximately 16 hours postoperatively (10). Risk factors for postoperative intracranial hypertension include glioblastoma resection, repeat surgery, and protracted surgery (greater than 6 hours). ICP monitoring performed in the supratentorial compartment may not accurately reflect pressures in the infratentorial compartment. During the first 12 hours postoperatively, monitored posterior fossa pressure was 50% greater than that of the supratentorial space (11). Following resection of a tumor at the cervical medullary junction, edema can cause upward transtentorial herniation, characterized by an abrupt decrease in the level of consciousness and impaired ventilation.

In addition to the possibility of cerebral edema or a postoperative hematoma, a change in a patient's level of alertness may signal the development of hyponatremia, alcohol withdrawal syndrome, hypoxia, sepsis, or the side-effects of high-dose corticosteroid administration. The development of obstructive hydrocephalus is a consideration following cranial base surgery.

Aggressive intraoperative cerebrospinal fluid drainage or diuretic administration can create a space between the dura and cranial vault as the cranial contents retract. CT scans reveal persistent intracranial air collections in the majority of patients 7 days following a craniotomy (12). A tension pneumocephalus may result, particularly if nitrous oxide has been part of anesthetic management. In the ICU, focal neurologic signs or a generalized decrease in alertness may signal the presence of a symptomatic tension pneumocephalus. Prompt placement of a burr hole to release trapped gases often results in an improved level of consciousness.

Peripheral nerve injuries related to surgical positioning may be initially recognized in the ICU. Sciatic nerve injury and brachial plexus injury have been attributed to intraoperative positioning. Corneal abrasions, either related to intraoperative damage to the fifth cranial nerve or to positioning, should be promptly suspected in patients who complain of eye pain.

Craniotomy patients remain particularly susceptible to complications such as deep venous thrombosis and pulmonary embolus. Pneumatic compression stockings reduce the incidence of these complications. Therapy for a pulmonary embolus is controversial because thrombolytic therapy is relatively contraindicated after craniotomy and many neurosurgeons prefer to wait 10 to 14 days following surgery before initiating systemic heparinization.

CEREBRAL VASCULAR LESIONS

Aneurysm

Increasingly, patients with subarachnoid hemorrhage (SAH) secondary to a ruptured cerebral aneurysm undergo surgery or interventional neuroradiologic management to isolate the aneurysm shortly after admission to the hospital (13). So-called "early surgery," which contrasts with the more traditional approach of waiting until the risk of posthemorrhage vasospasm has decreased, permits more aggressive treatment of delayed cerebral ischemia secondary to cerebral vasospasm.

TABLE 1. GRADES OF SUBARACHNOID HEMORRHAGE[a]

Grade	Description
0	Unruptured aneurysm
I	Asymptomatic, or minimal headache and slight nuchal rigidity
II	Moderate to severe headache, nuchal rigidity, no neurologic deficit other than cranial nerve palsy
III	Drowsiness, confusion, or mild focal deficit
IV	Stupor, moderate to severe hemiparesis, possibly early decerebrate rigidity and vegetative disturbances
V	Deep coma, decerebrate rigidity, moribund appearance

[a]Serious systemic disease such as hypertension, diabetes, severe arteriosclerosis, chronic pulmonary disease, and severe vasospasm seen on arteriography result in placement of the patient in the next less favorable category. Modified from Hunt WE, Hess RM. Surgical risk as related to time of intervention in the repair of intracranial aneurysms. *J Neurosurg* 1968;28:14–20, with permission.

After uncomplicated aneurysm clipping or endovascular occlusion, patients will most likely be extubated promptly if the preoperative neurologic grade was favorable (Hunt-Hess grades I through III) (Table 1). Intraoperative aneurysm rupture, acute hydrocephalus, brain swelling, significant hypothermia, administration of large doses of barbiturates, or hemodynamic instability may prompt a decision to delay extubation for a short interval postoperatively. In the ICU, problems that may require attention include management of cardiac output and blood pressure, rewarming from moderate hypothermia, identification and control of electrolyte abnormalities, treatment of hypovolemia, prophylaxis against seizures, identification of postoperative deficits related to surgical manipulation, recognition, and evacuation of postoperative intracranial hematomas.

Hemodynamic management of patients who have suffered SAH has generated considerable controversy. Before aneurysm obliteration, hypertension potentially can precipitate rebleeding, although hypervolemic, normotensive hemodilution may reduce cerebral ischemic symptoms. Once an aneurysm has been clipped, many surgeons add moderate hypertension to hypervolemic hemodilution in patients who have symptomatic vasospasm. Prophylactic hypervolemic hemodilution, with or without hypertension, may be used in asymptomatic patients. Most clinicians monitor either central venous pressure (CVP) or use a pulmonary arterial catheter to monitor cardiac output and pulmonary artery occlusion pressure (PAOP) in hemodiluted patients. While results in some series are encouraging, randomized prospective studies evaluating prophylactic hypervolemic therapy are lacking. Indeed, in patients with myocardial dysfunction, rapid expansion of volume may be detrimental, causing pulmonary edema and congestive heart failure. It has recently been recognized that more than one-half of patients who suffer aneurysm rupture also develop systemic complications that may adversely affect outcome (14). A high index of suspicion should be maintained for the development of thromboembolic events, fever, and pneumonia in particular.

Although SAH is associated with electrocardiographic changes suggestive of myocardial ischemia, those abnormalities do not accurately predict myocardial function as assessed by echocardiography (15). Myocardial dysfunction is more closely correlated with neurologic condition. Echocardiographic abnormalities can be induced in animals in experimental models of acute SAH. In previously healthy individuals after SAH, CVP correlates poorly with PAOP and cardiac performance. A PAOP of 14 mm Hg was associated with maximum cardiac performance without the use of inotropes in one clinical series (16).

Disturbances of cerebrospinal fluid circulation occur in most patients after SAH. While intracranial hypertension is related to the amount of intraventricular blood shown on CT scan, patients should be observed carefully in the ICU for decreases in level of consciousness. If an intraventricular drain is present, modest drainage of cerebrospinal fluid (CSF) may restore ICP to normal levels. Subacute hydrocephalus may be present on CT images performed in the first week following SAH, but often remains asymptomatic.

A syndrome of salt-wasting after SAH has been described. Hypovolemia, which may accompany relative hyponatremia in this group of patients, is often associated with the development of cerebral ischemia. Marked increases in atrial natriuretic peptide precede natriuresis while elevations of serum antidiuretic hormone levels are also reported (17).

After craniotomy for aneurysm clipping, patients must be observed for the development of seizures. Preoperative hypertension is a risk factor for epilepsy, and phenobarbital or phenytoin can be administered for prophylaxis. Finally, careful monitoring of the level of consciousness and ICP may alert the clinician to developing intracerebral hematomas, related to the operative site or to overzealous CSF drainage and tearing of the bridging dural veins.

Vasospasm after Subarachnoid Hemorrhage

Vasospasm causes delayed cerebral ischemic deficits in 20% to 30% of patients who survive SAH. While 70% of these patients develop radiographic evidence of vascular spasm, in many cases it is clinically asymptomatic (18).

Three to nine days after SAH, the patient with symptomatic vasospasm will characteristically become disoriented and drowsy over a period of hours. Focal deficits may follow. Vasospasm is presumed to be the etiology if repeat hemorrhage, mass lesion, intracranial hypertension, meningitis, or metabolic encephalopathy can be excluded through diagnostic studies.

Arteriography in patients who have vasospasm demonstrates luminal irregularities in large conducting vessels; however, CBF is not reduced until the angiographic diameter of the cerebral arteries is decreased by 50% or more compared to normal (19). Microscopic pathologic changes occur within the wall of the blood vessels within days of SAH. ICP and cerebral blood volume may actually increase during vasospasm owing to dilation of cerebral capacitance vessels (veins) and accumulation of tissue edema resulting from cerebral ischemia.

Positron emission tomography data indicate that in patients with focal deficits, CBF values are within the 10 to 20 mL per 100 g per minute range (50 mL per 100 g per minute being normal). In patients with regional CBF values less than 12 mL per 100 g per minute, clinical deficits are not reversible (20). Global CBF is markedly reduced (10 to 30 mL per 100 g per minute) in patients who are stuporous because of severe diffuse vasospasm (20).

The most common modality used clinically to confirm the presence of vasospasm is TCD ultrasonography, which measures blood flow velocity in the large extracerebral arteries. In the basal cerebral, middle cerebral, and internal carotid arteries, blood flow velocity and blood vessel diameter relate inversely. Theoretically, TCD should be able to confirm the presence of vasospasm in more than 90% of patients with anterior circulation aneurysms who have involvement of the basal vessels.

Serial TCD measurements are important. A *peak* flow velocity of 140 to 200 cm per second is defined as moderate spasm, while peak flow velocities greater than 200 cm per second are classified as severe (Fig. 1). Blood flow velocities, normal in the first 12 hours after ictus, tend to increase by the second postictal day, reach a plateau between days 6 and 9, and remain elevated for 15 to 30 days, depending upon the amount of blood in the basal cisterns on CT scan (21). A sharp rise in blood flow velocities (greater than 50 cm per second per 24 hours) is more predictive of impending spasm than a gradual increase in blood flow velocities over a period of days. In patients with severely elevated ICP, the diastolic component of large vessel flow is progressively lost; therefore, TCD ultrasonography using only *mean* flow velocities may inaccurately evaluate the severity and time course of vasospasm and can produce false-negative results. Some centers use intermittent xenon[133] measurements of CBF to complement TCD findings and identify patients with significant impairment of CBF before symptoms develop.

Cerebral vascular reactivity is impaired in patients who have vasospasm and in whom pressure autoregulation is ineffective. In patients with symptomatic vasospasm, the maximally dilated intraparenchymal resistance vessels are unable to dilate further in response to decreased perfusion pressure. Hypocapnia enhances vasospasm both in patients with severe diffuse vasospasm (Hunt-Hess grades III to IV) and in those with better neurologic grade (Hunt-Hess I to III) (22).

Cerebral infarction after the onset of vasospasm appears to correlate with the amount of blood seen on the patient's initial CT scan and with a history of hypertension (23). Chemical factors may also play a synergistic role with the anatomic degeneration seen with vasospasm. Oxyhemoglobin, released from lysis of subarachnoid red blood cells, is present in high concentrations in the CSF during vasospasm. This agent promotes the release of vasoactive eicosanoids and endothelin from the arterial wall, inhibits nitric oxide-mediated endothelium-dependent relaxation, and produces bilirubin and lipid peroxides that evoke an inflammatory response and cause damage to perivascular nerves (23).

Treatment modalities for vasospasm include fibrinolysis, angioplasty, calcium entry blockers, and hypervolemic hypertension. Fibrinolysis of the subarachnoid hematoma markedly reduces the effects of vasospasm. A continuous infusion of intracisternal recombinant tissue plasminogen activator has been used to promote clearance of blood from the subarachnoid space. While development of an intracranial hematoma is a risk, postoperative intracisternal administration of tissue plasminogen activator in serial doses is well tolerated, and appears to be effective in reducing the severity of delayed cerebral vasospasm (24).

When patients initially become symptomatic from vasospasm, angioplasty increases the caliber of spastic vessels and produces rapid clinical improvement while significantly reducing TCD

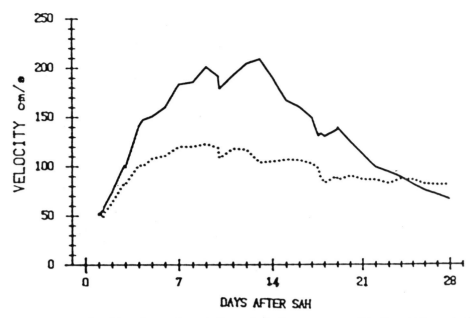

FIGURE 1. Data describing changes in peak flow velocity (in cm per second) in the middle cerebral artery in five patients with permanent neurologic deficits from cerebral infarction after subarachnoid hemorrhage. The *curve* shows the time course (in days) of severe symptomatic vasospasm. A peak flow velocity of 140 to 200 cm per second in the middle cerebral artery is defined as moderate spasm, while velocities greater than 200 cm per second are classified as severe. The *continuous line* is the side of the ruptured aneurysm. The *dotted line* is the unaffected side. (Modified from Seiler RW, Grolimund P, Aaslid R, et al. Cerebral vasospasm evaluated by transcranial ultrasound correlated with clinical grade and CT-visualized subarachnoid hemorrhage. *J Neurosurg* 1986;64:594–600, with permission.)

flow velocities in many patients (25). Transluminal angioplasty reportedly results in neurologic improvement in patients with refractory vasospasm in 60% to 70% of cases (25). The effects of dilation of vasospastic arteries appear stable, but early intervention is critical. Intraarterial papaverine infusion following endovascular dilation has achieved moderate success in selected patients with vasospasm.

Intracellular calcium (Fig. 2), known to mediate tension development in vascular smooth muscle, enters the cell through leakage, receptor-mediated channels, and voltage-mediated channels. A subtype of the voltage-mediated channel, the L-type calcium channel, which is abundant in cardiac, cerebral, and skeletal muscular vascular smooth muscle, is blocked by highly lipid-soluble, dihydropyridine drugs such as nimodipine and nicardipine. Clinical trials have demonstrated the efficacy of these drugs in ameliorating the effects of delayed cerebral ischemia related to vasospasm (26).

The initial report on the effectiveness of nimodipine was by Allen and coworkers (26), who administered oral nimodipine, 0.7 mg per kg loading dose, followed by 0.35 mg per kg every 4 hours, to a small group of patients in a randomized, double-blind prospective study. In these patients, who were Hunt-Hess grades I and II, nimodipine reduced the occurrence of severe neurologic deficits and mortality from vasospasm. Pickard found that oral nimodipine 60 mg every 4 hours reduced both the frequency of cerebral infarction and the percentage of patients with poor outcome in comparison to placebo treatment (26). Calcium antagonists, however, do not have a significant effect on the prevalence of angiographic vasospasm, but rather improve leptomeningeal pathways to increase collateral flow, enhance

microcirculation, and possibly exert a direct protective effect on neuronal cells by limiting calcium influx in marginally ischemic neurons. Nicardipine, which is available as an intravenous solution, decreased the incidence of delayed ischemic symptoms, but therapy made no difference in long-term outcome of patients in a recent prospective randomized trial (27). Agents of a new class of calcium antagonists that act to sequester intracellular calcium and inhibit protein kinase C, are more likely to affect the contractile properties of vascular smooth muscle. One such agent, AT877 reduced symptomatic and angiographic vasospasm in a prospective randomized trial (27).

As discussed previously, hypervolemic hemodilution has been advocated for prophylaxis and treatment of vasospasm in patients after SAH. Theoretic evidence supporting the need for volume expansion includes the observation that 10% to 33% of patients after SAH develop hyponatremia, associated with negative sodium balance and intravascular volume contraction (17). Hyponatremic patients are more likely to develop vasospasm. In one series, prophylactic volume expansion was associated with outcomes as good as those achieved with calcium-channel blocker prophylaxis (28). Although no large clinical trials have used a controlled, randomized design to compare volume expansion to other therapies for symptomatic vasospasm, many surgeons are convinced that patients demonstrate symptomatic improvement once blood volume has been expanded.

One algorithm for producing hypervolemia and increasing cerebral perfusion pressure consists of pulmonary artery catheterization and infusion of fluid, either saline or colloid, to increase the PAOP to 15 ± 3 mm Hg. Associated therapeutic goals include a CVP of 10 ± 2 mm Hg, a systolic blood pressure of

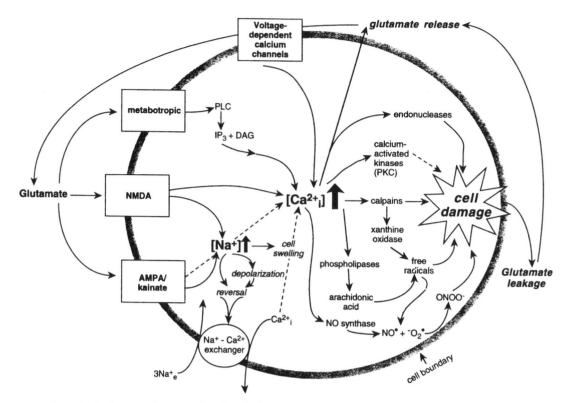

FIGURE 2. The possible mechanisms by which intracellular calcium may be increased in neurons during ischemia and the putative intracellular targets that may mediate cell damage and eventually cell death. Glutamate acts on n-methyl-d-aspartate (NMDA), α-amino-3-hydroxy-5-methyl-4-isoxazole propionate (AMPA)/kainate, and metabotropic receptors to produce an increase in cytosolic free Ca^{2+}. (Reprinted with permission from Gill R. The pharmacology of α-amino-3-hydroxy-5-methyl-4-isoxazole propionate (AMPA)/kainate antagonists and their role in cerebral ischaemia. *Cerebrovasc Brain Metab Rev* 1994;6:225–256.)

180 ± 10 mm Hg (a mean arterial pressure of 130 ± 10 mm Hg), and adequate arterial oxygen content, defined as a hemoglobin of 11 g per dL and an oxyhemoglobin saturation of 95% (Table 2) (29). If volume expansion does not achieve these hemodynamic goals, dopamine 5 to 10 μg per kg per minute is added to increase cardiac output greater than 6 to 8 L per minute. The combination of dobutamine and phenylephrine often increases cardiac output when dopamine proves ineffective. Using this protocol, most neurologic deficits attributed to vasospasm improve within 1 to 4 hours. Young patients with extremely high urinary output may require vasopressin or fludrocortisone acetate to maintain the desired intravascular fluid expansion.

While hemodilution is popular in some clinical centers, its clinical efficacy is unproven. Hematocrit values in the range

TABLE 2. HYPERVOLEMIC HYPERTENSIVE THERAPY FOR CEREBRAL VASOSPASM

Pulmonary artery occluded pressure: 15–18 mm Hg
Mean arterial pressure: 130 mm Hg
Hemoglobin: 11 g/dL
Oxygen saturation: >95%

Modified from Kirsch JR, Diringer MN, Borel CO, et al. Cerebral aneurysms: mechanisms of injury and critical care interventions. *Crit Care Clin* 1989;5:755–772, with permission.

of 35% to 50% are consistent with normal cerebral oxygen delivery. At higher values, an increase in oxygen capacity is offset by increased viscosity and decreased CBF. For hematocrit values below 35%, the decreased oxygen-carrying capacity is only partially offset by decreased viscosity and increased CBF.

Occasionally, hypertensive hypervolemic therapy is required for up to 3 weeks until neurologic status remains stable as treatment is tapered. A suggested protocol for weaning therapy involves 48 hours of intensive volume expansion and then gradual discontinuation of therapy while carefully monitoring clinical neurologic signs (29). Therapy may also be discontinued by weaning inotropic or vasoactive drugs to decrease mean arterial pressure in increments of 10 mm Hg every 4 to 6 hours until new neurologic symptoms appear, pretreatment blood pressure is achieved, or vasoactive drugs are stopped. Other investigators wean therapy when CBF increases and autoregulation or carbon dioxide responsiveness, determined by CBF measurements, becomes normal (30). Recurrent evidence of ischemic symptoms necessitates rapid return to previously effective levels of blood pressure.

Cardiac, hematologic, and pulmonary sequelae have been reported as consequences of volume expansion and induced hypertension. Recent evidence suggests that increases in cardiac index correlate with increases in PAOP but not with CVP. In patients with no history of heart disease, a PAOP of 14 mm Hg is associated with maximum cardiac performance (16).

ARTERIOVENOUS MALFORMATION (AVM)

Most aspects of the care of patients who have undergone craniotomy for resection of aneurysms and AVMs are similar. However, classic hemodynamic management after AVM resection emphasizes postoperative control of increases in mean arterial blood pressure. Patients who have undergone AVM resection are at risk for the development of a syndrome which can be deemed arteriocapillary-venous hypertension syndrome (particularly if the AVM was large and contained feeding vessels perforating deep into the brain) (31). Of a large surgical series, 5% of patients developed delayed neurologic deficits following AVM resection. Hemorrhage into the resected AVM nidus precipitated by increases in blood pressure occurred, and experimental evidence indicates that areas of brain immediately bordering large AVMs may be chronically ischemic, but hyperreactive to increases in $PaCO_2$ (32). After AVM resection, blood vessels that heretofore had been relatively hypoperfused become "hyperperfused." Vasomotor paralysis is unlikely, but reperfusion injury or intrinsic structural deficiencies of the capillaries may contribute to blood–brain barrier breakdown (33). Treatment may necessitate emergency reintubation, hyperventilation, administration of mannitol, and induction of barbiturate coma. Postoperative seizures after AVM resections are common and prophylaxis must be continued in the perioperative period.

Some complications following AVM resection are related to stagnation in former arterial feeders and venous outflow obstruction as originally proposed by Al-Rodhan and colleagues (34). This venous thrombosis causes edema and brain swelling. Finally, in patients where the AVM resection involved extensive manipulation of arteries at the base of the brain, symptomatic vasospasm has been described. The traditional hypertensive, hypervolemic hemodilution therapy may be inappropriate in postoperative patients where a fresh AVM nidus may predispose the patient to hemorrhagic risk.

SPECIFIC MANAGEMENT ISSUES

Decreased Level of Consciousness

Impaired consciousness is nonspecific; however, recognition of changing consciousness may signal a variety of treatable conditions, including intracranial hypertension, vasospasm after SAH, delayed posttraumatic intracranial hematomas, or systemic complications such as hyponatremia, hypoxemia, or hypercarbia. Focal neurologic findings often suggest a specific lesion (i.e., unilateral weakness or reflex changes developing after carotid endarterectomy suggest the possibility of carotid occlusion).

Frequent, accurately recorded neurologic examinations are an essential aspect of neurologic monitoring. Neurologic examination quantifies two key characteristics: changes in consciousness and focal brain dysfunction. The state of consciousness and the trend in neurologic function are the most important indications of the severity of neurologic disease and the most important predictors of survival. Assessment of consciousness is by two means, verbal response and response to pain. The former includes spontaneous speech: oriented, confused, inappropriate,

or incomprehensible. Response to pain is essential in assessing patients who make no verbal responses. Because consciousness waxes and wanes, the pain stimulus must be severe enough to elicit a response.

The Glasgow Coma Scale (GCS), originally developed as a prognostic tool for head-injured patients, has become popular as a brief estimate, with minimal interobserver variability, of level of consciousness in critically ill patients. The GCS score has been used successfully to stratify general ICU patients and predict mortality, although discrimination in the intermediate ranges (GCS scores 7 to 11) is poor. The GCS, which includes observations regarding eye opening, motor response in the "best" limb, and verbal responses, does not provide information regarding pupillary responses and brainstem functions.

An initial assessment of deteriorating neurologic status includes level of consciousness, best motor response, pupillary response, corneal responses, ocular muscle function, and respiratory function. Motor responses are lost in the following sequence: obeying commands, localization of pain, withdrawal to pain, flexion to pain, and extension to pain. The likelihood of severe morbidity and mortality increases substantially in patients who have abnormal posturing. In alert, cooperative patients, motor testing should include examination for pronator drift, often the first sign of an evolving hemiparesis.

Brainstem function (i.e., pupillary light responses) should also be tested in all comatose patients. In pharmacologically paralyzed, intubated patients, the pupillary reaction provides the only clinical neurologic assessment. In the course of transtentorial herniation, the superficial location of the parasympathetic fibers on the third nerve results in early compression, leading to ipsilateral pupillary dilation. Occasionally, moderate anisocoria and a sluggishly reactive pupil may signal uncal herniation in alert patients who retain full extraocular movements and a normal respiratory pattern. Bilateral dilated pupils constitute a grave prognostic sign. Corneal reflexes, important for protection of the eyes, are lost early after traumatic brain injury and have little prognostic significance.

Both the oculovestibular and the oculocephalic reflexes require the integrity of the third, fourth, and sixth cranial nerves, the medial longitudinal fasciculus, the eighth nerve afferents, and an intact brainstem. Impaired oculocephalic and oculovestibular reflexes are grave prognostic signs. The oculocephalic reflex requires movement of the neck and is relatively contraindicated in the presence of a cervical spine injury. The normal oculocephalic response, tested by abruptly rocking the head from right to left, is maintenance of the direction of gaze despite a shift in head position. If a normal oculocephalic ("doll's eyes") response cannot or should not be elicited, the normal vestibuloocular response of a comatose patient to irrigation of the external ear canal with 10 to 20 mL of ice-cold water should be tonic deviation of both eyes to the ipsilateral side (ice-water caloric). The oculovestibular response requires a patent external auditory canal. Initial syringing with measured cold saline should be performed with the patient's head in a neutral position if cervical spine injury is a consideration.

Neurologic examination may also suggest the possibility of intracranial hypertension. A patient able to follow simple commands, even if stuporous or lethargic, rarely has a raised ICP, whereas approximately 40% to 50% of head-injured patients with altered consciousness have intracranial hypertension. The symptoms and signs of raised ICP are not, however, uniformly reliable. In unconscious, head-injured patients, the probability of increased ICP is lower if the patient withdraws to painful stimuli, or moans or grimaces. A frankly raised ICP is likely to be encountered with GCS scores of 4 to 6 in head-injured patients. Severe increases in ICP may present as Cushing triad of hypertension, bradycardia, and respiratory irregularity; but the absence of Cushing triad does not rule out intracranial hypertension. Pupillary dilation may herald transtentorial herniation, but is a late manifestation of central herniation. Herniation, which could be a result of vascular insufficiency or direct compression and infarction of the brainstem, is a major catastrophe almost synonymous with imminent, extensive, and fatal brain damage. The presence of apnea is also a grave prognostic sign.

Cerebral Ischemia

Pharmacologic Management

After stroke, the therapeutic window for pharmacologic or other interventions has traditionally been thought to be narrow, but the concept of delayed neuronal cell death has extended the period to 48 hours in some studies (35). Few postoperative patients are candidates for acute thrombolytic therapy such as tissue plasminogen activator (TPA) or endovascular interventions such as carotid thromboendarterectomy. In addition to injury occurring during ischemia, experimental work suggests the likely occurrence of reperfusion injury, damage that occurs after restoration of flow in neural tissue or in the cerebral vasculature. Therapeutic interventions, even if initiated after restoration of perfusion, could perhaps decrease neurologic morbidity if the mechanisms underlying progressive injury can be identified and interrupted (36). Drugs that offer promise in ameliorating the effects of acute cerebral ischemia include calcium entry blockers, pentoxifylline, ancrod, thrombolytic agents, antagonists of excitotoxins, and gangliosides, although results from clinical phase III trials have often been disappointing to date (37).

Metaanalysis of five double-blind, placebo-controlled studies of the treatment of stroke with nimodipine, a calcium entry blocker that differentially dilates the cerebral vasculature, indicated that nimodipine improves mortality and outcome (38). Efficacy was particularly evident if nimodipine administration occurred within 12 hours of the onset of stroke or if the patient was more than 65 years of age. Adverse reactions, primarily hypotension, are relatively mild. Nimodipine is administered orally in a total daily dose of 120 mg, most often as four divided doses and is most efficacious if administered within 6 hours of the onset of neurologic symptoms.

Pentoxifylline is a methylxanthine that reduces blood viscosity increases in CBF in low-flow areas in patients with chronic cerebrovascular disease. If administered during the first few days after acute stroke, it produces clinical improvement that has not been sustained. It may be efficacious as an adjunct to other modalities in acute stroke.

Ancrod, a purified fraction of venom from the Malayan pit viper, enhances spontaneous fibrinolysis. The resulting hypofibrinogenemia lowers blood viscosity, thus increasing blood flow, and anticoagulates, thus inhibiting further thrombus formation (39). Ancrod also stimulates release of plasminogen activation. Neurologic outcome in patients with acute ischemic stroke may be improved if fibrinogen levels can be reduced by ancrod to 130 mg per dL or less within 6 hours (39). Enthusiasm for antithrombotic therapy is tempered in general by concern for the risk of hemorrhagic transformation of a cerebral infarction. New neuroimaging modalities such as diffusion weighted magnetic resonance imaging may serve to more accurately identify those patients at risk for this complication (40).

Cerebrovascular recanalization may improve CBF after acute thromboembolic events. TPA is a relatively thromboselective agent that promotes thrombolysis when administered by intravenous infusion. In recent studies of intravenous TPA, rates of recanalization ranged from 21% to 53%. Hemorrhagic transformation of the ischemic deficit is a concern, occurring in 4% to 11% of patients studied at 24 hours after treatment (41). Despite this fact, most patients demonstrated minimal change in clinical status after hemorrhagic infarction, and neurologic outcomes at 6 months were similar. Aspirin, 325 mg daily, appear to offer some benefit in virtually all ischemic stroke types, but caution is warranted in combining antithrombotic and antiplatelet agents (42).

Following stroke, the zone of ischemia can be limited by augmenting blood flow to the collateral circulation. Recommendations from the American Heart Association support maintenance of mean arterial blood pressure at levels $\leq$130 mm Hg and antihypertensive therapy, particularly in chronically hypertensive patients, only when the MAP is consistently $\geq$130 mm Hg (43). Labetalol (10 mg i.v.) is a good initial choice for therapy since it does not cause cerebral vasodilation. If imaging studies demonstrate that the patient has evidence of hemorrhagic transformation of a cerebral infarction, systolic blood pressure should be maintained at $\leq$170 mm Hg.

Maintenance of intravascular volume with nonglucose-containing fluids in stroke patients is crucial, and normovolemic hemodilution increases CBF and improves EEG activity (44). However, widespread clinical application has been impeded by concern regarding two physiologic risks. First, hypervolemia may produce cardiac failure or myocardial ischemia in patients who have coexisting cerebrovascular and coronary occlusive disease. Second, although flow may be slightly improved by moderate hemodilution, the reduction in oxygen-carrying capacity may prevent any improvement in local oxygen delivery. The Hemodilution in Stroke Study Group used invasive cardiovascular monitoring to guide hypervolemic hemodilution with pentastarch and increase cardiac output in patients with acute ischemic stroke. Among the actively treated patients, four of five deaths were due to cerebral edema (45). Although overall mortality and neurologic outcome were not superior in the hemodilution group, neurologic outcome was apparently improved in patients who were entered into the trial within 12 hours of the onset of stroke and those who had an increase of cardiac output $\geq$10% of baseline.

Acute Intracranial Hypertension

Control of increased ICP to maximize cerebral perfusion pressure and minimize cerebral ischemia depends on effective control of cerebral tissue volume, cerebral blood volume, and CSF volume. The therapy of intracranial hypertension must either decrease the volume of the component that caused the original problem (e.g., tumor or hematoma) or decrease the volume of one of the other components. On an emergent basis, intracranial hypertension is most quickly treated by reducing cerebral blood volume, often by intentionally using acute hyperventilation on a short-term basis to decrease CBF.

Brain tissue volume, often increased as a consequence of cerebral edema, can be reduced medically or surgically. Three types of cerebral edema have been described experimentally (46), although in individual patients more than one type of edema may be present. Interstitial edema occurs with hydrocephalus. Vasogenic edema, which accompanies intracranial tumors, is associated with opening of the blood–brain barrier to protein. The most clearly established use of glucocorticoids in neurologic intensive care is to treat the vasogenic edema associated with brain tumors and brain abscesses. Cytotoxic edema, which accompanies hypoxic or traumatic injury, is characterized by cellular swelling and is not responsive to glucocorticoids (46). Occasionally, decompressive craniectomy effectively relieves refractory intracranial hypertension.

Chronic fluid restriction does not effectively reduce brain tissue volume; however, diuretics are commonly used to reduce acute intracranial hypertension associated with cerebral edema. Mannitol and other osmotic diuretics reduce brain volume by osmotically removing water from uninjured brain in which the blood–brain barrier is intact. In addition, mannitol reduces blood viscosity and may improve microcirculatory flow (47). Mannitol reduces ICP for 3 to 4 hours. Small doses (0.25 to 0.5 g per kg) have been used effectively to maintain lower ICP in patients with closed head trauma but serum osmolality should not be allowed to increase above 310 mOsm per kg. Mannitol is less effective in patients with severe, diffuse brain injury because the integrity of the blood–brain barrier is compromised. Furosemide, 20 to 40 mg i.v., reduces ICP acutely in animal models and in patients (48). Although the initial effect is to reduce brain water, furosemide also inhibits the elaboration of CSF, thereby reducing another of the three components of intracranial volume. Diuretic therapy must be accompanied by the adequate assessment and maintenance of intravascular volume. In the presence of hypovolemia, cerebral perfusion pressure may decrease severely, provoking maximal vasodilation of arteriolar vessels, cerebral ischemia and deleterious increases in cerebral blood volume and ICP. Recently, hypertonic saline has been used in several small trials as rescue therapy for refractory intracranial hypertension (49).

Cerebral blood volume may be lowered by reducing CBF or facilitating cerebral venous drainage. Endotracheal intubation and mechanical ventilation maintain adequate gas exchange, thereby limiting the likelihood of inadvertent increases in CBF resulting from hypoxemia or hypercarbia. Adequate sedation and analgesia, by limiting the effects of brain stimulation on the cerebral metabolic rate for oxygen and CBF, are useful in the control of ICP. Hyperventilation has been commonly used to reduce CBF and cerebral blood volume, both as a sustained therapeutic measure and as an acute response to sudden increases in ICP; however, limited attention has been paid to the maintenance of adequate CBF during therapeutic hyperventilation. Mechanical

hyperventilation often reduces the internal jugular venous bulb oxygen saturation below acceptable average levels (50). Further studies are required to determine if monitoring of SjvO$_2$ or brain tissue oxygen levels in conjunction with monitoring of ICP and CBF can be used to improve outcome in patients with intracranial hypertension who require mechanical ventilation.

Blood pressure control represents a particularly difficult problem in patients with intracranial hypertension. Autoregulation is attenuated or abolished in areas of injured brain. Consequently, decreased systemic blood pressure may reduce CBF and worsen cerebral ischemia. Increased blood pressure where levels or cerebral perfusion pressure exceed 140 mm Hg may, in some patients, increase CBF and cerebral blood volume, thereby increasing ICP. Pharmacologic reduction of systemic blood pressure may have adverse effects on intracranial hemodynamics. SNP has been associated both with cerebral ischemia from rapid blood pressure reduction and with intracranial hypertension. Nitroglycerin, like SNP, may increase ICP (51). When SNP or nitroglycerin is used to reduce blood pressure in patients with intracranial lesions, the net effect on ICP is the result of reduced cerebral blood volume in injured areas that do not autoregulate and increased cerebral blood volume in intact regions where the drug therapy itself inhibits autoregulation. Labetalol, a combination β- and α-antagonist, causes little change in CBF in hypertensive patients (51).

CSF volume can be reduced mechanically, through systemic dehydration, or by pharmacologic intervention. CSF can be withdrawn through intraventricular catheters, which are placed more commonly in patients who have intraventricular hemorrhage and less commonly in other situations involving intracranial hypertension. Dehydration decreases the production of CSF. Drugs such as furosemide; acetazolamide, 250 mg orally or intravenously; and digoxin also reduce CSF production, although they are uncommonly used in acute situations.

Acute Intracerebral Hemorrhage

Spontaneous intracerebral hemorrhage accounts for approximately 10% of cerebrovascular disease. In patients who become comatose after intracerebral hemorrhage, mortality exceeds 50% (52). Usually related to chronic systemic hypertension, primary intracerebral hemorrhage most commonly occurs in penetrating vessels in the basal ganglia, subcortical white matter, thalamus, cerebellum, and pons. Although the abrupt onset of symptoms may suggest the cause of neurologic deterioration, CT scanning provides the definitive diagnosis (52). Increasingly, intracranial hemorrhage in young people is related to drug abuse, while hemorrhages related to the use of thrombolytics in stroke patients have a poor prognosis (53). The indications for surgical evacuation of intracerebral hematomas vary with the location and size of the lesion. Cerebellar hematomas exceeding 2 to 3 cm in diameter and large lobar hematomas often require emergency evacuation to prevent brainstem compression or herniation. Surgical evacuation of hemorrhages from the brainstem, thalamus, and putamen remains controversial.

ICP monitoring, control of intracranial hypertension, and maximizing cerebral perfusion may be useful in patients who present with or develop an altered sensorium. Treatment of primary intracerebral hemorrhage consists of intubation if coma is profound, seizure prophylaxis with phenytoin, control of blood pressure, and reduction of ICP (if necessary) with mannitol and CSF drainage. Glucocorticoids are not of benefit. Most patients are hypertensive, and mean arterial blood pressure levels between 90 and 130 mm Hg may be necessary in order to assure adequate cerebral perfusion. If diastolic pressures exceed 120 mm Hg, labetalol is particularly useful (52).

Meticulous care of postoperative neurosurgical patients is challenging and vital. Attention to a well-focused clinical examination remains the cornerstone of excellence in the delivery of critical care while technologies such as TCD, $SjvO_2$, and CBF measurements provide valuable information to guide specific therapy. The introduction and evaluation of new pharmacologic and neurointerventional therapies for cerebral ischemia promote optimism about the efficacy of care provided to patients with serious neurologic disease.

SUMMARY

Care of the neurosurgical patient can be especially challenging in the postoperative period. Good patient outcome often depends on prompt recognition and treatment of both frequent and infrequent complications. After carotid endarterectomy, careful monitoring is necessary to detect the occurrence of new neurologic deficits and to manage hemorrhage, hypertension, hypotension, and the hyperperfusion syndrome. The most common cause of perioperative mortality in carotid endarterectomy patients is myocardial infarction. After craniotomy, multiple challenges can arise related to hemodynamic control, ventilatory support, hematoma detection and treatment, pain management, and fluid therapy. Hypertension may be a sign of an evolving intracranial hematoma or other causes, including hypercarbia, pain, shivering, and bladder distention. After uncomplicated aneurysm clipping or endovascular occlusion, patients with favorable preoperative Hunt-Hess grades will likely be extubated promptly unless intraoperative complications or management decisions dictate continued intubation.

Cerebral infarction after onset of vasospasm appears to correlate with the amount of blood visualized on CT and with a history of hypertension. The most common modality used clinically to confirm the presence of vasospasm is TCD ultrasonography. After resection of a cerebral AVM, patients may develop a hyperperfusion syndrome, characterized by increased CBF in previously hypoperfused vessels. Control of acute intracranial hypertension can be accomplished by multiple interventions; hyperventilation is particularly valuable as temporizing therapy because it rapidly reduces CBF, cerebral blood volume, and ICP; however, sustained hyperventilation becomes ineffective and may be associated in some situations with poorer outcome.

KEY POINTS

The most common cause of perioperative mortality in carotid endarterectomy patients is myocardial infarction.

After uncomplicated aneurysm clipping or endovascular occlusion in patients with favorable preoperative Hunt-Hess grades, patients will likely be extubated promptly unless intraoperative complications or management decisions dictate continued intubation.

Cerebral infarction after onset of vasospasm appears to correlate with the amount of blood visualized on computed tomography and with a history of hypertension.

After resection of a cerebral arteriovenous malformation, patients may develop a hyperperfusion syndrome, characterized by increased cerebral blood flow (CBF) in previously hypoperfused vessels.

Control of acute intracranial hypertension can be accomplished by multiple interventions; hyperventilation is particularly valuable as temporizing therapy because it rapidly reduces CBF, cerebral blood volume, and intracranial pressure.

REFERENCES

1. Rigdon EE, Monajjem N, Rhodes RS. Criteria for selective utilization of the intensive care unit following carotid endarterectomy. *Ann Vasc Surg* 1997;11:20–27.
2. Carmichael FJ, McGuire GP, Wong DT, et al. Computed tomographic analysis of airway dimensions after carotid endarterectomy. *Anesth Analg* 1996;83:12–17.
3. Scuderi PE, Prough DS, Davis CH Jr, et al. The effects of regional and general anesthesia on blood pressure control after carotid endarterectomy. *J Neurosurg Anesth* 1989;1:41–45.
4. Lipsett PA, Tierney S, Gordon TA, et al. Carotid endarterectomy—is intensive care unit care necessary? *J Vasc Surg* 1994;20:403–410.
5. Sbarigia E, Speziale F, Giannoni MF, et al. Post-carotid endarterectomy hyperperfusion syndrome: preliminary observations for identifying at risk patients by transcranial Doppler sonography and the acetazolamide test. *Eur J Vasc Surg* 1993;7:252–256.
6. Levine TM. Swallowing disorders following skull base surgery. *Otolaryngol Clin North Am* 1988;21:751–759.
7. Beemer GH, Rozental P. Postoperative neuromuscular function. *Anaesth Intensive Care* 1986;14:41–45.
8. Kalfas IH, Little JR. Postoperative hemorrhage: a survey of 4992 intracranial procedures. *Neurosurgery* 1988;23:343–347.
9. Bullock R, Hannemann CO, Murray L, et al. Recurrent hematomas following craniotomy for traumatic intracranial mass. *J Neurosurg* 1990;72:9–14.
10. Constantini S, Cotev S, Rappaport ZH, et al. Intracranial pressure monitoring after elective intracranial surgery. A retrospective study of 514 consecutive patients. *J Neurosurg* 1988;69:540–544.
11. Rosenwasser RH, Kleiner LI, Krzeminski JP, et al. Intracranial pressure monitoring in the posterior fossa: a preliminary report. *J Neurosurg* 1989;71:503–505.
12. Reasoner DK, Todd MM, Scamman FL, et al. The incidence of pneumocephalus after supratentorial craniotomy. Observations on the disappearance of intracranial air. *Anesthesiology* 1994;80:1008–1012.
13. Lanzino G, Kassell NF. Surgical treatment of the ruptured aneurysm: timing. *Neurosurg Clin North Am* 1998;9(3):541–548.
14. Solenski NJ, Haley EC Jr, Kassell NF, et al. Medical complications of aneurysmal subarachnoid hemorrhage: a report of the multicenter,

cooperative aneurysm study. Participants of the Multicenter Cooperative Aneurysm Study. *Crit Care Med* 1995;23:1007–1017.

15. Davies KR, Gelb AW, Manninen PH, et al. Cardiac function in aneurysmal subarachnoid haemorrhage: a study of electrocardiographic and echocardiographic abnormalities. *Br J Anaesth* 1991;67:58–63.
16. Levy ML, Giannotta SL. Cardiac performance indices during hypervolemic therapy for cerebral vasospasm. *J Neurosurg* 1991;75:27–31.
17. Wijdicks EFM, Ropper AH, Hunnicutt EJ, et al. Atrial natriuretic factor and salt wasting after aneurysmal subarachnoid hemorrhage. *Stroke* 1991;22:1519–1524.
18. Bejjani GK, Bank WO, Olan WJ, et al. The efficacy and safety of angioplasty for cerebral vasospasm after subarachnoid hemorrhage. *Neurosurgery* 1998;42:979–987.
19. Voldby B, Enevoldsen EM, Jensen FT. Regional CBF, intraventricular pressure, and cerebral metabolism in patients with ruptured intracranial aneurysms. *J Neurosurg* 1985;62:48–58.
20. Powers WJ, Grubb RL Jr, Baker RP, et al. Regional cerebral blood flow and metabolism in reversible ischemia due to vasospasm. Determination by positron emission tomography. *J Neurosurg* 1985;62:539–546.
21. Lindegaard K-F. The role of transcranial Doppler in the management of patients with subarachnoid haemorrhage—a review. *Acta Neurochir* 1999;72[Suppl]:59–71.
22. Voldby B, Enevoldsen EM, Jensen FT. Cerebrovascular reactivity in patients with ruptured intracranial aneurysms. *J Neurosurg* 1985;62:59–67.
23. Weir B, Macdonald RL, Stoodley M. Etiology of cerebral vasospasm. *Acta Neurochir* 1999;72[Suppl]:27–46.
24. Findlay JM, Kassell NF, Weir BK, et al. A randomized trial of intraoperative intra-cisternal tissue plasminogen activator for the prevention of vasospasm. *Neurosurgery* 1995;37:168–176.
25. Newell DW, Elliott JP, Eskridge JM, et al. Endovascular therapy for aneurysmal vasospasm. *Crit Care Clin* 1999;15(4):685–699.
26. Gilsbach JM. Nimodipine in the prevention of ischaemic deficits after aneurysmal subarachnoid haemorrhage. An analysis of recent clinical studies. *Acta Neurochir Suppl* 1988;45:41–50.
27. Mayberg MR. Cerebral vasospasm. *Neurosurg Clin North Am* 1998;9(3):615–627.
28. Medlock MD, Dulebohn SC, Elwood PW. Prophylactic hypervolemia without calcium channel blockers in early aneurysm surgery. *Neurosurgery* 1992;30:12–16.
29. Kirsch JR, Diringer MN, Borel CO, et al. Cerebral aneurysms: mechanisms of injury and critical care interventions. *Crit Care Clin* 1989;5:755–772.
30. McKhann GM II, Le Roux PD. Perioperative and intensive care unit care of patients with aneurysmal subarachnoid hemorrhage. *Neurosurg Clin North Am* 1998;9(3):595–613.
31. Morgan MK, Sekhon LHS, Finfer S, et al. Delayed neurological deterioration following resection of arteriovenous malformations of the brain. *J Neurosurg* 1999;90:695–701.
32. Young WL, Solomon RA, Prohovnik I, et al. [133]Xe blood flow monitoring during arteriovenous malformation resection: a case of intraoperative hyperperfusion with subsequent brain swelling. *Neurosurgery* 1988;22:765–769.
33. Wong JH, Awad IA, Kim JH. Ultrastructural pathological features of cerebrovascular malformations: a preliminary report. *Neurosurgery* 2000;46:1454–1459.
34. Al-Rodhan NRF, Sundt TM Jr, Piepgras DG, et al. Occlusive hyperemia: a theory for the hemodynamic complications following resection of intracerebral arteriovenous malformations. *J Neurosurg* 1993;78:167–175.
35. Gomez CR, Wadlington VR, Terry JB, et al. Neuroendovascular rescue: nonthrombolytic approach to acute brain ischemia. *Crit Care Clin* 1999;15(4):755–776.
36. Jean WC, Spellman SR, Nussbaum ES, et al. Reperfusion injury after focal cerebral ischemia: the role of inflammation and the therapeutic horizon. *Neurosurgery* 1998;43:1382–1397.
37. De Keyser J, Sulter G, Luiten PG. Clinical trials with neuroprotective drugs in acute ischaemic stroke: are we doing the right thing? *Trends Neurosci* 1999;22:535–540.
38. Gelmers HJ, Hennerici M. Effect of nimodipine on acute ischemic stroke. Pooled results from five randomized trials. *Stroke* 1990;21:IV81–IV84.
39. The Ancrod Stroke Study Investigators. Ancrod for the treatment of acute ischemic brain infarction. *Stroke* 1994;25:1755–1759.
40. Beauchamp NJ Jr, Barker PB, Wang PY, et al. Imaging of acute cerebral ischemia. *Radiology* 1999;212:307–324.
41. Patel SC, Mody A. Cerebral hemorrhagic complications of thrombolytic therapy. *Prog Cardiovasc Dis* 1999;42:217–233.
42. Bednar MM, Gross CE. Antiplatelet therapy in acute cerebral ischemia. *Stroke* 1999;30:887–893.
43. Martin NA, Saver J. Intensive care management of subarachnoid hemorrhage, ischemic stroke, and hemorrhagic stroke. *Clin Neurosurg* 1999;45:101–112.
44. Wood JH, Polyzoidis KS, Epstein CM, et al. Quantitative EEG alterations after isovolemic-hemodilutional augmentation of cerebral perfusion in stroke patients. *Neurology* 1984;34:764–768.
45. Adams HP Jr, Brott TG, Crowell RM, et al. Guidelines for the management of patients with acute ischemic stroke. A statement for healthcare professionals from a special writing group of the Stroke Council, American Heart Association. *Stroke* 1994;25:1901–1914.
46. Rosenberg GA. Ischemic brain edema. *Prog Cardiovasc Dis* 1999;42:209–216.
47. Kelly BJ, Luce JM. Current concepts in cerebral protection. *Chest* 1993;103:1246–1254.
48. Cottrell JE, Robustelli A, Post K, et al. Furosemide- and mannitol-induced changes in intracranial pressure and serum osmolality and electrolytes. *Anesthesiology* 1977;47:28–30.
49. Allen CH, Ward JD. An evidence-based approach to management of increased intracranial pressure. *Crit Care Clin* 1998;14(3):485–495.
50. Robertson CS, Narayan RK, Gokaslan ZL, et al. Cerebral arteriovenous oxygen difference as an estimate of cerebral blood flow in comatose patients. *J Neurosurg* 1989;70:222–230.
51. Frank JI. Management of intracranial hypertension. *Contemporary Clin Neurol* 1993;77:61–76.
52. Gebel JM, Broderick JP. Intracerebral hemorrhage. *Neurol Clin* 2000;19(2):419–438.
53. McEvoy AW, Kitchen ND, Thomas DGT. Intracerebral hemorrhage in young adults: the emerging importance of drug misuse. *BMJ* 2000;320:1322–1324.

23

SUBARACHNOID HEMORRHAGE AND CEREBROVASCULAR ACCIDENT

LAUREN C. BERKOW
MAREK MIRSKI
JEFFREY R. KIRSCH

KEY WORDS

- Subarachnoid hemorrhage
- Aneurysm
- Arteriovenous malformation
- Vasospasm
- Hydrocephalus
- Hyperemia
- Edema
- Normal perfusion pressure breakthrough

INTRODUCTION

Three common cerebrovascular disease states can cause subarachnoid hemorrhage (SAH) at different phases of a patient's life. Arteriovenous malformations (AVMs) typically present in younger patients, while intracerebral aneurysms are more common in the middle-aged population. Hemorrhage due to cerebrovascular accident (i.e., stroke) is most common in older adults and is discussed in detail in Chapter 19. Other less common causes of SAH include trauma, and both benign and malignant neoplasms. Regardless of the etiology of SAH, intensive care management of these patients often begins before surgical intervention and continues postoperatively. This chapter will review the pathophysiology of SAH in order to provide a framework for more efficient and effective perioperative management. Although many good animal models of stroke exist, there is not a good animal model for either aneurysmal or AVM-induced SAH. While animal models have been developed to mimic the acute effects of SAH, including increases in intracranial pressure (ICP), they do not mimic the more delayed sequelae. Therefore, most of what will be discussed in this chapter is based on information from case series and clinical studies.

EPIDEMIOLOGY

Cerebral Aneurysm

Based on autopsy studies, approximately 2% to 5% of the population suffer an intracranial aneurysm. It is estimated that of this population, approximately 11 to 16 people per 100,000 per year experience rupture (1). SAH secondary to aneurysm rupture most often presents in patients between age 40 and 60, with a slightly increased incidence in females who are usually otherwise healthy.

As aneurysms increase in size, risk of rupture increases according to the law of Laplace. Aneurysms larger than 2.5 cm are considered giant aneurysms and are at high risk of rupture, unless internal clot has caused an artificial thickening of the aneurysm wall. Most aneurysms (approximately 95%) are found in the circle of Willis. Of these, approximately 40% occur at the anterior cerebral artery, 30% at the internal carotid artery, and 20% at the middle cerebral artery. It is not uncommon for a patient to present with multiple cerebral aneurysms (approximately 20%) or to present with a coexisting AVM. Aneurysms may also appear to run in families, though no definitive genetic link has been found.

Certain disease processes predispose to aneurysm or AVM formation. Aneurysms are more common in patients with coarctation of the aorta, polycystic kidney disease, Marfan syndrome, Ehlers-Danlos syndrome, and fibromuscular dysplasia, although no clear genetic link has been found to date. Patients who develop aneurysmal SAH are more likely to have a history of hypertension or substantial cigarette use (2).

Arteriovenous Malformations

AVMs tend to present earlier in life than aneurysms, although there is significant overlap. The detection rate for symptomatic lesions is approximately 1 per 100,000 person-years. The prevalence of detected, active (at-risk) AVM is difficult to estimate, but is probably 10 per 100,000 people. Of patients with AVMs, 4% to 10% have an associated aneurysm, often located on the arterial feeding vessel (3). Debate exists as to whether this finding is coincidental or is a result of AVM-associated increased flow. AVMs, especially involving the great vein of Galen, may present in infancy, and carry a significant mortality. The majority of AVMs are supratentorial, though they may also be of posterior fossa or dural origin. AVMs may arise from the cavernous, transverse, or sigmoid sinus, with significant potential for bleeding. Female gender, AVM size, and deep venous drainage have been shown to be significantly associated with neurologic deficits at in-hospital and long-term evaluation.

PATHOPHYSIOLOGY

Aneurysms

Aneurysms typically present at the branch points of vessels where the media layer of the vessel wall is thinnest. Most aneurysms cause no symptoms during a patient's life and are diagnosed incidentally at autopsy. Over time, degenerative changes in the muscular and elastic layers of the vessel wall may lead to aneurysm formation. A deficiency in type III collagen also may play a role in the evolution of aneurysm formation and eventual rupture.

Aneurysm rupture leads to sudden entrance of blood into the subarachnoid space or adjacent brain parenchyma, which leads to an increase in ICP and distorts structures in the brain. Blood in the subarachnoid space leads to meningeal irritation. Blood may also alter cerebrospinal fluid volume by blocking the normal circulatory pattern and outflow, leading to hydrocephalus. Alterations in consciousness may develop from elevation of ICP or from direct injury produced by blood extravasation into brain tissue. Focal neurologic deficits may develop from ischemia in specific locations because of compression of blood vessels by the aneurysm dome, clot, or tissue edema. Likewise, cranial nerve deficits may occur because of compression of these nerves by these same entities (i.e., aneurysm dome, clot, or edematous brain).

Arteriovenous Malformations

AVMs form during embryonic development, usually in the first 2 months of life *in utero*. A defect in the capillary system leads to direct connections between arteries and veins. A recent study suggests that abnormal expression of endothelial growth factor and Tie-2 receptors (which bind to angiopoietins) may be important in the ultimate formation of AVMs in patients (4). The resistance to flow supplied by the capillary bed is lost, resulting in a high-flow, low-resistance pathway. Over time, blood flows preferentially through this low resistance connection, causing the vessels to dilate and the AVM to enlarge and develop collaterals. These vessels are often poorly formed and, therefore, at increased risk of hemorrhage. As the AVM enlarges, normal brain parenchyma is displaced. Blood is supplied to the AVM through an arterial feeder, often from the middle cerebral artery, and drained by venous outflow channels. Smaller AVMs seem to carry a larger risk of hemorrhage, due to the higher perfusion pressure in the feeding vessels.

In addition to hemorrhage, the shunts caused by the AVMs can deprive surrounding normal brain tissue of adequate blood flow, leading to ischemia and neurologic deficits. In addition, it is thought that these relatively ischemic brain areas that surround the AVM develop impaired autoregulation and are unable to vasoconstrict in response to changes in blood flow (5). Shunts may become large enough to cause congestive heart failure, especially in younger patients.

DIAGNOSIS

Aneurysm

Although aneurysms usually are diagnosed as a result of rupture, unruptured aneurysms may be discovered incidentally during a neuroradiographic evaluation (e.g., computed tomography [CT] or magnetic resonance imaging [MRI]) of nonspecific symptoms (e.g., headache). As technology and access to health care continue to improve, larger numbers of patients with unruptured aneurysms are presenting for surgery. Occasionally, unruptured aneurysms may also cause symptoms due to mass effect or compression of structures such as cranial nerves (e.g., diplopia, unilateral cranial nerve III palsy). Aneurysms in certain locations can lead to specific patterns of symptoms. For example, a posterior communicating artery aneurysm can cause cranial nerve III compression, leading to ipsilateral ptosis, pupillary dilation, diplopia, and divergent strabismus. Cavernous sinus aneurysms may compress the optic chiasm or cranial nerves III, IV, V, or VI. An unruptured aneurysm may lead to an embolic event that leads to a neurologic deficit (e.g., giant aneurysm with internal clot).

Once ruptured, aneurysms may still be silent or only result in vague symptomatology. Patients who experience significant SAH, and who do not die at the time of rupture, often will experience the "worst headache of their life." The headache most often occurs during a time of exertion, as an increase in blood pressure with exertion is thought to be the initiating cause of an increased transmural pressure across the aneurysm wall and rupture. Care providers must always consider the possibility of SAH for patients who present for medical management of an acute (particularly severe) headache. Suspicion for SAH should be increased if the headache is associated with any other neurologic deficit, photophobia, or nuchal rigidity. Unfortunately, some patients who present for medical care are not evaluated for SAH and are discharged home with analgesics and the diagnosis of migraine headache. Untreated, patients with a ruptured cerebral aneurysm will likely present within a couple of days with complications related to rebleeding or vasospasm. With each subsequent episode of SAH it is estimated that the patient has approximately a 50% chance of immediate death.

Headache and meningeal signs (e.g., nuchal rigidity, photophobia) develop as a result of blood entering the subarachnoid space. This blood can be detected in several ways. The results of a lumbar puncture may be informative but risks related to lumbar puncture are significant. A lumbar puncture may reveal bloody cerebrospinal fluid that is a positive sign for SAH but does not confirm the presence or absence of an aneurysm (i.e., SAH may result from pathology other than an aneurysm). In addition, a positive tap for the presence of blood due to SAH must be differentiated from a "traumatic tap." In this regard SAH is confirmed by centrifuging the cerebrospinal fluid sample and observing xanthochromia, a breakdown product of lysed red blood cells that occurs in the cerebrospinal fluid over time in SAH. In a patient with an intracranial mass lesion, removing fluid from the lumbar subarachnoid space may cause a pressure difference between the structures in the cranium and spinal canal resulting in herniation of brain from the cranium and compression of important posterior fossa structures (e.g., brainstem, cranial nerves). Therefore, it is crucial to perform an imaging study prior to performing a lumbar puncture in any patient who presents with potential of neurologic compromise, to rule out the presence of a mass lesion. In addition, removal of cerebral spinal fluid from the lumbar subarachnoid space may result in an increase in transmural pressure and aneurysm rupture. Therefore, because of the potential risks and medicolegal implications, lumbar puncture is probably not the ideal first test for diagnosis of SAH.

A CT or MRI scan may demonstrate blood in the subarachnoid space, as well as hydrocephalus or intracranial hemorrhage, if present. The location of an aneurysm or AVM may be possible to infer by the location of the hemorrhage. Not all new SAHs are apparent with noninvasive imaging; approximately 4% of new hemorrhages are missed (6). Therefore, despite the risks, it may be necessary to perform lumbar puncture in patients with negative imaging studies in order to confirm the diagnosis of SAH. MRI scans can provide more detail than CT scans, and combined with MRI angiography, may identify the aneurysm itself. In addition, some AVMs are not visible by angiography but appear as a highly suggestive pattern on MRI scan.

Small aneurysms not visible on CT scan or MRI angiogram can be located using invasive angiography. Regardless of what is visualized on CT, MRI, or MRI angiography, complete traditional angiography of all four cerebral vessels (left and right internal carotid arteries and both vertebral arteries), should be obtained to rule out and/or identify multiple aneurysms. A single arteriogram will identify 80% of aneurysms and AVMs (7). In the presence of suspicious MRI or CT, suggestive clinical history or a lumbar puncture that is positive for blood, a negative initial angiogram has little value. Anomalies missed on the initial angiogram will usually be detected on repeat study (several weeks later). It is possible that an aneurysm could be missed on angiographic evaluation because of a poor quality examination (e.g., uncooperative patient and movement artifact), temporary compression of the aneurysm by surrounding edematous tissue, or poor perfusion of the aneurysm secondary to clot or vasospasm of the feeding blood vessel. Angiography is also useful for the diagnosis of arterial vasospasm, which will be discussed later in this chapter.

Arteriovenous Malformations

New onset seizure activity is a common presentation in patients with AVMs. These patients may also present with neurologic deficits, but this is a result of shunting of blood away from eloquent brain regions, rather than the occurrence of an embolic event, which is more common in cerebral aneurysm patients. Patients with large AVMs may also complain of vascular tinnitus and have a jugular venous bruit on physical examination. In infants and children with AVMs, the initial presentation may be congestive heart failure (because of the very high cardiac output that develops over time). Significant steal, either clinically or angiographically, or progressive neurologic deficits are poor prognostic indicators. Assessment of the degree of angiographic shunt preoperatively helps the surgeon determine whether the lesion should be removed in one or multiple stages.

Removal of a large AVM in a single stage is thought to put the patient at risk of developing severe postoperative cerebral edema. This may be a result of the normal brain effectively having an autoregulatory curve that is shifted far to the left because of the previous existence of such a large associated vascular shunt. With removal of the shunt (the large AVM) the normal brain is quickly exposed to much higher perfusion pressures than existed previous to surgery. In order to prevent the complications associated with single-stage removal of large lesions, the size of the shunt may be decreased in steps with a program of sequential preoperative embolization. Preoperative embolization with particulate material requires intervention of a specially trained neuroradiologist. As with surgery, care must be taken to not occlude too much of the AVM in one sitting, as this could lead to an acute increase in perfusion pressure to the surrounding normal brain and cerebral edema. Other complications from intravascular embolization include inadvertent embolization of blood vessels not included with the AVM, allergic reactions, emboli to the venous side of the central circulation, and retained catheter (8). In addition, although postangiogram evaluation may suggest complete occlusion of the AVM, without surgical intervention it is very likely that the AVM will reappear over time.

COMMON CLASSIFICATION SYSTEMS

Aneurysms

Several classification systems have been proposed to classify cerebral aneurysms (Table 1). Hunt and Hess developed a classification with which to grade aneurysms based on symptomatology (9). Another widely used system is the World Federation of Neurological Surgeon's grading scale, which utilizes the Glasgow Coma Scale and presence or absence of motor deficit to grade patients from I to V. More recent systems have been suggested using the patient's clinical status and Glasgow Coma Scale score (10). None of these classifications are universally accepted; while the Hunt-Hess system is widely recognized, it has been criticized for its significant interobserver variability.

Arteriovenous Malformations

While several grading systems for AVMs also exist, the system by Spetzler and Martin is most widely used (Table 2) (11). In general,

TABLE 1. COMPARISON OF HUNT-HESS AND WORLD FEDERATION OF NEUROLOGIC SURGEONS GRADING SCALES

Grade	Hunt-Hess Scale	World Federation of Neurologic Surgeons Scale
0	Unruptured aneurysm	Unruptured aneurysm
I	Asymptomatic or mild headache	Glasgow Coma Score of 15
II	Moderate to severe headache, nuchal rigidity, cranial nerve palsy	Glasgow Coma Score of 13 to 14 without focal deficit
III	Lethargy, confusion, mild focal deficit	Glasgow Coma Score of 13 to 14 with focal deficit
IV	Stupor, moderate to severe hemiparesis, early decerebrate rigidity	Glasgow Coma Score of 7 to 12
V	Deep coma, decerebrate rigidity, moribund	Glasgow Coma Score of 3 to 6

TABLE 2. SPETZLER-MARTIN GRADING SCALE FOR ARTERIOVENOUS MALFORMATIONS (AVM)[a]

Graded Feature	Points Assigned
AVM size:	
Small (<3 cm)	1
Medium (3–6 cm)	2
Large (>6 cm)	3
Eloquence of adjacent brain	
Noneloquent	0
Eloquent	1
Pattern of venous drainage	
Superficial only	0
Deep	1

[a]Grade = size points + eloquence points + venous drainage points.

grade is based on size, location, pattern of feeding and drainage vessels, degree of steal, and rate of flow. Proximity to an eloquent brain area (i.e., cortex, thalamus, hypothalamus, cerebellum) adds significant surgical morbidity.

PREOPERATIVE MANAGEMENT

Initial management depends upon the clinical status of the patient. Patients with an unruptured aneurysm or AVM should receive routine preoperative evaluation as well as preoperative angiography to identify the location of the abnormality and to determine the possibility of neuroradiologic intervention. All attempts should be made to optimize the patient's medical condition prior to surgery. In particular, any suggestion of significant cardiovascular or respiratory compromise should be addressed and all attempts should be made to optimize any existing impairment. Routine preoperative blood work will vary based on the presence of coexisting disease, but should always include a baseline hemoglobin concentration and assessment of blood type and blood group antibody screen. If the hemoglobin level is low (less than 9 mg per dL) or if significant intraoperative blood loss is possible (difficult surgical approach, large AVM or aneurysm), blood typing and crossmatch should be performed. In patients preoperatively treated with anticonvulsant medication, levels should be measured and doses adjusted if necessary.

Intensive care management of the SAH patient often begins prior to surgical intervention. Once the diagnosis of SAH is made, consideration should be given to transporting the patient directly to the intensive care unit (ICU) prior to angiography depending on their clinical grade (i.e., Hunt-Hess grade III or IV) and the presence of significant cardiovascular or respiratory comorbidities (i.e., hypertension or potential for airway compromise). Patients should be transferred to another facility if neuroradiology and/or an experienced vascular neurosurgeon are not available to provide patient care. If patient stability allows, four-vessel cerebral angiography should be performed as soon as possible to confirm the presence as well as the location of an aneurysm or AVM. Overall, the risk of re-rupture is approximately 6% to 8% during the first 24 hours following SAH and 1% to 1.5% per day for the initial 14 days, yielding a cumulative re-rupture risk during the first 2 weeks of 25%. Often the angiographic sheath is left in

place postangiography in anticipation of surgery, so appropriate precautions and care of the sheath should be undertaken.

Initial goals in the ICU, in addition to continuous monitoring of vital signs and airway protection, are to provide a quiet environment, as rebleeding from increases in transmural pressure is a major preoperative concern. (Law of Laplace: tension in the vessel wall is directly related to the difference in systemic blood pressure and ICP and vessel diameter and inversely related to wall thickness.) Sedatives and analgesics should be administered as needed while avoiding oversedation that might confound neurologic evaluation. In this regard, short-acting reversible agents should be chosen in the event of acute neurologic deterioration. If a short-acting reversible agent is used (e.g., narcotics and some benzodiazepines), determination of whether any subsequent deterioration is due to oversedation can be evaluated by patient assessment after administration of a specific antagonist (e.g., naloxone, flumazenil). However, such treatment should only be administered with great caution, as drug antagonism may result in an anxious, agitated patient with greater risk of labile blood pressure and ICP. Stool softeners, antireflux prophylaxis, and anticonvulsant therapy are commonly provided to patients with SAH (particularly from ruptured cerebral aneurysm) in order to prevent an increase in blood pressure that may occur during a Valsalva maneuver that will ultimately result in an increased transmural pressure. Likewise, in order to avoid unnecessary increases in blood pressure (and therefore, transmural pressure), invasive monitors should not be placed preoperatively unless needed based on the patient's overall clinical status.

Control of blood pressure is important to prevent re-rupture as well as to maintain cerebral perfusion pressure. Calcium channel blockers, usually nimodipine, have been shown to play a role in the prevention of clinical vasospasm as well as in blood pressure control (12).

Preoperative management may also include placement of a catheter in the lateral cerebral ventricle, if hydrocephalus is present. However, because acute, inadvertent drainage of cerebral spinal fluid may also result in an increase in transmural pressure and rebleeding, intraventricular catheters are not usually placed unless there is a significant impairment in neurologic function that is thought to be due to hydrocephalus. Intravenous glucocorticoid treatment is occasionally initiated if there is evidence of brain edema on CT scan. Although glucocorticoids have never been demonstrated to significantly reduce SAH-induced brain edema, treatment has been associated with fewer signs of meningeal irritation. This in turn may result in less discomfort, hypertension, and lower overall risk of rebleeding. When patients present to the hospital early following SAH (before 3 days) they are not typically at risk for suffering with complications related to vasospasm, and baseline transcranial Doppler studies of cerebral perfusion velocity are usually normal. However, early transcranial Doppler assessment may be helpful in subsequent diagnosis of vasospasm in that it allows for the establishment of the patient's own baseline values. Indeed, evolving data from our institution suggest there is great variability in baseline Doppler flow velocity that is age-dependent (13). Patients may present to the hospital hours or even days posthemorrhage. Therefore, frequent assessment of neurologic status is vital. Changes may develop gradually or suddenly, suggesting possible re-rupture, hydrocephalus, worsening edema, or vasospasm. Patients should be watched closely for any signs of seizure activity because the presence of blood in contact with the cerebral cortex is known to be a potent stimulus for seizures. Onset of seizures has been found to be an independent predictor of poor patient outcome following SAH (14). Vasospasm most commonly develops at any time between day 3 and 11 following SAH. The likelihood of developing vasospasm correlates with the degree of SAH and concentration of clot surrounding the basal arteries, and is much more common after aneurysmal SAH than after AVM-induced SAH. Based on the size of the hemorrhage, baseline medical status, and neurologic presentation, the patient may or may not be a surgical candidate. If the patient is deemed not appropriate for surgical intervention, the goal is routine intensive care, consideration of possible nonsurgical intervention (e.g., neuroradiologic for aneurysms and computer-directed radiation treatment), and prevention of the possible complications as discussed later in this chapter.

Timing of surgery remains controversial. Few studies have evaluated the role of timing of surgical intervention and outcome in patients with an AVM. Overall, there is no consensus as to when surgical intervention should take place in relationship to AVM size, when bleeding occurred, the extent of SAH, patient age, or AVM location. On the contrary, there have been many studies and significant debate regarding the timing of surgery for patients with an aneurysm.

Historically, neurosurgeons were of the opinion that surgery following aneurysm rupture should be delayed if the patient exhibited high clinical grade of SAH or developed any evidence of cerebral vasospasm. More recently, evidence has suggested that when the total risk of morbidity and mortality associated with SAH and surgery was taken into account, there was potentially a benefit to early surgical intervention. However, the International Cooperative Study on the timing of aneurysm surgery showed no difference between early and delayed surgery (15). Despite these mixed results, there has been a trend toward operative intervention within 48 hours of rupture.

OPERATIVE MANAGEMENT

General Considerations

The goals of operative management include avoidance of rebleeding and cerebral ischemia and successful repair of the aneurysm or AVM. Strict blood pressure control is mandatory throughout surgical intervention. Invasive arterial and central venous pressure monitors are placed routinely. These monitors may be placed before or after induction of anesthesia, depending on the patient's comorbidities. Many anesthesiologists will avoid placement of invasive monitoring modalities prior to induction, unless the preoperative presence of these monitoring modalities is considered essential to prevent complications in patients with significant coexisting disease. Reluctance to placing invasive monitors in patients with intracranial vascular lesions is based on avoiding excess noxious stimulation, potentially resulting in an increase in blood pressure, an increase in transmural pressure, and risk of blood vessel rupture. Likewise, anesthesia is induced with agents that will prevent any increase in blood pressure (and therefore transmural pressure) during tracheal intubation and placement of the

Mayfield head holder. If a femoral arterial sheath is not already present, one is often placed intraoperatively (after induction of anesthesia) to facilitate rapid procurement of an angiogram postclipping in patients with an aneurysm or postresection in patients with an AVM. A lumbar or ventricular drain may also be placed after induction of anesthesia to drain cerebrospinal fluid as needed during surgery and improve surgical exposure, particularly in patients who present with vascular lesions that are expected to be surgically difficult to approach. Use of a ventricular drain is most common (as compared to a lumbar drain) in patients who are known to have a large cisternal clot, because in this setting the incidence of obstructive postoperative hydrocephalus is high.

Early placement of an indwelling arterial catheter allows for beat-to-beat assessment of blood pressure and facilitates the avoidance of dangerous alterations in blood pressure. Depth of anesthesia should be increased in anticipation of surgical stimulation to avoid hypertension and increased transmural pressure. Additional monitors such as a precordial Doppler to monitor for venous air embolism may be desirable if the head position is significantly above heart level. Care must be taken to cushion all pressure points, especially if the final position is not supine.

After the patient has been draped, the patient's head and endotracheal tube are generally not easily accessible. It is important to ensure that the endotracheal tube is well secured and that all intravascular catheters, the stopcock for lumbar drain, and monitors are accessible prior to surgical incision. The surgeons should be notified if patient position hinders ventilation or access to important monitors and the lumbar drain. Once surgery has begun, the surgeons should be notified and asked to stop if it becomes necessary to alter patient position, the endotracheal tube, or monitors that are in contact with the patient.

Mannitol (0.25 to 1 g per kg) may be given to provide optimal operating conditions for the surgeons and to reduce brain edema. Concern that use of mannitol may acutely increase intravascular volume and increase the risk of rebleeding is unfounded. Moderate hyperventilation may be used to lower ICP and hypothermia may be employed to lower cerebral metabolic rate and provide for cerebral protection in the event that temporary clipping of a feeding vessel is needed. Surgeons commonly ask for the administration of prophylactic antibiotics prior to incision. However, the overall risk of infection without antibiotics is very low, making the need for prophylactic antibiotics questionable. Likewise, although corticosteroid administration is effective in decreasing brain edema resulting from some causes of vasogenic edema, their routine use in patients with an aneurysm or AVM remains unsupported. Pre- or intraoperative administration of anticonvulsants is appropriate in patients with blood in the subarachnoid space because blood in contact with the cerebral cortex is a potent inducer of seizures. Additional measures such as administration of loop diuretics, head-up position, added hyperventilation, or mannitol may be required if significant brain edema exists.

Aneurysms

Prior to placing a clip on the aneurysm neck, blood pressure should be maintained 10% to 20% below the patient's normal range. Although more intense controlled hypotension (mean arterial blood pressure 50 to 60 mm Hg) was advocated by neurosurgeons and neuroanesthesiologists in the past to minimize the intraoperative risk of rebleeding (and reduce tension in the aneurysm neck for safe clipping), lack of demonstrated benefit in controlled trials and the risks of systemic complications has greatly diminished the enthusiasm for this practice. Electroencephalogram (EEG) and somatosensory evoked potential monitoring are often used to assess adequacy of intraoperative cerebral perfusion. More recently, use of invasive brain tissue oxygen sensors, pH sensors, Pco_2 sensors, laser Doppler flowmetry devices, and microdialysis catheters have been advocated by some surgeons and anesthesiologists as monitors for adequacy of cerebral perfusion. This information assists the neurosurgeon and anesthesiologist during placement of temporary and permanent aneurysm clips to assure that cerebral blood flow has not been compromised to vital brain regions. For example, prior to placing a permanent clip to occlude the aneurysm, the surgeon may choose to temporarily clip feeding arteries to decrease the pressure in the aneurysm neck. When temporary clipping of the feeding blood vessels is used as a means of reducing the tension in the aneurysm neck prior to placing the permanent clip, inadequate perfusion to other vital areas of brain may occur. Therefore, in order to minimize the risk of ischemia during the period of temporary clipping, systemic blood pressure is increased to approximately 20% above baseline values to minimize the area of resulting ischemia.

Recent data in human subjects suggest that desflurane may be the most appropriate background anesthetic during aneurysm surgery (16). It has been hypothesized that desflurane is beneficial because it allows for improved perfusion to the area of brain at risk for reduced blood flow, thus decreasing the area of ischemia. Because most animal data suggest that ischemic neurologic injury may be accentuated by nitrous oxide, this agent should be avoided until all temporary clips have been removed and appropriate placement of the permanent clip is confirmed (17). Others have advocated administration of anesthetic agents (e.g., etomidate, propofol, thiopental) to the point of EEG burst suppression. Whereas each of these agents has been demonstrated to protect the ischemic brain in animal models, only thiopental has demonstrated efficacy in a clinical setting. Nonetheless, some centers still preferentially use etomidate because it is associated with hemodynamic stability or propofol because it has a short duration of action. The mechanism of action for each of these drugs is controversial. Because the use of any of these pharmacologic "neuroprotectants" may result in delayed awakening at the end of surgery, consideration should be given to using an anesthetic technique that uses only small amounts of narcotics and depends on a scalp block (using 0.5% bupivacaine or equivalent), placed at the end of surgery, to provide adequate postoperative analgesia.

The most exciting new area of research related to the intraoperative management of patients with cerebral aneurysms involves use of mild to moderate hypothermia (33° to 35°C) for neuroprotection. Significant evidence in animal models suggests that this degree of hypothermia protects the ischemic brain by decreasing the production of excitatory amino acids and other neurotoxic pathways. Currently, a multicenter study is underway to evaluate the benefits and disadvantages of administering mild to moderate hypothermia in patients having cerebral aneurysm surgery.

Arteriovenous Malformations

Maintenance of adequate mean arterial pressure as well as cerebral perfusion pressure are vital, especially for patients with large AVMs that may involve shunting of blood from normal areas. AVM resection is often associated with significant blood loss, especially if the AVM is linked to a large feeding vessel, a sinus, or dural vessels. In patients with a dural AVM, removal of the skull and opening of the dural layer can trigger significant bleeding. Re-rupture of the AVM prior to surgical exposure of the lesion often makes the lesion impossible to repair. Once the AVM has been successfully addressed, intraoperative angiography may be performed to confirm the results.

After removal of a large AVM, the surgeons may define a specific blood pressure range that they believe will reduce the likelihood of normal pressure cerebral edema. There is no scientific means of determining the optimal pressure range for an individual patient. Often, the pressure goal is defined at approximately 20% lower than the patient's average preoperative blood pressure. This blood pressure range is often maintained for the first 24 postoperative hours and then gradually allowed to return to baseline over the subsequent 24 hours, while carefully monitoring the patient for changes in neurologic function. Short-acting intravenous agents are advisable for blood pressure control (e.g., esmolol, nitroprusside, phentolamine).

At completion of surgery, the objective of the anesthesiologist is to extubate an awakening patient to permit a complete neurologic examination. A decreased level of consciousness demands distinction between surgical complication and residual anesthetic. If end-tidal inhaled anesthetic concentration is less than 0.2%, and the patient has impaired neurologic function, consideration should be given to the administration of narcotic and benzodiazepine reversal agents (if necessary, postoperative analgesia is provided with a scalp block). Naloxone should be titrated to produce the neurologic examination that proves to the care providers (neurosurgeons, anesthesiologists, nurses) that the patient does not have an underlying neurosurgical problem that needs rapid treatment (e.g., poorly positioned clip). Rapid administration of large doses of naloxone may produce significant cardiovascular stress, associated with myocardial ischemia in patients who are at risk. Observation in the ICU allows for continuous neurologic observation and early detection of complications.

Giant Aneurysms

Giant aneurysms may be clipped under routine general anesthesia or surgeons may request that the patient be managed with circulatory arrest to provide a bloodless field in which to isolate and control the aneurysm. Circulatory arrest is typically achieved with cardiopulmonary bypass. Barbiturate therapy, either by bolus dosing or continuous infusion, is used to achieve an EEG pattern of burst suppression. Hypothermia is added once EEG suppression is achieved to additionally lower cerebral metabolic requirements and to protect the ischemic brain by mechanisms that appear to be linked to a reduced production of excitatory amino acids. The goal of hypothermic arrest is 15° to 18°C.

Circulatory arrest is routinely limited to 60 minutes and requires systemic heparinization. To avoid the arrhythmias associated with profound hypothermia, the heart should be arrested either electrically with cardioversion or chemically with potassium chloride. Hemodilution by phlebotomy and replacement with crystalloid solutions may be employed to treat the increased blood viscosity associated with hypothermia. The patient should also be monitored for signs of hypothermia-induced coagulopathy and hyperglycemia. Patients with significant coexisting disease may not be candidates for circulatory arrest because of these risks.

Once the aneurysm is successfully clipped and meticulous hemostasis has been achieved, the patient is rewarmed. As the patient regains spontaneous circulation, heparinization is reversed. Phlebotomized blood may be returned to the patient, and any coagulopathy and electrolyte abnormalities should be corrected. Clipping under circulatory arrest routinely requires postoperative mechanical ventilation in the ICU, with extubation accomplished following emergence from the barbiturate therapy.

NEW TECHNIQUES

Aneurysms

Recently, alternatives to surgical clipping have been developed. Because of the development of high-quality microcatheters, it is now often possible to treat aneurysms, either ruptured or unruptured, with invasive neuroradiologic techniques. Early techniques dispensed microballoons into the aneurysm sac and assumed that endothelium would quickly cover the aneurysm orifice. Unfortunately, this was not reliable and many patients died with aneurysm rupture, either during or shortly following balloon placement. Thrombosis of some aneurysms can be performed using detachable coils placed into the aneurysm during angiography. Once each coil is in place in the aneurysm sac, an electrical charge is used to stiffen the coil, which in turn prevents its ability to leave the sac and produce a potentially lethal embolus. Small aneurysms with narrow necks as well as aneurysms that are difficult to access surgically may be candidates for this procedure. These patients should be monitored in an intensive care setting postprocedure because they carry the same postoperative risks as surgical candidates. Patients with multiple aneurysms may be treated with both coiling and surgery depending on the location and morphology of the aneurysms. In a prospective, randomized, single center study morbidity and mortality was similar for patients treated with endovascular versus surgical treatment of ruptured cerebral aneurysms (18). However, since this study is so recent, it is too early to determine the long-term influence on rebleeding rate.

Coiling of aneurysms in the neuroradiology suite is performed under general anesthesia with routine monitors plus invasive arterial blood pressure monitoring. Central venous monitoring may also be indicated in certain patients with significant coexisting disease. Continuous monitoring by anesthesia personnel is required, and a neurosurgical team needs to be available to provide backup support throughout the entire perioperative period should emergent surgical intervention become necessary.

Arteriovenous Malformations

The most common nonoperative approach that is used for patients with small AVMs is computer-directed radiosurgery.

Although relatively noninvasive, full treatment response using radiosurgery is not realized for months after initial treatment. Thus, a persistent rebleeding risk exists after radiosurgery, as compared with traditional surgical intervention. Some AVMs can be embolized using angiographic techniques, rarely for cure, but more commonly as an adjunct to surgery. Presurgical embolization can shrink the size of the AVM, allowing easier surgical repair as well as smaller risk of postoperative complications. The larger the AVM, the more shunt exists, which alters the blood flow patterns of the surrounding normal brain tissue. Embolization must be used cautiously in patients with a large AVM because excessive embolization in a single session may result in rapid transition of the shunt flow to the normal tissue with severe flow-mediated brain edema. Gradual embolization of a large AVM over several sessions allows these areas of brain to return to a normal perfusion pattern prior to surgery. These procedures are most often performed during general anesthesia to assure a cooperative patient during delicate manipulation of the microcatheters into the feeding AVM vessels.

COMPLICATIONS

Once an aneurysm ruptures, the risk of rebleeding is 25% during the first 2 weeks, and 50% of patients experience rebleeding within 6 months of the first hemorrhage. One year after the original hemorrhage, the risk of rebleeding is 3% per year for the remainder of the patient's life. The risk of rebleeding for patients with an AVM is much lower, approximately 6% in the first year. As stated, an aneurysm or AVM may rebleed intraoperatively at multiple stages of the procedure. Rupture may occur at induction, during placement of a lumbar or lateral ventricular drain, while placing the patient's head in a Mayfield head holder, during removal of the bone flap, or during dissection. Re-rupture prior to isolation of the aneurysm is usually catastrophic. If the rupture occurs after dissection is complete, it may be possible to gain control and complete the procedure, though outcome is usually still poor.

Cerebral edema as a result of surgical manipulation or ischemia can occur postoperatively and may present as a depression in the level of consciousness or a new neurologic deficit. Edema with accompanying mass shift can be identified on CT scan and is treated with ICP lowering agents such as mannitol or hypertonic saline. Glucocorticoids are also often administered in the setting of edema from a variety of different etiologies, without clear evidence for efficacy. In severe cases, invasive monitoring of ICP may be indicated. In life-threatening situations, the surgeons may decide to perform a craniectomy in an attempt to abort an evolving compartment syndrome or even remove brain tissue in noneloquent regions. Hydrocephalus may develop due to cerebrospinal fluid outflow obstruction by clotted blood or blood products. Clinically, the patient usually develops progressive obtundation. Treatment may include an intraventricular catheter (drain) or a ventriculoperitoneal shunt.

Seizures may also develop before or after surgical repair. Seizures are associated with rebleeding but it is controversial whether the rebleeding is the cause of the seizures or the seizures are the cause of the rebleeding. Some authors have suggested that abnormal movement in these patients is due to posturing, rather than seizure activity. Nonetheless, anticonvulsant therapy is routine following SAH in patients with an aneurysm or AVM. After recovery from surgical correction of the underlying cause of SAH, approximately 10% of patients will develop a chronic seizure disorder requiring long-term pharmacologic therapy.

Vasospasm

Although the syndrome of delayed neurologic deficits following aneurysmal SAH has been termed "vasospasm," the pathophysiology of this disease process is more likely related to excessive thickening of the arterial wall (mostly the media), rather than actual active spasm of the blood vessel. Vasospasm has also been demonstrated less often in patients with SAH following rupture of an AVM, as compared to patients with SAH following rupture of an aneurysm. This may be related to clot formation in the area of the major feeding arterial blood vessels following aneurysmal SAH. Because structural changes in the vessel wall underlie the pathology of vasospasm, onset of symptoms are delayed for at least 3 days following SAH. The peak incidence of symptoms related to vasospasm is from 4 to 14 days following SAH. Whereas as many as 70% of patients demonstrate evidence of cerebral arterial narrowing by angiography, clinically symptomatic vasospasm occurs in only approximately 30% of patients following aneurysmal SAH. Symptoms of vasospasm may be quite variable and subtle depending on the degree and location of arterial narrowing.

Any patient who develops neurologic deterioration without evidence of rebleeding or hydrocephalus (diagnosed by CT scan) should be suspected of having clinically relevant vasospasm. Symptoms develop gradually, and vary from increasing drowsiness or stupor to focal neurologic deficits. Cerebral ischemia develops due to inadequate cerebral blood flow to brain tissue as a result of vessel narrowing. Proximal narrowing of large conducting vessels is associated with vasodilation of distal vessels in the affected area, causing a paradoxic increase in blood volume and ICP. Brain edema also develops, contributing to more ischemia. Although angiography is the "gold standard" for establishing the diagnosis of vasospasm, transcranial Doppler studies may demonstrate increased cerebral blood flow velocity that correlate with angiographic vasospasm (19). In the presence of vasospasm, affected brain regions do not respond normally to hypoxia or hypercapnia. In fact, some investigators have determined when to stop their therapy for vasospasm in patients depending on when they exhibit return of normal vascular reactivity (using transcranial Doppler or xenon measurement techniques) in response to hypercapnia or a change in blood pressure.

Severity of vasospasm correlates with the amount of blood present in the subarachnoid space. Reduced perfusion appears to be most prominent in (but not entirely limited to) vascular territories with the largest accumulation of clot. Because blood is more likely to bathe the large cerebral blood vessels at the base of the brain, SAH following aneurysm rupture is more likely to be associated with the syndrome of delayed ischemic neurologic deficit than SAH following AVM bleeding. For this reason, neurosurgeons support early surgery and intraoperative removal of as much subarachnoid blood as soon as possible. Vasospasm is strongly linked to poor outcome and carries significant mortality and morbidity (2).

The mechanism of vasospasm remains controversial. Some believe that vessel wall thickening is due to an inflammatory vasculopathy that results in changes in the vessel wall morphology. A variety of morphologic changes in vasospastic vessel walls have been demonstrated in laboratory studies. Different factors have been linked to these changes, including oxygen free radicals, neutrophils, hemoglobin degradation products, prostaglandins, calcium, and other biologic peptides (20). Calcium channel blockers are used to treat vasospasm based on these studies, although their benefit probably relates to an ability to protect the ischemic brain, since administration does not result in changes in vessel diameter. Nonsteroidal antiinflammatory agents may also prevent vasculopathy via their effects on prostaglandins. Recently, a nonglucocorticoid 21-aminosteroid, tirilazad mesylate, has been demonstrated to improve outcome in men following aneurysmal SAH, suggesting that oxygen radicals may be important in the underlying mechanism of brain injury in this disease process (21).

Primary treatment of vasospasm revolves around prevention of its occurrence that is achieved by early surgery and removal of subarachnoid blood as well as early administration of calcium channel blockers to prevent the sequelae of ischemia. The use of antiinflammatory and antioxidant agents is becoming more common as a means of decreasing the intensity of vascular narrowing and brain injury associated with vasospasm, although clinically unproven. Once vasospasm has occurred, the goal is prevention of cerebral injury from the resulting ischemia. The therapies used in the treatment of vasospasm will be discussed further in the section on postoperative management in the ICU. If medical therapies do not succeed, attempts can be made to dilate the vessels endovascularly, either with balloon angioplasty or by direct infusion of vasodilatory agents such as papaverine. These techniques carry considerable risk, and often require multiple procedures, as the positive effects are short in duration.

HYPEREMIA AND NORMAL PERFUSION PRESSURE BREAKTHROUGH

After resection of an AVM and removal of the preexisting shunt, cerebral tissue subject to chronic hypoperfusion suddenly receives normal blood flow. These regions then may develop hyperemia, edema, or hemorrhage. Normal perfusion pressures lead to cerebral hyperemia, a phenomenon termed normal perfusion pressure breakthrough by Spetzler et al. (5). According to Spetzler's theory, chronically hypoperfused areas lose autoregulation and are unable to adapt to the increase in blood flow after the shunt is removed, leading to edema and hemorrhage. Patients with preoperative neurologic deficits secondary to shunting and those with an AVM greater than 4 cm in diameter (particularly those with a deep arterial supply) seem to have a higher incidence of this phenomenon. Staged removal of the AVM or surgery after preoperative embolization may allow chronically hypoperfused areas to regain normal autoregulation and prevent postoperative hyperemia.

Edema and hemorrhage may also occur as a result of venous outflow obstruction due to thrombosis secondary to decreases in blood flow after removal of the shunt. Surgical ligation of draining veins may also lead to outflow obstruction and hyperemia. Intraoperative hypothermia or deep barbiturate anesthesia may prevent postoperative hyperemic complications. Measurement of cerebral blood flow with xenon techniques demonstrates an increase in perfusion to affected areas of brain after removal of the AVM. Histologically, at least in animal models, blood vessels in brain regions adjacent to AVMs appear to have a decreased number of astrocytic foot processes, which is suggestive of an impaired blood–brain barrier function and higher likelihood of developing cerebral edema after removal of the AVM (22).

POSTOPERATIVE MANAGEMENT IN THE INTENSIVE CARE UNIT

Aneurysm

The goals of postoperative care are the prevention and treatment of the complications of SAH. Ischemia secondary to initial hemorrhage as well as posthemorrhage complications are main contributors to the morbidity and mortality associated with the condition. Postoperatively, the patient may still require endotracheal intubation and mechanical ventilation. The goal is extubation in a timely fashion if possible, as poor synchronization of the ventilator places the patient at risk of rebleeding (if unclipped aneurysms still exist) and increased ICP. Patients with low Glasgow Coma Scores and significant neurologic deficits often require prolonged mechanical ventilation and ultimately tracheostomy.

Blood pressure should be maintained within the normal range after surgical repair to prevent cerebral ischemia due to inadequate cerebral perfusion. Administration of vasopressor agents may be necessary to maintain cerebral perfusion pressure, and anticonvulsant therapy and antibiotics should be continued postoperatively. Calcium channel blockers such as nimodipine are often added to prevent symptoms of ischemia due to vasospasm-induced reduction in cerebral perfusion.

Any alteration in neurologic status should be aggressively investigated. A complete neurologic examination should be performed to identify any new focal deficits. A CT scan should be performed if patient stability permits to rule out hemorrhage, edema, or hydrocephalus. A new hemorrhage may be treated by surgical evacuation or with medical management depending on the size and location. Acute hydrocephalus may be treated with ventriculostomy and drainage, often with dramatic improvement of symptoms. Elevation in ICP as a consequence of brain edema can be treated acutely with mannitol, hypertonic saline, and hyperventilation (if the patient is mechanically ventilated).

If the above causes of neurologic deterioration have been excluded, vasospasm should be suspected. This is a diagnosis of exclusion since the presence of narrowed arterial blood vessels does not prove that this is the cause of the altered neurologic state. Increased cerebral blood flow velocities by transcranial Doppler flow studies may support the diagnosis. Vasospasm most commonly occurs 4 to 9 days posthemorrhage but can occur earlier, especially if the hemorrhage is large. Treatment focuses on trying to prevent ischemia (blood flow enhancement) and the sequelae of the evolving ischemia (e.g., calcium channel blockers, oxygen radical scavengers) until the vasospasm resolves.

Based on the assumption that the narrowed vessels result in decreased blood flow to brain tissue, volume expansion is employed to increase flow. It is assumed that the areas at risk have impaired autoregulation and, therefore, cerebral blood flow is dependent upon perfusion pressure. Crystalloids, colloids, and hypertonic saline are used to increase blood volume. Central venous pressure monitoring or pulmonary artery pressure monitoring, as well as arterial blood pressure monitoring, are essential to monitor intravascular volume as well as to watch for fluid overload.

Two problems may occur as a result of this treatment. Patients with normal kidney function may diurese the extra volume at the same rate or greater than the infusion, making it difficult to maintain goals. The diuresis may also cause the loss of essential electrolytes and related complications and, therefore, electrolyte concentrations should be closely monitored. Patients with heart disease or compromised renal function may develop congestive heart failure as a result of therapy. Strict monitoring of input and output is vital. Goals include cardiac output ranges of 6 to 8 L per minute and arterial occlusion wedge pressures in the range of 15 to 18 mm Hg. Fluid management in patients with SAH is further complicated by the common syndrome of cerebral salt-wasting in some patients and the less common syndrome of inappropriate antidiuretic hormone secretion in other patients (23). In addition, dilutional hyponatremia may also occur as a result of volume infusion so electrolytes must be monitored closely.

In addition to volume expansion, hypertension and hemodilution are employed. This is known as "triple H" therapy: hypertensive, hypervolemic, hemodilution. Hematocrit is maintained at approximately 25% to 30% to reduce blood viscosity and improve blood flow, while maintaining adequate oxygen carrying capacity.

Systemic blood pressure is elevated to increase cerebral blood flow and maintain perfusion pressure. In patients who have not undergone surgical clipping, induced hypertension should be more conservative to avoid re-rupture. Vasopressor agents such as phenylephrine or dopamine may be necessary in addition to volume expansion in order to maintain blood pressure goals. Volume expansion should be employed judiciously to avoid development of a dilutional coagulopathy. Once the goals of hypertensive, hypervolemic, hemodilution therapy are achieved, therapy should be continued until signs of vasospasm have resolved. Patients often show dramatic improvement in symptoms after therapy is initiated. Therapy should be weaned slowly as tolerated, as symptomatology may reappear with lowering of perfusion pressure. If symptoms do not improve with therapy, angioplasty techniques such as balloon dilation or direct injection of vasodilating agents may be attempted. The short-term benefits of these procedures must be weighed against the risk of vessel rupture.

Arteriovenous Malformations

Normal perfusion pressure breakthrough after AVM resection and postoperative hyperemia are treated by lowering blood pressure (consideration should be given to using nitroprusside, esmolol, labetalol, or phentolamine) and ICP (osmotic diuretics and head-up positioning). ICP monitoring may be useful for monitoring the progress of disease, particularly when there is a decrease in level of neurologic function. If neurologic function is significantly impaired, consideration should be given to securing the patient's airway. With increased ICP, more aggressive measures such as pharmacologic-induced coma to reduce cerebral blood flow and ICP may be required.

OUTCOME

With appropriate surgical and perioperative care many patients recover following SAH and continue to lead a productive life. Intensive care may be required for an extended period if vasospasm-induced cerebral ischemia persists. Recovery is often slow, and ultimately 30% of patients do not survive or remain severely disabled (15). Up to 50% of survivors have some level of psychosocial or cognitive deficit. Although mortality has decreased with earlier diagnosis and treatment, morbidity remains high.

FUTURE DEVELOPMENTS

Advances in endovascular technology will continue to expand therapeutic options for patients with an aneurysm or AVM. Although endovascular therapy has the same complications such as bleeding, rupture, and vasospasm, interventional neuroradiology does not require a craniotomy or a deep plane of anesthesia. Much of aneurysm research today focuses on the etiology of vasospasm and how to prevent its occurrence. Several recent studies have evaluated whether blocking some of the factors potentially linked to vasospasm with agents such as calcium channel blockers and antiinflammatories affect the time-course of vasospasm. Urokinase and t-PA therapy have been evaluated in the prevention of vasospasm through clot lysis (24). In addition, laboratory studies in rats using implantable controlled-release polymers containing ibuprofen have demonstrated inhibition of vasospasm (25). Early surgery, removal of clot from the subarachnoid space, and irrigation of the area to remove potential vasospastic factors have all been advocated.

SUMMARY

SAH as a result of cerebral aneurysm and AVM continues to be a significant cause of morbidity and mortality despite recent technological advances. Although improvements in surgical technique as well as preoperative and postoperative intensive care have allowed for earlier diagnosis and treatment, they have not alleviated the significant complications associated with this disease. Future research and development hopefully will be able to prevent or better treat the sequelae of SAH.

KEY POINTS

- Subarachnoid hemorrhage (SAH) due to cerebral aneurysm or arteriovenous malformation (AVM) is associated with significant morbidity and mortality that is due to increased intracranial pressure (initial hemorrhage and delayed hydrocephalus), blood-induced seizure activity, and delayed ischemic neurologic deficits (vasospasm).
- Surgical or neuroradiologic intervention is the treatment of choice for ruptured aneurysms or AVMs, as well as for symptomatic or larger unruptured aneurysms or AVMs.
- Although the exact mechanism of vasospasm is unclear, treatment involves blood flow promotion (e.g., angioplasty, hypertension, hemodilution, hypervolemia) and protection of the ischemic brain (e.g., calcium channel blockers, oxygen radical scavengers).
- Normal perfusion pressure breakthrough may occur after aggressive single-stage resection of an AVM and results in cerebral ischemia secondary to hyperemia in areas adapted to decreases in cerebral perfusion pressure.
- Meticulous medical management (e.g., control of blood pressure, electrolytes, respiratory variables) in the perioperative period is probably associated with improved neurologic outcome following SAH.

REFERENCES

1. Kirsch JR, Diringer MN, Borel CO, et al. Cerebral aneurysms: mechanisms of injury and critical care interventions. *Crit Care Clin* 1989;5:755–772.
2. Tamargo RJ, Walter KA, Oshiro EM. Aneurysmal subarachnoid hemorrhage: prognostic features and outcomes. *New Horizons* 1997;5:364–375.
3. Stein BM, Wolpert SM. Arteriovenous malformations of the brain. I. Current concepts and treatment. *Arch Neurol* 1980;37:1–5.
4. Hashimoto T, Emala CW, Joshi S, et al. Abnormal pattern of Tie-2 and vascular endothelial growth factor receptor expression in human cerebral arteriovenous malformations. *Neurosurgery* 2000;47:910–918.
5. Spetzler RF, Wilson CB, Weinstein P, et al. Normal perfusion pressure breakthrough theory. *Clin Neurosurg* 1978;25:651–672.
6. Kassell NF, Torner JC. The international cooperative study on timing of aneurysm surgery—an update. *Stroke* 1984;15:566–570.

7. Iwanaga H, Wakai S, Ochiai C, et al. Ruptured cerebral aneurysms missed by initial angiographic study. *Neurosurgery* 1990;27:45–51.
8. Sipos EP, Kirsch JR, Nauta HJ, et al. Intra-arterial urokinase for treatment of retrograde thrombosis following resection of an arteriovenous malformation. Case report. *J Neurosurg* 1992;76:1004–1007.
9. Hunt WE, Hess RM. Surgical risk as related to time of intervention in the repair of intracranial aneurysms. *J Neurosurg* 1968;28:14–20.
10. Oshiro EM, Walter KA, Piantadosi S, et al. A new subarachnoid hemorrhage grading system based on the Glasgow Coma Scale: a comparison with the Hunt and Hess and World Federation of Neurological Surgeons scales in clinical series. *Neurosurgery* 1997;41:140–148.
11. Spetzler RF, Zabramski JM. Grading and staged resection of cerebral arteriovenous malformations. *Clin Neurosurg* 1990;36:318–337.
12. Barker FG, Ogilvy CS. Efficacy of prophylactic nimodipine for delayed ischemic deficit after subarachnoid hemorrhage: a metaanalysis. *J Neurosurg* 1996;84:405–414.
13. Torbey M, Hauser TK, Bhardwaj A, et al. The effect of age on cerebral

blood flow velocities (CBFV) in patients with clinical vasospasm following subarachnoid hemorrhage (SAH). *J Neurosurg Anesth* 2000; 12:(4)404(abst).

14. Butzkueven H, Evans AH, Pitman A, et al. Onset seizures independently predict poor outcome after subarachnoid hemorrhage. *Neurology* 2000;14:1315–1320.

15. Kassell NF, Torner JC, Haley EC, et al. The international cooperative study on the timing of aneurysm surgery. Part 1: Overall management results. *J Neurosurg* 1990;73:18–36.

16. Hoffman WE, Wheeler P, Edelman G, et al. Hypoxic brain tissue following subarachnoid hemorrhage. *Anesthesiology* 2000;92:442–446.

17. Baughman VL, Hoffman WE, Thomas C, et al. The interaction of nitrous oxide and isoflurane with incomplete cerebral ischemia in the rat. *Anesthesiology* 1989;70:767–774.

18. Koivisto T, Vanninen R, Hurskainen H, et al. Outcomes of early endovascular versus surgical treatment of ruptured cerebral aneurysms: a prospective randomized study. *Stroke* 2000;31:2369–2377.

19. Sekhar LN, Wechsler LR, Yonas H, et al. Value of transcranial Doppler examination in the diagnosis of cerebral vasospasm after subarachnoid hemorrhage. *Neurosurgery* 1988;22:813–821.

20. Chyatte D, Sundt TM. Cerebral vasospasm after subarachnoid hemorrhage. *Mayo Clin Proc* 1984;59:498–505.

21. Kassell NF, Haley EC, Appersonhansen C, et al. Randomized, double-blind, vehicle-controlled trial of tirilazad mesylate in patients with aneurysmal subarachnoid hemorrhage—a cooperative study in Europe, Australia, and New Zealand. *J Neurosurg* 1996;84:221–228.

22. Sekhon LH, Morgan MK, Spence I. Normal perfusion pressure breakthrough: the role of capillaries. *J Neurosurg* 1997;86:519–524.

23. Diringer MN, Lim JS, Kirsch JR, et al. Suprasellar and intraventricular blood predict elevated plasma atrial natriuretic factor in subarachnoid hemorrhage. *Stroke* 1991;22:577–581.

24. Zabramski JM, Spetzler RF, Lee KS, et al. Phase I trial of tissue plasminogen activator for the prevention of vasospasm in patients with aneurysmal subarachnoid hemorrhage. *J Neurosurg* 1991;75:189–196.

25. Thai QA, Oshiro EM, Tamargo RJ. Inhibition of experimental vasospasm in rats with the periadventitial administration of ibuprofen using controlled-release polymers. *Stroke* 1999;30:140–147.

24

THE DIAGNOSIS AND MANAGEMENT OF BRAIN-DEAD AND NONHEART-BEATING ORGAN DONORS

JEFFREY S. PLOTKIN
MEGUMI NAKAMURA
AKE GRENVIK

KEY WORDS

- Brain death, diagnosis
- Brain scan
- Brainstem auditing evoked potentials
- Diabetes insipidus
- Electroencephalogram
- Hepatic transplantation
- Nonheart-beating organ donor
- Renal transplantation
- Transplantation

INTRODUCTION

Transplantation of abdominal and thoracic organs is an accepted and important therapeutic intervention in the treatment of end-stage organ disease. In 1999, 21,692 transplants were performed, while by October 20, 2000, 72,582 patients were waiting on all organ transplant lists combined (1).

The major obstacle to transplantation today is the limited supply of organs. An estimated 12,000 to 27,000 potential organ donors die by brain death each year in the United States. However, only 15% to 20% become actual donors (2). Although the number of patients on the waiting list increases every year, the number of donors has remained relatively constant. Therefore, it is incumbent upon the critical care physician to recognize and ensure sound physiologic management of the brain-dead organ donor to maximize the availability and optimal function of donated organs.

HISTORICAL PERSPECTIVES

The first successful solid-organ transplant was performed in 1954 by Murray and associates at the Peter Bent Brigham Hospital in Boston, with transplantation of a kidney from an identical twin to his brother (3). The recipient survived with a functioning kidney for 9 years. In 1956, Starzl and colleagues performed the first liver transplants in animals, and, in 1963, the first successful human

liver transplant (4). The first successful human lung transplant was performed by Hardy in 1963 (5), and the first human heart transplant by Barnard in Capetown, South Africa in 1967 (6).

Although previous reports have described the lethal cessation of cerebral blood flow due to trauma or disease, resulting in so-called "respirator brains" (2), the definition of brain death was first conceived by Mollaret and Goulon in 1959, when they described *coma dépassé* (literally translated as "beyond coma") as the loss of all reflex and electrical activity (7). The initial breakthrough in the legal concept of brain death came in August 1968 when the Harvard Committee, under the chairmanship of Beecher (former Chief of Anesthesiology at the Massachusetts General Hospital), published its definition of brain death (8). The term used, "irreversible coma," was obviously translated from Mollaret and Goulon's coma dépassé. The main Harvard criteria for brain death were summarized as: (a) unreceptivity and unresponsiveness, (b) absent movements or respirations, (c) absent reflexes, and (d) flat electroencephalogram (EEG). Also in 1968, the Uniform Anatomical Gift Act, now adopted by all 50 states, made organ donation possible by legalizing organ removal from a brain-dead, heart-beating cadaver.

The Uniform Determination of Death Act, jointly drafted by the American Bar Association and the American Medical Association in 1981 at the National Conference of Commissioners on Uniform State Laws, states that "an individual is dead if there is irreversible cessation of circulatory and respiratory functions, or if there is irreversible cessation of all functions of the entire brain, including the brainstem." When organ donation is not an issue, however, the traditional criteria for certification of death based on cessation of cardiopulmonary function are still the most commonly used.

The President's Commission on Ethical Problems in Medicine, also in 1981, published guidelines to define death (9). Included in this report are the following: (a) cerebral and brainstem functions must be absent, (b) the cause of death must be known and exclude recovery, and (c) cessation of all brain function must persist during a period of observation and treatment. Unlike the Harvard criteria, absent central nervous system (CNS) function is limited to the brain above the foramen magnum, since spinal cord reflexes often persist in brain death. The commission went on to state that criteria used to determine brain death should be explicit and accessible to verification, be adaptable to various clinical situations, avoid unreasonable delay, minimize errors classifying a dead person as alive, and, most important, eliminate errors classifying a living person as dead.

DETERMINATION AND DIAGNOSIS OF BRAIN DEATH

The technological and scientific advances of the twentieth century have made it possible to sustain cardiorespiratory function in the absence of neurologic survival. The Harvard Ad Hoc Committee, the President's Commission on Ethical Problems in Medicine, and the Uniform Determination of Death Act have made possible an earlier diagnosis of death based on neurologic criteria, while maintaining the possibility of certifying death based on traditional cardiorespiratory criteria. This distinction is necessary to provide for discontinuation of cardiorespiratory support in heart-beating, brain-dead cadavers, while, more important, permitting procurement of perfused, healthy organs for transplantation.

A distinction must be made between cerebral death, brainstem death, and whole-brain death. The United States accepts only whole-brain death, while the United Kingdom is satisfied with brainstem death as proof of death of the individual. No legal precedent, in any country, currently exists for equating cerebral death with brain death.

Equating life to function of the entire brain forms the foundation for the whole-brain concept of brain death. A person may, therefore, be declared dead only when it is proven that the function of the entire brain is permanently and irrevocably absent. Many groups have published whole-brain criteria for death. Common to all is that a careful neurologic examination must be performed, which must document no movement, including shivering, decorticate, and decerebrate posturing; no seizures; no

TABLE 1. CRITERIA FOR WHOLE-BRAIN DEATH

Loss of brainstem function
  Absent cranial nerve reflexes
    Pupillary light reflex
    Corneal reflex
    Oculocephalic reflex
    Oculovestibular reflex
    Gag reflex
    Cough reflex
  Absent respiratory brainstem reflex
    Apnea test
  Negative atropine test
Loss of cortical function
  No spontaneous movements
  No response to external stimuli
    Verbal
    Deep pain
Irreversibility
  Cause known and sufficient to account for brain death
  No improvement for 2 to 24 hrs

TABLE 2. CONDITIONS THAT CONFOUND THE DIAGNOSIS OF BRAIN DEATH

Shock	Hypothermia (<32°C)
Anesthetics	Paralytics
Methaqualone	Barbiturates
Diazepam	High-dose bretylium
Meprobomate	Mecloqualone
Trichloroethylene	Amitriptyline
Alcohols	Narcotics
Brainstem encephalitis	Guillain-Barré syndrome
Hepatic encephalopathy	Uremic encephalopathy
Hyperosmolar coma	Meningitis

response to verbal stimuli; no cranial nerve reflexes; and no respiratory efforts in the presence of hypercarbia. Table 1 lists specific neurologic criteria for certification of death. However, confounding conditions that may mimic brain death, listed in Table 2, may be present and necessitate confirmation of brain death through additional tests, such as four-vessel cerebral arteriography, discussed below.

As previously stated, a declaration of brain death requires that the function of the entire brain must be absent, and as such, also requires testing of brainstem and cortical function, as well as proof of irreversibility. Necessary clinical examinations and observations include:

1. Pupils are characteristically in the midposition (3 to 7 mm in diameter) and do not exhibit a pupillary light reflex to direct or consensual light. (It should be noted that this reflex may be altered by atropine, catecholamines, eye trauma or surgery, cataracts, scopolamine, and monoamine oxidase inhibitors.)
2. Corneal reflexes are absent.
3. The oculocephalic reflex (doll's eyes response) is absent (i.e., the eyes fail to cross the midline when the head is turned).
4. The oculovestibular reflex (cold water calorics test) is negative (i.e., 20 to 50 mL of ice water injected into the external ear canal fails to produce nystagmus). Of note, tricyclic antidepressants, anticholinergics, anticonvulsants, and some sedatives may alter this response.
5. Negative respiratory brainstem reflex (i.e., no respiratory efforts at a $PaCO_2$ greater than 60 mm Hg).
6. Failure of the heart rate to increase by more than 5 beats per minute after 1 to 2 mg of intravenous (i.v.) atropine, proving absence of vagal nuclear and, thus, vagal nerve function.

The respiratory brainstem reflex is tested using the apnea test. In practice, the patient should be preoxygenated with 100% oxygen for at least 5 minutes before disconnecting mechanical ventilation. During the period of apnea, oxygenation can be provided with 4 to 6 L per minute of oxygen via a tracheal tube cannula or T-piece to avoid hypoxemia with the attendant risks of hypotension, arrhythmias, and even cardiac arrest. Pulse oximetry is valuable as a monitoring device during this period. The test should be aborted if any of the above events occur. Lengthy test time is avoided if the patient is first hypoventilated to a $PaCO_2$ greater than 40 mm Hg (10). The atropine test should be performed before the apnea test to avoid the necessity of the apnea test should the former reveal an increase in heart rate.

Irreversible brain death is assumed if the cause of brain death is known and accepted to be sufficient to account for death. Further, irreversibility is assumed if the neurologic examination, as outlined previously, results in a diagnosis of brain death, and these results do not change on a subsequent examination, generally 2 to 12 hours later (the time between examinations varies among institutions). In cases in which the inciting event was anoxic in nature, the observation period is usually extended to 24 hours (10). Even when the patient meets all the aforementioned criteria, and is clinically and legally dead, some evidence of nerve cell function may exist. For example, not all patients become poikilothermic; spontaneous depolarizations may be detected by deeply placed electrodes despite an isoelectric EEG (11); and hypothalamic and pituitary function may continue despite no blood flow to the brain, as documented by four-vessel angiography.

Brainstem death, accepted since the mid-1970s by the United Kingdom as equaling death, requires only testing of brainstem reflexes to document death. This definition assumes that interruption of fibers within the reticular activating system in the pons and midbrain leads to a noncognitive state. Criteria set forth by the Conference of Medical Royal Colleges are otherwise almost identical to the brainstem criteria for the whole-brain definition of death used in the United States (Table 1) (12).

Cerebral death implies loss of neocortical function while brainstem function persists. Although not traditionally accepted as defining brain death, some aggressively advocate that it should (13). This proposal equates human life with cognition and awareness, thus implying that the loss of "personhood" defines death (14). Positron emission tomography, a relatively new technique to evaluate oxygen uptake and glucose metabolism in the brain, is one test that may be used to diagnose cerebral death, allowing objective measurement of absent cerebral metabolism. Those who oppose equating the persistent vegetative state with death question the ability to predict the permanence of such a state (15). Further, the so-called "slippery slope argument" implies the use of progressively less stringent criteria in response to societal pressures to diagnose death in patients in a persistent vegetative state. Although the proposal is possibly an attractive means of ending suffering and expense while simultaneously increasing the supply of donor organs, it seems very unlikely to become medically and legally acceptable in the near future.

A specific and controversial example of cerebral death (or, rather, cerebral absence) is anencephaly, a condition in which the newborn possesses a brainstem but no cerebrum. Each year in the United States, some 300 to 450 children need kidneys, while 400 to 600 need livers (16). These needs are not currently met by the number of brain-dead pediatric donors. If, however, anencephalic infants were used for organ donation, this problem might be solved (16). Anencephalic infants may breathe spontaneously owing to function of a rudimentary brainstem, but most die within 2 weeks from respiratory failure or infection (16). It should also be noted, however, that 20% have anomalies of other organs. Therefore, to be used as organ donors, these infants, with a functioning brainstem, would have to be resuscitated at birth and have their organs removed immediately. This sequence has occurred in Germany, where anencephalics are not considered to be alive human beings. Indeed, there is a report of successful kidney

transplantation from anencephalic donors in Germany (17). For this to become a reality in the United States, it would require a drastic redefinition of death to include those who are spontaneously breathing. It seems unlikely, however, that our society would consider breathing bodies dead and suitable for burial.

One of the controversies regarding the Harvard Criteria is whether they apply to infants and children. The brains of infants and young children appear to have greater resistance to damage although this issue is controversial and lacks convincing clinical documentation (18). Infants and young children may recover substantial brain function after periods of unresponsiveness that are longer than those from which adults can recover. The presence of open fontanelles and open sutures in young children makes the skull an expandable chamber. Therefore, intracranial pressure (ICP) does not exceed mean arterial pressure, and cerebral blood flow continues. In 1987, the Task Force for the Determination of Brain Death in Children endorsed the Determination of Death Act and offered the "Guidelines for the Determination of Brain Death in Children." The distinction from the criteria for adults are three separate longer observation periods depending on the child's age and the necessity of two agreeing EEGs or one EEG with confirming radionuclide angiography. However, multiple studies demonstrate that the adult criteria are applicable to infants and young children who are full term and more than 7 days of age (19–21), although there have been some reports criticizing this notion (22).

CONFIRMATORY TESTING FOR BRAIN DEATH

As stated earlier, additional testing may be necessary, in specific conditions (Table 2), to document loss of neuronal function or lack of cerebral blood flow. Having a definitive study such as a nuclear flow scan to confirm the diagnosis of brain death may help families with understanding and accepting brain death (23) (Table 3). Tests that have been used include EEG, evoked potentials (EP), nuclear blood flow studies, transcranial Doppler ultrasonography (TCD), and cerebral arteriography.

In many medical centers, EEG testing is no longer required for the diagnosis of brain death. Its value is severely limited by issues such as technical problems and inter-rater variability (24). Grigg and colleagues evaluated 56 clinically brain-dead patients and found diffuse widespread EEG activity in almost 20%,

TABLE 3. CONFIRMATORY TESTS FOR WHOLE-BRAIN CRITERIA

EEG
Evoked potentials
   Visual
   Somatosensory
   Brainstem auditory
Technetium-HMPAO scintigraphy
Transcranial Doppler
Xenon-enhanced computed tomography
Four-vessel angiography[a]

[a]"Gold standard."
EEG, electroencephalography.

reaffirming its diagnostic limitations. In addition, an isoelectric EEG confirms only loss of cerebral function, but gives no information regarding the brainstem or other deep brain structures (25).

EPs have been suggested by some as a confirmatory test for the diagnosis of brain death. Somatosensory and visual EPs are of no value in confirming brain death. Brainstem auditory evoked potentials (BAEPs), however, have shown limited value. In a study by Firsching and associates (26), absence of BAEPs confirmed brain death in only 31% of 85 patients studied. As this technique requires special equipment and training for interpretation, it appears to be of little clinical or economic value.

Xenon-enhanced computed tomography (CT) blood flow studies are of value in assessing the anterior cerebral circulation, but poorly visualize the posterior fossa and vertebral circulation. Technetium scintigraphy, on the other hand, shows some promise. Although free technetium does not cross the intact blood–brain barrier, the technetium-tagged tracer 99mTc-hexamethylpropylene amine oxime (^{99m}Tc-HMPAO) crosses it in proportion to tissue perfusion. In a study by Yatim and coworkers (27), ^{99m}Tc-HMPAO was compared with four-vessel angiography and yielded a 100% correlation in 17 cases. They further stated that no case had been published in the literature demonstrating persistence of cerebral blood flow by contrast angiography where ^{99m}Tc-HMPAO was negative. Kurtek and colleagues demonstrated that 19 of 23 patients who were clinically declared brain dead had no HMPAO cerebral uptake on the initial study (28). In the remaining four patients, the study showed a normal image in one, no cerebral flow but cerebellar flow in two, and no cerebellar flow but cerebral flow in one patient. This technique appears to be an easy, noninvasive alternative to four-vessel angiography. However, further studies will be required before adopting this test as a new "gold standard."

TCD is an attractive technique, since it can be performed noninvasively at the bedside and is easily learned. Feri and associates evaluated 37 patients consecutively. TCD revealed findings characteristic of brain death in 22 of the 37 patients with a clinical diagnosis of brain death, but not in the other 15 (29). Further studies are required, especially those comparing TCD to four-vessel angiography. TCD does, however, appear to be quite capable of documenting deteriorating cerebral perfusion pressure.

Nau and others (30) studied 50 patients with a clinical diagnosis of brain death, and subjected them to EEG, BAEP, TCD, and digital subtraction angiography (DSA). Agreement was reached in most cases, but some variation persisted, either due to true disparity of the test results or technical limitations. The authors concluded that the only reliable test to document brain death by whole-brain criteria remains four-vessel angiography.

Thus, four-vessel angiography still appears to be the "gold standard." This does not, however, imply the need for its routine use. Depending on state laws, clinical examination, in the absence of confounding factors, may be all that is required. If, however, any of the aforementioned confounding factors are present, angiography may be a way to diagnose brain death in a more timely fashion. In addition, with proper study and documentation, TCD or ^{99m}Tc-HMPAO scintigraphy may become the solution to prevent the need to transport unstable patients to the radiology department, as well as the need for i.v. dye, which may harm the potential donor kidneys.

PATHOPHYSIOLOGY AND INTENSIVE CARE UNIT MANAGEMENT

With the exception of extracranial malignancy, untreated sepsis, active tuberculosis, and human immunodeficiency virus (HIV) infection, all brain-dead patients should be considered potential organ donors. It is imperative that critical care physicians recognize all potential organ donors as rapidly as possible, since a delay in recognition can result in the loss of transplantable organs due to infection, shock, or even cardiac arrest leading to prolonged warm ischemia. It has been shown that 25% of potential donors are not recognized until 48 hours or more after development of brain death. This is a particular problem since 20% may suffer cardiovascular death within 6 hours and 50% within 24 hours of intensive care unit (ICU) admission (31). Knowledge of the conditions leading to brain death will alert the ICU physician to a potential donor. A study of 4,320 organ donors revealed the causes of brain death to be brain trauma in 55%, cerebral vascular accidents in 32%, asphyxiation or drowning in 4%, cardiovascular events in 2%, intoxication in 1%, and miscellaneous causes in 6% (32).

The initial management of these patients must revolve around protection of the injured brain to maximize the chances of meaningful neurologic recovery. Once the patient becomes recognized as brain dead and a potential organ donor, the management must shift to providing oxygen and blood delivery to transplantable organs. The critical care physician must, however, also demonstrate compassion when interacting with the families of organ donors to help them accept their loss and maximize the chances for organ donation and successful transplantation. In this regard, the first step must be to contact the local organ procurement agency to alert personnel to the possibility of an organ donor, and to obtain help in dealing with the families.

Standard management of these patients includes placement of intravascular catheters for hemodynamic monitoring, including radial arterial catheters, central venous or pulmonary arterial (PA) catheters, nasogastric tubes, urethral catheters, and large-bore i.v. catheters for volume replacement.

CARDIOVASCULAR EFFECTS AND INTERACTIONS

Significant cardiovascular changes occur during the development of, and immediately after, brain death. Novitzky and colleagues (33) described an "autonomic storm" occurring in baboons during sudden increases in ICP with abrupt onset of brain ischemia. Initially, a brief period of excessive parasympathetic activity occurred, manifested by marked bradycardia. Then a large increase in circulating catecholamines was noted, with epinephrine levels rising 11-fold, norepinephrine 3-fold, and dopamine 2-fold over baseline values within 5 minutes of the acute event. Ten minutes later, these levels had returned to baseline, and by the third hour, levels had fallen below baseline. A massive increase in systemic vascular resistance, produced by an extreme degree of peripheral vasoconstriction, occurred as a result of the catecholamine surge. Blood, therefore, redistributed to capacitance vessels and caused a rapid increase in venous return to the heart. The right heart was able to compensate for this tremendous increase in preload by increasing its output significantly, as demonstrated by a statistically significant increase in PA flow compared to aortic flow. However, the massive increase in systemic vascular resistance (SVR) led to temporary acute failure of the left ventricle (LV), resulting in transient mitral regurgitation and a steep increase in left atrial (LA) pressure. In fact, in most animals, LA pressure actually exceeded PA pressure for a few seconds during the period of peak peripheral vasoconstriction. One can easily envision how this would create increases in pulmonary capillary hydrostatic pressure, leading to sudden pulmonary edema and interstitial hemorrhage. These adverse effects actually occurred in 36% of the baboons, and may explain the phenomenon known as neurogenic pulmonary edema.

Novitsky and colleagues (33) further described five stages of ECG activity. Stage I consists of initial bradycardia, occasionally progressing to sinus arrest or a short period of atrioventricular dissociation, and lasting approximately 8 minutes. Stage II followed, with sinus tachycardia up to 160 beats per minute without ischemic changes, and lasted an average of 5 minutes. Stage III, lasting 15 minutes, was characterized by multifocal ventricular ectopic activity. This was followed by stage IV, which lasted approximately 2.5 hours. During stage IV, sinus tachycardia again became evident with the mean heart rate rising to 180 beats per minute and marked ischemic myocardial changes noted (Fig. 1). Finally, in stage V, heart rate returned to control levels or below. This stage lasted until the experiment was electively terminated at 17 hours. It should be noted, however, that 50% of the baboons continued to show QRS or ST segment abnormalities.

The authors also showed, in the same baboon model, that the catecholamine surge created coronary artery vasospasm, as evidenced by the presence of contraction bands in the smooth muscle of the arterial media and focal myocardial contraction band necrosis in 82%. These changes could be prevented by cardiac sympathectomy before induction of brain death, thereby strengthening the argument that these changes were, in fact, due to the catecholamine surge. Additional evidence of myocardial dysfunction is provided by Mertes and associates (34), who showed significant decreases in LV dp/dt in brain-dead pigs.

These animal studies were clinically correlated with human responses by Darracott-Cankovic and others (35). Using quantitative birefringence microscopy, they were able to show that despite similar sex, age, incidence of cardiac arrest, and level of inotropic support, 43% of donor hearts had impaired function before removal from the brain-dead donor, likely owing to the adverse oxygen supply/demand relationship already described. Impaired function was evidenced by primary nonfunction or the need for inotropic support after transplantation, although such malfunction may be caused by several factors.

After the hyperadrenergic state, severe hypotension often occurs and is multifactorial in origin. Destruction of pontine and medullary vasomotor centers, leading to total body vasoparalysis, secondary injury to the heart, volume depletion resulting from prior diuretic therapy, and other released hormones and chemicals are but a few explanations. The sequence of marked hypertension followed by extreme hypotension occurs in 50% of patients during the development of brain death (35).

Taking those consequences into account, and considering the need to minimize secondary myocardial injury during the hypercatecholamine phase, it would seem obvious to treat this hypertension and cardiac irritability with vasodilators and β-blockers that are both rapidly acting and rapidly metabolized. Sodium nitroprusside and esmolol, titrated as needed, are the recommended treatments. These infusions should be discontinued as

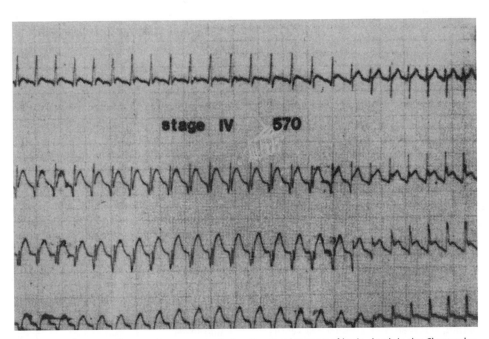

FIGURE 1. Electrocardiogram changes seen during the development of brain death in the Chacma baboon (stage IV, resembling acute myocardial infarction). (From Novitzky D, Harak A, Coope DK, et al. Electrocardiographic and histopathologic changes developing during experimental brain death in the baboon. *Transplant Proc* 1989;21:2567–2569, with permission.)

the hypercatecholamine state recedes, with preparations made to deal with the hypotension that may follow.

Initial therapy for hypotension should be volume expansion to attain a filling pressure (central venous pressure [CVP], pulmonary arterial occlusion pressure [PAOP]) of approximately 12 mm Hg. During fluid administration, one must consider the need for packed red blood cells to maintain a hematocrit of approximately 30% since this has been shown to maximize oxygen supply by optimizing the balance between oxygen content and blood flow related to changes in viscosity (36). Apart from these considerations, one must remember the possibility of the rapid loss of free water due to diabetes insipidus (see following) and choose fluids to avoid hypernatremia.

Vasopressors or inotropic agents are required in most donors (37). Dopamine has been the most widely used agent for the management of severe hypotension in these patients because it has the potential for maintaining or even increasing blood flow to the renal and mesenteric vasculature. Quesada and colleagues (37) show that as the dosage of dopamine increases, the chances of acute tubular necrosis in the grafted kidney increases. Interestingly, however, there is no difference in long-term graft survival. Furthermore, dopamine at 5 to 10 μg per kg per minute has been shown to sustain the arterial ketone body ratio (AKBR), indicating maintenance of the liver energy state, while maintaining mean arterial pressure (MAP). However, doses greater than 15 μg per kg per minute are associated with a decreased AKBR and increasing liver function test values (38). Other investigators have shown combinations of vasopressin and thyroid hormone (39) as well as vasopressin and epinephrine (40) to be beneficial in maintaining or improving AKBR and MAP. Based on these data, it seems safe to say that the agent chosen should promote blood flow while maintaining MAP (i.e., not a pure α-agonist), and should be used in as low a dose as possible.

Approximately 10% of brain-dead donors will experience cardiac arrest, usually preceded by bradycardia or ventricular fibrillation. Treatment should include a direct-acting β-agonist, such as epinephrine or isoproterenol, or transvenous or transcutaneous pacing. Atropine is ineffective, since destruction of the vagal nuclei in the brainstem abolishes the vagal response. If function is not promptly restored, one should proceed with open cardiac massage and emergent organ removal.

RESPIRATORY MANAGEMENT

The two goals of respiratory care in potential organ donors are to maintain optimal lung function for transplantation and adequate oxygen delivery to all other tissues. Ideally, the inspired oxygen concentration should be maintained below 50% to avoid the possibility of pulmonary oxygen toxicity, and certainly less than 100% to avoid absorption atelectases. Positive end-expiratory pressure (PEEP) should be kept at 5 cm H_2O, if possible, to avoid barotrauma (important if the lungs are to be transplanted) and prevent detrimental consequences with respect to venous return and cardiac output. Theoretically, a protective ventilation strategy should limit lung injury. Fluid resuscitation should be monitored closely to avoid overload, leading to pulmonary edema. Careful control of the cardiovascular system is essential to

avoid the possibility of neurogenic pulmonary edema secondary to the hypercatecholamine state since this usually precludes lung or heart-lung transplantation. Strict aseptic technique must be used when instrumenting the airway to avoid contamination.

Follette and coworkers report improved oxygenation and increased lung donor recovery using high-dose steroids (methylprednisolone, mean 14.5 $\pm$ 0.06 mg per kg) after brain death (41). The authors retrospectively analyzed 118 heart-beating, cadaveric, solid multiorgan donors, of whom 80 received steroids. The study showed no difference in most clinical or demographic variables, but a significant increase in oxygenation before aortic cross-cramping ($p = 0.01$). The number of procured lungs was markedly greater in the steroid-treated donors (25/80 patients versus 3/38; $p > 0.01$). However, the beneficial effect of steroids remains to be confirmed in larger prospective trials.

ENDOCRINE EFFECTS

The literature is abundant regarding endocrine function after brain death; however, the data are controversial at best, especially regarding thyroid function. Novitzky's group has documented the beneficial effects of a combination of triiodothyronine, insulin, and cortisol in animals (42) and humans (43). They show that this combination therapy is responsible for improvement in hemodynamics, myocardial function, and aerobic metabolism of the donor, as well as function of the donor organs after transplantation. These data, however, have not been reproduced in subsequent studies (44–47). In addition, the thyroid hormone abnormalities found (low T_3, low T_4, elevated T_3 replacement, and normal thyroid-stimulating hormone) define the euthyroid sick syndrome. Further, one study actually found that not only did T_3 replacement have no effect on myocardial function, it actually decreased myocardial blood flow (44).

The impact of T_3 at the cellular level is multifactorial. The initial effects are nongenomic and do not require RNA-protein synthesis. The observed hemodynamic effects occur within minutes.

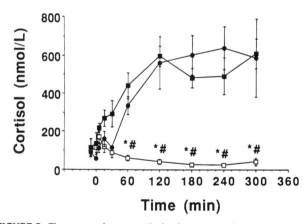

FIGURE 2. The mean plasma cortisol values versus time are presented as means $\pm$ SEM. The zero time denotes the brain death induction (*open boxes*), sham induction (*dark circles*), or the start of the clock for the time control (*dark boxes*). (From Huber TS, Nachreiner R, D'Alecy LG. Hormonal profiles in a canine model of the brain-dead organ donor. *J Crit Care* 1994;9:7–17, with permission.)

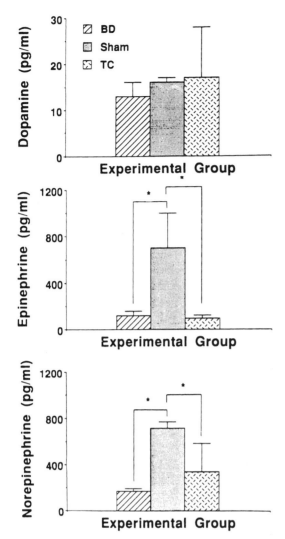

FIGURE 3. The mean dopamine, epinephrine, and norepinephrine values over the time interval of 30 to 300 minutes are presented for the three groups: BD, brain death; SHAM, sham brain-death induction (transient negative cerebral perfusion pressure); and TC, time control (no brain death). (From Huber TS, Nachreiner R, D'Alecy LG. Hormonal profiles in a canine model of the brain-dead organ donor. *J Crit Care* 1994;9:7–17, with permission).

There is a direct effect on mitochondria, stimulating the aerobic pathway and adenosine triphosphate production (48). T_3 has an extremely important role in intracellular Ca^{2+} homeostasis. T_3 activates the sarcoplasmic reticulum and sarcolemmal Ca^{2+} channels, which results in rapid Ca^{2+} mobilization from the cytosol into the mitochondria and the sarcoplasmic reticulum (49). Ca^{2+}-induced injury is avoided or reduced by this mechanism (50). Huber and coworkers (47) did, however, conclusively show, in a brain-dead canine model, an inability to increase serum cortisol, norepinephrine, and epinephrine levels 30 to 300 minutes after the induction of brain death (Figs. 2 and 3). They further postulated that these failures may account for the hemodynamic instability seen after brain death. The one hormone clearly shown to have low-to-nonexistent levels after brain death was arginine vasopressin (45). In fact, the incidence of diabetes insipidus in this group of human organ donors was 78%.

With the recent success of pancreatic transplantation, evaluation of the donor pancreas is essential. Hyperglycemia may be a significant problem in donor management. Masson and associates (51) evaluated 25 brain-dead organ donors prospectively to ascertain function of the endocrine pancreas. They found normal function in all 25 cases. Histologic and immunohistochemical examinations were available in 17 of the 25 cases and all were normal. Further, when hyperglycemia occurred, it was due to peripheral insulin resistance. They concluded that blood glucose concentrations are not a good predictor of endocrine pancreatic function before transplantation.

FLUIDS AND ELECTROLYTES

Once volume resuscitation is complete, maintenance fluid administration should consist of hypotonic saline titrated as needed to maintain blood pressure and CVP. In addition, glucose should be added as indicated to maintain adequate intrahepatic glucose stores. Brain-dead patients may develop a marked diuresis that is multifactorial in etiology. First, hyperglycemia, owing to peripheral insulin resistance, may be present and lead to osmotic diuresis. However, exogenous insulin should be used carefully since hypoglycemia may have detrimental consequences on hemodynamics and donor organ function. Second, these patients often have been treated with diuretics during the cerebral resuscitation phase of their care. Urinary output greater than 200 mL per hour should be replaced, milliliter for milliliter, with fluid that approximates the electrolyte content of the urine and should be guided by serum electrolytes. Third, as stated previously, diabetes insipidus is quite common in these patients. The diagnosis of diabetes insipidus is suspected when a brain-dead patient exhibits high urinary outputs, and is confirmed by the presence of hypernatremia (serum Na > 150 mEq/L), hyperosmolarity (serum osmolarity > 310 mOsm/L), and urinary hyposmolarity (<300 mOsm/L). Therapy is initially directed at volume replacement (usually in the form of free-water repletion), and is followed by the use of vasopressin, if necessary. Desmopressin, a synthetic analog of arginine vasopressin, can be used in doses of 0.5 to 2.0 μg i.v. every 8 to 12 hours, and may be the preferred preparation since it possesses a low pressor-antidiuretic ratio, with a longer duration of action. In a randomized controlled study, 97 brain-dead donors received desmopressin (1 μg bolus every 2 hours when diuresis was more than 300 mL per hour; $n = 49$), or no desmopressin ($n = 48$) (52). The authors found no significant differences between the two groups, except for final diuresis, which was lower in the desmopressin group. Hemodialysis requirement and serum creatinine concentrations did not differ in the first 15 days after transplantation. Long-term graft survival was similar in the two groups. Aqueous vasopressin, available as an i.v. infusion, can be started at a rate of 0.5 to 1.0 U per hour. This infusion is then titrated to maintain urinary output at 100 to 250 mL per hour. Its high pressor-antidiuretic ratio, however, may lead to regional organ ischemia.

High urinary output can rapidly lead to severe electrolyte abnormalities. Hypokalemia, hypomagnesemia, and hypophosphatemia should be aggressively evaluated and corrected. The overall loss of free water that occurs with osmotic diuresis or that is induced by diabetes insipidus can lead to a rapid rise in serum sodium. One must be careful to replace free water as needed to maintain serum sodium less than 155 mEq per L. Totsuka and colleagues indicate that the incidence of hepatic graft loss is increased to 33% with donor final serum sodium concentrations above 155 mEq per L compared with 11% at concentrations below 155 mEq per L (53).

TEMPERATURE REGULATION AND COAGULATION

Brain-dead patients, upon loss of hypothalamic function, lose the ability to thermoregulate, thus becoming poikilothermic. It is estimated that up to 86% of potential donors become hypothermic (less than 36°C), depending on the time interval between diagnosis and organ retrieval. In addition to confounding the diagnosis of brain death, hypothermia may lead to ventricular arrhythmias, coagulopathy, cold-induced diuresis, and regional vasoconstriction. Warming blankets, warmed i.v. fluids, and heated, humidified oxygen (40° to 46°C) via the mechanical ventilator may be required; however, overaggressive rewarming must be avoided, since oxygen consumption may increase.

Coagulopathy is usually due to hypothermia and dilution of clotting factors. Correction of severe coagulation abnormalities and clinical evidence of bleeding should be aggressively pursued to avoid major blood loss during the procurement procedure. Disseminated intravascular coagulopathy (DIC) has been found in as many as 88% of patients with severe head injury and is due to release of tissue thromboplastin from the injured brain. The concern over microvascular thrombosis makes the use of ϵ-aminocaproic acid in this situation controversial; its use is best avoided if possible.

ANESTHETIC MANAGEMENT

Anesthetic management is essentially a continuation of intensive care management in the operating room. The anesthesiologist, before transportation of the donor to the operating room, must first verify the appropriate medical and legal documentation regarding brain death and organ donation.

If not already in place, an arterial catheter must be placed in an upper extremity since the femoral vessels may be needed to facilitate organ preservation and removal. The need for a PA catheter is controversial; however, two studies have documented its utility based on extreme intraoperative hemodynamic heterogeneity and the desire to avoid the use of inotropes or vasopressors (54, 55). Arterial blood gases, acid-base status, and electrolyte and blood glucose levels should be assessed at least hourly. The same principles of fluid and electrolyte therapy stated previously hold true intraoperatively.

Ventilatory considerations are identical to those mentioned above with the exception of two points. First, if the lungs are not to be harvested, 100% oxygen should be used; if they are, 50% oxygen or less should be provided. Secondly, as the patient will be pharmacologically paralyzed during procurement to avoid reflex motor activity, oxygen consumption and carbon dioxide production will be significantly decreased. Therefore, "normal ventilation" will result in hypocapnia and a marked alkalosis. One must, therefore, adjust oxygen administration and ventilation accordingly.

Although the diagnosis of brain death requires loss of cerebral and brainstem function, spinal reflexes usually remain intact. Accordingly, to facilitate surgical exposure, neuromuscular blockade is routinely used. In addition to spinal reflexes, autonomic reflexes may remain intact. Specifically, a well-documented reflex pressor response to nociceptive stimuli may lead to excessive blood loss or poor perfusion to potentially transplantable organs. It is speculated that this is due to a possible spinal vasoconstrictor response, or even spinal stimulation of the adrenal glands. Afterload reduction by vasodilation is the mainstay of treatment, and may be provided by nitroglycerin, nitroprusside, or even isoflurane.

Principles of cardiovascular management in the ICU have been stated earlier and are directly applicable to the operating room. One specific difference is the absolute necessity of communicating any extreme changes in hemodynamic status to the surgeon to ensure rapid organ removal, if necessary.

Additional pharmacologic intervention may be required, depending on the given institutional protocols. Administration of mannitol (1 g per kg) or furosemide (40 to 100 mg) may be required before aortic cross-clamping. Furthermore, after aortic cannulation but before cross-clamping, 20,000 to 30,000 U heparin i.v. are given to prevent clotting in the donated organ vascular bed before flushing these vessels.

The organ procurement procedure involves an incision from the suprasternal notch to the symphysis pubis. As both the abdominal and thoracic cavities are exposed, there is the potential for marked hypothermia and extreme insensible fluid losses. The organs to be harvested are dissected until attached only by their vascular pedicles. The operation tends to be longer and bloodier if the pancreas is to be harvested. A special note should be made regarding heart-lung procurement: high endotracheal tube position must be confirmed with the harvesting surgeon to minimize mucosal injury in the area of future suture lines. Recently, however, this has become less of a concern as the technique of bilateral sequential lung transplantation (with bibronchial anastomoses) has been developed. Manipulation of the trachea, lungs, and esophagus may lead to significant hypotension based on mechanical factors, as well as problems with oxygenation and ventilation. Dopamine at doses of 5 to 10 μg per kg per minute may be required for blood pressure support, and a MAP of 60 mm Hg may have to be accepted for this short period. Once the aortic cross-clamp is applied and the cold cardioplegia solution is infused (as well as the cold preservation solution to the other organs), ventilation is stopped and the anesthetic management discontinued.

NONHEART-BEATING DONORS

The overall success of transplantation has led to our current predicament: an ever-increasing number of recipients waiting for organs with no corresponding increase in the number of brain-dead donors. Thus, organs from brain-dead donors cannot meet the demand that transplantation's success has created. Nonheart-beating donor (NHBD) organs, our only source of organs in the 1950s and 1960s, carry the concern of longer warm ischemic times, leading to graft dysfunction after transplantation; however, NHBDs are a means of increasing the organ pool and saving more lives. Presumed-consent policies outside the United States have facilitated rapid organ recovery from NHBDs and expanded the donor supply by 20% (56). Currently, 30 of the 61 active organ procurement agencies in the United States have official protocols on the use of NHBDs. According to the United Network for Organ Sharing (UNOS) database, 327 NHBDs were reported between 1994 and 1998 (1).

The NHBDs can be divided into four (Maastricht) categories (57). The first group, dead on arrival, are usually trauma patients or patients with myocardial infarction who are dead when they arrive at the emergency room. These patients may have aortic and inferior vena cava cannulae inserted for hypothermic *in situ* preservation, thus minimizing warm ischemic time while attempting to obtain consent for donation.

The second group includes patients who become asystolic and resuscitation is unsuccessful. If legally consented to ahead of time, an aortic cannula for infusion of cold preservation solution and an inferior vena cava cannula for drainage of blood are inserted upon certification of death. This procedure will serve to minimize warm ischemic time while preparations are made for procurement of donated organs.

The third group consists of terminally ill patients who are dependent on life-supporting treatment, usually a ventilator, and the treatment is deliberately withheld. These patients, upon signing donation consent forms, are taken to the operating room where weaning from mechanical ventilation is performed while assiduously avoiding suffering. Death is certified based on cardiorespiratory criteria after 2 to 5 minutes of circulatory arrest (ventricular fibrillation, electromechanical dissociation, or asystole), at which point procurement may proceed.

The fourth group consists of patients who are undergoing brain death evaluation but become asystolic before its completion. In these cases, cardiopulmonary resuscitation (CPR) is initiated and, if organ donation consent forms have been signed, the patient is swiftly moved to the operating room for emergent organ procurement. Certification of death is based on cardiorespiratory criteria and organ procurement can proceed only once the patient is pronounced dead. An alternative to this approach is to place these patients on cardiopulmonary bypass (CPB) for circulatory stabilization, a procedure that allows formal completion of brain-death evaluation.

The organ donor committee at the University of Pittsburgh has set another distinct category, which involves patients who die shortly after admission to the emergency department with unsuccessful CPR (32). These patients may be put on emergency CPB in a lifesaving attempt. They may recover all function, including heart function, and have CPB discontinued. If all organs, including the brain, are functional, but the heart remains dependent on CPB, a ventricular-assist device is considered as a bridge to potential heart transplantation. If brain death develops, the patient becomes an organ donor once consent is obtained from the next of kin. If both the heart and brain are failing, CPB may be discontinued in the operating room, provided that consent

for organ donation has been obtained and noncardiac organs are procured after certification of death based on cardiorespiratory criteria.

The University of Pittsburgh has reported the results of organ transplants from NHBDs for the period January 1989 to July 1994 (56). The function of 21 kidneys and 8 livers procured from 12 controlled NHBDs (i.e., donors who had life-sustaining therapy withdrawn in the operating room) was compared to the function of 22 kidneys and 6 livers from 14 uncontrolled NHBDs who developed unexpected cardiac arrest and underwent emergent organ procurement. The kidney recipients in both groups had a 95% 1-year survival with an 82% 1-year graft survival. Eight out of eight livers in the controlled group worked initially, but three were lost to complications, whereas only one out of six livers functioned from the uncontrolled group. Overall, livers from NHBDs showed a 21% incidence of vascular complications severe enough to require recipients to undergo retransplantation.

The University of Wisconsin has also reported experience from January 1993 to May 1994 (56). Five livers were obtained from controlled NHBDs, with one case of primary nonfunction. No arterial or biliary complications were noted, and 75% of the recipients were alive at 1-year follow-up. Six kidney-pancreas transplants were performed, and at 8 months, all patients were insulin-free, with only one requiring dialysis. Twenty-one kidney transplants were performed, and at 8 months, 19 had functioning grafts. Finally, one lung transplant was performed on a patient who had been on extracorporeal membrane oxygenation, which was discontinued 4 days later; the recipient survived.

Cho and colleagues analyzed the data from the Kidney Transplant Registry of the United Network for Organ Sharing (UNOS) comparing 229 kidney grafts from NHBDs with those of brain-dead donors (58). The study demonstrated a survival rate of 83% for grafts from NHBDs and 86% for grafts from brain-dead donors ($p = 0.26$). The authors concluded that transplantation of kidneys from NHBDs, especially those who died from trauma, is often successful, and the use of kidneys from such donors could increase the overall supply of cadaveric kidney transplants. Koostra reports use of kidneys from NHBDs could increase the supply of kidney transplants by a factor of 2 to 4.5 (59).

Overall, the results of transplants with NHBD organs are good, especially if the procurement occurs in a controlled situation. Strong ethical and moral issues, however, surround these cases. Significant problems regarding consent require each institution to develop policies after consultation with an institutional ethics committee.

THE FUTURE

The past 6 years has seen the number of brain-dead organ donors in the United States increase from 4,800 to 5,800 (i.e., by only 17%). Although the number of patients succumbing to brain death is at least double this number, the organ debt still would not be covered as the number of patients awaiting solid organ transplants has increased to 72,580 as of October 2000. Nonetheless, it is imperative to identify and properly manage all potential organ donors. Living-donor organ transplantation is increasing world-wide. In the United States alone, 4,690 such procedures were carried out in 1999 (kidneys, and partial livers and lungs). How-ever, ethical concerns and availability issues limit this resource as well. Immunosuppression, though more advanced now than at any time in the past, is still far from perfect. An understanding of the immune system and ways in which physicians can modu-late its activity may eliminate graft loss due to chronic rejection, thereby limiting the number of patients requiring retransplants.

Other possibilities to satisfy the ever-increasing organ demand include utilization of artificial organs and xenografting (trans-planting animal organs into humans). The next generation of the totally implantable artificial heart has recently been made available. Further, extracorporeal liver assist devices are actively studied as a bridge to liver transplantation. Experimentation with baboon organ transplantation is underway, and genetic engineer-ing of pigs to allow for organ acceptance is not far off. Successful xenotransplantation necessitates solving problems of hyperacute rejection and understanding the cellular immune responses that occur. Considerable progress has been made in our understanding of the molecular genetic basis of the rapid hyperacute antibody-mediated rejection mechanisms that occur in xenogeneic organ rejection. In parallel, strategies involving the use of transgenic animals expressing complement inhibitors are beginning to offer encouraging evidence that hyperacute rejection can be overcome. A greater understanding of cell-mediated immune interactions is required to achieve long-term xenograft survival. Current studies are focused on T cell receptor (TCR)/major histocompatibility complex (MHC) and costimulatory signals that activate human CD4 and CD8 T cells (60). However, ethical issues regarding animal sacrifice for human benefit may inhibit widespread accep-tance (60). Potential spread to xenograft recipients of nonhuman diseases is another risk factor.

It appears that no single solution will solve the organ shortage problem; however, the combination of multiple solutions may allow the day to come when no patient dies while awaiting trans-plantation.

SUMMARY

The success of transplantation has created an extreme short-age of donor organs relative to the ever-increasing demand by potential recipients. It is, therefore, incumbent upon all physi-cians to recognize the potential organ donor as early as possible and minimize the chances of damage to donor organs caused by hemodynamic, respiratory, and metabolic instability. Further, these physicians must become familiar with the pathophysiol-ogy of the brain-dead organ donor and the principles regarding their management to maximize the number of available donor organs.

Criteria for the diagnosis of brain death vary from center to center and country to country. Although whole-brain criteria are still used in the United States, it is conceivable that the future may see a switch to brainstem (as in the United Kingdom) or even cortical criteria.

Clinical criteria should generally be adequate for diagnosis; however, if confounding variables exist, confirmatory testing is es-sential. Four-vessel angiography is the "gold standard"; although, many noninvasive tests (TCD, technetium scintigraphy, etc.) now offer the promise of accuracy without risk.

Familiarity with NHBD organ procurement protocols and policies is essential for intensivists, anesthesiologists, surgeons, and emergency room personnel, since these patients must be recognized and treated immediately to minimize warm ischemic time and to optimize the function of grafted organs. In addition, knowledge of the categories of NHBDs and the outcomes of transplants performed with these organs may form the foundation upon which one may institute protocols for the procurement of such organs within a given institution.

KEY POINTS

The major obstacle to increasing transplantation in the United States today is the limited supply of donated organs.

The guidelines for the definition of death, according to the 1981 President's Commission on Ethical Problems in Medicine and Biomedical and Behavioral Research, include: (a) cerebral and brainstem functions must be absent; (b) the cause of death must be known and exclude recovery; and (c) cessation of all brain function must persist during a period of observation and treatment.

The apnea test, used to confirm brain death, consists of pre-oxygenation with 100% oxygen for 5 minutes, administration of oxygen, absence of mechanical ventilation, and demonstra-tion that there are no spontaneous respiratory efforts at a $PaCO_2$ greater than 60 mm Hg.

Confirmatory tests for brain death include four-vessel cere-bral angiography, isoelectric electroencephalogram, absent brainstem auditory evoked potentials, absent cerebral perfu-sion on brain scan with technetium-tagged HMPAO, and transcranial Doppler ultrasonography. The "gold standard" remains four-vessel angiography.

Once a patient becomes recognized as brain dead and as a potential organ donor, management must shift to providing oxygen and blood delivery to transplantable organs.

Management of hypotension in brain-dead patients await-ing harvest of transplantable organs consists of volume expan-sion and administration of vasopressors, ideally dopamine in doses of less than 10 μg per kg per minute.

Management of the lungs in a potential donor should avoid oxygen toxicity and high levels of positive end-expiratory pres-sure to avoid barotrauma, accompanied by careful fluid ad-ministration.

To control high urinary output in diabetes insipidus, desmopressin can be used in doses of 0.5 to 2.0 μg i.v. every 8 to 12 hours.

REFERENCES

1. United Network for Organ Sharing. Available at: http://www.unos.org. Accessed October 17, 2001.
2. Frist WH, Fanning WJ. Donor management and matching. *Cardiol Clin* 1990;8:55–71.
3. Merrill JP, Murray JE, Harrison JH, et al. Successful homotransplantation of the human kidney between identical twins. *JAMA* 1956;160:277–282.
4. Starzl TE, Marchioro TL, Von Kaulla KN, et al. Homotransplantation of the liver in humans. *Surg Gynecol Obstet* 1963;117:659–676.
5. Hardy JD, Webb WR, Dalton ML, et al. Lung homotransplantation in man. *JAMA* 1963;186:1065–1074.
6. Barnard CN. The operation. A human cardiac transplant: an interim report of a successful operation at Groote Schuur Hospital, Cape Town. *S Afr Med* 1967;41:1271–1274.
7. Mollaret P, Goulon M. Le coma dépassé. *Rev Neurol* 1959;101:3–15.
8. A definition of irreversible coma: ad hoc committee of the Harvard Medical School to examine the definition of brain death. *JAMA* 1968;205:337–340.
9. Guidelines for the determination of death: report of the medical consultants on the diagnosis of death to the President's Commission for the Study of Ethical Problems in Medicine and Biomedical and Behavioral Research. *JAMA* 1981;246:2184–2186.
10. Benzel EC, Mashburn JP, Conrad S, et al. Apnea testing for the determination of brain death: a modified protocol. Technical note. *J Neurosurg* 1992;76:1029–1031.
11. Pallis C. Brainstem death: the evolution of a concept. *Semin Thorac Cardiovasc Surg* 1990;2:135–152.
12. Diagnosis of brain death: statement issued by the honorary secretary of the Conference of Medical Royal Colleges and their Faculties in the United Kingdom on 11 October 1976. *Br Med J* 1976;2:1187–1188.
13. Truog RD, Fackler JC. Rethinking brain death. *Crit Care Med* 1992; 20:1705–1713.
14. Cranford RE, Smith DR. Consciousness: the most critical moral (constitutional) standard for human personhood. *Am J Law Med* 1987;13:233–248.
15. Young B, Blume W, Lynch A. Brain death and the persistent vegetative state: similarities and contrasts. *Can J Neurol Sci* 1989;16:388–393.
16. Harrison MR. Organ procurement for children: the anencephalic fetus as a donor. *Lancet* 1986;2:1383–1386.
17. Holzgreve W, Beller FK, Buchholz B, et al. Kidney transplantation from anencephalic donors. *N Engl J Med* 1987;316:1069–1070.
18. Medical Consultants on the Diagnosis of Death. Guidelines for the determination of death: Report of the Medical Consultants on the Diagnosis of Death to President's Commission for the Study of Ethical Problems in Medicine and Biomedical and Behavioral Research. *JAMA* 1981;246:2184.
19. Freeman JM, Ferry PC. New brain death guidelines in children: further confusion. *Pediatrics* 1988;81:301.
20. Ashwal S, Schneider S. Brain death in children. I. *Pediatr Neurol* 1987;3:5.
21. Ashwal S, Schneider S. Brain death in children. II. *Pediatr Neurol* 1987;3:69.
22. Scewmon DA. Brain death in children. *Neurology* 1988;38:1813.
23. Jenkins DH, Reilly PM, Schwab CW, et al. Improving the approach to organ donation: a review *World J Surg* 1999;23:644–649.
24. Buchner H, Schuchardt V. Reliability of electroencephalogram in the diagnosis of brain death. *Eur Neurol* 1990;30:138–141.
25. Grigg MM, Kelly MA, Celesia GG, et al. Electroencephalographic activity after brain death. *Arch Neurol* 1987;44:948–954.
26. Firsching R, Frowein RA, Wilhelms S, et al. Brain death: practicability of evoked potentials. *Neurosurg Rev* 1992;15:249–254.
27. Yatim A, Mercatello A, Coronel B, et al. ^{99m}Tc-HMPAO cerebral scintigraphy in the diagnosis of brain death. *Transplant Proc* 1991;23:2491.
28. Kurtek RW, Lai KK, Tauxe WN, et al. Tc-99 hexamethylpropylene amine oxime scintigraphy in the diagnosis of brain death and its implications for the harvesting of organs used for transplantation. *Clin Nucl Med* 2000;25:7–10.
29. Feri M, Ralli L, Felici M, et al. Transcranial Doppler and brain death diagnosis. *Crit Care Med* 1994;22:1120–1126.
30. Nau R, Prange HW, Klingelhofer J, et al. Results of four technical investigations in fifty clinically brain-dead patients. *Intensive Care Med* 1992;18:82–88.
31. Darby JM, Stein KS, Grenvik A, et al. Approach to management of the heartbeating brain-dead organ donor. *JAMA* 1989;261:2222–2228.
32. Grenvik A. Brain death and organ transplantation, a 40 year review. *Opusc Med* 1992;37:33–41.
33. Novitzky D, Wicomb WN, Cooper DKC, et al. Electrocardiographic, hemodynamic and endocrine changes occurring during experimental brain death in the Chacma baboon. *J Heart Transplant* 1984;4:63–69.
34. Mertes PM, Burtin P, Carteaux JP, et al. Changes in hemodynamic performance and oxygen consumption during brain death in the pig. *Transplant Proc* 1994;26:229–230.
35. Darracott-Cankovic S, Stovin PG, Wheeldon D, et al. Effect of donor heart damage on survival after transplantation. *Eur J Cardio Thoracic Surg* 1989;3:525–532.
36. Messmer K. Hemodilution. *Surg Clin North Am* 1975;55:659–678.
37. Quesada A, Teja JL, Rabanal JM, et al. Inotropic support in 50 brain-dead organ donors: repercussion on renal graft function. *Transplant Proc* 1991;23:2479–2480.
38. Okamoto R, Yamamoto Y, Lin H, et al. Influence of dopamine on the liver assessed by changes in arterial ketone body ratio in brain-dead dogs. *Surgery* 1990;107:36–42.
39. Washida M, Okamoto R, Manaka D, et al. Beneficial effect of combined 3,5,3′-triiodothyronine and vasopressin administration of hepatic energy status and systemic hemodynamics after brain death. *Transplantation* 1992;54:44–49.
40. Manaka D, Okamoto R, Yokoyama T, et al. Maintenance of liver graft viability in the state of brain death. Synergistic effects of vasopressin and epinephrine on hepatic energy metabolism in brain-dead dogs. *Transplantation* 1992;53:545–550.
41. Follette DM, Rudich SM, Babcock WD. Improved oxygenation and increased lung donor recovery with high-dose steroid administration after brain death. *J Heart Lung Transplant* 1998;17:423–429.
42. Cooper DKC, Novitzky D, Wicomb WN. Hormonal therapy in the brain-dead experimental animal. *Transplant Proc* 1988;20:51–54.
43. Novitzky D, Cooper DKC. Results of hormonal therapy in human brain-dead potential organ donors. *Transplant Proc* 1988;20:59–62.
44. Meyers CH, D'Amico TA, Peterseim DS, et al. Effects of triiodothyronine and vasopressin on cardiac function and myocardial blood flow after brain-death. *J Heart Lung Transplant* 1993;12:68–79.
45. Gramm HJ, Meinhold H, Bickel U, et al. Acute endocrine failure after brain death? *Transplantation* 1992;54:851–857.
46. Masson F, Thicoipe M, Latapie MJ, et al. Thyroid function in brain-dead donors. *Transplant Int* 1990;3:226–233.
47. Huber TS, Nachreiner R, D'Alecy LG. Hormonal profiles in a canine model of the brain-dead organ donor. *J Crit Care* 1994;9:7–17.
48. Novitzky D, Wicomb WN, Cooper DKC, et al. Improved cardiac function following hormonal therapy in brain dead pigs: relevance to organ donation. *Cryobiology* 1987;24:1.
49. Warnic PR, Davis FB, Cody V, et al. Proceedings of the Annual Meeting of the Endocrine Society, New Orleans:356(abst).
50. Segal J. In vivo effect of 3,5,3′-triiodothyronine on calcium uptake in several tissues in the rat: evidence for a physiological role for calcium as the first messenger for the prompt action of thyroid hormone at the level of the plasma membrane. *Endocrinology* 1990;127:17.
51. Masson F, Thicoipe M, Gin H, et al. The endocrine pancreas in brain-dead donors. A prospective study in 25 patients. *Transplantation* 1993;56:363–367.
52. Guesde R, Barrou B, Leblanc I, et al. Administration of desmopressin in brain-dead donors and renal function in kidney recipients. *Lancet* 1998;352:1178–1181.
53. Totsuka E, Dodson F, Urakami A, et al. Influence of high donor serum sodium levels on early postoperative graft function in human liver

transplantation: effect of correction of donor hypernatremia. *Liver Transpl Surg* 1999;5(5):421–428.

54. Pennefather SH, Dark JH, Bullock RE. Haemodynamic responses to surgery in brain-dead organ donors. *Anaesthesia* 1993;48:1034–1038.

55. Duke PK, Ramsay MAE, Paulsen AW, et al. Intraoperative hemodynamic heterogeneity of brain dead organ donors. *Transplant Proc* 1991;23:2485–2486.

56. UNOS Update (PO Box 13770, Richmond, VA 23225). November 1994;10(11).

57. Koostra G. Statement on non-heart-beating donor programs. *Transplant Proc* 1995;27:2965.

58. Cho YG, Terasaki PI, Cecka JM, et al. Transplantation of kidneys from donors whose hearts have stopped beating. *N Engl J Med* 1998;338:221–225.

59. Koostra G. The asystolic, or non-heartbeating donor. *Transplantation* 1997;63:917–921.

60. Bothwell AL. Characterization of the human antiporcine immune response: a prerequisite to xenotransplantation. *Immunol Res* 1999;19(2–3):233–243.

25

CARDIOGENIC SHOCK

ASHRAF M. GHOBASHY
MANUEL FONTES
ROBERTA L. HINES

> ### KEY WORDS
>
> - Acute mitral insufficiency
> - Cardiac tamponade
> - Cardiogenic shock
> - Mechanical assist devices
> - Myocardial infarction
> - Myocardial dysfunction
> - Myocardial performance
> - Revascularization
> - Ventricular free-wall rupture
> - Ventricular septal defect

INTRODUCTION

For purposes of this discussion, *cardiogenic shock* is defined as circulatory failure occurring as a result of either ventricular contractile dysfunction or cardiac rhythm disturbances. As with all forms of shock (regardless of cause), the principal metabolic derangements result from failure to maintain tissue perfusion and oxygenation. The first part of this review focuses on the determinants of cardiac function, the pathophysiology of myocardial infarction (MI), the evolution of pump failure, and management strategies. Next the pathophysiology and management goals for cardiogenic shock arising from mechanical complications of acute MI, namely, acute mitral regurgitation, cardiac tamponade, and septal or free-wall rupture, also are discussed. Finally, the pathophysiology and management of circulatory shock related to the alteration in right ventricle (RV) performance are presented.

CARDIAC FUNCTION

Traditionally, the variables that determine myocardial performance include heart rate (HR), preload, afterload, and contractility. These four intrinsic factors are interdependent, and derangements in one or more of these factors can result in inadequate cardiac function.

Heart Rate

Cardiac output (CO) is defined as the product of stroke volume (SV) and HR:

$$CO = SV \times HR$$

Therefore, HR is a critical determinant of ventricular performance; it establishes the time for both systole and diastole. HR can be influenced and regulated by the autonomic nervous system through sympathetic and vagal inputs, body temperature, and other metabolic processes (1). Extremes of HR impact negatively on cardiac performance by increasing myocardial oxygen consumption (*demand*) and reducing coronary perfusion time (*supply*). Such derangements can lead to myocardial ischemia and ventricular dysfunction, particularly in the setting of coronary artery disease (CAD). The left ventricle (LV) is most vulnerable to ischemic injuries because its extensive muscle mass receives perfusion only during diastole. In contrast, the RV (with significantly less muscle mass) receives blood flow during both systole and diastole.

Preload

Preload is defined as the loading state of the ventricle just prior to ventricular contraction. Myocardial fiber length at end diastole most accurately determines preload. For purposes of clinical management, however, the LV end-diastolic pressure (LVEDP) or its correlate, the pulmonary artery occlusion pressure (PAOP), is used to estimate preload. Fiber length depends in part on chamber compliance, which can be affected by ischemia, intrathoracic pressures, pericardial constraint, and other mechanical forces (2). Ventricular compliance (dV/dP) can be estimated by varying the end-diastolic volume (EDV) while measuring the corresponding change in LVEDP. As can be seen in Figure 1, the slope of the end-diastolic pressure–volume relationship (EDPVR) line defines compliance (Fig. 1). While contractility is maintained at a constant level, changes in preload are reflected by movement along the EDPVR line, resulting in similarly directed changes in stroke volume (3). Note that in the normal ventricle, ventricular filling is associated with minimal changes in ventricular pressure; however, as the ventricle becomes less compliant (i.e., "stiffer")

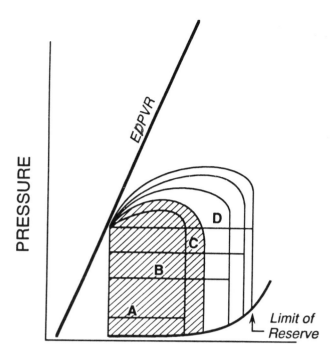

FIGURE 1. Representation of preload changes in the pressure–volume loop model. Changes in preload are reflected by movement along the end-diastolic pressure-volume relationship (EDPVR) line. Note that while contractility is maintained constant, changes in preload result in similarly directed changes in stroke volume until the limit of preload reserve (arrow) has been reached. The shaded loop represents normal, loop A, decreased preload; loops B, C, and D depict increased preload. (Adapted from Thomas JS, Kramer JL eds. *Manual of cardiac anesthesia*, 2nd ed. New York: Churchill Livingstone, 1993:11, with permission).

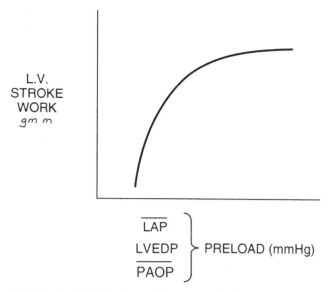

FIGURE 2. The Frank–Starling relation of chamber diastolic length [represented as left ventricular end-diastolic pressure (LVEDP), pulmonary capillary occlusion pressure (PAOP), or left atrial pressures (LAP)] and ventricular performance [cardiac output (CO), stroke volume (SV), cardiac index (CI), left ventricular (LV) stroke work]. With increasing diastolic muscle-fiber length (i.e., preload), both LV and right ventricular performance can increase steadily (3). However, once the limit of preload reserve is reached, myocardial performance cannot be enhanced further by augmenting SV.

secondary to hypertrophic or ischemic factors, the slope of the EDPVR becomes quite steep. In these settings, interpretation of pressure measurements as a direct assessment of ventricular volume may be unreliable.

In general, preload depends on venous return and in the absence of right or LV dysfunction it can be estimated by central venous pressure (CVP) measurement. That is, when biventricular compliance is normal, the CVP correlates well with the PAOP and can be used to estimate preload. In the setting of LV dysfunction, the CVP may underestimate the LVEDP. In contrast, when RV dysfunction exists, the CVP will overestimate the LVEDP.

The Starling relationship further states that with increasing preload (fiber length), the force of contraction increases, thereby augmenting SV. This relationship is operational until the limits of preload reserve, are reached; thus, SV cannot be increase further through preload augmentation (Fig. 2). However, caution must be exercised when attempting to maximize CO by excessive preloading. In these settings, significant increases in wall tension can precipitate myocardial ischemia.

Afterload

Afterload most often is defined as the impedance the ventricle must overcome to eject blood during systole. Systemic vascular resistance (SVR) and pulmonary vascular resistance (PVR) are used clinically to estimate afterload for the LV and RV, respectively. The variables used to calculate SVR [mean arterial pressure (MAP), CVP, and CO] are interdependent on HR, preload, and contractility. Thus, it would be important to consider the "global hemodynamic" picture when initiating or altering therapy based on SVR or PVR determinations. For example, the calculated SVR may be very high because of a low CO. In this situation, rather than using a vasodilator to affect the SVR as the primary therapy, other causes of reduced CO should be explored, that is, rhythm abnormality, contractile dysfunction, and inadequate ventricular filling.

Other variables used to define afterload include arterial impedance and wall tension (T). The former, although a more accurate measure of afterload, is extremely difficult to derive clinically. Wall tension or Laplace relation ($T = \text{Pr}/\text{h}$), where T is directly proportional to the product of intraventricular pressure and intracavitary radius (r) and inversely proportional to wall thickness (h), increases during isovolumetric contraction and decreases sequentially during ventricular ejection as volume and chamber radius diminish (4). The Laplace relation also suffers from lack of clinical utility because invasive cardiac catheterization and radiologic imaging are required to obtain values for ventricular pressure. Clinically, disease states that increase afterload also cause SV to decrease, whereas conditions that reduce afterload cause SV to increase. This concept is shown in Figure 3, where several pressure-volume loops generated by varying afterload while maintaining preload and contractility constant are displayed. Ventricular work generated in response to changes in preload and afterload is represented in Fig. 4.

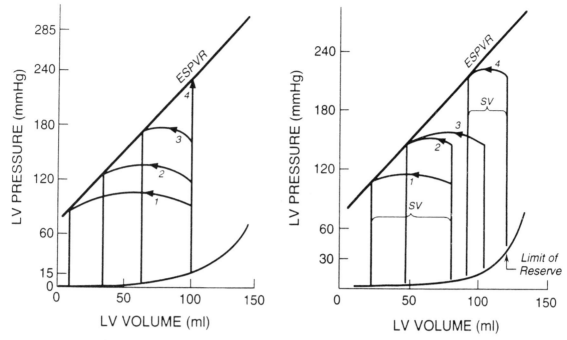

FIGURE 3. Illustration of pressure volume loops (**left**) and stress volume loops (**right**) of the left ventricle (LV) generated by altering preload or afterload. Loading conditions were altered by infusion of intravenous angiotensin to increase LV pressure or occlusion of the inferior vena cava to decrease LV pressure. The areas labeled as 1 in both groups represent control pressure–volume loops and stress–volume loops. At end systole, the points from each pressure–volume or stress–volume become linear [represented by the end systolic pressure–volume relationship (ESPVR) line]. Thus, the ESPVR line is load independent and its slope, dP/dV, is a reliable index of contractility. (Adapted from Ross J. Application and limitations of end-systolic measures of ventricular performance. *Fed Proc* 1984;43:2418–2422, with permission).

Contractility

There are various definitions for *contractility*, some load dependent (ejection fraction) and others load insensitive (preload recruitable stroke work) (5). In the isolated muscle preparation, contractility is defined simply as the velocity of fiber shortening at a given load. Although in the past this concept provided the physiologic foundation for studying contractility, it lacks clinical application. The first derivative of ventricular pressure with respect to time (dP/dt) is regarded by many as a marker of contractility. It increases with augmented venous return and with inotropic stimulation, whereas myocardial ischemia causes dP/dt to fall (1). It, too, suffers from the lack of direct clinical application.

Ventricular pressure–volume relationships can be used to access contractility as well as demonstrate the interdependence among preload, afterload, and contractility (Fig. 4). Using this technique, by sequentially increasing venous return, a family of pressure–volume loops related by a line connecting their intercept can be generated. The slope of this line expressed as (dP/dV) represents the elastance, *E*, which is a true index of contractility (6). The maximum elastance that can be achieved (E_{max}) represents the limit of ventricular systolic performance (7). Under normal conditions, ventricular filling begins with opening of the mitral valve. At end diastole, intraventricular pressure rises resulting in closure of the mitral valve. Next ventricular contraction begins (isovolumetric contraction). An abrupt rise in cavitary pressure develops and continues to build until aortic pressure (the

afterload) is surpassed, which forces the aortic valve to open, resulting in forward ejection. Systole ends with closure of the aortic valve, and a new cycle begins with diastolic isovolumetric relaxation.

MYOCARDIAL INFARCTION

Myocardial infarction is the leading cause of cardiogenic shock. The survival rate for cardiogenic shock consequent to an acute MI may be less than 20%. During the past two decades, several studies identified multiple predictors of perioperative MI (8). Only two variables, however, a recent history (<6 months) of MI and congestive heart failure (CHF), have been consistently shown to be associated with an adverse perioperative cardiac outcome (i.e., MI, cardiac death, and ventricular dysfunction).

Pathophysiology of Acute Myocardial Infarction

Plaque fissure resulting in exposure of subintimal collagen tissue to circulating platelet initiates the thrombotic processes, which leads to coronary artery thrombosis. Following acute occlusion and in the absence of collateral blood flow, cell death begins within 15 to 20 minutes. This process begins at the level of the subendocardium and progresses toward the epicardium. Studies demonstrated that at 3 and 6 hours after occlusion, 57% and

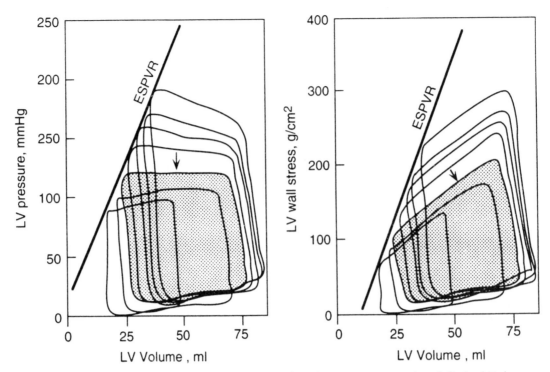

FIGURE 4. Depiction of left ventricular (LV) pressure-volume loops consequent to altered afterload. Each counterclockwise loop (arrow) indicates a given cardiac contraction. **Left,** With progressively increasing LV systolic pressure during ejection (beats 1, 2, and 3), stroke volume (SV) is reduced until finally at beat 4 ventricular systolic pressure is insufficient to open the aortic valve and an isovolumetric contraction ensues. **Right,** LV contraction cycles 1, 2 and 3 demonstrate that SV can be maintained in the presence of increased afterload with compensatory increase in end diastolic volume. However, further increase in afterload (cycle 4) results in a "mismatch" at the limit of preload reserve. In the setting of severe ventricular overdistension, the preload behaves as if it were fixed, and further increase in afterload results in reduced SV. (Adapted from Ross J. Surgical therapy for afterload mismatch. *J Am Coll Cardiol* 1985;5:811–826, with permission).

70% of the area at risk, respectively, have irreversible cell injury (9). Attempts at salvaging the myocardium using chemical thrombolysis, angioplasty, and surgical revascularization must be accomplished within 4 to 6 hours of onset of infarction.

Focal areas of necrosis are found frequently t autopsy in regions of the ventricle distant from the area of infarct (10). This finding is most consistent with a state of shock or from regional sympathetic catecholamine release (11). In addition, patients in cardiogenic shock often have a "piecemeal" necrosis marked by progressive myocardial necrosis from marginal extension of their infarct in an ischemic zone bordering on the infarction (12). Viability of the ischemic areas becomes highly dependent on collateral blood flow and coronary perfusion pressure (CPP). At autopsy, two-thirds of patients with cardiogenic shock have significant multivessel coronary artery stenosis of 75% or greater (12).

Evolution of Pump Failure

Myocardial injury affecting as little as 10% of ventricular mass can produce regional contractile dysfunction. Ejection fraction may remain unchanged; however, in the setting of preexisting ventricular dysfunction, SV can be significantly impaired. Cardiogenic shock ensues when contractile dysfunction involves 25% to 40% of the LV mass (8). The clinical picture may be further aggravated by mechanical factors such as acute mitral insufficiency from

a ruptured papillary muscle, perforation of the interventricular septum with left-to-right shunting, ventricular free-wall rupture resulting in cardiac tamponade, and persistent dysrhythmia.

Clinical Presentation

The onset and severity of symptoms associated with cardiogenic shock are directly related to the extent and amount of myocardial injury (Table 1). Typically, ischemic injury and cell death occur over the course of hours to days with subsequent progressive deterioration in ventricular performance. The clinical features may include mental obtundation, cool and clammy skin, thready rapid pulse, peripheral cyanosis, and others. Systolic blood pressure is often less than 90 mm Hg, and urine output may be negligible. Adequacy of pulmonary gas exchange will depend on the extent of pulmonary venous congestion and CO. Auscultation of the chest may reveal bilateral crackles of varying distribution throughout the lung fields; the heart sounds may be diminished, and ventricular gallops may be present. The electrocardiogram may demonstrate various types of arrhythmias, ischemic changes, and evidence of MI.

The hemodynamic profile in cardiogenic shock includes reduced arterial blood pressure, elevated PAOP of 20 to 25 mmHg, normal or elevated CVP, and a reduced cardiac index (CI) of less than 2.0 L per minute per M^2.

TABLE 1. CARDIOGENIC SHOCK: CLINICAL PRESENTATION

Central nervous systems
    Obtundation, irritability

Pulmonary
    Dyspnea, tachypnea, crackles, CXR positive for interstitial/alveolar
    edema

Cardiovascular
    Tachycardia, thready pulse, ventricular gallops (S_3 and S_4), JVD,
    ECG positive for ischemia or MI

Renal
    Oliguria or anuria, decreased urinary Na^+

Skin
    Cyanosis, cold and clammy

Hemodynamics
    BP <90 mm Hg systolic
    CVP variable (low to high), PAOP, usually >20 mm Hg,? V wave

CXR, chest roentgenogram; JVD, jugular venous distension; ECG, electrocardiograph; MI, myocardial infarction; NA^+, sodium; BP, blood pressure; CVP, central venous pressure; PAOP, pulmonary artery occlusion pressure.

MANAGEMENT OF CARDIOGENIC SHOCK

The first-line therapy for management of cardiogenic shock must be aimed at maximizing oxygen transport and delivery (Table 2). The major determinants of oxygen delivery to tissues are oxygen content in arterial blood and CO. Therefore, supplemental oxygen should be administered and adjusted based on arterial blood gas analysis. Endotracheal intubation and control of breathing remain a priority in the setting of shock states. Correction of acid–base and electrolyte disturbances as well as provision of anxiolytics are integral parts of the resuscitative effort.

TABLE 2. MANAGEMENT OF CARDIOGENIC SHOCK

Oxygen delivery
    Increase FIO_2; check arterial blood gas; check chest x-ray; intubate if
    indicated; correct acid-base; increase cardiac output

Cardiac function
  HR/rhythm
    Maintain normal sinus rhythm, avoid tachycardia (myocardial
    ischemia); for bradycardia, consider pacing or chronotropic
    drugs; monitor electrocardiogram (ischemia and arrhythmias)

  Preload
    Reduce increased preload with diuretics, venodilators
    (nitroglycerin, nitroprusside), monitor central venous pressure,
    pulmonary artery occlusion pressure, and stroke volume; obtain
    echocardiogram to rule out ischemia, valvular lesions,
    tamponade, intracardiac shunts; consider inotropes and/or
    intraaortic balloon pump

  Afterload
    Avoid increased afterload (wall tension), use vasodilators
    (nitroprusside); avoid hypotension; maintain coronary perfusion
    pressure; consider IABP or inotropes devoid of α-1
    effects (dobutamine, milrinone)

  Contractility
    Assess hemodynamics; obtain echocardiogram to assess heart
    function; use inotropes; consider vasodilators, intraaortic
    balloon pump, or ventricular assist devices; determine candidacy
    for thrombolytic therapy, angioplasty, or cardiac surgery

FIO_2, fraction of inspired oxygen; HR, heart rate; IABP, intraaortic balloon pump.

Specific therapeutic interventions to improve cardiac function require knowledge of the underlying cardiac pathology. To ensure an optimal clinical evaluation of cardiac function, invasive monitoring of arterial blood pressure; determination of CO; and measurement of central venous, pulmonary artery, and pulmonary capillary occlusion pressures are imperative. The diagnostic imaging by nuclear, two-dimensional echocardiography and Doppler ultrasound can provide invaluable information on ventricular function, acquired valvular diseases, aortic dissections, pericardial diseases, and intracardiac shunts resulting as complications of acute MI. The information derived from these monitors and imaging modalities can be used to refine clinical decisions and target therapeutic interventions.

Rate and rhythm disturbance occurs frequently during and after myocardial ischemia or MI. These abnormalities may be simple or complex and arising from either ventricular or supraventricular sites. Maintenance of normal sinus rhythm and rate and atrioventricular synchrony is critical to improving CO; therefore, the diagnosis and management of dysrhythmias are important for improving outcome (Chapter 27).

Cardiogenic shock may result from a reduction in SV caused by a derangement in one or more of the following elements of myocardial performance: HR, preload, afterload, and contractility. Therefore, specific management goals will be directed toward the pharmacologic or mechanical improvement of these variables.

Left ventricular preload (LVEDV) is invariably elevated in cardiogenic shock associated with an acute MI. In this situation, the PAOP is greater than 18 mm Hg and may be associated with marked pulmonary venous congestion. Initial therapy is aimed at reducing preload. Venodilation of the patient with nitrates, specifically, intravenous nitroglycerin, improves venous capacitance thereby reducing venous return and preload. This maneuver reduces wall tension and improves contractility and SV. In addition, coronary blood flow is augmented by reducing intracavitary pressure and coronary vascular resistance. The net result is improved myocardial performance, increased oxygen supply, and reduced oxygen demand.

Sympathoadrenal stimulation and release of catecholamines in response to the hemodynamic changes of shock can induce a vasoconstrictive state, which may increase demand on an already compromised ventricle. Consequently, the added afterload can significantly impede ventricular ejection. In these situations, afterload-reducing agents, most frequently sodium nitroprusside, alone or in combination with other vasodilators, may improve ventricular ejection and reduce myocardial oxygen consumption. With improved function of the ischemic myocardium, vasodilators also may impact the LV diastolic pressure–volume relationship by shifting it down and to the right. Concomitant unloading of the RV and reduction in the degree of pericardial restraint (consequent to vasodilator therapy) may further improve LV compliance. The potential for hypotension, however, may limit the use of vasodilator therapy in patients in cardiogenic shock. CPP is highly dependent on aortic pressures. In the presence of severe coronary artery stenosis, maintenance of normal to high normal mean aortic pressure is desirable. Hence, vasodilators must be used cautiously to ensure that coronary perfusion is maintained.

Afterload also can be reduced mechanically by placement of an intraaortic balloon pump (IABP). The IABP uses the technique of counterpulsation to maximize cardiac function during systole and diastole. Inflation of the balloon during diastole raises the aortic diastolic pressure, increasing CPP and myocardial oxygen delivery. Deflation of the balloon, just prior to ventricular ejection, creates a "pressure sink" or vascular void within the aortic root, thus mechanically reducing afterload. In summary, the advantages of IABP include systolic unloading, favoring a reduction in wall tension, myocardial oxygen consumption, preload and afterload, and diastolic augmentation, favoring myocardial oxygen supply.

In cardiogenic shock, reductions in SV result from defects in global contractility. Impairment of approximately 30% or more of ventricular mass can reduce cardiac performance markedly. Thus, the most effective way to improve cardiac performance is to augment contractility with positive inotropic agents alone or in combination with other vasoactive agents or ventricular assist devices. In addition, myocardial reperfusion techniques (pharmacologic thrombolysis, transluminal coronary angioplasty, or emergency coronary artery bypass surgery) may salvage myocardium at risk, thereby improving ventricular performance.

Sympathomimetic drugs (i.e., catecholamines) are pharmacologic agents capable of providing both inotropic and vasoactive effects. Regardless of their mode of action (direct or indirect), catecholamines exert *positive* inotropic action by stimulation of β_1-receptors. With the exception of norepinephrine and isoproterenol, catecholamines are capable of stimulating both α and β receptors (13). Of the adrenergic agents, dopamine is unique in its ability to also stimulate dopaminergic receptors (14).

The ultimate physiologic effect of an adrenergic agent is determined by the sum of its actions on α, β, or dopaminergic receptors. The effectiveness of any adrenergic agent will be influenced by the availability (i.e., density) and responsiveness (i.e., affinity) of adrenergic receptors. Stimulation and antagonism of these receptors induce reversible changes in receptor density. For example, chronically elevated levels of plasma catecholamines (such as occurs in CHF or hypertension) cause a downregulation in both the number and sensitivity of β receptors (15). The cellular and extracellular milieu also can affect the effectiveness of vasoactive and cardioactive drugs. Maintenance of normal acid–base status, normothermia, and electrolytes (including calcium and magnesium) improve the responsiveness to adrenergic receptor stimulation.

In an attempt to avoid the difficulties associated with adrenergic receptor density and number, noncatecholamine agents are frequently used. Noncatecholamine inotropic agents suggested for the management of cardiogenic shock include phophodiesterase inhibitors, thyroid hormone, and vasopressin.

Phosphodiesterase Fraction III Inhibitors

Phosphodiesterase (PDE) fraction III inhibitors (amrinone and milrinone) cause an increase in cyclic adenosine monophosphate (cAMP) independent of adrenergic receptor stimulation. By inhibiting the PDE III isoenzyme, this group of drugs blocks the breakdown of cAMP. In turn, cAMP accumulates intracellularly in both the myocardium and vascular smooth-muscle cells. In myocardial cells, accumulation of cAMP leads to an increase in intracellular calcium with a positive inotropic action. In vascular smooth muscle, cAMP accumulation has a vasodilator action

mediated by vascular smooth-muscle relaxation. The vasodilator action has both systemic and pulmonary vascular effects (16–18). Amrinone was the first PDE III introduced into clinical practice. Because of concerns regarding thrombocytopenia associated with prolonged amrinone administration, milrinone has become the PDE III of choice for use in both cardiac surgery and patients in the intensive care unit (ICU). Of note, milrinone is also 20 times more potent than amrinone. As these PDE III inhibitors affect through nonadrenergic mechanisms, their effectiveness is not altered in situations where β-receptor regulation is altered as previously described (15).

The literature is replete with numerous studies that demonstrate the ability of milrinone to augment ventricular performance in multiple settings, including CHF (19), ventricular dysfunction following cardiopulmonary bypass (CPB) (20,21), and in patients with a multisystem failure (22). Clinical investigation by Prielipp and colleagues assessed the ability of milrinone to increase CI and oxygen delivery in ICU patients (22). This study attempted to verify that a pharmacokinetic model previously developed in cardiac surgical patients to calculate dosing of milrinone (23) could be used to predict milrinone plasma concentrations in a medical–surgical ICU population. Their data confirmed that a milrinone loading dose of 50 μg per kilogram of body weight followed by an infusion of 0.5 μg per kilogram per minute achieved therapeutic plasma concentrations and significantly increase both CI and oxygen delivery in this mixed ICU patient population (22).

Data also suggest that milrinone may improve myocardial diastolic relaxation (positive "lusitropic" effect) and augment coronary perfusion. This action may be particularly beneficial in the management of diastolic dysfunction (24). The proposed mechanism for this effect on diastolic performance is that by decreasing LV wall tension, LV filling is enhanced. In addition, by decreasing LV wall tension and augmenting LV filling, myocardial blood flow and O_2 delivery are optimized. Because of the pharmacokinetic properties of milrinone, dosing studies were performed to validate the following administration technique. A loading dose of milrinone at 50 μcg per kilogram of body weight should be infused over 10 to 15 minutes. Because of the relatively short elimination half-life, the loading dose of milrinone should be followed by a continuous infusion of 0.5 μg per kilogram of body weight per minute to ensure optimal plasma levels. With this approach, the estimated half-life was approximately 50 minutes following CPB.

The PDE inhibitors also have unique effects on vascular tone, specifically vascular smooth muscle (25). The internal mammary artery and coronary arteries contain vascular endothelium, which may be injured by the mechanical effects of CPB and by cytokines released during CPB. The vasodilation associated with the PDE inhibitors produces significant vasodilation in these vascular beds. Salmenpera and Levy demonstrated the ability of milrinone to increase significantly internal mammary artery relaxation, which might prove valuable in the setting of coronary artery bypass grafting (CABG) (26).

A study by Lobato and colleagues compared epinephrine 0.03 μg per kilogram of body weight per minute to milrinone 50 μcg per kilogram on LV compliance following CPB (27). Milrinone increased LVEDA by 15%. Epinephrine failed to improve LV compliance.

Amrinone and Milrinone: Is There a Difference?

The principal reason that milrinone is the most frequently used PDE III inhibitor is based on its ability to preserve platelet function. To determine whether there were differences in clinical hemodynamic responses of these agents, a study by Rothwell and associates compared amrinone with milrinone in patients following elective cardiac surgery (28). In this study, 45 patients undergoing elective cardiac surgery at four centers received either amrinone or milrinone in a randomized blind fashion. Both amrinone and milrinone increased CI significantly (47% and 52%, respectively). Hemodynamic effects, including a decrease in systemic and PVR, were also similar. Therefore, these investigators concluded that the choice between agents should be based on nonhemodynamic considerations, such as cost and side effects.

Thyroid Hormone

Clinical and animal data suggest that reduced thyroid hormone concentrations may be one cause of decreased myocardial performance following CPBs as well as in patients with a clinical diagnosis of brain death. Of note, decreases in triiodothyronine (T_3) following CPB are out of proportion to the decreases that would be expected from hemodilution (by the pump priming solution) or from administration of heparin alone (29). The most dramatic decreases in T_3 are seen at the end of CPB and during the first hours after CPB; however, concentrations (T_3) gradually return toward normal values 12 to 24 hours after CPB.

The discovery of decreased circulating T_3 concentration during and after CPB prompted the investigation of its role in maintaining cardiac function. Novitzky and colleagues administered T_3 to ten patients prior to weaning from CPB (30,31). This resulted in an increase in mean arterial blood pressure and HR and a reduction in left arterial blood pressure and central venous blood pressure. In five other patients who initially could not be weaned from bypass, the administration of T_3 permitted CPB to be discontinued within 20 to 50 minutes.

The effects of T_3 in patients undergoing cardiac surgery and in patients with cardiogenic shock remain controversial. For example, studies by Klemperer and colleagues demonstrated a significant improvement in ventricular performance in patients who received T_3 following CPB (32). A subsequent study by Bennett-Guerrero and co-workers, however, was unable to show any significant changes in cardiovascular performance with the administration of supplemental T_3 (33). One possible reason for lack of change noted in this study is that a significant number of patients were receiving calcium-channel blockers, which would have interfered with the actions of T_3. Clearly, T_3 may have a role in select patients who develop LV dysfunction following CPB; however, it should not be used routinely in this patient population.

Thyroid hormone also has been used to improve the cardiac function of potential organ donors (i.e., patient with clinical signs of brain death). In one study, donors treated with an intravenous T_3 infusion (2 μg/hr) showed improved mean arterial blood pressure and HR, decreased CVP, and a reduced need for inotropic drug support compared with donors not receiving replacement (34).

In summary, *routine* administration of T_3 to patients undergoing cardiac surgery cannot be recommended at present; further studies will be needed to define more fully the role of T_3 in patients after CPB.

Arginine Vasopressin

Arginine vasopressin (AVP) is an endogenous peptide synthesized exclusively in the hypothalamus and released from the posterior pituitary (Table 3). Traditionally, AVP release is stimulated by changes in vascular volume and vascular time. Vasopressin is bound by two distinct types of receptors: vasomotor (V_1) and renal (V_2) (35).

Although under normal conditions AVP contributes little to blood pressure maintenance, recent investigations demonstrated the utility of AVP in certain refractory vasodilatory states (36–38), and it is now recommended for use in advanced cardiac life support (ACLS) algorithms. In a syndrome known as *postcardiotomy vasodilatory shock* [characterized by catecholamine resistance, SVR <650 dynes/sec/cm^5 (even with high norepinephrine infusion rates) and blood pressure <65 mm Hg], patients requiring LV assist devices were hemodynamically optimized using AVP (39–41). In these patients, the infusion of AVP significantly improved hemodynamics and reduced the need for norepinephrine infusion.

Subsequent investigators explored the role of AVP administration in the management of vasodilatory states in septic shock and following CPB (42,43). Although the precise mechanisms responsible for this vasodilatory state are unknown, patients experiencing those vasodilatory states are characterized by a significant reduction in circulating vasopressin. In these groups of patients, infusion of AVP in the range of 2 to 8 U per hour resulted in

TABLE 3. PRACTICAL GUIDE TO ADMINISTERING AVP

Manufacturing unit: Arginine vasopressin 20 U/2-mL bottles
Preparation: 100 U in 100 mL normal saline
Dose: 2–8 U/h
   Titrate until blood pressure improves
   Increasing >8 U/h provides little added vasopressor effect because of endogenous inhibitory mechanism

Indications
   Vasodilatory hypotension/shock resistant to high doses of catecholamines regardless of etiology
   Vasodilatory state requiring high doses of catecholamine vasopressors (eg, norepinephrine >8 μg/min to maintain mean blood pressure >65 mm Hg)
   Systemic vascular resistance <650 dynes s/cm^2 despite high dose catecholamine vasopressors
   Prophylactic use in vasodilatory shock states where the correction of AVP deficiency has been shown to be unique vasopressor (e.g., postcardiotomy shock, late-phase septic or hemorrhagic shock)

Contraindications
   Any form of hypertension/shock with a normal vascular resistance on no or minimal vasopressors

Complications
   None seen in our experience when used at 8 U/h or lower
   At > 10 U/h → decreased digital and cutaneous perfusion seen
   At > 20 U/h → intestinal ischemia, hepatic insufficiency, coronary spasm seen

AVP, arginine vasopressin.

significant hemodynamic improvements (ACLS guidelines calls for a single 40 U intravenous bolus for treatment of refractory hypotension). Increases in the infusion greater than 8 U per hour provided little added effect because of endogenous inhibitory mechanisms.

Combination Therapy

Because of the complex causes of pump failure in cardiogenic shock, multiple drug regimens are frequently used to optimize the desired therapeutic effects (43). Combination therapy enables greater selectivity of effect. The unwanted side effects of one drug can be avoided while supplementing its desired effects with another agent.

The rationale for combination therapy has evolved because of the fact that β stimulation is not always desirable, and α agonist action is not always undesirable. To maximize the desired effects of any particular combination of agents, however, frequent assessment of cardiac performance is a must. It is important to remember that the anticipated effects of any given agent will not necessarily be as expected when used in combination with others.

As intravenous catecholamines remain the primary modalities used clinically to augment ventricular performance, clinical studies performed over the past several years focused on defining the effect of combining these agents with Ca^{2+} and PDE III inhibitors (43–45). Are combinations of these drugs synergetic, additive, or antagonistic to catecholamines?

Clinical studies demonstrated the positive effect on cardiac performance using a technique that combines a β agonist with a PDE inhibitor. In theory, this practice makes pharmacologic sense because these agents work through different mechanisms. Prielipp and colleagues demonstrated an *additive* effect when epinephrine and amrinone were administered together in patients with low CO (44). In another study by the same authors, they showed that the combined administration of two β agonists (epinephrine and dobutamine) produced a *less* than additive effect (epinephrine functioned as a full agonist with dobutamine functioning as a partial agonist) (44). Another study evaluated the effect of combining Ca^+ with both catecholamines and the PDE III inhibitors. The administration of calcium chloride following CPB resulted in a refractiveness of the heart to catecholamines but not the PDE III inhibitors (45).

MECHANICAL COMPLICATIONS

Mechanical lesions resulting from complications of an MI include acute mitral valve regurgitation (papillary muscle dysfunction and rupture) and ventricular septal or free-wall rupture. Cardiac rupture accounts for approximately 15% of mortalities associated with acute MI.

Acute Mitral Regurgitation

Acute mitral regurgitation can occur as a result of pathologic changes involving the chordae tendineae or the papillary muscles from altered LV geometry secondary to myocardial ischemia or infarction.

Rupture of the posteromedial papillary muscle occurs five to ten times more commonly than rupture of the anterolateral papillary muscle. The former has a poorer and less reliable blood supply provided predominantly by the posterior descending branch of either the right or the left circumflex (depending on dominant system) artery. The papillary muscles are at risk of hypoxia as a result of their distant location from the epicardial vessels. Along with the increased intracavitary pressure that develops following an acute MI, this may lead to papillary muscle dysfunction or rupture. In the presence of either significant systolic or diastolic ventricular dysfunction, acute rupture of a papillary muscle may induce (or precipitate) cardiogenic shock. Clinical sequelae include elevated PAOP with peaked V waves, fulminant pulmonary edema, acute right ventricular failure, and systemic hypotension. In this situation, echocardiography coupled with Doppler flow studies can be instrumental in evaluating the severity of ventricular dysfunction and mitral regurgitation. Following papillary muscle rupture, cases of severe mitral regurgitation should be corrected by using surgical repair or replacement. CABG should be performed in addition as indicated. Without surgical intervention, the prognosis for death from complicated acute papillary muscle rupture is 50% in 24 hours and almost 100% within weeks. In contrast, early mitral valve surgery affords the best prognosis, with a 60% to 70% survival rate (46,47). Temporizing medical management goals for severe acute mitral regurgitation include the use of vasoactive drugs to reduce preload and afterload, cardioactive drugs to improve inotropy and chronotropy and placement of an IABP for reasons previously described.

Ventricular Septal Rupture

Rupture of the ventricular septal wall accounts for as many as 5% of all infarct-related deaths (48). Most cases of septal infarcts occur between 3 and 7 days following infarction. Clinical manifestations of this lesion depend on the size of the septal defect and the extent of the MI. In general, the pathophysiologic changes include a left-to-right shunt associated with increased pulmonary blood flow, systemic hypotension, reduced right ventricular performance, and evidence of systemic venous congestion. Early recognition and diagnosis can be made by Doppler echocardiographic examination or by right-sided heart catheterization. The classic finding attained by catheterization is a "step-up" in blood oxygen saturation from the right atrium to the RV or proximal pulmonary artery.

Survival with an acute septal rupture is less than 20% at 2 months and only 5% to 7% at 1 year with medical therapy (49); however, surgical repair of the defect, including myocardial revascularization, can dramatically alter outcome, with short-term survival approaching 75% in some series (48). Perioperative mortality is high for patients whose septal rupture is complicated by cardiogenic shock or by right ventricular infarction.

In preparation for surgery, aggressive medical management is aimed at improving CO using positive inotropic support alone or in combination with vasodilators to reduce both left and right ventricular afterload. Vasodilator therapy, however, may have undesirable hemodynamic effects by potentially aggravating systemic hypotension. Any modality that reduces blood flow to the myocardium also will produce further decreases in CPP.

Furthermore, increases in systemic vasodilation can reverse the intracardiac shunt (right-to-left shunting), resulting in marked arterial oxygen desaturation. Likewise, the use of inotropes and vasopressors may exacerbate left-to-right shunting with further increase in pulmonary blood flow and deterioration of RV function. Lastly, the IABP can be used in combination with vasoactive and cardioactive drugs to improve ventricular performance.

Free-wall Rupture

Acute free-wall rupture results from a transmural MI of the left ventricle; it affects the anterior and the inferior walls with equal frequency and accounts for up to 24% of all infarction-related deaths. It occurs most often between the second and the eighth day postinfarction (8). Death occurs almost instantaneously from hemopericardium resulting in cardiac tamponade and electromechanical dissociation. The lesion is incompatible with life, and most resuscitative efforts are unsuccessful except in the rare patient who has subacute form of this syndrome and may respond to therapy.

Cardiac Tamponade

Cardiac tamponade occurs when external pressures (e.g., intrapericardial pressure) to the heart impede venous return to the RV. Common causes of postsurgical cardiac tamponade include mediastinal bleeding, intrapericardial rupture from retrograde dissection of an aortic aneurysm, and hemopericardium related to free-wall rupture in the setting of a perioperative MI. Other causes of tamponade include excessive fluid or air accumulation within the pericardial sac or by extracardiac compression from distended lungs during positive pressure ventilation.

In the normal state, the pressure within the pericardium is just subatmospheric or zero. The pericardial pressure–volume relationship is such that any rapid accumulation of volume (blood, air, or serous fluid) causes an acute rise in intrapericardial pressure, which may exceed diastolic chamber pressure and impede venous return to the heart. Tamponade can occur with as little as 100 mL of volume in acute settings, whereas with gradual accumulation of fluid, up to 1,000 mL or more may be tolerated. The increased pericardial pressure resulting from this volume increase may produce dynamic changes in cardiac performance during inspiration and expiration. For example, during inspiration, intrathoracic pressure becomes more negative, favoring venous return to the RV. Thus, RVSV to the lungs is increased, whereas LVSV is reduced. The mechanisms for this observation include reduced venous return from the lungs secondary to the expansion of pulmonary vascular bed, bulging of the interventricular septum leftward impeding LV filling, and an increase in LV afterload from the effects of reduced intrathoracic pressure (50). During expiration, the cycle is reversed. Venous return to the LV is increased, the septum moves rightward, and RV filling is reduced. Alteration in arterial blood pressure waveform may demonstrate pulsus paradoxus.

Diagnosis of cardiogenic shock complicated by cardiac tamponade may be made clinically. The gold standard for diagnosing tamponade, however, is echocardiography. The physical findings in the Beck triad are hypotension, elevated CVP, and a quiet precordium on auscultation; these are infrequent. Electrocardiographic evidence of low voltage, electrical alternans, and diffuse ST-segment changes also lack sensitivity and specificity. Likewise, equalization of diastolic pressures (i.e., CVP = RVEDP = PAD = PAOP = LVEDP (where RVEDP represents right ventricular end-diastolic pressure and PAD equals pulmonary artery diastolic pressure) may be absent, especially after pericardiotomy for cardiac surgery. Two-dimensional echocardiographic imaging can demonstrate the presence, location, and amount of pericardial effusions, blood clot formation, ventricular dyssynergy, and signs of right atrial and ventricular collapse during diastole.

Management strategies for cardiogenic shock associated with cardiac tamponade include maintenance of rapid sinus rate and atrioventricular synchrony, preload augmentation (for hypovolemic patients), maintenance of afterload with vasoactive drugs to maintain CPP, and the addition of inotropes to augment contractility. The definitive therapy is surgical removal of blood clots and drainage of effusion or blood. Cardiac tamponade arising from ventricular free-wall rupture or from trauma requires immediate surgical intervention. Survival, however, is rare.

RIGHT VENTRICULAR DYSFUNCTION

Perioperative RV dysfunction associated with cardiogenic shock can be the result of either a single derangement or a combination of disturbances. Most notably, ischemia or infarction of the RV may be associated with 30% to 40% of cases of low-output hypotensive syndromes (8). Other factors that influence RV dysfunction include altered preload, afterload, LV performance, intrapericardial pressure, intrathoracic pressure, and interventricular septal kinetics.

Right Ventricular Infarction

Right ventricular infarctions were considered rare and clinically inconsequential by most clinicians until two decades ago. In fact, the entire RV was regarded as hemodynamically unimportant, functioning only as a volume conduit. With the advent of various diagnostic imaging techniques, however, allowing better characterization of RV function, there is now sufficient evidence to demonstrate that RV performance is essential because LV performance is highly dependent on RV function. Isolated RV infarction is rare, occurring in fewer than 3% of hearts with MIs examined at postmortem (51). In contrast, LV infarct involving the RV is far more common.

The right coronary artery (RCA) is the dominant artery that gives rise to the posterior descending artery (PDA) in 90% of humans. The PDA supplies the posterior walls of the right and left ventricles and the posterior third of the interventricular septum. Marginal branches of the RCA supply the RV free wall, whereas the anterior margin and anterior free-wall of the RV are supplied by the left anterior descending artery.

The thin-walled, compliant RV does not compensate well for increases in afterload. Even slight alterations in RV afterload produce dramatic decreases in RV performance. This is manifested by a progressive decline in RV ejection fraction, which is particularly deleterious if afterload increases acutely (Fig. 5). Increases

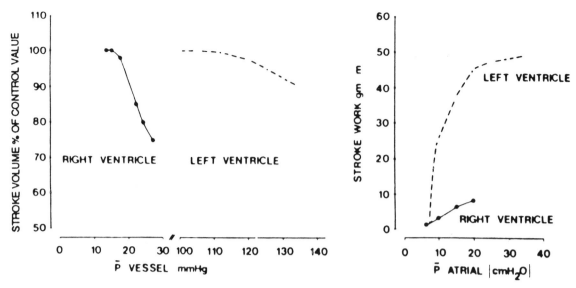

FIGURE 5. Varying effects of afterload (**left**) and preload (**right**) seen in ventricular function curves from the right and left ventricle. The right ventricle (RV) output is more afterload dependent and less preload dependent than the left ventricle (LV). (Reproduced from McFadden ER, Braunwald E. Cor pulmonale and pulmonary thromboembolism. In: Braunwald E, ed. *Textbook of cardiovascular medicine*. Philadelphia: WB Saunders, 1980:1643–1680, with permission.)

in RV afterload (i.e., PVR) can occur with positive-pressure ventilation, pulmonary emboli, acute respiratory distress syndrome (ARDS), and chronic obstructive lung disease (52).

Alterations in RV contractility have been observed with high levels of positive end-expiratory pressure (PEEP) (i.e., >20 cm H_2O), protamine administration, (both during and after cardiac surgery), and with RV ischemia (53). RV diastolic dysfunction is also evident at lower systolic blood pressures than under circumstances of normal coronary blood flow.

Abnormalities in LV function as a result of CAD, CHF, valvular heart disease, and systemic hypertension all impact on RV function, depending on the degree to which they affect RV diastolic volume, systolic function, and afterload.

Preoperative RV hypertrophy constitutes an additional problem in the perioperative maintenance of myocardial performance. RV hypertrophy caused by chronic pulmonary hypertension limits the ability of the RV to respond to even minimal increases in pulmonary resistance. In advanced stages of right ventricular hypertrophy, areas of relative ischemia often progress to ischemic cardiomyopathy. Postmortem studies show a high incidence of RV infarction in patients with RV hypertrophy.

Management of Right Ventricular Failure

The hemodynamics of RV failure include increased right atrial and RV end-diastolic pressures and decreased CO. Treatment strategies have emphasized volume loading, vasodilators, vasoconstrictors, inotropic support, maintenance of normal atrioventricular conduction, and mechanical assist devices. The appropriate sequence of these therapeutic measures depends largely on the status of PVR, that is, RV afterload and the contractility of both the RV and LV.

Volume expansion forms the basis of treatment when PVR and RV contractility are normal. An increased LVEDV maximizes contractility (fiber stretch) and maintains CO. RV dilation is the major compensatory mechanism for improving its contractility; however, treatment with volume expansion is limited by the pericardium to a ventricular filling pressure of approximately 12 mm Hg.

Right ventricular volume overload has been shown to distort the interventricular septum, leading to a reduction in both LV volume and septal contractility (53). Hence, a significant increase in RV volume may further decrease the already decreased LV compliance. In view of these facts, volume loading during acute RV infarction should be questioned. Inotropic support may be preferable for these patients because it maintains compliance of both ventricles.

Vasoconstrictive therapy, when indicated, can be used to treat RV dysfunction, particularly when RV ischemia occurs (54). Laver and colleagues produced RV dysfunction (in a canine model) by inducing myocardial ischemia with progressive occlusion of the main pulmonary artery. This was accompanied by a pronounced rise in RVEDP. The infusion of phenylephrine produced a dramatic increase in aortic diastolic pressure, thereby improving right ventricular perfusion (54). A vasoconstrictive dose of norepinephrine has been used successfully to increase afterload to treat ventricular dysfunction secondary to intracoronary air embolus during cardiac surgery (55).

When RV dysfunction occurs as a result of increased RV afterload, treatment should focus on agents that decrease pulmonary hypertension (Table 4). The management of RV dysfunction secondary to pulmonary hypertension remains an area of active clinical and laboratory investigation. Drug therapy is the primary modality for management of pulmonary hypertension, that is, drugs that demonstrate specificity for dilating the pulmonary vasculature versus the systemic vasculature (55).

Pulmonary vascular resistance is decreased, stimulating either cyclic guanosine monophosphate (cGMP) or cAMP. This

TABLE 4. IMPACT OF PULMONARY HYPERTENSION ON RIGHT VENTRICULAR FUNCTION

Increased right ventricular end diastolic and systolic pressure volume
Decreased right ventricular ejection fraction
Decreased movement and compliance of the septum
Increased risk of ischemia particularly in the face of right coronary artery disease

production is important for identifying which of these sites of actions is affected because studies suggest an additive effect when agents from different classes are combined. In a study by Hill and Pearl, combining inhaled nitric oxide (NO) with inhaled prostacyclin resulted in an additive effect in PVR (56).

Traditionally, pulmonary vasodilation was accomplished using nitroglycerin and sodium nitroprusside (SNP). Although both these modalities decrease PVR (predominantly by increased CO), the concomitant and often dramatic decrease in SVR (particularly with SNP) may result in systemic hypotension and often limits their clinical use. It is important to remember that ganglionic blockers do not affect PVR (57). Additional agents that have been used with variable success for pulmonary vasodilation include hydralazine and nifedipine (58,59). In addition, α-adrenergic blocking agents, such as tolazoline and phentolamine, have been used clinically to decrease PVR during NO administration (60).

Current research is aimed at identifying new drugs that have more specific pulmonary vasodilating effects mediated most likely by one of the two parallel cyclic nucleotide-dependent mechanisms responsible for controlling the tone of vascular smooth muscle. The best understood of these mechanisms is that of receptor-coupled adenylate cyclase, through which the β adrenergic receptor agonists (i.e., epinephrine and isoproterenol) promote pulmonary vasodilation (61). β-Agonist-stimulated adenylate cyclase produces cyclic AMP (cAMP), which results in activation of cAMP-dependent protein kinase, resulting in changes in the phosphorylation of myosin and relaxation of vascular smooth muscle. Some prostanoid receptors are also linked to the adenylate cyclase system. Agents, such as prostaglandin E_1 (PGE$_1$) and PGI$_2$ (prostacyclin), exert their vasodilator effects via this mechanism. PGE$_1$ effectively decreases PVR and augments RV performance in patients with pulmonary hypertension secondary to mitral valve disease (62). Data from animal models of pulmonary hypertension demonstrate that the pulmonary vasodilating effects of PGE$_1$ are more specific than those of β-agonist (isoproterenol or epinephrine), hydralazine, prostacyclin, or nifedipine (Fig. 6) (59).

Although all these agents decrease pulmonary artery pressure (PAP) and PVR, the hemodynamic effects differ among these various therapies. PGE$_1$ and isoproterenol result in the greatest degree of pulmonary specificity (i.e., pulmonary vasodilation). Prostacyclin demonstrated an intermittent pulmonary specificity (less than PGE but greater than isoproterenol or nifedipine). Nifedipine showed the smallest degree of pulmonary specificity and was the least effective in decreasing PAP.

The search for newer agents and delivery modalities led to the use of inhaled NO and prostacyclin, PDE III inhibitors, and adenosine (63–69) (Table 5).

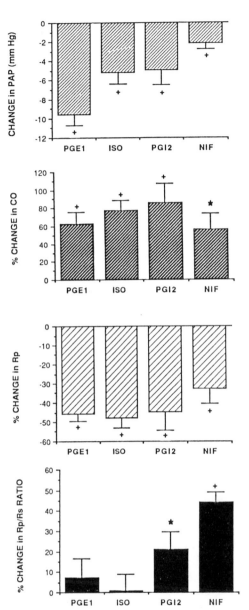

FIGURE 6. Data illustrating the change in mean pulmonary artery pressure (PAP), cardiac output (CO), pulmonary vascular resistance (Rp), and the ratio of the pulmonary to systemic vascular resistance (Rp/Rs). Variables are studied following the administration of prostaglandin (PGE$_1$), isoproterenol (ISO), prostacyclin (PGI$_2$), and nifedipine. PGE$_1$ and isoproterenol were the most selective pulmonary vasodilators. (Reproduced from Prielipp RC, Rosenthal MH, Pearl RG. Vasodilator therapy in vasoconstrictor induced pulmonary hypertension in sheep. *Anesthesiology* 1988;68:552, with permission.)

The discovery of NO provided an alternative mechanism for regulating vascular smooth-muscle tone. Although this pathway (mediated via cGMP) is not understood as well as the cAMP-dependent pathway, they are parallel in several ways. Activation of cytoplasmic guanylate cyclase by NO leads to an increase in cGMP, further activating a family of cGMP-dependent protein kineses, resulting in relaxation of the vascular smooth muscle (70).

When delivered as a gas into alveoli, exogenous NO diffuses into the adjacent vascular smooth muscle, where it activates guanylate cyclase, increasing cGMP and resulting in

TABLE 5. PHARMACOLOGIC MODALITIES FOR REDUCING PULMONARY VASCULAR RESISTANCE MECHANISM OF ACTION

cGMP	cAMP
Sodium nitroprusside	Adenosine
Nitroglycerin	β-agonists
	Prostaglandins
	Calcium channel blockers
	PDE-III Inhibitors

cGMP, cyclic guanosine monophosphate; cAMP, cyclic adenosine monophosphate; PDE-III, phosphodiesterase III.

smooth-muscle relaxation (Table 6). NO rapidly binds to hemoglobin (after diffusing into the intravascular space), forming nitrosylhemoglobin, which then is rapidly oxidized to methemoglobin, which is excreted by the kidney. It is this rapid binding of NO (yielding an inactive form) that impacts its specificity. Because all the NO is rendered inactive in the pulmonary circulation, the systemic effects (i.e., system vasodilation) are minimized.

Recent investigations focused on the potential for NO administration in patients with ARDS. Hypoxemia in ARDS is due to ventilation–perfusion mismatch and intrapulmonary shunting. Intravenous pulmonary vasodilator therapy with agents, such as nitroglycerin, nitroprusside, PGE_1, prostacyclin, and nifedipine, results in small decreases in PVR but large decreases in systemic blood pressure and arterial oxygenation. The adverse effects on oxygenation occur because the decrease in PVR is primary as a result of a reversal in hypoxic pulmonary vasoconstriction. NO can decrease PVR while improving oxygenation (71,72). The decreased shunt occurs because inhaled NO is distributed so that the associated vasodilation increases blood flow only to well-ventilated alveoli. Inhaled NO may reverse bronchoconstriction. Rossaint and co-workers investigated the effect of inhaled NO (18 ppm) on ten patients with ARDS (72). The results of NO therapy were compared with those obtained using an intravenous infusion of prostacyclin. Inhalation of NO (18 ppm) significantly reduced mm Hg from 37% ± 3% to 31% ± 5%. The PaO_2/FIO_2 ratio increased from 152 ± 15 to 199 ± 23. MAP and CO were unchanged. In the prostacyclin group, PAP decreased, but so did the PaO_2/FIO_2 and systemic arterial pressures. Intrapulmonary shunting increased. Seven patients in this study were treated with continuous inhalation of NO (3–20 ppm) for 3 to 35 days; six of seven patients survived.

TABLE 6. POTENTIAL CLINICAL APPLICATIONS OF INHALED NITRIC OXIDE

Pediatrics
  Persistent pulmonary hypertension of the newborn
Adults
  Acute respiratory distress syndrome
  Transplantation (cardiac, lung)
  Cardiac surgery
  Pediatric (congenital)
  Sickle cell disease

In a subsequent study, these same investigators demonstrated that inhaled concentration of only 60 to 250 ppb (much less than 1 ppm) were able to increase PaO_2 by 30% (73). These concentrations had little or no effect on PAP, however. Subsequent studies suggested that the optimal dose of NO in ARDS may be 2 ppm and that higher doses may decrease pulmonary hypertension but actually reverse oxygenation (74). The appropriate role of inhaled NO in ARDS remains to be elucidated. To date, no study has demonstrated improved survival in patients with NO.

Combining Nitrous Oxide with Phenylephrine: Does This Have Clinical Utility?

Doery and colleagues randomized patients with ARDS to receive intravenous phenylephrine, 50 to 200 μg per minute, titrated to a 20% increase in MAP, inhaled NO, and the combination of phenylephrine and NO. Phenylephrine significantly augmented the improvement in PaO_2 seen with inhaled NO (75). The result may reflect selective enhancement of hypoxic pulmonary vasoconstriction by phenylephrine, which complements the selective vasodilator action of NO.

Newer investigations are now focusing on the potential clinical applications of inhaled prostacyclin. Prostacyclin is a potent vasodilator primarily released from endothelial cells. Mechanistically, prostacyclin acts by binding to cell-surface receptors to activate adenylate cyclase probably via a protein (76). Prostacyclin also stimulates endothelial release of NO. It is a potent vasodilator, inhibits neutrophil activation, stabilizes cell membranes, and inhibits platelet aggregation.

The first clinical report of prostacyclin use was in 1980 by Watkins in a child with pulmonary hypertension (77). The use of systemic PGI_2 is severely limited by hypotension. Inhaled PGI_2 was used to treat pulmonary hypertension and RV failure (76). In this study, patients exhibited a mean decrease in PVR of 35% with a mean increase in CI of 26%. These changes were accompanied by a small (7%) but significant decrease in mean PAP and a 23% decrease in SVR. There were no significant changes in splenic arterial pressure or effective preload as measured by CVP or pulmonary capillary wedge pressure.

Because both NO and PGI_2 are potential inhaled therapies for pulmonary hypertension, it is important to realize that they have clinically significant differences. First, NO and PGI_2 act through different signaling pathways: NO via cGMP and PGI_2 via intracellular cAMP. As such, they appear to be additive in terms of their effects on pulmonary vasculature. PGI_2 is not actively bound on entering the vascular space as is NO and requires metabolic elimination in the liver. Thus, it has a significantly longer biologic half-life, which could predispose to systemic side effects.

Phosphodiesterase Inhibition: Direct and Indirect Pulmonary Vasodilation

The PDE III inhibitors combine both positive inotropic and vasodilatory effects that can have dramatic effects on the pulmonary vascular system. Early studies by Hess demonstrated the effects of amrinone (a bypridine PDE-III inhibitor) on pulmonary and systemic hemodynamics in patients with elevated PAP secondary to valvular heart disease (78). Data from this study demonstrated that amrinone decreases both PAP and PVR. Initially, this reduction was thought to be the result of an indirect effect of increasing cGMP levels with a subsequent reduction in PVR. In addition to these "indirect" pulmonary vasodilating effects, experimental data now indicate that the PDE III inhibitors also can cause the release of NO, resulting in more selective pulmonary vasodilation as well. In subsequent laboratory investigations, Morrary and colleagues were able to demonstrate a significant increase in the degree of relaxation of pulmonary vascular rings, which were bathed in amrinone when the vascular endothelium remained intact. In their experimental model, vascular relaxation was increased from 44% to 58% when the endothelium of the vessel was present (65).

Tanaka and associates demonstrated that in an animal model of embolism-induced pulmonary hypertension, milrinone increased CI and reduced PAP and PVR (67). These investigators studied the effects of two different milrinone infusions in animals following the development of pulmonary hypertension. Milrinone did not reduce PAP or PVR in normal dogs but did significantly decrease both PAP and PVR in the animals with pulmonary hypertension without any effect on mean arterial pressure.

Monrad et al. evaluated 18 patients with CHF [New York Heart Association (NYHA) class III–IV] and showed that, in addition to improving hemodynamics, milrinone also significantly decreased PVR (79). Benotti and co-workers also demonstrated a decrease in PVR (in patients with CHF) following milrinone administration (80).

Eichorn and colleagues evaluated the effects of milrinone and dobutamine on RV preload, afterload and systolic performance in patients with CHF (81). Although both drug regimens resulted in improvements in RV ejection fraction, only milrinone increased RV systolic function and reduced RV afterload. The changes that occurred secondary to dobutamine were predominantly due to enhanced RV inotropic activity.

In the European Multicenter Milrinone Trial (EMMT), 99 adult patients who had undergone either elective CABG surgery or valve replacement were studied (CI <2.5 L/min/M^2 and a PAOP ≤8 mm Hg) (82,83). All patients received a loading infusion of milrinone 50 μg per kilogram of body weight over 10 minutes, followed by a maintenance infusion of either 0.375, 0.5, or 0.75 μg per kilogram per minute for a period of 12 hours. In addition to significant improvements in systemic hemodynamics, milrinone also produced significant reductions in PAP and PVR. To target the group of patients who might receive the greatest benefit from a pulmonary vasodilator, the patients were stratified into the groups based on their post-bypass baseline PVR. Using this approach, the greatest changes in PVR occurred in patients with the higher pretreatment PVR (≥200 dynes/sec/cm^{-5}).

Adenosine is also being investigated as a potential agent for use in the treatment of pulmonary hypertension. Inbar and colleagues evaluated the effects of intravenous adenosine administered in combination with calcium-channel blockers in patients with primary pulmonary hypertension (84) (Table 7). The

TABLE 7. ADENOSINE AS A PULMONARY DILATOR

Dose	50 μg/kg/min
Hemodynamic effects	↓ Pulmonary vascular resistance, ↑ cardiac output
	± Mean arterial pressure
	No change in Pao$_2$
	↓ Pulmonary artery pressure

combination of adenosine and calcium-channel blockers (in the calcium-channel blocker responder group) reduced PVR by 49%, increased SV by 33%, and decreased PAP by 14%. Schrader and colleagues compared the effects of intravenous adenosine (50–500 μg/kg/min) with those of oral nifedipine (20 mg four times daily until a ≥20% decrease in PVR or systemic hypotension) in 15 patients with pulmonary hypertension (85). The maximal dose of adenosine (256 ± 46 μg/kg/min) produced a 2.4% reduction in the PAP [nonsignificant (NS)], a 37% decrease in PVR ($P < 0.001$), and a 57% increase in CI ($P < 0.001$). The administration of maximally effective doses of nifedipine (91 + 36 mg) produced a 15% reduction in PAP ($P < 0.005$) and an 8% increase in CI ($P = $ NS). Six patients (6 of 15) had significant reductions in PVR with adenosine but *not* with nifedipine.

Morgan and co-workers administered adenosine to seven patients with primary pulmonary hypertension (86). In all patients studied, there was a dose-dependent and significant reduction in PVR. SVR also decreased, but the ratio of PVR to SVR decreased by 10% ($P < 0.025$), indicating that adenosine exerts a higher vasodilator effect on the pulmonary circulation. Although results in the setting of primary pulmonary hypertension are promising, its application in treating patients with concomitant CAD remains controversial.

Because adenosine has potent negative inotropic, dromotropic, and chronotropic effects, concerns over sinoatrial (SA) and atrioventricular (AV) node dysfunction, coronary steal (with secondary ischemia), and hypotension have limited its use in patients with CAD (87). Fullerton and colleagues evaluated the affect of adenosine at 50 μg/kg/min to treat pulmonary hypertension (88). These investigators evaluated cardiac surgical patients with PAP greater than 30 mm Hg following the administration of adenosine (50 μg/kg/min). PAP dramatically decreased (from 36 to 28 mm Hg), and transpulmonary gradient decreased from 27 to 19, indicating a selective vasodilating effect.

When the principal factor affecting RV performance is depressed contractility, positive inotropic agents can be used to restore normal RV function. All the previously mentioned sympathomimetic agents are appropriate. Use of catecholamines such as dopamine, dobutamine, epinephrine, and isoproterenol has been successful. If RV dysfunction is precipitated by both reduced contractility and an increased afterload, treatment should include only those agents capable of both positive inotropic and pulmonary vasodilation (i.e., isoproterenol, epinephrine, milrinone, or amrinone). If, however, contractility is depressed as a result of low CPP (i.e., ischemia, CPB), agents such as norepinephrine can restore CPP; however, care must be taken to avoid elevating PVR.

The maintenance of normal atrioventricular conduction and contractility is essential to preserving normal RV function. Loss of sinoatrial activity is as detrimental to RV performance as is loss of atrial contractility to normal LV function. Similarly, correction of hypoxemia, hypercarbia, acid–base disturbance, and hypothermia can improve ventricular performance and lower PVR.

In addition to pharmacologic agents, the use of mechanical assist devices (right atrial to pulmonary artery pumps) has been suggested for the treatment of refractory RV dysfunction. This device was used initially to treat postpericardiotomy RV failure; however, it is effective only in increasing RV performance when PVR is normal. Pulmonary artery balloon counterpulsation has been used successfully by Higgins to wean patients with RV dysfunction secondary to pulmonary hypertension from CPB (89). It must be emphasized that both devices are merely temporary measures to be used as a bridge to cardiac transplantation.

SUMMARY

The management of cardiogenic shock is a complex process that relies for its success on the identification, diagnosis, and treatment of the underlying pathophysiology. Surgery induces a host of postoperative physiologic derangements that may impact negatively on the cardiovascular system. Patients with CAD or at risk for CAD account for the majority of cases of postoperative cardiogenic shock. Early recognition of myocardial ischemia or of MI and institution of myocardial reperfusion techniques (percutaneous balloon angioplasty or surgical revascularization) may salvage myocardium at risk and improve outcome. Mechanical complications of MI are associated with poor survival; prognosis may be improved in some cases with early surgical intervention. Cardiogenic shock also may arise from RV pathology and is best managed with pharmacologic agents.

KEY POINTS

Cardiogenic shock, which arises most often from massive myocardial infarction (MI) involving 25% to 40% of myocardial mass, complicates acute MI in 7.5% of cases and is associated with a mortality rate of 60% to 100%.

Early recognition and intervention (within 4–6 hours of onset of myocardial ischemia or MI) with specific aims of reducing the "area at risk" (with coronary angioplasty or surgical angioplasty or surgical revascularization) offer the best prognosis.

Cardiogenic shock arising from mechanical complications of MI (papillary–muscle rupture, ventricular–septal rupture,

free-wall rupture tamponade) occurs most often several days (3–7 days) after MI. Prompt diagnosis (echocardiographic) and surgical intervention may improve outcome.

RV infarction occurs in as many as 40% of LV infarctions. Management strategies are aimed at improving both RV and LV performance.

Mechanical-assist devices (intraaortic balloon counterpulsation and ventricular-assist devices) may be used in conjunction with vasoactive and cardioactive drugs to improve CO. In addition to reducing myocardial oxygen consumption, these devices can reduce myocardial stunning and extension of MI.

REFERENCES

1. Gleason WL, Braunwald E. Studies on the first derivative of ventricular pressure pulse. *Am J Clin Invest* 1962;41:80–91.
2. Milnor WR. *Cardiovascular physiology.* New York: Oxford University Press, 1990.
3. Thomas SJ. *Manual of cardiac anesthesiology,* 2nd ed. St. Louis: Mosby.
4. Strobeck JE, Sonnenblick EH. Myocardial and ventricular function. *Cardiovasc Rev* 1983;4:568–581.
5. Wallace AG, Skinner NS, Mitchell JH. Hemodynamic determinants of the maximal rate of rise of left ventricular pressure. *Am J Physiol* 1963;205:30–36.
6. Baan J, Van Der Velde ET. Sensitivity of end-systolic pressure-volume relation to type of loading interventions in dogs. *Circ Res* 1988;62:1247–1258.
7. Maughan WL, Oikawa RY. Right ventricular function. In: Scharf SM, Cassidy SS, eds. *Heart–lung interaction in health and disease.* New York: Marcel Dekker, 1989:179–220.
8. Cercek B, Shah PK. Complicated acute myocardial infarction, heart failure, shock, mechanical complications. *Cardiol Clin* 1991;9:569–593.
9. Mangano DT. Perioperative cardiac morbidity. *Anesthesiology* 1990;72:153–184.
10. Page DL, Caufield JB, Kastor J, et al. Myocardial changes associated with cardiogenic shock. *N Engl J Med* 1971;285:133.
11. Alonso DR, Scheidt S, Post M, et al. Pathophysiology of cardiogenic shock; quantification of myocardial necrosis, clinical, pathologic and electrocardiographic correlation. *Circulation* 1973;48:588.
12. Wackers FJ, Lie KL, Becker AE, et al. Coronary artery disease in patients dying from cardiogenic shock or congestive heart failure in the setting of acute myocardial infarction. *Br Heart J* 1976;38:906.
13. Mueller HS. Catecholamine support of the critically ill cardiac patient: inotropic agents versus vasopressors alpha- or beta-adrenergic agonists or both? *Intensive Crit Care Digest* 1986;5:36–39.
14. Goldberg LI, Rajfer SI. Dopamine receptors: applications in clinical cardiology. *Circulation* 1985;72:245.
15. Bristow MR, Ginsberg R, Minobe W, et al. Decreased catecholamine sensitivity and beta-adrenergic receptor density in failing human hearts. *N Engl J Med* 1982;307:205–211.
16. Benotti J, Grossman W, Braunwald E, et al. Hemodynamic assessment of amrinone: A new vasoactive agent. *N Engl J Med* 1978;299:1373–1377.
17. Honerjager P, Scafer-Korting M, Reiter M. Involvement of c-AMP in the direct inotropic effect of amrinone. *Naunym Schmiedebergs Arch Pharmacol* 1981;318:112–120.
18. Monrad ES, Baim DS, Smith HS, et al. Effects of milrinone on coronary hemodynamics and myocardial energetics in patients with congestive heart failure. *Circulation* 1985;71:972–979.
19. Benotti JR, Grossman W, Braunwald E, et al. Effects of amrinone on myocardial energy metabolism and hemodynamics in patients with severe congestive heart failure due to coronary artery disease. *Circulation* 1980;62:28–34.
20. Butterworth JF IV, Royster RL, Robertie PG, et al. Hemodyanamic effects of amrinone in patients recovering from aortocoronary bypass surgery. *Anesth Analg* 1990;70:S45(abst).
21. Prielipp RC, Butterworth JF IV, Zaloga GP, et al. Effects of amrinone on cardiac index, venous oxygen saturation and venous admixture in patients recovering from cardiac surgery. *Chest* 1991;99:820–825.

22. Prielipp RC, MacGregor DA, Butterworth JF, et al. Pharmacodynamics and pharmacokinetics of milrinone administration to increase oxygen delivery in critically ill patients. *Chest* 1996;109:1291–1301.

23. Bailey JM, Levy JH, Rogers HG, et al. Pharmacokinetics of amrinone during cardiac surgery. *Anesthesiology* 1991;75:961–968.

24. Doolan LA, Jones EF, Kalina J, et al. A placebo controlled trial verifying the efficacy of milrinone in weaning high risk patients from cardiopulmonary bypass. *J Cardiothorac Vasc Anesth* 1997;11:37–41.

25. Feneck RO. The European Milrinone Multicentre Trial Group: intravenous milrinone following cardiac surgery. II. Influence of baseline hemodynamics and patient factors on therapeutic response. *J Cardiothorac Vasc Anesth* 1992;6:563–567.

26. Salmenpera MT, Levy JN. The *in vivo* effect of phosphodiesterase inhibitors on the human internal mamary artery. *Anesth Anal* 1996;82:954–957.

27. Lobato EB, Gravenstein N, Martin TD. Milrinone not epinephrine improves left ventricular compliance after cardiopulmonary bypass. *J Cardiothorac Vasc Anesth* 2000;14:374–337.

28. Ratrmell J, Prielipp R, Butterworth J, et al. A multicenter, randomized, blind comparison of amrinone with milrinone after elective cardiac surgery. *Anesth Analg* 1999;86:683–690.

29. Teiger E, Menasche P, Mansier P, et al. Triiodothyronine therapy in open heart surgery: from hope to disappointment. *Eur Heart J* 1993;14:629–633.

30. Novitzky D, Cooper DKC, Barton CI, et al. Triiodothyronine as an inotropic agent after open heart surgery. *J Thorac Cardiovasc Surg* 1989;98: 972–978.

31. Noritsky E, Cooper OK, Swarepoel A. Inotropic effect of triiodothyrone (T3) following myocardial ischemia and cardiopulmonary bypass: irital experience in patients, undergoing open heart surgery. *Eur J Cardiothorac Surg* 1989;3:140–145.

32. Klemperer JD, Klein I, Gomez M, et al. Thyroid hormone treatment after coronary artery bypass surgery. *N Engl J Med* 1995;333:1522–1527.

33. Bennett-Guerrero E, Jimenez JL, White WD, et al. Cardiovascular effects of intravenous triiodothyronine in patients undergoing coronary artery bypass graft surgery: a randomized, double-blind, placebo-controlled trial. Duke T3 study group. *JAMA* 1996;275:687–692.

34. Jeevanandam V, Todd B, Hellman S, et al. Use of triiodothyronone replacement therapy to reverse donor myocardial dysfunction: creating a larger donor pool. *Transplant Proc* 1993;25:3305–3306.

35. Landry DW, Levin HR, Gallant EM, et al. Vasopressin deficiency contributes to the vasodilation of septic shock. *Circulation* 1997;95:1122–1125.

36. Michell RH, Kirk JC, Billah MM, et al. Hormonal stimulation of phosphatidylinositol breakdown with particular reference to the hepatic effects of vasopressin. *Biochem Soc Trans* 1979;7:861–865.

37. Morales DLS, Madigan J, Cullinane S, et al. Reversal by vasopressin of intractable hypotension in the late phase of hemorrhagic shock. *Circulation* 1999;100:226–229.

38. Argenziano M, Choudhri AF, Mozami N, et al. Vasodilatory hypotension after cardiopulmonary bypass: risk factors and potential mechanisms. *Circulation* 1997;96(Suppl 1):I–680.

39. Landry DW, Levin HR, Galian EM, et al. Vasopressin pressor hypersensitivity in vasodilatory septic shock. *Crit Care Med* 1997;25:1279–1282.

40. Argenziano M, Choudhri AF, Oz MC, et al. A prospective randomized trial of arginine vasopressin in the treatment of vasodilatory shock after left ventricular assist device placement. *Circulation* 1997;96:II–286–II–290.

41. Mellander S, Lewis David H. Effect of hemorrhagic shock on the reactivity of resistance and capacitance vessels and on capillary filtration transfer in cat skeletal muscle. *Circ Res* 1963;13:105–118.

42. Morales DLS, Gregg D, Helman DN, et al. Arginine vasopressin in the treatment of fifty patients with postcardiotomy vasodilatory shock. *Ann Thorac Surg* 1999 (*in press*).

43. Argeziano M, Chen JM, Choudhuri AF, et al. Management of vasodilatory shock after cardiac surgery: identification of predisposing factors and use of a novel progressor or agent. *J Thorac Cardiovase Surg* 1998;116:973–980.

44. Prielipp RC, MacGregor DA, Royster RL, et al. Dobutamine antago-

nizes epinephrine's biochemical and cardiotonic effects. *Anesthesiology* 1998;89:49–57.

45. Abernethy WB, Butterworth IV JF, Prielipp RC, et al. Calcium entry attenuates adenylyl cyclase activity: a possible mechanism for calcium-induced catecholamine resistance. *Chest* 1995;107:1420–1425.

46. Clements SD, Story WE, Hurst JW, et al. Ruptured papillary muscle, a complication of acute myocardial infarction: clinical presentation, diagnosis, and treatment. *Clin Cardiol* 1985;8:93.

47. Wei JY, Hutchins GM, Bulkley BH. Papillary muscle rupture in fatal acute myocardial infarction. *Ann Intern Med* 1979; 90:149.

48. Fox AC, Glassman E, Isom OW. Surgically remediable complications of myocardial infarction. *Prog Cardiovasc Dis* 1979;21:461.

49. Gray RJ, Sethna D, Matloff JM. The role of cardiac surgery in acute myocardial infarction with mechanical complications. *Am Heart J* 1983;106:723.

50. Ameli S, Shah P. Cardiac tamponade: pathophysiology, diagnosis, and management. *Cardiol Clin* 1991;9:665–673.

51. Andersen HR, Falk E, Nielsen D. Right ventricular infarction: frequency, size and topography in coronary heart disease: a prospective study comprising 107 consecutive autopsies from a coronary care unit. *J Am Coll Cardiol* 1987;10:1223.

52. Cabin HS. The pathophysiology of right ventricular myocardial infarction. *J Intensive Care Med* 1986;1:241.

53. Hines R. Perioperative management of patients with compromised left and right ventricular function. *Anesthesiol Clin North Am* 1991;9:637–656.

54. Laver MB, Strauss WH, Robost GM. Herbert Shubin Memorial Lectures. Right and left ventricular geometry: adjustment during acute respiratory failure. *Crit Care Med* 1985;7:509–516.

55. Ducas J, Duval D, Sasilva H, et al. Treatment of canine pulmonary hypertension: Effects of norepinephrine and isoproterenol on pulmonary vascular pressure flow characteristics. *Circulation* 1987;75:235–242.

56. Hill L, Pearl R. Combined inhaled nitric oxide and inhaled prostacyclin during experimental chronic pulmonary hypertension. *J Appl Physiol* 1999;86:1160–1164.

57. Lake C. Perioperative management of increased pulmonary vascular resistance. *Cardiothoracic and Vascular Anesthesia Update* 1990;13:1–21.

58. Lee KY, Molloy DW, Slykerman L, et al. Effects of hydralazine and nitroprusside on cardiopulmonary function when a decrease in cardiac output complicates a short term increase in pulmonary vascular resistance. *Circulation* 1983;689:1299–1303.

59. Prielipp RC, Rosenthal MH, Pearl RG. Hemodynamic profiles of prostaglandin E1, isoproterenol, prostacyclin, and nifedipine in vasoconstrictor pulmonary hypertension in sheep. *Anesth Analg* 1988;67:722–729.

60. Jones ODH, Shiore DF, Rigby ML, et al. The use of tolazoline hydrochloride as a pulmonary vasodilator in potentially fatal episodes of pulmonary vasoconstriction after cardiac surgery in children. *Circulation* 1981;64:134–139.

61. Hathaway DR, March KL, Lash JA, et al. Vascular smooth muscle: a review of the molecular basis of contractility. *Circulation* 1991;83:382–383.

62. D'Ambra MN, LaRaia PJ, Philbin DM, et al. Prostaglandin E$_1$: a new therapy for refractory right heart failure and pulmonary hypertension after mitral valve replacement. *J Thorac Cardiovasc Surg* 1985;89:567–572.

63. Frostell C, Fratacc MD, Wain JC, et al. Inhaled nitric oxide: a selective pulmonary vasodilator reversing hypoxic pulmonary vasoconstriction. *Circulation* 1991;83:2038–2047.

64. Morgan J, McCormack D, Griffiths, et al. Adenosine as a vasodilator in primary pulmonary hypertension. *Circulation* 1991;84:1415–l439.

65. Schranz D, Zepp F, Iversen S, et al. Effects of tolazoline and prostacyclin on pulmonary hypertension in infants after cardiac surgery. *Crit Care Med* 1992;20:1243–1249.

66. Morray J, Powers K, Clarke W. Amrinone reduces elevated pulmonary vascular resistance in isolated perfused rabbit lungs. *Anesthesiology* 1990;73:A1162.

67. Tanaka H, Tajimi K, Moritsune O, et al. Effects of milrinone on pulmonary vasculature in normal dogs with pulmonary hypertension. *Crit Care Med* 1991;1:68.

68. Schroeder R, Wood G. Plotkin J, et al. Intraoperative use of inhaled PGI$_2$ for acute pulmonary hypertension and right ventricular failure. *Anesth Analg* 2000;91:291–295.

69. Walmrath D, Schneider T, Schermuly R, et al. Direct comparison of inhaled nitric oxide and aerosolized prostacyclin in acute respiratory distress syndrome. *Am J Respir Crit Care Med* 1996;153:991–996.

70. Scarle A, Sahab E. Endothelial vasomotor regulation in health and disease. *Can J Anaesth* 1992;39:838–857.

71. Davidson D, Barefield E, Kattwinkel J, et al. Inhaled nitric oxide for the early treatment of persistent pulmonary hypertension of the newborn: a randomized, double masked, placebo conttrolled, dose response multicenter study. *Pediatrics* 1998;01:325–330.

72. Rossaint R, Falke KJ, Lopez FB, et al. Inhaled nitric oxide for the adult respiratory distress syndrome. *N Engl J Med* 1993;328:389–405.

73. Rossaint R, Gerlach H, Schmidt Ruhnke H, et al. Efficacy of inhaled nitric oxide in patients with severe ARDS. *Chest* 1995;107:1107–1115.

74. Manktelow C, Bigatello L, Hess D, et al. Physiologic determinents of the response to inhaled nitric oxide in patients with acute respiratory distress syndrome. *Anesthesiology* 1997;87:297–307.

75. Doery E, Hanson C, 3rd et al. Phenylephrine and inhaled nitric oxide and adult respiratory distress. *Anesthesiology* 1997;87:18–25.

76. Kerins DM, Murray R, Fitzgerald GA. Prostacyclin and prostaglandin E$_1$: molecular mechansism and therapeutic utility. *Prog Hemostasis Thrombosis* 1991;10:307–337.

77. Watkins WD, Peterson MB, Crone RK, et al. Prostacyclin and prostaglandin E$_1$ for severe idiopathic pulmonary artery hypertension [Letter]. *Lancet* 1980;1:1083.

78. Hess W. Effects of Amrinone on the right side of the heart. *J Cardiothorac Anesth* 1989;7:38–44.

79. Monrad ES, Baim DS, Smith HS. Effects of milrinone on coronary hemodynamics and myocardial energetics in patients with congestive heart failure. *Circulation* 1985;71:972.

80. Benotti JR, Lesko LJ, McCue JE, et al. Pharmacokinetics and pharmacodynamics of milrinone in chronic congestive heart failure. *Am J Cardiol* 1985;56:685–689.

81. Eichhorn EJ, Konstam MA, Weiland DS, et al. Differential effects of milrinone and dobutamine on right ventricular preload, afterload and systolic performance in congestive heart failure secondary to ischemic or idiopathic dilated cardiomyopathy. *Am J Cardiol* 1987;60:1329–1333.

82. Feneck RO, and the European Milrinone Multicentre Trial Group: Intravenous milrinone following cardiac surgery; I. Effects of bolus infusion followed by variable dose maintenance infusion. *J Cardiothor Vasc Anesth* 1992;6:554–562.

83. Feneck RO, and the European Milrinone Multicentre Trial Group. Intravenous milrinone following cardiac surgery; II. Influence of patient factors and baseline haemodynamics on therapeutic response. *J Cardiothor Vasc Anesth* 1992;6:563–567.

84. Inbar S, Schrader B, Kaufmann E, et al. Effects of adenosine in combination with calcium channel blockers in patients with primary pulmonary hypertension. *J Am Coll Cardiol* 1983;21:413–418.

85. Schrader B, Inbars S, Kaufman L, et al. Comparison of the effects of adenosine and nifedipine in pulmonary hypertension. *J Am Coll Cardiol* 1992;19:1060–1064.

86. Morgan JM, McCormack DG, Griffiths MJ, et al. Adenosine as a vasodilator in primary pulmonary hypertension. *Circulation* 1991;84:1145–1149.

87. Ogilby D, Abdulmassih S, Iskahdrian MD, et al. Effect of intravenous adenosine infusion on myocardial perfusion and function. *Circulation* 1992;86:887–895.

88. Fullerton DA, Jones SD, Grover FL, et al. Adenosine effectively controls pulmonary hypertension after cardiac operations. *Ann Thorac Surg* 1996;61:1118–1124.

89. Higgins RSD, Elefteriades J. Right ventricular assist devices and surgical treatment of right ventricular failure. *Cardiol Clin* 1992;10:185–192.

PERIOPERATIVE MYOCARDIAL ISCHEMIA

JAMES G. RAMSAY
GARY STOLOVITZ

KEY WORDS

- Coronary artery disease
- Heart
- Myocardial infarction
- Myocardial ischemia
- Perioperative cardiac morbidity
- Postoperative period

INTRODUCTION

Perioperative myocardial ischemia is associated with significant morbidity and mortality in the surgical population. It has been estimated that more than one-half of postoperative deaths are caused by cardiac events (1), most of which are ischemic in origin. Much attention in the cardiology literature has been given to the preoperative evaluation of patients at risk and in the anesthesiology literature to the perioperative detection of myocardial ischemia. These issues are discussed in this chapter, but the primary focus is on the perioperative management of ischemia, including its prevention and treatment.

PATHOPHYSIOLOGY

Myocardial ischemia is the result of an imbalance between myocardial oxygen supply and demand. Most commonly, ischemia results from a decrease in local blood supply resulting from coronary artery disease (CAD). Less commonly, global ischemia occurs secondary to a systemic reduction in supply such as occurs with severe hypotension. Ischemia also can result from an increase in oxygen demand in myocardium distal to coronary artery lesions. The classic determinants of oxygen demand are heart rate (HR), contractility, and wall tension; ischemia is most likely to occur when there is a concomitant rise in demand and decrease in supply. Perioperatively, the single hemodynamic abnormality most often associated with ischemia is tachycardia (2). Both an increase in demand and a reduction in supply (due to decreased diastolic filling time) are induced by rapid HR.

The clinical manifestations of myocardial ischemia range from asymptomatic or "silent" episodes to angina, arrhythmia, pulmonary congestion (from ventricular dysfunction), infarction, and sudden cardiac death. In the "ischemic cascade" (3), systolic (contractile) and diastolic (relaxation/filling) dysfunction occur first and are followed by electrocardiographic changes and, finally, although not predictably, by chest pain (Fig.1). The time course of this cascade is short. All events often occur in a period of less than 1 minute.

Chronic contractile dysfunction due to chronic hypoperfusion has been termed *hibernating myocardium*. Teleologically, this may be due to a matching of function and flow so that myocardial damage is avoided. It is characterized by a normalization of contractile function with restoration of blood flow. Inotropic stimulation of hibernating myocardium leads to anaerobic metabolism (4). In contrast, the term *stunned myocardium* refers to persistent contractile dysfunction after a short period of hypoperfusion despite full restoration of blood flow. Dysfunction may last hours to weeks. Clinical scenarios that have been associated with stunned myocardium include coronary-artery balloon angioplasty and cardioplegic arrest during cardiac operations. Potential mechanisms include damage to membranes and enzymes by free radicals, an increase in free cytosolic calcium during ischemia and reperfusion, and a lower sensitivity of myofibrils to calcium. Unlike hibernating myocardium, stunned myocardium responds to stimulation with inotropes without metabolic deterioration (5).

In the absence of CAD, coronary blood flow is autoregulated (i.e., maintained over a wide range of mean pressures). Flow becomes pressure dependent above and below the pressure limits of autoregulation (6) (Fig. 2). The difference between flow under normal conditions (line A) and flow in maximally dilated vessels (line D_1), as may occur with exercise or administration of coronary vasodilators, defines the concept of coronary-vascular reserve. The line D_2 represents the decrease in reserve that occurs in situations such as during tachycardia or increase in left-ventricular end-diastolic pressure (LVEDP). This reserve is first exhausted in the subendocardial zone when the distal pressure falls below about 55 mm Hg (7). Under normal conditions, the myocardium maximally extracts oxygen; any increase in demand must be satisfied by an increase in flow. In the presence of CAD, coronary flow cannot increase adequately because of the loss of pressure across fixed stenoses. Energy is lost when blood flows across a stenosis because of entrance effects, friction in the stenotic segment, and losses produced by turbulent distal eddies. This pressure drop is expressed by the following

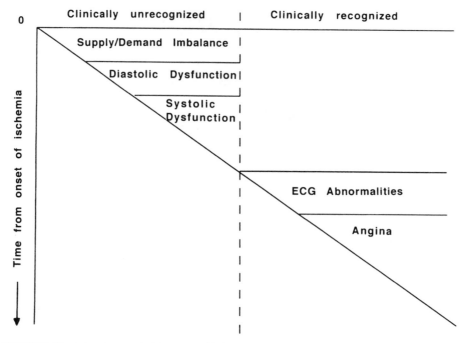

FIGURE 1. The ischemic cascade: The onset of ischemia is followed by left ventricular (LV) dysfunction, electrocardiographic changes, and angina, in that order. In the presence of ischemia, the absence of angina does not signify the absence of ventricular dysfunction. (Redrawn from Nesto RW, Kowalchuk GJ. The ischemic cascade: temporal sequence of hemodynamic, electrocardiographic and symptomatic expressions of ischemia. *Am J Cardiol* 1987;57:23C–30C, with permission.)

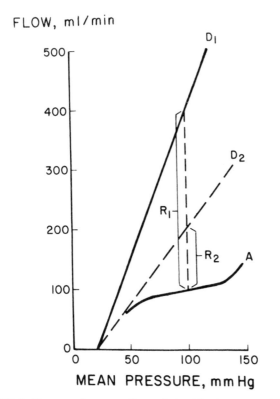

FIGURE 2. Diagram of pressure–flow relationships in autoregulated conditions (A) and maximally dilated vessels (D₁) in a normal heart. D₂ represents maximal flow in conditions such as coronary artery disease. R₁ and R₂ define the "coronary vascular reserve." (From Hoffman JI. Maximal coronary flow and the concept of vascular reserve. *Circulation* 1984;70:153–159, with permission.)

equation (8):

$$DP = fQ + sQ$$

in which *DP* is the pressure drop across the stenosis, *Q* is the blood flow, *f* is the factor accounting for frictional losses, and *s* is the factor accounting for separation losses caused by distal turbulence. Both factors *s* and *f* are inversely related to the cross-sectional area of the stenosis. Thus, conditions that increase myocardial blood flow, such as exercise, anemia, and pharmacologic vasodilation of the coronary arteriolar–resistance bed, cause a fall in distal perfusion pressure that rises exponentially with increases in flow. During exercise, this fall in distal pressure is somewhat but incompletely attenuated by an increase in systemic pressure. Thus, maintenance of adequate perfusion pressure and avoidance of conditions that worsen the pressure drop across a stenosis are important in preserving adequate myocardial oxygen supply.

The classic concept of a fixed coronary blood flow resulting from fixed coronary stenoses has been modified by an understanding of the complexity of various ischemic syndromes. In the same patient, varying degrees of exertion may cause angina at different times. Both transient ischemia and myocardial infarction (MI) display circadian variation, peaking in the early morning hours after awakening and declining in incidence as the day progresses (9). This phenomenon has been variably attributed to relatively increased HR and blood pressure (BP) in the morning hours, increased coronary tone, and increased platelet aggregation ability. The unifying mechanism appears to be increased sympathetic activity, which suggests that human coronary stenoses are dynamic. In fact, 70% of hemodynamically significant coronary stenoses are eccentric, with the lumen being circumscribed by an arc of at least 60 degrees of normal arterial wall (7). The stenotic segment is thus subject to the same stimuli of vasomotor tone as are normal segments. In addition, endothelial dysfunction in vessels with atheromata may result in impaired coagulation, altered vasomotor tone, and abnormal responses to stimuli (e.g., constriction versus dilation). In the perioperative setting, activation of the sympathetic nervous system and an increase in circulating procoagulants occur. When a patient has CAD, these factors alone can contribute to the development of myocardial ischemia.

Whereas perioperative myocardial ischemia is common in patients with CAD, its progression to unstable angina or infarction is much less frequent. The cause of these "acute coronary syndromes" is usually disruption of an atherosclerotic plaque with subsequent thrombus formation (10). Whereas severe stenoses (70% cross-sectional area reduction) tend to progress to complete stenoses about three times more frequently than do less-severe stenoses, occlusion of a severe stenosis infrequently leads to MI. This is because of the development of collateral blood flow over time. Occlusion of a less severe stenosis is more likely to result in MI as a result of the lack of collaterals.

Prinzmetal and colleagues described a syndrome of variant angina, emphasizing the role of coronary spasm in the generation of ischemia (11). They believe that spasm may occur in segments with atheromatous disease. More recently, angina has been described as occurring in patients with angiographically normal coronary arteries (*syndrome X*). This syndrome is characterized by a decreased vasodilator reserve to metabolic and pharmacologic stimuli. Its mechanism is unknown but is believed to be caused by an abnormality of the smooth muscle of the coronary microvasculature.

CLINICAL AND PERIOPERATIVE PRESENTATION

Patients with chronic stable angina who experience typical angina pectoris have frequent episodes of electrocardiographic (ECG) evidence of ischemia. These episodes are asymptomatic and most often are not accompanied by an increase in HR. Using positron emission tomography, Deanfield and co-workers (12) found that patients with ST-segment changes had perfusion defects both when exercising and at rest. They also noted that the presence of pain reflected only in part the duration and severity of ECG evidence of ischemia; a wide overlap occurred in the magnitude and duration of ST-segment depression between symptomatic and asymptomatic episodes. Chierchia and colleagues (13) observed that most patients with ST-segment evidence of ischemia demonstrated elevation in LVEDP or pulmonary artery (PA) diastolic pressures, as well as significant decreases in left ventricular (LV) dp/dt. Yeung and associates (14) observed that asymptomatic ischemia in patients with stable angina predicts death and MI for 2 years and all adverse events (including the need for revascularization) for 5 years.

Perioperative ST-segment deviations are common in surgical patients with CAD and have the same importance as in the medical setting. In a landmark study, Slogoff and Keats examined the incidence of intraoperative, pre-cardiopulmonary bypass (CPB) ischemia as defined by ST-segment depression in more than 1,000 patients undergoing myocardial revascularization (2). One-third

of the patients developed ischemia, and more than one half of the ischemic episodes occurred in patients without hemodynamic abnormalities [defined as HR $\geq$ 100 beats per minute (bpm) or systolic BP of $\geq$ 180 or BP $\leq$ 90 mm Hg]. Of the patients who developed tachycardia, however, 40% also developed ischemia. Ischemia was most likely to occur during intubation or surgical stimulation (skin incision or sternotomy) regardless of the presence or absence of hemodynamic abnormalities. Postoperative MI was three times more common in patients who had pre-CPB ischemia. In a subsequent study of 500 patients, the same investigators defined tachycardia as an increase of greater than 10 bpm above the resting HR and hypertension and hypotension as a greater than 20% change from resting systolic BP (15). Again, about one-half of new pre-CPB ischemic episodes were not associated with hemodynamic abnormalities. This follow-up study confirmed the earlier finding of a threefold increase in the occurrence of MI in patients with ischemia.

Knight and colleagues (16) expanded on the studies by Slogoff and Keats by investigating the incidence of ischemia in the preoperative, intraoperative, and postoperative periods in patients undergoing coronary artery bypass graft (CABG) operations; 42% had preoperative ST-segment evidence of ischemia, 18% had intraoperative episodes, and 40% had postoperative ST-segment changes. Episodes were preceded by a 20% increase in HR in a minority of cases during all three periods, and few intraoperative and postoperative episodes were preceded by an acute change in BP. In the postoperative period, however, the resting HR was increased to greater than 100 bpm in almost one-half of patients who developed ST-segment depressions. A diastolic BP of less than 50 mm Hg was present at the onset of ischemia in 33% of intraoperative episodes. These studies suggest that in cardiac surgical patients, whereas most ischemic episodes are not hemodynamically mediated, a low diastolic BP and tachycardia may predispose the patient to developing ischemia.

Similar patterns of ischemia have been observed in patients undergoing noncardiac operations. Mangano and co-workers (17) examined the association between perioperative myocardial ischemia and cardiac morbidity and mortality in 474 men with known CAD or at high risk for having CAD (Table 1). Of these

TABLE 1. PATIENTS WITH KNOWN CAD OR AT RISK

Definite CAD	Previous MI
	Typical angina
	Atypical angina with ischemic ECG response to exercise
	Scintigraphic evidence of a myocardial-perfusion defect
High risk for CAD	Vascular operation or at least 2 of the following:
	Age > 65 yr
	Hypertension
	Current smoker
	Serum cholesterol > 240 mg/dL
	Diabetes mellitus

CAD, coronary-artery-disease; ECG, electrocardiographic; MI, myocardial infarction.
Clinical variables suggesting definite coronary artery disease or high risk for CAD.
(From Mangano DT, Browner WS, Hollenberg M, et al. *N Engl J Med* 1990;323;1781–1788, with permission.)

patients, 41% had ECG evidence of ischemia postoperatively compared with 20% preoperatively and 25% intraoperatively. Only 23% of the postoperative episodes were preceded by an increase in HR greater than or equal to 20% above baseline. Similar to the findings of Knight's group, the mean HR was higher in the postoperative period (90 bpm versus 74 preoperatively and 72 intraoperatively). Multivariate analysis showed that only postoperative ischemia was an independent variable associated with postoperative ischemic events (cardiac death, MI, or unstable angina). In another study, 100 similar patients had follow-up for 1 week after a noncardiac operation (18). Most ischemic episodes occurred on days 2 and 3 postoperatively (Fig. 3), and 8 of the 13 adverse outcomes were preceded by ischemia. Tachycardia was most common on postoperative days 1 and 2 (Fig. 4). Finally, in a study of β-blocker prophylaxis with atenolol (19), patients who developed postoperative ischemia were more likely to die in the next 2 years than those who did not develop it, regardless of therapy (Fig. 5).

These studies indicate that in patients with CAD, perioperative ischemia is common and is associated with adverse outcome. In particular, postoperative ischemia occurs in almost one-half of such patients and is an independent predictor of adverse cardiac outcome. An important finding is that patients with risk factors (Table 1) had a similar incidence of ischemia and adverse outcome as did those with known disease. Clearly, it is incumbent on clinicians to take three crucial steps: (a) determine which patients are at risk for having CAD and developing ischemic events; (b) use techniques to detect myocardial ischemia in patients at risk; and (c) in these at-risk patients, attempt to reduce the risk of adverse outcome by implementing aggressive preventive and treatment modalities.

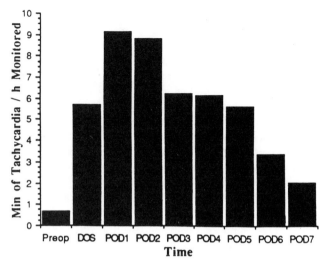

FIGURE 4. Pattern of postoperative tachycardia in patients undergoing noncardiac operations. For each postoperative day (POD), the average number of tachycardic (heart rate >100 beats per minute) minutes per hour monitored were calculated by dividing total minutes of tachycardia by total hours monitored. (From Mangano DT, Wong MG, London MJ, et al. Perioperative myocardial ischemia in patients undergoing noncardiac surgery-II: incidence and severity during the first week after surgery. The Study of Perioperative Ischemia Research Group. *J Am Coll Cardiol* 1991;17:851–857, with permission.)

CARDIAC RISK ASSESSMENT AND PREOPERATIVE EVALUATION

The goal of preoperative cardiac-risk assessment is to identify patients at risk for developing perioperative myocardial ischemia and MI to implement a treatment plan designed to decrease morbidity and mortality. Interventions based on this assessment may include preoperative medical optimization, preoperative coronary revascularization, or both. In addition, decisions regarding anesthetic and surgical techniques and the choice of hemodynamic monitors are often made based on the cardiac risk assessment. Whereas the validity and benefits of every step in this process remain controversial, there appears to be real potential for identification of high-risk patients and for therapy directed at reducing risk.

In 1996, the American College of Cardiology and the American Heart Association (ACC/AHA) published guidelines for perioperative cardiovascular evaluation (20). These guidelines, endorsed by the Society of Cardiovascular Anesthesiologists, have algorithms for relating preoperative risk factors or "predictors," functional capacity, and surgery-specific risks for individual patients. In a small number of patients, preoperative revascularization is indicated, usually only if this is also indicated independent of surgery. In another relatively small group of patients, the results of a specific test to elicit ischemia might affect the treatment (e.g., the inability to assess functional status in a patient with stable cardiac disease). As stated in the executive summary, "The overriding theme of these guidelines is that intervention is rarely necessary to lower the risk of surgery." The algorithm outlined in Fig. 6 provides a much more practical and satisfactory approach to the patient with heart disease than the older computational scoring systems described by Goldman and colleagues (21) and Detsky and associates (22). The reader is referred to these guidelines for a detailed explanation of how the algorithm was devised.

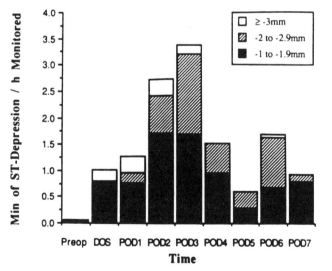

FIGURE 3. Pattern of postoperative ST-segment depression in patients undergoing noncardiac operations. For each postoperative day (POD), the total minutes of ST-segment depression were summed and then divided by the total duration of monitoring for all patients. The data were further divided into three groups: episode durations with maximal change from baseline −1 to −1.9 mm, −2 to −2.9 mm, and ≥ 3 mm. (From Mangano DT, Wong MG, London MJ, et al. Perioperative myocardial ischemia in patients undergoing noncardiac surgery-II: incidence and severity during the first week after surgery. The Study of Perioperative Ischemia Research Group. *J Am Coll Cardiol* 1991;17:851–857, with permission.)

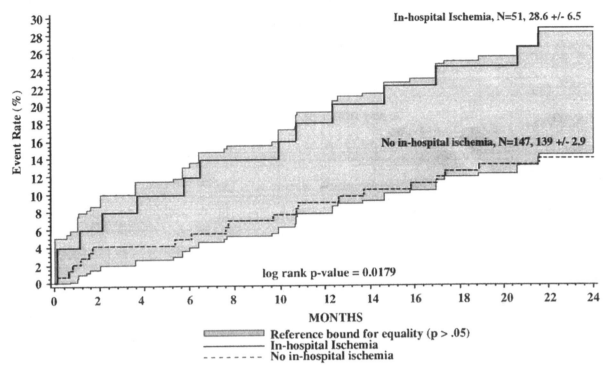

FIGURE 5. Kaplan–Meier event curves for death in patients with or without myocardial ischemia on postoperative day 0 to 2, as detected by Holter monitors. For this figure the patients who received perioperative atenolol versus those who did not are combined. (From Wallace A, Layug B, Tateo I, et al. Prophylactic atenolol reduces postoperative myocardial ischemia. *Anesthesiology* 1998;88:7–17, with permission.)

When the clinical assessment in conjunction with the anticipated risk of surgery suggests that there is a high risk of an ischemic event but there is no clear history of ischemia, then one of several noninvasive tests to elicit ischemia can be performed. These tests have a high negative predictive value, that is, a negative test suggests that coronary angiography is not indicated. Exercise testing assesses a patient's functional capacity: the ability to achieve a target HR (e.g., >100 bpm or 85% of the maximum predicted HR) without developing clinical or ECG evidence of ischemia predicts a low perioperative complication rate (23). Because patients with peripheral vascular disease are usually unable to exercise, other tests have been devised. The best studied of these are ambulatory electrocardiography (AECG), dipyridamole thallium scintigraphy (DTS), and dobutamine stress echocardiography (DSE). The relative merits of each technique continue to be studied and debated. Mantha and colleagues performed a meta-analysis on 20 studies to examine these tests and assign a relative risk to each test (the probability of adverse outcome when the test is positive divided by the probability of an adverse outcome when the test is negative) (24). Conceptually, a higher relative-risk score implies that a test is more effective at predicting cardiac events. Median relative risks were as follows: DSE 6.2, DTS 4.6, and AECG 2.7. Because of a wide overlap in the 95% confidence intervals, the data are not definitive in determining the optimal test. DSE is relatively fast, provides anatomic as well as functional data, and

compares favorably in most test comparisons. Boersma and associates (25) suggest that, used selectively in high-risk patients, DSE helps to identify patients who can undergo surgery with β-blockade (see later) versus those who need revascularization.

An elegant representation of the need to incorporate clinical data along with test data was made by Eagle and colleagues (26) in a study of cardiac risk assessment by combining clinical and DTS data (Table 2). In a multivariate analysis, they identified five clinical predictors of postoperative cardiac ischemic events: Q waves on the ECG, a history of ventricular ectopic activity, diabetes mellitus, age greater than 70 years, and angina. Those patients with none of these five predictors had few ischemic events. Those with three or more predictors had a high incidence of adverse outcome so that the DTS data provided little useful additional information. The test was most useful in risk assessment in patients with one or two of these clinical features. The rate of adverse events was 30% among patients who had redistribution on thallium scanning versus 3% for those without redistribution.

The utility of therapeutic interventions based on test data remains an enigma. Following the path of clinical evaluation, noninvasive testing and coronary catheterization often lead to a CABG operation. This course exposes the patient to three invasive procedures: angiography, coronary angioplasty or CABG, and the planned operation. Mason and colleagues (27) presented a "decision analysis" of revascularization strategies in patients

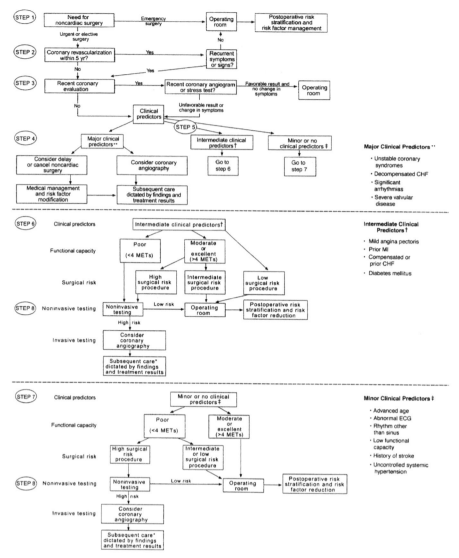

FIGURE 6. Stepwise approach to preoperative cardiac assessment. Individual steps are discussed in text of guidelines. Functional capacity is measured in "metabolic equivalents" or METs, ranging from 1 MET (barely able to care for self) to greater than 10 METs (vigorous sports). "Predictors" refers to predictors of perioperative cardiovascular risk, as determined by scientific evidence and expert opinion. "Subsequent care" may include cancellation or delay of surgery, coronary revascularization followed by non-cardiac surgery, or intensified medical care. (From Ritchie JL [Task Force Chair], et al. ACC/AHA Guidelines for Perioperative cardiovascular evaluation for noncardiac surgery. *Circulation* 1996;93:1280–1317, with permission.)

with positive DTS presenting for infrainguinal vascular surgery. They concluded that when the risk of angiography and CABG are added to the risk of the planned surgery, the cost would be greater and outcome possibly worse (depending on risk factors and local outcomes from CABG surgery) than simply proceeding with the elective surgery. This conclusion is strengthened by the work of Boersma and colleagues (25), who showed that perioperative β-adrenergic blockade alone in many patients with mildly positive DSE can confer a low and acceptable risk.

Few data are available on which to judge whether preoperative coronary angioplasty confers a benefit for the surgical patient. The AHA/ACC guidelines recommend angioplasty only for patients who require the procedure independent of planned surgery. In

1999, Posner and colleagues (28) reported that surgical patients with prior angioplasty had fewer cardiac outcomes than patients with untreated CAD but were twice as likely to have such outcomes as age-matched healthy patients. Of particular importance is that this study found no benefit to patients who had angioplasty less than 90 days before the planned surgery. For patients who have noncardiac surgery within 30 days of coronary stenting, outcomes may be dramatically worsened. Kaluza and colleagues (29) reported a high percentage of bleeding complications in patients who stayed on antiplatelet therapy as well as a high percentage of thrombotic complications (i.e., coronary occlusion) in patients who had this therapy discontinued for the surgery. Thirty-two percent of patients who underwent surgery within 2 weeks of angioplasty died of their complications.

TABLE 2. RISK OF ISCHEMIC EVENTS AFTER MAJOR VASCULAR OPERATION

No. of Clinical Variables[a]	Risk of Ischemic Event[b]
No clinical variables	3.1%
1 or 2 variables and (−) thallium redistribution	3.2%
1 or 2 variables and (+) thallium redistribution	29.6%
3 or more variables	50.0%

[a]Clinical variables: Q waves on the ECG; history of ventricular ectopic beats; diabetes mellitus; age > 70 years; angina.
[b]Ischemic events defined as unstable angina, ischemic pulmonary edema, myocardial infarction, or sudden postoperative death.
Modified from Eagle KA, Coley CM, Newell JB, et al. Combining clinical and thallium data optimizes preoperative assessment of cardiac risk before major vascular surgery. *Ann Intern Med* 1989;100:859–866, with permission.

ISCHEMIA

Prevention of Ischemia

The foregoing discussion clearly indicates that preoperative revascularization is not indicated in most patients with coronary disease. The AHA/ACC guidelines briefly discuss medical therapy, with the conclusion that β-blockers "may ultimately be shown to reduce risk of MI and death." Later in the same year, Mangano and colleagues published a landmark article demonstrating a reduction in mortality and the incidence of cardiovascular complications for 2 years after surgery (30) with the perioperative use of atenolol. The drug was given intravenously immediately before and after surgery and was continued for the duration of hospitalization. This publication resulted in a strong recommendation for the use of perioperative β blockade by the American College of Physicians (31). In a recent study from Europe, oral bisoprolol (a cardioselective β blocker) was administered orally for at least a week before surgery and perioperatively in patients with positive DSE (32). This study showed an even more impressive reduction in 30-day mortality rate and nonfatal MI than the study by Mangano et al. (Fig. 7). Unless there are contraindications, patients with known or suspected coronary disease should receive perioperative β blockade.

Unlike β blockade, the data for prophylactic use of other types of antianginal therapy in the perioperative period are either not supportive or conflicting. Whereas calcium-channel blocking drugs and nitrates are clearly indicated in the treatment of ischemia, their prophylactic use is not indicated. The AHA/ACC guidelines suggest use of nitroglycerin (i.e., intravenous infusion) only in high-risk patients who require this drug to control ischemia preoperatively and even then caution that the venodilation caused by nitrates may cause hypotension. Patients should, however, receive usual doses of all their antianginal drugs until surgery.

Monitoring for Ischemia

Early detection of myocardial ischemia should facilitate treatment and potentially decrease cardiac morbidity. Although no clinical trial has verified this assumption, it would be ethically impossible to conduct such a trial. Therefore, much interest has occurred in developing a sensitive, specific, and "user-friendly" monitor for ischemia in the perioperative setting. The three most commonly used monitors are the ECG, the PA catheter (PAC), and the transesophageal echocardiogram (TEE). ECG is widely available, simple to use, and inexpensive. ECG markers of ischemia include ST-segment depression or elevation, T-wave polarity changes, dysrhythmias (including sinus bradycardia or tachycardia), and atrioventricular blocks. Most of the literature regarding perioperative ischemia focuses on ST-segment changes. As with any test, the specificity of the ECG for detecting ischemia depends on the population being studied. Among patients with CAD or at risk for CAD, ST-segment changes are highly specific for ischemia, whereas other acute ECG changes are not. The classic criterion for ischemia is horizontal or downsloping ST-segment depression of greater than or equal to 0.1 mV (1 mm on a standard ECG with a calibrated amplitude signal of 1 mV = 1 cm) measured 80 msec from the "J" point (junction of S-wave and ST segment) (33). Downsloping ST-segment depression is more serious than is horizontal depression. ST-segment elevation in leads without Q waves is highly specific for detecting ischemia and localizes the site of severe ischemia resulting from proximal disease or spasm. ST-segment depression is also specific for detecting ischemia, but it poorly localizes the site of ischemia (34). New exercise-induced ST-segment elevation in leads with Q waves is less specific for ischemia and may reflect the presence of dyskinetic areas or a LV aneurysm. Some patients manifest "pseudonormalization" of the ECG, whereby abnormal ST segments at rest normalize in the presence of ischemia.

Lead selection is important to maximize the ECG as a monitor of ischemia. London and colleagues (35) showed that, when used in isolation, a V5 lead will detect 75% of intraoperative ischemic episodes that are seen in all 12 leads. Combining leads V4 and V5 increases sensitivity to 90%. Combining leads II (used because of its superiority in displaying the P wave) and V5 resulted in 80% sensitivity (Fig. 8).

Most ECG studies of perioperative ischemia have used continuous Holter monitors, the tapes from which are analyzed later. Several of these studies have shown that, despite the presence of an appropriately calibrated bedside monitor, caregivers failed to detect many episodes of ST-segment changes recorded by the Holter monitors. To address this problem, automated ST-segment analysis has been incorporated in modern operating room and intensive care unit (ICU) monitors to improve real-time detection of ischemia. These monitors display the ST-segment excursion in selected leads, allow trend graphing, and also have alarms. Some portable Holter and telemetry units have similar features. Whether the clinical use of these automated monitors is as sensitive as is the post hoc examination of Holter tapes has not been evaluated. Similarly, there are no published studies of the utility of this technique in early identification and intervention for myocardial ischemia.

The PAC has been advocated as a sensitive monitor of ischemia based on the observation that most patients in a coronary care unit with ECG evidence of ischemia demonstrate elevation in LVEDP (13). In a clinical report that has been widely quoted, Kaplan and colleagues suggested that, during CABG operations, an elevation in PA occlusion pressure (PAOP) may be a more sensitive monitor

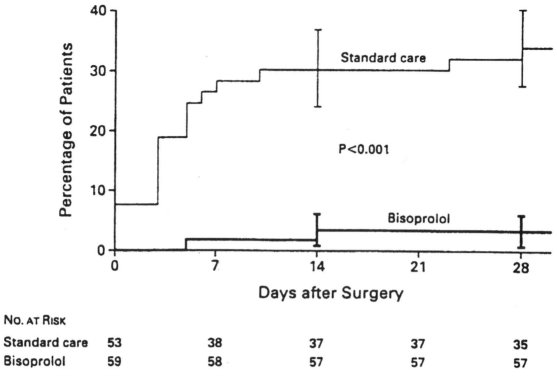

FIGURE 7. Kaplan–Meier estimates of the cumulative percentages of vascular surgery patients with positive preoperative dobutamine stress echocardiography tests who died of cardiac causes or had a nonfatal myocardial infarction during the perioperative period. Standard care excluded prophylactic β-adrenergic blockers; bisoprolol patients received oral bisoprolol for an average of 37 days before surgery and throughout the perioperative period. If patients were unable to take the drug orally or by nasogastric tube, intravenous metoprolol was given to keep the heart rate below 80 per minute. (From Poldermans D, Boersma E, Baxx JJ, et al. The effect of bisoprolol on perioperative mortality and myocardial infarction in high-risk patients undergoing vascular surgery. *N Engl J Med* 1999;341:1789–1794, with permission.)

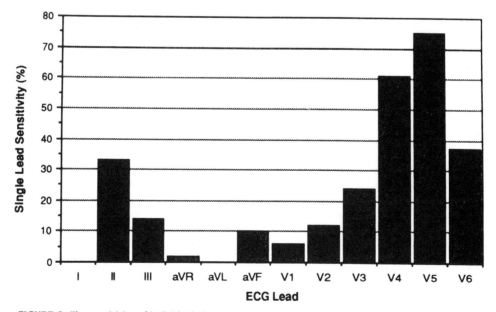

FIGURE 8. The sensitivity of individual electrocardiographic leads for ischemia is shown. Sensitivity is calculated by dividing the number of ischemic episodes detected by one lead by the total number of episodes detected by all leads. An assumption is made that all ST-segment changes are true positive. (From London MJ, Hollenberg M, Wong MG, et al. Intraoperative myocardial ischemia: localization by continuous 12-lead electrocardiography. *Anesthesiology* 1988;69:232–241, with permission.)

of ischemia than is the ECG (36). Other studies, however, report a low sensitivity of the PAC compared to other monitors, such as the ECG and TEE, for detecting ischemia (37).

The search for the "Holy Grail" of ischemia monitors continues with the introduction of echocardiographic assessment of ventricular-wall motion. When myocardial ischemia is induced in patients undergoing balloon angioplasty, LV dyssynergy appears earlier and more frequently than do ECG changes (38). Intraoperatively, abnormalities in ventricular wall motion seen by TEE are more common than are ECG changes and, in one study, were shown to predict adverse outcome better (39). Others found that the TEE, compared with preoperative clinical data and two-lead ECG (CC5 and CM5), adds little incremental clinical value in identifying patients at risk for developing adverse perioperative ischemic outcomes (40). Still others have questioned the sensitivity and specificity of new intraoperative segmental wall-motion changes (41). Similar to the issue of the post hoc evaluation of Holter ECG tapes, all the intraoperative studies quoted previously have used postoperative analysis of TEE tapes. Intraoperative real-time wall-motion assessment is operator dependent in its sensitivity and requires frequent or even constant attention to the TEE monitor. Automated border detection techniques (for wall-motion assessment) have not been validated in the perioperative setting. Postoperative use of the TEE as a monitor is not feasible. No study has evaluated real-time assessment of wall-motion changes in the perioperative setting.

Concordance among the various monitoring modalities in several studies is poor (40). This discordance can be attributed to technical issues regarding ECG lead selection or TEE imaging and to inherently different sensitivities and specificities of the techniques. Unfortunately, no "gold standard" for the clinical detection of myocardial ischemia exists, although most clinicians would consider the ECG the standard to which other techniques should be compared. The studies referred to in the foregoing show that perioperative ischemic changes on the ECG predict ischemic events for up to 2 years after surgery. Thus, it is possible to make the following recommendations: Perioperative ECG monitoring of leads II and V5 should be used on all patients at risk for having CAD. Use of monitors with automated ST-segment analysis should be considered. For patients with cardiac-conduction defects or paced rhythms that preclude ST-segment analysis, clinicians should consider using the PA catheter, TEE, or the PA catheter and TEE in the immediate perioperative period. The PA catheter probably should be reserved for use in patients in whom large fluid shifts are also anticipated (i.e., where other indications for this invasive monitor exist). In considering using the TEE, the clinician should keep in mind that stressful events such as induction of anesthesia, emergence from anesthesia, and the entire postoperative period are unmonitored.

Treatment of Ischemia

Because perioperative ischemia is associated with cardiac morbidity and mortality, suspected ischemia warrants prompt recognition and immediate treatment. Treatment may prevent the development of ischemic complications such as congestive heart failure (CHF) and dysrhythmias and may prevent the progression of myocardial ischemia to MI. Most episodes of perioperative myocardial ischemia do not lead to MI and do not appear to be "acute coronary syndromes" involving thrombosis. Rather than anticoagulant or thrombolytic therapy, which is indicated for the acute syndromes, therapeutic interventions are designed to improve oxygen supply to or reduce oxygen demand of the myocardium. Arterial oxygenation and hemoglobin concentration are the basis of oxygen delivery and must be measured in any patient experiencing ischemia. All patients with suspected ischemia or infarction should receive supplemental oxygen. The importance of maintaining an adequate coronary-perfusion pressure cannot be overemphasized. Myocardial oxygen demand is decreased by therapies that reduce HR, contractility, and ventricular-wall tension.

Determination of whether anginal pain or ECG changes in the postoperative setting are manifestations of chronic coronary disease or represent impending or acute infarction is a diagnostic dilemma. Short-lived symptoms or ECG changes that respond to antianginal therapy, accompanied by either no ECG changes or reversible ST segment/T wave changes, are most likely due to nonthrombotic supply- or demand-related ischemia. In addition to receiving aggressive therapy to improve the myocardial oxygen supply-to-demand ratio, such patients must have follow-up with repeated ECGs and serum markers to detect infarction (creatine phosphokinase myocardial band, or troponin I or T). In surgical patients, earlier markers such as myoglobin are universally elevated and of no help. New-onset chest pain or recurrent/refractory pain is more likely to represent an acute coronary syndrome, with the possibility of infarction. Even small elevations in troponin levels are associated with an increased incidence of adverse outcome; patients with new-onset, recurrent, or refractory pain require immediate cardiologic assessment because antithrombotic therapy with or without an interventional procedure may be indicated.

Nitrates and β-adrenergic receptor blockers are the mainstays of ischemia therapy, with calcium-channel entry blockers as adjuvant therapy. No role exists for the prophylactic administration of antiarrhythmic drugs, which may paradoxically increase mortality (42); however, decreased serum potassium and magnesium levels are associated with dysrhythmias, and levels of these ions should be supplemented as indicated. The intraaortic balloon pump (IABP) is an effective therapy for myocardial ischemia because it improves diastolic coronary-perfusion pressure and reduces afterload. The use of IABP is generally reserved for the patient who is having ischemia despite intensive medical therapy and, even then, only as a bridge to revascularization. A summary of common antianginal therapies is presented in Table 3.

Organic Nitrates

Organic nitrates have been used for more than 100 years and are effective in the management of both symptomatic and asymptomatic angina. Their mechanism of action is most likely related to venodilation, which results in a decrease in ventricular diastolic wall tension (a decrease in radius and intraventricular pressure). In higher doses, nitrates also reduce systemic pressure, which results in a decrease in ventricular systolic wall tension as well. Myocardial oxygen demand is therefore reduced. Myocardial oxygen supply is increased as a result of the ability of

TABLE 3. PHARMACOLOGIC TREATMENT OF ACUTE MYOCARDIAL ISCHEMIA

Therapy	How Supplied or Prepared	Usual Dose
Nitrates		
Nitroglycerin	50 mg in 250 mL (200 μg/mL)	Dose to effect (33–>300 μg/min)
Nitroglycerin sublingual	0.3 mg tablets 0.4 mg aerosolized metered dose	0.3–0.9 mg
β-adrenergic blockers		
Esmolol		
Bolus	10 mg/mL vial	10–100 mg. i.v.
Infusion	2.5g ampoule (dilute in 250 mL)	50–200 μg/kg/min
Metoprolol	1 mg/mL ampoule	0.5–5 mg. i.v.
Atenolol	1 mg/mL ampoule	1–10 mg. i.v.
Labetalol hydrochloride	5 mg/mL vial	2.5–25 mg. i.v.
Propranolol hydrochloride	1 mg/mL ampoule	0.5–1 mg. i.v.
Calcium-channel blockers		
Diltiazem hydrochloride		
Bolus	5 mg/mL vial	5–25 mg i.v.
Infusion	100 mg in 100 mL (1 mg/mL)	5–15 mg/h
Nicardipine hydrochloride		
Bolus	2.5 mg/mL (dilute before administering)	100–200 μg
Infusion	25 mg in 250 mL (100 μg/mL)	1–3 mg/h

i.v., intravenous.

nitrates to dilate selectively coronary-conductance vessels and, perhaps, also a result of a direct antiplatelet and antithrombotic effect (43). The biochemical mechanism appears to be the production of nitric oxide (NO). NO activates guanylate cyclase, which produces cyclic guanosine monophosphate (cGMP). Cyclic GMP production results in vasodilation by decreasing intracellular calcium concentration (44).

Intravenously administered nitroglycerin can be effectively titrated to the resolution of angina or monitored evidence of ischemia, such as the ECG findings. This drug should be first-line therapy for suspected perioperative ischemia. Tolerance to prolonged continuous nitrate therapy, resulting in attenuation of its hemodynamic and antiischemic effects, is well described but poorly understood. The clinical problem is best managed by allowing a daily nitrate-free interval. Otherwise, as with an unstable patient, the dose can be increased, or other therapy should be instituted. This problem is a compelling argument for avoiding nitroglycerin infusions in patients who do not have demonstrated ischemia. In the prethrombolytic era, nitrates were shown to reduce the incidence of death from acute MI by 35% (45). Current evidence suggests that, in the absence of recurrent angina or heart failure, nitrates are not indicated in acute MI.

β-Adrenergic Receptor Blockers

β-Adrenergic receptor blockers predominantly decrease myocardial oxygen demand by decreasing HR and contractility. A decreased HR increases the diastolic-filling period, thereby increasing myocardial oxygen supply. This effect is probably most important in extreme tachycardia. Propranolol antagonizes lipolysis induced by catecholamines, reducing the level of circulating free fatty acids and myocardial oxygen consumption (46). In the patient with stable angina, β-adrenergic blockers decrease the frequency of both clinical angina and silent ischemia (47). Exercise

tolerance and quality of life are greatly improved. As described previously, prophylactic β-adrenergic blockade reduces the incidence of adverse cardiovascular outcomes for up to 2 years after surgery.

Early treatment (within 24 hours) with β-adrenergic blockers in patients with clinically suspected MI may abort infarction in some patients. A review of studies addressing this issue concluded that the overall reduction in confirmed infarction among these patients is 13% (48). In a study of metoprolol in acute MI (MIAMI), metoprolol had a more pronounced effect when given less than 8 hours after onset of symptoms and to patients with elevated HR and systolic BP (49). In addition, the acute intravenous injection of metoprolol caused a prompt reduction in ST-segment elevation and the severity of chest pain. In a multicenter trial of intravenously administered atenolol following MI, almost all the reduction in mortality during the 7-day treatment period occurred on the day of admission or on the following day (50). Clinical evaluation and autopsy indicated a reduction in acute myocardial rupture to be the major mechanism for the early mortality reduction (51).

Overwhelming evidence exists that long-term β-adrenergic-blocker therapy following MI is beneficial (52). Mortality is reduced by about 20%, and the odds of nonfatal reinfarction are decreased by about 25%.

These studies in the nonsurgical population are strong evidence that perioperative patients experiencing ischemia or suspected infarction should receive aggressive treatment with β-blocking drugs. The availability of esmolol hydrochloride, an intravenously administered, short-acting, cardioselective, β-blocking drug has made it easier to administer this class of drug in acute or relatively unstable settings. The rapid onset and offset of this drug (half-life, 9 minutes) make it useful for the treatment of hemodynamic-mediated ischemia related to short-lived periods of stress and for administration to patients for whom the physician has concerns about hemodynamic stability. The use of longer-acting drugs such as metoprolol, atenolol, and propranolol hydrochloride is appropriate when a prolonged effect is desired.

Contraindications to the use of β blocker therapy do exist. Patients with bronchospastic pulmonary disease requiring β-agonist therapy, those with severe LV dysfunction, and those with high-grade atrioventricular block should not receive β-blocking agents. Most of the studies involving β-blockers mentioned earlier exclude patients who are hypotensive (usually systolic BP <100 mm Hg), bradycardic (usually <55 bpm), or who manifest clinical signs of CHF. With an LV ejection fraction below 35%, only 30% of patients without clinical CHF, and only 10% of those with clinical CHF will tolerate a full dose of a β-adrenergic blocker. In this group of patients who require treatment for ischemia, careful titration of low doses may be appropriate. It is also recognized that during acute ischemia clinical CHF may be precipitated by diastolic dysfunction. This syndrome may be amenable to therapy with β-blocking drugs. It is left to the clinician to distinguish between CHF secondary to diastolic dysfunction versus that due to systolic dysfunction. Distinguishing characteristics of diastolic dysfunction include the absence of an S3 heart sound, the absence of cardiomegaly, and the preservation of a normal ejection fraction with elevated ventricular end-diastolic pressures.

Calcium-channel Blockers

Despite theoretical expectations, the first-generation calcium-channel blockers diltiazem hydrochloride, nifedipine, and verapamil hydrochloride have been disappointing as first-line treatment for ischemia. Although these drugs decrease anginal symptoms and improve exercise tolerance, they are inferior to β-blocking drugs in the treatment of silent ischemia (48). In patients undergoing CABG operations, pre-CPB ECG evidence of ischemia is significantly more common in patients receiving calcium-channel blockers than in those patients receiving β-blockers. After an MI, verapamil appears to be of marginal benefit in decreasing mortality, and nifedipine, which increases HR, may increase reinfarction and mortality (53). Following non-Q-wave infarction, the use of diltiazem has been shown to decrease early reinfarction but not mortality (54). In the setting of ischemia or suspected MI, where nitrates and β-blockers are either ineffective or not tolerated, calcium-channel blocking drugs that slow the HR (verapamil and diltiazem) are recommended.

Calcium-channel blockers are the treatment of choice for patients with Prinzmetal or vasospastic angina. A history of chest pain at rest with reversible ST-segment elevation (presumably reflecting transmural ischemia) suggests the presence of this condition. Monotherapy with β-blocking drugs may precipitate ischemia in these patients, perhaps because of unopposed α-adrenergic activity. Intravenously administered nicardipine hydrochloride may be extremely useful in the acute management of ischemia in these patients.

Following CABG operations, spasm of native coronaries, the internal mammary graft, or vein grafts may lead to acute ischemia and sudden cardiovascular collapse. Events are most often heralded by hypotension and ST-segment elevation. Risk factors include patients with known vasospastic angina, withdrawal of calcium-channel blockers, respiratory alkalosis, and hypomagnesemia. Because intravenously administered nitrates are of marginal benefit, a calcium-channel antagonist should be administered, despite the presence of hypotension.

Drugs that Affect Coagulation

As discussed, unstable angina and MI are usually the result of atherosclerotic plaque disruption and subsequent thrombosis. These syndromes usually are separated into ST-segment elevation MI (STEMI) versus unstable angina/non-ST-segment elevation MI (UA/NSTEMI) categories, with the latter involving occlusive thrombus and the former less stable, less occlusive thrombus with a greater proportion of platelet aggregates. Antithrombotic therapy is now the cornerstone of therapy in these acute coronary syndromes. Because of the early, prominent role of platelets, aspirin therapy decreases the incidence of MI and death in patients presenting with unstable angina (55) and decreases mortality and reinfarction in patients presenting with all types of acute MI (56). The therapeutic action of aspirin in this setting is inhibition of cyclooxygenase-1 with prevention of thromboxane A_2 generation. This occurs with a dose of 80 to 160 mg. In the absence of contraindications (e.g., allergy, active bleeding, active peptic ulcer) aspirin should be given as soon as possible to all patients with suspected MI.

In the surgical patient, interventional cardiology should be involved early in the management of suspected MI. Angioplasty may be possible, but additional antiplatelet, antithrombin, or thrombolytic therapy beyond aspirin is problematic because of the high probablity of bleeding complications. Extensive research and ongoing developments in the cardiology literature have resulted in effective, evolving algorithms for the nonsurgical patient (57). For UA/NSTEMI syndromes, the addition of heparin (unfractionated or low-molecular weight) to aspirin provides a major risk reduction (58). In surgical patients, anticoagulation must only be undertaken in close consultation with the surgeon. In general, heparinization can be considered only some hours after surgery and probably longer for surgeries where bleeding can be catastrophic (e.g., neurosurgery). Hirudin is an alternative to heparin; however, this drug does not have an antagonist and offers no significant advantage in the surgical patient who has no other contraindication to heparin therapy.

Newer classes of antiplatelet drugs either inhibit adenosine diphosphate (ADP)-induced aggregation (the oral ADP receptor blockers ticlopidine and clopidigrel) or are specific glycoprotein (GP) IIb/IIIa receptor antagonists (intravenous abciximab, tirofiban, and eptifibatide). These drugs are of established benefit in keeping coronary arteries and stents open after angioplasty and in combination with aspirin (i.e., inhibit platelets by two mechanisms) in UA/NSTEMI. Whether or not the incidence of bleeding complications in surgical patients is different with these agents compared with heparin has not been determined.

For STEMI, thrombolytic therapy is clearly the established strategy of choice. Combining thrombolytic drugs with aspirin or heparin or one of the newer platelet receptor-blocking drugs gives improved coronary results at the price of increased bleeding complications. There is a growing literature that early angioplasty/stenting combined with GP IIa/IIIb inhibition may

TABLE 4. ANTICOAGULANT DRUGS USED EARLY IN ACUTE CORONARY SYNDROMES

Class of Drug/Name	Major Mechanism of Action	Indication[a]	Duration[b] of Action	Reversal Agent
Platelet inhibitors				
Aspirin (p.o.)	Inhibits production of thromboxane	All[c]	7–10 d[d]	No
Clopidogrel (p.o.)	ADP receptor blocker	Alternative to ASA	7–10 d[d]	No
Abciximab (i.v.)	Monoclonal antibody to GP IIb/IIIa receptor	UA/NSTEMI[e] (ongoing pain)	24–48 h[f]	No
Tirofiban (i.v.)	Nonpeptide, nonantibody GP IIb/IIA inhibitor	UA/NSTEMI[e] (ongoing pain)	2–3 h	No
Eptifibatide (i.v.)	Peptide GP IIb/IIIa inhibitor	UA/NSTEMI[e] (ongoing pain)	2–3 h	No
Thrombin inhibitors				
Unfractionated heparin (i.v.)	Binds to antithrombin	All[c]	2–3 h	Protamine
Low-molecular-weight heparins (s.c.)	Binds to antithrombin	Alternative to unfractionated heparin	12–24 h	No
Hirudin (i.v.)	Direct thrombin inhibitor	Heparin alternative	3–4 h	No

ASA, acetylsalicylic acid; UA/NSTEMI, unstable angina/non-ST segment elevation myocardial infarction; ADP, adenosine diphosphate; GP, glycoprotein; p.o., by mouth; i.v., intravenous; s.c., subcutaneous.
[a] Indications are evolving; therapy must be individualized.
[b] Normal renal and hepatic function.
[c] All patients without contraindications to the drug.
[d] Irreversible receptor blockade for life of platelet.
[e] One drug of this class should be given.
[f] Physiological half life far exceeds plasma half-life.

provide equivalent results to thrombolytic drugs, with a lower incidence of bleeding (59). This may be an option in surgical patients, in whom lytic drugs are contraindicated for at least one and probably 2 weeks postoperatively. Table 4 summarizes non-thrombolytic drugs affecting coagulation that are used early in the acute coronary syndromes.

Angiotensin-converting Enzyme Inhibitors

Initiation of angiotensin-converting enzyme inhibitors (ACE-I) therapy within days of an acute MI in patients with clinical CHF (60) or those with a LV ejection fraction of less than 40% but without overt CHF (61) have demonstrated a significant decrease in morbidity and mortality. Benefit was observed irrespective of administration of thrombolytic agents, aspirin, or β-blocking drugs. These results mirror the benefits of ACE-I for patients with chronic heart failure. Angiotensin II receptor antagonists have not been investigated in the setting of acute MI, but are expected to show similar benefits with fewer side effects. After β-blockade and aspirin, ACE-I should be considered in the setting of STEMI and, in persistently hypertensive patients with UA/NSTEMI. Intravenously administered enalaprilat is available but is not recommended for the acute treatment of ischemia; its use is indicated for the control of hypertension, especially in the presence of ventricular dysfunction.

ANESTHETIC MANAGEMENT

Patients at risk for developing myocardial ischemia should receive adequate premedication. On arrival in the operating-room area, sedation should be intensified, especially before painful or stress-

ful procedures. In patients who have central venous catheters inserted before cardiac operations, stress resulting from inadequate sedation may precipitate myocardial ischemia. In addition, the benefit of a psychologic approach to anxiety reduction in the form of an adequate preoperative visit cannot be overemphasized.

Intraoperative Period

Whereas most ischemia is not hemodynamically mediated, most studies have found that tachycardia is associated with ischemia. The use of anesthetic techniques that do not cause tachycardia, and aggressive treatment of tachycardia when it occurs, are recommended. Maintenance of relatively normal (i.e., resting, preoperative) BP and HR appears to be a reasonable goal. As described above, antianginal therapy should be maintained until the time of surgery, and β-blockade should be continued during surgery.

It is not possible to recommend definitively one technique of providing general anesthesia over another. Studies of different anesthetic techniques for CABG operations (opioid versus inhalational agents) do not show any effect on the incidence of adverse cardiac outcome. Early reports on the use of isoflurane suggested that this agent was associated with an increase in intraoperative myocardial ischemia because of its potential to cause coronary "steal." Several subsequent studies have refuted this concept and have demonstrated that when adequate coronary-perfusion pressure is maintained, risk does not increase. In a similar way, the first report of the use of desflurane during CABG operations suggested an increase in myocardial ischemia, but this finding has not been confirmed in other studies. The use of regional anesthesia has been advocated by some as a way to reduce myocardial ischemia and its complications. Enthusiasm is based on the ability of regional anesthesia to blunt sympathetic responses to the surgical procedure and to attenuate the hypercoagulable state that follows. Most studies have been conducted in vascular patients because this population is prone to ischemic outcomes secondary to concurrent coronary disease, and many vascular procedures can be performed with regional anesthesia. Vascular surgery patients have been shown to have platelets that are more easily activated and impaired fibrinolysis postoperatively (62). Regional anesthesia is associated with lower levels of serum catecholamines and other stress hormones (Fig. 9) (63) and beneficial effects on the coagulation system (64). Tuman and colleagues (64) observed a decrease in cardiovascular morbidity with the use of a regimen that included epidural anesthesia and analgesia. Baron and

colleagues, however, in a study of 176 patients (65), were unable to demonstrate such a benefit. In a report on 100 patients undergoing lower-extremity vascular operations, the effect of regional versus general anesthesia (including postoperative epidural fentanyl versus morphine administered via a patient-controlled-analgesia device) on arterial thrombotic complications was studied. No difference was found in the incidence of perioperative ischemia or infarction, but regional anesthesia appeared to reduce the need for reoperation for inadequate tissue perfusion (66). This latter effect was associated with the prevention of inhibition of fibrinolysis. Because no studies suggest worse outcomes with regional techniques, several suggest benefits, and postoperative epidural analgesia can be viewed as an advantage, regional and in particular epidural techniques should be considered in patients at risk for ischemia.

Pharmacologic attenuation of the "stress response" can be achieved with the use of centrally acting α-2 agonists. Numerous studies have shown that preoperative administration of clonidine reduces blood pressure, HR, and anesthetic requirements (Fig. 10) (67). Newer drugs of this class include mivazerol and dexmedetomidine. The former drug, given by infusion in a multicenter trial, reduced BP and HR as well as the incidence of myocardial ischemia, but cardiac outcomes were not affected (68). Studies with dexmedetomidine have had similar results; this drug is currently approved for sedation in critical care because it has a unique sedative profile.

Considerable interest has arisen in the use of adenosine-regulating drugs to prevent or modify ischemia. Adenosine is released into the myocardium during hypoxia, and inhibition of its reuptake has several beneficial effects, such as causing local vasodilation, free-radical scavenging, and decreased platelet aggregation. Acadesine is an adenosine-enhancing drug (exact mechanism of action is not known) that has been given as an infusion during CABG operations in several large trials, summarized in a meta-analysis that suggested a reduction in adverse cardiac outcomes (69). This drug is still investigational. Adenosine itself when given systemically interferes with atrioventricular–nodal conduction and is a potent vasodilator; therefore, it is unsuitable as an antiischemic drug.

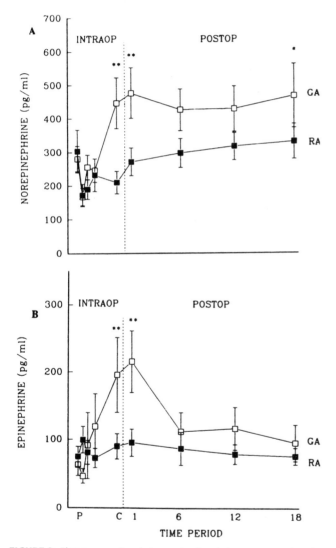

FIGURE 9. Plasma norepinephrine and epinephrine concentrations before induction of anesthesia (P), at skin closure (C), and 1, 6, 12, and 18 hours after lower-extremity revascularization. Data from patients receiving general anesthesia and parenteral morphine analgesia (GA) are contrasted with data from patients receiving epidural bupivacaine anesthesia and epidural fentanyl analgesia (RA). ****P** 0.01; ***P** 0.05 compared with RA group. Data are mean ± SEM. (From Breslow MJ, Parker SD, Frank SM, et al. Determinants of catecholamine and cortisol responses to lower extremity revascularization. The PIRAT Study Group. *Anesthesiology* 1993;79:1202–1209, with permission.)

Postoperative Period

In the postoperative period, patients often experience persistent tachycardia, elevated catecholamine levels, and a high incidence of ischemia that is associated with adverse outcome, as discussed. In noncardiac surgery patients at risk for ischemia, β-blockade needs to be continued for at least the duration of hospitalization. In CABG patients, the peak incidence of ischemia is the first 8 hours, and ischemia is a strong predictor of MI as determined by enzyme release or ECG plus enzyme criteria. There are no studies in the cardiac surgery literature that have evaluated prophylactic β-blockade to placebo in preventing postoperative ischemia; however, such patients frequently receive a drug of this class to reduce the incidence of atrial fibrillation. Control of postoperative pain and anxiety may help control the postoperative sympathetic nervous stimulation described previously. Administration of a sufentanil citrate infusion for 24 hours after CABG surgery

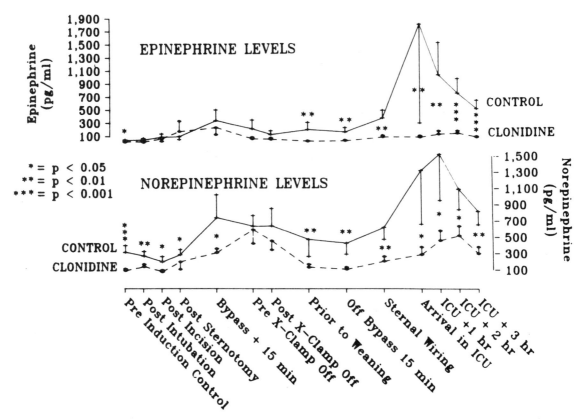

FIGURE 10. Mean values for perioperative (coronary artery bypass graft operation) plasma epinephrine (left ordinate) and norepinephrine (right ordinate) in a control group and in a study group receiving clonidine. At most sampling times, these values were significantly lower in the clonidine group. (From Flacke JW, Bloor BC, Flacke WE, et al. Reduced narcotic requirement by clonidine with improved hemodynamic and adrenergic stability in patients undergoing coronary bypass surgery. *Anesthesiology* 1987;67:11–19, with permission.)

(compared with intermittent morphine sulfate and midazolam hydrochloride) was associated with a reduced incidence of myocardial ischemia, but not of ischemic outcomes (70). A study of 12 hours of propofol sedation versus intermittent morphine and midazolam after CABG operations detected no difference in ischemia or outcome (71). Rather than using prolonged sedation after CABG operations, Cheng and associates (72) examined the incidence of ischemia and related outcomes after early extubation and found no difference when early extubation was compared with overnight sedation and ventilation. One could conclude from these studies that in CABG patients, factors other than adequacy of sedation or analgesia are responsible for postoperative ischemia.

As discussed previously, the use of epidural techniques to provide postoperative analgesia is associated with improved outcome in high-risk patients in several studies. There can be little doubt that epidural techniques provide the best possible postoperative pain control. Thoracic epidural analgesia (bupivacaine) can be used to control refractory angina, possibly by an effect on coronary arteries in addition to blockade of afferent pain fibers (73). Whether this finding can be used to promote the use of thoracic epidural analgesia in other settings is open to debate. In much of the literature on this topic, it is difficult to separate intraoperative from postoperative effects, and many aspects of this issue are left

unresolved (e.g., local anesthetic versus opioid technique, level of epidural, duration of use). The reader is referred to an excellent review of the possible role of epidural analgesia in perioperative outcome (74).

Postoperative hypothermia and anemia may contribute the incidence of myocardial ischemia. Vascular surgery patients arriving in the ICU with a core temperature less than 35°C have a higher incidence of postoperative myocardial ischemia than do patients who are warmer (75). Platelets may be more reactive at low temperatures, potentially explaining, in part, the hypercoagulability that is associated with hypothermia. Two groups reported increased ischemia, and in one case increased cardiac morbidity, with postoperative hematocrits less than 28% (76,77). These are important findings because other studies performed in critically ill patients *without* coronary disease support a lower transfusion threshold (78).

SUMMARY

Over the last 15 years, impressive developments have occurred in the understanding and treatment of myocardial ischemia and MI, and clinicians have become aware of the frequency of perioperative myocardial ischemia and its association with adverse outcome. Most ischemia is asymptomatic, highlighting the need to identify and treat patients prospectively. Whereas hemodynamics, especially tachycardia, contribute to the occurrence of ischemia, many episodes may represent a complex interaction between atherosclerotic plaques, coagulation, and sympathetic nervous stimulation. Preoperative risk assessment and management strategies are now well established, and perioperative β-adrenergic blockade has been definitively shown to be of benefit in reducing ischemic outcomes. The ECG remains the best-validated and most practical monitor for myocardial ischemia, especially in the postoperative period. The use of automated ST-segment analysis enhances the clinician's ability to identify and treat ischemia when it develops. Drugs used to treat ischemia in the medical setting are available in intravenous forms for acute perioperative therapy, with nitrates and β-blockers remaining first-line agents. The acute coronary syndromes (unstable angina or MI) should be

treated aggressively with antithrombotic or interventional therapy as permitted by the nature of surgery and the interval between surgery and the event. For the acute syndromes, aspirin should be given early, wherever possible, with other agents given in consultation with the surgeon and cardiologist. Developments in the fields of antiplatelet and antithrombotic therapy and interventional cardiology may make these modalities more available to surgical patients. The importance of sympathetic nervous system activation has led to investigation of therapies such as α_2-agonists and the potential for greater use of epidural anesthesia or analgesia techniques. Definitive studies demonstrating benefits from these techniques are lacking; however, there is consensus that benefit may exist. One of the greatest challenges will be to make cost-effective monitoring and timely therapy for myocardial ischemia widely available without the requirement for prolonging "intensive care" for the large population at risk.

KEY POINTS

Rather than the concept of fixed coronary stenosis leading to fixed coronary blood flow, a variety of ischemic syndromes, which are determined in part by the coronary anatomy, atheromatous disease, endothelial function, and sympathetic state, occur in patients with coronary-artery disease (CAD).

Most perioperative ischemia is clinically "silent," and its occurrence, particularly in the 3 days after the operation, is associated with adverse cardiac outcome. Most perioperative ischemia is not preceded by hemodynamic changes, although an association does exist between tachycardia and the occurrence of ischemia.

Clinical assessment of the risk for CAD is at least as important as sophisticated testing, and patients with risk factors appear to be just as likely to develop morbidity as are those patients with known CAD. The electrocardiogram (ECG) is the most validated and most practical monitor for perioperative myocardial ischemia.

In the absence of hemodynamic abnormalities (e.g., hypotension), intravenously administered nitroglycerin should be the first treatment for suspected myocardial ischemia. The role of nitroglycerin in the prevention of perioperative ischemia is questionable. Greater use of β-adrenergic-blocking drugs is warranted in the prevention and treatment of myocardial ischemia and in the setting of acute myocardial infarction (MI). Calcium-channel-blocking drugs can be effective in the treatment of myocardial ischemia and may be particularly useful in the setting of reperfusion after ischemia.

Increased use of antithrombotic drugs, such as aspirin and heparin, in the perioperative setting may help reduce the incidence of ischemia. The use of epidural anesthesia or analgesia may provide several benefits, including the reduction of the "stress response" and decreased inhibition of fibrinolysis.

REFERENCES

1. Mangano DT. Perioperative cardiac morbidity. *Anesthesiology* 1990; 72:153–184.
2. Slogoff S, Keats AS. Does perioperative ischemia lead to postoperative myocardial infarction? *Anesthesiology* 1985;62:107–114.
3. Nesto RW, Kowalchuk GJ. The ischemic cascade: temporal sequence of hemodynamic, electrocardiographic and symptomatic expressions of ischemia. *Am J Cardiol* 1987;57:23C–30C.
4. Ehring T, Schulz R, Heusch G. Characterization of "hibernating" and "stunned" myocardium with focus on the use of calcium antagonists in "stunned" myocardium. *J Cardiovasc Pharmacol* 1992;20(Suppl. 5):S25–S33.
5. Ehring T, Heusch G. Stunned myocardium and the attenuation of stunning by calcium antagonists. *Am J Cardiol* 1995;75:61E–67E.
6. Hoffman JI. Maximal coronary flow and the concept of vascular reserve. *Circulation* 1984;70:153–159.
7. Brown BG, Bolson EL, Dodge HT. Dynamic mechanisms in human coronary stenosis. *Circulation* 1984;70:917–922.
8. Nathan HJ. Coronary physiology. In: Kaplan JA, ed. *Cardiac anesthesia*, 3rd ed. Philadelphia: WB Saunders, 1993;235–260.
9. Stone PH. Triggers of transient myocardial ischemia: circadian variation and relation to plaque rupture and coronary thrombosis in stable coronary artery disease. *Am J Cardiol* 1990;66:32G–36G.
10. Fuster V, Badimon L, Badimon JJ, et al. The pathogenesis of coronary artery disease and the acute coronary syndromes. (first of two parts) *N Engl J Med* 1992;326:242–250.
11. Prinzmetal R, Kennamer R, Merliss R, et al. Angina pectoris: a variant form of angina pectoris: a preliminary report. *Am J Med* 1959;27:377.
12. Deanfield JE, Maseri A, Selwyn AP, et al. Myocardial ischemia during daily life in patients with stable angina: its relation to symptoms and heart rate changes. *Lancet* 1983;2:753–758.
13. Chierchia S, Lazzari M, Freedman B, et al. Impairment of myocardial perfusion and function during painless myocardial ischemia. *J Am Coll Cardiol* 1983;1:924–930.
14. Yeung AC, Barry J, Orav J, et al. Effects of asymptomatic ischemia on long-term prognosis in chronic stable coronary disease. *Circulation* 1991;83:1598–1604.
15. Slogoff S, Keats AS. Further observations on perioperative myocardial ischemia. *Anesthesiology* 1986;65:539–542.
16. Knight AA, Hollenberg M, London MJ, et al. Perioperative myocardial

ischemia: importance of the preoperative ischemic pattern. *Anesthesiology* 1988;68:681–688.

17. Mangano DT, Browner WS, Hollenberg M, et al. Association of perioperative myocardial ischemia with cardiac morbidity and mortality in men undergoing noncardiac surgery. The Study of Perioperative Ischemia Research Group. *N Engl J Med* 1990;323:1781–1788.

18. Mangano DT, Wong MG, London MJ, et al. Perioperative myocardial ischemia in patients undergoing noncardiac surgery-II: incidence and severity during the first week after surgery. The Study of Perioperative Ischemia Research Group. *J Am Coll Cardiol* 1991;17:851–857.

19. Wallace A, Layug B, Tateo I, et al. Prophylactic atenolol reduces postoperative myocardial ischemia. *Anesthesiology* 1998;88:7–17.

20. Ritchie JL (Task Force Chair), et al. ACC/AHA guidelines for perioperative cardiovascular evaluation for noncardiac surgery. *Circulation* 1996;93:1280–1317.

21. Goldman L, Caldera DL, Nussbaum SR, et al. Multifactorial index of cardiac risk in noncardiac surgical procedures. *N Engl J Med* 1977;297:845–850.

22. Detsky AS, Abrams HB, Forbath N, et al. Cardiac assessment for patients undergoing noncardiac surgery: a multifactorial clinical risk index. *Arch Intern Med* 1986;146:2131–2134.

23. Goldman L. Cardiac risk in noncardiac surgery: an update. *Anesth Analg* 1995;80:810–820.

24. Mantha S, Roizen MF, Barnard J, et al. Relative effectiveness of four preoperative tests for predicting adverse cardiac outcomes after vascular surgery: a meta-analysis. *Anesth Analg* 1994;79:422–433.

25. Boersma E, Poldermans D, Bax JJ, et al. Predictors of cardiac events after major vascular surgery. *JAMA* 2001;285:1865–1873.

26. Eagle KA, Coley CM, Newell JB, et al. Combining clinical and thallium data optimizes preoperative assessment of cardiac risk before major vascular surgery. *Ann Intern Med* 1989;110:859–866.

27. Mason JJ, Owens DK, Harris RA, et al. The role of coronary angiography and coronary revascularization before noncardiac vascular surgery. *JAMA* 1995;273:1919–1925.

28. Posner KL, Van Norman GA, Chan V. Adverse cardiac outcomes after noncardiac surgery in patients with prior percutaneous transluminal coronary angioplasty. *Anesth Analg* 1999; 89:553–560.

29. Kaluza GL, Joseph J, Lee JR. Catastrophic outcomes of noncardiac surgery soon after coronary stenting. *J Am Coll Cardiol* 2000;35:1288–1294.

30. Mangano DT, Layug EL, Wallace A, et al. Effect of atenolol on mortality and cardiovascular mortality after noncardiac surgery. *N Engl J Med* 1996;335:1713–1720.

31. Palda VA, Detsky AS. Perioperative assessment and management of risk from coronary artery disease. *Ann Intern Med* 1997;127: 313–328.

32. Poldermans D, Boersma E, Baxx JJ, et al. The effect of bisoprolol on perioperative mortality and myocardial infarction in high-risk patients undergoing vascular surgery. *N Engl J Med* 1999;341:1789–1794.

33. Fletcher GF, Froelicher VF, Hartley LH, Haskell WL, Pollock ML. Exercise standards. A statement for health professionals from the American Heart Association. *Circulation* 1990;82:2286–2322.

34. Mark DB, Hlatky MA, Lee KL, Harrell FE Jr, Califf RM, Pryor DB. Localizing coronary artery obstructions with the exercise treadmill test. *Ann Intern Med* 1987;106:53–55.

35. London MJ, Hollenberg M, Wong MG, et al. Intraoperative myocardial ischemia: Localization by continuous 12-lead electrocardiography. *Anesthesiology* 1988;69:232–241.

36. Kaplan JA, Wells PH. Early diagnosis of myocardial ischemia using the pulmonary arterial catheter. *Anesth Analg* 1981;60:789–793.

37. van Daele M, Sutherland GR, Mitchell MM, et al. Do changes in pulmonary capillary wedge pressure adequately reflect myocardial ischemia during anesthesia? A correlative preoperative hemodynamic, electrocardiographic, and transesophageal echocardiographic study. *Circulation* 1990;81:865–871.

38. Hauser AM, Gangadharan V, Ramos RG, Gordon S, Timmis GC. Sequence of mechanical, electrocardiographic and clinical effects of repeated coronary artery occlusion in human beings: echocardiographic observations during coronary angioplasty. *J Am Coll Cardiol* 1985;5:193–197.

39. Leung JM, O'Kelly B, Browner WS, Tubau J, Hollenberg M, Mangano DT. Prognostic importance of postbypass regional wall motion abnormalities in patients undergoing coronary artery bypass graft surgery. SPI Research Group. *Anesthesiology* 1989;71:16–25.

40. Eisenberg MJ, London MJ, Leung JM, et al. Monitoring for myocardial ischemia during noncardiac surgery. A technology assessment of transesophageal echocardiography and 12-lead electrocardiography. The Study of Perioperative Ischemia Research Group. *JAMA* 1992;268:210–216.

41. London MJ, Tubau JF, Wong MG, et al. The "natural history" of segmental wall motion abnormalities in patients undergoing noncardiac surgery. S.P.I. Research Group. *Anesthesiology* 1990;73: 644–655.

42. Teo KK, Yusuf S, Furberg CD. Effects of prophylactic antiarrhythmic drug therapy in acute myocardial infarction. An overview of results from randomized controlled trials. *JAMA* 1993;270:1589–1595.

43. Loscalzo J. Antiplatelet and antithrombotic effects of organic nitrates. *Am J Cardiol* 1992;70:18B–22B.

44. Cohn PF. Concomitant use of nitrates, calcium channel blockers, and beta blockers for optimal antianginal therapy. *Clin Cardiol* 1994;17:415–421.

45. Jugdutt BI, Warnica JW. Intravenous nitroglycerin therapy to limit myocardial infarct size, expansion, and complications. Effect of timing, dosage, and infarct location. *Circulation* 1988;78:906–919.

46. Mueller HS, Ayres SM. The role of propranolol in the treatment of acute myocardial infarction. *Prog Cardiovasc Dis* 1997;19:405.

47. Stone JG, Foëx P, Sear JW, et al. Myocardial ischemia in untreated hypertensive patients: effect of a single small dose of a beta-adrenergic blocking agent. *Anesthesiology* 1988;68:495–500.

48. Held PH, Yusuf S. Effects of b-blockers and calcium channel blockers in acute myocardial infarction. *Eur Heart J* 1993;14(Suppl F):18–25.

49. The MIAMI Trial Research Group. Metoprolol in acute myocardial infarction. Narcotic analgesics and other antianginal drugs. *Am J Cardiol* 1985;56:1G–57G.

50. First International Study of Infarct Survival Collaborative Group. Randomized trial of intravenous atenolol among 16 027 cases of suspected acute myocardial infarction:ISIS-1. *Lancet* 1986;2:57–66.

51. First International Study of Infarct Survival Collaborative Group. Mechanisms for the early mortality reduction produced by beta-blockade started early in acute myocardial infarction:ISIS-1. *Lancet* 1988;1:921–923.

52. Roberts R, Rogers WJ, Mueller HS, et al. Immediate versus deferred b-blockade following thrombolytic therapy in patients with acute myocardial infarction: results of Thrombolysis in Myocardial Infarction (TIMI) II-B study. *Circulation* 1991;83:422–437.

53. Yusuf S, Held P, Furberg C. Update of effects of calcium antagonists in myocardial infarction or angina in light of the second Danish Verapamil Infarction Trial (DAVIT-II) and other recent studies. *Am J Cardiol* 1991;67:1295–1297.

54. Gibson RS, Boden WE, Théroux P, et al. Diltiazem and reinfarction in patients with non-Q-wave myocardial infarction: results of a double-blind, randomized, multicenter trial. *N Engl J Med* 1986;315:423–429.

55. Lewis HD Jr, Davis JW, Archibald DG, et al. Protective effects of aspirin against acute myocardial infarction and death in men with unstable angina: results of a Veterans Administration Cooperative Study. *N Engl J Med* 1983;309:396–403.

56. ISIS-2. Second International Study of Infarct Survival Collaborative Group. Randomised trial of intravenous streptokinase, oral aspirin, both, or neither among 17,187 cases of suspected myocardial infarction. *Lancet* 1988;2:349–360.

57. Braunwald E, Antman EM, Beasley JW et al. ACC/AHA guidelines for the management of patients with unstable angina and non-ST segment elevation myocardial infarction: executive summary and recommendations: a report of the American College of Cardiology/American Heart Association Task Force on Practice Guidelines (Committee on Management of Patients with Unstable Angina). *Circulation* 2000;102:1193–1209).

58. Theroux P, Willerson JT, Armstrong PW. Progress in the treatment of acute coronary syndromes: a 50-year perspective (1950–2000). *Circulation* 2000;102:IV-2–IV-1).

59. Schomig A, Kastrati A, Dirshcinger J et al., for the Stent Versus Thrombolysis for Occluded Coronary Arteries in Patients with Acute

Myocardial Infarction Study investigators. Coronary stenting plus platelet glycoprotein IIb/IIIa blockade compared with tissue plasminogen activator in acute myocardial infarction. *N Engl J Med* 2000;343: 385–391.

60. The Acute Infarction Ramipril Efficacy (AIRE) Study Investigators. Effect of ramipril on morbidity and mortality of survivors of acute myocardial infarction with clinical evidence of heart failure. *Lancet* 1993;342:821–828.

61. Pfeffer MA, Braunwald E, Moyé LA, et al. Effect of captopril on mortality and morbidity in patients with left ventricular dysfunction after myocardial infarction. Results of the survival and ventricular enlargement trial. The SAVE Investigators. *N Engl J Med* 1992;327:669–677.

62. Samama MC, Thiry D, Elalamy I, et al. Perioperative activation of hemostasis in vascular surgery patients. *Anesthesiology* 2001;94:74–78.

63. Rutberg H, Hakanson E, Anderberg B, et al. Effects of the extradural administration of morphine, or bupivacaine, on the endocrine response to upper abdominal surgery. *Br J Anaesth* 1984;56:233–238.

64. Tuman KJ, McCarthy RJ, March RJ, et al. Effects of epidural anesthesia and analgesia on coagulation and outcome after major vascular surgery. *Anesth Analg* 1991;73:696–704.

65. Baron JF, Bertrand M, Barre E, et al. Combined epidural and general anesthesia versus general anesthesia for abdominal aortic surgery. *Anesthesiology* 1991;75:611–618.

66. Christopherson R, Beattie C, Frank SM, et al. Perioperative morbidity in patients randomized to epidural or general anesthesia for lower extremity vascular surgery. The Study of Perioperative Ischemia (SPI) Study Group. *Anesthesiology* 1993;79:422–434.

67. Flacke JW, Bloor BC, Flacke WE, et al. Reduced narcotic requirement by clonidine with improved hemodynamic and adrenergic stability in patients undergoing coronary bypass surgery. *Anesthesiology* 1987; 67:11–19.

68. McSPI-Europe Research Group. Perioperative sympatholysis: beneficial effects of the alpha 2-adrenergic agonist mivazerol on hemodynamic stability and myocardial ischemia. *Anesthesiology* 1997;86:346–363.

69. Mangano DT, for the McSPI Research Group. Effects of acadesine on myocardial infarction, stroke and death following surgery: a meta-analysis of the 5 international randomized trials. *JAMA* 1996;277:325–332.

70. Mangano DT, Siciliano D, Hollenberg M, et al. Postoperative myocardial ischemia. Therapeutic trials using intensive analgesia following surgery. The Study of Perioperative Ischemia (SPI) Study Group. *Anesthesiology* 1992;76:342–353.

71. Wahr JA, Ramsay JG, Jain U, and the McSPI Research Group. Incidence of myocardial ischemia in patients receiving propofol or morphine/midazolam for ICU sedation following coronary artery bypass graft surgery. *Anesthesiology* 1994;81:A256.

72. Cheng D, Karski J, Peniston C, et al. Safety of early extubation following coronary artery bypass graft (CABG) surgery: a prospective randomized controlled study of postop myocardial ischemia and infarction. *Anesthesiology* 1994;81:A81.

73. Blomberg S, Emanuelsson H, Kvist H, et al. Effects of thoracic epidural anesthesia on coronary arteries and arterioles in patients with coronary artery disease. *Anesthesiology* 1990;73:840–847.

74. Liu S, Carpenter RL, Neal JM. Epidural anesthesia and analgesia: their role in postoperative outcome. *Anesthesiology* 1995;82:1474–1506.

75. Frank SM, Beattie C, Christopherson R, et al. Unintentional hypothermia is associated with postoperative myocardial ischemia: the Study of Perioperative Ischemia (SPI) Study Group. *Anesthesiology* 1993;78:468–476.

76. Nelson AH, Fleisher LA, Rosenbaum SH. Relationship between postoperative anemia and cardiac morbidity in high-risk vascular patients in the intensive care unit. *Crit Care Med* 1993;21:860.

77. Hogue CW JR, Goodnough LT, Monk TG. Perioperative myocardial ischemic episodes are related to hematocrit level in patients undergoing radical prostatectomy. *Transfusion* 1998;38:924.

78. Hebert PC, Wells G, Blajchman MA, et al. A multicenter, randomized, controlled clinical trial of transfusion requirements in critical care. *N Engl J Med* 1999;340:409–417.

ACUTE THERAPY IN PATIENTS WITH CARDIAC ARRHYTHMIAS

ROGER D. WHITE

> ### KEY WORDS
>
> - Accessory pathways
> - Adenosine
> - Amiodarone
> - Arrhythmias
> - Atropine
> - Cardioversion
> - Defibrillation
> - Drug therapy
> - Ibutilide
> - Lidocaine
> - Pacing
> - Procainamide
> - Verapamil

INTRODUCTION

Treatment of patients with cardiac arrhythmias necessitates a knowledge of both pharmacologic and electric therapeutic approaches. In hemodynamically stable patients, drug therapy often is the first choice, but failure of drug therapy to terminate the arrhythmia mandates an electric intervention, such as cardioversion or pacing. In other situations, electric therapy is the treatment of first choice, with drugs needed for subsequent continued suppression of the arrhythmia. This chapter discusses both pharmacologic and electric therapy of arrhythmias. The interventions are discussed within the context of the arrhythmias for which treatment is likely to be needed on an urgent or semiurgent basis. Immediate diagnosis and intervention with appropriate therapy often will prevent degeneration of an arrhythmia into a life-threatening event, including cardiorespiratory arrest, affirming the necessity of the clinician's understanding of both diagnostic and therapeutic implications in the management of patients with cardiac arrhythmias.

This discussion is based on the "Guidelines 2000 for Cardiopulmonary Resuscitation and Emergency Cardiovascular Care" (1). This reference should be consulted for more detailed information regarding therapeutic options in algorithm format. These guidelines emphasize two critical points regarding management of patients with cardiac arrhythmias, particularly tachyarrhythmias. First, a diligent and informed effort should be made to secure the diagnosis, including review of a 12-lead electrocardiogram whenever possible and, second, tailoring therapy in accord with the patient's underlying cardiac function. Impaired function [congestive heart failure (CHF) or ejection fraction (EF) <

0.4] mandates alternative pharmacologic choices for almost all tachyarrhythmias.

BRADYARRHYTHMIAS

Slow heart rates in asymptomatic patients usually do not require any intervention. In symptomatic patients, a determination should be made that the patient's signs and symptoms are attributable to the slow heart rate. Symptoms and signs include hypotension, chest pain, dyspnea, altered level of consciousness, diaphoresis, and nausea and vomiting. In monitored patients in intensive care units (ICUs), decreased cardiac output may be evidence of the hemodynamic impact of the bradycardia.

Bradycardic rhythms include sinus bradycardia, atrioventricular (AV) junctional rhythm, and various forms of heart block. Regardless of the type or cause of the bradycardia, atropine sulfate is the first-line intervention for symptomatic patients. It is not necessary initially to define the type of bradycardic rhythm; the objective is to intervene quickly with a drug that is applicable to bradycardia of any type or cause. Atropine fulfills this role. The initial dose is 0.5 to 1.0 mg given as an intravenous bolus. When available, external or transvenous pacing should be used, if needed, after the initial dose of atropine because it provides more precise and controlled rate management without the risks of adverse drug effects. If pacing is not available, repeat 0.5- to 1.0-mg doses of atropine can be given at 3- to 5-minute intervals up to a total dose of 0.04 mg per kilogram of body weight, or approximately 2.5 to 3.0 mg. Pharmacologic alternatives in atropine-refractory patients include dopamine, starting at $5 \ \mu g \cdot kg^{-1} \cdot min^{-1}$ and titrated to a rate or pressure response or, in patients with severe hemodynamic compromise, epinephrine, beginning at 2 to 10 μg per minute. The use of isoproterenol is discouraged because the combined actions of increased myocardial oxygen demand, and peripheral vasodilation can provoke or worsen myocardial ischemia. Drugs that do not decrease coronary perfusion pressure are therefore preferred; however, isoproterenol can be used to achieve rapid correction of symptomatic bradycardia refractory to atropine and dopamine when pacing capability is not available. An infusion rate of 2 to 10 μg per minute is started and titrated to heart rate and rhythm response.

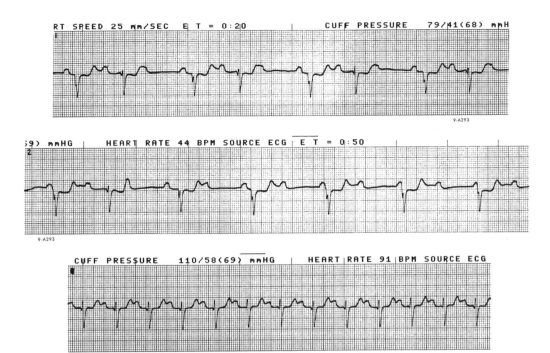

FIGURE 1. Symptomatic bradycardia in a postoperative patient. Initially, 3:2 Mobitz type I second-degree block was present **(upper)**. This progressed to high-grade atrioventricular (AV) block with a junctional escape rhythm **(middle)**. Following injection of 1.0 mg atropine, sinus rhythm was restored **(lower)**, with improvement in systemic arterial blood pressure as noted on upper and lower tracings.

Patients with sinus bradycardia, AV junctional rhythm, or Mobitz type I second-degree AV block [e.g., that accompanying an acute inferior myocardial infarction (MI)] may respond to atropine only, a response based on strong vagal tone, causing slow sinus-node discharge or impaired AV-nodal conduction (Fig. 1). This response also is often observed in patients with complete heart block and an AV junctional escape rhythm. Conversely, patients with Mobitz type II second-degree block or new-onset wide-QRS complex complete heart block are much less likely to respond to atropine. In these patients, infranodal block is usually present, and increased vagal tone is not a significant contributor. In rare circumstances, the vagolytic action of atropine can result in further slowing of heart rate in patients with a Mobitz type II block. This slowing results because atropine-induced, increased sinus discharge and enhanced AV-nodal conduction can stress further the already impaired infranodal conduction system, resulting in progression of the second-degree block to complete heart block with an idioventricular escape rhythm at a slow rate [e.g., 30–35 beats per minute (bpm)]. In patients with Mobitz II and new-onset wide-QRS complex complete heart block (infranodal disease), pacing is the treatment of choice. Even if these patients are asymptomatic, pacing electrode pads or a transvenous pacing electrode should be placed prophylactically. Mobitz type II block can progress unexpectedly to complete heart block with a resultant very slow and unstable idioventricular rhythm. In ICUs, transvenous pacing can be readily accomplished by passage of a pacing electrode into the right ventricle. If a pacing pulmonary artery (PA) catheter is in place, atrial and ventricular pacing electrodes can be inserted to permit atrial, ventricular, or AV sequential pacing. External pacing generators with dual-chamber sensing and pacing (DDD) capabilities are available to provide a spectrum of pacing options for optimizing hemodynamics with preservation of AV synchrony.

TACHYARRHYTHMIAS

Supraventricular Tachyarrhythmias

Supraventricular tachyarrhythmias are tachycardias that require the atria or AV junction for initiation and maintenance of the arrhythmia (2). Included in this discussion are tachycardias that have a reentrant circuit (AV-nodal reentrant tachycardia, sinus-node tachycardia, atrial flutter, and atrial fibrillation) and those arising from enhanced or abnormal automaticity [automatic (ectopic) atrial tachycardia and multifocal atrial tachycardia (MAT)].

Electrocardiographic distinction is frequently difficult, especially if the atrial mechanism is not evident. Tachyarrhythmias associated with the presence of accessory conduction pathways, most commonly seen in patients with the Wolff–Parkinson–White syndrome, will be considered separately because of the important therapeutic implications associated with these tachycardias when drugs are used. Although no drug can be considered truly selective in the termination of any of these tachycardias, it is important to be knowledgeable about the pharmacologic properties of those drugs whose mechanisms and sites of action make them most appropriate in the treatment of various supraventricular tachycardias.

The most common cause of paroxysmal supraventricular tachycardia (PSVT) is AV-nodal reentry. The therapeutic aim in this situation is to interrupt the reentrant circuit in the AV node by slowing either antegrade or retrograde conduction. Vagal maneuvers slow AV-nodal conduction and should be used initially in the treatment of supraventricular tachycardias in which the AV node is likely to be part of the reentrant circuit. Vagal stimulation is most effective when attempted immediately after the onset of the tachycardia, before reflex sympathetic tone competes with the increased vagal discharge. If vagal stimulation via carotid sinus massage or the Valsalva maneuver is ineffective, or if a vagal maneuver cannot be performed, adenosine, because of its efficacy as well as its safety, is the drug of first choice for pharmacologic conversion (3). Nearly 90% of PSVT episodes will terminate with one or two doses of adenosine. Its safety is accounted for largely by its very short half-life (6–10 seconds), a factor that also limits the duration of adverse effects.

An initial dose of adenosine should be injected into a relatively proximal vein, for example, an antecubital vein, or through a central vein, followed by a fluid bolus. For antecubital injection, the initial dose is 6 mg, followed if needed by 12 mg in 1 to 2 minutes. For central injection, 3 mg can be given, followed by a second dose of 6 mg. The rapid metabolic degradation of adenosine is likely to result in an inadequate concentration of the drug at the AV node if it is injected at a more distal site. The result can be a failure to terminate the tachycardia or paradoxical acceleration of the rate from the sympathoexcitatory effects of the drug (4). Transition of atrial flutter from 2:1 to 1:1 conduction has been observed after administration of adenosine (5).

The AV-nodal blocking action of adenosine is antagonized by methylxanthines such as theophylline; this action is secondary to competitive antagonism at adenosine receptors. In patients taking theophylline-containing medications, an initial adenosine dose of 9 mg can be given peripherally, or 5 to 6 mg can be given centrally. Conversely, the action of adenosine is enhanced by dipyridamole, which blocks the intracellular transport and metabolism of adenosine and thus maintains higher concentrations of adenosine at its active receptor sites. In patients taking dipyridamole, 2 mg of adenosine can be given peripherally or 1 mg centrally. Patients taking carbamazepine probably should also be given lower doses initially because this drug can produce impairment of AV-nodal conduction. Adenosine can induce bronchospasm in patients with underlying bronchospastic disorders and therefore probably should not be used in these patients.

In patients with preserved cardiac function in whom PSVT does not respond to adenosine or in whom it recurs after initial termination, verapamil (2.5–5.0 mg over 2 minutes, with repeat doses of 5 to10 mg every 15 to 30 minutes, if needed, to a total of 20 mg) or diltiazem can be used. Diltiazem is given as 0.25 mg per kilogram of body weight, followed by 0.35 mg per kilogram if needed. Neither drug should be used if the QRS complex is widened because of the possibility that the tachycardia is of ventricular origin, in which case, cardiovascular collapse may occur. Although, of course, it is possible that a tachycardia with a widened QRS complex is supraventricular in origin (aberrant conduction or a preexisting bundle-branch block), unless this is known with certainty, the safest course is to avoid both verapamil and diltiazem in any patient with a wide-QRS-complex tachycardia. Other therapeutic options in patients with normal cardiac function include β-blockers such as esmolol. Esmolol is given in a loading dose of 0.5 mg per kilogram of body weight, administered intravenously over 1 minute, followed by a mainte-

nance infusion of 50 μg per kilogram and increased as needed to a maximum of 300 μg per kilogram per minute. Supplemental bolus doses of 0.5 mg per kilogram can be given as the infusion rate is increased to the maximum.

Cardioversion always should be considered in patients who are unresponsive to pharmacologic interventions. If this cannot be used for any reason, then persistent or recurrent PSVT can be treated with procainamide or amiodarone. Procainamide is given intravenously at a rate of 20 mg per minute to a total of 17 mg per kilogram. In urgent situations, up to 50 mg per minute can be given. The maintenance infusion rate is 1 to 4 mg per minute. If hypotension or QRS widening occurs, the drug infusion should be terminated. Amiodarone is given intravenously in a dose of 150 mg over 10 minutes, followed by an infusion of 1 mg per minute for 6 hours and then 0.5 mg per minute. Supplementary 150-mg doses can be given, to a total dose of 2 g in 24 hours.

For patients with impaired ventricular function β-blocking and calcium-channel blocking drugs should be avoided. In this situation, amiodarone can be used as described previously. Digoxin also can be used in such patients, although its slow onset of action limits its usefulness.

As stated earlier, AV-nodal reentry is the most common cause of PSVT. Sinus-node reentrant tachycardia, as the name suggests, uses the sinus node for reentry. If P waves are visible on the electrocardiogram (ECG), they are nearly identical to those observed during sinus rhythm. As would be expected from the similarity of the electrophysiologic properties of the sinus and AV nodes, sinus-node-reentrant tachycardia can be terminated with adenosine as well as with vagal maneuvers and calcium-channel blockade. Therefore, if the atrial mechanism cannot be distinguished by the presence of visible P waves, adenosine can be expected to terminate the tachycardia if the sinus node rather than the AV node is the site of reentry.

The "Guidelines 2000" algorithm for management of patients with supraventricular tachycardia is shown in Figure 2.

For patients with atrial flutter or atrial fibrillation, the initial objective of therapy is often to control a rapid ventricular rate (6). Control can be accomplished with drugs, but in hemodynamically unstable patients, cardioversion is the treatment of choice. Atrial flutter is responsive to low-energy doses (e.g., starting with 50 J), whereas atrial fibrillation typically requires higher doses, such as 100 to 200 J initially. With rectilinear biphasic waveform cardioversion, energy doses in the range of 70 to 170 J have greater efficacy in termination of atrial fibrillation than the traditional 200-360 J with monophasic waveforms (7). Atrial flutter also can be treated with overdrive pacing using external generators with this feature. Pulse generators are available that incorporate high-rate atrial burst-pacing capability. Burst pacing should be at rates at least 30 bpm or faster than the tachycardia for 5 to 10 captured beats. Pacing at rates only slightly faster than the tachycardia rate can result in an increased tachycardia rate by fusion with paced beats, with failure to terminate the tachycardia and, possibly, hemodynamic compromise.

Several drugs are available for rate control in atrial flutter or atrial fibrillation (8). These drugs include the calcium channel blockers diltiazem and verapamil, β-adrenergic-blocking agents such as esmolol, digoxin, and amiodarone. Although it is not available in the United States, sotalol also has been shown to

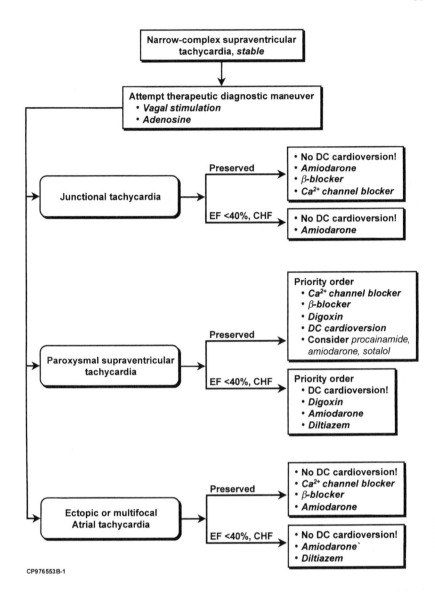

FIGURE 2. The Guidelines 2000 algorithm for supraventricular tachycardia. (Reprinted from the International Consensus of Science. Guidelines 2000 for cardiopulmonary resuscitation and emergency cardiovascular care. *Circulation* 2000;102(Suppl):I–162, with permission.)

be effective in rate control. Intravenous amiodarone has several electrophysiologic actions that are of therapeutic benefit in a spectrum of cardiac arrhythmias (9–11). It decreases heart rate, slows AV nodal conduction by both β-receptor and calcium-channel blockade, and slows intraventricular conduction by blockade of the sodium channel. In a sense, it can be considered a "broad-spectrum antiarrhythmic." The dosages are as described in the preceding information for PSVT. Because administration of amiodarone may convert atrial fibrillation to sinus rhythm, its use should be limited to patients within the first 48 hours of onset of the arrhythmia to prevent embolization unless transesophageal echocardiography confirms absence of thrombus. For patients with atrial fibrillation with duration of longer than 48 hours, intravenous heparinization followed by transesophageal echocardiography to exclude atrial clot can permit safe cardioversion within 24 hours (12). This is followed by 1 month of continued anticoagulation with warfarin.

Both amiodarone and sotalol have been effective in reverting new-onset atrial fibrillation (<24 hours' duration) to sinus rhythm compared with digoxin (13). In this prospective, random-ized, controlled study, a single intravenous dose of each drug was followed by 48 hours of orally administered drug. Compared with digoxin, there was a significant reduction in time to reversion to sinus rhythm in patients treated with sotalol or amiodarone, and at 48 hours those treated with the latter drugs were more likely to be in sinus rhythm than those treated with digoxin (95% versus 78%).

Ibutilide is a class III antiarrhythmic drug that prolongs the action potential duration and refractoriness primarily by blocking the delayed rectifier outward potassium current (14). It is indicated for pharmacologic conversion of atrial fibrillation or flutter of recent onset. Either effective anticoagulation or transesophageal echocardiographic confirmation of the absence of atrial thrombus is necessary for the treatment of atrial fibrillation or flutter present longer than 48 hours duration. The drug is effective in converting recent-onset atrial flutter in about 64% of patients, whereas in atrial fibrillation, the conversion rate is 32% (15). One study reported greater efficacy in both atrial flutter (76%) and atrial fibrillation (51%) when ibutilide was compared with procainamide (18%) (16) (Fig. 3).

***p = 0.005.

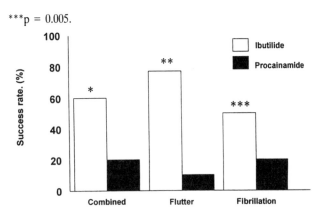

FIGURE 3. Rates of conversion of atrial fibrillation and atrial flutter in ibutilide and procainamide treatment groups. *P < 0.0001; **P = 0.0001; ***P = 0.005. (Reprinted from Volgman AS, Carberry PA, Stambler B, et al. Conversion efficacy and safety of intravenous ibutilide compared with intravenous procainamide in patients with atrial flutter or fibrillation. *J Am Coll Cardiol* 1998;31:1416, with permission.)

The initial dose of ibutilide is 1 mg given intravenously over approximately 8 minutes. If needed, a second dose of 1 mg can be given after 8 to 10 minutes. The drug should not be administered to patients with a prolonged QTc interval (>440 ms), to patients who are hypokalemic or hypomagnesemic, or to patients with severe left ventricular dysfunction (EF <0.3). The most serious adverse effect is polymorphic ventricular tachycardia, with an incidence of 4.3%. The risk is increased in the presence of any of the preceding abnormalities.

Ibutilide also has been shown to facilitate the termination of atrial fibrillation by transthoracic cardioversion. Cardioversion to sinus rhythm was observed in 36 of 50 patients (72%) who had not received the drug and in all 50 patients who were pretreated with 1 mg of intravenous ibutilide prior to cardioversion. In the

14 patients in whom cardioversion alone failed, sinus rhythm was restored with repeat cardioversion after injection of ibutilide (17).

Automatic (ectopic) atrial tachycardia is a non-reentrant narrow-complex tachycardia with P waves different from those during sinus rhythm, although often P waves are not discernible (Fig. 4). This tachycardia is caused by either enhanced automaticity in fully polarized atrial cells or by abnormal automaticity in partially depolarized atrial myocytes. The diagnosis is best confirmed by the presence of abnormal P wave morphology on the 12-lead ECG. Vagal stimulation or administration of adenosine may unmask the persistent atrial tachycardia after induction of AV block. Rate control or termination of the tachycardia can be achieved with β-blockers or calcium-channel blockers. Amiodarone also can be used and in the presence of impaired ventricular function, amiodarone, or diltiazem should be used.

Another supraventricular tachycardia that is non-reentrant and automatic in origin is multifocal atrial tachycardia (MAT) (18,19). Triggered automaticity is the most likely cause of this arrhythmia. It is diagnosed electrocardiographically by the presence of P waves of at least three different morphologies in the same lead, with a rate greater than 100 per minute (Fig. 5). The most common clinical association is chronic obstructive pulmonary disease, but MAT can occur in the presence of a variety of disorders, including acute myocardial ischemia or MI, catecholamine or theophylline excess, CHF, and hypokalemia. A high clinical awareness of this arrhythmia is necessary because it is often mistaken for atrial fibrillation and then followed by ineffective and possibly harmful therapy. Misdiagnosis as atrial fibrillation can lead to futile therapy with cardioversion, which does not terminate MAT. The therapeutic approach in this situation is obviously to treat the underlying disorder, if possible, and to control the rate if needed. A calcium-channel blocking drug (diltiazem or verapamil), a β-blocker, or amiodarone can be used.

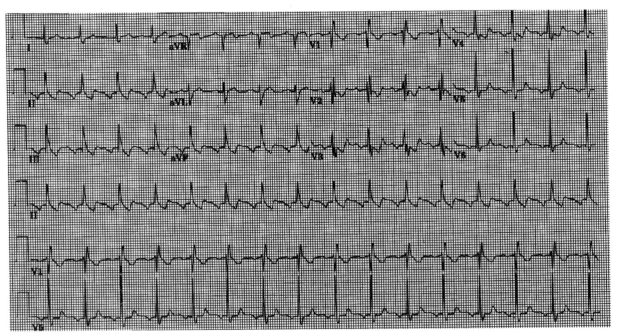

FIGURE 4. Automatic (ectopic) atrial tachycardia. Abnormal P waves are present at a rate of 190 per minute and 2:1 atrioventricular (AV) block is present.

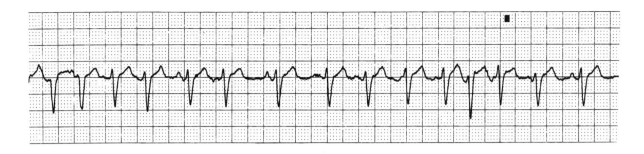

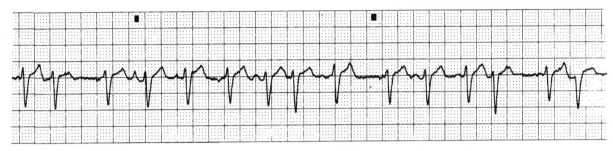

FIGURE 5. Multifocal atrial tachycardia (MAT). P waves of distinct and varying morphology are present, and the rhythm is irregular at a rate of 120 per minute. The irregular irregularity accounts for the frequent misdiagnosis of atrial fibrillation.

It must be emphasized that cardioversion is ineffective for both ectopic and multifocal atrial tachycardia. Thus, because MAT is often misdiagnosed as atrial fibrillation, the importance of establishing the correct diagnosis has important therapeutic implications.

Supraventricular Tachyarrhythmias in Patients with Accessory Pathways

Accessory conducting pathways can be present in many locations in the heart. Those pathways bridging the AV annulus are present in patients with Wolff–Parkinson–White syndrome. Other forms of accessory connections include antegradely conducting atriofascicular pathways connecting the anterolateral right atrium with the right ventricular apex close to the right bundle branch (Mahaim fibers) (Fig. 6) (20). Retrograde conduction in these tachycardias is via the AV node. If the diagnosis is certain from the 12-lead ECG, then adenosine, calcium-channel blockers, or β-blocking drugs can be used. If the diagnosis is uncertain, procainamide or amiodarone should be used. AV accessory connections may remain silent, or they may become manifest in the form of supraventricular tachyarrhythmias (SVT). These SVTs include orthodromic or antidromic AV-reciprocating tachycardia or atrial flutter or atrial fibrillation. Each of these is discussed and their therapeutic implications presented. In some studies, SVTs sustained by conduction through accessory pathways have been observed to occur with a frequency similar to that associated with AV-nodal reentry.

In patients with Wolff–Parkinson–White syndrome, the most common tachyarrhythmia is orthodromic AV-reciprocating tachycardia, in which the ventricles are depolarized via antegrade conduction through the AV node (21). Retrograde conduction to the atria is via the accessory pathway. Unless aberrant conduction or preexisting bundle-branch block is present, the resulting tachycardia is narrow complex, with retrograde inverted P waves sometimes visible following the QRS complex. Because the AV node is part of the circuit sustaining the tachycardia and typically is the weakest link in the arrhythmic circuit, drugs that make a pharmacologic "hit" by slowing AV conduction can be used to terminate the tachycardia. Adenosine is the drug of choice, in the doses and with the routes of administration discussed earlier. For the same reason, verapamil can also be used if adenosine is ineffective or if the tachycardia recurs. Precautions regarding the use of verapamil will be discussed subsequently.

Antidromic AV reciprocating tachycardia is seen much less frequently than is its orthodromic counterpart and is most likely to occur in patients with multiple rather than single accessory connections. It is characterized by a regular tachycardia with wide QRS complexes, thus resembling ventricular tachycardia. With antidromic AV reciprocating tachycardia, the ventricles are depolarized via the accessory connection, with retrograde return of the wave front to the atria through the AV node. The clinical history is important because, on the surface ECG, this tachycardia cannot be readily distinguished from ventricular tachycardia. As with orthodromic tachycardia, adenosine can be effective here also because the AV node is part of the tachycardia circuit. It should be used only if the diagnosis is certain, however. If the diagnosis is not certain, the arrhythmia should be treated as a wide-complex tachycardia. Procainamide can be used in the doses discussed earlier and with the same precautions during procainamide loading.

Atrial flutter or atrial fibrillation is the tachyarrhythmia of greatest concern for patients with Wolff–Parkinson–White

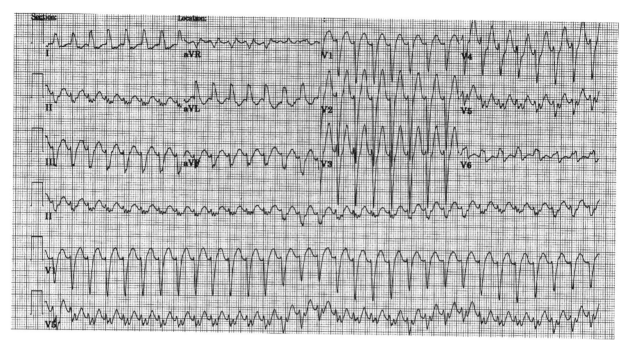

FIGURE 6. Mahaim-fiber tachycardia. The 12-lead electrocardiogram (ECG) in this tachycardia demonstrates a left bundle-branch block pattern, left-axis deviation, $<$ QRS $\leq$ 150 ms, an R wave in lead I, rS in V_1, and QRS transition at or after V_4.

syndrome and, fortunately, is the least common tachycardia. When atrial flutter or fibrillation occurs, the depolarizing wave fronts from the atria can be conducted antegradely into the ventricles over the accessory pathway, resulting in a wide-complex tachycardia with rapid ventricular rates (Fig. 7). The tachycardia may strikingly resemble ventricular tachycardia on the surface ECG, especially if intermittent narrow QRS complexes resulting

from antegrade AV-nodal conduction are present, resembling the capture/fusion complexes of ventricular tachycardia (Fig. 8). In the rare instance of sudden cardiac death in patients with Wolff–Parkinson–White syndrome, ventricular fibrillation results from rapid activation of the ventricles with the atrial fibrillation or flutter waves, resulting in increasing dispersion of recovery of ventricular excitability.

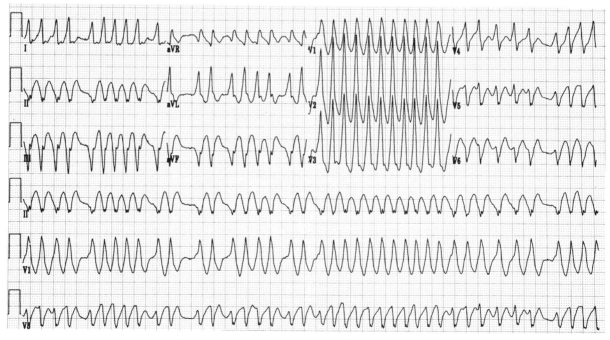

FIGURE 7. Atrial fibrillation in a patient with Wolff–Parkinson–White (WPW) syndrome.

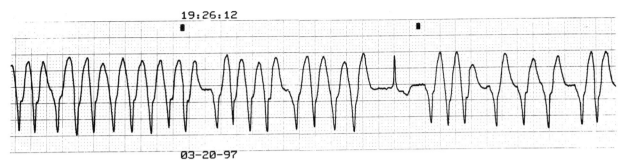

19:26:12

03-20-97

FIGURE 8. Rhythm strip in the same patient as in Figure 6. A normally conducted QRS complex is seen, resembling morphologically a capture beat as seen in ventricular tachycardia.

Cardioversion, using energy doses discussed earlier for atrial flutter and atrial fibrillation, is the treatment of choice for patients with this tachyarrhythmia. As in other causes of atrial fibrillation or flutter, cardioversion is a safe, effective option if the tachyarrhythmia has been present for less than 48 hours, which is likely to be the case in atrial fibrillation with rapid ventricular response over an accessory pathway. If atrial fibrillation has been present for more than 48 hours, anticoagulation is mandatory. Earlier cardioversion can be used if intravenous heparin is begun immediately and transesophageal echocardiography confirms the absence of atrial thrombus (12). For patients who are hemodynamically stable, procainamide or amiodarone can be used, but cardioversion should be used if at any time hemodynamic instability supervenes. Drugs that block AV-nodal conduction with little or no block of conduction over the accessory pathway must be avoided because further acceleration of the ventricular rate would be the result, risking precipitation of ventricular fibrillation. In this situation, atrial fibrillation or flutter wave fronts blocked in the AV node can be conducted rapidly into the ventricles over the accessory pathway, resulting in very fast ventricular rates. Three possible mechanisms can contribute to acceleration of the ventricular rate. First, some drugs, notably verapamil, can shorten the antegrade refractory period in the accessory pathway in some patients. Second, drug-induced vasodilation can result in reflex sympathetic discharge and, therefore, decreased accessory-pathway refractoriness. Finally, decreased AV-nodal conductance after drug injection can reduce concealed retrograde conduction into the accessory pathway and thus enhance antegrade conduction. Drugs to be avoided include digoxin, β-blockers, and calcium-channel blockers.

Ventricular Tachyarrhythmias

In intensive-care settings, ventricular tachycardia (VT) can occur as a consequence of a variety of disorders, including acute myocardial ischemia or MI; hypoxemia; electrolyte derangements, especially hypokalemia and hypomagnesemia; and CHF. Although it is true that VT can result in rapid cardiovascular collapse or degenerate into ventricular fibrillation (VF), it is often not appreciated that VT can be accompanied by hemodynamic stability, which is rate-related, as well as a consequence of compensatory sympathetic stimulation. The urgency of therapy is therefore dependent on the hemodynamic status of the patient and not simply because the tachycardia is ventricular in origin.

Monomorphic ventricular tachycardia (MVT) is characterized on the ECG by the presence of QRS complexes that are wide and of uniform morphology. ECG evidence that the wide-complex tachycardia is ventricular in origin includes the presence of intermittent P waves unrelated to the QRS complexes (AV dissociation) (Fig. 9) and fusion/capture complexes (Fig. 10). Other helpful ECG evidence is a QRS width greater than 140 ms and concordance of the QRS complexes across the precordium on a 12-lead ECG. Although these types of ECG evidence should be sought, they may not be present. It is important to recognize that clinical clues can provide strong support that the tachycardia is ventricular in origin: A clinical history of previous MI or coronary artery disease with angina is strongly indicative that the wide-complex tachycardia is ventricular (22). In fact, any wide-QRS tachycardia should initially be considered ventricular in origin until proven otherwise, and therapy should be directed with this consideration in mind.

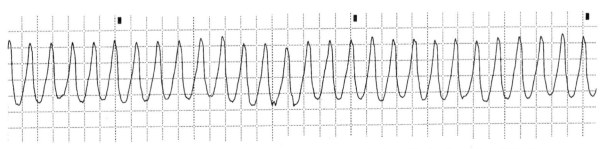

FIGURE 9. Ventricular tachycardia, confirmed by the presence of atrioventricular dissociation (P wave between the twelfth and thirteenth QRS complexes).

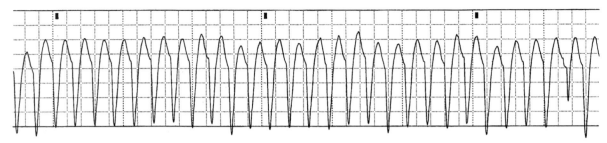

FIGURE 10. The diagnosis of ventricular tachycardia is confirmed by the presence of a capture beat (second complex from right).

In patients who are hemodynamically unstable following the onset of MVT or any other wide-QRS tachycardia, cardioversion is the intervention of choice. An initial energy dose of 100 J can be used, with stepwise increments as needed (100, 200, 300, and 360 J). If biphasic-waveform cardioversion is used, energy selection will be dependent on the specific waveform (7,23). Sedation, analgesia, or both, can be accomplished with any of several drugs, including a benzodiazepine, etomidate, an opioid, or ketamine hydrochloride. A general anesthetic with a thiobarbiturate such as thiopental or methohexital sodium is used frequently and provides complete amnesia; analgesia and recovery are rapid.

In hemodynamically stable patients with MVT with normal ventricular function, procainamide is the drug of choice, given in the doses discussed earlier. Amiodarone and lidocaine are considered acceptable alternatives in this setting. For patients with impaired cardiac function, amiodarone is recommended as the initial drug, with lidocaine an acceptable alternative. Cardioversion always should be considered an appropriate intervention for MVT, either initially or after failure to control the tachycardia with the selected drug. In fact, when drug therapy with a single antiarrhythmic drug is ineffective, it is best to proceed directly to cardioversion rather than to introduce yet another antiarrhythmic drug. The proarrhythmic potential of all these drugs must be appreciated when pharmacologic therapy is chosen for arrhythmia control.

Polymorphic ventricular tachycardia (PVT) is characterized by irregular and wide QRS complexes that vary in amplitude and twist about the isoelectric baseline (Fig. 11). PVT can occur in a variety of settings, such as acute MI, in which case therapy is as that described for MVT. If cardioversion is necessary for hemodynamic reasons, the energy doses recommended are those used in VF, that is, starting with 200 J, with monophasic shocks or lower energies with biphasic waveforms.

When accompanied by QT-interval prolongation, the PVT is defined as torsade de pointes ("twisting of the points" QRS complexes) (24–26). Torsade de pointes is a specific form of PVT with distinct diagnostic and therapeutic considerations (27,28).

In addition to the QRS morphologic features, the ECG shows evidence of prolonged repolarization, which manifests as lengthening of the QT-interval preceding and following the episodes of tachycardia. Clinical associations must be sought because correction of the underlying cause is essential for ultimate control of the arrhythmia. Magnesium may be useful in the treatment of torsade de pointes; the typical intravenous dose of magnesium sulfate in this case is 1 to 2 g over 1 to 2 minutes. If this drug does not control the arrhythmia, overdrive pacing, atrial or ventricular, can be used to suppress the prolonged repolarization giving rise to the torsade episodes. It is critical for successful treatment to identify the underlying cause of the repolarization abnormality while arrhythmia suppression is undertaken with magnesium sulfate or with overdrive pacing. Traditional ventricular antiarrhythmic therapy is not likely to be successful in controlling torsade de pointes. Certainly, awareness that class IA antiarrhythmic drugs, such as procainamide, disopyramide phosphate, and quinidine gluconate, can be the cause of torsade is essential. The major causes of prolonged repolarization associated with torsade de pointes are presented in Table 1.

The "Guidelines 2000" algorithm for treating patients with stable VT is shown in Fig. 12.

Ventricular tachycardia accompanying acute hyperkalemia may manifest by a sine-wave QRS pattern (Fig. 13). Again, the clinical suspicion or documentation of hyperkalemia can lead to prompt corrective therapy with sodium bicarbonate, calcium chloride, and glucose and insulin. A suggested therapeutic approach would include intravenously administered sodium bicarbonate, 1 to 2 mEq per kilogram of body weight; calcium chloride, 1 g; and glucose 1 g per kilogram with regular insulin 0.3 U per gram of glucose, the latter given over 1 hour.

Wide-Complex Tachyarrhythmias

When a wide-complex tachycardia is found, a concerted effort should be made to identify the specific diagnosis. This should include a search for AV dissociation on the 12-lead ECG or on

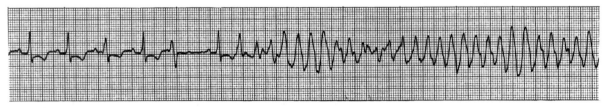

FIGURE 11. Polymorphic ventricular tachycardia accompanying an acute inferior myocardial infarction.

TABLE 1. CAUSES OF ACQUIRED PROLONGED REPOLARIZATION SYNDROMES

Drugs
  Procainamide
  Quinidine
  Disopyramide
  Sotalol
  Bepridil
  Amiodarone
  Probucol
  Phenothiazines (thioridazine, trifluoperazine, chlorpromazine)
  Tricyclic antidepressants (imipramine, amitriptyline, nortriptyline)
  Pentamidine
  Cisapride
  Organophosphate insecticides
  Terfenadine or astemizole (antihistamines) with
      ketoconazole or itraconazole (antimycotics), with
      erythromycin, clarithromycin or troleandomycin or
      severe hepatic disease

Electrolyte disorders
  Hypokalemia
  Hypomagnesemia
  Hypocalcemia
Intracranial hemorrhage or cerebrovascular accident
Bradycardia from any cause
Acute myocardial ischemia or infarction

tracings from the monitor. In some instances, an esophageal lead may be useful in identifying AV dissociation. The presence of AV dissociation is almost conclusive evidence that the tachycardia is ventricular in origin (Fig. 14). A clinical history of coronary or other heart disease supports a diagnosis of a ventricular origin of the tachycardia.

If, despite an attempt to define the mechanism of the tachycardia, one is left with a diagnosis of wide-complex tachycardia of uncertain origin, intervention will be determined by the patient's hemodynamic state (Fig. 15). In unstable patients, DC cardioversion should be considered first-line therapy. Otherwise, drug therapy can be used. Previously, lidocaine and adenosine were considered therapeutically or diagnostically useful. In fact, lidocaine has no diagnostic utility in this context and, as discussed earlier, it is now viewed as a second-line drug for VT, both monomorphic and polymorphic. Adenosine is not effective for the most common forms of VT and can be accompanied by several side effects, including chest pain, bronchospasm, and alarming acceleration of the ventricular rate in atrial fibrillation with accessory pathway conduction. Thus, neither of these drugs is recommended in the treatment of wide-complex tachycardia of uncertain origin. Instead, a "broad-spectrum" antiarrhythmic drug is recommended, such as procainamide or amiodarone. If

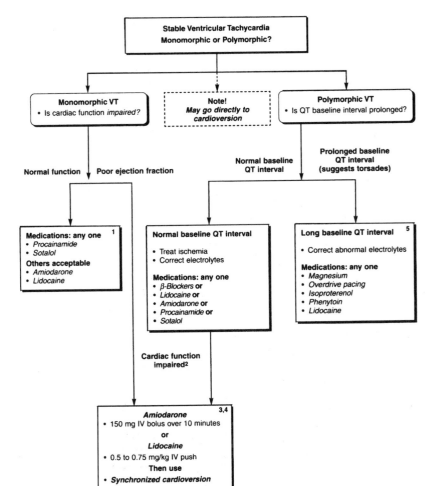

FIGURE 12. The "Guidelines 2000" algorithm for stable ventricular tachycardia. (Reprinted from International Consensus on Science. Guidelines 2000 for cardiopulmonary resuscitation and emergency cardiovascular care. *Circulation* 2000;102(Suppl):I–163, with permission.)

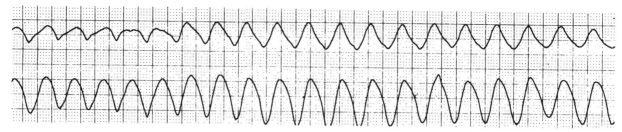

FIGURE 13. Hyperkalemic (sine-wave) ventricular tachycardia. The serum potassium was 7.9 mEq per liter.

impaired cardiac function is present, amiodarone is the drug of choice. Both drugs are effective in the treatment of SVT and VT, as discussed earlier, and thus become the drugs of choice when treating a hemodynamically stable patient with wide-complex tachycardia whose origin cannot be confirmed clinically or electrocardiographically.

Role of Lidocaine in the Treatment of Tachyarrhythmias

It is evident from the preceding discussion that lidocaine is no longer considered a first-line drug for the treatment of VT of wide-complex tachycardia of undetermined origin. The evidence evaluation process from which the "2000 Guidelines" were developed did not support the retention of lidocaine in its prior first-line position. Some studies have shown that lidocaine is not effective in termination of hemodynamically stable VT (29,30), and another study reported that lidocaine was less effective than procainamide (31). At this time, lidocaine is considered accept-

able therapy for stable MVT, but as a second-tier choice, with procainamide and amiodarone the drugs of first choice.

Pulseless VT and VF are forms of ventricular tachyarrhythmia that result in cardiorespiratory arrest and, therefore, require prompt interventions, beginning with defibrillation. Amiodarone has replaced lidocaine as the antiarrhythmic drug of first choice, given after epinephrine. Based on observations in the ARREST trial, the recommended dose of amiodarone in this setting is 300 mg initially, with 150-mg supplementary doses if needed (32). An infusion of 1 mg per minute for 6 hours can follow. Then doses of 0.5 mg per minute, up to a total 24-hour dose of 2 g, can be given. If torsade de pointes is present or hypomagnesemia is suspected or documented, magnesium sulfate should be injected as a 1- to 2-g bolus.

Epinephrine continues to be a mainstay in the treatment of all forms of cardiorespiratory arrest. The recommended initial intravenous dose is 1 mg. Thereafter, as long as the arrest persists, it is repeated at 3- to 5-minute intervals. In VT/VF arrest, a single dose of vasopressin 40 U administered intravenously is suggested as an alternative to epinephrine for the initial injection,

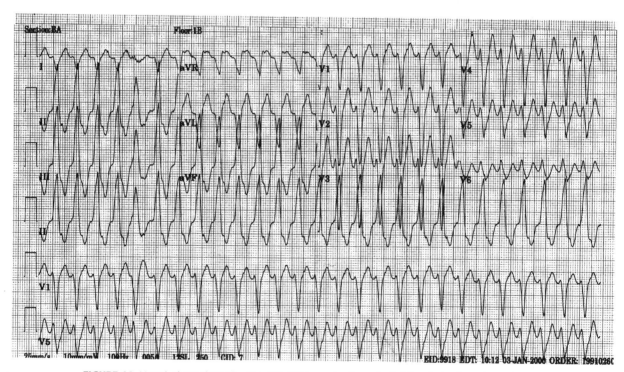

FIGURE 14. Ventricular tachycardia. The fifth QRS complex from the left is a fusion beat, best seen in lead I.

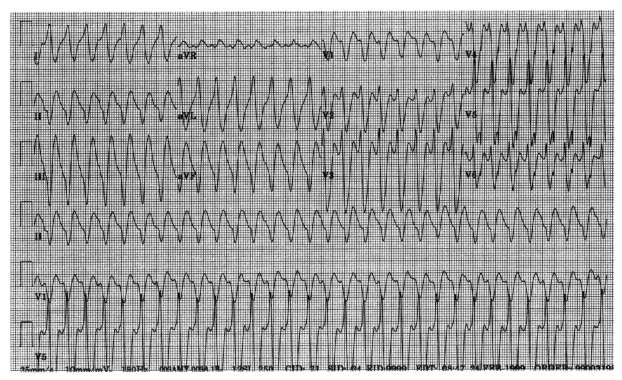

FIGURE 15. Wide-complex tachycardia. Atrioventricular dissociation is not seen, and the QRS morphology is not clearly diagnostic of the origin of the tachycardia.

followed by epinephrine at 3- to 5-minute intervals. Vasopressin has been demonstrated experimentally to increase cardiac and cerebral blood flow, with improved survival compared with epinephrine (33–35). In one study of shock-refractory VF in humans, patients who received vasopressin plus epinephrine had higher admission and 24-hour survival rates (36). Based on this admittedly limited evidence, a single dose of vasopressin is considered an acceptable alternative to the first dose of epinephrine in VT/VF arrest.

SUMMARY

Therapeutic decisions in caring for patients with cardiac arrhythmias are based on an assessment of the hemodynamic impact of the rhythm disturbance, the patient's underlying cardiac function, and the correct diagnosis of the arrhythmia. Both clinical examination and the ECG should be considered in making the diagnosis. Incorrect diagnosis can lead not only to ineffective therapy but also to potentially dangerous therapy, especially when wide-QRS tachyarrhythmias are present.

Symptomatic slow heart rates can be treated initially with atropine; in many forms of bradycardia, however, pacing, either external or transvenous, is the definitive therapy of choice. In some situations, including Mobitz type II second-degree block and in wide-QRS, new-onset complete heart block, external pacing can be used temporarily to bridge the patient over to transvenous pacing. The latter can be accomplished by passing a transvenous pacing electrode or by means of an atrial pacing electrode, a ventricular pacing electrode, or atrial and ventricular pacing electrodes inserted into a pacing PA catheter.

Adenosine is the drug of first choice in treating patients with PSVT. It is therapeutic in over 90% of patients with this tachyarrhythmia, in which AV-nodal reentry is the most common mechanism. In non-reentrant SVT, such as automatic (ectopic) atrial tachycardia or multifocal atrial tachycardia, adenosine may be useful in unmasking the underlying arrhythmia mechanism, but the 12-lead ECG should first be searched to define the mechanism of the arrhythmia. Other pharmacologic options include diltiazem and verapamil, β-blocking drugs, and amiodarone and digoxin. Ibutilide can be used for pharmacologic conversion of recent-onset atrial flutter or atrial fibrillation (<48 hours duration) or later after anticoagulation or transesophageal echocardiographic exclusion of atrial thrombus. Cardioversion should be considered if drug use is contraindicated or if the arrhythmia is not controlled with drug therapy.

Ventricular tachycardia can be monomorphic or polymorphic. When PVT is accompanied by prolonged repolarization, manifest as QT-interval lengthening on the ECG before or after episodes of tachycardia, the tachycardia is torsade de pointes, and its presence mandates specific diagnostic and therapeutic considerations. If the origin of a wide-QRS tachycardia cannot be confirmed clinically or electrocardiographically, amiodarone or procainamide, with amiodarone preferred in the presence of impaired cardiac function, should be used. In all situations, emergent cardioversion takes precedence if hemodynamic compromise is present or develops during drug therapy. Pulseless VT and VF are forms of ventricular tachyarrhythmia that require cardiac-arrest therapy with defibrillation and drugs, most importantly epinephrine, for maintenance of myocardial and cerebral blood flow during external chest compression or open-chest cardiac massage.

KEY POINTS

Acute-onset cardiac arrhythmias carry the potential of hemodynamic instability, including cardiovascular collapse.

Intervention necessitates knowledge of both electric and pharmacologic options for treatment. In turn, this requires an understanding not only of which therapeutic intervention to employ initially but how to use it.

In many situations, cardioversion or defibrillation is the initial intervention of choice, with drug therapy as follow-up in an attempt to prevent recurrence of the arrhythmia. In other more hemodynamically stable situations, drug therapy is used initially.

REFERENCES

1. International Consensus on Science. Guidelines 2000 for cardiopulmonary resuscitation and emergency cardiovascular care. *Circulation* 2000;102(Suppl):I-1–I-384.
2. Ganz LI, Friedman PL. Supraventricular tachycardia. *N Engl J Med* 1995;332:162–173.
3. Rankin AC, Brooks R, Ruskin JN, et al. Adenosine and the treatment of supraventricular tachycardia. *Am J Med* 1992;92:655–664.
4. Biaggioni I, Killian TJ, Mosqueda-Garcia R, et al. Adenosine increases sympathetic nerve traffic in humans. *Circulation* 1991;83:1668–1675.
5. Brodsky MA, Hwang C, Hunter D, et al. Life-threatening alterations in heart rate after the use of adenosine in atrial flutter. *Am Heart J* 1995;130:564–571.
6. Prystowsky EN, Benson DW, Fuster V, et al. Management of patients with atrial fibrillation. *Circulation* 1996;93:1262–1277.
7. Mittal S, Ayati S, Stein KM, et al. Transthoracic cardioversion of atrial fibrillation: comparison of rectilinear biphasic versus damped sine wave monophasic shocks. *Circulation* 2000;101:1282–1287.
8. Grant AO. Mechanisms of atrial fibrillation and action of drugs used in its management. *Am J Cardiol* 1998;82:43N–49N.
9. Kowey PR, Marinchak RA, Rials SJ, et al. Intravenous amiodarone. *J Am Coll Cardiol* 1997;29:1190–1198.
10. Desai AD, Chun S, Sung RJ. The role of intravenous amiodarone in the management of cardiac arrhythmias. *Ann Intern Med* 1997;127:294–303.
11. Connolly SJ. Evidence-based analysis of amiodarone efficacy and safety. *Circulation* 1999;100:2025–2034.
12. Silverman DI, Manning WJ. Role of echocardiography in patients undergoing elective cardioversion of atrial fibrillation. *Circulation* 1998;98:479–486.
13. Joseph AP, Ward MR. A prospective, randomized controlled trial comparing the efficacy and safety of sotalol, amiodarone, and digoxin for the reversion of new-onset atrial fibrillation. *Ann Emerg Med* 2000;36:1–9.
14. Murray KT. Ibutilide. *Circulation* 1998;97:493–497.
15. Stambler BS, Wood MA, Ellenbogen KA. Antiarrhythmic actions of intravenous ibutilide compared with procainamide during human atrial flutter and fibrillation: electrophysiological determinants of enhanced conversion efficacy. *Circulation* 1997;96:4298–4306.
16. Volgman AS, Carberry PA, Stambler B, et al. Conversion efficacy and safety of intravenous ibutilide compared with intravenous procainamide in patients with atrial flutter or fibrillation. *J Am Coll Cardiol* 1998;31:1414–1419.
17. Oral H, Souza JJ, Michaud GF, et al. Facilitating transthoracic cardioversion of atrial fibrillation with ibutilide pretreatment. *N Engl J Med* 1999;340:1849–1854.
18. McCord J, Borzak S. Multifocal atrial tachycardia. *Chest* 1998;113:203–209.
19. Schwartz M, Rodman D, Lowenstein SR. Recognition and treatment of multifocal atrial tachycardia: a critical review. *J Emerg Med* 1994;12:353–360.
20. Aliot E, de Chillou C, Revault d'Allones G, et al. Mahaim tachycardias. *Eur Heart J* 1998;19:E25–E31.
21. Bartlett TG, Friedman PL. Current management of the Wolff-Parkinson-White syndrome. *J Cardiovasc Surg (Torino)* 1993;8:503–515.
22. Baerman JM, Morady F, DiCarlo LA, et al. Differentiation of ventricular tachycardia from supraventricular tachycardia with aberration: value of the clinical history. *Ann Emerg Med* 1987;16:40–43.
23. Mittal S, Ayati S, Stein KM, et al. Comparison of a novel rectilinear biphasic waveform with a damped sine wave monophasic waveform for transthoracic ventricular defibrillation. *J Am Coll Cardiol* 1999;34:1595–1601.
24. Jackman WM, Friday KJ, Anderson JL, et al. The long QT syndromes: a critical review, new clinical observations and a unifying hypothesis. *Prog Cardiovasc Dis* 1988;31:115–172.
25. Greene TO, Spodick DH. Recognition and management of torsade de pointes. *Heart Disease and Stroke* 1992;1:383–390.
26. Horowitz LN. Polymorphic ventricular tachycardia, including torsade de pointes. In: Kastor JA, ed. *Arrhythmias.* Philadelphia: WB Saunders, 1994:376–394.
27. Cranefield PF, Aronson RS. Torsade de pointes and other pause-induced ventricular tachycardias: the short-long-short sequence and early after depolarizations. *PACE* 1988;11:670–677.
28. Leenhardt A, Coumel P, Slama R. Torsade de pointes. *J Cardiovasc Electrophysiol* 992;3:281–292.
29. Armengol RE, Graff J, Baerman JM, et al. Lack of effectiveness of lidocaine for sustained, wide QRS complex tachycardia. *Ann Emerg Med* 1989;18:254–257.
30. Nasir N Jr, Taylor A, Doyle TK, et al. Evaluation of intravenous lidocaine for the termination of sustained monophasic ventricular tachycardia in patients with coronary artery disease with or without healed myocardial infarction. *Am J Cardiol* 1994;74:1183–1186.
31. Gorgels AP, van den Dool A, Hofs A, et al. Comparison of procainamide and lidocaine in terminating sustained monomorphic ventricular tachycardia. *Am J Cardiol* 1996;78:43–46.
32. Kudenchuk PJ, Cobb LA, Copass MK. Amiodarone for resuscitation after out-of-hospital cardiac arrest due to ventricular fibrillation. *N Engl J Med* 1999;341:871–878.
33. Lindner KH, Prengel AW, Pfenninger EG, et al. Vasopressin improves vital organ blood flow during closed-chest cardiopulmonary resuscitation in pigs. *Circulation* 1995;91:215–221.
34. Prengel AW, Lindner KH, Keller A. Cerebral oxygenation during cardiopulmonary resuscitation with epinephrine and vasopressin in pigs. *Stroke* 1996;27:1241–1248.
35. Wenzel V, Lindner KH, Krismer AC, et al. Survival with full neurologic recovery and no cerebral pathology after prolonged cardiopulmonary resuscitation with vasopressin in pigs. *J Am Coll Cardiol* 2000;35:527–533.
36. Lindner KH, Dirks B, Strohmenger HU, et al. Randomized comparison of epinephrine and vasopressin in patients. *Lancet* 1997;349:535–537.

CARE OF THE HYPERTENSIVE PATIENT IN THE INTENSIVE CARE UNIT

BARRY A. HARRISON
MICHAEL J. MURRAY

KEY WORDS

- Joint National Committee (JNC) VI hypertension report
- Hypertensive emergency
- Hypertensive urgency
- Malignant hypertension
- Hypertensive encephalopathy
- Left ventricular failure
- Aortic dissection
- Perioperative hypertension
- Antihypertensive therapy

INTRODUCTION

Systemic arterial hypertension is a physical sign of diseases affecting the structure and function of the blood vessel. The blood-vessel wall, with its endothelium, smooth-muscle cells, and fibroblasts, constitutes one of the largest organ systems in the body. Approaching the blood vessel as an organ with its own biology aids the understanding of hypertension as it presents in the perioperative period and in the intensive care unit (ICU).

CLASSIFICATION OF HYPERTENSION

Community

Hypertension, defined as blood pressure (BP) greater than 140/90 mm Hg, affects more than 50 million Americans. Of this population, 25% are unaware and 72% have a BP of 140/90 mm Hg or higher. Additionally, most patients with hypertension have other cardiovascular risk factors, with 60% of the morbidity and mortality attributable to hypertension occurring in stage 1 of the disease. Because of these confounding factors, it is difficult to determine the relationship of perioperative hypertension to outcome.

In 1997, the Joint National Committee on Detection, Evaluation, and Treatment of High Blood Pressure published their latest recommendations on the diagnosis and treatment of hypertension (1). In this publication, hypertension is described as a continuum of elevated BP readings and is classified in stages (Table 1). The committee established new goals in the manage-ment of hypertension and recommended that isolated systolic hypertension be treated. The prescribed therapy should take into account the stage, the associated risk factors, and the presence of target organ damage.

For essential hypertension, the genetic abnormalities remain largely unknown; however, the associated factors based on population studies include obesity, insulin resistance, high salt intake, a sedentary lifestyle, stress, dyslipidemia, and low potassium or calcium intake (2). The cardiovascular, neurologic, and renal systems are the target organ systems that are most commonly involved.

Hospital

Reflecting the prevalence of hypertension in the community, up to 45% of hospitalized patients have preexisting hypertension, many of whom are admitted to the ICU with severe hypertension. The severity is based on both the absolute level and the associated end-organ damage. In this population, identifiable or secondary causes (Table 2) are found more commonly than in nonhospitalized patients with hypertension. Whether or not it has been previously diagnosed, hypertension is also an important problem in the perioperative period.

PATHOPHYSIOLOGY OF HYPERTENSION

Hemodynamics of Blood Pressure

Blood pressure is the product of cardiac output (CO) and systemic vascular resistance (SVR).

$$BP = CO \times SVR$$

Thus, an increase in either BP or CO without a compensatory decrease in the other will result in hypertension.

Cardiac Output

Although CO is dependent on preload, blood volume alone does not usually determine BP. Many older patients have arteriosclerosis with nondistensible blood vessels; any increase in CO, therefore, can lead to elevated systolic BP. In the perioperative period, increased filling volumes may cause or exacerbate hypertension.

TABLE 1. CLASSIFICATION OF BLOOD PRESSURE FOR ADULTS AGE 18 AND OLDER

Category	Systolic (mm Hg)		Diastolic (mm Hg)
Optimal[a]	<120	and	<80
Normal	<130	and	<85
High-normal	130–139	or	85–89
Hypertension			
Stage I	140–159	or	90–99
Stage II	160–179	or	100–109
Stage III	≥180	or	≥110

[a]Optimal blood pressure with respect to cardiovascular risk is below 120/80 mm Hg. However, unusually low readings should be evaluated for clinical significance.

Patients with fever, hyperthyroidism, and other conditions also can have elevated BP secondary to increases in CO.

Systemic factors that affect filling pressures and CO include sodium intake, aldosterone, glucocorticoids, atrial natriuretic factors, and thyroid hormone. Renal-related factors include pressure natriuresis, the renin angiotensin system, prostacyclin, and nitric oxide.

Systemic Vascular Resistance

The major hemodynamic abnormality in most hypertensive patients is increased SVR. Neurogenic factors, hormones, growth factors, and endothelial substances are the major regulators of SVR that determine vascular tone.

HYPERTENSION IN THE INTENSIVE CARE UNIT

Hypertensive Emergencies and Urgencies

Hypertensive emergencies and hypertensive urgencies require immediate diagnosis and management (Table 3). A *hypertensive emergency* is an increase in systemic arterial pressure that, if sustained over several hours, leads to irreversible end-organ damage. End-organ dysfunction is present at the time of diagnosis. A *hypertensive urgency* is an increase in systemic arterial pressure that, if sustained over several days, has the potential for irreversible end-organ damage (3). Management of these entities depends on the BP, extent of end-organ damage, and associated risk factors.

TABLE 3. BLOOD PRESSURE, TARGET ORGAN DAMAGE, TREATMENT FOR HYPERTENSIVE EMERGENCIES AND URGENCIES

	Diastolic Blood Pressure (mm Hg)	Target Organ Damage	Treatment Onset
Hypertensive emergencies	120–140	Yes	Intravenous (min)
Hypertensive urgencies	110–130	No	Oral (h)

The following conditions present with hypertensive emergencies and urgencies to the ICU.

Malignant Hypertension

Malignant hypertension (MHT), as defined by the World Heath Organization, is severe hypertension with bilateral retinal hemorrhages and exudates (4). There is no defined level of diastolic BP; however, the diastolic pressure is usually greater than 120 to 130 mm Hg. Papilledema is an insensitive sign of MHT, and its presence does not influence outcome. There is a higher incidence of MHT in men, African Americans, and in developing countries. The incidence is decreasing in developed countries, and in these countries it is estimated to account for fewer than 1% of all cases of HT.

Pathogenesis/Pathology

The degree of BP elevation and its acuity lead to MHT. Secondary factors include cigarette smoking, oral contraceptives, immunologic changes, intravascular coagulopathy, renal failure, and vasoactive agents. Subintimal cellular proliferation of the interlobular renal arteries is a common pathological finding and leads to vascular occlusion. Arteriolar fibrinoid necrosis also may be present.

Clinical Findings

Symptoms of MHT include headache, visual impairment, and gastrointestinal discomfort. Mild to severe renal impairment is present in approximately 60% of cases. Left ventricular hypertrophy (LVH) occurs commonly; cardiac failure has an incidence of about 30%. Encephalopathy occurs in up to 17% of cases.

TABLE 2. IDENTIFIABLE/SECONDARY CAUSES OF HYPERTENSION

Type of Hypertension	Effect	Cause	Associated Conditions or Predisposing Factors
Systolic with wide pulse pressure	Decreased aortic compliance	Arteriosclerosis	Age
	Increased stroke volume	Valvular heart disease, increased catecholamines	Aortic regurgitation, thyrotoxicosis, fever
Systolic and diastolic	Increased SVR	Unknown	Essential hypertension (>90%)
		Renal	Renovascular stenosis
		Endocrine	Pheochromocytoma, thyrotoxicosis
		Neurogenic	Increased ICP
		Miscellaneous	Coarctation medications (cyclosporine)

SVR, systemic vascular resistance; ICP, intracranial pressure.

Microangiopathic hemolytic anemia can be present. Secondary hyperaldosteronism occurs frequently and is manifested by hypokalemia and increased plasma renin levels. MHT is associated with a higher incidence of secondary hypertension resulting from renal and renovascular diseases.

Management

The goal of therapy is to lower the BP and to stop end-organ damage. MHT is treated as a medical emergency requiring admission to an ICU, intraarterial BP monitoring, and therapy with an intravenous agent such as sodium nitroprusside (SNP). Initially, the dose should be low, approximately 0.3 μg per kilogram per minute and titrated to effect. In uncomplicated MHT, however, oral atenolol 100 mg and nifedipine 40 mg decrease BP by an average of 20% to 30% within a few hours (5).

If the decrease in BP is too great, end-organ ischemia actually can be precipitated. The autoregulation set point, which maintains a constant blood flow independent of pressure, is set at a higher level in these patients, that is, a greater pressure is required to maintain flow. Therefore, patients may be less able to compensate for a sudden fall in BP. Cerebral infarction, particularly in the watershed areas of the brain, and blindness can result from a too aggressive and abrupt lowering of BP. Even orally administered antihypertensive agents may precipitate ischemic complications (6).

Outcome

In developed societies, 5-year survival has improved from 1% in 1939 to at least 75% in the 1990s. In developing countries, however, a 25% hospital mortality rate has been described.

Hypertensive Encephalopathy

Hypertensive encephalopathy is a serious but rare complication of hypertension. It is defined as an acute organic brain syndrome resulting from disruption of the blood–brain barrier.

Pathology

Hypertensive encephalopathy arises from sudden increase in BP either *de novo* or in patients with chronic HT. If BP exceeds the upper level of cerebral autoregulation, the blood–brain barrier is disrupted, precipitating plasma exudation and focal cerebral edema.

Clinical Features

Symptoms of hypertensive encephalopathy range from the common nonspecific symptoms of headache, nausea, and vomiting to severe and more specific signs of confusion, convulsions, transient hemiparesis, blindness, coma, and eventually, if untreated, irreversible brain damage and death.

Management

Management of hypertensive encephalopathy follows the same principles as in the management of complicated MHT. Intravenous SNP is a recommended first-line agent. Other therapies that have been used with success include β-blockers and calcium-channel blockers (nicardipine); fenoldopam is a novel therapy that may be of benefit (7). With appropriate BP control, hypertensive encephalopathy usually resolves within 12 hours after commencing treatment.

Hypertension and Left Ventricular Failure

Pathophysiology

Although LVH is a common finding even in mild hypertension, LVH is not a prerequisite for heart failure. Even in the absence of LVH, sudden BP increases may acutely overload the left ventricle, precipitating congestive heart failure (CHF). If there is concomitant renal impairment, fluid overload will aggravate the CHF.

In sustained HT, concentric LVH develops. Although the relationship between ejection fraction and wall stress is maintained, left ventricular relaxation is impaired. By itself, diastolic dysfunction can produce symptoms of dyspnea, chest pain, or syncope (8). In concentric LVH and diastolic dysfunction, the left ventricle is susceptible to acute volume and pressure overload. Later in the course of chronic hypertension, left ventricular systolic dysfunction occurs initially on exercise and eventually at rest.

Management

Pulmonary edema is treated in the usual clinical manner, that is, with supplemental oxygen and diuretics. SNP is used to decrease afterload and therefore to decrease preload and the hydrostatic pressure driving fluid into the lung.

Therapy in left ventricular failure with predominant diastolic dysfunction is difficult. It is important to avoid agents that unduly decrease preload and increase the heart rate. Treatment involves the cautious use of arterial vasodilators while maintaining an adequate left ventricular preload. SNP is an acceptable agent. Phentolamine has theoretical advantages because of possible positive inotropism, as does intravenous nicardipine, which has a less negative inotropic effect (9). Other calcium-channel blockers with a more negative inotropic effect are contraindicated for patients in pulmonary edema. β-Blockers are recommended for patients with hypertension and increasingly for patients with diastolic dysfunction (10), although they should be used with caution, if at all, in patients with pulmonary edema.

Hypertension and Myocardial Ischemia

Acute coronary insufficiency, unstable angina, and myocardial infarction are frequently associated with hypertension. In a meta-analysis, intravenous nitroglycerin and nitroprusside have been demonstrated to decrease mortality, independent of the level of BP (11).

Aortic Dissection

Aortic dissection has an incidence of 0.5 to 1 per 100,000 population, two to three times that of ruptured abdominal aortic aneurysm (12). Preexisting hypertension is common, as is coarctation of the aorta and a bicuspid aortic valve.

Pathophysiology

Controversy exists as to whether the initial event is an intimal tear, thus exposing the media to an elevated pulse pressure, which strips the intima from the adventitia, versus a hemorrhage into an abnormal media. The forces propagating the dissection are the BP and the rate of rise (dP/dt) of the pulse wave (13).

Clinical Features

The acute onset of severe ripping, tearing, or stabbing chest pain associated with restlessness is the classic symptom of dissection. Classic signs include decreased or absent peripheral pulses, new-onset aortic regurgitation, and neurologic complications (cerebral ischemia, peripheral neuropathy, and paraparesis). The differential diagnosis should include myocardial infarction. Chest roentgenography usually reveals an abnormal aortic outline in about 90% of patients. Aortography remains the gold standard for diagnosis and allows coronary angiography to be performed. Transesophageal echocardiography, however, has 100% specificity and sensitivity if done correctly. Computerized tomography is helpful, especially if it reveals no intimal flap, but no information can be obtained regarding the aortic valve or left ventricular function using this technique.

Management

Aortic dissection is a medical emergency that requires immediate diagnosis and treatment. Acute proximal dissection treated surgically has an 80% hospital survival, whereas acute distal dissection treated medically has a similar hospital survival. Treating pain, decreasing cardiac contractility (as measured by dP/dt), and controlling BP are the aims of treatment while maintaining tissue perfusion. Systolic BP should be decreased to 100 to 120 mm Hg by using SNP. Because this causes a reflex tachycardia and increased dP/dt, a β-blocking agent must be commenced before starting SNP. The adequacy of β-receptor inhibition is reflected by a heart rate of less than 60 beats per minute. If coexisting diseases increase the risks associated with a β-blocker, then a trial with esmolol, a cardioselective β-blocker with a short half-life, is indicated. Labetalol, with its α- and nonselective β-blocking effects, will decrease dP/dt while causing peripheral vasodilation. Calcium-channel blockers, with their vasodilator and negative inotropic effect, also may prove suitable. Hydralazine and diazoxide both increase dP/dt and thus should be avoided.

In proximal (type A) dissection, corrective surgery is classified as urgent. Although distal (type B) dissection therapy usually is managed medically, up to 50% of patients eventually will require an operation.

Hypertension and the Kidney

In the ICU, renal disease and hypertension are important coexisting diseases. Up to 30% of all end-stage renal disease is due to hypertension. Conversely, chronic renal disease is a common cause of secondary hypertension, and in turn the hypertension will accelerate the renal failure.

Renal Failure

Acute renal failure can result from MHT. Most of the other causes of acute renal failure are not associated with hypertension, and acute renal failure per se does not cause hypertension. End-stage renal disease, however, is associated with hypertension. Sodium and fluid retention are the obvious causes. Hypertension in postrenal transplantation patients may be related to treatment with cyclosporine or possibly posttransplant vascular stenosis.

Angiotensin-converting enzyme (ACE) inhibitors and calcium-channel blockers both have a role in managing the hypertension associated with renal disease; ACE inhibitors also may decrease the proteinuria associated with some forms of renal disease.

Pathophysiology

Glomerulonephritis, adult polycystic kidney disease, and chronic pyelonephritis are associated with an increased incidence of hypertension. Renovascular hypertension always should be considered in young women, in patients with MHT, in patients who have refractory HT, and especially patients who have advanced atherosclerosis or an abdominal bruit. Diagnostic tests are controversial, but renography stress tests with ACE inhibitors and furosemide are stated to have about 90% sensitivity and 96% specificity. Renin lateralization predicts beneficial responses in 90% of patients, but at least 50% of patients who do not lateralize respond to therapy.

Both ACE inhibitors and calcium-channel blockers are also effective agents in renovascular hypertension. With ACE inhibitors, there may be a marked reduction in renal blood flow through the kidney with the stenotic blood supply, and if this is the only kidney or if bilateral renovascular disease is present, reversible renal failure may be precipitated. ACE inhibition may worsen existing renal insufficiency or precipitate renal insufficiency if the patient is sodium- or volume-depleted (14). Calcium-channel blockers, because of their preglomerular vasodilatory effect, may maintain renal blood flow and still provide effective lowering of BP.

Hypertension in Pregnancy

Hypertension occurs in more than 5% of all pregnancies. The National High Blood Pressure Education Program Working Group on High Blood Pressure recommends four diagnostic categories of hypertension in pregnancy: chronic hypertension, preeclampsia–eclampsia, chronic hypertension with superimposed preeclampsia, and transient hypertension (15). Table 4 outlines antihypertensive drugs that are indicated in pregnancy. Use of ACE inhibitors has been demonstrated to cause renal failure in the newborn and should not be used in pregnancy or if a woman is attempting to become pregnant.

Hypertension and Neurologic Syndromes

Head injury and increased intracranial pressure often are associated with increased systemic arterial pressure. In acute stroke syndromes, the BP is often transiently elevated, but it usually returns to prestroke levels over the first 2 to 3 days following

TABLE 4. ANTIHYPERTENSIVE DRUGS IN PREGNANCY

Drug Class	Drug	Comments
α_2 blocker	Methyldopa	Extensive experience, safe
β-blocker	Atenolol/ metoprolol Labetalol	Safe and efficacious
Vasodilators	Hydralazine	Used parenterally
Calcium-channel blockers	Nifedipine	Promising studies, avoid when using magnesium
Diuretics	Thiazides	Gestational salt sensitive, not for preeclampsia when intravascular volume contracted

the event. If the hypertension is treated acutely, there is a possibility of decreasing perfusion pressure in the penumbra, an area of hypoperfusion surrounding the infarcted brain. Conversely, if a cerebral embolus undergoes spontaneous lysis, the former ischemic tissue now may be rendered hyperemic and with the associated HT hemorrhage may occur into the infarcted tissue. Treatment is mainly expectant, with treatment reserved for diastolic pressures greater than 130 mm Hg. If cerebral hemorrhage is the cause of the stroke, the hypertension should be treated only if the diastolic BP is greater than 120 mm Hg.

Hypertension and Excess Catecholamines

Sympathomimetic drugs stimulate vascular–endothelial α-receptors increasing SVR. The dose, route of administration, concurrent drug therapy, disease states, the patient's age and individual idiosyncrasy influence hypertension induced by sympathomimetics.

Monoamine oxidase inhibitors (MAOIs), which include isocarboxazid (Marplan), phenelzine (Nardil), pargyline (Eutonyl), and tranylcypromine (Parnate), form an irreversible stable complex with both forms (A and B) of the enzyme monoamineoxidase, thus inhibiting it. The effect is to increase intraneuronal levels of amine neurotransmitters (serotonin, norepinephrine, dopamine, epinephrine, octopamine).

The MAOIs interact with tyramine (alcohol, broad beans, caviar, cheese, chocolate). The uptake-1 mechanism transports tyramine into sympathetic nerve endings, where it releases stores of norepinephrine, resulting in vasoconstriction and hypertension.

Sympathomimetic drugs interact with MAOIs to produce an exaggerated response to pressor agents. Indirect, compared with direct, sympathomimetic drugs produce a greater reaction.

The MAOIs can interact with opioids such as meperidine to produce an excitatory (agitation, hypertension, headache, convulsions, and hyperpyrexia) or a depressive (respiratory, hypotension, coma) condition.

Newer MAOIs are relatively selective for either MAO A (moclobemide, clorgyline) or MAO B (selegiline) enzymes. Moclobemide is a reversible, short half-life inhibitor of MAO A. Its pressor response to tyramine and intravenous phenylephrine is decreased compared with the irreversible MAOIs.

Cocaine use can result in hypertension. Cocaine sensitizes cellular receptors to epinephrine and blocks the re-uptake of released epinephrine at peripheral nerve terminals. Toxicity results from excessive adrenergic stimulation both centrally (agitation, seizure) and peripherally (vasoconstriction). Moderate hypertension responds to sedation and nifedipine; however, severe HT will require parenteral therapy, usually phentolamine or SNP.

Autonomic hyperreflexia is a syndrome manifested by hypertension, bradycardia, and facial flushing that occurs in paraplegic and quadriplegic patients as a result of uncontrolled sympathetic discharge, usually in response to somatosensory or visceral stimulation. The hypertension may be severe, leading to neurologic effects. Autonomic hyperreflexia does not develop if the spinal cord deficit is below the seventh thoracic dermatome level.

PERIOPERATIVE HYPERTENSION

History and Definitions

Because of the prevalence of hypertension, about 25% of patients having a surgical procedure will carry a diagnosis of hypertension. Anesthetic drugs (ketamine) and techniques (endotracheal intubation) lead to acute increases in BP. Certain surgical procedures are associated with acute increases in BP-aortic cross-clamping, head and neck surgery, carotid endarterectomy, electroconvulsive therapy, and so on. It is not surprising, then, that hypertension in the perioperative period is a common problem that presents many clinical dilemmas.

In the 1970s, postoperative hypertension following coronary artery bypass grafting was described as an elevated BP without an obvious cause. A BP greater than 160/90 mmHg is a commonly accepted definition of perioperative HT, though some define it as a diastolic BP greater than 100 or 110 mmHg, while yet others describe it as a 20% increase in BP or a 30 mmHg increase in BP over preoperative values. The duration of the increase in BP also factors into whether or not a patient has perioperative hypertension; BP must be elevated for 10 or 15 minutes to meet the criteria for the diagnosis. Without an exact definition of this common problem, good clinical and outcome studies have been difficult to perform.

Several studies now describe an association of perioperative hypertension with myocardial ischemia, myocardial infarction, and mortality. Others have described perioperative hypertension as a relative risk factor for ICU admissions and for postoperative mortality. Similarly, postoperative hypertension has been shown to increase the incidence of strokes in carotid endarterectomy patients. Thus, there is an increased relative risk associated with perioperative hypertension; however, no randomized prospective trial has shown a correlation with treatment of HT with improved outcome.

In perioperative hypertension, the clinical approach should be as described by the JNC VI. The patient should be staged (I, II, III) based on the level of BP. Choice of therapy also should be based on comorbid risk factors and target organ damage. The aim of treatment is to reduce the incidence of cardiovascular and neurological events. Figure 1 outlines a JNC VI-based approach to perioperative hypertension.

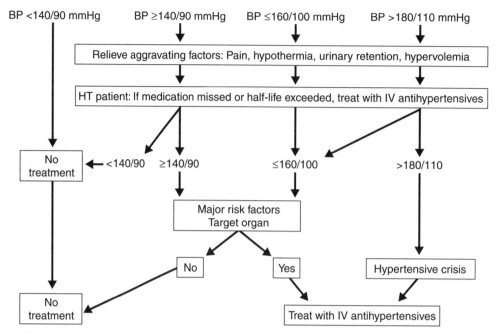

FIGURE 1. Treatment algorithm of perioperative hypertension. Risk factors include smoking, dyslipidemia, and diabetes. Target-organ damage: left ventricular hypertrophy, coronary artery disease, heart failure, stroke, nephropathy.

Preoperative

Preoperative Assessment of the Hypertensive Patient

A history and physical examination focused on the current medication(s), level of BP, identifiable causes of hypertension, the presence of target organ damage, and patient risk factors need to be performed on every hypertensive patient. BP must be measured with the patient supine or sitting; measurement is done using an appropriately sized BP cuff and correct technique. A review of the patient's BP readings will help determine the "baseline" BP, particularly important in the perioperative period. The lungs must be listened to for evidence of rales and bronchospasm, and the chest should be examined and heart auscultated for evidence of heart impulse displacement, heaves, and gallops. The abdomen is examined for pulsatile masses, enlarged kidneys, and bruits. The vascular examination should elicit signs of carotid bruits or discrepancies in pulses between the arms and legs. Neurologic examination ideally should include funduscopy. Failure to do a focused history and physical examination followed by an appropriate assessment increases the risk of inappropriate treatment and investigations.

The hypertensive stage, patient risk factors, and the presence of target organ damage should determine therapy. A BP of 180/110 mm Hg or greater is associated with a greater risk for perioperative ischemia (1). When possible, surgery should be delayed to bring BP down to a lower level (16).

Major risk factors include smoking, dyslipidemia, diabetes mellitus, age over 60 years, men and postmenopausal women, and a family history of coronary artery disease (CAD). Symptoms and signs of target organ damage affecting the cardiovascular system include left ventricular hypertrophy, CAD, and CHF. Vascular diseases include peripheral artery disease and hypertensive retinopathy. Neurologic diseases include stroke and transient ischemic attacks.

In the initial assessment of the hypertensive patient, only simple investigations are indicated. These include a complete blood count, sodium, potassium, creatinine, blood urea nitrogen, total and HDL cholesterol, fasting blood glucose, and a 12-lead electrocardiogram. Other tests are not cost effective in the initial workup of a patient with hypertensive.

Preoperative Antihypertensive Medication

Patients' comorbidities directly influence the initiation and goals of treatment and which antihypertensive drugs are indicated or contraindicated. In patients with CAD, a β-blocker or calcium-channel blocker is preferred, whereas in patients with severe CHF or with bradyarrhythmias, β-blockers and calcium-channel blockers may be contraindicated. In the latter circumstances, other vasoactive drugs and diuretics should be considered. In hypertrophic cardiomyopathy, diuretics and vasodilators are not recommended. β-Blockers should be used with caution in patients with reactive airways disease and in patients with chronic obstructive lung disease. In diabetic patients and in patients with renal disease, ACE inhibitors would be preferred. Chronic renal failure patients may benefit from loop diuretics and calcium-channel blockers.

Antihypertensive medication may influence the course of surgery and anesthesia. Clonidine attenuates the hypertensive and heart rate response seen in cardiovascular surgery. Clonidine also increases patients' sensitivity to phenylephrine; thus, smaller doses of phenylephrine are used with patients on clonidine who require a vasoconstrictor intraoperatively. Patients should be told to take their antihypertensive medications with a small sip of water the morning of surgery.

Cessation of clonidine can result in increases in BP above pretreatment levels. Other drugs resulting in a similar problem include α-methyldopa, guanethidine sulphate, and reserpine. Abrupt clonidine withdrawal may result in a syndrome similar to that seen with a pheochromocytoma.

The withdrawal of β-blocking drugs with no intrinsic sympathomimetic activity (ISA) in patients without ischemic heart disease is associated with hyperadrenergic symptoms [17]. There are no cases of rebound hypertension or hypertensive crisis associated with β-blocker withdrawal [18]. Withdrawal of β-blockers from patients with ischemic heart disease, however, leads to an increase in myocardial ischemic events and, in some cases, death [19].

Withdrawal phenomena are due to upregulation of receptors that occurs during exposure to the drugs. On withdrawal, increased sensitivity of the receptors to the normal agonists occurs.

Angiotensin-converting enzyme inhibitors play a prominent role in antihypertensive therapy, predominantly as second line agents, although in patients with HT and diabetes, they are first-line drugs. Patients on ACE inhibitors chronically display hypotension as a result of a decrease in cardiac output that occurs in up to 80% of patients. These hypotensive episodes are easily treated with intravenous fluid and vasopressors. Although significant problems can result, the advantages of continuing the ACE inhibitors outweigh the potential hypotensive effect. The same arguments apply to angiotensin-2 antagonists; patients taking these agents should be made euvolemic prior to the induction of anesthesia.

Medications Causing Hypertension

The parenteral use of nonsteroidal antiinflammatory drugs (NSAIDs) as analgesic supplements has become popular in both medical and surgical ICUs. Although it is still unclear whether NSAIDs induce hypertension, it is known that NSAIDs interact with many antihypertensives to reduce their effectiveness.

Cyclosporine is an important immunosuppressive agent used in transplantation and in some autoimmune disorders. The incidence of cyclosporine-induced hypertension varies from 50% in renal transplant patients to nearly 100% in heart transplant patients.

Erythropoietin induces hypertension. Erythropoietin-induced hypertension is associated with an elevation in SVR and a decrease in cardiac output. The hypertension is not related to the dose or rate of an increase in hematocrit.

Intraoperative Hypertension

Stress Response and Pathophysiology

The stress of surgery causes a hormonal and metabolic change that consists of increases in adrenocorticotropic hormone (ACTH), growth hormone, arginine vasopressin, cortisol, and aldosterone.

There is also hypothalamic activation of the sympathetic autonomic nervous system that results in increases in secretion of catecholamines from the adrenal medulla and norepinephrine from sympathetic nerve terminals. Renin is increased as a result of increased sympathetic efferent activity. The net result of these changes is to increase systolic BP and intravascular blood volume. With adequate or excessive fluid replacement, hypertension may result. These changes cause perioperative hypertension from an increased CO and SVR.

Measurement

Blood pressure is measured intraoperatively using oscillometry; measurement with an appropriately sized cuff is important. For the manual technique, an adequate-sized cuff is used, and for automatic measurement cuff size, arrhythmias and temperature all can influence the measurement. For invasive measurement of BP with an indwelling arterial catheter, the system should be neither overdamped nor underdamped because both will influence the measurement.

Induction

Induction and intubation of the trachea frequently are associated with an abrupt but short-lived increase in BP. Patients who cannot tolerate such an increase (i.e., patients with increased intracranial pressure, subarachnoid hemorrhage, aortic dissection, myocardial ischemia) should be adequately pretreated with an opioid (e.g., fentanyl, sufentanil) or a β-blocker (esmolol) before the trachea is intubated.

Maintenance

Certain surgical procedures are associated with a high incidence of intraoperative hypertension. Vascular surgical procedures in which a cross-clamp is placed on the aorta or other large blood vessels are associated with abrupt increases in BP secondary to the acute increase in left ventricular afterload. Carotid endarterectomy and head and neck procedures, because of stimulation of the carotid body, also are associated with hypertension. Patients undergoing nonsurgical procedures or cardiopulmonary bypass also have a high incidence of hypertension. Most anesthetized patients, however, who undergo other surgical procedures have an incidence of intraoperative hypertension that is less than 1% [20]. Whenever a patient develops an increase in BP intraoperatively, one must search for precipitating factors (i.e., hypoxia, hypercarbia, light anesthesia). If identified, they should be corrected before pharmacologic therapy is administered to treat the increased BP.

PARENTERAL PHARMACOLOGIC ANTIHYPERTENSIVE THERAPY

Diuretics

The loop diuretics, furosemide and bumetanide, can be given parenterally, and although they are not used routinely, they may be of benefit to patients with hypertensive emergencies. They are of use in select patients, especially those who have an expanded extracellular fluid volume, in patients with moderate to severe renal impairment, and in patients with resistant hypertension.

Peripheral Vasodilators

Hydralazine

Incubation of hydralazine with red cells generates nitric oxide (NO), activating guanyl cyclase and, therefore, increasing cytoplasmic levels of cyclic guanosine monophosphate (GMP). Hydralazine is dependent for action on an intact endothelium and is predominantly an arteriolar vasodilator. Hydralazine increases CO and heart rate with little or no decrease in pulmonary artery or right atrial pressure. It is given as an intravenous bolus of 5 to 20 mg; the onset of action is within 20 minutes. After 20 minutes, another bolus may be given if necessary. Although a lupus reaction may result with the use of oral hydralazine in patients who are "slow acetylators," this is not relevant with the short-term parenteral use of hydralazine titrated to effect.

Sodium Nitroprusside

Sodium nitroprusside is metabolized to NO and cyanide. The latter reacts with thiosulfates to form thiocyanate. Both SNP and thiocyanate are excreted through the kidney. The clearance of SNP is rapid resulting in a BP lowering half-life of less than a minute. Fifty milligrams is dissolved in 250 mL of 5% dextrose and water, with an initial intravenous infusion rate of 0.5 μg per kilogram per minute and is titrated to effect, up to a maximal dose of 10.0 μg per kilogram per minute. Because SNP is light sensitive, the infusion solution and tubing need to be protected from the light by aluminum foil. An important side effect is the development of cyanide or thiocyanate toxicity (21). Thiocyanate levels greater than 20 μg per milliliter are associated with symptoms of confusion, hyperreflexia, and convulsions. Excessive doses, prolonged infusions, and liver failure are associated with cyanide toxicity. The earliest signs of cyanide toxicity are metabolic acidosis and an increased mixed venous oxygen saturation. Monitoring the acid–base status and thiocyanate levels should be considered in patients with renal or hepatic failure or if SNP is infused for longer than 3 days or at high doses (10 μg/kg per minute for more than 8 hours). If cyanide toxicity develops, the SNP should be discontinued, and thiosulfate or nitrates should be administered to increase the conversion of cyanide to thiocyanate.

Nitroglycerin

Nitroglycerin is an exogenous NO donor that predominantly venodilates, although at higher doses, it also will dilate arterioles. In the ICU, it is not used for its antihypertensive effect, but rather it is used for myocardial ischemia or congestive cardiac failure. It is administered parenterally as a continuous infusion, at a concentration of 200 μg per milliliter. Its onset is within 1 to 2 minutes; the starting dose is 0.5 μg per kilogram per minute, titrating the dose to the desired effect.

Diazoxide

Diazoxide opens adenosine triphosphate (ATP)-sensitive potassium channels in vascular smooth muscle, dilating arterial but not venous resistance beds (22). Nearly 90% of diazoxide is protein bound, and most is excreted unchanged in the urine. Controlled intravenous infusions of 5 mg per kilogram of body weight at a rate of 15 mg per minute is safer than bolus administration. Because it is associated with fluid retention, diuretics often are given concomitantly. It is not often used for BP control because it can precipitate severe hypotension and is associated with glucose intolerance.

Side Effects of the Direct Vasodilators

Direct vasodilators are associated with severe hypotension if not carefully titrated to effect. They also induce a sympathetically mediated increase in heart rate secondary to their hypotensive effect.

Adrenergic Agents

β-Blockers

Cardioselectivity
Cardioselective or β_1 selective implies that the cardiac β_1 receptors would be inhibited (up to 65% of the β-receptors in the heart are β_1); however, the β_2 receptors in the bronchi and vasculature would remain unblocked. Because this effect is dose related, the effect is less at higher doses, and so even the most cardioselective drugs block β_2 receptors at high dose.

α_1-Blocking
Some β-blockers may block α_1-receptors resulting in vasodilation.

Intrinsic Sympathetic Activity (ISA)
Certain β-blockers (pindolol, practolol, and oxprenolol) manifest partial agonist activity, which results in preservation of resting heart rate and better preservation of ventricular function.

Membrane Stabilizing Effect
This effect refers to the local anesthetic effect of β-blockers on the cardiac action potential. It is of significance at high doses and its effect is unrelated to the β-adrenoreceptor.

Mechanism of Action

The predominant mechanism of action of β-blockers is to lower CO by decreasing heart rate. Other possible mechanisms include a central nervous system effect, inhibition of peripheral sympathetic nerve activity, stimulation of release of vasodilator prostaglandins, and an increase in atrial natriuretic factor.

Parenteral β-Blockers (Table 5)

Propranolol is the prototypical β-blocker. It has a relative potency of 1, is nonselective, has no ISA or α_1 blocking activity, but it does possess membrane-stabilizing activity. The β_1 effect decreases heart rate, conduction, and contractility (decreased chronotropy, ionotropy, and dromotropy, respectively), whereas the β_2 effect

TABLE 5. PARENTERAL β-BLOCKERS

	β_1 Potency Ratio	β_1 Selectivity	Intrinsic Sympathomimetic Activity	α_1-Blocking Activity	Dose	Onset (min)	Duration of Action
Propranolol	1.0	No	No	No	Bolus: 1–2 mg (0.1 mg/kg)	1–2 min	4 h
Atenolol	1.0	Yes	No	No	Bolus: 2–5 mg q 5–10 min Max: 5–10 mg	1–2 min	5–8 h
Metoprolol	1.0	Yes	No	No	Bolus: 2–5 mg q 5–10 min Max: 15 mg	1–2 min	<6 h
Esmolol	0.02	Yes	No	No	Loading: 0.5 mg/kg Continuous: 50–400 μg/kg/min	1–2 min	10–20 min
Labetalol	0.3	No	?Yes	Yes	Bolus: 20 mg q 10 min Max: 300 mg Continuous: 2 mg/min	5–10 min	3–6 h

β, beta-adrenoreceptor; q, every.

induces bronchoconstriction. The intravenous dose is 0.1 mg per kilogram of body weight and usually is titrated in 1.0-mg increments, with a maximum dose of 10.0 mg.

Atenolol and metoprolol have a relative potency of 1 and are cardioselective, atenolol being more so than metoprolol. They possess no ISA, membrane-stabilizing, or alpha$_1$ blocking activity. They are administered intravenously via bolus, atenolol at 5- to 10-mg increments and metoprolol at 5- to 15-mg increments.

Esmolol has a relative potency of 0.02, is cardioselective but has no ISA, membrane-stabilizing, or α_1 blocking activity. Esmolol is ultra–short acting with a half-life of 9 minutes. The recommended dose is a loading dose of 0.5 mg per kilogram followed by a maintenance infusion between 50 and 400 μg per kilogram per minute (23). It also can be given as an intravenous bolus dose of 20 to 50 mg to achieve an acute decrease in BP. The recovery time for the heart rate response is 30 minutes.

Labetalol has a relative potency of 0.3 and has an α_1-blocking effect that causes vasodilation. It is nonselective but may have ISA activity. In parenteral doses, it has a ratio of 7:1 with respect to its β:α_1 activity. It decreases BP via a decrease in SVR with little effect on CO. Parenteral doses are titrated to effect or until the development of complications. A suggested regimen is to administer doses of 0.25 mg per kilogram of body weight up to a total of 2.5 mg per kilogram (24). Continuous infusions of 0.2 mg per kilogram per hour have been described (25). Although labetalol is considered safe, there are case reports of serious hepatotoxicity associated with its oral use.

Selecting a β-Blocker

All β-blockers decrease BP, provided the dose is adequate. Therefore, the choice of agent is dependent on patients' comorbidities. β-Blockers with high ISA activity are suited for patients with left ventricular failure, high degree heart block, severe bradycardia, and variant (Prinzmetal) angina, whereas agents with little or no ISA activity are suited for patients with angina. Cardioselective β-blockers are indicated in chronic obstructive pulmonary disease and insulin-requiring diabetics. Vasodilating β-blockers are suggested for patients with left ventricular failure.

Relevant Adverse Reactions

Cardiovascular

As β-blockers impair the circulatory and metabolic response to exercise, the body's usual hemodynamic response to hypovolemia and sepsis with an intact cardiac reserve may not be seen. Patients with poor left ventricular function may develop CHF.

Sinus bradycardia is a common problem with β-blockers, but it is not a contraindication to their use. β-Blockers have not been found to exacerbate intermittent claudication (26).

Respiratory

About 50% of asthmatic patients will develop bronchospasm when given propranolol (27); however, patients with mild asthma may tolerate cardioselective β_1 blockers (28). Cardioselective β-blockers usually are tolerated well in patients with chronic obstructive pulmonary disease (29). As a general rule, β-blockers can be used if the patient is not actively wheezing.

Metabolic

Metabolic abnormalities associated with β-blockers include mild glucose intolerance and increased uric acid and potassium levels. As the symptoms and signs of hypoglycemia are in part manifested by the action of catecholamines on β-adrenoreceptors, β-blockers are relatively contraindicated in insulin dependent diabetics. If β-blockade is required, an agent that is cardioselective with a short half-life should be used.

Beta-blockers and calcium-channel entry blockers (diltiazem, verapamil) may have additive sinoatrial and atrioventricular node depressant effect. They also have an additive depressant effect on the left ventricle.

β-Blockers may increase serum levels of theophylline, lidocaine and chlorpromazine due to decreasing hepatic clearance.

α-Adrenoreceptor Agonists and Antagonists

α_2-Adrenoreceptors are located both prejunctionally and postjunctionally, whereas α_1-adrenoreceptors are postjunctional. Postjunctional α_2-adrenoreceptors are targets for circulating catecholamines and α_1-adrenoreceptors for catecholamines released from the neuronal terminal. Activity of peripheral postjunctional

α_2-adrenoreceptors helps maintain arteriolar tone. Several drugs block the α-receptor with a loss of α-vasoconstricting effect, blood vessels dilate and BP decreases. Phentolamine, a nonselective α-adrenoreceptor, blocks both α_1 and α_2-receptors. Currently, intravenous phentolamine is indicated in the management of pheochromocytoma or clonidine withdrawal. Parenteral phentolamine is administered via bolus dosing of 2 to 5 mg every 15 minutes until the BP is controlled.

Central-acting α_2 agonists also can be used to control BP. The prototypical drug in this context is clonidine. The difficulty with using clonidine is its slow onset and slow offset. Patients using clonidine preoperatively are at high risk for a hypertensive response if the clonidine is withdrawn acutely. Intraoperatively, although not yet approved in the United States for parenteral use, a 50-μg bolus of clonidine (Duraclon) can be given, with subsequent doses based on effect. At this time, intravenous clonidine has not been approved by the Food and Drug Administration (FDA) for routine therapy of hypertension.

Mivazerol, another α_2-agonist, has been given in Europe intravenously for the induction of anesthesia for up to 72 hours. The incidence of hypertension in the mivazerol group was 33% and in the placebo group, 39%, which was not statistically significant. It did not alter the rates of myocardial infarction and cardiac death in patients with CAD (30).

Another α_2-adrenergic agent, dexmedetomidine, is being used for sedation in the postoperative period. Because it is an α_2-agent, it is associated with hypotension during administration, but is not being administered specifically as an antihypertensive agent.

Peripheral Agonists: Dopamine Agonist Fenoldopam

Fenoldopam is a selective dopamine-1 receptor agonist. It has moderate affinity for α_2 receptors, but it does not have any significant α_2, β, or dopamine-2 activity. In normal and hypertensive subjects, fenoldopam decreases BP, SVR, and renal vascular resistance. Administration of fenoldopam results in increased left ventricular ejection fraction and a decrease in BP. It is recommended for management of hypertensive crisis and for patients with hypertension and to increase renal blood flow and urine output, but its cost may limit its use.

Calcium-channel Blockers

Background and Classification

Calcium-channel blockers inhibit second-messenger calcium systems in cardiovascular tissue. The first-generation calcium-channel blockers in order of appearance were verapamil (papaverine derivative), nifedipine (dihydropyridine), and diltiazem (benzothiadiazine). The second-generation blockers consist mainly of dihydropyrimidines. The three main classes of calcium-channel blockers (phenylalkylamine, dihydropyridine, and benzothiadiazine) not only differ in their structure but also their molecular action, their pharmacodynamics, and the sensitivity of the vasculature to their action.

Mechanism of Action

Calcium-channel blockers bind to a specific receptor of the L-type calcium channel, resulting in inhibition of the calcium channel. By preventing calcium-dependent contractions of vascular smooth muscle, they decrease SVR.

Calcium-channel Blockers

Verapamil is the prototypical calcium channel blocker (Table 6). Verapamil is used parenterally for the treatment of supraventricular arrhythmias. It is an arteriolar dilator and a direct negative inotrope.

Nifedipine, the prototypical 1,4 dihydropyridine calcium-channel blocker, is a powerful arteriolar vasodilator, thereby

TABLE 6. PARENTERAL/ORAL CALCIUM ENTRY BLOCKERS

Drug	Classification	Heart Rate	Myocardial Contractility	Nodal Conduction	Peripheral Vasodilatation	Dose	Onset	Duration of Action
Verapamil	Phenylalkylamine	Decreased	Decreased	Decreased	Increased	Bolus: 5–10 mg over 1 min repeated 10 min	Peaks 5 min (hypotensive effect only)	10–12 min (hypotensive effect only)
Nifedipine	Dihydropyridine	Increased/ unchanged	Decreased/ unchanged	Unchanged	Increased ++	Bolus: SL, "bite and swallow" 10–20 mg q 5–15 min	5–10 min	3–6 h
Diltiazem	Benzothiazepine	Decreased	Decreased	Decreased	Increased	Loading: 0.25 mg/kg over 2 min Continuous: 5–15 mg/h	2–5 min	1–3 h
Nicardipine	Dihydropyridine	Increased/ unchanged	Decreased/ unchanged	Unchanged	Increased	Initial: 5 mg/hr Increments: 1–2.5 mg/h q 15 min Max: 15 mg/h	10 min	30–60 min

q, every; SL, sublingual.

offsetting its direct negative inotropic effect. It has minimal effect on the atrioventricular node. The hemodynamic onset of nifedipine in the capsule form using the sublingual or "bite and chew" technique occurs within 5 minutes. It is almost fully absorbed after an oral dose, with peak blood levels occurring within 20 to 45 minutes, with a half-life of 3 hours. Nifedipine can be administered via the sublingual route, but absorption is variable.

Because of its oral pharmacokinetic properties, it is used by the sublingual route for hypertensive emergencies. Severe morbidity has been described with the oral and sublingual use of nifedipine, however, usually as a result of unexpected severe decreases in BP precipitating myocardial ischemia. The risk of unpredictable and uncontrolled responses of oral and sublingual nifedipine versus the ease of administration and efficacy needs to be assessed on an individual to individual basis.

Diltiazem is similar to verapamil, except it appears to have more activity on the sinus node and less on the atrioventricular node compared with verapamil. The parenteral form is used mainly for control of supraventricular arrhythmias.

Nicardipine is a second-generation calcium-channel blocker, with a structure similar to nifedipine. The proposed advantage over nifedipine is that nicardipine is vascular specific, having greater effect on arterial smooth muscle with a less negative inotropic effect (31). Importantly, nicardipine is water soluble without being light sensitive, which allows intravenous preparation and administration. The usual preparation is 25 mg in 250 mL of 5% dextrose or 0.9% NaCl (it is incompatible in sodium bicarbonate or lactated Ringer's solution).

Selecting a Calcium-channel Blocker

The choice of calcium-channel blocker depends on the indication for its use and the patient's comorbidities. For hypertension, nifedipine and nicardipine are agents of choice. In hypertensive patients with angina and unimpaired left ventricular function, verapamil or diltiazem may be indicated. If left ventricular function is impaired, then an assessment of the risk:benefit ratio should be made comparing the relatively less negative inotropic and more chronotropic effects of the 1,4 dihydropyridine agents with the more negative inotropic effect of verapamil (or diltiazem) but with less chronotropic properties.

If aortic stenosis or hypertrophic obstructive cardiomyopathy is present, then use of a 1,4 dihydropyridine is contraindicated. If sick-sinus syndrome or atrioventricular block is present, verapamil and diltiazem is contraindicated. With severe impairment of left ventricular function, all types of calcium-channel blockers are relatively contraindicated.

Relevant Adverse Reactions: Calcium-channel Blockers

The administration of parenteral verapamil and diltiazem can lead to atrioventricular block, asystole, and death. Factors potentiating these problems include rapid administration of large doses without adequate monitoring, preexisting sick sinus or atrioventricular block and concurrent β-blockade.

Excessive vasodilation usually occurs with the 1,4 dihydropyridine agents and usually consists of minor side effects, for example,

flushing, dizziness, headaches, and palpitations. Dependent edema resulting from local vasodilation is also a side effect. Major morbidity can occur with acute profound decreases in BP.

Angiotensin-converting Enzyme Inhibitors

Enalaprilat is the only parenterally available ACE inhibitor. Enalaprilat decreases BP as an indirect vasodilator. In contrast to other vasodilators, ACE inhibitors do not induce reflex sympathetic activation. Other antihypertensive effects of ACE inhibitors include decreased aldosterone secretion (inducing a natriuresis), specific renal vasodilation (also inducing a natriuresis), and decreasing inactivation of vasodilatory bradykinins. At the myocardial and vascular tissue level, they inhibit local formation of angiotensin II. Enalapril undergoes various degrees of metabolism before renal elimination. Other effects of ACE inhibitors include improvement in left ventricular end-diastolic function, maintenance of cerebral blood flow, and a renal protective effect resulting from preferential vasodilation. The suggested parenteral dose is initially 0.625 to 1.25 mg administered over a 5-minute period, although doses of up to 5 mg can be given. Although onset of action is approximately 15 minutes, its antihypertensive effect may take 6 hours. Doses can be repeated every 6 hours.

Side effects relevant to ICU patients include increased plasma potassium levels resulting from blunted potassium excretion, particularly in patients with renal impairment receiving potassium-sparing agents or potassium supplements. Preexisting volume depletion and renal artery stenosis may predispose to the development of renal impairment, which is usually reversible. Because angiotensin II is a major compensatory homeostatic mechanism to volume depletion, there is potential for patients with volume depletion receiving ACE inhibitors to develop marked hypotension. Angioedema possibly occurs with patients being treated with ACE inhibitors (32).

SUMMARY

Hypertension is a common disease that affects 20% of Americans. Intensivists need to be prepared to assess and manage patients admitted to the ICU because of hypertensive emergencies or MHT. They also must be familiar with how one treats hypertensive urgencies, that is, patients with elevated BP who are admitted to the ICU for other reasons and in whom BP can significantly affect their disease management. To manage a postoperative patient admitted to the ICU, one must treat precipitating factors such as hypercarbia, hypoxia, pain, and emergence excitement, but if BP remains elevated despite correction of these problems, one must be prepared to intervene with pharmacologic therapy.

Multiple pharmacologic agents are currently recommended. The JNC VI recommends diuretics and β-blockers as first-line agents. In an ICU setting, given the urgency of treating elevated BP, direct vasodilators such as SNP are often used, although β-blockers are ideal medications but unfortunately are frequently underused. In a select group of patients, calcium-channel blockers (e.g., in patients with dysrhythmias) or ACE inhibitors (for patients with renal failure) may be drugs of choice.

KEY POINTS

Hypertension is a common problem that affects more than 50 million Americans.

Hypertension was reclassified by the Joint National Committee on Detection, Evaluation, and Treatment of High Blood Pressure into three stages, with blood pressures greater than 140/90 mm Hg being abnormal.

The cause of hypertension is unchanged in that 90% of patients have essential hypertension.

Patients with malignant hypertension, that is, blood pressures typically greater than 200/120 mm Hg, are associated with organ dysfunction and damage. These patients require admission to an intensive care unit and intravenous therapy to decrease their blood pressure.

The cerebrovascular, the cardiovascular, and the renovascular systems are the organ systems most commonly affected by hypertension.

In evaluating a patient preoperatively, one must obtain an adequate history and perform a physical examination focusing on identifiable causes of hypertension, the presence of target organ damage, and patient risk factors.

For patients undergoing operative procedures, antihypertensive medications need to be continued preoperatively.

For patients with a past history of hypertension or who undergo certain procedures, that is, cardiovascular, cerebrovascular, and endocrine procedures (pheochromocytoma resection), intraoperative hypertension is common.

Patients with type B aortic dissections require intravenous antihypertensive therapy to normalize their blood pressure and improve outcome.

Before the administration of pharmacologic therapy in patients with hypertension either in the intensive care unit or in the operating room, other contributing factors need to be searched for, such as hypercarbia, hypoxia, distended bladder, and others.

Diuretics and β-blockers are the pharmacologic therapy of choice for treatment of hypertension, although patients with hypertensive emergencies and urgencies often require direct vasodilators.

Calcium-channel blockers and angiotensin-converting enzyme inhibitors are recommended for subgroups of patients with specific disorders, that is, for patients with dysrhythmias or hypertension and diabetes or for patients with renal vascular disease, respectively.

REFERENCES

1. National Institutes of Health, National Heart, Lung, and Blood Institute. *The Sixth Report of the Joint National Committee on Detection, Evaluation and Treatment of High Blood Pressure.* NIH Publication no. 98-4080, November 1997.
2. Carretero OA, Oparil S. Essential hypertension. Part I: definition and etiology. *Circulation* 2000;101:329–335.
3. Isles CG. Malignant hypertension and hypertensive encephalopathy. In: Swales JD, ed. *Textbook of hypertension.* Boston: Blackwell Scientific Publishers, 1994:1233–1247.
4. World Health Organization. Arterial Hypertension. *World Health Organ Tech Rep Ser* 1978;628:57.
5. Isles CG, Johnson AOC, Milne FJ. Slow release nifedipine and atenolol as initial treatment in blacks with malignant hypertension. *Br J Clin Pharmacol* 1986;21:377–383.
6. Grossman E, Messerli HF, Grodzicki T, et al. Should a moratorium be placed on sublingual nifedipine capsules given for hypertensive emergencies and pseudoemergencies? *JAMA* 1996;276:1328–1331.
7. Vaughan CJ, Delanty N. Hypertensive emergencies. *Lancet* 2000;356: 411–417.
8. Topol EJ, Traill TA, Fortuin NJ. Hypertensive hypertrophic cardiomyopathy of the elderly. *N Engl J Med* 1985;312:277–283.
9. Wallin JD. Intravenous nicardipine hydrochloride: treatment of patients with severe hypertension. *Am Heart J* 1990;119:434–437.
10. Metra M, Nodari S, D'Aloia A, et al. A rationale for the use of beta-blockers as standard treatment for heart failure. *Am Heart J* 2000; 139:511–521.
11. Lau J, Antman EM, Jimenez-Silva J, et al. Cumulative meta-analysis of therapeutic trials for myocardial infarction. *N Engl J Med* 1992;327:248–254.
12. Lilienfield DE, Gunderson PD, Sprafka JM, et al. Epidemiology of aortic aneurysms: I. Mortality trends in the United States, 1951 to 1981. *Arteriosclerosis* 1987;7:637–643.
13. Prokop EK, Palmer RF, Wheat MW Jr. Hydrodynamic forces in dissecting aneurysms: *in vitro* studies in a Tygon model and in dog aortas. *Circ Res* 1970;27:121–127.
14. Safian RD, Textor S. Renal artery stenosis. *N Engl J Med* 2001;344: 431–442.
15. Working Group Report on High Blood Pressure in Pregnancy. National Institutes of Health; National Heart, Lung, and Blood Institute; National High Blood Pressure Education Program. NIH Publication no. 00-3029, July 2000.
16. Eagle KA, Brundage BH, Chaitman BR, et al. Guidelines for perioperative cardiovascular evaluation for noncardiac surgery: Report of the American College of Cardiology/American Heart Association Task Force on Practice Guidelines. *J Am Coll Cardiol* 1996;27:910–948.
17. Hart GR, Anderson RJ. Withdrawal syndromes and the cessation of antihypertensive therapy. *Arch Intern Med* 1981;141:1125–1127.
18. Frishman WH. Beta-adrenergic blocker withdrawal. *Am J Cardiol* 1987;59:26F–36F.
19. Psaty BM, Koepsell, Wagner EH, et al. The relative risk of incident coronary heart disease associated with recently stopping the use of beta-blockers. *JAMA* 1990;263:1653–1657.
20. Forrest JB, Rehder K, Cahalan MK, et al. Multicenter study of general anesthesia. III: predictors of severe perioperative adverse outcomes. *Anesthesiology* 1992;76:3–15.
21. Friederich JA, Butterworth IV. Sodium nitroprusside: twenty years and counting. *Anesth Analg* 1995; 81:152–162.
22. Standen NB, Quayle JM, Davies NW, et al. Hyperpolarizing vasodilators activate ATP-sensitive K+ channels in arterial smooth muscle. *Science* 1989;245:177–180.
23. Gorczynski RJ, Quon CY, Krasula RW, et al. In: Criabine A, ed. *New drugs annual cardiovascular drugs*, vol 3. New York: Raven Press, 1985: 99–119.
24. Muzzi DA, Black S, Losassa TJ, et al. Labetalol and esmolol in the control of hypertension after intracranial surgery. *Anesth Analg* 1990;70:68–71.
25. Chauvin M, Deriaz H, Viars P. Continuous i.v. infusion of labetalol for postoperative hypertension. Haemodynamic effects and plasma kinetics. *Br J Anaesth* 1987;59:1250–1256.

26. Radack K, Deck C. Beta-adrenergic blocker therapy does not worsen intermittent claudication in subjects with peripheral arterial disease: a meta-analysis of randomized controlled trials. *Arch Intern Med* 1991;151:1769–1776.

27. Benson MK, Berrill WT, Cruickshank JM, et al. A comparison of four beta-adrenoreceptor antagonists in patients with asthma. *Br J Clin Pharmacol* 1978;5:415–419.

28. Sheppard D, DiStefano S, Byrd RC, et al. Effects of esmolol on airway function in patients with asthma. *J Clin Pharmacol* 1986;26:169–174.

29. Gold MR, Dec GW, Cocca-Spofford D, et al. Esmolol and ventilatory function in cardiac patients with COPD. *Chest* 1991;100:1215–1218.

30. Oliver MF, Julian DG, Holme I. Effect of mivazerol on perioperative cardiac complications during non-cardiac surgery in patients with coronary heart disease. *Anesthesiology* 1999;91:951–961.

31. Lambert CR, Pepine CJ. Effects of intravenous and intracoronary nicardipine. *Am J Cardiol* 1989;64:8H–15H.

32. Israili ZH, Hall WD. Cough and angioneurotic edema associated with angiotensin-converting enzyme inhibitor therapy: a review of the literature and pathophysiology. *Ann Intern Med* 1992;117:234–242.

PERIOPERATIVE MANAGEMENT OF THE CARDIAC SURGICAL PATIENT

J. G. REVES
STEVEN E. HILL
SAM THIO SUM-PING
JOHN V. BOOTH
IAN J. WELSBY

KEY WORDS

- Cardiopulmonary bypass
- Hemodynamics
- Complications
- Transfusion
- Accelerated recovery
- Risk factors

INTRODUCTION

Cardiac surgical patients are routinely admitted to the surgical intensive care unit (SICU) for monitoring of recovery from anesthesia, rewarming following cardiopulmonary bypass (CPB), optimization of hemodynamics, and weaning from ventilatory support. Traditionally, cardiac surgery patients remained in SICU for a few days before discharge to the ward. Over the past decade, ICU management has changed in response to changing patient populations, new surgical techniques, and the penetration of managed care. Patients presenting for surgery are older as the number of patients undergoing angioplasty and stenting increases. The number of percutaneous transluminal coronary angioplasty (PTCA) procedures increased 188% from 1987 to 1997 (1). Aggressive medical therapy and nonsurgical revascularization techniques also result in patients presenting for surgery at more advanced stages of disease. Moreover, with the advent of health maintenance organizations (HMOs) and other cost-containment strategies, there is an ongoing trend toward early withdrawal of ventilatory support and accelerated discharge from intensive care.

With the development of minimally invasive surgery, warm bypass, and off-pump bypass techniques, cardiac surgeons have altered the requirements for conventional postoperative recovery. Movement away from the opioid-based anesthetic techniques of the past to newer ones with shorter acting induction agents (propofol and etomidate), volatile agents (isoflurane and sevoflurane), and opioids (remifentanil) allow accelerated patient recovery from anesthesia. Consequently, it is incumbent on intensivists to develop strategies to manage this ever-changing patient population in an efficient and cost-effective manner while maintaining quality and minimizing morbidity and mortality. Although the majority of institutions utilize the SICU for postoperative care, avoidance of SICU admission altogether may be the future: some institutions utilize step-down units for the weaning process and high dependency care (2).

INITIAL ASSESSMENT AND MANAGEMENT

Once surgery is complete and the patient is stabilized in the operating room, the patient is transported to the SICU while still emerging from anesthesia. To improve comfort, the patient is often maintained on sedation with short-acting agents such as propofol or dexmedetomidine supplemented with morphine when needed. This allows the patient to wake up gradually in the SICU while necessary monitoring devices are being attached and the intensivist evaluates the patient. There is little evidence to support extubation in the operating room compared with early extubation in the ICU after 2 to 3 hours of stabilization (3).

Admission

During the transfer of care from the anesthesiologist to the intensivist, the latter must become familiar with the patient's entire medical history. Essential data include indication for surgery, preoperative cardiac function, cardiac catheterization findings, number of arterial and venous grafts, location of donor sites for the arterial grafts, bypass and cross-clamp times, difficulties weaning from the bypass pump, and postbypass cardiac assessment with pulmonary arterial catheter measurements or transesophageal echocardiography (TEE). It is also important to know the adequacy of hemostasis, the number and position of drains, whether cardiac pacing was required and whether the procedure was a "redo." "Redo" procedures (repeat sternotomy or thoracotomy) are technically more difficult and tend to result in greater blood loss and higher complication rates. The amount and type of fluids and any blood products administered should also be relayed to the intensivist.

Detailed initial and frequent examination of the postoperative cardiac patient should follow. The presence and position of invasive catheters, drains and the endotracheal tube should be confirmed. The patient's core and peripheral temperatures, the amount of drainage from the chest tubes, the patient's oxygen saturation (SpO_2) and end-tidal partial pressure of carbon dioxide ($PetCO_2$), fluid input and urinary output, and the patient's hemodynamic status need to be assessed. The extent of hemodynamic monitoring will depend on the patient's perioperative condition and anticipated complications during and after cardiac surgery. Patients should have an arterial line, a central venous pressure (CVP) line and a urinary catheter. There has been a recent trend away from pulmonary artery (PA) catheterization, partly as a result of work by Connors and colleagues (4) and partly because of the increased utilization of intraoperative TEE. The data derived from these monitors is sufficient to address the majority of clinical situations.

Immediate laboratory analysis includes arterial blood gases to assess acid-base status and alveolar-arterial oxygen gradient, and blood chemistry. Potassium and magnesium plasma levels need to be kept above 4.0 and 2.0 mmol per L, respectively, to minimize the incidence of dysrhythmias (5–8). Potassium repletion may not be successful without restoration of magnesium stores (6,9,10). A complete blood count is required to guide transfusion therapy and a coagulation profile is measured to assess potential clotting factor deficiency. An activated clotting time may also be used as a point of care test for adequate reversal of heparin given during surgery. At our institution, a new algorithm for blood transfusion (Table 1) was instituted recently and the number of blood products used has significantly diminished. A chest radiograph is

performed to assess lung volume and to exclude pneumothorax or parenchymal infiltrates as well as confirm correct position of the endotracheal tube, invasive catheters, and chest tubes. An electrocardiogram (ECG) is performed to exclude abnormal cardiac rhythm or evidence of new ischemia.

Stabilization Phase (First 4 Hours)

Perioperative hypothermia is associated with shivering (and thus increased oxygen utilization) and possibly ischemia (11), coagulopathies, and infection (12). Therefore an important part of early ICU management is rewarming the patient. Heated underblankets are now superseded by forced air warmers, which are more versatile (13). During rewarming, vasoconstriction and hypertension gradually give way to vasodilation and hypotension. During this phase, patients who initially require vasodilators such as nitroprusside may later require fluid and vasoconstrictors such as norepinephrine. Shivering is conventionally treated with meperidine (14).

It is rare for patients to be extubated in the operating room; most patients require ventilatory support for 4 to 8 hours. Initial ventilator settings are aimed to provide complete support of the work of breathing for the patient. The fraction of inspired oxygen (FIO_2) is normally set $\geq 60\%$ and is reduced quickly as appropriate. The arterial partial pressure of carbon dioxide ($PaCO_2$) should be maintained at 40 ± 2 mm Hg to maintain the CO_2-mediated stimulus to breathe.

Adequacy of cardiac output (CO) and perfusion can be assessed clinically with the evaluation of heart rate (HR), rhythm, blood pressure (BP), skin perfusion, and urine output. A patient with good skin perfusion and HR as well as BP and urine output in the normal range most probably has a normal CO. Systemic BP needs to be controlled, with a combination of nitroglycerin and nitroprusside infusion, to a mean BP range of 70 to 80 mm Hg in order to minimize surgical bleeding and myocardial oxygen demand. CO can be easily assessed utilizing a PA catheter with a target cardiac index (CI; equal to CO/body surface area) greater than 2.0 L per minute per M^2. Blood, crystalloid, or colloid may be infused to increase preload. CI can also be improved by optimizing afterload with a vasodilator such as nitroprusside. With an optimized preload and afterload, CI can sometimes be increased by pacing at a higher rate over the intrinsic HR. If preload and afterload are optimized, stroke volume (SV) would normally remain the same and a higher HR would increase CI.

If the target of a CI greater than 2 is not achieved with optimization of preload, afterload, and HR, infusion of an inotrope (Table 2) is usually required to improve cardiac contractility. There does not appear to be a significant difference among the commonly used inotropes, but personal preferences often exist among cardiac surgeons and intensivists depending on familiarity with the agent and clinical experience. One critical distinction to make in a hypotensive patient is between relative intravascular hypovolemia from vasodilation during warming and hypovolemia secondary to bleeding.

Hemostasis is assessed by measuring the amount of blood draining out of the chest tubes. Prothrombin time and aPTT are normally slightly elevated following cardiac surgery. Fresh frozen

TABLE 1. TRANSFUSION ALGORITHM

1. Unstable Patients
   Definition:
   Chest tube output > 200 mL/hr
   Cardiac index < 2.0 following optimized volume resuscitation and infusion of inotropes
   Mixed venous saturation ($S\bar{v}O_2$) <55% following optimized volume resuscitation and infusion of inotropes
   Arterial saturation < 92% with 100% oxygen and optimized ventilator settings
   Management: Transfuse blood and blood products as needed for intravascular volume replacement until patient is stable.

2. Stable Patients—High Risk
   Definition:
   Postcardiopulmonary bypass, ejection fraction < 35%
   Pulmonary restriction with FEV_1 <1.2
   Renal impairment with preoperative creatinine > 1.8 or an increase from normal to > 1.6
   Any end-organ dysfunction
   $S\bar{v}O_2$ < 55% with optimized volume resuscitation and infusion of inotropes
   Chest tube output > 75 mL/hr
   Clinical judgment of instability
   Management: Transfuse to maintain hematocrit $\geq$ 27%.

3. Stable Patients—Low Risk
   Definition:
   Patients with no high-risk criteria
   Management: Transfuse to maintain hematocrit $\geq$ 23%.

FEV_1, forced expiratory volume in 1 sec.

TABLE 2. RESPONSE TO COMMONLY USED INOTROPES

Inotrope	α1	β1	β2	PD-I[a]	Recommended Dose
Epinephrine	**	***	*	—	0.02–0.15 μg/kg/min
Norepinephrine	****	***	*	—	0.02–0.20 μg/kg/min
Dopamine	**	**	*	—	1.0–20.0 μg/kg/min
Dobutamine	*	***	*	—	1.0–20.0 μg/kg/min
Milrinone	—	—	—	***	0.35–0.75 μg/kg/min

[a]Phosphodiesterase inhibition.
* = relative activity.

plasma (FFP) is not required when there is no significant drainage from the chest tubes; if drainage from the chest tube exceeds 400 mL in the first 2 hours and 100 to 150 mL per hour after the first 2 hours, FFP is probably required to stop the bleeding. Infusion of 10 mL per kg of FFP normally restores the coagulation factors to an adequate level. It is also important to consider platelet transfusion in a bleeding patient after CPB even if the platelet count is over 100,000 per μL because the bypass pump can affect platelet function. The chest tubes need to be evaluated on a regular basis to avoid clogging by blood clots. When there is a sudden decrease in drainage from the chest tubes, the intensivist should exclude the possibility of concealed bleeding in the mediastinum and pericardial sac, which can lead to cardiac tamponade. If the response to the FFP and platelet infusion is not satisfactory, exploratory resternotomy should seriously be considered.

Urine output is usually not a problem for patients with a normal renal function prior to surgery. Most commonly, low urine output is due to hypovolemia and the patient needs either blood, crystalloid, or colloid to optimize the preload and CO. Patients with impaired renal function may be on a diuretic prior to surgery. If such a patient's urine output is still low with a sufficient preload and CO, they may need a diuretic such as furosemide to maintain adequate urine flow. The bladder catheter should also be checked for possible obstruction. It is common practice to start an infusion of renal dose dopamine for patients with marginal urine output, but there is at present no definitive evidence supporting a better outcome with this therapy (15). The use of fenoldopam, a new antihypertensive agent, may be helpful in protecting renal function in cases of marginal renal perfusion (16). Further studies are needed to confirm early findings.

Most patients will begin to emerge from anesthesia about 3 to 4 hours following admission to the SICU. A shorter wake-up time can be achieved by altering the anesthetic technique. Reported benefits of rapid emergence are somewhat controversial because the gradual wake-up period is generally spent on evaluation and preparing the patient for removal from cardiac and ventilatory support. Extubation prior to 2 hours following arrival in the ICU may not prove beneficial, except in selected low-risk patients, because of the value of stabilization in this patient population. No definitive studies to date have documented a significantly shorter ICU or hospital length of stay due to extubation of cardiac surgical patients in the operating room. Most patients receive an infusion of a short-acting sedative such as propofol or dexmedetomidine supplemented with an opioid when necessary as these drugs have no analgesic property. The pharmacokinetics of dexmedetomidine are similar to propofol. Other popular sedative agents include midazolam and fentanyl.

If there is no sign of emergence from anesthesia in 6 hours, all sedation should be stopped to exclude the possibility of overmedication. Upon recovery from anesthesia in the SICU, a brief neurologic examination should be performed to identify gross focal deficits or residual neuromuscular blockade. From 1% to 5% of patients develop major neurologic injury after cardiac surgery with between 25% and 80% of patients having subtle neurocognitive dysfunction (17,18).

Weaning Phase

Weaning from ventilatory support can start once the patient spontaneously breathes over the rate set on the ventilator. Weaning should not be aggressive until the patient is normothermic, has adequate pulmonary gas exchange and mechanical function, has emerged sufficiently from anesthesia, has no significant drainage from the chest tubes, has no residual neuromuscular blockade, and has stable cardiac function. A minimum acceptable level of oxygenation prior to weaning would be a PaO_2 higher than 70 mm Hg at FiO_2 of 0.5 or less. One method of weaning is to gradually reduce the rate set on the ventilator by two breaths per minute every 30 minutes until reaching a rate of zero with continuous positive airway pressure (CPAP) and 10 cm of water of pressure support. If the patient can maintain reasonable gas exchange and is not tachypneic after 30 minutes on CPAP, the patient is ready to have the endotracheal tube removed. Some intensivists prefer to evaluate the patient's pulmonary mechanics (Table 3) for further confirmation. Another weaning technique is to attempt CPAP trials every 30 minutes until a certain set criterion is satisfied (Table 3). Either method is safe and neither has any clear advantage over the other. However, many patients undergoing cardiac surgery have normal pulmonary function perioperatively and do not require a gradual wean from the ventilator. If the patient has remained stable during recovery from anesthesia and

TABLE 3. FACTORS PREDICTING WEANING SUCCESS

1. Mechanical
   Respiratory rate < 25/min
   Vital capacity > 12–15 mL/kg
   Maximal negative inspiratory pressure < –25 cm H_2O
   Minute ventilation ($\dot{V}$) < 10 L/min
   Maximal voluntary ventilation > 2 × resting $\dot{V}$
   Respiratory rate/tidal volume (L) ratio < 105

2. Gas Exchange
   PaO_2 > 60 mm Hg (FiO_2 < 0.4)
   PaO_2/FiO_2 ratio > 200
   Alveolar-arterial PO_2 gradient < 350 mm Hg

has no significant pulmonary disease, a rapid decrease in ventilator support to minimal levels can be safely instituted under close observation and the patient evaluated for extubation. The method of removal from ventilatory assistance varies between institutions depending on the characteristics of the individual ICU.

Postextubation Phase

Following successful extubation, the patient should participate in cough and deep breathing exercises with incentive spirometry. An arterial blood gas is normally checked about 30 to 45 minutes after extubation to evaluate the $Paco_2$ level and the acid-base balance and confirm sufficient oxygenation. An unacceptable blood gas analysis with a high $Paco_2$ or a large alveolar-arterial oxygen gradient is normally multifactorial. Factors to consider include partial airway obstruction; persistence of neuromuscular blockade; reduced central drive due to residual effects of anesthetic, sedative agents or opioids; pulmonary edema; and atelectasis. Atelectasis, predominantly in the base of the left lung, is common at this stage and can be improved with incentive spirometry and cough. Patients are often reluctant to cough at this stage because of pain. Patients should receive enough analgesics for pain control, but they should not be too sleepy to follow instructions. In many cases chest tubes are the main source of pain, and their removal helps the patient significantly. Hugging a pillow stabilizes the chest wall and may decrease pain during a coughing session.

Rehabilitation Phase

Soon after extubation, the patient should be able to communicate freely and be allowed sips of clear fluids. Preoperative medications should be restarted. Once the patient has been stable for 4 to 6 hours following extubation, invasive monitoring such as arterial, central venous, and PA catheters can be discontinued. Continuous ECG monitoring is the only modality required for stable patients. About 30% of cardiac patients develop atrial fibrillation (AF) between the second and third day following surgery. Most patients stay in the SICU for 24 hours or less and are then monitored by telemetry on a step-down unit. They typically start a normal diet the morning after surgery.

MANAGEMENT OF PERIOPERATIVE COMPLICATIONS

Hypotension

Hypotension has no concrete definition. There is general agreement that a systolic BP of less than 90 mm Hg or a mean arterial pressure (MAP) of less than 60 mm Hg denotes hypotension. However, the patient's baseline BP must be considered, as that determines the range of autoregulation for end-organs such as the brain or kidney. Provided the end-organ perfusion is sufficient for normal function, BP is adequate. With long-standing hypertension or atherosclerotic disease, a higher BP may be necessary to perfuse the renal or cerebral circulations. Monitoring of renal and cerebral function will provide the required information to guide that decision. Also, diastolic BP is a major determinant of myocardial blood flow, so attention must be paid to diastolic BP

if myocardial ischemia is evident. When diagnosing and treating hypotension, it is helpful to address the components defining BP:

$$MAP = CO \times SVR$$

where SVR = systemic vascular resistance.

CO is the product of HR and forward SV. The determinants of CO often need to be optimized in the perioperative period to achieve the target CI and enhance patient recovery.

Epicardial pacing is often used to ensure an HR of 80 to 90 beats per minute. Bradycardia can result in ventricular distension and subsequent failure in the fresh postoperative heart. Optimization of the atrioventricular (AV) interval can help improve ventricular filling, especially if diastolic function is impaired (19). An AV interval that is too short (under 0.10 seconds) can compromise the time for maximal left ventricular (LV) filling in response to the atrial kick. An AV interval that is too long (more than 0.225 seconds) may compromise the left atrial contribution to ventricular filling because of atrial contraction against a partially closed mitral valve. If the AV interval is normal, CO may best be improved by atrial pacing only with an increased HR.

Preload, contractility, and afterload determine SV. Inadequate LV preload is caused by hypovolemia, right ventricular (RV) failure, cardiac tamponade, or tension pneumothorax. Hypovolemia is the most common cause of hypotension in the postoperative patient. Peripheral rewarming causes vasodilation, requiring expansion of circulating blood volume for treatment. Ongoing bleeding requires intravascular volume replacement. Diagnosis of hypovolemia relies on both clinical observation (chest tube output) and invasive pressure measurements. Isolated measurements of CVP and pulmonary capillary occlusion pressure (PCOP) are less helpful than trends in these measurements or their response to a fluid bolus. Blood products, crystalloids, or artificial colloid solutions can be used to augment filling, depending on the hemoglobin level and coagulation status. Determination of which CVP, PCOP, or PA diastolic pressures correspond with adequate LV filling on intraoperative TEE is also helpful for postoperative management. These pressures will be low in the presence of hypovolemia and high in the presence of LV dysfunction. Preoperative cardiac catheterization data, particularly LV end-diastolic pressure, is a useful predictor of postoperative LV systolic or diastolic dysfunction.

Positive pressure ventilation can also produce relative hypovolemia, especially in patients with obstructive lung disease, by eliminating the normal venous pressure gradient for filling of the right atrium. The presence of "intrinsic positive end-expiratory pressure" is diagnostic of this condition. Adjustment of ventilator settings to increase expiratory time will help alleviate this problem. The development of a tension pneumothorax as the result of chest tube obstruction or occult intraoperative lung injury on a side not drained by a chest tube (usually the right) can also acutely compromise right heart filling. Assurance that breath sounds are present and symmetric on arrival in the SICU as well as scrutiny of the initial postoperative chest radiograph will identify this potential complication, which is easily remedied by tube thoracostomy (or needle thoracostomy followed by a chest tube in an emergency setting). Percussion of the chest will reveal tympany on the side of a tension pneumothorax and is sometimes helpful in the emergent diagnosis of tension pneumothorax.

RV dysfunction can be secondary to pulmonary hypertension, perioperative myocardial ischemia, or acute hypervolemia. It is important to avoid acidosis, hypoxia, high inflation pressures, or the use of nitrous oxide in this setting, which will all tend to exacerbate pulmonary hypertension. RV dysfunction in the presence of systemic hypotension will require more than simple pulmonary vasodilation with sodium nitroprusside (SNP), nitroglycerin (NTG), or prostaglandin E_1 (PGE_1). Supplementation with low-dose (less than 0.04 μg per kg per minute) epinephrine or norepinephrine may be needed to maintain adequate systemic pressures and provide inotropic support. Phosphodiesterase inhibitors such as milrinone (50 μg per kg load then 0.5 μg per kg per minute) act as inodilators but again may need catecholamines to support systemic pressures. Inhaled nitric oxide is a highly effective, selective pulmonary vasodilator (20) that does not cause systemic hypotension, but definitive data showing improved outcome sufficient to justify the expense and complexity of this mode of therapy have yet to be produced. Hypervolemia can result in ventricular distention with compromised systolic function and impaired CO. It can be treated with diuretics, NTG infusion, or phlebotomy.

When pharmacologic measures fail to correct RV dysfunction, mechanical support with RV assist devices (e.g., CardioWest Technologies, Inc., Thoratec, Corp., and Abiomed, Inc.) may be used if LV function is normal. Biventricular failure merits biventricular assistance. Use of intraaortic balloon pump (IABP) counterpulsation in the pulmonary circulation is possible but rarely used for right-sided failure.

Cardiac tamponade should be suspected in any unstable or acutely deteriorating patient, particularly if right-sided filling pressures are high. The presentation may not be classic (21) as the extracardiac collection may not be uniform (22), but identification of a compressing collection or diastolic right atrial collapse on TEE provides a definitive diagnosis. Chest reentry is performed in the ICU or in the operating room if conditions permit. The decision to reopen can be justified without definitive diagnosis, especially in the event of circulatory collapse. Closure of the chest may rarely result in a tamponadelike picture and under these circumstances, it is necessary to delay sternal approximation until the patient is stable (23).

Impaired myocardial contractility may be due to preexisting myocardial disease (systolic heart failure), reperfusion injury (myocardial stunning), or recurrent myocardial ischemia. Chronic systolic heart failure causes high circulating catecholamine levels, leading to depletion of myocardial norepinephrine stores and B_1 adrenoceptor downregulation. In practice, this makes epinephrine and norepinephrine first choice inotropes following cardiac surgery in this population of patients. Their effectiveness, however, may plateau. The addition of a phosphodiesterase inhibitor, such as milrinone or amrinone, produces a synergistic inotropic effect (24). This group of patients often requires the use of digoxin and continuation may be appropriate once electrolyte levels are stable and renal function determined. Thyroid hormone (T_3) has not proven beneficial in a cohort of euthyroid patients weaning from CPB (25), but its use should be considered if hypothyroidism is suspected or other therapies are ineffective.

Severity of postoperative myocardial dysfunction is variable and may represent ischemia from inadequate myocardial protection during aortic cross-clamping, reduction in available high-energy phosphates, injury from activated neutrophils, or high intracellular calcium levels. The decrement in myocardial performance usually peaks between 4 to 6 hours postbypass and will usually respond to inotropic support. It is often not possible to differentiate between preexisting myocardial damage and reversible perioperative myocardial dysfunction as a cause of poor contractility. If inotropes fail to reverse a low output state, an IABP can increase BP and CI with an LV assist device (LVAD) being used if the above fails. Biventricular assist is required if concurrent right-sided dysfunction or significant arrhythmias exist.

Postoperative myocardial ischemia as a result of incomplete revascularization or acute occlusion of either the native coronaries or the bypass grafts can result in a low output state. This condition is diagnosed by regional ECG changes or new segmental wall motion abnormalities on TEE. Inotropes tend to be less effective and are arrhythmogenic in ischemic areas. NTG, milrinone, or an IABP may sufficiently improve myocardial perfusion, but reexploration (with or without diagnostic angiography) remains the definitive approach for an occluded bypass graft.

Vasodilation post-CPB is commonly due to anesthetic drugs, peripheral rewarming, anemia, and variable degrees of a systemic inflammatory response to the extracorporeal circuit. Vasodilation, per se, is not undesirable and it is important to treat hypotension by addressing inadequate CO (preload, contractility, and HR) prior to increasing the SVR, except as a temporizing measure to maintain coronary perfusion while other therapy is initiated.

Increasing SVR can be achieved using inoconstrictors (dopamine, epinephrine, and norepinephrine) or pure vasoconstrictors (phenylephrine). CO measurements determine the appropriate drug. Vasoconstrictors reduce HR and CO. Of the inoconstrictors, norepinephrine produces the least increase in HR and CO.

Calcium increases BP without decreasing CO and has a negligible effect on HR. It is undesirable for ionized calcium levels to be abnormally high, so repeated administration should be guided by blood levels. Low blood levels may result from rapid blood product transfusion and can reduce vascular responsiveness to catecholamines. A normal ionized calcium level is the goal.

Postcardiotomy vasodilatory shock may be associated with unresponsiveness to catecholamines, particularly following LVAD implantation. When high-dose norepinephrine (greater than 0.1 μg per kg per minute) is required, or ineffective, arginine vasopressin (0.1 U per minute) has proven useful in increasing BP and reducing norepinephrine requirements (26). When using any vasoconstrictors for a prolonged period, it is essential to avoid hypovolemia as severe peripheral hypoperfusion with gangrene may result.

Electrocardiogram Changes

ST segment depression or elevation can occur intraoperatively or postoperatively. For intraoperative changes, transient causes include air in the coronary arteries and repolarization abnormalities during the washout of cardioplegia. Because of obligate coronary artery occlusion during off-pump coronary artery bypass grafting (CABG), ischemic ST segment depression or elevation arising from myocardium supplied by the artery being bypassed is often present. On completion of the graft, these changes should resolve following a short period of reperfusion.

Regardless of whether the bypass graft was performed with or without CPB, persistent changes following reperfusion call into question the patency of the coronary artery (native or graft) supplying the area of myocardium to which the ST changes localize. The development of new, focal segmental wall motion abnormalities seen on TEE confirm significant myocardial ischemia and the need to address the patency of the artery or bypass graft. Depending on the angiographic anatomy of the patient, the surgeon may proceed to further bypass grafting to better perfuse the ischemic area. Insertion of an IABP is an alternative means of improving coronary flow and may be required while further surgical intervention is considered.

Postoperatively, patients are monitored with continuous telemetry, mainly for detection of malignant dysrhythmias. However, if trends in ST segments are measured, telemetry can also serve as an effective monitor of ischemia. Bipolar leads can be as useful as chest leads for monitoring ischemia (27). Transient, postoperative ST changes may occur but their significance is unclear. If frequent, NTG infusion or β-blockade should be considered.

Persistent, postoperative ST segment changes should be investigated for acute myocardial ischemia/infarction with serial 12-lead ECG tracings, routine laboratory tests, cardiac enzymes (creatine phosphokinase [CK]-MB and troponin levels) and, when appropriate, ECG and possibly even angiography. Results of the above will dictate the need for revascularization, but immediate management should include oxygen, opioids, aspirin, β-blockers, and heparin unless contraindicated.

Marked reductions in the R-wave amplitude of V5 can occur on application of sternal spreaders and persist after sternal closure (28). In these circumstances, the size of ST segment changes needs to be considered relative to the reduction in R wave amplitude. Recovery of baseline R wave amplitude has been linked to improved outcome (29).

Widening of the QRS complex is commonly seen on initial infusion and washout of cardioplegia due to local hyperkalemia. This is short-lived on reperfusion, unless it represents an idioventricular complex in the presence of AV block or a ventricular-paced complex. New onset bundle-branch block is uncommon in the absence of ventricular pacing and may indicate ischemia or surgical interruption of the normal conduction pathways.

Dysrhythmias

Transient bradydysrhythmias are common following cardiac surgery and atrial and ventricular epicardial pacing wires are typically placed to facilitate temporary pacing in the immediate postoperative period. Optimal pacing modalities have been investigated (19); dual chamber pacing maximizes CO over a wide range of AV delay (100 to 225 milliseconds). Conditions impairing diastolic filling (ventricular hypertrophy, cardiomyopathy, fibrosis) may benefit by extending the AV delay.

Rate of pacemaker dependency varies between studies and is approximately 1% post-CABG, 2% post-primary valve replacement, 7% post-repeat valve replacement, and 10% post-orthotopic heart transplant (OHT) (30–32). Identified risk factors include perivalvular calcification, older age, preoperative left

bundlebranch block, and increased CPB time. Calcific aortic valve or tricuspid valve replacement may carry a 20% risk for permanent pacing, and there is an increased incidence of high-degree AV block following either mitral valve repair or replacement (31). Transseptal approaches to the mitral valve may cause sinus node dysfunction with resultant bradycardia or junctional dysrhythmias.

The etiology of bradydysrhythmia includes ischemia, edema, and irreversible surgical destruction of the conducting system. Recovery from the reversible causes can be considerably delayed. Permanent pacemakers are typically implanted for symptomatic sinus node dysfunction or AV block lasting beyond the fifth postoperative day. In the long term, up to 40% of patients with sinus node dysfunction and up to 100% of patients with complete AV block past day five remain pacemaker-dependent.

For heart transplant patients, chronotropic medication may avoid the need for a permanent pacemaker. Persistent sinus node dysfunction and high-degree AV block following OHT have been treated successfully with theophylline (33). However, concerns about safety without close monitoring outside the hospital have limited its use. Sinus node dysfunction is five times more likely than AV block to result in permanent pacemaker implantation in this group. Both types of dysfunction can be significantly reduced with bicaval rather than biatrial anastomoses (32).

Atrial dysrhythmias (primarily atrial fibrillation [AF]) are by far the most common dysrhythmias following CABG surgery with an overall incidence of approximately 30% (34). AF most commonly occurs 2 to 3 days after surgery and can increase hospital stay (34,35), risk of stroke, and mortality (36). The exact pathogenesis of postoperative AF is unclear. Structural changes in the atria, reduced threshold for dysrhythmia generation, and a hyperadrenergic state are all suggested as mechanisms. Associated risk factors for the development of AF include increasing age; prolonged CPB and aortic cross-clamp times; left atrial enlargement; cardiomegaly; chronic obstructive pulmonary disease; right coronary, SA or AV nodal artery disease; and hypomagnesemia and β-blocker withdrawal (34,35,37–39).

It seems logical to provide supplemental magnesium (38) and β-blockade (40) in the perioperative period to reduce the incidence of AF. While the use of β-blockade has generally been restricted to the postoperative period following establishment of hemodynamic stability, there is mounting evidence supporting intraoperative use, particularly before the catecholamine release that occurs on initiation of CPB.

Pharmacologic prophylaxis against AF is controversial. Digoxin has proved ineffective in this setting (40) and inconclusive results were obtained for prophylaxis with diltiazem, verapamil, and lower doses of magnesium. Effective reduction in postoperative supraventricular tachyarrhythmias (SVT) has been achieved with oral sotalol (41), intravenous and oral amiodarone (42,43), and intravenous procainamide (44). Adverse effects are uncommon but include: (a) hypotension, bradycardia, and torsade de pointes for sotalol; (b) hypotension and pulmonary toxicity for amiodarone; and (c) hypotension and enhanced AV conduction for procainamide.

Right and biatrial pacing are attractive options for suppressing postoperative SVT. Positive results (45,46) have been tempered with the finding that AAI mode pacing was ineffective and increased premature depolarizations in one study (47). Improved overdrive pacing algorithms and combination of atrial pacing and β-blockade (45,48) may increase the popularity of this technique. Biatrial pacing confers no advantage over the simpler right atrial pacing (45,49).

Current policy at our institution relies on intravenous metoprolol prior to initiation of CPB and oral metoprolol (25 mg b.i.d., if tolerated) postoperatively. The use of prophylactic procainamide or amiodarone is assessed based on existing risk factors.

Management of postoperative SVT depends on the patient's clinical condition. If appropriate, a 12-lead ECG and an atrial rhythm strip via the atrial pacing electrodes aid diagnosis of the exact rhythm. Hemodynamic instability merits immediate synchronized direct current (DC) cardioversion with an initial energy of 200 J for AF and 50 to 100 J for atrial flutter. Anteroposterior placement of defibrillator paddles may be more effective for conversion of atrial tachyarrhythmias. If the patient is hemodynamically stable, treatment focuses on rate control followed by pharmacologic or elective DC conversion to sinus rhythm.

Ventricular Dysrhythmias

Premature ventricular complexes are common after surgery and often associated with electrolyte imbalances. Sustained ventricular dysrhythmias after cardiac surgery are uncommon with an incidence of about 1% (49). Hemodynamic instability, electrolyte abnormalities, hypoxia, hypovolemia, ischemia, myocardial infarction, acute graft closure, reperfusion after cessation of CPB, prodysrhythmic effects of inotropic and antidysrhythmic drugs, and LV dysfunction are all associated with ventricular dysrhythmias (50). Prognosis of postoperative frequent premature ventricular complexes and nonsustained ventricular tachycardia in patients with good ventricular function is no different from controls (51). However, patients with nonsustained ventricular dysrhythmias and LV ejection fraction less than 40% demonstrate a 75% mortality rate at 15-month follow-up (50). Echocardiography can be used to identify this at-risk group.

Patients with sustained ventricular dysrhythmias have a poor short- and long-term prognosis with a hospital mortality rate of 50%. An additional 20% of the survivors have a cardiac death within 24 months (52). Such poor outcome merits aggressive therapy particularly in the higher risk patient with LV dysfunction. All electrolyte abnormalities should be corrected quickly. Ventricular fibrillation and pulseless ventricular tachycardia require defibrillation in accordance with advanced cardiac life support (ACLS) guidelines. Synchronized DC cardioversion with 200 to 360 J is used for symptomatic sustained ventricular tachycardia with a pulse. Stable sustained monomorphic ventricular tachycardia may be treated initially with intravenous antidysrhythmic medication. Procainamide may be infused at a rate of 30–50 mg per minute upto a maximum dose of 17 mg per kilogram or a widening of the QRS complex by 50%. The loading dose is followed by an intravenous continuous infusion of 1 to 4 mg per minute. Dose reductions are appropriate for older adult patients and patients with congestive heart failure or hepatic dysfunction. Lidocaine or amiodarone are good alternatives, especially in patients with LV dysfunction.

For patients with ventricular epicardial wires in place, conversion of stable ventricular tachycardia using overdrive ventricular pacing may be attempted by burst pacing the ventricle at rates above the native rate. Acceleration of the ventricular tachycardia may sometimes end in ventricular fibrillation and it is important to have a defibrillator immediately available.

Long-term management of patients with dysrhythmia depends on the severity of the condition. With sustained ventricular dysrhythmias, electrophysiologic testing is performed to evaluate whether antidysrhythmic medication or implantation of an implantable cardioverter (ICD)/defibrillator may be beneficial to the patient. A recent study demonstrated that ICD is superior to drug therapy for patients with hemodynamically significant ventricular dysrhythmias (53).

Infection

Infection rates in patients undergoing cardiac surgery tend to be higher due to a number of factors including prolonged operative time, presence of indwelling catheters, deleterious effects of CPB on the immune system, poor tissue perfusion, hyperglycemia, and implantation of foreign material. The magnitude of the problem is large with one series reporting 71% of perioperative site cultures in patients undergoing open heart procedures as positive (54). The overall incidence of postoperative infections has been quoted at between 2% and 20% (55), resulting in significantly prolonged hospitalization and substantial cost increases.

Severe infectious complications include sepsis and deep sternal wound infections (DSWI). Septic complications are difficult to predict or diagnose early in the immediate perioperative period after cardiac surgery. The proinflammatory cascade, triggered by CPB, induces a number of changes that mimic sepsis. Fever is common in the first 24 hours after cardiac surgery, and often represents a spectrum of physiologic insults such as basal atelectasis and activation of inflammatory cascades from CPB. There is some suggestion that Acute Physiologic and Chronic Health Evaluation II (APACHE II) scores may help predict a significant infection (56). Until the predictive value of APACHE scores is confirmed, it is reasonable to treat increased temperatures symptomatically in the first 24 hours after surgery.

DSWI represents one of the most devastating infectious complications of cardiac surgery. Clinical features of DSWI include redness and tenderness over the sternum, wound drainage or discharge (70% to 90% of cases), sternal instability, fever, and leukocytosis. Antibiotic therapy should be guided by culture results, but debridement and flap closure achieves healing in more than 90% of cases. Indications for surgery depend on depth and severity of infection. DSWIs are increased up to fivefold in the diabetic population, and present an area where improved perioperative care may reduce the incidence of this problem. A recent study suggested that uncontrolled hyperglycemia in diabetic patients after cardiac surgery, and not diabetes per se, is the true risk factor for DSWI (57). Furthermore, this study demonstrated that tighter control of blood glucose levels throughout the perioperative period (levels maintained below 200 mg per dL) independently decreased the risk of DSWI by 66%.

Oliguria

The incidence of acute renal failure (ARF) requiring dialysis following cardiac surgery is approximately 1%. Significant

TABLE 4. POSTOPERATIVE RISK FACTORS FOR RENAL INJURY

Low cardiac output
Excessive inotrope use
Prolonged ventilation
Sepsis
Cytomegaloviral infection

postoperative worsening of renal function is observed in approximately 7% of patients with approximately 15% of these patients requiring dialysis. In addition to increased morbidity, mortality, and perioperative cost, patients with renal injury have a fivefold longer SICU stay and a threefold longer hospital stay. They are also more likely to be discharged to an extended-care facility, with its associated financial and emotional costs (58).

In the absence of effective treatment strategies to reverse renal injury, major emphasis has focused on prevention. Identification of risk factors plays an important role in renal protection for cardiac surgery (Table 4). The most powerful postoperative predictor of renal dysfunction is depressed cardiac function following CPB. Postoperative evidence of myocardial dysfunction, including low CO state and need for inotropic support, is associated with a two- to fourfold increased risk of renal injury. Prolonged positive pressure ventilation, preexisting cytomegalovirus infection, and postoperative sepsis present additional risks for renal dysfunction and/or ARF.

Monitoring kidney function is not easy, and no single test evaluates all renal activity. Serum creatinine is the most commonly used test to assess perioperative renal function. Its major limitation is its nonlinear relationship with glomerular filtration rate (GFR), making it insensitive to GFR above 30 mL per minute. Plasma creatinine reflects a state of equilibrium between creatinine production and excretion and is influenced by gender, weight, and especially age. Creatine clearance and fractional excretion of sodium (FENa) (estimated as urine/plasma [U/P] sodium concentration divided by U/P creatinine) are probably better reflections of true renal function. However, they are rarely done because they are laborious and time-consuming.

In the absence of clinically proven renal protective drugs, current perioperative management of the cardiac surgical patient should include measures to ensure minimal renal stress such as maintenance of adequate intravascular volume and perfusion as well as avoidance of medullary hypoxia. While no firm evidence endorses the use of any drug to protect the kidney, several "renal protective" regimens remain popular. Activation of peripheral dopaminergic receptors (DA_1) has important effects on renal perfusion and tubular metabolism. Use of intravenous "renal dose" dopamine as a "protective" intervention is based largely upon the DA_1-mediated natriuretic, diuretic, and renal vasodilating properties of this drug at doses of 0.5 to 3.0 μg per kg per minute. While many animal models of renal stress demonstrate significant improvements in renal function, most human clinical studies have not shown a similar benefit. Dopamine increases global renal blood flow without augmenting medullary blood flow and therefore does not prevent medullary hypoxia. It has been used as prophylactic therapy in both patients with normal function as well as in those with significant preexisting renal injury. One must also keep in mind that use of intravenous

dopamine, even at low doses, may cause significant complications and any benefits from dopamine used solely for renal protection should be carefully considered against such complications (59). The potential usefulness of other clinically available DA_1-receptor agonists such as fenoldopam and dopexamine as renal protective agents, have yet to be determined. Fenoldopam does seem to have some promise (60). In the setting of the critical care unit, it has been shown to improve renal function. Current studies examining its role in the cardiac surgical patient are ongoing.

The rationale for use of diuretics as renal protective agents is that they induce a diuresis and natriuresis, potentially reducing the possibility of tubular obstruction following renal insult. While osmotic diuretics, such as mannitol, also reduce tubular swelling to achieve this goal, a secondary proposed protective property unique to loop diuretic agents, such as furosemide, is the reduction in medullary tubular oxygen consumption. Animal models of myoglobinuric and ischemic renal failure demonstrate a protective effect from mannitol. However, with the exception of usefulness in the setting of early myoglobinuric ARF and renal transplantation, clinical renal protective effects of mannitol have not been confirmed (58). There is similarly no convincing clinical evidence to advocate the use of furosemide as renoprotective. In contrast, both furosemide and mannitol have been incriminated in aggravating renal injury in some settings. A deleterious property common to the use of all diuretics is that they can induce dehydration if intravascular volume status is not carefully monitored. While there is some evidence that oliguric renal failure can be converted to nonoliguric renal failure by the use of diuretics, there is no proof that the reduced mortality seen with nonoliguric renal failure applies to patients receiving diuretics, or that "responders" do not simply represent a less injured subgroup of oliguric patients.

Neurocognitive Deficits

Central nervous system (CNS) dysfunction after CPB represents a continuum from neurocognitive deficits, occurring in approximately 25% to 80% of patients after CABG with CPB to overt stroke occurring in 1% to 5% of patients undergoing CABG (17,18). Successful strategies for perioperative cerebral protection begin with accurate individual patient risk assessment. Although studies differ somewhat as to all the risk factors, certain patient characteristics consistently demonstrate an increased risk for cardiac surgery-associated neurologic injury (Table 5). The factors representing key predictive variables in a recently validated model

TABLE 5. RISK FACTORS FOR NEUROLOGIC INJURY

Age
Symptomatic neurologic disease
Previous coronary artery bypass grafting
Triple vessel disease
Vascular disease
Unstable angina
Diabetes
Pulmonary disease
Aortic atherosclerosis
Normothermic (>35°C) cardiopulmonary bypass

include increasing age, history of symptomatic neurologic disease, prior CABG surgery, vascular disease, unstable angina, diabetes, and pulmonary disease (61).

Most current strategies aimed toward risk reduction involve intraoperative measures. However, tailoring anesthetic technique to allow earlier postoperative awakening may play a significant role in assessment and treatment of patients with postoperative neurologic dysfunction. Patients remaining comatose after surgery need early investigation. Metabolic abnormalities, drug side effect or overdose, or a primary CNS event need to be ruled out. An early computerized tomographic scan is warranted if the patient is hemodynamically stable. Early assessment may also allow intervention through pharmacologic or other methods.

Difficult Weaning from Ventilation

Most cardiac surgical patients are expeditiously weaned from mechanical ventilation. However, there remains a group of patients who present difficulty weaning from the ventilator. Identification of preoperative risk factors of this complication has been difficult. There is general agreement that patient factors play a major role and older patients, especially those with poor LV function, are extubated more slowly. Extubation imposes a significant stress on the cardiorespiratory system. The difference in oxygen consumption between spontaneous and total mechanical ventilation can be substantial (62). Intraoperative and postoperative predictors of failure to wean include prolonged CPB, high oxygen requirements, high ventilatory pressures, and low CO (63–65). There is a necessity to develop a set of risk factors that will aid physicians in matching patients to extubation criteria.

No weaning mode has proven superior for patients who are difficult to wean from the ventilator. T-piece trial, synchronized intermittent mandatory ventilation (SIMV), and pressure support ventilation (PSV) are equally effective for weaning. The best technique is likely to be the one most familiar to the ICU staff. Respiratory mechanics may also predict successful weaning. The respiratory rate/tidal volume (RR/V_T) ratio has been used with some success as a predictor of failure to wean. An RR/V_T ratio greater than 105 resulted in 95% of patients failing to wean, whereas an RR/V_T ratio less than 105 resulted in a weaning success of 80% (64). No single method of predicting failure to wean has been consistently successful, and close clinical monitoring is mandatory after extubation to determine those in need of reintubation.

One of the most common reasons for failure to wean is pulmonary edema, which worsens gas exchange and increases work of breathing. The correct diagnosis is made with a careful clinical examination, assessment of net fluid balance, and review of a chest radiograph. The etiology of the pulmonary edema will guide therapy. Aggressive diuresis may be indicated for patients with good cardiac function. Patients with poor cardiac function and pulmonary edema will need afterload reduction and/or inodilator therapy in combination with diuresis in preparation for successful extubation. It has been suggested that there is a "window" period during which extubation is easiest. This period starts as soon as the patient is stabilized in the SICU and normally occurs between 4 to 5 hours following admission. Most patients who have surgery in the morning are extubated in the late afternoon or early evening. Whether it is safer to extubate patients arriving late in the SICU

during the night or early the following morning depends on the availability of experienced staff in the middle of the night and the ability to safely and rapidly reintubate the patient if required. It is important to realize that prolonged intubation time may lead to respiratory tract mucociliary dysfunction, diminished clearing of secretions, additional sedation, and increased atelectasis (63).

Accelerated Recovery from Cardiac Surgery

Following open-heart surgery in the past, patients were traditionally maintained on sedation and mechanical ventilation until the morning after surgery. The belief was that cardiovascular and other organ systems needed recovery time from the profound physiologic disturbances induced by CPB. The idea of early extubation and minimization of ICU time, often termed "fast track," has been suggested for many years (66). Little attention was paid to the idea until the climate of cost containment and scarce ICU resources became a reality in the 1990s. The push toward improved cost-effectiveness in all areas of health care has resulted in a trend for early weaning from ventilator support and a shortened ICU and hospital length of stay (LOS) after cardiac surgery (67,68). This new trend is made possible with innovative surgical and anesthetic techniques as well as improved postoperative sedative and analgesic agents. Changes in surgical and anesthetic techniques include reduction in invasive monitoring, lower dosage of intraoperative opioids and benzodiazepines, and warmer core temperatures. Use of short-acting sedatives, such as propofol and dexmedetomidine, and nonsedating analgesics such as nonsteroidals for postoperative pain has hastened recovery from anesthesia and surgery. User-friendly system changes, such as preprinted management protocols and preauthorized transfer orders, have enabled rapid transit of patients through the ICU. Some centers avoid admitting patients to a conventional ICU altogether and use a cardiac recovery area instead (69).

The medical literature is mixed on the virtue of "fast-track" protocols. Opponents of accelerated recovery argue that patient outcome may be adversely affected. Disadvantages claimed are unrecognized morbidity from decreased monitoring intensity, possible delay in response to life-threatening scenarios, increase in reintubation rate, difficulties in selecting candidates for accelerated recovery, and potential patient and/or family displeasure with late evening or early morning patient transfers. While concern may exist that response time be prolonged for treatment of life-threatening complications in a lower acuity unit, evidence collected in studies of accelerated recovery has failed to confirm this fear. Life-threatening events remain an uncommon occurrence and can be minimized by strict criteria for removal from accelerated recovery protocols and a dedicated accelerated recovery team (70).

Reports conflict concerning the success of early extubation, and on morbidity following reintubation. Success rate varies from 60% (71) to 85% (73,74). Conventionally weaned patients who require reintubation have increased mortality (74) and morbidity including longer ICU LOS, ventilator dependency, a higher incidence of nosocomial pneumonia, and prolonged period of rehabilitation (75). However, fast-track patients requiring reintubation do not seem to experience the same morbidity (72,73), likely due to differences in the indication for reintubation in the two groups. Different approaches exist for selecting suitable fast-track patients. One approach is to set inclusion criteria. Preoperative patient characteristics alone tend to be imprecise (76). Other important considerations include the patient's clinical condition after weaning from CPB (77) and on arrival in the ICU (78). Others advocate considering all patients as fast-track candidates and setting perioperative criteria for excluding patients for accelerated recovery (79). Major factors associated with failure of early extubation include advanced age, requirement for inotropic or IABP therapy, persistent hypothermia, bleeding, and rapid atrial dysrhythmias.

During the initial phase of adoption of any fast-track protocol, monitoring for adverse effects is mandatory. Page and Washburn report a fourfold increase in the incidence of ARF following initiation of a fast-track protocol previously reported as successful (80). The problem was solved by screening for patients at highest risk for renal failure and targeting renal protection in this population. This intervention also decreased the overall incidence of perioperative renal dysfunction. This report emphasizes the importance of careful monitoring during the introduction of published patient care protocols, due to differences in institutions and patient populations.

Cost reduction is a major driving force behind accelerated recovery. One institution with fast-track recovery managed to decrease the average ICU and hospital costs per patient by 53% and 25%, respectively, without change in morbidity. Other benefits included a 15% increase in case volume and a decrease in cancellation (81). It is important to understand that new protocols alone do not result in real savings. A paradigm shift among all medical personnel involved is needed (70,82,83). Reengineering of the entire process, starting from the time the patient is scheduled for surgery until the patient's last postoperative outpatient visit, is required for any significant cost reduction to be realized. Whether such improvement will be seen nationwide or will have only a cost shifting effect without real savings in the overall care of patients undergoing CABG remains to be seen. Besides potential cost reductions, early extubation may offer increased patient satisfaction, earlier interaction between patient and relatives, earlier return to normal diet, improved pulmonary function with less postoperative pneumonia (84), earlier mobilization, and improved perioperative mental status (73).

MINIMALLY INVASIVE CARDIAC SURGERY

Minimally invasive cardiac surgery describes an expanding array of surgical procedures intended to lower costs, lessen postoperative pain, facilitate patient recovery, hasten hospital discharge, and speed return to a normal lifestyle. The combination of market forces driving cost reduction and the success of angioplasty techniques in relieving cardiac ischemia mandates reassessment of conventional coronary artery revascularization techniques. While the duration of patency for coronary arteries undergoing angioplasty does not tend to be as long as that achieved by conventional surgical revascularization, the initial cost of angioplasty is lower with lower initial morbidity for the patient (85). A surgical procedure that combines lower cost and lower patient morbidity may

compare favorably with angioplasty. Surgical techniques for coronary revascularization can be divided into five groups as outlined in Table 6.

Minimally Invasive Direct Coronary Artery Bypass

The main difference between minimally invasive direct coronary artery bypass (MIDCAB) and conventional CABG is the avoidance of complete sternotomy. The classic approach for MIDCAB is a left thoracotomy, but alternative incisions including right thoracotomy, partial sternotomy, and parasternal incisions have been used depending on the need for exposure. While avoidance of median sternotomy may hasten postoperative recovery, these potential benefits have not been conclusively demonstrated. There is also no decrease is cost compared with conventional CABG. As a result, MIDCAB is not as widely used as other "minimally invasive" techniques.

Port-Access Surgery

Port-access heart surgery also allows avoidance of median sternotomy. In the port-access technique, aortic occlusion is achieved with an endoaortic balloon introduced percutaneously in the right parasternal region of the first or second intercostal space, and right heart cannulation is accomplished via the femoral vein. Surgical incision can be a right or left anterior thoracotomy depending on the procedure planned. Advantages of port-access heart surgery include lower mediastinitis rates, lower AF rates, faster patient recovery, and avoidance of hazardous sternotomy for "redo" cardiac surgery. While coronary or valve surgery can be accomplished with the port-access technique, the right thoracotomy approach with full CPB is especially useful for mitral valve procedures. A recent trial of port-access mitral valve surgery revealed a significantly smaller skin incision and a faster return to normal patient activity (4 weeks versus 9 weeks) when compared with conventional median sternotomy (86). Other trials found shorter lengths of hospital stay, fewer blood transfusions, and lower rates of AF in the port-access group (87,88). Both MIDCAB and port-access surgery require CPB and heparinization. Therefore, epidural catheter placement is not recommended and postoperative management does not differ markedly from patients with conventional CABG.

Off-Pump Coronary Artery Bypass

Off-pump coronary artery bypass (OPCAB) procedures are CABG procedures performed with partial to full heparinization on the beating heart without support of CPB. Transfusion requirements for platelets and coagulation factors should be decreased with the avoidance of CPB and deliberate hypothermia. Lack of atriotomy may reduce the incidence of atrial dysrhythmias. Potential benefits of OPCAB procedures include a lower incidence of neurologic dysfunction, decreased pulmonary complications, fewer dysrhythmias, lower cost, and reduced transfusion requirements compared with conventional CABG (89–93). Postoperatively, patients can be extubated earlier as they have less bleeding and do not require further rewarming.

TABLE 6. COMPARISON OF MINIMALLY INVASIVE CARDIAC SURGICAL TECHNIQUES

Technique	Incision Site	Cannulation Site	Advantages	Disadvantages
Conventional CABG	Median sternotomy	Ascending aorta Right atrium	Excellent exposure Stable closure Extensive experience	Mediastinitis Slow recovery of upper extremity function Postoperative cough limited by pain
MIDCAB	Left thoracotomy Alt: paramedian or right thoracotomy Alt: partial sternotomy	Ascending aorta Right atrium	Avoids median sternotomy Useful for redo procedure Hasten recovery of upper extremity function[a]	Limited exposure No cost savings May require multiple incisions
Port-Access	Right anterior thoracotomy Alt: paramedian or left thoracotomy	Ascending aorta via right paramedian port Femoral vein	Avoids median sternotomy Avoids atriotomy Access to mitral valve Smaller skin incision Decreases hospital stay[a] Decreases atrial fibrillation incidence[a] Decreases transfusion[a] Decreases rehabilitation time[a]	Increased cost of equipment Contraindicated in patients with ascending aortic pathology Limited operative exposure Significant learning curve Unlikely to decrease cerebral emboli
OPCAB	Median sternotomy Alt: right or left thoracotomy Alt: partial sternotomy	None	Avoids aortic manipulation Avoids atriotomy and CPB Normothermia Decreases atrial fib incidence[a] Decreases transfusion[a] Decreases neurologic morbidity[b] Decreases pulmonary morbidity[b]	Cost of equipment Slow recovery of upper extremity function Mediastinitis Increases intraoperative ischemia Undetermined graft longevity
TMLR	Left thoracotomy	None	Decreases angina and increases quality of life for patients deemed inoperable Epidural analgesia safe Avoids median sternotomy Normothermia	Increased cost of equipment No immediate decrease of ischemia Decreases systolic function postoperatively Decreases diastolic function postoperatively Increases perioperative myocardial edema

[a]Limited supporting evidence exists.
[b]Proposed benefit.
CABG, coronary artery bypass grafting; MIDCAB, minimally invasive direct coronary artery bypass; CPB, cardiopulmonary bypass; OPCAB, off-pump coronary artery bypass; TMLR, transmyocardial laser revascularization.

Special considerations for OPCAB patients include concern for postoperative ischemia and the expectation of rapid recovery. During surgery, some patients are unable to tolerate OPCAB due to ischemia or cardiac failure and must be placed urgently on conventional CPB. These patients may suffer a significant decrement in ventricular function after CPB and may require aggressive inotropic or IABP support in the postoperative period. Although short-term patency of the left internal mammary artery graft is thought to be comparable to that of conventional grafts (90), evidence of postoperative myocardial ischemia warrants rapid intervention. Serial ECGs, serial myocardial enzyme levels, PA catheterization data, radionuclide stress testing, and coronary angiography could all be helpful in this evaluation. Pain management can be challenging in this fast-track patient population and aggressive respiratory therapy is required for prevention of postoperative pulmonary complications. Patient-controlled opioids can provide effective pain relief for these patients in a monitored setting of an ICU or step-down unit. Epidural analgesia is not commonly performed because of intraoperative heparinization.

Transmyocardial Laser Revascularization

Transmyocardial laser revascularization (TMLR) is a procedure designed to provide symptom relief and improved quality of life for patients with intractable myocardial ischemia not amenable to conventional CABG. This patient group often has undergone previous median sternotomy for bypass grafting and has recurrent coronary occlusion. The procedure uses myocardial microinjury induced by transmural laser passage through the myocardium from the epicardium to the LV cavity at multiple points over the LV surface. During the healing phase of the myocardial injury, the hope is that angiogenesis will occur with a net result of increased blood flow to the ischemic region over time. After recovery from TMLR, patients experience diminished anginal symptoms, increased exercise tolerance, increased survival free of cardiac events, and fewer cardiac-related rehospitalizations (94). The procedure is performed through a left thoracotomy with normothermia and a balanced anesthetic technique. The patients are either extubated in the operating room or shortly after arrival in the ICU.

TMLR does not immediately increase myocardial blood flow and myocardial ischemia is still a major concern in the early postoperative period. In fact, regional ischemia and impaired regional systolic function may be worsened with an increase in myocardial water content and impaired diastolic relaxation (95). Management with a PA catheter to monitor CO and intravascular volume together with the usual continuous monitoring of ECG, arterial pressure, oxygen saturation, and urine output is mandatory. The hemoglobin level should be maintained at 10 to 12 g per dL to optimize oxygen delivery. Inotropic support may be necessary for a low CO state. NTG is helpful in maximizing coronary and collateral blood flow. Afterload reduction and forced diuresis are often necessary to prevent LV failure. Care must be taken to avoid extreme depression of aortic diastolic pressure, which is the driving pressure for coronary perfusion. Tachycardia and diastolic dysfunction should be treated with cardioselective β-blockers, such as metoprolol or esmolol, to minimize myocardial depression. Effective pain management with thoracic epidural analgesia is extremely helpful in decreasing the stress on the compromised heart, and administration of local anesthetic through the epidural may improve postoperative angina. TMLR patients represent one of the most challenging patient groups in the cardiac SICU.

Minimally invasive cardiac surgery is a rapidly evolving field, and cardiac surgery will continue to change with economic and quality improvement pressures on the health care industry. The challenge to stay abreast of the changes in intraoperative management as they impact on postoperative management is one of great importance for the intensivist.

TRANSFUSION

Cardiac surgical patients are major consumers of blood bank resources. It is estimated that approximately 20% of all blood transfused in North America is associated with cardiac surgical procedures. There is a wide variation in transfusion practice nationwide. Depending on the institution, between 27% and 92% of CABG patients are transfused, and the number of units of packed cells received ranges from 0 to 4 (96).

Transfusion-related complications have decreased significantly in the last 10 to 15 years, but still remain a concern. Since the introduction of the hepatitis C test, the rate of viral infection has dropped to approximately 1 in 50,000. The risk of human immunodeficiency virus transmission is less than 1 in 500,000 and is no longer the main reason for avoiding blood transfusion (97). While the risk of major ABO incompatibility is less than 1 in 33,000, the incidence of minor transfusion reactions approaches 1 in 5 (98).

According to the American Society of Anesthesiologists (ASA), cost of transfusion therapy approaches 5 to 7 billion dollars per year in the United States, with up to 25% of red blood cell (RBC) transfusions judged to be unnecessary. The ASA strongly advocates judicious use of blood products and has published a set of practice guidelines (Table 7) (98). While it is important to remember that practice guidelines are imperfect and must not replace clinical judgment, the ASA guidelines provide a scientifically based model to assist decision-making. In the cardiac surgical patient population, the ASA guidelines fail to account for platelet dysfunction known to occur following CPB. When major bleeding occurs in this group, platelet transfusion is indicated even when platelet count is above 100,000 (99).

Unfortunately practice guidelines such as those from the ASA and the College of American Pathologists do not seem to change old transfusion habits, and inappropriate use of blood products has not been curtailed, especially in the cardiac surgical population (100). One possible reason for lack of success is the time delay for return of coagulation results from the laboratory, making directed transfusion therapy difficult in a bleeding patient. In response to this problem, several rapid assay devices are being developed. When combined with protocol-driven blood product

TABLE 7. AMERICAN SOCIETY OF ANESTHESIOLOGISTS TRANSFUSION PRACTICE GUIDELINES

Red blood cells should be transfused to increase oxygen delivery for patients at risk of developing complications from inadequate tissue oxygenation

Red blood cell transfusion should not be based on a single hemoglobin "trigger"

Red blood cell transfusion is rarely indicated when the hemoglobin concentration is greater than 10 g/dL

Red blood cell transfusion is almost always indicated when the hemoglobin concentration is less than 6 g/dL

Prophylactic platelet transfusion is not indicated in a nonbleeding patient when thrombocytopenia is due to increased platelet destruction

Surgical and obstetric patients usually require platelet transfusion if the platelet count is less than 50,000/1^{-6} and microvascular bleeding is present

Surgical and obstetric patients rarely require platelet transfusion if the platelet count is greater than 100,000/1^{-6}

Indications for fresh frozen plasma transfusion include:
1. Urgent reversal of warfarin therapy
2. Correction of factor deficiencies for which specific concentrates are unavailable
3. Correction of microvascular bleeding when prothrombin or partial thromboplastin times are >1.5 times normal

Fresh-frozen plasma is contraindicated for augmentation of plasma volume or albumin concentration

Indications for cryoprecipitate include:
1. von Willebrand disease unresponsive to desmopressin
2. Bleeding patients with von Willebrand disease
3. Bleeding patients with fibrinogen levels < 80–100 mg/dL

Adapted from American Society of Anesthesiologists Task Force on Blood Component Therapy, 1996. ASA, Park Ridge, IL, 1996# 249, with permission.

therapy, such "point-of-care" tests may serve to improve care and limit unnecessary transfusion (101,102).

Other strategies for limiting blood product requirements show some benefit in clinical trials. The use of antifibrinolytic therapy decreases the incidence of excessive postoperative bleeding due to coagulopathy (103,104). Effective antifibrinolytic agents include ϵ-aminocaproic acid, tranexamic acid and aprotinin. Intraoperative autologous hemodilution has also demonstrated a blood-sparing effect in some studies (105), but postoperative use of cell salvage has not proven to be effective in limiting use of blood products in cardiac surgery (106). Reinfusion of shed mediastinal blood may be associated with greater frequency of wound infection (107).

Several new products, designed to deliver oxygen and decrease dependence on allogeneic RBC transfusion, are under development and clinical trials. They can be divided into two main groups, perfluorocarbons and hemoglobin-based oxygen carriers. Perfluorocarbons are synthetic fluorinated hydrocarbons that increase the amount of dissolved oxygen in blood. At a given dose of perfluorocarbon, a linear relationship exists between the amount of oxygen dissolved and the Pa_{O_2}, with significant quantities of dissolved oxygen available for delivery for tissue use at high FI_{O_2}.

Hemoglobin-based oxygen carriers, either cross-linked or microencapsulated hemoglobin molecules, are extracted from human or bovine red cells. Human hemoglobin can also be produced from bacteria through genetic engineering technology. These products are sterilized by pasteurization, ultrafiltration, and chemical means, virtually eliminating the risk of bacterial or viral disease transmission. Since they have no cell-surface antigens, no need for typing or crossmatching exists. They also have a long shelf life. Side effects associated with hemoglobin-based oxygen carriers include complement fixation, toxic breakdown products such as hemin and iron, prooxidant activity, and nitric oxide scavenging with resultant hypertension and gastrointestinal dysmotility (108). Intramolecular crosslinking or encapsulation of the hemoglobin products reduces the associated side effects (109). While crosslinked hemoglobin products are undergoing advanced clinical trials, encapsulated hemoglobin molecules are still in the preclinical development stage.

RISK STRATIFICATION

The overall mortality for CABG has gradually decreased over the years and approaches 1% in low-risk patient populations (110). However, there is a subset of patients in whom morbidity and mortality remain high. Several risk scores have been developed to help identify this population of high-risk cardiac patients. The risk scores show excellent correlation with outcome for large groups of patients (76,111–114). Risk factors for adverse outcome common to these studies include advanced age, small patient size, female gender, prior cardiac surgery, hypoalbuminemia, emergent surgery, renal insufficiency, severe LV dysfunction, preoperative IABP, severe lung disease, and valvular dysfunction. The identified risk factors can be used for counseling patients as well as improving preparation for management of anticipated complications.

Other factors that influence outcome are intraoperative events. Duration of CPB, requirement for IABP following CPB, hemodynamic instability on ICU arrival, metabolic acidosis, and elevated alveolar-to-arterial oxygen gradient also predict increased morbidity and mortality (78). Combined preoperative and perioperative risk factors may be beneficial in predicting prolonged ICU stay and counseling surrogate decision makers for postoperative treatment decisions.

Risk stratification scores have also been developed for identifying patients at high risk of adverse neurologic outcome (61). The incidence of adverse neurologic outcome remains high with rates of type I adverse neurologic outcome (cerebral death, nonfatal stroke, or new transient ischemic attack [TIA]) reported to be up to 8.4% in patients undergoing intracardiac surgery combined with CABG (115). The incidence of less severe but persistent neurocognitive impairment following cardiac surgery with CPB is estimated to be between 22% (116) and 66% (117). The most-significant risk factors for adverse neurologic outcome relate to the formation of embolic material. These include proximal aortic atherosclerotic plaque, intracardiac thrombus, endocarditis, or repeated aortic cross-clamping (115). The preoperative risk factors included in the risk index by Newman and colleagues also correlate with the development of advanced atherosclerotic disease in the proximal aorta (61). The use of epiaortic ECG to further risk stratify patients with advanced ascending aortic plaque may allow intraoperative alteration of technique to avoid the diseased aorta. Limiting the procedure to off-pump coronary bypass techniques without aortic manipulation in this patient group may provide an opportunity to finally decrease the devastating neurologic complications associated with cardiac surgery.

While risk stratification scores correlate well with outcome in large groups of patients undergoing cardiac surgery, the sensitivity and specificity of these scores is inadequate to predict when an individual patient will have an adverse event (118). Therefore, these risk scores are mainly useful for comparison of anticipated outcome with actual outcome within an institution and between institutions as a guide for quality improvement. While helpful in establishing a patient as high risk or low risk for a procedure, a scoring system with higher predictive value is needed before risk stratification will be able to guide clinical decision making in the individual patient.

SUMMARY

The cardiac surgical patient population presents a unique opportunity for application of clinical acumen complemented by the use of advanced technology leading to improvement in patient outcome. This group of patients undergoes major physiologic stress with limited perioperative reserve, making effective supportive care essential to their recovery. As with other types of ICU patients, the key component of beneficence as well as nonmaleficence is attention to detail on the part of the ICU team. Knowledge of the patient's baseline condition, rapid and accurate assessment of the physiologic impact of perioperative events, effective management of trends in invasive monitoring data, and sound clinical judgment provide the framework for optimization of patient care. Ongoing research is seeking less invasive yet more effective techniques and attempting to identify patient populations for which the benefit of intervention far outweighs the risk. Such knowledge will empower practitioners to provide optimized patient care at acceptable cost with improved outcome.

KEY POINTS

- Perioperative hypothermia is associated with shivering, and possibly ischemia, coagulopathies, and infection.
- It is rare for patients to be extubated in the operating room; most patients require ventilatory support for 4 to 8 hours. Initial ventilator settings are aimed to provide complete support of the work of breathing for the patient.
- If the target of a cardiac index greater than 2 is not achieved with optimization of preload, afterload, and HR, infusion of an inotrope is usually required to improve cardiac contractility.
- Hemostasis is assessed by the amount of blood draining out of the chest tubes. If drainage from the chest tube exceeds 400 mL in the first 2 hours and 100 to 150 mL per hour after the first 2 hours, platelets and/or fresh frozen plasma are probably required to stop the bleeding.

- No definitive studies to date have documented a significantly shorter ICU or hospital length of stay due to extubation of cardiac surgical patients in the operating room. Most patients receive an infusion of a short-acting sedative such as propofol or dexmedetomidine supplemented with an opioid when necessary, as these drugs have no analgesic property. Other popular sedative agents include midazolam and fentanyl.

- Weaning from ventilatory support can start once the patient spontaneously breathes over the rate set on the ventilator, is normothermic, has adequate pulmonary gas exchange and mechanical function, has emerged sufficiently from anesthesia, has no significant drainage from the chest tubes, has no residual neuromuscular blockade, and has stable cardiac function.

- If the patient has remained stable during recovery from anesthesia and has no significant pulmonary disease, a rapid decrease in ventilator support to minimal levels can be safely instituted under close observation, and the patient evaluated for extubation.

- Cardiac tamponade should be suspected in any unstable patient or one whose condition is acutely deteriorating, particularly if right-sided filling pressures are high.

- Postoperative myocardial ischemia as a result of incomplete revascularization or acute occlusion of either the native coronaries or the bypass grafts can result in a low output state.

- Persistent, postoperative ST segment changes should be investigated for acute myocardial ischemia/infarction, with serial 12-lead electrocardiogram tracings, routine laboratory tests, cardiac enzymes (CK-MB and troponin levels), echocardiography, and angiography.

- Calcific aortic valve or tricuspid valve replacement may carry a 20% risk for permanent pacing and there is an increased incidence of high-degree arteriovenous block following either mitral valve repair or replacement.

- Atrial dysrhythmias (primarily atrial fibrillation) are by far the most common dysrhythmias following coronary artery bypass graft (CABG) surgery with an overall incidence of approximately 30%. Atrial fibrillation most commonly occurs 2 to 3 days after surgery and can increase hospital stay, risk of stroke, and mortality.

- Infection rates in patients undergoing cardiac surgery tend to be higher due to a number of factors including prolonged operative time, presence of indwelling catheters, deleterious effects of cardiopulmonary bypass (CPB) on the immune system, poor tissue perfusion, hyperglycemia, and implantation of foreign material.

- Significant postoperative worsening of renal function is observed in approximately 7% of patients with approximately 15% of these patients requiring dialysis.

- No firm evidence endorses the use of any drug to protect the kidney, yet several "renal protective" regimens remain popular.

- Central nervous system dysfunction after CABG represents a continuum from neurocognitive deficits, occurring in approximately 25% to 80% of patients after CABG with CPB, to overt stroke occurring in 1% to 5% of patients undergoing CABG.

- The main difference between minimally invasive direct coronary artery bypass (MIDCAB) and conventional CABG is the avoidance of complete sternotomy.

- Port-access heart surgery also allows avoidance of median sternotomy. In the port-access technique, aortic occlusion is achieved with an endoaortic balloon introduced percutaneously in the right parasternal region of the first or second intercostal space and right heart cannulation is accomplished via the femoral vein. Operative incision can be a right or left anterior thoracotomy depending on the procedure planned.

- Off-pump coronary artery bypass (OPCAB) procedures are CABG procedures performed with partial to full heparinization on the beating heart without support of CPB.

- Transmyocardial laser revascularization utilizes myocardial microinjury induced by transmural laser passage through the myocardium from the epicardium to the left ventricular (LV) cavity at multiple points over the LV surface. During the healing phase of the myocardial injury, the hope is that angiogenesis will occur with a net result of increased blood flow to the ischemic region over time.

- In unstable patients failing to respond to optimized volume resuscitation and infusion of inotropes, transfuse blood and blood products as needed for intravascular volume replacement until the patient is stable. In high-risk patients, hematocrit should be maintained at 27%, and in stable patients, at 23%.

REFERENCES

1. *2000 heart and stroke statistical update*. Dallas: American Heart Association, 2000.

2. Engoren M. Marginal cost of liberating ventilator-dependent patients after cardiac surgery in a stepdown unit. *Ann Thorac Surg* 2000;70(1):182.

3. Montes FR, et al. The lack of benefit of tracheal extubation in the operating room after coronary artery bypass surgery. *Anesth Analg* 2000;91(4):776–780.

4. Connors AF Jr, et al. The effectiveness of right heart catheterization in the initial care of critically ill patients. SUPPORT Investigators. *JAMA* 1996;276(11):889–897.

5. Casthely PA, Yoganathan T, Komer C, et al. Magnesium and arrhythmias after coronary artery bypass surgery. *J Cardiothorac Vasc Anesth* 1994;8(2):188–191.

6. Gulker H, Haverkamp W, Hindricks G. [Ion regulation disorders and cardiac arrhythmia. The relevance of sodium, potassium, calcium, and magnesium]. *Arzneimittel-Forschung* 1989;39(1A):130–134.

7. Baglin A, et al. Metabolic adverse reactions to diuretics. Clinical relevance to elderly patients. *Drug Safety* 1995;12(3):161–167.

8. Hollifield JW. Thiazide treatment of hypertension. Effects of thiazide diuretics on serum potassium, magnesium, and ventricular ectopy. *Am J Med* 1986;80(4A):8–12.

9. Ryan M. Interrelationships of potassium and magnesium homeostasis. *Mineral Electrolyte Metab* 1993;19:290–295.

10. Chadda KD. Clinical hypomagnesemia, coronary spasm and cardiac arrhythmia. *Magnesium* 1986 5(1):47–52.
11. Frank S, Beattie C, Christopherson R. Unintentional hypothermia is associated with postoperative myocardial ischemia. *Anesthesiology* 1993;78:468.
12. Kurz A, Sessler D, Lenhardt R. Perioperative normothermia to reduce the incidence of surgical-wound infection and shorten hospitalization. Study of Wound Infection and Temperature Group. *N Engl J Med* 1996;334(19):1209–1215.
13. Kurz A, Kurz M, Poeschl G. Forced-air warming maintains intraoperative normothermia better than circulating water mattresses. *Anesth Analg* 1993;77:89.
14. Wang J, et al. A comparison among nalbuphine, meperidine, and placebo for treating postanesthetic shivering. *Anesth Analg* 1999;88(3):686–689.
15. Perdue PW, Balser JR, Lipsett PA, et al. "Renal dose" dopamine in surgical patients: dogma or science? *Ann Surg* 1998;227(4):470–473.
16. Mathur V, et al. The effects of fenoldopam, a selective dopamine receptor agonist, on systemic and renal hemodynamics in normotensive subjects. *Crit Care Med* 1999;27(9):1832–1837.
17. Nussmeier NA, Arlund C, Slogoff S. Neuropsychiatric complications after cardiopulmonary bypass: cerebral protection by a barbiturate. *Anesthesiology* 1986;64(2):165–170.
18. Borowicz LM, et al. Neuropsychologic change after cardiac surgery: a critical review. *J Cardiothorac Vasc Anesth* 1996;10(1):105–11; quiz 111–112.
19. Durbin CG Jr, Kopel RF. Optimal atrioventricular (AV) pacing interval during temporary AV sequential pacing after cardiac surgery. *J Cardiothorac Vasc Anesth* 1993 7(3):316–320.
20. Frostell C, et al. Inhaled nitric oxide. A selective pulmonary vasodilator reversing hypoxic pulmonary vasoconstriction [published erratum appears in *Circulation* 1991;84(5):2212]. *Circulation* 1991 83(6):2038–2047.
21. Russo AM, O'Connor WH, Waxman HL. Atypical presentations and echocardiographic findings in patients with cardiac tamponade occurring early and late after cardiac surgery. *Chest* 1993;104(1):71–78.
22. Chuttani K, et al. Diagnosis of cardiac tamponade after cardiac surgery: relative value of clinical, echocardiographic, and hemodynamic signs. *Am Heart J* 1994;127(4 Pt 1):913–918.
23. Christenson JT, et al. Open chest and delayed sternal closure after cardiac surgery. *Eur J Cardiothorac Surg* 1996;10(5):305–311.
24. Royster RL, et al. Combined inotropic effects of amrinone and epinephrine after cardiopulmonary bypass in humans. *Anesth Analg* 1993;77(4):662–672.
25. Dyke C. The use of thyroid hormone in cardiac surgery. *Curr Opin Cardiol* 1996;11(6):603–609.
26. Morales DL, et al. Arginine vasopressin in the treatment of 50 patients with postcardiotomy vasodilatory shock. *Ann Thorac Surg* 2000;69(1):102–106.
27. Griffin RM, Kaplan JA. Myocardial ischaemia during non-cardiac surgery. A comparison of different lead systems using computerised ST segment analysis. *Anaesthesia* 1987;42(2):155–159.
28. Mark JB, et al. Electrocardiographic R-wave changes during cardiac surgery. *Anesth Analg* 1992 74(1):26–31.
29. Tsuda H, et al. QRS complex changes in the V5 ECG lead during cardiac surgery. *J Cardiothorac Vasc Anesth* 1992;6(6):658–662.
30. Jaeger FJ, et al. Permanent pacing following repeat cardiac valve surgery. *Am J Cardiol* 1994;74(5):505–507.
31. Brodell GK, et al. Cardiac rhythm and conduction disturbances in patients undergoing mitral valve surgery. *Cleve Clin J Med* 1991;58(5):397–399.
32. Grant SC, et al. Atrial arrhythmias and pacing after orthotopic heart transplantation: bicaval versus standard atrial anastomosis. *Br Heart J* 1995;74(2):149–153.
33. Haught WH, et al. Theophylline reverses high-grade atrioventricular block resulting from cardiac transplant rejection. *Am Heart J* 1994;128(6 Pt 1):1255–1257.
34. Creswell LL, et al. Hazards of postoperative atrial arrhythmias. *Ann Thorac Surg* 1993;56(3):539–549.
35. Mathew J, et al. Atrial fibrillation following coronary artery bypass graft surgery: predictors, outcomes, and resource utilization. MultiCenter Study of Perioperative Ischemia Research Group. *JAMA* 1996;276(4):300–306.
36. Almassi GH, et al. Atrial fibrillation after cardiac surgery: a major morbid event? *Ann Surg* 1997 226(4):501–511; discussion 511–513.
37. Leitch JW, et al. The importance of age as a predictor of atrial fibrillation and flutter after coronary artery bypass grafting. *J Thorac Cardiovasc Surg* 1990;100(3):338–342.
38. England MR, et al. Magnesium administration and dysrhythmias after cardiac surgery. A placebo-controlled, double-blind, randomized trial. *JAMA* 1992;268(17):2395–2402.
39. Salazar C, et al. Beta-blockade therapy for supraventricular tachyarrhythmias after coronary surgery: a propranolol withdrawal syndrome? *Angiology* 1979;30(12):816–819.
40. Kowey R, et al. Meta-analysis of the effectiveness of prophylactic drug therapy in preventing supraventricular arrhythmia early after coronary artery bypass grafting. *Am J Cardiol* 1992;69(9):963–965.
41. Gomes JA, et al. Oral d,l sotalol reduces the incidence of postoperative atrial fibrillation in coronary artery bypass surgery patients: a randomized, double-blind, placebo-controlled study. *J Am Coll Cardiol* 1999 34(2):334–339.
42. Butler J, et al. Amiodarone prophylaxis for tachycardias after coronary artery surgery: a randomised, double blind, placebo controlled trial. *Br Heart J* 1993 70(1):56–60.
43. Daoud EG, et al. Preoperative amiodarone as prophylaxis against atrial fibrillation after heart surgery. *N Engl J Med* 1997;337(25):1785–1791.
44. Laub GW, et al. Prophylactic procainamide for prevention of atrial fibrillation after coronary artery bypass grafting: a prospective, double-blind, randomized, placebo-controlled pilot study. *Crit Care Med* 1993;21(10):1474–1478.
45. Greenberg MD, et al. Atrial pacing for the prevention of atrial fibrillation after cardiovascular surgery. *J Am Coll Cardiol* 2000;35(6):1416–1422.
46. Blommaert D, et al. Effective prevention of atrial fibrillation by continuous atrial overdrive pacing after coronary artery bypass surgery. *J Am Coll Cardiol* 2000;35(6):1411–1415.
47. Chung MK, et al. Ineffectiveness and potential proarrhythmia of atrial pacing for atrial fibrillation prevention after coronary artery bypass grafting. *Ann Thorac Surg* 2000;69(4):1057–1063.
48. Gerstenfeld E, et al. Evaluation of right atrial and biatrial temporary pacing for the prevention of atrial fibrillation after coronary artery bypass surgery. *J Am Coll Cardiol* 1999;33(7):1981–1988.
49. Tam SK, Miller JM, Edmunds LH Jr. Unexpected, sustained ventricular tachyarrhythmia after cardiac operations. *J Thorac Cardiovasc Surg* 1991;102(6):883–889.
50. Huikuri HV, et al. Prevalence and prognostic significance of complex ventricular arrhythmias after coronary arterial bypass graft surgery. *Int J Cardiol* 1990;27(3):333–339.
51. Pinto R, et al. Prognosis of patients with frequent premature ventricular complexes and nonsustained ventricular tachycardia after coronary artery bypass graft surgery. *Clin Cardiol* 1996;19(4):321–324.
52. Topol EJ, et al. De novo refractory ventricular tachyarrhythmias after coronary revascularization. *Am J Cardiol* 1986;57(1):57–59.
53. A comparison of antiarrhythmic-drug therapy with implantable defibrillators in patients resuscitated from near-fatal ventricular arrhythmias. The Antiarrhythmics versus Implantable Defibrillators (AVID) Investigators. *N Engl J Med* 1997;337(22):1576–1583.
54. Kluge RM, et al. Sources of contamination in open heart surgery. *JAMA* 1974;230(10):1415–1418.
55. Nelson RM, Dries DJ. The economic implications of infection in cardiac surgery. *Ann Thorac Surg* 1986;42(3):240–246.
56. Kreuzer E, et al. Early prediction of septic complications after cardiac surgery by APACHE II score. *Eur J Cardiothorac Surg* 1992;6(10):524–528; discussion 529.
57. Furnary A, et al. Continuous intravenous insulin infusion reduces the incidence of deep sternal wound infection in diabetic patients after cardiac surgical procedures. *Ann Thorac Surg* 1999;67(2):352–360; discussion 360–362.
58. Mangano CM, et al. Renal dysfunction after myocardial revascularization: risk factors, adverse outcomes, and hospital resource utilization.

The Multicenter Study of Perioperative Ischemia Research Group. *Ann Intern Med* 1998;128(3):194–203.

59. Denton MD, Chertow GM, Brady HR. "Renal-dose" dopamine for the treatment of acute renal failure: scientific rationale, experimental studies and clinical trials. *Kidney Int* 1996;50(1):4–14.

60. Singer I, Epstein M. Potential of dopamine A-1 agonists in the management of acute renal failure. *Am J Kidney Dis* 1998;31(5):743–755.

61. Newman MF, et al. Multicenter preoperative stroke risk index for patients undergoing coronary artery bypass graft surgery. Multicenter Study of Perioperative Ischemia (McSPI) Research Group. *Circulation* 1996;94[9 Suppl]:II74–II80.

62. Nathan SD, et al. Prediction of minimal pressure support during weaning from mechanical ventilation. *Chest* 1993;103(4):1215–1219.

63. Higgins TL. Safety issues regarding early extubation after coronary artery bypass surgery. *J Cardiothorac Vasc Anesth* 1995;9[5 Suppl 1]:24–29.

64. Yang KL, Tobin MJ. A prospective study of indexes predicting the outcome of trials of weaning from mechanical ventilation. *N Engl J Med* 1991;324(21):1445–1450.

65. Wahba RW. Pressure support ventilation. *J Cardiothoracic Anesth* 1990;4(5):624–630.

66. Quasha AL, et al. Postoperative respiratory care: a controlled trial of early and late extubation following coronary-artery bypass grafting. *Anesthesiology* 1980;52(2):135–141.

67. Engelman RM, et al. Fast-track recovery of the coronary bypass patient. *Ann Thorac Surg* 1994;58(6):1742–1746.

68. Marquez J, et al. Cardiac surgery "fast tracking" in an academic hospital. *J Cardiothorac Vasc Anesth* 1995;9[5 Suppl 1]:34–36.

69. Westaby S, et al. Does modern cardiac surgery require conventional intensive care? *Eur J Cardiothorac Surg* 1993;7(6):313–318.

70. Cheng DC. Fast-track cardiac surgery: economic implications in postoperative care. *J Cardiothorac Vasc Anesth* 1998;12(1):72–79.

71. Reyes A, et al. Early vs. conventional extubation after cardiac surgery with cardiopulmonary bypass. *Chest* 1997;112(1):193–201.

72. Silbert BS, et al. Early extubation following coronary artery bypass surgery: a prospective randomized controlled trial. The Fast Track Cardiac Care Team. *Chest* 1998;113(6):1481–1488.

73. Cheng DC, et al. Morbidity outcome in early versus conventional tracheal extubation after coronary artery bypass grafting: a prospective randomized controlled trial. *J Thorac Cardiovasc Surg* 1996;112(3):755–764.

74. Epstein SK, Ciubotaru RL, Wong JB. Effect of failed extubation on the outcome of mechanical ventilation. *Chest* 1997;112(1):186–192.

75. Alexander WA, Cooper JR Jr. Preoperative risk stratification identifies low-risk candidates for early extubation after aortocoronary bypass grafting. *Tex Heart Inst J* 1996;23(4):267–269.

76. Higgins TL, et al. Stratification of morbidity and mortality outcome by preoperative risk factors in coronary artery bypass patients. A clinical severity score [published erratum appears in *JAMA* 1992;268(14):1860]. *JAMA* 1992;267(17):2344–2348.

77. Becker RB, et al. The use of APACHE III to evaluate ICU length of stay, resource use, and mortality after coronary artery by-pass surgery. *J Cardiovasc Surg* (Torino) 1995;36(1):1–11.

78. Higgins TL, et al. ICU admission score for predicting morbidity and mortality risk after coronary artery bypass grafting. *Ann Thorac Surg* 1997;64(4):1050–1058.

79. Serna DL, Chen JC, Milliken JC. Accelerated recovery after coronary artery bypass surgery in patients with poor left ventricular function: preliminary report. *Am Surg* 1998;64(10):942–946.

80. Page US, Washburn T. Using tracking data to find complications that physicians miss: the case of renal failure in cardiac surgery. *Jt Comm J Qual Improv* 1997;23(10):511–520.

81. Cheng DC, et al. Early tracheal extubation after coronary artery bypass graft surgery reduces costs and improves resource use. A prospective, randomized, controlled trial. *Anesthesiology* 1996;85(6):1300–1310.

82. Clark JA, Kotyra LG, Brocious T. Rapid progression following cardiac surgery. *Crit Care Nurs Clin North Am* 1999;11(2):159–175.

83. Hadjinikolaou L, et al. The effect of a 'fast-track' unit on the performance of a cardiothoracic department. *Ann R Coll Surg Engl* 2000;82(1):53–58.

84. London MJ, et al. Fast-track cardiac surgery in a Department of Veterans Affairs patient population. *Ann Thorac Surg* 1997;64(1):134–141.

85. Weintraub WS, et al. A comparison of the costs of and quality of life after coronary angioplasty or coronary surgery for multivessel coronary artery disease. Results from the Emory Angioplasty Versus Surgery Trial (EAST). *Circulation* 1995;92(10):2831–2840.

86. Glower DD, Landolfo K, Clements FM. Mitral valve operation via port access versus median sternotomy. *Eur J Cardiothorac Surgery* 1998;14[Suppl 1]:S143–S147.

87. Cohn LH. Minimally invasive aortic valve surgery: technical considerations and results with the parasternal approach. *J Cardiac Surg* 1998;13(4):302–305.

88. Cosgrove DM 3rd, Sabik JF, Navia JL. Minimally invasive valve operations. *Ann Thorac Surg* 1998;65(6):1535–8; discussion 1538–1539.

89. Benetti FJ, et al. Direct myocardial revascularization without extracorporeal circulation. Experience in 700 patients. *Chest* 1991;100(2):312–316.

90. Buffolo E, et al. Myocardial revascularization without extracorporeal circulation. Seven-year experience in 593 cases. *Eur J Cardiothorac Surg* 1990;4(9):504–507.

91. Pfister AJ, et al. Coronary artery bypass without cardiopulmonary bypass. *Ann Thorac Surg* 1992;54(6):1085–1091; discussion 1091–1092.

92. Puskas JD, et al. Off-pump multivessel coronary bypass via sternotomy is safe and effective. *Ann Thorac Surg* 1998;66(3):1068–1072.

93. Doty JR, et al. Cost analysis of current therapies for limited coronary artery revascularization. *Circulation* 1997;96[9 Suppl]:II-16–20.

94. Allen KB, et al. Comparison of transmyocardial revascularization with medical therapy in patients with refractory angina. *N Engl J Med* 1999;341(14):1029–1036.

95. Hughes GC, et al. Early postoperative changes in regional systolic and diastolic left ventricular function after transmyocardial laser revascularization: a comparison of holmium:YAG and CO_2 lasers. *J Am Coll Cardiol* 2000;35(4):1022–1030.

96. Stover E, et al. Variability in transfusion practice for coronary artery bypass surgery persists despite national consensus guidelines: a 24-institution study. Institutions of the Multicenter Study of Perioperative Ischemia Research Group. *Anesthesiology* 1998;88(2):327–333.

97. Goodnough LT, et al. Transfusion medicine. First of two parts—blood transfusion. *N Engl J Med* 1999;340(6):438–447.

98. American Society of Anesthesiologists. Practice guidelines for blood component therapy: a report by the American Society of Anesthesiologists Task Force on Blood Component Therapy. *Anesthesiology* 1996;84(3):732–747.

99. Development Task Force of the College of American Pathologists. Practice parameter for the use of fresh-frozen plasma, cryoprecipitate, and platelets. Fresh-frozen plasma, cryoprecipitate, and platelets administration practice guidelines. *JAMA* 1994;271(10):777–781.

100. Goodnough LT, Despotis GJ. Future directions in utilization review: the role of transfusion algorithms. *Transfus Sci* 1998;19(1):97–105.

101. Spiess BD, et al. Changes in transfusion therapy and reexploration rate after institution of a blood management program in cardiac surgical patients. *J Cardiothorac Vasc Anesth* 1995;9(2):168–173.

102. Shore-Lesserson L, et al. Thromboelastography-guided transfusion algorithm reduces transfusions in complex cardiac surgery. *Anesth Analg* 1999;88(2):312–319.

103. Wong BI, et al. Aprotinin and tranexamic acid for high transfusion risk cardiac surgery. *Ann Thorac Surg* 2000;69(3):808–816.

104. Levi M, et al. Pharmacological strategies to decrease excessive blood loss in cardiac surgery: a meta-analysis of clinically relevant endpoints. *Lancet* 1999;354(9194):1940–1947.

105. Nuttall GA, et al. Comparison of blood-conservation strategies in cardiac surgery patients at high risk for bleeding. *Anesthesiology* 2000;92(3):674–682.

106. Huet C, et al. A meta-analysis of the effectiveness of cell salvage to minimize perioperative allogeneic blood transfusion in cardiac and orthopedic surgery. International Study of Perioperative Transfusion (ISPOT) Investigators. *Anesth Analg* 1999;89(4):861–869.

107. Body SC, et al. Safety and efficacy of shed mediastinal blood transfusion after cardiac surgery: a multicenter observational study. Multicenter

Study of Perioperative Ischemia Research Group. *J Cardiothorac Vasc Anesth* 1999;13(4):410–416.

108. Remy B, Deby-Dupont G, Lamy M. Red blood cell substitutes: fluorocarbon emulsions and haemoglobin solutions. *Br Med Bull* 1999;55(1):277–298.

109. Chang TM. Modified hemoglobin-based blood substitutes: crosslinked, recombinant and encapsulated hemoglobin. *Vox Sang* 1998;74 [Suppl 2]:233–241.

110. Arom KV, et al. Safety and efficacy of off-pump coronary artery bypass grafting. *Ann Thorac Surg* 2000;69(3):704–710.

111. Parsonnet V, Dean D, Bernstein AD. A method of uniform stratification of risk for evaluating the results of surgery in acquired adult heart disease. *Circulation* 1989;79(6 Pt 2):I3–12.

112. Hannan EL, et al. Improving the outcomes of coronary artery bypass surgery in New York State. *JAMA* 1994;271(10):761–766.

113. Tremblay NA, et al. A simple classification of the risk in cardiac surgery: the first decade. *Can J Anaesth* 1993;40(2):103–111.

114. Tu JV, Jaglal SB, Naylor CD. Multicenter validation of a risk index for mortality, intensive care unit stay, and overall hospital length of stay after cardiac surgery. Steering Committee of the Provincial Adult Cardiac Care Network of Ontario. *Circulation* 1995;91(3):677–684.

115. Wolman RL, et al. Cerebral injury after cardiac surgery: identification of a group at extraordinary risk. Multicenter Study of Perioperative Ischemia Research Group (McSPI) and the Ischemia Research Education Foundation (IREF) Investigators. *Stroke* 1999;30(3):514–522.

116. Van Dijk D, et al. Neurocognitive dysfunction after coronary artery bypass surgery: a systematic review. *J Thorac Cardiovasc Surg* 2000;120(4):632–639.

117. Hogue CW Jr, et al. Neurological complications of cardiac surgery: the need for new paradigms in prevention and treatment. *Semin Thorac Cardiovasc Surg* 1999;11(2):105–115.

118. Weightman WM, et al. Risk prediction in coronary artery surgery: a comparison of four risk scores. *Med J Aust* 1997;166(8):408–411.

CURRENT CONCEPTS IN CARDIOPULMONARY RESUSCITATION

CHARLES W. OTTO

KEY WORDS

- Airway management
- Amiodarone
- Atropine
- Bretylium
- Calcium
- Chest compressions
- Defibrillation
- Epinephrine
- Lidocaine
- Postresuscitation care
- Prognosis
- Sodium bicarbonate
- Vasopressin
- Ventilation during cardiopulmonary resuscitation (CPR)

INTRODUCTION

Resuscitation from cardiac arrest in the hospital depends on the rapid response of a well-trained cardiopulmonary resuscitation (CPR) team, which usually includes physicians, nurses, respiratory care providers, and pharmacists. The critical care physician is usually a team member and often is expected to be the leader. The team must communicate readily and act in coordination. Providing the knowledge base and framework for effective teamwork are the goals of published CPR guidelines and widely taught courses in basic life support (BLS) and advanced cardiac life support (ACLS) (1). The critical care physician must be thoroughly familiar with ACLS protocols to function within the team. Team leadership also requires in-depth, current knowledge of physiology, pharmacology, and alternative CPR techniques. The purpose of this chapter is not to reiterate standard ACLS protocols but to provide the scientific background on which current CPR practice is based. It focuses exclusively on cardiopulmonary arrest. Other circumstances requiring cardiovascular support, such as shock (see Chapter 27) and dysrhythmias (see Chapter 28), are covered in other chapters. Do not resuscitate orders are discussed in Chapter 6.

Approximately 40% of patients suffering in-hospital cardiac arrest are resuscitated and 25% of these resuscitated patients survive to discharge (2). Excluding the operating room, the hospital setting with the best initial resuscitation rate is the intensive care unit (ICU), while the emergency department has the best survival rate. Success rates for in-hospital resuscitation and sur-

vival are similar to those associated with out-of-hospital arrest in cities with rapid response emergency medical systems (3). In out-of-hospital arrests, poor outcomes are associated with long duration of arrest before CPR is begun, prolonged ventricular fibrillation without definitive therapy, and inadequate coronary and cerebral perfusion during CPR (4). Optimum survival from ventricular fibrillation is obtained only if basic CPR is started within 4 minutes and defibrillation applied within 8 minutes (3). The very best outcome is achieved when defibrillation occurs within 1 minute (5). Survival rates decrease 7% to 10% for every minute that defibrillation for ventricular fibrillation is delayed (6). A better outcome might be expected for in-hospital arrests because of rapid response times and expert personnel. Intercurrent illnesses of hospitalized patients reduce the likelihood of survival and the arrest victim is more likely to be an older adult, a factor that may reduce survival. The cause of arrest associated with the best outcome and the most common cause of out-of-hospital arrest is ventricular fibrillation secondary to myocardial ischemia. This initiating event is less common in hospitalized patients. When applying CPR, attention to the details of effective resuscitation is important. Because CPR is only symptomatic therapy, so much attention should not be paid to the mechanics of CPR that the clinician fails to search for a treatable cause of the arrest.

AIRWAY MANAGEMENT

The goal of airway management during cardiorespiratory arrest is to provide a clear path for respiratory gas exchange while minimizing gastric insufflation and the risk of pulmonary aspiration. The most commonly used technique for opening the airway is the "head tilt/chin lift" method (Fig. 1). If this is ineffective, the "jaw thrust" maneuver is often helpful. Oropharyngeal and nasopharyngeal airways are useful for helping maintain an open airway in patients who are not intubated. Care must be used to ensure they are correctly inserted and do not worsen airway obstruction. Insertion in the semiconscious patient can induce vomiting or laryngospasm.

Effective airway management during CPR is a major problem, even for medical professionals. Many individuals cannot

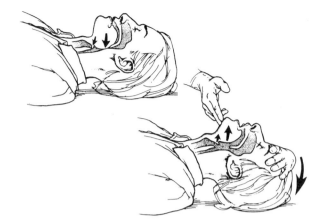

FIGURE 1. The jaw thrust maneuver as a method of opening the airway during cardiorespiratory arrest.

effectively manage a self-inflating resuscitation bag and mask. Larger tidal volumes at lower pressures are delivered by mouth-to-mouth or mouth-to-mask ventilation (7). The bag and mask apparatus is more effective if two individuals manage the airway: one to hold the mask and maintain the airway and one to squeeze the bag (8). In the hands of adequately trained personnel, the laryngeal mask airway (LMA) and esophageal tracheal Combitube (ETC) provide superior ventilation to the bag and mask apparatus and are recommended alternatives. Endotracheal intubation provides the best possible airway management. If a skilled laryngoscopist is available, endotracheal intubation should be carried out in all resuscitations lasting more than a few minutes. Intubation should not be performed until adequate ventilation by other means (preferably with supplemental oxygen) and circulation by chest compression have been established.

VENTILATION

If the airway remains patent, chest compressions cause substantial air exchange. Recent research suggests that when an arrest is witnessed, likely to be of cardiac (rather than respiratory) cause, and intubation will be available within a short time, closed chest compressions alone may be as efficacious as compressions and mouth-to-mouth ventilation (9–11). Current evidence indicates that chest compressions without mouth-to-mouth ventilation is significantly better than no CPR at all. Surveys have demonstrated that rescuers are reluctant to provide mouth-to-mouth ventilation because of the risk of infectious disease (12), although only 15 cases of CPR-related infections have been published since 1960, and no reports of human immunodeficiency virus (HIV), hepatitis B virus (HBV), hepatitis C, or cytomegalovirus have been found (13). If the preliminary ventilation studies are confirmed, basic life support teaching could be considerably simplified. Currently, airway management and ventilation remain the standard first steps of CPR. Chest compression-only CPR is recommended only when a rescuer is unwilling or unable to perform mouth-to-mouth ventilation and for use in telephone dispatcher-assisted CPR instruction where the simplicity of the technique improves bystander intervention.

Physiology of Ventilation during Cardiopulmonary Resuscitation

Insufflation of air into the stomach during resuscitation leads to gastric distension, impeding ventilation, and increasing the danger of regurgitation and gastric rupture. A useful aid in minimizing gastric insufflation is the use of cricoid pressure (Sellick maneuver). Pressure applied over the anterior arch of the cricoid cartilage can prevent air from entering the stomach at airway pressures up to 100 cm H_2O. In the absence of an endotracheal tube, the relative distribution of gas between the lungs and stomach during mouth-to-mouth or bag-valve-mask ventilation will be determined by the impedance to flow into each compartment. If gastric insufflation is to be avoided, inspiratory airway pressures must be kept low. A major cause of increased airway pressures and gastric insufflation is partial airway obstruction by the tongue and pharyngeal tissues. Meticulous attention to maintaining an open airway is necessary during rescue breathing. To cause an obvious rise in the chest of most adults, a tidal volume of 10 mL per kg (600 to 900 mL) will be needed. Even with an open airway, a relatively long inspiratory time is necessary to administer this volume at low pressure. Thus, rescue breaths should be given over 2 seconds during a pause in chest compressions.

Technique of Rescue Breathing

Using the head tilt/chin lift method of maintaining an open airway, mouth-to-mouth ventilation is administered by using the hand on the forehead to pinch the nose. When initiating resuscitation, two breaths should be given and breathing should be continued at a rate of 10 to 12 breaths per minute, watching for the chest to rise. For exhalation, the rescuer removes their mouth from the victim, listening for escaping air and taking a breath. During CPR, a pause for two breaths should be made after each 15 chest compressions whether there are one or two rescuers.

The best way to ensure adequate ventilation without gastric distension is endotracheal intubation, which is indicated during any prolonged resuscitation attempt. Other aspects of the resuscitation that might lead to a restoration of spontaneous circulation should not be delayed while efforts are made to place an endotracheal tube. Blood flow during CPR slows rapidly when chest compressions stop and recovers slowly when they restart. Consequently, following intubation, no pause should be made for ventilation and ventilation should be approximately 12 breaths per minute without regard for the compression cycle.

CIRCULATION
Physiology of Circulation during Closed Chest Compressions

Two theories have been proposed to explain the mechanism by which closed chest compressions cause blood to flow through the circulatory system (14,15). They are not mutually exclusive and continue to be investigated. With the original description of closed chest cardiac massage in 1960, Kouwenhoven and colleagues (14) suggested that the heart was compressed between the sternum and spine, resulting in increased intraventricular pressure, closing of the atrioventricular valves, and ejection of blood into the lungs and aorta. During the relaxation phase, negative intrathoracic pressure, caused by expansion of the thoracic cage, facilitates blood return and aortic recoil pressure results in aortic valve closure and coronary perfusion. This mechanism has come to be known as the cardiac pump theory of blood flow during CPR.

The publication of a case of "cough CPR" in 1976 (16) led to further investigations (17) and the thoracic pump theory of blood flow during CPR (15). According to this mechanism, all intrathoracic structures are compressed equally by the increase in intrathoracic pressure resulting from sternal compression. Backward flow through the venous system is prevented by valves in the subclavian and internal jugular veins and by dynamic compression of the veins at the thoracic outlet. Thicker, less compressible vessel walls prevent collapse on the arterial side. The heart acts as a passive conduit with the atrioventricular valves remaining open during chest compression.

Fluctuations in intrathoracic pressure play a significant role in blood flow during CPR, and the cardiac pump mechanism contributes under some circumstances, especially early during chest compressions. As the heart becomes less compliant during prolonged CPR, the thoracic pump becomes more important in maintaining flow. Which mechanism predominates probably varies from patient to patient and can vary even during the resuscitation of the same patient.

Distribution of Blood Flow during Cardiopulmonary Resuscitation

Whatever the actual mechanism of blood flow, cardiac output is severely reduced during closed chest compressions (ranging from 10% to 33% of prearrest values in experimental animals). Nearly all of the cardiac output is directed to organs above the diaphragm. Blood flow to the brain is 50% to 90% of normal, to the myocardium it is 20% to 50% of normal, and to the lower extremities and abdominal visceral it is less than 5% of normal. All flows tend to decrease with time but the relative distribution of flow does not change. Epinephrine and vasopressin improve flow to the brain and heart while flow to organs below the diaphragm is unchanged or further reduced.

Gas Transport during Cardiopulmonary Resuscitation

During the low flow state of CPR, excretion of carbon dioxide (CO_2) (mL of CO_2 per minute in exhaled gas) is decreased from prearrest levels approximately to the same extent as cardiac output is reduced. This reduced CO_2 excretion is due primarily to shunting of blood flow away from the lower half of the body. The exhaled CO_2 reflects only the metabolism of the part of the body that is being perfused. In the nonperfused areas, CO_2 accumulates during CPR. When normal circulation is restored, the accumulated CO_2 is washed out and a temporary increase in CO_2 excretion is seen.

Although CO_2 excretion is reduced during CPR, measurement of blood gases reveals an arterial respiratory alkalosis and a venous respiratory acidosis with a markedly elevated arterio-

venous CO_2 difference (18). The primary cause of these changes is the severely reduced cardiac output. Two factors account for the elevation of the venous partial pressure of CO_2 ($Pvco_2$). Buffering acid causes a reduction in serum bicarbonate, so that the same blood CO_2 content results in a higher $Pvco_2$. In addition, the mixed venous CO_2 content is elevated. When flow to a tissue is reduced, all the CO_2 produced fails to be removed and CO_2 accumulates, raising the tissue partial pressure of CO_2. This allows more CO_2 to be carried in each aliquot of blood and mixed venous CO_2 content increases. If flow remains constant, a new equilibrium is established where all CO_2 produced in the tissue is removed but at a higher venous CO_2 content and partial pressure. In contrast to the venous blood, arterial CO_2 content and partial pressure ($Paco_2$) usually are reduced during CPR. This reduction accounts for most of the observed increase in arteriovenous CO_2 content difference. Even though venous blood may have an increased CO_2, the marked reduction in cardiac output with maintained ventilation results in very efficient CO_2 removal.

Decreased pulmonary blood flow during CPR causes lack of perfusion to many nondependent alveoli. The alveolar gas of these lung units has no CO_2. Consequently, mixed alveolar CO_2 (i.e., end-tidal CO_2) will be very low and correlate poorly with arterial CO_2. However, end-tidal CO_2 does correlate well with cardiac output during CPR. As flow increases, more alveoli become perfused, there is less alveolar dead space, and end-tidal CO_2 measurements rise.

Technique of Closed Chest Compression

Standard chest compression technique consists of the rhythmic application of pressure over the lower half of the sternum. For compressions to be effective in providing blood flow to the brain and heart, the patient must be on a firm surface with the head level with the heart. The rescuer should stand or kneel at the side of the patient so that the hips are on a level with the patient's chest. The heel of one hand is placed on the lower sternum and the other hand placed on top of the first. Care must be taken that the xiphoid is not pressed into the abdomen. Pressure on the ribs or costal cartilages, rather than the sternum, increases the risk of rib fracture. The elbows should be locked in position with the arms straight and the shoulders over the hands. Using the weight of the entire upper body, the compression is delivered straight down with enough force to depress the sternum 3.5 to 5 cm. Following maximal compression, pressure is released completely from the chest but the hands stay in contact with the chest wall maintaining proper hand position for the next thrust.

Chest compressions, which should be performed at a rate of 100 per minute, are most effective if the compression and relaxation phases of the cycle are equal in length. This 50% compression time is easier to achieve at faster compression rates. Whether there are one or two rescuers, before intubation, it is recommended that 15 compressions be followed by a pause for two ventilations (2 seconds each) followed by 15 more compressions. In this scenario, fewer than 100 chest compressions will be delivered, but the rate should be a little less than two compressions per second when they are being delivered. When the airway is controlled by an endotracheal tube, breaths at a rate of 12 per minute should be interposed during chest compressions without a pause for ventilation.

Alternative Methods of Circulatory Support

A better understanding of circulatory physiology during CPR, especially involving the thoracic pump mechanism, has generated several proposals for alternative CPR techniques. Most alternative techniques are designed to provide better hemodynamics during CPR and, thus, extend the duration during which CPR can successfully support viability. Unfortunately, no new technique has proven to be reliably superior to standard techniques and no improvement in survival from cardiac arrest has been consistently demonstrated (19).

Closed-Chest Techniques

According to the thoracic pump theory, maneuvers that increase intrathoracic pressure during chest compression should improve blood flow and pressure (17). Several methods for raising intrathoracic pressure during CPR have been studied, including simultaneous ventilation and compression, abdominal binding with compression, and the pneumatic antishock garment. Early results indicated improved aortic pressures and carotid blood flows with these techniques (17). However, subsequent studies failed to demonstrate consistently improved resuscitation success or survival (20). None of these methods are currently recommended.

Other alternative techniques continue to be actively investigated. The pneumatic CPR vest relies entirely on the thoracic pump mechanism of blood flow (21). Animal studies have shown excellent hemodynamics and the ability to maintain viability for prolonged periods. Improved outcome from cardiac arrest has not been demonstrated in animals. One small clinical study found better aortic and coronary perfusion pressure with the vest compared to standard CPR but survival was not improved (22). Randomized human trials are now being conducted.

The technique of interposed abdominal compression-CPR (IAC-CPR) uses an additional rescuer to apply manual abdominal compressions during the relaxation phase of chest compressions (Fig. 2) (23). Abdominal pressure is released when chest compression begins. A large randomized trial of IAC-CPR in out-of-hospital cardiac arrest found no improvement in survival compared to standard CPR (24), but two in-hospital studies have reported improved survival (25). It is recommended as an alternative to standard CPR for in-hospital resuscitation. Further studies of IAC-CPR are needed to establish out-of-hospital efficacy.

Another proposed alternative technique is called active compression-decompression CPR (ACD-CPR) (26). With this method, CPR is performed with a suction device applied to the chest over the sternum allowing active decompression. Early out-of-hospital trials were discouraging, but more recent reports have had conflicting results. A large randomized trial in France found improved outcome from out-of-hospital arrest with the technique (27), but a large study in Canada of in-hospital and out-of-hospital arrests found no difference in immediate or late

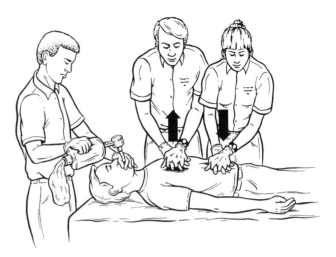

FIGURE 2. The technique of interposed abdominal compression-cardiopulmonary resuscitation (IAC-CPR).

survival (28). Two new devices are undergoing preliminary investigations. The impedance threshold valve lowers intrathoracic pressure, enhancing venous return during CPR. Phased chest and abdominal compression CPR is a combination of ACD-CPR and IAC-CPR.

Invasive Techniques

Much of the effort spent improving current CPR techniques and investigating new techniques was prompted by the hope that better blood flows would extend the time during which CPR can support viability. Unfortunately, the results have been disappointing. In spite of the occasional success of prolonged resuscitation efforts, it appears that closed chest compressions can sustain most patients for only 15 to 30 minutes. If successful restoration of spontaneous circulation has not occurred in that time, the results are dismal. In contrast to the closed chest techniques, two invasive maneuvers have been shown to be able to maintain cardiac and cerebral viability during long periods of cardiac arrest. In animal models, open-chest cardiac massage and cardiopulmonary bypass (through the femoral artery and vein using a membrane oxygenator) can provide better hemodynamics and myocardial and cerebral perfusion than closed chest techniques. Prompt restoration of blood flow and perfusion pressure with cardiopulmonary bypass can provide resuscitation with minimal neurologic deficit after 20 minutes of untreated fibrillatory cardiac arrest in canines. To be effective, however, these techniques must be instituted relatively early (probably within 20 to 30 minutes of cardiac arrest) (29). If open chest massage is begun after 30 minutes of ineffective closed chest compressions, the survival rates do not improve even though hemodynamics do improve (30). The necessary expertise may be available to apply these techniques during in-hospital arrest, but most rescuers are appropriately reluctant to apply such invasive maneuvers until it is clear that closed-chest techniques are ineffective. Unfortunately, invasive methods also may be unsuccessful at that point. Before invasive procedures can play a greater role in modern CPR, a method must be developed to predict early during resuscitation which patients can be successfully treated with closed chest compressions.

Assessing the Adequacy of Circulation during Cardiopulmonary Resuscitation

An obvious need exists to assess whether ongoing CPR is generating adequate myocardial and cerebral blood flow for viable resuscitation to occur. The traditional method is to palpate the carotid or femoral pulse during chest compressions. However, a palpable pulse primarily reflects systolic blood pressure. Mean blood pressure correlates better with cardiac output and diastolic pressure is the major determinant of coronary perfusion. Nevertheless, palpation of the pulse remains the only assessment tool available during BLS, but is not currently recommended for the layperson as they may not be experienced in detecting a pulse.

Successful resuscitation in experimental models is associated with myocardial blood flows of 15 to 30 mL per minute per 100 g (31). To obtain such flows, closed chest compressions must generate adequate cardiac output and coronary perfusion pressure. During CPR, coronary perfusion occurs primarily during the relaxation phase (diastole) of chest compression. In animal models, the critical myocardial blood flow is associated with aortic "diastolic" pressure of greater than 40 mm Hg and coronary perfusion pressure (aortic diastolic minus right atrial diastolic pressure) exceeding 25 mm Hg. One report, which confirmed similar findings in humans, noted that all patients with successful return of spontaneous circulation had coronary perfusion pressures higher than 15 mm Hg (32). Invasive pressure monitoring, when available during CPR, should be used to guide resuscitation efforts. If pressures are below the critical levels, adjustments should be made to improve chest compressions and additional vasopressor therapy should be considered. Vascular pressures below the critical levels are associated with poor results even in patients that may be able to be saved. However, obtaining pressures above the critical levels does not ensure success. Damage to the myocardium from underlying disease may preclude survival no matter how effective the CPR efforts.

Although invasive pressure monitoring may be the ideal, exhaled end-tidal CO_2 is an excellent noninvasive guide to the effectiveness of standard CPR. After intubation, CO_2 excretion during CPR is dependent primarily on blood flow rather than ventilation. Since alveolar dead space is large during low flow conditions, end-tidal CO_2 is very low (often less than 10 mm Hg). If cardiac output increases, more alveoli are perfused and end-tidal CO_2 rises (usually to more than 20 mm Hg during successful CPR). When spontaneous circulation resumes, the earliest sign is a sudden increase in end-tidal CO_2 to greater than 40 mm Hg. Within a wide range of cardiac outputs, end-tidal CO_2 during CPR correlates with coronary perfusion pressure, cardiac output, initial resuscitation, and survival. End-tidal CO_2 measured during human CPR has been used to predict outcome. Two studies have demonstrated that no patient with an end-tidal CO_2 less than 10 mm Hg could be successfully resuscitated (33). In the absence of invasive pressure monitoring, end-tidal CO_2 monitoring can be used to judge the effectiveness of chest compressions (34). Attempts should be made to maximize the value by alterations in technique or drug therapy. Sodium bicarbonate administration results in the liberation of CO_2 in the venous blood and a temporary rise in end-tidal CO_2. Therefore, end-tidal CO_2 monitoring will not be useful for judging the effectiveness of chest compressions for 3 to 5 minutes following bicarbonate administration.

DEFIBRILLATION

Duration and Electric Pattern of Fibrillation

Ventricular fibrillation is the most common electrocardiographic rhythm in adults experiencing cardiac arrest. The longer fibrillation continues, the more difficult is defibrillation and the less likely is successful resuscitation. The fibrillating heart has a high oxygen consumption, which increases myocardial ischemia and decreases the time to irreversible cell damage. The only effective treatment for this dysrhythmia is electric defibrillation, and the sooner defibrillation is applied, the higher the rate of successful resuscitation (3,35). Thus, conversion of ventricular fibrillation to a rhythm capable of restoring spontaneous circulation should be the first priority of any resuscitation attempt.

The amplitude and frequency (coarseness) of the fibrillatory waves on the electrocardiogram (ECG) may reflect the severity and duration of the myocardial insult and, thus, may have prognostic significance (36). Low voltage fibrillation is associated with poor outcome. Increasing myocardial ischemia results in less vigorous fibrillation, reduced amplitude electric activity, and more difficult defibrillation. Catecholamines with β-adrenergic activity, such as epinephrine, increase the amplitude of the electric activity but have no influence on defibrillation (35,37). Consequently, defibrillation should not be postponed for any other therapy but should be carried out as soon as the rhythm is diagnosed and the equipment available.

Defibrillators: Energy, Current, and Impedance

The defibrillator is a variable transformer that stores a direct current in a capacitor until discharged through the electrodes. Defibrillation is accomplished when the current passes through a critical mass of myocardium, causing simultaneous depolarization of the myofibrils. Optimum current flow and success of defibrillation is obtained by keeping transthoracic impedance as low as possible. Many of the important factors in minimizing impedance are under the rescuer's control. Resistance decreases with electrode size, so large paddles (greater than 8 cm diameter) should be used. The greatest reduction in impedance is obtained with the specially designed defibrillation gels or pastes applied to the paddles or self-adhesive defibrillation/monitor pads. Firm paddle pressure of at least 11 kg reduces resistance by improving electrode-skin contact and by expelling air from the lung. The reduction in transthoracic impedance that occurs with successive shocks may partially explain why additional shocks of the same energy may succeed when previous shocks did not. If relatively high-energy shocks (greater than 300 J) are used with reasonable attention to proper technique, resistance is probably of little clinical significance. For lower energy shocks, great care should be taken to minimize resistance. Defibrillators have been developed that measure transthoracic impedance prior to the shock by passing a low-level current through the chest during the charge cycle. Although not widely available, this technology may allow current-based defibrillation by adjusting the delivered energy for the measured resistance.

Energy Requirements and Adverse Effects

The incidence and severity of myocardial damage from defibrillation in humans is not clear. Repeated high-energy shocks in animals result in dysrhythmias, ECG changes, and myocardial necrosis. Whether such injuries occur in humans is unknown, although slight elevations in creatine kinase MB fractions have been reported after cardioversions with high energies. It would seem prudent to keep energy levels as low as possible during defibrillation attempts.

There is a general relationship between body size and energy requirements for defibrillation. Children need lower energies than adults, perhaps as low as 0.5 J per kg although the recommended pediatric dose is 2 J per kg. However, over the size range of adults, body size does not seem to be a clinically important variable. Multiple studies have demonstrated that using relatively low level initial shocks in adults is as successful as beginning with higher energy (38). Therefore, it is currently recommended that the initial shock be given at 200 J followed by a second shock at 200 to 300 J if the first is unsuccessful. If both fail to defibrillate the patient, additional shocks should be given at 360 J.

DRUG THERAPY (TABLE 1)

Catecholamines and Vasopressors

Mechanism of Action

The only drugs generally accepted as being useful during CPR are the vasopressors (39). Epinephrine has been used in resuscitation since the 1890s, and has been the vasopressor of choice in modern CPR since the studies of Redding and Pearson in the 1960s (40,41). The efficacy of epinephrine lies entirely in its α-adrenergic properties (42). Peripheral vasoconstriction leads to an increase in aortic diastolic pressure causing an increase in coronary perfusion pressure and myocardial blood flow. All strong α-adrenergic drugs and nonadrenergic vasopressors are equally successful in aiding resuscitation regardless of the β-adrenergic

potency. Beta-adrenergic agonists without alpha activity are no better than placebo. Alpha-adrenergic blockade precludes resuscitation while β-adrenergic blockade has no effect on the ability to restore spontaneous circulation. Although it is generally believed that epinephrine's ability to increase the amplitude of ventricular fibrillation (a β-adrenergic effect) makes defibrillation easier, studies have shown no effect of epinephrine on defibrillation success (35–37).

Beta-adrenergic stimulation is potentially deleterious during cardiac arrest. In the fibrillating heart, epinephrine increases oxygen consumption and decreases the endocardial-epicardial blood flow ratio, an effect not seen with methoxamine. Myocardial lactate production in the fibrillating heart is unchanged after epinephrine administration during CPR suggesting that the increased coronary blood flow does not improve the oxygen supply–demand ratio. In spite of these theoretical considerations, survival and neurologic outcome studies have shown no difference when epinephrine is compared to a pure α-agonist (methoxamine or phenylephrine) during CPR in animals or humans (43,44).

Epinephrine

Because epinephrine has been used for many years, it remains the vasopressor of choice in CPR. It should be administered whenever resuscitation has not occurred after adequate chest compressions and ventilation have been started and defibrillation attempted, if appropriate. When used in conjunction with chest compressions, epinephrine helps develop the critical coronary perfusion pressure necessary to provide enough myocardial blood flow for restoration of spontaneous circulation. If arterial diastolic pressure is less than 40 mm Hg or coronary perfusion pressure is less than 20 mm Hg, better chest compression technique, more epinephrine, or both are needed. If invasive vascular pressures are not available, the dose of epinephrine must be chosen empirically. The standard intravenous (i.v.) dose has been 0.5 to 1.0; animal studies in the 1980s suggested that higher doses of epinephrine might increase myocardial and cerebral perfusion and improve success of resuscitation. Case reports were published of return of spontaneous circulation (ROSC) when large doses (0.1 to 0.2 mg per kg) of epinephrine were given to patients who had failed resuscitation with standard doses.

Subsequent outcome studies prospectively comparing standard- and high-dose epinephrine have not demonstrated conclusively that higher doses will improve survival. Clinically, initial or escalating high-dose epinephrine has occasionally improved ROSC and early survival. However, eight adult prospective randomized clinical studies involving over 9,000 cardiac arrest patients have found no improvement in survival to hospital discharge or neurologic outcome, even in subgroups, when initial high-dose epinephrine is compared to standard doses (1).

High doses of epinephrine apparently are not needed as initial therapy for most cardiac arrests, and potentially could be deleterious under some circumstances. The cases of successful high-dose epinephrine use were in patients with prolonged CPR, and the high doses were given as "rescue" therapy when standard doses had failed; the use of higher doses of epinephrine may be appropriate under these circumstances. Current recommendations

TABLE 1. DRUGS USED IN CARDIOPULMONARY RESUSCITATION AND COMMON DOSAGES

Drug	Adult	Infant + Child
Epinephrine	1 mg	0.01 mg/kg
If dose fails, may consider	3–7 mg	0.1 mg/kg
Arginine vasopressin	40 units	Not recommended
Atropine sulfate	1 mg	0.02 mg/kg
Amiodarone hydrochloride	300 mg	5 mg/kg
Lidocaine hydrochloride	1.5 mg/kg	1 mg/kg
Bretylium tosylate[a]	5 mg/kg	5 mg/kg
Sodium bicarbonate	1 mEq/kg	1 mEq/kg
Calcium chloride	2–4 mg/kg	20 mg/kg

[a] No longer recommended in Advanced Cardiac Life Support (ACLS) algorithm.

are to give 1 mg i.v. every 3 to 5 minutes in the adult. If this dose seems ineffective, higher doses (3 to 8 mg) should be considered.

Vasopressin

The newest addition to the pharmacologic armamentarium in CPR is arginine vasopressin. It is administered as an alternative to epinephrine in a dose of 40 units i.v. Vasopressin is a naturally occurring hormone (antidiuretic hormone) that, when administered in high doses, is a potent nonadrenergic vasoconstrictor, acting by stimulation of smooth muscle V_1 receptors. It is usually not recommended for conscious patients with coronary artery disease because the increased peripheral vascular resistance may provoke angina. The half-life in the intact circulation is 10 to 20 minutes, and longer than epinephrine during CPR. Animal studies have demonstrated that vasopressin is as effective or more effective than epinephrine in maintaining vital organ blood flow during CPR. Repeated doses during prolonged CPR in swine were associated with significantly improved rates of neurologically intact survival compared to epinephrine and placebo. Postresuscitation myocardial depression and splanchnic blood flow reduction are more marked with vasopressin than epinephrine but they are transient and can be treated with low doses of dopamine. Preliminary clinical studies indicate that vasopressin is as effective as epinephrine, but have not definitively shown it to be superior. A small randomized, blinded study comparing vasopressin and standard-dose epinephrine in 40 patients with out-of-hospital ventricular fibrillation found improved 24-hour survival with vasopressin but no difference in ROSC or survival to hospital discharge (45). A larger, clinical trial of 200 inpatients found no difference between the drugs in survival for 1 hour or to hospital discharge (Ian Stiell, personal communication). In this study, response times were short, indicating that CPR outcome achieved with both vasopressin and epinephrine in short-term cardiac arrest may be comparable. The hemodynamic effects of vasopressin, compared to epinephrine, are especially impressive during long cardiac arrests. Thus, vasopressin may find most use in CPR during prolonged resuscitation.

Atropine

Atropine sulfate enhances sinus node automaticity and atrioventricular conduction by its vagolytic effects. Although atropine's primary use during CPR is when the ECG shows a pattern of asystole or slow idioventricular rhythm, neither animal nor human studies provide evidence that atropine actually improves outcome from asystolic or bradysystolic arrest (47,48). The predominant cause of asystole and slow ventricular rhythms is severe myocardial ischemia, and excessive parasympathetic tone probably contributes little to these rhythms during cardiac arrest. The most effective treatment for asystole or pulseless electric activity (PEA) is improvement in coronary perfusion and myocardial oxygenation with chest compressions, ventilation, and epinephrine. However, since cardiac arrest with these rhythms has a very poor prognosis and atropine has few adverse effects, it can be tried in patients when arrest is refractory to epinephrine and oxygenation. The recommended dose is 1 mg i.v., repeated every 3 to 5 minutes up to a total of 0.04 mg per kg. Following successful resuscitation,

full vagolytic doses may be associated with fixed mydriasis, which confounds neurologic examination. Sinus tachycardia following resuscitation occasionally may be due to use of atropine during CPR.

Amiodarone, Lidocaine, and Bretylium

Amiodarone, lidocaine, and bretylium are used during cardiac arrest to aid defibrillation when ventricular fibrillation is refractory to electric countershock therapy or when fibrillation recurs following successful conversion. Lidocaine, primarily an antiectopic agent with few hemodynamic effects, tends to reverse the reduction in ventricular fibrillation threshold caused by ischemia or infarction. It depresses automaticity by reducing the slope of phase-4 depolarization and reducing the heterogeneity of ventricular refractoriness. When ventricular tachycardia or ventricular fibrillation has not responded to or has recurred following epinephrine and defibrillation, lidocaine should be considered. To rapidly achieve and maintain therapeutic blood levels during CPR, relatively large doses are necessary. An initial bolus of 1 to 1.5 mg per kg should be given and additional boluses of 0.5 to 1.5 mg per kg can be given every 5 to 10 minutes during CPR up to a total dose of 3 mg per kg. Only bolus dosing should be used during CPR but an infusion of 2 to 4 mg per minute can be started after successful resuscitation.

Amiodarone is a pharmacologically complex drug with sodium, potassium, calcium, and α- and β-adrenergic blocking properties that is useful for treatment of atrial and ventricular dysrhythmias. Amiodarone can cause hypotension and bradycardia when infused too rapidly but less so than bretylium. This can usually be prevented by slowing the rate of drug infusion, or treated with fluids, vasopressors, chronotropic agents, or temporary pacing. There is a single randomized placebo controlled clinical trial demonstrating improved admission alive to hospital with amiodarone treatment although there was no difference in survival to discharge (46). This is more evidence of efficacy than exists for lidocaine or bretylium, suggesting that amiodarone should now be first-line treatment for shock-resistant fibrillation. In cardiac arrest, amiodarone is initially administered as a 300-mg rapid infusion. Supplemental infusion of 150 mg can be repeated as necessary for recurrent or resistant dysrhythmias to a maximum daily dose of 2 g.

Bretylium has been called a primary antifibrillatory drug because it reduces the chances for reentry to occur between ischemic and normal areas of myocardium. Like lidocaine, it reverses the reduction in fibrillation threshold caused by ischemia. Unlike lidocaine, bretylium has significant hemodynamic effects when administered i.v., causing the release of norepinephrine from adrenergic nerve endings. With a normal circulation, this results in tachycardia, hypertension, and increased contractility. After approximately 20 minutes, blockade of the uptake and release of norepinephrine from the nerve terminal begins, an effect that peaks 45 to 60 minutes after drug administration. This blockade can lead to profound hypotension. Although bretylium has some theoretical advantages over lidocaine for use during cardiac arrest, direct comparison of the drugs in clinical trials have found no differences in resuscitation success or survival. The initial dose is 5 mg per kg by i.v. bolus. The dose can be increased to 10 mg per kg and repeated at 5-minute intervals for a total dose of 30 to 35 mg per kg. Because of the side effects, the availability of other agents, and the limited supply of the drug, bretylium has been removed from the most recent ACLS treatment algorithms (1).

Sodium Bicarbonate

Although sodium bicarbonate was used commonly during CPR in the past, little evidence supports its efficacy. Current practice restricts sodium bicarbonate's use primarily to arrests associated with hyperkalemia, severe preexisting metabolic acidosis, and tricyclic antidepressant or phenobarbital overdose. It may be considered for use in protracted resuscitation attempts after other modalities have been instituted and failed. The use of sodium bicarbonate during resuscitation has been based on the theoretical considerations that acidosis lowers fibrillation threshold and acidosis impairs the physiologic response to catecholamines. But most studies have been unable to demonstrate improved success of defibrillation or resuscitation with the use of bicarbonate (49–51). The observation that metabolic acidosis develops very slowly during CPR may explain the absence of effect of buffer therapy; acidosis does not become severe until after 15 to 20 minutes of cardiac arrest (18,52,53).

Current recommendations for restricting sodium bicarbonate during CPR are based also on the documented complications from excessive use. Metabolic alkalosis, hypernatremia, and hyperosmolarity are well documented after administration of bicarbonate during resuscitation (53,54). These abnormalities are associated with low resuscitation rates and poor survival. However, if sodium bicarbonate is given judiciously according to standard recommendations, no significant metabolic abnormalities should occur. When bicarbonate is used during CPR, the usual dose is 1 mEq per kg initially with additional doses of 0.5 mEq per kg every 10 minutes. However, dosing of sodium bicarbonate should be guided by blood gas determination, whenever possible.

Calcium Salts

Results of several retrospective studies and prospective clinical trials that examined the efficacy of calcium during out-of-hospital human cardiac arrest showed that calcium was no better than placebo in promoting resuscitation and survival from asystole or PEA (55,56). Therefore, calcium may be helpful during cardiac resuscitation only if hyperkalemia, hypocalcemia, or calcium channel blocker toxicity is present. There are no other indications for its use during CPR. If calcium is administered, chloride salt (2 to 4 mg per kg) is recommended because it produces higher and more consistent levels of ionized calcium than other salts.

Routes of Administration

The preferred route of administration of all drugs during CPR is i.v. and the doses referred to in this chapter are for i.v. use. The most rapid and highest drug levels occur with administration into a central vein. Therefore, when a central venous catheter is available during a cardiac arrest, it should be used for drug therapy, but peripheral i.v. administration is also effective. The antecubital or

external jugular vein should be the site of first choice for starting an infusion during resuscitation because starting a central line usually requires stopping CPR. Sites in the upper extremities and neck are preferred because of the paucity of blood flow below the diaphragm during CPR. Drugs administered in the lower extremities may be extremely delayed or not reach the sites of action at all. Even when administered in the upper extremities, drugs may require 1 to 2 minutes to reach the central circulation. Onset of action may be speeded up if a drug bolus is followed by a 20- to 30-mL bolus of i.v. fluid. In children, the intraosseous route via the tibia is an effective alternative for administering i.v. medications.

Epinephrine, vasopressin, lidocaine, and atropine do not injure the lungs and can be absorbed from the tracheal mucosa; therefore, if i.v. access cannot be established, the endotracheal tube (following intubation) provides an alternative route for administration of these drugs. The time-to-effect and drug levels achieved are very inconsistent using this route during CPR. Studies have demonstrated that volumes of 5 to 10 mL need to be delivered to have reasonable uptake. Higher doses of the drugs are likely needed via this route; 2 to 2.5 times the i.v. dose is currently recommended. Studies conflict on whether deep injection is better than simple instillation in the tube. Sodium bicarbonate should not be given by this route.

POSTRESUSCITATION CARE

The major factors contributing to mortality following successful resuscitation are progression of the primary disease and cerebral damage suffered as a result of the arrest. During this postresuscitation period, the critical care physician may have the greatest impact on outcome. Active management following resuscitation appears to mitigate postischemic brain damage and improve neurologic outcome (57). Although significant numbers of patients have severe neurologic deficits following resuscitation, aggressive support does not increase the proportion surviving in a vegetative state. Most severely damaged patients die of multisystem failure within 2 weeks.

When blood flow to the brain is restored following a period of global brain ischemia, three stages of cerebral reperfusion are seen in the ensuing 12 hours. Multifocal areas of the brain have no-reflow immediately following resuscitation. Within an hour, global hyperemia occurs; prolonged global hypoperfusion quickly follows. Intracranial pressure elevation is uncommon following resuscitation from cardiac arrest, although severe ischemic injury can lead to edema during the following days.

Postresuscitation support is focused on providing oxygenation and stable hemodynamics in order to minimize any further cerebral insult. A comatose patient should be maintained on mechanical ventilation for several hours to ensure adequate oxygenation and ventilation. Restlessness, coughing, or seizure activity should be aggressively treated with appropriate medications including neuromuscular blocking agents, if necessary. The PaO_2 should be maintained above 100 mm Hg and moderate hypocapnia ($PaCO_2$ 30 to 35 mm Hg) may be helpful. A normal blood volume should be maintained and moderate hemodilution to a hematocrit of 30% to 35% may be useful. A brief 5-minute period of hypertension to mean arterial pressure of 120 to 140 mm Hg may help overcome the initial cerebral no-reflow. This often occurs secondary to the effects of epinephrine given during CPR. However, both prolonged hypertension (greater than 110 mm Hg) and hypotension are associated with a worsened outcome. Hyperglycemia during cerebral ischemia is known to result in increased neurologic damage; thus, it seems prudent to control glucose in the 100 to 180 mg per dL range.

In contrast to general supportive care, specific pharmacologic therapy directed at brain preservation has not been shown to have further benefit. Some animal trials of barbiturate therapy were promising but a large multicentered trial of thiopental found no improvement in neurologic status when this drug was given following cardiac arrest (57). Similar results have been found with calcium channel blockers. Initial animal studies were encouraging but a multicentered trial of lidoflazine treatment found no improvement in neurologic outcome (58). Currently, there is no evidence that any specific pharmacologic agent will improve neurologic outcome following resuscitation from cardiac arrest.

PROGNOSIS

For the comatose survivor of CPR, the question of ultimate prognosis is important. One retrospective study demonstrated that the neurologic examination of comatose victims upon admission to the ICU correlates highly with the likelihood of awakening (59). Patients without a pupillary light response and spontaneous eye movement who had no motor response or showed extensor posturing to pain had only a 5% chance of awakening. A companion study demonstrated that the chance of ever awakening fell rapidly in the days following arrest (60). If the patient was not awake within 4 days from the time of arrest, the chance of ever awakening was less than 20% and, in this study, all of the patients who did awaken had marked neurologic deficits. Most patients who completely recover show rapid improvement in the first 48 hours. A high correlation also exists between severity of neurologic injury and the level of creatine kinase-BB found in the cerebral spinal fluid (61,62). Peak values of 25 IU or more are associated with severe neurologic damage and are reached 48 to 72 hours following arrest.

SUMMARY

Cardiopulmonary resuscitation is an area in which critical care physicians must be well trained and must keep abreast of the latest developments, if better outcomes are to be obtained. The details of airway management and chest compressions, which ensure the adequacy of oxygenation, ventilation, and circulation during CPR, are key. However, so much attention should not be paid to these mechanics that a search for a treatable cause of the arrest is forgotten. Rapid defibrillation with appropriate energy and administration of appropriate drugs are important. It must always be remembered that ultimate outcome is critically dependent on aggressive, thorough postresuscitation care.

KEY POINTS

Successful resuscitation of a patient who has experienced a cardiopulmonary arrest is dependent on the knowledge and skills of the rescuers. Critical care physicians are expected to have these skills and to be able to lead the team performing resuscitation.

Airway management and ventilation is usually via an anesthesia mask and bag, although a laryngeal mask airway (LMA) or esophageal tracheal Combitube are acceptable alternatives. If the arrest is prolonged, the trachea should be intubated.

Two ventilations (2 seconds each) should be provided during a pause after every 15 chest compressions. When the trachea is intubated, ventilations should be provided at approximately 12 breaths per minute between chest compressions. If a rescuer is unwilling or unable to perform mouth-to-mouth ventilation, chest compression-only cardiopulmonary resuscitation (CPR) is recommended.

No alternative technique of chest compression has been shown to result in better survival than the standard technique, although several methods continue to be investigated.

Chest compression, to be effective in restoring spontaneous circulation, must provide a myocardial blood flow at least 15 to 30 mL per minute per 100 g. This flow is associated with generating a diastolic blood pressure of greater than 40 mm Hg.

Since most adult arrests are due to ventricular fibrillation, ultimate resuscitation depends on the duration of the arrest and timely defibrillation. The best chance for survival is rapid defibrillation with an automated external defibrillator or with a standard defibrillator at increasing energy shocks: 200 J, 200 to 300 J, 360 J, as necessary.

There is no ideal way to monitor the effectiveness of CPR, although invasive arterial blood pressure monitoring, when available, provides the best measure of adequacy of chest compressions and correlates with outcome. End-tidal CO_2 is an acceptable alternative when arterial pressure monitoring is not available. Arterial diastolic pressure should be greater than 40 mm Hg and end-tidal CO_2 should be greater than 20 mm Hg for best results.

Most successful resuscitations depend on basic life support and defibrillation, but several drugs may be useful during CPR. Epinephrine and vasopressin are the vasopressors of choice and the drugs most likely to be useful in helping resuscitate a patient in cardiorespiratory arrest. When there is ventricular irritability or recurrent episodes of fibrillation, amiodarone or lidocaine may be helpful in controlling the arrhythmia. Atropine has not been shown to improve outcome from arrest, but because of few adverse effects, can be give if a bradycardic rhythm requires therapy.

The routine administration of bicarbonate or calcium in cardiopulmonary arrest is no longer recommended, although circumstances exist in which these drugs may be appropriately used.

Administration of drugs during CPR should be intravenously, preferably through a central vein. When this route is not feasible, epinephrine, vasopressin, lidocaine, and atropine can be given via an endotracheal tube; sodium bicarbonate should not be administered by this route.

If initial resuscitation is successful, ultimate outcome may be dependent on the adequacy of postresuscitation care in the intensive care unit. Careful management to maintain hemodynamic stability and adequate arterial oxygenation and to minimize excessive cerebral oxygen consumption in the hours immediately following resuscitation is critical.

REFERENCES

1. American Heart Association. Guidelines 2000 for Cardiopulmonary Resuscitation and Emergency Cardiovascular Care: International Consensus on Science. *Circulation* 2000;102[Suppl]:I-1–I-384.
2. Taffet BE, Teasdale TA, Luchi RJ. In-hospital cardiopulmonary resuscitation. *JAMA* 1988;260:2069–2072.
3. Weaver WD, Hill D, Fahrenbruch CE, et al. Use of the automatic external defibrillator in the management of out-of-hospital cardiac arrest. *N Engl J Med* 1988;319:661–666.
4. Eisenberg MS, Bergner L, Hallstrom A. Cardiac resuscitation in the community. Importance of rapid provision and implications for program planning. *JAMA* 1979;241:1905–1907.
5. Hossack KF, Hartwig R. Cardiac arrest associated with supervised cardiac rehabilitation. *J Cardiac Rehab* 1982;2:402–408.
6. Eisenberg MS, Horwood BT, Cummins RO, et al. Cardiac arrest and resuscitation: a tale of 29 cities. *Ann Emerg Med* 1990;19:179–186.
7. Harrison RR, Maull KI, Keenan RL, et al. Mouth-to-mask ventilation: a superior method of rescue breathing. *Ann Emerg Med* 1982;11:74–76.
8. Hess D, Baran C. Ventilatory volumes using mouth-to-mouth, mouth-to-mask, and bag valve mask techniques. *Am J Emerg Med* 1985;3:292–296.
9. Van Hoeyweghen R, Bossaert L, Mullie A, et al. Quality and efficiency of bystander CPR. *Resuscitation* 1993;26:47–52.
10. Berg RA, Kern KB, Hilwig RW, et al. Assisted ventilation does not improve outcome in a porcine model of single-rescuer bystander cardiopulmonary resuscitation. *Circulation* 1997;95:1635–1641.
11. Berg RA, Kern KB, Hilwig RW, et al. Assisted ventilation during 'bystander' CPR in a swine acute myocardial infarction model does not improve outcome. *Circulation* 1997;96:4364–4371.
12. Locke CJ, Berg RA, Sanders AB, et al. Bystander cardiopulmonary resuscitation. Concerns about mouth-to-mouth contact. *Arch Intern Med* 1995;155:938–943.
13. Mejicano GC, Maki DG. Infections acquired during cardiopulmonary resuscitation: estimating the risk and defining strategies for prevention. *Ann Intern Med* 1998;129:813–828.
14. Kouwenhoven WB, Jude JR, Knickerbocker GG. Closed-chest cardiac massage. *JAMA* 1960;173:1064–1067.
15. Babbs CF. New versus old theories of blood flow during CPR. *Crit Care Med* 1980;8:191–195.
16. Criley JM, Blaufuss AH, Kissel GL. Cough-induced cardiac compression. Self-administered form of cardiopulmonary resuscitation. *JAMA* 1976;236;1246–1250.
17. Rudikoff MJ, Maughan WL, Effrom M, et al. Mechanisms of blood flow during cardiopulmonary resuscitation. *Circulation* 1980;61:345–352.
18. Weil MH, Rackow EC, Trevino R, et al. Difference in acid-base state between venous and arterial blood during cardiopulmonary resuscitation. *N Engl J Med* 1986;315:153–156.
19. Ewy GA. Alternative approaches to external chest compression. *Circulation* 1986;74[Suppl IV]:IV-98–IV-101.
20. Kirscher JP, Fine EG, Weisfeld ML, et al. Comparison of prehospital conventional and simultaneous compression-ventilation cardiopulmonary resuscitation. *Crit Care Med* 1989;17:1263–1269.
21. Criley JM, Niemann JT, Rosborough JP, et al. Modifications of cardiopulmonary resuscitation based on the cough. *Circulation* 1986;74[Suppl IV]:IV-42–IV-50.
22. Halpern HR, Tsitlik JE, Belfand M, et al. A preliminary study of cardiopulmonary resuscitation by circumferential compression of the chest with use of a pneumatic vest. *N Engl J Med* 1993;329:762–768.
23. Babbs CF, Tacker WA. Cardiopulmonary resuscitation with interposed abdominal compression. *Circulation* 1986;74(Suppl IV):IV-37–IV-41.
24. Mateer JF, Stueven HA, Thompson BM, et al. Pre-hospital IAC-CPR versus standard CPR: paramedic resuscitation of cardiac arrests. *Am J Emerg Med* 1985;3:143–146.
25. Sack JB, Kesselbrenner MB, Bregman D. Survival from in-hospital cardiac arrest with interposed abdominal counterpulsation during cardiopulmonary resuscitation. *JAMA* 1992;267:379–385.
26. Cohen TJ, Tucker KJ, Lurie KG, et al. Active compression-decompression: a new method of cardiopulmonary resuscitation. *JAMA* 1992;267:2916–2923.
27. Plaisance P, Lurie KG, Vicaut E, et al. A Comparison of standard cardiopulmonary resuscitation and active compression-decompression resuscitation for out-of-hospital cardiac arrest. *N Engl J Med* 1999;341:569–575.
28. Stiell IG, Herbert PC, Wells GA, et al. The Ontario trial of active compression-decompression cardiopulmonary resuscitation for in-hospital and pre hospital cardiac arrest. *JAMA* 1996;275:1417–1423.
29. Sanders AB, Kern KB, Atlas M, et al. Importance of the duration of inadequate coronary perfusion pressure on resuscitation from cardiac arrest. *J Am Coll Cardiol* 1985;6:113–118.
30. Kern KB, Sanders AB, Badylak SF, et al. Long-term survival with open-chest cardiac massage after ineffective closed-chest compression in a canine preparation. *Circulation* 1987;75:498–503.
31. Ralston SH, Voorhees WD, Babbs CF. Intrapulmonary epinephrine during prolonged CPR. Improved regional blood flow and resuscitation in dogs. *Ann Emerg Med* 1984;13:79–86.
32. Paradis NA, Martin GB, Rivers EP, et al. Coronary perfusion pressure and the return of spontaneous circulation in human cardiopulmonary resuscitation. *JAMA* 1990;263:1106–1113.
33. Sanders AB, Kern KB, Otto CW, et al. End-tidal carbon dioxide monitoring during cardiopulmonary resuscitation. A prognostic indicator for survival. *JAMA* 1989;262:1347–1351.
34. Kern KB, Sanders AB, Raife J, et al. A study of chest compression rates during cardiopulmonary resuscitation in humans. The importance of rate-directed compressions. *Arch Intern Med* 1992;152:145–149.
35. Yakaitis RW, Ewy GA, Otto CW, et al. Influence of time and therapy on ventricular defibrillation in dogs. *Crit Care Med* 1980;8:157–163.
36. Weaver SC, Cobb LA, Dennis D, et al. Amplitude of ventricular fibrillation waveform and outcome after cardiac arrest. *Ann Intern Med* 1985;102:53–55.
37. Otto CW, Yakaitis RW, Ewy GA. Effects of epinephrine on defibrillation in ischemic ventricular fibrillation. *Am J Emerg Med* 1985;3:285–291.
38. Weaver WD, Cobb LA, Copass MK, et al. Ventricular defibrillation—a comparative trial using 175-J and 320-J shocks. *N Engl J Med* 1982;307:1101–1106.
39. Otto CW. Cardiovascular pharmacology II. The use of catecholamines, pressor agents, digitalis, and corticosteroids in CPR and emergency cardiac care. *Circulation* 1986;74[Suppl IV]:IV-80–IV-85.
40. Redding JS, Pearson JW. Evaluation of drugs for cardiac resuscitation. *Anesthesiology* 1963;24:203–207.
41. Redding JS, Pearson JW. Resuscitation from ventricular fibrillation. Drug therapy. *JAMA* 1968;203:255–560.

42. Otto CW, Yakaitis RW. The role of epinephrine in CPR. A reappraisal. *Ann Emerg Med* 1984;13:840–843.

43. Brillman JC, Sanders AB, Otto CW, et al. A comparison of epinephrine and phenylephrine for resuscitation and neurologic outcome of cardiac arrest in dogs. *Ann Emerg Med* 1987;16:11–17.

44. Silvast T, Saarnivaara L, Kinnunen A, et al. Comparison of adrenaline and phenylephrine in out-of-hospital CPR: a double-blind study. *Acta Anaesthesiol Scand* 1985;29:610–613.

45. Lindner KH, Dirks B, Strohmenger HU, et al. Randomized comparison of epinephrine and vasopressin in patients with out-of-hospital ventricular fibrillation. *Lancet* 1997;349:535–537.

46. Kudenchuk PJ, Cobb LA, Copass MK, et al. Amiodarone for resuscitation after out-of-hospital cardiac arrest due to ventricular fibrillation. *N Engl J Med* 1999;341:871–876.

47. Coon GA, Clinton JE, Ruiz E. Use of atropine for brady-asystolic prehospital cardiac arrest. *Ann Emerg Med* 1981;10:462–467.

48. Stueven HA, Tonsfeldt DJ, Thompson BM, et al. Atropine in asystole: human studies. *Ann Emerg Med* 1984;13:815–817.

49. Guerci AD, Chandra N, Johnson E, et al. Failure of sodium bicarbonate to improve resuscitation from ventricular fibrillation in dogs. *Circulation* 1986;74[Suppl IV]:75–79.

50. Federiuk CS, Sanders AB, Kern KB, et al. The effect of bicarbonate on resuscitation from cardiac arrest. *Ann Emerg Med* 1991;20:1173–1177.

51. Vukmir RB, Bircher NG, Radovsky A, et al. Sodium bicarbonate may improve outcome in dogs with brief or prolonged cardiac arrest. *Crit Care Med* 1995;23:515–522.

52. Weil MH, Grundler W, Yamaguchi M, et al. Arterial blood gases fail to reflect acid-base status during cardiopulmonary resuscitation. A preliminary report. *Crit Care Med* 1985;13:884–885.

53. Bishop RL, Weisfeldt ML. Sodium bicarbonate administration during cardiac arrest. Effect on arterial pH, pCO_2, and osmolality. *JAMA* 1976;235:506–509.

54. Mattar JA, Weil MH, Shubin H, et al. Cardiac arrest in the critically ill. II. Hyperosmolal states following cardiac arrest. *Am J Med* 1974; 56:162–168.

55. Stueven HA, Thompson BM, Aprahamian C, et al. Calcium chloride: reassessment of use in asystole. *Ann Emerg Med* 1984;13:820–822.

56. Stueven HA, Thompson BM, Aprahamian C, et al. The effectiveness of calcium chloride in refractory electromechanical dissociation. *Ann Emerg Med* 1985;14:626–629.

57. Abramson NS, Safar P, Detre KM, et al. Randomized clinical study of cardiopulmonary-cerebral resuscitation: thiopental loading in comatose cardiac arrest survivors. *N Engl J Med* 1986;314:397–403.

58. Brain Resuscitation Clinical Trial II Study Group. A randomized clinical study of a calcium-entry blocker (lidoflazine) in the treatment of comatose survivors of cardiac arrest. *N Engl J Med* 1991;324:1225–1231.

59. Longstreth WT, Diehr P, Inui TS. Prediction of awakening after out-of-hospital cardiac arrest. *N Engl J Med* 1983;308:1378–1382.

60. Longstreth WT, Inui TS, Cobb LA, et al. Neurologic recovery after out-of-hospital cardiac arrest. *Ann Intern Med* 1983;98:588–592.

61. Mullie A, Lust P, Penninck J, et al. Monitoring of cerebrospinal fluid enzyme levels in post-ischemic encephalopathy after cardiac arrest. *Crit Care Med* 1981;9:399–400.

62. Edgren E, Terent H, Hedstrand U, et al. Cerebral spinal fluid markers in relation to outcome in patients with global cerebral ischemia. *Crit Care Med* 1983;11:4–6.

PERIOPERATIVE EVALUATION OF PULMONARY DISEASES AND FUNCTION

PETER J. PAPADAKOS

KEY WORDS

- Respiratory physiology
- Pulmonary function
- Chronic obstructive pulmonary disease (COPD)
- Chronic bronchitis
- Emphysema
- Bronchiectasis
- Cystic fibrosis
- Asthma
- Atelectasis

INTRODUCTION

Perioperative evaluation of pulmonary function and respiratory disease requires an understanding of the etiology, pathophysiology, and signs of the disease, thus leading to a plan of management, establishment of therapeutic goals, and a schedule for ongoing assessment in the operating room (OR) and intensive care unit (ICU). A knowledge of pulmonary physiology and pathophysiology combined with a complete history, physical examination, and the measurement of pulmonary function can alert the clinician to the need for perioperative interventions that can improve the outcome of surgery. The clinician must understand how the site and type of surgical procedure can alter pulmonary function and increase perioperative risk for a particular patient. The evaluation of pulmonary disease may require only a simple history and physical for low-risk patients. For moderate-risk patients, the addition of spirometric testing with arterial blood gas analysis provides a great deal of information at the lowest cost (1). More complex testing such as magnetic resonance imaging and nuclear medicine tests in combination with evaluation of the pulmonary circulation may be considered for patients undergoing pulmonary surgery or patients with debilitating pulmonary disease.

RESPIRATORY PHYSIOLOGY

Respiration is the combination of various physical and chemical processes by which oxygen is supplied to the living cell for its metabolic needs and carbon dioxide is removed. The main function of the respiratory system, the delivery of oxygen to the blood, is accomplished and regulated by an intricate set of structures. These structures include: (a) the lungs, which provide the gas exchange surface; (b) the conducting airways, which convey the air into and out of the lungs; (c) the thoracic wall, which acts as a bellows and supports and protects the lungs; (d) the respiratory muscles, which create the energy necessary for the movement of air into and out of the lungs; and (e) the respiratory centers with their sensitive receptors and communicating nerves, which control and regulate ventilation. Pathologic processes can affect any one of these functional components. The interactions of the cardiopulmonary, nervous, and musculoskeletal systems can be disrupted by disease and by surgery and anesthetic agents (3).

The respiratory system also acts as a major immune barrier by clearance of particles including viruses, bacteria, fungi, and inhaled environmental debris via a mucociliary escalator. The immune function also has been identified as a local cellular process that can lead to cytokine modulation (2). These structural and immunologic relationships determine physiologic function in the normal state (3,4).

Patient position plays an important role in pulmonary function. A change from the standing to the supine position causes a shift from mostly thoracic to predominantly diaphragmatic breathing. Surgery and pharmacologic agents can decrease pulmonary function by causing atelectasis and a decrease in functional residual capacity.

The neural regulation of respiration is complex. It is subject to voluntary and involuntary influences and involves medullary regulatory centers, central and peripheral chemoreceptors, cranial nerves, peripheral nerves, nociceptive mechanisms, and visceral reflexes that are consciously and unconsciously perceived. While resting bronchomotor tone is primarily influenced by parasympathetic nerves, multiple other bioactive molecules such as prostaglandins, nitric oxide, and catecholamines alter gas exchange and blood flow in the lungs. Neurologically mediated afferent and efferent activity influence some of the mechanisms that alter diaphragmatic function and the postoperative loss of lung volume. Age and multiple drugs diminish upper airway muscle tone and protective airway reflexes (3).

Functions of the lung not related to gas exchange include metabolic, secretory, and immunologic functions that are performed by specific groups of cells in the lungs. The vascular endothelium, Clara cells, K cells, type II pneumocytes, mast cells, and white cells all play a role in maintaining homeostasis in the lung (5).

PULMONARY PATHOLOGY

Lung disease is one of the most common diseases in the United States. Chronic lung disease affects over 28 million Americans (6). These diseases include asthma, chronic obstructive pulmonary disease (COPD), chronic bronchitis, pulmonary emphysema, bronchiectasis, cystic fibrosis, sarcoidosis, immunologic pneumonitis, and environmental lung diseases. An even larger number suffer from acute disorders such as infections, seasonal allergies, and occupational exposures. There are no data on the percentage of patients presenting for surgery or admitted to the ICU who have pulmonary disease.

Pulmonary pathology can be classified into two broad categories: restrictive ventilatory defects (RVDs) and obstructive ventilatory defects (OVDs). These categories are distinguished on the basis of clinical history, physical examination, and diagnostic tests, primarily spirometry. A detailed description of restrictive and obstructive lung diseases is provided in Chapter 34. RVDs are extrinsic if alveolar volume is reduced by external compression through a mass effect or decreased thoracic compliance. Common extrinsic RVDs include muscular dystrophy, pleural effusions, kyphoscoliosis, and atelectasis. Postoperative reductions in pulmonary function are also largely restrictive in nature. RVDs are intrinsic if alveoli are thickened or coated or otherwise present a barrier to gas diffusion. These intrinsic disorders include pulmonary fibrosis, alveolar proteinosis, interstitial lung disease, and acute respiratory distress syndrome (ARDS). ARDS can be precipitated by severe trauma, sepsis, smoke inhalation, metabolic disorders, drug toxicity, aspiration, hematologic disorders, and metabolic disorders (7). Estimates are that 150,000 cases of ARDS occur annually and that mortality ranges from 20% to 50% (7).

OBSTRUCTIVE LUNG DISEASE

OVDs are the most common category of respiratory pathology. In the United States COPD affects over 15 million individuals and is a common cause of death and disability in adults. Many patients with COPD have a combination of emphysema and chronic bronchitis. Asthma affects 12.4 million Americans, including 4.2 million under the age of 18 years. In total, over 42 million Americans have some form of OVD (6,8).

OVDs are characterized by obstruction to alveolar emptying. In emphysema there is a loss of alveolar elasticity and architecture, which results in alveolar closure and destruction of alveolar surface area. Air trapping and ventilation perfusion (V/Q) mismatching result. In COPD, small airway obstruction is secondary to mucosal inflammation, local edema, excess mucus production, decreased mucus clearance, and increased incidence of infection. Increased bronchomotor tone also is present in many OVDs. Asthma is a classic example of increased bronchomotor tone with increased reactivity of the airways, resulting in periodic wheezing, dyspnea, and cough. These clinical manifestations are the result of widespread narrowing of bronchi and bronchioles caused by mucosal inflammation, increased secretions, and smooth muscle contraction (9).

REVERSIBLE VERSUS IRREVERSIBLE DISEASE

One of the important preoperative evaluations is to discover if some component of RVDs and OVDs can be altered by lifestyle changes (smoking cessation) or pharmacologic management. Ongoing clinical evaluation, spirometry, and other pulmonary function tests are used to diagnose disease and to monitor therapeutic interventions. Spirometry is useful in distinguishing RVDs and OVDs, and in measuring reversible components of disease.

Classic spirometric tests measure the forced vital capacity (FVC) of the lungs after the patient inspires maximally to total lung capacity (TLC) and exhales maximally to residual volume (RV). Proper patient education and coaching by an experienced respiratory technologist are invaluable to getting proper data. The normal spirogram is a plot of exhaled lung volume against time. If the patient has a suspected or documented reversible disease or a history of bronchodilator use, the test is repeated after bronchodilator therapy.

Standard spirometric data include the total forced volume delivered into the spirometer (FVC) and specific volumes related to time during the forced expiration [forced expiratory volume at specific time (FEV_T)]. FVC is the volume of gas that can be exhaled as forcefully and rapidly as possible after a maximal inspiration. Normally, FVC = vital capacity (VC). In obstructive lung disease, however, FVC is reduced when compared to slow VC, indicating air trapping with forced exhalation. Forced expiratory volume timed (FEV_T), is the maximal volume of gas that can be exhaled over a specific period. The measurement is obtained from an FVC measurement. Commonly used time periods are 0.5, 1, 2, and 3 seconds with 1 second being the value most commonly used in preoperative evaluations. Normally, the percentages of the total volume exhaled during these time periods are as follows: $FEV_{0.5}$, 60%; FEV_1, 83%; FEV_2, 94%; and FEV_3, 97%. In obstructive disease, the time necessary to forcefully exhale a certain volume is increased (Fig. 1).

Another measure of airflow obstruction is flow rate during the VC maneuver. One of the most commonly used measurements is the forced expiratory flow rate measured between 25% and 75% of VC ($FEF_{25\%-75\%}$). This flow range is particularly important for the surgical patient because the ability to improve after bronchodilators correlates with improved postoperative outcome in some patients (11). Bronchodilators are the mainstay of evaluating the reversibility of bronchomotor tone. Other reversible components of pulmonary disease include infection, smoking, and obesity. Smoking and infection are extrinsic factors. Smoking cessation can improve lung function at any time (12). Proper treatment of pulmonary infection with antibiotics and pulmonary toilet can improve patient outcome.

Cardiac disease plays a major role in lung function. Improvement of cardiac function with diuretics, digoxin, and afterload reduction may greatly improve pulmonary function in congestive heart failure. Cardiac medications may alter bronchomotor tone (beta-adrenergic blockers) and diaphragmatic contractility (calcium channel blockers). Cardiac status should be optimized prior to elective surgery. Pulmonary hypertension should be evaluated and treated when present due to its high perioperative morbidity and mortality. Other factors such as age, gender, and previous

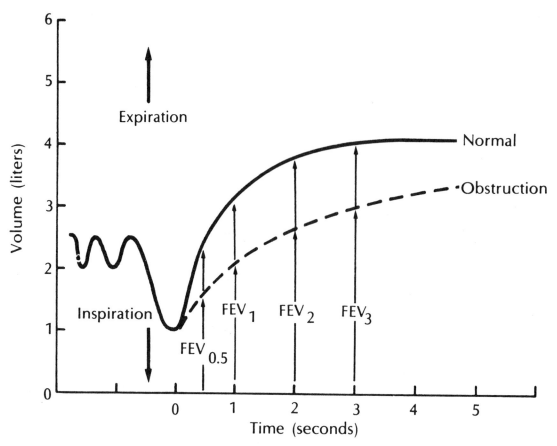

FIGURE 1. Forced expired volume timed (FEV$_T$). In obstructive pulmonary disease, more time is needed to exhale a specific volume. (From Des Jardins T, Burton GG, eds. *Clinical manifestations and assessment of respiratory disease.* St. Louis: Mosby–Year Book, 1995:34, with permission.)

medical conditions such as diabetes mellitus are also significant factors in pulmonary complications (12).

COMMON CHRONIC RESPIRATORY DISEASES

Chronic Bronchitis

The anatomic alterations of chronic bronchitis involve the primary conducting airways. Due to chronic inflammation, the

TABLE 1. PULMONARY FUNCTION FINDINGS—CHRONIC BRONCHITIS

A. Lung Volume and Capacity
  Tidal volume (TV) ↑
  Residual volume (RV) ↑
  Function residual capacity (FRC) ↑
  Total lung capacity (TLC) ↑/normal
  Vital capacity (VC) ↓/normal
  RV/TLC ratio ↑

B. Expiratory Maneuver Findings
  Forced vital capacity (FVC) ↓
  Forced expiratory volume at specific time (FEV$_T$) ↓
  FEV$_1$/FVC ratio ↓

C. Blood Gases
  Mild to moderate bronchitis
    pH ↑ Paco$_2$ ↓ HCO$_3$↑ (slightly) Pao$_2$ ↓
  Severe chronic bronchitis
    pH (normal) Paco$_2$ ↑ HCO$_3$ ↑ (significantly) Pao$_2$ ↓

bronchial walls are narrowed by vasodilation, congestion, and mucosal edema. The continued bronchial irritation causes the submucosal bronchial glands to enlarge and the number of goblet cells to increase, resulting in excessive mucus production. The number and function of cilia lining the tracheobronchial tree is diminished, and the peripheral bronchi are often partially or totally occluded by inflammation and mucus plugs, which in turn lead to hyperinflated alveoli.

Important etiologic factors in chronic bronchitis include cigarette smoking, atmospheric pollutants (sulfur dioxide, nitrogen oxide, and ozone), and infection. Patients demonstrate increased ventilatory rate due to stimulation of peripheral chemoreceptors and anxiety. Spirometry data are presented in Table 1.

In patients with chronic bronchitis, pharmacologic management should be optimized prior to surgery. Patients may receive mucolytic agents, sympathomimetics, parasympatholytics, xanthines, expectorants, antibiotics, and home oxygen. Elective surgery should be delayed in patients with active respiratory infection. Education by a respiratory therapist about mobilization of excessive mucus may play a role in the perioperative care of these patients (13).

Emphysema

The anatomic alterations of the lungs include permanent enlargement of the air spaces distal to the terminal bronchioles and

TABLE 2. PULMONARY FUNCTION FINDINGS IN EMPHYSEMA

A. Lung Volume and Capacity
  TV ↑
  Residual volume (RV) ↑
  Vital capacity (VC) ↓/normal
  Total lung capacity (TLC) ↑/normal
  RV/TLC Ratio ↑

B. Expiratory Maneuver Findings
  Forced vital capacity (FVC) ↓
  Forced expiratory flow (FEF)$_{25\%-75\%}$ ↓
  Forced expiratory volume at specific time (FEV$_T$) ↓
  FEV$_1$/FVC ratio ↓

C. Blood Gases
  Mild to moderate emphysema
    pH ↑ Paco$_2$ ↓ HCO$_3$ ↓ (slightly) Pao$_2$ ↓
  Severe (end-stage) emphysema
    pH (normal) Paco$_2$ ↑ HCO$_3$ ↑ (significantly) Pao$_2$ ↓

TABLE 3. PULMONARY FUNCTION FINDINGS IN BRONCHIECTASIS

A. Lung Volume and Capacity
  TV ↑
  Residual volume (RV) ↑
  Functional residual capacity (FRC) ↑
  Vital capacity (VC) ↓/normal
  Total lung capacity (TLC) ↑/normal
  RV/TLC ratio ↑

B. Expiratory Maneuver Findings
  Forced vital capacity (FVC) ↓
  Forced expiratory flow (FEF)$_{25\%-75\%}$ ↓
  Forced expiratory volume at specified time (FEV$_T$) ↓
  FEV$_1$/FVC ratio ↓

C. Blood Gases
  Mild to moderate bronchiectasis
    pH ↑ Paco$_2$ ↓ HCO$_3^-$ ↓ (slightly) Pao$_2$ ↓
  Severe bronchiectasis
    pH ↑ Paco$_2$ ↑ HCO$_3^-$ ↑ (significantly) Pao$_2$ ↓

destruction of the alveolar walls. As these structures enlarge and the alveoli coalesce, many of the adjacent pulmonary capillaries are also affected, resulting in a decreased area for gas exchange. The distal airways, weakened by emphysema, collapse during expiration in response to increased intrapleural pressure. This traps gas in the distal alveoli. There are two major types of emphysema: panacinar (panlobular) emphysema and centriacinar (centrilobular) emphysema. Spirometry data are presented, along with blood gas parameters for emphysema in Table 2.

In panacinar emphysema there is abnormal weakening and enlargement of all air spaces distal to the terminal bronchioles, alveolar ducts, alveolar sacs, and alveoli. The alveoli are enlarged and their septae are destroyed, resulting in significant loss of pulmonary parenchyma. Panacinar emphysema occurs throughout the lung but is primarily found in the lower and anterior lung fields. It has a high association with alpha$_1$-antitrypsin deficiency (14).

Centrilobular emphysema is the most common form of emphysema and is often associated with chronic bronchitis. This disease has a very strong association with smoking. In centrilobular emphysema, the lesion is in the center of the lobules, which corresponds to enlargement and destructive changes in the respiratory bronchioles. It usually involves the upper lung fields (15).

The general management of emphysema is similar to chronic bronchitis. Sympathomimetic, parasympatholytic, and xanthine agents are commonly prescribed to offset bronchial smooth muscle spasm. Replacement therapy with human alpha$_1$-proteinase inhibitor (Prolastin) may be helpful in patients suffering from alpha$_1$-antitrypsin deficiency.

Bronchiectasis

The anatomic alterations of the lung that characterize bronchiectasis are chronic dilation and distortion of one or more bronchi due to extensive inflammation and destruction of the bronchial wall cartilage, blood vessels, elastic tissue, and smooth muscle components. Bronchiectasis is commonly limited to a lobe or a segment and is often found in the lower lobes. There is a high correlation to persistent or intermittent bacterial colonization and infection, and the resultant inflammation seems to be the mechanism of perpetuating damage and dilation of bronchi.

Three forms or anatomic varieties have been described: varicose (fusiform), cylindrical (tubular), and saccular (cystic). Although bronchiectasis is seen in all ages, its onset is often in childhood. There is a strong genetic predisposition to bronchiectasis. Nearly half the cases are associated with cystic fibrosis (16). Several congenital conditions such as Kartagener syndrome and hypogammaglobulinemia predispose to bronchiectasis. Spirometry and blood gas data for bronchiectasis are presented in Table 3.

The basis of therapy of bronchiectasis is mobilization of mucus by postural drainage. Pharmacologic management is similar to chronic bronchitis. Supplemental oxygen may be required for hypoxemia.

Cystic Fibrosis (Mucoviscidosis)

Cystic fibrosis (CF) is a hereditary disease transmitted as a Mendelian recessive trait. Various mutations of a single gene located in the long arm of chromosome 7 are now recognized to be the cause of CF. The most common mutation, known as ΔF508, results in the deletion of the amino acid phenylalanine at position 508 of CF transmembrane conductance regulator (CFTR). CF is more common in whites than in blacks. Its incidence has been estimated to be one in 2,500 live births (17).

An increased concentration of sweat electrolytes and an abnormality of mucus secretion and elimination are the two distinct and well-recognized pathologic conditions in CF. The common basic pathogenic mechanism is the defective transport of chloride and sodium across the epithelial cell membrane as a result of abnormal CFTR protein production. Although the lungs of patients with CF appear normal at birth, abnormal structural changes develop quickly. Bronchial gland hypertrophy and metaplasia of goblet cells produce large amounts of thick tenacious mucus. Because the mucus is so thick, impairment of the normal mucociliary clearing ensues. Mucus plugging of small bronchi and bronchioles results in overdistension of the alveoli, and complete obstruction of small bronchi and bronchioles. Partial obstruction leads to overdistension of the alveoli. Complete obstruction produces patchy areas of atelectasis. The stagnant mucus in the tracheobronchial tree serves as an excellent culture medium for

TABLE 4. PULMONARY FUNCTION FINDINGS IN CYSTIC FIBROSIS

A. Lung Volume and Capacity
TV ↑
Residual volume (RV) ↑
Functional residual capacity (FRC) ↑
Vital capacity (VC) ↓/normal
Total lung capacity (TLC) ↑/normal
RV/TLC ratio ↑

B. Expiratory Maneuver Findings
Forced vital capacity (FVC) ↓
Forced expiratory flow (FEF)$_{25\%-75\%}$ ↓
Forced expiratory volume at specific time (FEV$_T$) ↓
FEV$_1$/FVC ratio ↓

C. Blood Gases
Mild to moderate cystic fibrosis
pH ↑ Paco$_2$ ↓ HCO$_3$ ↑ (significantly) Pao$_2$ ↓

TABLE 5. PULMONARY FUNCTION FINDINGS IN ASTHMA

A. Lung Volume and Capacity
TV ↑
Residual volume (RV) ↑
Functional residual capacity (FRC) ↑
Vital capacity (VC) ↓
Total lung capacity (TLC) ↑
RV/TLC ratio ↑

B. Expiratory Maneuver Findings
Forced vital capacity (FVC) ↓
Forced expiratory flow (FEF)$_{25\%-75\%}$ ↓
Forced expiratory volume at specific time (FEV$_T$) ↓
FEV$_1$/FVC ratio ↓

C. Blood Gases
Mild to moderate asthmatic episode
pH ↑ Paco$_2$ ↓ HCO$_3$ ↓ (slightly) Pao$_2$ ↓
Severe asthmatic episode (status)
pH ↓ Paco$_2$ ↑ HCO$_3$ ↑ (slightly) Pao$_2$ ↓

bacteria. Table 4 summarizes the pulmonary function tests and blood gas data for CF.

Early treatment in CF decreases the rate of lung volume loss and improves survival (18). Postural drainage and chest physiotherapy assists patients in clearing mucus plugs and acutely improves pulmonary function. Another important factor is secretion viscosity. The DNA of dying neutrophils is released into the sputum, increasing its viscosity. Breaking up the DNA with recombinant human deoxyribonuclease (DNase) improves sputum viscosity and clearance. Treatment with inhaled DNase decreases the frequency of exacerbations, improves FVC and pulmonary function, and reduces the need for antibiotic therapy (19,20). Additional therapies to assist in secretion management include airway oscillators, positive expiratory pressure (bilevel positive airway pressure/continuous positive airway pressure) mask therapy, and voluntary coughing.

Repeated lung infections are almost universal in patients with CF. These infections lead to destruction of lung tissue and loss of pulmonary function. Antibiotic therapy should be given whenever new symptoms develop. The initial choice of antibiotics should be targeted to infections commonly found in CF patients such as *Pseudomonas aeruginosa* and then adjusted based on sputum culture findings.

Heart–lung and bilateral lung transplantation have been used for patients with end-stage lung disease due to CF. Transplantation reverses the physiologic abnormalities that characterize CF, but its role is limited due to donor organ availability and the need for long-term immunosuppression (21). A new approach in the management of CF is to reverse the abnormal electrolyte transport. Early trials with aerosolized amiloride or triphosphate have been promising.

Asthma

Asthma involves increased reactivity of the airways resulting in periodic wheezing, dyspnea, and cough. The trachea and bronchi show an exaggerated sensitivity to the bronchoconstrictive effect of a variety of physical, pharmacologic, and biologic agents. In time, there is hypertrophy of the smooth muscle, the goblet cells, and the bronchial mucus glands. The airways become filled with thick, tenacious mucus, and extensive plugging may develop. The bronchial mucosa is edematous and infiltrated with eosinophils

and other inflammatory cells. The cilia become damaged and the basement membrane of the mucosa becomes thickened. Air trapping and hyperinflation of alveoli occur due to smooth muscle constriction, bronchial mucosal edema, and mucus hypersecretion. The anatomic alterations that occur during an asthmatic attack are completely reversible (10,11). Table 5 summarizes the pulmonary function tests and blood gas data for an asthmatic episode.

Depending on whether or not a specific external cause can be demonstrated, asthma is classified into extrinsic and intrinsic categories. Because extrinsic asthma is most often the result of an allergy, the terms allergic asthma and extrinsic asthma are often used interchangeably. Both extrinsic and intrinsic asthma may be precipitated by exposure to nonspecific stimulants such as exercise and cold air. Common atmospheric pollutants, including sulfur dioxide, nitric oxide, ozone, and aerosolized particulates can provoke or exacerbate asthma. More than 200 agents have been recognized to cause occupational asthma, including polyurethane, plastics, trimellitic anhydride, organic dusts, grain flours, and sawdust (22,23). While bacterial infections may cause asthma, viral upper airway infections are more predominant. This form of intrinsic asthma is commonly seen in children with respiratory syncytial virus, rhinovirus, and influenza virus.

Emotional factors and stress are known to affect asthma. The mechanism of effect of emotional factors on asthma is the result of complex interactions between the central nervous system (CNS) and the immune system. Proper premedication and sedation may greatly decrease attacks in these groups of patients during the perioperative period. Many asthmatic patients have more difficulty with their asthma in the late night and early morning hours. Precipitating factors associated with nocturnal asthma include gastroesophageal reflux, retained airway secretions, and exposure to allergens in the bedding and bedroom (24).

Sympathomimetic drugs, usually administered as aerosolized selective beta$_2$-agonists, are the most commonly used agents in the treatment of asthma. Inhaled drugs can be given with a jet or ultrasonic nebulizer or they can be more conveniently used from an MDI, either as propellant-generated aerosols or breath-activated devices for dry powder preparations. Salmeterol may be suitable for its preventive effect against exacerbations that occur at night, following exercise or prior to exposure trigger substances.

Corticosteroid preparations are playing an increasingly important role in the management of asthma. They decrease and prevent inflammation through the inhibition of various mediators. Corticosteroids also enhance and potentiate the effects of beta-adrenergic drugs and reduce mucus secretion. However, steroids may have negative long-term effects such as adrenal insufficiency and immunosuppression (25).

Zafirlukast (Accolate), an oral agent that opposes the bronchoconstrictive and inflammatory effects of leukotrienes, was recently approved for prophylactic and chronic treatment of asthma. Parasympatholytics are used to offset bronchial smooth muscle constriction. Cromolyn sodium and related compounds are antiinflammatory agents used for the preventive management of asthma. They work by inhibiting pulmonary mast-cell degranulation. They prevent bronchospasm induced by antigens, exercise, or occupational asthma.

General care of the patient with asthma should also include mobilization of bronchial secretions. Serial pulmonary function measurements such as FEV_1 can be used to monitor therapy.

EVALUATION OF THE PATIENT WITH RESPIRATORY DISEASE

Each patient with pulmonary disease should have a complete workup and risk assessment. A thorough clinical history and physical examination is the first step in functional assessment. The characteristics of the main complaint and associated symptoms should be ascertained, including the onset of symptoms, their severity and duration, the circumstances that lead to them or aggravate them, and the factors alleviating them. It is important to get a full picture of the patient's health prior to the present illness; previous diseases, surgeries, and injuries; occupational, environmental, and travel history; allergies, health of family, smoking and other habits; and a complete list of the patient's medications. The common and important symptoms of respiratory disease are limited in number. These symptoms are cough, expectoration, dyspnea, hemoptysis, chest pain, and wheezing (8). The goal of preoperative pulmonary assessment is to uncover any preexisting or potential pulmonary defects in order to identify patient factors, surgical factors, and anesthetic factors that can be controlled to limit perioperative pulmonary complications. While complex diagnostic studies can clarify a patient's health picture, clinical history and physical examination remain the most potent predictors of individual patient outcome (26,27).

The goal of preoperative pulmonary evaluation is to optimize the individual patient's pulmonary status in relation to the surgical and anesthetic risk factors. It should give insight to the level of monitoring required and the need for specialized postoperative care such as ICU admission and mechanical ventilation. The questions that need to be answered include whether or not there is a history of any of the following:

smoking;
acute, chronic, or recurrent upper or lower respiratory tract infection, including opportunistic infections, productive cough, wheezing, or dyspnea;

chronic lung disease;
cancer;
sarcoidosis;
industrial exposure;
radiation or chemotherapy to the lung or chest wall; and/or systemic diseases that can affect the lung.

A skilled and complete physical examination is highly important. The physical examination should consist of inspection, palpation, auscultation, and percussion of the head, neck, thorax, and abdomen. Close inspection of the upper airway and evaluation of difficulty in breathing is important (28). Assessment of the patient's voice quality gives information about vocal cord function, upper airway obstruction, and the gross ability to move air. The patient who cannot speak normally without dyspnea and hoarseness needs further evaluation.

The physical examination and evaluation of the patient should determine if the patient has a history of a difficult airway or evidence that this is likely to be a problem. A complete history and examination of the pulmonary system should address whether or not the patient has any of the following:

acute or chronic lung infections,
respiratory distress,
hypoxemia,
COPD,
restrictive lung disease,
congestive heart failure (CHF),
obesity,
scoliosis,
neuromuscular disease, and/or
other diseases that affect the respiratory system.

The patient is examined for clues of respiratory disease such as cyanosis, use of accessory muscles, nasal flaring, jugular venous distension, muscle wasting, obesity, peripheral edema, scoliosis, clubbing, arthritis, ascites, and evidence of prior surgery. Auscultation of the chest should include all lung fields. It can detect stridor, wheezing, rhonchi, crackles, asymmetry of breath sounds, focal consolidation, and defects in diaphragmatic excursion.

Breath sounds are highly important as a window to pathology. There are three types of breath sounds: tracheal, bronchovesicular, and vesicular. Tracheal breath sounds are heard directly over the trachea and are local and high-pitched. Tracheal breath sounds are produced by turbulent flow of air in the trachea and are relatively equal in both inspiration and expiration. Bronchovesicular breath sounds are heard around the sternum on the anterior chest wall and between the scapulae on the posterior chest wall. They are produced by turbulent flow in larger airways and are softer and not as high-pitched as tracheal sounds. Vesicular breath sounds are heard over the areas of the chest wall overlying lung parenchyma. They are produced by turbulent flow in larger airways but are softer and lower pitched than tracheal breath sounds and are primarily heard only on inspiration. They are low-pitched and softer because they represent the turbulent flow heard after the air has passed through normal lung tissue. The normal tissue acts as a filter and converts normal tracheal sounds to normal vesicular sounds.

Any lung disease that causes the parenchyma to become denser will result in less filtering of the turbulent flow sounds of the

TABLE 6. INTERPRETIVE NATURE OF LUNG SOUNDS

Name of Sound	Mechanism	Characteristics
Stridor	Upper airway narrowing	High-pitched
Bronchial breath sounds	Increased sound transmission	Equal inspiratory and expiratory components
Diminished breath sounds	Decreased sound transmission	Decreased sound transmission
Wheezes	Airflow through narrowed airway	Musical with a continuous pattern
Crackles	Sudden opening of closed airways or movement of airway secretions	Coarse inspiratory and expiratory

larger airways. This will make the sounds harsher and louder. Atelectasis, pulmonary fibrosis, and pneumonia can cause harsh sounds over the affected area. Disorders of the lung, which cause loss of density such as emphysema, result in excessive filtration of the turbulent flow sounds. This will make normal sounds very hard to hear. Rapid airflow through a site of obstruction is believed to cause the airway wall to flutter rapidly between a partially open and closed position. This will produce a wheeze. Wheezing is most often heard during exhalation because the intrathoracic airways are narrow. Some clinicians have referred to low-pitched wheezes as rhonchi. Discontinuous lung sounds are termed crackles. They represent the opening and closing of lung parenchyma. The term rales is used to describe several abnormal lung sounds but has been abandoned in that it is nonspecific. Partial upper airway obstruction can cause a wheezing-type sound heard during inspiration and is referred to as stridor. It is important to remember that not all patients with upper airway obstruction present with stridor. Fatigue and the use of sedative and narcotic agents will reduce the degree of air movement past the obstruction and cause an absence of stridor.

The interpretive nature of lung sounds is summarized in Table 6. Once physical assessment is complete, rational decisions about diagnostic testing can proceed.

Chest Radiograph and Other Imaging Techniques

The chest radiograph is the most common test of preoperative pulmonary function. The difference in the density of various structures allows for excellent delineation on the x-ray film. The air-containing lungs have the least density and do not significantly interfere with the passage of roentgen rays, causing dark punts on the film. The bony structures have the highest density and therefore impede x-rays and prevent their impression on film, which remains white. The heart and soft tissue, which have density greater than air but less than bone, cause differing shades of white and gray on the radiograph.

The standard PA projection, which is the cornerstone of radiographic examination of the chest, is obtained by placing the patient in front of the radiographic film so that the patient's chest touches the film and the x-ray tube is behind the patient. However, in the typical supine portable film taken in the ICU, the x-ray tube is above the patient and the patient is lying on top of

the film. The chest radiograph can be used to evaluate atelectasis, effusions, pneumothorax, pneumonia, chronic changes, cardiovascular changes, and lung collapse. The radiograph should not be used in isolation (29). Preoperative chest radiographs should be considered for patients with known pulmonary, cardiovascular, or malignant disease, chest trauma, on mechanical ventilation, or heavy smoking history.

Computed tomography (CT) is an imaging technique in which radiologic and computer technologies are combined to generate cross-sections of the body as thin slices. Thoracic CT scan is supplementary to standard radiographic studies. It is useful for delineation of mediastinal and hilar structures, intrapulmonary nodules, and pleural diseases, for staging intrathoracic malignancies and for evaluating the vascular structures in the chest. Great progress has been made with CT scanning in our understanding of ARDS (30).

Magnetic resonance imaging (MRI) is based on characteristics of nuclei of atoms of certain elements in the body tissues that can be magnetized when placed in a strong magnetic field. MRI is superior to CT for imaging soft tissue masses and lymph node structures in the chest and is helpful in evaluating neoplastic disease.

Imaging techniques are discussed in detail in Chapter 63.

Arterial Blood Gas Studies

Arterial blood gas (ABG) analysis provides a "snapshot" of preoperative resting pulmonary function. The main function of the respiratory system is to maintain arterial blood oxygen and CO_2 tensions within a physiologic range. ABG analysis includes the direct measurement of partial pressure of oxygen (Pa_{O_2}), partial pressure of carbon dioxide (Pa_{CO_2}), and pH and calculation of serum bicarbonate. Hemoglobin saturation may be directly measured or estimated from a nomogram.

Pa_{O_2} and Pa_{CO_2} can change dramatically during the perioperative period due to a variety of physiologic stresses (31). The Pa_{O_2} parallels the decreases in FRC and FVC that occur following abdominal surgeries, trauma, and thoracic surgery. Mild hypoxemia is present when the Pa_{O_2} is below normal for the age of the patient but above 59 mm Hg. Moderate hypoxemia is present when the Pa_{O_2} is between 40 mm Hg and 50 mm Hg. Typical ABG values for specific diseases were reviewed earlier in this chapter. For patients on supplemental oxygen, the severity of the oxygenation abnormality is often assessed by the Pa_{O_2}/F_{IO_2} ratio; values below 200 are part of the definition of ARDS. Use of pulse oximetry for arterial hemoglobin saturation is now a monitoring standard in the ICU and OR. ABG analysis is used to titrate mechanical ventilation and can act as a marker of lung recruitment. CO_2 retention can be a marker of pulmonary failure even though there is no prospective study of the value of elevated Pa_{CO_2} for predicting acute respiratory failure. Discovery of a reversible cause of hypercarbia such as improper sedation or inappropriate ventilator settings is important.

Normal preoperative resting ABGs do not ensure a good perioperative pulmonary outcome, but abnormal ABGs can lead to bad outcome if not acted upon. They are one of the most important adjuncts in patient management in the ICU.

A useful noninvasive method to rapidly estimate Pa_{CO_2} is the use of capnometry to measure end-tidal P_{CO_2} by spectrometry

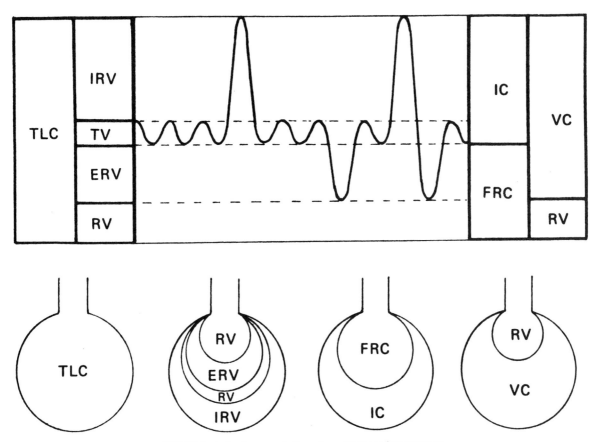

FIGURE 2. A classic presentation of a pulmonary function test.

or infrared analysis. It is continuous and can be used to evaluate patients in real time. An important use of end-tidal P_{CO_2} is to evaluate proper placement of an endotracheal tube (32). It can also be used in the ICU to aid in ventilator weaning.

Pulmonary Function Testing

Pulmonary function tests (PFTs) can help characterize preoperative pulmonary health and help predict postoperative pulmonary failure. The classic way to present pulmonary function is in graphic form (Fig. 2). PFTs provide an assessment of baseline function, which can be used to grade the patient to known standards for specific pulmonary diseases. PFTs can assess response to bronchodilator therapy which can be used to manage patients in the operating room and in the postoperative period. The typical effects of different respiratory disorders on PFTs were reviewed earlier in the chapter.

Routine PFTs may be performed with simple spirometric devices or by advanced instrumentation in modern pulmonary function laboratories. As lung volumes and flow rates are usually the most useful and informative parameters to be measured, simple spirometry will suffice in most situations. FRC is an important measurement that is being used by intensive care physicians to predict the speed of weaning. Decreases in FRC makes the patient more prone to respiratory complications.

The prognostic value of PFTs for surgical patients is controversial. They are helpful in patients with underlying disease or patients undergoing major surgery of the chest or abdomen. They may not add any information in patients without pulmonary disease as risk factors.

In contrast to spirometry, the flow of gas over time intervals is useful in some specific diseases. In some studies, these flows predicted pulmonary complications in thoracotomy patients (33). Values less than 50% of predicted value were associated with high mortality and morbidity. It is also useful to grade specific pulmonary diseases as outlined earlier in the chapter (Fig. 3).

Flow Volume Loops

The FVC maneuver can be used to record flow versus volume instead of volume versus time, and to graphically display the response to bronchodilators. In general, plotting flow versus volume and volume versus time produces similar spirometric data. When combined with maximum inspiratory effort at the end of the FVC maneuver, however, the flow-volume loop provides important additional data on upper-airway function. Partial or fixed airway obstruction will manifest as changes in the loop. Intrathoracic airway obstruction is most evident during expiration, whereas extrathoracic upper-airway obstruction is most evident during inspiration. Flow-volume loops depict a number of measures of pulmonary function that are not captured by regular pulmonary function spirometry. In addition to FVC and FEV_1, flow volume loops allow visual recognition of peak expiratory flow rate (PEFR), $FEF_{25\%-75\%}$, and various patterns of airway

Total lung capacity is the volume of air at the end of a maximum inspiration and it is made up of four volumes:

 A. Residual Volume (RV) is the volume of air that remains in the lungs after maximum expiration.

 B. Expiratory Reserve Volume (ERV) is the maximum volume of air that can be exhaled after expiration of tidal volume.

 C. Tidal Volume (TV) is the volume of air inspired and expired with each normal breath.

 D. Inspiratory Reserve Volume (IRV) is the maximum volume of air that one can breathe in after inspiration of tidal volume.

By combining two or more of these volumes, we have the following four lung capacities.

 A. Functional Residual Capacity (FRC) is the total of RV and ERV. It is the volume remaining in the lung at the end of expiration of TV.

 B. Inspiratory Capacity (IC) is the sum of TV and IRV. It is the maximum volume of air that can be inspired from a resting state.

 C. Vital Capacity (VC) is the total of ERV, TV, and IRV, or the sum of ERV and IC. It is the maximum volume of air that can be forcefully exhaled after a maximum inspiration.

 D. Total lung capacity (TLC) is the sum of RV, ERV, TV, and IRV or the sum of VC and RV or the sum of IC and FRC.

FIGURE 3. A review of the basic technique of pulmonary function testing.

obstruction. For instance, a "square" loop results when fixed intrathoracic and fixed extrathoracic sources of obstruction coexist. In contrast, loops are "squared" only in inspiration or expiration when extrathoracic or intrathoracic obstruction exists, respectively. As with spirometry, flow-volume loops are useful in assessing prebronchodilator and postbronchodilator performance. As with PFTs, improvements of 10% or greater indicate a salutary response to bronchodilators.

ANESTHETIC FACTORS

Anesthetic factors have a variable influence on respiratory illnesses. Anesthesia can be classified as topical, regional, neuraxial, or general. Conscious (moderate) sedation is often used in conjunction with techniques other than general anesthesia.

Local anesthesia is generally safe unless toxic limits are exceeded. Neuraxial and general anesthesia both present risks to patients with lung disease. Neuraxial anesthesia includes subarachnoid anesthesia that may compromise pulmonary function by altering abdominal muscle and thoracic muscle function, thereby creating dependence on diaphragmatic breathing. Epidural anesthesia carries the same risks but is often regarded as safer and more controllable than subarachnoid anesthesia.

Evidence exists that in high-risk patients, epidural anesthesia with analgesia extended into the postoperative period can reduce the risk of pulmonary failure requiring endotracheal intubation and the risk of infection related to intraoperative endotracheal intubation. However, patients undergoing lower-extremity vascular surgeries under either epidural anesthesia or general anesthesia showed no difference in either pulmonary failure or infection rate (35).

General anesthesia affects lung function with a 10% decrease in FRC, a 20% to 90% decrease in FVC, small-airway collapse from decreased lung volumes, altered mucociliary function with increased risk of pulmonary infection, V/Q mismatch resulting in a widened alveolar-to-arterial oxygen difference (A-a gradient), and central hypoventilation from residual anesthetic agents, muscle relaxants, opioids, or a combination of these. It is important that patients be closely monitored in the perioperative period because they will be prone to respiratory events.

Other factors can adversely affect postoperative pulmonary function. Postoperative pain alters breathing patterns and curtails the patient's normal tendency to breathe deeply, sigh, and cough. Opioid analgesics may alleviate pain but may also alter central respiratory drive, breathing patterns, and upper-airway function. Length and type of surgery and anesthesia also correlate with respiratory events. Other variables which play a role in postoperative pulmonary function include incisional site, abdominal distension, patient position, and restrictive bandages.

ATELECTASIS

One of the most important aspects of lung function is atelectasis. It not only affects gas exchange, but new data suggest that it may affect the incidence of organ failure through the release of cytokines (34). This has led to the concept of the "open lung" (35). Every effort must be made to recruit and maintain lung volumes throughout the perioperative period. Use of such procedures may decrease complications and time to wean (36,37). This is discussed in greater depth elsewhere in the book.

SUMMARY

It is imperative that the clinician has an understanding of the various diseases of the lung and how they affect gas exchange and pulmonary function. Complete evaluation of the patient should include a complete history and physical examination supported by specific tests as needed. Through proper understanding, we can develop care plans that will decrease mortality and morbidity. No test or evaluation by itself can completely predict outcomes.

KEY POINTS

- Proper evaluation and workup of chronic respiratory diseases will decrease mortality and morbidity in the perioperative period.
- A background knowledge of asthma, emphysema, cystic fibrosis, bronchiectasis, and bronchitis will aid in the management of these conditions.
- Proper workup with pulmonary function testing and blood gas evaluation aids in the perioperative management of the complex patient.
- Pulmonary pathophysiology is a highly important predictor of anesthesia and critical care problems.
- The most important tests in pulmonary disease are spirometry and pulmonary function test.

REFERENCES

1. Tisi GM. Perioperative evaluation of pulmonary function. Validity, indications, and benefits. *Am Rev Respir Dis* 1979;119:293–310.
2. Tremblay K, Valenza F, et al. Injurious ventilatory strategies increase cytokines and C-fos M-RNA expression in an isolated rat lung model. *J Clin Invest* 1997;99:944–952.
3. Stoelting RK. *Pharmacologic and physiology in anesthetic practice*, 2nd ed. Philadelphia: JB Lippincott, 1991.
4. Hemmings H Jr, Hopkins P. *Foundations of anesthesia: basic clinical sciences*. London: Mosby Harcourt, 2000.
5. Gillis CN. Pharmacological aspect of metabolic processes in the pulmonary microcirculation. *Ann Rev Pharmacol Toxicol* 1986;26:183–200.
6. Lung disease data: 1995. New York: American Lung Association, 1995.
7. Villar J, Petty TL, Slutsky AS. ARDS in the middle age. What we learned. *Appl Cardiopulmonary Pathophysiol* 1998;7:167–172.
8. Farzan S, Farzan D. *A concise handbook of respiratory diseases*, 4th ed. Stamford, CT: Appleton & Lange, 1997.
9. Wilkins RL, Dexter JR. *Respiratory disease: a case study approach to patient care*, 2nd ed. Philadelphia: FA Davis Company, 1998.
10. Des Jardins T, Burton GC. *Clinical manifestations and assessments of respiratory disease*, 3rd ed. St. Louis: Mosby–Year Book, 1995.
11. Gracey DR, Divertie MN, Didiez EP. Preoperative pulmonary preparation of patients with chronic obstructive pulmonary disease. A prospective study. *Chest* 1979;76:123–129.
12. Rose DK, Cohen MM, Wigglesworth DF, et al. Critical respiratory events in the post-anesthesia care unit. Patient, surgical, and anesthetic factors. *Anesthesiology* 1994;81:410–418.
13. Ferguson GT, Cherniack RM. Management of chronic obstructive pulmonary disease. *N Engl J Med* 1993;328:1017–1022.
14. Proteases and antiproteases. *Am J Respir Crit Care Med* 1994;150 [6 Suppl]:S109–S189.
15. Snider GL. Chronic obstructive pulmonary disease: risk factors, pathophysiology, and pathogenesis. *Am Rev Med* 1989;40:411–429.
16. Nicotra MB. Bronchiectasis. *Semin Respir Infect* 1994;9:31–40.
17. Aitkin ML, Fiel SB. Cystic fibrosis. *Dis Mon* 1993;39:1–52.
18. Dankert-Roelse, JE, te Meerman GT. Long-term prognosis of patients with cystic fibrosis in relation to early detection by neonatal screening. *Thorax* 995;50:712–720.
19. Fuchs HJ, Borowitz DS, Christensen DH, et al. Effect of aerosolized recombinant human DNase on exacerbation of respiratory symptoms and on pulmonary function in patients with cystic fibrosis. *N Engl J Med* 1994;331:637–642.
20. Marshall SG, Ramsey BW. Aerosol therapy in cystic fibrosis: DNase, tobramycin. *Semin Respir Crit Care Med* 1994;15:434–438.
21. Egan TM. Lung transplantation in cystic fibrosis. *Semin Respir Crit Care Med* 1996;17:137–147.
22. American Thoracic Society. Progress at the interface of inflammation and asthma. *Am J Respir Crit Care Med* 1995;152:385–424.
23. Chan-Yeung M, Malo IL. Occupational asthma. *N Engl J Med* 1995; 333:107–112.

24. Weersink EJM, Postma DS. Nocturnal asthma: not a separate disease entity. *Respir Med* 1994;88:483–491.

25. Barnes PJ, Pedersen S. Efficacy and safety of inhaled corticosteroids in asthma. *Am Rev Respir Dis* 1993;148:S1–S26.

26. Zibrak JD, O'Donnell CR, Marton K. Indications for pulmonary function testing. *Ann Intern Med* 1990;112:763–771.

27. Kopp VJ, Arora SK, Boysen PG. Perioperative evaluation of pulmonary function. In: Murray DB, Coursin RG, Pearl D, et al, eds. *Critical care medicine: perioperative management.* Philadelphia: Lippincott Raven, 1997.

28. Benumof JL. Management of the difficult adult airway with emphasis on awake intubation. *Anesthesiology* 1991;75:1087–1110.

29. McPherson DS. Preoperative laboratory testing: should any tests be routine before? *Med Clin North Am* 1993;77:289–308.

30. Gattinoni L, Pesenti A, Bombino N, et al. Relationships between lung-computed tomographic density, gas exchange, and PEEP in acute respiratory failure. *Anesthesiology* 1988;69:824–832.

31. Boysen PG. Evaluation of pulmonary function tests and arterial blood gases. In: Kaplan JA, ed. *Thoracic anesthesia,* 2nd ed. New York: Churchill Livingstone, 1991:1–18.

32. Schnapp LM, Cohen NH. Pulse oximetry: uses and abuses. *Chest* 1990;98:1244–1250.

33. Crapo RO. Pulmonary function testing. *N Engl J Med* 1994;331:25–30.

34. Tremblay L, Valenza F, Ribeiro SP, et al. Injurious ventilatory strategies increase cytokines and C-fos M-RNA expression in an isolated rat lung model. *J Clin Invest* 1997;99:944–952.

35. Christopherson R, Bettie C, Frank SM, et al. Perioperative morbidity in patients randomized to epidural or general anesthesia for lower extremity vascular surgery. Perioperative Ischemia Randomized Anesthesia Trial Study Group. *Anesthesiology* 1993;79:422–434.

36. Lachmann B. Open up the lung and keep the lung open. *Intensive Care Med* 1992;18:319–321.

37. Amato MBP, Barbas CS, Medeiros D, et al. Beneficial effects of the open lung approach with low distending pressures in acute respiratory distress syndrome: a prospective randomized study on mechanical ventilation. *Am J Respir Crit Care Med* 1995;152:1835–1846.

PNEUMONIA

C. WILLIAM HANSON, III

INTRODUCTION

Pneumonia has been characterized as "the old man's friend." It is not the physician's friend, however. It is a disease that is difficult to diagnose or characterize in many instances, difficult to treat in certain patient populations, and a major source of morbidity and mortality in the United States and the world. The National Center for Health Statistics indicates that there are over 90,000 deaths attributable to pneumonia per year in the United States, making it the sixth leading cause of death. There are 4.8 million cases of pneumonia per year in the U.S. and it is responsible for 1.2 million emergency department visits annually.

Community-acquired pneumonia (CAP) is often managed on an outpatient basis, but may necessitate hospital or intensive care unit (ICU) admission. Nosocomial pneumonia (NP) and ventilator-associated pneumonia (VAP) are complications in the hospitalized patient and the leading cause of death among patients with hospital-acquired infections (1). The terms are often used interchangeably although the latter is technically a subset of the former. NP is a hospital-acquired infection of lung parenchyma. VAP is an NP that occurs in mechanically ventilated patients, typically in the intensive care unit (ICU).

COMMUNITY-ACQUIRED PNEUMONIA

CAP represents two-thirds of the overall incidence of the disease and accounts for 10% of adult admissions to hospitals in the United States (2–5). There is an increasing tendency to treat CAP on an outpatient basis, and guidelines have been developed by the Patient Outcomes Research Team (PORT) to standardize the decision regarding treatment site (6). This chapter will not address outpatient management of CAP.

Diagnosis

The diagnosis of CAP is relatively uncomplicated. CAP is defined as pneumonia developing in an ambulatory, nonhospitalized patient. While the disease may develop in healthy individuals in adults, it is more typically seen in older patients and those with comorbid illnesses or as a result of local epidemiologic factors. The organism responsible for CAP is virtually never determined (less than 2% of the time) in those treated as outpatients and is only determined about half the time in hospitalized patients (7). Causative organisms include *Staphylococcus pneumoniae* (which accounts for two-thirds of all bacteremic pneumonia cases), *Haemophilus influenzae*, *Legionella* species, *Chlamydia*, *Mycoplasma*, viruses, and fungal organisms. Other gram-positive, gram-negative, and anaerobic bacteria are reported infrequently in CAP.

There are seasonal variations in the incidence of pneumonia relating to the etiologic pathogen. *S. pneumoniae*, *H. influenzae*, and influenza pneumonia occur primarily during the winter months. *Chlamydia* pneumonia occurs throughout the year. *Legionella* pneumonia outbreaks are more likely during the summer.

A variety of epidemiologic associations characterize different pathogens (Table 1). Pneumococcal pneumonia, for example, is commonly found in patients with compromised immune function, such as alcoholics, smokers, and nursing home residents. Herald symptoms include rigors and pleurisy. In addition to pneumococcal pneumonia, smokers commonly develop *H. influenzae* or *Moraxella catarrhalis* pneumonia.

Factors that increase susceptibility to pneumonia include impaired lymphocyte function in older adults (secondary to thymic involution), mechanical factors (e.g., decreased cough, impaired ciliary function), and comorbid illnesses. A scoring system has been developed from the work of the pneumonia PORT (Table 2) to determine the risk of death from CAP and guide the decision regarding whether or not to hospitalize a patient with CAP. Patients are classified into one of five severity groups. Class I patients are less than 50 years of age, have a normal mental status, relatively normal vital signs, and none of five major comorbid conditions (neoplastic disease, liver disorder, congestive heart failure, cerebrovascular disease, or renal disease). Classes II through V are determined by a scoring system based on demographics, comorbid diseases, physical examination, and laboratory and/or radiographic findings. Class I and II patients have a mortality risk less than 1%. Class III patients have a mortality risk of 2.8%; class IV,

TABLE 1. EPIDEMIOLOGIC ASSOCIATIONS FOR ORGANISMS CAUSING COMMUNITY-ACQUIRED PNEUMONIA

Epidemiology	Organism
Alcoholism	*Streptococcus pneumoniae*, anaerobic organisms
COPD, smoking	*S. pneumoniae, Haemophilus influenzae, Mycoplasma catarrhalis, Legionella* spp.
Dental caries	Anaerobic organisms
Previous recent hospitalization or nursing home residency	*S. pneumoniae*, gram-negative rods, *Staphylococcus aureus, H. influenzae*
HIV infection	Mycobacterium, pneumocystis, cryptococcus
Animal exposure	
Bats	*Histoplasma capsulatum*
Birds	*Chlamydia psittaci*
Rabbits	*Francisella tularensis*
Farm animals, cats	*Coxiella burnetii*
Structural lung disease (cystic fibrosis)	*Pseudomonas aeruginosa, P. cepacia, S. aureus*

COPD, chronic obstructive pulmonary disease; HIV, human immunodeficiency virus.

TABLE 2. PATIENT OUTCOMES RESEARCH TEAM (PORT) FOR CLASSES II–V

Patient Characteristic	Points
Demographic factors	
Age	
Male	Years of age
Female	Years of age − 10
Nursing home resident	10
Comorbid disease	
Cancer	30
Liver disease	20
Congestive heart failure	10
Cerebrovascular disease	10
Renal disease	10
Physical finding	
Altered mental status	20
Respiratory rate > 30 bpm	20
Systolic BP < 90 mm Hg	20
Temperature < 35°C or > 40°C	15
Pulse > 125 bpm	10
Laboratory or radiographic finding	
Arterial pH < 7.35	30
Blood urea nitrogen > 30 mg/dL	20
Sodium < 130 mEq/L	20
Glucose > 250 mg/dL	10
Hematocrit < 30%	10
Arterial po_2 < 60 mm Hg on room air	10
Pleural effusion on chest radiograph	10

		Mortality %
Class II	< 71 points	
Class III	71–90 points	2.8
Class IV	91–130 points	8.2
Class V	> 130 points	> 29

BP, blood pressure; bpm, breaths per minute.

8.2%; and class V, more than 29%. Classes I and II are generally treated as outpatients. Class III can be treated on an outpatient basis or with a brief (i.e., 23-hour) inpatient stay. Classes IV and V are typically admitted for therapy.

The diagnosis of CAP should be suspected in patients with new lower respiratory tract symptoms (cough, sputum production, dyspnea), fever, and auscultatory signs of pneumonia (crackles, altered breath sounds). While upper respiratory tract infections are often viral in origin and do not require empiric treatment, lower respiratory tract infections warrant antibiotic therapy. A chest radiograph is sensitive, although not specific. Sputum Gram's stain and cultures, blood cultures, a hematologic panel, and specific tests for individual organisms (e.g., *Mycobacteria, Legionella*) are typically acquired. Additional tests may be indicated (Table 3). The choice and intensity of diagnostic studies vary among experts. The rationale supporting empiric treatment and minimal testing in most cases of CAP managed on an outpatient basis is the cost of diagnostic studies and the lack of specificity of most studies. Rationales for testing include the ability to refine the choice of antibiotics, identify new organisms (i.e., Hantavirus), track the emergence of resistant organisms, and improve the cost efficiency of therapy.

Invasive diagnostic tests are performed in specific circumstances. Possible tests include transtracheal aspiration, bronchoscopy with protected brush sampling, bronchoalveolar lavage (BAL) with or without balloon protection, direct needle aspiration of the lung, thoracentesis (in the presence of a pleural effusion), and open lung biopsy. While these procedures are not typically indicated in the routine patient with CAP, invasive testing is appropriate in certain subsets, such as the immunologically compromised patient with a high risk of mortality.

The etiology of CAP can be ascertained with varying degrees of confidence depending on available diagnostic information (8). A definite etiology is established in the setting of a compatible clinical syndrome plus the recovery of a probable etiologic organism from an uncontaminated specimen such as blood, pleural fluid, or transtracheal or transthoracic aspirate. Alternatively the recovery of a likely pathogen from the upper airway supports the diagnosis in the appropriate setting. The diagnosis is believed to be probable in the appropriate clinical setting when a likely pulmonary pathogen is recovered from respiratory secretions in significant quantities (moderate to heavy growth).

Treatment

The decision as to the site of treatment (inpatient versus outpatient) is typically guided by clinical prediction rules such as those described by the pneumonia PORT. Outpatient treatment for CAP is typically empiric and initiated with doxycycline, a

TABLE 3. ADDITIONAL TESTS FOR COMMUNITY-ACQUIRED PNEUMONIA

1. Thoracentesis with fluid analysis (Gram stain, culture, pH determination and differential)
2. Upper respiratory aspirates (i.e., nasotracheal suctioning, induced sputum)
3. Bronchoscopic sampling
4. Transtracheal sampling

fluoroquinolone, or a macrolide antibiotic. Empiric inpatient therapy is usually initiated with a beta-lactam and macrolide or fluoroquinolone antibiotic. The regimen may be refined subsequently based on tests acquired prior to treatment. Inpatient therapy is typically initiated with intravenous antibiotics.

Recommendations from the Infectious Diseases Society of North America suggest treatment of *S. pneumoniae* until the patient is afebrile for approximately 72 hours, treatment of mycoplasmal or chlamydial pneumonia for 14 days, and treatment of organisms that cause necrosing pneumonia for at least 14 days. There are a variety of reasons to transition from intravenous to oral therapy as early as possible. Earlier transition results in lower drug costs and shorter hospital stays. A number of randomized, controlled studies support this approach (9). The transition to oral therapy is appropriate once the patient is improving clinically, hemodynamically stable, and able to ingest and digest oral agents. These conditions are often met within 3 days.

The patient's response to treatment is determined by the appropriateness of the initial antibiotic choice, host factors (i.e., age, immunologic competence), and the severity of the illness. Subjective response to appropriate treatment can be expected to occur within the first 3 days of therapy. Objective signs such as defervescence may take from 2 to 7 days depending on the presence of bacteremia and age. Blood cultures are typically sterile in initially bacteremic patients after 24 to 48 hours of treatment.

The chest film may actually progress despite appropriate therapy and is typically the slowest objective indicator to show a response to treatment. The chest film may show infiltrates up to 4 weeks following the initiation of antibiotics in healthy patients with pneumococcal pneumonia, and well after that in older adult or immunocompromised patients.

Patients who fail to respond within the expected time period may have been diagnosed incorrectly and have some alternative cause for clinical findings consistent with pneumonia such as pulmonary embolism, inflammatory lung disease, acute respiratory distress syndrome (ARDS), and so forth. Alternatively, the patient may have pneumonia and fail to respond because inappropriate antibiotics were prescribed. The patient may not respond despite appropriate antibiotics due to underlying host factors or the organism may be resistant to the prescribed regimen (drug-resistant strain). In the event of treatment failure, further evaluation may involve radiologic imaging, ventilation–perfusion studies, and/or bronchoscopy.

A variety of complications may eventuate from the original infection. These include metastatic infections such as meningitis, pericarditis, arthritis, endocarditis, peritonitis, and empyema. Renal failure, congestive heart failure, multiple organ dysfunction syndrome, and sepsis with ARDS are ominous complications of CAP.

HOSPITAL-ACQUIRED OR NOSOCOMIAL PNEUMONIA

Hospital-acquired pneumonia (HAP), NP, and VAP are a series of interrelated terms applied to pneumonia that arises in the hospitalized patient (10). HAP and NP are equivalent terms, defined as pneumonia occurring more than 48 hours after admission, while VAP is an NP developing in mechanically ventilated patients

TABLE 4. CENTERS FOR DISEASE CONTROL AND PREVENTION DEFINITIONS FOR NOSOCOMIAL PNEUMONIA

Definition: Must meet at least one of the following criteria:
Criterion 1: Patient has crackles or dullness to percussion on physical examination of the chest and at least one of the following:
  a. new onset of purulent sputum or change in character of sputum
  b. organisms cultured from blood
  c. isolation of an etiologic agent from a specimen obtained by transtracheal aspirate, bronchial brushing, or biopsy

Criterion 2: Patient has a chest x-ray examination that shows new or progressive infiltrate, consolidation, cavitation, or pleural effusion and at least one of the following:
  a. new onset of purulent sputum or change in character of sputum
  b. organisms cultured from blood
  c. isolation of an etiologic agent from a specimen obtained by transtracheal aspirate, bronchial brushing, or biopsy
  d. isolation of virus from or detection of viral antigen in respiratory secretions
  e. diagnostic single antibody titer (immunoglobulin M) or fourfold increase in paired sera (immunoglobulin G) for pathogen
  f. histopathologic evidence of pneumonia

and is discussed more extensively under "Ventilator-Associated Pneumonia" later in the chapter. The Centers for Disease Control and Prevention (CDC) definition of NP requires the (adult) patient to meet specific criteria (Table 4). These infections are typically more serious than CAP and have higher mortality rates.

The available data suggest that the incidence of NP is 5 to 10 per 1,000 hospital admissions. The incidence increases by 6- to 20-fold in mechanically ventilated patients. Pneumonia is the second most common nosocomial infection in the United States. It has the highest morbidity and mortality of the nosocomial infections tracked by the CDC, and the diagnosis is associated with the prolongation of hospital stays by 7 to 9 days. The crude mortality rate for NP may be as high as 70%, although not all of these deaths are directly attributable to NP. Studies have estimated that one-third to one-half of the NP deaths are directly attributable to the disease.

A number of mechanisms have been postulated to explain the development of NP. The final common pathway is the failure of host defense mechanisms. This typically results from one or more factors: (a) impaired host defenses, (b) the inoculum of a sufficient quantity of organisms into the lower respiratory tract that overwhelms host defenses, or (c) the presence of a highly virulent organism.

The pathogenic organism can enter the lung from a variety of sources. Microaspiration or macroaspiration of oropharyngeal, esophageal, or gastric contents is one direct route by which bacteria enter the respiratory tract. Inhalation of infected aerosols, as from a contaminated humidifier, is an alternative direct route. Bacteria can enter the lung hematogeneously, as from an infected tricuspid valve, or exogenously, as from an infected pleural space. Intubated patients are susceptible to direct inoculation of pathogens into the airway by ICU personnel. Finally, translocation of bacteria from the gastrointestinal (GI) tract has been postulated as a potential mechanism of infection.

As with CAP, host factors such as preexistent comorbid diseases and advanced age predispose the patient to the development of NP. The hospitalized patient is at additional risk both from issues pertaining to the acute process necessitating hospitalization, as well as proximity to the type (more virulent) and quantity of organisms found in hospitals. The use of a number of drugs predisposes the patient to the development of NP. These include immunosuppressive agents (corticosteroids, cytotoxic agents), antacids (which may lead to bacterial overgrowth in the stomach), and empiric broad-spectrum antibiotics. Devices such as surgical drains, intravenous lines, endotracheal tubes, and nasogastric tubes are routes by which pathogens can bypass host defenses.

NP is often described as a postoperative infection. Early studies indicated that up to 75% of NPs occur in surgical patients; patients undergoing thoracoabdominal procedures are at greatest risk. More recent studies have shown that older adult patients (over 70 years of age), patients undergoing endotracheal intubation and mechanical ventilation, patients with depressed mental status (particularly closed head injury), patients with preexistent lung disease, and patients with previous large-volume aspirations are also at risk. Additional factors include hospitalization during the fall or winter, stress-ulcer prophylaxis, presence of a nasogastric tube, severe trauma, and administration of antimicrobials.

The organisms that cause NP differ from those that cause CAP. The distribution differs among hospitals due to inherently differing flora, different patient populations, and different approaches to diagnosis. Bacteria are the predominant pathogen, fungi rare, and viruses extremely rare. The bacteria are typically aerobic, probably due both to a real predominance of those organisms and the difficulty in or failure to obtain anaerobic cultures. Some evidence suggests that up to half of NPs are polymicrobial (1,11,12), with predominantly gram-negative species. *Staphylococcus aureus* (often resistant to methicillin) and *S. pneumoniae*, as well as other gram-positive organisms, are increasingly prevalent.

Diagnosis

Diagnostic studies are ordered to determine whether or not a patient has pneumonia (as an explanation for a particular constellation of signs and symptoms), to identify an etiologic organism, and to define the severity of illness. NP can be diagnosed clinically (13–16) based on symptoms, signs, and noninvasive studies, or with invasive testing (using needle aspiration or bronchoscopic techniques). A purely clinical diagnostic approach may be excessively sensitive; however, the cost, the risk of complications, the requirement for specialized laboratory and procedural skills, and the potential insensitivity of invasive tests are problematic.

All patients suspected to have NP should have a history and physical examination, chest radiograph, and hematologic, electrolyte, and organ-specific laboratory studies including an arterial blood gas analysis. Sputum is commonly collected for Gram stain and culture as well as organism-specific assays (i.e., acid-fast staining). Additional studies may include thoracentesis when an effusion is present. Invasive studies may be performed when they are deemed appropriate by the clinician. Some of the risks associated with bronchoscopic evaluation are less relevant in the intubated patient who has already assumed the risks associated with instrumentation of the airway. The specific issues particular to VAP will be described more extensively below.

Patients with NP can be readily divided into three groups with unique spectra of pathogens. The first are patients lacking unusual

TABLE 5. ORGANISMS IN NOSOCOMIAL PNEUMONIA

Core organisms
  Streptococcus pneumoniae
  Enterobacter (*Escherichia coli*, *Klebsiella* spp. *Proteus* spp., *Serratia marcescens*)
  Haemophilus influenzae
  Methicillin-sensitive *Staphylococcus aureus*
Additional organisms
  Anaerobic organisms
  Legionella spp.
  Pseudomonas spp.
  Acinetobacter spp.
  Methicillin-resistant *S. aureus*

risk factors who present with mild-to-moderate NP, with onset at any time during hospitalization or patients with early-onset severe NP. The second group are those patients with risk factors (i.e., coexisting illness) and mild-to-moderate NP. The final group of patients have severe NP with early onset and risk factors or late onset with or without risk factors. Patients in the first group are at risk for the core organisms listed in Table 5. Patients in the other two groups are at risk from the core organisms as well as the additional organisms listed in Table 5.

Prevention

Because of the morbidity, mortality, and cost associated with NP, a variety of interventions have been investigated for their ability to prevent the disease. These range from those that are available and probably efficacious to those that are unproven and still under evaluation.

Specific vaccines, hand washing, and the isolation of patients with resistant or virulent organisms are examples of interventions that may prevent NP. Vaccines against *S. pneumoniae* and influenza are available and potentially effective in preventing the spread of these organisms to and among hospitalized patients. Hand washing is demonstrably effective in preventing the spread of organisms and, unfortunately, often neglected (17). Patient isolation is controversial, but probably efficacious in reducing the spread of organisms within the hospital or ICU. Enteral nutrition is associated with lower rates of NP than parenteral nutrition (18–20), particularly when the enteral formula is delivered to the distal gut. This may be due to improved barrier function and reduced bacterial translocation in the lower GI tract.

A number of studies have suggested that treatment with H_2 blockers is associated with higher rates of NP, although other studies have shown contradictory results. The use of sucralfate as an alternative has been shown to be superior to H_2 blockers in preventing NP. Selective digestive decontamination (SDD) is another approach designed to prevent bacterial translocation in the small gut by reducing bacterial load. While it has been studied extensively, SDD has not demonstrably lowered the incidence or improved the outcome of NP.

Treatment

Depending on the risk stratification of the patient described earlier, different antibiotic regimens should be prescribed. NP should be treated with an antibiotic regimen most appropriate for core organisms (e.g., a second or third generation [nonpseudomonal] cephalosporin plus a beta-lactamase inhibitor or a fluoroquinolone). Clindamycin and vancomycin (when there is a significant incidence of methicillin-resistant *S. aureus*) should be added to the foregoing regimen in patients with mild to moderate NP. Finally, patients with severe NP should be treated with an aminoglycoside or ciprofloxacin plus one of the following agents: antipseudomonal penicillin, beta-lactam/beta-lactamase inhibitor, ceftazidime, cefoperazone, imipenem, or aztreonam. Vancomycin can be added to this regimen when appropriate.

The initial regimen may require modification when the results of cultures become available. Modifications may be necessary to cover unsuspected or resistant organisms. Alternatively it is often possible to refine a regimen by the deletion of antibiotics when expected (i.e., *Pseudomonas aeruginosa* or *S. aureus*) organisms are not recovered. A more problematic situation is the decision to change a regimen because the patient fails to respond to an empiric regimen. Because there is not a commonly accepted "natural course" for NP, it is difficult to recognize when a patient is behaving unexpectedly. Confounding factors include variable approaches to the diagnosis of the process or variations in the course of NP (or what is presumed to be NP) depending on what disease process is actually present. The clinical response to treatment may also vary depending on patient-related factors such as age and coexistent illnesses, on bacterial factors relating to drug resistance and virulence, and on the course of the illness precipitating hospital admission.

While treatment failure is difficult to define, a positive response to treatment is suggested by improvement in indicators such as fever, leukocytosis, organ failure, and sputum purulence. As with CAP, improvement in radiographic appearance is likely to lag behind clinical improvement.

The nonresponding or deteriorating patient will often require endotracheal intubation and mechanical ventilation. While these patients do not technically meet the definition of VAP, the diagnostic interventions required in the former population are relevant to both groups.

VENTILATOR-ASSOCIATED PNEUMONIA

VAP is defined as a parenchymal lung infection occurring more than 48 hours after initiation of mechanical ventilation. It occurs in 10% to 25% of patients intubated for longer than 48 hours and, according to some studies, it is the most common acquired infection in ICU patients (21). VAP has an associated mortality rate of 25% to 70%. Risk factors include prolonged mechanical ventilation and reintubation after failed extubation. A large Canadian study of 1,014 patients found that the primary diagnosis of burn injury, trauma, central nervous system disease, respiratory tract disease, cardiac disease, or witnessed aspiration was independently predictive of VAP. The same study showed that the risk of VAP rose daily for the first 5 days of mechanical ventilation and declined thereafter and that systemic antibiotic therapy had a protective effect. Other factors that have been associated with VAP include low endotracheal tube cuff pressure, transport outside of the ICU, and supine patient position.

As with CAP and NP, the pathogenesis of VAP relates to host and pathogen factors. The specific host factors in VAP include the presence of an endotracheal "foreign body," the endotracheal tube. This provides an abnormal conduit between the upper and the lower airway. As a result, secretions from the airway and the stomach are in continuity with the pool of secretions that invariably accumulates above the cuff of the endotracheal tube. These secretions are aspirated into the trachea, form a biofilm lining the endotracheal tube and the upper airway, and are then disseminated into the lung with each inspiration and with suctioning (Fig. 1). Because normal oral flora are rapidly replaced by nosocomial organisms (i.e., gram-negative rods, resistant *S. aureus*) in ICU patients, it is these bacteria that are ultimately dispersed throughout the lungs and therefore the typical cause of VAP.

- Antibiotic therapy and antacid therapy alters the milieu of the mouth and stomach

- Oropharyngeal and gastric colonization by pathogenic, gram-negative organisms

- Development of subglottic secretion pool

- Aspiration of pooled secretions around the cuff of the endotracheal tube

- Aerosolization of the aspirated secretions during the inspiratory phase of the ventilator cycle

- Dispersion of the aerosolized bacteria into the lung

- Development of ventilator-associated pneumonia

FIGURE 1. Mechanisms of ventilator-associated pneumonia.

Autopsy studies of patients with VAP have shown three distinct patterns of infection. They are tracheobronchitis, bronchopneumonia, and bronchiolitis. Because pneumonia (confirmed histologically in the untreated patient) is associated with a bacterial burden of greater than 10^3 colony-forming units (CFUs) per gram of lung tissue, which corresponds to greater than 10^3 CFUs per mL, this threshold is typically used as a quantitative threshold for the diagnosis of VAP.

Diagnosis

The traditional "gold standard" for the diagnosis of VAP is an open lung biopsy, which is rarely employed and is susceptible to confounding factors such as sampling error. Standard sampling tests include tracheobronchial aspirates, protected specimen brush, and bronchoalveolar lavage (both conventional and protected). These tests may be blind or directed to presumed areas of infection.

The invasive tests include bronchoscopic protected brush sampling, in which a bacterial count of 10^3 CFUs per mL is used to diagnose VAP. Alternatively BAL, in which a bacterial count of 10^4 CFUs per mL is commonly used as a threshold for VAP, permits immediate Gram stain. The performance of these studies requires competence both on the part of the physician who performs the procedure and the microbiology laboratory. Bronchoscopy is also costly and time-intensive.

An alternate approach advocated by some involves the acquisition of protected brush or BAL specimens using catheters inserted directly through the endotracheal tube. These approaches can be safely performed by respiratory therapists or nurses but do require specialized catheters. An even less specialized approach is quantitative cultures of suctioned sputum, which reportedly is as sensitive, although less specific, than invasive approaches.

A recent postmortem study comparing histologic and microbiologic sampling methods for VAP reached the conclusion that the diagnostic performance of different diagnostic techniques depends to a great degree on the reference used to compare approaches, and that "all techniques for detecting VAP are of limited value." The authors concluded that the diagnosis typically relies on a balance between "clinical judgment and microbiological

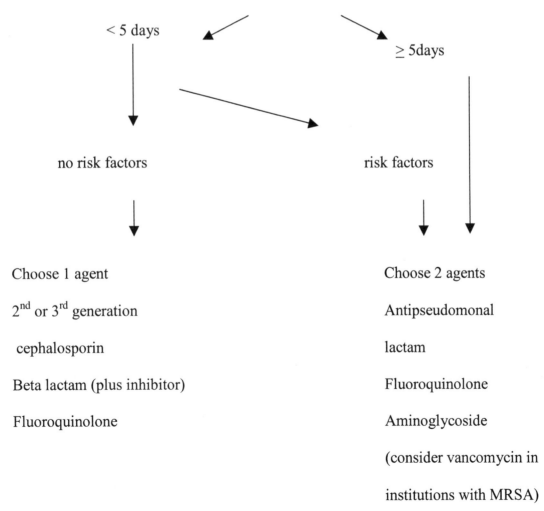

FIGURE 2. Therapeutic flow chart for ventilator-associated pneumonia (VAP).

results." Clinical diagnosis of VAP appears to be the most common approach in the U.S. (whereas many European clinicians prefer invasive methods).

Prevention

A number of approaches have been evaluated for their ability to reduce the incidence of VAP. They include many of the measures detailed in the section on NP such as hand washing and isolation procedures, as well as enteral feeding and selective decontamination of the gut (or portions of the gut). None of these studies have persuasively shown gut organisms to be a major source of VAP.

A number of other investigations have evaluated airway management practices. A reduction in the incidence of VAP has resulted from routine suctioning of supraglottic secretions using specially designed catheters. VAP has also been reduced by avoidance of the supine position in critically ill patients, probably because the head-up position minimizes aspiration. Noninvasive ventilation obviates the diagnosis of VAP and has been shown to reduce the incidence of NP. While this solution is not appropriate for the majority of critically ill patients, its use has increased in recent years.

Respiratory therapy practices that have been shown to alter the incidence of VAP include kinetic bed therapy and the use of heat and moisture exchangers. Ventilator circuit changes more often than every 7 days may be associated with a higher incidence of VAP. Finally, closed endotracheal suctioning systems do not decrease the incidence of VAP.

Treatment

The organisms that are associated with VAP vary widely both among hospitals and ICUs within an individual hospital. Gram-negative and polymicrobial infections appear to be the most common based on published series. While anaerobic infections were previously thought to be common, recent autopsy studies have failed to show anaerobes in postmortem specimens from patients with VAP (22,23). *Legionella* outbreaks have occurred in ICUs where water sources are contaminated.

Because of the uncertainties associated with the diagnosis of VAP, empiric therapy is typically instituted using an array of antibiotics that will cover all likely pathogens isolated from lower respiratory tract secretions. Recent studies indicate that therapy should be initiated soon after VAP is suspected and that the therapy should address all likely organisms. These studies have shown that the need to broaden therapy after culture data become available correlates with higher mortality in that patient subgroup.

One major branch point in the determination of antibiotic regimen has to do with the likelihood that a resistant organism is involved (e.g., *P. aeruginosa, Acinetobacter, Stenotrophomonas maltophilia*). The best predictors of these resistant organisms are the preceding duration of mechanical ventilation and previous broad-spectrum antibiotic therapy. The American Thoracic Society recommends coverage of these organisms for patients with suspected VAP who have been hospitalized for longer than 5 days prior to onset, have received antibiotics, have been treated with corticosteroids, have structural lung disease, or are immunosuppressed.

Empiric antibiotic selection should be informed by patient-related risk factors and by institutional resistance patterns. In patients with a low likelihood of drug-resistant VAP, monotherapy is reasonable (Fig. 2). Patients at risk for VAP due to a resistant organism should be treated with combination therapy (i.e., extended spectrum cephalosporin plus an aminoglycoside). In institutions where methicillin-resistant *S. aureus* is prevalent, vancomycin should be considered as a component of empiric therapy in at-risk patients.

Recent data indicate that the emergence of multiply resistant bacteria is now a major problem in the United States (24) and that the problem is particularly prevalent in the intensive care setting. Several therapeutic strategies have been used to combat the problem. They include: (a) restricted use of certain antibiotics (to prevent indiscriminate use of new drugs); (b) scheduled changes in the classes of agents used for empiric therapy; (c) refinement of antibiotic therapy once culture and sensitivity data become available; and (d) discontinuation of antibiotics when VAP is excluded.

SUMMARY

Pneumonia is a challenging problem for the intensivist. It is difficult to diagnose, is attended by substantial morbidity and mortality, and has major economic consequences. New interventions that improve the accuracy and speed of diagnosis or improve the probability of cure are likely to have a significant, positive impact on a diverse group of patients including the very young, the hospitalized, the immunosuppressed, or older adult patients.

KEY POINTS

- Nosocomial pneumonia (NP) and ventilator-associated pneumonia (VAP) are the leading causes of death among patients with hospital-acquired infections.
- Community-acquired pneumonia (CAP) represents two-thirds of the overall incidence of all pneumonia and accounts for 10% of adult admissions to hospitals in the United States.
- Factors that increase susceptibility to pneumonia include impaired lymphocyte function in older adult patients, mechanical factors, and comorbid illnesses.
- Outpatient treatment for CAP is typically empiric and initiated with doxycycline, a fluoroquinolone, or a macrolide antibiotic.
- Hospital-acquired pneumonia (HAP) is pneumonia occurring more than 48 hours after admission; VAP is an NP that develops in mechanically ventilated patients.

- NP typically results from impaired host defenses, the inoculum of a sufficient quantity of organisms into the lower respiratory tract that overwhelms host defenses, or the presence of a highly virulent organism.
- Seventy-five percent of NPs occur in surgical patients; patients undergoing thoracoabdominal procedures are at greatest risk.
- Patients with NP should have a history and physical examination, chest radiograph, and hematologic, electrolyte, and organ-specific laboratory studies including an arterial blood gas analysis.
- Specific vaccines, hand washing, and the isolation of patients with resistant or virulent organisms are examples of interventions that may prevent NP.
- NP should be treated with an antibiotic regimen most appropriate for core organisms (e.g., second or third generation [nonpseudomonal] cephalosporin plus a beta-lactamase inhibitor or a fluoroquinolone).
- VAP is defined as a parenchymal lung infection occurring more than 48 hours after initiation of mechanical ventilation.
- Risk factors for VAP include prolonged mechanical ventilation and reintubation after failed extubation.

- Secretions from the airway and the stomach are in continuity with the pool of secretions that invariably accumulates above the cuff of the endotracheal tube. In VAP, these secretions are aspirated into the trachea.
- The traditional "gold standard" for the diagnosis of VAP is an open lung biopsy. Standard sampling tests include tracheobronchial aspirates, protected specimen brush, and bronchoalveolar lavage.
- A bacterial count of 103 colony-forming units per mL is used to diagnose VAP.
- VAP has also been reduced by avoidance of the supine position in critically ill patients.
- Empiric therapy for VAP is typically instituted using an array of antibiotics that will cover all likely pathogens isolated from lower respiratory tract secretions.
- The best predictors of these resistant organisms is the duration of mechanical ventilation and previous broad-spectrum antibiotic therapy.
- In patients with a low likelihood of drug-resistant VAP, monotherapy is reasonable. Patients at risk for VAP due to a resistant organism should be treated with combination therapy (i.e., extended spectrum cephalosporin plus an aminoglycoside).

REFERENCES

1. Craven DE, Steger KA. Epidemiology of nosocomial pneumonia. New perspectives on an old disease [Review]. *Chest* 1995;108:1S–16S.
2. Niederman MS. Community-acquired pneumonia: a North American perspective. *Chest* 1998;113:179S–182S.
3. Niederman MS. Severe community-acquired pneumonia: what do we need to know to effectively manage patients? [Editorial; comment]. [Review]. *Intensive Care Med* 1996;22:1285–1287.
4. Niederman MS, Bass JBJ, Campbell GD, et al. Guidelines for the initial management of adults with community-acquired pneumonia: diagnosis, assessment of severity, and initial antimicrobial therapy. American Thoracic Society. Medical Section of the American Lung Association. *Am Rev Respir Dis* 1993;148:1418–1426.
5. Niederman MS, McCombs JS, Unger AN, et al. The cost of treating community-acquired pneumonia. *Clin Therapy* 1998;20:820–837.
6. Fine MJ, Auble TE, Yealy DM, et al. A prediction rule to identify low-risk patients with community-acquired pneumonia. *N Engl J Med* 1997;336:243–250.
7. Bartlett JG, Breiman RF, Mandell LA, et al. Community-acquired pneumonia in adults: guidelines for management. The Infectious Diseases Society of America. *Clin Infect Dis* 1998;26:811–838.
8. Bartlett JG, Mundy LM. Community-acquired pneumonia [Review]. *N Engl J Med* 1995;333:1618–1624.
9. Fine MJ, Medsger AR, Stone RA, et al. The hospital discharge decision for patients with community-acquired pneumonia. Results from the Pneumonia Patient Outcomes Research Team cohort study. *Arch Intern Med* 1997;157:47–56.
10. Anonymous. Hospital-acquired pneumonia in adults: diagnosis, assessment of severity, initial antimicrobial therapy, and preventive strategies. A consensus statement, American Thoracic Society, November 1995 [Review]. *Am J Respir Crit Care Med* 1996;153:1711–1725.
11. Rouby JJ, Martin DL, Poete P, et al. Nosocomial bronchopneumonia in the critically ill. Histologic and bacteriologic aspects. *Am Rev Respir Dis* 1992;146:1059–1066.
12. Rouby JJ, Rossignon MD, Nicolas MH, et al. A prospective study of protected bronchoalveolar lavage in the diagnosis of nosocomial pneumonia. *Anesthesiology* 1989;71:679–685.
13. Niederman MS. Bronchoscopy in nonresolving nosocomial pneumonia [Review]. *Chest* 2000;117:212S–218S.
14. Chastre J, Fagon JY. Invasive diagnostic testing should be routinely used to manage ventilated patients with suspected pneumonia. *Am J Respir Crit Care Med* 1994;150:570–574.
15. Chastre J, Fagon JY, Bornet-Lecso M, et al. Evaluation of bronchoscopic techniques for the diagnosis of nosocomial pneumonia. *Am J Respir Crit Care Med* 1995;152:231–240.
16. Chastre J, Fagon JY, Trouillet JL. Diagnosis and treatment of nosocomial pneumonia in patients in intensive care units [Review]. *Clin Infect Dis* 1995;21[Suppl 3]:S226–S237.
17. Gilmour J, Hughes R. Handwashing: still a neglected practice in the clinical area [Review]. *Br J Nurs* 1982;6:1278–1280.
18. Moore FA, Moore EE, Jones TN, et al. TEN versus TPN following major abdominal trauma–reduced septic morbidity. *J Trauma-Injury Infect Crit Care* 1989;29:916–922.
19. Moore FA, Moore EE, Kudsk KA, et al. Clinical benefits of an immune-enhancing diet for early postinjury enteral feeding. *J Trauma-Injury Infect Crit Care* 1994;37:607–615.
20. Moore FA, Moore EE, Poggetti R, et al. Gut bacterial translocation via the portal vein: a clinical perspective with major torso trauma. *J Trauma-Injury Infect Crit Care* 1991;31:629–636.
21. Morehead RS, Pinto SJ. Ventilator-associated pneumonia [Review]. *Arch Intern Med* 2000;160:1926–1936.
22. Torres A, El-Ebiary M. Bronchoscopic BAL in the diagnosis of ventilator-associated pneumonia [Review]. *Chest* 2000;117:198S–202S.
23. Torres A, Fabregas N, Ewig S, et al. Sampling methods for ventilator-associated pneumonia: validation using different histologic and microbiological references. *Crit Care Med* 2000;28:2799–2804.
24. Archibald L, Phillips L, Monnet D, et al. Antimicrobial resistance in isolates from inpatients and outpatients in the United States: increasing importance of the intensive care unit. *Clin Infect Dis* 1997;24:211–215.

PERIOPERATIVE MANAGEMENT OF OBSTRUCTIVE AND RESTRICTIVE PULMONARY DISEASES

STEPHEN J. RUOSS

INTRODUCTION

The optimal perioperative management of patients with significant lung disease requires an understanding of the nature and extent of any lung disease present, as well as the development and execution of a clear plan for both preoperative and postoperative care.

The study of perioperative risk assessment and management has historically focused on cardiac disease and its associated risks, and considerable effort has been devoted to the identification and reduction of risk factors for perioperative cardiac morbidity and mortality. However, recent studies reveal that the incidence of postoperative pulmonary complications is often greater than that for cardiac complications, and these pulmonary complications result in greater morbidity and prolongation of hospital stay than do cardiac complications (1,2).

Given the presence of underlying comorbid pulmonary problems in surgical candidates, the risk of pulmonary complications will continue to be an important issue in perioperative patient management. However, the presence of significant, even severe, lung disease can still allow for the successful execution of surgery. There will always be a complex and varying balance between the relevant surgical risks and the potential benefits of the proposed surgery, coupled with the desires of the patient.

This chapter reviews risk considerations for perioperative pulmonary complications, the methods of assessing risk, and an approach to the reduction and management of these complications in patients with obstructive and restrictive pulmonary diseases.

OBSTRUCTIVE AND RESTRICTIVE PULMONARY DISEASES

Obstructive pulmonary diseases are the most common chronic pulmonary disease category. The clinical range of obstructive pulmonary disease is quite diverse, including genetically determined diseases such as cystic fibrosis; diseases with genetic and environmental foundations, such as asthma; and acquired diseases, including tobacco smoking-related chronic obstructive pulmonary disease (COPD). The majority of significant pulmonary complication risk is associated with COPD, although other obstructive diseases clearly need to be considered.

Restrictive pulmonary diseases are a less frequent perioperative consideration but, when present, warrant special consideration. The restrictive pulmonary diseases include fibrotic interstitial lung diseases of unknown cause (such as idiopathic pulmonary fibrosis); secondary fibrotic lung disease associated with connective tissue diseases including scleroderma, systemic lupus, and rheumatoid arthritis; and inhalational or toxic exposure diseases including hypersensitivity pneumonitis, pneumoconioses, or drug-related pneumonitis. The latter category warrants a special note of perioperative caution in the case of bleomycin-induced pneumonitis, where exposure to supplemental oxygen is associated with an increased risk of amplifying the lung injury and fibrosis, particularly in the 6 to 12 months following bleomycin therapy. Additional disease-specific issues of potential concern for perioperative evaluation and management include esophageal dysmotility and chest wall restrictive disease. Esophageal dysmotility is often seen in patients with scleroderma and associated with increased reflux and aspiration risk, while chest wall restrictive defects are often encountered in patients with ankylosing spondylitis and require careful airways management and secretion control due to the patients' compromised neck extension and cough capacity.

Many aspects of perioperative consideration are common to both restrictive and obstructive lung diseases. Special considerations unique to the disease states will be addressed where relevant.

TABLE 1. CLINICAL RISK FACTORS FOR POSTOPERATIVE PULMONARY COMPLICATIONS

Potential Risk Factor	Type of Surgery	Incidence of Pulmonary Complications		Unadjusted Relative Risk Associated with Factor
		When Factor was Present (%)	When Factor was Absent (%)	
Smoking	Coronary bypass	39	11	3.4
	Abdominal	15–46	6–21	1.4–4.3
ASA class > II	Unselected	26	16	1.7
	Thoracic or abdominal	26–44	13–18	1.5–3.2
Age >70 yr	Unselected	9–17	4–9	1.9–2.4
	Thoracic or abdominal	17–22	12–21	0.9–1.9
Obesity	Unselected	11	9	1.3
	Thoracic or abdominal	19–36	17–27	0.8–1.7
COPD	Unselected	6–26	2–8	2.7–3.6
	Thoracic or abdominal	18	4	4.7

ASA, American Society of Anesthesiologists; COPD, chronic obstructive pulmonary disease.
Modified and reproduced with permission from Smetana GW. Preoperative pulmonary evaluation. *N Engl J Med* 1999;340:937–944.

CLINICAL RISK FACTORS FOR PERIOPERATIVE PULMONARY COMPLICATIONS

Multiple patient clinical characteristics have been associated with an increased risk of perioperative pulmonary complications (Table 1; also see Chapter 35). These include overall general health status and age, in addition to smoking and/or the presence of significant airways obstruction, or both. Obesity, while often assumed to confer an increased operative risk for pulmonary complications, does not appear to be a significant independent risk factor.

General Health and Cardiovascular Status

The measurement of general health status is an important tool for defining the risk of overall complications, as well as pulmonary and postoperative complications. The two principal methods for general health assessment are the American Society of Anesthesiologists (ASA) index and the Goldman cardiac risk index (3). Both of these prediction tools have been demonstrated to predict increased perioperative pulmonary morbidity as well as overall postoperative mortality (Table 1), although their use has not been uniformly demonstrated. The ASA index has been found to be an accurate predictor of overall postoperative morbidity and mortality (4,5). The Goldman cardiac risk index can also accurately assess risk for overall morbidity and mortality, but its principal utility is in predicting postoperative cardiac complications (3). Prause and colleagues examined a large cohort of patients being evaluated for elective surgery to assess the predictive use of the ASA physical status index and the Goldman cardiac risk index (6). The data from their group of 16,227 patients supported the use of both indices for prediction of overall postoperative mortality. They did not assess the predictive use of these indices for postoperative pulmonary complications. In contrast, a subsequent study of 845 patients scheduled for noncardiac thoracic surgery confirmed the risk prediction validity of the ASA index, but found that the Goldman cardiac risk index provided no prediction use for overall postoperative mortality (7).

The ASA index is useful for predicting postoperative pulmonary complications in patients with obstructive lung diseases,

including asthma and COPD (8). In patients with severe COPD who are undergoing abdominal, thoracic, and cardiac surgeries, operative complication rates increased as a function of ASA classification, from a 10% complication rate in ASA class II to a 46% complication rate in ASA class IV patients (8). The Goldman cardiac risk index also has independent predictive use for postoperative pulmonary complications, for both abdominal and noncardiac thoracic surgery (9,10).

Age

Increasing age is associated with higher risk for perioperative pulmonary complications, although this association is not uniformly seen in studies (Table 1) and appears principally to be a function of comorbid medical conditions rather than age alone (11,12). In studies of patients with severe obstructive pulmonary disease, age was not a predictor of pulmonary complications (8). However, while age was not a useful predictor of pulmonary complications in both these studies, the ASA class was a significant predictor. This association of increased ASA class (class = ≥ 3) with pulmonary complications has also been noted in other studies which examined age as a risk factor (11,13). Thus, caution should be used when assigning operative risk on the basis of age, as the use of this approach may be limited. The most substantial data in support of the validity of age as an independent and significant predictor of pulmonary complications come from a recent publication of the National Veterans Administration Surgical Quality Improvement Program (2). This prospective cohort study of 81,700 patients developed a respiratory failure risk index from a simplified logistic regression model and found age, along with operative anatomic site, selected metabolic parameters, airways obstruction, and overall functional status, to be predictive of postoperative respiratory failure in a subsequent validation patient cohort of 99,300 patients. Although this study suggests an independent association of advancing age with postoperative respiratory complications, clinicians should consider the increasingly frequent comorbidities that accompany advanced age when determining operative candidacy.

Smoking

Smoking has long been known to be a very significant risk factor for perioperative pulmonary complications. A substantial body of literature confirms smoking as a leading cause of perioperative complications (2,12,14,15) (Table 1). The risk of complications is greatest in patients with significant obstructive lung disease and in active smokers. Smoking cessation is associated with reduced risk of complications, but the duration of cessation is important for complication risk. Cessation of smoking within 1 month of surgery is not associated with any reduction in the incidence of pulmonary complications, and might even increase the complication rate (16). A period of at least 8 weeks of smoking cessation is necessary before the incidence of complications is significantly reduced over that for active smokers (17,18). Abstinence for at least 6 months affords additional risk reduction over more recent smoking cessation (18).

Obstructive Lung Disease

Patients with COPD have a documented increased risk of perioperative pulmonary complications (2,8,11,13,19,20). The use of spirometry as a predictor of postoperative complications is less clear. In multiple studies, spirometry does not appear to independently predict postoperative pulmonary complications in patients undergoing elective abdominal surgery (10,21). A recent retrospective nested case-control study by Lawrence and associates in a large patient cohort analyzed preoperative clinical variables by multivariate analysis to identify predictors of postoperative respiratory complications (10). Neither the overall severity of COPD nor any individual spirometry parameter predicted postoperative complications in this study, although abnormal findings on preoperative lung examination did predict complications. These results would appear to argue for exclusion of pulmonary function testing from the preoperative evaluation and planning strategy for patients with smoking and/or obstructive lung disease histories, as has been advocated by some authors. However, two additional comments are relevant. First, there are conflicting data that have found that some pulmonary function test (PFT) parameters (including a reduced forced expiratory volume-1 [FEV_1] percentage) are predictors of increased postoperative pulmonary risk (11). Hypoxemia and hypercapnia have also been identified as predictors of postoperative pulmonary complications. Second, the simple use of PFT parameters as predictive tools for postoperative pulmonary complications does not address the more important question, namely whether treating any identified abnormal spirometry findings is effective in reducing postoperative pulmonary complications. It certainly is reasonable to expect that, in a selected population of preoperative patients who have a high suspicion of significant obstructive lung disease, a management strategy that combines spirometry testing and appropriate therapy to optimize lung function may produce significant perioperative benefit. This question has not yet been adequately addressed in prospective studies.

A summary recommendation for the consideration of PFTs in the preoperative evaluation of patients with COPD should reasonably include the following: (a) obtain PFTs in any patients with known or suspected significant obstructive lung disease, and (b) treat any significant abnormalities identified, particularly reversible airflow obstruction or hypoxemia.

None of these considerations can be an absolute determinant of surgical candidacy of any individual patient with obstructive lung disease. Although operative morbidity and mortality are increased in the presence of severe obstructive lung disease (8), most patients still have good surgical outcomes. The decision to proceed with surgery also needs to take into consideration the purpose of the proposed surgery and the clinical outcome in the absence of surgery.

Asthma does not appear to be associated with an increased incidence of postoperative pulmonary complications *in patients with adequate disease control* (22). However, poor disease control or active exacerbations of asthma are associated with increased postoperative complications. Current active symptoms, including nocturnal wheezing and awakening; any recent disease flare-up requiring systemic corticosteroids and/or hospitalization; and comorbid cardiac disease are all associated with an increased risk for perioperative complications (22). It is imperative that an adequate asthma evaluation and therapy plan be executed before surgery is undertaken for any patients with a significant asthma history. Spirometry or peak expiratory flow rate (PEFR) determination is an indispensable part of preoperative evaluation for asthma patients. The goal of preoperative evaluation and management of asthma patients should be to attempt to achieve an FEV_1 or PEFR which is 80% of the predicted normal value, or at least 80% of the patient's personal best measured values (22).

Obesity

Obesity can be associated with significant changes in respiratory and cardiac function, including reduced lung volumes, alveolar hypoventilation with hypoxia and hypercapnia, poor respiratory secretion clearance, and pulmonary hypertension with compromised right ventricular performance. These physiologic effects of obesity may contribute to an increased risk for perioperative pulmonary complications. Despite these concerns, there is not a consistent significantly increased postoperative complication rate associated with obesity, including morbid obesity (Table 1). A review of ten studies of morbidly obese patients undergoing gastric bypass revealed an incidence of postoperative pneumonia and atelectasis of 3.9%, not significantly different than the accompanying rates reported in nonobese patients (23). There is not, however, a uniform exclusion of obesity as a significant risk factor for postoperative pulmonary complications. Studies of vascular and nonvascular abdominal surgical case series have noted an increased postoperative pulmonary complication rate associated with obesity (11,24). The complication risk may be greater in patients with weights above 150% of ideal body weight (11). There may be multiple additional considerations that are significant but have not been uniformly considered in the existing studies. These include possible cardiac comorbidities; the duration, type, and location of surgery; and anesthetic method and agents employed.

It should also be noted that the presence of obstructive sleep apnea, common in morbidly obese patients (though very often not clearly identified), is associated with a substantially increased incidence of significant pulmonary hypertension (25) which can potentially have an impact on perioperative cardiac function. Consideration should be given to preoperative echocardiographic evaluation in morbidly obese patients, including assessment of right ventricular function and estimation of pulmonary arterial systolic pressure. Evaluation is likely to be most important in those patients who have evidence of right heart overload and decompensation, with chronic lower extremity edema and possible ascites or hepatic congestion ("cor pulmonale").

SURGICAL AND ANESTHETIC CONSIDERATIONS FOR PERIOPERATIVE PULMONARY COMPLICATIONS

Perioperative pulmonary complications can be significantly influenced by specific aspects of surgical and anesthetic management. It is important to understand and consider these issues when planning the perioperative care of patients with existing lung disease.

Surgical Anatomic Site, Technique, and Duration

Perioperative pulmonary complications are related to a number of surgical as well as anesthesia considerations, some of which are outlined in Tables 2 and 3. The surgical anatomic site is an important determinant of postoperative pulmonary complications. Abdominal and thoracic operations are associated with a substantial risk for pulmonary complications (21), with thoracic and upper abdominal sites carrying the greatest risk owing to their proximity to the diaphragm and consequent high risk for perioperative and postoperative ventilatory compromise due to structural and/or functional compromise of the diaphragm (Table 2). The use of laparoscopic surgical techniques appears to substantially decrease perioperative pulmonary complication rates when compared to open surgery at similar anatomic sites (26,27) (Table 2).

With the advent of laparoscopic abdominal surgery, an additional perioperative concern is the risk of hypercapnia and respiratory acidosis as a consequence of peritoneal cavity CO_2 insufflation during laparoscopic surgery. Patients with COPD are

at greatest risk for this complication. The presence of significant airflow obstruction with FEV_1 less than 70% of predicted and a reduced pulmonary diffusion capacity less than 80% of predicted are associated with increased risk for developing perioperative hypercapnia and acidosis (28).

Prolonged surgical procedure duration (greater than 2 to 3 hours) is also associated with an increased incidence of pulmonary complications, especially in patients with smoking history (11,14,18,21).

Operative Anesthetic Techniques

There have been conflicting data regarding the benefits of epidural anesthesia for prevention of pulmonary complications (Table 3). A metaanalysis published in 2000 of 141 prior studies concluded that epidural or spinal anesthesia reduces postoperative morbidity and mortality (29). Benefits included reductions in the incidence of total mortality, thromboembolic disease, and bleeding, in addition to postoperative pneumonia. Endotracheal anesthesia can offer the potential advantage of better airway and secretion control, and may be preferred in some situations. General anesthesia may be required for the surgical anatomic site or due to the surgical method such as laparoscopy. In the specific instance of laparoscopic surgery in patients with severe COPD, general anesthesia should be used since peritoneal cavity inflation with CO_2 can cause decreased ventilation due to abdominal distension.

The use of epidural analgesia in postoperative management has demonstrated benefit in reducing postoperative complications. A recent metaanalysis concluded that the use of epidural analgesia is associated with a significant improvement in postoperative outcomes (30). This included reductions in the incidence of postoperative infections as well as overall pulmonary complications.

Perioperative Neuromuscular Blockade

The selection and use of neuromuscular blocking agents is important, as residual neuromuscular blockade is associated with increased postoperative complications. The use of the longer-acting neuromuscular blocker pancuronium is associated with an increased rate of pulmonary complications compared with the

TABLE 2. SURGICAL SITE AND INCIDENCE OF PULMONARY COMPLICATIONS

		Type of Surgery				
		Upper Abdominal	Lower Abdominal	Laparoscopic Cholecystectomy	Thoracic	All Other
Study	Year	% of Cases with Complications (Total No. of Cases)				
Gracey, et al. (74)[a]	1979	25 (57)	0 (7)		19 (21)	17 (72)
Garibaldi, et al. (75)[b]	1981	17 (201)	5 (208)		40 (102)	
Pedersen (13)	1990	33 (419)	16 (200)			3 (6687)
Southern Surgeons Club (26)	1991			0.3 (1518)		
Philips, et al. (76)	1994			0.4 (841)		
Brooks-Brunn (21)	1997	28 (238)	15 (162)			

[a]Patients had chronic obstructive pulmonary disease.
[b]Complication was defined as pneumonia.
Modified and reproduced with permission from Smetana GW. Preoperative pulmonary evaluation. *N Engl J Med* 1999;340:937–944.

TABLE 3. OPERATIVE RISK FACTORS

Risk Factor	Type of Surgery	Incidence of Pulmonary Complications		Unadjusted Relative Risk Associated with Factor
		When Factor was Present (%)	When Factor was Absent (%)	
Surgery lasting > 3 hr	Unselected	10–53	3–15	1.6–5.2
	Thoracic or abdominal	40	11	3.6
General anesthesia	Unselected	8–19	0–17	1.2–∞
	Thoracic, abdominal, or vascular	28–32	11–12	2.2–3.0
Intraoperative pancuronium	Unselected	17[a]	5	3.2

[a]The value is the incidence among patients with residual neuromuscular blockade.
Modified and reproduced with permission from Smetana GW. Preoperative pulmonary evaluation. *N Engl J Med* 1999;340:937–944.

shorter-acting agents atracurium and vecuronium (13). Monitoring with train-of-four motor nerve stimulation can decrease the frequency of prolonged neuromuscular weakness after therapy, although this surveillance method has significant limitations when being used to assess the adequacy of ventilatory muscle strength (31). When long-acting neuromuscular blocking agents are used, regular and frequent (at least every 6 hours) testing with train-of-four nerve stimulation should be employed to avoid excess drug administration.

Preoperative Patient Education and Training

As will be discussed later in the chapter, the introduction of deep breathing and incentive spirometry methods to patients *before* surgery can reduce postoperative pulmonary complication rates. The use of these patient education activities is greatest in patients with significant underlying obstructive lung disease. This makes it important to identify active pulmonary disease, and supports the selective use of preoperative pulmonary function testing.

ASSESSMENT OF PERIOPERATIVE PULMONARY RISK

Preoperative Tests

Pulmonary Function Tests

Any discussion of the use of preoperative PFTs should consider the following points:

1. Obstructive lung disease is associated with an increased risk of postoperative pulmonary complications.
2. PFTs are more accurate and sensitive in detecting lung disease than is the combination of history and physical examination.
3. The identification of PFT abnormalities in patients at risk for postoperative pulmonary complications is only likely to be of use if management strategies that can alter those risks are applied in an appropriate preoperative clinical context. A test that does not result in any change in patient management is unlikely to have any associated use.

The first two of the above points are more often addressed in the literature, while the third point is often neglected in favor of an unstated assumption that the act of simply identifying the presence of lung disease, whether by PFTs or by patient history and physical examination, will be sufficient to reduce postoperative pulmonary complications and improve outcome. This is not only an unreasonable expectation, but has little or no support in the literature.

A rational approach to optimal preoperative pulmonary management should include the identification of any significant pulmonary disease and aggressive treatment of any identified problems. This approach is likely to achieve optimal preoperative patient status, and reduce the risk of postoperative pulmonary complications. The potential use of preoperative PFTs lies in their capacity to identify and measure physiologic pulmonary impairment so that treatment can improve a patient's physiologic status, and hopefully the postoperative course as well. A major limitation of studies that have examined the use of preoperative PFTs for predicting postoperative complications is that they have not evaluated the use of the combination of preoperative testing *and* treatment. Until studies are undertaken which assess the benefit of combined preoperative diagnosis and treatment, it is unlikely that we will have a full and clear understanding of the potential use of preoperative PFTs.

As discussed previously, the presence of COPD is associated with an increased risk of postoperative pulmonary complications in both thoracic and nonthoracic surgery. One might reasonably conclude from this that if COPD is a significant risk factor for postoperative complications, it should then logically follow that preoperative PFTs would be useful for predicting and/or reducing postoperative pulmonary complications. Despite this expectation, routine preoperative PFTs have not clearly been shown to have predictive use for postoperative pulmonary complications, particularly in nonthoracic surgery (32–36) (Table 4). Interpretation of these studies is complicated by the differing surgical procedures and anesthesia methods considered, by variations in the patient clinical characteristics, and by a lack of uniform definitions of pulmonary complications. There is also a considerable range in the validity of clinical research methods of the studies, making a clear and uniform interpretation of the data difficult.

A systematic analysis of abdominal surgery performed before spirometry studies published through 1987 found significant methodologic flaws in all 22 studies examined (32). On the basis of the identified methodologic problems, Lawrence and coworkers concluded that the predictive use of spirometry for postoperative pulmonary complications after abdominal surgery

TABLE 4. SPIROMETRY AND THE RELATION WITH POSTOPERATIVE PULMONARY COMPLICATIONS

| | | | Incidence of Pulmonary Complications | | |
| | | | Among Patients with Abnormal Spirometric Findings | Among Patients with Normal Spirometric Findings | RR Associated with Abnormal Findings (95% CI)[a] |
Study	Year	Type of Surgery	% (Total No. of Cases)		
Fogh, et al. (77)	1987	Abdominal	27 (22)	16 (100)	1.7 (0.8–3.9)
Poe, et al. (78)	1988	Cholecystectomy	34 (38)	11 (171)	3.3 (1.8–6.1)
Svensson, et al. (37)[a,b]	1991	Aortic	49 (47)	32 (44)	1.5 (0.9–2.6)
Kispert, et al. (38)	1992	Vascular	23 (62)	6 (85)	3.8 (1.5–10.1)
Kroenke, et al. (19)[c]	1993	Abdominal and thoracic	52 (52)	39 (52)	1.4 (0.9–2.1)
Bando, et al. (79)[b]	1997	Cardiac	11 (67)	10 (301)	1.0 (0.5–2.2)

RR, relative risk; CI, confidence interval.
[a]Abnormal findings were defined as a forced expiratory volume (FEV_1) < 73% of predicted.
[b]Complication was defined as the need for mechanical ventilation for > 48 hrs.
[c]Abnormal findings were defined as an FEV_1 of 50%–79% of predicted and an FEV_1:forced vital capacity (FVC) ratio < 70%.
Modified and reproduced with permission from Smetana GW. Preoperative pulmonary evaluation. *N Engl J Med* 1999;340:937–944.

was unproven (32). Despite these limitations, a 1990 systematic review of the literature for all preoperative pulmonary evaluations (33), and an accompanying consensus statement from the American College of Physicians (34), found sufficient data on which to base recommendations for preoperative testing of patients as a function of surgical site and the proposed procedure.

Recommendations for Preoperative Pulmonary Function Tests

The following guidelines for obtaining preoperative PFTs are based on the analysis and recommendations from both a 1990 American College of Physicians consensus panel (33,34), and a 1995 American Thoracic Society consensus panel statement (20). While there are significant limitations to these guidelines, largely due to the incomplete data available to address some of the pertinent issues, these recommendations remain a useful and appropriate guide.

1. Patients' pulmonary symptomatic history (principally the presence of dyspnea, wheezing, or cough) and physical examination findings (wheezing, prolonged expiratory phase, or focal crackles) may be useful in identifying patients with significant underlying lung disease who would benefit from preoperative PFT and optimal pulmonary medical therapy to reduce their postoperative complication risk. Although data are limited, there is support for these evaluation steps (10,33).

2. There are no PFT parameters that should, by themselves, exclude a patient from consideration for surgery. PFT results can at best define only a relative risk for postoperative complications (Table 4), not any specific patient's absolute risk. Ultimately, the decision to proceed with surgery should be made on the basis of careful clinical assessment including, but not limited to, PFT results where appropriate.

3. Thoracic surgical candidates for lung resection should be considered for preoperative pulmonary evaluation, including spirometry and arterial blood gas analysis. Available evidence supports the use of PFTs for the prediction of postoperative pulmonary complications in thoracic surgical patients (33,34,36).

4. Patients with severe COPD are at a much increased risk for complications after thoracic surgery (8,19). There are, however, no validated PFT criteria that can exclude patients from surgery simply on the basis of preoperative pulmonary function evaluation. Preoperative exercise study parameters, including maximal oxygen uptake, may be of help in identifying patients with limited functional reserve and a very high operative risk (36), but these data have not been validated in careful prospective trials.

5. Cardiac surgery patients with underlying COPD who are to undergo open thoracic surgery have an increased incidence of postoperative complications. There are no data to support the unselected use of preoperative PFTs for cardiac surgical patients (33). It is prudent to test patients who have a significant smoking history or known COPD, or who have symptoms or examination findings suggestive of obstructive lung disease.

6. For abdominal surgery candidates, conflicting data exist for the predictive use of preoperative PFTs (32) (Table 4). A careful review of the literature has not found strong support for routine preoperative PFTs, this despite the notable increased risk of postoperative pulmonary complications in patients undergoing abdominal surgery, specifically upper abdominal surgery. Patients with a smoking history or a history of dyspnea or wheezing on examination should have preoperative PFTs and an arterial blood gas measurement. In addition, patients with known or suspected obstructive lung disease who are to undergo extensive or prolonged abdominal surgery, even if it is not on an upper abdominal site, should have preoperative PFTs.

7. Major vascular surgeries are, by virtue of the anatomic sites involved, associated with an increased incidence of pulmonary complications. Preoperative PFTs have been found to be useful in identifying patients at higher risk for postoperative pulmonary complications (37,38) (Table 4).

8. For simple surgeries not involving the abdomen or thorax, the limited but available evidence does not support the need for routine preoperative PFTs.

Nonspirometric pulmonary function parameters may have predictive use for postoperative pulmonary complications in some limited clinical circumstances. In a retrospective study of patients undergoing major abdominal surgery, a longer history of cigarette smoking and a lower preoperative PaO_2 were associated with greater risk for postoperative mechanical ventilation, while preoperative FEV_1 did not predict need for mechanical ventilation (39). Historically, the presence of hypercapnia, with a PCO_2 of greater than 45 mm Hg has been associated with increased postoperative pulmonary complications, which might be expected as there is significant concordance of severe COPD with hypercapnia. However, the predictive use of hypercapnia has not been supported in a more recent investigation (40). At present there are insufficient data to support the use of arterial blood gas analysis as a routine predictive screening tool. The presence of hypercapnia should, however, be considered when providing supplemental oxygen support, as hypercapnia is associated with an increased risk of respiratory decompensation with oxygen supplementation (41). Elevated pulmonary vascular resistance and pulmonary hypertension have been associated with increased postoperative pulmonary complications, though there are conflicting data on this issue (42). There are at present no data to support the screening of patients for pulmonary hypertension, although the presence of severe pulmonary hypertension is associated with increased perioperative mortality.

Exercise Testing

Preoperative pulmonary exercise testing has been advocated as a useful tool for assessing risk of postoperative pulmonary complications. While this approach appears to be of use in selected patients with COPD who are being considered for thoracotomy and lung resection, or abdominal surgery (9,43,44), the use of exercise testing has not been confirmed in all instances where it has been studied (45). In addition, exercise testing is cumbersome, expensive, and has not yet been prospectively validated in nonthoracic surgery studies. In studies demonstrating a predictive use from preoperative exercise testing, the parameter with the greatest utility appears to be a reduced maximum oxygen consumption (36). An increased postoperative complication incidence has also been associated with a reduced stair climbing capacity. Multiple studies have noted an increased operative risk of pulmonary complications in thoracotomy patients who were unable to climb more than two flights of stairs (36).

PREDICTION TOOLS FOR THE ESTIMATION OF POSTOPERATIVE PULMONARY OUTCOME

A number of clinical tools have been developed for the prediction of postoperative pulmonary complications (40,45). These prediction tools were derived from prospective data in patient cohorts undergoing thoracic surgery. These assessment tools support the use of specific clinical parameters to identify patients at increased risk for pulmonary complications. It is important to note that these studies are not concordant regarding the clinical parameters of greatest predictive use. Epstein and colleagues (45) developed a combined pulmonary risk index that includes a pulmonary history and symptoms composite, a decreased FEV_1/forced vital capacity ratio of less than 70%, a $PaCO_2$ greater than 45 mm Hg,

and a modification of the Goldman cardiac risk index (3) to predict increased risk for pulmonary complications after lung resection surgery. In contrast, the study by Kearney and coworkers prospectively collected clinical parameters, then retrospectively analyzed these clinical parameters, as well as derived a formula for predicting postoperative FEV_1 (40). Their study did not find any predictive use from the presence of an elevated $PaCO_2$, while it did support the pulmonary complication risk assessment use of their derived formula for predicting the postoperative FEV_1. It is also important to note that neither of these risk assessment methods has been validated by independent prospective use, and thus they both remain unproven as clinically useful tools.

Arozullah and associates recently published a clinical index for predicting postoperative respiratory failure (2). These investigators examined the records of a surgical cohort of 88,719 patients in the Veterans Affairs system to develop a prediction model for postoperative respiratory failure. Respiratory failure in this study was defined as either a requirement for mechanical ventilation for more than 48 hours postoperatively, or the need for reintubation and mechanical ventilation after initial postoperative extubation. A prediction index was derived and then subsequently prospectively validated in a separate cohort of 99,390 preoperative Veterans Affairs system patients. The index is computed from multiple clinical factors including type of surgery (abdominal aortic aneurysm repair, thoracic surgery, neurosurgery, upper abdominal surgery, peripheral vascular surgery, neck surgery, and emergency surgery); albumin level less than 30 g per L; blood urea nitrogen level more than 30 mg per dL; dependent functional status; COPD; and age (2). This index is easy to apply in clinical context, and has the advantage over prior models in that it has been prospectively validated in an independent patient cohort, which is not the case for other risk prediction tools (24,40,45,46).

PERIOPERATIVE PULMONARY MANAGEMENT: STRATEGIES FOR RISK REDUCTION

Preoperative Phase

Although it has long been accepted as obvious and reasonable to attempt to optimize patients' pulmonary status before surgery so as to reduce complication rates, it is only relatively recently that a substantial body of literature has emerged to highlight and support this concept. This concept is very important for multiple aspects of perioperative pulmonary evaluation and care, including smoking cessation, treatment of active lung disease, and preoperative pulmonary rehabilitation training (Table 7).

Smoking Cessation

Preoperative smoking cessation should be strongly recommended for all elective surgeries. Cessation of smoking before surgery has significant demonstrated benefit (15,17,47). Smoking cessation coupled with institution of bronchodilators and improved pulmonary secretion clearance also reduces postoperative pulmonary complications (20). Even acute cessation 12 to 18 hours before surgery may have benefits, including the reduction of nicotine and carboxyhemoglobin levels, which can improve oxygenation and possibly reduce perioperative cardiac and pulmonary morbidity. The promise of prompt and significant benefit from smoking cessation immediately before surgery has not, however, been borne out in studies. Cessation of smoking within 1 month of surgery has not been associated with a reduction in postoperative pulmonary complications, and might even increase the complication rate (16). Smoking abstinence for at least 8 weeks before surgery significantly reduces the incidence of perioperative pulmonary complications over that of active smokers, and smoking abstinence for at least 6 months is associated with additional risk reduction compared with more recent smoking cessation (18).

Although the decision to cease or continue smoking before surgery clearly remains with the patient, the goals and likely benefits of surgery and the relative risk of complications will need to be weighed by the surgeon before proceeding with an elective surgery in a patient with significant lung disease who chooses to continue smoking.

Optimal Preoperative Medical Therapy for Obstructive Lung Diseases

The recent clinical practice guidelines position paper published in the *Annals of Internal Medicine* advocates combined agent treatment of patients with COPD (48). This multidrug therapy approach is strongly supported by available literature. Appropriate therapy for COPD should include the use of inhaled short-acting beta-agonist and anticholinergic bronchodilator medications; a second agent can be added to the regimen of patients who are on maximal doses of an initial inhaled agent (48). The use of theophylline may have significant benefit on airways function, but the toxicity profile and low therapeutic index makes theophylline use potentially hazardous, particularly in the perioperative period. The concomitant administration of other drugs, including multiple different antibiotics, or cardiac drugs such as propranolol, verapamil, and mexiletine can substantially increase serum theophylline levels. Theophylline can also alter responses to other drugs, including increasing arrhythmia risk with halothane, and lowering seizure threshold when used with ketamine. If theophylline has been used by patients, and has proven beneficial, particularly in patients with more severe disease, the prudent approach may be to continue its use through the perioperative period, though close monitoring of serum levels and careful consideration of possible adverse drug interactions should be undertaken.

Systemic corticosteroid treatment, in short courses, improves spirometry and reduces relapse rates in COPD (48). Surgical outcomes are not adversely affected by the preoperative administration of corticosteroids to patients with asthma (49,50), and patients should be treated with increased steroid therapy if it is clinically indicated. It is not the preoperative or perioperative use of systemic steroids that poses the greater postoperative complication risk in patients with obstructive lung disease, but rather the suboptimal treatment of any active lung disease. The presence of signs and symptoms of active airways obstruction which is inadequately treated represents a more significant risk for pulmonary complications than does the perioperative use of corticosteroids (49,50). Corticosteroids are also safe and reasonable for preoperative use in COPD patients where treatment is clinically indicated. Recent metaanalyses support the use of corticosteroids for exacerbations of COPD (48,51), and this should be considered when planning surgery in patients with COPD.

Pulmonary Rehabilitation and Incentive Spirometry Training

Inspiratory training maneuvers to improve lung volumes are not only effective in the postoperative period, but have additional use when initiated preoperatively (14,52,53). The benefits from inspiratory training have been reported in both chest and abdominal surgical series. Breathing training initiated in patients in a rehabilitation program before upper abdominal surgery was found to produce a substantial reduction in the incidence of postoperative respiratory complications in a population of patients undergoing elective abdominal surgery (14). The incidence of complications, including pneumonia and respiratory failure, was highest in patients with significant pulmonary disease history and duration of surgery longer than 120 minutes. The benefit of preoperative deep breathing training was greatest in those patients with moderate and high risk of complications (14).

The optimal inspiratory training strategy is not clear, although deep breathing, incentive spirometry device use, and intermittent positive pressure breathing (IPPB) have all been reported to be helpful. A prospective trial comparing incentive spirometry, IPPB, and deep breathing training in abdominal surgery patients found significant (approximately 50%) reductions in pulmonary complication rates for all three intervention arms compared with the control population (52). No statistically significant difference was seen among the three intervention arms with respect to pulmonary complications. However, the incentive spirometry intervention group had a significantly shorter hospital stay than did the control group, and this was not observed in the other interventions.

The available literature clearly supports the use of breathing maneuver training for patients undergoing thoracic or abdominal surgery. The choice of specific method to achieve improved lung volume can be made on the basis of local experience and availability.

Perioperative and Postoperative Phase

Anesthesia Choice

As previously outlined, the relevant literature does not clearly support the superiority of either regional or general anesthesia over the other for reducing the incidence of postoperative pulmonary complications. A prudent approach to the selection of regional or general anesthesia should focus on the particular circumstances of the patient's medical problems, including lung disease and the surgery that is planned. Instances where one anesthetic choice might be favored over the other can be identified, such as intubation and general anesthesia for better airways management or for patients with severe COPD who are to undergo laparotomy and might be at risk for hypercapnic respiratory decompensation after CO_2 inflation of the peritoneal cavity. Epidural analgesia should be considered for postoperative pain management, and is of benefit in reducing postoperative complications (30).

Surgical Techniques

As has been discussed earlier in this chapter, the choice of surgical approach can also alter the risk of postoperative complications. Limiting operative duration to less than 2 hours, when possible, can reduce the risk of postoperative respiratory complications. Another aspect of surgical approach to emphasize is the selection of patients for laparoscopic surgery. There is a very real risk that peritoneal cavity inflation with CO_2 can precipitate hypercapnic acidosis and respiratory failure in patients with severe COPD. The risk of this complication warrants particular caution and close monitoring when laparoscopic surgery is performed in COPD patients. Given the inability of either oximetry or end-tidal CO_2 monitoring to adequately assess changes in ventilation in patients with severe COPD, arterial blood gas monitoring is appropriate when laparoscopic surgery is undertaken in this patient group.

Postoperative Deep-Breathing Maneuvers

Postoperative deep-breathing maneuvers, including incentive spirometry, spontaneous deep-breathing training, or IPPB are all beneficial in reducing postoperative pulmonary complications, especially in identified high-risk patients (52,54). The benefit of the three different methods appears to be equivalent (54). These methods should be used routinely in the postoperative course.

Oxygen Supplementation

Supplemental oxygen therapy is of significant benefit to patients with hypoxemia and exacerbations of COPD. This subject has recently been reviewed in detail, and remains a fundamental and important recommended adjunctive therapy for COPD (48). Caution should be exercised in the delivery of oxygen to patients with COPD, as hypercapnia (including with respiratory failure) can complicate oxygen therapy (41). The mechanisms for supplemental oxygen-induced hypercapnia are likely multiple and include altered ventilation–perfusion matching and/or depressed central ventilatory drive. This physiologic consideration is particularly important in the postoperative period, where the use of inhalational anesthetics and opiate analgesics can significantly alter ventilation–perfusion relationships and/or ventilatory drive.

Attempts have been made to prospectively identify patients at greatest risk for developing hypercapnic respiratory decompensation after oxygen supplementation. Bone and colleagues, in a study of 50 patients with COPD exacerbation, derived a prediction function for the identification of patients at risk for respiratory failure after supplemental oxygen therapy (41). The derived prediction equation (pH = $7.66 - [0.0091 \times Pao_2]$) had a sensitivity, in both the original patient cohort and in a subsequent validation cohort, of approximately 80%. Despite these data, this prediction tool is very infrequently used in clinical circumstances.

In summary, the substantial use of oxygen therapy in COPD exacerbations favors treatment, but the risk of respiratory compromise has to be considered. Patients who are placed on oxygen therapy, particularly those with substantial obstructive lung disease, need to be monitored closely for compromise of ventilation and acid-base status.

Venous Thromboembolism Prophylaxis

Venous thromboembolism remains a common and major clinical problem in surgical patients. The incidence of deep venous thrombosis, reviewed in the recent American College of Chest

TABLE 5. VENOUS THROMBOEMBOLISM PROPHYLAXIS RECOMMENDATIONS

Levels of Risk Examples	Incidence of Disease without Prophylaxis (%)				Successful Prevention Strategies
	Calf DVT	Proximal DVT	Clinical PE	Fatal PE	
Low risk Minor surgery in patients < 40 yr with no additional risk factors	2	0.4	0.2	0.002	No specific measures Aggressive mobilization
Moderate risk Minor surgery in patients with additional risk factors; nonmajor surgery in patients aged 40–60 yr with no additional risk factors; major surgery in patients < 40 yr with no additional risk factors	10–20	2–4	1–2	0.1–0.4	LDUH q12h, LMWH, ES, or IPC
High risk Nonmajor surgery in patients > 60 yr or with additional risk factors; major surgery in patients > 40 yr or with additional risk factors	20–40	4–8	2–4	0.4–1.0	LDUH q8h, LMWH, or IPC
Highest risk	40–80	10–20	4–10	0.2–5	LMWH, oral anticoagulants, IPC/ES + LDUH/LMWH, or ADH

DVT, deep venous thrombosis; PE, pulmonary embolism; ADH, adjusted-dose heparin; ES, elastic stockings; IPC, intermittent pneumatic compression devices; LDUH, low-dose unfractionated heparin; LMWH, low-molecular-weight heparin.
Modified and reproduced with permission from Geerts WH, et al. Prevention of venous thromboembolism. *Chest* 2001;119:132S–175S.

Physicians consensus statement on prevention of venous thromboembolism (VTE) (55), ranges from less than 5% in low-risk patients to approximately 20% in patients with multiple risk factors. The incidence of pulmonary embolism is less, but can be as high as 10% in high-risk patient populations (55). Optimal postoperative patient management should consider the substantial risks of venous thromboembolism in surgical patients, and include evaluation for VTE where clinical suspicion is present. Postoperative patients should, except where their use is contraindicated, be treated with VTE prophylaxis measures (Table 5).

The safety and benefit of VTE prophylaxis measures is well established in general surgical patients as well as in specialty surgical groups including orthopedic, trauma, urologic, and neurosurgical patients (55). Despite documented efficacy, effective prophylaxis measures are often substantially underprescribed (55,56). In a random survey of surgeons conducted by the American College of Surgeons, 86% claimed they used prophylaxis in 1993, with this proportion rising to 96% by 1997. However, a study of 2,000 patients hospitalized at 16 acute-care hospitals in the United States showed that only one-third of these patients actually received prophylaxis despite the presence of multiple VTE risk factors that warranted prophylaxis (55). The use of DVT prophylaxis is higher in teaching hospitals than in nonteaching hospitals (55). In addition, appropriate diagnostic tests are often not performed in appropriate high-risk patient populations (56).

Appropriate perioperative VTE prophylaxis management should be administered to all patients with significant risk, with the specific prophylaxis measures selected for patients in accordance with demonstrated use and any clinical restrictions (Table 5). Unfractionated heparin remains a proven therapy. Low-molecular-weight heparins are at least as effective as unfractionated heparin for prophylaxis as well as active VTE therapy, and have the advantage of lower incidence of bleeding complications (57,58). Pneumatic sequential compression devices have VTE relative risk reduction rates comparable to heparin or warfarin in most clinical circumstances, and have the advantage of no bleeding risk (55).

POSTOPERATIVE MANAGEMENT OF RESPIRATORY DECOMPENSATION

Noninvasive Ventilatory Assistance

The development and availability of noninvasive positive pressure ventilation (NPPV) devices have provided an important ventilatory therapy option for patients with respiratory compromise. The current widely available NPPV options include continuous positive airway pressure (CPAP) and bilevel positive airway pressure (BiPAP), the latter allowing for independent adjustment of inspiratory and expiratory pressures. Both modalities can be delivered by either standard ventilators or by small portable bedside devices and can be used with either full-face or nasal mask delivery, thus making this therapy an attractive option for patients with respiratory decompensation. The use of NPPV therapy has not, however, been demonstrated to be uniformly beneficial nor necessarily safe in all clinical circumstances. The selection of patients for treatment with NPPV should be based on the patients' clinical characteristics and status, and the goals of NPPV (Table 6).

TABLE 6. CONSIDERATIONS FOR NONINVASIVE POSITIVE PRESSURE VENTILATION (NPPV)

Conditions where NPPV has a demonstrated benefit:
  Hypoxemic respiratory failure
  Hypercapneic respiratory failure
  Chronic obstructive pulmonary disease with acute severe exacerbations

Conditions where NPPV may have benefit:
  Neuromuscular diseases
  Chest wall compliance problems

Conditions where NPPV therapy has not been shown to be beneficial:
  Primary acute lung injury, including acute pneumonia

Exclusion criteria:
  Intolerance of mask devices
  Altered level of consciousness
  High aspiration risk; esophageal dysfunction
  Severe hypoxemia
  High-grade cardiac arrhythmias

Therapy considerations:
  Therapy advantage of nasal vs. face mask currently uncertain
  Frequent patient checks for mask-related skin injury
  Nasogastric tube drainage for patients using full-face mask
  No enteral feeding during NPPV treatment
  Stress ulcer prophylaxis during treatment

Clinical benefit has been demonstrated for NPPV in selected circumstances. There is demonstrated use of NPPV over conventional care in COPD exacerbations (59–62). In a randomized prospective study by Kramer and colleagues in patients with acute severe exacerbations of COPD, the use of nasal BiPAP was associated with a reduced need for intubation (60). The rate of intubation was reduced from 67% in the control population (treated with standard therapy, including oxygen and inhaled bronchodilators) to 9% in the BiPAP-treated arm. Similarly, a study by Brochard and associates (59) in a selected population of patients with acute exacerbations of COPD demonstrated benefit from the application of BiPAP, with reduction in need for intubation from 74% in the control group to 26% in the BiPAP-treated group. Of note, this study excluded many patients, including those with demonstrated pneumonia, which limits the ability to generalize these results to an NPPV recommendation for all patients with acute exacerbation of COPD. The use of NPPV for respiratory failure from non-COPD causes is less certain than for COPD. While some studies have found no use for NPPV in acute respiratory failure without COPD (63), others have shown benefit, with a reduced rate of intubation with use of NPPV (62,64).

Delclaux and others examined the use of CPAP in acute hypoxemic nonhypercapnic patients (63). This study examined 123 consecutive intensive care unit (ICU) admissions for acute lung injury in patients without a history of COPD. The study found early benefit in oxygenation at 1 hour of therapy when comparing the NPPV group with the oxygen-treated group. The study did not, however, find any subsequent benefit from NPPV, including for patient intubation rates, length of ICU stay, or hospital mortality (63). This study points out some important limitations of NPPV therapy. The NPPV therapy used in this trial was CPAP, which can be physiologically different than BiPAP, as the latter has the capacity to use increased inspiratory pressures. Whether BiPAP has a greater use than CPAP in acute respiratory decompensation is not clear at the present time. In addition, the study examined NPPV use in a patient cohort with acute lung injury, not COPD, and acute lung injury may not be as amenable to NPPV therapy. The potential advantage of BiPAP over CPAP was explored in a prospective study using BiPAP in a population of patients with both COPD-related and non-COPD-related causes for acute respiratory failure (62). This study found that patients with hypoxemic non-COPD acute respiratory failure had a benefit from BiPAP over conventional medical therapy, with a lower intubation rate, although the ICU mortality rates between the two groups were not statistically different.

For selected forms of hypoxemic acute respiratory failure other than acute lung injury (including cystic fibrosis, opportunistic pneumonia in patients with acquired immunodeficiency syndrome, candidates for lung transplantation, and postbronchoscopy or postextubation respiratory distress), there may be an advantage to the use of NPPV (64). However, insufficient data exist to clearly delineate all appropriate candidates.

Cardiogenic pulmonary edema should be distinguished from acute lung injury when considering NPPV since NPPV appears to be effective in cardiogenic pulmonary edema (65,66). Whether BiPAP offers an advantage over CPAP for therapy in cardiogenic pulmonary edema is not yet clear.

NPPV is associated with a decreased risk and incidence of nosocomial pneumonia compared with patients receiving standard endotracheal intubation and mechanical ventilation (67). In patients with severe respiratory failure from COPD, NPPV is associated with a reduced cost of care compared with intubation and mechanical ventilation.

NONINVASIVE POSITIVE PRESSURE VENTILATION IN POSTOPERATIVE PATIENTS

The use of NPPV specifically in postoperative circumstances has not been systematically studied. In a subset of patients with acute respiratory failure associated with solid organ transplant there is a clear benefit from NPPV in avoiding intubation and mechanical ventilation (68). This study prospectively compared the use of NPPV with standard supportive oxygen therapy. The use of NPPV was associated with statistically significant reductions in the rate of endotracheal intubation (20% versus 70%), the rate of fatal complications (20% versus 50%), length of ICU stay in survivors (mean $\pm$ SD days: 5.5 $\pm$ 3 versus 9 $\pm$ 4), and ICU mortality (20% versus 50%). There was no difference in hospital mortality (68). In a recent study by Martin and colleagues (62), postoperative patients composed a subset of the patient cohort with acute respiratory failure, but this population was not analyzed separately. This study did find an overall benefit of BiPAP in reducing the intubation rate for acute respiratory failure, particularly in non-COPD patients whose causes for respiratory failure included neuromuscular disease, postextubation status, and hypoxemic pulmonary disease (62). These data are limited in scope, and do not clarify the limits of use of NPPV for postoperative patients, but do argue effectively for consideration of NPPV as an adjunct for respiratory support in cases of respiratory decompensation in the perioperative period.

Problems associated with the use of NPPV include mask (nasal or full-face) pressure-related skin abrasion or necrosis, mask intolerance due to discomfort, and transient hypotension (62); significant hemodynamic compromise has not been associated with the use of BiPAP. The alternative to NPPV, endotracheal intubation and mechanical ventilation, can cause hypotension, particularly in patients with significant airways obstruction, where air-trapping, hyperinflation, and compromised central venous return may occur. These data have been incorporated in the recommendations of multiple authors (69,70), and are summarized in Table 6.

MECHANICAL VENTILATION STRATEGIES FOR PATIENTS REQUIRING ENDOTRACHEAL INTUBATION

The strategy for patients who require intubation and mechanical ventilation is dependent upon the underlying clinical disease state. The most important recent advance in mechanical ventilation strategy involves the ventilation of patients with acute lung injury or acute respiratory distress syndrome (ARDS). From a study conducted by the National Institutes of Health-sponsored ARDS research network, there is now strong clinical trial evidence to support the use of a small tidal volume (6 mL per kg) ventilation strategy in patients requiring mechanical ventilation for ARDS (71). The ARDS Network study revealed a striking 22% reduction in mortality when comparing 6 mL per kg with 12 mL per kg tidal volume. The question of the optimal level of positive end-expiratory pressure (PEEP) to be used in treating ARDS has not yet been fully answered. The ARDS Network trial used higher average PEEP (greater than 9 cm H_2O), arguing this would help avoid atelectasis and additional ventilator-related lung injury. Whether PEEP levels higher than these might achieve greater benefit is not yet known.

An additional important consideration in mechanically ventilated patients is the avoidance of ventilator-associated pneumonia (VAP). VAP is associated with significantly increased length of ICU stay and an attributable mortality of approximately 20% to 30% (72). Risk factors for developing VAP include underlying cardiorespiratory disease, neurologic injury, and trauma. Important modifiable VAP risk factors include supine body position, witnessed aspiration, paralytic agents, and antibiotic exposure. Attention to these modifiable risk factors, including the use of semirecumbent positioning of patients and avoidance of paralytic agents, can improve outcome (72).

PERIOPERATIVE CONSIDERATIONS FOR RESTRICTIVE PULMONARY DISEASE

The assessment of perioperative risk in patients with restrictive lung diseases is not as well investigated as it is in obstructive lung disease. A number of points about restrictive lung disease are pertinent, and may help with the evaluation and management of these patients in the perioperative period.

Risk Factor Assessment

The most common causes of restrictive ventilatory conditions are interstitial fibrotic lung diseases, which include primary idiopathic pulmonary fibrosis as well as interstitial lung diseases associated with systemic, most commonly rheumatologic, diseases. It is important to appreciate this, as it is often the associated extrapulmonary organ involvement that can contribute to perioperative problems. The presence of esophageal motility problems, very common in patients with scleroderma and mixed connective tissue diseases, can substantially increase aspiration risk and thus perioperative risk. Motility problems should be identified preoperatively, and optimal medical therapies undertaken prior to surgery. Attention should also be placed on maintaining optimal patient positioning to minimize aspiration. Elevating the head of the bed has substantial use in reducing the risk of VAP, although the application of this simple and effective maneuver is commonly neglected (72).

The other major category of patients with restrictive ventilatory defects to be considered for careful perioperative management are those with chest wall deformities and/or chronic neuromuscular diseases that compromise ventilation. Patients with neuromuscular diseases need not have intrinsic lung or chest wall structural abnormalities to have compromised lung volumes and ventilatory capacity; significant neuromuscular weakness can be sufficient to limit lung volumes and ventilation at baseline, with decompensation then precipitated by surgery or medications. Pulmonary gas exchange may be adequate in the preoperative period, but may be severely altered by position changes and/or the use of sedative and analgesic agents.

The utility of preoperative PFTs for patients with restrictive pulmonary disease is uncertain. No substantial prospective study data are available to support obtaining routine preoperative PFTs in these patients. It is very important, however, to consider the major limitations and associated physiology of interstitial lung disease to minimize the risk of postoperative problems. Progressive ventilatory compromise in interstitial lung disease can produce progressive hypercapnia, which can be magnified by surgery and postoperative analgesic therapy. Preoperative arterial blood gas determination will identify patients who have baseline hypercapnia and can guide closer postoperative ventilation surveillance and pain management.

Pulmonary hypertension is common in patients with interstitial lung disease and can substantially increase perioperative risks. Preoperative echocardiography and/or pulmonary artery catheterization can diagnose the magnitude of pulmonary hypertension and any cardiac compromise. These studies are not advocated routinely for all patients with interstitial lung disease. However, clinicians should maintain a high index of suspicion for concomitant pulmonary hypertension in patients with interstitial lung disease. In cases where severe pulmonary hypertension is identified, consideration should be given to pulmonary vasodilator therapy. Inhaled nitric oxide can produce selective pulmonary vasodilation in the perioperative period. Continuous intravenous epoprostenol (prostacyclin) is rarely initiated in the immediate perioperative period but can have substantial benefits with long-term administration (73).

Perioperative Ventilatory Support

The management of perioperative ventilatory support for patients with restrictive ventilatory defects should, as for patients with obstructive lung disease, include consideration of NPPV. There are limited data to support the use of perioperative NPPV for restrictive diseases, but NPPV can play a role in the management of respiratory failure in restrictive disease, and should be considered (64). In patients with interstitial lung disease who are to be treated with NPPV, the possibility of concomitant esophageal motility problems should be considered, as this can increase the aspiration risk. Options for management include nasogastric tube evacuation of the stomach and consideration of alternative ventilatory strategies including endotracheal intubation to protect the airway from aspiration events.

SUMMARY

Chronic obstructive pulmonary disease (COPD) is associated with an increased risk of perioperative and postoperative complications, and can be associated with increased surgical mortality. Well-recognized risk factors for postoperative pulmonary complications include overall health status and smoking history, in addition to obstructive lung disease. Surgical site is also a significant risk factor for postoperative pulmonary complications, with thoracic and upper abdominal surgery carrying the greatest risks. Surgical risks include prolonged operation time and the use of neuromuscular blocking agents. The presence of airways obstruction on PFTs is associated with increased postoperative risk, but the predictive use of PFTs is limited. A decision to proceed with surgery should be based on a composite analysis of the status of preoperative clinical problems, including pulmonary problems; the goals of surgery; and an estimate of perioperative risks. An outline for perioperative management to optimize surgical outcome is found in Table 7.

Appropriate recognition of significant pulmonary disease is essential to achieving optimal preoperative management, which

TABLE 7. PERIOPERATIVE RISK MANAGEMENT STRATEGY

Preoperative period
  Smoking cessation, preferably for at least 8 wks before surgery
  Obtain spirometry in patients with significant airway obstruction, or who are to undergo thoracic or upper abdominal surgery
  Treat any significant airflow obstruction:
      bronchodilator therapy
      inhaled steroids as indicated
      systemic steroids if needed
  Antibiotics for acute respiratory infections
  Initiate lung expansion methods training
  Venous thromboembolism prophylaxis

Perioperative period
  Limit surgical time when possible
  Consider laparoscopic vs. open procedure where feasible
  Regional anesthesia with spinal or epidural anesthesia if possible
  Avoid longer-acting neuromuscular blocking agents
  Consider epidural analgesia for thoracic or complex abdominal surgery
  Venous thromboembolism prophylaxis

Postoperative period
  Incentive spirometry
  Venous thromboembolism prophylaxis

can reduce the risk of perioperative pulmonary complications. Preoperative PFTs should be performed on patients who have known or suspected pulmonary disease, or who are to undergo thoracic or significant abdominal surgery, and should be based in part on the clinical context. Preoperative patient care should focus on optimal and aggressive medical treatment for any identified lung disease, and introduction to deep-breathing training, particularly for thoracic and abdominal surgery candidates. Planning of the surgical approach should include efforts to identify and minimize intraoperative risk factors. Postoperative ancillary management should include deep-breathing maneuvers and thromboembolism prophylaxis. Careful pain management should focus on avoiding respiratory compromise. Epidural analgesia has significant use for pain control after thoracic and abdominal surgery. The options for postoperative ventilatory support, if needed, include NPPV as well as intubation and mechanical ventilation. Noninvasive ventilatory support provides benefit in selected conditions, including atelectasis, COPD exacerbations, and instances of acute hypoxemic respiratory failure. Caution should be exercised to avoid complications associated with noninvasive ventilatory support, including aspiration.

Decisions regarding perioperative evaluation and management of patients with restrictive lung diseases are not based on such substantial literature as is the case for obstructive pulmonary disease, but should consider the physiologic problems encountered in this patient population. Given the predominance of multiorgan involvement in many of the diseases that cause restrictive pulmonary defects, special attention should be given to identification and management of any concomitant nonpulmonary organ dysfunction, such as esophageal problems and pulmonary hypertension, which can increase the risk of perioperative complications.

KEY POINTS

- Chronic obstructive and restrictive pulmonary diseases are associated with an increased risk of perioperative complications.
- Risk factors for postoperative pulmonary complications in patients with chronic obstructive pulmonary disease (COPD) include overall health status, smoking history, surgical site, and prolonged operation time.
- The presence of airways obstruction on pulmonary function tests (PFTs) is associated with increased postoperative risk, but the predictive use of PFTs is limited.
- Preoperative patient care should focus on optimal and aggressive medical treatment for any identified lung disease.

- Epidural analgesia has significant use for pain control after thoracic and abdominal surgery.
- Noninvasive ventilatory support provides benefit in selected conditions, including atelectasis and COPD exacerbations, and in some patients with acute hypoxemic respiratory failure.
- In patients with restrictive lung disease, special attention should be given to identification and management of any concomitant nonpulmonary organ dysfunction, such as esophageal problems and pulmonary hypertension, which can increase the risk of perioperative complications.

REFERENCES

1. Lawrence VA, Hilsenbeck SG, Mulrow CD, et al. Incidence and hospital stay for cardiac and pulmonary complications after abdominal surgery. *J Gen Intern Med* 1995;10:671–678.
2. Arozullah AM, Daley J, Henderson WG, et al. Multifactorial risk index for predicting postoperative respiratory failure in men after major noncardiac surgery. The National Veterans Administration Surgical Quality Improvement Program. *Ann Surg* 2000;232:242–253.
3. Goldman L, Caldera DL, Nussbaum SR, et al. Multifactorial index of cardiac risk in noncardiac surgical procedures. *N Engl J Med* 1977;297:845–850.
4. Wolters U, Wolf T, Stutzer H, et al. ASA classification and perioperative variables as predictors of postoperative outcome. *Br J Anaesth* 1996;77:217–222.
5. Hall JC, Tarala RA, Hall JL, et al. A multivariate analysis of the risk of pulmonary complications after laparotomy. *Chest* 1991;99:923–927.
6. Prause G, Ratzenhofer-Comenda B, Pierer G, et al. Can ASA grade or Goldman's cardiac risk index predict peri-operative mortality? A study of 16,227 patients. *Anaesthesia* 1997;52:203–206.
7. Prause G, Offner A, Ratzenhofer-Komenda B, et al. Comparison of two preoperative indices to predict perioperative mortality in non-cardiac thoracic surgery. *Eur J Cardio-Thorac Surg* 1997;11:670–675.
8. Kroenke K, Lawrence VA, Theroux JF, et al. Operative risk in patients with severe obstructive pulmonary disease. *Arch Intern Med* 1992;152:967–971.
9. Gerson MC, Hurst JM, Hertzberg VS, et al. Prediction of cardiac and pulmonary complications related to elective abdominal and noncardiac thoracic surgery in geriatric patients. *Am J Med* 1990;88:101–107.

10. Lawrence VA, Dhanda R, Hilsenbeck SG, et al. Risk of pulmonary complications after elective abdominal surgery. *Chest* 1996;110:744–750.
11. Calligaro KD, Azurin DJ, Dougherty MJ, et al. Pulmonary risk factors of elective abdominal aortic surgery. *J Vasc Surg* 1993;18:914–920.
12. Dales RE, Dionne G, Leech JA, et al. Preoperative prediction of pulmonary complications following thoracic surgery. *Chest* 1993;104:155–159.
13. Pedersen T. Complications and death following anaesthesia. A prospective study with special reference to the influence of patient-, anaesthesia-, and surgery-related risk factors. *Dan Med Bull* 1994;41:319–331.
14. Chumillas S, Ponce JL, Delgado F, et al. Prevention of postoperative pulmonary complications through respiratory rehabilitation: a controlled clinical study. *Arch Phys Med Rehab* 1998;79:5–9.
15. Moores LK, Pearce AC, Jones RM, et al. Smoking and postoperative pulmonary complications. An evidence-based review of the recent literature. *Clin Chest Med* 2000;21:139–146, ix–x.
16. Bluman LG, Mosca L, Newman N, et al. Preoperative smoking habits and postoperative pulmonary complications. *Chest* 1998;113:883–889.
17. Pearce AC, Jones RM, Crowe JM, et al. Smoking and anesthesia: preoperative abstinence and perioperative morbidity. *Anesthesiology* 1984;61:576–584.
18. Warner MA, Offord KP, Warner ME, et al. Role of preoperative cessation of smoking and other factors in postoperative pulmonary complications: a blinded prospective study of coronary artery bypass patients. *Mayo Clin Proc* 1989;64:609–616.
19. Kroenke K, Lawrence VA, Theroux JF, et al. Postoperative complications after thoracic and major abdominal surgery in patients with and without obstructive lung disease. *Chest* 1993;104:1445–1451.
20. American Thoracic Society. Standards for the Diagnosis and Care of

Patients with Chronic Obstructive Pulmonary Disease. *Am J Respir Crit Care Med* 1995;152:S77–S120.

21. Brooks-Brunn JA. Predictors of postoperative pulmonary complications following abdominal surgery. *Chest* 1997;111:564–571.

22. *Guidelines for the Diagnosis and Management of Asthma*. National Asthma Education Program. Expert Panel Report. National Heart, Lung and Blood Institute, National Institutes of Health. Publication No. 91-3042, August, 1991.

23. Pasulka PS, Bistrian BR, Benotti PN, et al. The risks of surgery in obese patients. *Ann Intern Med* 1986;104:540–546.

24. Brooks-Brunn JA. Validation of a predictive model for postoperative pulmonary complications. *Heart Lung* 1998;27:151–158.

25. Bady E, Achkar A, Pascal S, et al. Pulmonary arterial hypertension in patients with sleep apnoea syndrome. *Thorax* 2000;55:934–939.

26. Southern Surgeons Club. A prospective analysis of 1518 laparoscopic cholecystectomies. The Southern Surgeons Club. *N Engl J Med* 1991;324:1073–1078.

27. Nguyen NT, Lee SL, Goldman C, et al. Comparison of pulmonary function and postoperative pain after laparoscopic versus open gastric bypass: a randomized trial. *J Am Coll Surg* 2001;192:469–476.

28. Wittgen CM, Naunheim KS, Andrus CH, et al. Preoperative pulmonary function evaluation for laparoscopic cholecystectomy. *Arch Surg* 1993;128:880–885.

29. Rodgers A, Walker N, Schug S, et al. Reduction of postoperative mortality and morbidity with epidural or spinal anaesthesia: results from overview of randomised trials. *BMJ* 2000;321:1493.

30. Ballantyne JC, Carr DB, deFerranti S, et al. The comparative effects of postoperative analgesic therapies on pulmonary outcome: cumulative meta-analyses of randomized, controlled trials. *Anesth Analg* 1998;86:598–612.

31. Eriksson LI. Ventilation and neuromuscular blocking drugs. *Acta Anaesthesiol Scand Suppl* 1994;102:11–15.

32. Lawrence VA, Page CP, Harris GD. Preoperative spirometry before abdominal operations. A critical appraisal of its predictive value. *Arch Intern Med* 1989;149:280–285.

33. Zibrak JD, O'Donnell CR, Marton K. Indications for pulmonary function testing. *Ann Intern Med* 1990;112:763–771.

34. Preoperative pulmonary function testing. American College of Physicians. *Ann Intern Med* 1990;112:793–794.

35. Smetana GW. Preoperative pulmonary evaluation. *N Engl J Med* 1999;340:937–944.

36. Reilly JJ Jr. Evidence-based preoperative evaluation of candidates for thoracotomy. *Chest* 1999;116:474S–476S.

37. Svensson LG, Hess KR, Coselli JS, et al. A prospective study of respiratory failure after high-risk surgery on the thoracoabdominal aorta. *J Vasc Surg* 1991;14:271–282.

38. Kispert JF, Kazmers A, Roitman L. Preoperative spirometry predicts perioperative pulmonary complications after major vascular surgery. *Am Surg* 1992;58:491–495.

39. Jayr C, Matthay MA, Goldstone J, et al. Preoperative and intraoperative factors associated with prolonged mechanical ventilation. A study in patients following major abdominal vascular surgery. *Chest* 1993;103:1231–1236.

40. Kearney DJ, Lee TH, Reilly JJ, et al. Assessment of operative risk in patients undergoing lung resection. Importance of predicted pulmonary function. *Chest* 1994;105:753–759.

41. Bone RC, Pierce AK, Johnson RL Jr. Controlled oxygen administration in acute respiratory failure in chronic obstructive pulmonary disease: a reappraisal. *Am J Med* 1978;65:896–902.

42. Reilly JJ Jr. Benefits of aggressive perioperative management in patients undergoing thoracotomy. *Chest* 1995;107:312S–315S.

43. Walsh GL, Morice RC, Putnam JB, et al. Resection of lung cancer is justified in high-risk patients selected by exercise oxygen consumption. *Ann Thorac Surg* 1994;58:704–710; discussion 711.

44. Melendez JA, Fischer ME. Preoperative pulmonary evaluation of the thoracic surgical patient. *Chest Surg Clin North Am* 1997;7:641–654.

45. Epstein SK, Faling LJ, Daly BD, et al. Predicting complications after pulmonary resection. Preoperative exercise testing vs. a multifactorial cardiopulmonary risk index. *Chest* 1993;104:694–700.

46. Melendez JA, Carlon VA. Cardiopulmonary risk index does not predict complications after thoracic surgery. *Chest* 1998;114:69–75.

47. Warner MA, Divertie MB, Tinker JH. Preoperative cessation of smoking and pulmonary complications in coronary artery bypass patients. *Anesthesiology* 1984;60:380–383.

48. Bach PB, Brown C, Gelfand SE, et al. Management of acute exacerbations of chronic obstructive pulmonary disease: a summary and appraisal of published evidence. *Ann Intern Med* 2001;134:600–620.

49. Pien LC, Grammer LC, Patterson R, et al. Minimal complications in a surgical population with severe asthma receiving prophylactic corticosteroids. *J Allergy Clin Immunol* 1988;82:696–700.

50. Kabalin CS, Yarnold PR, Grammer LC, et al. Low complication rate of corticosteroid-treated asthmatics undergoing surgical procedures. *Arch Intern Med* 1995;155:1379–1384.

51. Snow V, Lascher S, Mottur-Pilson C. Evidence base for management of acute exacerbations of chronic obstructive pulmonary disease. *Ann Intern Med* 2001;134:595–599.

52. Celli BR, Rodriguez KS, Snider GL. A controlled trial of intermittent positive pressure breathing, incentive spirometry, and deep breathing exercises in preventing pulmonary complications after abdominal surgery. *Am Rev Respir Dis* 1984;130:12–15.

53. Castillo R, Haas A. Chest physical therapy: comparative efficacy of preoperative and postoperative in the elderly. *Arch Phys Med Rehabil* 1985;66:376–379.

54. Thomas JA, McIntosh JM. Are incentive spirometry, intermittent positive pressure breathing, and deep breathing exercises effective in the prevention of postoperative pulmonary complications after upper abdominal surgery? A systematic overview and meta-analysis. *Physical Therapy* 1994;74:3–10; discussion 10–16.

55. Geerts WH, Heit JA, Clagett GP, et al. Prevention of venous thromboembolism. *Chest* 2001;119:132S–175S.

56. Cook D, Attia J, Weaver B, et al. Venous thromboembolic disease: an observational study in medical-surgical intensive care unit patients. *J Crit Care* 2000;15:127–132.

57. Kakkar VV. Effectiveness and safety of low molecular weight heparins (LMWH) in the prevention of venous thromboembolism (VTE). *Thromb Haemost* 1995;74:364–368.

58. Gould MK, Dembitzer AD, Doyle RL, et al. Low-molecular-weight heparins compared with unfractionated heparin for treatment of acute deep venous thrombosis. A meta-analysis of randomized, controlled trials. *Ann Intern Med* 1999;130:800–809.

59. Brochard L, Mancebo J, Wysocki M, et al. Noninvasive ventilation for acute exacerbations of chronic obstructive pulmonary disease. *N Engl J Med* 1995;333:817–822.

60. Kramer N, Meyer TJ, Meharg J, et al. Randomized, prospective trial of noninvasive positive pressure ventilation in acute respiratory failure. *Am J Respir Crit Care Med* 1995;151:1799–1806.

61. Antonelli M, Conti G, Rocco M, et al. A comparison of noninvasive positive-pressure ventilation and conventional mechanical ventilation in patients with acute respiratory failure. *N Engl J Med* 1998;339:429–435.

62. Martin TJ, Hovis JD, Costantino JP, et al. A randomized, prospective evaluation of noninvasive ventilation for acute respiratory failure. *Am J Respir Crit Care Med* 2000;161:807–813.

63. Delclaux C, L'Her E, Alberti C, et al. Treatment of acute hypoxemic nonhypercapnic respiratory insufficiency with continuous positive airway pressure delivered by a face mask: a randomized controlled trial. *JAMA* 2000;284:2352–2360.

64. Meduri GU, Turner RE, Abou-Shala N, et al. Noninvasive positive pressure ventilation via face mask. First-line intervention in patients with acute hypercapnic and hypoxemic respiratory failure. *Chest* 1996;109:179–193.

65. Bersten AD, Holt AW, Vedig AE, et al. Treatment of severe cardiogenic pulmonary edema with continuous positive airway pressure delivered by face mask. *N Engl J Med* 1991;325:1825–1830.

66. Pang D, Keenan SP, Cook DJ, et al. The effect of positive pressure airway support on mortality and the need for intubation in cardiogenic pulmonary edema: a systematic review. *Chest* 1998;114:1185–1192.

67. Carlucci A, Richard JC, Wysocki M, et al. Noninvasive versus con-

ventional mechanical ventilation. An epidemiologic survey. *Am J Respir Crit Care Med* 2001;163:874–880.

68. Antonelli M, Conti G, Bufi M, et al. Noninvasive ventilation for treatment of acute respiratory failure in patients undergoing solid organ transplantation: a randomized trial. *JAMA* 2000;283:235–241.

69. Hillberg RE, Johnson DC. Noninvasive ventilation. *N Engl J Med* 1997;337:1746–1752.

70. Keenan SP. Noninvasive positive pressure ventilation in acute respiratory failure. *JAMA* 2000;284:2376–2378.

71. Ventilation with lower tidal volumes as compared with traditional tidal volumes for acute lung injury and the acute respiratory distress syndrome. The Acute Respiratory Distress Syndrome Network. *N Engl J Med* 2000;342:1301–1308.

72. Cook D. Ventilator associated pneumonia: perspectives on the burden of illness. *Intensive Care Med* 2000;26:S31–S37.

73. Gaine S. Pulmonary hypertension. *JAMA* 2000;284:3160–3168.

74. Gracey DR, Divertie MB, Didier EP. Preoperative pulmonary preparation of patients with chronic obstructive pulmonary disease: a prospective study. *Chest* 1979;76:123–129.

75. Garibaldi RA, Britt MR, Coleman ML, et al. Risk factors for postoperative pneumonia. *Am J Med* 1981;70:677–680.

76. Phillips EH, Carroll BJ, Fallas MJ, et al. Comparison of laparoscopic cholecystectomy in obese and non-obese patients. *Am Surg* 1994; 60:316–321.

77. Fogh J, Willie-Jorgensen P, Brynjolf I, et al. The predictive value of preoperative perfusion/ventilation scintigraphy, spirometry and x-ray of the lungs on postoperative pulmonary complications. A prospective study. *Acta Anaesth Scand* 1987;31:717–721.

78. Poe RH, Kallay MC, Dass T, et al. Can postoperative pulmonary complications after elective cholecystectomy be predicted? *Am J Med Sci* 1988;295:29–34.

79. Bando K, Sun K, Binford RS, et al. Determinants of longer duration of endotracheal intubation after adult cardiac operations. *Ann Thorac Surg* 1997;63:1026–1033.

ACUTE LUNG INJURY AND ACUTE RESPIRATORY DISTRESS SYNDROME

MICHAEL A. MATTHAY
JEANINE P. WIENER-KRONISH
IVAN CHENG
MICHAEL A. GROPPER

KEY WORDS

- Acute respiratory distress syndrome
- Alveolar epithelium
- Endothelial injury
- Lung
- Acute lung injury
- Multiple-organ dysfunction syndrome
- Pneumothorax
- Pulmonary edema
- Respiratory failure
- Sepsis syndrome

INTRODUCTION

Acute lung injury and the acute respiratory distress syndrome (ALI/ARDS) frequently develop in patients with already established nonpulmonary organ failure (1,2). Furthermore, the clinical course of patients with ALI/ARDS often is complicated by the development or worsening of nonpulmonary organ dysfunction (1). Mortality in patients with ALI/ARDS is increased in patients with nonpulmonary organ dysfunction, especially hepatic dysfunction (1,3). Although several clinical disorders are associated with the development of ALI/ARDS (4), sepsis is the most common and the most lethal cause, probably because the lung injury is more severe (5,6) and the extent of nonpulmonary organ dysfunction is greater (1,2). This chapter considers recent advances in definitions, clinical features, pathogenesis, resolution, and treatment of ALI/ARDS.

DEFINITION

An international conference was convened in 1994 to develop uniform definitions that would facilitate clinical care, clinical research, and testing of potential therapeutic strategies for the prevention and treatment of ALI/ARDS. The conference included clinicians and academicians from North America and Europe (6). This group recognized that the adult respiratory distress syndrome develops in children; so the term for the clinical syndrome was changed to the acute respiratory distress syndrome.

The consensus conference also made a distinction between ALI and ARDS (Fig. 1). ALI is characterized by an acute onset; a partial pressure arterial oxygen (Pa_{O_2})/fraction of inspired oxygen (F_{IO_2}) below 300, regardless of the presence or absence of positive end-expiratory pressure (PEEP); bilateral infiltrates on chest radiograph; and a pulmonary artery occlusion pressure (PAOP) of less than 19 mm Hg when measured; or no clinical evidence of left atrial hypertension. ARDS was diagnosed using all of these criteria, except the Pa_{O_2}/F_{IO_2} was less than 200, regardless of the presence or absence of PEEP. Although there are some limitations to these definitions (7), they have worked remarkably well in facilitating clinical research and clinical trials in the last 8 years. Interestingly, the initial severity of oxygenation is not a major independent predictor of outcome. Patients who develop ALI with a Pa_{O_2}/F_{IO_2} ratio between 200 and 300 have a similar mortality rate to patients who present with a Pa_{O_2}/F_{IO_2} less than 200 (2,3), with the possible exception of patients with lung injury from trauma (8). A meeting of the American-European Consensus group was held in Barcelona in September 2000 and recommended specifying the presence or absence of nonpulmonary organ dysfunction and the inciting clinical disorder when the diagnosis of ALI/ARDS is made.

CLINICAL PRESENTATION

The initial clinical presentation of ARDS was first described by Petty and co-workers (9,10). The patient usually has tachypnea with a respiratory rate greater than 20 breaths per minute and is frequently cyanotic if not receiving supplemental oxygen. The chest radiograph shows patchy opacities that may not be symmetric (Fig. 2). Measurement of arterial blood gases, in particular the Pa_{O_2}/F_{IO_2} ratio, is required to establish the diagnosis of ALI or ARDS. Other pulmonary abnormalities in patients with ALI/ARDS include an increased shunt fraction (Q_S/Q_T) and increased dead-space ventilation (V_D/V_T). Recent preliminary work from our institution indicates that the dead-space fraction is elevated to almost 60% on the first day of diagnosis, and a markedly elevated dead space fraction may

Criteria for ALI/ARDS
American/European Consensus Conf.

Timing: acute
CXR: bilat infiltrates
WP: <19 mm Hg
(or no clinical CHF)

PaO₂/FiO₂: <300   <200

ALI   ARDS

FIGURE 1. Criteria of the American–European Consensus Conference for the diagnosis of acute lung injury or adult respiratory distress syndrome. CXR, chest x-ray; WP, wedge pressure; CHF, congestive heart failure. (From Schuster DP. What is acute lung injury? What is ARDS? *Chest* 1995;107:1721–1726, with permission.)

identify patients who are less likely to survive (11). As lung injury and edema progress, pulmonary compliance decreases. Measurement of the pulmonary arterial occlusion pressure may be needed in some patients to differentiate ALI/ARDS from cardiogenic pulmonary edema. A pulmonary arterial occlusion pressure greater than 19 mm Hg suggests that the respiratory failure and pulmonary edema may be from cardiac insufficiency or intravascular volume overload.

PREDISPOSING FACTORS

Numerous predisposing factors have been associated with ALI/ARDS (12). Depending on the nature of the reporting hospital, the most common causes of ALI/ARDS are pneumonia, sepsis, aspiration of gastric contents, and major trauma (13). Other less common causes include major surgery with multiple blood product transfusions, fat emboli, acute pancreatitis,

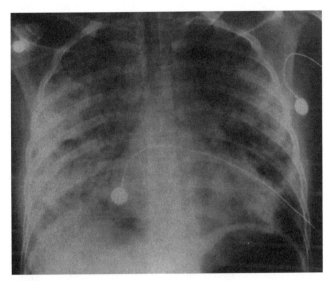

FIGURE 2. Chest radiograph from a patient with acute respiratory distress syndrome (ARDS) secondary to sepsis syndrome. Note the bilateral diffuse infiltrates. The heart size is normal, suggesting noncardiogenic pulmonary edema.

TABLE 1. PREVIOUS DIAGNOSIS AND INCIDENCE OF ARDS DEVELOPMENT IN ICUs IN TWO U.S. LOCATIONS

Previous Diagnosis	Incidence of ARDS (%)[a]	
	Washington	Colorado
Aspiration of gastric contents	7/23 (30)	16/45 (36)
Sepsis		
Bacteremia	9/239 (4)	—
Sepsis syndrome	5/13 (35)	—
Multiple transfusions		
10 U in 24 h	—	9/197 (5)
10 U in 6 h	4/17 (24)	—
Pneumonia in the ICU	—	10/84 (12)
Pulmonary contusion	5/19 (17)	—
Cardiopulmonary bypass	—	4/237 (2)
Fracture	1/12 (8)	2/38 (5)
Near drowning	2/3 (67)	—
Burn	—	2/87 (2)
Pancreatitis	1/1 (100)	—
Disseminated intravascular coagulopathy	—	2/9 (22)
Prolonged hypotension	0/1 (0)	—

ARDS, acute respiratory distress syndrome; ICU, intensive care unit.
[a]Number of patients who develop ARDS/number of patients with original diagnosis.
Modified from Wiener-Kronish JP, Gropper MA, Matthay MA. The adult respiratory distress syndrome: definition and prognosis, pathogenesis and treatment. *Br J Anaesth* 1990;65:107–129, with permission.

drug overdoses, and smoke inhalation and major burns. When a patient has more than one risk factor for developing ALI/ARDS, the incidence increases significantly (12). Pepe and colleagues examined which clinical syndromes were associated with the development of ARDS (12). As illustrated in Table 1, sepsis syndrome and gastric aspiration were identified as two conditions frequently associated with ALI/ARDS. From 20% to 40% of patients with sepsis syndrome will progress to develop ARDS. The inciting factor leading to clinical lung injury in sepsis syndrome is probably endothelial injury. Rubin and colleagues (1) found that an elevated circulating von Willebrand factor-antigen (vWf-Ag), a marker of endothelial-cell injury, was 92% sensitive and 77% specific for predicting lung injury. If vWf-Ag was elevated and the patient had nonpulmonary organ failure, there was an 80% positive predictive value that the patient would develop clinical lung injury and would not survive.

PATHOLOGY AND PATHOGENESIS

Pathologically, ALI/ARDS is characterized by protein-rich edema fluid. This fluid usually is associated with a large influx of neutrophils into the interstitium and distal airspaces of the lung (14). There is injury to the lung endothelium and often evidence of alveolar epithelial injury as well. The pathology is described as diffuse alveolar damage, which includes alveolar epithelial cell injury, acute inflammatory cell infiltration, proteinaceous alveolar and interstitial edema fluid, alveolar hyaline membranes, type II pneumocyte proliferation, and, later in the syndrome, varying degrees of intraalveolar and interstitial fibrosis (15). Cellular damage occurs in ALI/ARDS with the influx of inflammatory cells and damage to the endothelium and epithelium (Fig. 3).

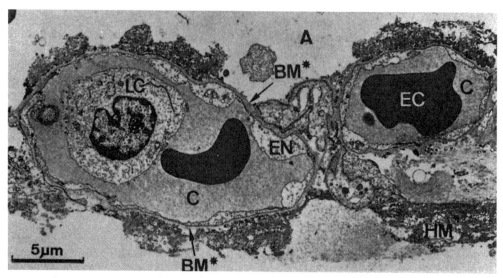

FIGURE 3. Electron micrograph of a lung specimen from a 19-year-old woman who died after 4 days of fulminant capillary leakage as a result of septicemia. Note the irregularly swollen and damaged endothelium. Also note that there is loss of the epithelial cell lining in some areas where the basement membrane is exposed to the alveolar space. A, alveolar space; BM, denuded basement membrane; C, capillary; EC, intravascular erythrocyte; EN, swollen endothelial cell; HM, hyaline membrane; LC, intravascular leukocyte. (From Gropper MA, Wiener-Kronish JP. The adult respiratory distress syndrome: diagnosis, pathophysiology, and treatment. In: Hanowell FJ, ed. *Pulmonary care of the surgical patient.* Mount Kisco, NY: Futura Publishing, 1994, with permission.)

The importance of endothelial injury and permeability to the formation of pulmonary edema in ALI/ARDS has been well established for many years. More recently, the critical importance of epithelial injury to both the development of and recovery from ALI/ARDS has been better appreciated (5). The degree of alveolar epithelial injury is an important predictor of outcome in ALI/ARDS (16,17). The normal alveolar epithelium is composed of two cell types. Flat alveolar epithelial type I cells constitute 90% of the alveolar surface area and are easily injured. Cuboidal alveolar type II cells constitute the remaining 10% of the alveolar surface area and seem to be more resistant to injury. The currently recognized functions of type II cells include surfactant production, ion transport, and proliferation and differentiation to regenerate type I cells after injury.

The loss of epithelial integrity in ALI/ARDS has several major consequences. First, under normal conditions, the epithelial barrier is much less permeable than the endothelial barrier (18). Thus, epithelial injury contributes to alveolar flooding. Second, loss of epithelial barrier integrity and injury to type II cells disrupts normal epithelial ion and fluid transport function, impairing the removal of edema fluid from the alveolar space (19). Third, injury to type II cells reduces surfactant production and turnover, contributing to the surfactant abnormalities characteristic of ALI/ARDS (20). Fourth, loss of epithelial barrier properties in pneumonia can lead to septic shock (21). Finally, if injury to the alveolar epithelium is severe, disorganized or insufficient epithelial repair may lead to a fibrosing alveolitis.

Neutrophil-dependent Lung Injury

Many clinical and experimental studies have provided evidence for neutrophil-mediated injury in ALI/ARDS (22). Histologic studies of early ALI/ARDS show a marked accumulation of neutrophils in the lung (14,15); neutrophils predominate in the pulmonary edema fluid and bronchoalveolar lavage fluid from ARDS patients (21). Many animal models of ALI are neutrophil dependent.

New evidence raises the question of whether neutrophilic inflammation in ALI/ARDS is the cause or the result of lung injury. ALI/ARDS may develop in patients with profound neutropenia, and some animal models of ALI are neutrophil independent. Clinical trials using granulocyte colony-stimulating factor (G-CSF) to increase the numbers and activation state of circulating neutrophils in severe pneumonia did not increase lung injury (23). Also, the neutrophil plays a critical role in host defense in ALI/ARDS, especially in pneumonia and sepsis. This may explain, in part, why treatments that use antiinflammatory strategies have been largely unsuccessful. In some causes of ALI, such as from aspiration of gastric contents, experimental studies strongly support a major role for the neutrophil in the initial phase of lung injury (24). The role of the neutrophil is less clear in other causes of lung injury.

Other Proinflammatory Mechanisms

Cytokines

A complex network of cytokines and other proinflammatory compounds initiate and amplify the inflammatory response in ALI/ARDS. Proinflammatory cytokines may be produced locally in the lung by inflammatory cells, lung epithelial cells, or fibroblasts (21). Regulation of cytokine production by extrapulmonary factors also has been described. Macrophage inhibitory factor is a regulatory cytokine produced by the anterior pituitary that is found in high concentrations in the bronchoalveolar lavage fluid of patients with ALI/ARDS (25). This cytokine increases production of the proinflammatory cytokines interleukin-8 (IL-8) and tumor necrosis factor-α (TNF-α) and can override glucocorticoid-mediated inhibition of cytokine secretion.

Newer evidence indicates that it is not simply the production of proinflammatory cytokines that is important in ALI/ARDS, but rather the balance between proinflammatory and antiinflammatory mediators. Several endogenous inhibitors of proinflammatory cytokines have been described, including IL-1 receptor antagonist, soluble TNF receptors, autoantibodies to IL-8, and antiinflammatory cytokines such as IL-10 and IL-11. A better understanding of the role of cytokines in ALI/ARDS will be gained in the future through studies of the biologic activity of specific cytokines (26,27) rather than by measuring static levels by immunologic methods.

Ventilator-induced Lung Injury

Experimental evidence indicates that mechanical ventilation at high volumes and pressures can injure the lung, causing increased permeability pulmonary edema in the uninjured lung (28) and enhanced edema formation in the injured lung (5). Initial theories to explain these deleterious effects focused on capillary stress failure resulting from alveolar overdistension. More recently, cyclic opening and closing of atelectatic alveoli during mechanical ventilation has been shown to cause lung injury independent of alveolar overdistension. Alveolar overdistension coupled with the repeated collapse and reopening of alveoli can initiate a proinflammatory cytokine cascade (29).

In patients with ALI/ARDS, ventilation at traditional tidal volumes (10–15 mL/kg) may overdistend noninjured alveoli, perhaps promoting further lung injury, inhibiting resolution, and contributing to multisystem organ failure (5,29). The failure of traditional ventilatory strategies to prevent end expiratory closure of atelectatic alveoli also may contribute to lung injury. These concerns stimulated a number of clinical trials of protective ventilatory strategies to reduce alveolar overdistension and improve recruitment of atelectatic alveoli (5). Interestingly, a recent study found that a protective ventilatory strategy could reduce both the pulmonary and systemic cytokine response in patients with ALI/ARDS (13).

Other Mechanisms of Injury

Like any form of inflammation, ALI/ARDS is a complex process in which multiple pathways can propagate or inhibit lung injury (5). For example, abnormalities of the coagulation system often develop with small-vessel platelet–fibrin thrombi and impaired fibrinolysis (5,15). This pathway is of particular interest in view of the recent report that pharmacologic inhibition of the coagulation cascade with activated protein C can diminish mortality in patients with sepsis. Also, abnormalities of surfactant production, composition, and function probably contribute to alveolar collapse and gas exchange abnormalities (19).

Fibrosing Alveolitis

Following the acute or exudative phase of ALI/ARDS, some patients have an uncomplicated course with rapid resolution (16,17). Others progress to fibrotic lung injury, which is observed histologically as early as 5 to 7 days after the onset of ALI/ARDS (30). The alveolar spaces become filled with mesenchymal cells and their products along with new blood vessels (30). The biopsy finding of fibrosing alveolitis correlates with an increased mortality from ALI/ARDS (31), and patients dying of ALI/ARDS usually have a marked accumulation of collagen and fibronectin in the lung.

Recent studies suggest that the process of fibrosing alveolitis begins early in the course of ALI/ARDS and is promoted by early proinflammatory mediators such as IL-1 (32). Levels of procollagen III peptide, a precursor of collagen synthesis, are elevated in the alveolar compartment very early in the course of ALI/ARDS, even at the time of intubation and mechanical ventilation (26). Furthermore, the early appearance of procollagen III in the alveolar space identifies patients with a higher mortality (33).

RESOLUTION

Strategies that enhance resolution ultimately may be as important as treatments that attenuate early inflammatory lung injury. Alveolar edema is removed by the active transport of sodium and chloride from the distal airspaces into the lung interstitium (34). Water follows passively, probably through transcellular water channels, the aquaporins, located primarily on type I cells (34,35). The presence of water channels is not required, however, to maximize the rate of alveolar fluid clearance (36). In clinical studies of ALI/ARDS, alveolar fluid clearance occurs surprisingly early, often measurable within the first few hours after intubation and mechanical ventilation (16). Intact alveolar fluid clearance portends a better outcome as measured by oxygenation, duration of mechanical ventilation, and survival (16,17) (Fig. 4).

A considerable quantity of both soluble and insoluble protein must be removed from the airspaces. The removal of insoluble protein is particularly important because hyaline membranes provide a framework for the growth of fibrous tissue. Soluble protein appears to be removed primarily by diffusion between alveolar epithelial cells. Insoluble protein may be removed by endocytosis, transcytosis by alveolar epithelial cells, and phagocytosis by macrophages.

The alveolar epithelial type II cell serves as the progenitor cell for reepithelialization of a denuded alveolar epithelium. Type II cells proliferate to cover the denuded basement and then differentiate into type I cells, restoring the normal alveolar architecture and increasing the fluid transport capacity of the alveolar epithelium (37). The proliferation is controlled by epithelial growth factors, including keratinocyte and hepatocyte growth factors. The ability of the epithelial cells to migrate and spread over the denuded epithelium is regulated in part by autocrine and paracrine production of transforming growth factor-α, epidermal growth factor, and provisional matrix components such as fibronectin (27,38,39).

The mechanisms underlying the resolution of the inflammatory cell infiltrate and fibrosis are incompletely understood. Apoptosis, the process of programmed cell death, is thought to be a major mechanism for clearance of neutrophils from sites of inflammation and may be important in neutrophil clearance from the injured lung. In one study of bronchoalveolar lavage

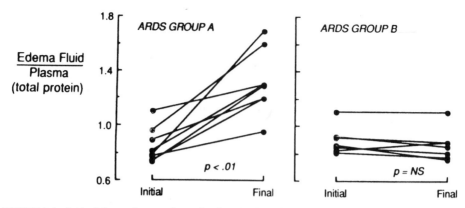

FIGURE 4. Individual data points are shown for the initial and final alveolar edema fluid to plasma total-protein-concentration ratio in nine patients with acute respiratory distress syndrome (ARDS) who improved clinically (group A) compared with seven patients with ARDS who did not improve clinically (group B). The interval between the initial and final alveolar fluid sample was similar in group A (6.8 ± 5.1 hours) compared with group B (5.4 ± 4.1 hours) patients. The mortality rate was lower in the group A patients, suggesting that the early ability to remove some of the alveolar edema fluid indicated an intact alveolar epithelial barrier function, with an improved prognosis for recovery. (From Matthay MA, Wiener-Kronish JP. Intact epithelial barrier function is critical for the resolution of alveolar edema in humans. *Am Rev Respir Dis* 1990:1250–1257, with permission.)

fluid from ALI/ARDS patients, however, the numbers of apoptotic neutrophils were low, perhaps because of the presence of antiapoptotic factors such as G-CSF and granulocyte–macrophage colony-stimulating factor (GM-CSF) (40). Nevertheless, high levels of markers of apoptosis are present in the pulmonary edema fluid of ALI/ARDS patients, and bronchoalveolar lavage fluids of patients with ALI/ARDS can promote epithelial cell apoptosis (41). These are potentially important observations because the mechanisms that alter epithelial barrier integrity need to be identified. The role of proapoptotic and antiapoptotic mechanisms in both injury and repair is an important area for future research.

Treatment

Improvement in the supportive care of ALI/ARDS patients may have contributed to the recent decline in mortality (Table 2) (42,43). Care of any ALI/ARDS patient should include a careful search for the underlying cause with particular attention to treatable infections such as sepsis or pneumonia. Appropriate treatment with antimicrobial agents or surgical treatment of abdominal infections should be promptly instituted. Prevention and early treatment of nosocomial infections are critical because patients frequently die of uncontrolled infection. Adequate nutrition with enteral feeding is preferred because this route does not carry the serious risk of line sepsis from parenteral nutrition. Prevention of gastrointestinal bleeding and thromboembolism are also important.

Improved understanding of the pathogenesis of ALI/ARDS has led to testing of several novel treatment strategies. Although many specific therapies have not proven beneficial, the quality of ALI/ARDS clinical trials is improving. An important advance has been the establishment of the National Institutes of Health (NIH)-supported ALI/ARDS Network, which now includes 20 university medical centers (5). This network has established the infrastructure for implementing well-designed, multicenter, randomized trials of potential new therapies.

Mechanical Ventilation

The most appropriate mode of mechanical ventilation in ARDS has been controversial since the syndrome was first described. Although tidal volume in normal persons at rest is 6 to 7 milliliters per kilogram of body weight, historically 12 to 15 milliliters per kilogram was recommended in ALI/ARDS, in part because higher tidal volumes were associated with an improvement in arterial oxygenation. Use of this relatively high tidal volume in conjunction with elevated airway pressures, however, has been implicated in propagating the lung injury in ALI/ARDS. Interestingly, the possibility of ventilator associated lung injury was first considered in the 1970s, leading to the 1974 extracorporeal membrane oxygenation trial in which ventilation was reduced to 8 to 10 milliliters per kilogram, although there were no specific guidelines for limiting airway pressures (44). This strategy failed to improve mortality, however, as did a later trial of extracorporeal carbon dioxide removal (45).

Recently, a multicenter trial of 6 milliliter per kilogram of body weight compared with 12 milliliters per kilogram tidal volume in 861 patients was completed by the NIH ALI/ARDS Network (13). In the low tidal-volume arm, plateau pressure was limited to 30 cm H_2O, and a detailed protocol was used to adjust F_{IO_2} and PEEP levels in all patients. Mortality was significantly reduced by 22% in the low-tidal-volume arm. This constitutes the first large multicenter trial with convincing evidence that a specific therapy for ARDS can reduce mortality. In addition, the trial provides evidence for the clinical significance of ventilator associated lung injury and establishes a well-defined protocol for ventilating patients with ALI/ARDS against which future ventilator strategies can be compared.

The results of this network trial differ from two previous negative studies of low tidal volume: a Canadian (120 patients) (46) and a European study (116 patients) (47). There are several possible explanations for the discrepant results. First, the NIH Network study had both the largest difference in tidal volume between groups and the lowest tidal volume in the low tidal

TABLE 2. RESULTS OF PRIOR TRIALS OF SEVERAL PHARMACOLOGIC TREATMENTS FOR ALI/ARDS

Treatment	Year	How Studied	No. of Patients	Comments
Glucocorticoids (acute)	1984	Phase 3	87	No benefit
	1988	Phase 3	59	No benefit
Prostaglandin E$_1$				
Intravenous	1989	Phase 3	100	No benefit.
Liposomal	Unpublished	Phase 3		Stopped for lack of benefits
Surfactant (Exosurf)	1996	Phase 3	725	No benefit. New preparations and modes of delivery are being studied
Glucocorticoids (late)	1998	Phase 3	24	Decreased mortality but small study
Inhaled nitric oxide	1998	Phase 2	177	No benefit
	1999	Phase 3	203	No benefit
Ketoconazole	1999	Phase 2	234	No benefit
Procysteine	Unpublished	Phase 3		Stopped for lack of efficacy
Lisofylline	2001	Phase 2/3	234	Stopped for lack of efficacy

ALI, acute lung injury; ARDS, acute respiratory distress syndrome.

volume arm when the tidal volumes are compared using the same calculation of ideal body weight. Thus, the NIH study may have been better able to show a difference between the treatment arms. Second, the NIH Network study provided more aggressive treatment of respiratory acidosis associated with alveolar hypoventilation and hypercapnia. Conceivably, respiratory acidosis had deleterious effects in the low-tidal-volume arms of the other studies. Finally, the other studies were underpowered compared with the much larger NIH study.

There has also been considerable interest in the optimal level of PEEP in ALI/ARDS. It was noted decades ago that application of PEEP in ALI/ARDS patients could improve oxygenation, allowing a reduced F$_{IO_2}$ (10,48). The best-documented effect of PEEP on lung function is an increase in functional residual capacity (48), probably from recruitment of collapsed alveoli (49). Although lung injury could be prevented in rats using PEEP, the prophylactic use of 8 cm H$_2$O PEEP in patients at risk for ARDS was not successful (50).

More recently, Amato and colleagues used an open lung approach to ventilate patients with ALI/ARDS (51). In addition to a low tidal volume and pressure-controlled inverse ratio ventilation, the protocol included raising the level of PEEP above the lower inflection point on a pressure–volume curve for each patient in an attempt to ensure adequate recruitment of atelectatic lung. With this approach, mortality was reduced. Adoption of this mode of ventilator care, however, cannot yet be recommended for several reasons. First, this study was small and involved only a single center. Second, mortality in the conventional ventilation arm was unusually high (71%), suggesting that this high-tidal-volume arm may have been especially injurious. Furthermore, the mortality difference was only apparent at 28 days; survival to hospital discharge was equivalent. Third, reliable measurement of the lower inflection point on the pressure volume curve is technically difficult and requires sedation and paralysis. Despite these issues, the Amato study raises the possibility that improved alveolar recruitment with higher lev-

els of PEEP than were used in the NIH Network study might further reduce ventilator associated lung injury. Several alternative approaches to conventional mechanical ventilation have been proposed, including prone ventilation (5,52), but none has yet proved beneficial. Future trials of low tidal volume combined with higher levels of PEEP will be important to assess the potential value of increasing lung recruitment in the presence of the low-tidal-volume approach. Also, some investigators would like to test the value of intermittent recruitment maneuvers designed to inflate periodically the lungs of patients with ALI/ARDS.

Fluid and Hemodynamic Management

The rationale for restricting fluid administration in patients with ALI/ARDS is to decrease pulmonary edema. Animal studies indicated there was less edema fluid formation in ALI if left atrial pressure was lowered. Several clinical studies have supported this hypothesis (53,54). Currently, a randomized trial of fluid management based on pulmonary artery catheter versus central venous pressure monitoring is being carried out by the NIH ARDS Network. While awaiting these results, a reasonable objective is to maintain the intravascular volume at the lowest level consistent with adequate systemic perfusion as assessed by metabolic acid–base balance and renal function. If systemic perfusion cannot be maintained with restoration of intravascular volume, as in septic shock, vasopressors are indicated to restore end-organ perfusion and normalize oxygen delivery. Based on several negative clinical trials, however, supranormal levels of oxygen delivery cannot be recommended (55,56).

Surfactant Therapy

Because of the success of surfactant replacement in the neonatal respiratory distress syndrome, surfactant replacement has been proposed as a treatment for the surfactant abnormalities of ALI/ARDS. A synthetic surfactant preparation (Exosurf), however, had no impact on oxygenation, duration of mechanical ventilation, or survival (57). There are several possible explanations for the negative results. First, the surfactant was delivered as an aerosol, and less than 5% may have reached the distal airspaces. Also, Exosurf, a protein-free phospholipid preparation, may not be the most appropriate surfactant replacement in ALI/ARDS. Evaluation of newer surfactant preparations that contain recombinant surfactant proteins is under way, and new modes of instillation are being tested, including tracheal instillation and bronchoalveolar lavage.

Inhaled Nitric Oxide and Other Vasodilators

Nitric oxide is a potent vasodilator that can be delivered to the pulmonary vasculature by inhalation without causing systemic vasodilation. Although observational studies suggest that inhaled nitric oxide might be beneficial in ALI/ARDS (58), randomized, double-blinded studies have been discouraging. In a phase 2 study, no difference was found in mortality or number of days alive and off mechanical ventilation with inhaled nitric oxide in ALI/ARDS (59). Improvements in oxygenation were modest and not sustained, and pulmonary arterial pressure showed only a minor decrease on the first day of treatment. A recent phase 3 study of inhaled nitric oxide for ALI/ARDS showed no effect on mortality or the duration of mechanical ventilation (60). Thus, inhaled nitric oxide cannot be recommended for routine treatment of ALI/ARDS but may be useful as a rescue therapy in patients with refractory hypoxemia. Several less selective vasodilators also have not been beneficial, including nitroprusside, hydralazine, prostaglandin E_1, and prostacyclin (5).

Glucocorticoids and Other AntiInflammatory Strategies

Recognition of the inflammatory nature of the lung injury in ALI/ARDS prompted interest in antiinflammatory treatments, particularly glucocorticoids. However, when given before the onset of or early in the course of ALI/ARDS glucocorticoids had no benefit (61,62). More recently, glucocorticoids have been used to treat the later fibrosing alveolitis stage. Encouraging results were reported in preliminary studies and in a small randomized trial of 24 patients (63). A larger randomized, multicenter trial by the NIH ARDS Network of high-dose methylprednisolone for ALI/ARDS of at least 7 days' duration has enrolled more than 125 patients. Because high-dose methylprednisolone may increase the incidence of infection, routine corticosteroid treatment of patients with established ALI/ARDS cannot be recommended until results of a large multicenter trial are available. A short course of high-dose glucocorticoids could be considered as rescue therapy for patients with severe nonresolving ALI/ARDS. In addition to glucocorticoids, other antiinflammatory interventions designed to interrupt the process of ALI have been investigated without success. The failure of these antiinflammatory strategies may reflect the complexity and redundancy of the inflammation in ALI

or the inability to deliver these agents early enough in the course of ALI/ARDS.

Acceleration of Resolution

Recognition of the importance of the resolution phase of ALI/ARDS has stimulated interest in strategies to hasten recovery from lung injury. Experimentally, removal of pulmonary edema fluid from the alveolar space can be enhanced by both catecholamine-dependent and catecholamine-independent mechanisms, including inhaled and systemic β agonists (34). One recent experimental study demonstrated that inhaled β agonists can accelerate the resolution of alveolar edema in sheep and rats with hydrostatic pulmonary edema (64) as well as in animal models of lung injury (65). The β agonists are appealing for clinical ALI/ARDS because they are already in wide clinical use and lack serious side effects, even in critically ill patients. Also, preliminary data from our institution indicate that aerosolized beta agonists in mechanically ventilated patients result in therapeutic levels in the pulmonary edema fluid (66). The β agonists also may increase surfactant secretion and perhaps exert an antiinflammatory effect, thus helping to restore normal lung vascular permeability (67).

An additional approach to enhancing resolution of ALI/ARDS is to accelerate reepithelialization of the injured alveolar barrier. Alveolar epithelial type II cell proliferation is under the control of a number of epithelial growth factors, including keratinocyte growth factor. Experimentally, administration of keratinocyte growth factor can protect against lung injury (68,69), probably in part because of enhanced alveolar type II cell proliferation, increased alveolar fluid clearance, antioxidant effects, and a reduction in lung endothelial injury. These findings raise the question of whether an epithelial specific growth factor could be used to accelerate the resolution of ALI/ARDS.

SUMMARY

In the last 5 years, major progress has been made in the treatment of ALI/ARDS. A lung-protective ventilatory strategy with a low tidal volume (mL/kg predicted body weight) in conjunction with a plateau pressure limit of 30 cm of H_2O attenuated the severity of clinical lung injury and reduced mortality by 22% (13). Ironically, after all the years of searching for antiinflammatory treatments for ALI/ARDS, it turns out that a lung protective ventilatory strategy has proved to be the most efficacious antiinflammatory treatment ever discovered for ALI/ARDS. It is still possible, however, that pharmacologic treatments also may enhance survival. The recent report that mortality in sepsis can be reduced with a pharmacologic treatment that inhibits the coagulation system makes it clear that it may be possible to reduce the early inflammatory lung injury in ALI/ARDS with lung-protective ventilatory strategies and pharmacologic treatment (70,71). Also, therapy directed at hastening the resolution of lung injury by increasing the functional recovery of the alveolar epithelium may be of value, both in diminishing the fibroproliferative phase of ALI/ARDS as well as accelerating the resolution of alveolar edema.

KEY POINTS

Major progress has been made in establishing uniform, workable clinical definitions for clinical acute lung injury (ALI) and the acute respiratory distress syndrome (ARDS). The use of these definitions has facilitated the testing of several new therapeutic strategies for patients with ALI/ARDS. Although some minor refinements in the definitions may be needed, the diagnosis of clinical ALI can be made by determining the degree of hypoxemia and the presence of bilateral pulmonary infiltrates on a chest radiograph in a patient who does not have evidence of cardiac failure or intravascular volume overload. The most important clinical disorders associated with the development of ALI/ARDS are sepsis, pneumonia, aspiration of gastric contents, and major trauma.

Progress has been made in understanding the pathogenesis of clinical ALI, particularly by neutrophil-dependent and -independent mechanisms as well as the contribution of ventilator-associated lung injury in propagating the severity of initial lung injury. It is also clear that the fibrosing alveolitis that occurs in some ALI/ARDS patients is initiated early in the course of lung injury, perhaps by a preponderance of proinflammatory cytokines that stimulate fibroblast proliferation. The critical role of the alveolar epithelium to the resolution of lung injury has been established, both as an important source of surface-active material to stabilize the injured alveolus and also because the alveolar epithelium provides the ion and water transport pathways for the removal of alveolar edema fluid. Impaired alveolar epithelial fluid clearance is associated with worse clinical outcomes.

The first major breakthrough in the treatment of ALI/ARDS occurred recently, when an NIH sponsored randomized clinical trial of 861 patients demonstrated that a lung-protective ventilator strategy using a low tidal volume and a plateau pressure limit reduced mortality by 22%. Additional trials with both lung-protective strategies and new pharmacologic treatments are under way, raising hope that mortality may be further reduced in the near future in this important cause of acute respiratory failure in critically ill patients.

REFERENCES

1. Rubin DB, Wiener-Kronish JP, Murray JF, et al. Elevated von-Willebrand factor antigen is an early plasma predictor of impending acute lung injury and death in non-pulmonary sepsis syndrome. *J Clin Invest* 1990;86:474–480.
2. Doyle RL, Szaflarski N, Modin GW, et al. Identification of patients with acute lung injury: predictors of mortality. *Am J Respir Crit Care Med* 1995;152:1818–1824.
3. Zilberberg MD, Epstein SK. Acute lung injury in the medical ICU: comorbid conditions, age, etiology and hospital outcome. *Am J Respir Crit Care Med* 1998;157:1159–1164.
4. Murray JF, Matthay MA, Luce JM, et al. An expanded definition of the adult respiratory distress syndrome. *Am Rev Respir Dis* 1988;138:720–723.
5. Ware LB, Matthay MA. The acute respiratory distress syndrome. *N Engl J Med* 2000;342:1334–1349.
6. Bernard GR, Artigas A, Brigham KL, et al. The American–European Consensus Conference on ARDS: definitions, mechanisms, relevant outcomes, and clinical trial coordination. *Am J Respir Crit Care Med* 1994;149:818–824.
7. Abraham E, Matthay MA, Dinarello CA, et al. Consensus conference definitions for sepsis, septic shock, acute lung injury, and acute respiratory distress syndrome: time for a reevaluation. *Crit Care Med* 2000;28:232–235.
8. Eberhard L, Morabito D, Matthay M, et al. Initial severity of metabolic acidosis predicts the development of acute lung injury in severely traumatized patients. *Crit Care Med* 2000;28:125–131.
9. Ashbaugh DG, Bigelow DB, Petty TL, et al. Acute respiratory distress in adults. *Lancet* 1967;2:319–323.
10. Petty TL, Ashbaugh DG. The adult respiratory distress syndrome: clinical features, factors influencing prognosis and principles of management. *Chest* 1971;60:273–279.
11. Nuckton T, Alonso J, Kallet R, et al. In early ARDS wasted ventilation predicts mortality. *Am J Respir Crit Care Med* 2001;(abst) (*in press*).
12. Pepe PE, Potkin RT, Reus DH, et al. Clinical predictors of the adult respiratory distress syndrome. *Am J Surg* 1982;144:124–130.
13. ARDS Network. Ventilation with low tidal volumes as compared with traditional tidal volumes for acute lung injury and the acute respiratory distress syndrome. *N Engl J Med* 2000;342:1301–1308.
14. Anderson WR, Thielen K. Correlative study of adult respiratory distress syndrome by light, scanning, and transmission electron microscopy. *Ultrastruct Pathol* 1992;16:615–628.
15. Tomashefski JF. Pulmonary pathology of acute respiratory distress syndrome. *Clin Chest Med* 2000;21:435–466.
16. Ware LB, Matthay MA. Alveolar fluid clearance is impaired in the majority of patients with acute lung failure and acute respiratory distress syndrome. *Am J Respir Crit Care Med* 2001;163:1376–1383.
17. Matthay MA, Wiener-Kronish JP. Intact epithelial barrier function is critical for the resolution of alveolar edema in humans. *Am Rev Respir Dis* 1990;142:1250–1257.
18. Pittet JF, MacKersie RC, Martin TR, et al. Biochemical markers of acute lung injury: prognostic and pathogenetic significance. *Am J Respir Crit Care Med* 1997;155:1187–1205.
19. Sznajder JI. Strategies to increase the alveolar epithelial fluid removal in the injured lung. *Am J Respir Crit Care Med* 1999;160:1441–1442.
20. Lewis JF, Jobe AH. Surfactant and the adult respiratory distress syndrome. *Am Rev Respir Dis* 1993;147:218–233.
21. Kurahashi K, Kajikawa O, Sawa T, et al. Pathogenesis of septic shock in *Pseudomonas aeruginosa* pneumonia. *J Clin Invest* 1999;104:743–750.
22. Matthay MA. Conference summary: acute lung injury. *Chest* 1999;116:119S–126S.
23. Nelson S, Belknap SM, Carlson RW, et al. A randomized controlled trial of filgrastim as an adjunct to antibiotics for treatment of hospitalized patients with community-acquired pneumonia. CAP Study Group. *J Infect Dis* 1998;178:1075–1080.
24. Folkesson HG, Matthay MA, Herbert CA, et al. Acid aspiration induced lung injury in rabbits is mediated by interleukin-8 dependent mechanisms. *J Clin Invest* 1995;96:107–116.
25. Donnelly SC, Haslett C, Reid PT, et al. Regulatory role for macrophage migration inhibitory factor in the acute respiratory distress syndrome. *Nat Med* 1997;3:320–323.
26. Pugin J, Verghese G, Widmer M-C, et al. The alveolar space is the site of intense inflammatory and profibrotic reactions in the early phase of ARDS. *Crit Care Med* 1999;27:304–312.

27. Geiser T, Jarreau PH, Atabai K, et al. Interleukin-1B augments *in vitro* alveolar epithelial repair. *Am J Physiol* 2000;279:L1184–L1190.

28. Dreyfuss D, Soler P, Basset G, et al. High inflation pressure pulmonary edema. Respective effects of high airway pressure, high tidal volume, and positive end-expiratory pressure. *Am Rev Respir Dis* 1988;137:1159–1164.

29. Slutsky AS, Tremblay LN. Multiple system organ failure: is mechanical ventilation a contributing factor? *Am J Respir Crit Care Med* 1998;157:1721–1725.

30. Fukuda Y, Ishizaki M, Masuda Y, et al. The role of intraalveolar fibrosis in the process of pulmonary structural remodeling in patients with diffuse alveolar damage. *Am J Pathol* 1987;126:171–182.

31. Martin C, Papazian L, Payan MJ, et al. Pulmonary fibrosis correlates with outcome in the adult respiratory distress syndrome. *Chest* 1995;107:196–200.

32. Lindroos PM, Coin PG, Osornio-Vargas AR, et al. Interleukin-1b (IL-1b) and the IL-1b alpha 2-macroglobulin complex upregulate the platelet-derived growth factor alpha on rat pulmonary fibroblasts. *Am J Respir Cell Mol Biol* 1995;13:455–465.

33. Clark JG, Milberg JA, Steinberg KP, et al. Type III procollagen peptide in the adult respiratory distress syndrome. *Ann Intern Med* 1995;122:17–23.

34. Matthay MA, Folkesson HG, Verkman AS. Salt and water transport across alveolar and distal airway epithelia in the adult lung. *Am J Physiol* 1996;270:L487–L503.

35. Dobbs LG, Gonzalez R, Matthay MA, et al. Highly water-permeable type I alveolar epithelial cells confer high water permeability between the airspace and vasculature in rat lung. *Proc Natl Acad Sci U S A* 1998;95:2991–2996.

36. Folkesson HG, Matthay MA, Westrom BR, et al. Alveolar epithelial clearance of protein. *J Appl Physiol* 1996;80:1431–1445.

37. Folkesson HG, Nitenberg G, Oliver BL, et al. Upregulation of alveolar epithelial fluid transport after subacute lung injury in rats from bleomycin. *Am J Physiol* 1998;275:L478–L490.

38. Kheradmand F, Folkesson HG, Shum L, et al. Transforming growth factor-α (TGF-α) enhances alveolar epithelial cell repair in a new *in vitro* model. *Am J Physiol* 1994;267:728–738.

39. Garat C, Kheradmand F, Albertine KH, et al. Soluble and insoluble fibronectin increase alveolar epithelial wound healing in vitro. *Am J Physiol* 1996;271:L844–L853.

40. Matute-Bello G, Liles WC, Radella F II, et al. Neutrophil apoptosis in the acute respiratory distress syndrome. *Am J Respir Crit Care Med* 1997;156:1969–1977.

41. Matute-Bello G, Liles WC, Steinberg KP, et al. Soluble Fas-ligand induces epithelial cell apoptosis in humans with acute lung injury (ARDS). *J Immunol* 1999;163:2217–2225.

42. Milberg JA, Davis DR, Steinberg KP, et al. Improved survival of patients with acute respiratory distress syndrome (ARDS): 1983–1993. *JAMA* 1995;273:306–309.

43. Abel SJC, Finney SJ, Brett SJ, et al. Reduced mortality in association with the acute respiratory distress syndrome. *Thorax* 1998;53:292–294.

44. Zapol WM, Snider MT, Hill JD, et al. Extracorporeal membrane oxygenation in severe acute respiratory failure. *JAMA* 1979;242:2193–2196.

45. Morris AH, Wallace CJ, Menlove RL, et al. Randomized clinical trial of pressure-controlled inverse ratio ventilation and extracorporeal CO₂ removal for adult respiratory distress syndrome. *Am J Respir Crit Care Med* 1994;149:295–305.

46. Stewart TE, Meade MO, Cook DJ, et al. Evaluation of a ventilation strategy to prevent barotrauma in patients at high risk for acute respiratory distress syndrome. *N Engl J Med* 1998;338:355–361.

47. Brochard L, Roudot-Thoraval F, Roupie E, et al. Tidal volume reduction for prevention of ventilator-induced lung injury in acute respiratory distress syndrome. *Am J Respir Crit Care Med* 1998;158:1831–1838.

48. Falke KH, Pontoppidan H, Kumar A. Ventilation with end-expiratory pressure in acute lung disease. *J Clin Invest* 1972;51:2315–2323.

49. Gattinoni L, Pesenti A, Bombino M. Relationship between lung computed tomographic density, gas exchange, and PEEP in acute respiratory failure. *Anesthesiology* 1988;69:824–832.

50. Pepe PE, Hudson LD, Carrico CJ. Early application of positive end-expiratory pressure in patients at risk for the adult respiratory distress syndrome. *N Engl J Med* 1984;311:281–286.

51. Amato MB, Barbas CS, Medeiros DM, et al. Effect of a protective-ventilation strategy on mortality in the acute respiratory distress syndrome. *N Engl J Med* 1998;338:347–354.

52. Nakos G, Tsangaris I, Kostanti E, et al. Effect of prone position on patients with hydrostatic pulmonary edema compared with patients with acute respiratory distress syndrome and pulmonary fibrosis. *Am J Respir Crit Care Med* 2000;161:360–368.

53. Humphrey H, Hall J, Sznajder I, et al. Improved survival in ARDS patients associated with a reduction in pulmonary capillary wedge pressure. *Chest* 1990;97:1176–1180.

54. Mitchell JP, Schuller D, Calandrino FS, et al. Improved outcome based on fluid management in critically ill patients requiring pulmonary artery catheterization. *Am Rev Respir Dis* 1992;145:990–998.

55. Yu M, Levy MM, Smith P, et al. Effect of maximizing oxygen delivery on morbidity and mortality rates in critically ill patients: a prospective, randomized, controlled study. *Crit Care Med* 1993;21:830–838.

56. Hayes MA, Timmins AC, Yau EHS, et al. Elevation of systemic oxygen delivery in the treatment of critically ill patients. *N Engl J Med* 1994;330:1717–1722.

57. Anzueto A, Baughman RP, Guntupalli KK, et al. Aerosolized surfactant in adults with sepsis-induced acute respiratory distress syndrome. *N Engl J Med* 1996;334:1417–1421.

58. Rossaint R, Falke KJ, Lopez F, et al. Inhaled nitric oxide for the adult respiratory distress syndrome. *N Engl J Med* 1993;328:399–405.

59. Dellinger RP, Zimmerman JL, Taylor RW. Effects of inhaled nitric oxide in patients with acute respiratory distress syndrome: results of a randomized phase II trial. *Crit Care Med* 1998;26:15–23.

60. Payen D, Vallet B, and the Genoa Group. Results of the French prospective multicentric randomized double-blind placebo-controlled trial on inhaled nitric oxide in ARDS. *Intensive Care Med* 1999;25:S166.

61. Bernard GR, Luce J, Sprung C. High-dose corticosteroids in patients with the adult respiratory distress syndrome. *N Engl J Med* 1987;317:1565–1570.

62. Luce JM, Montgomery BA, Marks JD, et al. Ineffectiveness of high-dose methylprednisolone in preventing parenchymal lung injury and improving mortality in patients with septic shock. *Am Rev Respir Dis* 1988;136:62–66.

63. Meduri GU, Headley AS, Golden E, et al. Effect of prolonged methylprednisolone therapy in unresolving acute respiratory distress syndrome: a randomized controlled trial. *JAMA* 1998;280:159–165.

64. Frank JA, Wang Y, Osorio O, et al. Beta-adrenergic agonist therapy accelerates the resolution of hydrostatic pulmonary edema in sheep and rats. *J Appl Physiol* 2000;89:1255–1265.

65. Saldias F, Comellas A, Ridge KM, et al. Isoproterenol increases edema clearance in rat lungs exposed to hyperoxia. *J Appl Physiol* 1999;87:30–36.

66. Atabai K, Ware L, Snider M, et al. Aerosolized beta-2 agonists achieve therapeutic levels in the pulmonary edema fluid of ventilated patients. *Am J Respir Crit Care Med* 2001;(abst) (*in press*).

67. Ye RD. Beta-adrenergic agonists regulate NFkB activation through multiple mechanisms. *Am J Physiol* 2000;23:L615–L618.

68. Yano T, Deterding RR, Simonet WS, et al. Keratinocyte growth factor reduces lung damage due to acid instillation in rats. *Am J Respir Cell Mol Biol* 1996;15:433–442.

69. Wang Y, Folkesson HG, Jayr C, et al. Alveolar epithelial fluid transport can be simultaneously upregulated by both KGF and beta-agonist therapy. *J Appl Physiol* 1999;87:1852–1860.

70. Bernard GR, Vincent JL, Laterre PF, et al. Efficacy and safety of recombinant human activated protein C for severe sepsis. *N Engl J Med* 2001;344:699–709.

71. Matthay MA. Severe sepsis—a new treatment with both anticoagulant and antiinflammatory properties. *N Engl J Med* 2001;344:759–762.

PERIOPERATIVE CARE OF THORACIC SURGICAL PATIENTS

JOANNE MEYER
BRIAN P. KAVANAGH

KEY WORDS

- Air leak
- Atelectasis
- Bronchial leak
- Bronchoscopy
- Dysrhythmias
- Esophageal airway
- Mediastinal shift
- Myasthenia gravis
- Pleural effusion
- Pneumothorax
- Reduction resection
- Thoracic surgery
- Thoracoscopy
- Thymectomy
- Transplantation

INTRODUCTION

Thoracic operations involve many unique perioperative assessment issues, technical manipulations, and acute physiologic changes, which are not readily appreciated or understood from managing the care of general-surgical or critical-care patients. Furthermore, the postoperative respiratory, fluid, and analgesic management requires knowledge and skills that are specific, in many cases, to thoracic operations.

ASSESSMENT, INDICATIONS, AND INTRAOPERATIVE CONSIDERATIONS FOR THORACIC OPERATIONS

Bronchoscopy

Fiberoptic bronchoscopy is performed in intubated or nonintubated patients for bronchial hygiene, diagnostic lavage, bronchial brushings, endobronchial biopsy, or transbronchial biopsy. In nonintubated patients, topical anesthesia with cocaine hydrochloride and/or lidocaine hydrochloride permits adequate examination with minimal sedation. Pretreatment with antisialagogues (e.g., glycopyrrolate 0.2–0.4 mg) may reduce the airway secretions and improves visibility through the bronchoscope. In intubated patients with controlled ventilation, sedation and analgesia are limited only by the patient's hemodynamic status. Use of a larger (7.5–8.5 mm) endotracheal tube permits easier access and ventilation. Careful monitoring of oxygenation, ventilation, and hemodynamics is important in all cases.

Rigid Bronchoscopy

Rigid bronchoscopy can be performed in the intensive care unit (ICU) or in the operating room. In most cases, this procedure requires deep anesthesia and paralysis but can be performed with light anesthesia and spontaneous ventilation if excellent topical airway anesthesia has been achieved. Maintenance of ventilation in these cases is either by intermittent jet ventilation or intermittent manual ventilation with occlusion on the proximal end of the bronchoscope and completion of the anesthetic circuit. Procedures involving direct or indirect laryngoscopy have similar implications to bronchoscopy.

Laser Bronchoscopy

The use of laser bronchoscopy has expanded the treatment options for patients with obstructive airway malignancies. The laser beam is introduced through a flexible fiberoptic bronchoscope. For proximal airway lesions, a shielded endotracheal tube with a saline-filled cuff may be used to control ventilation and the laser beam introduced beside it. Patients undergoing laser bronchoscopy are frequently hypoxemic before the operation and may develop profound episodic hypoxemia related to bleeding, aspiration of tumor debris, and hypoventilation during the procedure. As with all laser operations involving the airway, precautions, including eye protection (for the patient and surgical team), use of low concentrations of oxygen during resection [maximum fraction of inspired oxygen (F_{IO_2}) < 0.3], avoidance of nitrous oxide, use of moist towels to dissipate heat, and safe application of the laser beam all serve to reduce the risk of airway fires and damage to normal tissue. Hypoxemia is treated by ventilating with an F_{IO_2} of 1.0, removing debris, coagulating bleeding vessels, and advancing the rigid bronchoscope distal to the obstructing mass to allow effective ventilation.

Pulmonary Resection

Assessment of patients before thoracic operations depends largely on the type of operation planned and on the patient's physiologic state. Two questions must be answered. First, is the disease surgically curable? Second, assuming the disease is resectable, does the patient's physiologic reserve permit the proposed intervention?

For pulmonary neoplasms, the principal staging procedures involve a history and physical examination; chest radiograph; bronchoscopy; computed tomographic (CT) scan of the thorax; and, occasionally, mediastinoscopy. Staging systems are TNM based (T is the primary tumor diameter and local extension, N is extent of lymph node involvement, and M is presence of systemic metastasis). The stage at diagnosis yields an approximately linear relationship to postoperative survival. Approximately 30% of non–small-cell neoplasms are considered resectable preoperatively, but this percentage falls to about 20% following thoracotomy and direct local inspection and biopsy. Approximately 10% of patients with small-cell neoplasms are considered suitable candidates for an operation, with chemotherapy playing a major role as an adjunct to operation or as sole therapy in the vast majority of cases.

The thoracic surgery patient often has both pulmonary and cardiac disease. In determining the patient's ability to withstand the operation, the clinician must focus on two issues. First, does the patient's overall cardiovascular status allow for the performance of a major operation with acceptable risks of perioperative cardiac events (1,2) (see also Chapter 1)? Second, does the patient's pulmonary status allow the proposed resection (3)?

The consideration of perioperative cardiac risk is similar to preoperative cardiac assessment for patients undergoing any other major surgical intervention. Various risk assessment scores have been developed to help predict adverse cardiac events (1,2). Clinical criteria such as history of angina or myocardial infarction, congestive heart failure, diabetes, or abnormalities on electrocardiogram (ECG) may identify patients who need further risk stratification with thallium imaging or angiography. Patients with severe or unstable cardiovascular or other reversible systemic disease should be treated medically, and their condition should be optimized before the thoracic operation is performed; lung resections are virtually never emergent. If coronary revascularization is required, it is best performed before the thoracotomy but can be performed as a combined procedure.

The unique aspect of assessment for lung resection surgery involves preoperatively predicting the patient's pulmonary status following resection of lung tissue. In an effort to ensure that the patient has sufficient postoperative pulmonary reserve following lung resection, a wide variety of pulmonary-function indexes have been developed and standardized. The preoperative assessments (see Chapter 31) include grade of dyspnea, resting arterial blood gas (ABG) profile, forced expiratory volume at 1 second (FEV_1), forced vital capacity (FVC), diffusion capacity (DLCO), maximum voluntary ventilation (MVV), exercise oximetry, ventilation perfusion scanning, assessment of pulmonary vascular resistance (PVR), and determination of maximal oxygen consumption (VO_2) (4).

If the patient is fully fit and has excellent exercise tolerance, further evaluation will contribute little, and the patient could undergo pneumonectomy or lobectomy with good postoperative pulmonary function. Although most surgical candidates have some clinical pulmonary impairment, if they are able to climb stairs without experiencing arterial oxygen desaturation or dyspnea to the point of speechlessness, they almost certainly can undergo pulmonary resection. Those at higher risk for pneumonectomy include those with a high baseline $Paco_2$, FVC less than 50% of predicted, FEV_1 less than 50% of FVC or an absolute value less than 2 L, DLCO less than 50% of predicted, and a MVV less than 50% predicted (5,6). Specific prediction of postoperative pulmonary function centers on the degree of baseline pulmonary impairment (actual value or percentage of predicted value) and on the extent of functional pulmonary resection. The most common method of predicting postoperative functional lung tissue is to assess the FEV_1 with preoperative spirometry ($FEV_1 Pre$), perform a V/Q study to estimate the fraction of perfusion in the area to be resected (FqResect), and calculate $FEV_1 Post$ by multiplying $FEV_1 Pre$ and (1-FqResect) (6). If $FEV_1 Post$ is greater than 40% of the FEV_1 predicted value, on the basis of the patient's age, sex, and height, the patient should have adequate pulmonary reserve following the planned lung resection. The aim is to leave a patient with a final FEV_1 of at least 40% of the predicted value (>800 mL on average) on the basis of age, sex, and height. If a patient's ability to tolerate the operation is still in question or if there is significant pulmonary hypertension, a pulmonary artery (PA) catheter can be inserted to stratify further risk based on high PVR or decreased maximum VO_2.

Once the lung resection patient goes to the operating room, monitoring, as for all patients undergoing general anesthesia, includes continuous ECG monitoring, intermittent blood pressure monitoring by noninvasive cuff, pulse oximetry, and end-tidal carbon dioxide determination. Arterial lines and Foley catheters are commonly used in larger thoracic operations, whereas central venous lines and pulmonary artery catheters are generally limited to patients with significant cardiac or other comorbid disease.

Operations for Major Airway Obstruction

Operations usually are undertaken in this context to obtain tissue for diagnosis (bronchoscopy, with or without mediastinoscopy) or to relieve acute airway obstruction (laser bronchoscopy). Preoperative assessment centers around formulating a plan to secure the patient's airway and developing contingency plans in the event that securing the airway proves to be difficult. In patients with airway lesions or foreign bodies, increased obstruction may occur with supine body position or muscle relaxation induced by sedating premedications or anesthetics. The key issue before inducing anesthesia is knowledge of the anatomy of the airway. Although history, physical examination, spirometry, chest radiograph, thoracic inlet radiograph, and flow–volume loop analysis may yield useful information, the definitive investigation is a CT scan examining the entire airway. The critical questions are as follows: Is the airway compressed or involved? What is the extent of the mass? How high above the carina is the mass? In cases of doubt, it is imperative that the patient be breathing spontaneously for intubation and that the distal end of the endotracheal tube be confirmed by flexible fiberoptic bronchoscopy to be distal to any airway mass or compression before inducing anesthesia or paralysis (7). Backup strategies include the availability of skilled help, rigid bronchoscopy, and possible femorofemoral cardiopulmonary bypass (CPB). Additional considerations for patients with mediastinal-mass lesions include the presence of vascular compression, namely, superior vena caval compression or pericardial or cardiac involvement.

Tracheal Resection

Tracheal resection is undertaken for treating tracheal disease, tumor, or stenosis that is not amenable to dilation. The stenosed or diseased portion of the trachea is resected, and the proximal and distal ends are anastomosed. The procedure involves careful preoperative assessment of the airway and intraoperative ventilation of the lungs through the distal trachea through a breathing circuit introduced through the operative field.

T-tube Insertion and Changes

Montgomery T-tubes (silicone, three-limb, T-shaped tubes) are used to allow the tracheal anastomosis to heal, without worsening stenosis, while also allowing ventilation. The tube is placed using a rigid bronchoscope with the patient under general anesthesia, using the oropharyngeal route across the anastomosis. The superior limb lies cephalad in the trachea toward the larynx, the inferior limb is directed distally into the trachea, and the third limb is directed percutaneously to the exterior. The difficulties with these devices usually occur during initial placement or, subsequently, during replacement with a similar tube.

Video-assisted Thoracoscopic Surgery

Video-assisted thoracoscopic surgery (VATS) has been used for a number of years in patients undergoing thoracic operations. The aim of this procedure is to perform interpleural inspection, biopsy, or pulmonary resection, with a decreased need for postoperative analgesia and without the respiratory implications of a full thoracotomy incision. The procedure is carried out using single-lung anesthesia; CO_2 can be insufflated into the chest cavity to ensure deflation of the lung and optimization of visibility. No randomized controlled clinical trials document the precise role of this technique, but preliminary evidence suggests a potential for reduction in the length of hospital stay and improved postoperative recovery profile (8).

Lung-volume Reduction Surgery

Lung-volume reduction surgery (LVRS) was introduced in the 1950s but was not widely accepted because of its high morbidity and mortality rates. With improvements in surgical technique and postoperative care, LVRS has reemerged as a potentially beneficial operation in patients with severe emphysematous lung disease. Further study is required to define appropriate patient selection. The mechanism of benefit from this operation has not been clearly defined but is likely based on the physiologic alterations that occur secondary to significant thoracic hyperinflation. These patients breathe at lung volumes that are greatly in excess of normal. The pressure–volume relationships of the lungs are abnormal, with the result that the inspiration–expiration cycle is occurring on the uppermost, flattened portion of the pressure–volume curve. The work of breathing is increased and contributes to respiratory failure. When the operation reduces the resting volume of the lungs, they occupy a more favorable position on the pressure–volume curve, and the work of breathing is decreased. Improvement persists to at least 6 months. (9). Patients are extu-

bated postoperatively as soon as possible to reduce barotrauma. In the event of an unsuccessful operation, respiratory failure may rapidly ensue due to suboptimal resection technique or ongoing air leaks.

Lung Transplantation

The clinical development of lung transplantation has accelerated over the past 10 years with the emergence of several centers performing large numbers of procedures (10). The transplantation of a single lung into a patient with pulmonary fibrosis in 1983 marked the resurgence of the current interest in pulmonary transplantation. Patient outcome is now significantly improved, paralleling advances in surgical technique, anesthetic management, and postoperative immunosuppression and critical care. Double-lung transplantation using a single tracheal anastomosis was developed 5 years later. This technique required CPB, and tracheal anastomotic-healing difficulties frequently occurred. Since then, the technique of sequential single-lung transplantation (SSLT), a procedure in which the two lungs are transplanted in sequence, has been developed and remains the technique of choice in current practice for double-lung transplantation. By late 1993, more than 2,000 lung-transplantation procedures were completed. Double-lung transplantation procedures are now usually completed as SSLT, and the frequency of single-lung transplantations has markedly diminished. Lung transplantation is reviewed in Chapter 54.

Myasthenia Gravis and Thymoma

Myasthenia gravis (MG) is an immunologic condition caused by the development of autoantibodies against skeletal-muscle cholinergic receptors and clinically is characterized by muscle weakness and fatigue, which increase with muscle use. This condition has several clinical presentations, and the clinical classification (groups I–V) focuses on the predominant muscle groups involved, the chronicity of the presentation, and the presence of muscular atrophy (11). The incidence of MG is approximately 3 per 100,000; presentation usually occurs at between 20 and 30 years; and, like most autoimmune diseases, it is more common in women than in men. The ocular muscles are most often involved, and the disease may remain confined to these muscles. The key clinical features of MG are muscle fatigability, an absence of sensory involvement, and improvement with anticholinesterase therapy.

In contrast, patients with the Eaton–Lambert syndrome, which may be associated with small-cell carcinoma of the lung, show significant improvement of strength with repetitive muscle stimulation, demonstrate predominant proximal limb–muscle involvement, do not have pathogenic antiacetylcholine-receptor antibodies in large quantities, and show good responses to guanidine hydrochloride.

The treatment of MG consists of four management strategies: anticholinesterase medication, thymectomy, immunologic manipulation, and supportive therapy (mechanical ventilation, airway protection, and nutrition). Anticholinesterase medication consists of oral pyridostigmine bromide or neostigmine methylsulfate; however, pyridostigmine has a longer duration of action and is associated with fewer muscarinic adverse effects, such as abdominal cramps and excessive salivation. This first-line therapy for all patients with MG shows initial effects within hours, but optimization of doses may take weeks.

Thymectomy is a highly effective treatment for many patients with MG, but the precise role of thymic tissue in the pathogenesis is unclear. Approximately 10% of patients with MG have a thymoma. Staging is determined by the extent of local invasion and whether there are distant metastases. The response of MG to thymectomy is poor in patients with a thymoma or in patients with only ocular symptoms. Thymectomy is performed in patients with thymoma to prevent local spread or as surgical treatment for a malignant tumor (approximately 10% of thymomas). Large thymomas may lead to airway compression, and the same considerations as mentioned previously regarding intubation and anesthesia for patients with airway obstruction should apply. Thymectomy results in a clinical cure in up to 80% of patients who do not have a thymoma, but this may require 3 to 4 years.

Immunologic therapy includes corticosteroids, azathioprine, and plasma exchange. Steroid therapy begins at moderate doses to induce an initial remission with subsequent tapering to low doses. Steroid use may decrease the requirement for anticholinesterase medication. The role for steroids in current practice is to prepare patients before they undergo thymectomy and to treat patients in whom thymectomy is either not indicated or has not resulted in sufficient clinical improvement. To reduce the adverse effects associated with steroids, or in the event of steroid failure, azathioprine may be used. The clinician should determine the adequacy of perioperative steroid coverage of patients who have received steroid treatment. Plasma exchange is currently used to obtain short-term improvement in patients preoperatively or in those who are acutely ill. It does not appear to have long-term benefits as chronic therapy.

Supportive therapy for patients with MG consists of endotracheal intubation for airway protection, mechanical ventilation for respiratory failure, and enteral nutrition. Intubation should be performed early in the management of a patient with MG while treatment is being optimized. Delays in intubation result in aspiration, greatly worsening the patient's clinical course. As long as the diagnosis of MG is definite, intubation with succinylcholine chloride (1.0–1.5 mg/kg) may be performed as per the clinical practice of the anesthesiologist. In critically weak patients, neuromuscular blocking agents are frequently not required.

POSTOPERATIVE CARE AND COMPLICATIONS

Most patients who undergo thoracic operations are extubated in the operating room and transported with chest tubes unclamped to the postanesthetic care unit or to the ICU for monitoring. General assessment and management should occur as for any postoperative patient, giving attention to the possibility of specific complications. Appropriate care includes ECG, blood pressure and arterial saturation monitoring, management of the thoracostomy–drainage tube (see Chapter 14) and fluid balance, provision of adequate analgesia, and attention to overall ventilatory status. The postoperative chest radiograph should

be examined for correct placement of the thoracoscopy tube, lung expansion, centrality of the mediastinum, optimum central-line placement, and subsegmental atelectasis on the operative side.

Fluid Management

Fluid management should aim for the minimum amount compatible with adequate end-organ perfusion and maintenance of electrolyte balance (see Chapters 16). Hypoxemia may occur secondary to increased postoperative pulmonary capillary permeability and is exacerbated by excessive fluid administration. In most patients with normal hemodynamics, maintenance of a urinary output of 0.5 to 1.0 mL per kilogram per hour is adequate.

Dysrhythmias

Dysrhythmias are common in patients undergoing thoracic operations, and atrial fibrillation occurs following thoracotomy in 15% to 25% of patients. The pathogenesis of these dysrhythmias is unclear but may be related to atrial trauma, atrial distention, altered gas exchange, pain, and excessive sympathetic activity. In the thoracic surgical patient, the occurrence of atrial dysrhythmias adversely affects prognosis (12).

The standard approach to treatment of dysrhythmias does not require modification for thoracic surgery patients (see Chapter 29). Prophylaxis with digoxin or calcium-channel blockade is not of clear benefit.

Atelectasis and Mediastinal Shift

Atelectasis is a common complication following thoracic surgical procedures. It is usually multifactorial as a result of secretions, splinting, bronchospasm, intraoperative trauma, and hypoventilation. Patients may be asymptomatic or may present with fever or with symptoms and signs of varying degrees of respiratory compromise. The chest radiograph should delineate the area of the lung involved and may show evidence of tracheal deviation. Mediastinal shift toward the involved hemithorax to compensate for volume loss occurs after any pulmonary resection. This shift is most marked after pneumonectomy, when elevation of the diaphragm also occurs. Any mediastinal shift should not encroach on the functioning lung, and excessive shift is suggestive of volume loss on the operated side and is usually due to atelectasis. Simple measures to reduce atelectasis include early ambulation, incentive spirometry, humidified oxygen, maintaining adequate systemic hydration, bronchodilators, and adequate analgesia. Aggressive chest physiotherapy and suctioning and even fiberoptic bronchoscopy are indicated if moderate to severe atelectasis occurs. Excessive secretions associated with extensive collapse or lack of lung reexpansion, especially if the secretions are thick and tenacious, may require endotracheal intubation for suctioning and ventilatory support. Less commonly, pneumothorax or hydropneumothorax of the contralateral (not operated on) pleural space may produce a mediastinal shift and should be excluded by clinical examination and radiography.

Airway Obstruction

Airway obstruction following thoracic surgery may be due to laryngeal or tracheal edema, retained secretions, blood in the airway, or bilateral recurrent laryngeal nerve palsy. Early recognition is key to timely and appropriate management. Upper-airway problems usually manifest as stridor, whereas lower lesions cause wheezing or rhonchi. Respiratory distress and hypoxia may occur. Careful appraisal of the patient by the thoracic surgeon and intensivist should determine the likelihood of anticipated problems.

Trauma to the larynx or trachea causing edema may occur after endotracheal intubation for any procedure. Extra trauma to these structures may occur in thoracic surgery as a result of passage of larger-bore or double-lumen tubes, bronchial blockers, rigid bronchoscopes, and frequent reintubations. Patients who have tracheal surgery or resection are at particular risk of obstruction. These patients usually are extubated in the operating room and are maintained in a semirecumbent position, with their necks flexed to reduce tension on the tracheal anastomosis. Strong skin sutures, extending from beneath the mandible to the level of the sternum, can be inserted before the patient emerges from anesthesia and serve to maintain the neck in flexion. Early recognition of obstruction is key to management. Initial management includes 100% oxygen. Racemic epinephrine can be given via nebulizer to reduce airway edema. If the patient can achieve adequate oxygenation with an FIO_2 of 0.3 or 0.4, a mixture of helium and oxygen (Heliox) can be used. The replacement of nitrogen with helium in this mixture allows a more laminar flow of air through the stenosed airway and thereby decreases the obstruction. If there is any question about maintaining an adequate airway or if respiratory failure supervenes, careful tracheal intubation—with minimal sedation and no paralysis and possibly use of the fiberoptic bronchoscope—may be the management of choice.

Tracheobronchial obstruction may be caused by blood, blood clots, secretions, or aspirated gastric contents, especially large particulate matter. Lung separation and isolation (double-lumen endotracheal tube) will help to prevent single-lung pathology from affecting both lungs and will allow frequent suctioning of each tracheobronchial tree. If there has been excessive secretions or blood suctioned from the airway or if there is clinically significant tracheobronchial obstruction, aggressive suctioning is required and bronchoscopy (fiberoptic or rigid bronchoscopy) may be necessary prior to extubation.

T-Tube Insertion and Changes

If a patient with a T-tube develops a difficulty with airway patency or with respiratory drive (e.g., residual sedation or neuromuscular blockade), the exterior limb of the T-tube can be occluded, and ventilation can be assisted initially with a face mask and oxygen. Alternatively, the proximal limb of the T-tube can be occluded with a bronchial blocker, and the patient can be ventilated through the exterior limb by using a 6.0 to 7.5 mm endotracheal-tube connecting piece to couple the T-tube to an anesthesia bag or ventilator.

As always in patients following airway operations, airway manipulations should be approached with extreme caution. The physician should be fully knowledgeable about the precise nature of the patient's lesion and about any experienced or anticipated difficulties; this information should be obtained through a direct report from the surgeon and anesthesiologist involved in the case. These personnel should ideally be directly involved in the postoperative care of patients who have undergone T-tube insertions. The ability to intubate the trachea directly via the oral or nasal routes, or the ability to expeditiously obtain a percutaneous or surgical airway, never should be assumed.

Bronchoscopy

Complications associated with bronchoscopy include bronchospasm, hypoxemia, airway trauma, dental trauma, endobronchial bleeding, pneumothorax, and complications associated with excessive sedation. Careful assessment and oxygen supplementation usually are required, and chest radiography is indicated if transbronchial biopsy has been performed.

Mechanical Ventilation

The need for mechanical ventilation following thoracotomy usually results from unexpected intraoperative events, excessively prolonged operative time, massive fluid or blood-product administration, incomplete reversal of neuromuscular blockade, hypothermia, or an analgesia-associated complication. Mechanical ventilation (discussed in depth in Chapter 47) is relatively straightforward in these patients. If mechanical ventilation is likely to be greater than several hours in duration, double-lumen or Univent tubes should be exchanged for single-lumen tubes. These single-lumen tubes are easier to manage and may be associated with fewer tracheal-pressure-related complications. Positive-pressure ventilation provides ventilatory support, ideally with ventilator settings that are associated with low or moderate peak airway pressures (<30 cm H_2O) and low levels of positive end-expiratory pressure (PEEP). Settings resulting in high peak airway pressures or excessive levels of PEEP jeopardize the integrity of the bronchial anastomosis and can result in bronchopleural fistula development.

Patients with obstructive airway diseases have a tendency to develop high levels of intrinsic PEEP, which can be attenuated by use of minimal tidal volumes, low respiratory rates, and low inspiratory-to-expiratory (I:E) ratios (maximizing time in expiration). Patients with restrictive lung diseases have little propensity to develop intrinsic PEEP, and the principal problem is high airway pressures for a given tidal volume. The solution here is to reduce tidal volumes and inspiratory flow rates and to maintain minute ventilation through increased respiratory rate and increased I:E ratio (maximizing time in inspiration).

Respiratory insufficiency may be irreversible after resection if the patient has been left with inadequate pulmonary reserve. This should be avoided by preoperative evaluation of pulmonary function.

Air Leakage

Air leakage is common initially after lobectomy or segmental resection because small airways are commonly transected and most pulmonary fissures are not complete. With satisfactory thoracostomy-tube drainage (two pleural thoracostomy tubes placed anterior and posterior at the level of the diaphragm going to the apex), moderate underwater-seal suction (20–30 cm H_2O), physiotherapy, and ambulation, initial air leakage normally stops in 3 to 4 days. Persistent air leakage is more likely to occur if adhesions are present between the lung and chest wall. If moderate air leakage is present after 7 days, removal of the thoracostomy tube—to allow the lung to collapse moderately—and reinsertion of a new tube often correct the leak. Major segmental or bronchial air leaks typically do not occur early and are related to operations for bullous disease or severe complications such as bronchial-stump disruption or bronchopleural fistula development. Mechanical ventilatory support after lung resection, if necessary, is usually satisfactory, even with a relatively large air leak because volume-limited ventilators can be adjusted to cope with the leak; however, positive-pressure ventilation, especially with the use of PEEP, may prolong air leaks, increasing the risk of pneumothorax and infection.

Pneumothorax

A pneumothorax may occur with or without an accompanying air leak. The first step in management is to ensure proper chest-tube function using a closed system with adequate underwater seal and a patent tube. A persistent pneumothorax may respond to increasing suction on the drainage system or may require a new tube if the area is loculated.

Tension pneumothorax may occur if an air leak occurs and is not adequately drained from the chest cavity (no chest tube in place or the chest tube is obstructed). Positive-pressure ventilation increases the chance that a pneumothorax will develop under tension. Mediastinal shift, decreased venous return, hypotension, and respiratory insufficiency (increased inflation pressures with positive-pressure ventilation) are the principal features. Reestablishing the thoracostomy-tube patency or prompt insertion of a large-bore needle into the anterior pleural space (second intercostal space, midclavicular line) usually relieves the tension, after which more definitive management with a thoracostomy tube is carried out.

Bronchopleural Fistula

Bronchial-stump disruption is a serious complication. The development of a major bronchopleural fistula is associated with a 20% mortality rate. Satisfactory initial closure of the stump should be tested intraoperatively by filling the hemithorax with saline and maintaining the pressure in the anesthesia breathing circuit at 40 cm H_2O. If no bubbles appear, the stump has been properly closed. Fistulae appearing within a few days of the operation usually are related to technical errors (poor suturing or stapling techniques or bronchial ischemia resulting from inappropriate dissection before closure). An abrupt increase in the air leak from the thoracostomy tube, hemoptysis, and radiographic changes showing a pneumothorax with or without an air-fluid level and partial lung collapse are signs of the development of a bronchopleural fistula. Prompt reoperation and

closure of the fistula are recommended for early bronchial-stump disruption. A bronchopleural fistula that appears after the first postoperative week usually is caused by ischemia and necrosis because of an inadequate blood supply, infection, or tumor in the bronchial stump. Poor healing due to preoperative radiation ($\geq 3,000$ rads) also may influence the development of a bronchopleural fistula. Late breakdown usually occurs in patients who are severely debilitated and are at high risk for requiring reoperation; therefore, prolonged thoracostomy-tube drainage will be required. Bronchopleural fistulae following lobectomy are usually well managed by thoracostomy-tube drainage and suction until pleurodesis occurs, at which time suction can be discontinued and the tube can be left in place until only a small tube tract is left. These fistulae usually close spontaneously over several months. The development of a bronchopleural fistula following pneumonectomy is a much more severe complication. The fistula usually becomes apparent within 7 to 10 days and is related to technical problems or devascularization. Patients may complain of sudden copious, blood-stained or watery sputum, which represents drainage of pneumonectomy fluid into the airway. Radiographic findings are diagnostic if the postpneumonectomy air-fluid level has dropped to a lower level than was seen on previous films. Immediate drainage with the affected side down is required so as to not empty pleural space contents into the tracheobronchial tree. Pleural fluid should be cultured and broad-spectrum antibiotics should be administered. Bronchoscopy will allow assessment of the size and location of the fistula. In stable patients, immediate closure is justified, but technical difficulties preclude routine surgical closure in patients who are more than 10 days postpneumonectomy. Immediate closure involves the application of a large, well-vascularized muscle or omental pedicle. If immediate closure is not selected, wide, open drainage on a long-term basis is necessary. This drainage is best achieved by the creation of a Claggett window (rib resection) or Eloesser flap when the patient is stable and the mediastinal contents are relatively fixed. Granulation and spontaneous closure of the fistula are long-term aims. Long-term ventilation with double-lumen tubes may present difficulties because of the tubes' relatively large size, but modern polyvinyl chloride nonirritant double-lumen tubes with high-volume, low-pressure cuffs may be left *in situ*, if necessary, for several days. With a left-sided bronchopleural fistula, double-lumen-tube positioning may be more difficult because the right-upper-lobe bronchus may be obstructed by a right-sided double-lumen endotracheal tube. High-frequency ventilation may be successful in this circumstance. A bronchopleural fistula that develops after sleeve resection requires emergency bronchoscopy to assess the integrity of the bronchial anastomosis. If disruption is present or suspected, pneumonectomy is considered (7).

Intrapulmonary Hemorrhage

Significant bleeding into the tracheobronchial tree characteristically occurs postoperatively as a complication of bronchoscopic biopsy of an adenoma or of a vascular malignancy or occasionally as the result of pulmonary artery catheterization. Management is directed at stopping the bleeding, keeping the airway clear of blood, and maintaining ventilation. Rigid bronchoscopy and tamponade of the bleeding site with vasoconstrictor-soaked pledgets may stop the bleeding, but if this procedure fails, immediate thoracotomy or bronchial embolization is necessary to control the bleeding site. Rapid control of the bleeding is essential with preservation of airway patency the overriding concern. If possible, a double-lumen tube should be inserted, but this may not be possible in the setting of massive hemorrhage. Blockage of the affected bronchus with packing or a Fogarty catheter (bronchial blocker) through the rigid bronchoscope and intubation with a single-lumen endotracheal tube after removal of the bronchoscope is an alternative approach.

Interpleural Hemorrhage

Bleeding from the lung surface usually decreases rapidly in the first 12 hours postoperatively. Some blood loss is expected but should not exceed 500 mL in 24 hours. Sustained blood loss in excess of 150 to 200 mL per hour suggests surgical bleeding. Pleural-space bleeding is more common after repeat thoracotomy or previous pleural infection. Potential sources of severe hemorrhage include bleeding from divided pulmonary arteries and veins due to inadequate ligature or staple placement. Pulmonary circulation bleeding is rare but can be catastrophic. Rapid blood loss requires immediate reexploration to control the hemorrhage. Monitoring of pleural-space bleeding can be performed using thoracostomy-tube drainage and serial chest radiography. The use of large-bore thoracostomy tubes is very important in this situation because excessive bleeding will form clots in the chest and may obstruct smaller chest tubes. A clotted hemothorax may require repeat thoracotomy for evacuation. Adequate fluid and blood replacement should be instituted before reexploration is undertaken. Excessive bleeding that occurs for longer than 24 hours after the thoracic operation is quite unusual and is often secondary to vessel erosion by infection at a suture line or pressure from a cut rib or thoracostomy tube.

Pleural Effusion

A persistent or increasing effusion, when combined with signs of sepsis, may indicate an empyema. Pleural infection may be related to an air leak, failure of the remaining lung to fill the hemithorax, operative contamination, or preexistent pulmonary infection. Identification of the source of infection (bronchopleural fistula, chest-wall infection, or gastrointestinal fistula), immediate and possibly prolonged drainage, and the administration of antibiotic medications are important factors in the treatment of the empyema. Rib resection (Claggett window) and thoracoplasty may be necessary in some patients. Chylothorax occurs more commonly on the left rather than on the right after thoracotomy because the development of a chylothorax is related to surgical dissection between the aorta and esophagus. Disruption of the thoracic duct or one of its main branches results in escape of chyle into the pleural space. Chyle is sterile and bacteriostatic, and, thus, infection is uncommon. Thoracostomy-tube drainage is necessary for 1 to 2 weeks until the leak closes; leaks that

continue beyond this time may require an operation with oversewing of the leaking lymphatics.

Torsion or Infarction

Torsion or infarction is possible if the blood vessels of the remaining lobe or segment become twisted as the lung reexpands to occupy the cavity after excision. Following lobectomy, structures that hold the lobes of the lung in place are disrupted or excised, that is, adjacent lobes, the inferior pulmonary ligament, and incomplete fissures. Extensive hilar and mediastinal dissection produces additional mobility. The middle lobe and lingula are most susceptible to torsion. Torsion usually occurs within the first 48 hours postoperatively. The higher-pressure pulmonary and bronchial arteries remain open, but the lower-pressure pulmonary veins collapse with venous outflow obstruction. The engorgement and enlargement of the lung area drained by the involved veins may result in tissue infarction. Serial chest radiographs will show a homogeneous density that is enlarging and is associated with hemoptysis, pyrexia, dyspnea, and tachycardia. Bronchoscopy is diagnostic; instead of a mucus plug, a distorted compressed bronchus will be seen. Immediate reexploration of the surgical site is indicated, with possible further excision required if nonviable lung is found.

Cardiac Herniation

Cardiac herniation is a rare complication of pulmonary resection. Wide surgical excision of the pericardium (to ensure adequate margins for tumor removal) plus excision of supporting lung tissue may allow the heart to herniate into the hemithorax (especially after pneumonectomy). Herniation occurs after chest closure in the early postoperative period and may be related to differential pressures in the two hemithoraxes pushing (or pulling) the heart through the defect. Although symptoms and signs may be sudden in onset and dramatic (decreased venous return, hypotension, and cardiovascular collapse, absent apical impulse, myocardial ischemia, dysrhythmias, obstruction to ventricular outflow, and myocardial infarction), the diagnosis may not be obvious if herniation is limited. Signs and symptoms may be much more profound with right-sided herniation compared with left-sided herniation because of the ease with which vena caval compression can occur. On the left side, herniation may cause no immediate signs or symptoms, although the apical impulse may be elevated to the second intercostal space. In severe cases, the chest radiograph will show protrusion of the heart into the operative hemithorax, and the electrocardiogram will demonstrate abnormal rotation of the electrical axis, dysrhythmias, and ST-segment and T-wave abnormalities. Immediate reoperation with correction of the herniation and pericardial patching should be undertaken. Temporizing measures (discontinuation of suction, placing the patient in the lateral decubitus position with the operative hemithorax uppermost, and controlling coughing) may help as the patient is prepared and transported to the operating room. For intubated patients, minimizing airway pressures and discontinuing PEEP are indicated in anticipation of operative correction.

Postoperative Infections

Pulmonary, pleural, or systemic infections can occur in a variety of conditions following thoracotomy. Critical issues here include the timing of the infection, the pattern of pulmonary involvement, intercurrent antibiotic use, ambient infections in the ICU, and the patient's immunologic status. Investigation and management are as outlined in Chapter 20.

Lung Transplantation

The major issues relating to the postoperative lung-transplant recipients are mechanical ventilation, hemodynamic and fluid management, tissue rejection, nutrition, and sepsis (see Chapter 75 for further discussion) (10). Weaning from mechanical ventilation commences when the patient's hemodynamic and gas-exchange statuses are stable. We usually use pressure-support weaning in conjunction with aggressive chest physiotherapy; typically, patients are extubated within 2 to 5 days.

Hemodynamic management is the same as for other postoperative patients but with minimization of fluid intake. Patients frequently demonstrate a hyperdynamic picture with elevated cardiac index and a depressed systemic vascular resistance (SVR). If the patient has systemic hypotension or a low cardiac output state, fluid boluses should be judiciously used and the clinician should be aware that a diagnosis of tamponade is possible. Tamponade may be caused by blood or fluid in the pericardium or from elevated intrathoracic pressure as a result of either graft edema and swelling or an excessively large graft. In some cases, right ventricular function may be critically dependent on adequate right coronary artery perfusion pressure, which may be best maintained by the use of vasopressors.

Tissue rejection may be acute or chronic. *Acute* rejection usually presents on the fourth or fifth day following the operation and presents as worsened gas exchange, pulmonary infiltrates, fever, and pulmonary hypertension. Definitive diagnosis requires a transbronchial or, rarely, an open-lung biopsy. In cases of acute graft dysfunction, characterized by V/Q mismatch, pulmonary hypertension, and elevated PVR, the use of inhaled nitric oxide (NO) has been shown to improve the gas exchange and selectively reduce PVR and pulmonary hypertension while not altering SVR (13). It is unclear whether NO changes outcome.

Nutrition is a key issue in lung-transplant recipients. In general, patients can receive enteral nutrition when gastrointestinal function returns, thereby maintaining a state of positive nitrogen balance. For patients with cystic fibrosis, enteral nutrition may not be possible, and osmotic cathartics can be used to prevent the development of bowel obstruction secondary to a meconium-ileus equivalent.

Sepsis is a considerable problem in this population. The issue of infection (pulmonary or systemic) in the immunocompromised host is reviewed in Chapter 51. The temporal pattern of pulmonary infiltrates gives the clinician an initial clue to the likely diagnosis, with bacterial pneumonia occurring on days 2 and 3, acute rejection on days 4 through 6, and cytomegalovirus (CMV) pneumonitis on week 4 following the operation. Prophylaxis is standard in many programs, focusing on bacterial, viral, and fungal pathogens. Antibacterial agents are administered according to the results of bacterial cultures from donor lungs. After 1 month, trimethoprim–sulfamethoxazole is given in prophylactic doses against *Pneumocystis carinii*; acyclovir against herpes simplex virus; and CMV-hyperimmune globulin against CMV. In addition, ganciclovir sodium is given to recipients of CMV-mismatched grafts.

Myasthenia Gravis

Following thymectomy for the treatment of MG, patients may require ventilatory support. Factors that suggest the likely need for postoperative ventilatory support include long duration of disease, coexisting respiratory disease, high requirement for anticholinesterase medication, and an FVC of less than 2.9 L. The need for postoperative mechanical ventilatory support also may depend on the specific type of operation—transsternal versus transcervical thymectomy—and additional coexisting patient factors. In our practice, we have not found scoring systems useful. We concentrate on ensuring absence of residual neuromuscular blockade and titrate anticholinesterase medication to the patient's clinical response. The single best marker for determining the need of intubation, or the likely success of extubation, is the result of sequential FVC measurements.

Patients with MG may develop acute deteriorations in their clinical strength, which may be a result of worsening of the MG process itself, insufficient medication, or excess effects of anticholinesterase medication. If the crisis is such that the airway or ventilation is compromised, the initial management is endotracheal intubation and ventilatory support, followed by medical interventions (optimization of anticholinesterase and antiinflammatory agents and plasmapheresis). Clinical signs and symptoms to distinguish between "cholinergic crisis" (excessive anticholinesterase medication) and "myasthenia crisis" are unreliable, and the issue is best determined by the patient's response to small doses (2 mg, followed by 8 mg if no response occurs) of intravenously administered edrophonium chloride. The use of edrophonium will result in an improvement in strength in a myasthenic crisis but will not have a significant impact on a cholinergic crisis.

Postthoracotomy Analgesia

Provision of effective analgesia for patients following thoracic operations is difficult for many reasons. First, the pain is among the most severe of any operative procedure. Second, the neuronal pathways involved in the transmission of pain are multiple and may involve the phrenic and intercostal nerves. Third, the nature of the injury producing the pain syndrome is complex and involves intentionally incised tissues as well as traumatically interrupted intercostal nerves, broken ribs, crushed parenchyma, and pleural disruption. Fourth, the pain is exacerbated by the presence of thoracostomy tubes. These factors contribute to the complexity and severity of postthoracotomy pain and may make optimal therapy difficult (14).

SYSTEMIC ANALGESIA

Several approaches may provide analgesia for patients following thoracic operations. Systemically administered opioids have traditionally served as the basis for postthoracotomy analgesia and are usually the therapy against which all other modalities are compared. These agents may be delivered by intravenous, transdermal, subcutaneous, or intramuscular routes and are limited by adverse effects, which include nausea, vomiting, somnolence, and respiratory depression. Superior analgesia, with reduced adverse effects, may be observed when systemically administered opioids are delivered using a patient-controlled system, but clinical studies have not provided verification.

In addition to the use of opioids, systemic administration of ketamine (15) has been associated with excellent analgesia. The main adverse effects of ketamine in this context are hallucinations and delirium, but at doses in the range of 1.0 mg/kg, these effects have not been noted.

Multiple studies have documented the efficacy of nonsteroidal antiinflammatory drugs (NSAIDs) in the treatment of postthoracotomy analgesia. The benefits of NSAID use in this context are demonstrated by decreased opioid consumption with a concomitant reduction in patient-reported pain scores (16,17). The pharmacologic basis for the clinical use of these agents has been described (18). The potential problems associated with the use of NSAIDs include gastrointestinal bleeding, decreased platelet function, and renal insufficiency. When NSAIDs are used on a short-term basis, these issues are unlikely to cause problems in low-risk patients (those patients without gastrointestinal bleeding or coagulopathy and who have normal renal function). The modes of NSAID administration to patients following thoracic operations depend on the agents chosen and the available preparations. Parenteral ketorolac, rectal indomethacin, rectal piroxicam, intravenous lysine acetyl salicylate, and rectal diclofenac sodium all have been shown to be efficacious in providing analgesia to patients after thoracic operations. Although this class of agents is clearly useful as an adjunct to systemically administered opioid analgesia, the efficacy of these drugs as additions to comprehensive epidural regimens is unclear.

Intercostal Analgesia

Intercostal analgesia involves blockade of the intercostal nerves by the injection of local anesthetic solutions (19). The modes of administration of these agents include direct injection intraoperatively before wound closure, percutaneous postoperative injection, or instillation through one or more implanted indwelling intercostal catheters. From the postoperative critical care perspective, the most useful method is to inject 3 to 5 mL of solution into the intercostal space containing the surgical incision and to inject the solution into the two spaces above and the two spaces below the incision. After careful aspiration, the clinician injects the solution close to and inferior to the rib. The systemic absorption is high with this technique, but clinical toxicity is seldom a problem. Pneumothorax is not a problem in this patient population because patients routinely have thoracostomy tubes in place. The overall role of this technique in postthoracotomy analgesia

is difficult to define, but continuous infusions and intermittent injections appear to be useful; little overall benefit is derived from the routine use of single preincisional intercostal injections. Patients recovering from general anesthesia who develop respiratory depression as a result of systemically administered opioids frequently benefit from the use of intercostal blockade.

Interpleural Analgesia

Interpleural analgesia is another alternative analgesic modality for this patient population (20,21). For this technique, local anesthetics are administered into the pleural space through a catheter, either as a continuous infusion or by intermittent injections. The precise mechanisms of action are unclear, but the clinical toxicity is low. This technique does provide temporary improvement in pain control, but it does not have a clear impact on the overall analgesic management of the patient following a thoracic operation.

Intrathecal Opioids

Intrathecal opioids have been used in patients for postthoracotomy analgesia (22), but adequately controlled studies are insufficient. The technique involves the lumbar intrathecal administration of a small dose of a long-acting opioid, usually morphine sulfate, either before or after the operation. The potential advantages include ease of administration and fewer adverse effects from the systemic analgesia because of dose-sparing effects; however, the important issues of respiratory depression and patient selection remain to be defined in this population.

Epidural Analgesia

Epidural analgesia has a long and somewhat controversial history in the provision of analgesia following thoracic operations. The mechanisms of action, clinical techniques, and potential complications involved with epidural analgesia have been discussed (23–26). Epidural analgesia may be administered by the thoracic or lumbar routes and may consist of local anesthetics, opioids, or a combination of both. Controversy exists regarding the most appropriate route of delivery of epidural opioids. No evidence shows that either route is definitely superior, but there is agreement on some facts. Lipid-soluble agents, such as fentanyl, are equally effective in this population, whether administered through the intravenous or lumbar–epidural routes (27). Thoracic–epidural administration of lipid-soluble opioids is probably superior, in terms of efficacy, compared to intravenous administration. Little rationale exists for the administration of thoracic, as opposed to lumbar, epidural lipophobic opioids (morphine or hydromorphone). Lumbar–epidural administration of morphine has clear benefits over intravenously administered morphine (28). No role exists for the concomitant use of either intravenously or epidurally administered opioid antagonists, or for opioid agonist-antagonist compounds, with epidural administration of opioids in patients after thoracotomy operations. When opioids are combined with local anesthetics and administered through the thoracic–epidural route, the resultant analgesia is frequently excellent. Combining the agents reduces the required doses of the individual agents, and using the thoracic, as opposed to the epidural site, may further decrease the amounts of drug required.

No role exists for the use of lumbar–epidural administration of local anesthetics, ostensibly administered in an attempt to provide dense thoracic analgesia, because the resultant hypotension is usually significant and the efficacy is limited. The administration of epidural analgesia, which usually begins in the operating room before the commencement of the operation, has the advantages of safe insertion of the catheter in the awake patient and allows the clinician to confirm the adequacy of the blockade. The catheters also can be easily inserted in the ICU, provided the usual precautions are taken with respect to consent, the physical insertion of the needle and catheter, and careful titration of epidural drugs in a potentially somnolent patient whose condition may be unstable.

Paravertebral Blockade

Paravertebral blockade can provide analgesia and neural blockade equivalent to that of a unilateral epidural block (29,30). In this regard, paravertebral blockade provides a particularly attractive method of postthoracotomy analgesia. With this technique, the sympathetic blockade is unilateral, and, thus, the adverse effects of sympathectomy may be reduced. The doses of local anesthetic solution are decreased, potentially resulting in less toxicity. The major complication of the technique is ipsilateral pneumothorax, which is usually not a significant problem in the context of an *in situ* ipsilateral thoracostomy drainage tube. The exact place of paravertebral blockade in providing postthoracotomy analgesia is unclear, however, and the optimum doses and combinations of agent remain to be determined.

Transcutaneous Electric Nerve Stimulation

Transcutaneous electric nerve stimulation (TENS) is a technique in which an electrical current is applied to the skin, resulting in diminished nociception through a mechanism that is unclear. Although the technique has been used in a variety of settings, the studies in postthoracotomy patients are inconclusive. The use of TENS is associated with virtually no significant adverse effects other than skin irritation and potential interference with the functioning of an electronic pacemaker.

SUMMARY

The critical care management of patients before and after thoracic operations is a diverse practice involving pathophysiologic alterations in a variety of systems and demands a wide range of skills. Optimum care of these patients is challenging, but in modern practice and with appropriate patient selection, excellent outcome in terms of morbidity, mortality, patient comfort, and resource use can be achieved.

KEY POINTS

Innovative therapies have expanded our ability to assess patients with pulmonary disease; provide broader care alternatives, frequently with less physiologic transgression; potentially improve or reverse progressive disease; and care for older or more compromised patients.

Patients who undergo thoracic surgical procedures have unique perioperative needs. They require focused evaluation of their baseline respiratory mechanics, gas exchange, and cardiopulmonary reserve to determine whether they are likely to have adequate postoperative function to allow surgical intervention. Furthermore, judicious perioperative fluid balance, respiratory therapy, and pain management are required to provide optimal care.

Patients undergoing operations for major airway obstruction require anatomic and physiologic definition of the problem. Critical preoperative issues include the presence of airway compression or invasion, the extent of the lesion, the exact location of obstruction, and the presence of vascular or cardiac compromise.

Lung-reduction operations continue to be evaluated as a means to improve the quality of life of selected patients who are severely restricted by emphysema and thoracic hyperinflation. The goal is to reduce resting lung volume to improve the pressure–volume position of the lung and limit the work of breathing of the patient. Early extubation is recommended to avoid barotrauma and pulmonary complications.

Improved immunosuppression and surgical techniques, such as single-lung or sequential single-lung transplants, have aided the growth of lung transplantation. Further application of this therapy is limited by organ availability; challenges in organ preservation; and infection, rejection, and the delayed development of bronchiolitis obliterans in the transplanted lung.

Myasthenia gravis is an autoimmune disease caused by autoantibodies against skeletal-muscle cholinergic receptors. It develops most commonly in younger women who characteristically have muscle weakness and fatigue with muscle use. Thymectomy is highly effective in selected patients with myasthenia. Patients undergoing thymectomy require careful dosing of their anticholinesterase and steroid therapy and assessment of postoperative respiratory function.

Bronchial-stump disruption may occur within a few days of pulmonary resection, usually from technical difficulty or surgical error. Delayed disruption tends to occur a week or even later after the operation and occurs in more debilitated patients who developed ischemia and necrosis of the stump. Disruption causes a large bronchopleural fistula and is associated with a 20% mortality rate.

Postthoracotomy pain is frequently intense and is exacerbated by respiration and the presence of a thoracostomy tube. Although epidural analgesia is a popular choice from the many options available to treat postthoracotomy pain, optimal use of this technique remains controversial.

REFERENCES

1. Goldman L, Caldera D, Nussbaum, et al. Multifactorial index of cardiac risk in noncardiac surgical procedures. *N Engl J Med* 1977;297:845–850.

2. Detsky AS, Abrams HB, Forbath N, et al. Cardiac assessment for patients undergoing non-cardiac surgery: a multifactorial clinical risk index. *Arch Int Med* 1986;146:2131–2134.

3. Harman E, Lillington G. Pulmonary risk factors in surgery. *Med Clin North Am* 1979;63:1289–1298.

4. Petty TL. Pulmonary function testing: a practical approach. In: Pearson FG, Deslauriers J, Ginsberg RJ, et al., eds. *Thoracic surgery.* New York: Churchill Livingstone; 1995:57–68.

5. Markos J, Mullan BP, Hillman DR, et al. Preoperative assessment as a predictor of mortality and morbidity after lung resection. *Am Rev Respir Dis* 1989:902.

6. Miller JI Jr. Physiologic evaluation of pulmonary function in the candidate for lung resection. *J Thorac Cardiovasc Surg* 1993;105:347.

7. Sandler AN. Anesthesia. In: Pearson FG, Deslauriers J, Ginsberg RJ, et al., eds. *Thoracic surgery.* New York: Churchill Livingstone, 1995:85–112.

8. Lewis R, Caccavale RJ, Sisler GE. Video-assisted thoracic surgery. In: Pearson FG, Deslauriers J, Ginsberg RJ, et al., eds. *Thoracic surgery.* New York: Churchill Livingstone, 1995:917–929.

9. Cooper JD, Trulock EP, Triantafillon AN, et al. Bilateral pneumonectomy (volume reduction) for chronic obstructive pulmonary diseases. *J Thorac Cardiovasc Surg* 1995;109:106.

10. Patterson GA, Cooper JD. Lung transplantation. In: Pearson FG, Deslauriers J, Ginsberg RJ, et al., eds. *Thoracic surgery.* New York: Churchill Livingstone, 1995:931–959.

11. Finley JC, Pascuzzi RM. Rational therapy of myasthenia gravis. *Semin Neurol* 1990;10:70–82.

12. Krowka MJ, Pairolero PC, Trastek VF, et al. Cardiac dysrhythmia following pneumonectomy: clinical correlates and prognostic significance. *Chest* 1987;91:490.

13. Kavanagh BP, Pearl RG. Inhaled nitric oxide in anesthesia and critical care medicine. *Int Anesthesiol Clin* 1995;33:181–210.

14. Kavanagh BP, Katz J, Sandler AN. Pain control after thoracic surgery: a review of current techniques. *Anesthesiology* 1994;81:737–759.

15. Dich-Nielsen JO, Svendsen LB, Berthelsen P. Intramuscular low-dose ketamine versus pethidine for postoperative pain treatment after thoracic surgery. *Acta Anaesthesiol Scand* 1992;36:583–587.

16. Keenan DJM, Cave K, Langdon L, et al. Comparative trial of rectal indomethacin and cryoanalgesia for control of early postthoracotomy pain. *BMJ* 1983;287:1335–1337.

17. Perttunen K, Kalso E, Heinonen J, et al. IV diclofenac in postthoracotomy pain. *Br J Anaesth* 1992;68:474–480.

18. Dahl JB, Kehlet H. Non-steroidal anti-inflammatory drugs: rationale for use in severe postoperative pain. *Br J Anaesth* 1991;66:703–712.

19. Chan VWS, Chung F, Cheng DCH, et al. Analgesic and pulmonary effects of continuous intercostal nerve block following thoracotomy. *Can J Anaesth* 1991;38:733–739.

20. Camporesi EM. Interpleural analgesia: a new technique [Editorial]. *J Cardiothorac Anesth* 1989;3:137–138.

21. Covino BG. Interpleural regional analgesia [Editorial]. *Anesth Analg* 1988;67:427–429.

22. Gray JR, Fromme GA, Nauss LA, et al. Intrathecal morphine for postthoracotomy pain. *Anesth Analg* 1986;65:873–876.

23. Cousins MJ, Mather LE. Intrathecal and epidural administration of opioids. *Anesthesiology* 1984;61:276–310.

24. Cousins MJ, Bromage PR. Epidural neural blockade. In: Cousins MJ, Bridenbaugh PO, eds. *Neural blockade in clinical anesthesia and management of pain,* 2nd ed. Philadelphia: JB Lippincott, 1988:252–360.

25. Bridenbaugh PO, Green NM. In: Cousins MJ, Bridenbaugh PO, eds. *Neural blockade in clinical anesthesia and management of pain,* 2nd ed. Philadelphia: JB Lippincott, 1988:213–251.

26. Etches RC, Sandler AN, Daley MD. Respiratory depression and spinal opioids. *Can J Anaesth* 1989;36:165–185.

27. Sandler AN, Stringer D, Panos L, et al. A randomized, double-blind comparison of lumbar epidural and intravenous fentanyl infusions for postthoracotomy pain relief. Analgesic, pharmacokinetic, and respiratory effects. *Anesthesiology* 1992;77:626–634.

28. Shulman M, Sandler AN, Bradley JW, et al. Postthoracotomy pain and pulmonary function following epidural and systemic morphine. *Anesthesiology* 1984;61:569–575.

29. Conacher ID, Kokri M. Postoperative paravertebral blocks for thoracic surgery: a radiological appraisal. *Br J Anaesth* 1987;59:155–161.

30. Matthews PJ, Govenden V. Comparison of continuous paravertebral and extradural infusions of bupivacaine for pain relief after thoracotomy. *Br J Anaesth* 1989;62:204–205.

RESPIRATORY CARE

WILLIAM T. PERUZZI
BARRY A. SHAPIRO

INTRODUCTION

Respiratory support encompasses a wide range of prophylactic, therapeutic, and diagnostic interventions. These range from simple oxygen-delivery systems to invasive and complicated interventions such as bronchoscopy and airway-pressure therapy. The application of the correct modality at the appropriate time often results in a favorable outcome with minimal risks. Inappropriate or delayed application of the necessary modality may result in serious clinical deterioration and the need for more invasive and more expensive supportive measures later. It is important to understand not only the types of respiratory care modalities available but also the organization of a respiratory care department, the role of respiratory therapists, and how these paradigms are changing in the current socioeconomic environment.

OXYGEN THERAPY
Disorders Of Oxygenation

Hypoxemia can be defined as a relative deficiency of oxygen in the arterial blood. *Hypoxia* exists when oxygen tension at the cellular level is inadequate. Distinguishing the terms is important because either one may exist without the other. For example, it is not uncommon for a patient with acute or chronic lung disease to have an arterial oxygen tension (PaO_2) of 65 mm Hg. This level clearly represents hypoxemia, but, in the absence of dyspnea, acidosis, or cardiac arrhythmias, there is no evidence of tissue oxygen deprivation; thus, the patient is not hypoxic. Conversely, a patient with a PaO_2 of 90 mm Hg, a cardiac index (CI) of 1.5 L

per minute per M^2, hypotension, and metabolic acidosis is demonstrating hypoxia resulting from decreased oxygen delivery; however, the patient is not hypoxemic.

The alveolar partial pressure of oxygen (PaO_2) results from a dynamic equilibrium between oxygen delivery to the alveolus and oxygen extraction from the alveolus. As Figure 1 schematically illustrates, oxygen delivery to the alveolus is a function of the minute ventilation (V_E) and the inspired oxygen fraction (FIO_2), whereas oxygen extraction from the alveolus is a function of the deoxygenation status of blood presented to the alveolus ($SvO_2 \times Hgb = C_{VO_2}$) and the capillary blood flow (Qc). If the factors that determine oxygen extraction remain constant, a decrease in alveolar ventilation or FIO_2 will result in less oxygen delivery to the alveolus. Because the alveolar contents of nitrogen and water vapor remain essentially unchanged, the PaO_2 must decrease; therefore, the capillary blood will equilibrate with a lower PaO_2.

If factors determining alveolar oxygen delivery remain constant, a decrease in pulmonary artery (PA) oxygen content (C_{VO_2}) or an increase in capillary blood flow will result in more oxygen extraction from the alveolus. There are three major reasons for mixed venous blood to have decreased oxygen content. First, an increase in metabolic rate increases oxygen consumption ($\dot{V}O_2$). If there is no increase in perfusion, the tissues will extract more oxygen from each deciliter of blood and thereby decrease the venous blood oxygen content. Second, decreased cardiac output (CO) at a constant ($\dot{V}O_2$) requires the tissues to extract more oxygen from each deciliter of blood, thereby decreasing the venous blood oxygen content. Third, a decreased arterial oxygen content will result in a lower venous oxygen content after the normal extraction of oxygen by the tissues. Obviously, a compensatory mechanism for all three scenarios is an increase in CO. The preceding presentation has attempted to express the specific gas-exchange factors that are traditionally referred to as the *ventilation–perfusion* (V/Q) relationship. Low V/Q refers to perfusion in excess of ventilation, leading to a decreased alveolar oxygen tension and hypoxemia. It is important to recognize that changes in FIO_2 and SvO_2 can change the alveolar PO_2 without changing the V/Q relationship. Therefore, arterial oxygenation deficits must be considered beyond the scope of V/Q relationships.

Anatomic shunting is defined as blood that goes from the right side to the left side of the heart without traversing pulmonary capillaries. *Capillary shunting* is defined as blood that goes from

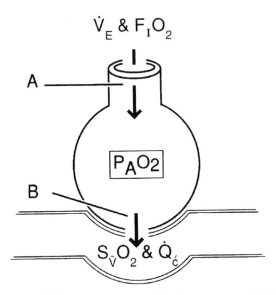

FIGURE 1. Alveolar oxygen tension (Pa_{O_2}) is determined from the dynamic equilibrium established between the alveolar oxygen delivery (arrow A) and the alveolar oxygen extraction (arrow B). Alveolar oxygen delivery is a function of the minute ventilation (V_E) and the inspired oxygen fraction ($F_{I_{O_2}}$). Alveolar O_2 extraction is a function of the pulmonary arterial oxygenation status (Sv_{O_2}) and the capillary blood flow (Qc). (From Shapiro BA, Peruzzi WT, Templin R. *Clinical application of blood gases*, 5th ed. St. Louis: Mosby–Year Book, 1994;48, with permission.)

the right side to the left side of the heart by traversing pulmonary capillaries that are adjacent to unventilated alveoli. In both circumstances, right heart blood enters the left heart without an increase in oxygen content. This phenomenon is traditionally referred to as *zero* V/Q, or *true shunting*, because the blood does not interact with alveolar gas. Shunting and hypoxemia are not synonymous terms, nor do they have linear relationships. The hypoxemic effect of any shunt will depend both on the size of the shunt and on the oxygenation status of the blood that shunts. A small shunt in a patient with a low Sv_{O_2} may have profound hypoxemic effects, whereas a large shunt in patient with a high Sv_{O_2} may cause only mild hypoxemia.

Oxygen diffusion defects, resulting from edema fluid or fibrous tissue between the alveolar epithelium and the capillary endothelium, can impose a significant impediment to oxygen diffusion and inhibit equilibration between pulmonary capillary and alveolar oxygen tensions. This impaired oxygen exchange is worsened as blood transit time decreases (blood transverses the lung more rapidly). Arterial hypoxemia secondary to diffusion defects is not common but is responsive to an increase in alveolar Po_2.

A V/Q mismatch can result from retained bronchial secretions, bronchospasm, obstructive endobronchial lesions, chronic obstructive pulmonary disease (COPD), pulmonary edema, or other pulmonary pathology. The hallmark of hypoxemia due to V/Q mismatch is that it is responsive to oxygen therapy. To determine oxygen responsiveness, an appropriate oxygen challenge must be given (1). If, at sea level, the $F_{I_{O_2}}$ is increased by 0.2 (i.e., from 0.2 to 0.4 or from 0.3 to 0.5), the Pa_{O_2} of all ventilated alveoli should increase by at least 90 to 100 mm Hg. Subsequently, the Pa_{O_2} will increase by significantly more than 10 mm Hg if less than 15% true shunt is present; however, it will increase by

significantly less than 10 mm Hg if greater than 30% true shunt exists.

True shunt can result from several different pathologic conditions: intracardiac shunt, alveolar collapse as occurs in acute lung injury (ALI), pulmonary consolidation associated with lung infections, segmental or lobar lung collapse resulting from retained secretions or other lung pathology, pulmonary arterial–venous malformations or pulmonary-capillary dilation as sometimes seen in liver disease, and large vascular lung tumors. Oxygen therapy is of limited benefit with true shunt. The reason is that, regardless of the $F_{I_{O_2}}$ or Pa_{O_2}, oxygen transfer cannot occur when blood does not come into contact with functional alveolar units. Therefore, true shunt pathology is refractory to oxygen therapy. For several types of pathology resulting in true shunt, there is little or no available therapy; antibiotics or surgical interventions may help other types of true shunt-producing disease. The type of lung pathology that is the most responsive to therapy is that involving diffuse or focal lung collapse. Segmental or lobar lung collapse often can be reversed with appropriate bronchial hygiene or removal of the source of obstruction.

Diffuse alveolar collapse often results from destabilization of the alveolar architecture resulting from disruption of the surfactant layer and alveolar epithelial damage associated with ALI (2,3). This type of pathology is responsive to positive endexpiratory pressure (PEEP) (4). PEEP levels of 5 to 10 cm H_2O will increase alveolar size and redistribute interstitial lung water from the interstitial regions between the alveolar epithelium and pulmonary-capillary endothelium to the peribronchial and hilar regions of the lung. (5,6) PEEP levels of 15 cm or greater of H_2O no longer increase alveolar size; rather, these levels of PEEP "recruit" nonfunctional collapsed alveoli to expanded and functional alveolar units (7).

Oxygen Administration

When dealing with lung pathology that is potentially amenable to treatment with oxygen administration, the indications for oxygen therapy and the available methods of oxygen administration must be considered. To understand the indications for oxygen therapy, the physiologic responses to hypoxemia and hypoxia must be appreciated. First, there is an increase in minute ventilation, which increases alveolar ventilation and the work of breathing. Second, there is an increase in CO, which maintains oxygen delivery in the face of a decrease in arterial oxygen content but increases the stress placed on the cardiovascular system. Therefore, the goals of oxygen therapy are to improve arterial oxygen content and subsequently decrease the work of breathing and myocardial stress.

Oxygen Content

Oxygen content is determined by the concentration of hemoglobin (Hgb) in the blood, the percentage of the Hgb that is saturated with oxygen, the maximal amount of oxygen that can be bound to Hgb (constant of 1.34 mL O_2/g hemoglobin), and the amount of oxygen dissolved in the plasma (0.003 mL O_2/mm Hg). Thus,

$$Ca_{O_2} = [Hgb] \cdot [Sa_{O_2}] \cdot [1.34] + [Pa_{O_2}] \cdot [0.003]$$

It should be obvious that the primary determinant of oxygen content is the Hgb concentration (g/dL) and the degree of Hgb saturation (expressed as a decimal). At atmospheric pressure, the amount of oxygen dissolved in the plasma ($[PaO_2]$ [0.003]) is usually negligible. The value of 1.34 mL per gram of Hgb represents the amount of oxygen that can be bound to Hgb contained within a red-blood-cell membrane; a value of 1.39 mL per gram of Hgb sometimes is used and represents the amount of oxygen that can be bound by stroma-free Hgb, which occurs when cells are lysed during co-oximetry measurements (8).

Oxygen-delivery Systems

There are three basic types of gas delivery systems: rebreathing systems, nonrebreathing systems, and partial rebreathing systems. Rebreathing systems collect exhaled gases into a reservoir on the expiratory limb of the system, which contains a carbon-dioxide absorber (permitting the reentry of expiratory gases into the inspiratory gas flow without rebreathing of carbon dioxide). This system is used primarily for the delivery of anesthetic gases to conserve expensive volatile anesthetics. Such systems have little or no use in current critical care settings.

A partial rebreathing system is one in which the initial portion of the expired gases, consisting mainly of gas from the anatomic dead space, is expired into a reservoir while the latter portions of the expiratory gases are vented to the atmosphere through one-way valves. The expiratory gases from the anatomic dead space contain little carbon dioxide and therefore can be rebreathed without significant consequences. The reservoir also receives fresh inspiratory gas flow; thus, the patient breathes both expiratory gas, containing little carbon dioxide, and fresh inspiratory gas.

Most oxygen-delivery systems are nonrebreathing systems in that all expiratory gases are vented in such a fashion that exhaled carbon dioxide is not rebreathed during subsequent breaths. This is often accomplished with one-way valves to prevent mixing of inspired and expired gases.

Nonrebreathing systems are divided into high-flow (fixed performance) and low-flow (variable performance) systems. A *high-flow* system means that the inspiratory gas flow rate delivered by the system is sufficient to meet the peak inspiratory-flow demands of the patient. Thus, all inspiratory gas is supplied by the oxygen delivery system and the FIO_2 is both known and stable. To accomplish this, the inspiratory gas flows must be three to four times the measured minute ventilation (9). The use of high-flow oxygen-delivery systems is indicated whenever there is a need for a consistent and predictable FIO_2, especially in patients with unstable ventilatory patterns.

Conversely, a *low-flow* system delivers a fixed amount of oxygen to the patient, and entrainment of room air is necessary to meet the patient's peak inspiratory-flow rates. In this setting, the FIO_2 is variable and unpredictable if the patient has an abnormal or changing pattern of ventilation. If the patient has a stable, normal pattern of ventilation, however, low-flow oxygen-delivery systems can deliver a predictable and consistent FIO_2 (Table 1).

It must be understood that use of a low-flow oxygen-delivery system does not imply delivery of low oxygen concentrations. For example, it is possible to calculate the FIO_2 for a low-flow system, such as a nasal cannula, if certain assumptions are made as follows: (a) the anatomic reservoir (nose, nasopharynx, and

TABLE 1. FLOW RATES AND FIO_2, WITH LOW-FLOW OXYGEN-DELIVERY DEVICES

Low-Flow System	Oxygen Flow Rates (L/min)	FIO_2
Nasal cannula	1	0.24
	2	0.28
	3	0.32
	4	0.36
	5	0.40
	6	0.44
Simple face mask	5–6	0.40
	6–7	0.50
	7–8	0.60
Partial-rebreathing mask	6	0.60
	7	0.70
	8	0.80
	9	0.80+
	10	0.80+
Nonrebreathing mask	10	0.80+
	15	0.90+

Predicted FIO_2 values for low-flow systems assume a normal and stable pattern of ventilation.
Modified from Shapiro BA, Peruzzi WT, Templin R. *Clinical application of blood gases*, 5th ed. Chicago: Mosby-Year Book, 1994, with permission.

oropharynx) is approximately 50 mL or one-third of the anatomic dead space (150 mL); (b) the oxygen flow rate is 6 L per minute (100 mL/sec) via the nasal cannulae; (c) the patient's respiratory rate of 20 breaths per minute results in a 1-second inspiratory phase and a 2-second expiratory phase; and (d) there is negligible gas flow during the terminal 0.5-second of the expiratory phase, thus allowing the anatomic reservoir to completely fill with oxygen. Using the preceding assumptions, the FIO_2 can be calculated for variable tidal volumes (V_T) (Table 2). This variability in FIO_2 at 6 L per minute of oxygen flow clearly demonstrates the effects of a changing ventilatory pattern on FIO_2. In general, the larger the V_T or the faster the respiratory rate, the lower the FIO_2. The smaller the V_T or lower the respiratory rate, the higher the FIO_2. With a stable, unchanging ventilatory pattern and oxygen-flow rate, low-flow systems can deliver a relatively consistent FIO_2.

Low-flow Systems

Low-flow oxygen devices are the most commonly used oxygen-delivery systems because of their simplicity, ease of use, health

TABLE 2. VARIABILITY IN FIO_2 WITH LOW-FLOW OXYGEN-DELIVERY SYSTEMS AND VARIABLE PATTERNS OF VENTILATION

	V_T = 500 mL	V_T = 250 mL
Anatomic reservoir	50 mL O_2	50 mL O_2
Inspiratory phase (1 sec)	100 mL O_2	100 mL O_2
Entrained room air	350 mL	100 mL
O_2 from entrained room air (21% oxygen)	70 mL O_2	20 mL O_2
Total volume O_2/V_T	220 mL/500 mL	170 mL/250 mL
FIO_2	0.44	0.68

V_T, tidal volume; FIO_2, inspired oxygen concentration.
Modified from Vender JS, Spiess BD. *Post anesthesia care*. Philadelphia: WB Saunders, 1992, with permission.

care providers' familiarity with the systems, economics, and patient acceptance. In most clinical situations, low-flow systems are acceptable and preferable.

Nasal Cannula

The nasal cannula is the most frequently used oxygen-delivery device because of its simplicity, ease of use, and comfort. To be effective, the patient's nasal passages must be patent to allow filling of the anatomic reservoir; however, the patient does not need to breathe through the nose. Oxygen will be entrained from the anatomic reservoir even in the presence of mouth breathing. If the oxygen flow rate exceeds 4 L per minute, the gases should be humidified to prevent drying of the nasal mucosa. Flows greater than 6 L per minute will not increase the F_{IO_2} significantly above 0.44 and often are poorly tolerated by the patient.

Simple Face Mask

A simple face mask consists of a mask with two side ports. The mask provides an additional 100- to 200-mL oxygen reservoir and will provide a higher F_{IO_2} than will a nasal cannula. The open ports in the sides of the mask allow entrainment of room air and venting of exhaled gases. A minimum flow of 5 L per minute is necessary to prevent carbon-dioxide accumulation and rebreathing. Flow rates greater than 8 L per minute will not increase the F_{IO_2} significantly above 0.6.

Partial-rebreathing Mask

A partial-rebreathing mask (Fig. 2A) is similar in construction to the simple face mask, but it also incorporates a 600- to 1,000-mL reservoir bag into which fresh gas flows. The first one-third of the patient's exhaled gas fills the reservoir bag. Because this gas

is primarily from anatomic dead space, it contains little carbon dioxide. With the next breath, the patient inhales a mixture of the exhaled gas and fresh gas. If the fresh gas flows are equal to or greater than 8 L per minute and the reservoir bag remains inflated throughout the entire respiratory cycle, adequate carbon dioxide evacuation and the highest possible F_{IO_2} should occur. The rebreathing capacity of this system allows some degree of oxygen conservation, which may be useful while transporting patients with portable oxygen supplies.

Tracheostomy Collars

Tracheostomy collars are used primarily to deliver humidity to patients with artificial airways. Oxygen may be delivered with these devices, but, similar to other low-flow systems, the F_{IO_2} is unpredictable, inconsistent, and depends on the ventilatory pattern.

High-flow Systems

Although high-flow systems are more complex, more labor intensive to initiate and maintain, and more expensive, clinical situations in which it is important to deliver a precise F_{IO_2} require their use.

Venturi Mask

These masks entrain air using the Bernoulli principle and constant pressure-jet mixing (10). This physical phenomenon is based on a rapid velocity of gas (e.g., oxygen) moving through a restricted orifice (Fig. 3). This movement produces viscous shearing forces, which create a subatmospheric pressure gradient downstream relative to the surrounding gases. This pressure gradient causes room air to be entrained until the pressures are equalized. In this manner, flows high enough to meet the patient's

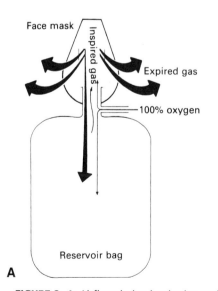
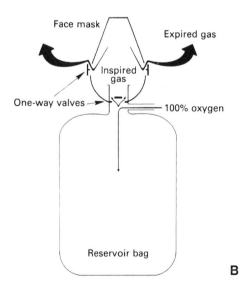

FIGURE 2. A: Airflow during inspiration and expiration through a partial-rebreathing mask. Note the first part of the exhaled gas from the anatomic dead space enters the reservoir bag to be inspired with the next breath. **B:** Airflow during inspiration and expiration through a nonrebreathing mask. Note that all expired gas exits through one-way valves on the sides of the mask and is precluded from entering the reservoir bag by an additional one-way valve. (From Shapiro BA, Kacmarek RM, Cane RD, et al. *Clinical application of respiratory care*, 4th ed. St. Louis: Mosby–Year Book, 1991:127, with permission.)

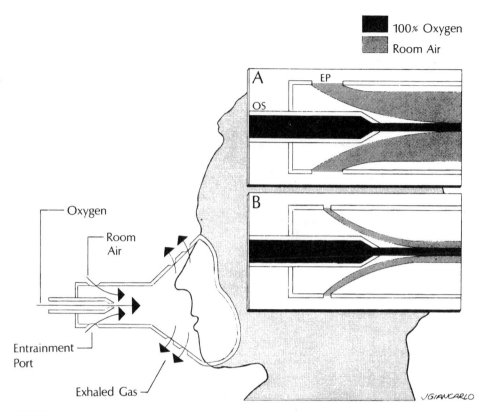

FIGURE 3. Principle of an air-entrainment device. Pressurized oxygen is forced through a constricted orifice; the increased gas velocity distal to the orifice creates a shearing effect that causes room air to be entrained through the entrainment ports. The high flow of gas fills the mask; holes allow both exhaled and delivered gases to escape. Insets A and B illustrate that the size of the entrainment ports (EP) determines the amount of room air to be entrained; OS is the oxygen source. Large ports (**A**) result in relatively low F_{IO_2}; small ports (**B**) result in relatively higher F_{IO_2}. For any size EP, the F_{IO_2} is stable; however, the total gas flow will vary with the pressurized oxygen flow (see text). (From Burton GG, Hodgkin JE, Ward JJ, eds. *Respiratory care*, 3rd ed. Philadelphia: JB Lippincott, 1991, with permission.)

peak-inspiratory demands can be generated. As the desired F_{IO_2} increases, the air-to-oxygen-entrainment ratio decreases with a net reduction in total gas flow. Therefore, the probability of the patient's needs exceeding the total flow capabilities of the device increases with higher F_{IO_2} settings. Occlusion of or impingement on the exhalation ports of the mask can cause back pressure and can alter gas flow (*Venturi stall*). In addition, the oxygen-injector port can become clogged, especially with water droplets. Therefore, aerosol devices should not be used with Venturi masks; if humidity is necessary, a vapor-type humidifier should be used.

There are two basic types of Venturi systems: (a) a fixed F_{IO_2} model, which requires specific color-coded inspiratory attachments with labeled jets that produce a known F_{IO_2} with a given flow, and (b) a variable-F_{IO_2} model, which has graded adjustments of the air-entrainment port that can be set to allow variation in delivered F_{IO_2}.

Non-rebreathing Mask

A non-rebreathing mask (Fig. 2B) is similar to a partial rebreathing mask but with the addition of three unidirectional valves. Two of the valves are located on opposite sides of the mask. They permit venting of exhaled gas and prevent entrainment of room air. The remaining unidirectional valve is located between the mask and the reservoir bag and prevents exhaled gases from entering the fresh-gas reservoir. As with the partial-rebreathing mask, the reservoir bag should be inflated throughout the entire ventilatory cycle to ensure adequate carbon dioxide clearance from the system and the highest possible F_{IO_2}.

To avoid air entrainment around the mask and dilution of the delivered F_{IO_2}, masks should fit snugly on the face, but excessive pressure should be avoided. If the mask is fitted properly, the reservoir bag should respond to the patient's inspiratory efforts. Unfortunately, if fresh-gas flows and the volume of the reservoir bag are insufficient to meet inspiratory demands, the patient's well-being could be compromised. Therefore, masks may be fitted with a spring-loaded tension valve that will open and allow entrainment of room air as needed to meet inspiratory demands. If such a valve is not present, another option is to remove one of the unidirectional valves that prevent room-air entrainment. If the total ventilatory needs of the patient are met by the nonrebreathing system, the system then functions as a high-flow system. If room air entrainment occurs, then it is functioning as a low-flow system.

Aerosol Mask and T-Piece

An F_{IO_2} greater than 0.40 with a high-flow system is best provided with a large-volume nebulizer and wide-bore tubing. Aerosol masks, in conjunction with air-entrainment nebulizers or air/oxygen blenders, can deliver a consistent and predictable FIO_2 regardless of the patient's ventilatory pattern. A T-piece is used in place of an aerosol mask for patients with an endotracheal or tracheostomy tube. An air-entrainment nebulizer can deliver an FIO_2 of 0.35 to 1.0, produce an aerosol, and generate flow rates of 14 to 16 L per minute. As with Venturi masks, a higher FIO_2 results in less room-air entrainment and lower flow rates. If a greater total flow is required, two nebulizers can feed a single mask and increase the total flow. Air/oxygen blenders can deliver a consistent FIO_2 in the range of 0.21 to 1.0, with flows up to 100 L per minute. These devices are usually used in conjunction with humidifiers.

COMPLICATIONS OF OXYGEN THERAPY

Suppression of Respiratory Drive

When patients who retain carbon dioxide receive oxygen therapy, they may exhibit a depression in their respiratory drive. The resultant decrease in minute ventilation produces an increase in the $PaCO_2$, carbon dioxide narcosis, and further depression of the respiratory drive. Oxygen should be administered with caution to patients who retain carbon dioxide. More recent studies indicate that the increase in $PaCO_2$ is often due to an increase in V_D/V_T with oxygen therapy rather than to a decrease in respiratory drive.

Oxygen-absorption Atelectasis

Absorption atelectasis occurs when high alveolar oxygen concentrations cause alveolar collapse. Normally, nitrogen, which is at equilibrium with the blood, remains within the alveoli and "splints" alveoli open. When a high FIO_2 is administered, nitrogen is "washed out" of the alveoli, and the alveoli are filled primarily with oxygen. In areas of the lung with reduced V/Q ratios, oxygen will be absorbed into the blood faster than ventilation can replace it. The alveoli then become progressively smaller until they reach the critical volume at which surface-tension forces cause alveolar collapse. This phenomenon is precipitated primarily by the administration of an FIO_2 greater than 0.5 and is illustrated in Figure 4.

Oxygen Toxicity

A high FIO_2 can be injurious to the lungs. The mechanism of oxygen toxicity is related to production of oxygen free radicals such as superoxide anions ($O_2 \cdot^-$), hydroxyl radicals ($OH \cdot$), hydrogen peroxide (H_2O_2), and singlet oxygen ($^1O_2$). These radicals affect cell function by inactivating sulfhydryl enzymes, interfering with DNA synthesis, and disrupting the integrity of cell membranes. During periods of lung-tissue hyperoxia, the normal oxygen-radical-scavenging mechanisms are overwhelmed, and toxicity results (11). The FIO_2 at which oxygen toxicity becomes important is controversial and variable depending on the animal species, degree of underlying lung injury, ambient barometric pressure, and duration of exposure. In general, it is best to avoid exposure to an FIO_2 of greater than 0.5 for more than 24 hours.

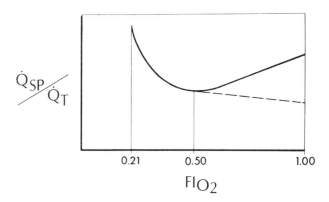

FIGURE 4. The general relationship between intrapulmonary shunt fractions (QSP/QT) and increasing inspired oxygen concentration (FIO_2). The shunt fraction diminishes as the FIO_2 is increased from 0.21 (room air) toward 0.50. This diminution is readily attributed to the decreasing hypoxemic effect of low ventilation perfusion (V/Q) as the alveolar PO_2 increases. As the FIO_2 is increased from 0.50 toward 1.0, the shunt fraction increases. Broken line depicts what would be anticipated if all low V/Q alveoli remained open as the FIO_2 increased. The observed increase in shunt fraction must be attributed to increased zero V/Q. (From Shapiro BA, Peruzzi WT, Templin R. *Clinical application of blood gases,* 5th ed. St. Louis: Mosby–Year Book, 1994, with permission.)

AIRWAY-CLEARANCE TECHNIQUES

Bronchial hygiene is useful and effective when the patient is carefully evaluated, the goals of therapy are clearly defined, and the appropriate modalities are applied.

Prophylactic Versus Therapeutic

Prophylactic bronchial hygiene therapy is administered to patients who are essentially free of acute pulmonary pathology with the intent of preventing inadequate bronchial hygiene. Therapeutic bronchial hygiene therapy is aimed at reversing preexisting inadequate bronchial hygiene, specifically the mobilization of retained secretions and the reinflation of atelectatic lung regions.

Humidification

Air inspired through the nose is warmed and nearly 90% humidified by the time it passes through the pharynx. The administration of dry oxygen lowers the water content of the inspired air, and the use of artificial airways bypasses the nasopharynx and oropharynx, where the humidification of inspired gases primarily takes place. If adequate humidification of inspired gases is not provided before the gas enters the trachea, the deficit of humidity is provided by moisture from the mucous blanket of the tracheobronchial tree. Thus, both oxygen administration and the use of artificial airways can increase the demands on the lung to humidify inspired gases. If humidification of inspired gases is not appropriately addressed, drying of the tracheobronchial tree, ciliary dysfunction, impairment of mucus transport, inflammation and necrosis of the ciliated pulmonary epithelium, retention of dried secretions, atelectasis, bacterial infiltration of the pulmonary mucosa, and pneumonia may occur. To prevent these complications, a humidifier or nebulizer should be used to increase the water content of inspired gases. A humidifier increases the water vapor in a gas. Humidification can be accomplished by passing gas over heated water (heated passover humidifier); by fractionating gas into tiny bubbles as gas passes through water (bubble humidifiers); by allowing gas to pass through a chamber that contains a heated, water-saturated wick (heated-wick humidifier); or by vaporizing water and selectively allowing the vapor to mix with the inspired gases (vapor-phase humidifier).

A nebulizer increases the water content of the inspired gas by generating aerosols (small droplets of particulate water) of uniform size, which become incorporated into the delivered gas stream and then evaporate into the inspired gas as it is warmed in the respiratory tract. There are two basic types of nebulizers. Pneumatic nebulizers operate from a pressurized-gas source and are either jet or hydronomic. Electric nebulizers are powered by an electric source and are referred to as *ultrasonic*. There are several varieties of the above nebulizers, which are more dependent on design differences than on the power source.

Incentive Spirometry

The incentive spirometer is an effective and inexpensive prophylactic bronchial hygiene tool. This device provides a visual goal or "incentive" for the patient to achieve and sustain a maximal inspiratory effort. When performed on an hourly basis, this modality provides optimal lung inflation, distribution of ventilation, and an improved cough. Thus, atelectasis and the retention of bronchial secretions are prevented. Incentive spirometry also can be helpful in the diagnosis of acute pulmonary pathology in that a sudden decrease in a patient's ability to perform at a previously established level may herald the onset of severe atelectasis, pneumonia, or other pulmonary pathology. For incentive spirometry to be effective, several conditions must exist: The patient must be cooperative, motivated, and well instructed in the technique (by the respiratory therapist, nurse, or physician); the patient must be able to obtain a vital capacity greater than 15 mL per kilogram or an inspiratory capacity greater than 12 mL per kilogram; and the patient should not be tachypneic or receiving a high F_{IO_2}.

Chest Physical Therapy

Chest physical therapy (CPT) techniques can be classified into those that promote bronchial hygiene, those that improve breathing efficiency, or those that promote physical reconditioning. The CPT techniques considered here are those concerned with bronchial hygiene.

Postural Drainage

Postural drainage is a technique that uses different body positions to facilitate gravitational drainage of mucus from various lung segments (Fig. 5). Diseases that are amenable to postural drainage therapy include cystic fibrosis, bronchiectasis, COPD, acute atelectasis, lung abscess, and others. In hospitalized patients, the basilar lung regions often benefit from postural drainage because most hospital-bed positions do not permit adequate drainage of

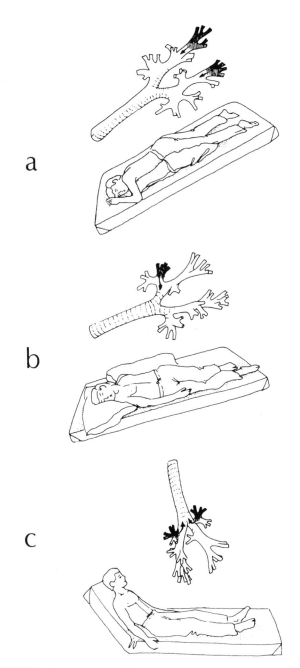

FIGURE 5. Common postural drainage positions for **a**, posterior basilar segments; **b**, middle lobe and lingula; and **c**, apical segments of upper lobes. (From Shapiro BA, Kacmarek RM, Cane RD, et al. *Clinical application of respiratory care*, 4th ed. St. Louis: Mosby–Year Book, 1991, with permission.)

these segments. When performing postural drainage of unilateral lung disease, it is best to follow with drainage of the contralateral lung. The reason for this is that cross-contamination of the nondiseased lung is always a possibility. It is important to avoid inappropriate positioning during postural drainage. Patients with increased intracranial pressure (ICP) or congestive heart failure (CHF) may not tolerate head-down positioning to facilitate drainage of the basilar lung segments. Also, it is important to avoid direct pressure on sites of injury, operations, or burns.

Percussion and Vibration

External manipulation of the thorax, in the form of percussion and vibration, is used to facilitate the process of postural drainage. Chest percussion and vibration are techniques used to loosen and mobilize secretions that adhere to bronchial walls (12). The purpose of percussion is intermittently to apply kinetic energy to the chest wall and lung. Chest percussion is accomplished by rhythmically striking the thorax with cupped hands or a mechanical device placed directly over the lung segment to be drained. This force generates a mechanical energy wave that is transmitted through the chest wall to the lung tissue and loosens adherent mucus (12,13). Mechanical percussion devices are available and have some theoretic advantages in that they apply vibratory or percussive forces in a more consistent, uniform fashion and are not subject to fatigue.

No convincing evidence, however, has demonstrated the superiority of one method over the other (14); health care providers who perform percussion and drainage must adhere to standard techniques to ensure the success of the maneuver.

Vibration normally follows percussion and involves the application of a fine tremorous action that is manually performed by pressing in the direction of the ribs and soft tissue of the chest. Chest vibration is accomplished by placing the hands on the chest wall and generating a rapid vibratory motion in the arms, from the shoulders, and gently compressing the chest wall in the direction that the ribs normally move during exhalation (12,15,16). Vibrations should be delivered over the draining area during the patient's expiration for optimal effect.

Indications and Contraindications

Indications for the use of CPT are the inability or reluctance of a patient to change body position (i.e., during mechanical ventilation or in paralyzed patients); the presence of segmental atelectasis; physical evidence of retained secretions; and the presence of diseases, such as cystic fibrosis, bronchiectasis, or cavitating lung disease, that result in increased mucus production. Contraindications to the use of CPT include situations in which proper positioning cannot be safely accomplished, when a patient's injuries would preclude appropriate percussion or vibratory maneuvers, or when preexisting disease processes could be exacerbated during the procedure (16). Specifically, contraindications to the Trendelenburg position include increased ICP, recent neurosurgical procedures, unclipped cerebral-artery aneurysms; uncontrolled hypertension, pulmonary edema associated with CHF, abdominal distention, increased risk for gastroesophageal reflux or aspiration (e.g., esophageal operation, altered airway-protective reflexes, or decreased mental status), ongoing epidural opioid or anesthetic infusion, and a recent eye operation. The reverse trendelenburg position is contraindicated for use in patients with hypotension or other hemodynamic instability. External manipulation of the thorax, such as percussion and vibration, is contraindicated in patients with subcutaneous emphysema; a recent skin graft or myocutaneous-flap procedures on the thorax; thermal injuries, open wounds or skin infections of the thorax; flail chest or fractures, osteomyelitis, or osteoporosis of the ribs; soft-tissue injuries to the thorax or complaints of chest-wall pain attributable to other causes; temporary transvenous pacemakers or recently inserted permanent pacemakers; suspected pulmonary tuberculosis, pulmonary embolism (PE), pulmonary contusions, or a bronchopleural fistula; large pleural effusions or an undrained empyema; increased ICP or other unstable intracranial pathology; unstable spine injuries or recent spine operation; active hemorrhage with hemodynamic instability; severe or uncontrolled coagulopathies; and confused or combative patients who do not tolerate physical manipulation.

Another hazard associated with CPT is the development of hypoxemia during the procedure. In many cases, hypoxemia can be treated by initiating oxygen therapy or increasing the inspired oxygen concentration during CPT. The decision to use CPT requires that the physician assess potential benefits versus potential risks and limitations. Therapy should be provided no longer than is necessary to obtain the desired therapeutic results.

Alternative Airway-clearance Techniques

In addition to the traditional CPT techniques, alternative airway-clearance methods, such as positive-expiratory-pressure (PEP) therapy, forced-expiratory technique (FET), and autogenic drainage (AD), recently gained support in the literature and are widely used in Europe (12,17–19). These techniques either serve as replacement for the traditional CPT or are used in conjunction with CPT to remove retained secretions and promote aerosol deposition. These techniques focus on controlled breathing and modified coughing techniques, but patients require significant training before they can adequately master the various maneuvers. Patients who actively participate in alternative airway-clearance methods are usually those with long-standing pulmonary processes, such as cystic fibrosis patients who can cooperate and tolerate the maneuvers. Patients in the intensive care unit (ICU) or patients with short-term pulmonary complications are not good candidates for treatment with alternative airway-clearance methods.

Intermittent Positive-pressure Breathing

Intermittent positive pressure breathing (IPPB) is the application of inspiratory positive pressure to the airway in order to provide a significantly larger tidal volume than the patient can produce spontaneously. IPPB should not be confused with positive-pressure ventilation delivered with a mechanical ventilator, which is intended to provide ventilatory support. IPPB is most useful in disease states in which the patient's depth of breathing is limited. This type of therapy is very expensive; therefore, for this mode of therapy to be indicated, the patient's vital capacity should be less than 15 ml/kg and the IPPB treatment should augment this volume by at least 100%. In addition, some endpoint should be planned for the therapy. The use of IPPB should be limited to those patients with severely compromised respiratory reserves who are suffering an acute illness or an exacerbation of a chronic condition that causes a temporary deterioration in their overall respiratory state. Patients with more severe and chronic ventilatory-reserve limitations often require a chronic artificial airway (i.e., tracheostomy) to maintain consistent bronchial hygiene.

Suctioning

Removal of bronchial secretions via suction is a commonly used bronchial-hygiene technique. Performed appropriately, this procedure is safe and effective. Performed without appropriate caution, it can result in significant complications or death. Airway suctioning can be accomplished safely in patients with artificial airways (endotracheal or tracheostomy tubes) in place. In these circumstances, the patient should be ventilated with a manual resuscitation bag and a high FIO_2. This "preoxygenation" will minimize the hypoxemia that is induced by removing the patient from an oxygen source and applying suction to the airways. A sterile suction catheter then should be placed into the airway and advanced, without the application of vacuum, beyond the tip of the artificial airway until the catheter can no longer be easily advanced. The catheter should be withdrawn slightly before suction is applied. Suctioning then can be accomplished by the intermittent application of vacuum and gradual withdrawal of the catheter in a rotating fashion. The duration of the entire procedure should not exceed 20 seconds. Following completion of suctioning, the patient should be manually ventilated with an oxygen-enriched atmosphere to ensure adequate lung reexpansion and oxygenation. The patient should be monitored for signs of distress, bronchospasm, hemodynamic instability, or arrhythmias throughout the entire procedure.

In the mechanically ventilated patient whose condition creates concerns of infection, either to the patient or to the health care professional who is rendering care, a closed-system suction catheter may be of benefit (20). Unlike open-system suction catheters, the closed-system suction catheters can be reused and physically incorporated into the patient's ventilator circuit at the connection between the ventilator circuit and the artificial airway. This system also may be used when any disconnection from mechanical ventilation or intermittent discontinuation of high levels of PEEP may result in compromise. In the closed system, the catheter itself is shrouded in a protective sleeve that allows the versatility of advancing or retracting the catheter in the patient's airway without interrupting mechanical ventilation. Unlike open-system suctioning, closed-system suctioning does not require the patient to be preoxygenated with a manual resuscitator; hypoxemia can be avoided by temporarily increasing the FIO_2 to 100% shortly before and during the suction maneuver. When fully retracted, the closed-system suction catheter does not create airway interference or obstruction and can be left in line for extended periods, usually 24 to 48 hours or as determined by an institution's infection-control policy.

Suctioning of the tracheobronchial tree without an artificial airway in place (i.e., nasotracheal suctioning) is practiced in many centers but carries several risks. Because the patient cannot be manually ventilated and "preoxygenated" before the procedure, hypoxemia and hemodynamically significant arrhythmias can occur (21,22). In addition, passing the suction catheter through the vocal cords can result in laryngospasm or vocal-cord injury with subsequent airway obstruction. In many patients who have

impaired but reasonable ventilatory reserves, this technique is often carried out without significant problems; however, patients with extremely marginal ventilatory reserves are at the greatest risk for the aforementioned complications.

Suctioning of the tracheobronchial tree should only be undertaken when appropriately indicated. The primary indication is the presence of bronchial secretions that can be identified visually or on auscultation. Rising airway pressures in mechanically ventilated patients may also indicate the presence of retained bronchial secretions. Mucosal irritation, trauma, and bleeding can be precipitated by frequent and aggressive suctioning in the absence of bronchial secretions. "Routine" suctioning of the airway should be discouraged except in neonates, in whom small airways can be acutely obstructed by a small accumulation of secretions.

Bronchoscopy

Bronchoscopy can be used for both diagnostic and therapeutic purposes in various clinical settings. In the critical care setting, the indications for bronchoscopy tend to be focused on diagnosing infections, removing retained secretions or foreign bodies, and assessing and controlling hemoptysis. Additionally, in the ICU, the procedure is often performed on patients undergoing mechanical ventilatory support and necessitates a different approach than that taken with awake, stable, spontaneously ventilating patients. Observation of the patient during bronchoscopy is essential and should be delegated to personnel other than the bronchoscopist or the immediate assistant. It is often best to have a respiratory therapist provide manual ventilation during the procedure and also monitor the patient for adverse physiologic effects. Introduction of a bronchoscope into the airways of a mechanically ventilated patient often results in increased airway pressures, interference with distribution of ventilation, and inhibition of ventilator function. Manual ventilation of the patient by a respiratory therapist during bronchoscopy can be useful because the therapist can instantly feel changes in airway resistance, alter the pattern of ventilation to compensate for the problem, inform the bronchoscopist that a problem exists, and assist with maneuvers that will alleviate the compromising situation before a deterioration in the patient's condition can occur.

There are several relative contraindications to bronchoscopy, but no absolute contraindications exist. The decision to perform the procedure must be based on the balance of potential risks and benefits. Considerations that should be taken into account include the following: (a) the hemodynamic stability of the patient; (b) the patient's respiratory status, including oxygenation, ventilation, PEEP level, airway pressures, and so on; (c) the presence of coagulopathies and the potential for their correction or amelioration before the procedure; and (d) the patient's mental status during the procedure.

Therapeutic bronchoscopy is indicated for clearance of secretions when radiographic studies show evidence of segmental or lobar atelectasis and the patient's clinical condition requires urgent intervention or when atelectasis is persistent despite aggressive bronchial-hygiene maneuvers (i.e., postural drainage, percussion, and vibration) and is likely to result in detrimental sequelae, such as pneumonia or lung abscess. In such circumstances,

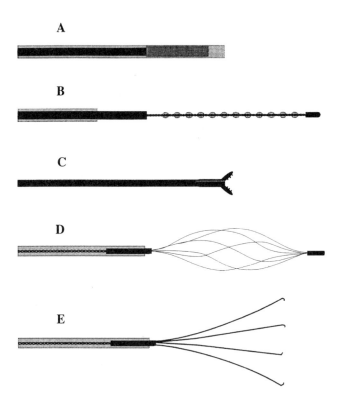

FIGURE 6. A: Protected bronchial microbiology brush in the retracted position with the protective diaphragm in place. **B:** Protected bronchial microbiology brush in the extended sampling position before retraction into the protective sleeve. **C:** Foreign-body-retrieval forceps with "teeth." **D:** Retrieval basket for grasping irregularly shaped or difficult-to-grasp objects from the bronchial tree. **E:** Retrieval device for grasping large, soft objects from the bronchial tree.

ment needed to alleviate bronchial obstruction resulting from tumor or collapse (24).

In the critical care setting, diagnostic bronchoscopy is useful for the detection and characterization of bacterial and opportunistic lung infections. The use of bronchoscopy for the diagnosis of nosocomial pneumonia, however, especially ventilator-associated pneumonia, is controversial. The methods by which cultures are obtained, the use of quantitative or semiquantitative culture techniques, the threshold of bacterial growth necessary for the diagnosis of pneumonia versus colonization, and other factors that are most useful in differentiating bacterial colonization from pneumonia in different patient populations are all debated (25–27). There are several reasons to perform bronchoscopy for the diagnosis of lung infections. Cultures of endotracheal aspirates may not yield results consistent with the pathologic organism because of oropharyngeal contamination or tracheal colonization. The use of clinical (fever, leukocytosis, and purulent secretions) and radiographic (focal infiltrates) criteria for differentiation of pneumonia from airway colonization is generally limited, especially in intubated patients (25–27). Microbiologic specimens obtained from localized areas of the lung, especially if they include samples of alveolar contents, provide more specific information regarding the pathologic process (28); however, the sensitivity and specificity for the diagnosis of pneumonia can be influenced greatly by the type of pathology present, the bronchoscopic technique, and interpretive thresholds (25,29).

Bronchoscopy permits direct visualization of the airways so that anatomic abnormalities, such as tumors or aberrant bronchial anatomy, which can predispose the patient to developing airway obstruction and infection, can be detected. Occasionally, it is important to obtain tissue samples by transbronchial biopsy to elucidate further the pathologic process when culture results alone are insufficient.

The diagnosis of lung infections can be accomplished by using various bronchoscopic techniques, including protected bronchial brushing, bronchoalveolar lavage (BAL) (protected or unprotected), or transbronchial biopsy. Each of these methods has indications and limitations that must be considered when planning diagnostic procedures. Protected bronchial brushing is useful for the diagnosis of bacterial pneumonia because this technique permits the avoidance of contaminated upper-airway secretions and more select sampling of the region of lung of interest. This technique has limitations because the potential for contamination with upper-airway secretions continues, but it is much more likely that positive cultures from the area of lung in question will be representative of the pathologic process. The type of protected brush (Fig. 6A,B) and the methods used to obtain samples will vary, but it is primarily the ability to obtain quantitative cultures (30) that justifies the risks and expense of this procedure. This technique allows the retrieval of 0.001 to 0.01 mL of lung secretions (31). The level of bacterial growth used to diagnose a ventilator-associated pneumonia with protected bronchial brushing is generally accepted as more than 10^3 colony-forming units (cfu) per milliliter (32) (Table 3).

Bronchoalveolar lavage also permits sampling from a specific region of lung and has several added advantages compared with protected bronchial brushing. BAL samples a large area of the distal airways and alveoli, is appropriate for all types of microbiologic

inspired bronchial secretions may not be effectively mobilized by any means other than direct visualization, lavage, and manual removal. Therapeutic bronchoscopy is also useful in the retrieval of aspirated foreign bodies. Such foreign bodies may range from particulate food material, which may not be evident on chest radiograph, to any number of inanimate objects. The degree of difficulty encountered with the location and removal of a foreign body depends on several factors, such as its size, shape, consistency, location, and the duration of time it has been in the bronchial tree. Various foreign-body-retrieval tools (Fig. 6C–E) are designed to be passed through the suction channel of the bronchoscope and grasp or snare objects of various size, shape, and consistency.

The localization and control of bleeding in the airways are some of the most difficult challenges in bronchoscopy for several reasons. Depending on the severity of the bleeding, visualization is often difficult. One of the risks of bronchoscopy is mucosal injury and its associated additional hemorrhage. Once located, the source of bleeding may not be amenable to control by bronchoscopic techniques. Despite these problems, bronchoscopy can be important in obtaining information that is useful in the planning of procedures necessary to diagnose and control sites of pulmonary hemorrhage, such as localizing the bleeding to a specific lung, lobe, or segment for more rapid angiographic location and intervention. Bronchoscopy is also useful in the diagnosis and treatment of retained clots in the airway (23) and for stent place-

TABLE 3. SENSITIVITY AND SPECIFICITY OF MICROBIOLOGIC STUDIES FROM BAL

	Sensitivity	Specificity	Remarks
Acute bacterial pneumonia in immunocompetent patients	Up to 80%	Up to 100%	Quantitative culture with a cutoff point of $\geq 10^4$ cfu/mL is usually used
Nosocomial bacterial pneumonia in mechanically ventilated patients	Remains a challenge; up to 87%	Remains a challenge; up to 100%	Quantitative culture with a cutoff point of $\geq 10^4$ cfu/mL is usually used The presence of intracellular organisms within cells of BAL may provide a sensitive and specific means for early and rapid diagnosis of pneumonia
Mycobacterium tuberculosis	Up to 92%	100%	If the amount of antigen 5 is $\geq 1,000$ μg/mL, the diagnosis of tuberculosis is specifically established Gen-Probe Amplified *Mycobacterium tuberculosis* Direct Test is used for rapid detection of tuberculosis in research laboratories
CMV pneumonia	Culture: 85.7%–100%	Culture: up to 70%	A positive culture and positive cytology of BAL can virtually establish the diagnosis; negative culture may rule it out
	Detection of CMV inclusions: up to 21% *In situ* DNA hybridization: 90%	Detection of CMV inclusions: 98% *In situ* DNA hybridization: 63%	*In situ* DNA hybridization is a rapid diagnostic method Immunocytochemistry studies are useful when a patient has a positive culture and negative cytologic examination. Amplification of CMV-DNA by polymerase chain reaction is the most sensitive method
Pneumocystis carinii	Up to 90%	100%	Different staining may be used, including: Gram-Weigert, Papanicolaou's, methenamide silver, Grocott's, and Diff-Quick

BAL, bronchoalveolar lavage; CMV, cytomegalovirus.
From Emad A. Bronchoalveolar Lavage: a useful method for diagnosis of some pulmonary disorders. *Rest Care* 1997;97:768, with permission.

diagnoses [bacterial, fungal, *Pneumocystis carinii* (PCP), and others], and provides a sample volume that is adequate for a large number of tests (27). BAL can be performed either in a nonprotected or a protected manner. The nonprotected technique involves isolating the bronchus of interest from the remainder of the tracheobronchial tree by wedging the tip of the bronchoscope into an airway lumen and lavaging with a large volume (approximately 120–200 mL in 5 to 10 aliquots) of nonbacteriostatic saline. One may expect to obtain return of less than 50% of the lavage fluid, which will contain approximately 1 mL of actual lung secretions (27). The first lavage sample is likely to be contaminated with central-airway secretions and often is discarded or treated as bronchial washings (33). Protected BAL has been developed to decrease the potential contamination of the lavage fluid with secretions contained within the lumen of the bronchoscope. This technique uses a protected transbronchoscopic balloon-tipped catheter to lavage from the level of third-generation bronchi following expulsion of the protective polyethylene-glycol diaphragm and occlusion of the bronchi with the air-filled balloon (34). When using BAL, the level of bacterial growth accepted as being consistent with a ventilator-associated pneumonia is 10^4 cfu per milliliter because of dilution of the alveolar secretions (25,32). Some clinicians would use a higher diagnostic threshold (10^5 cfu/mL) with nonprotected BAL because of the increased chance of sample contamination and would accept the fact that this threshold will increase the specificity but decrease the sensitivity

of the test. The use of "blind" (nonbronchoscopic), nonprotected BAL to monitor and diagnose ventilator-associated pneumonia in trauma patients has been advocated (35). Whereas this use may be generally appropriate and cost effective for pneumonia surveillance in this group of patients, the results may be misleading in patients with chronic lung disease or in immunocompromised patients. Thus, the patient population must be considered carefully in choosing diagnostic bronchoscopic techniques.

A special non-bronchoscopic catheter for BAL has been developed and proven to be useful in the diagnosis of PCP (36). This device is also useful in circumstances, such as during mechanical ventilation with high PEEP, when the risks of bronchoscopy are considered too high; however, bleeding and pneumothorax can occur with the use of this device. The use of transbronchial biopsy in the critical care setting is most often not necessary and is frequently contraindicated, especially for patients who are being treated with positive-pressure ventilation. Bronchoscopy remains a valuable diagnostic tool in the following clinical settings: (a) immunocompromised patients [i.e., human immunodeficiency virus (HIV)-infected and organ-transplant patients], (b) ventilator-associated pneumonia, and (c) severe persistent community- or hospital-acquired pneumonia. Fiberoptic bronchoscopy is especially useful in the diagnosis of atypical pneumonia (i.e., cytomegalovirus, *Mycobacterium tuberculosis*, *Pneumocystis carinii*) (29). Again, risks and benefits must be weighed before choosing the diagnostic technique.

The administration of antibiotic therapy before obtaining bronchoscopic bacterial cultures has been shown both to decrease sensitivity (likely because of the inhibition of growth) and to decrease specificity (probably due to increased airway colonization) (27). Obviously, the preferred method is to obtain culture samples before instituting antibiotic therapy, but if antibiotics already have been administered, the only recourse is to interpret the culture results accordingly. When lidocaine is used during a bronchoscopy from which bacterial cultures are to be obtained, the lidocaine may inhibit the growth of some microorganisms (37), but this finding has not been noted when lidocaine is used in nebulization (27,38).

AEROSOL THERAPY

An aerosol is a suspension of fine particles of a liquid in a gas. Aerosols have three basic applications in respiratory care: as an aid to bronchial hygiene, to humidify inspiratory gases, and to deliver medications. When dealing with medical aerosols for inhalation, particle size should be 5 μm or smaller for gravitational effects to be sufficiently small to permit deposition in the pulmonary tree (39).

Bland-aerosol Therapy

When used as an aid to bronchial hygiene, water is one of the most important physically active agents. Aerosol therapy can be useful in the hydration of dried, retained secretions and the restoration and maintenance of the mucous blanket. This hydration, in conjunction with appropriate cough mechanisms and other bronchial-hygiene techniques, will permit the mobilization of retained secretions. Care must be taken, however, because bland (i.e., without medication) aerosols used for these purposes can result in the patient's clinical deterioration due to either increased airway resistance (bronchospasm) or swelling and expansion of dried secretions (40). These detrimental effects may be ameliorated by the administration of a bronchodilator or the use of techniques to mobilize the expanding secretions. Although bland-aerosol therapy is widely used, evidence to support the utility of such therapy is not available (41,42). Generally, it appears that there is a need to reassess the clinical utility of this modality.

The major indication for nebulized saline, either hypotonic or hypertonic, is for induction of sputum specimens. The administration of high-volume aerosolized saline for 30 minutes via a continuous ultrasonic aerosol is appropriate to achieve a sputum induction, provided the patient has a strong effective cough and there is sputum in the airways that can be mobilized and expectorated. Obtaining sputum specimens for the diagnosis of PCP in immunocompromised individuals requires a special procedure. The diagnosis is confirmed by visualization of the organisms in samples of sputum, BAL fluid, or lung tissue obtained on biopsy. Sputum samples should be obtained after the patients have brushed their teeth and rinsed their mouths. The patient inhales an ultrasonic nebulization of 3% sodium chloride through his or her mouth to promote a vigorous cough and produce a

sample containing alveolar cells and contents. With this technique, the diagnosis can be obtained in 50% to 80% of patients with PCP due to the acquired immunodeficiency syndrome (AIDS) (43–45). This diagnostic yield may be decreasing in light of current inhaled and systemic antibiotic prophylaxis of PCP.

Complications associated with ultrasonically nebulized aerosols include wheezing or bronchospasm, infection, overhydration, and patient discomfort. Other persons in the room may be exposed to droplet nuclei of *Mycobacterium tuberculosis* or other airborne infections produced as a consequence of coughing, particularly during sputum induction. The use of sputum induction for diagnostic purposes is effective only if the patient has a productive cough and is able to produce a "deep specimen" that is not contaminated. Success in obtaining quality sputum specimens is best accomplished early in the morning after the patient has been supine for several hours. In the presence of an effective cough and adequate hydration, which is possible after using an ultrasonic nebulizer for 30 minutes, a patient should, in most cases, successfully mobilize any retained secretions to the level where an adequate specimen can be expectorated, collected, and sent to the laboratory for analysis.

Aerosolized Medications

The delivery of medications for the reversal and prevention of bronchoconstriction is an important application of aerosol therapy. Table 4 provides data on the most commonly used aerosolized pharmacologic agents. These medications include β-agonists, anticholinergic agents, and antiinflammatory agents. The β-agonists and anticholinergic agents act primarily by enhancing bronchodilation through increases in intracellular cyclic adenosine monophosphate (cAMP) levels or decreases in intracellular cyclic guanosine monophosphate (cGMP) levels. The use of antiinflammatory agents has gained popularity in the treatment of bronchospastic disorders because the disease processes have been demonstrated to be of an inflammatory nature.

When delivered in aerosolized form, antibiotic medications, such as pentamidine isoethionate and amphotericin B, have been found to be effective for the prophylaxis and treatment of opportunistic pulmonary infections such as PCP and pulmonary aspergillosis (46–49). Nebulized pentamidine decreases the frequency, severity, and occurrence of PCP in patients with AIDS (50). Pentamidine aerosolization should generate particles with a mass median aerodynamic diameter (MMAD) of less than 3.0 μm to ensure adequate penetration to the lung parenchyma and to minimize the irritation associated with deposition in the airways. The currently recommended dosage regimen for prophylaxis is 60 mg administered by an ultrasonic nebulizer (Fisoneb) every 24 to 72 hours for a total of 5 doses over a 2-week period and 60 mg every 2 weeks thereafter. If using a jet-type nebulizer (Respirgard II), the dose of pentamidine is 300 mg every 4 weeks (50,51). Invasive pulmonary fungal infections are significant problems in immunocompromised patients, especially those undergoing bone marrow transplantation during their neutropenic stages. Aerosolization and inhalation of amphotericin B have been investigated as a method to provide prophylaxis against pulmonary fungal infections while minimizing the adverse side effects of the drug (48,52). Aerosolized amphotericin appears to be well tolerated and has minimal systemic absorption (47,53); however, well-controlled outcome data are not available. Aerosolized antibiotic therapy for infections associated with cystic fibrosis also has been explored but was found to be of equivocal efficacy (54). Ribavirin has been recommended for the treatment of respiratory syncytial virus (RSV) in children, especially those with congenital heart disease, immunodeficiency, or bronchopulmonary dysplasia (54). This drug also has been used in certain immunocompromised adults; however, because of the high expense of treatment and the rarity of severe RSV infections in adults, the diagnosis of RSV infection should be confirmed by rapid laboratory testing before commencing therapy. The United States Food and Drug Administration (FDA) has recommended the small-particle aerosol generator (SPAG) for aerosolization of ribavirin for the treatment of RSV in children, but SPAG also can be used for adults if such therapy is deemed appropriate. The SPAG system will generate particles with an MMAD of less than 1.5 μm. The delivery of bronchodilators and antibiotics and the use of aerosolization are being investigated as means by which to deliver other drugs, such as insulin (55), that otherwise require chronic parenteral administration.

Unfortunately, a high incidence of bronchospastic reactions is associated with the administration of aerosolized antibiotics and other medications. These reactions necessitate either pretreatment or concurrent treatment with an aerosolized β-agonist. In addition, these agents potentially have toxic effects for health care-delivery personnel who are administering the treatments; therefore, appropriate exhaust, scavenging, or filtering systems should be used during administration of the treatments.

Small-volume Nebulizers, Metered-dose, and Dry-powder Inhalers

The delivery of medications by small-volume nebulizers (SVN) historically has been the standard for aerosol-medication delivery. Small and relatively easy to use, the SVN does require a gas source that can produce a flow of 5 to 10 L per minute. Optimal gas-source flow settings and specific design characteristics of a particular SVN are variables that determine aerosol particle size. As such, this method of drug delivery is expensive and potentially inefficient (56) and requires a significant time commitment on the part of the respiratory therapist. Recent variations in the SVN design that incorporate a reservoir bag to collect and suspend aerosol particles of desired therapeutic size and the addition of a PEP valve to promote better aerosol deposition have been engineered to improve SVN efficiency. Advocates of these design changes suggest that the result is better aerosol-particle size, less systemic absorption of medication, and more medication targeted and deposited to the airways; however, no published clinical studies have supported this claim.

A functional alternative to the SVN is the metered-dose inhaler (MDI). The MDI is a device that permits the patient to rapidly self-administer an inhaled drug. The delivery of drug to the lower airways, with appropriate use of the MDI, has been demonstrated to be approximately 10% of the total dose and is comparable to that attained with the SVN (57–59). In contrast

to the SVN, with which 66% of the drug is deposited in the apparatus and 2% is deposited in the mouth and stomach, MDI administration results in only 5% to 10% of drug deposition in the apparatus with 80% deposited in the mouth and stomach (57,60). This factor carries implications pertaining to local side effects and tissue toxicity (i.e., oral thrush associated with inhaled-steroid use) (57). In terms of clinical effects, no differences between MDI and SVN therapy have been found for peak expiratory-flow rates or severity of symptoms in stable patients treated with either modality (61). In addition to having clinical efficacy equal to that of SVN devices, administering bronchodilator therapy with MDI devices requires less manpower and offers significant cost savings to the hospital (62). Studies suggest that there can be substantial benefit from the increased use of MDI with a spacer and a percentage of patients can replace SVN with MDI using a spacer device (41–43,63). The effective use of an MDI requires that the patient meet certain clinical criteria. The patient must be able to position and actuate the device appropriately, inspire deeply, and coordinate the inspiratory effort with the device actuation (Table 4).

To ensure efficacious use, a successful coordination of efforts is necessary, which requires appropriate instruction, training, and practice (64). Problems with proper technique are especially pronounced with younger or older patients (65). To ameliorate some of the problems associated with MDI use, "spacer devices" have been developed (66). A spacer effectively acts as a reservoir into which the drug is discharged by attaching and actuating the MDI device (Fig. 7). The use of a spacer eliminates the need for significant coordination of hand, mouth, and breathing functions and improves delivery of the drug to the airways.

A breath-activated variation to the MDI is the Autohaler. This device addresses concerns related to particle deposition and coordination issues inherent in the use of conventional MDI devices (67). Objectively comparing the conventional MDI devices and the Autohaler is difficult because the Autohaler is limited to use with one drug (pirbuterol acetate) in the United States. As do conventional MDI devices, the Autohaler uses chlorofluorocarbons (CFC) as a propellant, a factor that is of environmental concern and strictly regulated by the government. A comparison of therapy with an MDI-spacer system versus SVN treatments indicated that a greater spirometric response was initially obtained with SVN, but this response equalized over the time of hospitalization (68). A study comparing MDI versus SVN delivery of albuterol in mechanically ventilated patients indicated equal clinical responses in both groups (69). In light of such information, it is reasonably clear that SVN administration of bronchodilators should be reserved for patients who are unstable or otherwise incapable of using an MDI device. Patients can be assigned to MDI-spacer therapy if they meet the following criteria (70):

1. Respiratory rate less than 25 breaths per minute
2. Ability to hold the breath for 5 seconds or longer
3. Vital capacity more than 15 mL per kilogram
4. Ability to understand verbal and visual instructions
5. Appropriate hand-mouth-inspiratory coordination
6. Peak expiratory flow rates of 150 L per minute or greater for women and 200 L per minute or greater for men

TABLE 4. AEROSOLIZED BRONCHODILATORS AND ANTIASTHMATIC DRUGS

Drug	Device delivery	Adult dosages[a]	Frequency	Effects	Mechanisms of action
Inhaled β-agonists					
Epinephrine	SVN	0.25–0.5 mL (2.5–5.0 mg)	q.i.d.	Bronchodilation, tachycardia	β-Agonist
	MDI	0.2 mg/puff	q.i.d.		
Racemic epinephrine	SVN	0.25–0.5 mL (5.625–11.25 mg)	q.i.d.	Bronchodilation	$\beta_2 > \beta_1$
Isoproterenol 0.5% (Isoprel)	SVN	0.25–0.50 mL (1.25–2.5 mg)	q2–4h	Bronchodilation, tachycardia, vasodilation, flushing	Prototype β-agonist; significant β_1 side effects
	MDI	131 μg/puff	2 puffs q.i.d.		
Isoetharine hydrochloride 1%	SVN	0.25–0.50 mL (2.5–5.0 mg)	q2–4h	Bronchodilation, tachycardia	β_2-Agonist, increase in cAMP
	MDI	340 μg/puff	1–2 puffs q.i.d.		β_1
Terbutaline 0.1% (Brethane, Bricanyl)	MDI	200 μg/puff	2 puffs q4–6h	Bronchodilation	$\beta_2 > \beta_1$
Metaproterenol 5%	SVN	0.3 mL (15 mg)	t.i.d.–q.i.d.	Bronchodilation	$\beta_2 > \beta_1$
	MDI	650 μg/puff	2–3 puffs t.i.d. to q.i.d.		
Albuterol 0.5%	SVN	0.3 mL (15 mg)	t.i.d.–q.i.d.	Bronchodilation	$\beta_2 > \beta_1$
	MDI	90 μg/puff	2 puffs, tid or q.i.d.		
	DPI	200 μg/cap	1 cap q4–6h		
Bitolterol	SVN	1.25 mL (2.5 mg)	b.i.d.–q.i.d.	Bronchodilation	$\beta_2 > \beta_1$
	MDI	370 μg/puff	2 puffs, q8h		
Pirbuterol	MDI	200 μg/puff	2 puffs, q4–6h	Bronchodilation	$\beta_2 > \beta_1$
Salmeterol	MDI	21 μg/puff	2 puffs, b.i.d.	Bronchodilation	$\beta_2 > \beta_1$
Levalbuterol	SVN	0.625 mg 1.25 mg	6 to 8 t.i.d.	Bronchodilation	$\beta_2 > \beta_1$
Anticholinergic drugs					
Atropine sulfate 2% or 5%	SVN	0.025 mg/kg up to 2.5 mg in 2–5 mL	q6–8h	Bronchodilation	Cholinergic blocker, decreases cGMP
Ipratropium bromide 0.02%	SVN	0.5 mg in 2.5 mL	t.i.d. or q.i.d.	Bronchodilation	Cholinergic blocker, decreases cGMP
	MDI	18 μg/puff	2 puffs, t.i.d. to q.i.d.		
Inhaled corticosteroids and antiallergy agents					
Beclomethasone acetonide	MDI	42–84 μg/puff 48 μg/puff	2 puffs, q6 2 puffs, q6	Antiinflammatory	Antiinflammatory; inhibits leukocytes
Budesonide	DPI	200 & 400 μg	1–2 caps b.i.d.	Antiinflammatory	Antiinflammatory; inhibits leukocytes
Flunisolide	MDI	250 μg/puff	2 puffs b.i.d.	Antiinflammatory	Antiinflammatory; inhibits leukocytes
Fluticasone propionate	MDI	44, 110, 220 μg/puff	2 puffs b.i.d.	Antiinflammatory	Antiinflammatory; inhibits leukocytes
	DPI	50, 100, 250 μg/disk	1 disk b.i.d.		
Triamcinalone acetonide	MDI	100 μg/puff	2–4 puffs, b.i.d. to q.i.d.	Antiinflammatory	Antiinflammatory; inhibits leukocytes
Dexamethasone sodium phosphate	MDI	0.1 mg/puff	3 puffs t.i.d. or q.i.d.	Antiinflammatory	Antiinflammatory; inhibits leukocytes
Cromolyn sodium	SVN	20 mg (2–4 mL)	q6h	Stabilization of mast cell membranes	Suppression of mast cell response

SVN, small-volume nebulizer; q.i.d., four times daily; MDI, metered dose inhaler; cAMP, cyclic adenosine monophosphate; t.i.d., three times daily; DPI, dry-powder inhaler; cGMP, cyclic guanosine monophosphate; b.i.d., twice daily; Ag–ab, antigen antibody.

[a]Dosages may vary.

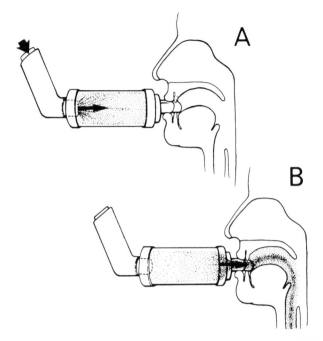

FIGURE 7. Illustration of a spacer with a metered-dose inhaler (MDI). **A:** The aerosol suspension dispersing equally in the gas volume within the spacer following ejection from the MDI. **B:** The patient takes a deep, slow inhalation of the medication. (From Shapiro BA, Kacmarek RM, Cane RD, et al. *Clinical application of respiratory care*, 4th ed. St. Louis: Mosby–Year Book, 1991, with permission.)

Patients should be instructed in MDI-spacer use by a properly trained respiratory therapist. Before patients completely switch to this device, their technique should be evaluated, and additional training should be given if necessary.

Delivery of bronchodilators to patients undergoing mechanical ventilation can be effective but is also problematic. The use of an SVN to deliver bronchodilators during mechanical ventilation can result in bacterial contamination of the ventilator circuit, alteration in the delivered V_T, increased work of breathing during patient-initiated modes of ventilation, and damage to flow-measurement devices incorporated into some ventilator circuits (71). In addition, administration of aerosols by an endotracheal tube will reduce penetration to the lower airways (72). MDIs, in conjunction with mechanical ventilatory supports, have been evaluated for use in delivery of bronchodilators and have been shown to be comparable to SVN delivery systems, without the associated problems (71). The use of MDI devices with spacers has undergone nonclinical bench testing with evidence of increased aerosol delivery; however, trials to document an improvement in clinical response are not yet available (71). Improved aerosol delivery also can be accomplished by adapting a nozzle-extension system to the MDI and extending the nozzle tip beyond the end of the endotracheal tube (73,74). Again, clinical studies to support the improved efficiency of this method of aerosol delivery are lacking, and the results of animal studies indicate that tracheal epithelial injury may occur when this system is used (71,75).

Another method of inspired-drug delivery is the dry-powder inhaler (DPI). DPIs create aerosols by drawing air through an aliquot of dry powder. The powder contains either micronized

(<5 μm in diameter) drug particles bound into loose aggregates or micronized drug particles that are loosely bound to large (>30 μm in diameter) lactose or glucose particles (1). Patients using a DPI must be able to generate an inspiratory flow rate greater than 30 to 60 L per minute to be effective. DPIs are not recommended for patients in acute bronchoconstriction or for children under the age of 6. DPIs are recommended for prophylactic and maintenance therapy because of the inspiratory flow requirements (76). These devices have two major advantages over SVN or MDI devices: They are activated by the patient's inspiratory effort and therefore do not require a high degree of hand-mouth-inspiratory-effort coordination, and they do not use CFC propellants.

This drug-delivery method appears to have equal efficacy compared with MDI and SVN delivery systems (57). The use of these devices may increase as the concern for environmental protection results in the elimination or severe restriction of CFC propellants (39). Although patients can find DPIs more convenient and easier to use than MDIs, one report suggests that as many as 25% of patients may use DPIs improperly (39). Clinicians must understand the required technique involved with DPIs and provide the necessary instruction and periodic review of technique for patients to receive the benefits of medication delivery utilizing a DPI (40,41,42).

Continuous Positive Airway Pressure

A typical continuous-flow, continuous positive airway pressure (CPAP) system includes a medium-volume, high-compliance reservoir bag (5–10 L) and maintains system flow in excess of the patient's peak inspiratory flow demands (Fig. 8). Characteristically, system continuous flows are maintained at 60 to 90 L per minute. The adequacy of continuous flow is evaluated by observing gas continuously exiting from the system, even during peak inspiratory-flow periods. A system-pressure manometer and, ideally, an oxygen analyzer should be included in all CPAP circuits. Finally, a pressure pop-off valve is included in all systems to prevent excessive pressure (such as occurs with system obstruction or when the patient coughs with a high-flow resistance PEEP device) from building up in the system. With all circuits, some fluctuations in system pressure are noted, with the acceptable range being about ±2 cm H_2O. Fluctuations of greater magnitude during inspiration can be corrected by increasing system flow, increasing the size of the circuit reservoir, or increasing the flow and the size of the reservoir. Changes in baseline pressure during exhalation are affected primarily by the flow-resistance properties of the PEEP device.

The use of CPAP applied by full-face mask or nasal mask has been used for respiratory support in patients with various types of pulmonary pathology, ranging from CHF to obstructive sleep apnea. The primary respiratory effects of CPAP are that it increases functional residual capacity; improves distribution of ventilation, lung compliance, and oxygenation; and decreases the work of breathing. CPAP applied with a nasal mask is more comfortable, often better tolerated, and allows the patient to communicate more effectively than does CPAP applied with a full-face mask. Additionally, if vomiting occurs, nasal-mask CPAP does not present an obstacle to airway clearance. In severely

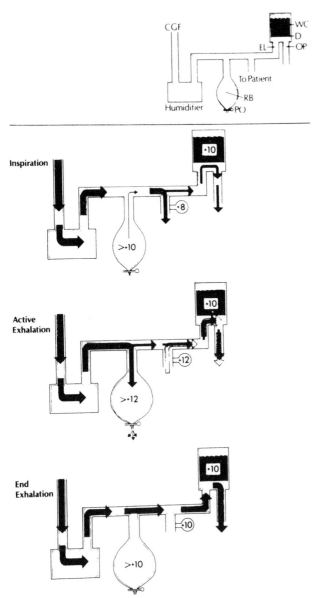

FIGURE 8. Schematic representation of a continuous positive airway pressure (CPAP) device. CGF, continuous gas flow source; RB, elastic reservoir bag; PO, pop-off mechanism, which is an open nipple with an adjustable clamp; WC, water column determining the threshold pressure of +10 cm H$_2$O; D, diaphragm of the positive end-expiratory pressure (PEEP) device; EL, exhalation line of the patient circuit; OP, outlet port of the PEEP device. The continuous gas flow must be great enough to force some gas continuously to enter the reservoir bag except during peak inspiratory flow. Through adjustment of the pop-off mechanism, the pressure in the bag is maintained equal to or greater than the threshold pressure. Thus, gas will always flow through the outlet port of the PEEP device. Note that the patient's airway pressure fluctuates no more than ±2 cm H$_2$O of the threshold pressure. Inspiration: Most of the gas flow will enter the patient's airway without added impedance; the remainder of the gas flows through the outlet port of the PEEP device. Note that at the moment of the patient's peak inspiratory flow, a small amount of gas may enter the patient circuit from the reservoir bag. Active exhalation: Airway pressure is greater than threshold, causing more of the continuous gas flow to enter the reservoir bag. The increased expiratory flow may create increased pressure if the PEEP device has orificial resistor properties and thus increase the work of breathing. End exhalation: The continuous gas flow and reservoir bag maintain the circuit pressure at the threshold pressure. (From Shapiro BA, Kacmarek RM, Cane RD, et al. *Clinical application of respiratory care*, 4th ed. St. Louis: Mosby–Year Book; 1991, with permission.)

hypoxemic patients, however, nasal CPAP may not permit a seal sufficient to sustain the airway pressure necessary to maintain oxygenation.

Biphasic-airway-pressure (BiPAP) therapy is effectively the combination of CPAP with pressure-support augmentation of spontaneous inspiration. This method permits mechanical support of spontaneous ventilatory efforts without the need for intubation. This method of "noninvasive" ventilatory support has been demonstrated to be efficacious in patients demonstrating hypoxemia, hypercapnia, or hypercapnia and hypoxemia due to COPD, CHF, ARDS, and PCP (77–79). Although pressure injury to the nose has been reported with the use of biphasic airway pressure, the potential complications of gastric distention and aspiration do not appear to be significant. Of course, this mode of ventilatory support would not be appropriate for patients with a compromised ability for airway protection or glottic pathology (i.e., supraglottic thermal injury, or laryngeal edema). Additionally, patients must be observed carefully to ensure that the device does not become displaced and that spontaneous ventilation continues.

ORGANIZATION OF A RESPIRATORY CARE DEPARTMENT

The leadership of a respiratory care department is, by necessity, a dichotomous one. The hospital administration is responsible for the provision of the personnel, equipment, and supplies necessary to meet the patient-care needs and the goals of the respiratory care department. The role of the medical director of respiratory care is to ensure that the departmental policies and procedures, which govern the administration of therapy, provide for safe and appropriate patient care. The successful respiratory care department balances the provision of high-quality care with cost-effective methods and management. This balance necessitates a cooperative relationship between cost-conscious hospital administrative personnel and a quality-oriented medical director.

The organization of a respiratory care department requires different personnel responsible for various functions, such as financial planning, organization, personnel management, technical support, education, and patient care. In the past, it was possible to have several layers of management to fulfill many of these functions; however, under current cost-containment measures, departments must be much more streamlined and cost effective. In light of the fact that personnel costs are usually the greatest costs for any organization of significant size, versatility of personnel at all levels is the key to the future success of respiratory care departments.

The current trend in the health care marketplace is that of multitasking or job sharing in order to become more cost effective or value conscious. In this circumstance, persons trained in traditional roles are also trained to perform tasks that are outside of their normal purview. For example, respiratory therapists or nurses may be trained to perform ECGs rather than using an entirely separate technical staff to fulfill this need. This cross-training allows persons who have a broader scope of training to become more versatile and efficient while maintaining

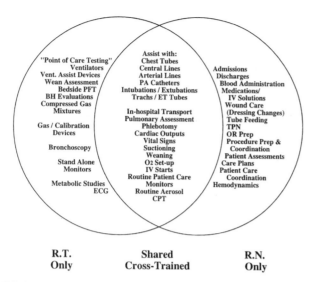

R.T.
Only
Shared
Cross-Trained
R.N.
Only

FIGURE 9. A sample of assigned and shared responsibilities between respiratory therapists and nurses in a "team-approach" critical care model.

high-quality, cost-effective patient care. This concept becomes increasingly more important as the increasing acuity of inpatient care shifts the focus of hospital care toward the costly critical care setting and technologic advances (e.g., point-of-care testing, hemodynamic monitoring, and respiratory support). Figure 9 illustrates the concept of cost-effective multitasking between respiratory care and nursing personnel in an ICU. In addition to personnel efficiency, the maintenance of cost-effective health care requires that therapy be tailored to provide only the care that is necessary and efficacious.

Respiratory therapy is generally poorly understood, overprescribed, and among the most expensive care provided by hospitals; therefore, a trend has evolved in which therapist-driven systems assign and deliver respiratory care (80). Such systems permit persons who have the most detailed knowledge of the care that is being delivered to play an active role in the allocation of therapy that is necessary and the elimination of therapy that is superfluous (81). The success of such programs requires strong medical direction and clear guidelines or protocols for the implementation of therapy (82).

SUMMARY

The practice of respiratory care has always been integral to the practice of critical care medicine. The advancements of technology and medical science have made this role even more important but also more complex and difficult. These advancements require appropriate training and understanding of the equipment now used to deliver state-of-the-art respiratory care. Also, the complexity of patients requiring critical care necessitates the inclusion of persons capable of making complicated clinical assessments and decisions. The complexity of this situation will only increase as medical science advances. Therefore, the training and capabilities of respiratory care practitioners must advance to keep pace with these changes.

THE FUTURE

Many changes are currently taking place and are being planned for future respiratory care practices. Medication delivery is an active area of research and development. Work is being done to determine improved ways to deliver medications that are currently administered through the airways and to develop more medications to be delivered via inhalation therapy. Bronchial-hygiene therapy is an extremely costly aspect of health care today. In light of the current medical and economic milieu, there must be a serious focus on efficacy, cost-effectiveness, and outcomes associated with various respiratory care interventions. Bronchoscopy is an important diagnostic and therapeutic tool. Techniques that improve the diagnostic capabilities in terms of detection and identification of infectious processes are continually being evaluated. This is especially important in the care of immunocompromised patients. Finally, the role of the respiratory care practitioner is rapidly evolving from one in which respiratory care workers perform focused duties to one in which their skills and functions are expanded into a broader range of unconventional duties. This evolution includes the development of respiratory therapist–nursing teams in the ICU, expansion of clinical duties (i.e., electrocardiography and point-of-care testing), and a focus on the delivery of cost-effective, high-quality patient care.

KEY POINTS

This chapter addresses several important aspects of respiratory care. The first aspect is the general topic of oxygenation. In this section, disorders of oxygenation, the concept of oxygen content, methods of oxygen delivery, and complications of oxygen therapy are discussed. The second area of importance is that of bronchial-hygiene therapy. Here the difference between prophylactic and therapeutic bronchial-hygiene therapy is presented. Methods of bronchial hygiene, ranging from incentive spirometry through various types of chest physical therapy, are addressed. Other topics, such as humidification and intermittent positive-pressure breathing, also are considered. The third major area of consideration is

that of bronchoscopy. Both therapeutic and diagnostic bronchoscopic procedures are presented. The fourth major topic of consideration is aerosol therapy, which includes delivery of bronchodilators and antibiotics and the various methods of delivery, including small-volume nebulizers, metered-dose inhalers, and dry-powder inhalers.

Continuous positive airway pressure (CPAP) delivered by face mask is another advance in respiratory care, and this section includes a discussion of nasal-mask CPAP and biphasic airway pressure therapy. Finally, the general structure and organization of a respiratory care department are discussed.

REFERENCES

1. Shapiro BA, Kacmarek RM, Cane RD, et al. Limitations of oxygen therapy. In: Shapiro BA, Kacmarek RM, Cane RD, et al., eds. *Clinical application of respiratory care,* 4th ed. St. Louis: Mosby–Year Book, 1991:135–150.

2. Solliday NH, Shapiro BA, Gracey DR. Adult respiratory distress syndrome: clinical conference in pulmonary disease from Northwestern University-McGaw Medical Center, Chicago. *Chest* 1976;69:207–213.

3. Lamy M, Fallat RJ, Koeniger E, et al. Pathologic features and mechanisms of hypoxemia in adult respiratory distress syndrome. *Am Rev Respir Dis* 1976;114:267–284.

4. Shapiro BA, Cane RD, Harrison RA. Positive end-expiratory pressure in acute lung injury. *Chest* 1983;83:558–563.

5. Shapiro BA, Cane RD. Metabolic malfunction of the lung: noncardiogenic edema and adult respiratory distress syndrome. *Surg Ann* 1981;13:271–298.

6. Miller WC, Rice DL, Unger KM, et al. Effect of PEEP on lung water content in experimental noncardiogenic pulmonary edema. *Crit Care Med* 1981;9:7–9.

7. Shapiro BA, Cane RD, Harrison RA. Positive end expiratory pressure therapy in adults with special reference to acute lung injury: a review of the literature and suggested clinical correlations. *Crit Care Med* 1984;12:127–141.

8. Shapiro BA, Peruzzi WT, Templin R. Arterial oxygenation. In: *Clinical application of blood gases,* 5th ed. St. Louis: Mosby–Year book, 1994:33–53.

9. Schacter EN, Littner MR, Luddy P, et al. Monitoring of oxygen delivery systems in clinical practice. *Crit Care Med* 1980;8:405–409.

10. Scacci R. Air entrainment masks: jet mixing is how they work; the Bernoulli and Venturi principles are how they don't. *Respir Care Clin N Am* 1979;24:928–931.

11. Deneke SM, Fanberg BL. Normobaric oxygen toxicity of the lung. *N Engl J Med* 1980;303:76–86.

12. Hardy AK. A review of airway clearance: new techniques, indications, and recommendations. *Respir Care Clin N Am* 1994;39:440–452.

13. Eid N, Buchheit J, Neuling M, Phelps H. Chest physiotherapy in review. *Respir Care Clin N Am* 1991;36:270–282.

14. Maxwell M, Redmond A. Comparative trial of manual and mechanical percussion technique with gravity-assisted bronchial drainage in patients with cystic fibrosis. *Arch Dis Child* 1979;54:542–544.

15. Shapiro BA, Kacmarek RM, Cane RD, et al. Applying and evaluating bronchial hygiene therapy. In: Shapiro BA, Kacmarek RM, Cane RD, et al., eds. *Clinical application of respiratory care,* 4th ed. St. Louis: Mosby–Year Book, 1991:85–108.

16. AARC clinical practice guideline: postural drainage therapy. *Respir Care Clin N Am* 1991;36:1418–1426.

17. Lieberman JA, Cohen NH. Evaluation of a fixed orifice device for the delivery of positive expiratory pressure to non-intubated patients. *Anesthesiology* 1992;77:A587.

18. Mahlmeister M, Fink J, Hoffman G, et al. Positive-expiratory-pressure mask therapy: theoretical and practical considerations and a review of the literature. *Respir Care Clin N Am* 1991;36:1218–1229.

19. Van Hengstum M, Festen J, Beurskens C, et al. Effect of positive expiratory pressure mask physiotherapy (PEP) versus forced expiration technique (FET/PD) on regional lung clearance in chronic bronchitis. *Eur Respir J* 1991;4:651–654.

20. Sloan HE. Vagus nerve in cardiac arrest; effect of hypercapnia, hypoxia and asphyxia on reflex inhibition of heart. *Surg Gynecol Obstet* 1950;91:257–264.

21. Crimlisk JT, Paris R, McGonagle EG, et al. The closed tracheal suction system: implications for critical care nursing. *Dim Crit Care Nurs* 1994;13:292–300.

22. Shim C, Fine N, Fernandez R, Williams MH Jr. Cardiac arrhythmias resulting from tracheal suctioning. *Ann Intern Med* 1969;71:1149–1153.

23. Arney KL, Judson MA, Sahn SA. Airway obstruction arising from blood clot: three reports and a review of the literature. *Chest* 1999;115:293–300.

24. Hautmann H, Bauer M, Pfeifer KJ, et al. Flexible bronchoscopy: a safe method for metal stent implantation in bronchial disease. *Ann Thorac Surg* 2000;69:398–401.

25. Bonten MJM, Gaillard CA, Wouters EFM, et al. Problems in diagnosing nosocomial pneumonia in mechanically ventilated patients: a review. *Crit Care Med* 1994;22:1683–1691.

26. Garrard CS, A'Court CD. The diagnosis of pneumonia in the critically ill. *Chest* 1995;108:17S–25S.

27. Baselski VS, Wunderink RG. Bronchoscopic diagnosis of pneumonia. *Clin Microbiol Rev* 1994;7:533–558.

28. Cook DJ, Fitzgerald JM, Guyatt GH. Evaluation of the protected brush catheter and bronchoalveolar lavage in the diagnosis of nosocomial pneumonia. *J Intensive Care Med* 1991;6:196–205.

29. Emad A. Bronchoalveolar lavage: a useful method for diagnosis of some pulmonary disorders. *Respir Care* 1997;42:765–790.

30. Pollack HM, Hawkins EL, Bonner JR, et al. Diagnosis of bacterial pulmonary infections with quantitative protected catheter cultures obtained during bronchoscopy. *J Clin Microbiol* 1983;17:25559.

31. Wimberley N, Faling LJ, Bartlett JG. A fiberoptic bronchoscopy technique to obtain uncontaminated lower airway secretions for bacterial culture. *Am Rev Respir Dis* 1979;119:337–343.

32. Baselski, VS, Robison MK, Pifer LW, et al. The standardization of criteria for processing and interpreting laboratory specimens with suspected ventilator-associated pneumonia. *Chest* 1992;102:571S–579S.

33. Davis GS, Giancola MS, Costanza MC, et al. Analyses of sequential bronchoalveolar lavage samples from healthy human volunteers. *Am Rev Respir Dis* 1982;126:611–616.

34. Meduri GU, Beals DH, Maijub AG, et al. Protected bronchoalveolar lavage. A new bronchoscopic technique to retrieve uncontaminated distal airway secretions. *Am Rev Respir Dis* 1991;143:855–864.

35. Pugin J, Auckenthaler R, Mili N, et al. Diagnosis of ventilator-associated pneumonia by bacteriologic analysis of bronchoscopic and nonbronchoscopic "blind" bronchoalveolar lavage fluid. *Am Rev Respir Dis* 1991;143:1121–1129.

36. Bustamante EA, Levy H. Sputum induction compared with bronchoalveolar lavage by Ballard catheter to diagnose Pneumocystis carinii pneumonia. *Chest* 1994;105:816–822.

37. Wimberley N, Willey S, Sullivan N, Bartlett JG. Antibacterial properties of lidocaine. *Chest* 1979;6:37–40.

38. Kirkpatrick MB, Bass JB Jr. Quantitative bacterial cultures of bronchoalveolar lavage fluids and protected brush catheter specimens from normal subjects. *Am Rev Respir Dis* 1989;139:546–548.

39. Aerosol consensus statement. Consensus conference of aerosol delivery. *Chest* 1991;100:1106–1109.

40. Kuo CD, Lin SE, Wang JH. Aerosol, humidity and oxygenation. *Chest* 1991;99:1352–1356.

41. Hess D. The open forum: reflections on unanswered questions about aerosol therapy delivery techniques [Editorial]. *Respiratory Care* 1988;33:19–20.

42. Ward JJ, Helmholz HF Jr. Applied humidity and aerosol therapy. In: Burton GG, Hodgkin JE, Ward JJ, eds. *Respiratory care: a guide to clinical practice,* 3rd ed. Philadelphia: JB Lippincott Co, 1991; 355–396.

43. Bigby TD, Margolskee D, Curtis JL, et al. The usefulness of induced sputum in the diagnosis of Pneumocystis carinii pneumonia in patients with the acquired immunodeficiency syndrome. *Am Rev Respir Dis* 1986;133:515–518.

44. Kovacs JA, Ng VL, Masur H, et al. Diagnosis of Pneumocystis carinii pneumonia: improved detection in sputum with use of monoclonal antibodies. *N Engl J Med* 1988;318:589–593.

45. Masur H, Gill VJ, Ognibene FP, et al. Diagnosis of *Pneumocystis pneumonia* by induced sputum technique in patients without the acquired immunodeficiency syndrome. *Ann Intern Med* 1988;109:755–756.

46. Leoung GS, Hopewell PC. *Pneumocystis carinii* pneumonia: therapy and prophylaxis. In: Cohen PT, Sande MA, Volberding PA, eds. *The AIDS knowledge base,* 2nd ed. Boston: Little, Brown 1994:6.17-1–6.17-35.

47. Myers SE, Devine SM, Topper RL, et al. A pilot study of prophylactic aerosolized amphotericin B in patients at risk for prolonged neutropenia. *Leuk Lymphoma* 1992;8:229–233.

48. Hertenstein B, Kern WV, Schmeiser T, et al. Low incidence of invasive fungal infections after bone marrow transplantation in patients

receiving amphotericin B inhalations during neutropenia. *Ann Hematol* 1994;68:21–26.

49. Niki Y, Bernard EM, Edwards FF, et al. Model of recurrent pulmonary aspergillosis in rats. *J Clin Microbiol* 1991;29:1317–1322.

50. Hardy WD. Prophylaxis of AIDS-related opportunistic infections (OIs). Current status and future strategies. *AIDS Clin Rev* 1991:145–180.

51. Newman SP, Simonds AK. Aerosol therapy in AIDS. *Lung* 1990;168 Suppl:685–691.

52. Schmitt HJ. New methods of delivery of amphotericin B. *Clin Infect Dis* 1993;17(Suppl 2):S501–S506.

53. Beyer J, Barzen G, Risse G, et al. Aerosol amphotericin B for prevention of invasive pulmonary aspergillosis. *Antimicrob Agents Chemother* 1993;37:1367–1369.

54. Ziment I. Drugs used in respiratory therapy. In: Burton GG, Hodgkin JE, Ward JJ, eds. *Respiratory care: a guide to clinical practice*, 3rd ed. Philadelphia: JB Lippincott, 1991:411–448.

55. Laube BL, Georgopoulos A, Adams GK III. Preliminary study of the efficacy of insulin aerosol delivered by oral inhalation in diabetic patients. *JAMA* 1993;269:2106–2109.

56. Newman SP. Aerosol deposition considerations in inhalation therapy. *Chest* 1985;88:152S–160S.

57. Kacmarek RM, Hess D. The interface between patient and aerosol generator. *Respir Care Clin N Am* 1991;36:952–976.

58. Newman SP, Pavia D, Moren F, et al. Deposition of pressurized aerosols in the human respiratory tract. *Thorax* 1981;36:52–55.

59. Spiro SG, Singh CA, Tolfree SE, et al. Direct labeling of ipratropium bromide aerosol and its deposition pattern in normal subjects and patients with chronic bronchitis. *Thorax* 1984;39:432–435.

60. Lewis RA, Fleming JS. Fractional deposition from a jet nebulizer: how it differs from a metered dose inhaler. *Br J Dis Chest* 1985;79:361–367.

61. Jenkins SC, Heaton RW, Fulton TJ, et al. Comparison for domiciliary nebulized salbutamol and salbutamol from a metered-dose inhaler in stable chronic airflow limitation. *Chest* 1987;91:804–807.

62. Bowton DL, Goldsmith WM, Haponik EF. Substitution of metered-dose inhalers for hand-held nebulizers. Success and cost savings in a large, acute-care hospital. *Chest* 1992;101:305–308.

63. Camargo CA, Kenney PA. Assessing costs of aerosol therapy. *Respir Care Clin N Am* 2000;45:756–763.

64. Roberts RJ, Robinson JD, Doering PL, et al. A comparison of various types of patient instruction in the proper administration of metered inhalers. *Drug Intell Clin Pharm* 1982;16:53–59.

65. Armitage JM, Williams SJ. Inhaler technique in the elderly. *Age Ageing* 1988;17:275–278.

66. Sackner MA, Kim CS. Recent advances in the management of obstructive airways disease. Auxiliary MDI aerosol delivery systems. *Chest* 1985;88:161S–170S.

67. Chapman KR, Love L, Brubaker H. A comparison of breath-activated and conventional metered-dose inhaler inhalation techniques in elderly subjects. *Chest* 1993;104:1332–1337.

68. Morley TF, Marozsan E, Zappasodi SJ, et al. Comparison of beta-adrenergic agents delivered by nebulizer vs metered dose inhaler with InspirEase in hospitalized asthmatic patients. *Chest* 1988;94:1205–1210.

69. Gay PC, Patel HG, Nelson SB, et al. Metered dose inhalers for bronchodilator delivery in intubated, mechanically ventilated patients. *Chest* 1991;9:66–71.

70. Leiner GC, Abramowitz S, Small MJ, et al. Expiratory peak flow rate standard values for normal subjects. Use as a clinical test of ventilatory function. *Am Rev Respir Dis* 1963;88:644–651.

71. Hess D. Inhaled bronchodilators during mechanical ventilation: delivery techniques, evaluation of response, and cost-effectiveness. *Respir Care Clin N Am* 1994;39:105–122.

72. Ahrens RC, Ries RA, Popendorf W, Wiese JA. The delivery of therapeutic aerosols through endotracheal tubes. *Pediatr Pulmonol* 1986;1:19–26.

73. Niven RW, Kacmarek RM, Brain JD, et al. Small bore nozzle extensions to improve the delivery efficiency of drugs from metered dose inhalers: laboratory evaluation. *Am Rev Respir Dis* 1993;146:1590–1594.

74. Taylor RH, Lerman J, Chambers C, et al. Dosing efficiency and particle-size characteristics of pressurized metered-dose inhaler aerosols in narrow catheters. *Chest* 1993;103:920–924.

75. Spahr-Schopfer IA, Lerman J, Cutz E, et al. Airway mucosal damage induced by high dose aerosol in rabbits (abstract). *Am Rev Respir Dis* 1992;145:A364.

76. Fink JB: Aerosol device selection: evidence to practice. *Respir Care* 2000;45:874–885.

77. Meduri GU, Conoscenti CC, Menashe P, et al. Noninvasive face mask ventilation in patients with acute respiratory failure. *Chest* 1989;95:865–870.

78. Brochard L, Isabey D, Piquet J, et al. Reversal of acute exacerbations of chronic obstructive lung disease by inspiratory assistance with a face mask. *N Engl J Med* 1990;323:1523–1530.

79. Pennock BE, Kaplan PD, Carlin BW, et al. Pressure support ventilation with a simplified ventilatory support system administered with a nasal mask in patients with respiratory failure. *Chest* 1991;100:1371–1376.

80. Weber K, Milligan S. Therapist-driven protocols: the state-of-the-art (Conference report). *Respir Care Clin N Am* 1994;39:746–756.

81. Hart SK, Dubbs W, Gil A, et al. The effects of therapist-evaluation of orders and interaction with physicians on the appropriateness of respiratory care. *Respir Care Clin N Am* 1989;34:185–190.

82. Shapiro BA, Cane RD, Peterson J, et al. Authoritative medical direction can assure cost-beneficial bronchial hygiene therapy. *Chest* 1988;93:1038–1042.

37

BASIC PRINCIPLES AND NEW MODES OF MECHANICAL VENTILATION

NEIL R. MACINTYRE

KEY WORDS

- Acute respiratory distress syndrome
- Alveolar recruitment
- High-frequency ventilation
- Patient-ventilator interactions
- Positive end-expiratory pressure
- Pressure-targeted ventilation
- Respiratory failure
- Tidal volume
- Ventilator-induced lung injury
- Ventilator management protocol
- Volume-targeted ventilation

INTRODUCTION

Mechanical ventilation is the process of using devices to provide, either totally or partially, O_2 and CO_2 transport between the environment and the pulmonary capillary bed. The desired effect of mechanical ventilation is to maintain appropriate levels of oxygen and CO_2 in arterial blood while also unloading the ventilatory muscles. Although negative pressure chambers or wraps and extracorporeal circuits might fulfill this definition, this discussion focuses on the use of positive airway pressure to provide mechanical ventilatory support.

The use of positive pressure mechanical ventilation is widespread. In the United States, estimates range from one to three million patients annually requiring mechanical ventilatory support outside the operating room (1). In the United States, this support is supplied by an installed base of about 50,000 positive-pressure ventilators. Traditionally, this support has been provided in intensive care unit settings, but there are trends toward expanding the venues to subacute facilities, long-term care facilities, and the home. As the aged population expands and as more aggressive surgical and immunosuppressive therapies are developed, the need for mechanical ventilation is likely to expand (1,2).

DESIGN PRINCIPLES

Most modern ventilators use piston or bellows systems or controllers of high-pressure sources to drive gas flow (3,4). Tidal breaths are generated by this gas flow and can be controlled either entirely by the ventilator or can be interactive with patient efforts. Generally, pneumatic, electronic, or microprocessor systems provide for various breath types. These systems can be classified by what initiates the breath (*trigger variable*), what controls gas delivery during the breath (*target or limit variable*), and what terminates the breath (*cycle variable*) (4,5). Trigger variables are either patient effort (detected by the ventilator as a pressure or flow change, pressure and flow triggers, respectively) or a set machine timer. Target or limit variables are generally either a set flow or a set inspiratory pressure. Cycle variables are generally a set volume, a set inspiratory time, or a flow rate. Figure 1 uses this classification scheme to describe the most common breath types available on the current generation of mechanical ventilators.

The availability and delivery logic of different breath types define the "mode" of mechanical ventilatory support (4,5). The mode controller is an electronic, pneumatic, or microprocessor based system that is designed to provide the proper combination of breaths according to set algorithms and feedback data (conditional variables). Table 1 describes the common modes of mechanical ventilation according to the breath types available.

In general, volume and pressure assist or control modes of ventilation are designed to provide "total" support in that there should be minimal or no muscle loading. Modes that supply partial support are of two types: modes that allow spontaneous breaths that are (a) either interspersed between machine breaths [intermittent mandatory ventilation (IMV), synchronized intermittent mandatory ventilation (SIMV)] or are superimposed over the machine breath (airway pressure release ventilation [APRV]); and (b) modes that supply partial support with every breath, such as pressure support, pressure assist, or proportional assist ventilation (PAV; see below).

In recent years, newer designs have incorporate advanced monitoring and feedback functions into these controllers to allow for limited forms of "closed-loop" ventilator control (6). Design features are summarized in Table 2. Although these newer modes have been verified to perform as designed in the clinical setting, it

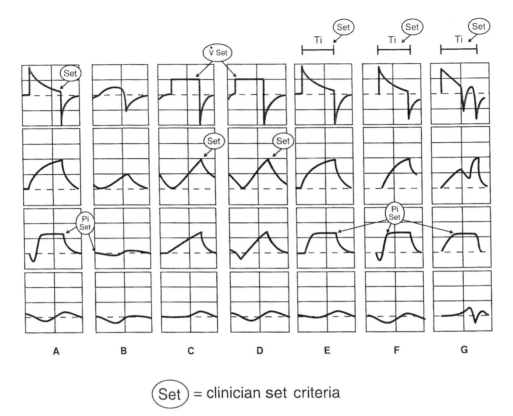

$\boxed{\text{Set}}$ = clinician set criteria

FIGURE 1. Common breath types available on modern mechanical ventilators. The upper panel is flow, the second panel is volume, the third panel is airway pressure, and the bottom panel is esophageal pressure (a reflection of pleural pressure). The circled parameters are those set by the clinician. Breaths are classified by their trigger, target, and cycle variables. **Breath A** is a pressure support (PS) breath (patient triggered, pressure targeted, flow cycled), **breath B** is a spontaneous (SP) breath with only the baseline airway pressure clinician set, **breath C** is a volume control (VC) breath (machine triggered, flow targeted, volume cycled), **breath D** is a volume assist (VA) breath (patient triggered, flow targeted, volume cycled), **breath E** is a pressure control (PC) breath (machine triggered, pressure targeted, time cycled), **breath F** is a pressure assist (PA) breath (patient triggered, pressure targeted, time cycled). **Breath G** is a pressure relief (PR) breath, a variation of the pressure control breath that incorporates a pressure relief mechanism to allow spontaneous breathing during the inflation time period.

is important to note that none has been assessed in any meaningful clinical outcome studies. Claims that these new approaches reduce lung injury, shorten the duration of mechanical injury, or automatically wean patients are thus unwarranted at this time.

VENTILATION AND RESPIRATORY SYSTEM MECHANICS

Equation of Motion

Lung inflation during mechanical ventilation occurs when pressure and flow are applied at the airway opening. These applied forces interact with respiratory system compliance (both lung and chest-wall components), airway resistance, and, to a lesser extent, respiratory system inertia and lung-tissue resistance to produce gas flow (4,7,8). For simplicity, because inertia and tissue resistance are relatively small, they can be ignored such that the interactions of pressure, flow, and volume with respiratory system mechanics can be expressed by the simplified equation of motion:

Driving pressure = (flow × resistance)

+ (volume/system compliance)

In the mechanically ventilated patient, this relationship is expressed as

$$\Delta Pao = (V' \times R) + (V_T / CRS)$$

where ΔPao is the change in pressure above baseline at the airway opening, V' is the flow into the patient's lungs, R is the resistance of circuit, artificial airway and natural airways, V_T is the tidal volume, and CRS is the respiratory system compliance.

By performing an inspiratory hold at end inspiration (i.e., no-flow conditions: $V' = 0$), the components of ΔPao required for flow and for respiratory system distension can be separated. Specifically, when $V' = 0$ at end inspiration, ΔPao is referred to as a "plateau" pressure and reflects the static system compliance ($CRS = V_T / \Delta Pao$, plateau). Calculating the difference in ΔPao during flow and during no-flow (the "peak to plateau difference") allows for a calculation of inspiratory airway resistance [$R = (\Delta Pao, \text{peak} - \Delta Pao, \text{plateau}) / V'$].

Separating the two components of respiratory system compliance (chest wall and lung compliance, C_{CW} and C_L, respectively) during a passive machine-controlled positive-pressure breath requires an esophageal pressure measurement (Pes) to approximate

TABLE 1. COMMON MODES OF MECHANICAL VENTILATION ACCORDING TO BREATH TYPES

Modes	Breath Types Available						
	VC	VA	PC	PA	PS	PR	SP
Volume assist control	x[a,b]	x					
Pressure assist control			x[a–c]	x[c]			
Volume SIMV	x	x			x		x
Pressure SIMV			x	x	x		x
APRV (BiPAP)						x[b]	x
PSV					x[d]		

VC, volume control; VA, volume assist; PC, pressure control; PA, pressure assist; PS, pressure support; PR, pressure relief; SP, spontaneous breath; SIMV, synchronized intermittent mandatory ventilation; APRV, airway pressure release ventilation; BiPAP, bilevel positive airway pressure; PSV, pressure-supported ventilations.
[a]Rate of control breaths can be automatically adjusted according to minute ventilation criteria and called such things as apnea ventilation, minimum minute ventilation, etc. Rate can also be turned to 0 to provide a pure assist mode of support.
[b]When inspiratory times of these breaths are extended beyond expiratory time, the term "inverse ratio ventilation" is often used.
[c]Inspiratory pressure can be automatically adjusted according to tidal volume or minute ventilation criteria on some machines (pressure-regulated volume control).
[d]Inspiratory pressure can be automatically adjusted according to tidal volume or minute ventilation criteria on some machines (volume support, pressure augmentation, volume assured pressure support).

pleural pressure. With this measurement, the inspiratory change in Pes (ΔPes) reflects C_{CW} and can be used in the following calculations:

$$C_{CW} = V_T/\Delta Pes$$

and

$$C_L = V_T/(\Delta Pao, plateau - \Delta Pes)$$

In patients with near-normal chest walls, C_{CW} has only a small effect on measured Pao (i.e., ΔPes is quite small) such that ΔPao, plateau is a reasonable reflection of C_L and lung distention. In the setting of stiff chest walls (e.g., edema, abdominal distention, surgical dressings, obesity), however C_{CW} can have considerable effects on measured Pao, and this must be considered when using only ΔPao, plateau to assess lung distention.

Pressure Targeted Versus Flow/Volume Targeted Breaths

Currently, there are two basic approaches to delivering positive pressure breaths: pressure targeting and flow/volume targeting. With pressure targeting, the clinician sets an inspiratory pressure target (with either time or flow as the cycling criteria) such that flow and volume are dependent variables (i.e., varying with lung mechanics and patient effort to maintain the flow and volume targets). With flow/volume targeting (breaths C and D in Fig. 1), the clinician sets an inspiratory flow and cycling volume such that airway pressure is the dependent variable. Changes in compliance or resistance will cause a change of tidal volume (but not Pao) with the pressure-targeted breath. In contrast, similar changes in compliance or resistance will change Pao (but not flow or volume) with a volume-targeted breath. These design characteristics need to be considered in choosing a pressure or a flow/volume targeted

breath for a given patient. Specifically, if CO_2 clearance is more important than limiting lung distension (e.g., mild lung injury in a head-injury patient), volume guarantee with volume cycled breaths would be the best choice. In contrast, if regional overdistension is more of a concern than CO_2 clearance (e.g., in severe lung injury with high ventilatory pressures), assuring a maximal distending pressure limit with a pressure targeted breath would be the best choice (see "Lung Stretch Injury" to follow). In addition, if a patient's spontaneous flow demand is high during patient triggered breaths, the variable flow of the pressure-targeted breath may be more synchronous than the fixed flow of the flow/volume targeted breath (see "Interactions" to follow).

Intrinsic Positive End-Expiratory Pressure and the Ventilatory Pattern

Measured Pao during breath delivery depends on both the ΔPao as well as the baseline pressure (both applied and intrinsic positive end-expiratory pressure, or PEEP). Intrinsic PEEP is determined by three factors: minute ventilation, the expiratory time fraction, and the respiratory system's expiratory time constant (the product of resistance and compliance) (9). If minute ventilation increases, expiratory time fraction decreases, or the time constant lengthens (i.e., higher R or C values), the potential for intrinsic PEEP to develop increases. An additional factor affecting intrinsic PEEP is gas density; so a low-density gas (heliox) in patients with severe airflow obstruction may facilitate lung emptying and reduce intrinsic PEEP.

The development of intrinsic PEEP will have different effects on pressure-targeted compared with flow/volume-targeted ventilation. In flow/volume-targeted ventilation, the constant delivered volume in the setting of a rising intrinsic PEEP will increase the peak and plateau Pao to maintain a constant ΔPao. In contrast, in pressure-targeted ventilation, the set Pao limit coupled with a rising intrinsic PEEP level will decrease ΔPao and thus the delivered tidal volume (and minute ventilation).

In the passive patient, intrinsic PEEP can be assessed in two additional ways. First, when an inadequate expiratory time is producing intrinsic PEEP, analysis of the flow graphic will show that expiratory flow has not returned to zero before the next breath is initiated. Second, intrinsic PEEP in alveolar units that have patent airways can be quantified during a prolonged expiratory hold maneuver that permits equilibration of the intrinsic PEEP throughout the ventilator circuitry (10).

Distribution of Ventilation

A positive-pressure tidal breath must distribute itself among the millions of alveolar units in the lung (11). Factors that affect this distribution include regional resistances, compliances, functional residual capacities, and the delivered flow pattern (including inspiratory pause). In general, delivered ventilation will tend to distribute more to units with high compliance and low resistance (Fig. 2), which creates the potential for regional overdistension of healthier lung units, even in the face of "normal"-sized tidal volumes (see "Lung Stretch Injury").

Flow pattern also can affect ventilation distribution (11,12). Specifically, slower flows will tend to distribute more evenly in

TABLE 2. PARTIAL CLOSED-LOOP MODES OF VENTILATORY SUPPORT

Mode Name	Design Principles	Putative Advantage	Comments
Mandatory minute ventilation (MMV), automatic minute ventilation (AMV)	SIMV mode (Table 1) with capability of increasing/ decreasing mandatory breath rate depending on minute ventilation	Provide guaranteed minimum minute ventilation in patients with unreliable ventilatory drives.	If desired minute ventilation set inappropriately, inappropriate levels of support would be provided.
Pressure-regulated volume control (PRVC)[a], autoflow, variable pressure control	Pressure-targeted time cycled breaths with capability of automatically adjusting pressure on subsequent breaths to guarantee volume	Decelerating, variable flow pattern provides synchrony/gas mixing effects of a pressure targeted breath with the volume guarantee of the volume cycled breath during high levels of ventilatory support.	Since pressure will adjust with the changing respiratory system mechanics, this mode does not set a pressure limit.
Volume support (VS)[a], variable pressure support	Pressure-targeted flow cycled breaths with capability of automatically adjusting pressure on subsequent breaths to guarantee volume	Decelerating, variable flow pattern provides synchrony/gas mixing effects of a pressure targeted breath with the volume guarantee of the volume cycled breath during weaning.	Since tidal volume (V_T) is the main controller, inappropriate V_T selection may lead to inappropriate pressure adjustments as patients recover.
Volume-assured pressure support (VAPS), pressure augmentation	Pressure-targeted flow cycled breaths with the capability of adding a backup set flow during the breath to guarantee volume	Decelerating, variable flow pattern provides synchrony/gas mixing effects of a pressure targeted breath with the volume guarantee of the volume cycled breath.	Does not provide a pressure limit and, if V_T selection is inappropriately high, may give inappropriately high pressures as patients recover.
Adaptive support ventilation (ASV)	Automatic frequency-tidal volume combination set based on clinician set level of support (% of alveolar ventilation provided by ventilator) and respiratory system mechanics (compliance and resistance to set the "minimal work" pattern (Otis), adequate expiratory time to avoid auto PEEP).	Automatic "default" settings with ability to adjust to patient mechanics and effort	"Minimal work" assumptions have not been tested in sick patients.

SIMV, spontaneous intermittent mandatory ventilation; PEEP, positive end-expiratory pressure.
[a]Automode is a technique that switches back and forth from PRVC and VS depending on the adequacy of patient triggering efforts.

obstructive inhomogeneities (although consequent shorter expiratory times may worsen air trapping), whereas faster flows (especially decelerating flows) will tend to distribute more evenly in compliance inhomogeneities. In addition, rapid initial flows (a consequence of set decelerating flow profiles or pressure targeted breaths) pressurize the lung most rapidly and thus produce the highest mean inspiratory alveolar pressure for a given end inflation pressure. Finally, inspiratory pauses can also allow pendelluft action to inflate, slowly filling alveoli (Fig. 2, resistance abnormality).

It should be noted that more uniform ventilation distribution does not necessarily mean better ventilation–perfusion (V/Q) matching (i.e., more even ventilation distribution may actually worsen V/Q matching in a lung with perfusion inhomogeneities). Because of all these considerations, predicting which flow pattern will optimize ventilation-perfusion matching is difficult and often an empirical trial and error exercise.

ALVEOLAR RECRUITMENT AND GAS EXCHANGE

Infiltrative lung disease produces severe V/Q mismatching through alveolar flooding and collapse (13,14). In many (but not all) of these disease processes, these collapsed alveoli can be recruited during a positive-pressure ventilatory cycle (15,16). Two specific techniques to maintain this recruitment are the application of PEEP and manipulations of the inspiratory–expiratory time relationships.

Positive End-Expiratory Pressure

Defined as an elevation of transpulmonary pressures at the end of expiration, PEEP can be produced by either expiratory circuit valves (*applied* PEEP) or as a consequence of ventilator settings interacting with respiratory system mechanics (*intrinsic* PEEP).

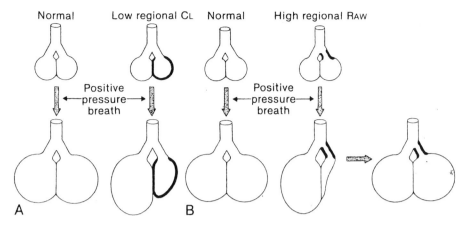

FIGURE 2. Schematic effects of the distribution of ventilation in two-unit lung models with homogeneous mechanical properties (**left breath**), with abnormal compliance distribution (**middle breath**), and abnormal resistance distribution (**right breath**). (From MacIntyre NR, Mechanical ventilatory support. In: Dantzker DR, ed, *Comprehensive respiratory care*. Philadelphia: WB Saunders, 1995, with permission.)

Note that expiratory muscle contraction can raise intrathoracic pressures at end expiration, but this should not be considered PEEP because it is not a transpulmonary pressure (i.e., alveolar–pleural pressure).

Alveoli prevented from "de-recruiting" by PEEP provide several patient benefits. First, recruited alveoli improve V/Q matching and gas exchange (13–16). Second, as discussed in more detail later, recruited alveoli throughout the ventilatory cycle are not exposed to the risk of injury from the shear stress of repeated opening and closing (16,17). Third, PEEP prevents surfactant breakdown in collapsing alveoli and thus improves lung compliance (18). PEEP, however, also can be detrimental. Because the tidal breath is delivered above the baseline PEEP, end-inspiratory pressures are raised by PEEP application. This must be considered if the lung is at risk for stretch injury (see "Lung Stretch Injury"). Moreover, alveolar injury in lung disease is often quite heterogeneous; therefore, appropriate PEEP in one region may be suboptimal in another and yet excessive in another. Optimizing PEEP is thus a balance between recruiting the recruitable alveoli in diseased regions without overdistending already recruited alveoli in healthier regions. Another potential detrimental effect of PEEP is that it also raises mean intrathoracic pressure, which can compromise cardiac filling in susceptible patients (see "Cardiac Effects" to follow).

Criteria for determining the appropriate PEEP setting can be based on either gas-exchange or mechanical goals. Gas-exchange goals are the traditional approach to setting PEEP (15). When using gas-exchange goals, the idea is to use the fraction of inspired oxygen (FIO_2 requirements), PaO_2, or the calculated shunt fraction as the target. An example would be to apply whatever PEEP is necessary to attain a minimally acceptable PaO_2 at the lowest possible FIO_2. A more aggressive gas-exchange goal would be to normalize (or at least minimize) shunt fraction. This approach, however, may require very high levels of PEEP (i.e., sometimes in excess of normal maximal transpulmonary pressure). This approach is not commonly used today out of concern that overdistending healthier lung regions is probably an unacceptable trade-off for aggressive shunt reduction. Moreover, some of the apparent shunt reduction that occurs with high PEEP levels may be a con-

sequence of reduced cardiac output from the high intrathoracic pressures.

Mechanical goals for PEEP applications have the appeal of setting ventilator pressures in accordance with respiratory system mechanical behavior. This approach actually dates back several decades when "best compliance" was proposed as a reasonable way to set proper PEEP (19). Today, the goal is similar but is often more specifically focused on static pressure–volume (PV) relationships (20) (Fig. 3). One approach is to use the lower inflection point on a static PV curve (Fig. 3, point A) as the marker for an optimal pressure that prevents de-recruitment. A variation on this approach would be to use the lower inflection point on the deflation limb of the static PV curve. Because of respiratory system compliance hysteresis (21), this deflation limb value is generally several centimeters of H_2O lower than the value on the inflation limb and may be a better representation of the true critical de-recruitment pressure. A corollary to both these approaches is that it may be beneficial to first perform a "volume-recruitment" maneuver (e.g., a 1-minute period of 35–40 cm H_2O inflation hold) before returning to the desired PEEP level (22).

Inspiratory Flow Pattern and Inspiratory–Expiratory Time Manipulations

Inspiration during a positive pressure breath consists of a tidal volume and a flow profile that, as noted, can affect ventilation distribution (and thus V/Q). Inspiratory time (and the relationship of inspiratory to expiratory (I:E) time can be particularly important. Prolonging inspiratory time, generally by adding a pause or using a rapid decelerating flow (i.e., pressure targeted) breath can substantially increase mean inflation pressure and will lengthen gas-mixing time in the lung. Moreover, if the resultant expiratory time is inadequate for the lung to return to its relaxed volume (i.e., functional residual capacity, or FRC), intrinsic PEEP develops.

There are several physiologic effects of prolonging inspiratory time (23–25). First, the increased gas mixing time may improve V/Q matching in infiltrative lung disease. Second, the development of intrinsic PEEP can have similar effects to that of applied PEEP (see preceding). Indeed, much of the improvement in gas

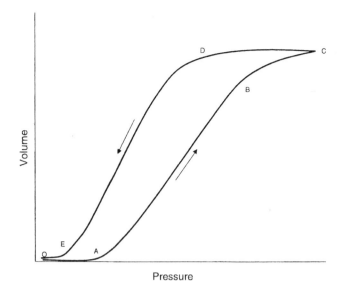

FIGURE 3. A schematic pressure-volume plot in a patient with infiltrative lung disease and alveolar collapse in end expiration (**Point O**). On the vertical axis is delivered volume and on the horizontal axis is distending pressure, ideally the alveolar-to-pleural pressure gradient under static conditions. Both inflation (up arrow) and deflation (down arrow) phases of the breath are illustrated. **Point A** is the lower inflection point during inflation and represents the point when the bulk of recruitable alveoli begin to be opened. **Point B** is the upper inflection point during inflation and represents that point when recruitable alveoli begin to be overdistended and compliance falls. **Point C** is the maximal pressure and volume during the maneuver. **Point D** is the upper inflection point during deflation when alveoli begin to empty. **Point E** is the lower inflection point during deflation when alveoli begin to collapse or de-recruit. Operating on the concept that positive end-expiratory pressure (PEEP) should be used to maintain recruitment and that the PEEP/tidal volume (V_T) combination should not produce overdistension, there are two conceptual approaches to setting the PEEP/V_T combination using this plot. One is to set the PEEP just above Point A and keep the PEEP/V_T combination below Point B (inflation curve settings). A second is to do a volume recruitment maneuver to Point C and set the PEEP/V_T combination between Points D and E (deflation curve settings). (From MacIntyre NR. *Principles of mechanical ventilation.* In: Murray M, ed. *Respiratory diseases*, 3rd ed. Philadelphia: WB Saunders, 2000, with permission.)

exchange associated with long inspiratory time strategies may be merely a PEEP phenomenon. It should be noted, however, that the distribution of intrinsic PEEP (most pronounced in lung units with long time constants) may differ from that of applied PEEP, and thus V/Q effects also may differ. Third, because these long inspiratory times significantly increase total intrathoracic pressures, cardiac output may be affected (see "Cardiac Effects" below). Finally, I:E ratios that exceed 1:1 (inverse ratio ventilation, or IRV) are uncomfortable and patient sedation/paralysis is often required.

Generally, inspiratory time prolongation is reserved for patients in whom the plateau pressure from the PEEP/tidal volume combination has approached 35 cm H_2O and potentially toxic concentrations of FIO_2 are being used without meeting arterial oxygenation saturation or oxygen delivery goals.

LUNG INJURY FROM POSITIVE-PRESSURE VENTILATION

The lung can be injured when it is stretched excessively by positive-pressure ventilation. The most obvious injury is that of alve-

olar rupture presenting as extraalveolar air in the mediastinum (pneumomediastinum), pericardium (pneumopericardium), subcutaneous tissue (subcutaneous emphysema), pleura (pneumothorax), and vasculature (air emboli). The risk for extraalveolar air increases as a function of the magnitude and duration of alveolar overdistension.

In experimental animals, a parenchymal lung injury not associated with extraalveolar air also can be produced by mechanical ventilation strategies that stretch the lungs beyond the normal maximum (i.e., transpulmonary distending pressures of 30–35 cm H_2O). Pathologically, this manifests as diffuse alveolar damage (16,17,26,27) and is associated with cytokine release (27) and bacterial translocation (28). It also appears that this injury is potentiated by a shear stress phenomenon that occurs when injured alveoli are repetitively opened and collapsed during the ventilatory cycle (16,17,27).

This injury may occur clinically when low-resistance/high-compliance units receive a disproportionately high regional tidal volume in the setting of high alveolar distending pressures (Fig. 2) and appears to be potentiated in atelectatic units that do not receive levels of PEEP adequate to prevent collapse. As in the animal studies, overdistension and underrecruitment during positive-pressure ventilation also can release inflammatory cytokines into the circulation, which can produce multiorgan dysfunction (27). The recently reported National Institutes of Health ARDS (acute respiratory distress syndrome) Network study showing improved mortality when using smaller tidal volumes (6 ml/kg) to limit overdistension (ARDSnet) attests to the importance of limiting end inspiratory stretch (29).

Concern about overdistension/underrecruitment injury is the rationale for using mechanical measurements of the lung to guide ventilator management in a "lung-protective" approach (30,31). The simplest guide to limiting overdistension is to manage patients below the normal maximal transpulmonary pressure of 35 cm H_2O (in a patient with near-normal chest-wall compliance, end-inspiratory transpulmonary pressure is approximated by the airway plateau pressure) (29,30). Conceptually, however, the most direct way to determine lung-protective ventilator settings mechanically would be to use the static PV curve as described in Figure 3. Using this approach, one study showed impressive improvement in ARDS outcome (31).

Because static pressure volume curves are time consuming and often require heavy sedation or paralysis of the patient, simpler ways of determining inflection points are being investigated. Potential approaches include a very slow constant flow (i.e., 10 L/minute) breath and recording of a single dynamic PV curve (32). Under these circumstances, flow is so slow that flow resistive pressure is minimized and the curve approximates a static curve. Corrections for endotracheal tube resistive pressure can be subtracted mathematically, or pressures can be recorded from the distal end of the endotracheal tube. The addition of an esophageal pressure tracing to account for chest-wall effects (see preceding) also might be important in patients with abnormal chest-wall compliance.

It is important to note that reducing the risk of stretch injury may require the use of small tidal volumes and lower minute ventilations (29,30). This may cause PCO_2 elevation and a respiratory acidosis. This willingness to accept a respiratory acidosis to prevent lung overstretch is sometimes referred to as *permissive hypercapnia* (33). Increases in CO_2 levels seem to be tolerated in increments of about 10 mm Hg per hour, and most patients can tolerate pH values in the 7.1 to 7.2 range (33). It should be noted, however, that allowing acidosis should be done with caution in patients with increased intracranial pressure or unstable hemodynamics (vasopressor dependence or dysrhythmias). An interesting adjunct to help deal with CO_2 clearance in low tidal-volume ventilation is tracheal gas insufflation (TGI). This experimental technique uses a 6 to 10 L per minute flow of fresh gas through a small-bore catheter placed at the distal end of the endotracheal tube to wash the endotracheal tube free of CO_2 during exhalation and thereby reduce dead space (34).

An interesting ventilatory strategy focused on lung "protection" is high-frequency ventilation (HFV), which refers to ventilatory strategies using higher than normal breathing frequencies (i.e., 60–500 breaths per minute in the adult) (35,36). With this breathing pattern, tidal volumes are often smaller than anatomic dead space, and thus gas transport mechanisms other than convective flow must be invoked (e.g., "augmented" diffusion, asymmetric flow profiles, Taylor dispersion, and pendelluft) (37). Conventional ventilators are incapable of responding this quickly, and thus either jet devices or high-frequency oscillators must be used. The theoretical advantage to HFV in infiltrative lung disease is that the high delivered minute ventilation and short expiratory time will produce substantial intrinsic PEEP, whereas the small delivered tidal volumes will limit maximal pressures and distending volume. The lung will thus be recruited and ventilated in the optimal portion of the pressure volume curve (i.e., between C and D in Fig. 3). In infants at high risk for barotrauma, HFV has been shown to be safe and effective in reducing long-term lung injury (38). Adult experience is less, and clinical trials are needed before widespread application can be recommended.

PATIENT–VENTILATOR INTERACTIONS

Mechanical ventilation modes that permit spontaneous ventilatory activity are termed *interactive* modes in that patients can affect various aspects of the ventilator's functions. These interactions can range from simple triggering of mechanical breaths to more complex processes affecting delivered flow patterns and breath timing. Interactive modes allow for muscle "exercise," which, when done at nonfatiguing or physiologic levels, may prevent muscle atrophy and facilitate fatigue recovery (39). In addition, permitting spontaneous patient ventilatory activity and using comfortable interactive modes may reduce the need for the sedation or neuromuscular blockers often required to prevent patients from "fighting" the ventilator (40).

Interactive modes can be either synchronous or dyssynchronous with patient efforts. *Synchronous* interactions mean that the ventilator is sensitive to the initiation, modulation, and termination of a patient's ventilatory effort. Synchrony is considered during the three phases of interactive breath delivery: breath triggering, ventilator flow delivery, and breath cycling.

Ventilator Breath Triggering

Interactive mechanical ventilation needs to sense a spontaneous effort (either an airway pressure drop or airway flow change) to trigger a mechanical response. Even with modern sensors, however, there is unavoidable dyssynchrony in the triggering process (41). First, a certain level of insensitivity must be put in the sensor to avoid artifacts triggering the ventilator (i.e., "autocycling"). Second, even when the patient effort has been sensed, demand valve systems have an inherent delay (up to 100 msec or more) before they physically open and achieve target flow into the airway (system responsiveness). Both these factors can result in significant "isometric-like" pressure loads on the ventilatory muscles during the triggering process (41). In addition, in the setting of air trapping (intrinsic PEEP), the elevated alveolar pressure at end expiration can serve as a significant triggering threshold load on the ventilatory muscles (42,43).

Several strategies can be used to minimize the magnitude of the dyssynchrony induced during breath triggering. First, using ventilators with microprocessor flow controls can result in significantly better valve characteristics than that obtained with older-generation ventilators. Second, continuous-flow systems superimposed on the demand systems can improve demand system responsiveness in patients with high ventilatory drives (although such flows can reduce sensitivity in patients with very weak ventilatory drives). Third, flow-based triggers can produce a more sensitive and responsive breath triggering process (41). Fourth, a small amount of applied inspiratory pressure support usually increases the ventilator's initial flow delivery and can thereby improve response characteristics of the demand valve system. Fifth, in obstructive-disease patients with an inspiratory threshold load induced by intrinsic PEEP, setting applied PEEP below the intrinsic PEEP level can help equilibrate the end-expiratory alveolar and circuit pressures and improve triggering (42,43). Finally, sensors in the pleural space or on the phrenic nerve may improve trigger performance on future systems.

Ventilator-delivered Flow Pattern

During an interactive breath, ventilatory muscles are contracting (44,45), and the ventilator flow delivery should be adequate to meet one of three goals: (a) to unload fully the contracting ventilatory muscles in patients with severely overloaded and fatigued muscles; (b) to unload partially the contracting ventilatory muscles in patients recovering from muscle fatigue; or (c) not to affect the loads (i.e., add no imposed loads) on contracting ventilatory muscle in patients during spontaneous breathing trials. Synchronous flow interactions can be defined accordingly.

Breaths Designed to Fully Unload Ventilatory Muscles

For an interactive breath to unload ventilator muscles fully, the patient should be required to trigger only the ventilator and then have the ventilator supply all of the work of the breath. The goal of synchrony during a fully unloading breath is thus to deliver adequate flow over the entire inspiratory effort to unload totally the contracting muscles. Achieving this goal can be assessed by comparing the pressure pattern of the patient-triggered breath with a machine-triggered breath (i.e., a breath occurring without patient activity). Synchronous flow delivery should

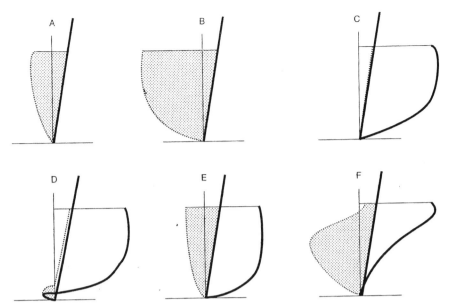

FIGURE 4. Pressure–volume plots depicting various patient–ventilator interactions for a constant tidal volume. In each plot, volume is on the vertical axis and pressure is on the horizontal axis. Machine pressures are depicted by solid lines; esophageal pressures are depicted by dashed lines. The solid angled line directed upward and to the right from the origin reflects passive inflation esophageal pressure (chest-wall compliance). The shaded area reflects patient work. **Breath A** depicts a normal unloaded spontaneous (unsupported/unassisted) breath. **Breath B** depicts an abnormally loaded spontaneous breath. **Breath C** depicts a machine controlled breath in the abnormal patient. **Breath D** depicts a synchronous assisted breath designed to unload totally the abnormal patient (only triggering load is evident). **Breath E** depicts a synchronous assisted breath designed to unload partially the abnormal patient. Under these circumstances, *synchrony* is defined as a smooth airway pressure "bias" that converts the patient's loading pattern to a more normal configuration (i.e., resembling Breath A). **Breath F** depicts a dyssynchronous assisted breath in the abnormal patient. High-pressure patient loads exist through much of this breath because of inappropriate ventilator flow delivery. (From MacIntyre NR. *Principles of mechanical ventilation*, in Murray M, ed. *Respiratory diseases*, 3rd ed. Philadelphia: WB Saunders, 2000, with permission.)

produce nearly identical airway pressure waveforms and only evidence of triggering in the pleural/esophageal pressure waveforms (Fig. 4, Breath D). This is usually accompanied by a near-normal spontaneous respiratory frequency. Generally, a pressure-targeted breath with its variable flow feature will be easier to synchronize with an active patient demand than a fixed flow breath (46,47).

Breaths Designed To Partially Unload Ventilatory Muscles

For an interactive breath to unload partially ventilatory muscles, the patient and the ventilator need to "share" the work of the breath. *Synchrony* then is defined as having the ventilator provide a constant pressure "bias" on the ventilatory muscles such that their PV configuration normalizes and "nonphysiologic" high pressure–low volume breaths are avoided (Fig. 4: the abnormal load pattern in breath B is "normalized" in breath E but not in breath F) (46,47). Synchronous partially unloaded breaths thus will have a similar airway pressure waveform shape (although less magnitude) as a controlled breath, whereas the pleural/esophageal pressure waveforms will resemble a normal loading pattern (Fig. 4: breath E). In addition, flow synchrony usually is associated with a near-normal spontaneous breathing frequency. On current systems, variable flow, pressure-targeted breaths are better designed for partial unloading than are fixed-flow breaths.

Breaths Designed Not to Affect Ventilatory Muscle Loads

For an interactive breath not to affect loads on the ventilatory muscles (and not impose loads), the ventilator must supply flow sufficient only to keep the distal airway pressure constant (continuous positive airway pressure, or CPAP). Under these conditions, flow synchrony is defined as flow that maintains a pleural–esophageal pressure waveform that would mimic that of an extubated patient.

In recent years, three developments have occurred to enhance flow synchrony under all three conditions listed previously: tracheal pressure targeting, pressure rise-time adjustments, and proportional assist ventilation (PAV).

Tracheal-pressure targeting uses pressure at the distal end of the endotracheal tube to govern gas flow during pressure targeted breaths (48,49). The inherent lag introduced by the high-resistance endotracheal tube on the pressure–flow control algorithm of the ventilator during interactive breaths is thus eliminated. Tracheal pressure targeting can use either a tracheal pressure-sensing catheter or mathematic calculations to estimate tracheal pressure from circuit pressure, delivered flow, and endotracheal tube dimensions (automatic tube compensation, or ATC). The problem with direct pressure sensing is the difficulty with catheter reliability in an airway containing mucus and moisture. The problem with mathematic models is that they have difficulty accounting for kinked tubes, mucus/moisture within the tube and the angle between the tube opening and the airway.

Pressure rise-time adjusters allow the clinician to adjust the rate of rise of pressure during pressure-targeted breaths (50). Very rapid rates of rise are helpful in meeting flow demands of patients with very vigorous inspiratory flow demands. In contrast, much slower rates of rise are needed in patients with less vigorous inspiratory flow demands. In practice, adjustment of the rate of rise should be aimed at creating a smooth "square wave" of airway pressure because this is the setting that provides the most comfort and flow synchrony (50). It also should be remembered that the rate of rise also will affect breath cycling with pressure support algorithms using a percent of peak flow as a cycle criteria. Specifically, a rapid rate of rise will produce breath cycling at high inspiratory flows, whereas a much slower rate of rise will produce breath cycling at much lower inspiratory flows.

PAV is an experimental technique that uses "gain" settings on patient flow and volume demand to govern ventilator gas flow (51,52). Operationally, the ventilator calculates patient compliance and resistance, and the clinician selects a proportion of the total compliance/resistance load that is to be assisted by the ventilator. As the patient begins an inspiratory effort, the ventilator adjusts pressure and flow to provide the desired level of support for a given flow and volume demand. Unlike pressure support, which increases flow but holds pressure constant for increased demand, PAV will increase both pressure and flow for increased demand. In clinical studies, PAV performs as designed (52), but clinical outcome studies remain to be done.

Breath Cycling

Cycling dyssynchrony can occur in one of two ways. First, if the breath lasts beyond patient effort, an inadequate expiratory time may develop (along with air trapping) or patient expiratory efforts may be required to terminate the breath (53). Second, if the breath terminates before the patient effort is finished, the patient may be left demanding additional flow without any being delivered. Significant imposed loading or double-breath triggering may result. With either type of cycle dyssynchrony, it is important that the clinician recognize it and make appropriate adjustments to the cycling criteria.

POSITIVE-PRESSURE VENTILATION AND CARDIAC FUNCTION

In addition to affecting ventilation and ventilation distribution, intrathoracic pressure applications from positive-pressure ventilation can also affect cardiovascular function (54–56). In general, as mean intrathoracic pressure is increased, right ventricular filling is decreased and results in decreased cardiac output and pulmonary perfusion. Volume expansion is therefore required to maintain cardiac output in the setting of high intrathoracic pressure. The effect of reduced cardiac filling on cardiac output may be partially counteracted by better left ventricular function because elevated intrathoracic pressures effectively decrease left ventricular afterload.

Intrathoracic pressures also can influence distribution of perfusion. The relationship of alveolar pressures to perfusion pressures is described by the three-lung-zone model (57). Specifically, the supine human lung is generally in a zone 3 (distension) state. As intraalveolar pressures rise, however, zone 2 and zone 1 regions can appear, creating high V/Q units. Indeed, increases in dead space (i.e., a zone 1 lung) can be a consequence of ventilatory strategies that use high ventilatory pressures (e.g., IRV).

Positive-pressure ventilation can affect other aspects of cardiovascular function. Specifically, dyspnea, anxiety, and discomfort from inadequate ventilatory support can lead to stress-related catechol release with subsequent increases in myocardial oxygen demands and dysrhythmias (58). In addition, coronary blood vessel oxygen delivery can be compromised by inadequate gas exchange from the lung injury coupled with low mixed venous PO_2 due to high oxygen consumption demands by the ventilatory muscles.

NON–PRESSURE-RELATED COMPLICATIONS OF MECHANICAL VENTILATION

Oxygen Toxicity

Oxygen concentrations approaching 100% are known to cause oxidant injuries in airways and lung parenchyma (59). Much of the data supporting this concept, however, have come from animals that often have quite different tolerances to oxygen than humans. It is thus not clear what the "safe" oxygen concentration or duration of exposure is in sick humans. Most consensus groups have argued that FIO_2 values less than 0.4 are safe for prolonged periods and that FIO_2 values greater than 0.80 should be avoided if at all possible. As noted, this means that tradeoffs among high PEEP/plateau pressures, high inspired oxygen concentrations, and the minimal arterial oxygen content goal must occur in the management of patients with severe gas-exchange abnormalities.

Patient Ventilator Interface Complications

The patient–ventilator interface includes the ventilator circuitry and the artificial airway. The most important complications associated with this apparatus are ventilator disconnections (including artificial airway dislodgment). This has been reported to occur in up to 8% to 13% of ventilated patients (60) and, if left uncorrected, can be fatal. Because circuit pressure and flow still can occur with the ventilator disconnected from the patient (e.g., the airway is in the esophagus or the disconnected circuit is only partially occluded as it lays on the patient's chest), it is critical that carefully set, redundant (i.e., pressure and flow) alarms are present. Other complications of the patient–ventilator interface include obstructions from secretions, circuit leaks, airway injury from inadequate heat and humidity, tracheal injury from the artificial airway, and loss of delivered tidal volume in a compliant circuit.

Pulmonary Infectious Complications

Mechanically ventilated patients are at risk for pulmonary infections for several reasons (61,62). First, the natural glottic closure protective mechanism is compromised by an endotracheal tube. This permits continuous seepage of oropharyngeal material into the airways. Second, the endotracheal tube itself impairs the cough reflex and serves as an additional potential portal for pathogens to enter the lungs. This is particularly important if the circuit is contaminated. Third, airway and parenchymal injury from both the underlying disease as well as management complications noted previously make the lung prone to infections. Fourth, the intensive care unit environment, with its heavy antibiotic use and presence of very sick patients in close proximity, is itself a risk.

Preventing ventilator-associated pneumonias is critical because length of stay and mortality are heavily influenced by their development (61,62). Hand washing and carefully chosen antibiotic regimens for other infections can have important beneficial effects. Management strategies that avoid breaking the integrity of the circuit (i.e., circuit changes only when visibly contaminated) also appear to be helpful. Finally, continuous drainage of subglottic secretions may be a simple way to reduce lung contamination from oropharyngeal material .

Ventilator Management Protocols

Both total and partial forms of ventilator support are amenable to being performed by skilled nonphysician persons under protocols. Indeed, properly designed protocols not only optimize ventilator settings but have been shown in several randomized controlled trials to reduce the duration of mechanical ventilation (63,64).

In a protocol for total support of a patient in acute respiratory failure, the three important "drivers" for decision making are the pH, the PO_2, and the plateau pressure. The pH is determined by the frequency–tidal volume settings, the Pa_{O_2} is determined by the PEEP and FIO_2 settings, and the plateau pressure is determined by the tidal volume and the PEEP (both intrinsic and applied). Breath types and mode selection will depend on whether pressure-limiting or volume guarantee is more important and whether patient–ventilator synchrony is an issue.

In a protocol for partial support of a patient with stable or recovering respiratory failure, patient–ventilator synchrony is a particularly important issue, and proper mode selection and breath characteristics can have significant impact on patient comfort and sedation use. Perhaps more important during partial support, however, is the need for regular clinical assessments for discontinuation potential.

An example of a well-designed protocol for both total and partial support is the one used by the National Institutes of Health ARDS Network for its clinical trials (29). This protocol has been adapted for general clinical use and is presented in the Appendix. Although designed for patients with ARDS, the fundamentals of this protocol can be modified and used for any patient requiring mechanical ventilatory support. Modifications for patients with obstructed airways might include an emphasis on longer expiratory times and permissive hypercapnia to minimize intrinsic PEEP. The PEEP FIO_2 table also might be adjusted for patients with obstructed airways to minimize unnecessary applied PEEP. In contrast, protocol modifications for patients with neuromuscular problems (including postanesthesia) might include more generous tidal volumes to improve comfort because excessive plateau pressure measurements are less likely in this population.

APPENDIX: MODIFIED VENTILATORY SUPPORT PROTOCOL USED BY THE NATIONAL INSTITUTES OF HEALTH ACUTE RESPIRATORY DISTRESS SYNDROME (ARDS) NETWORK

Full-support Ventilation Orders

1. Patient height (inches) = _____
2. Patient predicted body weight (PBW) = _____
   Male: 50 + 2.3 (Height in inches − 60)
   Female: 45.5 + 2.3 (Height in inches − 60)

Full Vent Support

Mode:	Assist control (A/C)
Tidal volume (V_T)	Set V_T initially to 8 mL/kg PBW, then reduce by 1 mL/kg at intervals < 2 h until V_T = target V_T of 6 mL/kg PBW
Rate:	Set respiratory rate (RR) to match minute ventilation prior to enrollment, not to exceed 35 breaths per minute (bpm)
Note:	Adjust V_T and RR to achieve arterial pH and end-expiratory plateau pressure goals

pH Goals: 7.30–7.45

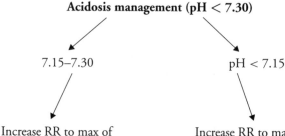

Acidosis management (pH < 7.30)

7.15–7.30   pH < 7.15

Increase RR to max of 35, or until pH > 7.30 or Pa_{CO_2} < 25 If RR = 35 consider buffer

Increase RR to max of 35. Consider buffer. If above fails V_T may be increased in steps of 1 mL/kg PBW until pH > 7.15 (plateau pressure may be exceeded).

Alkalosis management (pH > 7.45)

Decrease RR if possible

Plateau Pressure Goals: Plateau Pressure ≤ 30 cm H_2O

Check plateau pressure (0.5 sec inspiratory hold), SpO_2, and V_T at least q4h and after each change in PEEP or V_T.

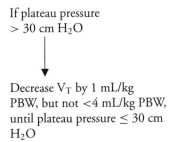

If plateau pressure
> 30 cm H$_2$O

↓

Decrease V$_T$ by 1 mL/kg
PBW, but not <4 mL/kg PBW,
until plateau pressure ≤ 30 cm
H$_2$O

Inspiration: Expiration (I : E) Ratio Goals: I : E = 1 : 1 to 1 : 3

Inspiratory flow rate and waveform are not collected directly by the protocol rules. Instead, inspiratory flow and waveform should be adjusted to achieve I:E = 1:1 to 1:3. Adjustments to inspiratory flow or waveform may be necessary to maintain this target range when RR changes. Please check and make appropriate adjustments.

Oxygenation Goals:

55 mm Hg ≤ Pa$_{O_2}$ ≤ 80 mm Hg

or

88% ≤ Sp$_{O_2}$ ≤ 95%

LOWER POSITIVE END-EXPIRATORY RATE (PEEP)/HIGHER FRACTION OF EXPIRED OXYGEN (F$_{IO_2}$) TREATMENT GROUP

F$_{IO_2}$	PEEP	F$_{IO_2}$	PEEP
30	5	80	14
40	5	90	14
40	8	90	16
50	8	90	18
50	10	100	18–24
60	10		
70	10		
70	12		
70	14		

Weaning

Patients will be assessed for the following criteria between 0600–1000 (if a patient procedure, test, or other extenuating circumstance prevents assessment during this time, then the assessment and initiation of the weaning procedure may be delayed for up to 4 h):

F$_{IO_2}$ ≤ 0.40
Values of both PEEP and F$_{IO_2}$ ≤ values from previous day
Not receiving neuromuscular blocking agents and without evidence of neuromuscular blockade
Patient exhibiting inspiratory efforts. Ventilator rate will be decreased to 50% of baseline level for up to 5 min if necessary to detect inspiratory efforts if no efforts are evident at baseline ventilator rate
Systolic arterial pressure >90 mm Hg without vasopressor support

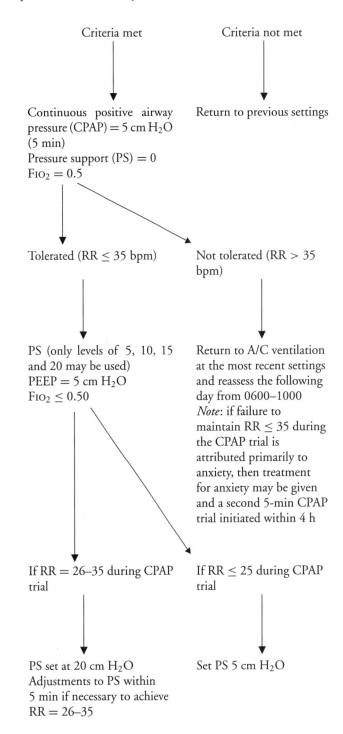

Criteria met   Criteria not met

↓   ↓

Continuous positive airway   Return to previous settings
pressure (CPAP) = 5 cm H$_2$O
(5 min)
Pressure support (PS) = 0
F$_{IO_2}$ = 0.5

Tolerated (RR ≤ 35 bpm)   Not tolerated (RR > 35 bpm)

↓

PS (only levels of 5, 10, 15   Return to A/C ventilation
and 20 may be used)   at the most recent settings
PEEP = 5 cm H$_2$O   and reassess the following
F$_{IO_2}$ ≤ 0.50   day from 0600–1000
                                Note: if failure to
                                maintain RR ≤ 35 during
                                the CPAP trial is
                                attributed primarily to
                                anxiety, then treatment
                                for anxiety may be given
                                and a second 5-min CPAP
                                trial initiated within 4 h

If RR = 26–35 during CPAP   If RR ≤ 25 during CPAP
trial   trial

↓   ↓

PS set at 20 cm H$_2$O   Set PS 5 cm H$_2$O
Adjustments to PS within
5 min if necessary to achieve
RR = 26–35

Assessment for tolerance

1. Total RR ≤ 35 bpm (≤5 min at RR > 35 may be tolerated)
2. Sp$_{O_2}$ ≥ 88% (<5 min at <88% may be tolerated)
3. No respiratory distress (two of the following)
   HR > 120% of the 0600 rate (≤5 min at >120% may be tolerated)
   Marked use of accessory muscles
   Abdominal paradox
   Diaphoresis
   Marked subjective dyspnea

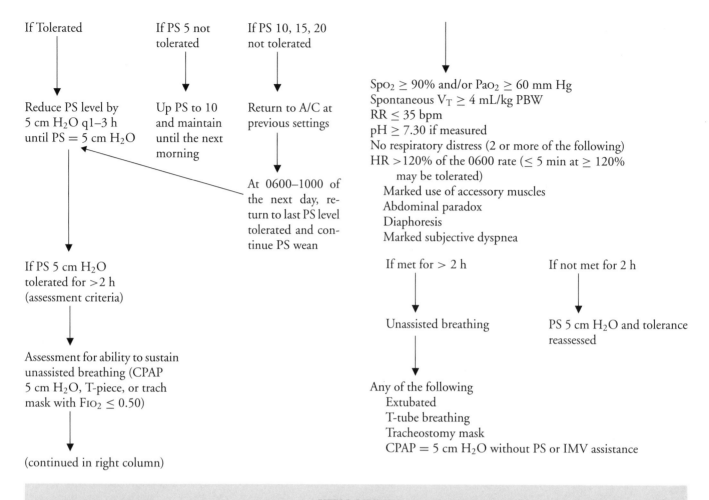

If Tolerated

↓

Reduce PS level by 5 cm H_2O q1–3 h until PS = 5 cm H_2O

↓

If PS 5 cm H_2O tolerated for >2 h (assessment criteria)

↓

Assessment for ability to sustain unassisted breathing (CPAP 5 cm H_2O, T-piece, or trach mask with $F_{IO_2} \leq 0.50$)

↓

(continued in right column)

If PS 5 not tolerated

↓

Up PS to 10 and maintain until the next morning

If PS 10, 15, 20 not tolerated

↓

Return to A/C at previous settings

↓

At 0600–1000 of the next day, return to last PS level tolerated and continue PS wean

$Sp_{O_2} \geq 90\%$ and/or $Pa_{O_2} \geq 60$ mm Hg
Spontaneous $V_T \geq 4$ mL/kg PBW
RR ≤ 35 bpm
pH ≥ 7.30 if measured
No respiratory distress (2 or more of the following)
HR >120% of the 0600 rate (≤ 5 min at $\geq 120\%$ may be tolerated)
  Marked use of accessory muscles
  Abdominal paradox
  Diaphoresis
  Marked subjective dyspnea

If met for > 2 h

↓

Unassisted breathing

↓

Any of the following
  Extubated
  T-tube breathing
  Tracheostomy mask
  CPAP = 5 cm H_2O without PS or IMV assistance

If not met for 2 h

↓

PS 5 cm H_2O and tolerance reassessed

KEY POINTS

Modes of mechanical ventilation are classified by the trigger variable, the target or limit variable, and the cycle variable.

Mechanical ventilation may provide complete or only partial support of the work of breathing.

Positive end-expiratory pressure (PEEP) may produce alveolar recruitment and prevent ventilator-induced lung injury.

Ventilator-induced lung injury results from alveolar overdistention and cyclical stretching.

Newer modes of mechanical ventilation may improve patient–ventilator interactions and improve weaning.

Ventilator management protocols can be performed by nonphysicians and may improve outcome.

REFERENCES

1. MacIntyre NR. Scope of mechanical ventilation and the need for innovations. *Semin Respir Crit Care Med* 2000.
2. MacIntyre NR. Mechanical ventilation: the next 50 years. *Respir Care Clin N Am* 1998;43:490–493.
3. Branson RD, Hess DR, Chatburn RL. *Respiratory care equipment.* Philadelphia: Lippincott–Williams & Wilkins, 1999.
4. MacIntyre NR, Branson RD. *Mechanical ventilation.* Philadelphia: WB Saunders, 2000.
5. American Respiratory Care Consensus Group. Essentials of a mechanical ventilator. *Respir Care Clin N Am* 1992;37:1000–1008.
6. MacIntyre NR, ed. Innovations in mechanical ventilation. *Semin Respir Crit Care Med* 2000.
7. Truwit JD, Marini JJ. Evaluation of thoracic mechanics in the ventilated patient. Part I, primary measurements. *J Crit Care* 1988;3:133–150.
8. Truwit JD, Marini JJ. Evaluation of thoracic mechanics in the ventilated patient. Part II, applied mechanics. *J Crit Care* 1988;3:192–213.
9. Marini JJ, Crooke PS. A general mathematical model for respiratory dynamics relevant to the clinical setting. *Am Rev Respir Dis* 1993;147:14–24.
10. Pepe PE, Marini JJ. Occult positive end-expiratory pressure in mechanically ventilated patients with airflow obstruction. *Am Rev Respir Dis* 1982;126:166–170.
11. Milic-Emili J, Henderson JAN, Dolovich MB, et al. Regional distribution of inhaled gas in the lung. *J Appl Physiol* 1966;21:749–759.
12. Macklen PT. Relationship between lung mechanics and ventilation distribution. *Physiology* 1973;16:580–588.
13. Beydon L, Lemaire F, Jonson B. Lung mechanics in ARDS: compliance and pressure-volume curves. In: Zapol WM, Lemaire F, eds. *Adult respiratory distress syndrome.* New York: Marcel Dekker, 1991:139–161.
14. Salmon RB, Primiano FP, Saidel GM, et al. Human pressure-volume relationships: alveolar collapse and airway closure. *J Appl Physiol* 1981;51:353–362.
15. Benito S, Lemaire F. Pulmonary pressure-volume relationship in acute

respiratory distress syndrome in adults: role of positive and expiratory pressure. *J Crit Care* 1990;5:27–34.

15. Gattinoni L, Pelosi P, Crotti S, et al. Effects of positive end expiratory pressure on regional distribution of tidal volume and recruitment in adult respiratory distress syndrome. *Am J Respir Crit Care Med* 1995;151:1807–1814.

16. Webb HJH, Tierney DF. Experimental pulmonary edema due to intermittent positive pressure ventilation with high inflation pressures: protection by positive end-expiratory pressure. *Am Rev Respir Dis* 1974;110:556–565.

17. Dreyfus D, Saumon G. Ventilator induced lung injury; lessons from experimental studies. *Am J Respir Crit Care Med* 1998;157:294–323.

18. Wyszogrodski I, Kyei-Aboagye K, Taaeusch HW Jr, et al. Surfactant inactivation by hyperventilation: conservation by end-expiratory pressure. *J. Appl Physiol* 1975;38:461–466.

19. Suter PM, Fairley HB, Isenberg MD. Optimum end-expiratory pressure in patients with acute pulmonary failure. *N Engl J Med* 1975;292: 284–289.

20. Servillo G, Svantesson C, Beydon L, et al. Pressure volume curves in acute respiratory failure. *Am J Respir Crit Care Med* 1997;155:1629–1636.

21. Sharp JT, Johnson FN, Goldbert NB, et al. Hysteresis and stress adaptation in the human respiratory system. *J Appl Physiol* 1967;23:487–97.

22. Van der Kloot TE, Blanch L, Youngblood AM, et al. Recruitment maneuvers in 3 experimental models of acute lung injury: effect on lung volume and gas exchange. *Am J Respir Crit Care Med* 2000;161:1485–1495.

23. Abraham, E, Yoshihara, G. Cardiorespiratory effects of pressure controlled ventilation in severe respiratory failure. *Chest* 1990;98:1445–1449.

24. Cole AGH, Weller SF, Sykes MD. Inverse ratio ventilation compared with PEEP in adult respiratory failure. *Intensive Care Med* 1984;10: 227–332.

25. Armstrong, BW, MacIntyre NR. Pressure controlled inverse ratio ventilation that avoids air trapping in ARDS. *Crit Care Med* 1995;23:279–285.

26. Kolobow T, Morentti MP, Fumagalli R, et al. Severe impairment in lung function induced by high peak airway pressure during mechanical ventilation. *Am Rev Respir Dis* 135:312–315, 1987.

27. Ranieri VM, Suter PM, Totorella C, et al. Effects of mechanical ventilation on inflammatory mediators in patients with acute respiratory distress syndrome. *JAMA* 1999;282:54–61.

28. Nahum A, Hoyt J, Schmitz L, et al. Effect of mechanical ventilation strategy on dissemination of intratracheally administered E coli in dogs. *Crit Care Med* 1997;25:1733–1743.

29. NIH ARDS Network. Ventilation with lower tidal volumes as compared to traditional tidal volumes in acute lung injury and acute respiratory distress syndrome. *N Engl J Med* 2000;342:1301–1308.

30. Slutsky AS. ACCP Consensus Conference: Mechanical Ventilation. *Chest* 1993;104:1833–1859.

31. Amato MB, Barbas CSV, Medeivos DM, et al. Effect of a protective-ventilation strategy on mortality in the acute respiratory distress syndrome. *N Engl J Med* 1998;338:347–354.

32. Servillo G, Svantesson C, Beydon L, et al. Pressure volume curves in acute respiratory failure: automated low flow inflation versus occlusion. *Am J Respir Crit Care Med* 1997;155:1629–1636.

33. Fiehl F, Perret C. Permissive hypercapnia–how permissive should we be? *Am J Respir Crit Care Med* 1994;150:1722–1737.

34. Hess DR, MacIntyre NR. Tracheal gas insufflation: overcoming obstacles to critical implementation. *Resp Care* 2001;46:198–199.

35. Froese AB. High frequency oscillatory ventilation for ARDS–let's get it right this time. *Crit Care Med* 1998;25:906–908.

36. MacIntyre NR. High frequency ventilation. In: Tobin M, ed. *Principles and practice of mechanical ventilation.* New York: McGraw Hill, 1994.

37. Chang HK. Mechanisms of gas transport during high frequency ventilation. *J Appl Physiol* 1984;56:553–563.

38. Keszler M, Donn SM, Bucciarelli RL, et al. Multicenter controlled trial comparing HFJV with conventional ventilation in newborns with PIE. *J Pediatr* 1991;119:85–93.

39. Marini JJ. Exertion during ventilator support: how much and how important? *Respir Care* 1986;31:385–387.

40. Hansen-Flaschen J, Brazinsky S, Bassles C, et al. Use of sedating drugs and neuromuscular blockade in patients requiring mechanical ventilation for respiratory failure. *JAMA* 1991;266:2870–2875.

41. Sassoon CSH. Mechanical ventilator design and function: the trigger variable. *Respir Care Clin N Am* 1992;37:1056–1069.

42. Gay PC, Rodarte JR. Hubmayr RD. The effects of positive expiratory pressure on isovolume flow and dynamic hyperinflation in patients receiving mechanical ventilation. *Am Rev Respir Dis* 1989;139:621–626.

43. MacIntyre NR. McConnell R, Cheng KC. Applied PEEP reduces the inspiratory load of intrinsic PEEP during pressure support. *Chest* 1997;111:188–193.

44. Flick GR, Belamy PE, Simmons DH. Diaphragmatic contraction during assisted mechanical ventilation. *Chest* 1989;96:130–135.

45. Marini JJ, Smith TC, Lamb VJ. External work output and force generation during synchronized intermittent mechanical ventilation. *Am Rev Respir Dis* 1988;138:1169–1179.

46. Haas CF, Branson RD, Folk LM, et al. Patient determined inspiratory flow during assisted mechanical ventilation. *Respir Care Clin N Am* 1995;40:716–721.

47. MacIntyre NR, McConnell R, Cheng KC, Sane A. Pressure limited breaths improve flow dys-synchrony during assisted ventilation. *Crit Care Med* 1997;25:1671–1677.

48. MacIntyre NR. What is tracheal pressure triggering?—do we need it? *Resp Care* 1996;41:524–528.

49. Branson RD. Techniques for automated feedback control of mechanical ventilation. *Semin Respir Crit Care Med* 2000;21:203–210.

50. Ho L, MacIntyre NR. Effects of initial flow rate and breath termination criteria on pressure support ventilation. *Chest* 1991;99:134–38.

51. Younes M. Proportional assist ventilation, a new approach to ventilatory support. *Am Rev Respir Dis* 1992;145:114–120.

52. Grasso S, Ranieri VM. Proportional assist ventilation. *Semin Respir Crit Care Med* 2000;21:161–166.

53. Jubran A, Van de Graaf WB, Tobin MJ. Variability of patient ventilator interactions with pressure support ventilation in patients with chronic obstructive pulmonary disease. *Am J Respir Crit Care Med* 1995;152: 129–136.

54. Marini JJ, Culver BH, Butler J. Mechanical effect of lung inflation with positive pressure on cardiac function. *Am Rev Respir Dis* 1979;124:382–386.

55. Scharf SM, Caldini P, Ingram RH Jr. Cardiovascular effects of increasing airway pressure in the dog. *Am J Physiol* 1977;232:1135–1143.

56. Pinsky MR, Summer WR. Cardiac augmentation by phasic high intrathoracic pressure support in man. *Chest* 1983;84:370–375.

57. Wagner PD. Ventilation-perfusion relationships. *Annu Rev Physiol* 1980;42:233–247.

58. Lemaire F, Teboul JL, Cinotti L, et al. Acute left ventricular dysfunction during unsuccessful weaning from mechanical ventilation. *Anesthesiology* 1988;69:171–179.

59. Jenkinson SG. Oxygen toxicity. *New Horizons* 1993;1:504–511.

60. Zwillich C, Pierson DJ, Creagh C, et al. Complications of mechanical ventilation: a prospective study of 354 consecutive episodes. *Am J Med* 1974;57:161–170.

61. Langer M, Mosconi P, Cigada M, et al. Long-term respiratory support and risk of pneumonia in critically ill patients. *Am Rev Respir Dis* 1989;140:302–305.

62. Fagon J, Chastre J, Domart Y, et al. Nosocomial pneumonia in patients receiving continuous mechanical ventilation. *Am Rev Respir Dis* 1989;139:877–884.

63. Ely EW, Baker AM, Dunagan DP, et al. Effect on the duration of mechanical ventilation of identifying patients capable of breathing spontaneously. *N Engl J Med* 1996;335:1864–1869.

64. Kollef MH, Shapiro SD, Silver P, et al. A randomized controlled trial of protocol directed versus physician directed weaning from mechanical ventilation. *Crit Care Med* 1997;25:567–574.

38

WEANING FROM MECHANICAL VENTILATORY SUPPORT

E. WESLEY ELY

KEY WORDS

- Respiration, artificial
- Respiratory insufficiency
- Mechanical ventilation
- Ventilator weaning
- Critical care
- Respiratory therapy
- Clinical protocols
- Intensive care unit

- Outcomes
- Trauma
- Perioperative management
- Sedatives
- Analgesics
- Neuromuscular blockade

New York (Reuters Health)—"Hospital intensive care units could save more than $1.4 billion dollars annually if they followed the practices of the nation's best ICUs. Better-performing hospitals seem to be making more attempts to *standardize* the care given in the ICU. The top hospitals make their care consistent and still allow flexibility to try new treatments that produce better and better outcomes."
February 2001

—http://web1.po.com/html/reuters/archive/ec020611.nws.shtml

INTRODUCTION

One of the recent advances in critical care medicine has been the advent of efforts to organize or "protocolize" decision making by talented health care professionals who work diligently to care for our sickest patients. The importance of clinical experience cannot be overemphasized, but we now know that such clinical expertise can be greatly enhanced by incorporating evidence-based guidelines to streamline decision making. This is the new paradigm for critical care, and an abundance of data specific to weaning from mechanical ventilation (MV) show that patient-centered outcomes can be dramatically improved via protocols. Despite the popularity of the term *weaning*, one of the most important concepts to arise from recent prospective, randomized, controlled trials (RCTs) is that the standard gradual reduction in ventilator support may unnecessarily delay extubation in up to two-thirds of patients who have recovered from respiratory failure (1–6).

A strong impetus to liberate patients from the ventilator at the earliest possible time comes from the relationship between duration of MV and survival. In a recent report, proportional

hazards analysis of "time until in-hospital death" confirmed the relationship between duration of MV and survival even after adjustment for differences in severity of illness, age, race, gender, diagnosis, and treatment assignment (Fig. 1) (7). This observation supports long-standing anecdotal impressions and the findings of a multicenter registry of acute respiratory distress syndrome (ARDS) patients in which 85% of the nonsurvivors had died by the fourth week, and the subsequent mortality rate was lower than that of the population as a whole (8). With these facts in mind, numerous investigators have attempted to reduce the duration of MV.

Economic and organizational pressures have encouraged physicians to be more effective and efficient in the management of patients. In this chapter, we use an evidence-based approach to discuss establishing a protocolized approach to mechanically ventilated patients. Whereas each institution must make adjustments even to validated protocols, important general concepts can ease the process of implementation and enhance success.

WEANING FROM THE VENTILATOR: RANDOMIZED CONTROLLED TRIALS

Despite numerous efforts to determine the best method of weaning patients from MV, it was not until 1994 that any RCT showed one method (i.e., pressure support ventilation, or PSV) to be superior to others (9). Yet, within a year, another well-performed RCT showed seemingly conflicting results, with spontaneous breathing trials (SBTs) leading to earlier extubation in mechanically ventilated patients (4). Although these investigations reached contradictory conclusions, these trials showed that (a) weaning strategies influence the duration of MV; (b) the specific criteria used to initiate changes in ventilatory support influence outcome; and (c) the most ineffective approach was intermittent mandatory ventilation, a previously widely used strategy.

Several lines of evidence suggest that physicians do not efficiently discontinue MV. In the cited studies (4,9), 69% to 76% of patients evaluated for enrollment were judged ready for immediate extubation. In addition, as many as half of patients who extubate themselves prematurely do not require reintubation within 24 hours (10,11). Physicians' predictions of whether patients can have MV successfully discontinued are inaccurate,

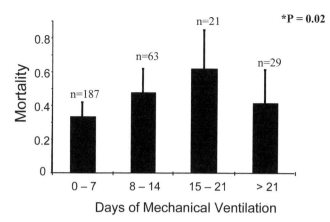

FIGURE 1. Duration of mechanical ventilation and survival. There was a significant relationship between the number of days of mechanical ventilation and survival ($P = 0.02$). The mortality rate increased steadily from 1 to 3 weeks of ventilator use, and then it dropped for those requiring more than 21 days of mechanical ventilation. Proportional hazards analysis of time until in-hospital death confirmed the relationship between survival and duration of mechanical ventilation even after adjustment for differences in the severity of illness, age, race, gender, diagnosis, and treatment assignment ($P = 0.001$).

with positive and negative predictive values of only 50% and 67%, respectively (12).

Because the aforementioned studies did not include a control (not protocolized) group, clinicians still could argue that "their" way of weaning was better than a standardized protocol. To answer the question of whether or not standardizing weaning with a protocol would benefit patients, we enrolled 300 mechanically ventilated medical and nonsurgical cardiac patients into an RCT in which the treatment group was "weaned" to extubation using a two-step process of screening by respiratory care practitioners (RCPs) followed by SBTs when recovery was sufficient to "pass" the daily screen (DS) (5). The DS and SBT are defined in Table 1. Because of the difficulty in having busy clinicians change practice patterns, we also incorporated a written and verbal physician prompt into the treatment arm, which notified them when a patient had successfully passed an SBT.

The physicians involved in our investigations were all board-certified intensivists or cardiologists operating in "closed" intensive care units (ICUs). A survey taken prior to initiating the investigation indicated that most (68%) doubted that their practice style could be improved by routine objective measurements along with increased input from respiratory care practitioners. The outcomes of the investigation included removal from MV 2 days earlier in the protocol-directed group despite a higher severity of illness, 50% fewer complications, and a reduction in the cost of ICU stay by $5,000 per patient (Table 2) (5). Kaplan-Meier survival analysis (Fig. 2) and Cox proportional-hazards model demonstrated that subjects assigned to the intervention group had MV successfully discontinued earlier (relative rate of successful extubation of 2.13, 95% confidence interval, 1.58 to 2.86; $P < 0.0001$).

The protocol encouraged extubation as soon as recovery was documented, and we expected a higher rate of complications (particularly reintubation) in the intervention group. In fact, the risk of nonlethal complications was lower in the intervention

TABLE 1. THE DAILY SCREEN AND THE SPONTANEOUS BREATHING TRIAL (SBT)

Daily Screen (DS)
Takes only about 2 min; patient should pass all five criteria:
1. Patient coughs when suction catheter passed, intact gag reflex.
2. Patient not receiving any vasopressor or sedative infusions drips. Dopamine allowed if dose $\leq 5\ \mu$g/kg/min, and intermittent dosing of sedatives allowed
3. $PaO_2/FIO_2 \geq 200$, e.g., PaO_2 of 100/FIO_2 of 0.5 = 200, higher is better
4. PEEP set ≤ 5 cm H_2O
5. Respiratory rate / tidal volume ratio (f / V_T) ≤ 105. This is also known as the rapid shallow breathing index (RSBI); lower is better

   Measured after 1 min of spontaneous breathing with ventilator rate set to 0 and pressure support set to 0.

   Average V_T calculated by dividing f into V_E ($V_T = V_E/f$), alternatively: $f/V_T = f^2/V_E$.

   e.g., rate (f) of 20, V_E of 10 L/min: (20 × 20) divided by 10 = f/V_T of 40.

Spontaneous Breathing Trial (SBT)
What is an SBT and who gets one?
  A trial of spontaneous breathing for 120 min with "flow-by" mode, ventilator rate set to 0 and pressure support set to 0.
  A patient who passes the DS is a candidate for an SBT.
Who performs the spontaneous trial? It's a TEAM EFFORT . . .
  Respiratory therapist performs daily screen (DS) and prompts doctor to order an SBT.
  Respiratory therapist initiates a trial, monitors the patient during the trial in conjunction with the nurse, and reinitiates MV if criteria for trial termination are met.
  ICU nurse monitors the patient for criteria for trial termination and notifies the respiratory therapist if they are met.
When is a spontaneous trial terminated?
  If the patient successfully tolerates it for 2 h
  When one of the following conditions is met:
    Respiratory rate > 35 for > 5 min
    $SaO_2 < 90\%$ during > 30 sec of good quality measurement
    20% increase or decrease in heart rate for > 5 min
    SBP > 180 or SBP < 90 during at least 1 min of continuous recording or repeated measurements
    Agitation, anxiety, or diaphoresis confirmed as a change from baseline and present for > 5 min
What does it mean if a patient passes an SBT?
  Successful completion of a 2-h SBT indicates a 90% chance of successfully staying off of MV for 48 h

PaO_2, partial-pressure arterial oxygen; FIO_2, fraction of inspired oxygen; PEEP, positive end-expiratory pressure; MV, mechanical ventilation; SBP, systolic blood pressure.
Adapted from Ely EW, Baker AM, Dunagan DP, et al. Effect on the duration of mechanical ventilation of identifying patients capable of breathing spontaneously. *N Engl J Med* 1996;335:1864–1869.

group. The reintubation rate in our institution prior to the initiation of this investigation was 8%, comparable to that seen in our controls. The intervention group experienced a lower rate of reintubation (4%), perhaps because of careful objective screening prior to extubation. Because reintubation is associated with an increased risk of nosocomial pneumonia (13), this finding may prove especially important if confirmed. The reintubation rates in this trial compare favorably with those rates in two recent large weaning trials: 7.3% (9) and 17.7% (4). Subsequent implementation of this protocol in 530 patients at another large medical center was associated with a similar reintubation rate (i.e., 6%) and no increased risk of mortality (14).

It has been recommended that ICUs either adopt or adapt the methods of this validated protocol or establish their own

TABLE 2. OUTCOMES FROM PROTOCOL-DRIVEN WEANING VERSUS INTENSIVISTS' BEST CARE

	Intervention (n = 149)	Control (n = 151)	P value
APACHE II score	19.8	17.9	0.01
Weaning days	1	3	0.0001
Ventilator days	4.5	6	0.003
Reintubation (%)	6 (4)	15 (10)	0.04
Mech Vent >21 d (%)	9 (6)	20 (13)	0.04
Any complication (%)	30 (20)	62 (41)	0.001
Total ICU costs	$15,740	$20,890	0.03

APACHE, acute physiology and chronic health evaluation score; ICU, intensive care unit.
Adapted from Ely EW, Baker AM, Dunagan DP, et al. Effect on the duration of mechanical ventilation of identifying patients capable of breathing spontaneously. *N Engl J Med* 1996; 335:1864–1869, with permission.

protocols with similar goals (15). Use of the protocol to manage just four patients would result in one person being off MV after 48 hours who otherwise would not have been. In addition, if the protocol were used in six patients, one fewer complication would be expected. Because the techniques and measurements require no special monitoring or equipment, no additional expenditures beyond staffing, and no laboratory studies (arterial blood gases were optional), we believe this protocol to be broadly applicable in both university and community hospital settings.

Simultaneously, Kollef and colleagues (16) were conducting another RCT (n = 357) of protocol-directed versus physician-directed weaning in four ICUs (two medical and two surgical). This investigation incorporated three separate "weaning" protocols because of difficulty in achieving consensus among different units. The protocol-directed group incorporated an amalgam of SBTs, PSV, and synchronized intermittent mandatory ventilation protocols and demonstrated an earlier initiation of weaning ef-

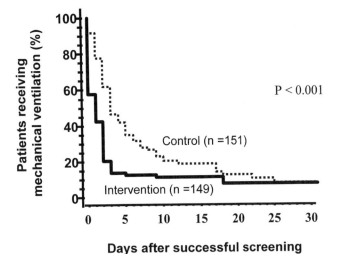

FIGURE 2. Kaplan-Meier curves of the risk of remaining mechanically ventilated in protocol versus control groups. After adjusting for baseline characteristics using co-variants that described severity of illness (acute physiology and chronic health evaluation score, or APACHE II), age, gender, race, intensive care unit (ICU) location, and duration of intubation prior to enrollment, a Cox proportional-hazards analysis demonstrated that subjects in the protocol group were removed from mechanical ventilation more rapidly than controls (relative rate of successful extubation = 2.13, 95% confidence interval, 1.55 to 2.92, P < 0.001).

forts and a median duration of MV of 35 hours versus 44 hours in the physician-directed group. In a more recent RCT that included 385 patients (~50% surgical, predominantly trauma), Marelich and colleagues showed that the use of a weaning protocol shortened the duration of mechanical ventilation from 124 hours to 68 hours (P = 0.001) (17). In the investigations by both Kollef et al. (16) and Marelich et al. (17), the benefits of the weaning protocols on duration of mechanical ventilation were evident in Kaplan-Meier curves that looked nearly identical to that of Ely and colleagues shown in Figure 2.

Daily Screening Techniques

Many institutions have now incorporated various DS techniques as the first step of weaning protocols and to accelerate progress toward extubation. Such screens are important because physicians often fail to identify patients who can be successfully extubated and tend to underestimate the probability of successful discontinuation of MV (18). In one investigation, physicians' clinical judgment had a specificity of 35% and a likelihood ratio of 1.5 (12), values that indicate little clinical utility without the use of objective monitoring parameters. Perhaps the most important reason to continue some form of daily screening (individualized to the specific patient population) is to identify specific and treatable issues that are causing a delay in patient readiness for liberation from the ventilator.

Many weaning parameters have been proposed to identify patients ready for extubation and range from simple maneuvers [e.g., counting and measuring breaths (19)] to more complicated techniques requiring the insertion of esophageal or gastric balloons (20,21) or use of computerized decision support models (18). Eloquently performed investigations of difficult-to-wean patients determined that, in addition to the frequency/tidal volume ratio (f/V_t) (19), physiologic measurements, including an airway occlusion pressure at 0.1 second ($P_{0.1}$) above 4.5 cm H_2O (10,22,23) and a tension-time index above 0.15 (24,25) are helpful determinants of diaphragmatic fatigue and weaning failure. In general, these tests confirm that the load imposed on the inspiratory muscles is in excess of the neuromuscular capacity. Historic reliance on such measures is appealing because of their scientific basis and the theoretical potential to limit risks to the patient. In most patients, however, these technically demanding tests are neither necessary nor practical for widespread use within the confines of a protocol. Until recently, no RCT had documented that application of any tools produced better outcomes than physician judgment alone (5).

Manthous and colleagues (2) arrived at the following summary statements regarding three commonly used weaning parameters: (a) maximal inspiratory pressure or negative inspiratory force has a poor predictive value with an area under a receiver-operating-characteristic (ROC) curve (i.e., sensitivity versus 1− specificity) of 0.61 to 0.68; (b) spontaneous minute ventilation shows even poorer predictive combination, with ROC curve area of 0.40 to 0.54 and (c) f/V_T or Rapid Shallow Breathing Index yielded an ROC curve area of 0.75 to 0.89. Jaeschke et al. (26) discussed a process to determine whether these parameters are useful clinically. The f/V_T threshold level of 105 breaths/min/L chosen by Yang and Tobin (19) has a relatively high ROC curve area and appeared useful in our screening partly because it is followed by a second step of SBTs. In fact, many patients with a ratio between 80 and 105 may fail SBTs (23,26). Possible alterations in the diagnostic thresholds for different components of the DS (e.g., the best "cutoff" for the f/V_T) are discussed below in "Subgroups of Patients."

After review of the literature, we chose a set of five simple parameters to use as a DS to be obtained on all patients (Table 1). Medical ICU and critical care unit (CCU) patients required an average of 2 to 3 days to pass the DS (5), and subsequent data derived from surgical patients yielded similar findings (27). Whereas 75% of our patients eventually passed the screen, another recent report found that 290 of 537 (54%) patients passed the same screening tool (14). During DS assessments in more than 1,500 patients, there were no complications, such as temporally associated self-extubation, prolonged desaturation, or hemodynamic instability. During our hospital-wide implementation of the protocol, once patients passed the DS (n = 722), 41% (n = 298) consistently passed the DS, whereas 59% (n = 424) fluctuated between passing and not passing the DS (27). When the DS was passed and an SBT was obtained, patients would pass the SBT 75.4% of the time, a rate that did not vary over the 12-month period of implementation or among services and units.

Overly rigid interpretation of the "rules" of the protocol seemed counterproductive. For example, determining on consecutive days that a patient failed the DS because the PaO_2/FIO_2 ratio was 198 (rather than being >200) or their f/V_T was 107 (rather than being <105) was considered inappropriate because some patients do not fit within the confines of specified "cutoffs" or thresholds (26,28–30). Continuing to advance patients through the protocol at this point and assessing their ability to breathe with an SBT may prove successful in many of these circumstances. Ongoing investigations are randomizing patients to a screen followed by an SBT versus going straight to an SBT each day (see next section). For clinicians modifying protocols to fit their institutional preferences, an important take-home message is to make daily screens inclusive rather than exclusive. That is, having false-positive screens that push patients further along in the protocol is preferable to holding patients back due to overly rigid criteria.

Spontaneous Breathing Trials

Because of the heterogeneity of patients with respiratory failure and the dynamic interplay of multiple factors determining their need for ventilatory support, we believe there are inherent limitations of all current measures used to determine whether the patient is ready for extubation. Rather, allowing the patient to breathe spontaneously for a predetermined time trial during close monitoring (i.e., an SBT) is the optimum confirmation of the patient's readiness for extubation. In fact, the joint American College of Chest Physicians (ACCP)/Society of Critical Care Medicine (SCCM)/American Association for Respiratory Care (AARC) clinical practice guidelines on protocols and weaning give a daily assessment of the patient's ability to sustain spontaneous breathing the highest level 1/grade A recommendation based on available data (6). Unfortunately, an international survey of mechanical ventilation showed that fewer than 20% of patients currently receive an SBT while weaning, and this number is less than 10% in the United States (31).

An SBT is a trial of spontaneous breathing for a predetermined amount of time (e.g., 30–120 minutes) using "flow-by" mode or T-piece, with no ventilator rate and no pressure support. RCPs or nurses perform screening and then either initiate an SBT or prompt a physician to do so. The same health care professionals then monitor the patient during the trial and reinitiate MV if criteria for trial termination are met. Criteria for termination or failure of an SBT include any of the following: (a) respiratory rate greater than 35 breaths per minute for more than 5 minutes; (b) SaO_2 below 90% during more than 30 seconds of quality measurement; (c) a 20% increase or decrease in heart rate for longer than 5 minutes; (d) SBP greater than 180 or SBP below 90 during 1 minute of continuous recording or repeated measurements; (e) agitation, anxiety, or diaphoresis confirmed as a change from baseline and present for more than 5 minutes. If a patient without significant neurologic disease (to be discussed later) successfully completes an SBT, this indicates at least an 85% to 90% chance of successfully staying off of MV for 48 hours (5).

The described SBT was used in the aforementioned investigations (4,5) and further validated by other investigators (23). In a preliminary report, Wood and colleagues (14) found that of 275 patients passing the DS who were selected for an SBT, 264 (96%) passed, with 232 of 264 (88%) extubated and 217 of these patients (94%) remaining extubated for 3 days. This experience confirms the low reintubation rates described previously. Esteban and the Spanish Lung Failure Collaborative Group defined practical aspects of the SBT and showed in an RCT of 526 patients that successful extubation was achieved equally effectively with SBTs lasting 30 minutes or 120 minutes (32). In a previous study, they documented that the SBT could be conducted with either a low level of PSV or a T-piece (33). In our studies, SBTs were performed with either standard T-tube circuits or flow-triggered openings of the demand valve without additional support. Incorporating flow-triggering during the SBT was a convenience that minimized respiratory therapist involvement and had not been investigated by others. Taken together, these investigations support institutional variations in the specific method of conducting an SBT. In fact, individual physicians may wish to tailor the technique and duration of SBTs for individual patients.

Not only is passing an SBT clinically important, but also failing an SBT has major prognostic implications. Most patients who failed a breathing trial did so fairly early, with a median duration of the SBT until failure of around 20 minutes (32). Vallverdu and associates (23) studied outcomes of a 2-hour T-piece trial and found that the mean time to failure (among those who could not sustain 120 minutes of spontaneous breathing) was 39 minutes; however, 36% of patients failed after the first 30 minutes of successfully breathing on their own. None of seven weaning parameters consistently predicted time to failure. Because of the morbidity and mortality associated with reintubation, indices need to be developed to identify patients who can sustain spontaneous breathing without distress but nonetheless will require reintubation after extubation (32).

Implementation of a Protocol

The implementation process itself is challenging and is discussed later. The protocol offered here is not meant as a stand-alone device to implement directly. Rather, these tools will need to be modified according to institutional needs.

The level of institutional commitment to improving outcomes as well as the team's leadership, persistence, and consistency in implementation will determine the ultimate success of any management protocol. Protocolized care has been advocated in many facets of medicine, but relinquishing control of the patient's management often creates resentment and frustration on the part of physicians. Even when the evidence clearly supports change, it is difficult to get physicians to alter their management styles (34) because what is really required is a change of culture. In certain circles of physicians within some institutions, there may be a low "readiness to change," and these professionals may require either motivational interventions or consultation with respected opinion leaders (34,35). Important considerations that may increase the chances of successfully changing the behavior of health care professionals include education, timely feedback, participation by physicians in the effort to change, administrative interventions, and even financial incentives and penalties (34).

Few data document the feasibility or steps necessary in implementing such protocols on a large scale with monitoring of protocol compliance. We sought to monitor prospectively and to describe the institution-wide implementation of our previously validated approach. We made slight modifications and reintroduced the protocol *without* daily supervision of a weaning team, physician, or RCP supervisor to test its feasibility as a therapist-driven protocol (TDP) (27). Compliance with the protocol was monitored closely by using a daily data-collection tool. RCP completion of the DS varied little on average throughout the year, with an overall completion above 95% ($P = 0.35$). Correct interpretation of the DS was also high (95% overall correct) ($P = 0.42$). Once the DS was completed and passed, the next step of the protocol was to assess the patient's ability to pass an SBT. Overall compliance rates in obtaining an SBT were initially low, but these rates increased in the fifth and sixth months and remained fairly stable thereafter. To determine whether the frequency of ordering SBTs differed in relation to physician specialty, we compared medical and surgical performance. Across the year of implementation, SBTs more often were ordered on the medicine services (81% versus 63%, $P = 0.001$).

Throughout the year, 75% of patients who were assessed with SBTs (after having passed a DS) successfully passed their SBTs. Although one patient had temporally associated hypotension and desaturation, no other complications were noted from SBTs. A potentially important, but unmeasured, complication of failed SBTs is the possibility that respiratory muscle fatigue would adversely impact the next SBT. Mechanical ventilator-associated complications included a reintubation rate of 14%, tracheostomy rate of 18%, and prolonged duration of MV (>21 days) of 13%. The current investigation did not compare management with this TDP with that of a control group, nor was it our purpose to restudy the efficacy and cost savings of the protocol. Rather, we attempted to appraise the complicated interplay of program implementation and the challenges of effecting changes in physician and nonphysician behavior. Important differences from the original investigation that precluded a direct comparison of outcomes measures included a major shift in the patient population,

TABLE 3. SUGGESTIONS FOR IMPLEMENTATION OF A WEANING PROTOCOL

How to maximize the likelihood of success in achieving both a change of behavior and long-term protocol implementation:
  Identify the patient-care issue as a high priority item (e.g., ventilator weaning and timely extubation)
  Obtain baseline data (e.g., lengths of stay and complication rates)
  Base the program on medical evidence, but also reviews of other programs and obtaining local expert opinion
  Acknowledge the need for a "change in culture" on the part of both physicians and nonphysician healthcare professionals
  Work hard to attain "buy-in" and participation of key opinion leaders/physicians
  Establish a team including the hospital administration, respiratory care practitioners, nurses/nurse practitioners, potentially ethicists, and physicians
  As a team, establish goals and set objective definitions of success and failure
  Structure a graded, staged implementation process which provides all of the following:
  Education
  Timely feedback
  Compliance monitoring
  Tracking of appropriate outcomes (including cost) via daily data collection
  Avoid complicated plans aimed at perfection; rather, remain practical and useful
  Consider the entire process to be dynamic not fixed; incorporate innovative changes over time to respond to lessons learned
  Avoid changing personnel too often
  Avoid overly rigid interpretation of the "rules" of the protocol
  Do not remove clinical judgment on part of any team members
  Acknowledge the need for and plan to have periodic refresher implementation processes to avoid the otherwise inevitable "regression to baseline"

over one-third of whom were trauma and other surgical patients; lack of prospectively recorded severity of illness indicators; and marked expansion in the participating staff of physicians, RCPs, and nurses. That the protocol was successful and safe in surgical ICU patients and accepted 63% of the time by surgeons overall during the first year is important new information, extending the relevance of this approach beyond the medical and coronary ICUs.

Respiratory care practitioners competently performed and interpreted the DS, and both RCPs and physicians improved their compliance rates in using SBT assessments in their patients who had recovered from respiratory failure. It became clear from this experience that a commitment to the implementation of the TDP was essential on the part of the hospital and its administration to ensure its success. The initial outlay of resources by the institution, including dedicated monitoring staff, computer support, and the time of RCPs to attend in-services, was key. Several practical barriers to protocol implementation also became apparent. Although some aspects of this experience are unique to our medical center, many observations have important implications for institutions currently dealing with the need for a more systematic approach to MV (Table 3).

Varying sizes and administrative structures of both academic and community medical centers might be expected to present intrinsic challenges in implementation of this and other protocols. Differences in the number of RCPs and RCP experience could have dramatic differences on the results. Protocol implementation (and acceptance) might be considerably easier in smaller, self-contained units with fewer staff and more direct communication channels. As in other circumstances in which new care modalities are introduced, obtaining the "buy in" of key physicians, RCPs, and nurses (i.e., the opinion leaders) is a major element of successful protocol implementation (34,36) and was a factor in our experience. Avoiding personnel changes as much as possible is also desirable. Devoting to a unit the same therapists who are knowledgeable of the protocol and who interact with the physicians and nurses in a comfortable and consistent manner appears helpful (37). It is also apparent that overly rigid interpretation of the "rules" of the protocol seems counterproductive.

Through diligence and the passage of time, an ongoing change of culture can be achieved that allows protocol implementation and appropriate modification of bedside behavior for both physicians and RCPs. When this vigorous reinforcement through educational interventions was discontinued, however, recidivism to previous baseline level of performance was observed. A more in-depth discussion of these implementation issues and barriers to success is included elsewhere (27).

CONTROLLING THE DELIVERY OF SEDATIVES TO REDUCE TIME ON THE VENTILATOR

It seems reasonable that if protocolizing decisions regarding the liberation from the ventilator can enhance outcomes, then standardizing the delivery of paralytic agents, analgesics, and sedatives also may be of benefit to patients. Indeed, this is the most recent development in the area of protocolization and weaning. One randomized, controlled investigation that used a nursing-implemented protocol to manage the delivery of sedation showed a reduction in the duration of mechanical ventilation by 2 days ($P = 0.008$), decreased length of stay in the ICU by 2 days ($P < 0.0001$), and a lower tracheostomy rate among the treatment group (6% versus 13%, $P = 0.04$) (38). In another recently published controlled trial, of 128 patients receiving mechanical ventilation in the ICU, those in whom sedative infusions were interrupted daily had a shorter duration of mechanical ventilation and earlier discharge from the ICU than patients in whom infusions were not interrupted (39). These two studies monitored only the "arousal component of consciousness" and tracked relatively few adverse events, none of which included patients' distress during awakening, recollections of discomfort after their stay in the ICU, delirium, or persistent neuropsychological outcomes. Emerging work in the area of "content of consciousness" is yielding exciting interactions between the development of delirium and outcomes, including the duration of mechanical ventilation, success rates in weaning, and duration of stay in the hospital, as well as long-term neuropsychological outcomes (40,41). In addition, the pharmacoeconomic impact of guidelines for analgesia, sedation, and neuromuscular blockade appear favorable and are receiving more attention in the medical literature (42). Specific to the perioperative patient, it is important to mention that prior to extubation, the effects of anesthesia (such as ongoing neuromuscular blockade and sedation) should be adequately resolved to prevent undue complications.

PATIENT SUBGROUPS

Many physicians believe that different patient groups should be managed differently. Groups who might require modified strategies include (a) chronic obstructive pulmonary disease (COPD) patients; (b) congestive heart failure (CHF), myocardial infarction, and cardiothoracic surgical patients; (c) neurosurgical patients and closed head trauma patients; (d) older patients; and (e) patients requiring prolonged mechanical ventilation or designated as "failure to wean." In our first investigation of primarily medical patients (5), neither increased complication rates nor prolonged MV was found among those within any of these diagnostic groups (including persons with acute myocardial infarction or COPD). The following discussion will outline the literature concerning these subgroups and whether particular adjustments in weaning protocols in these groups are needed.

Chronic Obstructive Pulmonary Disease

Episodes of acute respiratory failure requiring MV in patients with COPD are associated with ICU and hospital mortality rates ranging from 1% to 16% and 11% to 46%, respectively (43–45). Whereas numerous investigations have been performed to help predict the need for MV in patients with COPD (46–48) or to estimate the likelihood of survival (43,44,49,50), many physicians are unaware that most COPD patients who require MV survive and that their mortality is not necessarily increased over that of other medical patients requiring such support. Our COPD patients' survival ((Fig. 3) (51) was comparable to that in the published literature (43–45) and to that of patients with other causes of respiratory failure. In a recent multivariate analysis (43), the need for MV in COPD patients did not influence short-term or long-term outcome after adjusting for severity of illness.

Others have reported that conventional weaning criteria may be inadequate in COPD patients (52). In our ICUs, the predictive characteristics of the DS worked as well for COPD patients as for persons with other diagnoses (51). Whereas airway occlusion pressure at 0.1 second (i.e., $P_{0.1}$) has been shown repeatedly to be especially worthwhile in COPD patients (23,52–54), it has been neither widely accepted nor applied generally due to technical demands and high interindividual and intraindividual variability of this measure. As newer mechanical ventilators will begin including the $P_{0.1}$ into their software, more clinicians may examine the incorporation of this parameter into weaning protocols for COPD patients.

A multicenter RCT by Nava and colleagues (55) investigated the use of a weaning protocol incorporating noninvasive PSV after extubation in patients with respiratory failure due to COPD. At 48 hours after intubation, a T-piece weaning trial (i.e., SBT) was attempted in 50 patients. If this failed, two methods of weaning were compared: (a) extubation and application of noninvasive PSV (i.e., BiPAP) by a face mask versus (b) further invasive PSV by endotracheal tube. The average PSV in the noninvasive group was 19 ± 2 cm H_2O, whereas the invasive group received 17.6 ± 2.1 cm H_2O. Importantly, both groups of COPD patients received at least two SBT attempts daily. The criteria to

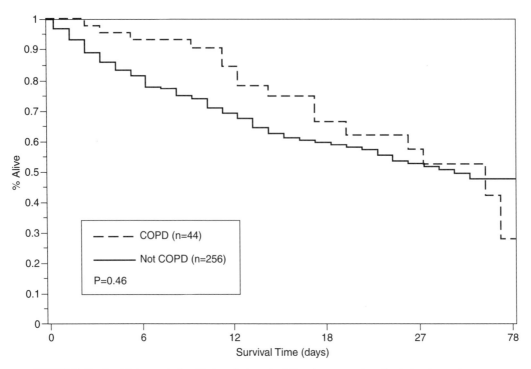

FIGURE 3. Kaplan-Meier analysis of in-hospital survival time between chronic obstructive pulmonary disease (COPD) patients and other patients. Censoring of patients at time of death and hospital discharge was performed for this analysis. There was no difference in survival between the two groups ($P = 0.46$) by Cox proportional hazards analysis.

pass the SBTs were similar to those in our investigations (5,27), except the duration of successful spontaneous breathing was 3 hours, and a pH greater than or equal to 7.35 was required. Outcomes of this important investigation included reduced weaning time and ICU stay, fewer instances of nosocomial pneumonia, and improved 60-day survival rates in the noninvasive group (Table 4) (55).

Congestive Heart Failure and Myocardial Infarction Patients

Our original investigation included 73 medical and nonsurgical cardiac patients with significant comorbidities (5), differing from other studies, which have included a surgical or mixed population or excluded patients with acute coronary disease. We subsequently enrolled 123 coronary patients with myocardial infarction (MI) and CHF, and 95 patients in the cardiothoracic

surgical ICU (27). The latter were only enrolled if they remained on MV for over 24 hours, as they are routinely managed during the first day with a rapid "wean-to-extubation" protocol, and thus represented a select group. Cardiac surgical patients often have many aspects of their care (especially weaning from MV), directed by nonphysicians under protocol guidance (56,57). Importantly, none of these nearly 300 patients with cardiac diseases had a higher rate of detectable complications, suggesting that broad application of this strategy to cardiac patients is safe and effective. Although others showed that some patients have electrocardiographic changes consistent with ischemia during weaning trials (58), no prospective studies have documented clinically important ischemic events resulting from management by a weaning protocol. Using this experience of safety, intensivists and surgeons must take care to avoid delaying extubation unnecessarily and realize that even cardiothoracic surgical patients (when not able to wean rapidly the first day) may benefit from enrollment in standard weaning protocols.

Neurosurgery Patients and Closed Head Trauma

Recognizing the vastly different neuromuscular and cardiopulmonary status of neurosurgical and trauma patients receiving MV, we have begun a series of investigations in this patient population (59,60). In our initial attempts at protocolizing the care of these patients, compliance on the part of the neurosurgeons with extubation after a patient had passed an SBT presented a particularly interesting dilemma. The most common reason cited for not extubating a spontaneously breathing neurosurgical

TABLE 4. NONINVASIVE VENTILATION IN WEANING COPD PATIENTS

Outcome	Invasive (n = 25)	BiPAP (n = 25)	P value
Ventilator days	17 ± 12	10 ± 7	0.02
ICU days	24 ± 14	15 ± 5	0.005
Pneumonia	7	0	0.02
Success at 2 mo	68%	88%	NS
Survival at 2 mo	72%	92%	0.009

BiPAP, bilevel positive airway pressure; COPD, chronic obstructive pulmonary disease; ICU, intensive care unit.

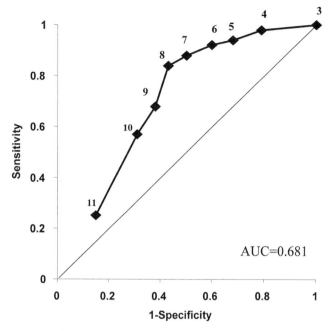

FIGURE 4. Receiver operating characteristic (ROC) Curve of Glasgow Coma Scale (GCS) as a predictor of successful extubation in neurosurgical patients. In these 100 mechanically ventilated neurosurgical patients, the GCS score was the best predictor of successful extubation, with an area under the curve of 0.681 (*P* < 0.0001).

patient was a depressed mental status, consistent with observations published by Coplin et al. (61). In contrast to Coplin and colleagues, however, we did find an association between the Glasgow Coma Scale (GCS) and the need for reintubation (*P* = 0.0001) (60), a finding that others have seen as well (62). Of 109 extubation attempts, only 53% occurred without any complications or reintubations. Multivariate analysis demonstrated that GCS (*P* <0.0001) and PaO_2/FIO_2 ratio (*P* <0.0001) were independent predictors of successful extubation. GCS greater than 8 was associated with success in 67% of patients, whereas only 21% with a GCS less than 8 had successful extubation (*P* < 0.0001) (Fig. 4) (60). This observation supports the concerns of neurosurgeons regarding early liberation of patients from the ventilator. Future investigations of neurosurgical patients should appraise whether the coupling of mental status measures, sedations scales, and GCS as part of the DS and SBT assessments can optimize the decision to extubate these patients or perhaps make a decision for early tracheostomy.

In support of this last concept (i.e., the importance in some patient subgroups of coupling neurologic screening assessments with standard cardiopulmonary screening), Vallverdu and colleagues (23) studied weaning indices and MV liberation in 46 neurologic patients, including ischemic stroke, intracerebral hemorrhage, subarachnoid hemorrhage, head trauma, encephalitis, metabolic encephalopathy, and brain tumor. Although their average reintubation rate was 15%, fifteen (33%) neurologic patients needed reinstitution of invasive MV, but only 6% of the 171 other patients with acute respiratory failure and COPD required reintubation. Most predictors of weaning success lacked discriminatory ability in these patients. Interestingly, f/V_T and $P_{0.1}$ had their lowest accuracy in neurologic patients (65% and

63%, respectively) and did not discriminate among weaning failure and success patients (23). Only maximal inspiratory pressure (MIP, *P* = 0.05) and expiratory pressure (MEP, *P* = 0.001) differed among successfully extubated neurologic patients. In this group, the ability to cough and clear secretions, objectively reflected by the MEP, may help in clinical decision making. Because the need for reintubation was neither clinically nor physiologically suspected, these researchers concluded that other tools need to be developed and prospectively validated to determine the optimum time to extubate patients who have mental status changes and neurologic impairment. Finally, simple maneuvers such as placing ventilated patients in the semirecumbent position to decrease the risk of pneumonia should be adhered to as part of any mechanical ventilation protocol (63).

Trauma patients are often younger and have less comorbidity than older patients. As a result, they can often be removed from the ventilator readily after demonstrating success on relatively short SBTs (i.e., 30 minutes). In fact, Marelich and colleagues found that the predominant benefit of a weaning protocol in their subgroup of trauma patients was seen during the first 96 hours (17). In that study, trauma patients managed with a protocol were less likely to develop ventilator-associated pneumonia (6% versus 15%, *P* = 0.06) (17). In the older patients with blunt trauma, however, consideration of the likelihood of comorbid conditions is imperative. If an older patient does have a condition such as coexistent cardiac, pulmonary, or neurologic disease, then we consider all the issues discussed in the appropriate subgroup sections of this chapter. Specific data on age itself, however, are discussed below.

Older Patients

The number of adults 85 years and older is estimated to be about 4 million and is expected to double by the year 2030 (64). Over the same period, costs of care for older persons will account for 74% of total U.S. health care expenditures. One approach to decreasing health care costs might be to limit or ration the intensive care provided to the aged (65–68). Indeed, recent data demonstrated that older patients do receive less aggressive management for some medical illnesses (69), and data from the SUPPORT investigators showed that age (especially above 70 to 75 years) has great importance on the intensity of care given to patients (70–72).

Age has been considered an important prognostic indicator of hospital outcome (67,73). A recent report showed that many prior investigations of MV in older persons were limited by their retrospective design and the absence of adjustment for confounding factors, such as severity of illness (74). The diversity of the design and conclusions of these investigations has served only to fuel the controversy over whether age has an independent impact on the outcomes of patients treated with MV. In our prospectively followed cohort of 300 mechanically ventilated patients, we found that patients 75 years or older remained on MV a median of 4 days (interquartile ranges, 2–9) versus 6 days (3–11) for patients younger than 75 years (*P* = 0.14) (74). Older patients actually had a greater likelihood of passing a daily screen of weaning parameters (as a marker of recovery from respiratory failure) and did so earlier than younger patients [risk ratio 1.58 (95%

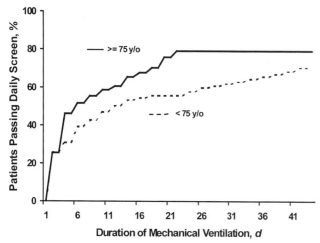

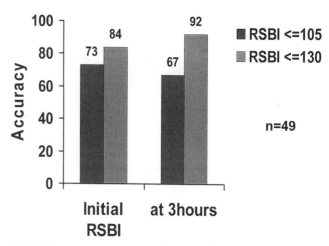

FIGURE 5. Kaplan-Meier analysis of the rate of recovery of respiratory failure by age. This analysis used the percent of patients passing a daily screen of weaning parameters as a surrogate marker of "recovery," and adjustments were made for sex, race, and severity of illness at baseline using a modified acute physiology and chronic health evaluation (APACHE II) score, excluding age. The distribution of times until passing the daily screen suggested that patients aged more than 75 years achieved this recovery milestone earlier than did those less than 75 years of age (risk ratio 1.58, 95% confidence interval 1.13–2.22, $P = 0.03$).

FIGURE 6. Accuracy of rapid shallow breathing index (RSBI) in older patients. Histogram demonstrating that in this group of older patients (i.e., more than 70 years of age), the threshold for the rapid shallow breathing index (i.e., f/V_T) of 130 yielded a higher accuracy in predicting successful extubation than the conventional threshold of 105. Furthermore, measuring the index at 3 hours enhanced the accuracy beyond that of measurements taken at the onset of spontaneous breathing.

confidence interval, 1.13–2.22), $P = 0.03$] (Fig. 5). The ICU cost of care was lower [$12,822 ($9,821–$26,313) versus $19,316 ($9,699–$39,950)] in older patients ($P = 0.03$). Median hospital costs tended to be lower in the older group, although not significantly so ($21,292 versus $29,049, $P = 0.17$). Using multivariate logistic regression analysis to adjust for race, gender, and severity of illness, patient age of 75 years or older was predictive of approximately 1 day less on the ventilator, but this was not statistically significant (95% confidence interval, 2.8 to 1.2 days). Multivariate analyses also confirmed that ICU and hospital length of stay did not differ after adjustment ($P > 0.1$), but ICU and hospital costs were lower for older patients ($P = 0.02$). These outcomes were not explained by differences in mortality because in-hospital mortality among the older patients was 38% versus 39% among younger patients ($P = 0.98$), and Cox proportional-hazards analysis confirmed there was no difference in survival between the two groups (relative risk for older patients was 0.82, 95% confidence interval 0.52–1.29).

Because of differences in access to health care in women (75) and differences among physicians in their practice styles (including the vigor of their approaches to liberation from the ventilator), further prospective analyses of gender differences in outcomes from MV are needed. Gender, associated body dimensions, and age are appropriate considerations that may affect not only outcome from MV but also objective measures of readiness to discontinue MV. Female gender, smaller endotracheal tube size (≤ 7 mm), and older age have been associated with an elevated f/V_T ratio (29,30), and it may be appropriate to adjust the "passing" threshold for this measurement in these instances to avoid erroneously regarding a patient as still requiring MV (Fig 6).

Certain pitfalls regarding decision making in older persons should be recognized and avoided. These include the premature application of predictive equations (76) or anecdotal experiences.

Further prospective investigations are needed to define "physiological age" and to determine whether or not it is truly more important than chronological age (77,78). In the absence of validated measures of "physiological age," the current observations suggest that an overreliance on chronological age is inappropriate. By using multivariate analysis to adjust for severity of illness and other variables, we found that the older (i.e., over the age of 75 years) spent an amount of time on the mechanical ventilator comparable to that of younger patients but had a lower cost of ICU and in-hospital care. Accordingly, the decision to use MV should not be based on age alone, and the appropriate use of ventilatory support in older patients requires further prospective evaluation.

PROLONGED MECHANICAL VENTILATION AND FAILURE TO WEAN

It is difficult to identify the patients in whom prolonged MV will be necessary. Patients who require prolonged MV are best managed in a long-term, acute-care facility (LTAC). Scheinhorn and colleagues reported successful weaning in 56% of 1,123 LTAC patients requiring prolonged MV, with 1-year survival rates of 38% among discharged patients. (79). The management of chronically ventilated patients beyond their acute stay in the ICU has been addressed in other reports (80,81), including a consensus statement by the ACCP (82). In the most recent report from the Barlow Respiratory Hospital, Scheinhorn and colleagues compared 252 consecutive patients (9,135 patient ventilator days) admitted for weaning with a control group of 238 historical controls. Using a 19-step protocol that was therapist implemented and patient specific (TIPS), they showed a decrease in median time of weaning from 29 to 17 days ($P < 0.001$). The same number of successfully weaned patients was present in both groups ($\sim$55%), and the mortality rates were similar in the TIPS group

This mnemonic is not meant to be all inclusive; rather, it is meant to be an aid in considering the possible reasons why a patient might have difficulty being liberated from mechanical ventilation:

*W*heezes
*H*eart disease, hypertension
*E*lectrolytes
*A*nxiety, Airway abnormalities, aspiration, alkalosis (metabolic)
*N*euromuscular disease (including diaphragm dysfunction and prior use of neuromuscular blockers)
*S*epsis, Sedation
*N*utrition (over and under feeding)
*O*piates, Obesity
*T*hyroid disease

(27.4%) versus the historical controls (30.7%). Such long-term acute-care facilities are an important component of the care algorithm for difficult to wean patients.

It is important to make every effort to define and correct problems that prevent extubation. Special considerations in weaning failure patients include reactive airways disease or COPD, cardiac diseases such as ischemic disease, CHF, uncontrolled systemic hypertension contributing to pulmonary edema, metabolic disturbances such as electrolyte disturbances or metabolic alkalosis, uncontrolled anxiety or pain, ongoing aspiration and secretion problems, neuromuscular disorders including prior use of neuromuscular blockers or diaphragmatic dysfunction, ongoing sepsis or other infections such as pneumonia, malnutrition or overfeeding, sedation imbalance with overuse of narcotics or sedative/hypnotics, obesity, hypothyroidism, and the need to position the patient upright or sitting in the bed to use gravity to maintain tidal volume. This list is long, but it is imperative that any clinician caring for mechanically ventilated patients be aware of these commonly found reasons for failure to wean. We have devised the pneumonic "WHEANS NOT" (Table 5) to simplify the approach to the "difficult-to-wean" patient.

REINTUBATIONS

Distinguishing Causes

Despite the rigor with which a team of health care professionals evaluates their patients and uses evidence based decision making and clinical experience in determining liberation from MV, some patients will require reintubation and go on to develop complications. Reintubation may simply be a marker of illness (23,83), but this event is associated with an eight times higher odds ratio for nosocomial pneumonia (13) and a sixfold to 12-fold increase in mortality (32,33,62,84). During the past few years, it has become clear that the most important determinants of the morbidity associated with reintubation relate to distinguishing its cause in each patient (i.e., extubation failure resulting from airway compromise versus true weaning or "pump" failure) and the time to reintubation (83). Aspects of failed liberation from MV that have inherent relationships to weaning approaches include the following: (a) reintubation rates, (b) unplanned extubation, (c) failed extubation attributable to airway causes, and (d) weaning failure implying cardiopulmonary limitations. Each of these is

relevant to implementing and monitoring the outcomes of weaning protocols.

Reintubation Rates

Reported reintubation rates range from 4% to 20% for different ICU populations (4,5,9,27,33,83–85) and may be as high as 33% in patients with mental status changes and neurologic impairment (23). The marked variability in reintubation rates probably reflects multiple factors, including differences in both patient populations and physician decision making. Whereas hospitals often track reintubation as a quality assurance measurement, the optimal rate is not known. A reintubation rate of 0% would indicate that the managing physicians were not "pushing" vigorously to liberate patients at the earliest possible time. Alternatively, an excessively high reintubation rate might suggest reckless decision making or a very high-risk population (e.g., neurosurgical patients). We hypothesized that an aggressive weaning protocol might increase reintubation rates; we found the opposite. Our protocol was the first RCT to our knowledge that documented a lower reintubation rate than in controls (4% versus 10%, $P = 0.04$) (5). Although this rate may have been perceived initially as "too low," another investigation of more than 500 patients reported a 6% reintubation rate when incorporating the same two-step protocol (14). Interestingly, when patients with neurologic disease were excluded from analysis of the investigation by Vallverdu and co-workers (23), only 8 of 125 patients (6%) required reintubation after successfully passing a similar two-step process. Two important points must be made: (a) we initially investigated only medical and coronary ICU patients, not those in postsurgical ICUs; and (b) the protocol allowed clinical decision making rather than having extubation be an automatic step, and this may have allowed a slightly lower reintubation rate. When the protocol was implemented hospital wide in the "out-of-study setting" and changed to a TDP (without direct supervision by a managing physician), compliance decreased and reintubation rates increased to 14% (27).

Unplanned Extubation

This category of events in the liberation from MV may occur accidentally or as the result of the patient's deliberate self-extubation (86,87). It has been known for some time that when self-extubation occurs, patients require reintubation only about 50% of the time (10,11), a fact that should further motivate physicians to adopt proactive protocols directed toward earlier extubation (interestingly, we noted only a 1% self-extubation rate among intervention patients) (5). Three prospective investigations focused on unplanned extubation and included 1,584 patients in more than a dozen European ICUs (62,88,89). The overall unplanned extubation rate from this entire experience was 10.8%, and 47% of the 171 self-extubated individuals were reintubated. Chevron and colleagues (62) prospectively studied their unplanned extubations and found a total of 66 of 414 (16%) mechanically ventilated patients over a 15-month period. Eighty-seven percent of self-extubations were deliberate. Multivariate analysis showed inadequate sedation and oral intubation to be risk factors for unplanned extubation. Risk factors for reintubation in 37% were

TABLE 6. UNPLANNED EXTUBATION: IMPORTANT FEATURES AND PREVENTIVE MEASURES

1. Unplanned extubation occurs in approximately 11% of patients receiving mechanical ventilation (62,88,89), although some institutions have experienced rates less than 5% (5,11)
2. Important features associated with unplanned extubation are as follows (62,88):
   - Chronic respiratory failure
   - Poor endotracheal tube fixation
   - Orotracheal intubation
   - Inadequate intravenous sedation
   - Although inadequate nursing staff and occurrence during procedures have been reported, neither has been statistically associated with unplanned extubation
3. Complications reported in patients following unplanned extubation (86–88):
   - Reintubation
   - Nosocomial pneumonia
   - Vocal cord trauma
   - Death has been reported, but most authors have not found a higher mortality among those with unplanned versus planned extubation
4. Reintubation is required in 50% of patients after unplanned extubation (10,11,62,88,89)
5. Important features associated with need for reintubation after unplanned extubation are as follows (62,83,88,89):
   - Accidental rather than deliberate extubation
   - Occurrence before active weaning has begun
   - Depressed mental status
   - PaO_2/FIO_2 ratio below 200 mm Hg
6. Evidence-based suggestions for reducing the likelihood of unplanned extubation and reintubation (5,62,83,88):
   - Vigilance during procedures at the patient's bedside (anecdotal, not shown in investigations to be statistically associated)
   - Adequate sedation of agitated patients and possible use of sedation protocol
   - Particular attention to orally intubated patients
   - Strong fixation of the endotracheal tube
   - Daily screening and assessment of patients' readiness for liberation from mechanical ventilation

PaO_2, partial-pressure arterial oxygen; FIO_2, fraction of inspired oxygen.

depressed mental status (GCS < 11), accidental nature of extubation rather than deliberate, and a PaO_2/FIO_2 ratio less than 200 torr (62). Betbese and colleagues (89) reported an unplanned endotracheal extubation rate in 59 of 750 patients. Twenty-seven of these 59 patients (46%) required reintubation, and the need for reintubation was not associated with survival. The two most striking factors associated with the need for reintubation were an accidental rather than deliberate unplanned extubation ($P = 0.01$) and the event occurring in patients who had not yet begun weaning ($P = 0.001$) (89). Lastly, Boulain and colleagues (88) completed a multicenter prospective investigation that followed up on 420 patients over 2 months and found 46 unplanned extubations, of whom 28 (60.8%) were reintubated. Multivariate analysis allowed the researchers to determine the following four factors associated with unplanned extubation: (a) chronic respiratory failure, (b) poor endotracheal tube fixation, (c) orotracheal intubation, and (d) inadequate intravenous sedation. These important observational studies have allowed us to summarize important features and formulate provisional recommendations for reducing the occurrence of unplanned extubations (Table 6).

Extubation Versus Weaning Failure

There is an important distinction between reintubation required because of airway compromise vs. non-airway precipitants. Epstein and Ciubotaru performed an analysis of prospectively collected data in 74 medical ICU patients who required reintubation within 72 hours of extubation (83). They classified the causes for reintubation as airway related (upper airway obstruction, aspiration, or excess pulmonary secretions) or non-airway related (respiratory failure, CHF, encephalopathy, or other). The mortality rate was 42% (31 of 74) and was highest in patients for whom failure was because of non-airway factors (53% versus 17%, $P < 0.01$). This group tended to undergo reintubation earlier by about 10 hours (mean 21 versus 31 hours), and their mortality increased with longer interval between extubation and reintubation ($P < 0.05$). Using logistic regression, both the cause of extubation failure and the increased length of time to reintubation were associated with hospital mortality (83). These researchers concluded that identification of patients having non-airway problems ought to occur as early after extubation as possible, with timely reinitiation of ventilatory support. These patients have a true "weaning failure," whereas the other patients ought to be considered "airway failures." The optimum strategies of renewed liberation efforts are likely to differ in these groups.

As demonstrated by numerous investigators, most patients will come off MV without special techniques or interventions. We need reliable indices that identify patients who are able to sustain spontaneous breathing but who require reintubation. These patients are likely to have long stays on the ventilator and to consume an inordinate amount of resources. If an airway problem is suspected prior to extubation, one might conduct a "leak test" to help determine the likelihood of postextubation stridor (90). When the cuff was deflated in this investigation, patients who developed postextubation stridor (i.e., airway failures) had a smaller difference between the inspiratory and expiratory tidal volumes. The authors used ROC curve analysis to determine that 105 mL was the best predictive cutoff for development of postextubation stridor.

SUMMARY

Many advances have been made regarding the optimal methods of removing patients from MV. These efforts are important because MV is associated with considerable morbidity, mortality, and cost (7,51). On the other hand, premature removal from MV can contribute to failed extubation, nosocomial pneumonia, or increased mortality rates (33,83). Until recent years, physicians most often have approached the discontinuation of MV through a gradual reduction in ventilatory support, reflected in universally applied, but varying forms of "weaning." We now know, from recent prospective, randomized, controlled trials, that this gradual approach may unnecessarily delay extubation of patients who have recovered from respiratory failure. With better recognition of the complications of MV, and increasing attention placed on the considerable resources consumed during the care of patients with respiratory failure, a change in the culture of weaning is well supported in the literature. Evidence supports the concept of liberation from MV (4,5) so that the timely recognition of patients having recovered from respiratory failure is more important than manipulation of MV in an attempt to accelerate recovery. Furthermore, using the talents of nonphysician health care professionals can improve the outcomes of patients. It is imperative that protocols not be put in place to supplant clinical judgment. Protocols are meant as guides for patient management,

not as a set of rules "engraved in stone." Likewise, protocols should be viewed as dynamic tools, which should be modified periodically to accommodate new data or health care professionals' preferences. Incorporating new information as it becomes available will increase protocol acceptance by all medical care professionals involved in the care of critically ill, mechanically ventilated patients.

KEY POINTS

CLINICAL PRACTICE GUIDELINES—EVIDENCE-BASED WEANING RECOMMENDATIONS

Nonphysician health care professionals can provide protocol-based care that enhances outcomes for patients with respiratory care needs [not limited to liberation from mechanical ventilation (MV)].

Randomized controlled trials demonstrate that protocols for liberating patients from MV driven by nonphysician health care professionals can result in improved clinical outcomes.

Daily screening of patients, often considered the "first step" in a weaning protocol, should be tailored to be inclusive, not exclusive, so that patients will be advanced within the protocol if at all possible. Perhaps the most important reason to continue some form of daily screening (individualized to the specific patient population) is to identify specific and perhaps treatable issues that are causing a delay in patient readiness for liberation from the ventilator.

An empiric approach to a trial of weaning (spontaneous breathing trial) is safe and indicated.

When a patient appears to be improving, but can either not oxygenate or ventilate adequately when breathing spontaneously, we recommend the following:

That all remediable factors to enhance the prospects of successful liberation from MV be addressed (e.g., electrolyte

derangements, bronchospasm, malnutrition, excess secretions, and so on).

That the patient be placed on a comfortable, safe, and well-monitored mode of MV, such as pressure support ventilation, synchronized intermittent mandatory ventilation with pressure support ventilation, or extubation with support using noninvasive positive pressure ventilation.

That few data support multiple manipulations of ventilator settings each day in an effort to wean or "train" the patient. In fact, these efforts may be viewed as a waste of precious resources (both person-power and time). Strategies that incorporate periodic "resting" of the patient for varying intervals on control mode MV have been advocated by some researchers but have not been associated with superior outcomes. For clinicians who prefer to continue stepwise reductions in MV, it appears that multiple daily spontaneous breathing trials or pressure support ventilation are superior to intermittent mandatory ventilation (9). Whichever mode is used, at least a once-daily spontaneous breathing trial should be incorporated, as mentioned.

Patients' abilities to breathe spontaneously should be assessed at the risk of failure, but in the face of repeated failures, clinicians must consider longer-term options, including both tracheotomy and a chronic or step-down ventilator facility.

The decision to extubate the patient must be guided by objective information combined with clinical acumen to reduce unnecessary reintubations and self-extubations.

REFERENCES

1. Weinberger SE, Weiss JW. Weaning from ventilatory support. *N Engl J Med* 1995;332:388–389.
2. Manthous CA, Schmidt GA, Hall JB. Liberation from mechanical ventilation: a decade of progress. *Chest* 1998;114:886–901.
3. Hall JB, Wood LD. Liberation of the patient from mechanical ventilation. *JAMA* 1987;257:1621–1628.
4. Esteban A, Frutos F, Tobin MJ, et al. A comparison of four methods of weaning patients from mechanical ventilation. *N Engl J Med* 1995;332:345–350.
5. Ely EW, Baker AM, Dunagan DP, et al. Effect on the duration of mechanical ventilation of identifying patients capable of breathing spontaneously. *N Engl J Med* 1996;335:1864–1869.
6. Ely EW, Meade M, Haponik EF, et al. Mechanical ventilator weaning protocols driven by non-physician health care professionals: clinical practice guidelines of the ACCP, SCCM, and AARC. *Chest* 2001; (in press).
7. Ely EW, Baker AM, Evans GW, et al. The prognostic significance of passing a daily screen of weaning parameters. *Intensive Care Med* 1999; 25:581–587.
8. Sloane PJ, Gee MH, Gottleib JE, et al. A multicenter registry of patients with acute respiratory distress syndrome: physiology and outcome. *Am Rev Respir Dis* 1992;146:419–426.
9. Brochard L, Rauss A, Benito S, et al. Comparison of three methods of gradual withdrawal from ventilatory support during weaning from mechanical ventilation. *Am J Respir Crit Care Med* 1994;150:896–903.
10. Listello D, Sessler C. Unplanned extubation: clinical predictors for reintubation. *Chest* 1994;105:1496–1503.
11. Tindol GA Jr, DiBenedetto RJ, Kosciuk L. Unplanned extubations. *Chest* 1994;105:1804–1807.
12. Stroetz RW, Hubmayr RD. Tidal volume maintenance during weaning with pressure support. *Am J Respir Crit Care Med* 1995;152:1034–1040.
13. Torres A, Gatell JM, Aznar E. Re-intubation increases the risk of nosocomial pneumonia in patients needing mechanical ventilation. *Am J Respir Crit Care Med* 1995;152:137–141.
14. Wood KE, Flaten AL, Reedy JS, et al. Use of a daily wean screen and weaning protocol for mechanically ventilated patients in a multidisciplinary tertiary critical care unit. *Crit Care Med* 1999;27:A94.
15. Luce JM. Reducing the use of mechanical ventilation. *N Engl J Med* 1996;25:1916–1917.

16. Kollef MH, Shapiro SD, Silver P, et al. A randomized, controlled trial of protocol-directed versus physician-directed weaning from mechanical ventilation. *Crit Care Med* 1997;25:567–574.

17. Marelich GP, Murin S, Battistella F, et al. Protocol weaning of mechanical ventilation in medical and surgical patients by respiratory care practitioners and nurses: Effect on weaning time and incidence of ventilator-associated pneumonia. *Chest* 2000;118:459.

18. Strickland JH Jr, Hasson JH. A computer-controlled ventilator weaning system: a clinical trial. *Chest* 1993;103:1220–1226.

19. Yang KL, Tobin MJ. A prospective study of indexes predicting the outcome of trials of weaning from mechanical ventilation. *N Engl J Med* 1991;324:1445–1450.

20. Mohsenifar Z, Hay A, Hay J, et al. Gastric intramural pH as a predictor of success or failure in weaning patients from mechanical ventilation. *Ann Intern Med* 1993;119:794–798.

21. Gluck EH, Barkoviak MJ, Balk RA, et al. Medical effectiveness of esophageal balloon pressure manometry in weaning patients from mechanical ventilation. *Crit Care Med* 1995;23:504–509.

22. Sassoon CS, Mahutte CK. Airway occlusion pressure and breathing pattern as predictors of weaning outcome. *Am Rev Respir Dis* 1993;148:860–866.

23. Vallverdu I, Calaf N, Subirana M, et al. Clinical characteristics, respiratory functional parameters, and outcome of a two-hour T-piece trial of patients weaning from mechanical ventilation. *Am J Respir Crit Care Med* 1999;158:1855–1862.

24. Bellemare F, Grassino A. Effect of pressure and timing of contraction on human diaphragm fatigue. *J Appl Physiol* 1982;53:1190–1195.

25. Vassilakopoulos T, Zakynthinos S, Roussos C. The tension-time index and the frequency/tidal volume ratio are the major pathophysiologic determinants of weaning failure and success. *Am J Respir Crit Care Med* 1998;158:378–385.

26. Jaeschke RZ, Meade MO, Guyatt GH, et al. How to use diagnostic test articles in the intensive care unit: Diagnosing weanability using f/Vt. *Crit Care Med* 1997;25:1514–1521.

27. Ely EW, Bennett PA, Bowton DL, et al. Large scale implementation of a respiratory therapist-driven protocol for ventilator weaning. *Am J Respir Crit Care Med* 1999;159:439–446.

28. Epstein SK. Etiology of extubation failure and the predictive value of the rapid shallow breathing index. *Am J Respir Crit Care Med* 1995;152:545–549.

29. Epstein SK, Ciubotaru RL. Influence of gender and endotracheal tube size on preextubation breathing pattern. *Am J Respir Crit Care Med* 1997;154:1647–1652.

30. Krieger BP, Isber J, Breitenbucher A et al. Serial measurements of the rapid-shallow-breathing index as a predictor of weaning outcome in elderly medical patients. *Chest* 1997;112:1029–1034.

31. Esteban A, Anzueto A, Alia I, et al. How is mechanical ventilation employed in the intensive care unit. *Am J Respir Crit Care Med* 2000;161:1450–1458.

32. Esteban A, Alia I, Tobin M, et al. Effect of spontaneous breathing trial duration on outcome of attempts to discontinue mechanical ventilation. *Am J Respir Crit Care Med* 1999;159:512–518.

33. Esteban A, Alia I, Gordo F, et al. Extubation outcome after spontaneous breathing trials with T-tube or pressure support ventilation. *Am J Respir Crit Care Med* 1997;156:459–465.

34. Greco PJ, Eisenberg JM. Changing physicians' practices. *N Engl J Med* 1993;329:1271–1273.

35. Main DS, Cohen SJ, DiClemente CC. Measuring physician readiness to change cancer screening: preliminary results. *Am J Preventive Med* 1995;11:54–58.

36. Soumerai SB, McLaughlin TJ, Gurwitz JH, et al. Effect of local medical opinion leaders on quality of care for acute myocardial infarction: a randomized controlled trial. *JAMA* 1998;279:1358–1363.

37. Cohen IL. Weaning from mechanical ventilation—the team approach and beyond. *Intensive Care Med* 1994;20:317–318.

38. Brook AD, Ahrens TS, Schaiff R, et al. Effect of a nursing implemented sedation protocol on the duration of mechanical ventilation. *Crit Care Med* 1999;27:2609–2615.

39. Kress JP, Pohlman AS, O'Connor MF, et al. Daily interruption of sedative infusions in critically ill patients undergoing mechanical ventilation. *N Engl J Med* 2000;342:1471–1477.

40. Ely EW, Margolin R, Francis J, et al. Delirium in the ICU: measurement and outcomes. *Am J Respir Crit Care Med* 2000;161:A506.

41. Ely EW, Inouye S, Bernard G, et al. Delirium in mechanically ventilated patients: validity and reliability of the confusion assessment method for the intensive care unit (CAM-ICU). *JAMA* 2001;286:2703–2710.

42. Mascia MF, Koch M, Medicis JJ. Pharmacoeconomic impact of rational use guidelines on the provision of analgesia, sedation, and neuromuscular blockade in critical care. *Crit Care Med* 2000;28:2300–2306.

43. Seneff MG, Wagner DP, Wagner RP'JE, et al. Hospital and 1-year survival of patients admitted to intensive care units with acute exacerbation of chronic obstructive pulmonary disease. *JAMA* 1995;274:1852–1857.

44. Hudson LD. Survival data in patients with acute and chronic lung disease requiring mechanical ventilation. *Am Rev Respir Dis* 1989;140:S19–S24.

45. Brochard L, Mancebo J, Wysocki M, et al. Noninvasive ventilation for acute exacerbations of chronic obstructive pulmonary disease. *N Engl J Med* 1995;333:817–822.

46. Vitacca M, Clini E, Porta R, et al. Acute exacerbations in patients with COPD: predictors of need for mechanical ventilation. *Eur Respir J* 1996;9:1487–1493.

47. Jeffrey AA, Warren PM, Flenley DC. Acute hypercapnic respiratory failure in patients with chronic obstructive lung disease: risk factors and use of guidelines for management. *Thorax* 1992;47:34–40.

48. Moran JL, Green JM, Homan SD, et al. Acute exacerbations of chronic obstructive pulmonary disease and mechanical ventilation: a reevaluation. *Crit Care Med* 1998;26:71–78.

49. Menzies R, Gibbons W, Goldberg P. Determinants of weaning and survival among patients with COPD who require mechanical ventilation for acute respiratory failure. *Chest* 1989;95:398–405.

50. Anthonisen NR. Prognosis in chronic obstructive pulmonary disease: Results from multicenter clinical trials. *Am Rev Respir Dis* 1989;140:S95–S99.

51. Ely EW, Baker AM, Evans GW, et al. The cost of respiratory care in mechanically ventilated patients with chronic obstructive pulmonary disease. *Crit Care Med* 2000;28:408–413.

52. Conti G, DeBlasi R, Pelaia P, et al. Early prediction of successful weaning during pressure support ventilation in chronic obstructive pulmonary disease patients. *Crit Care Med* 1992;29:366–371.

53. Sassoon CSH, Te TT, Mahutte CK, et al. Airway occlusion pressure: an important indicator for successful weaning in patients with chronic obstructive pulmonary disease. *Am Rev Respir Dis* 1987;135:107–113.

54. Sassoon CSH, Light RW, Lodia R, et al. Pressure-time product during continuous positive airway pressure, pressure support ventilation, and T-piece during weaning from mechanical ventilation. *Am Rev Respir Dis* 1991;143:469–475.

55. Nava S, Ambrosino N, Clini E, et al. Noninvasive mechanical ventilation in the weaning of patients with respiratory failure due to chronic obstructive pulmonary disease: a randomized controlled trial. *Ann Intern Med* 1998;128:721–728.

56. Wood G, MacLeod B, Moffatt S. Weaning from mechanical ventilation: physician-directed vs a respiratory-therapist-directed protocol. *Respir Care* 1995;40:219–224.

57. Kollef MH, Horst HM, Prang L, et al. Reducing the duration of mechanical ventilation: three examples of change in the intensive care unit. *New Horizons* 1998;6:52–60.

58. Chatila W, Ani S, Guaglianone D, et al. Cardiac ischemia during weaning from mechanical ventilation. *Chest* 1996;109:1577–1583.

59. Ely EW, Namen AM, Tatter S, et al. Impact of a ventilator weaning protocol in neurosurgical patients: a randomized, controlled trial. *Am J Respir Crit Care Med* 1999;A370.

60. Namen AM, Ely EW, Tatter S, et al. Predictors of successful extubation in neurosurgical patients. *Am J Respir Crit Care Med* 2001;163:658–664.

61. Coplin WM, Pierson DJ, Cooley KD et al. Implications of extubation delay in brain-injured: patients meeting standard weaning criteria. *Am J Respir Crit Care Med* 2000;161:1530–1536.

62. Chevron V, Menard J, Richard J, et al. Unplanned extubation: risk factors of development and predictive criteria for reintubation. *Crit Care Med* 1998;26:1049–1053.

63. Drakulovic MB, Torres A, Bauer TT, et al. Supine body position as a risk factor for nosocomial pneumonia in mechanically ventilated patients: a randomised trial. *Lancet* 1999;354:1851–1858.

64. Hobbs F, Damon BL, Taeuber CM. Sixty-Five Plus in the United States. 1996. Washington, DC: U.S. Department of Commerce, Economics, and Statistics Administration, Bureau of the Census.

65. Shaw AB. Age as a basis for healthcare rationing: support for ageist policies. *Drugs Aging* 1996;9:403–405.

66. Baltussen R, Leidl R, Ament A. The impact of age on cost-effectiveness ratios and its control in decision making. *Health Econ* 1996;5:227–239.

67. Sage WM, Hurst CR, Silverman JF, et al. Intensive care for the elderly: outcome of elective and nonelective admissions. *J Am Geriatr Soc* 1987;35:312–318.

68. Singer PA, Lowy FH. Rationing, patient preferences, and cost of care at the end of life. *Arch Intern Med* 1992;152:478–480.

69. Giugliano RP, Camargo CA, Lloyd-Jones DM, et al. Elderly patients receive less aggressive medical and invasive management of unstable angina. *Arch Intern Med* 1998;158:1113–1120.

70. Hamel MB, Philips RS, Teno JM, et al. Seriously ill hospitalized adults: do we spend less on older patients? *J Am Geriatr Soc* 1996;44:1043–1048.

71. Hakim RB, Teno JM, Harrell FE, et al. Factors associated with do-not-resuscitate orders: patients' preferences, prognoses, and physicians' judgments. SUPPORT Investigators. The Study to Understand Prognoses and Preferences for Outcome and Risks of Treatments. *Ann Intern Med* 1996;125:284–293.

72. Hamel MB, Teno JM, Goldman L, et al. Patient age and decisions to withhold life-sustaining treatments from seriously ill, hospitalized adults. *Ann Intern Med* 1999;130:116–125.

73. Knaus WA, Draper EA, Wagner DP, et al. An evaluation of outcome from intensive care in major medical centers. *Ann Intern Med* 1986;104:410–418.

74. Ely EW, Evans GW, Haponik EF. Mechanical ventilation in a cohort of elderly patients admitted to an intensive care unit. *Ann Intern Med* 1999;131:96–104.

75. Yuen EJ, Gonnella JS, Louis DZ, et al. Severity-adjusted differences in hospital utilization by gender. *Am J Medical Qual* 1995;10:76–80.

76. Cohen IL, Lambrinos J, Fein IA. Mechanical ventilation for the elderly patient in intensive care: incremental changes and benefits. *JAMA* 1993;269:1025–1029.

77. Boult C, Dowd B, McCaffrey D, et al. Screening elders for risk of hospital admission. *J Am Geriatr Soc* 1993;41:811–817.

78. Goldberg AI. Life-sustaining technology and the elderly: prolonged mechanical ventilation factors influencing the treatment decision. *Chest* 1988;94:1277–1282.

79. Scheinhorn DJ, Chao DC, Stearn-Hassenpglug M, et al. Post-ICU mechanical ventilation. Treatment of 1,123 patients at a regional weaning center. *Chest* 1997;111:1654–1659.

80. Scheinhorn DJ, Hassenpflug M, Artinian BM, et al. Predictors of weaning after 6 weeks of mechanical ventilation. *Chest* 1995;107:500–505.

81. Scheinhorn DJ, Chao DC, Stearn-Hassenpflug M, et al. Outcomes in post-ICU mechanical ventilation: a therapist-implemented weaning protocol. *Chest* 2001;119:236–242.

82. Make BJ, Hill NS, Goldberg AI, et al. Mechanical ventilation beyond the intensive care unit: report of a consensus conference of the American College of Chest Physicians. *Chest* 1998;113:289S–344S.

83. Epstein SK, Ciubotaru RL. Independent effects of etiology of failure and time to reintubation on outcome for patients failing extubation. *Am J Respir Crit Care Med* 1998;158:489–493.

84. Epstein SK, Ciubotaru RL, Wong JB. Effect of failed extubation on the outcome of mechanical ventilation. *Chest* 1997;112:186–192.

85. Burrowes P, Wallace C, Davies JM, et al. Pulmonary edema as a radiologic manifestation of venous air embolism secondary to dental implant surgery. *Chest* 1992;101:561–562.

86. Coppola DP, May JJ. Self-Extubation: a 12-month experience. *Chest* 1990;98:165–169.

87. Vassal TN, Anh GD, Gabillet JM, et al. Prospective evaluation of self-extubations in a medical intensive care unit. *Intensive Care Med* 1993;19:340–342.

88. Boulain T, and the Association des Reanimateurs du Centre-Ouest. Unplanned extubations in the adult intensive care unit: a prospective multicenter study. *Am J Respir Crit Care Med* 1998;157:1131–1137.

89. Betbese AJ, Perez M, Rialp G, et al. A prospective study of unplanned endotracheal extubation in intensive care unit patients. *Crit Care Med* 1998;26:1180–1186.

90. Miller RL, Cole RP. Association between reduced cuff leak volume and postextubation stridor. *Chest* 1996;110:1035–1040.

ACUTE ABDOMINAL CONDITIONS IN THE PERIOPERATIVE INTENSIVE CARE PATIENT

BRUCE M. POTENZA

KEY WORDS

- Acute abdomen
- Abdominal compartment syndrome
- Colitis: ischemic, infectious, and inflammatory
- Cholecystitis
- Diarrhea
- Ileus
- Obstruction
- Pancreatitis
- Perforation
- Peritonitis: primary, secondary, and tertiary
- Sepsis

INTRODUCTION

Abdominal complications in the perioperative patient represent a wide range of potential morbidity and mortality. The diagnosis of an acute abdominal process may be challenging to establish due to the incapacitated state of the patient, the complexity of the surgical procedure performed, or the multiplicity of involved organ systems. The shared symptoms of many disease entities encountered in the critically ill may further complicate the diagnosis of an evolving process. Diagnostic laboratory results and imaging studies may be inconclusive. The physician rendering care not only must be adept with general critical care supportive measures, but be cognizant of the potential postoperative problems as well as the timing and most appropriate means to evaluate these complications. The approach to many postoperative events continues to evolve. Improved image resolution, dynamic computed tomography (CT) scanning and enhanced duplex arterial and venous imaging have aided in the diagnostic quest. New and superior therapies, such as percutaneous intraabdominal drainage, vascular stenting, and embolization are changing the way we approach some abdominal pathologies. Diagnostic and therapeutic endoscopy continues to evolve and provide valuable assistance in the management of some of these issues. Yet, in the end, the physician must synthesize all of the pieces of incomplete data and formulate a diagnostic and therapeutic plan for the patient. Results of the therapy must be constantly reevaluated to ensure the patient is making progress. Should the patient regress, the plan may need to be adapted or redesigned to meet the patient's needs.

ANATOMY AND PHYSIOLOGY

The abdomen is a coelomic cavity bounded by the diaphragm superiorly, pelvic floor inferiorly, abdominal wall anteriorly, and retroperitoneum posteriorly. Intraabdominal organs include the liver, stomach, and small and large bowel. The retroperitoneal organs include the kidney and adrenal glands, aorta and cava, and duodenum. The right and left colon have posterior attachments to the retroperitoneum and are relatively fixed within the abdomen, whereas the jejunum and ileum are on a movable mesentery within the abdomen. In the female, the uterus, ovaries, and fallopian tubes lie within the abdomen, but the vagina lies beneath the pelvic floor. These anatomic relationships are important to understand as they help define the spread of disease within the abdomen. For example, a posterior perforation of the duodenum will be confined initially within the retroperitoneum, whereas an anterior perforation will spread into the abdominal cavity. A missed penetrating injury to the posterior left colon may initially be confined and develop into a retroperitoneal abscess, whereas an anterior penetrating left colonic injury is free to leak into the peritoneal cavity, resulting in pancreatitis. Another important set of relationships to consider are the potential spaces within the abdominal cavity. These are areas of the abdominal cavity that are bound by surrounding organs and tend to be in dependent positions within the abdomen. These areas include the bilateral subphrenic spaces, the subhepatic space or Morison pouch, the lesser sac, the right and left paracolic gutters, and the pelvis (1, 2). Fluid from a perforated viscus may sequester in these areas and develop into an abscess (3). These are prime sites to search for an infected fluid collection.

The greater omentum is attached superiorly along the transverse colon and is freely mobile. In the event of an inflamed or injured organ, the omentum will attempt to adhere and cover or "wall off" the inflamed tissue. Likewise, in the event of a hollow viscus perforation, the omentum will attempt to seal off this area to contain the spillage. This situation may be seen in a perforated appendix or diverticulum. Although the omentum may succeed in containing the infection, prompt drainage, antibiotics, and surgery may be needed.

The abdomen is a dynamic space lined by a mesothelial membrane called peritoneum. This single layer lines the abdomen and is composed of the parietal and visceral peritoneum. The parietal peritoneum lines the anterior and lateral abdominal walls as well as the retroperitoneum, pelvic floor, and diaphragm. The visceral peritoneum covers the intraperitoneal organs and mesentery.

The peritoneum is a semipermeable membrane that permits the passage of fluid and solutes along a concentration gradient. In an adult, the total area of the peritoneum is approximately 1.7 mm^2. By comparison, the surface area of the peritoneum closely approximates total body surface area of the skin. As a result of the combination of large surface area and permeability characteristics, large fluid shifts may occur into and out of the peritoneal cavity during illness and injury. These fluid shifts must be taken into account in the management of critically ill patients.

Within the abdomen, a small amount of fluid is normally present to act as a lubricant for the intraabdominal organs. The normal respiratory movement of the diaphragm produces a gentle circular flow of the ascitic fluid throughout the abdomen (4). This facilitates the resorption of the fluid into the diaphragmatic lymph channels. In times of disease, the production of abdominal fluid may exceed the ability to resorb the fluid. Ascites then develops. The ascitic fluid may become infected as seen in primary bacterial peritonitis or it may become infected due to a perforation of an intraabdominal structure, resulting in secondary peritonitis.

Parietal and visceral nerves innervate the abdomen. Parietal peritoneal afferent nerves travel via somatic nerve fibers and follow the corresponding anatomic dermatome distribution. As such, the somatosensory innervation is highly localized (4). Pain from right lower quadrant appendicitis will be localized to the appropriate cutaneous dermatome once the appendiceal inflammation reaches the peritoneum. Thus an inflamed appendix adherent to the lateral abdominal wall will cause pain in the corresponding cutaneous dermatome of the right lower quadrant. In another patient, appendicitis may cause pain in the right inguinal area if the appendix is adherent to the right pelvic structures. If the appendix is retrocecal and cephalad in location, the pain might seem to be in the right upper quadrant. Visceral afferent fibers travel via the autonomic nervous system. Common visceral afferent pathways include the celiac, superior, and inferior mesenteric plexus and the pelvic nerve plexus. Pains from these fibers reflect stretching, distension, and contractions of the abdominal viscera and organs. The pain tends to be poorly localized and may be perceived in the epigastrium, the periumbilical area, and the suprapubic area. To complicate matters further, the visceral afferent nerve fibers stimulate both the right and left side of the spinal cord making attempts at localization more difficult. Pain from a small bowel obstruction tends to present with a more diffuse picture of abdominal pain. Thus, pain from a segment of strangulated small bowel, localized in the left upper quadrant, may seem to originate in the epigastrium. Referred pain is the result of the convergence of diseased organ afferent nerve stimulation with shared nerve fibers of nondiseased organs. An example would be the right upper shoulder discomfort associated with the right upper quadrant pain of biliary colic.

ETIOLOGY

The critically ill patient may present with any abdominal pathology, but certain disease entities are more common in these patients (5). Diseases such as acalculous cholecystitis, pancreatitis, peritonitis, ileus, and colitis are often seen in the critically ill (6,7). Associated factors such as hemorrhagic shock, septic shock, hypoxemia, and cardiac bypass procedures are predisposing factors to the development of these entities. Recent surgical procedures such as gastric and bowel resection, vascular bypass grafting, and exonerative oncologic procedures all carry potential complication. Comorbid disease combined with pharmacologic paralysis and sedation greatly hinder our ability to evaluate the perioperative patient.

In addition to the normal intensive care course of a postoperative patient, a physician must have a familiarity with complications associated with a particular surgical procedure (8) (Table 1). Knowledge of the timing and presentation of these events is essential for the prompt recognition, identification and treatment. It is imperative to consider the patient's disease process within the context of the recent surgical procedure. Entities such as bleeding, anastomotic breakdown, biliary leak or intraabdominal abscess may occur as a result of a surgical procedure. Additional disease entities may be a result of an exacerbation of a patient's co-morbid disease. Cardiac arrhythmias, intestinal ischemia due to a low cardiac output state or pulmonary insufficiency may be due to a worsening of the patients underlying pathophysiology rather than a direct complication of a recent surgical procedure.

An obvious site of a complication in one patient may be elusive in the next. For example, a postoperative patient admitted to the ICU who complains of abdominal pain will focus the clinician's attention on this area. On the other hand, the same postoperative patient may develop sepsis. Within this context, the abdomen is but one of several potential sites of infection. Postoperative problems in immunosuppressed patients such as transplant, cancer, and human immunodeficiency virus/acquired immunodeficiency syndrome (HIV/AIDS) patients may be particularly difficult to diagnose. The clinical signs and symptoms may be late in manifesting or underestimate the severity of the complication.

SPECIFIC DISEASE ENTITIES

Diarrhea

Diarrhea is a common development in postoperative patients. It may be related to dystonic gastrointestinal (GI) motility, infection, or inflammation. For example, a hypermotile segment of sigmoid colon due to an adjacent pelvic abscess may lead to diarrhea. Intraluminal infection with bacteria, virus, or protozoa may result in diarrhea. Inflammatory diseases such as Crohn disease or ulcerative colitis may lead to diarrhea. Bloody diarrhea may be due to a GI bleed or an intrinsic bowel process such as inflammatory bowel disease or ischemic colitis. Bloody diarrhea seen after an abdominal aortic aneurysmectomy may represent ischemic colitis secondary to ligation of the inferior mesenteric artery. Occasionally, diarrhea is due to a fecal impaction. More commonly in the ICU, enteral tube feed intolerance may precipitate diarrhea. Atrophy of the enterocyte during critical illness

TABLE 1. COMMON SURGERIES AND ASSOCIATED ABDOMINAL COMPLICATIONS

Problem	Etiology	Complication	S & S	Timing	Therapy
Anastomotic breakdown or leak	Poor blood supply—hypotension Tension on suture line Infected perianastomotic tissues	Leakage or breakdown of anastomosis Spillage of luminal contents—infection or abscess formtion	Fever, ↑ WBC Abdominal pain, distension, ileus	Usually 5–7 days postoperatively Late breakdown >10 days due to poor healing, nutrition, or steroid usage	Drainage and intestinal diversion in most cases Possible anastomotic resection In some instances, drain and TPN
Small bowel obstruction	Adhesions Hernia Luminal obstruction Intussusception Volvulus	Partial bowel obstruction Possible intestinal ischemia due to vascular compromise	Abdominal distension and pain +/− ↑ WBC Intolerance of feedings Obstipation Fluid sequestration	Early (2–3 d), tends to be a mechanical operative lesion Late (>2 wks), from adhesions	Nasogastric suctioning Intravenous fluid replacement Observation Operative intervention in some cases
Vascular anastomosis problems	Suture line failure Thrombosis Infection	Rupture or leak Pseudo- or mycotic aneurysm Ischemia of distal tissues	Pain, pallor, poor distal perfusion Pulsatile mass Signs of infection Hematoma formation ↓ HCT	Leaks may occur immediately Thrombosis anytime Aneurysm late >2 wks	Simple leak; reverse anticoagulation Simple suture line repair Aneurysm—excise
Major vessel thrombosis	Aortic or mesenteric grafting Extremity grafting	Ischemia	Pain, paresthesia, pulselessness, pallor, bloody diarrhea	Immediate to anytime	Thrombosis; embolectomy, thrombectomy, or lytic therapy
Ileus	Bowel manipulation, resection, reanastomosis	Functional obstruction of the bowel due to GI hypomotility	Abdominal distension, increased fluid requirements, hypoactive bowel sounds	Immediately postoperative After systemic disease or hypotension	Supportive care Nutritional support Exclude obstructive lesions Prokinetic agents
Missed traumatic injury	Bowel perforation, bleeding, ductile disruption	Spillage of bowel contents, infarcted bowel, ductile leakage	Hypovolemia, HCT drop Ileus, infection, or sepsis	Bleeding; immediate to days Perforation; 4–7 d	
Solid organ resection	Transection of major blood vessels or ducts	Bleeding from the dissection Ductile leak	Hemorrhage Pancreatic fistula, biloma, uroma	Immediate to days	Fluids, blood, Drainage and reoperation in some cases

S & S, signs and symptoms; WBC, white blood cells; TPN, total parenteral nutrition; HCT, hematocrit; GI, gastrointestinal.

and prolonged periods of nothing by mouth contribute to this predicament. Simple adjustment of the rate or the concentration of the enteral feeds will usually correct this cause of diarrhea. Potential etiologies of a primary infectious diarrhea include *Salmonella, Shigella,* or *Yersinia.* Unless the patient was a reservoir for these organisms prior to admission, infections diarrhea is unlikely to develop while the patient is in the ICU. Likewise, enteric viruses may induce diarrhea, but this is uncommon in the ICU. In the immunocompromised patient, opportunistic infections due to *Cryptosporidium* or cytomegalovirus may develop.

The use of broad-spectrum antibiotics may induce an antibiotic-associated colitis. Simple cessation of the antibiotics will permit the normal bowel flora to recolonize, and the diarrhea will abate. A more serious extension of this problem is overgrowth of *Clostridium difficile,* and pseudomembranous colitis with profound diarrhea, resulting in severe fluid and electrolyte abnormalities. Toxic megacolon may develop in some patients. If signs of systemic toxicity are present and the patient is

unresponsive to fluid resuscitation and appropriate antibiotic therapy, a subtotal colectomy is indicated. Intraoperative improvement of the systemic symptoms may be seen as soon as the colon has been removed. Stool cultures, fecal leukocyte, serum toxin levels, or endoscopic demonstration of pseudomembranes aid in the diagnosis of *C. difficile* colitis. Two-week treatments with Flagyl 500 mg p.o. t.i.d. or vancomycin 125 mg p.o. q.i.d. or cholestyramine 4 g p.o. t.i.d. are effective in eradicating *C. difficile.* If the patient is too ill for oral medications, then metronidazole 500 mg intravenous (i.v.) q.i.d. may be administered. If the patient has distal colonic involvement, a high-colonic vancomycin enema may be administered.

Ileus

An ileus is due to an alteration of normal GI motility resulting in a functional obstruction of the GI tract. Ileus may be associated with neurogenic disorders, pharmacologic agents, metabolic disturbances, severe systemic disease, trauma, or recent abdominal surgery. If one section of the GI tract is either hypotonic or atonic, this will render the more proximal portions functionally obstructed. The distal segments may evacuate giving a false sense of security that the GI tract is beginning to function. An ileus may be localized or due to diffuse disease of the GI tract. Examples of a localized ileus are adjacent organ inflammation in pancreatitis or trauma, whereas a diffuse ileus may be seen in the postoperative period or accompanying sepsis (9). Resolution of an ileus tends to parallel the resolution of the underlying disease process with postoperative ileus usually occurring in 3 to 7 days.

Physical examination will reveal abdominal distension, hypoactive bowel sounds, and tenderness to deep palpation. There are no localized peritoneal findings, and tenderness is due to the compression of the underlying distended bowel. The white blood cell count may be slightly elevated and the patient may be intravascularly depleted due to third space fluid sequestration. Therapy is directed at correcting the precipitating event and is accompanied by nasogastric suction, fluid replacement, and supportive care. Prokinetic agents such as erythromycin, cisapride, metoclopramide, or neostigmine have limited effectiveness in resolving an ileus. Cisapride has recently been taken off the market due to cardiac arrhythmias secondary to QT prolongation.

Occasionally, an isolated colonic ileus may develop and is referred to as an acute colonic pseudoobstruction or Ogilvie syndrome (10). This tends to preferentially involve the more proximal colon, particularly the cecum and ascending colon. Secondary areas of involvement include the transverse colon and the splenic flexure. Ogilvie syndrome occurs more in older adults and chronically debilitated patients. Antecedent events include major abdominal surgery, systemic sepsis, and major trauma or cardiopulmonary bypass procedures. A major contributing factor is medication that inhibits GI motility. Drugs such as opiates for postoperative pain, calcium channel blockers, phenothiazines, and beta-blockers have been implicated. Although the exact etiology of this disease is unknown, it has been postulated that there is an imbalance between an excess of sympathetic tone or a decrease in the parasympathetic tone within the large bowel. This may result in an adynamic colonic segment. The proximal bowel maintains its function and can propel air into the adynamic segment resulting in massive colonic distension (11).

The patient may develop abdominal distension and pain. The bowel sounds may be normal in the early phase of the pseudoobstruction, but become hypotonic and quiet in the latter phases. Typically there are small amounts of air distal to the affected large bowel segment and a small amount of air in the rectum. As the disease progresses, the distal air may evacuate giving a false sense that bowel function is returning. Repeat radiographs demonstrate evacuation of the distal colon with continued pseudoobstruction in the proximal colon. It is important to consider the combination of the absolute colonic distension in combination with the rate of distension. For example in the cecum, dilation to 12 cm is worrisome, but equally important is the rate in which the dilation occurred. If this was rapid (24 to 48 hours) a more aggressive approach is mandated, whereas if this occurred over days, a more conservative approach may be advisable. In some institutionalized patients or patients on medications that inhibit normal bowel contractility, cecal dilation to 15 to 16 cm may be seen on plain films without serious consequences. Concern for bowel wall distension, secondary ischemia, necrosis, and perforation are paramount, as mortality rates of 40% have been reported in the face of perforation. Nasogastric suction, fluid replacement, replacement of a rectal tube to bypass the external anal sphincter, and endoscopic decompression are the mainstays of therapy. Colonoscopy will decompress 60% to 90% of these effectively, but there is a 40% recurrence rate requiring a second endoscopy. More recently, neostigmine, a potent acetylcholinesterase inhibitor, has been studied and shown to reverse the pseudoobstruction in some patients (12,13). The dose used is 2.5 mg i.v. over 3 minutes (14). Transient cardiovascular monitoring for bradycardia is indicated, as there will be a number of older adult patients who may develop bradycardia or heart block. Flatus or bowel movements may be seen within 30 minutes. If there is no resolution of the pseudoobstruction, the neostigmine may be repeated in 20 minutes. Failure to relieve the pseudoobstruction may necessitate surgical intervention. If there is no suspicion of bowel wall ischemia or necrosis, a simple cecostomy will suffice. This may be performed through an oblique right lower quadrant incision, midline incision, or via laparoscopy. If there is significant ischemia to the bowel, then resection of the affected colonic segment and proximal diversion are the mainstays of treatment. Laparoscopy may have a role in the management of this disease in that it permits examination of the colon and the placement of a colonic diversion to vent the affected segment. Close inspection of the bowel is imperative to exclude focal areas of bowel ischemia.

Mechanical Obstruction

Mechanical obstruction may affect the GI tract anywhere. Sources of upper GI (foregut) obstruction include esophageal obstruction due to tumor, stricture, or esophageal webs. Gastric obstructions may be seen at the pylorus and are usually due to longstanding peptic ulcer disease with pyloric scarring and edema. Occasionally, tumor will obstruct the gastric outlet. Symptoms for these patients include nausea, vomiting, and early satiety. The vomitus is generally composed of partially digested material and gastric secretions. Relief is through placement of a nasogastric (NG) tube to suction and keeping the patient n.p.o. Plain abdominal radiographs reveal a distended gastric bubble. Oral contrast imaging will aid in demonstrating the level and characteristics of the obstruction. Definitive care depends upon the exact etiology of the lesion and is usually surgical. The patient can be maintained on NG suction and i.v. fluids or total parenteral nutrition (TPN) while endoscopy and/or CT evaluation are performed.

Small bowel obstruction is by far a more common occurrence in the ICU. Factors such as adhesions due to prior surgery, internal or external hernias, and neoplasm are common precipitating events. Prior documentation of a hernia in the premorbid state is a valuable piece of information for the physician attempting to evaluate a mass recently discovered in the patient's groin or midline abdomen. In the obtunded or sedated patient, differentiating between an incarcerated hernia and a strangulated hernia may be difficult. If the patient's condition permits a conservative approach with nasogastric decompression, i.v. fluid infusion and surgical consultation are attempted. Abdominal radiographs may demonstrate dilated loops of proximal small bowel with diminishing distal bowel gas. Bowel sounds may initially be present as the distal bowel evacuates gas. As the obstruction becomes more advanced, the bowel sounds may become hyperactive and demonstrate a tinkling sound. As the obstruction becomes more longstanding, bowel sounds may be absent. This is an ominous sign and usually indicates failure of conservative management. Further indications that conservative management is not succeeding include failure to decompress the proximal bowel, fever, rising white blood cell count, or abdominal tenderness. Surgical intervention may be indicated. One must remember that the findings are insensitive indicators of the presence of a compromised segment of bowel and should be viewed within the context of the patient's clinical condition (15).

The etiology of large bowel obstruction differs from that of small bowel obstruction because the ascending and descending colon are attached to the retroperitoneum. Common etiologies of large bowel obstruction include volvulus, fecal impaction, tumor, or complications of inflammatory bowel or diverticular disease (16). Occasionally, the sigmoid colon may herniate through an inguinal hernia defect and become incarcerated. A sigmoid volvulus may occur when a large redundant sigmoid colon usually twists, in a counterclockwise motion, upon its mesentery and creates a closed loop obstruction. The radiographic appearance of this is a dilated loop of large bowel with both ends of the loop anchored in the pelvis. If a contrast enema is obtained, there is the classic beaked bird deformity seen at the site of the obstruction. Attempts at colonoscopic or contrast enema decompression may be considered in stable patients with an early presentation. Surgical intervention is mandated if these therapeutic modalities fail, the patient has a late clinical presentation, or has a course that is suspicious for bowel compromise. In the acute setting, this involves proximal diversion and resection of any compromised bowel. Reanastomosis is not favored due to the nonprepped bowel and the generally dilated proximal colonic segment. Patients with a strangulated sigmoid volvulus have a mortality rate of 33% to 80% (17).

The cecum may be attached to a long mesentery and twist and rotate 90 degrees in a clockwise fashion to form a bowel obstruction. Colonoscopy may be attempted to decompress the volvulus. Contrast enemas may also be attempted with Gastrografin; however, they are less effective for pathology on the right side of the colon than on the left. Further rotation causes complete bowel obstruction with proximal small bowel dilation. If these methods are unsuccessful, or the patient appears toxic, surgery is indicated. Mortality rates with a cecal volvulus range from 14% if the bowel is viable, to 41% in the presence of gangrene or perforation.

Large bowel obstruction due to an advanced carcinoma usually presents with a more benign course of increasing abdominal distension, signs and symptoms of worsening obstruction, and dehydration. Complicated diverticular disease may be seen in the ICU. Whereas perforation is a more common problem with diverticulitis, obstruction may also be seen in patients with diverticular disease. In fact, obstruction may be due to diverticular perforation as well as chronic stricturing. In the case of acute diverticulitis, symptoms of left and occasionally right lower quadrant pain, fever, leukocytosis, and signs of constipation or obstipation herald this process. A CT scan may demonstrate diverticula, mesenteric fat stranding, bowel wall edema, proximal colonic dilation, localized abscess formation, or diffuse peritonitis. In

patients with colonic obstruction due to an exacerbation of diverticular disease, initial conservative therapy consists of bowel rest, an n.p.o. status, and i.v. antibiotics. The edema of the bowel and the obstruction may resolve with time. A stricture of the colon secondary to diverticulitis requires surgical resection. Attempts should be made to prepare and cleanse the colon for surgery, if possible, so that a one-stage operative procedure may be performed. In the case of a nearly complete bowel obstruction, an endoscopically placed small lumen stent may allow for proximal colonic decompression. A subsequent gentle mechanical bowel preparation may permit a one-stage bowel resection and reanastomosis. In complicated cases of diverticulitis with a pericolonic abscess, percutaneous drainage may be used. In a small number of patients with loculated or multiple abscesses or diffuse peritonitis, surgery is indicated with proximal diversion and diverticular resection. A two-stage procedure is required in these patients.

Acute Cholecystitis

In the general population, acute cholecystitis is due to cystic duct obstruction by biliary stones in 90% of affected patients. In the remaining 10% of the cases, acalculous cholecystitis is seen. In the ICU, more than 50% of postoperative cholecystitis is acalculous (18). The pathophysiology of acalculous cholecystitis is thought to be secondary to gallbladder ischemia. Precipitating factors include hypotension, systemic illness such as sepsis, coagulopathies, abdominal trauma, or abdominal compartment syndrome (19). Complications of acalculous cholecystitis include gallbladder ischemia, infarction, and perforation. Most perforations are walled off by the omentum and form localized abscesses; however, in some cases, free peritoneal perforations occur, leading to a secondary peritonitis.

Signs and symptoms of acalculous cholecystitis may be typical with right upper quadrant abdominal or epigastric pain, nausea, or vomiting with fever and leukocytosis. In the critically ill patient, the disease may present in an insidious fashion. Nonsurgical sources of referred abdominal pain may complicate the diagnostic process (Table 2). An unexplained fever, leukocytosis, intolerance to an enteral diet, or the development of an unexpected ileus should raise the suspicion of this process and may be the only clues to the underlying problem. Serum chemistries are often misleading. In calculous cholecystitis with obstruction of the common bile duct, a rise in the total bilirubin and alkaline phosphatase characterizes the disease process. Secondary elevation of the transaminases may be seen if the obstruction remains for a longer period of time. In acalculous cholecystitis, no elevation of these enzymes tends to be the rule rather than the exception.

Imaging studies include ultrasonography (US), which is noninvasive and portable, and the CT scan. Both can usually visualize the gallbladder and hepatobiliary tree; however, resolution for biliary stones is greater with the ultrasound. Important findings include a gallbladder wall thickness of more than 3.5 mm, gallbladder distension (more than 5 cm), pericholecystic fluid accumulation, gallbladder sludge or gas within the gallbladder and, of course, biliary stones. Nuclear scans such as the HIDA are not usually helpful. Frequent false-positive scan results may be seen in patients who are fasting or on TPN. Likewise, false-negative results may be seen in the presence of focal gallbladder wall

TABLE 2. NONSURGICAL ETIOLOGIES OF ABDOMINAL PAIN

Cardiac	Pulmonary	Gastrointestinal
Myocardial ischemia	Lower lobe pneumonia	Hepatitis
Myocardial infarction	Pulmonary emboli	Gastroenteritis
Pericarditis	Pulmonary infarction	Limited and nonperforated peptic ulcer disease
Aortic dissection	Pleuritis	Hepatosplenomegaly
		Spontaneous bacterial peritonitis
		Pancreatitis
		Esophageal spasm
Genitourinary	**Gynecologic**	**Metabolic**
Pyelonephritis	Ectopic pregnancy	Acute porphyria
Renal calculi	Ovarian torsion	Sickle cell crisis
Renal infarction	Ovarian cysts	Acute adrenal insufficiency
Hydronephrosis	Pelvic inflammatory disease	Diabetic ketoacidosis
		Familial Mediterranean fever

involvement or may be seen if the gallbladder wall is completely necrotic but the cystic duct is patent.

The preferred treatment of both calculus and acalculous cholecystitis is laparoscopic or open cholecystectomy. If the patient is too ill to undergo surgery, temporizing measures such as a percutaneous cholecystostomy may be undertaken. Aspiration of a suspected acalculous cholecystitis gallbladder will yield positive cultures in only 50% of specimens. Thus, no growth of bile aspirate does not exclude the diagnosis of acalculous cholecystitis. Fifty percent of the patients with acalculous cholecystitis develop gangrene while 10% to 20% progress to perforation. There is a 33% mortality rate (20).

Complicated hepatobiliary stone disease with distal common bile duct stone results in a gallstone pancreatitis. Conservative therapy consisting of fluid replacement and antibiotics while waiting for a rapid decrease in total bilirubin, transaminases, and amylase is prudent. If within 24 to 48 hours there is no biochemical evidence of a rapid decrease in the aforementioned enzymes, endoscopic retrograde cholangiopancreatography (ERCP) is indicated (21). The endoscopist may be able to retrieve the impacted stone as well as perform a sphincterotomy, if indicated. An elective cholecystectomy may be performed when the patient's enzymes normalize.

Pancreatitis

Acute severe pancreatitis may be the primary reason for the ICU admission or the patient may develop pancreatitis as a complication of another disease, surgical procedure, or trauma. In the former case, the patient may be able to give an accurate history consisting of epigastric pain with radiation into the back, fever, nausea, and vomiting. On the other hand, a postoperative patient who suddenly develops increasing fluid requirements, becomes intolerant to tube feedings, and develops an ileus should have pancreatitis considered in the differential diagnosis. While severe pancreatitis accounts for only 10% of all patient episodes of pancreatitis, it carries a mortality rate of 30% (22). Those patients who die from severe pancreatitis do so as a result of infection (80%), pulmonary complications such as acute respiratory distress syndrome (ARDS), or hemodynamic collapse.

Common etiologies of pancreatitis include calculous hepatobiliary disease, alcohol, trauma, drugs, and ischemia to the pancreas such as that seen in cardiopulmonary bypass (20,22–25). Elevations of the serum lipase and amylase coupled with dynamic abdominal CT scanning are the mainstays of establishing the diagnosis. The CT scan may demonstrate pancreatic enlargement, edema, or necrosis. It may also demonstrate a peripancreatic fluid collection, retroperitoneal edema or hemorrhage, mesenteric stranding and edema, transverse colonic bowel wall thickening, or potential infarction. A CT grading system has been developed to attempt to stratify the radiographic findings based upon the severity of pancreatic injury (26). Other grading systems such as the Ranson criteria for stone and nonstone disease as well as the Acute Physiologic and Chronic Health Evaluation (APACHE) II and III scores have been used to stratify and prognosticate patients with pancreatitis with varying results (21,27). If biliary stone disease is suspected as the etiology, US is a good test to establish the diagnosis. Ultrasound is not as accurate in pancreatic imaging due to the problem of overlying gas filled loops of bowel that obscure the visualization of the pancreas.

Therapy is initially directed at fluid resuscitation as these patients demonstrate large fluid losses due to vomiting, third space edema, or fluid sequestration within the bowel lumen. Aggressive and continued fluid administration is necessary to prevent secondary organ dysfunction such as acute tubular necrosis (ATN) or gut hypoperfusion. NG suction and Foley catheterization are necessary. Early intubation and respiratory support may be necessary. Meticulous critical care is the mainstay of treatment. Determination of potentially reversible causes of pancreatitis should be sought. These include obstructive common bile duct or pancreatic ductal pathologies or medications. Traumatic injuries of the pancreas may require conservative care, drainage, or pancreatic resection. These injuries are often initially missed in the early phase of the trauma workup. Early ERCP should be used only when a biliary or pancreatic tract obstruction is suspected. In nonobstructive pancreatitis, early ERCP has been associated with increased mortality. If the CT scan demonstrates evidence of peripancreatic fluid collections, the vexing question of a sterile versus infected fluid collection must be answered. In the presence of a stable afebrile patient, observation, serial leukocyte counts, and amylase levels may be sufficient, as these may represent early sterile pancreatic pseudocysts. In an unstable patient with an unexplained fever and leukocytosis, diagnostic fluid aspiration may be needed to determine the presence of a pancreatic abscess (27). Likewise, the spectrum of pancreatic ischemia and necrosis presents an interesting challenge to the surgeon. The difficult questions as to when and how much pancreatic tissue to debride remain unresolved. Fine-needle aspiration may be needed to sample pancreatic tissue of questionable viability to determine the presence of infection (28). There is an inherent sampling error that might yield a normal, uninfected pancreatic sample when an infected pancreatic area is not sampled. An erroneous conclusion of no pancreatic infection may be made. Gas within the pancreas or retroperitoneum is a clear sign of infection, which will need surgical debridement. The timing of these surgical procedures is unclear. Infected pancreatic tissue, abscess, or large areas of necrosis should be considered for early debridement. In general, the literature supports a more conservative approach to pancreatic debridement in the absence of infection (29). Necrosectomy is reserved for patients not improving with conservative measures or who have complicating intraabdominal problems such as transverse colonic infarction or hemorrhage due to erosion into the splenic or splanchnic arteries or veins. Interventional radiology may be of assistance with delineation or embolization of the bleeding vessel.

Infectious complications of pancreatitis account for 80% of all deaths, yet the use of empiric antibiotics remains controversial (30–32). Imipenem and fluoroquinolones both have good penetration into pancreatic tissue. A comprehensive analysis concerning the role of antibiotics in acute pancreatitis may be found in a review by Banks (27).

Nutritional support is paramount and the decision about TPN versus enteral feedings must be made. Patients with an ileus secondary to the pancreatitis or abdominal complication, which prohibits enteral feeding, require TPN. For those with GI motility and no contraindications, enteral feeding distal to the ampulla of Vater is well tolerated, does not worsen the underlying pancreatitis, and may inhibit bacterial translocation.

Mesenteric Ischemia

Mesenteric ischemia is a difficult problem to diagnose because the symptoms are often protean. Pathophysiologic events leading to bowel ischemia include low cardiac output, focal or diffuse arteriosclerosis, emboli, thrombosis, venous insufficiency, or trauma. Sudden intolerance to enteral feedings should raise the question of intestinal ischemia. There are numerous case reports of patients developing ischemic bowel when fed enterally in the presence of hypotension, vasopressor therapy, or severe burns (33).

Signs and symptoms of mesenteric ischemia include mild diffuse abdominal pain and tenderness. Typically, the pain appears out of proportion to the physical examination. There may be an elevated temperature to 101° to 102°F, a leukocytosis and, in the later stages of bowel ischemia, a rising lactate level and worsening base deficit. Abdominal radiographs may demonstrate an edematous and thickened bowel wall, distension, pneumatosis, and an abrupt cut-off sign. Findings on abdominal CT with bolus contrast include bowel wall thickening, mesentery thickening or streaking, pneumatosis, or free fluid. A late finding is air in the hepatobiliary tree or in the portal vein. Abnormalities in CT contrast enhancement may be limited in the affected segments or reflect regional or global splanchnic hypoperfusion. In cases of venous thrombosis, CT may be 70% to 90% accurate with the actual occlusive segment delineated and associated with mesenteric engorgement (34). An arteriogram may be diagnostic in acute arterial insufficiency or demonstrate a prolonged arterial phase with venous occlusive disease problem. It may outline the site of arterial obstruction and extent of disease, and help define the collateral circulation. Arteriography can distinguish between arterial embolus, arterial thrombus, venous thrombosis, and nonocclusive ischemia. Endoscopy may visualize areas of ischemic changes in the bowel wall. Although not precise, the color changes and extent of edema visualized with colonoscopy may be used to estimate the depth of bowel wall involvement.

The spectrum of findings range from mucosal hyperemia to purpuric deeper involvement to the white ischemic appearance of full thickness ischemia.

Therapy is directed at the precipitating event. Improving perfusion in a low flow state with volume loading or vasopressor or inotropic agents may be necessary. Embolectomy or thrombectomy are indicated in appropriate candidates. Arterial insufficiency is primarily managed surgically with bypass. There is a limited role for angioplasty of proximal stenotic lesions. Anticoagulation in the face of limited venous occlusion may be instituted in the absence of infarcted bowel.

The determination of ischemic versus infarcted bowel has always been a dilemma. Only abdominal exploration will yield the answer in some cases and early operation is the key to patient survivability in this disease process. In some cases, the time to obtain diagnostic studies closes the envelope to perform revascularization. Intraoperative decisions as to the viability of bowel segments can also be challenging. Use of the Doppler or examination under ultraviolet light after injection with fluorescein may aid in the determination of viability.

Acute Abdominal Compartment Syndrome

This is a syndrome that is characterized by an acute rise in intraabdominal pressure that results in impaired intraabdominal organ perfusion (35). Although primarily seen in acute traumatic injury to the abdomen, it may be seen in postoperative abdominal surgical patients, burn patients, or patients receiving massive fluid resuscitation (36). The common pathophysiologic pathway is an acute rise in the pressure within the abdominal cavity. This results in impairment of the perfusion of intraabdominal and extraabdominal organs and may lead to multiple organ dysfunction (37).

Normal intraabdominal pressure is less than 10 mm Hg. Increases in this pressure due to intraabdominal hemorrhage, surgical packing, or third-space fluids may cause a rise in the intraabdominal pressure (38). In many of these patients, the bowel mesentery and the bowel walls are very thickened and edematous. The increase in pressure within the abdomen has both direct and indirect effect on organ perfusion (18,39). For example, in the kidney there may be direct compression of the renal artery or vein resulting in impaired perfusion. Additional organ hypoperfusion is due to the increased intraabdominal pressure that impairs venous return to the heart and results in decreased cardiac output. Splanchnic perfusion is diminished, which may result in mesenteric ischemia. Additional increases in the intraabdominal pressure result in an upward movement of the diaphragm, impairing pulmonary mechanics and causing reduction in the functional residual capacity and vital capacity. The peak and mean airway pressures rise, contributing to difficulty in ventilation. Intracranial pressure elevations are also described, resulting in decreased cerebral perfusion (37,40).

A simple method to measure the intraabdominal compartment pressure is via measurement of the bladder pressure. To perform this test, simply instill 100 cc of sterile water into the bladder via the Foley catheter. Then, clamp the Foley catheter just distal to the rubber aspiration port. A central venous monitoring line attached to a 16-gauge needle is then inserted into the Foley aspiration port. After zeroing the central line to the level of the symphysis pubis, the bladder pressure can be interpreted. Other

TABLE 3. ACUTE ABDOMINAL COMPARTMENT SYNDROME—PHYSIOLOGIC CONSEQUENCES AND TREATMENT

	Grade 1	Grade 2	Grade 3	Grade 4
	0–15 mm Hg	16–25 mm Hg	26–35 mm Hg	>36 mm Hg
Cardiovascular	Stable	Mild instability, ↓ preload, ↑ SVR	Unstable, tachycardia, ↓ preload, ↓ cardiac output	Circulatory collapse, ↓ contractility Cardiac output marginal
Pulmonary	Stable	↓ Tidal volumes ↑ Pulmonary vascular resistance	↑ Peak and mean ↑ Airway pressure, pleural pressures	Inability to ventilate Hypercarbia and hypoxemia
Splanchnic	Normal splanchnic blood flow	Mild ↓ in blood flow	Severe ↓ in blood flow and ischemia	Marked perfusion abnormalities
Renal	Normal urine output	↓ Urine output ↓ Renal blood flow ↓ Glomerular filtration rate	Oliguria	Anuria
Therapy	Maintain adequate intravascular volume	Intravascular volume expansion	Volume expansion and decompression	Volume expansion, decompression and reexploration

SVR, systemic vascular resistance.
Adapted from Saggi BH, Sugerman HJ, Ivatury RR, et al. Acute abdominal compartment syndrome in the critically ill. *J Intensive Care Med* 1999;207–219; and Meldrum DR, Moore FA, Moore EE, et al. Prospective characterization and selective management of the abdominal compartment syndrome. *Am J Surg* 1997;174;667–973, with permission.

forms of intraabdominal pressure monitoring are available, but are more difficult to use.

A grading system has been proposed that attempts to quantify the physiologic responses to increasing pressure (Table 3). Intraabdominal pressures of 10 to 15 mm Hg are only modest increases and the resultant minor physiologic deficits are easily corrected by volume loading with crystalloids. Increases in the pressure to 16 to 25 mm Hg primarily result in mild instability of the patient and manifest as decreases in urinary output, mild hypotension, and elevations in peak airway pressures. Hypovolemic resuscitation is indicated. At pressures of 26 to 35 mm Hg, severe intraabdominal and extraabdominal organ dysfunction is present. The treatment is surgical decompression. Pressures of greater than 35 mm Hg are treated with reexploration and decompression. The degree of mesenteric and bowel edema is often profound and prohibits the closure of the abdominal wall. Temporary closures with a sterile 2 liter i.v. bag (Bogota bag) or a vacuum packing technique are methods to address this problem. Formal abdominal wound closure can be facilitated at a later time when the edema has resolved. In summary, correction of the underlying abdominal pathology along with temporary abdominal closure techniques is the mainstay of treatment. Prompt recognition of the abdominal compartment syndrome and appropriate management of these patients are the only methods to combat the insidious progression of this disease entity. Appropriate therapy including fluids, reoperation, and decompression, when indicated, is the mainstay of treatment.

The Abdomen as an Occult Source of Infection

There are many disease processes by which the abdomen may become a source of occult infection or sepsis (41). While sepsis remains one of the leading causes of death in the ICU, the determination of an intraabdominal infectious source may be difficult (42). Unlike other parts of the body that lend themselves to easier examination and imaging, the abdomen may harbor pathology with little or no clinical signs or symptoms. Therefore, our ability to diagnose or exclude an intraabdominal process is often challenging (7).

An appreciation of the pathophysiologic processes and presentation of abdominal infection aids in directing the physician in the workup of a decompensated ICU patient. On the most basic level, an intraabdominal infection may be from a primary abdominal process. Likewise, it may be due to spread from a secondary source. The spread may be hematogenous, such as septic emboli lodging in the spleen or liver. It may be contiguous, such as a pleuroperitoneal fistula due to a subpulmonic empyema. The infection may be due to a foreign body such as a peritoneal dialysis catheter or one introduced by a break in sterile technique in using the dialysis catheter. The abdomen may also be a site for a tertiary or disseminated nosocomial infectious process. The primary sources of infection are restated for emphasis in this section.

A hollow viscus may perforate, as in the case of a gastric or duodenal ulcer. Diverticula of the colon or an acute appendicitis may perforate. A segment of bowel may become ischemic, necrotic, and then perforate. A traumatic injury may perforate at the time of injury or become necrotic in a delayed fashion. An example of this would be a degloving injury to bowel or a mesenteric hematoma or compromise that would leave a segment of bowel ischemic (43). With time, this segment may become necrotic and in 2 to 4 days the bowel may perforate (44). Iatrogenic injuries from a flexible sigmoidoscopy, colonoscopy, or percutaneous aspiration or biopsy may lead to perforation.

A hollow viscus may also leak. A recent bowel anastomosis is most likely to breakdown and leak 5 to 7 days' postoperatively. A partially torn segment of bowel wall from a traumatic injury might be seen with a large tear of the serosa, a transmural hematoma of the bowel wall, or a missed penetrating injury to the abdomen (44). Inflammatory or infectious conditions of the bowel may cause direct abdominal infection, as develops with complicated appendicitis or diverticulitis. Inflammation or infection may lead to systemic toxicity as in infectious colitis. A segment of inflammatory bowel may perforate or fistulize, resulting in a local, regional, or systemic infectious process. Toxic megacolon may develop into a systemic inflammatory response without an actual infectious process. An ischemic process will likely have an adverse systemic metabolic consequence as well as result in local bowel wall ischemia, necrosis, or perforation. The solid organs of the abdomen may become a nidus of infection. Examples include a splenic or liver abscess, pyelonephritis, or a tuboovarian abscess. Advanced pelvic inflammatory disease may result in occult abdominal infection.

Any of these "perforating or leaking" processes may develop into an abscess or diffuse peritonitis. The peritoneum itself may develop a primary bacterial peritonitis in individuals with ascites (45). Likewise, a secondary peritonitis may present due to intraabdominal pathology. A tertiary peritonitis, usually due to hematogenous spread of nosocomial, less virulent organisms, may develop (41). Vascular grafts and anastomosis may harbor infection, causing a latent presentation. Primary graft infection may result in graft loss, localized graft infection, mycotic aneurysm, or disruption of the anastomosis. The latter will present with a loss of vascular continuity and brisk hemorrhage. Localized infection can be a source of fever of unknown origin.

Identification of the etiology of fever, sepsis, or the systemic inflammatory response in ICU patients can be very difficult. Multiple disease entities such as ventilator-assisted pneumonia, sinusitis, catheter infection, and urinary tract infections are common to ICU patients (6,46). All may lead to adverse systemic physiologic response. If the diagnosis remains elusive, the clinician must consider the presence of an intraabdominal disease process. The key question becomes, "What is the likelihood of an intraabdominal process causing the patient's demise?" (47). The second question centers around how best to achieve "source control of the infection."

The approach to this question has changed over the last 25 years. With the advent of ICU care in the 1970s, many patients appeared to be septic or developed multisystem organ failure without an obvious etiology. In an effort to exclude the abdomen as a potential source, exploratory abdominal surgery was performed (43). Results were mixed with some authors reporting up to a 50% discovery of an intraabdominal source of infection. Others were less impressed by this approach. Sutherland and colleagues attempted to stratify those factors that preoperatively would predict a high likelihood of finding intraabdominal pathology (48). The morbidity of a negative laparotomy in an ICU patient is not insignificant and needed to be weighed against routine exploratory laparotomies. Norwood and Civetta (49) examined the use of CT scanning to detect occult abdominal infection. Two of their conclusions are important to consider. First, CT scans provided little useful information if performed before the eighth postoperative day. Second, CT scans should be used to search for a septic abdominal focus only if the information will help direct patient care. In the setting of recent abdominal surgery, Bunt (50) examined the use of abdominal reoperation to look for a source of sepsis. He reported that "nondirected" laparotomies yielded only a 13% positive rate and that a negative laparotomy was associated with a 93% mortality rate. This led him to develop a management protocol for the use of abdominal reexploration. Indications for reexploration included: (a) patients with signs and symptoms referable to abdominal pathology; (b) young patients (less than 50 years of age) with worsening signs of multisystem

organ failure; and (c) older patients with an unreliable abdominal examination due to a neurologic deficit or steroid-induced changes in presentation.

If an intraabdominal source of infection is identified, control of the infectious process is mandated (51). Antibiotics alone will not treat most infections if there is an undrained infectious focus. Control of further bowel spillage or control of a fistula may be accomplished by proximal diversion. Percutaneous drainage may temporize the situation and facilitate the effectiveness of antibiotics. This may permit a delayed one-step surgical procedure instead of a multistaged procedure (6).

The newer, fourth-generation CT scanners with dynamic contrast injection have greatly enhanced the ability to image the abdomen. Conventional and duplex US also greatly assist in the imaging of the hepatobiliary system. Both CT and US can be used to percutaneously drain intraabdominal fluid collections. White blood cell-tagged nuclear scans have a limited efficacy in the ICU (52). In selected patients, laparoscopy is an effective modality to examine the abdomen without the attendant morbidity of a formal laparotomy. Laparoscopic inspection of the abdomen may not be as complete as a laparotomy; however, major pathology is usually excluded (53). Contraindications to laparoscopy include massive bowel distension, inability of the patient to tolerate abdominal pressure increases to 15 mm Hg, or the inability of the patient to tolerate general anesthesia. Newer gasless laparoscopic techniques are being developed and bedside laparoscopy is being studied.

In the end, it is an increased index of suspicion of an intraabdominal disease process that directs the patient's evaluation and management. A pragmatic approach to the identification of occult intraabdominal infection combines the patient's presentation, laboratory data, and diagnostic studies. A thorough understanding of the potential complications of an operative procedure as well as the expected timing of these complications aids in management. A directed or guided approach to the abdomen as an occult source of infection, sepsis, or multisystem organ failure appears to be the most prudent approach (54).

SUMMARY

There are multiple complications that might affect the postoperative patient. Familiarity with the type of operative procedures and associated complications aid in the management of these patients. Anticipation of perioperative complications not only facilitates prevention, but assists in establishing the diagnosis. In this manner, the treating physician anticipates the potential complications against a postoperative "time line." Thus, at certain postoperative days the clinician looks for specific complications to arise. Certain disease processes are common to ICU patients. Evaluation of these patients should be a directed or guided approach. Likewise, surgical reoperation is a guided procedure. An exploratory reoperative surgery is better termed "a guided second look surgery." If the patient is too ill intraoperatively, it is prudent to perform only those measures necessary to save the patient's life. Attempts to stop major bleeding and control further bowel spillage, combined with packing and a temporary abdominal closure, assist in reducing cases of the abdominal compartment syndrome.

REFERENCES

1. Nance FC. Diseases of the peritoneum, mesentery and omentum. In: Bockus J, ed. *Gastroenterology*, 4th ed. Philadelphia: WB Saunders, 1985:vol 7;4177–4179.
2. Levison ME, Bush LM. Peritonitis and other intra-abdominal infection. In: Mandell GL, Bennet JE, Dolin R, eds. *Principles and practice of infectious disease*, 5th ed. New York: Churchill Livingston; 2000:821–848.
3. Rolandelli R, Roslyn JJ. Surgical management of gastrointestinal fistulas. *Surg Clin North Am* 1996;76(5):1111–1122.
4. Glasgow RE, Mulvihill SJ. Abdominal pain, including the acute abdomen In: Feldman M, Sleisenger MH, Scharschmidt BF, eds. *Gastrointestinal and liver disease*. Philadelphia: WB Saunders, 1998: 80–84.
5. Spirit MJ. *Acute care of the abdomen*. Baltimore: Williams & Wilkins, 1998:163–186.
6. Marik PE. Fever in the ICU. *Chest* 2000;117(3):627–639.
7. Diethelm AG, Stanley RJ, Robbin ML. Evaluating the acute abdomen. In: Civetta JM, Taylor RW, Kirby KK, eds. *Critical care*, 3rd ed. Philadelphia: Lippincott-Raven, 1997:1099–1108.
8. Lubin MF, Walker HK, Smith RB. *Medical management of the surgical patient*. Boston: Butterworth, 1988:489–789.
9. Resnik J, Greenwald DA, Brandt LJ. Delayed gastric emptying and post operative ileus after non-gastric abdominal surgery, part I. *Am J Gastroenterol* 1997;92(5):751–762.
10. Snape Jr. WJ. Pathogenesis, diagnosis, and treatment of acute colonic ileus. Gastroenterology, Oct. 12, 1999. Available at: http://www.medscape.com. Accessed October 25, 2001.
11. Vanek VW, Al-Salti M. Acute pseudo-obstruction of the colon (Ogilvie's syndrome)—an analysis of 400 cases. *Dis Colon Rectum* 1986;29(3):203–210.
12. Ponec RJ, Saunders MD, Kimmey MB. Neostigmine for the treatment of acute colonic pseudo-obstruction. *N Engl J Med* 1999;341(3):137–141.
13. Paran H, Silverberg D, Mayo A, et al. Treatment of acute colonic pseudo-obstruction with neostigmine. *J Am Coll Surg* 2000;190:315–318.
14. Trevisani GT, Hyman NH, Church JM. Neostigmine safe and effective treatment for acute colonic pseudo-obstruction. *Dis Colon Rectum* 2000;43:599–603.
15. Richards WO, Williams LF Jr. Obstruction of the small and large intestine. *Surg Clin North Am* 1988;68(2):355–376.
16. Lopez-Kostner F, Hool GR, Lavery IC. Management and causes of acute large-bowel obstruction. *Surg Clin North Am* 1997;77(6):1265–1290.
17. Bubrick MP. Volvulus of the colon. In: Gordon PH, Nivatvongs S, eds. *Principles and practice of surgery for the colon, rectum and anus*, 2nd ed. St. Louis: Quality Medical Publishing Inc, 1992:799–816.
18. Liolios A, Oropello JM, Benjamin E. Gastrointestinal complications in the intensive care unit. *Clin Chest Med* 1999;20(2):329–345.
19. Barie PS, Fischer E. Acute acalculous cholecystitis. *J Am Coll Surg* 1995;180(2):232–244.
20. Ratschko M, Fenner T, Lankisch PG. The role of antibiotic prophylaxis in the treatment of acute pancreatitis. *Gastroent Clin* 1999;28(3):641–659.
21. Tsiotos GG, Mullany CJ, Zietlow S, et al. Abdominal complications following cardiac surgery. *Am J Surg* 1994;167:553–557.
22. Baron TH, Morgan DE. Acute necrotizing pancreatitis. *N Engl J Med* 1999;340(18):1412–1417.
23. Ohri SK, Desai JB, Gaer JAR, et al. Intra-abdominal complications after cardiopulmonary bypass. *Ann Thorac Surg* 1991;52:826–831.
24. Mercado PD, Farid H, O'Connell TX, et al. Gastrointestinal complications associated with cardiopulmonary bypass procedures. *Am Surg* 1994;60:789–792.
25. Lubetkin EI, Lipson DA, Palevsky HI, et al. GI complications after orthotopic lung transplantation. *Am J Gastroent* 1996;91(11):2382–2390.
26. Baktgazar EJ. Imaging and intervention in acute pancreatitis. *Radiology* 1994;193(2):297–306.

27. Banks PA. Practice guidelines in acute pancreatitis. *Am J Gastroenterol* 1997;92(3):377–386.
28. Traverso WL, Kozarek RA. Interventional management of peripancreatic fluid collections. *Surg Clin North Am* 1999;79(4):745–757.
29. Beger H, Isenmann R. Surgical management of necrotizing pancreatitis. *Surg Clin North Am* 1999;79(4):783–800.
30. Runzi M, Layer P. Acute and chronic pancreatitis—nonsurgical management of acute pancreatitis. *Surg Clin North Am* 1999;79(4):759–765.
31. Reed RL II. Contemporary issues with bacterial infection in the intensive care unit. *Surg Clin North Am* 2000;80(3):895–910.
32. Runzi M, Layer P. Nonsurgical management of acute pancreatitis. Use of antibiotics. *Surg Clin North Am* 1999;79(4):759–765.
33. Schunn CDG, Daly JM. Small bowel necrosis associated with post operative jejunal feeding. *J Am Coll Surg* 1988;180:410–416.
34. Cappell MS. Gastrointestinal disorders and systemic disease, part II—intestinal (mesenteric) vasculopathy I. *Gastroenterol Clin* 1998;27(4):783–814.
35. Ertel W, Oberholzer A, Platz A, et al. Incidence and clinical pattern of the abdominal compartment syndrome after "damage-control" laparotomy in 311 patients with severe abdominal and/or pelvic trauma. *Crit Care Med* 2000;28(6):1747–1753.
36. Ivatury RR, Sugerman HJ. Abdominal compartment syndrome: a century later, isn't it time to pay attention? *Crit Care Med* 2000;28(6):2137–2138.
37. Saggi BH, Sugerman HJ, Ivatury RR, et al. Acute abdominal compartment syndrome in the critically ill. *J Intensive Care Med* 1999;14(5):207–219.
38. Burch JM, Moore EE, Moore FA, et al. The abdominal compartment syndrome. *Surg Clin North Am* 1996;76(4):833–842.
39. Ivatury RR, Deibel L, Porter JM, et al. Intra-abdominal hypertension and the abdominal compartment syndrome. *Surg Clin North Am* 1997;77(4):783–800.
40. Meldrum DR, Moore FA, Moore EE, et al. Prospective characterization and selective management of the abdominal compartment. *Am J Surg* 1997;174(6):667–672.
41. Sleeman D, Norwood SH. The complicated post operative abdomen. In: Civetta JM, Taylor RW, Kirby RR, eds. *Critical care*, 3rd ed. Philadelphia: Lippincott-Raven 1997;1109–1120.
42. Norwood SH, Civetta MD. Evaluation of sepsis in critically ill patients. *Chest* 1987;92(1):137–144.
43. Wilson RF, Walt AJ, Dulchavsky S. Injuries to the colon and rectum. In: Wilkson RF, Walt AJ eds. *Management of trauma—pitfalls and practice.* Baltimore: Williams & Wilkins 1996;534–553.
44. Espinoza R, Rodriguiez A. Traumatic and nontraumatic perforation of hollow viscera. *Surg Clin North Am* 1997;77(6):1291–1300.
45. Farber MS, Abrams JH: Abdominal emergencies: has anything changed? Antibiotics for the acute abdomen. *Surg Clin North Am* 1997;77(6):1396–1417.
46. Sosa JL, Reines HD. Evaluating the acute abdomen. In: Civetta JM, Taylor RW, Kirby RR, eds. *Critical care*, 3rd ed. Philadelphia: Lippincott-Raven, 1997;1099–1108.
47. Merrell RC. The abdomen as source of sepsis in critically ill patients. *Crit Care Clin* 1995;11(2):255–272.
48. Sutherland FR, Temple WJ, Snodgrass T, et al. Predicting the outcome of exploratory laparotomy in ICU patients with sepsis or organ failure. *J Trauma* 1989;29(2):152–157.
49. Norwood SH, Civetta JM. Abdominal CT scanning in critically ill surgical patients. *Am J Surg* 1985;202 (2) :166–175.
50. Bunt TJ. Non-directed re laparotomy for intra-abdominal sepsis—a futile procedure. *Am Surg* 1986;52(5):294–298.
51. Jimenez MF, Marshall JC. Source control in the management of sepsis. *Intensive Care Med* 2001:27:S49–S62.
52. Bearcroft PW. Leucocyte scintigraphy or computed tomography for the post-operative patient? *Eur J Radiol* 1996;23(2):126–129.
53. Martin RF, Flynn P. Abdominal emergencies: has anything changed? The acute abdomen in the critically ill patient. *Surg Clin North Am* 1997;77(6):1455–1462.
54. Deitch EA, Goodman ER. Trauma care in the new millennium—prevention of multiple organ failure. *Surg Clin North Am* 1999;79(6):1471–1485.
55. Anderson JD, Fearon KCH, Grant IS. Laparotomy for sepsis in the critically ill. *Br J Surg* 1996;85:525–539.

GASTROINTESTINAL HEMORRHAGE IN THE CRITICALLY ILL

DOUGLAS B. COURSIN
KENNETH E. WOOD

KEY WORDS

- Upper- and lower-gastrointestinal bleeding
- Peptic ulcer disease
- Portal hypertension
- Variceal bleeding
- Transjugular intrahepatic portosystemic shunt (TIPS)
- Stress-related erosive syndrome
- Gastrointestinal prophylaxis;

- H2-antagonists, proton-pump inhibitors, and sucralfate
- Mallory-Weiss tear
- Arteriovenous malformation
- Diverticular bleeding
- Ischemic colitis
- Mesenteric vasculopathy
- Protocol: Gastrointestinal bleed

INTRODUCTION

Gastrointestinal hemorrhage (GIH) remains a common reason for intensive care unit (ICU) admission and a major cause of morbidity and mortality in critically ill patients (1–3). Patients with GIH are increasingly older and more commonly have significant comorbid pathology. GIH is empirically divided into upper-GI and lower-GI pathologies. Emergent therapy of life-threatening hemorrhage requires rapid identification of the bleeding site, adequate resuscitation with fluids and packed red cells, correction of concurrent coagulopathy, and definitive intervention whenever possible. GIH can be characterized as primary or secondary. The former defines the bleeding event as the reason for ICU admission while the latter refers to bleeding that develops consequent to the admission for another critical illness. Various groups have identified markers such as host factors, patient course, and endoscopic findings that aid in risk stratification of patients presenting with primary upper-GI bleeding (4). Risk stratification is useful in admission triage decisions, allocation of critical resources such as intensive care, and facilitation of preemptive recognition of patients who are at increased risk for significant morbidity and mortality and may need re-endoscopy, interventional x-ray procedures, or surgery. Risk stratification also provides definitions of parameters, which enhance clinical research in patients with GIH.

Stress-related erosive syndrome (SRES) (also known as stress ulceration) has been identified as a major cause of secondary GIH in critically ill patients (5). The proper identification of patients at risk for SRES, the optimal means of prophylaxis and management, and risk of side-effects from prophylaxis, such as the incidence of nosocomial pneumonia, are ongoing areas of investigation. Recent metaanalyses and data from prospective trials provide guidance in identifying those patients at risk for SRES, those patients who appear to benefit from prophylaxis, and the optimal means of limiting and treating this potentially lethal complication of critical illness (5,6). The course in patients who develop SRES is reflective of the severity of illness and underlying comorbidities. It is often associated with multiple-organ dysfunction syndrome (MODS), which explains the much greater mortality (upward of 30%) reported in secondary GIH compared to primary.

UPPER GASTROINTESTINAL BLEEDING

Upper gastrointestinal (UGI) bleeding is a significant cause of morbidity and mortality (7% to 10%) and results in more than 300,000 hospitalizations at a cost in excess of $2.5 billion per year in the United States (2). It is defined as bleeding proximal to the ligament of Treitz. This common medical problem may be the result of a variety of pathologic processes (Table 1).

Initial Triage of Patients with Acute Upper Gastrointestinal Bleeding

With increasing economic pressures to limit ICU resource allocation, effective use of these diminishing resources requires scrutiny of common ICU admission diagnoses for appropriateness. Recent data estimate that 25% of ICU upper gastrointestinal bleeding (UGIB) admissions are low risk and could be triaged to non-ICU locales (7). Clinical characteristics of UGIB patients with a poor outcome are well recognized. Early incorporation of GI endoscopy in the evaluation of patients with known or suspected UGIB has evolved to play a pivotal role in the approach to these patients. The integration of endoscopic findings and patient clinical characteristics allows for risk stratification and evidence-based

TABLE 1. CAUSES OF UPPER GASTROINTESTINAL BLEEDING

Peptic ulceration
Portal hypertension
   Varices
   Congestive or portal gastropathy
Stress-related erosive syndrome (stress ulceration)
Mallory-Weiss syndrome
Mucosal erosive diseases
Vascular enteric fistulas
Vascular anomalies
   Vascular ectasias
   Arteriovenous malformation
Dieulafoy lesion
Tumors
   Leiomyoma
   Leiomyosarcoma
   Adenocarcinoma
   Lymphoma
Miscellaneous
   Hemobilia
   Whipple disease
   Vasculitis

outcome prediction that provides a paradigm for UGIB triage (8) (Fig. 1 and Table 2).

High- and low-risk patients can be differentiated based upon known clinical characteristics associated with poor outcomes (4,9). High risk includes age above 60, significant comorbid disease, coagulopathy, hemodynamic instability, evidence of ongoing bleeding, and secondary bleeding associated with another primary diagnosis. These patients should be considered for ICU admission and emergent diagnostic/therapeutic endoscopy. Surgical services and interventional radiology should be alerted for possible evaluation.

Low-risk patients can be triaged to a non-ICU setting for urgent endoscopy. Rockall combined clinical factors with endoscopic findings to generate a score for risk stratification and outcome prediction that has been prospectively validated (8) (Table 2). Scores equal to 2 are associated with a 5.3% risk of rebleed and a 0.2% mortality. These patients can be considered for a short period of observation and/or early discharge. Prospectively validated models have defined criteria for outpatient treatment and early hospital discharge (10,11). Patients with Rockall scores equal to 3 are at greater risk for poor outcome and require an assessment for the likelihood of rebleeding. Predicting the risk of rebleeding is crucial because it allows the endoscopist to define candidates for endoscopic therapeutic intervention and populations that warrant continued ICU observation. Stigmata of recent hemorrhage such as active bleeding, a visible vessel, or adherent clot are established predictors of rebleeding and associated with a 50% probability of continued bleeding or rebleeding if therapeutic endoscopy is not undertaken. Ulcers on the proximal lesser curvature of the stomach and the posterior surface of the duodenum have a greater propensity to rebleed as a consequence of arterial proximity (4).

Similar to the Rockall Score, the Baylor Bleeding Score is a prospectively validated predictor that is based upon clinical variables (age, number, and severity of comorbid illnesses) and endoscopic findings and can be applied to predict rebleeding after

initial endoscopy. Stratification of patients into high-risk (score greater than 10) and low-risk (score equal to 5 or less) categories was associated with rebleeding rates of 31% and 0%, respectively (12). Failure of endoscopy to control bleeding is also associated with shock and ulcers equal to or more than 2 cm in diameter (13). In patients with failed therapeutic endoscopy, it is important that surgery or interventional radiology procedures are urgently considered. Patients with cessation of bleeding and a low risk of rebleeding can be considered for transfer out of the ICU, whereas those with a high risk of rebleeding should be observed in the ICU.

Peptic Ulcer Disease

Peptic ulcer disease accounts for approximately 50% of UGI bleeding (1). Approximately 20% of patients diagnosed with bleeding ulcers present with melena, 30% with hematemesis, and 50% with both. As many as 5% of patients will present with hematochezia. Melena may result from the presence of as little as 50 to 100 mL of blood in the UGI tract. More than 1,000 mL of blood in the UGI tract is almost always associated with hematochezia. Bleeding from peptic ulcer disease ceases spontaneously in 75% to 80% of cases, and most patients have an uneventful recovery without specific intervention (1,2).

Pathogenesis

Although the exact cause of peptic ulcer disease is not known, the imbalance between provocative factors (namely acid and pepsin) and defensive mechanisms (including mucosal blood flow, mucosal secretion of bicarbonate and mucus, integrity of the cell membrane, production of prostaglandins, and cellular regeneration) appears to play a key role. The use of nonsteroidal antiinflammatory drugs (NSAIDs) and infection with *Helicobacter pylori* are important risk factors for bleeding ulcers. NSAIDs may cause both gastric and duodenal ulcers (14).

Diagnosis

Patients with acute UGI bleeding should undergo early endoscopic examination. The initial studies that assessed the outcome effect of diagnostic endoscopy failed to demonstrate improvement. However, the introduction of therapeutic endoscopy using laser, electric cautery, heat probe, or injection techniques that facilitate control of hemorrhage, has clearly been shown to decrease rebleeding, limit the need for surgical intervention, and improve outcome in patients with active bleeding or visible vessels (12,15,16). Therefore, early endoscopy allows for risk stratification and treatment in triaging patients and obtaining biopsy material (1,2,15,16).

Treatment

The initial management of the patient with UGI bleeding involves hemodynamic assessment (blood pressure, pulse, and postural changes), and institution of appropriate resuscitative measures (Table 3). A nasogastric (NG) tube is often placed to aid in the assessment of the site, volume, and severity of UGI bleeding. Unless the patient has massive bleeding or severe nausea and

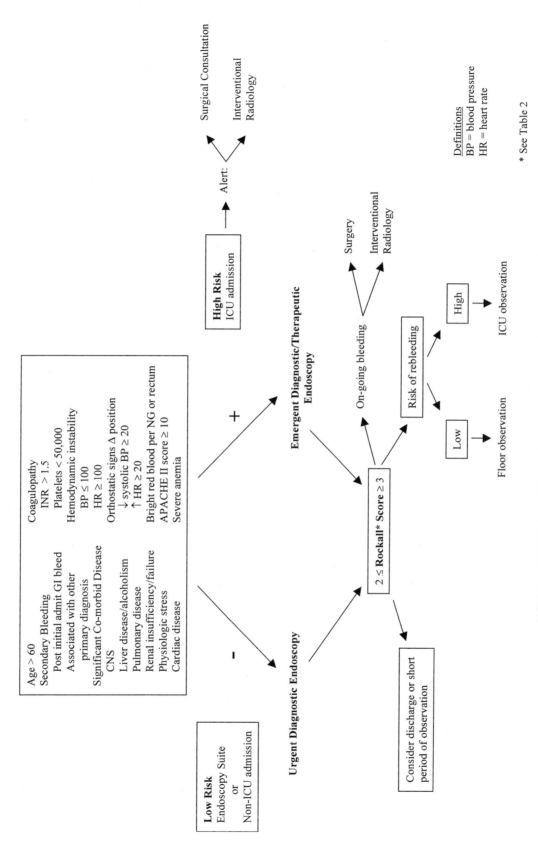

FIGURE 1. Intensive care unit triage for presumed upper gastrointestinal bleeding.

Age > 60
Secondary Bleeding
Post initial admit GI bleed
Associated with other
  primary diagnosis
Significant Co-morbid Disease
  CNS
  Liver disease/alcoholism
  Pulmonary disease
  Renal insufficiency/failure
  Physiologic stress
  Cardiac disease

Coagulopathy
  INR > 1.5
  Platelets < 50,000
Hemodynamic instability
  BP ≤ 100
  HR ≥ 100
Orthostatic signs Δ position
  ↓ systolic BP ≥ 20
  ↑ HR ≥ 20
Bright red blood per NG or rectum
APACHE II score ≥ 10
Severe anemia

Low Risk
Endoscopy Suite
  or
Non-ICU admission

High Risk
ICU admission

Alert:

Surgical Consultation

Interventional
Radiology

Urgent Diagnostic Endoscopy

**Emergent Diagnostic/Therapeutic
Endoscopy**

2 ≤ **Rockall* Score** ≥ 3

Consider discharge or short
period of observation

On-going bleeding

Surgery

Interventional
Radiology

Risk of rebleeding

High

Low

ICU observation

Floor observation

Definitions
BP = blood pressure
HR = heart rate

* See Table 2

TABLE 2. ROCKALL SEVERITY SCORE[a]

	Points			
Variable	0	1	2	3
Age	<60 yr	60–79 yr	>80 yr	
Shock	No shock			
	Systolic BP >100	Systolic BP ≥100	Systolic BP ≤100	
	HR ≤100	HR ≥100		
Comorbidity	No major comorbidity		Cardiac failure	Renal failure
			Ischemic heart disease	Liver failure
			Any major comorbidity	Disseminated malignancy
			Malignancy in upper GI tract	
Diagnosis	Mallory-Weiss tear	All other diagnoses		
	No lesion identified and no signs of recent hemorrhage			
Major signs of recent hemorrhage	None or dark spot only		Blood in upper GI tract, adherent clot, visible or "spurting" vessel	

BP, blood pressure; HR, heart rate; GI, gastrointestinal.
[a]Rockall Severity Score equals the summation of points from individual variables. The scoring range is 0–10 points.

vomiting, the NG tube is removed to limit catheter-induced mucosal injury or perforation. Acute loss of up to 10% of blood volume is rarely associated with systemic signs. Orthostatic changes in blood pressure (greater than 20 torr decrease in systolic or 10 torr in diastolic with standing) and pulse (greater than 20 beat increase with standing) indicate an acute loss of at least 20% of the intravascular blood volume, while hypovolemic shock indicates an acute blood loss of 40% or more of blood volume. The development of orthostasis or significant changes in vital signs may be affected by age (greater in older adults), medication (use of beta- or calcium channel blockers, vasodilators), and comorbidity (diabetic-induced autonomic neuropathy). In the setting of rapid hemorrhage, the magnitude of blood loss may be underestimated by the initial preresuscitation hematocrit since equilibrium with extravascular fluid compartment requires several hours.

There is no evidence to support the belief that lavage with cold fluid or vasoconstrictors is beneficial. Ice lavage may dele-

TABLE 3. RESUSCITATION PROTOCOL FOR UPPER GASTROINTESTINAL BLEEDING

Obtain adequate intravenous access
    Two large-bore intravenous cannulas
    Central venous access when necessary
    Consider pulmonary artery catheter if significant myocardial ischemia or infarction
Insert urinary bladder catheter
Replace intravascular volume
Serially monitor:
    Blood pressure and orthostatic changes (consider invasive blood pressure monitoring)
    Heart rate
    Hematocrit
    Urinary output
    Central venous pressure/cardiac output, when available
Transfuse blood products as necessary
Obtain gastroenterologic consultation
Consider surgical consultation
Consider interventional radiologic procedure or consultation as needed

teriously lower body temperature, induce shivering, and compromise platelet function and coagulation (2). Since most UGI bleeding lesions are amenable to therapy with acid suppression, empiric therapy is initiated with intravenous H2-receptor antagonists, often by continuous infusion. Many advocate the routine administration of a proton-pump inhibitor (PPI) instead of an H2-receptor antagonist. Pantoprazole is now available as the first injectable PPI in the United States (17–19).

Endoscopic hemostasis is the most effective nonsurgical modality in the treatment of bleeding ulcers. Prospective, randomized trials have shown that both bipolar electrocoagulation and heater probes are highly effective in reducing blood transfusion, rebleeding, hospital stay, and the need for urgent surgery (1,2,20). An even less costly modality than thermal contact is injection therapy. Epinephrine, polidocanol, absolute alcohol, and hypertonic saline have been documented to provide effective hemostasis (21).

Alternatively, interventional angiography allows for specific localization of the bleeding site and opportunity to perform embolization during the same session. This approach is particularly applicable if surgery poses an extremely high risk and endoscopic therapy has been unsuccessful or is unavailable (22). Intraarterial infusion of vasopressin may stop bleeding in 50% of cases, but this is not appreciably better than systemic vasopressin or octreotide (2). Success rates of up to 80% with arterial embolization with absorbable gelatin sponge, autologous clot, tissue adhesives, or mechanical occlusive devices have been reported (1,23).

Endoscopic findings associated with an increased need for surgery include a flat pigmented spot, an adherent clot, a visible vessel, or active bleeding (1). Although there has been a striking reduction in the frequency of ulcer surgery over the past 30 years, surgery continues to remain the most appropriate and effective treatment for approximately 10% of patients (24). Surgery is currently reserved for patients who do not respond to endoscopic therapy or when such therapy is not available. Endoscopic and radiographic techniques to identify the source and initiate therapy often facilitate optimal surgical care. A detailed discussion of the types of surgical procedures used to treat bleeding ulcers is well reviewed elsewhere (24). Surgical

TABLE 4. SURGICAL THERAPY OF BLEEDING ULCER

Oversewing and vagotomy pyloroplasty
Billroth I
Wedge resection of ulcer and vagotomy or pyloroplasty

management includes classic approaches outlined in Table 4 and the application of newer techniques using minimally invasive laparoscopic techniques (24).

Recurrence of peptic ulcer disease and bleeding is fairly common. The long-term treatment strategy targets the elimination of defined risk factors. These include the use of NSAIDs and infection with *H. pylori*. Documentation of infection with *H. pylori* is recommended before institution of therapy. This can be accomplished by biopsies and culture of the gastric body (the gold standard test), stool analysis, or noninvasive tests such as urea breath analysis. The treatment of choice for *H. pylori* varies among experts, but usually consists of a 7- to 14-day combination drug regimen that includes an acid suppressant (usually a PPI or H2-antagonist) to increase gastric pH and facilitate antimicrobial activity against *H. pylori*. Acid suppression is combined with two or three oral antibiotics such as amoxicillin or clarithromycin with metronidazole and tetracycline. Bismuth subsalicylate is also administered in various protocols (25,26).

Despite many clinical advances over the past 30 years, the mortality rate from bleeding peptic ulcer has remained at 6% to 7% (2). Explanations for this lack of improvement are the increasing age of affected patients and the prevalence of concurrent severe illnesses. Currently, mortality is not directly related to hemorrhage, but results from MODS (27).

Portal Hypertension

Esophagogastric varices are responsible for 10% to 20% of UGI bleeding (28–30), but GI variceal bleeding develops in only one-third of patients with portal hypertension. Almost 90% of variceal bleeding presents with hematemesis, with or without melena. Mortality after a variceal bleed is substantial (greater than 25%) and is greater for esophageal than gastric varices. Child's criteria are the most widely used clinical criteria for quantifying the severity of liver disease (Table 5). In the setting of variceal bleeding, patients in Child's class A have a mortality of 10% or less with each bleed; the expected mortality in Child's class B is 30% to 40%; while patients in Child's class C probably have at least a 70% mortality with each bleed (31).

TABLE 5. CHILD CLASSIFICATION OF LIVER DISEASE[a]

	Class A	Class B	Class C
Serum bilirubin (mg/dL)	<2.0	2.0–3.0	>3.0
Serum albumin (g/dL)	>3.5	3.0–3.5	<3.0
Encephalopathy	None	Minimal	Advanced
Ascites	None	Easily controlled	Poorly controlled
Nutrition	Excellent	Good	Poor
Surgical risk	5%	10%	50%

[a]See reference 13 for further details.

Pathogenesis

The hepatic sinusoids are a low-resistance vascular bed; therefore, portal venous pressure is normally low (5 to 10 mm Hg). Portal hypertension (defined as a portal pressure greater than 10 to 15 mm Hg), is most commonly secondary to intrahepatic disease (cirrhosis), but may also result from extrahepatic disorders (e.g., hepatic vein thrombosis [Budd-Chiari syndrome], portal vein thrombosis). Although portal pressure must be elevated for varices to develop, there is only poor correlation between portal pressure and the incidence of variceal bleeding (30). In other words, patients with relatively low pressures may sustain variceal hemorrhage while some with very high pressures may not.

Diagnosis

UGI endoscopy is the most important diagnostic modality in the assessment of a bleeding patient in whom portal hypertension is suspected. Visualization of bleeding esophageal varices confirms the diagnosis of variceal hemorrhage, but it is important to remember that 30% to 50% of patients with known varices actually bleed from another source. In the presence of portal hypertension, even bleeding resulting from other causes, such as gastritis or ulceration, is more profuse secondary to gastric congestion and accompanying coagulopathy. Rebleeding after an initial esophageal variceal bleed is a major risk for increased morbidity and mortality. It usually occurs within 48 hours of the initial hemorrhage. Those patients at greatest risk for a rebleed are older than 60 years of age and/or those with large varices, red signs on varices, significant initial bleeds, ascites, or renal failure (30).

Treatment

As with gastric or duodenal ulcer bleeding, initial resuscitation of the patient is of paramount importance. In addition, protection of the airway, particularly in patients with encephalopathy or massive bleeding, is crucial. Some authors advocate hemodynamic monitoring with a pulmonary artery (PA) catheter to ensure prompt volume replacement and avoid overfilling, since this may precipitate rebleeding. The right atrial (RA) pressure ideally should be maintained between 4 and 8 mm Hg (32).

Diagnostic endoscopy offers the earliest opportunity for definitive treatment of variceal bleeding. Injection sclerotherapy controls bleeding in up to 80% to 90% of esophageal varices, but does not reduce portal pressure. Sclerotherapy often requires several treatments and reduces in-hospital rebleeding, but it is associated with a 10% to 20% incidence of severe complications such as perforation, bleeding, or infection. Banding ligation is another alternative for endoscopic management of acute variceal hemorrhage. Although banding is relatively cumbersome and time consuming to perform, there is speculation that it is more beneficial than sclerotherapy (30). The optimal endoscopic treatment for bleeding gastric varices remains to be defined. If the expertise for early interventional endoscopy is not available, other options include drug treatment and balloon tamponade (i.e., Sengstaken-Blakemore tube).

Vasopressin was widely used (with and without nitroglycerine to limit coronary vasoconstriction) and controlled variceal bleeding in 60% to 70% of patients. Systemic side effects as a consequence of intense vasoconstriction and ischemia occur in 20% to 30% of patients, predominantly affecting the myocardial and cerebral circulation (33). Vasopressin has been largely supplanted by the infusion of octreotide, a long-acting analog of somatostatin, or terlipressin (currently unavailable in the United States). Octreotide reduces splanchnic blood flow and decreases hepatic venous pressure while preserving cardiac output and systemic blood pressure. It is particularly advantageous in controlling vigorous variceal bleeding in hemodynamically unstable patients. This control often enables other effective therapy to be safely performed with fewer side effects than reported with vasopressin (2,34).

Balloon tamponade controls variceal bleeding by direct pressure on varices. With experience, it is highly effective and controls bleeding in 90% of cases. However, up to 50% of patients rebleed when the tube is deflated, and there is a complication rate of 25% to 30% (asphyxiation, aspiration, viscus or tracheal rupture, displaced balloons). The balloon should not remain inflated for more than 48 hours. Alternative, definitive treatment must be available when the balloon is deflated (32).

Portal decompression by transjugular intrahepatic portosystemic stent-shunt (TIPS) effectively controls variceal bleeding in patients with portal hypertension (35,36). TIPS is indicated in active variceal hemorrhage when emergent endoscopy fails, recurrent bleeds occur despite adequate endoscopy, or bleeding is isolated to gastric fundal varices. Contraindications to TIPS include peritonitis, sepsis, severe cardiopulmonary decompensation (e.g., cardiomyopathy, pulmonary hypertension), marked elevation in bilirubin (greater than 15 mg per dL), or severe, intractable coagulopathy. Malinchoc and colleagues have established a risk score for patients potentially undergoing TIPS (37).

At experienced centers, TIPS placement is successful in 90% of patients. Shunt stenosis may occur in up to 15% of patients and may progress to occlusion in 10% of cases, with an associated risk of bleeding. A universal rise in serum ammonia level has been noted in patients for the first 3 days after TIPS, with encephalopathy developing in up to 20% of patients during short-term follow-up (36). Additional acute complications after TIPS include bleeding, cardiac decompensation, and increased pulmonary shunting (36).

Surgical intervention is now confined to those patients who continue to bleed despite aggressive measures. Current surgical techniques include esophageal transection, with or without devascularization or portosystemic shunting, which carries a high mortality rate (greater than 35%) when performed emergently.

Stress-Related Erosive Syndrome

Critically ill patients commonly develop stress-related erosive syndrome (SRES). This syndrome manifests as superficial mucosal lesions predominantly in the acid-producing portion of the stomach. The incidence of SRES is reported to be declining because of improved monitoring and support of the critically ill and, to a lesser extent, the use of pharmacologic prophylaxis. However, the incidence depends largely on how SRES is defined and reported. Severe hemorrhage is reported in 1% to 7% of the ICU population (38,39). Clinically significant SRES bleeding is defined as overt hemorrhage in combination with orthostasis, a 2 g/dL drop in hemoglobin, 2 U packed red blood cell transfusion within 24 hours, or need for surgical intervention to control bleeding (5). The development of significant SRES is associated with increased morbidity and mortality in critically ill patients.

Pathogenesis

It is speculated that mucosal ischemia (e.g., during sepsis, hypotension) and gastric acidity play major roles in the pathogenesis of SRES, which increase the propensity of SRES to cause significant hemorrhage. Indeed, platelet aggregation is decreased at a gastric pH less than 6.9 and absent at a gastric pH less than 5.9 (40).

Diagnosis

Endoscopy is the most sensitive diagnostic procedure in identifying SRES. The lesions are usually multiple and are located in the stomach, with sparing of the antrum. The earliest abnormality on endoscopy is a pattern of alternating pallor and hyperemia. More severe changes consist of subepithelial hemorrhages, erosions, and, less often, acute ulcers.

Treatment

Therapy for SRES hemorrhage is similar to that for peptic ulcer bleeding. With attention to metabolic parameters, adequate resuscitation and appropriate prophylaxis, uncontrolled hemorrhage from SRES is rarely seen today. H2-blockers or PPI are the most commonly used agents for prophylaxis. Enteral feeding has also been shown to lower the incidence of SRES (5). Although the risk–benefit ratio for the prophylactic use of these agents is favorable, providing prophylaxis to the majority of ICU patients is expensive and labor-intensive. Cook and colleagues report that prophylaxis can be safely withheld from many critically ill patients unless they have a coagulopathy or require prolonged mechanical ventilation (41). Contentious debate continues with respect to whether the type of prophylaxis used to limit the development of SRES alters the incidence of nosocomial or ventilator-associated pneumonia (5).

Mallory-Weiss Syndrome

Mallory-Weiss tears of the esophagogastric junction are present in 5% to 15% of patients with acute UGI bleeding (28). Hematemesis is almost always the presenting manifestation. Mallory-Weiss syndrome occurs twice as often in men as compared to women. A recent history of alcohol abuse is common and a history of vomiting or retching is reported in 85% of patients with this disorder. Bleeding ceases spontaneously in 80% to 90% of cases, with less than a 10% chance of rebleed.

Pathogenesis

Mallory-Weiss tears occur within 2 cm of the gastroesophageal junction and are usually associated with a hiatal hernia. Mucosal laceration is believed to be caused by tremendous increase in the pressure gradient across the wall of the esophagogastric junction.

Diagnosis

The Mallory-Weiss tear is diagnosed endoscopically. Single or multiple short, shallow tears may be found at the esophagogastric junction.

Treatment

Usually, no specific therapy is necessary because bleeding stops spontaneously. Profuse bleeding due to this lesion may be controlled endoscopically with injection therapy or application of a heater probe. Selective intraarterial or intravenous infusion of vasopressin is also effective in cases of uncontrolled bleeding. In the rare patient with exsanguinating hemorrhage, surgical intervention is required.

Aortoenteric Fistulas

A fistula between the aorta and the GI tract is a relatively rare but often fatal process. Bleeding can present as hematemesis, melena, or hematochezia. Patients often present with a "herald bleed," followed by massive GIH. The distal portion of the duodenum (followed by jejunum, ileum, colon, stomach, appendix, and rectum) is the most likely site of hemorrhage for both primary and secondary aortoenteric fistulas.

Pathogenesis

Primary aortoenteric fistulas occur between the native aorta and the GI tract. Causes of primary aortoenteric fistulas include abdominal aortic aneurysm, infectious aortitis, penetrating peptic ulcer, tumor invasion, and trauma. Secondary fistulas occur between an aortic graft and the gastrointestinal tract. The incidence of such a fistula after aortic reconstructive surgery has been reported to be 0.6% to 1.5%, with the interval between the surgery and onset of GI bleeding ranging from a few days to years (42).

Diagnosis

The diagnosis of aortoenteric fistula must be considered in any patient who has had aortic reconstructive surgery, or has an abdominal aortic aneurysm. Failure to diagnose and treat this disease is uniformly fatal. UGI endoscopy probably identifies less than one-half of patients with aortoenteric fistula. If endoscopy fails to demonstrate an aortoenteric fistula or another convincing source of bleeding, other potential diagnostic options include abdominal computed tomography, aortography, barium contrast radiography, and exploratory laparotomy.

Treatment

After initial resuscitation, survival is dependent on early surgical intervention. Even in surgically treated patients, postoperative mortality approaches 60% (42). In patients with an aortoenteric fistula involving an aortic graft, removal of the entire graft, with alternative bypass construction, is preferred to patching or closing the defect.

Mucosal Erosive Disease

Esophagitis is increasingly recognized as a cause of acute UGI bleeding (43,44). Bleeding induced by erosive gastritis occurs in response to irritant material such as ethanol or NSAIDs, and infrequently causes acute, massive UGI bleeding. When the bleeding is acute, the most common presentation is hematemesis.

Pathogenesis

Contributing factors to peptic esophagitis include gastroesophageal reflux, esophageal dysmotility, and decreased ability of the esophagus to clear acids. Less common causes of esophagitis include infection (cytomegalovirus, *Candida albicans,* herpes simplex) or corrosive esophagitis (secondary to the ingestion of alcohol, caustic substances, and various medications, including tetracycline, quinidine, and potassium).

Diagnosis

When mucosal lesions are visualized during esophagoscopy, a number of different tests confirm the diagnosis (e.g., biopsy, cytology, pH monitoring, manometry).

Treatment

Whenever possible, the offending agent should be eliminated. Acute bleeding will usually cease spontaneously without specific intervention. For NSAID-induced damage, an H2-receptor antagonist or misoprostol (a synthetic prostaglandin E_1 analog) reduces the incidence of mucosal lesions.

Vascular Anomalies

Although abnormal or aberrant vascular structures are an unusual cause of UGI hemorrhage, up to 25% to 35% of patients with chronic renal failure have UGI bleeding secondary to vascular malformations (45). GI telangiectasia is associated with the Osler-Weber-Rendu and CREST (calcinosis, Raynaud syndrome, esophageal dysmotility, scleroderma, and telangiectasia) syndromes. Vascular ectasia may present with chronic or recurrent acute bleeding. Arteriovenous malformations or Dieulafoy lesions most commonly present with major acute hemorrhages. If untreated, such lesions often rebleed.

Pathogenesis

The exact mechanism of formation of vascular anomalies is unclear. Postulated causes include congenital vascular abnormalities, disorders of connective tissues, chronic low-grade venous obstruction, and local mucosal hypoxia (45).

Diagnosis

Diagnosis of these lesions is made endoscopically, but most cannot be reliably differentiated based upon their endoscopic features. Endoscopically detected UGI tract vascular lesions are most commonly found in the stomach and proximal duodenum.

Treatment

Treatment

Endoscopic thermal therapy is generally regarded as the initial therapy of choice for bleeding vascular anomalies. The traditional approach for definitive cure of Dieulafoy lesion is subsequent resection. Surgical resection may be required for widespread ectasias if thermal therapy is unsuccessful. If a patient is at particularly high risk for developing surgical complications, estrogen therapy has been anecdotally reported to control recurrent hemorrhage.

Tumors

A wide variety of mesenchymal neoplasms, such as leiomyomas, leiomyosarcomas, neurofibromas, and lymphoma, rarely cause UGI bleeding.

LOWER GASTROINTESTINAL BLEEDING

It is important to remember that massive UGI bleeding may manifest itself as hematochezia in up to 15% of cases. Although there are many causes (Table 6) of lower gastrointestinal (LGI) bleeding, diverticular disease and angiodysplasia are the most common causes.

Colonic Diverticulosis

The incidence of diverticula increases with age and affects 20% to 50% of the population over the age of 60. Involvement of the entire colon with diverticulosis occurs in 10% of patients. Overt LGI bleeding occurs in about 5% of patients with diverticulosis (46,47). Therefore, diverticular bleeding is one of the most common causes of hematochezia in this age group. The bleeding is usually painless and not accompanied by diverticulitis. In most instances, the bleeding stops spontaneously with a 25% chance of rebleed. The risk of rebleeding after the second episode is almost 50%.

Pathogenesis

Diverticulosis of the large bowel results from protrusions of mucosa through muscular layers, generally at the site of nutrient

TABLE 6. CAUSES OF LOWER GASTROINTESTINAL BLEEDING

Upper gastrointestinal bleeding
Diverticular disease
Vascular anomalies
Hemorrhoids
Vascular enteric fistulas
Ischemic colitis
Inflammatory bowel disease
Infectious colitis
Neoplasm and polyps
Miscellaneous
    Radiation colitis
    Vasculitis
    Ulcers of colon and rectum

vessels. The formation of diverticula is believed to be secondary to segmental pressure gradients in different parts of the colon. Diverticula are most common in the sigmoid colon and, to a lesser extent, in the proximal colon.

Diagnosis

When patients present with massive LGI bleeding, colonoscopy may be difficult because large amounts of blood in the lumen obscure visualization. In such cases, either a nuclear bleeding scan or angiogram can more precisely localize the site. For the angiogram to demonstrate the active site, the rate of bleeding must be at least 1 to 2 mL per minute, while nuclear bleeding scans can detect blood loss at the rate of 0.1 to 0.5 mL per minute or greater.

Treatment

The first steps in the therapy of patients with diverticular bleeding are fluid resuscitation, maintaining adequacy of perfusion, urinary output, and hematocrit, with identification and correction of coagulopathy. Most cases of mild or moderate hemorrhage stop spontaneously with conservative measures. When uncontrolled bleeding occurs, infusion of vasopressin intravenously or intraarterially through the angiographic catheter may effectively control bleeding. Angiographic-guided embolization may be used in select patients. Persistent bleeding, despite medical therapy, can usually be treated with segmental colectomy after localization of the bleeding site.

Vascular Anomalies

Angiodysplasia is the source of approximately 25% of LGI bleeding in patients over 50 years of age. Bleeding usually manifests as bright red blood per rectum or as maroon-colored stool. However, up to 10% of patients may have only occult blood loss. Bleeding is typically brief, but continued hemorrhage may occur. The rate of GI bleeding is a function of the size and number of angiodysplasias bleeding at a given time. Angiodysplasia and diverticular diseases are the most likely sources of lower GIH.

Pathogenesis

Although the pathogenesis of colonic angiodysplasia, a degenerative lesion consisting of tortuous submucosal vessels within the wall of the colon, is not known, it is believed that with age, degenerative changes occur within the wall of the colon. Angiodysplasia is most common after age 50. The lesions are usually multiple and found primarily in the cecum and ascending colon (46).

Diagnosis

Colonoscopy often localizes the site of bleeding, but on occasion, mesenteric angiography may be necessary to visualize the lesion.

Treatment

Endoscopic hemostasis or embolization during angiography is highly successful. Persistent recurrent bleeding requires surgical therapy. Most authors advocate hemicolectomy after the site of blood loss is established by angiography or technetium 99-labeled red cell scan.

Ischemic Colitis/Mesenteric Vasculopathy

In patients who develop lower gastrointestinal bleeding while in the intensive care unit, mesenteric ischemia deserves particular attention. Ischemia of the colon, like other vascular diseases, most often affects older adults.

Pathogenesis

In this disorder, hemodynamic and systemic abnormalities may predispose older patients to developing functional intestinal ischemia with or without preexisting anatomic vascular obstruction (5). With occlusive or nonocclusive interruption of blood flow to a segment of colon, ischemia may develop. Ischemic colitis is almost always nonocclusive. Most commonly, ischemic colitis involves the left colon, the splenic flexure, and sigmoid colon, which are the watershed areas between the distribution of the superior and inferior mesenteric arteries and the inferior mesenteric and iliac arteries.

Diagnosis

Clinical characteristics of this disorder include sudden onset of abdominal pain and bleeding out of proportion to physical findings. In most instances, abdominal pain precedes bleeding. Interestingly, the abdomen is usually soft to palpation despite the intense abdominal pain. Unexplained acidosis and minimal radiographic findings are common. Sigmoidoscopy is usually valuable in establishing the diagnosis of ischemic colitis.

Treatment

The initial steps in management of ischemic colitis include the determination and correction of predisposing factors (i.e., replace intravascular volume, augment cardiac output, reverse hypotension). The use of broad-spectrum antibiotics is indicated if peritonitis is suspected. Most patients respond to conservative medical management. Occasionally, surgical intervention is required to remove infarcted bowel in fulminant ischemic colitis.

SUMMARY

GI hemorrhage occurs commonly as a presenting or secondary process in critically ill patients. The overall outcome is probably improved for many patients, but significant morbidity and mortality are related to increasing age at presentation and associated end-organ dysfunction. Patients with GIH require prompt evaluation, aggressive resuscitation, and definitive medical or surgical therapy. Evidence from prospectively validated trials can be used to define risk stratification, and an algorithmic approach to triage patients with UGI bleeding predicts complications such as rebleeding or need for additional intervention. SRES is a major cause of secondary GI bleeding; however, the patient populations that should routinely receive SRES prophylaxis and the optimum means of prevention remain controversial despite multiple studies and metaanalyses. LGI bleeding should be differentiated from massive UGI bleeding with rapid transit time.

KEY POINTS

GI bleeding continues to be a common reason for ICU admission or complication in critically ill patients. GIH is empirically divided into upper or lower GI in origin. Despite advances in critical care, interventional therapies such as endoscopy, angiography, and TIPS, GI hemorrhage has a significant associated morbidity and mortality with certain populations at increased risk for rebleeding. The overall outcome is probably improved for many patients, but significant morbidity and mortality are related to increasing age at presentation and associated end-organ dysfunction. Applying an algorithm as outlined in the text can effect triage of UGI hemorrhage. ESUS is a common cause of secondary hemorrhage in critically ill patients, especially head-injured and mechanically ventilated patients, and patients with coagulopathy or renal insufficiency. The optimal means of preventing stress ulceration remains under investigation, but PPI may be the most advantageous. Diverticular disease or angiodysplasia most commonly causes LGI bleeding.

REFERENCES

1. Laine L, Peterson WL. Bleeding peptic ulcer. *N Engl J Med* 1994; 331:717–727.
2. Kupfer Y, Cappell MS, Tessler S. Acute gastrointestinal bleeding in the intensive care unit: The intensivist's perspective. *Gastroenterol Clin North Am* 2000;28:275–308.
3. Lewis JD, Shin EJ, Metz DC. Characterization of gastrointestinal bleeding in severely ill hospitalized patients. *Crit Care Med* 2000;28:46–50.
4. Hussain H, Lapin S, Cappell MS. Clinical scoring systems for determining the prognosis of gastrointestinal bleeding. *Gastroenterol Clin North Am* 2000;29:445–464.
5. Beejay U, Wolfe WW. Acute gastrointestinal bleeding in the intensive care unit: the gastroenterologist's perspective. *Gastroenterol Clin North Am* 2000;29:309–336.
6. Cook DJ, Reeve BK, Guyatt GH, et al. Stress ulcer prophylaxis in critically ill patients. Resolving discordant meta-analyses. *JAMA* 1996;275:308–314.
7. Kollef MH, Canfield DA, Zuckerman GR. Triage considerations for patients with gastrointestinal hemorrhage admitted to a medical intensive care unit. *Crit Care Med* 1995;23:1048–1054.
8. Rockall TA, Logan RFA, Devlin HB, et al. Risk assessment after upper gastrointestinal haemorrhage. *Gut* 1996;38:316–321.
9. Kollef MH, O'Brien JD, Zuckerman GR, et al. BLEED: a classification tool to predict outcomes in patients with acute upper and lower gastrointestinal hemorrhage. *Crit Care Med* 1997; 25:1125–1132.

10. Longstreth GF, Feitelberg SP. Outpatient care of sedated patients with acute non-variceal upper gastrointestinal haemorrrhage. *Lancet* 1995; 345:108–111.

11. Hay JA, Maldonado L, Weingarten SR, et al. Prospective evaluation of a clinical guideline recommending hospital length of stay in upper gastrointestinal tract haemorrrhage. *JAMA* 1997;278:2151–2156.

12. Saeed ZA, Ramirez FC, Hepps KS, et al. Prospective validation of the Baylor bleeding score for predicting the likelihood of rebleeding after endoscopic hemostasis of peptic ulcers. *Gastrointest Endo* 1995; 41:561–565.

13. Brullet E, Calvet X, Campo R, et al. Factors predicting failure of endoscopic injection therapy in bleeding duodenal ulcer. *Gastrointest Endo* 1996;43:111–116.

14. Holvoet J, Terriere L, Van Hee W, et al. Relation of upper gastrointestinal bleeding to non-steroidal anti-inflammatory drugs and aspirin: a case control study. *Gut* 1991;32: 730–734.

15. de Dombal FT, Clarke JR, Clamp SE, et al. Prognostic factors in upper G.I. bleeding. *Endoscopy* 1986;18:6–10.

16. Branicki FJ, Boey J, Fok PJ, et al. Bleeding duodenal ulcer. A prospective evaluation of risk factors for rebleeding and death. *Ann Surg* 1990;211:411–418.

17. Welage LS, Berardi RR. Evaluation of omeprazole, lansoprazole, pantoprazole, and rabeprazole in the treatment of acid-related diseases. *J Am Pharm Assoc* 2000;40:52–62.

18. Howden CW. Use of proton-pump inhibitors in complicated ulcer disease and upper gastrointestinal tract bleeding. *Am J Health Syst Pharm* 1999;56:S5–S11.

19. Levy MJ, et al. Comparison of omeprazole and ranitidine for stress ulcer prophylaxis. *Dig Dis Sci* 1997;42:1255–1259.

20. Cook DJ, Guyatt GH, Salena BJ, et al. Endoscopic therapy for acute nonvariceal upper gastrointestinal hemorrhage: a meta-analysis. *Gastroenterology* 1992;102:139–148.

21. Laine L. Multipolar electrocoagulation versus injection therapy in the treatment of bleeding peptic ulcers. A prospective, randomized trial. *Gastroenterology* 1990;99:1303–1306.

22. Lefkovitz Z, Cappell MS, Kaplan M, et al. Radiology in the diagnosis and therapy of gastrointestinal bleeding. *Gastroenterol Clin North Am* 2000;29:489–512.

23. Lang EK. Transcatheter embolization in management of hemorrhage from duodenal ulcer: long-term results and complications. *Radiology* 1992;182:703–707.

24. Stabile BE, Stammos MJ. Surgical management of gastrointestinal bleeding. *Gastroenterol Clin North Am* 2000;29:189–222.

25. Laheij RJF, van Rossum LGM, Jansen JMBJ, et al. Evaluation of treatment regimens to cure *Helicobacter pylori* infection: a meta-analysis. *Aliment Pharmacol Ther* 1999;13:857–864.

26. Megraud F, Marshall BJ. How to treat *Helicobacter pylori*. First-line, second-line, and future therapies. *Gastroenterol Clin North Am* 2001; 29759–29773.

27. Segal WN, Cello JP. Hemorrhage in the upper gastrointestinal tract in the older patient. *Am J Gastroenterol* 1997; 92:42–46.

28. Gilbert DA, Silverstein FE, Tedesco FJ, et al. The national ASGE survey on upper gastrointestinal bleeding, III. Endoscopy in upper gastrointestinal bleeding. *Gastrointest Endosc* 1981; 27:94–102.

29. Rigau J, Bosch J, Bordas JM, et al. Endoscopic measurement of variceal pressure in cirrhosis: correlation with portal pressure and variceal hemorrhage. *Gastroenterology* 1989;96:873–880.

30. Luketic VA, Snayl AJ. Esophageal varices: I. Clinical presentation, medical therapy, and endoscopic therapy. *Gastroenterol Clin North Am* 2000: 29:337–386.

31. Hoefs JC. Portal hypertension. In: Gitnick G, ed. *Principles and practice of gastroenterology and hepatology*. Norwalk, CT: Appleton & Lange; 1994:837–879.

32. Williams SG, Westaby D. Management of variceal hemorrhage. *BMJ* 1994;308:1213–1217.

33. Navarro VJ, Garcua-Tsao G. Variceal hemorrhage. *Crit Care Clin* 1995;11:391–414.

34. Cello JP, Chan MF. Octreotide therapy for variceal hemorrhage. *Digestion* 1993;54:20–26.

35. Rossle M, Haag K, Ochs A, et al. The transjugular intrahepatic portosystemic stent-shunt procedure for variceal bleeding. *N Engl J Med* 1994;330:165–171.

36. Luketic VA, Sanyal AJ. Esophageal varices: II. TIPS (transjugular intrahepatic portosystemic shunt and surgical therapy. *Gastroenterol Clin North Am* 2000; 29:387–420.

37. Malinchoc M, Kamath PS, Gordon FD, et al. A model to predict poor survival in patients undergoing transjugular intrahepatic portosystemic shunts. *Hepatology* 2000;31:864–871.

38. Schuster DP, Rowley H, Frinstein S, et al. Prospective evaluation of the risk of upper gastrointestinal bleeding after admission to a medical intensive care unit. *Am J Med* 1984;76:623–630.

39. Cook D, Heyland D, Griffith L, et al. Risk factors for clinically important upper gastrointestinal bleeding in patients requiring mechanical ventilation. *Crit Care Med* 1999;27; 2812–2817.

40. Green FW Jr, Kaplan MM, Curtis LE, et al. Effect of acid and pepsin on blood coagulation and platelet aggregation. A possible contributor to prolonged gastroduodenal mucosal hemorrhage. *Gastroenterology* 1978;74:38–43.

41. Cook DJ, Fuller HD, Guyatt GH, et al. Risk factors for gastrointestinal bleeding in critically ill patients. *N Engl J Med* 1994;330:377–381.

42. Nagy SW, Marshall GB. Aortoenteric fistulas. Recognizing potentially catastrophic causes of gastrointestinal bleeding. *Postgrad Med* 1993;93:211–222.

43. Wilmer A, et al. Duodenogastroesophageal reflux and esophageal mucosal injury in mechanically ventilated patients *Gastroenterology* 1999;116:1293–1299.

44. Plaiser PW, van Buuren HR, Bruining HA. An analysis of upper GI endoscopy done for patients in surgical intensive care: high incidence of and morbidity from reflux esophagitis. *Eur J Surg* 1997;163:903–907.

45. Lichtentein DR, Berman MD, Wolfe MM. Approach to the patient with acute upper gastrointestinal hemorrhage. In: Taylor MB, ed. *Gastrointestinal emergencies*. Baltimore: Williams & Wilkins, 1992:92–116.

46. Reinus JF, Brandt LJ. Vascular ectasias and diverticulosis. Common causes of lower intestinal bleeding. *Gastroenterol Clin North Am* 1994;23:1–20.

47. Savides TJ, Jensen DM. Therapeutic endoscopy for nonvariceal gastrointestinal bleeding. *Gastroenterol Clin North Am* 2000; 29:465–487.

CARE OF THE PATIENT WITH FULMINANT HEPATIC FAILURE

CHRISTOPHER J. JANKOWSKI
MARK T. KEEGAN
DAVID J. PLEVAK

KEY WORDS

- Coagulopathy
- Fulminant hepatic failure
- Hepatic encephalopathy
- Hepatorenal syndrome
- Intracranial hypertension
- Liver transplantation
- Bioartificial liver-assist device

DEFINITION AND TERMINOLOGY

Fulminant hepatic failure (FHF) is one of the most catastrophic conditions in medicine. Patients with the disease can become extremely ill very rapidly and require all the sophisticated support systems available in a modern intensive care unit (ICU). FHF is characterized by severe liver dysfunction, hepatic encephalopathy, and coagulopathy in a patient without preexisting liver disease (1). FHF is estimated to affect 2,000 individuals annually in the United States (2,3). Since this disease affects previously healthy individuals, the rapid progression and severity of the illness is often alarming to families and physicians alike. As recently as the 1980s, mortality for patients with FHF was as high as 94% (4). However, improved intensive care and the advent of transplantation for the treatment of end-stage liver disease have improved survival. Yet even in this modern era of transplantation, bioartificial liver-assist devices, and invasive intracranial monitoring, the 1-year patient survival rates are no better than 63% (5). Since many patients with FHF never have an opportunity to receive a cadaveric liver graft, today's research is focused on preserving the remaining hepatocytes, improving hepatocyte regeneration, and developing novel methods of hepatocyte transplantation.

ETIOLOGY

FHF can occur from a variety of hepatocyte insults. The underlying causes of FHF differ around the world, with drug-induced acute liver failure playing a large role in Europe and the United States. In contrast, developing countries have little drug-induced FHF, other than for an occasional case associated with isoniazid toxicity.

Acetaminophen, with more than one billion pills sold annually, is now the most common cause of FHF in the United States, just as it has been for many years in the United Kingdom (6). Other drugs that can cause FHF include isoniazid, tricyclic antidepressants (7), volatile anesthetics, and nonsteroidal antiinflammatory drugs (8). Toxins are responsible for a small number of cases of FHF and include *Amanita phalloides* (9), carbon tetrachloride (10), and aflatoxin (11).

Hepatitis A and B are the most often identified viruses causing FHF. Hepatitis D and E account for a variable, but usually small proportion of cases in Western countries. Hepatitis C very rarely, if ever, is the cause of FHF. Other nonhepatotropic viruses, such as Epstein-Barr virus (12), cytomegalovirus (13), adenoviruses (14), and herpes simplex virus can also cause FHF, but these causes of FHF are exceedingly rare. In many instances (up to 38%), an infectious agent cannot be identified; however, the clinical picture appears to be very much like infection-induced acute hepatic failure. In these instances, the assumed etiologic agent is usually identified as being non-A, non-B, and non-C hepatitis (3).

Miscellaneous causes of FHF include liver cell necrosis secondary to shock, obstruction of hepatic veins (Budd-Chiari syndrome [15] or venoocclusive disease [16]), Wilson disease (17), hyperthermia (18), autoimmune hepatitis, surgical hepatectomy (19), or microvesicular steatosis (acute fatty liver of pregnancy [20] or Reye syndrome [21]).

CLINICAL PRESENTATION

FHF is not merely a disease involving the liver. The sudden loss of hepatocyte function results in protean manifestations of multiorgan system failure (22). Because patients with FHF characteristically are well until the abrupt onset of their illness, they typically do not have the stigmata that are often associated with chronic liver disease. Usually absent are external signs of malnutrition, spider angioma, and marked ascites. Hepatic encephalopathy is the hallmark feature of FHF. Although hepatic encephalopathy does occur in patients with chronic liver disease, it does not have the diagnostic or prognostic implications that it has in the patient with FHF.

The pathogenesis of multiorgan failure in FHF is complex and not well elucidated. In addition to the loss of hepatocyte function, the release of large quantities of cellular debris including actin, mediators (interleukin-1, endotoxin, interleukin-6), and tumor necrosis factor are involved. In addition, as the liver's function declines, it is increasingly unable to perform host defense functions. The opsonic capability of proteins such as fibronectin, C-reactive protein, and α_1-antitrypsin are inhibited and the clearance of gut-derived translocated bacteria and endotoxin is decreased.

NEUROLOGIC COMPLICATIONS

The biochemical cause of encephalopathy in FHF, as in cirrhotic patients, remains unclear. Recent attention is given again to ammonia as a possible etiologic agent by virtue of the excellent correlation of arterial ammonia levels with the presence of cerebral edema (23). Unlike cirrhotic patients, FHF patients may become agitated prior to onset of deeper grades of coma and the transition to advanced stages of coma occurs very rapidly in most patients (Table 1). Also, in contrast to cirrhosis, cerebral edema is a common complication of FHF and occurs in up to 80% of patients with grade 4 hepatic coma (24). In addition, cerebral edema accounts for 34% to 80% of FHF-associated mortalities on autopsy studies. Cerebral edema has been documented in 48% to 86% of patients with FHF when intracranial pressure (ICP) monitoring is used. Since cerebral blood flow can be either increased or decreased in these patients (25) and loss of cerebral autoregulation can occur (26), the brain is more susceptible to cardiovascular lability. By detecting cerebral edema and increased ICP, the clinician can affect overall outcome of these patients with therapies directed at increasing cerebral perfusion pressure by lowering the ICP or raising mean arterial blood pressure. Therapies directed at the treatment of intracranial hypertension include head elevation, hyperventilation, diuretic therapy (including mannitol), pharmacologically induced coma, and the use of moderate hypothermia.

The value of ICP monitoring in diagnosing intracranial hypertension and directing treatment is still debated and its use is limited to certain transplant centers. Controlled trials have not been performed to fully evaluate the use of this monitor. Certainly these coagulopathic and immunocompromised patients

TABLE 1. CLINICAL GRADING OF HEPATIC ENCEPHALOPATHY

Grade of Encephalopathy	Neurologic Findings
1	Behavioral changes without changes in level of consciousness
2	Gross disorientation, slowing of mentation, occasional decrease in level of consciousness
3	Suppressed level of consciousness but responsive to painful stimuli, no meaningful communication
4	Unresponsive to pain, decerebrate posturing

are at risk for complications. However, ICP monitoring has been reported to be relatively safe in an analysis combining the experience of 68 centers and 262 patients (27). In this report, ICP monitoring had an incidence of intracranial hemorrhage of 3.1% with epidural monitors and 18% with subdural bolts. The incidence of fatal hemorrhages was 1.3% and 5%, respectively. Infectious complications were minimal and malfunction that required repositioning occurred in 7.4% patients.

When Lidofsky and coworkers integrated ICP monitoring into their care of patients with FHF, they achieved an overall survival rate of 56.6% (92% in those receiving liver transplantation) (28). This rate is compared to a 26% survival rate found in a survey of numerous other centers.

For patients with preserved renal function, the use of loop diuretics and mannitol has been effective in reducing cerebral edema in FHF patients. However, the use of these agents is limited by the hyperosmolarity that results after repeated dosing. Infusions of barbiturates have been shown to be effective in treating refractory intracranial hypertension and are especially valuable in those situations where renal function is not preserved. Barbiturates reduce the oxygen requirements of the brain and decrease cerebral blood flow, leading to a decrease in the volume of the intracranial contents and hence a fall in ICP. Infusions of propofol may also be effective in treating increased ICP in FHF, but clinical experience is more limited. Recently, the use of moderate hypothermia (32° to 33°C) has been applied to patients with uncontrolled intracranial hypertension from acute hepatic failure. In this investigation, four patients who were candidates for liver transplantation were successfully bridged to transplantation with a mean of 13 hours of hypothermia. In contrast, three patients who were unsuitable candidates for liver transplantation died from cerebral edema after systemic warming.

In addition to using ICP monitoring to direct the use of therapies intended to reduce cerebral edema, these monitors can also be used to make decisions regarding the timing and advisability of transplantation. Lidofsky and coworkers noted that if intracranial hypertension was responsive to medical management, liver transplantation could be applied without neurologic sequelae (28). However, intracranial hypertension refractory to medical management was an excellent predictor of brainstem herniation. Noninvasive means have been used to attempt to detect cerebral edema and make decisions regarding the advisability of liver transplantation in patients with FHF. In the past, many have believed that cerebral edema, as noted on computed tomography (CT) scan of the head, occurs too late in the course of the disease to be of much diagnostic assistance. However, Wijdicks and associates looked retrospectively at CT scans of patients with FHF (29). They were able to identify those patients with high-grade encephalopathy on the basis of subtle findings of edema on CT scan. Hence, CT scanning, especially when used in serial fashion, may be useful in identifying early evidence of cerebral edema.

CARDIOVASCULAR COMPLICATIONS

Similar to patients with chronic liver disease, patients with FHF also have a hyperdynamic circulatory state. In 1953, Kowalski and Abelmann first described depressed systematic vascular resistance in patients with liver dysfunction (30). The etiology of this hemodynamic condition is unknown. However, it has been suggested that this condition may result from a supply-dependent oxygen delivery, similar to that which occurs in septic shock (31). An additional or alternative cause of the hyperdynamic circulatory state could be the failing liver's inability to remove vasoactive mediators. It may be inaccurate to state that the hyperdynamic circulatory state is a "complication" of liver disease since the elevated cardiac output appears to facilitate the supply of blood and oxygen to failing vital organs. In fact, if the hyperdynamic circulatory state is absent, the clinician should investigate the cause of the patient's inability to generate a high cardiac output. Complications of the hyperdynamic circulatory state may occur in older adults or those with underlying cardiac disease. These individuals may not be able to meet the demands of the hyperdynamic circulatory state, and thus, develop cardiac failure.

PULMONARY COMPLICATIONS

Patients with chronic liver disease often develop hypoxemia from hepatopulmonary syndrome (32). However, this condition of pulmonary vascular dilation and shunting has only been described in one patient with FHF. When hypoxemia occurs in the patient with FHF, it usually is the result of pulmonary infiltrates from fluid overload (often the result of the transfusion of multiple coagulation products), acute respiratory distress syndrome (ARDS), or pneumonia. These patients are immune-compromised and prone to infectious complications (see "Infectious Complications" later in this chapter). The hyperdynamic circulatory state can result in mild pulmonary hypertension in patients with FHF. However, severe pulmonary hypertension, which can occur in patients with chronic liver disease (portopulmonary hypertension), has not been described.

Many patients with FHF require endotracheal intubation and mechanical ventilation. These interventions are usually made for airway management and the application of hyperventilation in the treatment of increased ICP.

COMPLICATIONS OF COAGULATION

The presence of severe coagulopathy often precedes hepatic coma in patients with FHF. Loss of clotting factors II, V, VII, IX, and X, due to decreased hepatic synthesis, results in marked prolongation of both the prothrombin time (PT) and activated partial thromboplastin time (aPTT). Intermittent measurement of the PT is the best available guide to hepatic recovery or deterioration, since changes in the international normalized ratio (INR) reflect hepatic synthesis (unless influenced by large doses of fresh frozen plasma). Consumption of coagulation factors is difficult to distinguish from synthetic dysfunction, as the liver is compromised in its abilities to remove activated clotting factors and circulating fibrinolysins (33).

Platelet counts are usually depressed in patients with liver disease. Thrombocytopenia in patients with chronic liver disease most typically results from portal hypertension and splenic se-

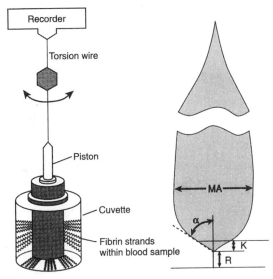

FIGURE 1. A schematic of the thromboelastogram. As the blood sample clots, a graphic recording of the strength of the clot over time is produced. Altered function in various components of the coagulation cascade yields characteristic tracings. Quantitative data also can be derived from the tracings. Parameters include the reaction time (*R*), coagulation time (*K*), alpha angle (*α*), and the maximum amplitude (*MA*). (Reprinted with permission from Tuman K, Spiess B, McCarthy R, et al. Effects of progressive blood loss on coagulation as measured by thromboelastography. *Anesth Analg* 1987;66:856.)

questration. This etiology of thrombocytopenia is rare in patients with FHF. Most of the thrombocytopenia seen in these patients results from an ongoing disseminated intravascular coagulopathy (DIC) and fibrinolysis. When disorders of platelet function occur in FHF, they are usually associated with the occurrence of renal insufficiency.

The treatment of the multifactorial coagulopathy of FHF can be extremely difficult. Although laboratory studies, such as platelet counts, PT, aPTT, and fibrinogen levels provide information regarding the status of individual aspects of the coagulation cascade, they do not provide an overall assessment of this complex and interdependent process. Tests that provide a global view of coagulation status are invaluable to the clinician in guiding transfusion therapy. The thromboelastogram (TEG) provides such a view. The TEG has been used over the past two decades in the intraoperative care of patients undergoing liver transplantation (34). Its use can be easily transferred to the ICU (35). A TEG is performed by placing a small amount of blood into a cuvette and stirring the blood with an agitator connected to a strain gauge (Fig. 1). As the movement of the agitator is inhibited, the strain gauge provides a graphic representation of the strength of the ensuing clot. Based on the morphology of the plotted information, the clinician can determine if there are qualitative or quantitative deficiencies in coagulation factors, platelets, or fibrinogen. The TEG also can indicate the presence of fibrinolysis (Fig. 2).

INFECTIOUS COMPLICATIONS

Patients with FHF are susceptible to infections. Their increased risk results from decreased opsonin function and complement

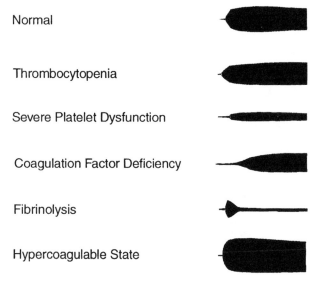

Normal

Thrombocytopenia

Severe Platelet Dysfunction

Coagulation Factor Deficiency

Fibrinolysis

Hypercoagulable State

FIGURE 2. Characteristic thromboelastogram tracings. (From Mark JB, Slaughter TF, Reves JG. Cardiovascular monitoring. In: Miller RD, Miller ED Jr, Reeves JG, eds. *Anesthesia,* 5th ed. Philadelphia: Churchill Livingstone, 2000:1192.)

deficiency, leukocyte dysfunction, impaired Kupffer cell function, bacterial gut translocation, and the release of immunosuppressive cytokines and endotoxin (36). In addition, there are potential iatrogenic causes of infections in these patients, including the presence of indwelling catheters, ICP monitors, and endotracheal tubes. Infections worsen the outcome of these patients and, along with cerebral edema, are common causes of death. Bacterial infection occurs in 50% of patients with FHF. The sources of these bacteria are blood, respiratory tract, urinary tract, or skin (wounds or intravascular catheters). *Staphylococcus aureus* is the most common organism isolated, followed by *S. epidermidis* and streptococcal species. Fungal infections occur in one-third of patients (often together with bacterial infections) and typically appear late in the course of the disease, after antibiotic therapy. *Candida albicans* is the most frequent fungal organism found. In some institutions, *Aspergillus* species infection occurs with considerable frequency. Fungal infection from any organism is a bad prognostic sign and may preclude transplantation.

GASTROINTESTINAL COMPLICATIONS

Gastrointestinal (GI) hemorrhage often occurs in patients with FHF. However, GI hemorrhage is usually not the result of varices, as is often the case in patients with chronic liver disease. Instead, it is the result of stress ulceration with a significant contribution from an underlying coagulopathy. Pancreatitis is a common complication of FHF. In one series, 35 patients who died with FHF and had an autopsy performed had documented pancreatitis. The cause of this high incidence of pancreatitis is speculative but may include circulating cytokines, inflammatory cells, and possibly, intermittent systemic hypotension.

MALNUTRITION

Malnutrition, especially protein malnutrition, is a significant consequence of both acute and chronic liver failure. In patients with FHF, protein malnutrition is primarily evidenced by a significant decrease in circulating proteins (albumin, transferrin, prealbumin, and others) because these patients usually have not had adequate time to significantly reduce their skeletal muscle mass (37). The edema that sometimes accompanies FHF may provide an illusion of adequate nourishment. Previous investigations of patients with chronic liver disease have demonstrated a catabolic state with significant protein metabolism (38). It can be assumed that such a situation is present and possibly even more severe in those patients with FHF.

METABOLIC DISORDERS

Disorders of glucose metabolism often occur in patients with liver disease. Hyperglycemia is the usual finding in patients with liver dysfunction. However, hypoglycemia can occur, especially in patients with end-stage FHF. Because the ability to generate glucose through gluconeogenesis is one of the last hepatic functions to fail, hypoglycemia is an ominous sign of an impending terminal situation. In patients with chronic liver disease (especially those with portal hypertension), common metabolic findings include hypokalemia and intravascular volume constriction with metabolic alkalosis. In contrast, patients with FHF may develop hyperkalemic anion-gap metabolic acidosis from both their acute liver failure and their developing renal insufficiency. Hypocalcemia will usually occur in patients with FHF. Since serum albumin levels are usually low, ionized calcium can be normal. Ionized serum magnesium levels can be either high or low in these patients, depending on the presence or absence of renal insufficiency.

Lactic acidosis occurring late in the course of FHF is a bad prognostic sign (39).

RENAL DYSFUNCTION AND FAILURE

Renal dysfunction occurs commonly in patients with liver disease. Renal dysfunction and failure occur primarily by two mechanisms: acute tubular necrosis and hepatorenal syndrome. Acute tubular necrosis can result from hypotensive episodes, the influence of nephrotoxic antibiotics, and sepsis.

Hepatorenal syndrome has recently been divided into two clinical types. Type 1 is characterized by rapidly progressive renal failure (a doubling of the initial serum creatinine to a level greater than 2.5 mg per dL in less than 2 weeks). Type 2 hepatorenal syndrome is renal insufficiency that does not have a rapidly progressive course. Both type 1 and type 2 hepatorenal syndrome are characterized by overly avid sodium retention, with extremely low urine sodium and fractional excretion of sodium (FENa < 1%). Once the hepatorenal syndrome occurs, the use of intravascular volume expansion, renal dose dopamine, or fenoldopam may temporarily improve the situation. However, in type 1 hepatorenal syndrome, deterioration is progressive despite these fluid and pharmacologic therapies.

Hemodialysis needs to be employed in many patients with FHF. Unfortunately, increased cerebral edema and herniation have occurred with intermittent hemodialysis. The use of continuous hemodialysis methods is preferred, especially in those patients with high-grade hepatic encephalopathy or evidence of cerebral edema. A novel dialysis variant has recently been introduced which uses an albumin-containing dialysate to remove substances thought to contribute to the onset and progression of hepatorenal syndrome (40). Additional controlled randomized trials, with more robust clinical endpoints, need to be accomplished before this device is introduced into mainstream practice.

TREATMENT

Patients with FHF should be admitted to a liver transplant center. History, physical examination, and laboratory analysis can usually elucidate the etiology of the liver failure. The physical examination, in addition to identifying stigmata of chronic liver disease, should be directed at discerning signs of multiorgan involvement, especially of the central nervous system, renal system, coagulation, and nutritional status. Laboratory evaluation should include electrolytes, complete blood count (CBC), liver function tests, coagulation screen, arterial blood gas, viral hepatitis serology, copper studies, uric acid, plasma glucose, blood urea nitrogen, creatinine, drug and toxicology screens, and arterial ammonia.

Specific therapies for FHF are limited to antidotes for mushroom poisoning and *N*-acetylcysteine for acetaminophen overdose. Aggressive supportive management and liver transplantation in selected patients remains the backbone of therapy of patients with FHF.

Selective bowel decontamination is a protocol that sterilizes the patient's bowel of potentially pathogenic organisms (aerobic bacteria and fungi) while preserving potentially protective anaerobic flora (41). The loss of the liver's ability to clear gut-derived translocated bacteria and endotoxin can result in the circulation of these and other inflammatory mediators, and theoretically could initiate the systemic inflammatory response syndrome and multisystem organ failure. Some liver transplant centers have administered nonabsorbable antibiotics for selective bowel decontamination perioperatively. The results of bowel decontamination in these varied patient groups have been mixed.

Based on our data in patients with chronic liver disease and our clinical experience with patients with FHF, we recommend that protein supplementation be initiated in the early phases of illness. However, close attention needs to be paid to the patient's neurologic and renal status to limit exacerbation of hepatic encephalopathy and uremia secondary to protein supplementation. The use of branch-chain amino acids to promote protein anabolism and aid in the treatment of hepatic encephalopathy remains controversial.

All patients with FHF should receive vitamin-K supplementation (10 mg enterally for 3 days), gastric ulcer prophylaxis, and appropriate blood product transfusion to minimize bleeding complications. The use of sedative medication should be minimized to allow intermittent evaluation of neurologic status. Some data suggest that hepatic encephalopathy is enhanced by γ-aminobutyric acid (GABA) receptor stimulation. Flumazenil, a benzodiazepine and GABA antagonist, has been used with some success in providing temporary (minutes to hours) improvement in mental status in patients with FHF (42). Flumazenil administration may be useful as a diagnostic and prognostic tool. In one report, no patient who died within 48 hours of flumazenil challenge had improvement in mental status when flumazenil was administered.

Several transplant centers use grade of encephalopathy (Table 1) as a means of directing therapy. At our institution, with the development of grade 2 hepatic encephalopathy, the patient is transferred to an ICU. A baseline head CT scan is obtained and lactulose is administered. Parenteral or enteral nutrition is initiated, while plasma glucose is closely monitored. The patient is then systemically cultured and given selective bowel decontamination. Renal function is monitored (serum urea, creatinine, urine output), and volume status optimized with central venous pressure or pulmonary artery catheter monitoring. In patients with developing renal insufficiency, dopamine or fenoldopam might be helpful in supporting renal function. For patients in renal failure, hemodialysis is initiated in those who are candidates for liver transplantation.

If grade 3 hepatic encephalopathy develops, the patient's trachea is intubated, the head is placed in a midposition and elevated 30 degrees, and the neurosurgical service is contacted for ICP monitor placement. Current recommendations for ICP monitoring are a fiberoptic catheter placed epidurally or intraparenchymally. Following placement of the monitor, efforts should be made to maintain the ICP below 20 and the cerebral perfusion pressure above 60. If renal failure is not present, diuretic therapy (mannitol and furosemide) can be used until hyperosmolality (greater than 310 to 320 mOsm) is achieved. After hyperosmolality develops, or in the presence of renal failure, therapeutic options include hyperventilation (43), drug-induced coma (44), and moderate systemic hypothermia (45). Daily head CT scans should be obtained when feasible to rule out severe cerebral edema or intracranial hemorrhage.

If the patient progresses to grade 4 hepatic encephalopathy (Table 1), efforts should be made to detect evidence of irreversible brain injury. The monitors include ICP monitoring (recalcitrant intracranial hypertension), CT scanning (catastrophic lesion), electroencephalography, radiolabeled cerebral blood flow studies (no cerebral flow), and cerebral angiography (no intracranial flow).

MEDIATOR THERAPY

The failing liver resides in an environment of circulating soluble mediators, including cytokines, arachidonic-acid metabolites, and products of cytokine-activated cells, such as nitric oxide (46). Further hepatotoxicity results when these mediators are improperly cleared. Therapy for these patients, in whom these inflammatory substances are present in increased amounts, remains in an experimental phase. However, in the future, immunotherapies and receptor blockers against lipopolysaccharide, tumor necrosis factor, interleukin-1, and neutrophil surface antigens may have a role in the treatment of FHF. The inhibition of nitric oxide synthesis with arginine analogs may assist in the treatment of the failing liver and possibly may ameliorate the damaged liver's effect on other organ systems.

Selective bowel decontamination can be viewed as an indirect form of mediator therapy because the resultant reduction in bacterial translocation can reduce circulating endotoxemia. Another indirect form of mediator therapy is the new liver dialysis system. This device is modeled after charcoal hemoperfusion systems of years past (47). The device is specifically designed to remove mediators and toxins, including aromatic amino acids, fatty acids, phenols, mercaptans, and endogenous benzodiazepines. This device has been approved by the U.S. Food and Drug Administration and is currently undergoing clinical trials. Additionally, the extracorporeal albumin dialysis machine, previously discussed under "Renal Dysfunction and Failure," removes toxins which are thought to precipitate hepatorenal failure.

LIVER-SUPPORT DEVICES

In addition to the two devices discussed under "Mediator Therapy," whose primary purpose is the removal of mediators and toxins, there are two other machines currently under investigation, which have the potential of providing synthetic liver function. The device developed by Demetriou uses preserved porcine hepatocytes to provide detoxifying synthetic functions (48). This bioartificial liver machine recently underwent a controlled randomized trial, the results of which have not yet been published. However, the end result of this 162-patient multicenter trial is that, although there were differences in survival between the patients who were treated with the machine and those who were not, it did not reach statistical significance. In the future, a modified porcine bioartificial liver device will require reevaluation before it can be offered for general clinical use.

The second type of bioartificial liver device currently under investigation uses immortalized human hepatocytes. This device is currently undergoing multicenter investigation, the results of which are not yet available.

When an effective artificial liver-support device becomes available for clinical practice, it will be used primarily for patients with acute liver disease (FHF and primary nonfunction after unsuccessful liver transplantation). The device will be used as a bridge to allow time for liver regeneration or transplantation to occur.

LIVER TRANSPLANTATION

Orthotopic liver transplantation remains the treatment of choice for long-term survival in most patients with FHF. The United Network for Organ Sharing (UNOS) has published a 1-year patient survival rate of 63% for those receiving liver transplants for FHF (5). Survival figures from the pretransplant era ranged from 6% to 19%. Thus, despite the absence of a randomized control trial between liver transplantation and conservative medical management for patients with FHF, current data suggest that

liver transplantation has made an important contribution in the care of patients with this illness. The dilemma for the clinician caring for the patient with FHF is not only if, but when, to transplant. The goal is to allow enough time for liver regeneration to occur, while not waiting so long as to significantly compromise the patient's clinical status before transplantation (49–52). In one investigation, when transplantation was accomplished before the patient achieved grade 4 hepatic encephalopathy, 91% of the patients survived; if they achieved grade 4 encephalopathy, the survival rate was only 25% (53). A decision regarding liver transplantation must be made by a liver transplant team after discussions with the patient (if possible) and the patient's family and should be based on the patient's underlying disease and stage of hepatic encephalopathy.

An additional dilemma that the clinician caring for a patient with FHF often encounters is that of obtaining a liver after the decision to transplant has been made. FHF receives highest priority under the current UNOS guidelines. However, with growing liver transplant candidate lists across the United States, the availability of organs is decreasing. In fact, of the estimated 2,000 individuals who develop FHF annually in the United States, only 200 to 300 receive a liver transplant. Hence, alternatives to orthotopic liver transplantation as the treatment of choice must be developed. Potential alternatives include hepatocyte transplantation (54), xenografting, and living-related liver transplantation. Hepatocyte transplantation is currently in the experimental stage with human subjects. Xenografting has been attempted with some temporary success (55). Genetic strategies are being explored that would alter the immunogenetic character of laboratory animals to make them more useful for transplantation in the future. Living-related liver transplantation is a procedure that is currently being implemented with some success (56). This concept was developed in Japan where cadaveric transplantation was not possible until very recently. Living-related donation uses a right lobe hepatectomy from the donor with transplantation orthotopically to the recipient. Thus far, results have been satisfactory for both donor and recipient when this technique is used in cases of chronic and acute hepatic failure.

SUMMARY

Patients with FHF provide the intensivist with the challenge of caring for a patient who, in the best of circumstances, may have a 63% chance for survival. Although there are some similarities between FHF and chronic liver disease, the differences are extremely important to understand. The goal of the intensivist is to diligently support what function the failing liver has, while meticulously caring for the other organs at risk of failure. The patient would benefit most from a situation that would allow a proper amount of time for liver regeneration to occur (possibly with the help of liver-support devices), and yet, not permit so much time as to allow for the development of multiorgan system failure, which would greatly complicate liver transplantation. Orthotopic transplantation remains the best opportunity for long-term survival for most patients with FHF. Future long-term alternatives will be required as cadaveric organ pools are depleted by an overwhelming demand.

KEY POINTS

Fulminant hepatic failure (FHF) is a catastrophic condition that progresses more quickly and virulently than an exacerbation of chronic hepatic dysfunction. FHF is a multiorgan disease. In addition to the hepatic system, it may involve the cardiovascular, renal, pulmonary, neurologic, immunologic, and hematologic systems. Intracranial hypertension is a frequent cause of mortality. Orthotopic liver transplantation remains the treatment of choice for long-term survival. With depletion of the cadaveric organ pool, alternative therapies will need to be developed for long-term survival.

REFERENCES

1. Trey C, Davidson CS. The management of fulminant hepatic failure. In: Popper H, Schaffner F, eds. *Progress in liver diseases.* Vol III. New York: Grune & Stratton, 1970;282–298.
2. Lee WM. Acute liver failure. *N Engl J Med* 1993;329:1862–1872.
3. Hoofnagle JH, Carithers RL, Shapiro C, et al. Fulminant hepatic failure: summary of a workshop. *Hepatology* 1995;21:240–252.
4. Rakela J, Lange SM, Ludwig J, et al. Fulminant hepatitis; Mayo Clinic experience with 34 cases. *Mayo Clin Proc* 1985;60:289–292.
5. United Network for Organ Sharing (UNOS). Available at: http://www.unos.org. Accessed October 17, 2001.
6. Schiodt FV, Rochling FG, Casey DL, et al. Acetaminophen toxicity in an urban county hospital. *N Engl J Med* 1997;337:1112–1117.
7. Danan G, Bernuau J, Moullot X, et al. Amitriptyline-induced fulminant hepatitis. *Digestion* 1984;30:179–184.
8. Rabinovitz M, Van Theil DH. Hepatotoxicity of nonsteroidal, anti-inflammatory drugs. *Am J Gastroenterol* 1992;87:1696–1704.
9. Floersheim GL. Treatment of human amatoxin mushroom poisoning. Myths and advances in therapy. *Med Toxicol* 1987;2:1–9.
10. Ruprah M, Mant TGK, Flanagan RJ. Acute carbon tetrachloride poisoning in 19 patients: implications for diagnosis and treatment. *Lancet* 1985;1:1027–1029.
11. Ngindu A, Johnson BK, Kenya PK, et al. Outbreak of acute hepatitis caused by aflatoxin poisoning in Kenya. *Lancet* 1982;1:1346–1348.
12. Markin RS, Linder J, Zuerlein K, et al. Hepatitis in fatal infectious mononucleosis. *Gastroenterology* 1987;93:1210–1217.
13. Shusterman NH, Frauenhoffer C, Kinsey MD. Fatal massive hepatic necrosis in cytomegalovirus mononucleosis. *Ann Intern Med* 1978;88:810–812.
14. Purtilo DT, White R, Filipovich A, et al. Fulminant liver failure induced by adenovirus after bone marrow transplant [Letter]. *N Engl J Med* 1985;312:1707–1708.
15. Sandle GI, Layton M, Record CO, et al. Fulminant hepatic failure due to Budd-Chiari syndrome. *Lancet* 1980;1:1199.
16. Woods WG, Dehner LP, Nesbit ME, et al. Fatal veno-occlusive disease of the liver following high dose chemotherapy, irradiation and bone marrow treatment. *Am J Med* 1980;68:285–290.
17. Roche-Sicot J, Benhamou J-P. Acute intravascular hemolysis and acute liver failure associated as a first manifestation of Wilson's disease. *Ann Intern Med* 1977;86:301–303.
18. Larner AJ, Dyer RG, Burke DA, et al. Fulminant hepatic failure complicating exertional heatstroke with rhabdomyolysis. *Eur J Gastroenterol Hepatol* 1993;5:55–58.
19. Yamanaka N, Okamoto E, Kuwata K, et al. A multiple regression equation for prediction of posthepatectomy liver failure. *Ann Surg* 1984;200:658–663.
20. Amon E, Allen SR, Petrie RH, et al. Acute fatty liver of pregnancy associated with preeclampsia: management of hepatic failure with postpartum liver transplantation. *Am J Perinatol* 1991;8:278–279.
21. Crocker JFS. Reye's syndrome. *Semin Liver Dis* 1982;2:340–352.
22. Beal AL, Cerra FB. Multiple organ failure syndrome in the 1990s. *JAMA* 1994;271:226–233.
23. Clemmesen JO, Larsen FS, Kondrup J, et al. Cerebral herniation in patients with acute liver failure is correlated with arterial ammonia concentration. *Hepatology* 1999;29:648–653.
24. Ware AJ, D'Agostino AN, Combes B. Cerebral edema: a major complication of massive hepatic necrosis. *Gastroenterology* 1971;61:877–884.
25. Aggarwal S, Kramer D, Yonas H, et al. Cerebral hemodynamic and metabolic changes in fulminant hepatic failure: a retrospective study. *Hepatology* 1994;19:80–87.
26. Strauss G, Hansen BA, Kirkegaard P, et al. Liver function, cerebral blood flow autoregulation, and hepatic encephalopathy in fulminant hepatic failure. *Hepatology* 1997;25:837–839.
27. Blei AT, Olafsson S, Webster S, et al. Complications of intracranial pressure monitoring in acute liver failure. *Lancet* 1993;341:157–158.
28. Lidofsky SD, Bass NM, Prager MC, et al. Intracranial pressure monitoring and liver transplantation for fulminant hepatic failure. *Hepatology* 1992;16:1–7.
29. Wijdicks EFM, Plevak DJ, Rakela J, et al. Clinical and radiologic features of cerebral edema in fulminant hepatic failure. *Mayo Clin Proc* 1995;70:119–124.
30. Kowalski HJ, Abelmann WH. The cardiac output at rest in Laennec's cirrhosis. *J Clin Invest* 1953;32:1025–1033.
31. Bihari D, Gimson AE, Waterson M, et al. Tissue hypoxia during fulminant hepatic failure. *Crit Care Med* 1985;13:1034–1039.
32. Krowka MJ. Clinical management of hepatopulmonary syndrome. *Semin Liver Dis* 1993;13:414–422.
33. Pernambuco JRB, Langley PG, Hughes RD, et al. Activation of the fibrinolytic system in patients with fulminant liver failure. *Hepatology* 1993;18:1350–1356.
34. Kang Y. Coagulation and liver transplantation. *Transplant Proc* 1993;25:2001–2005.
35. Plevak D, Divertie G, Carton E, et al. Blood product transfusion therapy after liver transplantation: comparison of the thromboelastogram and conventional coagulation studies. *Transplant Proc* 1993;25:1838.
36. Callery MP, Kamei T, Mangino MJ, et al. Organ interactions in sepsis: host defense and the hepatic-pulmonary macrophage axis. *Arch Surg* 1991;126:28–32.
37. DiCecco SR, Wieners EJ, Wiesner RH, et al. Assessment of nutritional status of patients with end-stage liver disease undergoing liver transplantation. *Mayo Clin Proc* 1989;64:95–102.
38. Plevak DJ, DiCecco SR, Wiesner RH, et al. Nutritional support for liver transplantation: identifying caloric and protein requirements. *Mayo Clin Proc* 1994;69:225–230.
39. Bihari D, Gimson A, Lindridge J, et al. Lactic acidosis in acute liver failure. Some aspects of pathogenesis and prognosis. *J Hepatol* 1985;1:405–416.
40. Mitzner SR, Stange J, Klammt S, et al. Improvement of hepatorenal syndrome with extracorporeal albumin dialysis MARS: results of a prospective, randomized, controlled clinical trial. *Liver Transpl* 2000;6:277–286.
41. Heyland DK, Cook DJ, Jaeschke R, et al. Selective decontamination of the digestive tract: an overview. *Chest* 1994;105:1221–1229.
42. Ferenci P, Grimm G. Benzodiazepine antagonist in the treatment of human hepatic encephalopathy. *Adv Exp Med Biol* 1990;272:255–265.
43. Ede RJ, Gimson AES, Bihari D, et al. Controlled hyperventilation in the prevention of cerebral oedema in fulminant hepatic failure. *J Hepatol* 1986;2:43–51.
44. Forbes A, Alexander GJM, O'Grady JG, et al. Thiopental infusion in the treatment of intracranial hypertension complicating fulminant hepatic failure. *Hepatology* 1989;10:306–310.

45. Jalan R, Damink SWMO, Deutz NEP, et al. Moderate hypothermia for uncontrolled intracranial hypertension in acute liver failure. *Lancet* 1999;354:1164–1168.
46. Curran RD, Billiar TR, Stuehr DJ, et al. Multiple cytokines are required to induce hepatocyte nitric oxide production and inhibit total protein synthesis. *Ann Surg* 1990;212:462–471.
47. Silk DBA, Trewby PN, Chase RA, et al. Treatment of fulminant hepatic failure by polyacrylonitrile-membrane haemodialysis. *Lancet* 1977;2:1–3.
48. Watanabe FD, Mullon CJ-P, Hewitt WR, et al. Clinical experience with a bioartificial liver in the treatment of severe liver failure: a phase I clinical trial. *Ann Surg* 1997;225:484–494.
49. Shakil AO, Kramer D, Mazariego GV, et al. Acute liver failure: clinical features, outcome analysis and applicability of prognostic criteria. *Liver Transpl* 2000;6:163–169.
50. Karvountzis GG, Redeker AG. Relation of alpha-fetoprotein in acute hepatitis to severity and prognosis. *Ann Intern Med* 1974;80:156–160.
51. Lee WM, Galbraith RM, Watt GH, et al. Predicting survival in fulminant hepatic failure using serum Gc protein concentrations. *Hepatology* 1995;21:101–105.
52. O'Grady JG, Alexander GJM, Hayllar KM, et al. Early indicators of prognosis in fulminant hepatic failure. *Gastroenterology* 1989;97:439–445.
53. Daas M, Plevak DJ, Wijdicks EFM, et al. Acute liver failure: results of a 5-year clinical protocol. *Liver Transpl Surg* 1995;1:210–219.
54. Bilir BM, Guinette D, Karrer F, et al. Hepatocyte transplantation in acute liver failure. *Liver Transpl* 2000;6:32–40.
55. Starzl TE, Fung J, Tzakis A, et al. Baboon-to-human liver transplantation. *Lancet* 1993;341:65–71.
56. Miwa S, Hashikura Y, Mita A, et al. Living-related liver transplantation for patients with fulminant and subfulminant hepatic failure. *Hepatology* 1999;30:1521–1526.

42

PERIOPERATIVE RENAL PROTECTION

H.T. LEE
ROBERT N. SLADEN

KEY WORDS

- Adenosine
- Angiotensin-converting enzyme (ACE) inhibitors
- Atrial natriuretic peptide (ANP)
- Autoregulation
- Calcium channel blockers
- Creatinine
- Cyclosporin A
- Dialysis
- Diuretics: loop; furosemide; mannitol
- Dopamine/dopexamine
- Fenoldopam
- Nitric oxide
- Norepinephrine
- Tubular function tests: creatinine clearance; fractional excretion of sodium
- Vasomotor nephropathy
- Vasopressin

INTRODUCTION

Perioperative acute renal failure (ARF) remains one of the most feared entities in the intensive care unit (ICU) (1–3). Modern dialytic techniques are extremely efficient in controlling uremia, hyperkalemia, acidosis, and fluid overload with relative hemodynamic stability. Despite therapeutic advances, the mortality and morbidity of ARF have changed little over the last three decades despite intensive research focus in both basic and clinical sciences. Several factors may be responsible.

The pathophysiology of ARF is extremely complex and is only partially understood. The surgical population consists of a steadily increasing proportion of older adult patients who have major comorbidity. Surgical interventions are increasingly radical (e.g., ventricular-assist devices as a bridge to cardiac transplantation) so that the severity of insults is increasing in the perioperative and ICU setting. Consequently, ARF as a single disease entity is becoming rarer; it is often associated with or progresses into multiple-organ dysfunction syndrome.

Experimental models in basic research may be too simple. For example, nitric oxide (NO) has been shown to have a renal protective role *in vivo* via its favorable renovascular effects (4). However, NO induces apoptosis *in vitro* and NO antagonists are actually renal protective *in vitro* (5,6). This exemplifies the problems associated with applying clear-cut basic research into more complex clinical problems. Renal protection remains our best weapon to prevent the enormous impact on resources, morbidity, and mortality caused by ARF.

ETIOLOGY AND PATHOPHYSIOLOGY OF PERIOPERATIVE ACUTE RENAL FAILURE

Etiology of Acute Renal Failure

The etiology of perioperative ARF is outlined in Table 1. Ischemic or nephrotoxic acute tubular necrosis (ATN) accounts for about 80% to 90% of perioperative renal failure (7). Renal vascular injury is usually secondary to blunt trauma. Markedly increased intraabdominal tension dramatically reduces renal blood flow (RBF) and glomerular filtration rate (GFR) (8–12). Bilateral arterial thrombosis occurs in the setting of diffuse atherosclerosis, while bilateral renal vein thrombosis is associated with intraabdominal malignancy and hypercoagulable states. Atheromatous or cholesterol renal artery embolization occurs in older, diabetic males when friable plaque is dislodged by arteriography, aortic cross-clamp, or even simple coughing (13).

Preexisting renal insufficiency (GFR 25 to 50 mL per minute) may deteriorate into ARF with relatively minor hemodynamic perturbations. A preoperative plasma creatinine (P_{Cr}) greater than 2.0 mg per dL is a highly significant predictor of postoperative ARF following major surgery (14,15). Subclinical renal involvement in systemic diseases (e.g., vasculitides, systemic lupus erythematosus, sickle cell anemia) may become overt with the stress of trauma or surgery. Acute interstitial nephritis is uncommon, but may be induced by nonsteroidal antiinflammatory drugs (NSAIDs) or by hypersensitivity to certain antibiotics (e.g., ampicillin, rifampicin), with serum sickness and eosinophilia. Acute poststreptococcal glomerulonephritis is rare, but a similar entity has been described after staphylococcal or gram-negative infections.

Pathogenesis of Acute Renal Failure

Paradigms of Renal Injury and Failure

The pathophysiology of ARF is described in terms of paradigms (models) based on physiological and biochemical concepts that provide the rationale for prophylactic and therapeutic interventions.

TABLE 1. ETIOLOGY OF PERIOPERATIVE ACUTE RENAL FAILURE (ARF)

Acute tubular necrosis (ATN)
  Ischemic
  Nephrotoxic

Vasomotor nephropathy (refractory prerenal syndromes)
  Septic shock
  Hepatorenal syndrome

Renal vascular injury
  Traumatic
  Abdominal compartment syndrome (venous hypertension)
  Thromboembolism
    Arterial thrombosis
    Venous thrombosis
    Atheromatous embolism

Acute or chronic renal failure
Systemic disease
  Vasculitis, systemic lupus erythematosus, sickle cell anemia

Acute interstitial nephritis
Acute glomerulonephritis

The most well-established model is the hemodynamic–nephrotoxic paradigm, which dictates that renal injury is caused by direct ischemic or nephrotoxic insults, and that optimization of blood flow to the kidney and urine flow is important in protecting against ARF (3). A modification of this is the oxygen supply-demand paradigm (16), which highlights the imbalance of intrarenal blood flow between the renal cortex (which has an ample blood supply) and medulla (which has a precarious blood supply). ARF results when there is increased oxygen consumption (VO_2) and/or decreased oxygen delivery (DO_2) in the most hypoxia-susceptible portion of the kidney. In addition, there are two closely related syndromes that exacerbate hemodynamic and nephrotoxic injury: vasomotor nephropathy (pathologic renal vasoconstriction) and loss of autoregulation (pathologic systemic vasodilation).

The cell fate paradigm focuses on the fate of an individual polarized tubular cell after it is injured and reveals a cascade of events that occur within a cell and determines whether its fate will be apoptotic (programmed) or necrotic (disruptive) cell death. An understanding of these intracellular events could lead to the development of alternative therapeutic strategies (17). The interactive cell biology paradigm dictates that the kidney is an anatomically and physiologically complex organ and renal cells interact with each other when challenged with injury (3).

Pathogenesis of Acute Tubular Necrosis

The Hemodynamic Paradigm

Initiation of Injury. Experimental animal models of ATN often use an intraarterial infusion of norepinephrine or interruption of renal arterial blood flow. The nature of the resulting ischemic injury is related to the duration of renal vasoconstriction or renal ischemia. An infusion of short duration (less than 60 minutes) or minimal ischemic time (less than 25 minutes) results in oliguria but no anatomic damage to the renal tubules, and subsequently renal function returns to normal (1). This is akin to "prerenal failure" (i.e., hemodynamically mediated oliguria which is re-

versed by restoration of normal RBF). An intermediate duration (60 to 120 minutes) infusion or more severe ischemic time (25 to 45 minutes) causes ischemic damage to the metabolically active tubular cells, although the basic renal architecture remains preserved. Oliguria persists and progressive azotemia follows. This is analogous to the clinical entity of ATN. Although oliguria is not reversed by restoring RBF to normal, full renal recovery can occur after several days in the absence of further insults. A prolonged infusion (greater than 120 minutes) or ischemia (greater than 60 minutes) causes renal infarction, cortical necrosis, and irreversible ARF.

A long-standing debate among nephrologists regarding the primacy of vasoconstriction versus tubular dysfunction in the genesis of ATN remains unsettled. Proponents of the latter point out that a sustained reduction in RBF to 40% to 50% of normal is sufficient to induce ATN, but GFR declines to less than 10% of normal, and remains low when normal RBF is restored (18). The luminal cells of the proximal tubule (especially the S3 segment) are highly metabolically active and susceptible to ischemic injury (19). Necrotic cells slough and obstruct the tubular lumen, causing proximal intraluminal hypertension which impedes glomerular filtration. Ischemic damage to the tubular basement membrane induces back-leak of filtrate into the renal interstitium, which correlates closely with the severity of the renal insult (1,20).

Perpetuation of Injury. After the initial tubular insult, a state of low GFR is sustained by vasoconstriction mediated by tubuloglomerular feedback via the juxtaglomerular apparatus. Tubuloglomerular feedback modulates blood pressure, salt and water homeostasis, and renal autoregulation (21,22). In ATN, active reabsorption in the medullary thick ascending limb of the loop of Henle (mTAL) is impaired and intratubular chloride concentration increases. Chemoreceptor cells in the macula densa of the distal tubule (which abuts on the afferent arteriole) trigger the release of renin. Renin cleaves angiotensinogen to angiotensin I, which in turn is hydrolyzed to the octapeptide angiotensin II by angiotensin-converting enzyme (ACE). Angiotensin II constricts the afferent arterioles and the mesangial cells of the glomerular tuft, which decreases glomerular surface area and GFR.

Elevated plasma renin activity is a marker for protracted renal failure requiring dialysis (23). On the other hand, renin-induced reductions in GFR decrease tubular oxygen consumption (VO_2), induce oliguria, conserve intravascular volume, and protect the organism from dehydration in ATN, a response referred to as "acute renal success" (24).

The Oxygen Supply-Demand Paradigm

Brezis and colleagues have postulated an alternative hypothesis for the pathogenesis of ATN (25) based on the observation that the renal medulla receives only 6% of the total RBF, extracts about 80% of delivered oxygen (DO_2), and has a very low tissue oxygen tension. Medullary blood flow is maintained by adenosine-mediated vasoconstriction in the cortex and prostaglandin and NO-induced vasodilation in the medulla. The mTAL contains the energy-dependent, sodium-potassium adenosine triphosphatase (ATPase) pump responsible for medullary hypertonicity. It is therefore very vulnerable to medullary hypoxemia, which may occur even when cortical blood flow is marginally reduced.

The initial response to renal hypoperfusion is increased mTAL sodium chloride absorption to attempt to restore intravascular volume, which increases tubular VO_2 in the face of decreased tubular DO_2. Continued mTAL hypoxia impairs active sodium chloride absorption and results in the tubuloglomerular feedback described above.

In experimental ATN, the prior administration of saline, diuretics (mannitol, furosemide), or vasodilators (dopamine, prostaglandins) attenuates ischemic injury to the kidney. Tubular injury and back-leak is considerably less; oliguria does not occur and recovery is relatively rapid (18). Nonoliguric ARF is the most common form of ATN: in most clinical situations the kidney is subjected to multiple lesser insults in a protected environment. Moreover, "conversion" of oliguric into nonoliguric ARF significantly eases the management of patients with ARF. Unfortunately, current clinical outcomes of both oliguric and nonoliguric forms of ARF are both poor.

Gelman suggests that therapeutic interventions in renal insufficiency should be directed at enhancing mTAL oxygen balance (26). Tubular DO_2 should benefit from increased cardiac output, RBF, and arterial oxygen content, while tubular VO_2 could be decreased by inhibition of the ATP-consuming sodium pump with diuretics, such as furosemide. However, it appears that renal DO_2 and VO_2 differ markedly from global circulatory indices. Decreased renal DO_2 did not cause tubular damage in septic sheep, perhaps because the decrease in GFR decreased mTAL work and VO_2, thereby maintaining medullary oxygen balance (27).

Vasomotor Nephropathy

The term vasomotor nephropathy implies renal dysfunction due to impaired renal vasomotor control, although intrinsic renal injury can be a late consequence. In some conditions (e.g., ARF [28], severe sepsis [29], and possibly cardiopulmonary bypass [30]), autoregulation is lost or attenuated. Thus, hypotension results in a dramatic decrease in RBF that is restored by normalization of renal perfusion pressure, even if achieved by vasoconstrictor therapy.

Acute Renal Failure. In established ARF there is an almost complete loss of renal autoregulation (28). Thus, when intermittent hemodialysis causes hypotension, it represents an intermittent ischemic renal insult that may delay or even prevent renal recovery from ATN. There is animal evidence that the renal vasculature is relatively unresponsive to the vasoconstrictor effect of norepinephrine in ATN (31). The implication is that perfusion pressure should be maintained by vasoconstrictor drugs during hemodialysis (see below). Hemodynamically unstable patients in ARF should receive continuous venovenous hemodialysis (CVVHD) so as to minimize further insults to the kidney and increase the likelihood of renal recovery.

Septic (Vasodilated) Shock. Elevated cardiac index and peripheral vasodilation characterize sepsis. However, endotoxin and activated mediators, including tumor necrosis factor, endothelin, thromboxane A_2, prostaglandin F_2, and leukotrienes induce afferent arteriolar constriction and direct nephrotoxic injury (32). This results in an intense prerenal state with oliguria and very low urinary sodium (U_{Na}) excretion. The severity of vasomotor

nephropathy correlates with the severity of sepsis and plasma renin activity (33). Loss of autoregulation in severe sepsis is implicated by the dramatic improvement in oliguria and renal function that may be observed when hypotension is reversed by vasopressor therapy.

Similar responses may be seen in states of vasodilated shock induced by contact activation of the inflammatory cascade by protracted cardiopulmonary bypass (CPB) or insertion of a ventricular-assist device (VAD).

Liver Failure (Hepatorenal Syndrome). Patients with end-stage liver failure often develop oliguria and progressive renal insufficiency, termed hepatorenal syndrome. Hepatocellular failure results in portosystemic endotoxemia and renal vasoconstriction. Thus, like sepsis, a prerenal syndrome occurs in the face of elevated cardiac index and decreased systemic vascular resistance (SVR) (i.e., oliguria with a U_{Na} less than 10 mEq per L). However, unlike sepsis, vasopressor therapy may exacerbate renal function, perhaps because renal injury is also related to ascites, which decreases intravascular volume and increases renal vein pressure. Fluid loading, inotropic support, and portosystemic shunting improve renal function. Interestingly, kidneys from donors dying in liver failure function successfully when transplanted into recipients with normal liver function, indicating that this is a disorder of renal milieu rather than primary renal disease (34). Ultimately, renal recovery is dependent on improvement of liver function or orthotopic liver transplantation (35).

Nephrotoxic (Drug-Induced) Vasomotor Nephropathy. The intrarenal vasodilator prostaglandins, PGE_2 and prostacyclin (PGI_2), counteract the vasoconstrictor and salt-retaining actions of the renin-angiotensin-aldosterone axis and have a protective role during renal stress (36). NSAIDs such as indomethacin, ibuprofen, naproxysyn, and ketorolac reversibly inhibit cyclooxygenase and intrarenal vasodilator prostaglandin synthesis for 8 to 24 hours. (Aspirin irreversibly acetylates cyclooxygenase but the kidney restores it within 24 to 48 hours.) Inhibition of prostaglandin synthesis decreases medullary perfusion and creates the potential for mTAL ischemia. Even so, nephrotoxic renal injury is extremely rare with an isolated nephrotoxin in a hemodynamically stable state (e.g., a young, healthy, well-hydrated patient). The risk of renal injury increases exponentially with an increasing number of nephrotoxic insults in a hemodynamically compromised environment (e.g., an older adult, dehydrated patient with chronic renal insufficiency) (37).

ACE inhibitors (e.g., captopril, enalapril, lisinopril) or angiotensin-II receptor antagonists (e.g., losartan) suppress compensatory efferent arteriolar constriction induced by angiotensin II with hypovolemia or decreased RBF. Administration of these agents to patients with hypotension, renal insufficiency, or unilateral renal artery stenosis risks acute deterioration in GFR and hyperkalemia (38). It is prudent to avoid their use for the treatment of hypertension or for afterload reduction in the immediate perioperative period in patients who have evidence of inadequate intravascular volume or renal insufficiency.

Immunosuppression with cyclosporin A inevitably results in some degree of hypertension and renal vasoconstriction mediated in part through sympathetic activation. Achievement of adequate immunosuppression requires acceptance of chronic mild to moderate renal insufficiency (i.e., serum creatinine 1.5 to 2.0 mg per dL). The vasomotor basis for cyclosporin A nephrotoxicity is supported by evidence of renal protection conferred by vasodilator therapy with calcium blockers (diltiazem) (39) or dopaminergic agonists (dopamine, fenoldopam) (40).

Natural History of Perioperative Acute Renal Failure

Hemodynamic events that precipitate ischemic ATN include hypovolemic, cardiogenic, and septic shock, circulatory arrest, cardiopulmonary bypass, and aortic cross-clamping. Any stress resulting in activation of the sympathoadrenal and renin-angiotensin systems may induce cortical and tubular ischemia. The kidney is relatively devoid of beta$_2$-receptors so that the alpha-adrenergic effects of endogenous or exogenous epinephrine induce unopposed vasoconstriction. Sympathoadrenal responses may be a compensatory attempt to redistribute blood flow to the relatively hypoxic renal medulla, but at the expense of inducing cortical ischemia (25). Coexistent nephrotoxic insults exacerbate tubular ischemic injury and hasten the onset of ATN (Table 2).

Myers and Moran postulated three clinical patterns of postoperative renal injury (Fig. 1) (23). Pattern A describes a single, limited episode of complete renal ischemia (e.g., suprarenal aortic cross-clamping). A short-lived, attenuated form of ATN may develop, but renal recovery follows after 24 to 48 hours. In pattern B, renal function declines and recovers in parallel with improved cardiac output (e.g., in a patient with reversible myocardial dysfunction after cardiac surgery). In pattern C, renal recovery is interrupted by superadded ischemic and nephrotoxic insults, particularly sepsis, resulting in dialysis-dependent ARF and a high mortality. The clinical corollary is that appropriate renal protection could prevent prerenal failure developing into ATN or even cortical necrosis, thus avoiding dialysis and its attendant morbidity and mortality. Using the Myers model, the analogy would be to prevent pattern A or B from deteriorating to pattern C. However, in many situations we have little control over the degree of renal injury.

TABLE 2. NEPHROTOXINS

Endogenous Nephrotoxins	Exogenous Nephrotoxins
Bilirubin[a]	Radiocontrast dyes
Myoglobin[a]	Fluoride (methoxyflurane, enflurane)
Hemoglobin (red cell stroma)[a]	Aminoglycoside antibiotics
Uric acid	Cyclosporin A
	Cisplatinum
	Amphotericin B
	Low molecular weight dextrans
	NSAIDs

[a]Pigment nephropathy.
NSAIDs, nonsteroidal antiinflammatory drugs.
Note: The risk of nephrotoxicity is low with a single insult in a healthy, well-hydrated patient, but increases exponentially with the number of nephrotoxic insults and the number of renal risk factors (e.g., diabetes, congestive heart failure, chronic renal insufficiency, hypovolemia, etc.).

IDENTIFICATION OF THE HIGH-RISK PATIENT

The primary goal of preoperative assessment is to identify the patient who is at high risk for perioperative ARF (41).

Preexisting Renal Insufficiency

In the presence of preexisting renal insufficiency (Table 1) relatively mild insults can precipitate ARF. Renal reserve is depleted in patients with one kidney, but preoperative blood urea nitrogen (BUN) and P_{Cr} may be normal. GFR declines progressively with advancing age, from about 125 mL per minute in young adults to about 80 mL per minute at age 60 and about 60 mL per minute at age 80. However, P_{Cr} does not usually increase until GFR falls below 50 mL per minute. In older adult or cachectic patients with depleted muscle mass, creatinine generation is so slight that P_{Cr} remains subnormal despite a GFR as low as 25 mL per minute (42).

After cardiac surgery the incidence of ARF increases from 2% to 4% to more than 10% when preoperative P_{Cr} is 1.9 mg per dL or greater (14). An even greater increase in the incidence of postoperative ARF with preoperative renal dysfunction is seen in patients undergoing suprarenal aortic cross-clamping (43). Patients who developed ARF had an in-hospital mortality of 63.2%, compared with 3% in patients without ARF.

Genetic Polymorphism and Predisposition to Acute Renal Failure

Certain patients may be genetically predisposed to (or protected from) the development of perioperative ARF. A recent study of cardiac surgical patients at Duke University (44) found that individuals with the epsilon-4 allele of apolipoprotein E (APOE) had lower postoperative peak P_{Cr} (but higher risk of neurologic abnormalities) compared with those with the epsilon-2 and epsilon-3 allele. This suggests that genetic polymorphism may play a role in determining the organ response to ischemic insults.

High-Risk Procedures and Events (Table 3)

Cardiac Surgery

ARF is uncommon in patients with previously normal renal function who have uncomplicated surgery and good cardiac function after CPB. The mortality in patients who develop hemodialysis-dependent ARF, however, is formidable (45). In a study at Duke University on 2,672 consecutive patients undergoing coronary revascularization, fewer than 0.7% developed hemodialysis-dependent ARF, but in these patients mortality increased from 1.8% to 28% (46). Development of postoperative renal dysfunction alone appears to be associated with a significantly worse outcome (46,47); in the Duke study a postoperative increase in P_{Cr} of ≥ 1.0 mg per dL above baseline was associated with a 14% mortality.

Cardiopulmonary bypass implies low renal perfusion pressure, nonpulsatile blood flow, release of renal vasoconstrictors (e.g., angiotensin, thromboxane), and tubular enzymuria. This suggests that CPB may consistently induce a subclinical renal injury not

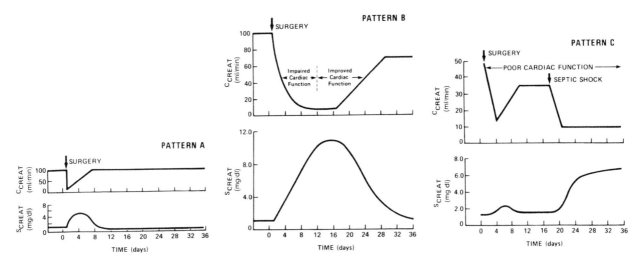

FIGURE 1. Patterns of postoperative acute renal failure. These three diagrams illustrate pattern types of renal dysfunction after surgery. In each case, C_{creat} indicates creatinine clearance in mL per minute and S_{creat} indicates serum creatinine in mg per dL. **Pattern A:** The diagram indicates the renal insult typically provided by suprarenal cross-clamping (i.e., abbreviated acute renal failure). There is an abrupt (step) decrement in creatinine clearance followed by a linear (ramp) incremental recovery over the next 7 days. Note that serum creatinine is still rising on days 3 and 4, while renal function is actually recovering. This emphasizes the usefulness of measuring creatinine clearance as a prognostic indicator of renal function. Renal recovery is complete. **Pattern B:** Renal dysfunction secondary to impaired cardiac function (e.g., after complex cardiac surgery). There is an exponential decrement in creatinine clearance associated with a linear increase in serum creatinine on days 1 to 12. After day 12, cardiac function recovers and results in a ramp increment in creatinine clearance and a sigmoidal decline in the serum creatinine. Renal recovery is incomplete, but dialysis is not required. **Pattern C:** Multiple renal insults. Creatinine clearance undergoes a ramp decrement after surgery because of poor cardiac function. From days 4 to 10, partial recovery occurs, but it is interrupted by the onset of septic shock on day 18. A further ramp decrement in creatinine clearance results in protracted acute renal failure, which requires dialysis. In this situation, mortality is between 60% and 90%. (From Myers BD, Moran SM. Hemodynamically mediated acute renal failure. *N Engl J Med* 1986;314:97–105, with permission.)

modified by hypothermia or mannitol (48). Nevertheless, the most important determinants of ARF after CPB are preexisting renal insufficiency (14), and postoperative low cardiac output states (49). Pulsatile CPB flow (which decreases plasma renin activity) (50) or low-dose dopamine (51) does not prevent tubular enzymuria or appear to have any protective effect in patients with previously normal renal function (50,52,53). Anecdotal reports suggest a favorable effect of pulsatile CPB in the presence of renal

insufficiency (54), but controlled studies in high-risk patients are necessary.

Vascular Surgery

Patients undergoing major vascular surgery often have coexistent renovascular disease with a mean preoperative creatinine clearance (C_{Cr}) of about 60 mL per minute (55). Preoperative angiography exposes patients to the danger of nephrotoxicity from intravascular contrast dyes, which induce an osmotic diuresis that worsens hypovolemia and delays diagnosis. The risk is exacerbated by diabetes, hypovolemia, congestive heart failure, and myeloma (56). Patients who develop radiocontrast-induced ARF after interventional or diagnostic procedures have had a mortality rate as high as 34% (57). Renal protection may be provided by nonionic low osmolality contrast dyes, hydration (58), intravenous mannitol (59), calcium blocking agents (60), oral N-acetylcysteine (61), or by deferring elective surgery at least 3 to 5 days after radiocontrast studies.

Suprarenal aortic cross-clamping induces a time-dependent ischemic renal injury. The incidence of ARF is not affected by pump bypass, atriorenal bypass, perfusion with cold Ringer lactate, or ACE inhibitors, although renal endarterectomy does protect patients with preexisting renal dysfunction (43). In a study using mannitol protection, GFR was still only 23 mL per minute 2 hours after suprarenal cross-clamp release, compared with 60 mL per minute in patients undergoing infrarenal

TABLE 3. RISK FACTORS FOR PERIOPERATIVE RENAL FAILURE

Advanced age
Preexisting renal insufficiency
  Congestive heart failure
  Diabetic nephropathy
  Hypertensive nephropathy
  Liver failure (hepatorenal syndrome)
  Pregnancy-induced hypertension
  Systemic disease (e.g., scleroderma, systemic lupus erythematosus)

Sepsis
Shock
High-risk procedures
  Renal revascularization
  Aortic cross-clamping
  Cardiopulmonary bypass
  Urologic procedures
  Transplantation

Nephrotoxins (see Table 2)

cross-clamping. GFR remained depressed for 48 hours, with evidence of tubular injury suggesting an attenuated form of ATN (55). The authors infer that mannitol pretreatment prevents a more severe renal injury. However, in animal studies, saline-loading, mannitol, dopamine, or a mannitol-dopamine combination was unable to prevent a 30% to 50% decrease in renal function after thoracic aortic cross-clamping (62).

Infrarenal aortic cross-clamping may also adversely affect renal function. Palpation of the renal arteries to detect stenosis may itself induce reflex spasm. During aortic dissection prior to infrarenal cross-clamping, GFR decreases as much as 30% from baseline (55). With cross-clamping RBF decreases about 40% and urine flow about 25% even without significant systemic hemodynamic changes, probably through renin-angiotensin activation (63). Infrarenal aortic cross-clamping increases SVR about 40%, which is well tolerated in patients with normal left ventricular function. However, in patients with impaired cardiac function or myocardial ischemia aortic cross-clamping is associated with a significant increase in pulmonary artery occluded pressure (PAOP) and decrease in cardiac output, which could result in decreased RBF (64).

Several other mechanisms of renal injury occur in major vascular surgery. Ulcerating atherosclerotic intimal plaque can be dislodged into the renal arteries by adjacent cross-clamping or surgical manipulation and cause embolic renal infarction and irreversible ARF (13). Hemodynamic instability caused by aneurysmal rupture, prolonged hypotension after aortic cross-clamp release ("declamping shock"), myocardial ischemia, or bleeding appears to be the most important predictors of postoperative ARF after major vascular surgery (43). Oliguric ARF occurs in about one-third of patients after ruptured aortic aneurysm, either as an immediate consequence of circulatory shock, or as a later component of sequential multiorgan system failure and sepsis. When this occurs, in-hospital mortality approaches 90%.

Biliary Tract and Hepatic Surgery

Preoperative obstructive jaundice or established liver failure are important risk factors for postoperative renal dysfunction. The gut excretion of bile salts, which bind and inactivate endotoxins, effectively ceases in the presence of severe cholestasis (i.e., conjugated bilirubin greater than 8 mg per dL). Endotoxin is absorbed into the portal circulation and induces intense renal vasoconstriction (vasomotor nephropathy). Preoperative oral administration of bile salts (e.g., sodium taurocholate) or intravenous mannitol appears to limit renal impairment in surgical patients with obstructive jaundice (65). Endotoxin-induced vasomotor nephropathy likely also accounts for the renal dysfunction associated with liver failure (hepatorenal syndrome). Progressive azotemia is associated with urine sodium concentration equal to 20 mEq per L, suggesting intact renal tubular function and prerenal failure.

Patients with severe hepatic disease are very susceptible to relatively minor renal insults, including diuretic-induced hypovolemia or vasoconstrictor therapy. Patients who present for liver transplantation with severe liver failure are at particular risk of perioperative ARF. Some degree of hepatorenal syndrome may be coexistent. Circulatory instability is more likely because of coag-

ulopathy and bleeding, and all patients receive the nephrotoxic immunosuppressive agent, cyclosporin A.

Urogenital Surgery and Complicated Obstetrics

Surgical or traumatic disruption of the urogenital tract predisposes to partial or complete obstruction and urinary tract infection. Peripartum causes of ARF include circulatory shock, which may complicate peripartum hemorrhage or amniotic fluid embolism, or pregnancy-induced hypertension (PIH, preeclampsia). In the latter, renal involvement is characterized by diffuse vascular constriction and fibrinoid necrosis of arterioles. The classic triad of PIH is hypertension, edema, and proteinuria, but the degree of renal insufficiency is quite variable. Of note, in the third trimester cardiac output is increased, C_{Cr} may reach 150 to 180 mL per minute, and BUN is normally 5 to 8 mg per dL and P_{Cr} is 0.5 mg per dL. "Normal" values such as BUN 12 mg per dL or P_{Cr} 1 mg per dL indicate early renal insufficiency.

Trauma, Intraabdominal Hypertension, and Rhabdomyolysis

ARF is a relatively uncommon, but crucial complication of major trauma. It may occur as a result of direct renal trauma, hemorrhagic shock, rhabdomyolysis, mismatched transfusion, elevated intraabdominal pressure, or as a component of trauma-induced systemic inflammatory response syndrome (SIRS) and multiple-organ dysfunction. In a review of 72,757 admissions to nine trauma centers, only 78 patients developed dialysis-dependent ARF, an incidence of 0.01%; however, the overall mortality was 58% (66). About one-third of patients developed ischemic ARF within 1 week. In the remainder it occurred later, at about 3 weeks, associated with multiorgan system failure, which accounted for 82% of all deaths. Older adult patients with preexisting medical conditions had a higher mortality than their healthier counterparts, developed ARF with a lower Injury Severity Score, and had a high incidence of fatal multiorgan system failure.

Severe abdominal distension, usually caused by bleeding, may be associated with oliguria and deteriorating renal function. In animal models elevation of intraabdominal pressure greater than 20 mm Hg sharply decreases cardiac output, RBF, and GFR to about 25% of normal (9). Renal dysfunction is probably due to direct compression of the kidneys or increases in renal vein pressure (67). Intraabdominal pressure may be indirectly measured at the bedside by transducing it via a filled and clamped Foley catheter. The finding of a high pressure may be an indication for laparotomy and abdominal decompression, which quickly restores renal function (8,10–12).

Major crush injury, thermal injury, or compartment syndromes often cause muscle edema, ischemia and necrosis (rhabdomyolysis). Rhabdomyolysis also occurs with acute muscle ischemia, prolonged immobilization, protracted fever, status epilepticus, myoclonus, severe exercise, acute pancreatitis, and in association with acute alcohol or cocaine intoxication. Rhabdomyolysis results in the release of myoglobin, about one-fourth the size of hemoglobin and rapidly filtered by the glomerulus. Nephrotoxic ATN may occur when myoglobin precipitates in the proximal tubule under conditions of hypovolemia (i.e., low tubular flow) and acidic urine (pH less than 6). Acidity alters myoglobin from an anion to a cation, increasing its glomerular filtration and conversion to acid hematin, which reacts with tubular protein and precipitates in the proximal tubule (68).

Unless there is a high index of suspicion, rhabdomyolysis and myoglobinemia may not be diagnosed before causing irreversible renal damage, which is more likely to occur in a well-muscled individual with normal GFR than in a cachectic patient with low GFR. The affected muscle may appear obviously ischemic, or swollen, painful, and edematous, and urine may be red. However, all these signs may be absent. The test for urine myoglobin is qualitative, not quantitative, and may intermittently become negative because myoglobin is so rapidly cleared by the kidney. Quantitative studies of myoglobin indicate that a serum myoglobin of greater than 400 μg per L, urine myoglobin of greater than 1,000 ng per mL, and myoglobin clearance of less than 4 mL per minute are predictors of myoglobinemic ARF (69). Serial estimations of total creatinine phosphokinase (CPK) are a useful guide to the severity and progress of rhabdomyolysis and potential for renal damage (70). We have rarely encountered renal dysfunction when total CPK is less than 10,000 U per dL.

DETECTION OF RENAL DYSFUNCTION IN THE INTENSIVE CARE UNIT

Urine Flow Rate and Oliguria

Urine flow rate is not a reliable index of renal function: ARF may occur without oliguria, and oliguria may occur without ARF. Although oliguria is the most important clinical sign of renal dysfunction, it is a normal response to hypovolemia. In the ICU, oliguria should be assumed to be hemodynamically mediated and potentially reversible (i.e., prerenal) until proven otherwise. Complete cessation of urinary flow suggests mechanical obstruction of the urinary tract or catheter system.

Oliguria itself is a relative term. Oliguric ARF is defined by a urine flow of less than 400 mL per day (15 mL per hour). Functional oliguria, in the sense of the lowest acceptable urine flow rate, is usually defined as less than 0.5 mL per kg per hour. However, in many situations a much higher urine flow rate is anticipated or desired. For example, after mannitol has been administered during cardiac or neurosurgery, urine flow should exceed 2.0 mL per kg per hour—lower flow could be considered relative oliguria.

Tubular Function Tests and the Evaluation of Oliguria

Tests of renal tubular function may help to differentiate prerenal oliguria (i.e., relative or absolute hypovolemia) from ATN (Table 4). Volume depletion stimulates normal renal tubules to conserve water and salt, resulting in concentrated urine with low sodium. When tubular conserving function is lost, the urine becomes dilute and high in sodium. However, in nonoliguric ARF urine, studies are intermediate between ATN and prerenal azotemia. In vasomotor nephropathy due to the hepatorenal syndrome or sepsis, a prerenal syndrome occurs despite a

TABLE 4. EVALUATION OF OLIGURIA

	Prerenal	ATN
U:P osmolality	>1.4:1	1:1
U:P creatinine	>50:1	<20:1
Urine Na (mEq/L)	<20	>80
FENa (%)	<1	>3
C_{Cr} (mL/min)	15–20	<10

U:P, urine:plasma; Na, sodium; FENa, fractional excretion of sodium; ATN, acute tubular necrosis; C_{Cr}, creatinine clearance.

hyperdynamic circulation, and is very resistant to attempts to enhance intravascular volume.

Potent diuretics (e.g., furosemide, mannitol, low-dose dopamine) may overcome tubular conserving function and render urine studies unable to be interpreted. However, a study on hydrated and nonhydrated patients prior to cardiac surgery demonstrated striking differences in the renal response to low-dose dopamine (71). Patients hydrated with intravenous saline before anesthesia had expected increases in urine volume, sodium excretion, and free water clearance, but fluid-restricted patients did not respond to dopamine at all. Urine osmolality in the nonhydrated group was 749 mOsm per kg compared with 374 mOsm per kg in the hydrated group, suggesting that tubular conservation mechanisms induced by preoperative fluid restriction can overcome the saliuretic effect of low-dose dopamine.

Tubular Concentrating Ability

Tubular concentrating ability, as measured by the urine to plasma osmolar ratio (U:P Osm), is a sensitive index of tubular function. In prerenal oliguria the U:P Osm exceeds 1.5:1; whereas isosthenuria (U:P Osm = 1.0) suggests established ATN. The ability to concentrate urine may be lost 24 to 48 hours before serum creatinine or BUN starts to increase.

Free water clearance (CH_2O) expresses tubular concentrating ability by incorporating clearance techniques, but does not really provide any more information than U:P Osm and requires a timed urine collection.

The urine to plasma creatinine ratio (U:P$_{Cr}$) is another useful and simply derived index of tubular function, and represents the proportion of water filtered by the glomerulus that is abstracted by the distal tubule, normally about 98%. In prerenal states U:P$_{Cr}$ may be as high as 100:1, but in ATN the ratio declines to less than 20:1. For example, a P$_{Cr}$ of 2.0 mg per dL and a urinary creatinine (U$_{Cr}$) of 100 mg per dL suggest that oliguria is prerenal (U:P$_{Cr}$ = 50:1). If the U$_{Cr}$ were only 20 mg per dL, it would suggest ATN (U:P$_{Cr}$ = 10:1).

Sodium Conservation

In prerenal states the urine sodium (U$_{Na}$) declines to less than 20 mEq per L. In established ATN, the ability to conserve sodium is lost, and U$_{Na}$ exceeds 60 to 80 mEq per L. Diuretic therapy given in a prerenal state may overwhelm tubular sodium conservation, resulting in a high U$_{Na}$ despite normal tubular function. However, U$_{Na}$ may remain low despite low-dose dopamine administration in hypovolemic patients, testifying to the avidity of tubular sodium reabsorption.

The fractional excretion of sodium (FE_{Na}) expresses sodium clearance as a percentage of C_{Cr}:

$$FE_{Na} = U_{Na}/P_{Na} \times 100\%/U_{Cr}/P_{Cr} \qquad (Eq.\ 1)$$

where U_{Na} = urine sodium, P_{Na} = plasma sodium, U_{Cr} = urine creatinine, and P_{Cr} = plasma creatinine. Thus, the FE_{Na} may be calculated from a spot sample of blood and urine.

During dehydration or hypovolemia, sodium clearance and FE_{Na} decrease to less than 1% of C_{Cr}. In ARF the tubular ability to conserve sodium is lost and FE_{Na} increases to greater than 3%. However, an increased FE_{Na} is a normal response to diuretic therapy and postoperative salt and water mobilization. Sequential increases in FE_{Na} associated with declining C_{Cr} more reliably indicate deteriorating renal function than an isolated, high FE_{Na}.

Creatinine Clearance

Creatinine, an end-product of creatine phosphate metabolism, is normally generated from muscle at a uniform rate and is primarily filtered by the glomerulus. When renal function is stable, P_{Cr} is a useful clinical guide to the GFR, but it becomes unreliable when renal function is rapidly changing (72). The P_{Cr} represents the equilibrium between endogenous creatinine production and urinary excretion. If creatinine excretion were to suddenly cease (i.e., GFR = zero), P_{Cr} would initially appear normal, then rise at a variable rate dependent on its production. After a transient renal insult (e.g., suprarenal aortic cross-clamping), P_{Cr} may increase for a few days while GFR is actually recovering (55).

The relationship between P_{Cr} and GFR is inverse and exponential. P_{Cr} usually does not rise above normal until the GFR declines less than 50 mL per minute. An apparently innocuous increase in serum creatinine from 0.8 to 1.6 mg per dL implies a 50% decrease in GFR. Even with steady-state renal function, P_{Cr} may be a misleading index of GFR. Perioperative fluid administration increases total body water and dilutes P_{Cr}. In a cachectic patient with low muscle mass, P_{Cr} may remain less than 0.9 mg per dL in the face of a GFR less than 25 mL per minute (42).

Nomograms such as the Cockroft-Gault equation use age, weight, gender, and P_{Cr} to estimate GFR (73):

$$GFR\ (males) = (140 - age) \times weight\ (kg)/(P_{Cr} \times 72)$$
$$(Eq.\ 2)$$

$$GFR\ (females) = above \times 0.85 \qquad (Eq.\ 3)$$

In obese or edematous patients, the Cockroft-Gault equation overestimates GFR because total body weight is greater than lean body mass. In cachectic patients with depleted lean body mass, P_{Cr} less than 1.0 mg per dL may also result in overestimated GFR. Accuracy is improved by using calculated ideal body weight and correcting low P_{Cr} to 1.0 mg per dL (74). However, the Cockroft-Gault equation is subject to the same limitations as P_{Cr} in tracking rapid changes in GFR.

C_{Cr} is defined as the virtual volume of plasma cleared of creatinine per unit time, in mL per minute:

$$C_{Cr} = U_{Cr} \times V/P_{Cr} \qquad (Eq.\ 4)$$

TABLE 5. CREATININE CLEARANCE

Value[a]	Implication
150–180	Last trimester, compensated sepsis, early trauma
120	Normal (healthy 20-year-old)
80	Normal (healthy 60-year-old)
25–50	S_{Cr} may become abnormal,[b] adjust drug dosages
15–25	Prerenal uremia, nonoliguric ARF
<10	Oliguric ARF

S_{Cr}, serum creatinine; ARF, acute renal failure
[a]Usually expressed as mL/min/1.73M^2.
[b]Note that creatinine clearance may decrease by more than 50% from baseline before S_{Cr} starts to rise above normal values. In cachectic patients with low creatinine production, S_{Cr} may not increase above normal until creatinine clearance decreases to less than 30 mL/min/M^2.

where V = urinary flow rate in mL per minute. Note that C_{Cr} incorporates the creatinine excretion rate ($U_{Cr} \times V$).

In clinical practice, the 2-hour C_{Cr} provides a rapid and useful bedside assessment of GFR, particularly when renal function is changing (Table 5). It is not the duration of urine collection that is critical to the C_{Cr}, but its precise timing and volume measurement (75). Two-hour C_{Cr} in catheterized patients with urine flow greater than 15 mL per hour correlates well with values obtained with 12- to 24-hour urine collections (42,76) (Fig. 2). The C_{Cr} provides earlier warning of renal dysfunction than the P_{Cr} and is a reliable prognostic guide. In trauma patients undergoing surgery, Shin and associates (as cited by Bjornsson) found that a 1-hour C_{Cr} less than 25 mL per minute within 6 hours was the most reliable predictor of subsequent renal dysfunction or failure (72).

Normal C_{Cr} shows considerable fluctuation, including diurnal variation, and creatinine generation varies with muscle mass, physical activity, protein intake, and catabolism (77,78). Loss of variation is characteristic of renal dysfunction. Substances and drugs that interfere with creatinine assay by the Jaffe reaction

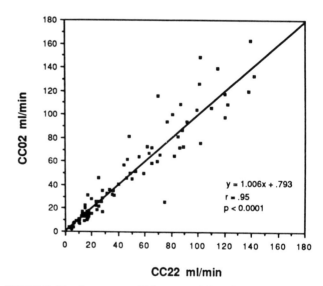

FIGURE 2. Two-hour versus 22-hour creatinine clearance. There is a close and significant correlation in creatinine clearance estimation from a 2-hour and 22-hour urine collection. *CC02*, 2-hour urine collection; *CC22*, 22-hour urine collection. (From Sladen RN, Endo E, Harrison T. Two-hour versus 22-hour creatinine clearance in critically ill patients. *Anesthesiology* 1987;67:1013–1016, with permission.)

include glucose, protein, ketones, ascorbic acid, barbiturates, cephalosporins, trimethoprim, and H2-antagonists. Because creatinine is secreted by the proximal tubule, C_{Cr} overestimates GFR by about 20%. As the GFR declines, tubular secretion of creatinine increases so that when GFR is less than 40 mL per minute the error may exceed 100% (72). When P_{Cr} is very high, it is excreted into the gut and undergoes metabolism by intestinal organisms. Nonetheless, serial estimations of C_{Cr} provide a useful clinical guide to alterations in renal function. At low levels of GFR even a 200% disparity between C_{Cr} and actual GFR (e.g., 12 versus 6 mL per minute), would require little change in clinical management.

STRATEGIES TO PREVENT OR TREAT RENAL INJURY

Potential strategies for renal protection are summarized in Table 6. They include enhancement of renal DO_2 to vulnerable regions, suppression of reflex vasoconstrictor responses, pharmacologic renal vasodilation, maintenance of tubular flow, and decreased tubular VO_2. When renal autoregulation is lost, restoration and maintenance of normal renal perfusion pressure is essential.

Of all these approaches, the simplest and most effective is the suppression of reflex vasoconstrictor responses by intravenous volume expansion. This helps to maintain cardiac output, the most important determinant of renal perfusion, since 25% of the cardiac output goes to the kidneys. Also, atrial distension secondary to fluid administration results in the release of endogenous atrial natriuretic peptide (ANP), an inducer of salt and water excretion and potential renal protective agent (2,3).

Early institution of appropriate hemodynamic and urinary monitoring is essential to identify and treat intravascular hypovolemia and oliguria. A urine flow rate of at least 0.5 to 1.0 mL per kg per hour is desirable. Oliguria is a normal response to intravascular hypovolemia and postoperative oliguria should be considered to be prerenal until otherwise proven. In fact, probably 75% of cases of ARF in the ICU are nonoliguric (urine flow rate 15 to 80 mL per hour). Thus, oliguria does not imply ARF and a

TABLE 6. STRATEGIES FOR RENAL PROTECTION

- Enhance RBF[a]
  Increase DO_2 to vulnerable regions
- Suppress reflex vasoconstrictor responses
  Stimulate endogenous ANP release by fluid challenge
- Pharmacologic renal vasodilation
  Dopaminergic agents, calcium channel blockers, ANP
- Maintain tubular flow and prevent tubular obstruction
  Fluid administration, mannitol
- Decrease tubular VO_2 and enhance oxygen balance
  Loop diuretics (suppress Na-ATPase pump)
- Restore renal perfusion pressure when autoregulation impaired/lost
  Norepinephrine, vasopressin

RBF, renal blood flow; DO_2, oxygen delivery; ANP, atrial natriuretic peptide; VO_2, oxygen consumption; Na, sodium; ATP, adenosine triphosphate.
[a]Enhance RBF by enhancing cardiac output, because 25% of the cardiac output goes to the kidneys.

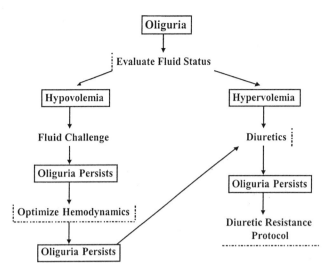

FIGURE 3. Management of oliguria. Steps in the management of oliguria should follow a logical progression. Evaluation of fluid status should incorporate clinical assessment (e.g., mucous membranes, orthostasis, neck veins, etc.), urinalysis (urine specific gravity, urine sodium, etc.), chemistry (blood urea nitrogen:creatinine ratio), and invasive hemodynamic monitoring, if present.
Evidence (or suspicion) of hypovolemia warrants serial fluid challenges. If oliguria persists, hemodynamics should be optimized with the aid of invasive monitoring (central venous, pulmonary artery catheter) if necessary. The goal is to maximize cardiac output by stabilizing rate and rhythm, optimizing preload and applying inotropic support. If afterload is excessive, it should be decreased by inodilator or vasodilator therapy. If it is inadequate (i.e., vasodilated shock), it should be normalized by vasoconstrictors. If oliguria persists in the face of normal hemodynamic function, administer a diuretic (dopaminergic agents, loop diuretics). If oliguria persists, initiate the Diuretic Resistance Protocol outlined in Table 7.
If evaluation of fluid status reveals normal or hypervolemic intravascular volume status, administer a diuretic (dopaminergic agents, loop diuretics). If oliguria persists, initiate the Diuretic Resistance Protocol outlined in Table 7. (From Sladen RN. Oliguria in the ICU. Systematic approach to diagnosis and treatment. *Anesth Clin North Am* 2000;18:739–752, with permission.)

"normal" urinary flow rate does not exclude it. A clinical algorithm for the management of oliguria is illustrated in Fig. 3.

Pulmonary artery catheterization is indicated when close monitoring of intravascular volume status is vital or difficult to interpret by central venous pressure (CVP) alone. Examples include preexisting renal dysfunction, respiratory failure, congestive heart failure, severe lung disease, capillary leak syndromes, septic shock, major trauma, and after prolonged CPB. Standard principles of hemodynamic management should be applied: normalization of cardiac rhythm and rate, augmentation of preload by adequate maintenance and replacement fluids, judicious use of inotropic support, and afterload reduction with vasodilator or inodilator agents.

Pharmacologic Interventions

Diuretics

Loop Diuretics
Loop diuretics, such as furosemide, may confer renal protection by decreasing the metabolic work of the mTAL, by inducing renal cortical vasodilation, and by "flushing" obstructing tubular casts

TABLE 7. STRATEGIES FOR DIURETIC RESISTANCE

- Restore normal hemodynamics (CO, RBF, perfusion pressure)
- Administer higher doses of diuretic agents
    Example: furosemide 80–120 mg, bumetanide 2.5–5 mg i.v.
    (doses of furosemide $\geq$240 mg i.v. induce venodilation and
    increase the risk of ototoxicity)
- Concomitant administration of human albumin
    Useful in hypoalbuminemia—albumin is necessary for furosemide
    delivery to the tubules
- Continuous diuretic infusion
    Maintains tubular drug concentration just above diuretic threshold,
    avoiding evanescent peaks (and potential toxic effects) associated
    with bolus dosing
    Example: furosemide 40 mg i.v. load, followed by 2–10 mg/h
    infusion (requires close monitoring to avoid hypovolemia,
    electrolyte imbalance)
- Segmental nephron blockade (loop diuretic + thiazide)
    Loop diuretic blocks Na^+ reabsorption at mTAL, thiazide blocks
    compensatory reabsorption downstream at DT
    Example: bumetanide 5 mg i.v. + metolazone 5 mg p.o.
    (metolazone, a thiazide-type diuretic, has unpredictable GI
    absorption and should be administered at least 1 h prior to the
    parenteral loop diuretic)

CO, cardiac output; RBF; renal blood flow; mTAL, medullary thick ascending limb; DT, distal tubule; GI, gastrointestinal.

through the nephron. Loop diuretics can increase U_{Na} and water excretion even in the presence of marked renal impairment (79).

In animal models, prior administration of furosemide provides protection against ischemic or nephrotoxic insults (18), probably by renal cortical vasodilation or decreased preglomerular vascular resistance through inhibition of tubuloglomerular feedback. Increased tubular flow may "wash out" nephrotoxins and cellular debris and prevent tubular obstruction. Inhibition of the mTAL sodium-potassium-ATP pump, which decreases active tubular sodium chloride transport and tubular VO_2, may confer resistance against ischemic insults.

In clinical practice, loop diuretics are usually given *after* rather than before a renal insult. For any therapeutic effect to be obtained they must be given within 18 hours of the ischemic and/or toxic event. In states of low GFR, delivery of furosemide to the renal tubules is impaired, so high doses are required to effect a diuresis (80); this may defer or even avoid the need for dialysis. In 1977, Anderson and colleagues reported that 18 of 54 patients had converted from oliguric to nonoliguric ARF after receiving high-dose (2 to 10 mg per kg) furosemide intravenously, with a reduction in mortality from 50% to 26% (81). However, patients with shock and perioperative ARF were specifically excluded, and it has not been demonstrated that high-dose furosemide alters the natural history of ARF once dialysis is required (3,82).

In fact, there is no clinical evidence that loop diuretics alter the outcome of perioperative ARF (83). Conversion of oliguric ARF to nonoliguric ARF may ease ICU patient management by attenuating volume overload and hyperkalemia, and allow more fluid (e.g., total parenteral nutrition) to be given to the patient. Although the conversion does not alter the natural history of the disease, it suggests that patients who respond to furosemide may simply have a less severe renal injury.

Administration of large doses of furosemide to a patient with oliguria due to hypoperfusion may have several unwanted effects.

Furosemide may worsen radiocontrast-induced ARF (84). Severe systemic venodilation may cause hypotension. Any diuresis evoked will exacerbate hypovolemia. Nephrotoxins (e.g., aminoglycosides) are concentrated at the renal tubule. High-dose furosemide (greater than 1 g per day i.v.) may cause ototoxicity and the large infusion volume may precipitate pulmonary edema (3). Use of furosemide to maintain high tubular flow rates is less controversial in situations where cellular debris or pigments may cause tubular obstruction and damage (e.g., intravascular hemolysis or rhabdomyolysis).

Mannitol

Mannitol is an "inert" sugar that is not metabolized, remains largely confined to intravascular space, and is directly excreted by the kidneys. It may confer renal protection by several mechanisms, but for greatest effect it should be present at the time of the insult. Its potent osmotic activity expands the intravascular volume and increases ventricular preload, cardiac output, RBF, and GFR. Atrial distension stimulates ANP (85). By preventing water reabsorption in the proximal tubules, mannitol diminishes tubular obstruction. Osmotic hemodilution may protect against the "no-reflow" phenomenon caused by swelling of ischemic endothelium and red cell aggregation (86). Mannitol may attenuate reperfusion injury by scavenging free radicals, and increase the activity of vasodilator intrarenal prostaglandins, notably prostacyclin (PGI_2) (87). On the other hand, mannitol may increase renal tubular oxygen demand because osmotic diuresis increases solute delivery to the renal tubules.

In high-risk situations, 6.25 to 12.5 g (25 to 50 mL of a 25% solution) is given 10 to 20 minutes prior to a defined insult (for example, aortic cross-clamping) and repeated if necessary every 4 to 6 hours. Alternatively, a continuous infusion of 5% to 10% mannitol may be given at 50 mL per hour. The solution must be warmed if crystallization has occurred. Rapid administration can precipitate pulmonary edema by excessive expansion of the intravascular space. To avoid a hyperosmolar syndrome (serum osmolality greater than 320 mOsm per kg), the maximum cumulative dose in a 24-hour period should be no greater than 1.5 g per kg (88).

Prophylactic administration of mannitol prior to aortic cross-clamping has been widely used for nearly 30 years. However, in a saline-loaded canine model of thoracic aortic cross-clamping, neither mannitol, dopamine, or a mannitol-dopamine combination prevented a 50% to 70% decline in GFR and RBF after release of the cross-clamp (62). Gamulin and colleagues continuously infused 20% mannitol at 100 mL per hour in 12 patients undergoing infrarenal aortic cross-clamping (63). Despite mannitol, a 38% decrease in RBF and a 75% increase in calculated renal vascular resistance persisted 1 hour after cross-clamp release. Urine flow decreased from 4 to 3 mL per minute. Since there were no controls, it is not known whether mannitol prevented renal injury. In mannitol-protected patients, Myers and associates demonstrated that suprarenal cross-clamping caused a "mini-ATN," with decreased GFR and loss of tubular concentrating ability (55). One to two hours after cross-clamp release, GFR was still only 23 mL per minute, compared with 60 mL per minute in patients undergoing infrarenal cross-clamping. This lesion took about 48 hours to resolve. The authors inferred that mannitol pretreatment prevented more severe and sustained renal injury.

CPB entails low perfusion pressure and nonpulsatile blood flow, which elicit the release of renal vasoconstrictors, including catecholamines, vasopressin, renin-angiotensin, and thromboxane. The presence of microalbuminuria and tubular enzymuria suggest that CPB induces a subclinical renal injury (48). Nonetheless, the incidence of ARF after uncomplicated CPB in patients with previously normal renal function is only 1% to 3%. The two most important risk factors for ARF after cardiac surgery are a preoperative P_{Cr} greater than 1.9 mg per dL (14) and postoperative cardiac dysfunction. The routine addition of mannitol to the CPB prime for renal protection washes out the hypertonic renal medulla and renders the kidney incapable of concentrating urine. In the early postoperative period an osmotic diuresis of 200 to 400 mL per hour may ensue, exacerbating hypovolemia and hypokalemia. Persistence of isosthenuria for more than a few hours indicates tubular injury and predicts postoperative renal dysfunction.

Osmotic diuresis with mannitol has been advocated for many years to protect against nephrotoxic injury, including that associated with radiocontrast dyes (59), rhabdomyolysis, and obstructive jaundice. However, if the intravascular volume lost is not repleted, osmotic diuresis with mannitol may actually exacerbate nephrotoxic injury (84).

In experimental glycerol-induced myoglobinuric ARF, mannitol confers renal protection through osmotic diuresis and increased tubular flow (89). In the clinical treatment of rhabdomyolysis, mannitol is used with intravenous hydration (with or without furosemide) to keep urine flow greater than 100 mL per hour. Urinary alkalinization (pH greater than 5.6) decreases the conversion of myoglobin to toxic acid hematin.

In severe cholestasis the excretion of bile salts, which bind and inactivate gut organism endotoxins, effectively ceases, resulting in portal septicemia and renal damage (90). The risk of postoperative renal dysfunction is particularly high when preoperative jaundice is greater than 8 mg per dL (90). In a review of 12 surgical series including over 2,000 patients with obstructive jaundice, the incidence of postoperative ARF ranged from 4% to 18%, with a mean mortality of 76% (91). Preoperative oral administration of the bile salt sodium taurocholate appears to be as effective as mannitol in preventing renal impairment (65).

In summary, mannitol may have a role in protecting kidneys when added to preservation solutions during renal transplantation (87). It may improve outcome in crush injury and subsequent myoglobin-induced renal dysfunction when administered early. However, mannitol administration is contraindicated in volume-depleted patients (unless volume is aggressively restored) and in patients with poor left ventricular function (where it may precipitate pulmonary edema).

Dopaminergic Agonists

For many years, it was believed that there were two subtypes of dopamine (DA) receptors, termed DA_1 and DA_2 (51). However, molecular cloning has demonstrated that there are at least two subtypes of DA_1 and three subtypes of DA_2 receptors (92). Stimulation of DA_1 receptors situated in the renal and splanchnic vas-

culature causes vasodilation and increased RBF and GFR. In the proximal tubules, DA_1 receptors activate adenylate cyclase and phospholipase C, which culminates in inhibition of active sodium reabsorption leading to natriuresis and diuresis (93). Stimulation of DA_2 receptors, situated on the presynaptic terminal of postganglionic sympathetic nerves innervating renal blood vessels, inhibits release of norepinephrine and blunts vasoconstriction. Based on the receptor subtypes, dopaminergic agonists and antagonists may be categorized as selective or nonselective. For example, dopamine is a mixed DA_1 and DA_2 agonist; fenoldopam is a selective DA_1 agonist; and haloperidol, chlorpromazine, and metoclopramide are nonselective dopaminergic antagonists (94).

Dopamine

Low-dose dopamine (0.5 to 3.0 μg per kg minute) acts as a nonselective dopaminergic agonist (95). At moderate doses (3 to 10 μg per kg per minute) its beta$_1$-adrenergic effect may induce unwanted tachycardia and at doses greater than 10 μg per kg per minute its alpha-adrenergic effect causes progressive renal vasoconstriction. Its favorable effects on renal function may be mediated by renal vasodilation (DA_1, DA_2 effect) or increased cardiac output (beta$_1$ effect), but its predominant clinical action appears to be as a tubular saliuretic (DA_1 effect) (96).

In equiinotropic doses after cardiac surgery, dopamine and dobutamine had similar effects on GFR and RBF; however, dopamine caused greater urine flow (2.8 versus 1.0 mL per minute) and FE_{Na} (2.5% versus 0.7%), suggesting stimulation of tubular DA_1 receptors (97). In hemodynamically stable patients with normal renal function, low-dose dopamine (200 μg per minute) appeared to have only a diuretic effect, without an improvement in C_{Cr} (96). In contrast, low-dose dobutamine (175 μg per minute) consistently improved C_{Cr} without a diuretic effect, presumably through its inotropic action.

Dopamine is indicated as a diuretic whenever urine output is low (less than 0.5 mL per kg per hour), despite restoration of stable systemic hemodynamics. As a saliuretic, dopamine could protect the renal tubules by suppressing the sodium pump, decreasing VO_2, and increasing tubular flow. However, there are relatively few data that suggest that prophylactic administration of low-dose dopamine protects the kidney from injury, although it increases renal clearance of aminoglycosides (98), reverses low RBF caused by oral cyclosporin A (79), and counteracts the renal damage induced by recombinant interleukin-2 therapy for metastatic urologic cancer.

The role of dopamine in protecting against renal injury in aortic or cardiac surgery is more equivocal. Low-dose dopamine did not improve RBF, GFR, or urine flow during thoracic aortic cross-clamping in dogs (62). In humans, mannitol and dopamine substantially increased urine flow and sodium excretion during infrarenal cross-clamping, but had no better effect on GFR depression than fluid loading to a PAOP of 12 to 15 mm Hg (99). In 37 euvolemic patients with normal renal function after elective, major vascular abdominal surgery, who were given sufficient crystalloid to maintain a urine flow greater than 1 mL per kg per hour, adding low-dose dopamine did not confer any additional benefit (100).

The prophylactic administration of low-dose dopamine during CPB in patients with normal or mildly abnormal preoperative renal function undergoing uncomplicated coronary revascularization has not been demonstrated to enhance urine flow, C_{Cr}, or CH_2O, or prevent transient renal impairment and enzymuria (53,101). The conclusion has been that low-dose dopamine is ineffective in patients with renal dysfunction undergoing cardiac surgery (102). However, it must be acknowledged that because the incidence of postoperative ARF is less than 2% in low-risk patients, most studies on normal patients are underpowered to detect a significant benefit conferred by dopamine.

In a retrospective study on patients undergoing orthotopic liver transplantation, prophylactic low-dose dopamine decreased the incidence of dialysis-dependent ARF from 27% to 9.5% of patients (103). In contrast, a subsequent controlled, prospective study failed to find that it had any benefit on intraoperative urine flow, postoperative C_{Cr}, ARF, or mortality (104). Grundmann and coworkers randomized 50 cadaveric kidney graft recipients into two equal groups; one received 2 μg per kg per minute dopamine for 4 days (105). Although the dopamine group had higher urine flow, C_{Cr} and requirement for dialysis were identical. Moreover, dopamine often caused tachycardia.

When potent inotropic agents (e.g., epinephrine, norepinephrine) are administered to septic or other hemodynamically unstable patients, low-dose dopamine is often given concurrently in the belief that this confers renal protection. There is some animal evidence to support this practice. In anesthetized dogs given a norepinephrine infusion (0.2 to 1.6 μg per kg per minute), the addition of a dopamine infusion (4.0 μg per kg per minute) increased RBF by 40% to 50% above that with norepinephrine alone (106).

Low-dose dopamine has often been added to furosemide therapy in patients with unresponsive oliguria, but most studies have been anecdotal and uncontrolled. In a review of nine such studies encompassing 144 subjects published between 1970 and 1984, dopamine (1.0 to 4.0 μg per kg per minute) increased mean urine flow from 15 to 80 mL per hour (107). To be effective, it appears that dopamine must be administered within 24 hours of the onset of oliguria (108). In 15 adult patients after cardiac surgery with oliguria (urine flow $\sim$20 mL per hour) and mild renal dysfunction ($C_{Cr} \sim$ 65 mL per minute), low-dose dopamine increased urine flow to $\sim$50 mL per minute and C_{Cr} to $\sim$110 mL per minute (109). In 19 surgical ICU patients who remained oliguric despite fluid resuscitation to stable hemodynamics, low-dose dopamine did not change hemodynamics, but increased mean urinary output from 0.29 to 1.04 mL per kg per hour (110). Urine flow decreased when dopamine was stopped and increased when it was restarted.

In patients with chronic renal disease, dopamine has a diuretic effect, but does not significantly increase GFR or RBF when the baseline GFR is less than 50 mL per minute per 1.73 M^2 (110).

Recent reviews have discouraged the routine use of low-dose dopamine (92). After cardiac surgery dopamine, even at low-doses, increases the incidence of supraventricular and ventricular arrhythmias (111). It is now apparent that this is due to the wide interindividual variability in the pharmacologic handling of dopamine. In a study in human volunteers, MacGregor and associates found a 27-fold variability in the range of plasma dopamine levels (112). In some individuals, infusion of "low-dose" dopamine resulted in plasma levels in the alpha-adrenergic range. Thus, it is likely that when a clinical benefit is seen, it is as much due to dopamine's inotropic effect in increasing renal blood flow and perfusion pressure as it is to its dopaminergic effect.

In conclusion, low-dose dopamine may have a role in increasing urine flow in early oliguric renal failure. Although it is a useful diuretic and/or inotropic agent, it has no proven efficacy in preventing or improving renal outcome in the perioperative period.

Dopexamine

Dopexamine, a synthetic analog of dopamine, is a potent beta$_2$-agonist with about one-third the dopaminergic effect of dopamine. Unlike dopamine, dopexamine has minimal effect at beta$_1$-adrenoceptors and no alpha-adrenoceptor activity. It increases heart rate and acts as an inodilator (inotropic agent with arterial vasodilation). Used in the dose range of 1 to 5 μg per kg per minute, dopexamine provides left and right ventricular afterload reduction in acute and chronic heart failure, while augmenting RBF through its dopaminergic and beta$_2$-adrenergic effects (113). Tachycardia is common, but tachyarrhythmias are not. The drug is not yet approved for use in the United States.

Fenoldopam

Fenoldopam, a dopamine analog, is a selective DA$_1$-receptor agonist. It has potential pharmacologic advantages over dopamine in attenuating renal dysfunction. Fenoldopam activates presynaptic and postsynaptic DA$_1$-receptors, but had no effect on DA$_2$, beta-adrenoreceptors, or alpha-adrenoreceptors (114). It produces vasodilation in the renal and mesenteric vascular beds and increases RBF at doses that do not affect blood pressure. At higher doses, fenoldopam lowers blood pressure but still maintains renal perfusion. Fenoldopam exerts a natriuretic effect via DA$_1$ receptors in the proximal convoluted tubule. Given by intravenous infusion at 0.1 to 0.5 μg per kg per minute, it has a rapid onset and offset of effect with an elimination half-life (t 1/2) of 10 minutes. In laboratory studies, fenoldopam induces hypotension while maintaining RBF, relaxes norepinephrine-induced arterial vasoconstriction, and reverses cyclosporine-induced nephrotoxicity (40).

In hypertensive patients in the emergency room setting, fenoldopam provides dose-dependent reduction in blood pressure, with a mild reflex tachycardia, and marked increases in RBF, urine flow, and saliuresis, but little change in GFR (115). In 1998, fenoldopam received approval from the U.S. Food and Drug Administration for short-term (48-hour) parenteral control of hypertension. However, its role in the management of perioperative hypertension and in providing perioperative renal protection has not been established.

Calcium Channel Blockers

Calcium channel blockers prevent ischemic renal injury by a number of mechanisms, including the prevention of reflow-induced vasoconstriction after ischemia, inhibition of angiotensin action in the glomerulus, and decrease in circulating interleukin-2 receptors (60). They may reduce the accumulation of oxygen free radicals and reperfusion injury through prevention of intracellular calcium influx and the calcium/calmodulin-dependent conversion of xanthine dehydrogenase to xanthine oxidase.

However, calcium channel blockers may overcome renal autoregulation and worsen renal function when they induce hypotension. Administration of nifedipine to patients with renal insufficiency has been reported to cause nonoliguric renal failure, which improved when the drug was discontinued (116). In contrast, in hypertensive patients, diltiazem and nifedipine promoted natriuresis and increased RBF and GFR (117).

Calcium channel blockers confer important protection against nephrotoxins, such as cyclosporin A, cisplatinum, and radiocontrast dyes (60,118,119). In patients undergoing cadaveric renal transplantation, diltiazem was added to the graft-preservative solution, infused into the donor for 48 hours, and then given orally (119). The incidence of transplant ATN decreased from 41% to 10%, and when ARF did occur, hemodialysis requirement was significantly less. Diltiazem impairs cyclosporin A metabolism so that plasma cyclosporin A levels are higher with fewer episodes of early acute rejection, but it protects against cyclosporin A nephrotoxicity (118). Cyclosporin A dosage may be reduced by 30% to achieve the same drug levels, representing a substantial cost saving to patients.

Angiotensin-Converting Enzyme Inhibitors

Renin secretion from the afferent arteriole is stimulated by hypovolemia, which may be absolute (hemorrhage, diuresis, sodium loss or restriction) or relative (positive pressure ventilation, congestive heart failure, sepsis, or cirrhosis with ascites). Renin cleaves off a decapeptide, angiotensin I, from circulating angiotensinogen. In the kidney and lung, angiotensin I is converted to an octapeptide, angiotensin II, by endothelial-based ACE (120). Modest levels of angiotensin II predominantly constrict efferent arterioles and maintain GFR during mild to moderate decreases in RBF or perfusion pressure. High levels of angiotensin II constrict afferent arterioles and the glomerular mesangium and decrease RBF and GFR (23).

The consequences of ACE inhibition or angiotensin-II receptor blockade depend on the patient's volume status, systemic hemodynamics, baseline renal function, and presence of renovascular stenoses. In the long-term treatment of hypertension and congestive heart failure, especially in diabetics, the administration of ACE inhibitors decreases renal vascular resistance and appears to benefit renal function. Preliminary data suggest that short-term pretreatment with captopril may prevent a decrease in RBF and GFR and preserve sodium excretion during CPB (121). However, as previously noted, deterioration in renal function may occur in hemodynamically unstable patients (38), and it is prudent to avoid the use of ACE inhibitors in the immediate postoperative period.

Nitric Oxide Donors

Sodium nitroprusside (SNP), an activator of soluble guanylate cyclase and nitric oxide (NO) donor, may increase RBF by en-

hancing cardiac output. However, SNP overrides renal autoregulation, and RBF and GFR decrease in proportion to the decrease in mean arterial pressure (MAP). Moreover, reflex renin-angiotensin activation prevents return of RBF to normal when the drug is discontinued. Although the vascular effects of NO and NO donors may have renal therapeutic effects, the toxic cellular effect of high levels of NO may limit their use in the clinical setting (3). In isolated renal cells, such as proximal tubules, NO induces apoptotic death and is directly cytotoxic (4). In fact, NO antagonists are protective in *in vitro* experiments.

Atrial Natriuretic Peptide

Atrial natriuretic peptide (ANP) is released from electron-dense granules in atrial myocytes in response to local wall stretch and increased atrial volume, and causes a prompt, sustained increase in GFR, even when RBF is not increased or when arterial pressure is decreased (120). This suggests that it causes afferent arteriolar dilation with or without efferent arteriolar constriction. The action of ANP on vascular smooth muscle appears to be mediated by guanylate cyclase activation and increased cyclic guanosine monophosphate (cGMP). It reverses constriction induced by norepinephrine (a competitive block) or angiotensin II (a noncompetitive block).

There is a close interaction between the activation of vasoconstrictor responses, which result in salt retention (and protect against hypovolemia and hyponatremia) and the activation of vasodilator responses, which result in salt excretion (and protect against hypervolemia and hypernatremia). For example, hypovolemia triggers the release of angiotensin, aldosterone, and antidiuretic hormone (ADH). If sufficient salt and water accumulate to induce intravascular volume expansion and atrial stretch, ANP is released.

ANP opposes the renin-angiotensin-aldosterone-ADH system and endothelin-induced vasoconstriction. It inhibits renin secretion, thereby decreasing angiotensin production. ANP decreases both angiotensin-stimulated and direct aldosterone release from the zona glomerulosa of the adrenal cortex, and blocks the salt-retaining action of aldosterone at the distal tubule and collecting duct. ANP inhibits ADH secretion from the posterior pituitary and antagonizes its effect on the V_2-receptor in the collecting duct. Exogenous administration of ANP decreases systemic blood pressure, probably through venodilation and decreased cardiac preload. It increases GFR and induces natriuresis, and can also reverse renovascular hypertension.

In animal studies, ANP administration has consistently reversed functional impairment in ischemic and nephrotoxic ARF, with improvement in RBF, GFR, natriuresis, azotemia, and histologic damage (122–124). Early human studies also showed promise. A pilot study in patients with newly established ARF examined the addition of ANP infusion to high-dose diuretic therapy. Mean C_{Cr} doubled (10 to 21 mL per minute in 24 hours) and the incidence of dialysis was halved compared to control patients (23% versus with 52%) (125).

Subsequently a large (504 patients), randomized multicenter study was designed (126). Patients were prospectively identified as having oliguric (urine output less than 400 mL per day) or nonoliguric ATN, and assigned to a 24-hour infusion of anaritide (a synthetic analog of ANP) or placebo. Patients with oliguric ATN who received anaritide had significantly better dialysis-free survival (27% versus 8%). However, in patients with nonoliguric ATN, survival was actually worse after anaritide (48% versus 59%). The authors observed a fall in blood pressure and urine flow rate after anaritide in the nonoliguric patients, but not in the oliguric patients. One possible explanation for these findings is that nonoliguric ATN represents a lesser renal insult, more nephrons are preserved, and renovascular responsiveness is not as attenuated as it is in oliguric ATN (123). The intact vasomotor response to ANP and ensuing hypotension may have injured intact or partially damaged nephrons, especially if renal autoregulation was impaired (28).

As a consequence, another multicenter, randomized, double-blind, placebo-controlled trial was designed, this time to assess the effect of a 24-hour infusion of anaritide in 222 patients with oliguric ATN only (127). There was no difference in dialysis-free survival rates (21% for ANP and 15% for placebo) or 60-day mortality (60% versus 56%). Almost all patients developed systolic hypotension (less than 90 mm Hg) during the anaritide infusion, which may have negated its beneficial effect. The authors concluded that ANP is of no benefit in established ARF.

ANP has also been disappointing in prophylaxis against nephrotoxic injury in humans. Administration of ANP, to patients with existing renal insufficiency (C_{Cr} 1.5 to 1.8 mg per dL), had no impact on the incidence of radiocontrast-induced nephropathy (128).

In summary, endogenous ANP appears to play an essential renal protective role in the response to stress. However, its promise as a renal "rescue agent" in animal models of ATN has not been fulfilled in large-scale human studies.

Renal Ischemic Preconditioning and Adenosine

It is a well-known paradox that organs subjected to sublethal ischemic events develop profound resistance to subsequent, more severe ischemic insults. In 1986, Murry and coworkers first described the protective effects of "ischemic preconditioning" in cardiac muscle. Multiple brief ischemic periods prior to a prolonged ischemic insult lessened myocardial dysfunction and infarction size after reperfusion (129). Subsequently, ischemic preconditioning was demonstrated in noncardiac tissues, such as skeletal muscle, brain, and liver (130). Renal protective effects of ischemic preconditioning *in vivo* have also been described (131,132). In anesthetized rats, 4 cycles of 8 minutes of global renal ischemia separated by 5 minutes of reperfusion protected renal function against 45 minutes of global, warm ischemia. The application of renal preconditioning to clinical situations, such as supraaortic cross-clamping, awaits human studies.

Adenosine

Adenosine is an endogenous degradation product of ATP and is produced by every mammalian cell type. In the kidney, it plays an essential role in regulating intrarenal distribution of blood flow, renin release and electrolyte transport. At present, there are four known subtypes of adenosine receptors, A_1, A_{2a}, A_{2b}, and A_3 (133). Activation of the A_1-adenosine receptor induces cortical vasoconstriction and fosters blood flow to the oligemic medulla. It also decreases renin release and inhibits diuresis and natriuresis. In contrast, A_{2a}-adenosine receptors increase medullary renal blood flow, renin release, diuresis, and natriuresis.

These actions confer adenosine with potentially protective effects in renal ischemic reperfusion injury. Renal VO_2 might be diminished by a decrease in cortical blood flow, GFR, and sympathetic tone (A_1-adenosine receptor), while renal DO_2 might be increased by increased medullary blood flow (A_2-adenosine receptor). In addition, adenosine induces cytoprotection and increases cellular resistance to ischemia in many organ systems including the heart, brain, and kidneys. It is the key mediator of ischemic preconditioning in the heart and brain.

Lee and Emala (131,132) recently characterized the role of adenosine receptor subtypes in an *in vivo* model of ARF. In anesthetized rats, preischemic administration of adenosine, as well as selective A_1-adenosine receptor activation, protects renal function against global renal ischemic reperfusion injury. Selective A_3-receptor activation actually worsens ischemic injury. Selective A_{2a}-adenosine receptor stimulation has the greatest renal protective effects, even if delayed until the early reperfusion period after termination of renal ischemia.

In summary, these findings suggest that pharmacologic development of a safe, specific A_{2a}-adenosine receptor agonist could have far-reaching implications for protection against renal ischemic injury. The primary caveat (recalling the experience with ANP) is that success in animal models does not necessarily translate into clinical efficacy in patients.

Vasopressor Therapy in Vasodilated Shock

Norepinephrine

The beneficial effects of norepinephrine on renal function when normal renal perfusion pressure is restored in patients with oliguric septic shock are well established (29,134). In the original study by Desjars and colleagues, a group of hypotensive septic patients who were oliguric despite volume resuscitation and dopamine (15 μg per kg per minute) were infused with norepinephrine to increase MAP from 50 to 70 mm Hg (29). Urinary flow rate tripled and C_{Cr} doubled. Norepinephrine increased the SVR with little change in cardiac index or DO_2.

The use of low-dose norepinephrine to maintain MAP greater than 60 mm Hg in sepsis appears to improve cardiac function (increased stroke volume, decreased heart rate) and GFR without adversely affecting cardiac index, oxygen extraction, or oxygen delivery.

Arginine Vasopressin

Landry and coworkers first observed that there is a remarkable sensitivity to the vasoconstrictor effects of infused arginine vasopressin (AVP) in patients with septic shock with profound hypotension despite catecholamine infusion. Infusion of AVP at rates as low as 2 to 6 U per hour increased systolic blood pressure from a mean of about 90 mm Hg to about 145 mm Hg, and catecholamine infusions could be discontinued. This was associated with a tripling of urine flow rate in some patients (135).

Landry and coworkers also noted that plasma AVP levels are remarkably low in patients in septic shock (~3 pg per mL versus 20 pg per mL in patients in cardiogenic shock) (136). This is attributed to sustained baroreceptor-mediated AVP release during the initial hypotensive stages of sepsis. When patients are admitted to the ICU because of hypotension, the posterior pituitary stores are probably exhausted of AVP. Simple restoration of normal circulating AVP and reactivation of the V_1-receptor could thus explain the "sensitivity" to AVP. There is also some evidence that AVP overcomes the loss of vascular responsiveness to norepinephrine induced by massive release of NO by activation of inducible NO synthase in sepsis.

Infusion of AVP may benefit renal function by enhancing renal perfusion pressure in the face of abnormal autoregulation. It may also occur because AVP preferentially constricts the efferent arteriole, improving the filtration fraction and GFR (137).

In our current clinical practice, we administer an infusion of AVP (1 to 6 U per hour) in all forms of vasodilatory shock (i.e., hypotension), despite increasing doses of norepinephrine and high cardiac index (≥ 2.5 L per minute per M^2). These forms include sepsis, high-dose inodilator therapy (i.e., milrinone) for severe right ventricular failure, and the inflammatory response to VAD implantation (138). The goal is to decrease (but not eliminate) norepinephrine dosage, thereby enhancing its inotropic effect. Infusion of AVP is not beneficial in doses exceeding 12 U per hour or to treat hypotension secondary to low cardiac output.

In these situations it can induce severe acral cyanosis and even gangrene.

SUMMARY

Despite advances in supportive care and dialytic techniques, ARF continues to be a devastating perioperative problem. This is related, in part, to the age and premorbid pathology in the patients who develop ARF and to the growth of aggressive surgical interventions and life support devices. ARF is associated with a high morbidity and mortality despite multiple innovative therapies. Unfortunately, many of these have failed to provide anticipated benefits. Renal ischemia and nephrotoxins cause the majority of ARF.

Various paradigms have been explored to facilitate the understanding of the course of ARF and aid in the development of effective interventions. These models include: hemodynamic, O_2 supply-demand, and vasomotor. The natural history of postoperative ARF has been described as one of three types. Type A is short lived and follows a single insult. Type B follows the course of cardiac function with recovery of renal function as cardiac output recovers. Type C is due to multiple renal insults. Secondary insults such as shock, sepsis, nephrotoxins, and even supportive therapies such as dialysis may exacerbate it. Recovery may be limited with type C ARF and it has a high morbidity and mortality.

Various potential strategies for renal protection exist. They include enhancement of renal DO_2 to vulnerable regions, suppression of reflex vasoconstrictor responses, pharmacologic renal vasodilation, maintenance of tubular flow, and decreased tubular VO_2. Suppression of reflex vasoconstriction is the easiest to reverse since it is often amenable to appropriate volume repletion. Pharmacologic therapy is applied widely with varying degrees of supportive evidence and benefit.

KEY POINTS

Although effective dialytic therapies exist to treat acute renal failure (ARF), it remains a major cause of intensive care unit morbidity and mortality. In the past, ARF was considered a single entity, but now it seems to be a common effect/indicator of multisystem organ failure. ARF is not easily prevented due to its presence in older adult patients with ischemic or nephrotoxic acute tubular necrosis. Animal data demonstrate the potential of numerous treatments, but few drug therapies have been effective in human studies.

Clinicians have constructed various paradigms to unravel the complexity of acute renal failure; to study the condition comprehensively requires many approaches to its various facets. The study of acute tubular necrosis and vasomotor nephropathy has led to greater understanding of the association with liver failure, septic shock, and other ARF-related complications.

Certain patient characteristics such as preexisting renal insufficiency or a genetic predisposition to renal pathology, base-line hepatic insufficiency, cardiac dysfunction, diabetes mellitus, and advanced age increase the risk of postoperative ARF. A number of procedures have been identified as "high risk" in regard to the development or progression to ARF. These include patients who undergo major cardiac, vascular, and hepatic surgery.

Just as there are many aspects and complications of ARF, there is also a spectrum of potential treatments. Prevention and treatment range from simple reflex vasoconstrictor response suppression (through volume expansion) to administration of loop diuretics and mannitol in order to prevent sustained, prolonged renal damage. Many methods exist, but few have proven useful by themselves. The administration of calcium channel blockers, angiotensin-converting enzyme inhibitors, nitric oxide donors, adenosine, norepinephrine, and arginine vasopressin have been postulated as potential therapies, but so far none have proven useful as broad-based treatments for ARF.

REFERENCES

1. Aronson S, Blumenthal R. Perioperative renal dysfunction and cardiovascular anesthesia: concerns and controversies. *J Cardiothorac Vasc Anesth* 1998;12:567–586.
2. Lameire N, Vanholder R. Pathophysiologic features and prevention of human and experimental acute tubular necrosis. *J Am Soc Nephrol* 2001;12[Suppl 17]:S20–S32.
3. Star RA. Treatment of acute renal failure. *Kidney Int* 1998;54:1817–1831.
4. Goligorsky MS, Noiri E. Duality of nitric oxide in acute renal injury. *Semin Nephrol* 1999;19:263–271.
5. Noiri E, Peresleni T, Miller F, et al. In vivo targeting of inducible NO synthase with oligodeoxynucleotides protects rat kidney against ischemia. *J Clin Invest* 1996;97:2377–2383.
6. Yu L, Gengaro PE, Niederberger M, et al. Nitric oxide: a mediator in rat tubular hypoxia/reoxygenation injury. *Proc Natl Acad Sci U S A* 1994;91:1691–1695.
7. Thadhani R, Pascual M, Bonventre JV. Acute renal failure. *N Engl J Med* 1996;334:1448–1460.
8. Cullen D, Coyle J, Teplick R, et al. Cardiovascular, pulmonary and renal effects of massively increased intra-abdominal pressure in critically ill patients. *Crit Care Med* 1989;17:118–121.
9. Harmann P, Kron I, McLachlan H, et al. Elevated intra-abdominal pressure and renal function. *Ann Surg* 1982;196:594–597.
10. Kron I, Harmann P, Nolan S. The measurement of intra-abdominal pressure as a criterion for abdominal re-exploration. *Ann Surg* 1984;199:28–30.
11. Platell C, Hall J, Dobb G. Impaired renal function due to raised intraabdominal pressure. *Intensive Care Med* 1990;16:328–329.
12. Richards W, Scavell W, Shin B, et al. Acute renal failure associated with increased intra-abdominal pressure. *Ann Surg* 1983;197:183–187.
13. Castleman B, Scully RE, McNeely BU. Case records of the Massachusetts General Hospital: Case 8–1972. *N Engl J Med* 1972;286:422–428.
14. Higgins TL, Estafanous FG, Loop FD, et al. Stratification of morbidity and mortality outcome by preoperative risk factors in coronary artery bypass patients. A clinical severity score. *JAMA* 1992;267:2344–2348.
15. Mangano CM, Diamondstone LS, Ramsay JG, et al. Renal dysfunction after myocardial revascularization: risk factors, adverse outcomes, and hospital resource utilization. The Multicenter Study of Perioperative Ischemia Research Group. *Ann Intern Med* 1998;128:194–203.
16. Brezis M, Rosen S. Hypoxia of the renal medulla—its implications for disease. *N Engl J Med* 1995;332:647–655.
17. Lieberthal W, Koh JS, Levine JS. Necrosis and apoptosis in acute renal failure. *Semin Nephrol* 1998;18:505–518.
18. Myers B. Pathogenesis of postischemic acute renal failure in man. *Kidney Int* 1983;16:37–41.
19. Lieberthal W, Nigam SK. Acute renal failure. I. Relative importance of proximal vs. distal tubular injury. *Am J Physiol* 1998;275:F623–F631.
20. Myers B, Chui F, Hilberman M, et al. Transtubular leakage of glomerular filtrate in human acute renal failure. *Am J Physiol* 1979;237(4):F319–F325.
21. Levens NR, Peach MJ, Carey RM. Role of the intrarenal renin-angiotensin system in the control of renal function. *Circ Res* 1981;48:157–167.
22. Stanton BA, Koeppen BM. Elements of renal function. In: Berne RM, Levy MN, eds. *Physiology*, 3rd ed. St Louis: Mosby–Year Book, 1993:719–753.
23. Myers BD, Moran SM. Hemodynamically mediated acute renal failure. *N Engl J Med* 1986;314:97–105.
24. Thurau K, Boylan JW. Acute renal success: the unexpected logic of oliguria in acute renal failure. *Am J Med* 1976;61:308–315.
25. Brezis M, Rosen S, Epstein F. The pathophysiologic implications of medullary hypoxia. *Am J Kidney Dis* 1989;13:253–258.
26. Gelman S. Preserving renal function during surgery. *Anesth Analg* 1992;74[Suppl 1]:88–92.
27. Weber A, Schwieger IM, Poinsot O, et al. Sequential changes in renal oxygen consumption and sodium transport during hyperdynamic sepsis in sheep. *Am J Physiol* 1992;262(6 Pt 2):F965–F971.
28. Kelleher SP, Robinette JB, Miller F, et al. Effect of hemorrhagic reduction in blood pressure on recovery from acute renal failure. *Kidney Int* 1987;31:725–730.
29. Desjars PH, Pinaud M, Bugnon D, et al. Norepinephrine has no deleterious renal effects in human septic shock. *Crit Care Med* 1989;17:426–429.
30. Mackay JH, Feerick AE, Woodson LC, et al. Increasing organ blood flow during cardiopulmonary bypass in pigs: comparison of dopamine and perfusion pressure. *Crit Care Med* 1995;23:1090–1098.
31. Conger JD, Hammond WS. Renal vasculature and ischemic injury. *Renal Fail* 1992;14:307–310.
32. Badr KF. Sepsis-associated renal vasoconstriction: potential targets for future therapy. *Am J Kidney Dis* 1992;20:207–213.
33. Cumming AD. Sepsis and acute renal failure. *Renal Fail* 1994;16:169–178.
34. Epstein M. Hepatorenal syndrome: emerging perspectives of pathophysiology and therapy. *J Am Soc Nephrol* 1994;4:1735–1753.
35. Detroz B, Honore P, Monami B, et al. Combined treatment of liver failure and hepatorenal syndrome with orthotopic liver transplantation. *Acta Gastroenterologica Belgica* 1992;55:350–357.
36. Levenson DJ, Simmons CEJ, Brenner BM. Arachidonic acid metabolites, prostaglandins and the kidney. *Am J Med* 1982;72:354–374.
37. Clive D, Stoff J. Renal syndromes associated with nonsteroidal antiinflammatory drugs. *N Engl J Med* 1984;310:563–572.
38. Bender W, La France N, Walker W. Mechanism of deterioration of renal function in patients with renovascular hypertension treated with enalapril. *Hypertension* 1984;6[Suppl 1]:I193–I197.
39. Neumayer HH, Kunzendorf U. Renal protection with the calcium antagonists. *J Cardiovasc Pharmacol* 1991;18[Suppl 1]:S11–S118.
40. Brooks DP, Drutz DJ, Ruffolo RRJ. Prevention and complete reversal of cyclosporine A-induced renal vasoconstriction and nephrotoxicity in the rat by fenoldopam. *J Pharmacol Exp Ther* 1990;254:375–379.
41. Novis BK, Roizen MF, Aronson S, et al. Association of preoperative risk factors with postoperative acute renal failure. *Anesth Analg* 1994;78:143–149.
42. Wilson RF, Soullier G. The validity of two-hour creatinine clearance studies in critically ill patients. *Crit Care Med* 1980;8:281–284.
43. Svensson LG, Coselli JS, Safi HJ, et al. Appraisal of adjuncts to prevent acute renal failure after surgery on the thoracic or thoracoabdominal aorta. *J Vasc Surg* 1989;10:230–239.
44. Chew ST, Newman MF, White WD, et al. Preliminary report on the association of apolipoprotein E polymorphisms, with postoperative peak serum creatinine concentrations in cardiac surgical patients. *Anesthesiology* 2000;93:325–331.
45. Chertow GM, Levy EM, Hammermeister KE, et al. Independent association between acute renal failure and mortality following cardiac surgery. *Am J Med* 1998;104:343–348.
46. Conlon PJ, Stafford-Smith M, White WD, et al. Acute renal failure following cardiac surgery. *Nephrol Dial Transplant* 1999;14:1158–1162.
47. Mangano CM, Diamondstone LS, Ramsay JG, et al. and the Multicenter Study of Perioperative Ischemia Group. Renal dysfunction after myocardial revascularization: risk factors, adverse outcomes, and hospital resource utilization. *Ann Intern Med* 1998;128:194–203.
48. Ip-Yam PC, Murphy S, Baines M, et al. Renal function and proteinuria after cardiopulmonary bypass: the effects of temperature and mannitol. *Anesth Analg* 1994;78:842–847.
49. Hilberman M, Derby GC, Spencer RJ, et al. Sequential pathophysiological changes characterizing the progression from renal dysfunction to acute renal failure following cardiac operation. *J Thorac Cardiovasc Surg* 1980;79:838–844.
50. Canivet JL, Larbuisson R, Damas P, et al. Plasma renin activity and urine beta 2-microglobulin during and after cardiopulmonary bypass: pulsatile vs non-pulsatile perfusion. *Eur Heart J* 1990;11:1079–1082.
51. Goldberg L, Rajfer S. Dopamine receptors: applications in clinical cardiology. *Circulation* 1985;72:245–248.

52. Badner NH, Murkin JM, Lok P. Differences in pH management and pulsatile/nonpulsatile perfusion during cardiopulmonary bypass do not influence renal function. *Anesth Analg* 1992;75:696–701.

53. Myles PS, Buckland MR, Schenk NJ, et al. Effect of "renal-dose" dopamine on renal function following cardiac surgery. *Anesth Intensive Care* 1993;21:56–61.

54. Matsuda H, Hirose H, Nakano S, et al. Results of open heart surgery in patients with impaired renal function as creatinine clearance below 30 ml/min. The effects of pulsatile perfusion. *J Cardiovasc Surg* 1986;27:595–599.

55. Myers BD, Miller DC, Mehigan JT, et al. Nature of the renal injury following total renal ischemia in man. *J Clin Invest* 1984;73:329–341.

56. Parfrey PS, Griffiths SM, Barrett BJ, et al. Contrast material-induced renal failure in patients with diabetes mellitus, renal insufficiency or both. A prospective, controlled study. *N Engl J Med* 1989;320:143.

57. Levy EM, Viscoli CM, Horwitz RI. The effect of acute renal failure on mortality. A cohort analysis. *JAMA* 1996;275:1489–1494.

58. Eisenberg RL, Bank WO, Hedgecock MW. Renal failure after major angiography can be avoided with hydration. *Am J Radiol* 1981;136:859.

59. Snyder HE, Killen DA, Foster JH. The influence of mannitol in toxic reactions to contrast angiography. *Surgery* 1968;64:640.

60. Neumayer HH, Gellert J, Luft FC. Calcium antagonists and renal protection. *Renal Fail* 1993;15:353–358.

61. Tepel M, van der Giet M, Schwarzfeld C, et al. Prevention of radiographic-contrast-agent-induced reductions in renal function by acetylcysteine. *N Engl J Med* 2000;343:180–184.

62. Pass L, Eberhart R, Brown J, et al. The effect of mannitol and dopamine on the renal response to thoracic aortic cross-clamping. *J Thorac Cardiovasc Surg* 1988;95:608–612.

63. Gamulin Z, Forster A, Morel D, et al. Effects of infra-renal aortic cross-clamping on renal hemodynamics in humans. *Anesthesiology* 1984;61:394–399.

64. Meloche R, Pottercher T, Audet J, et al. Hemodynamic changes due to clamping of the abdominal aorta. *Can Anaesth Soc J* 1977;24:20–34.

65. Plusa SM, Clark NW. Prevention of postoperative renal dysfunction in patients with obstructive jaundice: a comparison of mannitol-induced diuresis and oral sodium taurocholate. *J Royal Coll Surg Edinburgh* 1991;36:303–305.

66. Morris JA Jr, Mucha P Jr, Ross SE, et al. Acute posttraumatic renal failure: a multicenter perspective. *J Trauma* 1991;31:1584–1590.

67. Laver MB. Dr. Starling and the "ventilator" kidney. *Anesthesiology* 1979;50:383–386.

68. Clyne DH, Kant KS, Pesce AJ, et al. Nephrotoxicity of low molecular weight serum proteins. Physicochemical interactions between myoglobin, hemoglobin, Bence-Jones protein and Tamm-Horsfall mucoprotein. *Curr Probl Clin Biochem* 1979;9:299.

69. Wu AH, Laios I, Green S, et al. Immunoassays for serum and urine myoglobin: myoglobin clearance assessed as a risk factor for acute renal failure. *Clin Chem* 1994;40:796–802.

70. Ellinas PA, Rosner F. Rhabdomyolysis: report of eleven cases. *J National Med Assoc* 1992;84:617–624.

71. Bryan AG, Bolsin SN, Vianna PTG, et al. Modification of the diuretic and natriuretic effects of a dopamine infusion by fluid loading in preoperative cardiac surgical patients. *J Cardiothorac Vasc Anesth* 1995;9:158–163.

72. Bjornsson TD. Use of serum creatinine concentrations to determine renal function. *Clin Pharmacokinetics* 1979;4:200–222.

73. Cockroft DW, Gault MH. Prediction of creatinine clearance from serum creatinine. *Nephron* 1976;16:31–41.

74. Robert S, Zarowitz BJ, Peterson EL, et al. Predictability of creatinine clearance estimates in the critically ill. *Crit Care Med* 1993;21(10):1487-1495.

75. Tobias GJ, McLaughlin RF, Hopper J. Endogenous creatinine clearance: a valuable clinical test of glomerular filtration and a prognostic guide in chronic renal disease. *N Engl J Med* 1962;266:317–323.

76. Sladen RN, Endo E, Harrison T. Two-hour versus 22-hour creatinine clearance in critically ill patients. *Anesthesiology* 1987;67:1013–1016.

77. Shin B, Mackenzie C, Helrich M. Creatinine clearance for early detection of posttraumatic renal dysfunction. *Anesthesiology* 1986;64:605–609.

78. Wesson LG, Lauler DP. Diurnal cycle of glomerular filtration rate and sodium and chloride excretion during responses to altered salt and water balance in man. *J Clin Invest* 1961;40:1967–1977.

79. Memoli B, Libetta C, Conte G, et al. Loop diuretics and renal vasodilators in acute renal failure. *Nephrol Dial Transplant* 1994;4:168–171.

80. Krasna M, Scott G, Scholz P, et al. Postoperative enhancement of urinary output in patients with acute renal failure using continuous furosemide therapy. *Chest* 1986;89:294–295.

81. Anderson R, Linas S, Berns A, et al. Nonoliguric acute renal failure. *N Engl J Med* 1977;296:1134–1137.

82. Lassnigg A, Donner E, Grubhofer G, et al. Lack of renal protective effects of dopamine and furosemide during cardiac surgery. *J Am Soc Nephrol* 2000;11:97–104.

83. Conger JD. Interventions in clinical acute renal failure: what are the data? *Am J Kidney Dis* 1995;26:565–576.

84. Solomon R, Werner C, Mann D, et al. Effects of saline, mannitol, and furosemide to prevent acute decreases in renal function induced by radiocontrast agents. *N Engl J Med* 1994;331:1416–1420.

85. Laragh J. Atrial natriuretic hormone, the renin-angiotensin axis, and blood-pressure electrolyte homeostasis. *N Engl J Med* 1985;313:1330–1340.

86. Mason J. The pathophysiology of ischemic acute renal failure. A new hypothesis about the initiation phase. *Renal Physiol Basel* 1986;9:129–147.

87. Better OS, Rubinstein I, Winaver JM, et al. Mannitol therapy revisited (1940–1997). *Kidney Int* 1997;52:886–894.

88. Gennari F, Kassirer J. Osmotic diuresis. *N Engl J Med* 1974;291:714–720.

89. Zager RA, Foerder C, Bredl C. The influence of mannitol on myoglobinuric acute renal failure: functional, biochemical, and morphological assessments. *J Am Soc Nephrol* 1991;2:848–855.

90. Bailey ME. Endotoxin, bile salts and renal function in obstructive jaundice. *Br J Surg* 1976;63:774–778.

91. Wait RB, Kahng KU. Renal failure complicating obstructive jaundice. *Am J Surg* 1989;157:256–263.

92. Denton MD, Chertow GM, Brady HR. "Renal-dose" dopamine for the treatment of acute renal failure: scientific rationale, experimental studies and clinical trials. *Kidney Int* 1996;50:4–14.

93. Lokhandwala MF, Amenta F. Anatomical distribution and function of dopamine receptors in the kidney. *FASEB J* 1991;5:3023–3030.

94. Goldberg L, Volkman P, Kohli J. A comparison of the vascular dopamine receptor with other dopamine receptors. *Ann Rev Pharmacol Toxicol* 1978;18.

95. Hollenberg N, Adams D, Mendell P, et al. Renal vascular responses to dopamine: hemodynamic and angiographic observations in normal man. *Clin Sci Mol Med* 1973;45:733–742.

96. Duke GJ, Briedes JH, Weaver RA. Renal support in critically ill patients: low-dose dopamine or low-dose dobutamine? *Crit Care Med* 1994;22:1919–1925.

97. Hilberman M, Maseda J, Stinson E, et al. The diuretic properties of dopamine in patients after open-heart operation. *Anesthesiology* 1984;61:489–494.

98. Kirby MG, Dasta JF, Armstrong DK, et al. Effect of low-dose dopamine on the pharmacokinetics of tobramycin in dogs. *Antimicrob Agent Chemother* 1986;29:168–170.

99. Paul MD, Mazer CD, Byrick RJ, et al. Influence of mannitol and dopamine on renal function during elective infrarenal aortic cross-clamping in man. *Am J Nephrol* 1986;6:427–434.

100. Baldwin L, Henderson A, Hickman P. Effect of postoperative low-dose dopamine on renal function after elective major vascular surgery. *Ann Intern Med* 1994;120:744–747.

101. Bellomo R, Chapman M, Finfer S, et al. Low-dose dopamine in patients with early renal dysfunction: a placebo-controlled randomised trial. Australian and New Zealand Intensive Care Society (ANZICS) Clinical Trials Group. *Lancet* 2000;356:2139–2143.

102. Lassnigg A, Donner E, Grubhofer G, et al. Lack of renoprotective effects of dopamine and furosemide during cardiac surgery. *J Am Soc Nephrol* 2000;11:97–104.

103. Polson RJ, Park GR, Lindop MJ, et al. The prevention of renal impairment in patients undergoing orthotopic liver grafting by infusion of low dose dopamine. *Anaesthesia* 1987;42:15–19.

104. Swygert TH, Roberts LC, Valek TR, et al. Effect of intraoperative low-dose dopamine on renal function in liver transplant recipients. *Anesthesiology* 1991;75:571–576.

105. Grundmann R, Kindler J, Meider G, et al. Dopamine treatment of human cadaver kidney graft recipients: a prospectively randomized trial. *Lancet* 1980;ii:827–828.

106. Schaer GL, Fink MP, Parrillo JE. Norepinephrine alone versus norepinephrine plus low-dose dopamine: enhanced renal blood flow with combination pressor therapy. *Crit Care Med* 1985;13:492–496.

107. Schwartz LB, Gewertz GL. The renal response to low-dose dopamine. *J Surg Res* 1988;45:574–588.

108. Graziani G, Cantaluppi A, Casati A, et al. Dopamine and furosemide in oliguric acute renal failure. *Nephron* 1984;37:39–42.

109. Davis RF, Lappas DG, Kirklin JK, et al. Acute oliguria after cardiopulmonary bypass: renal functional improvement with low-dose dopamine infusion. *Crit Care Med* 1982;10:852–836.

110. Flancbaum L, Choban PS, Dasta JF. Quantitative effects of low-dose dopamine on urine output in oliguric surgical intensive care unit patients. *Crit Care Med* 1994;22:61–68.

111. Chiolero R, Borgeta A, Fisher A. Postoperative arrhythmias and risk factors after open heart surgery. *Thorac Cardiovasc Surgeon* 1991;39:81–84.

112. MacGregor DA, Smith TE, Prielipp RC, et al. Pharmacokinetics of dopamine in healthy male subjects. *Anesthesiology* 2000;92:338–346.

113. Ghosh S, Gray B, Oduro A, et al. Dopexamine hydrochloride: pharmacology and use in low cardiac output states. *J Cardiothorac Vasc Anesth* 1991;5:382–389.

114. Garwood S. New pharmacologic options for renal preservation. *Anesthesiol Clin North Am* 2000;18:753–771.

115. Murphy MB, Elliott WJ. Dopamine and dopamine receptor agonists in cardiovascular therapy. *Crit Care Med* 1990;18:S14–S18.

116. Diamond J, Cheung J, Fang L. Nifedipine-induced renal dysfunction. *Am J Med* 1984;77:905–909.

117. Bauer J, Sunderrajan S, Reams G. Effects of calcium entry blockers on renin-angiotensin-aldosterone system, renal function and hemodynamics, salt and water excretion and body fluid composition. *Am J Cardiol* 1985;56:62H–67H.

118. Neumayer HH, Kunzendorf U, Schreiber M. Protective effects of calcium antagonists in human renal transplantation. *Kidney Int* 1992;36[Suppl]:87–93.

119. Wagner K, Albrecht S, Neumayer H-H. Prevention of post-transplant acute tubular necrosis by the calcium antagonist diltiazem: a prospective, randomized study. *Am J Nephrol* 1987;7:287–291.

120. Ballerman BJ, Zeidel ML, Gunning ME, et al. Vasoactive peptides and the kidney. In: Brenner BM, Rector FCJ, eds. *The kidney,* 4th ed. Philadelphia: WB Saunders, 1991:510–583.

121. Colson P, Ribstein J, Mimran A, et al. Effect of angiotensin converting enzyme inhibition on blood pressure and renal function during open heart surgery. *Anesthesiology* 1990;72:23–27.

122. Atanasova I, Girchev R, Dimitrov D, et al. Atrial natriuretic peptide and dopamine in a dog model of acute renal ischemia. *Acta Physiologica Hungarica* 1994;82:75–85.

123. Conger JD, Falk SA, Hammond WS. Atrial natriuretic peptide and dopamine in established acute renal failure in the rat. *Kidney Int* 1991;40:21–28.

124. Seki G, Suzuki K, Nonaka T, et al. Effects of atrial natriuretic peptide on glycerol induced acute renal failure in the rat. *Japan Heart J* 1992;33:383–393.

125. Rahman SN, Kim GE, Mathew AS, et al. Effects of atrial natriuretic peptide in clinical acute renal failure. *Kidney Int* 1994;45:1731–1738.

126. Allgren RL, Marbury TC, Rahman SN, et al. Anaritide in acute tubular necrosis. *N Engl J Med* 1997;336:828–834.

127. Lewis J, Salem MM, Chertow GM, et al. and the Anaritide Acute Renal Failure Study Group: Atrial natriuretic factor in oliguric acute renal failure. *Am J Kidney Dis* 2000;36:767–774.

128. Kurnik BR, Allgren RL, Genter FC, et al. Prospective study of atrial natriuretic peptide for the prevention of radiocontrast-induced nephropathy. *Am J Kidney Dis* 1998;31:674–680.

129. Murry CE, Jennings RB, Reimer KA. Preconditioning with ischemia: a delay of lethal cell injury in ischemic myocardium. *Circulation* 1986;74:1124–1136.

130. Lee HT. Adenosine pretreatment of human myocardium and ischemic preconditioning. *Circulation* 1998;97:2279.

131. Lee HT, Emala CW. Protective effects of renal ischemic preconditioning and adenosine pretreatment: role of A$_1$ and A$_3$ receptors. *Am J Physiol Renal Physiol* 2000;278:F380–F387.

132. Lee HT, Emala CW. Protein kinase C and G$_{i/o}$ proteins are involved in adenosine- and ischemic preconditioning-mediated renal protection. *J Am Soc Nephrol* 2001;12:233–240.

133. Fozard JR, Hannon JP. Adenosine receptor ligands: potential as therapeutic agents in asthma and COPD. *Pulm Pharmacol Ther* 1999;12:111–114.

134. Dasta JF. Norepinephrine in septic shock: renewed interest in an old drug. *DICP* 1990;24:153–156.

135. Landry DW, Levin HR, Gallant EM, et al. Vasopressin pressor hypersensitivity in vasodilatory septic shock. *Crit Care Med* 1997;25:1279–1282.

136. Landry DW, Levin HR, Gallant EM, et al. Vasopressin deficiency contributes to the vasodilation of septic shock. *Circulation* 1997;95:1122–1125.

137. Edwards RM, Rizna W, Kinter LB. Renal microvascular effects of vasopressin and vasopressin antagonist. *Am J Physiol* 1989;256:F526–F534.

138. Argenziano M, Choudri AF, Oz MC, et al. A prospective randomized trial of arginine vasopressin in the treatment of vasodilatory shock after left ventricular assist device placement. *Circulation* 1997;96:II286–II290.

MANAGEMENT OF ACUTE RENAL FAILURE IN THE CRITICALLY ILL PATIENT

MICHELLE A. HLADUNEWICH
RICHARD A. LAFAYETTE

KEY WORDS

- Acute intermittent peritoneal dialysis (AIPD)
- Acute renal failure (ARF)
- Acute tubular necrosis (ATN)
- Continuous renal replacement therapy (CRRT)
- CRRT controversies
- Dialysis
- Dialysis complications
- Intermittent hemodialysis (IHD)
- Medical management of ARF
- Sustained low-efficiency dialysis (SLED)

INTRODUCTION

Acute renal failure (ARF) is defined as an increasing creatinine due to a sustained decline in the glomerular filtration rate (GFR). It is often associated with decreased urine output. The reported incidence of ARF in the intensive care settings ranges from 7% (1) to 15% (2). However, the true incidence is difficult to ascertain given the variable definitions of ARF. It is likely that incidence will increase with an aging population, with increased comorbidities, and an increased number of patients being supported through multisystem organ failure (MSOF). A study, which followed the natural history of patients with culture-positive septic shock, found the incidence of ARF to be 51% (3).

Despite advances in supportive care and renal replacement therapy, mortality in the critically ill patient with ARF remains alarmingly high. Mortality rates as high as 79% have been reported in patients requiring renal replacement therapy in the intensive care unit (ICU) (4). Even when more conservative definitions of renal failure are used, the mortality remains excessive. A study of patients undergoing bone marrow transplantation revealed mortality rates of 17% for patients with preserved renal function, 37% for those who doubled their creatinine, and 87% for patients requiring dialysis (5). Similarly, a recent large study, which used a definition of renal insufficiency that did not include dialysis, reported a mortality rate of 62% as compared to 15% in critically ill patients with preserved renal function (6).

Whether renal failure itself is an independent predictor of a poor outcome or merely another component of MSOF remains controversial. ARF associated with increased mortality has been well documented in the cardiac and vascular surgery literature. The most recent study by Chertow and colleagues revealed a 63.7% mortality for patients requiring dialysis following cardiac surgery versus 4.3% for patients with intact renal function, even after adjusting for comorbidities and postoperative complications (7). On the other hand, investigators have found determination of an Acute Physiologic and Chronic Health Evaluation (APACHE) II Score at the initiation of dialysis predictive of patient survival and recovery of renal function (8). In addition, studies using multivariate regression techniques have identified hypoalbuminemia, mechanical ventilation, and elevated bilirubin and lactate levels as predictors of mortality in patients with ARF, suggesting outcome may be related more to the severity of the underlying disease than to the severity of renal dysfunction (9,10).

In the critically ill patient, the most common cause of renal insufficiency lies along a continuum of hemodynamic compromise. This ranges from prerenal insufficiency to acute tubular necrosis (ATN) to the irreversible state of bilateral cortical necrosis, which based on a series of autopsy findings in Japan occurred in 20% of postoperative patients who died with renal failure (11). Renal hypoperfusion, as a result of insufficient cardiac output, hypovolemia, and/or vasodilation, often coupled with other nephrotoxic insults, is the most common cause of ATN. A prospective multicenter study conducted in Madrid (12) revealed that out of 253 ICU cases with ARF, 75.9% were secondary to ATN, 17.8% had a prerenal cause, and only two cases (0.8%) were due to obstruction. Although cited as rare causes of renal insufficiency in this patient population (12), glomerulonephritis remains the most common cause of end-stage renal disease worldwide, and acute interstitial nephritis (AIN) accounts for up to 15% of ARF cases. In patients with ATN, 23.4% were multifactorial in origin. Brivet and associates (1) looked more closely at the causes of ATN to find that the majority were due to sepsis (48%) and the remainder were secondary to other causes of hemodynamic compromise (32%) and toxic insults (20%).

Some nephrotoxic insults are particularly common in this patient population and deserve mention. Due to their often compromised hemodynamic state, ICU patients are at particular risk of renal injury from angiotensin-converting enzyme (ACE) inhibitors and nonsteroidal antiinflammatory drugs (NSAIDs), which can further compromise renal perfusion by blocking angiotensin II-mediated efferent vasoconstriction and afferent vasodilatory prostaglandins, respectively. Toxic nephropathy from radiocontrast dye, as well as antibiotics, such as gentamicin and amphotericin remain prevalent in the ICU setting. Although hemoglobinuric renal failure has become rare as a result of improved surgical and blood banking techniques, pigment nephropathy secondary to rhabdomyolysis is seen following crush injuries, extremity ischemia, seizures, and various intoxications. Disseminated intravascular coagulation (DIC) following surgical catastrophes or sepsis may contribute to ATN and cortical necrosis. Finally, atheroembolic disease must be entertained as a possible cause of ARF following vascular surgery proximal to the renal arteries, use of intraaortic balloon pumps, or angiographic procedures.

The purpose of this chapter is to address preventive strategies and the general medical management of the critically ill patient with ARF. In addition, the indications for renal replacement therapy, fundamental principles of dialysis, available modes of therapy, as well as the potential complications of dialytic therapy will be discussed. Finally, controversies surrounding the initiation and proper use of various renal replacement options will be addressed.

PREVENTION AND GENERAL MEDICAL MANAGEMENT OF ACUTE RENAL FAILURE

Despite a better understanding of the pathogenesis of ARF secondary to ATN, management remains largely supportive. To date, many treatment options have looked promising in the animal literature (Table 1). Unfortunately, the agents that have been studied in humans with ARF have not demonstrated any benefit. Thus, recognition of the patient at significant risk for renal insufficiency and efforts aimed at prevention are of utmost importance in the critical care setting.

TABLE 1. AGENTS STUDIED IN ANIMALS FOR THE PREVENTION AND/OR MANAGEMENT OF ACUTE RENAL FAILURE

Mannitol
Loop diuretics
Low-dose dopamine
Fenoldopam
Calcium channel blockers
Natriuretic peptides (atrial natriuretic peptide, urodilatin, etc.)
Growth factors (GF) (insulinlike GF, epidermal GF, hepatocyte GF)
Endothelin receptor antagonists
Adenosine receptor antagonists (theophylline)
Thyroxine
Monoclonal antibodies to intracellular adhesion molecules (ICAM—1mAb, etc.)
Free radical scavengers
Thromboxane receptor antagonists
Platelet-activating factor inhibitors

Maintenance of Renal Perfusion Pressure

Prerenal insufficiency is completely reversible if renal perfusion and glomerular ultrafiltration pressure are rapidly restored. Invasive hemodynamic monitoring is often required to guide the resuscitative effort which, at least initially, involves the optimization of preload and cardiac output by the administration of fluids. However, in many patients, fluid resuscitation alone is insufficient for maintaining an adequate mean arterial pressure (MAP), mandating the addition of either an inotropic or vasopressor agent.

The kidney receives 20% of the cardiac output, the highest amount of blood flow in the body relative to organ weight. In the intact kidney, GFR is maintained over a wide range of renal perfusion pressures due to an intrinsic system of autoregulation. However, a MAP persistently below 60 to 80 mm Hg impairs the kidney's ability to perform the autoregulatory functions necessary to maintain GFR (13,14). Bersten and colleagues demonstrated that normal GFR and renal perfusion are maintained with a MAP above 80 mm Hg, whereas a MAP of 67 mm Hg reduced GFR by 33% (15). Additional work in septic sheep by the same group demonstrated that at clinically relevant doses of epinephrine, renal blood flow (RBF) decreased transiently (15 minutes), but subsequently increased to 36% above baseline with the improved MAP and cardiac output (16). Another study found that norepinephrine and phenylephrine did not reduce RBF except when used in healthy dogs with intact autoregulation or at higher than usual doses in septic animals (17). Although human data establishing the optimal MAP for renal perfusion do not exist, acceptance of a lower MAP for fear of renal vasoconstriction during vasopressor administration appears unwarranted.

Renal Dose Dopamine and Fenoldopam

Despite being the subject of much controversy and debate for many years, low-dose dopamine is used extensively in the ICU setting. At a dose of 1 to 3 μg per kg per minute, "renal dose dopamine" is thought to increase RBF by inducing afferent arteriole vasodilation via the dopaminergic-1 (DA-1) receptor. The expected increase in GFR and urine output has been variable, and many argue that the increased urine output is simply due to the natriuretic and diuretic effects of the drug, which occur due to decreased sodium reabsorption primarily by the proximal tubule. In addition to its use as a therapeutic option for the improvement of renal function, renal dose dopamine has been used to ameliorate the vasoconstrictor effects of agents like epinephrine, norepinephrine, and phenylephrine. However, this practice is once again controversial, as the studies are small and uncontrolled (18,19). In addition, as already mentioned, data do not demonstrate any significant permanent detriment to RBF when these pressors were used at clinically relevant doses (15–17). Recently, two controlled trials reexamined the ongoing "renal dose dopamine" saga. The first revealed that any observed benefit to diuresis or creatinine clearance disappeared after 48 hours (20). Moreover, a placebo-controlled, randomized study failed to show any clinically significant renal protection from a continuous infusion of low-dose dopamine in ICU patients with either oliguria or increased serum creatinine (21). Thus, despite the attractive theoretical rationale for using "renal dose dopamine," clinicians should refrain from using it either as a sole therapeutic agent or in combination with other pressors for the treatment or prevention of ARF, as the drug is not without cardiac and metabolic side effects.

Fenoldopam selectively activates the renal dopamine D-1 receptor without the nonselective effects upon other dopamine and adrenergic receptors. Again, the rationale for its potential success is increased renal blood flow, enhanced natriuresis, and improved urine output resulting in renal protective effects without the potential cardiac side effects. To date, no compelling human data exist to support its use for this purpose.

Loop Diuretics and Mannitol

Loop diuretics are thought to be beneficial in preventing or minimizing proximal tubular obstruction by increasing urine flow. Furosemide also increases vasodilator prostaglandin formation, which may dilate the renal afferent arteriole improving renal perfusion. Mannitol, in addition to its diuretic benefits, may preserve mitochondrial function by minimizing postischemic swelling. Thus, in experimental animal models of ARF, loop diuretics and mannitol have appeared promising as protective agents when given at the time of ischemic injury. Unfortunately, both have failed to impact renal function or outcome in human studies (22). In fact, loop diuretics may actually predispose high-risk patients with diabetes or chronic renal insufficiency to further renal injury (23). Nevertheless, loop diuretics are still commonly used for the purpose of converting oliguric to nonoliguric renal insufficiency, which aids in the management of fluid overload and hyperkalemia. Instead of actually improving outcome, response to diuretic administration likely implies less severe kidney failure.

Other Medical Therapies

The increased knowledge of pathogenesis has led to trials of multiple agents in animal models of ARF. Oxygen radical scavengers, amino acids, antiintercellular adhesion molecule-1 antibodies, antiinflammatory neuropeptides, atrial natriuretic peptide (ANP), and various growth factors have all showed promise in experimental studies. Unfortunately, recent randomized controlled trials of two therapies in humans failed to show any significant benefit. The first trial, which examined a 24-hour infusion of ANP in critically ill patients with ATN, did not show improvement in the overall rate of dialysis-free survival compared to placebo (24). The second trial, which involved injections of human insulinlike growth factor I in patients with ARF, failed to show enhanced recovery of renal failure when compared to placebo (25). Both studies concluded that the late administration of these drugs in human trials, as compared to animal trials, might have contributed to the lack of a beneficial effect.

Avoidance of Nephrotoxicity

Without effective treatment, the mainstay of management of patients with ARF remains preventive and supportive. As an example, up to 30% of aminoglycoside nephrotoxicity occurs at "therapeutic levels" (26). Thus, nephrotoxic agents should be avoided or minimized when possible. Certain treatments have been shown to be effective at limiting toxicity. Adequate saline hydration prior to amphotericin B administration, as well as the use of the liposomal formulation, which limits kidney exposure to the drug, are significantly renal protective (27). In patients with chronic stable renal failure, a randomized controlled trial comparing saline hydration alone to saline hydration in conjunction with either furosemide or mannitol prior to the administration of contrast found the rise in serum creatinine to be the least in the patients receiving saline hydration alone (23). Although lower osmolality and nonionic contrast agents offer little advantage in patients with normal renal function, their use should be considered in patients with renal insufficiency, especially with accompanying diabetes mellitus (28). A recent study demonstrated an additional protective effect of acetylcysteine in patients with moderate renal insufficiency who received saline hydration as well as a low-osmolality, nonionic contrast agent (29). Saline hydration with forced diuresis and possibly alkalinization may limit heme pigment toxicity. Finally, it is critical that all medications whose pharmacodynamics are altered by renal dysfunction be appropriately dose-adjusted (Table 2).

TABLE 2. DOSAGE ADJUSTMENTS FOR COMMONLY USED MEDICATIONS IN THE INTENSIVE CARE UNIT

Medication	GFR 10–50 mL/min	GFR <10 mL/min	CRRT
Amikacin	7.5 mg/kg q24–48h	7.5 mg/kg q48–72h	7.5 mg/kg q24–48h
Tobramycin	1.7 mg/kg q24–48h	1.7 mg/kg q48–72h	1.7 mg/kg q24–48h
Gentamicin	1.7 mg/kg q24–48h	1.7 mg/kg q48–72h	1.7 mg/kg q24–48h
Vancomycin	1 g q24–96h	1g q4–7d	1 g q24–96h
Ceftazidime	1–2 g q24–48h	1–2 g q48h	1–2 g q24–48h
Ceftriaxone	1 g q12h	1 g q12h	1 g q12h
Cefotaxime	1 g q8–12h	1 g q24h	1 g q12h
Ciprofloxacin	400 mg q12–24h	400 mg q24h	200 mg q12h
Imipenem	1 g q12h	1 g q24h	1 g q12h
Piperacillin	3–4 g q6–8h	3–4 g q8h	3–4 g q6–8h
Metronidazole	7.5 mg/kg q6h	7.5 mg/kg q12h	7.5 mg/kg q6h
Digoxin	0.25–0.5 mg q36h	0.25–0.5 mg q48h	0.25–0.5 mg q36h
Phenytoin	1 g load; 300 mg q24h	1 g load; 300 mg q24h	1 g load; 300 mg q24h
Theophylline	6 mg/kg load; then 9 mg/kg q24h	6 mg/kg load; then 9 mg/kg q24h	6 mg/kg load; then 9 mg/kg q24h

GFR, glomerular filtration rate; CRRT, continuous renal replacement therapy.

Fluid and Electrolyte Management

Many complications of ARF can be managed medically without the institution of dialytic therapy. Hypervolemia can be limited by salt and water restriction and the judicious use of diuretics. Maintenance fluids should be discontinued and all medications maximally concentrated. Serum potassium typically increases by 0.5 mmol per L per day in oliguric renal failure, and the metabolism of dietary protein produces 50 to 100 mmol per day of nonvolatile acids, which must be excreted for acid-base homeostasis. Potassium supplementation should be avoided unless the patient is significantly depleted. In addition to diuretics, potassium-binding resins are often used to control hyperkalemia. Sodium bicarbonate supplementation can be used for the control of acidosis while paying close attention to intravascular volume status.

Nutritional Support

Enteral feeds are always preferred, but parenteral nutrition should not be denied due to concerns regarding excess volume in the oliguric patient. Severely ill patients, especially those with renal failure, are extremely catabolic requiring a caloric intake of approximately 35 kcal per day with 1 to 1.2 g of protein per kg per day; adequate nutritional support should be provided even if increased nitrogenous waste or fluid overload necessitates earlier dialysis (30). Once some form of renal replacement therapy has been initiated, larger amounts of protein supplementation may be necessary. Intermittent hemodialysis increases the metabolic rate by 15% to 20% (30) and continuous hemodiafiltration has been shown to result in 10 to 15 g of amino acid loss daily (31). Thus, an increase to as high as 1.5 g of protein per kg per day has been recommended for patients on renal replacement therapy (32). To date, no evidence exists for further escalation in protein or caloric intake in terms of overall survival or hastened renal recovery (33). Profound deficiencies of fat-soluble vitamins, other than vitamin K, have been documented in patients with ARF (34). In addition, dialysis removes water-soluble vitamins. Thus, adequate vitamin supplementation is required as well.

Anemia

The anemia that occurs in critically ill patients, including those with ARF, is typically multifactorial in origin. Low serum erythropoietin (EPO) levels have been documented in critically ill patients with and without renal failure (35). Animal studies using EPO in ischemic ARF showed a rapid and significant increase in the serum hematocrit (36). A recent human trial in critically ill patients documented increased reticulocyte counts, increased hemoglobin concentrations, and a decreased number of red blood cell transfusions in critically ill patients randomized to EPO (35).

INDICATIONS FOR RENAL REPLACEMENT THERAPY

Despite optimal medical management of the complications of ARF, renal replacement therapy is often necessary. As renal replacement therapy has its own complications, it must be instituted

TABLE 3. ABSOLUTE INDICATIONS FOR RENAL REPLACEMENT THERAPY

Conditions refractory to medical management:
    Volume overload
    Hyperkalemia
    Metabolic acidosis
Uremic complications:
    Encephalopathy (coma, seizure, multifocal myoclonus)
    Pericarditis (friction rub, tamponade)
    Bleeding diathesis (platelet dysfunction)

with caution. However, there are a number of absolute indications for initiating dialysis therapy (Table 3), including fluid overload, hyperkalemia or metabolic acidosis refractory to medical management, and severe uremic symptoms. The critically ill patient may manifest a change in mental status, asterixis, multifocal myoclonus, or seizure activity as a sign of uremic encephalopathy. Uremic pericarditis presents with a pericardial friction rub or other signs of effusion or tamponade. Finally, bleeding secondary to uremic platelet dysfunction may serve as an urgent indication for renal replacement therapy. Less common urgent indications for renal replacement therapy include intoxications (e.g., lithium, salicylates, alcohols, etc.), hypercalcemia, hyperphosphatemia, or hyperuricemia.

In the absence of an absolute indication, the decision to begin renal replacement therapy rests on clinical judgment. Typically, a sustained decline in kidney function with a blood urea nitrogen (BUN) level approaching 100 mg per dL results in the initiation of dialysis. The origin of the seemingly arbitrary level of 100 mg per dL stems from trials conducted in the 1950s and 1960s, where patients who had dialysis initiated at a BUN level of 150 mg per dL or less had decreased mortality, compared to patients who had dialysis initiated when the BUN exceeded 200 mg per dL (37,38). The BUN, however, is often difficult to interpret in the critically ill patient. The catabolic state, gastrointestinal (GI) bleeding, the use of medications (steroids), or a significant prerenal component to the renal insufficiency may result in elevations of the BUN relative to the serum creatinine. Similarly, poor nutrition or liver disease may hamper urea generation, such that uremic symptoms become evident at significantly lower serum urea levels. Thus, a creatinine clearance below 10 to 15 mL per minute may be a better indicator of the need for renal replacement therapy.

FUNDAMENTAL PRINCIPLES OF WATER AND SOLUTE REMOVAL BY DIALYSIS

During dialysis, solute removal can occur either by diffusion or convection. Water, in contrast, moves freely through the membrane and equilibrates on both sides based on osmotic forces. The rate of diffusion of water-soluble, nonprotein-bound solutes smaller than 5,000 daltons is determined by the surface area and solute permeability of the dialysis membrane, as well as the concentration gradient of solute between plasma and the dialysate. Passage of a given solute across a semipermeable membrane is greatest when the concentration gradient between the two solutions for that particular solute is highest. The blood and dialysate flow rates maintain this concentration gradient between the two compartments. Hemodialysis, as well as some continuous forms of renal replacement therapy, including continuous arteriovenous hemodialysis (CAVHD) and continuous venovenous hemodialysis (CVVHD) operate on this principle, wherein the countercurrent flow of dialysate maintains the solute concentration gradient across the membrane.

Ultrafiltration is responsible for the bulk removal of water, as hydrostatic and osmotic forces push it through a semipermeable membrane. With convective transport, solvent drag carries small and intermediate-sized solutes with the water through the membrane. The rate of ultrafiltration is determined by the hydrostatic and oncotic pressure gradients, as well as the membrane's permeability to water, as defined by the equation:

$$\text{Filtration rate} = \text{Kuf} \left[(P\text{ blood} - P\text{ filtrate}) - \sigma (\pi\text{ blood} - \pi\text{ filtrate}) \right]$$

The permeability of the membrane to water is indicated by its ultrafiltration coefficient (Kuf), which is defined as the number of mL of fluid per hour that will be transferred across the membrane per mm Hg pressure gradient. The transmembrane hydrostatic pressure gradient (P blood − P filtrate) provides the driving force for ultrafiltration. The pressure in the blood compartment is generated by the patient's blood pressure in continuous arteriovenous hemofiltration (CAVH) or by an external pump in continuous venovenous hemofiltration (CVVH), whereas the resistance to flow across the membrane is dependent on the pressure in the dialysate compartment. An oncotic pressure gradient (π blood − π filtrate) opposes the hydrostatic pressure gradient. As water is filtered from the plasma, proteins are concentrated in the remaining plasma, raising blood oncotic pressure. The reflection coefficient (σ) for modern membranes is 1.0 and π filtrate is typically zero. Thus, the oncotic pressure gradient is defined by π blood. The maintenance of an adequate blood flow through the dialysis pump as well as predilution of the blood by replacement fluid minimizes this potential counterproductive effect of an elevated blood oncotic pressure.

TECHNIQUES OF RENAL REPLACEMENT THERAPY

Intermittent Hemodialysis

Intermittent hemodialysis is the most common mode of renal replacement therapy, applied both in the acute and chronic setting. Acute hemodialysis usually requires placement of a double-lumen, 13 to 19 cm, 8 to 12 F catheter into a femoral or internal jugular vein. If possible, the subclavian vein should be avoided due to higher rates of thrombosis and stenosis, as well as possible technical complications, including superior vena cava perforation with a stiff catheter or difficult to tamponade bleeding in patients with uremic platelet dysfunction (39–41). A roller pump pushes blood into the dialysis circuit. Dialysate flows in a countercurrent manner on the other side of the dialysis membrane, allowing solutes to move along their diffusion gradient.

Daily or alternate-day conventional hemodialysis is the standard dialytic regimen for the hemodynamically stable patient

with severe ARF. Compared to intermittent peritoneal dialysis and the slow continuous modes of renal replacement therapy, hemodialysis offers the advantage of more rapid removal of solute and water, with an hourly urea clearance rate of approximately 160 mL per minute. However, hypotension often complicates the use of intermittent hemodialysis in the critically ill, hemodynamically unstable patient despite techniques to augment blood pressure, such as administration of mannitol or hypertonic saline, increased dialysate calcium concentration, and lower dialysate temperature.

Continuous Renal Replacement Therapy

As discussed previously, continuous renal replacement therapy (CRRT) uses either dialysis with diffusion-based solute removal (CAVHD and CVVHD), filtration with convection-based solute removal (CAVH and CVVH), or a combination of both principles (continuous arteriovenous hemodiafiltration [CAVHDF] and continuous venovenous hemodiafiltration [CVVHDF]). With slower rates of water and urea removal, CRRT offers the advantage of better hemodynamic stability.

Most forms of CRRT require replacement fluid to prevent iatrogenic metabolic derangement. The amount and type of replacement fluid must be guided by frequent serum electrolyte evaluations, as well as hemodynamic/volume assessments. Frequent clotting of the dialysis filter is the most significant technical problem. In contrast to intermittent hemodialysis, where anticoagulation can be omitted in certain situations, the need for some form of anticoagulation is universal for CRRT. Even in the patient with significant coagulation deficiencies, frequent filter clotting will occur. The desire to prevent frequent clotting and the potential for insufficient therapy must be balanced by the increased risk of bleeding in the face of anticoagulation. Adequate anticoagulation can be achieved systemically or regionally using heparin or with regional citrate. With systemic heparinization, a loading dose followed by a continuous infusion is administered, and serum partial thromboplastin time is monitored. Regional heparinization involves neutralization with protamine as blood leaves the dialysis circuit. Citrate infused prior to the dialysis filter lowers ionized calcium, which is necessary for the clotting process. The process is subsequently reversed by infusing calcium into the dialysis outflow track, preventing the development of low levels of ionized calcium in the patient. Serum-ionized calcium levels must be monitored closely and the infusion adjusted as necessary. As citrate is metabolized into bicarbonate, metabolic alkalosis, sometimes severe, can develop.

There are a variety of CRRT procedures, which are classified by the nature of their vascular access, as well as the principal method of solute and water removal employed (Table 4).

Continuous Venovenous Hemofiltration

Continuous venovenous hemofiltration (CVVH) uses only venous access and therefore requires an external blood pump to maintain blood flow through the circuit. Volume removal and solute clearance are achieved by ultrafiltration rates of 1 to 2 L per hour. This requires ongoing replacement of fluid losses to prevent iatrogenic hypovolemia and electrolyte depletion.

TABLE 4. CONTINUOUS RENAL REPLACEMENT THERAPIES

Technique	Clearance Method	Access	Blood Pump
Continuous venovenous hemofiltration (CVVH)	Ultrafiltration	Venous	Yes
Continuous venovenous dialysis (CVVHD)	Slow ultrafiltration and diffusion	Venous	Yes
Continuous venovenous hemodiafiltration (CVVHDF)	Ultrafiltration and diffusion	Venous	Yes
Continuous arteriovenous hemofiltration (CAVH)	Ultrafiltration	Arterial	No
Continuous arteriovenous hemodialysis (CAVHD)	Slow ultrafiltration and diffusion	Arterial	No
Continuous arteriovenous hemodiafiltration (CAVHDF)	Ultrafiltration and diffusion	Arterial	No
Slow continuous ultrafiltration (SCUF)	Slow ultrafiltration	Either	Either

Typically, adequate clearance of solute is achievable, in addition to fluid removal as daily convective clearance ranges from 25 to 50 L.

Continuous Venovenous Hemodialysis

Continuous venovenous hemodialysis (CVVHD) is similar to CVVH in that a venous access is used with a blood pump. However, a slow flow of dialysate runs in a countercurrent direction to the blood flow. The ultrafiltration rate is typically decreased to match daily fluid intake or achieve a slightly negative fluid balance. With 30 to 50 L per day of urea clearance, CVVHD is often employed in the very catabolic patient with inadequate metabolic control using CVVH alone.

Continuous Venovenous Hemodiafiltration

Continuous venovenous hemodiafiltration (CVVHDF) combines the principles of diffusion to remove small solutes and convection to remove larger solutes using a venous access and a blood pump. In contrast to CVVHD the ultrafiltration rate exceeds that necessary to maintain euvolemia, necessitating aggressive fluid replacement. The additional fluid infused and filtered adds significantly to urea clearance and solute removal.

Continuous Arteriovenous Hemofiltration (CAVH), Continuous Arteriovenous Hemodialysis (CAVHD) and Continuous Arteriovenous Hemodiafiltration (CAVHDF)

The arteriovenous modes of renal replacement therapy are similar in principle to each of the corresponding venovenous modes. However, they all require arterial catheterization and depend on the patient's blood pressure to drive the system, as opposed to an external blood pump. For both those reasons, they are rarely employed in the ICU. Typically, the femoral artery and vein are cannulated with 8 F catheters. Appreciable rates of hemorrhage and atheroembolism exist, and these modes are relatively contraindicated in patients with peripheral vascular disease or coagulopathies. In addition, a MAP greater than 80 mm Hg is often necessary to drive the system, a goal not realized in many ICU patients.

Slow Continuous Ultrafiltration

Slow continuous ultrafiltration (SCUF) is designed to remove 5 to 7 L of fluid per day in patients with volume overload, but without significant uremia or other metabolic derangements. Solute removal is minimal with this technique owing to extremely slow ultrafiltration without dialysis or replacement fluid. SCUF can be accomplished via arteriovenous or venovenous access.

Sustained Low-Efficiency Daily Dialysis

Sustained low-efficiency daily dialysis (SLED) is a hybrid form of dialysis with characteristics of both intermittent hemodialysis and CRRT. It has been used for the treatment of hemodynamically unstable patients in institutions without access to CRRT due to high machinery costs or lack of nursing expertise for a CRRT program. The institutions which use this method of renal replacement therapy claim it to be more economical and effective since it avoids the frequent interruptions to standard CRRT secondary to time out of unit for diagnostic and therapeutic procedures, as well as the frequent extracorporeal machinery failure of CRRT.

Like CRRT, lower levels of solute clearance are maintained for longer periods of time. However, standard hemodialysis machines are used with lower blood and dialysate flow rates. Due to the slower blood flow rate, heparin is typically necessary to prevent clotting. The amount of time dialyzed per day varies based on the institution. To date, a handful of small clinical studies have revealed adequate metabolic control with this method, but no definitive outcome data are available (42,43).

Acute Intermittent Peritoneal Dialysis

Peritoneal dialysis is a rarely used alternative to hemodialysis for the treatment of ARF, yet is a viable option in select patients, particularly those with hemodynamic instability. Acute intermittent peritoneal dialysis (AIPD) is simple to use, requires no extracorporeal circuit or anticoagulation, and therefore is less labor-intensive than CRRT. Because fluid and solute removal are slow, it is associated with minimal risk of cardiovascular instability or disequilibrium syndrome, but it has limited application in the severely fluid-overloaded, hyperkalemic, or catabolic patient. Other limitations include the risk of bowel perforation, peritoneal infection, obligatory protein loss, and the need for an intact peritoneal cavity and membrane. In addition, the raised intraabdominal pressure from fluid instillation may interfere with respiratory mechanics or increase the risk of aspiration.

AIPD removes solutes by simple diffusion from the blood perfusing the peritoneum. Solutes move down the concentration gradient from plasma to peritoneal dialysate. Fluid removal is achieved by raising the osmolality of the dialysate (i.e., by adding glucose to a level greatly exceeding plasma glucose).

The technique of AIPD involves placement of a catheter in the peritoneal space, usually in the midline, between the umbilicus and symphysis pubis. One to two liters of peritoneal dialysis fluid are introduced over 30 to 60 minutes. The fluid is allowed to approach equilibrium with plasma and is then drained by gravity over 30 to 120 minutes. The larger the volume and the more frequent the turnover of dialysate, the more effectively the concentration gradients are maintained and the more rapid the solute removal. Use of AIPD has diminished owing to improved hemodialysis techniques, better dialysis membranes, and the introduction of CRRT.

COMPLICATIONS OF ACUTE DIALYTIC THERAPIES

Dialytic therapies in the treatment of ARF have been safe and remarkably well tolerated in patients with trauma, shock, sepsis, or multiorgan failure. Nevertheless, patients on dialysis may develop emergent situations that require prompt attention.

Sudden Death During Dialysis

Sudden death during dialysis is extremely unusual. Some of the causes for this uncommon response to dialysis include brain herniation, due to an acute elevation of intracranial pressure seen with intermittent hemodialysis (IHD); air embolism; acute cardiac tamponade; acute myocardial infarction (MI); acute hemorrhage (noniatrogenic or iatrogenic due to machine malfunction or disconnection of blood lines); cardiac arrhythmias from electrolyte abnormalities; or complications of dialysis line placement.

Hypotension

Hypotension occurring at the onset of dialysis may be related to multiple factors. The absence of definitive etiologies for hypotension (i.e., sepsis, MI, cardiac tamponade, or arrhythmia) suggests the possibility of excessive ultrafiltration or occult hemorrhage. Hypotension during the early phase may be associated with complement activation by bioincompatible membranes (cuprophane) or, rarely, with an allergic response to any component of dialysis equipment. Appropriate responses include termination or slowing of fluid removal or dialysis, fluid administration, and administration of vasopressors. Maneuvers to reduce the incidence of hypotension include recognition of hypovolemia, withholding antihypertensive medications before dialysis, avoidance of cuprophane and cellulose dialyzers, and treatment of cardiac dysfunction. In addition, increasing the sodium concentration of the dialysate, adding calcium, and cooling of the dialysate bath may limit dialysis-related hypotension.

Hypoxemia

Dialysis has been associated with hypoxemia owing to a variety of factors, including hypoventilation, pulmonary sequestration of leukocytes, and complement activation. Hypoventilation can occur with either an acetate bath due to hypocapnia from loss of carbon dioxide to the dialysis solution or with a bicarbonate bath due to alkalosis. The existence of leukocyte sequestration secondary to complement activation from a nonbiocompatible membrane is controversial. Oxygen supplementation is typically administered to ameliorate hypoxemia.

First-Use Syndrome

First-use syndrome, which occurs shortly after starting dialysis with a new dialyzer, is mediated by complement activation. Symptoms include acute pruritus, back pain, hypoxia, and hypotension. Most often seen with cuprophane or cellulose dialyzers, the syndrome does not usually occur with more biocompatible membranes. These symptoms decrease with reuse of dialyzers. Acute anaphylaxis with bronchospasm, vasodilation, and circulatory collapse may occur at the start of dialysis due to hypersensitivity to ethylene oxide used to sterilize equipment, and is generally prevented by thorough rinsing of the dialyzer.

Dialysis Disequilibrium Syndrome

The dialysis disequilibrium syndrome is a central nervous system (CNS) disorder that is now rare, but remains important. It is characterized by neurologic symptoms of varying severity, which in its most severe form includes seizures, obtundation, coma, and death. Milder symptoms of the dialysis disequilibrium syndrome include hypertension, headache, nausea, vomiting, arrhythmias, blurred vision, muscle twitching, and tremors. It is thought to result from either acute changes in cerebrospinal (CSF) fluid pH or cerebral edema. The generation of idiogenic osmoles and/or relatively slow urea clearance from the CSF compared to plasma may lead to a shift of fluid to the CSF. Patients who are undergoing initial hemodialysis are at greatest risk, particularly if the BUN is markedly elevated (above 175 mg per dL). Other predisposing factors include severe metabolic acidosis, extremes of age, and the presence of other CNS diseases, such as a preexisting seizure disorder.

Prevention of dialysis disequilibrium may be achieved by avoiding rapid dialysis during the initiation phase of dialysis and by pretreatment with osmotically active compounds, such as mannitol, to prevent osmolar shifts due to urea loss during dialysis. Anticonvulsants, such as phenytoin, have been used both to prevent and treat dialysis disequilibrium in patients who are to undergo their first dialysis and in whom BUN is extremely high. Acute treatment of seizures should be the same as in other conditions.

Fever during Dialysis

Febrile reactions during dialysis are not uncommon, and may be secondary to either infection or a pyrogenic reaction to the dialysate. An important source of bacteremia in this patient population is an infected temporary vascular access site. Typically, these patients are febrile prior to commencing dialysis, but occasionally they develop fever and chills only while on dialysis.

An infected hemodialysis catheter is managed in the same fashion as any other infected line in a critically ill patient. Fever occurring about an hour after starting dialysis and resolving spontaneously after completion of dialysis usually results from pyrogens introduced by the dialysate. Treatment consists of antipyretics and removal of the source. Occasionally, overheating the dialysate (51°C or higher) can cause a pyrogenic response, which can result in hemolysis and fatal hyperkalemia. In the event of such a reaction, dialysis should be stopped immediately, blood in the system should not be returned to the patient, and the patient should be monitored closely for hemolysis and hyperkalemia.

Air Embolism

Air embolism, although rare with modern machines, is a potentially catastrophic complication. The most common sites of air entry include the arterial needle, arterial tubing, or a central catheter inadvertently left open. Symptoms of air embolism depend on the amount of air introduced as well as patient position. If the patient is sitting, air will migrate upward into the cerebral venous system resulting in seizures, loss of consciousness, and possibly death. If the patient is supine, air becomes trapped in the right ventricle. The foam generated may pass into the lungs, causing dyspnea, cough, and chest tightness. It may also pass into the left ventricle, decreasing cardiac output and causing shock.

When air embolism is suspected, the venous lines of the dialyzer should be clamped immediately and the blood pump stopped. The maneuver of placing the patient in the left lateral decubitus and Trendelenburg positions attempts to trap the air in the apex of the right heart. Cardiorespiratory support with 100% oxygen should be provided. Aspiration of air via an existing central venous catheter or a percutaneously inserted needle may be attempted.

Hemorrhage

Spontaneous hemorrhage is common in dialysis patients. Sites include subdural or epidural hematomas, uremic hemopericardium and tamponade, retroperitoneal hemorrhage, GI hemorrhage, anterior chamber bleeding into the eyes, and hemorrhagic pleural effusion. Bleeding usually is associated with heparinization or defective platelet function due to uremia. Prompt recognition of bleeding disorders may prevent morbidity and mortality.

CONTROVERSIES SURROUNDING RENAL REPLACEMENT THERAPY IN THE CRITICALLY ILL

A number of controversies surround the provision of renal replacement therapy to the critically ill patient. A closer examination of these issues including the mode, initiation, and adequacy of renal replacement therapy, as well as membrane biocompatibility, should help one to understand why decisions regarding renal replacement therapy vary among clinicians. In addition, the use of CRRT as a means of cytokine removal for the systemic inflammatory response syndrome is reviewed.

Mode of Renal Replacement Therapy: The Continuous Renal Replacement Therapy versus Intermittent Hemodialysis Controversy

Since its advent in 1977, CRRT has been considered an alternative form of renal replacement therapy for the hemodynamically unstable patient. Due to slower fluid and solute removal, CRRT has been used successfully in patients who could not tolerate IHD (44). Over the course of 24 hours, CRRT removes quantities of small solutes similar to those removed in shorter intervals of conventional hemodialysis. By 48 hours, solute removal exceeds that of a conventional 4-hour hemodialysis session. CVVHDF has been demonstrated to provide superior control of azotemia within 48 hours compared to alternate-day IHD (45). In addition, CRRT is the preferred method of therapy in patients with severe hyperphosphatemia or raised intracranial pressure. Continuous removal of phosphate prevents the rebound increase in plasma concentration seen following IHD. Rapid solute removal with IHD may shift water into the brain and cause acute hypotension, which can aggravate raised intracranial pressure and reduce cerebral perfusion pressure.

Despite the theoretical benefits of CRRT over IHD in the critically ill patient population, prospective trials have failed to show a mortality benefit (46,47). A prospective randomized study of 166 patients reported overall ICU and in-hospital mortalities of 50.6% in the IHD group to 56.6% in the CRRT group. Although the randomization failed to control for severity of illness with an overrepresentation of severe cases in the CRRT group, attempts to control for the unbalanced randomization through stratification based on APACHE scores resulted in the same conclusion (46). A second study, which followed their patient population prospectively without randomization to a treatment modality, did not find any difference in survival after adjusting for severity of illness (47). Results of retrospective analyses tend to marginally favor CRRT or find the two modalities equivalent after adjusting for severity of illness (48–50).

Given the exorbitant cost of renal replacement therapy in the ICU, the time to renal recovery is of paramount importance. Due to impaired autoregulation, ischemic renal damage is potentiated by further bouts of hypotension, which occur more often in patients being treated with IHD. To date, studies have demonstrated a shorter time to renal recovery in patients treated with CRRT (46,48). In the prospective randomized trial, renal recovery was achieved in more patients treated with CRRT than IHD (92.3% versus 59.4%, $p = 0.01$) despite more severely ill patients being randomized to the CRRT group. However, this finding was limited to a smaller subgroup of patients who received an adequate trial of therapy with no crossover (n = 99). Similarly, van Bommel and colleagues report a statistically significant decrease in the time to renal recovery by 7 days in patients treated with CRRT compared to IHD (48).

Without a convincing trend toward a survival benefit for CRRT, most clinicians regard the two modalities as equivalent, reserving CRRT for those patients who are hemodynamically unstable, in whom renal recovery may be enhanced by its use.

Initiation and Adequacy of Renal Replacement Therapy in the Intensive Care Unit

As already discussed, the only evidence of a survival benefit for early or "prophylactic" dialysis originates from studies conducted decades ago (37,38). In these retrospective analyses, initiating dialysis earlier to maintain the BUN less than 150 mg per dL afforded patients a survival benefit. A similar study conducted in the 1960s demonstrated that the observed mortality benefit could be attributed to fewer deaths from GI bleeding and sepsis (51). The first prospective studies, which attempted to elucidate whether more intensive dialysis resulted in a survival benefit, were not adequately powered to demonstrate significance (52,53). In one study, an impressive survival benefit of 44% in patients whose BUN was maintained below 70 mg per dL compared to those whose BUN was maintained below 150 mg per dL did not reach statistical significance due to small sample sizes (52).

More recently, investigators have attempted to study adequacy of renal replacement therapy using the same markers typically applied to chronic dialysis. This clearance marker known as the Kt/V is the amount of plasma cleared of urea divided by the volume of distribution of urea. As this marker of dialysis adequacy was developed to monitor patients in a steady state, its applicability to the critically ill patient is not clear. However, a recent study linked Kt/V to outcome in the ICU (54). For patients with intermediate severity of illness scores, a higher dose of delivered dialysis was associated with a significant reduction in mortality. However, this mortality benefit did not apply to patients with either low or high severity of illness scores, whose survival was independent of their dialysis dose. As a marker of renal replacement therapy adequacy, it is unclear what defined level of Kt/V should be applied to the critically ill. In chronic dialysis patients, a Kt/V of 1.2 constitutes minimal adequate therapy. However, it has been shown that 68% of patients with ARF fail to meet this minimum requirement due to underprescribed dialysis in the catabolic patient, poor blood flow and recirculation through temporary access catheters, and frequent filter clotting from insufficient anticoagulation (55).

For both IHD and CRRT, it has been suggested that more is better. A study published only in abstract form randomized 72 ICU patients to daily IHD versus alternate-day IHD found survival to be significantly reduced in the daily dialysis group (21% versus 47%, *p* less than 0.025) (56). In the realm of CRRT, a recent study randomized 425 patients to CVVH with either 25 mL per hour per kg, 35 mL per hour per kg, or 45 mL per hour per kg of ultrafiltration (57). They found a significantly higher mortality rate in the group who received the least ultrafiltration, but no significant difference in mortality between the two groups who received higher levels of ultrafiltration.

Dialyzer Membrane Biocompatibility

While more dialysis may prove to be better in terms of survival, there is concern that the dialysis therapy itself may delay renal recovery. Discussed previously is the possibility that dialysis-induced hypotension further damages the ischemic kidney. Although thought to be more common with IHD, CRRT can result in hypotension from overly aggressive ultrafiltration.

Another possible mechanism for dialysis-induced renal damage is a possible inflammatory response from exposure to the dialysis membrane, which theoretically could be worse for CRRT due to longer periods of exposure. Animal studies revealed that dialysis with a bioincompatible membrane (cuprophane) results in complement activation and deposition of neutrophils into the kidney where they cause further ischemic and direct inflammatory damage.

Two initial studies comparing the older bioincompatible membranes to newer more compatible cellulose and synthetic membranes showed both a survival advantage as well as more rapid renal recovery in the patients dialyzed with biocompatible membranes (58,59). In the first study, however, the survival advantage was limited to nonoliguric patients (58). Theoretically these patients have more functioning nephrons with better preserved renal blood flow, and therefore may be more susceptible to complement activation. Similarly, in the second study, a larger fraction of nonoliguric patients were rendered oliguric following dialysis with the nonbiocompatible membrane (59). However, this study incorporated data from the first study. Later studies failed to demonstrate any benefit for the use of biocompatible membranes, in terms of either survival or renal recovery (60,61). Although the earlier studies have been criticized for their randomization techniques, none of the later studies have been adequately powered to show a 25% survival advantage, if one exists, and have been criticized for not comparing the extremes of membrane bioincompatibility. Thus, the issue remains unresolved with most centers choosing biocompatible membranes despite the increased costs.

Continuous Renal Replacement Therapy Removal of Cytokines in the Systemic Inflammatory Response Syndrome

The systemic inflammatory response syndrome (SIRS) is thought to contribute to MSOF through the uncontrolled production of multiple inflammatory cytokines. However, therapies aimed at modulating various aspects of the cytokine cascade in critically ill patients have been largely unsuccessful. As hemofiltration is capable of removing the larger "middle molecules" with molecular weights up to 30,000 daltons, removal of cytokines like tumor necrosis factor, interleukins, complement anaphylatoxins, platelet-activating factor, and endotoxin is theoretically possible.

In canine and porcine animal models of SIRS, both low (1 L per hour) and high (6 L per hour) volume hemofiltration have demonstrated improvements in cardiovascular and pulmonary parameters (62–64). In addition, the filtrate removed from affected animals resulted in hemodynamic instability when infused into healthy animals (62). Similarly, human data demonstrate successful removal of inflammatory mediators by ultrafiltration, although serum concentrations remain unaltered (65,66). Although promising uncontrolled observations exist for the use of hemofiltration in SIRS, controlled trials have not demonstrated any survival benefit (67,68).

Reasons for the discordance between animal and human data are numerous. The majority of animal studies have used significantly higher volumes of ultrafiltration than are typically provided in current clinical settings, and the most efficacious rate of ultrafiltration remains to be determined. In addition, even the most biocompatible membranes become quickly saturated with the highest rates of cytokine removal occurring during the first hour and declining steadily thereafter (69). How often membranes may need to be changed and the cost implications of such a maneuver are unknown. Finally, data are lacking regarding the generation rates and half-lives of many cytokines, as well as the impact of removing potentially beneficial cytokines.

SUMMARY

Acute renal failure (ARF) is an unfortunately common event in the ICU with dramatic rates of morbidity and mortality. Careful attention to maintaining volume and hemodynamic stability, as well as avoiding potential nephrotoxins, can prevent many cases.

Once developed, ARF can be medically managed to prevent life-threatening fluid, electrolyte, and uremic complications. Renal replacement therapy routinely saves the lives of patients with severe metabolic disturbances. However, the ideal modality, regimen, and even solute removal goals of renal replacement therapy are still uncertain. Efforts to prevent fluid, electrolyte, and uremic complications, while limiting dialytic complications such as hypotension and hemorrhage remain the current standard of care. Research continues to provide important lessons, such as the inability of dopamine to prevent renal injury or to speed recovery in established renal failure. Likewise, hopes that standard CRRT would improve mortality rates in ARF and sepsis have thus far been unfulfilled. It is hoped that ongoing studies will provide insights into improving outcomes in ICU patients with ARF.

KEY POINTS

Acute renal failure (ARF) results when the body retains an excess of creatinine after a prolonged decline in glomerular filtration rate, most commonly secondary to renal hypoperfusion. The current mortality rate for patients with ARF remains high despite modern therapy. Due to its relation to advanced age, septic shock, and multisystem organ failure, it is unknown whether ARF is a truly independent predictor of mortality.

The treatment of ARF is mainly supportive with appropriate fluid and electrolyte management and nutrition. Multiple innovative therapies have been proposed to improve survival. Despite initial promise in animal models, human studies have not been as successful in altering the natural history of ARF. Various investigations have shown a lack of beneficial impact on recovery from ARF with low-dose dopamine infusion, as well as loop diuretics, mannitol, oxygen radical scavengers, and other therapies.

Where drug and gene therapies have proven generally unhelpful, numerous dialytic techniques are useful in fluid management and blood detoxification. Techniques are generally grouped as either intermittent or continuous forms of dialysis. The main categories are divided into venovenous (necessitating an external blood pump) and arteriovenous (relying on the patient's blood pressure). In addition, there are various forms of hemofiltration, ultrafiltration, hemodialysis, and hemodiafiltration. Peritoneal dialysis plays a relatively minor role in the management of the critically ill.

A number of complications may arise from dialysis, including reaction to membranes, air emboli, dialysis disequilibrium, infection, hypotension, hypoxemia, fever, hemorrhage, and, rarely, sudden death. Many controversies surround dialytic therapy and the search for the ideal treatment for renal failure continues.

REFERENCES

1. Brivet FG, Kleinknecht DJ, Loirat P, et al. Acute renal failure in intensive care units—causes, outcome, and prognostic factors on hospital mortality: a prospective, multicenter study. *Crit Care Med* 1996:24:192–198.
2. Menashe PI, Ross SA, Gottlieb JE. Acquired renal insufficiency in critically ill patients. *Crit Care Med* 1988:16:1106–1109.
3. Rangel-Frausto M, Pittet D, Costigan M, et al. The natural history of the systemic inflammatory response syndrome (SIRS). *JAMA* 1995:273:117–123.
4. Cosentino F, Chauff C, Piedmonte M. Risk factors influencing survival in ICU renal failure. *Nephrol Dial Transplant* 1994:9:S179–S182.
5. Zager RA, O'Quigley J, Zager BK, et al. Acute renal failure following bone marrow transplantation: a retrospective study of 272 patients. *Am J Kidney Dis* 1989:13:210–216.
6. Guerin C, Girard R, Selli JM, et al. Initial versus delayed acute renal failure in the intensive care unit. A multicenter prospective epidemiological study. *Am J Respir Crit Care Med* 2000:161:872–879.
7. Chertow GM, Levy EM, Hammermeister KE, et al. Independent association between acute renal failure and mortality following cardiac surgery. *Am J Med* 1998:104:343–348.
8. Parker RA, Himmelfarb J, Tolkoff-Rubin N, et al. Prognosis of patients with acute renal failure requiring dialysis: results of a multicenter study. *Am J Kidney Dis* 1998:32:432–443.
9. Chertow GM, Lazarus JM, Paganini EP, et al. Predictors of mortality and the provision of dialysis in patients with acute tubular necrosis. The Auriculin Anaritide Acute Renal Failure Study Group. *J Am Soc Nephrol* 1998:9:692–698.
10. Sasaki S, Gando S, Kobayashi S, et al. Predictors of mortality in patients treated with continuous hemodiafiltration for acute renal failure. *ASAIO J* 2001:47:86–91.
11. Hida M, Saitoh H, Satoh T. Autopsy findings in postoperative acute renal failure patients, collected from the annuals of pathological autopsy cases in Japan. *Tokai J Exper Clin Med* 1984:9:349–355.
12. Liano F, Junco E, Pascual J, et al. The spectrum of acute renal failure in the intensive care unit compared with that seen in other settings. *Kidney Int* 1998:53:S16–S24.
13. Shipley RE, Study RS. Changes in renal blood flow, extraction of inulin, glomerular filtration rate, tissue pressure and urine flow with acute alterations in renal artery pressure. *Am J Physiol* 1951;167:676–688.
14. Schmid HE, Garrett RC, Spencer MP. Intrinsic hemodynamic adjustments to reduced renal perfusion pressure gradients. *Circ Res* 1964:14[Suppl]:I170–177.

15. Bersten AD, Holt AW. Vasoactive drugs and the importance of renal perfusion pressure. *New Horizons* 1995:3:650–661.

16. Bersten AD, Rutten AJ, Summersides G. Epinephrine infusion in sheep: systemic and renal hemodynamic effects. *Crit Care Med* 1994:22:994–1001.

17. Hellbrekers LJ, Liard JF, Laborde AL, et al. Regional autoregulatory responses during infusion of vasoconstrictor agents in conscious dogs. *Am J Physiol* 1990:259:H1270–H1277.

18. Hoogenberg K, Smit AJ, Girbes ARJ. Effects of low dose dopamine on renal and systemic hemodynamics during incremental norepinephrine infusion in healthy volunteers. *Crit Care Med* 1998:26:260–265.

19. Richer M, Robert S, Lebel M. Renal hemodynamics during norepinephrine and low dose dopamine infusions in man. *Crit Care Med* 1996:24:1150–1156.

20. Ichai C, Passeron C, Carles M, et al. Prolonged low-dose dopamine infusion induces a transient improvement in renal function in hemodynamically stable, critically ill patients: a single blind, prospective, controlled study. *Crit Care Med* 2000:28:1329–1335.

21. Australian and New Zealand Intensive Care Society Clinical Trials Group. Low-dose dopamine in patients with early renal dysfunction: a placebo-controlled randomized trial. *Lancet* 2000:356:2139–2143.

22. Conger JD. Interventions in clinical acute renal failure: what are the data? *Am J Kidney Dis* 1995;26:565–576.

23. Solomon R, Werner C, Mann D, et al. Effects of saline, mannitol and furosemide on acute decreases in renal function induced by radiocontrast agents. *N Engl J Med* 1994:331:1416–1420.

24. Allgren RL, Marbury TC, Rahman SN, et al. Anaritide in acute tubular necrosis. *N Engl J Med* 1997:336:828–834.

25. Hirshberg R, Kopple J, Lipsett P, et al. Multicenter clinical trial of recombinant human insulin-like growth factor I in patients with acute renal failure. *Kidney Int* 1999:55:2423–2432.

26. Brady HR, Brenner BM, Clarkson MR, et al. Acute renal failure. In: Brenner BM, Rector FC, eds. *The kidney,* 6th ed. Philadelphia: WB Saunders, 2000:1201–1262.

27. Sawaya BP, Briggs JP, Schnermann J. Amphotericin B nephrotoxicity. The adverse consequences of altered membrane proteins. *J Am Soc Nephrol* 1995:6:154–164.

28. Rudnick MR, Goldfarb S, Wexler L, et al. Nephrotoxicity of ionic and nonionic contrast media in 1196 patients: a randomized trial. *Kidney Int* 1995:47:254–261.

29. Tepel M, van der Giet M, Schwartzfeld C, et al. Prevention of radiographic-contrast induced reductions in renal function by acetylcysteine. *N Engl J Med* 2000:343:180–184.

30. Leverve X, Barnoud D. Stress metabolism and nutritional support in acute renal failure. *Kidney Int* 1998:53:S62–S66.

31. Frankenfield DC, Reynolds HN. Nutritional effect of continuous hemodiafiltration. *Nutrition* 1995;11:388–393.

32. Marcias WL, Alaka KJ, Murphy MH, et al. Impact of the nutritional regimen on protein catabolism and nitrogen balance in patients with acute renal failure. *J Parent Enteral Nutr* 1996:20:56–62.

33. Bellomo R, Seacombe J, Daskalakis M, et al. A prospective comparative study of moderate versus high protein intake for critically ill patients with acute renal failure. *Renal Fail* 1998:20:545–547.

34. Druml W, Schwarzenhofer M, Apsner R, et al. Fat-soluble vitamins in patients with acute renal failure. *Miner Electrolyte Metab* 1998:24:220–226.

35. Corwin HL, Gettinger A, Rodriguez RM, et al. Efficacy of recombinant human erythropoietin in the critically ill patient: a randomized, double-blind, placebo-controlled trial. *Crit Care Med* 1999;27:2346–2350.

36. Nemoto T, Yokota N, Keane WF, et al. Recombinant erythropoietin rapidly treats anemia in ischemic acute renal failure. *Kidney Int* 2001:59:246–251.

37. Parsons FM, Hobson SM, Blagg CR, et al. Optimum time for dialysis in acute reversible renal failure: description and value of improved dialyzer with large surface area. *Lancet* 1961:1:129–134.

38. Fischer RP, Griffen WOJ, Reiser M, et al. Early dialysis in the treatment of acute renal failure. *Surg Gynecol Obstet* 1966:123:1019–1023.

39. Treotola SO, Kuhn-Fulton J, Johnson MS, et al. Tunneled infusion catheters: increased incidence of symptomatic venous thrombosis after subclavian versus internal jugular venous access. *Radiology* 2000:217:89–93.

40. Hernandez D, Diaz F, Rufino M, et al. Subclavian vascular access stenosis in dialysis patients: natural history and risk factors. *J Am Soc Nephrol* 1998:9:1507–1510.

41. Kappes S, Towne J, Adams M, et al. Perforation of the superior vena cava. A complication of subclavian dialysis. *JAMA* 1983:249:2232–2233.

42. Schlaeper C, Amerling R, Manns M, et al. High clearance continuous renal replacement therapy with a modified dialysis machine. *Kidney Int* 1999:72:S20–S23.

43. Kumar VA, Craig M, Depner TA, et al. Extended daily dialysis: a new approach to renal replacement for acute renal replacement in the intensive care unit. *Am J Kidney Dis* 2000:36:294–300.

44. Paganni P, O'Hara P, Nakamoto S. Slow continuous ultrafiltration in hemodialysis resistant oliguric acute renal failure patients. *Trans Am Soc Artif Intern Organs* 1984:30:173–178.

45. Bellomo R, Farmer M, Bhonagiri S, et al. Changing acute renal failure treatment from intermittent hemodialysis to continuous hemofiltration: impact on azotemic control. *Int J Artif Organs* 1999:22:145–150.

46. Mehta R, McDonald B, Gabbai F, et al. A randomized clinical trial of continuous versus intermittent dialysis for acute renal failure. *Kidney Int* 2001;60:1154–1163.

47. Rialp G, Roglan A, Betbese AJ, et al. Prognostic indexes and mortality in critically ill patients with acute renal failure treated with different dialytic techniques. *Renal Fail* 1996:18:667–675.

48. van Bommel E, Bouvy ND, So KL, et al. Acute dialytic support for the critically ill: intermittent hemodialysis versus continuous arteriovenous hemodiafiltration. *Am J Nephrol* 1995:15:192–200.

49. Swartz RD, Messana JM, Orzol S, et al. Comparing continuous hemofiltration with hemodialysis in patients with severe acute renal failure. *Am J Kidney Dis* 1999:34:424–432.

50. Bellomo R, Boyce N. Continuous venovenous hemodiafiltration compared with conventional dialysis in critically ill patients with acute renal failure. *ASAIO J* 1993:39:M794–M797.

51. Kleinknecht D, Jungers P, Chanard J, et al. Uremic and non-uremic complications in acute renal failure: evaluation of early and frequent dialysis on prognosis. *Kidney Int* 1972:1:190–196.

52. Conger JD. A controlled evaluation of prophylactic dialysis in post-traumatic acute renal failure. *J Trauma* 1975:15:1056–1063.

53. Gillum DM, Dixon BS, Yanover MJ, et al. The role of intensive dialysis in acute renal failure. *Clin Nephrol* 1986:25:249–255.

54. Paganini EP, Tapolyai M, Goormastic M, et al. Establishing a dialysis therapy/patient link in intensive care unit acute dialysis for patients with acute renal failure. *Am J Kidney Dis* 1996:28:S81–S89.

55. Evanson JA, Himmelfarb R, Wingard S, et al. Prescribed versus delivered dialysis in acute renal failure patients. *Am J Kidney Dis* 1998:32:731–738.

56. Schiffl H, Lanf SM, Koing A, et al. Dose of intermittent hemodialysis and outcome of acute renal failure: a prospective randomized study. *J Am Soc Nephrol* 1997:8:291A.

57. Ronco C, Bellomo R, Homel P, et al. Effects of different doses in continuous veno-venous haemofiltration on outcomes of acute renal failure: a prospective randomized trial. *Lancet* 2000:356:26–30.

58. Hakim RM, Wingard RL, Parker RA. Effect of the dialysis membrane in the treatment of patients with acute renal failure. *N Engl J Med* 1994:331:1338–1342.

59. Himmelfarb J, Tolkoff-Rubin NT, Chandran P, et al. A multicenter comparison of dialysis membranes in the treatment of acute renal failure requiring dialysis. *J Am Soc Nephrol* 1998:9:257–266.

60. Jorres A, Gahl GM, Dobis C, et al. Haemodialysis-membrane biocompatibility and mortality of patients with dialysis-dependent acute renal failure: a prospective randomized multicenter trial. *Lancet* 1999;354:1337–1341.

61. Gastaldello K, Melot C, Kahn RJ, et al. Comparison of cellulose diacetate and polysulphone membranes in the outcome of acute renal failure. A prospective randomized study. *Nephrol Dial Transplant* 2000;15:224–230.

62. Grootendorst AF, van Bommel EF, van Leengoed LA, et al. Infusion of ultrafiltrate from endotoxemic pigs depresses myocardial performance in normal pigs. *J Crit Care* 1993:8:161–169.

63. Gomez A, Wang R, Unruh H, et al. Hemofiltration reverses left ventricular dysfunction during sepsis in dogs. *Anesthesiology* 1990:73:671–685.

64. Rogiers P, Zhang H, Smail N, et al. High volume hemofiltration improves hemodynamics in experimental endotoxic shock. *Intensive Care Med* 1996:22:S396.

65. Schetz M, Ferdinande P, Van den Berghe G, et al. Removal of pro-inflammatory cytokines with renal replacement therapy: sense or nonsense? *Intensive Care Med* 1995:21:169–176.

66. Bellomo R, Tipping P, Boyce N. Continuous veno-venous hemofiltration with dialysis removes cytokines from the circulation of septic patients. *Crit Care Med* 1993:21:522–526.

67. Braun N, Rosenfeld S, Giolai M, et al. Effect of continuous hemodiafiltration on IL-6, TNF-alpha, C3a, and TCC in patients with SIRS/septic shock using two different membranes. *Contrib Nephrol* 1995;116:89–98.

68. Bellomo R, Farmer M, Wright C, et al. Treatment of sepsis-associated severe acute renal failure with continuous hemodiafiltration: clinical experience and comparison with conventional dialysis. *Blood Purif* 1995:13:246–254.

69. De Vriese AS, Colardyn FA, Philippe JJ, et al. Cytokine removal during continuous hemofiltration in septic patients. *J Am Soc Nephrol* 1999:10:846–853.

AN APPROACH TO VENOUS THROMBOEMBOLISM/PULMONARY EMBOLISM IN THE CRITICALLY ILL

KENNETH E. WOOD

KEY WORDS

- Pulmonary embolism
- Hemodynamics
- Shock
- Electrocardiogram
- Arterial blood gas
- D-dimer
- Echocardiogram
- Ventilation perfusion scan
- Angiogram
- Heparin
- Thrombolytic therapy
- Embolectomy
- Cardiac arrest
- Venous thromboembolism

Venous thrombosis is always a severe disease and is often fatal, because fragments of the thrombi may detach and occlude branches of the pulmonary artery ... the occlusion of the main branches of the pulmonary artery causes a striking rise in blood pressure in these vessels. This rise—which the right heart must fight in order to ensure circulation—may sometimes lead to cardiac arrest.

— Picot 1884, Lecons de Clinique Médicale

INTRODUCTION

Although significant advances have been made in the prophylaxis, diagnostic modalities, and therapeutic options for pulmonary embolism (PE), it remains a commonly underdiagnosed and lethal entity. It is estimated that PE occurs in more than 600,000 patients per year and is reported to cause or contribute to 50,000 to 200,000 deaths (1). The incidence of PE causing, contributing, or accompanying death in hospitalized patients has remained remarkably constant at about 15% over the past 40 years (2). Similarly, the antemortem diagnosis of fatal PE has not changed appreciably over the same period and remains fixed at approximately 30% (3). Recent large, contemporary observational studies of PE have reported an overall 3-month mortality of 17% (4) and an in-hospital mortality of 31% when PE was associated with hypotension (5). Mortality directly attributed to PE was 45% and 91% in the respective groups (4,5). Thus, PE remains common, underdiagnosed, and lethal. In cases of fatal PE, two-thirds of the patients die within 1 hour of presentation (3), and anatomically massive PE will account for only one-half of those deaths, with the remainder ascribed to smaller submassive or recurrent emboli (6,7). Traditionally, life-threatening PE has been equated with anatomically massive PE obstructing 50% to 60% of the pulmonary vasculature (8). Therefore, it seems reasonable to propose that outcome from PE is a function of the size of the embolism and the underlying cardiopulmonary status (CPS) of the patient. Similar hemodynamic and clinical outcomes will manifest from a massive PE in a patient with adequate CPS and a submassive PE in a patient with a compromised CPS. Figure 1 depicts the proposed relationship between mortality and severity as characterized by a combination of embolism size and CPS. Progressive increments in severity are associated with a relatively constant low mortality, provided therapeutic anticoagulation is achieved. The combination of embolism size and CPS necessary to produce hypotension is associated with a mortality of 30% (5). A minimal increase in severity produces cardiac arrest, which has a mortality of at least 70% (5,9). It has been suggested that the term *major* be used to define any combination of embolus size and CPS that results in a hemodynamically significant event (10). The combination of embolism size and CPS that produces the mortality inflection point remains elusive. Although the presence of right ventricular (RV) dysfunction has been proposed to signify this point, this remains controversial because the vast majority of patients with PE and RV dysfunction will survive (11). It is crucial to reconcile the predictors necessary to establish this critical inflection point because it will define the threshold at which patients are deemed at sufficient risk with conventional therapy to justify the risk and potential benefits of more aggressive and costly therapies.

Hypotension secondary to RV failure resulting from a combination of embolism size and CPS is thought to be a more accurate indicator of the magnitude of the PE than the degree of angiographic obstruction (12). The presence of hemodynamic decompensation or shock is associated with a threefold to sevenfold increase in mortality (4,12,13). Thus, the presence of hypotension provides an early and readily available discriminator between potential survivors and nonsurvivors and provides the rationale to devise a physiologic approach to the diagnosis and management

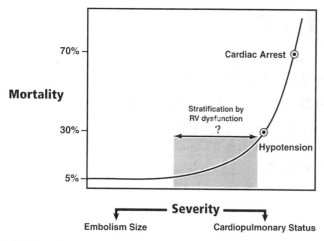

FIGURE 1. Outcomes in pulmonary embolism: relationship between mortality and severity.

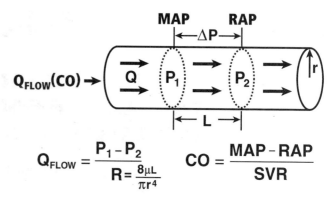

FIGURE 2. Poiseuille's Law representing the relationship between flow, pressure, and resistance.

of PE. The spectrum of PE that the intensivist most frequently encounters is predominately confined to two scenarios: (a) the patient presenting with shock or respiratory failure in whom the diagnosis of PE is a consideration and (b) the established intensive care unit (ICU) patient in whom PE develops post admission. In either scenario, the diagnosis and management of PE in the ICU are particularly challenging because differentiating PE from other life-threatening illness is frequently difficult, logistical constraints can impair definitive diagnostic testing, and hemorrhagic risks can compromise the ability to anticoagulate or undertake thrombolysis. This chapter reviews a structured physiologic approach to the diagnosis, resuscitative and therapeutic strategies, as well as discuss issues specifically germane to PE encountered in the ICU. Similar to the "golden hour" of trauma, myocardial infarction (MI), and stroke, there exists a "golden hour" of major PE, during which time an expeditious approach to diagnosis and therapy can potentially affect outcome.

SHOCK MODEL AND PATHOPHYSIOLOGY

The care of the critically ill, hemodynamically unstable patient frequently proceeds along two parallel paths: physiologic resuscitation and differential diagnosis generation. Use of a universally applicable model of the circulation that enables an expeditious application of diagnostic and resuscitative strategies is desirable. The conventional approach to hemodynamics uses Poiseuille's law to conceptualize the circulatory system as a cylindrical conduit. *Flow* (cardiac output) is defined as a function of pressure gradients (mean arterial pressure, right atrial pressure) (Fig. 2). Because flow is pulsatile, it is necessary to incorporate a hydraulic pump into the model. A hydraulic model of the circulation more accurately presents the circulatory system as two hydraulic pumps (right and left sides of the heart), each with its own *capacitance* (volume reservoir) and *impedance* (resistive element) (Fig. 3). Consequent to this series in hydraulic alignment, cardiac output cannot exceed venous return and vice versa; for practical purposes, both pumps can be conceptualized as a single hydraulic unit. Therefore, the circulatory system can be defined as

a three-compartment model, a capacitance bed that provides volume to a hydraulic pump that generates flow into an impedance bed. Any hemodynamic abnormality can be characterized by a disturbance(s) of one or more of these variables. The surrogates for venous capacitance pressure, hydraulic pump function, and impedance are right atrial pressure (RAP), cardiac output (CO), and systemic vascular resistance (SVR), respectively. Frequently, invasive monitoring is not established on initial presentation, and it is prudent to use the available physical examination surrogates to define model variables. Estimation of the RAP from the internal jugular vein approximates pressure in the venous capacitance bed; pulse character and temperature of the extremities approximate impedance (resistance). Warm, flushed extremities with a wide pulse pressure indicate low impedance (resistance), whereas cool constricted extremities with a narrow thready pulse suggest high impedance (resistance). In shock patients, flow and resistance are almost universally reciprocal ($Q \times R = \Delta P$ or $CO \times SVR = BP$); therefore, the initial assessment of impedance (resistance) allows for inferential derivation of hydraulic flow (CO). Given the potential consideration for thrombolytic therapy in this population, invasive monitoring should be reserved for circumstances when the model variables cannot be well characterized from the physical examination. Representative examples are illustrated in Table 1.

The impaction of embolic material on the pulmonary outflow tract precipitates the vicious pathophysiologic cycle of events depicted in Figure 4. Mechanical obstruction and neurohumoral factors combined with the underlying CPS will increase pulmonary impedance, creating a pressure load on the RV. An escalating pressure load will decrease RV output and initiate RV decompensation and dilatation. These pressure and volume loads can increase RV wall stress, precipitating RV ischemia. RV dilatation will limit left ventricular (LV) distensibility through a septal shift and via pericardial restraint, thereby decreasing LV preload and cardiac output. The subsequent decrease in mean arterial pressure (MAP) will decrease the RV coronary perfusion pressure gradient, further compounding the potential for ischemic insult and RV decompensation (14). Translation of the pathophysiology into the previously discussed three compartmental model is shown in Figure 5. Model variables would reveal an increased RAP, decreased CO, and increased SVR, which would be clinically correlated with jugular venous distention, a thready pulse,

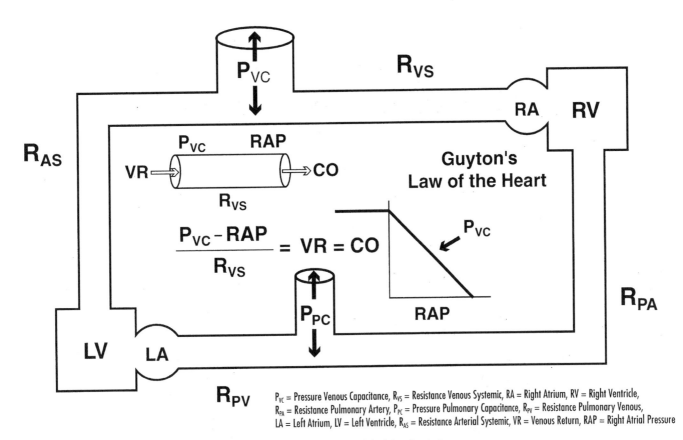

$$\frac{P_{VC} - RAP}{R_{VS}} = VR = CO$$

P_{VC} = Pressure Venous Capacitance, R_{VS} = Resistance Venous Systemic, RA = Right Atrium, RV = Right Ventricle, R_{PA} = Resistance Pulmonary Artery, P_{PC} = Pressure Pulmonary Capacitance, R_{PV} = Resistance Pulmonary Venous, LA = Left Atrium, LV = Left Ventricle, R_{AS} = Resistance Arterial Systemic, VR = Venous Return, RAP = Right Atrial Pressure

FIGURE 3. Hydraulic model of the circulation.

and cool extremities, respectively. With relatively clear lungs as determined by auscultation and chest radiograph, the hydraulic lesion localizes to the right side of the heart with the differential diagnosis as shown in Figure 5.

It is instructive to review the clinical manifestations of PE in patients who have an adequate CPS to assess the pure effects and compensations of the disease. In this population, the physiologic and clinical manifestations are directly correlated with the embolism size (15). The degree of angiographic obstruction is directly related to the mean pulmonary artery pressure (mPAP), RAP, and PaO$_2$. The mPAP will begin to rise only when 25% to 30% or more of the pulmonary vascular bed is occluded, and, despite obstruction of 50% or more, the normal RV cannot generate an mPAP greater than or equal to 40 mm Hg. Elevations of mPAP of 40 mm Hg or more represent either underlying

cardiopulmonary disease or recurrent emboli with RV hypertrophy. At high levels of mPAP (30–40 mm Hg), either elevations or depressions of CO are observed, suggesting that the range of RV failure is narrow and that mPAP of 30 to 40 mm Hg in patients with adequate CPS should be considered to represent severe pulmonary hypertension. The mPAP can be less than expected in the presence of anatomically massive embolism if the RV is failing and cannot generate forward flow [mPAP = CO × pulmonary vascular resistance (PVR)]. Increases in the RAP are directly related to the mPAP but are unusual until the mPAP is 30 mm Hg or greater and the obstruction is 35% to 40% or greater. RAP can be elevated without a diminution in CO with PE; however, a decrease in CO without an increase in RAP should suggest an alternative non-PE diagnosis. An elevated RAP can be used to assess the extent of encroachment on RV reserve. Characteristically, the CO in patients with an adequate CPS will be elevated as a consequence of the hypoxically mediated sympathetic response. Inadequacy of the preceding compensatory mechanisms will result in cardiac failure characterized by RV dilatation with an increased mPAP, RAP, and heart rate (HR). Systemic hypotension will ensue when sympathetic vasoconstriction is inadequate to generate pressure in response to diminished flow (BP = CO × SVR). Thus, in patients with an adequate CPS, there appears to be a hierarchical series of compensations, with systemic hypotension defining the exhaustion and failure of the available compensatory measures. In contrast, patients with a compromised CPS will manifest a more marked degree of cardiopulmonary impairment with a lesser degree of angiographic obstruction (15,16). With an

TABLE 1. HYDRAULIC CIRCULATORY SHOCK MODEL

Impedance (SVR)	Capacitance (RAP)	Hydraulic Pump (CO)	Diff Dx
↑	↓	↓	Hypovolemia
↑	↑	↓	Cardiogenic
↓↓	→	↑	Vasogenic/ sepsis
↑	↑	↓	Pulmonary embolism

SVR, systemic vascular resistance; RAP, right atrial pressure; CO, cardiac output; Diff Dx, differential dignosis.

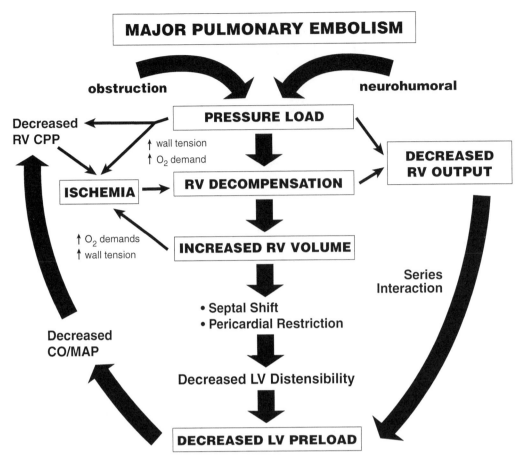

FIGURE 4. Pathophysiologic cycle of major pulmonary embolism.

average angiographic obstruction of only 23% (which is below the threshold to elicit elevations in mPAP in healthy patients), patients with a compromised CPS have an average mPAP of 40 mm Hg. CO is uniformly depressed, and the RAP and PaO$_2$ are unreliable indicators of the degree of angiographic obstruction. There appears to be no consistent relationship between the magnitude of the cardiopulmonary impairment and the degree of angiographic obstruction, which clearly illustrates the role of the underlying CPS in this population. The preceding overview suggests that PE can be characterized on the basis of CPS and embolism size. The focus of the remainder of the chapter is on major PE, which is the spectrum of the disease most likely to confront the intensivist.

INCIDENCE AND PRESENTATION

The Virchow triad of stasis, vessel trauma, and hypercoagulability represents the fundamental risk factors for venous thromboembolism (VTE). Specific clinical states are depicted in Table 2. Although uncommon in outpatients, VTE is common in hospitalized patients; it is estimated that PE will occur in 1% of all hospital admissions (17). For a hospital admitting 36,000 patients per year, this would translate into one PE per day. In addition to age and a previous history of VTE, certain clinical circumstances

are associated with an unusually high risk. Insofar as it has long been recognized that PE and deep venous thrombosis (DVT) are a continuum of the same disease process and that 90% of PE arises from DVT in lower extremities, it is instructive to review the incidence of DVT in certain high-risk populations. Patients undergoing major general surgery as defined by abdominal operations requiring general anesthesia for 30 minutes or longer have an overall 25% incidence of DVT when no prophylaxis is used; 9% of patients will have clinically detectable DVT, and 7% will have proximal DVT. The incidence of PE in this population is 1.6%, one-half of which will be fatal. Similarly, in patients for whom no prophylaxis is used who undergo elective hip surgery, the incidence of DVT is 50%, with 23% clinically detectable and 20% proximal. PE will occur in 5% to 10% and will be fatal in one-half (18). In patients with major trauma who did not receive prophylaxis, DVT was found in 58%, proximal DVT in 18%. In this study, the incidence of DVT in major categories of trauma was reported as follows: face, chest, or abdomen (50%); major head injury (54%); spinal injuries (62%); lower-extremity orthopedic injury (69%); pelvic fractures (61%); femoral fractures (80%); and tibial fractures (77%) (19). The incidence of DVT in critically ill medical patients who do not receive prophylaxis is reported to be 15% (20). Given the staggering incidence of DVT in high-risk patients who do not receive prophylaxis, DVT prophylaxis has become a standard of care for this population.

Major Pulmonary Embolism
Hydraulic Model

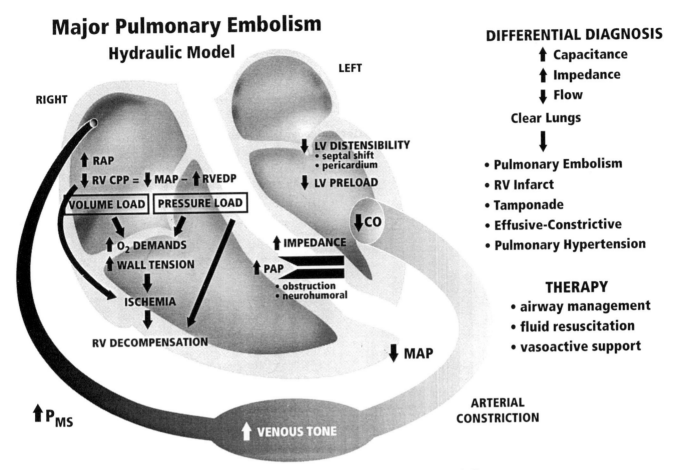

FIGURE 5. Pathophysiologic model of major pulmonary embolism.

Meta-analysis and large series have clearly shown that DVT prophylaxis significantly diminishes the incidence of DVT and reduces fatal PE (18,21–23). Although VTE is often thought to develop as a result of the omission of standard DVT prophylaxis, it is crucial to recognize that VTE frequently occurs also in patients who have received appropriate prophylaxis. A recent large series reported that more than 50% of patients with VTE had received appropriate prophylaxis (24). In a study of medical ICU patients, of whom 92% received appropriate prophylaxis, DVT was documented by ultrasound in 12% (25). Therefore, the presence of DVT prophylaxis should not dissuade the clinician from

considering VTE if the clinical suspicion is high. A comprehensive review of the spectrum of DVT prophylaxis is beyond the scope of this chapter, and the reader is referred to the recent ACCP antithrombotic consensus statement (26). Table 3 provides guidelines for high-risk patients likely to be encountered in the ICU.

It has been estimated that hemodynamically unstable major PE constitutes approximately 10% of all PE presentations (10). Given the potential for lethality within the first hour and the exclusion of patients with hemodynamic instability or contraindications to thrombolytic therapy in many clinical trials, the true percentage may be higher. In the Urokinase Pulmonary Embolism Trial (UPET) (13) and Urokinase-Streptokinase Pulmonary Embolism Trials (USPET) (27), 19% of patients without underlying cardiopulmonary disease presented with cardiovascular collapse characterized by shock or syncope. In the largest observational study of major PE (1,001 patients), which required right-sided heart failure or pulmonary hypertension as entry criteria, Management Strategy and Prognosis of Pulmonary Embolism Registry (MAPPET) reported 59% of patients as having hemodynamic instability on presentation, 18% with cardiac arrest, 10% with shock requiring vasopressor support, and 31% with an arterial pressure of 90 mm Hg or lower not requiring pressors (5). Syncope represents a clinical intermediate between hypotension and cardiac arrest because patients who recover consciousness have a high incidence of hypotension, whereas failure

TABLE 2. RISK FACTORS FOR VENOUS THROMBOEMBOLIC DISEASE

Age	Oral contraceptives
Malignancy	Hormonal replacement
Surgery	Pregnancy
Trauma	Protein C, S deficiency
Immobilization	Antithrombin III deficiency
History of venous thromboembolism	Factor V Leiden
Congestive heart failure	
Myocardial infarction	
Stroke	

TABLE 3. VENOUS THROMBOEMBOLISM PROPHYLAXIS

Category	Recommendation
General surgery	
Low risk	No specific prophylaxis
Minor procedures	
≤40 yr old	
No VTE risk factors	
Moderate risk	LDUH, LMWH, ES, or IPC
Minor procedures with VTE risk	
Nonmajor surgery	
40–60 yr old	
No VTE risk	
Major operations	
≤40 yr old	
No VTE risk	
Higher risk	LDUH, LMWH, or IPC
Nonmajor surgery	
≥60 yr old or VTE risk	
Major surgery	
≥40 yr old or VTE risk	
Very high risk with multiple risk factors	LDUH or LMWH combined with ES or IPC
Neurosurgery	IPC ± ES
Trauma	LMWH if no contraindication
	IPC ± ES if LMWH contraindicated
	High risk with suboptimal prophylaxis; consider duplex screen
	IVC filter *not* recommended for primary prophylaxis
Spinal cord injury	
Acute phase	LMWH if not contraindicated
	LDUH, ES, IPC ineffective
	IPC/ES possibly beneficial if combined with LMWH or LDUH or if anticoagulants are contraindicated
Rehabilitation phase	LMWH or warfarin
Medical conditions	
Acute myocardial infarction	LDUH or IV heparin
Ischemic stroke	LDUH or LMWH if not contraindicated
	ES or IPC if LDUH/LMWH contraindicated
General medical with VTE risks	LDUH or LMWH

VTE, venous thromboembolism; LMWH, low molecular weight heparin; LDUH, low-dose unfractionated heparin; ES, elastic graduated compression stockings; IPC, intermittent pneumatic compression; IVC, intravenous catheter
Adapted form ACCP Consensus Conference on Antithrombotic Therapy. *Chest* 2001;119:S132–S175, with permission.

TABLE 4. SIGNS AND SYMPTOMS OF MAJOR PULMONARY EMBOLISM IN PATIENTS WITHOUT CARDIOPULMONARY DISEASE (N = 40)

	Circulatory Collapse	
	Shock (%)	Syncope (%)
Tachycardia ≥100/min	86	58
Tachypnea ≥20/min	81	89
Dyspnea	71	89
Apprehension	71	74
Accentuated P_2	62	79
Rales	48	47
Fever (≥37.5°C)	43	21
Pleuritic pain	38	63
Cough	33	42
Deep venous thrombosis	19	42
Hemoptysis	10	5

Adapted from Stein PD. *Am J Cardiol* 1981;47:218–222, with permission.

evidence of cor pulmonale (28). The incidence of cardiac arrest is difficult to define, although it reportedly occurred in 29% (29) of Miller's series of anatomically massive PE and in 18% of MAPPET patients (5). The signs and symptoms of major PE in patients from UPET and USPET are compiled in Table 4. In the series by Miller and associates of patients with cardiac catheterization–documented PE shock, 87% experienced the sudden onset of dyspnea, 70% manifested cardiovascular collapse, and 22% had chest pains simulating MI. In 48% of patients, there were signs and symptoms of minor PE within the week preceding the major presentation (29). In MAPPET, 70% of patients had an acute onset of symptoms 48 hours or sooner prior to presentation, 96% were dyspneic, and 70% were tachycardic (5).

DIAGNOSTIC FINDINGS

The early generation of a differential diagnosis usually depended on elements derived from the history, physical examination, and the basic but readily available diagnostic studies: ECG, chest radiograph (CXR), and arterial blood gas (ABG). Rarely are definitive studies for PE available in the first hour of clinical presentation; therefore, recognizing the manifestations of major PE from the preceding is crucial to ensure that PE is appropriately incorporated into the differential diagnosis. By using the previously described hydraulic model of the circulation, major PE can be defined by a characteristic pattern and differential diagnosis, as depicted in Figure 5. An increase in pressure in the venous capacitance bed (elevated RAP) with high impedance and low flow (narrow pulse pressure and cool extremities) against the background of clear lungs isolates the hydraulic lesion to the right side of the heart with the differential diagnosis as depicted. Physical findings of RV dysfunction could include RV S3, RV heave, increased P_2, and the inspiratory accentuation of a systolic murmur at the right base consistent with tricuspid regurgitation. Prominent findings by the Miller group included an arterial pulse that was sharp and of low volume, tachycardia, clinical RV failure with an elevated RAP, an RV gallop rhythm,

to recover consciousness is associated with cardiac arrest. Although not a presentation commonly associated with PE, syncope has been reported in 13% of patients in large trials and series (13,27,28). In the series by Thames and colleagues, syncope was reported to be recurrent, prominent in presentations from outside the hospital, and associated with higher degrees of angiographic obstruction, cardiac arrest, elevations in RAP, lower PaO_2 and cardiac index, and electrocardiographic (ECG) and an accentuated P_2. The intensity of the physical findings diminished with time (29). In the Prospective Investigation of Pulmonary Embolism Diagnosis (PIOPED) study, the following associations were noted between physical findings and hemodynamics: third heart sound (mPAP 39 mm Hg; RAP 12 mm Hg), RV heave (mPAP 29 mm Hg; RAP 8 mm Hg), palpitations (mPAP 27 mm Hg; RAP 6 mm Hg), and diaphoresis (mPAP 26 mm Hg; RAP 8 mm Hg) (17). Invasive monitoring may be in place at the onset and should complement the preceding hydraulic model characterization and physical findings: elevated RAP, mPAP, and SVR and decreased CI. The pulmonary capillary wedge pressure (PCWP) should be low but may be normal as a consequence of the possible distortion of the LV pressure–volume relationship induced by the septal shift (30). Patients with a compromised CPS can manifest similar findings but frequently have complex findings dominated by their underlying disease.

The initial description of the ECG manifestations of PE was reported by McGinn and White in 1935, when they described the $S_I Q_{III} T_{III}$ ECG correlate of acute cor pulmonale (31). A normal ECG is uncommon in PE; in UPET and PIOPED patients with an adequate CPS, a normal ECG was reported in 14% and 30%, respectively (32,33). Rhythm disturbances are rare; atrial fibrillation or flutter is reported in 0% to 5%, and first-, second-, or third-degree heart block or ventricular dysrhythmias are uncommon (32,33). The ECG correlate of acute cor pulmonale [right-axis deviation, complete or incomplete right bundle-branch block (RBBB), $S_I Q_{III} T_{III}$, P pulmonale] occurred in 32% of patients with anatomically massive PE in UPET (32). In the series by Miller and colleagues of PE shock patients, abnormalities of conduction or repolarization of the RV were found in 78%, RBBB in 22%, $S_I Q_{III} T_{III}$ in 27%, and a normal ECG in 17% (34). In UPET, nonspecific T-wave changes occurred in 42% of patients and ST segment depression or elevations occurred in 42% (32). In PIOPED, 49% of patients had ST-T abnormalities (33). Isolated T-wave inversions are the most common abnormalities reported in other series (35).

The ECG manifestations of PE are related to the angiographic and lung-scan magnitude of the PE. UPET patients with ST segment abnormalities, T-wave inversion, right axis and incomplete RBBB had larger perfusion defects (32). Recently, the anterior T-wave inversions in the precordial leads were shown to represent the ECG finding most correlative with PE severity, occurring in 85% with massive PE versus 19% in nonmassive PE. When this finding is present, 90% of patients had an obstruction of 50% or greater, and 81% had an mPAP of 30 mm Hg or greater. Early appearance on day 1 was associated with an obstruction of 69% compared with 52% where the finding developed after day one. Normalization of the inverted T-wave pattern correlated with physiologic resolution in patients who received thrombolytics (35). As a consequence of increased myocardial wall stress and decreased coronary perfusion pressure, MI in the presence of normal coronaries has been reported (36).

Although it is nonspecific, the CXR can contribute to the diagnostic assessment of PE by excluding diseases that mimic PE, defining abnormalities that mandate further evaluation, and providing a crude estimate of severity (37). A normal CXR is unusual in PE and occurred in 16% of PIOPED patients, whereas

TABLE 5. DIAGNOSTIC FINDINGS IN PULMONARY EMBOLISM

Electrocardiogram (ECG)
  Anterior T-wave inversions
  Abnormalities in the ST-T segment, elevation or depression
  ECG correlate of acute cor pulmonale
    Complete or incomplete RBBB
    $S_I Q_{III} T_{III}$

Chest x-ray

Hilar dilatation	Elevated hemidiaphragm
Pulmonary artery dilatation	Pleural effusion
Relative pulmonary vascular oligemia	Pulmonary infarction
Cardiomegaly	

atelectasis or a pulmonary parenchymal abnormality occurred in 68% of patients. Pleural effusions were seen in 48% of patients and were confined to blunting of the costophrenic angle as none occupied one-third or more of the hemithorax (33). In UPET patients with an adequate CPS, a normal CXR was observed in 34% with parenchymal (elevated hemidiaphragm 46%, consolidation 39%, pleural effusion 30%, and atelectasis 28%) and vascular (decreased pulmonary vascularity 22%, prominent central pulmonary artery 21%) signs present in 67% and 37% of patients, respectively. Vascular signs were more common in massive PE (38). An association between PE severity and the radiographic findings was also evident in PIOPED patients. The lowest mPAP and lowest $P(A-a)O_2$ measurements were found in patients with a normal CXR, whereas the highest levels were seen in patients with cardiomegaly, decreased pulmonary vascularity (Westermark's sign), and a prominent pulmonary artery (37). Oligemia is common with anatomically massive PE and is reported to correlate with angiographic oligemia in 80% of cases (39). Findings in PE patients with shock or collapse are depicted in Table 5.

Abnormalities in gas exchange are complex and a function of the size and character of the embolic material, the extent of the obstruction, the underlying CPS, and the time since embolization. Hypoxia has been ascribed to an increase in dead space, right-to-left shunting, ventilation–perfusion (V/Q) inequality, and a low mixed venous O_2 (40). Although somewhat counterintuitive, low V/Q ratios account for a majority of the observed hypoxia. Redistribution of blood flow away from the embolized area results in the overperfusion of the nonembolized lung regions. Atelectasis that initially develops distal to the embolized area, followed by early reperfusion and flow through a patent foramen ovale, are also thought to account for the low V/Q ratio (40). Despite this impressive list of physiologic mechanisms, several caveats regarding hypoxia in PE should be recognized. First, hypoxia is not uniformly present. A PaO_2 of 80 mm Hg or greater was seen in 12% of UPET and 19% of PIOPED patients (41,42). Second, even a normal $P(A-a)O_2$ gradient does not exclude PE (33). Third, a close relationship has been recognized between the extent of the vascular obstruction and the degree of hypoxia (43). Although not uniformly available, the role of the D-dimer assay is rapidly evolving in the initial evaluation of suspected PE. Elevated levels of D-dimer are found in VTE and many other conditions in which fibrin cross-links are cleaved by plasmin, which accounts for the low reported specificity. The high sensitivity and corresponding negative predictive value potentially make it an ideal test to exclude PE (44).

DIAGNOSTIC APPROACH

Heparin should be initiated at therapeutic doses until the PE has been excluded, provided there are no contraindications to anticoagulation. The efficacy of heparin is attributed to an impairment of clot propagation and prevention of recurrent PE. The risk of recurrent venous thromboembolism is highest immediately after a PE (45); because recurrent PE is reported to be the most common cause of death in hemodynamically stable patients (11), it is necessary to achieve a therapeutic level of anticoagulation rapidly. The failure to establish an early therapeutic activated partial thromboplastin time (aPTT) level is associated with a high rate of recurrence (46). The use of a weight-based heparin nomogram has been shown to facilitate the optimal achievement of a therapeutic aPTT more rapidly and effectively to prevent recurrent thromboembolism (47). It has been clearly demonstrated that a 4- to 5-day course of heparin with warfarin initiated on day 1 is as effective as a traditional 10-day heparin course (48). This course has not, however, been studied in patients who have hemodynamically unstable major PE, and it is recommended that heparin be used for 7 to 10 days with the initiation of warfarin delayed until the aPTT has been therapeutic for 3 days (49). Heparin dosing requirements for patients with massive PE are reportedly higher, and substantial amounts of heparin may be required to ensure that adequate anticoagulation is rapidly achieved and sustained. Anti-factor Xa heparin levels are recommended when heparin dosing is greater than 40,000 U per day (50). Low-molecular-weight heparin (LMWH) has proved effective in treating submassive PE with proximal DVT, but its use in major PE remains unstudied at this time (51).

The presence of shock in acute PE, either as the consequence of massive PE in patients with an adequate CPS or submassive PE in patients with a compromised CPS, represents the failure of available compensatory mechanisms to sustain tissue perfusion and is associated with a significant increase in mortality. Therefore, the presence of shock defines an early, readily available, and reliable discriminator between survivors and nonsurvivors. The presence of shock is associated with a threefold to sevenfold increase in mortality (4,12,13). Tables 6 and 7 illustrate the relationship between shock, embolism size, and outcome reported in large series. Traditionally, massive PE is defined by angiographic obstruction of greater than 50% (1). The vast majority of patients with anatomically massive PE, however, do not present with shock (12,13,52–54). It is crucial to recognize that hemodynamically stable nonshock patients with submassive or massive PE have similar mortality rates (12,13). Unless accompanied by shock and hemodynamic instability, massive PE is not associated with an increased mortality (12,13,52–54). As illustrated in Table 7, several large series reported a 0% mortality in patients with anatomically massive PE without shock (55,56,57). The preceding finding is best exemplified in the original series from Alpert and colleagues and the UPET study, in which the shock vs. nonshock mortality rates were reported as 25% versus 5% and 36% versus 5%, respectively (12,13). It is interesting to note that the mortality rate for submassive (9.8%) was higher than that for massive (6.7%) cases in UPET because all the patients with submassive embolism and shock died (13). Using the presence of shock as an algorithmic discriminator, a diagnostic approach to the patient with suspected major PE is presented in Figure 6. In the nonshock patient, death within the first hour is unlikely. The tempo of the evaluation is less urgent than in the shock patient. In the nonshock population, the patient can be heparinized and transported to the confirmatory study of choice. Alternatively, the shock patient is much more likely to die within the first hour, and the speed of the evaluation must be expeditious. Although the pace of the evaluation for these two patient populations is different, the confirmatory studies are similar and will be discussed jointly using the shock patient as the prototype. In the patient with shock, the ideal diagnostic evaluation should begin in the area where the patient can be optimally resuscitated and stabilized. Duplex venous ultrasound is appealing because it is readily available and has excellent sensitivity and specificity for DVT in symptomatic patients. A positive finding subsequently can exploit the identical treatment for DVT and PE. It is crucial, however, to recognize that the sensitivity of Doppler ultrasound in an asymptomatic patient population has been reported to be less than 50% (58), as evidenced in studies where venogram-documented DVT was reported in 70% to 90% of PE patients (59), whereas documentation of DVT by ultrasound occurred in fewer than 50% of PE patients (60). Therefore, the absence of DVT by ultrasound does not preclude PE, nor does its presence confirm PE as the primary cause because the DVT may be incidental to another life-threatening process. Consequently, Doppler ultrasound is of somewhat limited use in the initial evaluation of shock patients, but it may be useful in the decision to place an inferior vena

TABLE 6. RELATIONSHIP BETWEEN SHOCK, EMBOLISM SIZE, AND OUTCOME

Study and Treatment	No. of Patients	% Shock Mortality	% Nonshock Mortality	% Massive in Shock Mortality	% Nonmassive in Shock Mortality	% Massive in Nonshock Mortality	% Nonmassive in Nonshock Mortality
UPET (13); heparin	160	9	91	12	4	88	96
or urokinase		36	6	18	100	5	6
Alpert et al. (12);	136	21	79	38	11	62	90
heparin		25	5	32	11	7	4

UPET, Urokinase Pulmonary Embolism Trial.

TABLE 7. ANATOMICALLY MASSIVE PULMONARY EMBOLISM RELATIONSHIP BETWEEN SHOCK AND OUTCOME

Study	Treatment	% Shock	% Mortality	% Nonshock	% Mortality
Miller et al., 1977 (29)	Heparin, lysis embolectomy	60	22	40	7
Marini et al., 1988 (55)	Urokinase/heparin	None	None	100	0
Verstraete et al., 1988 (52)	rt-PA	21	14	79	4
Tilsner, 1991 (54)	Urokinase	11	40	89	2
Diehl et al., 1992 (53)	rt-PA	33	22	68	3
Sors et al., 1994 (56)	rt-PA	None	None	100	0
Meneaveau et al., 1988 (57)	rt-PA streptokinase	None	None	100	0

rt-PA, recombinant tissue-type plasminogen activator.

cava (IVC) filter or in independently identifying an indication for anticoagulation.

Echocardiography (ECHO) is of enormous potential use in the shock patient because it is readily available and repeatable, useful in the recognition and differentiation of PE, and capable of assessing severity and response to therapy (61). In hemodynamically compromised patients, ECHO is reported to be the most frequent diagnostic procedure (5). Although used predominantly to characterize the degree and extent of RV pressure overload, a transthoracic (TTE) or transesophageal (TEE) ECHO has the ability to detect emboli in transit or define alternative diagnoses,

such as pericardial disease, hypovolemia, aortic dissection, myocardial dysfunction, and valvular insufficiency (62). Table 8 depicts the ECHO findings of PE-induced RV pressure overload. RV dilatation is the most common finding and is reported to occur in 50% to 100% of cases (63). Similar to the extent of obstruction required to induce elevations in mPAP, it appears that an obstruction greater than 30% is required to produce RV dilatation (64). Minor PE, defined by an obstruction of less than 20% or an mPAP of less than 20 mm Hg, does not characteristically produce ECHO of RV pressure overload or RV dilatation (65). The presence of a normal echocardiogram without signs

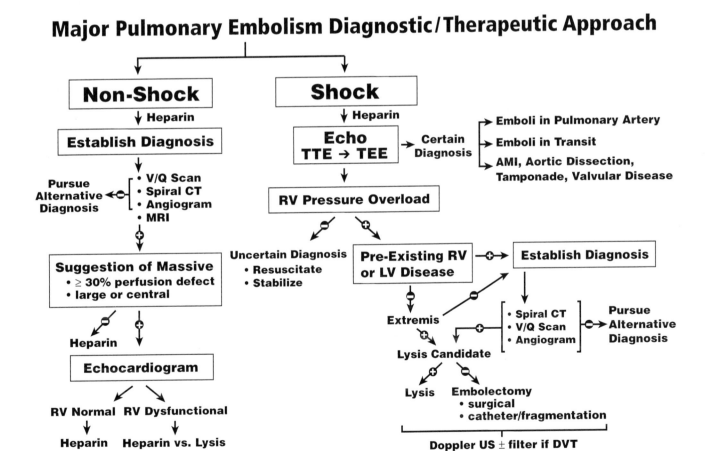

FIGURE 6. Diagnostic–therapeutic approach to major pulmonary embolism.

TABLE 8. ECHOCARDIOGRAPHY IN THE DIAGNOSTIC EVALUATION OF PULMONARY EMBOLISM

Pulmonary Embolism	Alternative Diagnosis
Right-sided emboli in transit	Acute MI
RV pressure overload	Tamponade
RV dilatation/hypokinesis	Aortic dissection
Increased RV/LV diameter ratio	Valvular disease
Paradoxical septal shift	Hypovolemia
Tricuspid regurgitation	
PA dilatation	
Loss of inspiratory collapse of the IVC	

MI, myocardial infarction; RV, right ventricle; LV, left ventricle; EF, ejection fraction; PA, pulmonary artery; IVC, intravenous catheter.

of right ventricular pressure overload effectively mitigates against PE as a cause of the shock state. In that circumstance, further resuscitation, stabilization, and diagnostic alternatives should be considered.

The presence of RV dilatation is not specific for PE. In patients with a previous cardiopulmonary disease RV dilatation may be representative of a spectrum of diseases ranging from RV infarct with myocardial dysfunction to cor pulmonale with pulmonary hypertension. Several echocardiographic findings have been reported to be useful in differentiating PE from these other conditions. Characteristically, acute PE is associated with a septal shift and minimal collapse of the IVC with inspiration and should not be accompanied by RV hypertrophy (62). The maximal velocity of the tricuspid regurgitant jet (TRjet) is directly proportional to the peak systolic pressure gradient between the RV and the RA and can be reliably used to estimate pulmonary artery pressure. It appears that the velocity of the TRjet in acute PE is intermediate between the low TRjet velocity associated with RV infarct and cardiomyopathy (2.5–2.8 m per second) and the elevated TRjet (3.5–3.7 m per second) seen in a chronically hypertrophied right ventricle (62).

Unless the embolus in transit is directly visualized, TTE provides only indirect evidence of PE. When acute PE is associated with RV dilatation, it is almost uniformly bilateral and, in most cases, is located in the central proximal pulmonary vessels, which can be reliably imaged by TEE (66,67). Several large series reported sensitivities of 80% to 96% and specificity of 84% to 100% for TEE performed immediately after RV dilatation is documented by TTE (66,67). Comparable sensitivity to spiral computed tomography (CT) has been attributed to the ability of PE to visualize the proximal extending mobile parts of more distally impacted thrombi.

When ECHO cannot be performed or documents RV pressure overload without direct evidence of thrombus, it is necessary to pursue confirmatory studies. Given the unstable nature and potential lethality of major PE, it is crucial to undertake an expeditious approach to defining the definitive diagnosis. Hospital, culture, expertise, experience, and availability frequently will define the choice of a confirmatory study. Traditionally, the V/Q scan has been considered the first-line study; unfortunately, it is diagnostic in only a minority of cases. In PIOPED, most patients with PE (59%) did not have a high probability scan. Most V/Q scans are nondiagnostic intermediate (39%) and low probability (34%). Scan interpretations of normal (15%) or high probability

(13%) are rare (68). This is further magnified in patients with chronic obstructive pulmonary disease (COPD), in which cases normal scans (5%) and high-probability scans (5%) are even less common and nondiagnostic intermediate scans (60%) predominate (69). It should be recognized, however, that the positive predicted value of high, intermediate, and low or normal scans is preserved in patients with or without cardiopulmonary disease, COPD, and critical illnesses (70,71). The combination of clinical probability and scan probability enhances the predicted value such that combinations of high clinical probability and high scan probability or low clinical probability and low scan probability are considered definitive for the diagnosis or exclusion of PE. Unfortunately, these combinations occur in only a minority of patients (68). Therefore, using the traditional approach will necessitate that most patients subsequently require angiography as the definitive confirmatory study. Although recognized as the gold confirmatory standard, angiography is expensive, invasive, requires a skilled and experienced staff to perform it; also, it is not uniformly available. Complications are common in critically ill patients from ICUs and in patients with pulmonary hypertension (72). In the MAPPET series of patients with PE-related RV dysfunction and hypotension, angiography was performed in only 14% of patients (5). Therefore, given the potential for a delay in diagnosis and associated complications, alternative approaches have been suggested. Spiral or helical CT is appealing because it is readily available, noninvasive, and, similar to TTE/TEE, it can provide alternative diagnosis (73). When spiral CT is compared with angiography for PE in the central pulmonary arteries, pooled analyses of large series report excellent sensitivity (94%), specificity (94%), and positive predictive value (93%) (74). The low sensitivity for spiral CT in some series has been attributed to the inability of the spiral CT to detect vessels at the subsegmental level. Given the infrequent nature of subsegmental PE and the variable interobserver angiographic agreement of its presence, the clinical significance of subsegmental PE is uncertain and therefore unlikely to precipitate shock. Similar to spiral CT, magnetic resonance imaging (MRI) accurately visualizes central vessels and provides alternative diagnoses; reportedly, MRI has comparable sensitivity and specificity. MRI offers the additional advantages of eliminating the use of nephrotoxic contrast material and making it possible to undertake MRI venography at the same session (75). Unfortunately, contraindications to MRI, patient isolation, and duration of the examination most likely will limit the utility of MRI in critically ill patients. Independent of which confirmatory strategy is used, the documented presence of PE in a hemodynamically unstable patient defines an indication for aggressive intervention with thrombolysis or, when thrombolysis is contraindicated, surgical or catheter embolectomy.

THERAPEUTIC APPROACH

Throughout the diagnostic evaluation period, patients with suspected major PE frequently require aggressive resuscitation and ongoing stabilization. Hemodynamic stability is often maintained by an intense catecholamine surge. Vasoconstriction of the arterial system provides for perfusion pressure gradients to ensure adequate flow to critical organs. The PE-induced increase in

TABLE 9. RESOLUTION OF PULMONARY EMBOLISM WITH THROMBOLYTIC THERAPY

| | Early | | | | |
Study	Angio	Scan	Hemodyn	Echo	Late
UPET, 1970 (13)	↑ 24 h	↑ 24 h	↑ 24 h	—	Scan equal day 5
Tibbutt, et al., 1974 (99)	↑ 72 h	—	↑ 72 h	—	Limited
Arnesen, et al., 1978 (100)	↑ 72 h	—	—	—	—
Ly, et al., 1978 (101)	↑ 72 h	—	—	—	No difference -1 yr
Marini, et al., 1988 (55)	→ 7 day	→ 24 h	→ 7 day	—	No difference
PIOPED, 1990 (68)	→ 2 h	→ 24, 48 h	↑ PVR 1.5 h	—	Scan equal day 3
Giuntini, et al., 1984 (102)	—	↑ 24 h	—	—	Scan equal day 7
Levine, et al., 1990 (103)	—	↑ 24 h	—	—	Scan/angio equal day 7
Dalla-Volta, et al., 1992 (104)	↑ 2 h	→ 7 day	↑ 2 h PAP-CI	—	—
Goldhaber, et al., 1993 (11)	—	↑ 24 h		↑ 3, 24 h	—

Angio, angiography; Hemody, hemodynamic; Echo, echocardiogram; UPET, Urokinase Pulmonary Embolism Trial; PIOPED, Prospective Investigation of Pulmonary Embolism Diagnosis; PAIMS, *Plasminogen Activator Italian* Multicenter Study; PVR, pulmonary vascular resistance; PAP, pulmonary artery pressure; CI, cardiac index; —, not studied; h, hour; ↑, improved thrombosis compared to heparin; →, no difference in thrombosis compared to heparin.

RAP necessitates venoconstriction to increase the pressure in the venous capacitance bed to maintain a perfusion pressure gradient for venous return (Fig. 5). With escalating oxygen requirements or refractory hypoxia, patients with suspected major PE frequently require intubation and mechanical ventilation. Intubation can provoke cardiovascular collapse for multiple reasons: (a) sedative–hypnotics used to facilitate intubation can abolish the catecholamine surge on which the patient is dependent for vasoconstriction; (b) overzealous initial lung inflation can further impair venous return; and (c) mechanical ventilation can further increase the PVR and precipitate a decline in RV function. Therefore, intubation should be undertaken judiciously and preferentially use a technique that involves a conscious, awake patient and use of topical or local anesthesia and etomidate to preserve the hemodynamic status. Recognizing that atelectasis or pulmonary consolidation is the most common finding on chest x-ray, positive-pressure ventilation has been shown to improve oxygenation in PE (76). Patients with major PE frequently require vasoactive support to maintain blood pressure. Traditionally, volume expansion is the initial treatment for hypotension associated with RV dysfunction. With PE-induced RV dysfunction and high RV pressures contributing to RV ischemia/wall stress and a septal shift impairing left ventricular compliance, additional fluid may compound the preceding problems and precipitate further RV deterioration (77). As such, when cavitary pressures are high or there is documented severe right ventricular dysfunction, fluids should be given judiciously and consideration given to the early use of vasopressors. It appears that norepinephrine is the preferred vasopressor of choice in patients with PE-induced shock, given its ability to maintain aortic pressure to provide adequate coronary flow to the stressed right ventricle. Additionally, norepinephrine possesses β_1-inotropic properties that provide complementary enhancement of RV function. Dobutamine increases CO and overall oxygen transport but may alter ventilation perfusion relationships and decrease the PaO_2. Additionally, dobutamine can cause peripheral vasodilatation through a β_2 effect, which leads to the recommendation that dobutamine be considered in moderate hypotension with appropriate monitoring and that norepinephrine be used for severe shock (78). Limited data exist on

unloading the RV with pulmonary vasodilators in patients with incipient or overt RV failure, as an adjunct to thrombolysis, in patients with contraindications to thrombolysis or in patients awaiting embolectomy. Inhaled prostacyclin (PGI_2) and nitric oxide have been reported to increase cardiac output and decrease pulmonary pressures while improving gas exchange in severe PE (79,80).

Despite the absence of definitive mortality data, thrombolytic therapy is uniformly acknowledged to be the treatment of choice for patients with hemodynamically unstable PE (81). Several points regarding thrombolytic therapy and major PE should be stressed. First, when assessed by angiogram, perfusion scan, hemodynamics, or echocardiography, thrombolytic therapy produces more rapid clot lysis compared with heparin in virtually all trials except two (Table 9) (55,81). No trial has reported any difference in the previously outlined physiologic parameters with respect to the degree of embolic resolution after 5 to 7 days. Given the hyperbolic relationship between PVR and vascular obstruction, it is evident that very small decreases in obstruction to less than 60%, as would be anticipated with thrombolysis, can reduce the PVR appreciably and alleviate right ventricular wall stress (82). However appealing the rapid resolution of embolic obstruction might be, only one trial demonstrated a mortality benefit (83). This small trial of only eight patients should be viewed with caution because all the patients randomized to thrombolytics were treated within hours of presentation, whereas those randomized to heparin previously failed heparin therapy and sustained recurrent PE, provoking severe respiratory failure. Table 10 reviews the comparative outcome studies. Second, it does not appear that there is any difference in thrombolytic agents, provided they are given in equivalent doses over the same time frame (84). Third, bolus therapy with recombinant tissue plasminogen activator (rt-PA) at 0.6 mg per kilogram of body weight over 15 minutes appears to be equivalent to the tradiional 100 mg over 2 hours (84). Fourth, intravenous rt-PA appears to be the equivalent of intrapulmonary rt-PA (52). Fifth, bleeding complications from thrombolytic therapy are common and, from pooled analysis, it appears that the overall incidence of major hemorrhage associated with PE thrombolysis is between

TABLE 10. OUTCOME OF THROMBOLYSIS VERSUS HEPARIN IN RANDOMIZED CLINICAL TRIALS FOR PULMONARY EMBOLISM

Study	No. of Patients	Heparin		Lysis	
		Mortality (%)	Recurrent (%)	Mortality (%)	Recurrent (%)
UPET, 1970 (13)	160	7	19	9	15
Tibbutt, et al., 1974 (99)	30	8	—	0	—
Ly, et al., 1978 (101)	20	9	—	0	—
Marini, et al., 1988 (55)	30	0	0	0	0
PIOPED, 1990 (68)	13	0	—	11	—
Levine, et al., 1990 (103)	58	0	0	3	0
Goldhaber, et al., 1993 (11)	101	4	9	0	0
Jerjes-Sanchez, et al., 1995 (83)	8	100	—	0	0

UPET, Urokinase Pulmonary Embolism Trial; PIOPED, Prospective Investigation of Pulmonary Embolism Diagnosis.

8.4% and 11.9%. The profile is similar among thrombolytic agents (84). Fatal hemorrhage is reported to occur in 2.2% of patients, and the incidence of intracranial hemorrhage ranges from 1.2% to 2.1% and is fatal in 50% of cases (84).

For patients with contraindications to thrombolytic therapy, failure of maximum medical therapy or ongoing/intermittent cardiac arrest, surgical embolectomy should be considered. Availability and expertise are limited and, in the modern era of medical embolectomy with thrombolytic therapy, surgical embolectomy is rarely performed (85). In MAPPET, only 1% of 594 patients with shock or cardiac arrest underwent the procedure (5). It has been suggested that diagnostic confirmatory studies can delay definitive treatment and contribute to mortality for patients considered for surgical embolectomy (86). It appears that cardiopulmonary bypass is the preferred operative technique and is associated with improved survival compared with venous inflow occlusion and normothermic circulatory rest (59% versus 48%) (87). Partial cardiopulmonary bypass has been advocated for circulatory support in moribund patients requiring angiography. Mortality in embolectomy series has declined progressively since the 1960s to 26% in contemporary series (86). Higher mortality rates are reported in series with a predominance of cardiac arrest patients (86). Catheter embolectomy and fragmentation are alternatives to patients not in cardiac arrest. Catheter embolectomy can reverse systemic hypotension, decrease PAP, improve CO, and have a mortality comparable to surgical embolectomy in patients without cardiac arrest (88). Indications to place an IVC filter include failure of anticoagulation and inability to anticoagulate or tolerate a subsequent embolic event. The placement of an IVC filter in patients with a free-floating thrombus in the lumen of a femoral or iliac vein is controversial in patients who are not hemodynamically compromised. IVC filter placement reduces the frequency of recurrent PE in the first 12 days of treatment and should strongly be considered in patients with RV compromise and a documented residual DVT (89).

SPECIAL CONSIDERATIONS

Right-sided heart emboli in transit have been increasingly recognized because of the widespread availability and increasing application of ECHO in the diagnostic evaluation of PE. Emboli in transit have been classified into two major categories with different morphologies, causes, and clinical significance. Type A thrombi are long, thin, extremely mobile emboli, characteristically found in the right atrium; they originate in the deep venous system. In a large series of patients with massive PE and cardiovascular instability, right-sided heart emboli were detected in 18% of patients; 84% of the emboli were in the RA and measured between 2 and 10 cm in 92% of cases, with prolapse into the RV in 83% of cases (90). Type A patients were a high-risk group characterized by severe PE, which was fatal in one-third of the patients within 24 hours of diagnosis. Overall, early mortality (≤8 days) was 44% and uniformly related to PE. The mortality rate was in excess of 60% in patients treated with anticoagulation alone, 40% with thrombolysis, and 27% in surgically treated patients. This European Cooperative Study concluded that type A thrombi should be considered an absolute surgical emergency.

Type B thrombi are usually smaller, round or oval, less mobile, and commonly associated with RV thrombogenic abnormalities. They are common in patients with congestive heart failure, pacemaker electrodes, or foreign bodies, and they resemble LV thrombus. PE is reported to occur in about 40% of these patients but is rarely fatal and is associated with a good prognosis independent of the treatment type (90). In contrast, a large meta-analysis of 119 cases reported that morphologic characteristics were not related to survival. Overall mortality was 31%, and there was no difference between attached and unattached thrombi. Factors predicting survival were the presence of PE and the treatment type. The probability of survival was less in patients with documented PE compared with patients without documented PE. There appeared to be no difference in outcome related to treatment with heparin, thrombolytic agents, or surgical embolectomy. The authors of this meta-analysis concluded that the efficacy of these three treatment approaches was similar, and they advocated that heparin be the best choice for patients who are stable (91).

Cardiac arrest will occur within 1 to 2 hours of onset of symptoms in two-thirds of fatal PE cases (1) and acute MI/PE reportedly accounts for 70% of nontraumatic cardiac arrests (92). Therefore, cardiac arrest should be considered a risk for all patients with major PE, and PE should be considered as a diagnosis for all patients with cardiac arrest. In arrested patients undergoing resuscitation and stabilization, it is imperative to establish a diagnosis and initiate therapy rapidly. TEE has been reported to be of diagnostic utility when performed in cardiac arrest (9,93). In a series of patients with cardiac arrest, of whom 13% had PE, TEE confirmed the diagnosis in 27 of 31 patients for whom a definitive diagnosis was established from reference standards. In 31% of the cases, major decisions were based on the TEE findings (93). In a recent cardiac arrest series studied with TEE, the incidence of PE was 25% and occurred in 56% of patients with pulseless electrical activity (PEA) and in 64% of patients with RV enlargement without LV enlargement (9). Cardiac arrest caused by PE almost uniformly is due to pulseless PEA and usually follows shock, but it may occur spontaneously and is at least momentarily reversible in a third of the cases. When reversible, the heart rate is frequently normal or high with normal QRS complexes. Therapy for suspected PE in cardiac arrest consists of cardiopulmonary resuscitation (CPR), which can mechanically fracture the embolus, and thrombolysis or embolectomy. An evolving body of European literature suggests that thrombolytic therapy can be given safely during cardiac arrest without a significant risk of bleeding complications (94). Thrombolysis in these reported series is commonly administered as a bolus of urokinase, streptokinase, or rt-PA. It should be noted that survival for patients in MAPPET presenting in cardiac arrest was 35% (5), which is more than double the reported 14% survival for CPR in general (95) and suggests that these patients should be treated aggressively.

Right ventricular dysfunction has long been recognized as a poor outcome marker for patients with PE, especially in those with hemodynamic instability (12,16). More recently, RV dysfunction in hemodynamically stable patients has been identified as a predictor of worst outcome in virtually all studies and appears to be related to recurrent PE (4,11). Recognizing that approximately 50% of all PE patients have signs of RV dysfunction, there appears to be a subset within this population with mortality exceeding those with normal RV function but substantially less than shock patients (4,96). It has been reported that 10% of hemodynamically stable patients with RV dysfunction will deteriorate into shock, with a 50% mortality rate attributed to recurrent PE (97). Thrombolysis has been proposed to be a benefit in this group, based on the observation from two series (11,96), although one trial reported a worse outcome (98). In MAPPET, hemodynamically stable patients with RV dysfunction who were treated with thrombolysis had a lower mortality (4.7% versus 11.1%), reduced rate of recurrent PE (7.7% versus 18.7%), and an increased frequency of major bleeding (21.9% versus 7.8%) compared with heparin. The heparin group was significantly older and had a higher incidence of congestive heart failure and chronic pulmonary disease, which makes this observational study difficult to interpret (96). A registry of 128 consecutive patients compared thrombolysis with heparin in patients with RV dysfunction and hemodynamic stability; thrombolysis was associated with a significantly higher mortality (6.25% versus 0%), severe bleeding (9.4% versus 0%), and intracranial bleeding (4.7% versus 0%) (98). Even though the vast majority of patients with hemodynamically stable PE and RV will survive (11), it is imperative to define more precisely the subset of patients with RV dysfunction who will benefit from thrombolysis, given the substantial costs and risk of bleeding. Insofar as it is recognized that recurrent PE against the background of RV dysfunction appears to be a mechanism for worse outcome, the identification of substantial residual DVT may be a discriminator for the use of thrombolytic therapy in this patient population.

SUMMARY

Pulmonary embolism remains a common, lethal, and underdiagnosed process. It occurs even in patients who have had appropriate prophylaxis and frequently manifests its lethality within the first hour of presentation. The diagnosis and management of PE in the ICU are particularly challenging because differentiating PE from other life-threatening illness is frequently difficult. Logistic constraints impair definitive diagnostic testing, and hemorrhagic risks can compromise the ability to anticoagulate or undertake thrombolysis. A structured physiologic approach to diagnostic evaluation, resuscitation, stabilization, and definitive therapy is necessary to achieve an optimal outcome in this lethal disease. Echocardiography is an ideal diagnostic tool because it is transportable and capable of differentiating shock states and recognizing the characteristic features of PE. Spiral CT is evolving to replace angiography as a confirmatory study in this population. Thrombolytic therapy is acknowledged as the treatment of choice, with embolectomy reserved for those in whom thrombolysis is contraindicated.

KEY POINTS

Pulmonary embolism (PE) remains common, underdiagnosed, and lethal. Deep venous thrombosis and PE can occur in patients who have had appropriate prophylaxis and should be considered in the differential diagnosis if risks and clinical suspicion remain high.

The combination of embolism size and cardiopulmonary status resulting in hypotension is associated with a fivefold increase in mortality. The presence of hypotension provides a readily available discriminator to differentiate survivors and nonsurvivors and structure the diagnostic-therapeutic approach.

Echocardiography is an ideal tool to assess the shocked patient with suspected PE because it is readily available, useful in the recognition and differentiation of PE, and capable of assessing severity and response to therapy. Spiral computed tomography is evolving to replace ventilation–perfusion (V/Q) scans and angiography.

Thrombolytic therapy is the treatment of choice in the hypotensive patient, with embolectomy reserved for those in whom thrombolysis is contraindicated or failing.

REFERENCES

1. Dalen JE, Alpert JS. Natural history of pulmonary embolism. *Prog Cardiovasc Dis* 1975;17:259–270.
2. Nordström M, Lindblad B. Autopsy-verified venous thromboembolism with a defined urban population—the city of Malmö, Sweden. *APMIS* 1998;106:378–384.
3. Stein PD, Henry JW. Prevalence of acute pulmonary embolism among patients in a general hospital and at autopsy. *Chest* 1995;108:978–981.
4. Goldhaber SZ, Visani L, DeRosa M. Acute pulmonary embolism: clinical outcomes in the international cooperative pulmonary embolism registry (ICOPER). *Lancet* 1999;353:1386–1389.
5. Kasper W, Konstantinides S, Geibel A, et al. Management strategies and determinants of outcome in acute major pulmonary embolism: results of a multicenter registry. *J Am Coll Cardiol* 1997;30:1165–1171.
6. Morpurgo M, Schmid C. The spectrum of pulmonary embolism clinicopathologic correlations. *Chest* 1995;107:185–205.
7. Morgenthaler TI, Ryu JH. Clinical characteristics of fatal pulmonary embolism in a referral hospital. *Mayo Clin Proc* 1995;70:417–424.
8. Dalen JE, Dexter L. Diagnosis and management of massive pulmonary embolism. *Disease a Month* August 1967;(Aug):1–34.
9. Comess KA, DeRook FA, Russell ML, et al. The incidence of pulmonary embolism in unexplained sudden cardiac arrest with pulseless electrical activity. *Am J Med* 2000;109:351–356.
10. Hoagland PM. Massive pulmonary embolism. In: Goldhaber SZ, ed. *Pulmonary embolism and deep vein thrombosis.* Philadelphia: WB Saunders, 1985:179–208.
11. Goldhaber SZ, Haire WD, Feldstein ML, et al. Alteplase versus heparin in acute pulmonary embolism: randomized trial assessing right ventricular function and pulmonary perfusion. *Lancet* 1993;341:507–511.
12. Alpert JS, Smith R, Carlson J, et al. Mortality in patients treated for pulmonary embolism. *JAMA* 1976;236:1477–1480.
13. Urokinase Pulmonary Embolism Trial. Phase I results: a cooperative study. *JAMA* 1970;214:2163–2172.
14. Vlahakes GJ, Turley K, Hoffman JE. The pathophysiology of failure in acute right ventricular hypertension: hemodynamic and biochemical correlations. *Circulation* 1981;63:87–95.
15. McIntyre KM, Sasahara AA. The hemodynamic response to pulmonary embolism in patients without prior cardiopulmonary disease. *Am J Cardiol* 1971;28:288–294.
16. McIntyre KM, Sasahara AA. Determinants of right ventricular function and hemodynamics after pulmonary embolism. *Chest* 1974;65:534–543.
17. Stein PD. Prevelance in a general hospital. In: Stein PD, eds. *Pulmonary embolism.* Baltimore: Williams & Wilkins, 1996:3–11.
18. Clagett GP, Anderson FA, Levine MN, et al. Prevention of venous thromboembolism. *Chest* 1992;102:391S–407S.
19. Geerts WH, Code KI, Jay RM, et al. A prospective study of venous thromboembolism after major trauma. *N Engl J Med* 1994;331:1601–1606.
20. Samama MM, Cohen AT, Darmon JY. A comparison of enoxaparin with placebo for the prevention of venous thromboembolism in acutely ill medical patients. *N Engl J Med* 1999;341:793–800.
21. Claggett GP, Reisch JS. Prevention of venous thromboembolism in general surgical patients. Results of meta-analysis. *Ann Surg* 1988;208:227–240.
22. Collins R, Scrimgeour A, Yusuf S, et al. Reduction in fatal pulmonary embolism and venous thrombosis by peri-operative administration of subcutaneous heparin: overview of results of randomized trials in general, orthopaedic and urologic surgery. *N Engl J Med* 1988;18:1162–1173.
23. Prevention of fatal postoperative pulmonary embolism by low doses of heparin: an International multicentre trial. *Lancet* 1975;2:45–51.
24. Goldhaber SZ, Dunn K, MacDougall RC. New onset of venous thromboembolism among hospitalized patients at Brigham and Women's Hospital is caused more often by prophylaxis failure than by withholding treatment. *Chest* 2000;118:1680–1684.
25. Marik PE, Andrews L, Maini B. The incidence of thrombosis in ICU patients. *Chest* 1997;111:661–664.
26. Geerts WH, Heit JA, Claggett GP, et al. Prevention of venous thromboembolism. *Chest* 2001;119:S132–5175.
27. Urokinase-Streptokinase Embolism Trial. Phase 2 results: a cooperative study. *JAMA* 1974;229:1606–1613.
28. Thames MD, Alpert JS, Dalen JE. Syncope in patients with pulmonary embolism. *JAMA* 1977;238:2509–2511.
29. Miller GAH, Hall RJC, Paneth M. Pulmonary embolectomy, heparin and streptokinase: their place in the treatment of acute massive pulmonary embolism. *Am Heart J* 1977;93:568–574.
30. Machida K, Rappaport E. Left ventricular function in experimental pulmonary embolism. *Jpn Heart J* 1971;12:221–232.
31. McGinn S, White PD. Acute cor pulmonale resulting from pulmonary embolism. *JAMA* 1935;104:1473–1480.
32. Stein PD, Dalen JE, McIntyre KM, et al. The electrocardiogram in acute pulmonary embolism. *Prog Cardiovasc Dis* 1975;17:247–257.
33. Stein PD, Terrin ML, Hales CA, et al. Clinical, laboratory, roentgenographic and electrocardiographic findings in patients with acute pulmonary embolism and no pre-existing cardiac or pulmonary disease. *Chest* 1991;100:598–603.
34. Miller GAH, Sutton GC. Acute massive pulmonary embolism: clinical and hemodynamic findings in 23 patients studied by cardiac catheterization and pulmonary arteriography. *Br Heart J* 1970;32:518–523.
35. Ferrari E, Imbert A, Chevalier T, et al. The ECG in pulmonary embolism: predictive value of negative T waves in precordial leads—80 case reports. *Chest* 1997;111:537–543.
36. Oram S. Acute pulmonary embolism mimicking coronary artery disease. *Lancet* 1962;2:1076–1079.
37. Stein PD, Athanasoulis C, Greenspan RH, et al. Relationship of plain chest radiographic findings to pulmonary artery pressure and arterial blood oxygen levels in patients with acute pulmonary embolism. *Am J Cardiol* 1992;69:394–396.
38. Stein PD, Willis PW III, DeMets DL, et al. Plain chest roentgenogram in patients with acute pulmonary embolism and no pre-existing cardiac or pulmonary disease. *American Journal of Noninvasive Cardiology* 1987;1:171–176.
39. Laur A. Roentgen diagnosis of pulmonary embolism and its differential from myocardial infarction. *AJR Am J Roentgenol* 1963;90:632–637.
40. D'Alonzo GE, Dantzker DR. Gas exchange alterations following pulmonary embolism. *Clin Chest Med* 1984;5:411–419.
41. Urokinase Pulmonary Embolism Trial. *Circulation* 1973;47(Suppl II):1–108.
42. Stein PD, Goldhaben SZ, Henry JW, et al. Arterial blood gas analysis in the assessment of suspected acute pulmonary embolism. *Chest* 1996;109:78–81.
43. Stein PD, Goldhaber SZ, Henry JW. Alveolar-arterial oxygen gradient in the assessment of acute pulmonary embolism. *Chest* 1995;107:139–143.
44. Brill-Edwards P, Lee A. D-dimer testing in the diagnosis of acute venous thromboembolism, thrombosis and hemostasis. *State of the Art* 1999;82:688–694.
45. Hull R, Delmore T, Genton E, et al. Warfarin sodium versus low-dose heparin in the long term treatment of venous thrombosis. *N Engl J Med* 1979;301:855–858.
46. Hull RD, Raskob GE, Hirsh J. Continuous intravenous heparin compared with intermittent subcutaneous heparin in the initial treatment of proximal-vein thrombosis. *N Engl J Med* 1986;315:1109–1114.
47. Raschke RA, Reilly BM, Guidry JR, et al. The weight-based heparin dosing nomogram compared with a "standard care nomogram." *Ann Intern Med* 1993;119:874–881.
48. Hull RD, Raskob GE, Rosenbloom D, et al. Heparin for 5 days as compared with 10 days in the initial treatment of proximal venous thrombosis. *N Eng J Med* 1990;322:1260–1264.
49. Bates SM, Hirsh J. Treatment of venous thromboembolism, thrombosis and hemostasis. *Sems Thromb and Hemost* 1999;82:870–877.
50. Levine MN, Hirsh J, Gent M. A randomized trial comparing the activated thromboplastin time with heparin assay in patients with acute venous thromboembolism requiring large daily doses of heparin. *Arch Intern Med* 1994;154:49–56.

51. Hull RD, Raskob GE, Brant RF, et al. Low molecular weight heparin vs. heparin in the treatment of patients with pulmonary embolism. American-Canadian thrombosis study group. *Arch Intern Med* 2000;160:229–236.

52. Verstraete M, Miller GAH, Bounameaux H, et al. Intravenous and intrapulmonary recombinant tissue-type plasminogen activator in the treatment of acute massive pulmonary embolism. *Circulation* 1988;77:353–360.

53. Diehl JL, Meyer G, Ignal J, et al. Effectiveness and safety of bolus administration of alteplase in massive pulmonary embolism. *Am J Cardiol* 1992;70:1477–1480.

54. Tilsner V. Thrombolytic therapy in fulminant pulmonary thromboembolism. *Thorac Cardiovasc Surg* 1991;39:357–359.

55. Marini C, Di Ricco G, Rossi G, et al. Fibrinolytic effects of urokinase and heparin in acute pulmonary embolism: a randomized clinical trial. *Respiration* 1988;54:162–173.

56. Sors H, Pacouret G, Azarian R, et al. Hemodynamic effects of bolus vs. 2-h infusion of alteplase in acute massive pulmonary embolism: a randomized controlled multicenter trial. *Chest* 1994;106:712–717.

57. Meneveau N, Schiele F, Metz D. Comparative efficacy of a two-hour regimen of streptokinase versus alteplase in acute massive pulmonary embolism: immediate clinical and hemodynamic outcome and one year follow-up. *J Am Coll Cardiol* 1998;31:1057–1063.

58. Kearn C, Ginsberg JS, Hirsh J. The role of venous ultrasonography in the diagnosis of suspected deep venous thrombosis and pulmonary embolism. *Ann Intern Med* 1998;129:1044–1049.

59. Hull RD, Hirsch J, Carter CJ, et al. Pulmonary angiography, ventilation lung scanning and venography for clinically suspected pulmonary embolism and abnormal perfusion lung scan. *Ann Intern Med* 1983;98:891–899.

60. Girard P, Musset D, Parent F, et al. High prevalence of detectable deep venous thrombosis in patients with acute pulmonary embolism. *Chest* 1999;116:903–908.

61. Come PC. Echocardiographic evaluation of pulmonary embolism and its response to therapeutic interventions. *Chest* 1992;101:1515–1625.

62. Torbicki A, Tramarin R, Morpurgo M. Role of echo/Doppler in the diagnosis of pulmonary embolism. *Clin Cardiol* 1992;15:805–810.

63. Konstantinides S, Geibel A, Kasper W. Role of cardiac ultrasound in the detection of pulmonary embolism. *Sem Respir Crit Care Med* 1996;17:39–49.

64. Kasper W, Geibel A, Tiede N, et al. Echocardiography in the diagnosis of lung embolism. *Herz* 1989;14:82–101.

65. Kasper W, Geibel A, Tiede N. Distinguishing between acute and subacute massive pulmonary embolism by conventional and Doppler echocardiography. *Br Heart J* 1993;70:352–356.

66. Pruszczyk P, Torbicki A, Kuch-Wocial A, et al. Non-invasive diagnosis of suspected severe pulmonary embolism: transesophageal echocardiography vs. spiral CT. *Chest* 1997;112:722–728.

67. Wittlich N, Erbel R, Eichler A, et al. Detection of central pulmonary artery thromboembolism by transesophageal echocardiography in patients with severe pulmonary embolism. *J Am Soc Echocardiogr* 1992;5:515–524.

68. PIOPED Investigators. 1990. Value of ventilation-perfusion scan in acute pulmonary embolism: results of the prospective investigation of pulmonary embolism diagnosis (PIOPED). *JAMA* 1990;263:2753–2759.

69. Lesser BA, Leeper KV, Stein PD, et al. The diagnosis of acute pulmonary embolism in patients with obstructive pulmonary disease. *Chest* 1992;102:17–22.

70. Stein PD. Application of ventilation/perfusion lung scans in specific populations of patients. *Sem Resp Crit Care Med* 1996;17:23–29.

71. Henry JW, Stein PD, Gottschalk A, et al. Scintigraphic lung scans and clinical assessment in critically ill patients with suspected acute pulmonary embolism. *Chest* 1996;109:462–466.

72. Stein PD, Athanasoulis C, Alavi A. Complications and validity of pulmonary angiography in acute pulmonary embolism. *Circulation* 1992;85:462–469.

73. Cross JJL, Kemp PM, Walsh CG, et al. A randomized trail of spiral CT and ventilation perfusion scintigraphy for the diagnosis of pulmonary embolism. *Clin Radiol* 1998;53:177–182.

74. Stein PD, Hull RD, Pineo GF. The role of newer diagnostic techniques in the diagnosis of pulmonary embolism. *Curr Opin Pulm Med* 1999;5:212–215.

75. Meany J, Weg J, Chenevert T, et al. Diagnosis of pulmonary embolism with magnetic resonance angiography. *N Engl J Med* 1997;336:1422–1427.

76. Caldini P. Pulmonary hemodynamics and arterial oxygen saturation in pulmonary embolism. *J Appl Physiol* 1965;20:184–190.

77. Ducas J, Prewitt RM. Pathophysiology and therapy of right ventricular dysfunction due to pulmonary embolism. *Cardiovasc Clin* 1987;17:191–202.

78. Layish DT, Tapson VT. Pharmacologic hemodynamic support in massive pulmonary embolism. *Chest* 1997;111:218–224.

79. Webb SAR, Stott S, Van Heerden PV. The use of inhaled aerosolized prostacyclin IAP in the treatment of pulmonary hypertension secondary to pulmonary embolism. *Intensive Care Med* 1996;22:353–335.

80. Capellier G, Jacques T, Balvay P. Inhaled nitric oxide in patients with pulmonary embolism. *Intensive Care Med* 1997;23:1089–1092.

81. PIOPED Investigators. Tissue plasminogen activator for the treatment of acute pulmonary embolism. *Chest* 1990;97:528–533.

82. Petitpretz P, Simmoneau G, Cerrina J, et al. Effects of a single bolus of urokinase in patients with life-threatening pulmonary emboli: a descriptive trial. *Circulation* 1984;70:861–866.

83. Jerjes-Sanchez C, Ramirez-Rivera A, Garcia M de L, et al. Streptokinase and heparin versus heparin alone in massive pulmonary embolism: a randomized controlled trial. *J Thromb Thrombolysis* 1995;2:227–229.

84. Arcasoy SM, Kreit JW. Thrombolytic therapy of pulmonary embolism. a comprehensive review of current evidence. *Chest* 1999;115:1695–1707.

85. Doerge HC, Schoendube FA, Loeser H. Pulmonary embolectomy: review of a 15 year experience and role in the age of thrombolytic therapy. *Eur J Cardiothorac Surg* 1996;10:952–957.

86. Stulz P, Schläpfer R, Feer R, et al. Decision making in the surgical treatment of massive pulmonary embolism. *Eur J Cardiothorac Surg* 1994;8:188–193.

87. Del Campo C. Pulmonary embolectomy: a review. *Can J Surg* 1985;28:111–113.

88. Greenfield LJ, Proctor MC, Williams DM, et al. Long term experience with transvenous catheter pulmonary embolectomy. *J Vasc Surg* 1993;18:450–457.

89. Decousus H, Leizorovicz A, Parent F, et al. A clinical trial of vena caval filters in the prevention of pulmonary embolism in patients with proximal deep-vein thrombosis. *N Engl J Med* 1998;338:409–415.

90. Kronik G. The European working group on echocardiography: the European cooperative study on the clinical significance of right heart thrombi. *Eur Heart J* 1989;10:1046–1059.

91. Kinney EL, Wright RJ. Efficacy of treatment of patients with echocardiographically detected right-sided heart thrombi: a meta-analysis. *Am Heart J* 1989;118:569–573.

92. Bottiger BW. Thrombolysis during cardiopulmonary resuscitation. *Fibrinolysis and Proteolysis* 1997;11(Suppl 2):93–100.

93. Van der Wouw PA, Koster RW, Delemarre BJ, et al. Diagnostic accuracy of transesophageal echocardiography during cardiopulmonary resuscitation. *J Am Coll Cardiol* 1997;30:780–783.

94. Bottiger BW, Bohrer H, Bach A, et al. Bolus injection of thrombolytic agents during cardiopulmonary resuscitation for massive pulmonary embolism. *Resuscitation* 1994;28:45–54.

95. Ballew KA, Philbrick JT. Causes of variation in reported in-hospital CPR survival: a critical review. *Resuscitation* 1995;30:203–215.

96. Konstantinides S, Geibel A, Olschewski M, et al. Association between thrombolytic treatment and the prognosis of hemodynamically stable patients with major pulmonary embolism. *Circulation* 1997;96:882–888.

97. Grifoni S, Olivotto I, Cecchini P, et al. Short-term clinical outcome of patients with acute pulmonary embolism, normal blood pressure and echocardiographic right ventricular dysfunction. *Circulation* 2000;101:2817–2822.

98. Hamel E, Pacouret G, Djoffal-Vinoentelli D, et al. Thrombolysis or heparin in the treatment of non-life threatening massive pulmonary

embolism with right ventricular dilatation: Results from 128 consecutive patient monocentre register. *Eur Heart J* 1998;19:A1399.

99. Tibbutt DA, Davies JA, Anderson JA et al. Comparison by controlled clinical trial of streptokinase and heparin in the treatment of life-threatening pulmonary embolism. *BMJ* 1974;1:343–347.

100. Arnesen H, Heilo A, Jakobsen E, et al. A prospective study of streptokinase and heparin in the treatment of deep vein thrombosis. *Acta Med Scand* 1978;203(6):457–463.

101. Ly B, Arnesen H, Eie H, et al. A controlled trial of streptokinase and heparin the treatment of major pulmonart embolism. *Acta Med Scand* 1978;203:465–470.

102. Giuntini C, Marini C, Di Ricco G, et al. A controlled clinical trial on the effect of heparin infusion and two regimens of urokinase in acute pulmonary embolism. *G Ital Cardiol* 1984;14(Suppl 1): 26–29.

103. Levine M, Hirsh J, Weitz J, et al. A randomized trial of a single bolus dosage regimen of recombinant tissue plasminogen activator in patients with acute pulmonary embolism. *Chest* 1990;98:1473–1479.

104. Dalla-Volta S, Palla A, Santolicandro A, et al. PAIMS 2: alteplase combined with heparin versus heparin in the treatment of acute pulmonary embolism; plasminogen activator Italian multicenter study 2. *J Am Coll Cardiol* 1992;20:520–526.

45

PERIOPERATIVE HEMOSTASIS AND COAGULOPATHY

CAROL A. DION
KATHLEEN H. CHAIMBERG
ANDREW GETTINGER
D. DAVID GLASS

KEY WORDS

- Activated clotting time
- Disseminated intravascular coagulation
- D-dimer
- Fibrinogen-degradation products
- HELLP (hemolysis, elevated liver

- transaminases, low platelets) syndrome
- Heparin-induced thrombocytopenia
- Lupus anticoagulant
- Massive transfusion
- Thromboelastograph
- Vitamin K

NORMAL HEMOSTASIS

Normal hemostasis is a balance between the simultaneous, opposing processes of clot formation and fibrinolysis, the latter of which limits clot formation to the site of injury. For a clot to form normally, there must be functioning endothelium, platelets with adequate number and function, and sufficient coagulation factors. *Primary* hemostasis refers to formation of the platelet plug, a process that occurs within 1 to 3 minutes of injury. When endothelium is injured, von Willebrand factor (vWF) bridges platelets to the damaged subendothelium. The platelet granules subsequently release mediators that promote further platelet aggregation at the site of injury, and the platelet plug is formed. *Secondary* hemostasis refers to the action of the coagulation cascade to form clot. The platelet membrane is rich in phospholipid, which provides the surface on which many of the inactive proenzyme forms of the coagulation factors are activated. The final step in the coagulation cascade is the formation of fibrin, a polypeptide that then polymerizes on the surface of the platelets to stabilize the platelet plug. This stable clot is formed within 3 to 10 minutes of injury.

The coagulation factors are glycoproteins that are synthesized in the liver and circulate in the inactive proenzyme form. Factors V and VIII are also synthesized in extrahepatic sites. The synthesis of factors II, VII, IX, and X is dependent on vitamin K. The

contribution of vitamin K deficiency to clinical coagulopathies is addressed below (see "Vitamin K Deficiency"). Once coagulation has been initiated, the factors are modified to serine proteases, each of which sequentially activates another factor, ending with the formation of fibrin. The coagulation cascade consists of the intrinsic and extrinsic pathways, both of which lead to factor X activation, and the common pathway in which the activated X (Xa) thus formed leads to fibrin formation (Fig. 1). The intrinsic and extrinsic pathways are not entirely distinct *in vivo*, but considering them as separate pathways facilitates understanding the events of coagulation. The extrinsic pathway, also called the *tissue-factor pathway*, is initiated when tissue or vessels are injured and tissue factor (TF), a receptor on cell surfaces, is exposed to blood. TF binds trace amounts of circulating factor VII, and this complex autocatalyzes the rapid conversion of more VII to VIIa. Factor VIIa then initiates the common pathway by activating factor X in the presence of calcium and phospholipid (Fig. 1).

The *intrinsic pathway*, which starts with factor IX, can be initiated by either of two routes: the *extrinsic* pathway or the *contact-activation* pathway (Fig. 1). The TF/VIIa complex, which activates VII in the extrinsic pathway, also directly catalyzes the activation of IX. Alternatively, in the contact-activation pathway, XII binds to negatively charged surfaces of exposed damaged subendothelium. High-molecular-weight kininogen (HMWK) facilitates the conversion of XII to XIIa by kallikrein. Factor XIIa activates XI, and XIa initiates the intrinsic pathway. Using VIIIa as a cofactor, IX initiates the common pathway. The contact activation pathway is not required for the rapid formation of fibrin clot *in vivo* because patients with deficiencies of the contact activation proteins do not have a bleeding tendency. Both intrinsic and extrinsic pathways converge at X activation, a process that requires calcium and a phospholipid surface, the platelet membrane. Note that factor VIII is unique to the intrinsic pathway, and VII is the key factor in the extrinsic pathway, facts that are relevant to the evaluation of the prothrombin time (PT) and activated partial thromboplastin time (aPTT) tests, discussed later.

Important points about the common pathway are that Xa, in the presence of calcium, phospholipid, and Va, activates prothrombin to thrombin (factor II) and that thrombin

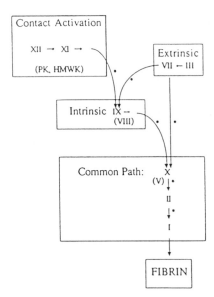

FIGURE 1. Coagulation protein activation sequence. Asterisks denote participation of calcium ion. Roman numerals correspond to coagulation factors. PK, prekallikrein; HMWK, high-molecular-weight kininogen. (From Horrow J. Management of coagulation and bleeding disorders. In Kaplan J, ed. *Cardiac anesthesia*, 3rd ed. Philadelphia: WB Saunders, 1993:952, with permission.)

sequentially cleaves fibrinogen into fibrin monomer and polypeptide fragments, termed *fibrinopeptides A and B*. The fibrin monomers associate to form polymers, which then are covalently cross-linked to form an insoluble clot. Thrombin not only cleaves fibrinogen but also stimulates platelets to aggregate and release their granule contents, which, in turn, attracts more platelets and promotes clot formation. This action of thrombin is just one example of how the pathways are amplified during clot formation.

The self-limiting aspects inherent to the cascade and that serve to prevent widespread clot formation when coagulation is initiated can be divided into two categories: (a) specific serine protease inhibitors such as antithrombin III (AT-III), thrombin, and protein C and S; and (b) the fibrinolytic system. AT-III inactivates thrombin by binding to it in a 1:1 ratio, and this binding is enhanced by a factor of 1,000 in the presence of heparin. About 75% of the thrombin formed is inactivated by AT-III, whereas the remaining 25% is inactivated by other minor inhibitors. AT-III also inhibits the activity of at least five other factors in the pathways and the fibrinolytic enzyme plasmin (see later discussion on plasmin). Thrombin itself has a role in limiting coagulation by activating protein C, a vitamin-K-dependent inhibitor that inactivates Va and VIIIa. Protein S is a vitamin-K-dependent cofactor of protein C. So potent is the coagulation system that patients deficient in protein C frequently suffer recurrent thrombosis. The substantial roles of thrombin and AT-III in promoting and limiting coagulation, respectively, are central in the pathophysiology of disseminated intravascular coagulation (DIC) (see section on "Disseminated Intravascular Coagulation").

Fibrinolysis is the process of limiting clot formation to the site of injury, remodeling clot, and removing thrombus once healing has occurred. Fibrinolysis is carried out by the serine protease plasmin. Plasmin is capable of degrading many substrates, including fibrin monomer, cross-linked fibrin clot, fibrinogen, and

others. Under normal circumstances, plasmin mainly degrades cross-linked fibrin clot. The proenzyme form, plasminogen, is synthesized in the liver and circulates throughout the bloodstream. The processes of clot formation and fibrinolysis are limited to the site of injury because plasminogen is concentrated at the clot by binding noncovalently to fibrin strands. Plasminogen bound in the clot is activated to plasmin whenever coagulation is initiated. For example, when the contact activation pathway is initiated, prekallikrein, HMWK, and XII are each capable of activating plasminogen. Plasminogen is also activated by the release of tissue plasminogen activator (t-PA) or urokinase plasminogen activator (u-PA) from stimulated endothelium. To prevent diffuse fibrinolysis throughout the vasculature, a scavenging protein (α-2-antiplasmin) avidly consumes plasmin at the site of injury. In addition, fibrinolysis is limited by plasminogen activator inhibitor, which is secreted from endothelial cells and platelets and irreversibly inhibits t-PA and u-PA.

In certain disease states, such as severe liver disease or disseminated neoplasm, in which the plasmin inhibitor α-2-antiplasmin has been depleted, plasmin freely degrades native fibrinogen (*fibrinogenolysis*) and non-cross-linked fibrin. The initial product of fibrinogenolysis is termed the *X fragment*, which subsequently is processed into a nonfunctional *Y fragment*. The latter is finally cleaved into *D* and *E fragments*, which are the antigens detected by currently used assays for fibrinogen-degradation products (FDPs). Certain antigens are common between these fibrinogen degradation products and products of fibrin degradation. Hence, most current tests for degradation products cannot distinguish between the two. The abbreviation FDPs, therefore, refers to products of either fibrinogen or fibrin cleavage by plasmin. When plasmin degrades cross-linked fibrin clots, the detectable product is a complex that includes two joined D fragments, known as the *D-dimer*.

In summary, normal hemostasis consists of clot formation and processes that limit clot formation to the site of injury. For these two opposing systems to balance, adequate levels and activity of coagulation factors, platelets, vWF, serine protease inhibitors, plasmin, and plasmin inhibitors must be present. A significant derangement in any one of these areas may result in clinical hemorrhage or thrombosis.

LABORATORY METHODS

The laboratory workup of bleeding includes an assessment of primary hemostasis, that is, platelet number and function and secondary hemostasis (i.e., the coagulation proteins).

Tests of Primary Hemostasis

Tests pertinent to primary hemostasis are the platelet count, the bleeding time, and platelet aggregation studies. The platelet count is performed as part of the automated blood-cell profile and, with currently used instruments, is reliable even with counts as low as 20,000 per microliter. Very low platelet counts, however, should be confirmed by direct examination of the peripheral smear. Thrombocytopenia is empirically defined as a platelet count less than 100,000 per microliter.

The bleeding time is a test of platelet plug formation. The time is prolonged with qualitative abnormalities in platelet function and also with deficiencies or qualitative abnormalities of plasma proteins necessary for platelet adhesion and aggregation. These proteins include vWF and fibrinogen. The test is independent of the platelet count above 100,000 per microliter, but it is linearly prolonged as the platelet count falls from 100,000 to 10,000 per microliter (1). The bleeding time is theoretically helpful, but it is difficult to standardize in practice because the measurement is affected by many uncontrolled variables, such as the experience of the operator, the depth of the incision, and the patient's skin temperature and hematocrit level. An assessment of bleeding time is indicated to work up hereditary bleeding disorders, especially von Willebrand disease; to help determine the cause of ongoing bleeding; and to monitor the effects of antiplatelet therapy. No evidence exists that the bleeding time predicts surgical hemorrhage, and the test should not be used as a preoperative screen in this manner (2,3). Some causes of a prolonged bleeding time are listed in Table 1.

Platelet-aggregation and -release studies test platelet function *in vitro*, and thus an abnormal result is more specific for a platelet abnormality as the cause of bleeding. These tests are most useful in the workup of inherited thrombocytopathies. Briefly, light transmission through platelet-rich plasma is monitored as platelet aggregation proceeds over time in response to several stimulators of platelet aggregation and release. The light-transmission pattern generated by the patient's plasma then is compared with normal patterns. Defects in primary platelet aggregation, platelet release, and secondary aggregation can be detected.

From tests of whole blood clotting (see "The Thromboelastograph and Sonoclot"), one can derive further information regarding platelet number and function.

TABLE 1. CAUSES OF A PROLONGED BLEEDING TIME

Drugs
von Willebrand disease
Inherited platelet-function defects
    Glanzmann's thrombasthenia
    Bernard-Soulier syndrome
    Storage-pool deficiencies
    Cyclo-oxygenase deficiency
    Other
Bone-marrow disorders
    Leukemias
    Myelodysplastic syndromes
    Polycythemia vera
    Essential thrombocythemia
Afibrinogenemia
Uremia
Paraproteinemia
Disseminated intravascular coagulopathy
Cardiopulmonary bypass
Foods (Szechwan purpura, fish oils)
Other

Adapted from Santoro SA. Laboratory evaluation of hemostatic disorders. In: Hoffman R, Benz EJ, Shahil SJ, et al., eds. *Hematology: basic principles and practice.* New York: Churchill Livingstone; 1991:1266–1276, with permission.

Tests of Secondary Hemostasis

To understand the tests of secondary hemostasis, recall from looking at Figure 1 and reading the earlier discussion on normal coagulation that the contact-activation pathway consists of prekallikrein, HMWK, and factors XII and XI, and the intrinsic pathway consists of IX and VIII. The extrinsic pathway consists of TF and factor VII. The common pathway consists of V, X, prothrombin, and fibrinogen.

It is imperative that the blood specimen be obtained from a nontraumatic venipuncture or from an indwelling line from which heparin has been thoroughly cleared. Citrate is the anticoagulant routinely used in blood tubes for coagulation tests. From the blood sample, the laboratory personnel prepare platelet-free, citrated plasma by centrifugation.

The PT tests the extrinsic and common pathways. Normal values are about 12 seconds. The PT is performed by measuring the clotting time of platelet-poor plasma after adding excess calcium (to overwhelm the citrate) and thromboplastin. Thromboplastin provides both the phospholipid surface for the calcium-phospholipid-dependent steps in the coagulation cascade and the tissue factor that initiates the extrinsic pathway via activation of factor VII. In the past, when crude extracts of rabbit brain or human placenta were the only source of thromboplastin, wide intralaboratory and interlaboratory variations in PT results were significant problems and complicated patient management. The international normalized ratio (INR) was developed by the World Health Organization (WHO) in the early 1980s to reduce such variability by accounting for the differential sensitivity of the commercially available thromboplastin sources to factor VII (4). Each thromboplastin source is assigned an International Sensitivity Index (ISI); a number that describes its sensitivity in reference to a standard thromboplastin. So that the PT may be compared among laboratories that use different thromboplastins, the result is reported as the absolute time in seconds and also as the INR, the ratio of the patient's PT to the PT of a control plasma raised to the power of the ISI (5).

The PT detects abnormalities of factors VII, X, V, II (thrombin), fibrinogen, or the presence of a factor inhibitor. Note that three of the four vitamin-K-dependent coagulation factors are measured by the PT; including VII, the factor with the shortest half-life. Reduction of factors V, VII, or X to 50% of normal significantly prolongs the PT. Depression of fibrinogen to 60 to 80 mg per deciliter may be the sole cause of a prolonged PT (6).

The partial thromboplastin time (PTT) tests the intrinsic and common pathways. A phospholipid source (partial thromboplastin) and excess calcium are added to the patient's citrated plasma, and time to clot formation is measured. The glass test tube provides the surface that activates the contact factors. Alternatively, kaolin, ellagic acid, or celite may be added to provide a negatively charged surface that improves contact activation. The latter method is the aPTT. Normal values are 25 to 40 seconds. The aPTT detects abnormalities in prekallikrein; HMWK; factors XII, XI, IX, VIII, X, V, and II; fibrinogen; or inhibitors of these. The aPTT is prolonged if the level of one of these factors is decreased to 20% to 30% of normal or if there is an inhibitor to one of these factors.

The thrombin time (TT) tests clot formation from fibrinogen. Exogenous thrombin is added to citrated plasma, and the time to clot formation is measured. Normal values are less than 10 seconds. The TT is prolonged if fibrinogen is low or functionally abnormal or if heparin or FDPs are present in the patient's plasma. The TT is not affected by levels of any other coagulation factors. The reptilase time is similar to the TT except that the reptilase time test uses a snake-venom enzyme that is not inhibited in the presence of heparin.

Factor inhibitors are acquired or inherited circulating macromolecules that interfere with a coagulation-factor reaction. Patients with an inhibitor present with a prolonged coagulation time, usually the aPTT. The presence of an inhibitor is distinguished from a factor deficiency by mixing a sample of the patient's plasma with normal plasma. Significant correction of the aPTT indicates a factor deficiency, whereas poor correction indicates the presence of an inhibitor. The most common clinically important inhibitors are the lupus anticoagulant and inhibitors of factor VIII. Inhibitors of factor VIII are autoantibodies that are acquired, usually developing in elderly patients or patients with autoimmune disease. Both men and women are affected. The lupus anticoagulant (misnamed because it is more often found in patients without lupus and because it is associated with thrombosis rather than bleeding) is an immunoglobulin G (IgG) or immunoglobulin M (IgM) antibody that binds to phospholipid and prolongs the phospholipid-dependent steps in the coagulation cascade. Clinical conditions associated with the presence of the lupus anticoagulant are chronic autoimmune disorders, certain medications (e.g., hydralazine hydrochloride, procainamide hydrochloride, quinidine, phenothiazine), human immunodeficiency virus infection, recurrent fetal wastage, venous or arterial thrombotic events, and recent acute viral infection. Although the appropriate antithrombotic therapy may vary, depending on the patient's specific presentation, unfractionated or low-molecular-weight heparin (LMWH) may be most effective because most patients with antiphospholipid thrombosis syndrome will experience thrombosis again while on warfarin (7). The use of heparin, together with low-dose aspirin, is suggested for the treatment of pregnant women with a history of recurrent fetal loss (8). Testing for the lupus anticoagulant is complex, and the preferred method differs among published authors. The factor VIII inhibitor is easier to demonstrate. In general, assays for the specificity of an inhibitor for a particular factor (e.g., VIII) and assays for the amount of inhibitor activity present consist of incubating the patient's plasma with normal plasma for 2 to 4 hours and showing that the activity of the factor under question in the mixture decreases over time. The Bethesda assay and Oxford assay are two tests in which this method is used.

Tests of Fibrinolysis

The euglobulin-clot-lysis time is a commonly used qualitative test to diagnose a state of increased fibrinolysis. Briefly, the test involves mixing plasma and fibrinogen, plasminogen, and plasminogen activators, allowing clot to form, and then measuring the time until the clot lyses. A shortened clot-lysis time indicates abnormally increased fibrinolysis. The test is qualitative only, and the degree of shortening of the clot-lysis time does not correlate with the degree of increased fibrinolysis.

As discussed previously under "Normal Hemostasis," the products of plasmin's action on either fibrinogen or non-cross-linked fibrin are FDPs. These products are detected in a patient's serum by a latex agglutination assay. Elevated FDPs may be the result of primary fibrinolysis, as in severe liver disease or secondary fibrinolysis, as in DIC. The D-dimer is an antigen that is formed when plasmin digests cross-linked fibrin. In the D-dimer assay, a commercially available antibody to the D-dimer antigen recognizes the antigen in the patient's serum. D-dimer is uniquely formed during clot lysis and indicates the presence of DIC rather than primary fibrinolysis (9,10).

Activated Clotting Time

The activated coagulation time (ACT) is a general test of coagulation. It is performed by combining 1 to 2 mL of whole blood with an activator (glass particles, kaolin, or diatomaceous earth, otherwise known as *celite*) that speeds the first step in the intrinsic pathway, contact activation of XII to XIIa. The time to clot formation is measured. A normal ACT is 110 to 120 seconds. Clinically, the ACT is used most often to assess the adequacy of heparinization in vascular and cardiac operations. In these settings, very large doses of heparin are used. The aPTT is too sensitive to heparin effect to be useful at such high doses. Although practices at individual institutions vary, in general, an ACT of 480 seconds is desired prior to commencing cardiopulmonary bypass (CPB). Young and colleagues demonstrated that above an ACT of 400 seconds, no fibrin monomer was observed on pump materials. Above an ACT of 500, linearity between the ACT and heparin dose no longer holds (11). As discussed later (see section regarding bleeding post-CPB), the celite-activated ACT is prolonged by aprotinin to a greater degree than the kaolin-activated ACT.

Thromboelastograph and Sonoclot

The thromboelastograph (TEG) and Sonoclot are two ways to measure the viscoelastic strength of whole blood as clot is formed over time. The TEG is generated by a piston rotating in a cuvette of heated whole blood. As the blood clots, the rotation of the piston changes, and these changes generate curves on a chart recorder. The curves are analyzed by measurement of many geometric parameters, each of which reflects some aspect of clot formation or lysis, such as the speed of fibrin cross-linking and the absolute strength of the fibrin clot. Opinions differ regarding the usefulness of the TEG in either predicting or managing the patient who develops a post-CPB bleeding diathesis (12,13). Advocates argue that the TEG offers a number of advantages, including results that are obtainable during CPB (allowing earlier identification and treatment of abnormalities) and information regarding platelet-fibrin interactions that are not obtainable from routine clotting tests (14). The TEG is probably most useful in helping to diagnose ongoing fibrinolysis in the post-CPB state. With fibrinolysis, the TEG has a characteristic teardrop shape (Fig. 2). The TEG has been used effectively to monitor the changing coagulation status throughout hepatic transplantation (15). Implementation of the TEG in the intensive care unit (ICU) will require more widespread acquisition of the technology and expertise required to perform and interpret the test.

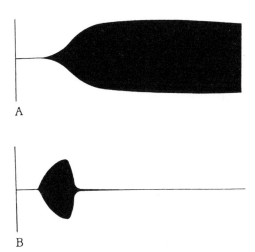

FIGURE 2. A: Normal post-bypass thromboelastography tracing. **B:** Thromboelastography tracing consistent with fibrinolysis in the postbypass period. The horizontal axis is time, and the vertical axis is clot formation. (From Spiess BD, Tuman KJ, McCarthy RJ, et al. Thromboelastography as an indicator of post-cardiopulmonary bypass coagulopathies. *J Clin Monit* 1987;3:25–30, with permission.)

The Sonoclot piston vibrates in a small blood sample, and as the blood clots, impedance to vibration is measured and recorded. The tracing generated is known as the *Sonoclot signature*. The shape of the curves reflects the kinetics of fibrinogen conversion to fibrin and of clot retraction. The shape of the "signature" depends significantly on the number and function of platelets. Although the Sonoclot has been used by some to assess platelet function after CPB or to monitor patients with a hypercoagulable state, the test has not gained wide acceptance.

Because "normal" tracings differ among individuals, both the TEG and Sonoclot are more useful when a patient's baseline TEG or Sonoclot signature has been established preoperatively for comparison.

BEDSIDE ASSESSMENT

Common causes of perioperative bleeding in patients in the ICU are listed in Table 2. The evaluation of coagulopathy begins with a thorough history and physical examination. These should be directed toward determining whether the coagulopathy (a) results from a defect in primary or secondary hemostasis, (b) is preexisting and chronic versus acutely developing in the perioperative or posttraumatic setting, (c) results from a primary hematologic disorder or is secondary to another pathologic process, (d) is localized to a surgical site or is diffuse throughout the microvasculature, or (e) is accompanied by signs of arterial or venous thrombosis.

Because of the condition of the critically ill patient, the history may be obtainable only from the family and medical records. A history of spontaneous gingival or other mucosal bleeding or epistaxis and easy bruising points to a platelet lesion, whereas a history of large-vessel bleeding, such as hematoma formation and hemarthroses, points toward a defect in the coagulation cascade. The patient should be questioned about bleeding or the need for transfusions with prior procedures, especially tonsillectomy, dental extractions, or vaginal delivery. In addition, a

TABLE 2. COMMON CAUSES OF PERIOPERATIVE BLEEDING

Disseminated intravascular coagulopathy
Liver disease
Vitamin K deficiency
Hypothermia
The post–cardiopulmonary bypass state
Massive transfusion
Purpura
Heparin-induced thrombocytopenia
Inadequate surgical hemostasis
Drug-induced platelet dysfunction

history of previous transfusions or pregnancies may point to an immune mechanism for subsequent bleeding. The presence of acute or chronic renal failure predisposes the patient to developing platelet dysfunction. A history of malignancy treated with chemotherapy or radiation therapy would indicate bone-marrow suppression as a cause of thrombocytopenia. Nutritional deficiencies, liver disease, fat-malabsorption syndromes, or antibiotic therapy may cause vitamin K deficiency and prolongation of coagulation times. The patient should be questioned in detail about all medications, especially over-the-counter preparations that include aspirin or nonsteroidal antiinflammatory agents. Specific query should be directed toward the patient's use of herbal remedies because evidence suggests that some (e.g., feverfew, garlic, ginkgo biloba) may negatively impact platelet function, particularly when taken in combination with conventional medication (16). Further, many patients do not regularly disclose their use of herbal products to their physician without being specifically asked (17).

Physical examination of the patient with a coagulopathy should be aimed first at determining whether bleeding is localized to an anatomic site with inadequate surgical hemostasis or whether there is diffuse oozing from all venipuncture sites and mucous membranes. Petechiae, purpura, and splenomegaly are signs associated with thrombocytopenia. Signs of infection or sepsis may support DIC as the cause of bleeding. Signs of end-organ dysfunction that may result from microvascular thrombosis are consistent with DIC or thrombotic thrombocytopenic purpura (TTP). Signs of liver failure, such as ascites, angiomata, and jaundice should be sought. The presence or absence of hypothermia should be established. After obtaining the history and performing a physical examination, the clinician should order a laboratory screen.

LABORATORY ASSESSMENT
Coagulation Studies

The initial laboratory screen should consist of the aPTT, PT, and platelet count. Some practitioners also advocate inclusion of the TT in the initial screen. If only the aPTT is prolonged, abnormalities of the intrinsic pathway to which VIII is unique should be considered. Conditions consistent with prolongation of only the aPTT are (a) hemophilia A or B, (b) factor XI deficiency, (c) heparin therapy, (d) lupus anticoagulant, and (e) acquired anti-VIII antibodies.

If only the PT is prolonged, abnormalities of the extrinsic pathway to which VII is unique should be considered. Because the synthesis of VII is vitamin K dependent and has the shortest half-life, VII is the first factor to decrease in these situations: (a) early liver disease, (b) early vitamin K deficiency, and (c) early Coumadin (warfarin) therapy. An isolated prolonged PT is also consistent with congenital factor VII deficiency. If both the aPTT and the PT are prolonged, one of three conditions may exist: (a) multiple factors in both pathways are affected, (b) there is a selective decrease in one or more of the common pathway factors, or (c) fibrinogen level is less than 60 to 80 mg per deciliter.

The differential diagnosis of prolonged aPTT and PT includes liver disease; DIC; renal disease; Coumadin therapy; large-dose heparin therapy; primary fibrinolysis; and, rarely, congenital deficiencies of factors I, II, V, or X. The previous choices may be distinguished by a fibrinogen level. In this setting, a normal fibrinogen level is consistent with Coumadin therapy, heparin therapy, vitamin K deficiency, and neoplasia. A low fibrinogen level (60–80 mg/dL) is consistent with hepatic failure or DIC. (However, as addressed under the section covering DIC, a normal fibrinogen level also may be consistent with a diagnosis of DIC). In DIC, the FDPs and the D-dimer are elevated, and thrombocytopenia is almost always present. A more in-depth discussion of DIC follows. A prolonged TT (indicating elevated FDPs, low fibrinogen, or abnormal fibrinogen) is consistent with liver disease, DIC, or a dysfibrinogenemia. A prolonged TT in the setting of a normal reptilase time indicates a heparin effect.

Primary fibrinolysis is associated with certain clinical conditions, including urinary tract operations or disease, trauma to or operations of the liver or oral cavity, and the post-CPB state. A shortened euglobulin-clot-lysis time establishes a state of increased fibrinolysis. The euglobulin-clot-lysis time is a nonspecific finding, however, and the clinician must distinguish primary fibrinolysis from fibrinolysis that is secondary to DIC. The presence of the D-dimer confirms that both thrombin and plasmin are activated and, therefore, favors the diagnosis of DIC. As discussed under the section on DIC, profragment 1 + 2 (PF 1 + 2) and fibrinopeptide A (FPA) are elevated in DIC but not in primary fibrinolysis. Antifibrinolytic therapy may be helpful in the treatment of fibrinolysis but is safe only if DIC is not present.

Platelet Count

Workup of the platelet phase of clotting includes checking the platelet count and function. The platelet count should be addressed first because the bleeding time, the easiest screen of platelet function, is affected by thrombocytopenia. *Thrombocytopenia* is empirically defined as a platelet count less than 100,000 per microliter. Bleeding with trauma or moderately invasive operations usually is not seen until the platelet count is less than 50,000 per microliter, and spontaneous bleeding usually is not seen until the count is less than 10,000 to 15,000 per microliter. In general, the mechanisms of thrombocytopenia can be categorized as decreased bone-marrow production, altered distribution, and increased destruction. Common causes of thrombocytopenia are summarized in Table 3.

The first step in distinguishing among these possibilities is to assess the platelet size [mean platelet volume (MPV)] and the peripheral smear. A large MPV indicates increased platelet turnover and circulation of young platelets; a small MPV indicates decreased platelet production. If the smear reveals red

TABLE 3. CAUSES OF THROMBOCYTOPENIA

Decreased production
  Bone-marrow suppression
    Chemotherapy or radiation
    Viral illness
    Human immunodeficiency virus infection
    Drugs (thiazides, ethanol, cocaine, cimetidine, some
      penicillins and cephalosporins, estrogens)
    Sepsis
  Bone-marrow replacement
    Tumor
    Myelofibrosis
  Other
    Late vitamin-B_{12} and folate deficiency
Altered distribution
  Splenic sequestration
  Hypothermia
  Dilution in massive transfusion
Increased destruction
  Immune
    Thrombotic thrombocytopenia purpura
    Hemolytic-uremic syndrome
    Idiopathic thrombocytopenic purpura
    Systemic lupus erythematosus
    Human immunodeficiency virus infection
    Drugs (quinine, quinidine, sulfonamides, gold salts,
      heparin, some penicillins and cephalosporins, H_2
      antagonists)
    Sepsis
    Posttransfusion purpura
  Nonimmune
    Consumption (DIC)
    Mechanical destruction (CPB, prosthetic cardiac valves)
    Severe hyperthermic syndromes
  Mechanism unknown
    Rejection of renal or hepatic allografts
    Gestational thrombocytopenia
    Hemolysis, elevated liver transaminases, low platelets

DIC, disseminated Intravascular coagulopathy; CPB, cardiopulmonary bypass.

cell fragments, thrombocytopenia may be part of a microangiopathic process such as TTP or the hemolytic uremic syndrome (HUS) (See "Thrombocytopenia with Microangiopathic Hemolysis: TTP, HUS, and HELLP Syndrome"). If all three cell lines are decreased, a bone marrow examination is indicated. Idiopathic thrombocytopenic purpura (ITP), TTP, HUS, hypothermia, and DIC can each affect either platelet count or function and are discussed in detail in separate sections.

Qualitative Platelet Disorders

When the platelet count is above 100,000 per microliter and the patient reports a history of easy bruising, petechiae, or purpura, then a measurement of the bleeding time is indicated to establish a diagnosis of platelet dysfunction. Causes of qualitative platelet disorders that are commonly encountered in the critically ill patient are listed in Table 4.

It is thought that in uremia, circulating metabolites interfere with platelet function. In support of this theory is the fact that platelet function improves after dialysis. Cryoprecipitate (a source of vWF) or 1-deamino-8-D-arginine vasopressin (DDAVP),

TABLE 4. QUALITATIVE PLATELET DISORDERS

Metabolic causes
  Uremia
  Stored whole blood
  Circulating fibrin-degradation products or fibrinogen
    degradation products in DIC and liver disease
  Hypothyroidism
Pharmacologic causes
  Antiinflammatory agents
    Aspirin
  Nonsteroidal antiinflammatory agents
  Antibiotics
    Penicillins
    Cephalosporins
    Nitrofurantoin
Phosphodiesterase inhibitors
  Dipyridimole
  Methylxanthines
Cardiac medications
  ß-blocking agents
  Calcium-channel blockers
  Furosemide
  Nitrates
  Sodium nitroprusside
  Quinidines

Psychiatric medications
  Tricyclic antidepressants
  Phenothiazines

Chemotherapeutic agents
  Vincristine sulfate
  Vinblastine sulfate

Other medications
  Local anesthetics
  Dextran
  Hydroxyethyl starch
  Hydrocortisones
  Methylprednisolone
  Cyclosporin A
  Antihistamines

DIC, disseminated intravascular coagulopathy.

which increases factor VIII levels and causes the release of vWF from endothelial cells, may improve platelet adhesion by increasing the VIII:vWF complex, which bridges platelets at the site of injury. Platelet transfusions should be given for life-threatening hemorrhage.

Aspirin and Other Drugs

Aspirin irreversibly inhibits platelet cyclooxygenase, an enzyme necessary for the synthesis of thromboxane A2. The defect lasts for the life of the platelet, about 7 to 10 days. Nonsteroidal antiinflammatory agents reversibly inhibit the same enzyme, and platelet function returns to normal 24 hours after the last dose. Cephalosporins, many penicillins (ampicillins, penicillins, carbenicillin indanyl sodium, nafcillin sodium, and ticarcillin disodium), dextran, hydroxyethyl starch, tricyclic antidepressants, alcohol, and some local anesthetics interfere with platelet membrane or receptor function. Furosemide, verapamil hydrochloride, sodium nitroprusside, and trimethaphan camsylate can induce platelet dysfunction.

Hereditary Thrombocytopathies

In addition to these causes of platelet dysfunction, multiple hereditary thrombocytopathies present with easy bruising and mucosal bleeding and are characterized by abnormal aggregation and release studies. The Bernard–Soulier syndrome is an autosomal trait in which platelet-membrane receptors are lacking and adhesion is abnormal. In Glanzmann thrombasthenia, platelets are unable to bind to vWF and thus are defective in aggregation. In hereditary storage-pool diseases, the platelet granules are deficient, and secondary aggregation is unreliable. DDAVP is helpful in controlling bleeding in the storage pool disorders and may be helpful in the other hereditary disorders. The laboratory approach to assessing bleeding in the postoperative patient is summarized in Figure 3.

DISSEMINATED INTRAVASCULAR COAGULATION

Disseminated intravascular coagulation is a syndrome of systemic hemorrhage and thrombosis. Thrombosis may be either microvascular or in large vessels and is responsible for ischemia and end-organ damage. The syndrome may be acute and severe, or it may be chronic and compensated. The acute form is more likely to be predominantly hemorrhagic, whereas the chronic form is more likely to be predominantly thrombotic (9). Each form is associated with certain well-defined clinical settings (Table 5). The chronic form may convert to the fulminant form. The diagnosis of DIC requires evidence of activation of both the procoagulant and fibrinolytic systems, consumption of inhibitors, and evidence of damage to, or failure of, end organs. In contrast to normal coagulation, in which thrombosis and fibrinolysis are confined to the site of injury, DIC is characterized by the systemic activation of both circulating thrombin and circulating plasmin, a process that results in diffuse thrombosis and hemorrhage throughout the circulation. The syndrome of DIC is the final common pathway in many pathophysiologic states in which thrombin and plasmin are systemically activated.

Simultaneous thrombosis and hemorrhage are the result of the actions of thrombin and plasmin, respectively. Circulating thrombin cleaves fibrinogen to fibrin monomer with two main consequences: (a) the fibrin monomer polymerizes to form clot in the microcirculation, and (b) the diffuse fibrin clots trap platelets and contribute to thrombocytopenia.

Unlike thrombin, circulating plasmin cleaves both fibrinogen and cross-linked fibrin. The three results are (1) fibrinogen degradation by-products bind to fibrin monomer to create soluble fibrin monomer, which is unable to participate in clot formation; (2) fibrinogen degradation products coat platelet membranes to render the platelets dysfunctional; and (3) cross-linked fibrin is degraded, releasing D-dimer. The first two results impair clot formation, the third degrades clot, and the sum is a tendency toward hemorrhage.

The physical examination should be directed toward assessing signs of diffuse hemorrhage and thrombosis. Common findings are petechiae, purpura, or subcutaneous hematomas; oozing from operative wounds and from venipuncture and intravascular catheter sites; and signs of end-organ ischemic injury from

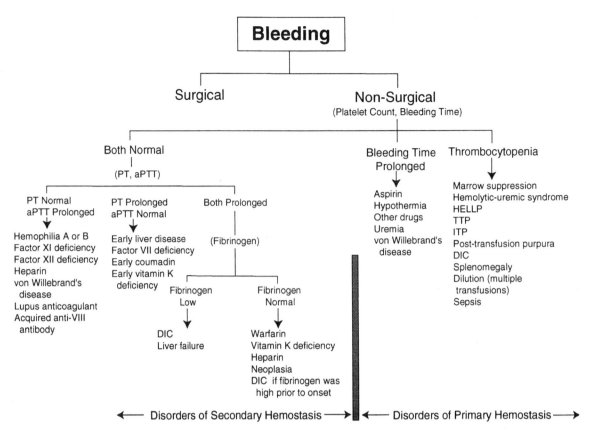

FIGURE 3. Laboratory approach to abnormal perioperative bleeding. Once anatomic sources of bleeding have been excluded, disorders of primary and secondary hemostasis are investigated as described in the text. PT, prothrombin time; aPTT, activated partial thromboplastin time; DIC, disseminated intravascular coagulation; TTP, thrombotic thrombocytopenic purpura; ITP, idiopathic thrombocytopenic purpura; HELLP, hemolysis, elevated liver transaminases, low platelets. (Adapted from Pohlman TH, Carrico CJ. Evaluation of bleeding in the surgical patient. In: Civetta JM, Taylor RW, Kirby RR, eds. *Critical care*, 2nd ed. Philadelphia: JB Lippincott, 1992:627–639, with permission.)

TABLE 5. CLINICAL SETTINGS ASSOCIATED WITH DISSEMINATED INTRAVASCULAR COAGULOPATHY

Sepsis, especially meningococcemia
Obstetric complications
  Eclampsia
  Amniotic-fluid embolism
  Placental abruption
  Retained-dead-fetus syndrome
  Hypertonic-saline abortion

Malignancy, especially acute promyelocytic leukemia
Liver disease
Pancreatitis
Trauma, especially head injury
Fat-embolism syndrome
Burns
Near-drowning in fresh water
Intravascular hemolysis
Massive transfusion
Prosthetic devices
  Intraaortic balloon assist device
  LeVeen shunt

Aortic aneurysm
Giant hemangioma

vascular thrombosis. The cardiac, pulmonary, renal, hepatic, and central nervous systems are likely to be affected.

Little consensus has been reached regarding which laboratory criteria are necessary to diagnose DIC. It is important when interpreting laboratory tests to consider whether an abnormal result can be attributed to the pathophysiology of the underlying clinical condition, such as with hypofibrinogenemia in liver disease. In addition, test results differ in acute, hemorrhagic DIC and chronic, compensated DIC. Traditionally, screening tests have consisted of the aPTT, PT, TT, fibrinogen, and platelet count. Of these, the PT and aPTT are prolonged in only slightly more than 50% of patients with DIC. A possible mechanism for normal or shortened values is the generalized circulation of all the clotting factors in their activated forms, a state that may accelerate fibrin formation (9). Seventy percent of patients with acute hemorrhagic DIC have a fibrinogen level less than 150 mg per deciliter. Because fibrinogen is an acute-phase reactant, however, a normal level or a recent decrease from an elevated level is consistent with DIC. Similarly, a low level may result from other conditions, such as liver disease, and alone is not diagnostic of DIC. The TT may be normal with fibrinogen levels as low as 75 mg per deciliter but is prolonged if circulating FDPs and hypofibrinogenemia are present in great enough magnitude to retard clot formation. The TT may be of additional usefulness if the clot formed *in vitro* is observed for clot lysis, a process that indicates the presence of significant plasmin activity. Clot lysis within 10 minutes confirms plasmin activation.

A peripheral smear reveals a low platelet count in more than 90% of cases of DIC, but the specificity of thrombocytopenia for DIC is only 48% because thrombocytopenia is often caused by the underlying clinical disorder. The smear may show predominantly large young platelets resulting from shortened survival secondary to entrapment in fibrin mesh. In DIC, the platelet count ranges from 2,000 to 100,000 per microliter, with an average count of 60,000 per microliter. Tests of platelet function, such as the bleeding time and aggregation studies, are invariably abnormal in DIC because the FDPs coat the platelets, and, therefore, these tests add little. Schistocytes are present on the peripheral smear in 50% of cases of DIC.

More sensitive and specific than these tests are ones that demonstrate concomitant thrombosis and fibrinolysis inherent to DIC. FDPs are elevated in more than 85% of cases of DIC.

Because FDPs are formed from plasmin degrading fibrinogen as well as fibrin, however, their presence alone does not prove lysis of fibrin clot. D-dimer is a unique antigen that is formed when plasmin digests cross-linked fibrin. The presence of D-dimer indicates that clot has formed and has been digested by plasmin. A positive D-dimer assay has a sensitivity of 85% and a specificity of 97% for predicting DIC. Combined, the FDP and D-dimer assays have a sensitivity of 100% and a specificity of 97% (18).

In addition to the previous tests, a few other assays may be helpful in establishing the diagnosis of DIC in that they provide evidence of coagulation, fibrinolysis, or consumption of inhibitors. PF 1 + 2 is cleaved from prothrombin during its activation to thrombin by Xa. FPA is the fragment that thrombin cleaves from fibrinogen. Both PF 1 + 2 and FPA, measured by enzyme-linked immunosorbent assay (ELISA), are usually elevated in DIC, and a positive assay confirms procoagulant activity. AT-III, a natural inhibitor of thrombin, Xa, IXa, and XIIa, binds readily and irreversibly to the large quantities of these activated proteases in DIC. Because AT-III is bound irreversibly, measures of its remaining functional activity are reduced in DIC. Plasminogen is usually low and plasmin high in DIC, findings that demonstrate activation of the fibrinolytic system. In addition, the complex of plasmin and its naturally occurring inhibitor, α-2-antiplasmin, is usually elevated during DIC and normalizes as the syndrome resolves. Free α-2-antiplasmin is decreased in DIC.

The single most important treatment for DIC is management of the underlying disease process that triggered it. Supportive therapies that correct hypovolemia and acidosis also should be carried out promptly. If clinical bleeding is present, or if an operation is necessary, replacement with blood components should be considered. In general, a platelet count above 50,000 per microliter to 100,000 per microliter is recommended for patients undergoing operations; the desired level depends on the degree of invasiveness of the procedure. A fibrinogen level below 150 mg per deciliter can be corrected with cryoprecipitate. A fibrinogen level below 75 mg per deciliter will prolong the PT and TT and should be corrected with cryoprecipitate before fresh frozen plasma (FFP) is given to normalize the PT and aPTT. Theoretically, the infusion of FFP and cryoprecipitate can worsen DIC by

further activating coagulation factors and by providing substrate (fibrinogen) for thrombin to produce more FDPs. Such worsening is likely to occur in patients with low AT-III levels. In patients with low AT-III levels or clinical evidence of ongoing DIC, only components devoid of fibrinogen and other factors should be used (9). Safe components are washed packed red blood cells, platelets, AT-III concentrate, albumin, and hydroxyethyl starch. If levels of AT-III are normal, however, it is safe to replace fibrinogen and factors with cryoprecipitate and FFP. FFP itself contains natural inhibitors to the serine proteases of the coagulation cascade.

Low levels of AT-III correlate with poor survival in patients with DIC and septic shock (19). Preliminary studies support the potential efficacy of AT-III administration in reducing mortality rates for patients with severe sepsis (20). The desired level of AT-III proposed by Bick (9) is 125% of normal or greater. Further research is warranted to confirm the beneficial effects of AT-III and to define its optimal timing and dosage in the clinical setting (21).

The use of heparin may be beneficial in treating patients with DIC that is primarily thrombotic. Inactivation of thrombin by AT-III is enhanced a thousand-fold in the presence of heparin. After heparin administration, fibrinogen levels rise, FDP levels fall, and microvascular thrombosis is reduced. Heparin use may be particularly helpful in controlling thrombosis in patients with acral and dermal ischemia and necrosis (22). Patients deficient in AT-III are resistant to heparin until repletion of AT-III levels. Heparin is infused intravenously at a rate of 5 to 7 U · kilogram per hour without a loading dose (18). One researcher recommends subcutaneous heparin in a dose of 80 to 100 U every 4 to 6 hours, a regimen he believes is less likely to exacerbate hemorrhage (9). Within 4 hours, the fibrinogen should increase, and the FDPs and D-dimer should decrease. The success of heparin therapy is assessed by serial determinations of these three laboratory values. A prolongation of the aPTT after initiation of heparin therapy indicates that the dose is too high and should be decreased. Clinical conditions in which there is either low-grade or localized DIC, and in which heparin may be beneficial are the retained-dead-fetus syndrome, giant hemangiomas, acute promyelocytic leukemia, and solid tumors (23). The use of heparin is contraindicated in patients with fulminant hemorrhagic DIC and other clinical situations such as central nervous system hemorrhage (9). Overall, heparin use decreases the consumption of clotting factors but also increases the risk of hemorrhage.

In a very small percentage of patients, hemorrhage is perpetuated by ongoing fibrinolysis. This state is characterized by elevated plasmin levels, a deficiency of α-2-antiplasmin, or both. Treatment may include the use of an antifibrinolytic agent such as ϵ-aminocaproic acid (EACA, Amicar) or tranexamic acid in combination with heparin. In patients with DIC, the antifibrinolytic agents never should be used without heparin, or diffuse, unopposed thrombosis may occur. EACA is given in a loading dose of 3 to 4 g, followed by continuous infusion at 1 g per hour until the α-2-antiplasmin is greater than 40% of normal.

Newer methods of treating DIC have yet to be proved in large-scale clinical trials. In one study, the use of LMWH was shown to ameliorate DIC (24). There is some evidence to indicate that LMWH is as effective as unfractionated heparin but may be associated with a lower risk of bleeding complications (25).

Recombinant hirudin is a direct thrombin inhibitor; its activity, in contrast to heparin, is independent of AT-III. Hirudin, which has been used for prophylaxis of deep venous thrombosis and during extracorporeal circulation, may be of clinical utility in treating DIC. It was recently been shown to have a beneficial role in the treatment of endotoxin-induced DIC both in animals as well as in an experimental human model (26,27). In isolated cases, administration of purified human protein C has improved DIC (28,29).

In summary, DIC is a syndrome of systemic thrombosis and hemorrhage that results from the simultaneous activation of thrombin and plasmin in the setting of a known predisposing clinical condition. Common laboratory findings are a prolonged PT, aPTT, and TT and a decreased fibrinogen and platelet count. The diagnosis is confirmed by an elevated FDP and D-dimer assay. The most important and immediate therapy is treatment of the underlying condition. If DIC is predominantly hemorrhagic and the AT-III level is normal, factors and fibrinogen can be replaced with FFP and cryoprecipitate. If AT-III is low, replacement is restricted to components free of fibrinogen. In DIC that is primarily thrombotic, subcutaneous or intravenously administered heparin may be helpful. If DIC occurs with deficient α-2-antiplasmin, EACA in combination with heparin may decrease fibrinolysis. AT-III, recombinant hirudin, LMWH heparin, and protein C have all shown promise as potential therapies but have yet to be proved in large-scale, randomized trials.

LIVER DISEASE

Patients with hepatic disease who are in the ICU commonly develop coagulopathies. The cause is multifactorial and includes decreased synthesis of coagulation proteins, decreased clearance of FDPs, and increased fibrinolysis.

In cirrhosis, the reduction in factor levels parallels the impairment of parenchymal cell function. Factor VII, which has a half-life of only 4 to 6 hours, and protein C are the first to fall. The result of a low factor VII level is a prolonged PT. Next, the remaining vitamin-K-dependent factors (II, IX, and X) decrease, and the aPTT is prolonged. The fibrinogen level is usually maintained until end-stage disease. Because of impaired synthetic function, however, the factors and fibrinogen that are produced may be functionally abnormal. Severe cirrhosis is associated with increased fibrinolysis, which may be either primary in etiology or secondary to concomitant DIC. The distinction can be made by finding an elevated D-dimer, which favors the diagnosis of DIC. In patients with portal hypertension with splenomegaly, splenic sequestration contributes to thrombocytopenia. In addition, the impaired reticuloendothelial system of the liver fails to clear FDPs, and the FDPs circulate and interfere with platelet function. Ethanol itself may inhibit thromboxane A2 synthesis and reduce platelet-storage-pool ADP, and both these lesions impair platelet function. *In vitro* aggregometry is abnormal. Patients with alcoholic cirrhosis often bleed from varices or gastric or duodenal ulcers. While these mechanical causes are examined, the patient should be supported with components that replace deficient and dysfunctional factors and platelets: FFP and platelet concentrates. DDAVP (0.3 μg per kilogram, infused intravenously over

20 minutes) may improve platelet function. Antifibrinolytics (EACA and tranexamic acid) are safe only if DIC is not present.

In acute toxic or infectious hepatitis, impairment of coagulation correlates with the severity of the parenchymal cell damage. Coagulation may be normal, or factor levels may be slightly decreased. Thrombocytopenia, if present, is usually mild. The coagulopathy of fulminant hepatitis mimics that of severe cirrhosis with reduced fibrinogen levels, DIC, and possibly hyperfibrinolysis (30).

A particular challenge is the perioperative management of the patient who has undergone liver transplantation. These patients have a preoperative coagulopathy related to liver failure, a large intraoperative transfusion requirement, and excessive fibrinolysis that is stimulated during the anhepatic and reperfusion phases of transplantation. Clinical studies comparing intraoperative antifibrinolytic therapy to placebo have demonstrated reduced transfusion requirements in treated patients undergoing liver transplantation (31,32).

In summary, the coagulopathy of liver disease is multifactorial in etiology. Unlike the situation in other types of coagulopathy, the coagulation factors and fibrinogen may be dysfunctional because of abnormal hepatic synthetic function, and the platelets may be rendered dysfunctional by circulating FDPs that the liver fails to clear. Treatment of the bleeding patient with liver disease consists of replacement of deficient components and administration of DDAVP to enhance platelet function.

VITAMIN K DEFICIENCY

A critical late step in the synthesis of factors II (prothrombin), VII, IX, and X (and proteins C and S) is dependent on vitamin K. In this step, an enzyme (γ-glutamyl carboxylase) carboxylates several glutamic-acid residues at the amino terminal end of these factors. The presence of the carboxyl moiety is essential for these factors to bind calcium ion, an action without which the calcium–phospholipid-dependent steps in the coagulation cascade do not take place. The active form of vitamin K, vitamin K hydroquinone, is the cofactor for γ-glutamyl carboxylase. During the carboxylation reaction, vitamin K is oxidized to vitamin K epoxide. The latter is subsequently reduced in a two-step enzymatic process that regenerates the biologically active hydroquinone form (Fig. 4). The mechanism of warfarin anticoagulation is inhibition of the two enzymes that regenerate vitamin K. Deficiency of vitamin K, whether from inadequate intake or pharmacologic antagonism by warfarin, results in hypocarboxylated, dysfunctional coagulation proteins and consequent slowed clot formation.

Vitamin K deficiency is the most common cause of a prolonged PT among patients in the ICU. Deficiency is usually multifactorial. Because the vitamin is fat soluble, absorption from the gastrointestinal tract is decreased in biliary obstruction and in fat malabsorption syndromes. Antibiotics that inhibit gut flora decrease the amount of vitamin K ordinarily supplied by these organisms. Deficiency by the latter mechanism usually occurs in the geriatric or pediatric populations after at least 2 weeks of antibiotic therapy. Malnutrition or administration of total parenteral nutrition without added vitamin K can cause deficiency.

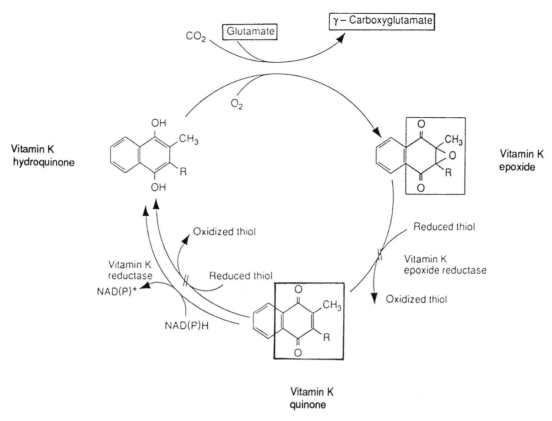

FIGURE 4. Vitamin-K-dependent carboxylation of coagulation factors. Vitamin K hydroquinone is a cofactor in the carboxylation reaction. Warfarin interferes with the regeneration of the hydroquinone by inhibiting vitamin K epoxide reductase and vitamin K reductase. (Adapted from Furie BC, Furie B. Vitamin K: metabolism and disorders. In: Hoffman R, Benz EJ, Shattil SJ, et al., eds. *Hematology: basic principles and practice*, 2nd ed. New York: Churchill Livingstone, 1995:1739, with permission.)

Because factor VII has the shortest half-life of the vitamin-K-dependent factors, the PT is the most sensitive early indicator of vitamin K deficiency. For example, antibiotic therapy combined with malnutrition can render the PT abnormal in 2 to 3 days. The aPTT is not prolonged until much later in vitamin K deficiency, when the other vitamin-K-dependent factors, especially IX, become affected.

The treatment of acute hemorrhage in a patient who has been taking warfarin or who is deficient in vitamin K is replacement of the vitamin-K-dependent factors with FFP. If the patient is not hemorrhaging acutely, the treatment of the coagulopathy is vitamin K replacement with 1 to 10 mg administered intravenously or subcutaneously for 3 days. During treatment with vitamin K, normalization of the PT should occur within 24 hours in a healthy person and within 72 hours in a critically ill person. Large parenteral or oral vitamin K doses, including excessive dietary intake, antagonize the action of subsequently administered warfarin. Therefore, if only temporary reversal of warfarin therapy is desired, as for a surgical procedure, FFP, rather than vitamin K, should be given.

In summary, vitamin K deficiency from malnutrition and antibiotic therapy is common in critically ill patients, and the earliest, most sensitive indicator is a prolonged PT. Emergent therapy is infusion of FFP, and nonemergent therapy is vitamin K replacement.

HYPOTHERMIA

Hypothermia may be encountered in patients in the ICU postoperatively, particularly in patients who have undergone lengthy procedures with large incisions and significant transfusion requirements, or in patients who have been exposed to cold environmental conditions.

Hypothermia affects hemostasis in several ways. Hypothermia enhances fibrinolysis, and the FDPs formed then interfere with platelet aggregation. Hypothermia slows the enzymatic cleavage of proenzymes to activated clotting factors. A specific heparin-like inhibitor of Xa is generated during hypothermia, and this inhibitor is not reversed by protamine. Hypothermia induces a transient platelet dysfunction characterized by decreased aggregation and thromboxane synthesis. In addition, platelet counts fall during hypothermia, probably as a result of splenic sequestration, and they recover after rewarming. Measures should be taken to warm to normal temperature any patient who is hypothermic and bleeding.

POST–CARDIOPULMONARY BYPASS

Multiple factors may contribute to bleeding in a patient who has undergone CPB. These patients have often taken antiplatelet and anticoagulant medications such as aspirin and warfarin preoperatively. A patient undergoing emergent coronary revascularization for treatment of an MI may have received a thrombolytic agent. Increasing numbers of patients undergoing percutaneous coronary intervention are receiving one of several of the recently developed platelet glycoprotein IIb-IIIa inhibitors. Persistent effects of these drugs may contribute to postoperative hemorrhage.

When assessing the patient, one should first investigate anatomic sources of bleeding. Chest-tube drainage in excess of 10 mL per kilogram in the first hour, or 20 mL per kilogram over the first 3 hours, or any sudden increase to 300 mL per hour in an adult suggests inadequate surgical hemostasis. Hypertension from pain or agitation or inadequate antihypertensive therapy promotes bleeding from vein-graft sites. Retained mediastinal clot may trigger DIC.

Once anatomic sources have been excluded, other etiologies should be investigated. If the patient's core temperature is lower than 35°C, the patient usually will benefit from warming. Next, the many ways that CPB itself can trigger a coagulopathy should be addressed. Most importantly, the heparin given for bypass may not have been adequately reversed with protamine. Persistent heparin effect can be demonstrated by finding an elevated ACT, and this effect can be corrected by titrating small additional doses of protamine until the ACT is less than 130. Caution is advised with repeated administration, however, because protamine overdosage has been found to alter *in vitro* adenosine diphosphate (ADP)-induced platelet aggregation in a dose-dependent manner and may predispose patients to further bleeding as a result (33,34). Other ways in which heparin can contribute to bleeding are heparin-induced thrombocytopenia, discussed separately, and heparin rebound. The latter refers to clinical bleeding with a prolonged ACT that occurs one or more hours after adequate reversal of heparin with protamine. The mechanism of rebound may be delayed release of administered heparin bound to tissues. It is possible that administration of FFP, which contains AT-III, may contribute to heparin rebound.

The fibrinolytic pathway is probably activated during CPB in response to fibrin formation in the extracorporeal circuit. If α-2-antiplasmin is overwhelmed, a systemic fibrinolytic state may occur. The TEG may demonstrate clot lysis, and FDPs are elevated. Ordinarily, this CPB-induced fibrinolysis resolves spontaneously, but rarely it can be the cause of postoperative bleeding. The intraoperative use of antifibrinolytic therapy has been shown to be effective in reducing postoperative bleeding following cardiac surgery (35). Doses of antifibrinolytics are EACA, 100 to 150 mg per kilogram (approximately 7 to 10 g) as a loading dose, followed by an infusion of 10 mg/kg/h to 15 mg per kilogram per hour (approximately 1 g per hour) or tranexamic acid 10 mg per kilogram as a loading dose, followed by an infusion of 1 mg per kilogram per hour.

Aprotinin, a polypeptide derived from bovine lung, is a nonspecific inhibitor of serine proteases, including plasmin. Multiple clinical trials involving aprotinin have demonstrated its efficacy in reducing blood loss and rates of blood product transfusion when used during open heart surgery (36). Both "high" (280 mg, intra-venous loading dose and 280 mg into the bypass prime volume, followed by 70 mg per hour infusion) and "low" (140 mg, intravenous loading dose and 140 mg into the bypass prime volume, followed by 35 mg per hour infusion) doses reduced blood loss, but the difference in blood lost between the two dosing schedules was not significant (37). Aprotinin also significantly reduced the volume of blood lost in patients who had been taking aspirin preoperatively (38). Although its efficacy has been established, the mechanism by which aprotinin reduces perioperative bleeding in cardiac surgery remains inconclusive (39). Whereas antifibrinolysis through plasmin inhibition certainly plays a role, considerable debate has centered around a potential beneficial effect on platelet function (40–42). Practical disadvantages of aprotinin include its greater expense over alternative antifibrinolytics and its potential to induce allergic reactions, including anaphylaxis (43). One further practical issue related to the clinical use of aprotinin relates to the appropriate method of monitoring the adequacy of heparin-induced anticoagulation during CPB. Aprotinin prolongs the diatomaceous earth (celite)-based ACT to a greater degree than it affects the kaolin-based ACT (44). This may be secondary to the greater potency of kaolin to activate coagulation (45) or kaolin's ability to bind aprotinin, thus interfering with aprotinin's inhibition of contact activation *in vitro* (46). Hence, an alternative dosage regimen for giving heparin should be used, or the target ACT should be altered. A controversial issue is whether patients who receive aprotinin have a higher incidence of early saphenous vein graft occlusion. Results from the International Multicenter Aprotinin Graft Patency Experience (IMAGE) trial suggested a higher occlusion rate after aprotinin versus placebo in the European, but not the United States, patient population. These researchers attributed this geographic difference to a higher incidence in the European patients of predisposing factors known to promote graft occlusion (47).

Platelets are affected by CPB in at least three ways: (a) the circuit induces a platelet-aggregation defect, the severity of which is proportional to the duration of CPB; (b) hypothermia causes transient thrombocytopenia secondary to sequestration; and (c) platelets are destroyed at blood–gas interfaces in cardiotomy suction and bubble oxygenators. In addition, many patients presenting for open heart surgery have had recent exposure to a variety of agents that can negatively affect platelet function (e.g., heparin, aspirin, glycoprotein IIb/IIIa inhibitors). The circuit is an artificial surface that activates platelets and thereby causes depletion of γ-granule contents. Platelet-membrane-glycoprotein receptor IIb/IIIa, necessary for platelet-plug formation, is reduced during bypass. These qualitative platelet defects normally resolve within 2 to 4 hours after CPB has ended (48). In addition, intraoperative blood loss replaced with platelet-free components contributes to a dilutional thrombocytopenia. Similarly, clotting factors may be decreased by denaturation at blood–gas interfaces or dilution during transfusion. Platelets and factors should be replaced if deficiencies persist after adequate heparin reversal. Iloprost, a synthetic analog of prostacyclin, may protect platelets from the effects of the CPB circuit. DDAVP probably is not helpful in treating bleeding after CPB (49) unless the patient had been taking aspirin preoperatively (50). Sodium nitroprusside and nitroglycerin, agents that are commonly used intraoperatively and postoperatively, exert their vasodilating effects via nitric oxide, which is a potent inhibitor of platelet aggregation. These vasodilators prolong the bleeding time, although it is unclear whether *in vivo* the mechanism is inhibition of platelet aggregation or a result of direct vasodilation.

In summary, evaluation of bleeding in a patient after CPB involves investigating anatomic and nonsurgical sources of bleeding, including a heparin effect, ongoing fibrinolysis, and deficiency of platelets or factors. Other factors that may contribute to bleeding in the patient who has undergone a cardiac operation are hypothermia, massive transfusion, and DIC. In addition to the usual laboratory tests (PT, aPTT, TT, platelet count, fibrinogen, and D-dimer), the ACT and TEG are useful in detecting persistent heparin effect and ongoing fibrinolysis, respectively.

MASSIVE TRANSFUSION

Massive transfusion is defined as the replacement of one or more blood volumes in a 24-hour period. One blood volume in a 70-kg adult is about 5 L of blood lost, or a transfused volume of 10 U of packed red blood cells (PRBCs). Likely settings for massive transfusion are significant gastrointestinal hemorrhage, trauma, and large surgical resections, including removal of neoplasms, aortic operations, and some transplant operations. Common complications of massive transfusion are dilutional coagulopathy, DIC and fibrinolysis, hypothermia, citrate toxicity, hypokalemia, hyperkalemia, and infection.

Dilutional thrombocytopenia is the most significant cause of bleeding after massive transfusion. If ongoing blood loss is replaced with only PRBCs, the platelet count falls nearly exponentially. The splenic platelet pool is mobilized and counteracts loss during hemorrhage. If the patient's platelet count was high preoperatively, the remaining number of platelets may be adequate to prevent bleeding. If the count was normal or low to start, however, dilution usually results in a count below 50,000 to 100,000 per microliter and may contribute to clinical bleeding. Repletion of platelets enhances the function of the coagulation factors as well as platelet-plug formation. Platelets provide the surface on which many of the factors are activated and fibrin strands form. Further, platelets release vWF and fibrinogen locally at the site of injury. Platelets are more likely than are factors to be rendered dysfunctional as a result of the hypoxia and acidosis that often accompany the clinical setting in which massive transfusion is necessary.

Coagulation-factor levels fall exponentially during massive transfusion of PRBCs. About 40% of factors remain after transfusion of one blood volume; 3% to 15% of blood-clotting activity remains after two blood volumes; and less than 5% remains after three blood volumes. Because only 10% to 30% of normal factor activity is required for adequate hemostasis, replacement of factors with FFP is less urgent than transfusion of platelets. The use of cryoprecipitate is indicated if fibrinogen levels are very low.

When cells injured by diffuse ischemia and hypoperfusion release procoagulant substances, DIC can be initiated. In addition, endothelial cells injured during hypoperfusion may release t-PA, which stimulates concomitant fibrinolysis. Hypothermia results if blood products and crystalloid solutions are transfused without using warming devices.

Citrate is added to banked blood to chelate calcium and thus prevent clotting during storage. After transfusion, citrate is metabolized by the liver to bicarbonate. If blood is infused very rapidly or if the patient has liver disease, is hypothermic, or has a metabolic alkalosis, the serum-ionized calcium level may decrease secondary to chelation by citrate. Another likely setting for hypocalcemia is the anhepatic phase of liver transplantation when no metabolism of citrate occurs. Although calcium is a required cofactor for the vitamin-K-dependent steps in the coagulation cascade, significant hypocalcemia generally warrants correction for reasons related to cardiovascular stability prior to it being a major contributor to coagulopathy. Calcium repletion is suggested if the patient is hypotensive during the anhepatic phase of liver transplantation or if the ionized-calcium level falls to or below 50% of baseline (51). If calcium repletion is vigorously undertaken, rebound hypercalcemia may occur when perfusion is restored and citrate is metabolized.

Both hyperkalemia and hypokalemia are associated with massive transfusion. In stored blood, there is a progressive decline in the function of the red-cell ADP pump and a resultant leak of potassium out of cells such that the extracellular potassium concentration in the stored blood increases at a rate of about 1 mEq per liter daily. Because the actual volume of plasma in a unit of whole blood is small—approximately 300 mL—the total amount of potassium transfused per unit of blood is only 4 to 7 mEq. In other words, only 70 mEq of potassium is gained during the transfusion of 10 U of whole blood. Hyperkalemia during massive transfusion is more likely a result of metabolic acidosis from hypoperfusion. Following resuscitation, hypokalemia often results from two mechanisms: as transfused cells become metabolically active, they take up substantial potassium; as citrate is metabolized to bicarbonate, the ensuing metabolic alkalosis causes an intracellular shift of potassium.

Laboratory abnormalities seen in massive transfusion are prolonged PT, aPTT, TT; decreased platelet count; and decreased fibrinogen. FDPs are not usually increased unless concomitant DIC is present. The patient with coagulopathy from massive transfusion presents clinically with diffuse oozing from surgical and venipuncture sites.

In summary, massive transfusion may be accompanied by a number of complications. Coagulopathy secondary to dilutional thrombocytopenia and factor deficiency should be anticipated, and platelets and factors should be replaced in that order. Whereas hypocalcemia may occur during very rapid infusion of blood, repletion in adults is rarely necessary except during the anhepatic phase of liver transplantation. Hyperkalemia may be seen with the lactic acidosis accompanying hypovolemia, and hypokalemia may follow with the metabolic alkalosis that develops during metabolism of citrate. Therapy is supportive.

THROMBOCYTOPENIA

Although thrombocytopenia is arbitrarily defined as a platelet count of 100,000 per microliter, the clinician should judge the adequacy of a given patient's level in light of the clinical setting. Points to consider are the presence or risk of ongoing bleeding, the rate of decrease in the platelet count, and the need for an urgent and invasive surgical procedure. Some types of thrombocytopenia encountered in the critically ill patient are addressed in the following section.

Heparin-induced Thrombocytopenia

Thrombocytopenia develops in 3% to 7% of all patients receiving intravenous heparin. Low platelet counts also may be seen in patients receiving only subcutaneous heparin or heparin flushes for catheters or in patients with indwelling heparin-bonded catheters. Heparin-induced thrombocytopenia (HIT) is associated more frequently with heparin species of high-molecular-weight and of low antithrombin affinity.

There are two types of HIT: HIT types I and II. HIT type I usually occurs within the first few days of heparin therapy. It is characterized by a mild, transitory, and asymptomatic reduction in the platelet count, rarely to less than 100,000 per microliter. This form results when heparin binds to platelet membranes causing ADP release and platelet aggregation with a consequent reduction in the number of circulating platelets. HIT type I is self-limited and reversible; heparin therapy need not be discontinued.

In contrast, HIT type II leads to a severe, progressive reduction in the platelet count, often to less than 100,000 per microliter. Fewer than 5% of patients receiving heparin develop HIT II. This form usually begins after 5 to 14 days of heparin therapy. A patient with previous exposure to heparin may develop the syndrome within hours of reexposure, however. The mechanism is thought to be immune mediated (52). Platelet factor 4 (PF4) binds to the heparin molecule. IgG antibodies then are generated; these recognize and bind the heparin/PF4 complex. The anti-heparin/PF4 IgG immunocomplex then leads to further platelet activation and aggregation, resulting in thrombocytopenia. In addition, platelet aggregates may provoke an endothelial lesion, generating thrombin *in vivo*. Approximately 20% to 30% of patients will develop the heparin-induced thrombocytopenia and thrombosis syndrome (HITTS), characterized by arterial and venous thromboses with associated morbidity and mortality rates of 30% and 80%, respectively (53). The most common presentation of HITTS is lower-extremity ischemia, although MI, cerebrovascular accident, and pulmonary embolism all have been reported.

Heparin-induced thrombocytopenia should be suspected when platelet counts fall after heparin therapy has been started. Diagnosis is made by demonstrating that the patient's serum induces platelet aggregation and serotonin release in the presence of heparin. Documenting platelet-associated IgG alone is not specific for the diagnosis of HIT II because many other agents and conditions induce antiplatelet antibodies. Type I will resolve spontaneously, but the diagnosis of type II mandates the immediate discontinuation of all heparin therapy, including that used to flush central and arterial lines. Although these patients are thrombocytopenic, hemorrhagic events are not frequent. Platelet transfusions should be given with caution and only as indicated for intractable bleeding, as repleting platelets may worsen intravascular thrombosis.

If anticoagulation is indicated for an underlying condition in the patient with HIT II, an alternative agent must be selected. Although the cautious use of LWMH or the heparinoid danaproid has been suggested, the therapeutic use of these drugs in HIT II should be preceded by exclusion of *in vitro* antibody cross-reactivity. Studies suggest cross-reactivity rates near 10% for danaproid and greater than 80% for the LMWHs (54,55). Man-

agement strategies for the patient who must undergo a surgical procedure that requires systemic anticoagulation have included the use of heparin preceded by either antiaggregative therapy, for example, aspirin and dipyridamole (56) or iloprost (57), or plasmapheresis to remove antiplatelet antibodies (58). A unique challenge is the patient who must undergo CPB, particularly on an emergent basis. Recent case series describe the use of recombinant hirudin in this situation (59,60). Advantages of hirudin include a lack of cross-reaction with heparin-induced antibodies, an immediate onset and relatively short half-life, and the availability of an adequate measure of anticoagulant activity (60). Another alternative may include the use of ancrod, an investigational agent derived from the venom of Malaysian pit vipers. Ancrod converts fibrinogen into soluble fibrin products, thereby decreasing plasma fibrinogen and blood viscosity. It has been used successfully in patients with HIT undergoing cardiac surgery with CPB (61). As ancrod depletes normal fibrinogen, replacement with cryoprecipitate may be needed postoperatively.

In summary, the clinician should have a high suspicion for HIT in patients who demonstrate a falling platelet count after the initiation of heparin therapy. Thrombocytopenia may be mild and may not require alteration of heparin therapy or may be severe and associated with life-threatening intravascular thrombosis. In the latter case, heparin should be discontinued immediately, but platelet transfusions should be given with caution and only if there is clinical bleeding.

IDIOPATHIC THROMBOCYTOPENIC PURPURA

Idiopathic thrombocytopenic purpura (ITP), more accurately known as *autoimmune thrombocytopenic purpura*, is primarily a disorder of increased platelet destruction. Autoantibodies form that bind to platelet surface receptors and cause the premature removal of platelets from the circulation by the reticuloendothelial system (RES). ITP can be seen at any age; among adults, it is most frequent in the 20- to 40-year-old group. Women are three times more likely than men to be affected. In children, ITP is usually an acute, self-limited disorder that resolves spontaneously. In adults, it is typically a chronic disorder with a more insidious onset. ITP may be associated with systemic lupus erythematosus or human immunodeficiency virus infection.

Practice guidelines for the diagnosis and management of ITP in adults were published by the American Society of Hematology in 1997 (62). Little scientific evidence exists regarding the accuracy or reliability of laboratory tests for diagnosis. Therefore, ITP is largely a clinical diagnosis made by confirming the presence of isolated thrombocytopenia while excluding concurrent causes. In addition to a thorough history and physical examination, a complete blood count with examination of the peripheral blood smear is recommended. Because adult patients with moderate to severe thrombocytopenia generally begin treatment soon after diagnosis, data on the natural history of untreated disease are lacking. Optimal therapy for chronic ITP has yet to be established. Treatments options most commonly recommended include glucocorticoids, intravenous IgG, anti-D immune globulin, and splenectomy. Other treatments reportedly used for refractory cases include azathioprine, danazol, combination chemotherapy, and vinca alkaloids, among others. In patients who do not respond to therapy, the principal cause of death from ITP is intracranial hemorrhage.

POSTTRANSFUSION PURPURA

Posttransfusion purpura is an immune-mediated thrombocytopenia. It is seen particularly in older women who have had prior pregnancies or transfusions that have stimulated the production of antiplatelet antibodies. Profound thrombocytopenia and hemorrhage occur approximately 1 week after a blood transfusion. The mechanism is antibody-mediated destruction of native platelets. Administration of intravenous gamma globulin and plasmapheresis are both effective treatments.

THROMBOCYTOPENIA WITH MICROANGIOPATHIC HEMOLYSIS

Thrombotic thrombocytopenic purpura (TTP), hemolytic uremic syndrome (HUS), and the HELLP syndrome (hemolysis, elevated liver transaminases, low platelets) are among several syndromes of thrombocytopenia and microangiopathic hemolytic anemia without consumption of coagulation factors. Others include severe vasculitides, gastric carcinoma, and malignant hypertension. Common to these entities is platelet aggregation in arterioles and capillaries and consequent ischemic end-organ damage. Intravascular hemolysis results from red-blood-cell entrapment in platelet thrombi.

Left untreated, TTP, a syndrome of severe thrombocytopenia, leads to progressive deterioration and death. Not all patients present with the classic clinical pentad of fever, thrombocytopenia, and hemolytic anemia with renal and neurologic impairment. In more than 50% of patients, severe thrombocytopenia (platelets <20,000/μL) results from "consumption" of platelets as they aggregate in the microcirculation. Neurologic signs may fluctuate and include headache, paresthesias, paresis, visual disturbances, seizures, and coma. Hematuria and proteinuria are common, but only a few patients have severe renal impairment. TTP occurs in women about twice as often as in men, and the incidence peaks in the fourth decade. The triggering event is unknown, although as many as one-half of patients admit to a prodromal viral-like illness. It has been suggested that unusually large vWF multimers (ULvWF) are secreted in excess and induce platelet aggregation (63). The diagnosis is distinguished from DIC by its accompanying normal coagulation times. Other typical laboratory findings are a markedly elevated serum lactate dehydrogenase (LDH; five to ten times normal), elevated unconjugated bilirubin, decreased or absent haptoglobin, and schistocytes and reticulocytes on the peripheral smear. Treatment consists of plasma exchange with FFP. Platelet transfusions may worsen thrombosis. Infrequent relapses (intermittent TTP) occur in 10% to 30% of survivors. A rare form that begins in childhood recurs frequently at regular intervals (chronic relapsing TTP).

Hemolytic uremic syndrome occurs mainly in children and presents with the triad of hemolysis, renal failure, and thrombocytopenia. The mortality rate is much lower than that in TTP.

Hemolysis and thrombocytopenia are less severe than in TTP, but acute renal failure is more severe and frequently requires dialysis. Neurologic signs are not as prominent as in TTP, although uremic encephalopathy may complicate the course of the disease. Most cases are preceded by an episode of bloody diarrhea caused by *Shigella dysenteriae* or *Escherichia coli*. These species release an exotoxin that probably directly damages glomerular endothelial cells, an insult leading to ULvWF multimer release and platelet aggregation. Chemotherapy or total-body irradiation also can precipitate HUS. Although plasma exchange has been used in the treatment of HUS, controlled trials have yet to be performed. The clinical course is usually a single, nonrecurrent episode, although chronic renal failure and hypertension may result.

In normal pregnancy, there may be a decrease in platelets of about 20% by term. Preeclampsia is the syndrome of hypertension, generalized edema, and proteinuria associated with increased placental production of thromboxane A2. Preeclampsia progresses to eclampsia when the patient manifests seizure activity without other precipitating cause. Thrombocytopenia commonly occurs in both preeclampsia and eclampsia. The mechanism of thrombocytopenia is not known but may be immune-mediated destruction or platelet adhesion to exposed collagen at sites of damaged endothelium. The magnitude of thrombocytopenia correlates with the severity of preeclampsia or eclampsia and with maternal and fetal morbidity. In particular, there is increased risk of maternal intracranial hemorrhage. The treatment is delivery of the fetus; the platelet count routinely returns to normal within 3 to 4 days postpartum. Although preeclampsia itself is not associated with red-blood-cell hemolysis, the course in up to 15% of patients may progress to the HELLP syndrome. Most patients with HELLP present in the third trimester with malaise and epigastric or right-upper-quadrant pain resulting from subcapsular hepatic edema or hemorrhage. As in TTP and HUS, intravascular platelet deposition and microangiopathic hemolytic anemia occur. Thrombocytopenia may progress rapidly to counts below 50,000 per microliter; it typically nadirs 24 to 48 hours postpartum and may persist for up to 7 days. Hemolysis generally resolves within 48 hours postpartum. Laboratory investigation yields a low platelet count, elevated transaminases, and positive tests for intravascular hemolysis (elevated LDH, decreased haptoglobin, unconjugated hyperbilirubinemia, and schistocytes on peripheral smear). Fulminant DIC may develop. Patients with HELLP are at increased risk for developing hepatic rupture, which often presents with the sudden onset of upper abdominal pain, nausea, vomiting, fever, and hypotension. Definitive treatment for HELLP syndrome is delivery of the fetus. If thrombocytopenia is protracted postpartum, plasma exchange may be efficacious. TTP and HUS may occur during pregnancy and should be included in the differential diagnosis of HELLP. DIC may occur concomitantly with TTP, HUS, or HELLP, but is not a component of these syndromes. These syndromes differ from DIC in that the PT, aPTT, fibrinogen, and D-dimer are usually normal.

In summary, TTP, HUS, and HELLP are similar syndromes of thrombocytopenia and microangiopathic hemolysis. HUS differs in that it tends to affect children, impairs renal function more than TTP and HELLP do, and has milder hematologic involvement. The natural courses of TTP and HELLP are more severe and rapidly progressive than is the course of HUS. Plasma exchange with FFP improves TTP, whereas prompt delivery improves HELLP.

SUMMARY

The balance between coagulation and clot lysis is crucial to maintaining homeostasis, responding to tissue insult and facilitating normal repair of vascular injury. It is predicated on appropriate activation of platelets (*primary hemostasis*) with adhesion, aggregation, and contraction of the initial platelet plug. The platelet plug then acts as a template for activation of circulating coagulation factors (*secondary hemostasis*), followed by the final phase, which consists of fibrin polymerizing on the platelet surface.

Excessive clot propagation is limited by AT-III, protein C (which depends on its cofactor, protein S), and thrombin. Fibrinolysis limits clot formation at normal endothelium and promotes clot remodeling and lysis as healing proceeds. The serine protease, plasmin, is formed when plasminogen, which is intercalated in the clot, is activated. This results in breakdown of cross-linked fibrin. Binding to α-2-antiplasmin rapidly clears plasmin.

Abnormal hemostasis and lysis is encountered regularly in medical and surgical ICU patients as either a primary or secondary process. This includes inadequate production of platelets, excessive sequestration of platelets, increased destruction of platelets, or severe dysfunction of platelets. Insufficient coagulation factor production is routinely present in patients with advanced liver disease, whereas vitamin K deficiency is a common occurrence in critically ill patietns. DIC is frequently identified in patients with significant inflammation or sepsis. This may result in a bleeding diathesis but more commonly is associated with microvascular thrombosis. The treatment of DIC remains controversial, but modulation of the coagulation cascade with activated protein C, tissue factor pathway inhibitor, and AT-III is under intense investigation.

A host of laboratory tests are available to assess the coagulation cascade. These tests, combined with careful history, physical examination, and appropriate consultation with a hematologist/transfusion specialist, allow for rapid intervention with appropriate blood products and drugs that modulate or enhance hemostasis or lysis.

KEY POINTS

Both surgical and medical patients who are critically ill are predisposed to developing coagulation disorders for a number of reasons, including preexisting disease, nutrition deficiencies, sepsis, and massive transfusion. Although the causes of coagulopathy in the intensive care population are diverse, a systematic approach that considers abnormalities of platelet number and function and abnormalities of the coagulation proteins should lead to the correct diagnosis. This approach requires an understanding of the laboratory methods used and the clinical signs and symptoms associated with abnormal platelet function, factor deficiencies, and microvascular thrombosis. Current therapies are mainly supportive, consisting of correcting the underlying disease process and repletion of deficiencies when ongoing hemorrhage is clinically significant.

REFERENCES

1. Kjeldsberg CR, Swanson J. Platelet satellitism. *Blood* 1974;43:831–836.
2. Peterson P, Hayes TE, Arkin CF, et al. The preoperative bleeding time test lacks clinical benefit. *Arch Surg* 1988;133:134–139.
3. Gewirtz AS, Miller ML, Keys TF. The clinical usefulness of the preoperative bleeding time. *Arch Pathol Lab Med* 1996;120:353–356.
4. Riley RS, Rowe D, Fisher LM. Clinical utilization of the international normalized ratio (INR). *J Clin Lab Anal* 2000;14:101–114.
5. Bussey HI, Force RW, Bianco TM, et al. Reliance on prothrombin time ratios causes significant errors in anticoagulation therapy. *Arch Intern Med* 1992;152:278–282.
6. Santoro SA. Laboratory evaluation of hemostatic disorders. In: Hoffman R, Banz EJ Jr, Shattil SJ, eds. *Hematology: basic principles and practice.* New York: Churchill Livingstone; 1991:1267.
7. Bick RL, Baker WF. Antiphospholipid syndrome and thrombosis. *Semin Thromb Hemost* 1999;25:333–350.
8. Caruso A, De Carolis S, Di Simone N. Antiphospholipid antibodies in obstetrics: new complexities and sites of action. *Hum Reprod Update* 1999;5:267–276.
9. Bick RL. Disseminated intravascular coagulation: objective criteria for diagnosis and management. *Med Clin North Am* 71994;8:511–543.
10. Parker RI, Farmer JC. Coagulation: essential physiologic concerns. In: Civetta JM, Taylor RW, Kirby RR, eds. *Critical care*, 2nd ed. Philadelphia: JB Lippincott, 1992:1705.
11. Cohen JA. Activated coagulation time method for control of heparin is reliable during cardiopulmonary bypass. *Anesthesiology* 1984:60:121–124.
12. Nuttall GA, Oliver WC, Ereth MH, et al. Coagulation tests predict bleeding after cardiopulmonary bypass. *J Cardiothorac Vasc Anesth* 1997;11:815–823.
13. Williams GD, Bratton SL, Riley EC, et al. Coagulation tests during cardiopulmonary bypass correlate with blood loss in children undergoing cardiac surgery. *J Cardiothorac Vasc Anesth* 1999;13:398–404.
14. Shore-Lesserson L, Manspeizer HE, DePerio M, et al. Thromboelastography-guided transfusion algorithm reduces transfusions in complex cardiac surgery. *Anesth Analg* 1999;88:312–319.
15. Kang YG, Martin D, Marquez J, et al. Intraoperative changes in blood coagulation and thromboelastographic monitoring in liver transplantation. *Anesth Analg* 1985;64:888–897.
16. Miller LG. Herbal medicinals: selected clinical considerations focusing on known or potential drug-herb interactions. *Arch Intern Med* 1998;158:2200–2211.
17. Eisenberg DM, Davis RB, Ettner SL, et al. Trends in alternative medicine use in the United States, 1990-1997: results of a follow-up national survey. *JAMA* 1998;280:1569–1575.
18. Schmaier AH. Disseminated intravascular coagulation: pathogenesis and management. *Intensive Care Med* 1991;6:209–228.
19. Fourrier F, Chopin C, Goudeman J, et al. Septic shock, multiple organ failure, and disseminated intravascular coagulation: compared

patterns of antithrombin III, protein C, and protein S deficiencies. *Chest* 1992;101:816–823.

20. Eisele B, Lamy M, Thijs LG, et al. Antithrombin III in patient with severe sepsis. *Intensive Care Med* 1998;24:663–672.

21. Balk R, Emerson T, Fourrier F, et al. Therapeutic use of antithrombin concentrate in sepsis. *Semin Thromb Hemost* 1998;24:183–194.

22. Spicer TE, Rau JM. Purpura fulminans. *Am J Med* 1976;61:566–571.

23. Feinstein DI. Treatment of disseminated intravascular coagulation. *Semin Thromb Hemost* 1988;14:351–362.

24. Oguma Y, Sakuragawa N, Maki M, et al. Clinical effect of low molecular weight heparin (Fragmin) on DIC: a multicenter cooperative study in Japan. *Thromb Res* 1990;59:37–49.

25. de Jonge E, Levi M, Stoutenbeek CP, et al. Current drug treatment strategies for disseminated intravascular coagulation. *Drugs* 1998;55:767–777.

26. Munoz MC, Montes R, Hermida J, et al. Effect of the administration of recombinant hirudin and/or tissue-plasminogen activator (t-PA) on endotoxin-induced disseminated intravascular coagulation model in rabbits. *Br J Haematol* 1999;105:117–121.

27. Pernerstorfer T, Hollenstein U, Hansen JB, et al. Lepirudin blunts endotoxin-induced coagulation activation. *Blood* 2000;95:1729–1734.

28. Gerson WT, Dickerman JD, Bovil EG, et al. Severe acquired protein C deficiency in purpura fulminans associated with disseminated intravascular coagulation: treatment with protein C concentrate. *Pediatrics* 1993;91:418–422.

29. Rintala E, Seppala O, Kotilainen P, et al. Protein C in the treatment of coagulopathy in meningococcal disease. *Lancet* 1996;347:1767.

30. Mammen EF. Coagulation defects in liver disease. *Med Clin North Am* 1994;78:545–554.

31. Porte RJ, Molenaar IQ, Begliomini B, et al. Aprotinin and transfusion requirements in orthotopic liver transplantation: a multicentre randomised double-blind study. *Lancet* 2000;355:1303–1309.

32. Boylan JF, Klinck JR, Sandler AN, et al. Tranexamic acid reduces blood loss, transfusion requirements, and coagulation factor use in primary orthotopic liver transplantation. *Anesthesiology* 1996;85:1043–1048.

33. Mochizuki T, Olson PJ, Szlam F, et al. Protamine reversal of heparin affects platelet aggregation and activated clotting time after cardiopulmonary bypass. *Anesth Analg* 1998;87:781–785.

34. Barstad RM, Stephens RW, Hamers MJ, et al. Protamine sulphate inhibits platelet membrane glycoprotein Ib-von Willebrand factor activity. *Thromb Haemost* 2000;83:334–337.

35. Munoz JJ, Birkmeyer NJ, Birkmeyer JD, et al. Is epsilon-aminocaproic acid as effective as aprotinin in reducing bleeding with cardiac surgery? a meta-analysis. *Circulation* 1999;99:81–89.

36. Davis R, Whittington R. Aprotinin: a review of its pharmacology and therapeutic efficacy in reducing blood loss associated with cardiac surgery. *Drugs* 1995;49:954–983.

37. Cosgrove DM 3d, Heric B, Lytle BW, et al. Aprotinin therapy for reoperative myocardial revascularization: a placebo-controlled study. *Ann Thorac Surg* 1992;54:1031–1038.

38. Murkin JM, Lux J, Shannon NA, et al. Aprotinin significantly decreases bleeding and transfusion requirements in patients receiving aspirin and undergoing cardiac operations. *J Thorac Cardiovasc Surg* 1994;107:554–561.

39. Segal H, Hunt BJ. Aprotinin: pharmacological reduction of perioperative bleeding. *Lancet* 2000;355:1289–1290.

40. Shigeta O, Kojima H, Jikuya T, et al. Aprotinin inhibits plasmin-induced platelet activation during cardiopulmonary bypass. *Circulation* 1997;96:569–574.

41. Wahba A, Black G, Koksch M, et al. Aprotinin has no effect on platelet activation and adhesion during cardiopulmonary bypass. *Thromb Haemost* 1996;75:844–848.

42. van Oeveren W, Eijsman L, Roozendaal KJ, et al. On the mechanism of platelet preservation during cardiopulmonary bypass by aprotinin. *Lancet* 1988;1:655.

43. Cohen DM, Norberto J, Cartabuke R, et al. Severe anaphylactic reaction after primary exposure to aprotinin. *Ann Thorac Surg* 1999;67:837–838.

44. Despotis GJ, Filos KS, Levine V, et al. Aprotinin prolongs activated and nonactivated whole blood clotting time and potentiates the effect of heparin *in vitro*. *Anesth Analg* 1996;82:1126–1131.

45. Wendel HP, Heller W, Gallimore MJ, et al. The prolonged activated clotting time (ACT) with aprotinin depends on the type of activator used for measurement. *Blood Coagul Fibrinolysis* 1993;4:41–55.

46. Dietrich W, Dilthey G, Spannagl M, et al. Influence of high-dose aprotinin on anticoagulation, heparin requirement, and celite- and kaolin-activated clotting time in heparin-pretreated patients undergoing open-heart surgery: a double-blind, placebo-controlled study. *Anesthesiology* 1995;83:679–689.

47. Alderman E, Levy JH, Rich JB, et al. Analyses of coronary graft patency after aprotinin use: results from the international multicenter aprotinin graft patency experience (image) trial. *J Thorac Cardiovasc Surg* 1998;116:716–727.

48. Pohlman TH, Carrico CJ. Evaluation of bleeding in the surgical patient. In: Civetta JM, Taylor RW, Kirby RR, eds. *Critical care*, 2nd ed. Philadelphia: JB Lippincott, 1992:637.

49. Hackmann T, Gascoyne RD, Naiman SC, et al. A trial of desmopressin (1-desamino-8-D-arginine vasopressin) to reduce blood loss in uncomplicated cardiac surgery. *N Engl J Med* 1989;321:1437–1443.

50. Dilthey G, Dietrich W, Spannagl M, et al. Influence of desmopressin acetate on homologous blood requirements in cardiac surgical patients pretreated with aspirin. *J Cardiothorac Vasc Anesth* 1993;7:425–430.

51. Dzik W. Massive transfusion. In: Churchill WH, Kaitz SR eds. *Transfusion medicine*. Boston: Blackwell Scientific, 1988:225.

52. Fabris F, Luzzatto G, Stefani PM, et al. Heparin-induced thrombocytopenia. *Haematologica* 2000;85:72–81.

53. Slaughter TF, Greenberg CS. Heparin-associated thrombocytopenia and thrombosis: Implications for perioperative management. *Anesthesiology* 1997;87:667–675.

54. Vun CM, Evans S, Chong BH. Cross-reactivity study of low molecular weight heparins and heparinoid in heparin-induced thrombocytopenia. *Thromb Res* 1996;81:525–532.

55. Adarmes CA, Windisch PA. *Technology report: anticoagulant options in heparin-induced thrombocytopenia*, 1st ed. Oak Brook, IL: University Health System Consortium, 1988:47–48.

56. Smith JP, Wall JT, Muscato MS, et al. Extra corporeal circulation in a patient with heparin-induced thromboyctopenia. *Anesthesiology* 1985;62:363–365.

57. Corbeau JJ, Jacob JP, Moreau X, et al. Iloprost (Ilomedine) and extracorporeal circulation with conventional heparinization in a patient with heparin-induced thrombocytopenia. *Ann Fr Anesth Reanim* 1993;12(1):55–59

58. Salmenpera MT, Levy JH. Pharmacologic manipulation of hemostasis-anticoagulation. In: Lake CL, Moore RA, eds. *Blood*, 1st ed. New York: Raven Press, 1995:105–117.

59. Latham P, Revelis AF, Joshi GP, et al. Use of recombinant hirudin in patients with heparin-induced thromboyctopenia with thrombosis requiring cardiopulmonary bypass. *Anesthesiology* 2000;92:263.

60. Koster A, Kuppe H, Hetzer R, et al. Emergent cardiopulmonary bypass in five patients with heparin-induced thrombocytopenia type II employing recombinant hirudin. *Anesthesiology* 1998;89:777–780.

61. Spiess BD, Gernsheimer T, Vocelka C, et al. Hematologic changes in a patient with heparin-induced thrombocytopenia who underwent cardiopulmonary bypass after ancrod defibrinogenation. *J Cardiothorac Vasc Anesth* 1996;10:918–921.

62. The American Society of Hematology ITP Practice Guideline Panel. Diagnosis and treatment of idiopathic thrombocytopenic purpura: recommendations of the American Society of Hematology. *Ann Intern Med* 1997;126:319–326.

63. Moake JL. Thrombotic thrombocytopenic purpura and the hemolytic uremic syndrome. In: Hoffman R, Benz EJ, Shattil SJ, et al. *Hematology: basic principles and practice*, 2nd ed. New York: Churchill Livingstone, 1995;1881.

TRANSFUSION MEDICINE FOR THE INTENSIVIST

EDUARDO N. CHINI
NIKI M. DIETZ
RONALD J. FAUST

KEY WORDS

- Autologous transfusion
- Blood substitutes
- Fresh frozen plasma
- Ischemic optic neuropathy
- Massive transfusion; complications: coagulopathy, metabolic
- Platelets
- Red blood cells
- Transfusion: reaction, risk, routine
- Transfusion-related acute lung injury

INTRODUCTION

The American National Red Cross refers to blood donation as the "gift of life." The acquired immunodeficiency syndrome (AIDS) epidemic, however, significantly changed the public's and heath care professionals' perception of blood transfusion (1,2). In the last two decades, the safety and indications for blood component transfusion have been a topic of intense debate. Among the issues that have been reevaluated are thresholds for transfusion at which benefits outweigh risks (1,2). The American Society of Anesthesiologists (ASA) and other groups have attempted to define guidelines for perioperative blood component use (2). As the clinical indications for the use of blood components become better clarified, not only will risks to patients be reduced, but also significant monetary savings could be accrued. These considerations are of major importance to the intensivist because both anemia and blood component transfusion are common in the management of critically ill patients admitted to the intensive care unit (ICU).

TRANSFUSION RISKS

Adverse reactions during blood-component therapy are multiple (Table 1) and occur in about 1% to 3% of transfusions. The most common are nonhemolytic febrile reactions, which do not present a major risk to the patient's well-being. Transmission of blood-borne pathogens and hemolytic transfusion reactions are the most severe complications of blood component therapy (1). Current practice in transfusion medicine has been very effective in reducing the risks of blood transfusion. Indeed, as of the year 2000, the blood supply in the United States is safer than ever, and the risk of dying from a blood-component transfusion is very remote (1,3,4). As with any other therapy, however, complications of blood-component transfusion must be considered when evaluating the risk-to-benefit ratio of treatment with blood products.

Risk of Transmission of Infectious Diseases

Advances in donor education, selection, and screening and the introduction of new laboratory tests had a major impact on the risk of blood transfusion (3–5). At present, the risk of transfusion-transmitted viral infections is extremely low (Table 2) (1,3,5).

The AIDS epidemic significantly transformed transfusion practice in the 1980s. Almost 30,000 patients were transfused with human immunodeficiency virus (HIV)-positive blood before screening for the virus became available in 1985 (6). After implementation of HIV-antibody testing in March 1985, only a few cases of transfusion-related HIV infections per year were reported to the Centers for Disease Control and Prevention (CDC). Recently, using mathematical models, the overall risk of transfusion-transmitted AIDS was estimated to be 1 in 200,000 to 1 in 2,000,000 (Table 2). Most transfusion-related HIV infections appear to occur during the so-called window period (1,4), that is, the time between infection and seroconversion, now estimated to be between 18 to 25 days (1,4). This window period and the risk of HIV-transmission are expected to decrease even further as a result of implementation of DNA-based polymerase-chain-reaction assay for detection of HIV in blood donors (4,5).

Transfusion-related non-A, non-B hepatitis occurred in about 7% to 12% of all blood transfusions (7,8) until hepatitis C virus (HCV) was identified in 1989 and laboratory testing for the detection of this virus was implemented in 1990 (7–10). The estimated risk of HCV transmission by blood-component transfusion is now believed to be 1 in 30,000 to 150,000 U transfused (9,10). Indeed, although blood transfusion accounted for

TABLE 1. TRANSFUSION RISKS

Infectious
  Viruses
    CMV
    Hepatitis A, B, C, Delta
    HIV, type 1 and type 2
    HTLV-I and -II
    Epstein–Barr virus
  Bacteria
    Staphylococcus spp
    Yersinia enterocolitica
    Pseudomonas spp
    Enterobacter spp
    Klebsiella spp
    Bacillus spp
    Coagulase-negative staphylococci
    Salmonella spp
    Escherichia coli
    Serratia marcescens
  Spirochetes
    Syphilis
    Lyme disease
  Parasites
    Malaria
    Chagas disease
    Toxoplasmosis
    Babesiosis
    Filariasis
    Kala-azar
    Trypanosomiasis
    Visceral leishmaniasis
  Prion disease
Immune-mediated transfusion reactions
    Mild allergic
    Anaphylactic
    Febrile, nonhemolytic (FNHTR)
    Hemolytic
      Acute
      Delayed
  Transfusion-related acute lung injury (TRALI)
  Posttransfusion purpura
Controversial immunosuppressive risks
  Increased spread of malignancy
  Decreased resistance to infection

CMV, cytomegalovirus; HIV, human immunodeficiency virus; HTLV, human T-cell lymphotrophic virus.

a substantial number of HCV infections in the past, now it is a rare cause of infection (8–10). However, because about 80% of HCV-infected patients will develop chronic hepatitis, 20% will have cirrhosis of the liver, and in about 5% the HCV infection will lead to development of hepatocellular carcinoma (8–10).

The introduction of hepatitis B virus (HBV) surface antigen screening markedly reduced the risk of transfusion-transmitted HBV (Table 2), and now hepatitis B accounts for fewer than 10% of all cases of posttransfusion hepatitis (11). The risk of hepatitis A (HAV) transmission through blood components is very remote because there is no carrier state for this virus (Table 2) (1,11).

Human T-lymphotrophic viruses I and II (HTLV-I/II) are retroviruses associated with development of adult T-cell leukemia (ATL) and a form of myelopathy (1,11). Although HTLV can be transmitted by blood transfusion in up to 50% of recipients of infectious donor blood, only one case of transfusion-transmitted

ATL has been reported to date (1,11). Since 1989, however, it has been routine to test donated blood for HTLV (1,11).

Cytomegalovirus (CMV) is a herpes virus very common in the general population. CMV can be transmitted by transfusion (11). Posttransfusion CMV infection is asymptomatic in most recipients. In fact, in the United States, donated blood is not routinely screened for CMV (11), although susceptible patients (including neonates who weigh less than 1,200 g and immunodepressed recipients of bone marrow transplantation) can develop an often fatal CMV infection (11). Blood donor leukocytes appear to be the reservoir of infectious CMV. To prevent transfusion-related CMV infection in susceptible recipients, leukocyte-depleted blood components or screened CMV negative units can be used (11).

Recent experimental studies raised the possibility of transmission of prion diseases, such as Creutzfeldt–Jakob disease (CJD), through blood transfusion (12). It is impossible, however, to prove whether or not blood transfusion in humans can indeed transmit CJD (12). Additionally, the U.S. Food and Drug Administration (FDA) developed guidelines to decrease the rather theoretical risk of transfusion-transmitted CJD (5,12). These include indefinite deferral of donors that have relatives with CJD and donors that spent at least 6 months in the United Kingdom from 1980 to 1996 (5).

Septic reactions associated with transfusion were greatly reduced when plastic closed blood-collection systems were introduced in the 1960s. Although rare, transfusion-related sepsis continues to occur (Table 2). The highest risk of bacterial growth is found in platelet concentrates because these concentrates are stored at room temperature (Table 2). In fact, because the risk of bacterial contamination increases with storage time, platelet concentrate shelf life is limited to 5 days (1,11). The clinical presentation of transfusion-related sepsis is variable, ranging from mild fever, to acute septic shock, to death in about 25% of patients (1). The pathogens involved in transfusion-associated sepsis are frequently the same as those implicated in catheter-related sepsis (1,11), including *Staphylococcus aureus, Klebsiella pneumonia,* and *Staphylococcus epidermidis* (1,11). Red blood cells (RBCs) also can produce transfusion-related sepsis (Table 2). *Yersinia enterocolitica,* an organism that grows best under refrigeration in an iron-rich medium, has been implicated often in the development of sepsis caused by transfusion of RBCs (1,11). Recipients of *Yersinia*-infected RBCs have a 50% mortality rate (1,11). In any patient who spikes a high fever or shows signs of sepsis after undergoing a transfusion, the possibility of contaminated blood components has to be investigated, and empirical antibiotic therapy should be considered (1,11).

As described in Table 1, several other viruses, bacteria, and parasites not covered in the preceding discussion can be transmitted by blood transfusion. At present, however, the risk of transmission of infectious diseases through transfusion is very low (1,3,5). Patients should be reassured that the risk of undertransfusion might be higher than the risk of acquiring a transfusion-related infection; nevertheless, it is possible to anticipate the development of new variants of retroviruses, protozoa, and other infectious agents that may not be detected by current screening methods. In this regard, clinicians must weigh the risks and benefits of blood-component transfusion before ordering this therapy.

TABLE 2. RISKS OF BLOOD TRANSFUSION

Viral Infection	Risk Per Unit Transfused	Window Period (d)
Hepatitis A	1/1,000,000	—
Hepatitis B	1/30,000–1/250,000	59
Hepatitis C	1/30,000–1/150,000	82
HIV	1/200,000–1/2,000,000	22
HTLV	1/250,000–1/2,000,000	51
Bacterial contamination		
RBCs	1/500,000	
Platelets	1/12,000	
Acute hemolytic reactions	1/1,000,000	
Delayed hemolytic reaction	1/1,000	
Transfusion-related acute lung injury	1/5,000	

HIV, human immunodeficiency virus; HTLV, human T-cell lymphotrophic virus; RBCs, red blood cells.
Modified from Goodnough LT, Brecher ME, Kanter MH, et al. Transfusion medicine (first of two parts): blood transfusion. *N Engl J Med* 1999;340:438–447, with permission.

Allergic and Febrile Reactions

Mild allergic and febrile reactions are the most common transfusion-related complications. Allergic reactions usually manifest as an urticarial rash and occur in about 1% to 4% of transfused patients. Not technically part of the symptoms of a hemolytic reaction, a mild rash should not prevent completion of transfusion unless a patient presents with associated signs of anaphylaxis. When present, pruritus can be treated symptomatically with diphenhydramine hydrochloride (11).

Febrile nonhemolytic transfusion reaction (FNHTR) occurs in about 0.5% to 1% of blood recipients (11). FNHTR may be mediated by leukoagglutinins in the recipient and by cytokines present in stored blood products (11). FNHTRs are usually self-limited, but because fever can be a sign of hemolytic reaction or sepsis, blood transfusion should be interrupted when the patient develops fever. On notification, the blood bank will assist in confirming the presence or absence of a hemolytic or septic reaction (Table 3). The shift to leukocyte-reduced blood components is expected to reduce further the incidence of FNHTR (11).

Hemolytic Transfusion Reaction

Although rare, acute hemolytic transfusion reaction (HTR) still is the most frequent noninfectious cause of transfusion-associated fatalities, occurring in 1 of 250,000 to 1 of 1,000,000 transfusions (Table 2) (1,13). Most of these reactions are caused by ABO-incompatible blood transfused to the wrong patient through misidentification. The risk may be higher in the operating room and in the ICU because unconscious patients cannot identify themselves before transfusion. In fact, ICU patients rely totally on the personnel caring for them to adhere scrupulously to identification practices.

Shock, disseminated intravascular coagulation (DIC), and acute renal failure are the three major pathophysiologic sequelae of acute HTR (14). This reaction is mediated by many substances, including complement, interleukins, and cytokines, such as tumor necrosis factor (TNF) (14). Indeed, this pathophysiologic process bears many similarities to sepsis syndrome (14). The clinical severity of HTR is proportional to the volume of incompatible blood infused; thus, transfusion must be stopped as soon as HTR is suspected (11). Signs and symptoms include fever, chills, chest and lumbar pain, nausea, hypotension, tachycardia, hemoglobinuria, and coagulopathy (11). Several laboratory tests are helpful in diagnosing HTR, including free serum and urinary hemoglobin, serum haptoglobulin, positive direct antiglobulin test, and elevated bilirubin (11). Aggressive fluid therapy and monitoring of the cardiovascular and coagulation systems in the intensive care setting are recommended (11). The institution of large-bore venous accesses and pulmonary artery (PA) catheterization permits aggressive monitoring of volume status and fluid replacement to treat shock and renal vascular ischemia. The use of "renal" dose dopamine is recommended by some authorities to

TABLE 3. EVALUATION OF TRANSFUSION REACTIONS

Mild allergic
  Monitor for any signs of anaphylaxis

Febrile
  Stop the transfusion
  Rule out acute hemolysis, transfusion-associated sepsis

Hemolytic transfusion reaction
  Stop the transfusion
  Investigate for clerical error
  Coombs test
  Serum haptoglobin
  Institute large-bore venous access and hemodynamic monitoring
  Monitor patient for coagulopathy
  Treat respiratory failure as indicated

Transfusion-associated sepsis
  Stop the transfusion
  Culture patient's blood
  Culture suspected unit or satellite samples

Transfusion-related acute lung injury
  Supportive therapy for recipient
  Chest x-ray
  Evaluate for fluid overload
  Review gender of donors of all components transfused within 6 h
  Evaluate female donors for leukoagglutinins and
    anti-HLA antibodies

Anaphylaxis
  Stop all components
  Treat hemodynamics appropriately
  Evaluate for anti-IgA antibody

HLA, human leukocyte antigen; IgA, immunoglobulin A.

improve renal blood flow even in normotensive patients. Use of the diuretic furosemide is also indicated. Although controversial, heparin anticoagulation may be used for the treatment of DIC in the setting of HTR.

Anaphylactic Reaction

Some patients can develop acute severe anaphylaxis in response to transfusion of blood products (11). Some of those patients are IgA deficient and produce anti-IgA antibodies that can react with IgA antibodies present in donor RBCs, platelets, and plasma. In IgA-deficient recipients, anaphylactic reactions can be prevented by using RBCs or platelets washed to remove IgA and by using plasma components from immunoglobulin A (IgA)-deficient blood donors (11).

Transfusion-related Acute Lung Injury

Transfusion-related acute lung injury (TRALI) is an acute severe respiratory distress syndrome with an incidence estimated to be 1 in 5,000 transfusions (Table 2) (15). TRALI is characterized by development of noncardiogenic pulmonary edema 2 to 4 hours after blood transfusion (15).

Donor leukoagglutinins and donor antibodies to human leukocyte antigens (HLA), which react with recipient leukocytes and monocytes, are hypothesized to cause this reaction. This reaction results in complement activation, which in turn leads to neutrophil aggregation and increased permeability of the pulmonary microcirculation (15). Multiparous female donors most often carry these leukoagglutinins. To establish the diagnosis, suspected donors must be contacted and the presence of these antibodies evaluated (15). Recently, lipid products, generated during blood storage, also were implicated in the pathogenesis of TRALI (16).

Intensivists should be well aware of this life-threatening reaction. In one review, acute pulmonary edema was listed as the second most common cause of noninfectious transfusion-related death (15). Volume overload is the most frequent cause of pulmonary edema after blood transfusion; however, the development of respiratory distress should raise the possibility of TRALI reaction. Indeed, if a PA catheter is in place and the PA pressure and the occlusion pressure (PAOP) are found to be normal, the diagnosis of TRALI is likely. The usual clinical presentation of TRALI includes hypoxemia, bronchospasm, and acute respiratory distress. The chest radiograph usually shows bilateral pulmonary infiltrates. Therapy is supportive, including supplemental oxygen, endotracheal intubation, mechanical ventilation, and positive end-expiratory pressure (PEEP) as indicated (Table 3). TRALI reaction usually resolves in 24 to 48 hours, and at least 90% of the patients experience a complete recovery (15).

Immunomodulation

Blood transfusion has been shown to cause immunosuppression (17). Immunomodulation appears to be mediated by exposure of recipient to donor leukocytes; however, the clinical significance of this immunosuppression is the subject of great debate (17). Indeed, several studies attempted to determine the correlation between allogeneic blood transfusion and the recurrence

TABLE 4. ADVANTAGES AND DISADVANTAGES OF PREOPERATIVE AUTOLOGOUS BLOOD DONATION

Advantages
  Decrease infectious risks
  Decrease risks of clerical error
  Avoid alloimmunization
  Avoid other types of reactions and immunomodulation
Disadvantages
  Increase expenses
  Waste of units that are not transfused
  Risk of volume overload
  Infection and administration errors not totally eliminated
  Increase preoperative anemia

of cancer and the susceptibility to infection (17). These studies generated conflicting data. Although available evidence raises the possibility that allogeneic blood transfusion may increase the risk of perioperative infections and recurrence of cancer, no definitive conclusion can be drawn at present (17).

AUTOLOGOUS TRANSFUSION

Autologous blood has been considered the safest blood available, and autotransfusion is the most effective way to avoid the risks associated with allogeneic blood transfusion (18–20). Although it is safe, autologous blood transfusion is not risk free. Indeed, in one study, the likelihood that 1 U of autologous blood would be transfused to the wrong patient was estimated to be 1 in 30,000 to 50,000 U (18). Table 4 summarizes the advantages and disadvantages of autologous blood compared with allogeneic blood transfusion (20,21). The four types of autologous blood donation include preoperative donation, acute normovolemic hemodilution (ANH), intraoperative salvage, and postoperative salvage (20,21).

Preoperative Autologous Blood Donation

Although preoperative donation is the simplest form of autologous transfusion and requires the least equipment, studies in the late 1980s found it to be far underused; up to 97% of patients scheduled for some orthopedic procedures could avoid allogenic blood transfusion through predeposited autologous blood (18). Some studies, however, suggested that autologous blood donation increases the risk of postoperative anemia and the likelihood of overall transfusion (20). Furthermore, the cost of autologous blood donation is greater then that of allogeneic blood (20), and it does not fit within the usual range of medical procedures thought to be cost-effective when risk-to-benefit ratios are analyzed (20). It is possible that the cost-effectiveness of preoperative autologous blood donation could be improved by the development of algorithms to determine which patients would benefit the most from it.

Nuttal and colleagues, in a retrospective analysis of 165 patients undergoing primary total hip arthroplasty (THA), determined clinical predictors for preoperative autologous blood donation and proposed guidelines to increase its cost-effectiveness

(22). These researchers proposed that male patients with hemoglobin of less than 14.7 would benefit from autologous donation (22). Similar guidelines could be used to select which patients benefit the most from autologous blood donation and could be extended to other types of surgeries if specific transfusion patterns are analyzed.

Acute Normovolemic Hemodilution

Acute normovolemic hemodilution involves removal of a patient's whole blood and replacement with large volumes of crystalloid or colloid solutions at the start of surgery. After anesthetic induction, blood is withdrawn from an arterial or a large central venous cannula. Collected blood is stored at room temperature in the operating room. The patient then is reinfused with his or her own blood when necessary. This has been recommended for patients in whom the surgical blood loss is expected to exceed 20% of the intravascular volume, and preoperative hemoglobin is more than 10 g per deciliter (23). ANH should not be performed in patients with severe cardiac disease (23).

Acute normovolemic hemodilution lowers the patient's hemoglobin at the start of surgery so that fewer RBCs are lost intraoperatively. In addition, one of the advantages of ANH is the provision of fresh autologous blood containing platelets and coagulation factors for reinfusion. Also, because collected blood remains in the operating room, the possibility of clerical error in patient identification and the risk of ABO incompatibility are decreased. Few randomized studies actually show that this technique reduces the need for allogeneic blood transfusion (20). Because of the necessary crystalloid and colloid replacement, ANH exaggerates intraoperative fluid shifts when blood loss is small. When intraoperative blood loss is high, the limited number of units provided by ANH is inadequate to prevent transfusion of allogeneic blood.

Intraoperative Blood Salvage

This technique is widely used in cardiovascular and orthopedic surgeries and in other types of operations where moderate or high blood loss is expected. Intraoperative salvage is the only type of autologous transfusion that might allow avoidance of allogeneic blood in emergency surgery and when blood loss is high (20). A recent meta-analysis of 27 randomized clinical trials concluded that cell salvage decreases the rate of perioperative allogeneic blood transfusion in orthopedic surgery (24). Although expensive equipment is used to wash surgical debris and anticoagulant from blood salvaged in a continuous-flow centrifuge, this technique is thought to be cost-effective if 2 or more units of RBCs are collected (7).

The effects of intraoperative blood salvage on coagulation have been well studied. An early salvage device was thought to cause disseminated intravascular coagulation (DIC). Cell washing should prevent this complication by removing fibrin-degradation products collected from the wound and produced by the salvage device itself. Anticoagulant used in the collection process is also a concern. Heparin (30,000 U/L) or 3.9% trisodium citrate solutions are mixed with blood as it is collected from the wound. Virtually all anticoagulant is removed during the washing process. Although washing systems provide a cellular product that is free of anticoagulants, they also wash out soluble coagulation factors and platelets. Thus, intraoperative blood salvage provides a product that is deficient in platelets and coagulation factors.

As with other strategies of autologous blood donation, intraoperative blood salvage appears to be very safe, but it is not risk free. For instance, four deaths related to air embolism during intraoperative blood salvage were reported to the New York Department of Health from 1990 to 1995 (25). Furthermore, cell-washing devices do not effectively remove bacteria. Autologous units frequently yield positive cultures, with skin contaminants the most frequently identified organisms. Intraoperative cell salvage is generally considered contraindicated in cases where there is pus or spillage of bowel contents.

Although malignancy is also considered a contraindication to the use of intraoperative blood salvage, one group used this technique during radical cystectomy for carcinoma of the bladder and found no increase in cancer recurrence (26).

Postoperative Salvage

In certain types of surgeries, such as total knee replacement and cardiac operations, significant blood loss is experienced postoperatively. Postoperative blood salvage involves collection of blood from surgical drains for autologous transfusion. As with other forms of autologous transfusion, cost-effectiveness and whether this technique actually reduces the need for allogeneic blood are somewhat controversial (27). In one report, the amount of blood collected postoperatively represented only 8.7% and 16.8% of perioperative blood loss for patients undergoing hip and knee arthroplasty, respectively (27); only 3 of 31 patients lost the equivalent of 1 U of RBCs postoperatively (27). Development of criteria to determine which patients will benefit from postoperative blood salvage is needed. In fact, selection of postoperative salvage in surgeries in which large postoperative blood loss is anticipated could improve efficacy. Blood loss is often difficult to predict, however.

RED BLOOD CELLS

Colloquially referred to as "packed cells" (to distinguish them from the component–whole blood), the component RBCs are prepared from 450 mL of donor blood collected into citrate phosphate dextrose adenine (CPDA-1) anticoagulant. When Adsol is used, 100 mL of an additive solution containing adenine, saline, and mannitol are added to the cells collected in CPDA-type solution. Adsol prolongs the shelf life of RBCs to 42 days and decreases viscosity, yielding a product with a hematocrit level of approximately 55%. Blood stored by freezing is referred to as RBCs *deglycerolized*. Glycerol (20%–40%) is used to prevent cell damage during the freezing process. Cells must be washed after thawing to remove glycerol; deglycerolized RBCs outdate within 24 hours. Washed RBCs also can be prepared from unfrozen blood to remove granulocytes, leukoagglutinins, and proteins, which may cause reactions in some recipients. For patients with a history of previous FNHTR, leukocyte-reduced RBCs can be prepared more efficiently by filtration through leukocyte-depletion filters.

TABLE 5. ASA RECOMMENDATIONS FOR RBCs

1. Transfusion is rarely indicated when the hemoglobin concentration is greater than 10 g/dL and is almost always indicated when it is less than 6 g/dL.
2. Whether intermediate hemoglobin concentrations (6–10 g/dL) justify or require RBC transfusion should be based on the patient's risk.
3. The use of a single hemoglobin "trigger" for all patients is not recommended.
4. Perioperative autologous transfusion and measures to decrease blood loss should be employed where appropriate.
5. The indications for autologous RBCs may be more liberal than for allogeneic RBCs.

ASA, American Society of Anesthesiologists; RBCs, red blood cells.

Guidelines for RBC Transfusion

Although it is simple to say that the indication for RBC transfusion is to enhance oxygen-carrying capacity, the decision as to which patients need improved oxygen-carrying capacity is usually complex (28). Substantial rates of unnecessary transfusion have been documented, and a number of groups have prepared guidelines to assist clinicians in making decisions on when or when not to transfuse RBCs (Table 5) (1,2). Figure 1 illustrates how medical conditions affect the ideal hemoglobin levels for a given patient; determination of patient risk factors requires good medical judgment.

Transfusion of RBCs is crucial in the treatment of trauma and major blood losses. In less extreme situations, however, the efficacy of allogeneic RBC transfusion has been challenged (21,29,30). Indeed, a limited capacity of allogeneic RBCs older than 7 days to increase oxygen carrying capacity has been described in animal models (29,30). Recently, determination of ideal hemoglobin level in critically ill patients and transfusion triggers have been a subject of intense debate (31,32).

Few randomized, controlled studies of transfusion "threshold" are available. In fact, it is not known at which level of hemoglobin critically ill patients may benefit from transfusion. Hebert and colleagues reported the first prospective, randomized, controlled clinical trial of transfusion requirements in critically ill patients. They evaluated at what hemoglobin level patients would benefit from RBC transfusion in a large number of patients (32) by comparing outcomes of 838 critically ill patients empirically maintained at two different levels of normovolemic anemia. Patients were randomly assigned to one of two groups. The first was a restrictive transfusion strategy group in which RBCs were transfused if the hemoglobin concentration dropped below 7.0 g per deciliter, and the hemoglobin concentrations were maintained between 7.0 to 9.0 g per deciliter. The other patients were assigned to a liberal strategy group, in which transfusion was triggered when the hemoglobin concentration was below 10.0 g per deciliter, and the hemoglobin level was maintained at 10.0 to 12.0 g per deciliter. The 30-day mortality rate was similar in the two groups (32). The mortality rates were significantly lower, however, with the restrictive transfusion strategy among a subgroup of patients who were younger and less ill (32). Furthermore, maintaining the hemoglobin levels between 7.0 and 9.0 also decreased the average number of RBCs transfused by 54% and decreased the exposure to any RBC transfusion by 33% (32). These results indicate that a transfusion threshold as low as 7.0 g per deciliter of hemoglobin is as safe as, or safer than, the traditional 10.0 g per deciliter threshold in critically ill patients. Furthermore, the diversity of patient population included in this study indicates that this conclusion may be generalized to most critically ill patients, with the possible exception of patients with acute "ongoing" bleeding or active coronary ischemic disease. Indeed, some recent studies support this conclusion (33,34).

In 1995, Vichinsky and associates reported a comparison of conservative and aggressive transfusion regimens in the

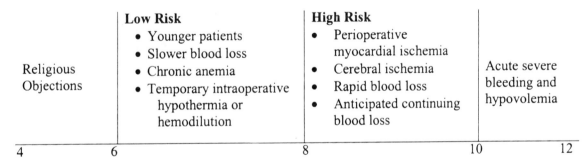

| Religious Objections | **Low Risk**
• Younger patients
• Slower blood loss
• Chronic anemia
• Temporary intraoperative hypothermia or hemodilution | **High Risk**
• Perioperative myocardial ischemia
• Cerebral ischemia
• Rapid blood loss
• Anticipated continuing blood loss | Acute severe bleeding and hypovolemia |

4   6   8   10   12

Target Hemoglobin Concentration (g/dL)

FIGURE 1. Factors that affect the clinical judgment to transfuse red blood cells (RBCs) perioperatively are depicted along a baseline showing a range of target hemoglobin concentrations. For patients with hemoglobin levels below 6 g per deciliter, a lack of patient consent, usually based on religious objections, is the only reason not to transfuse. Hemoglobin levels can be allowed to drop to anemic levels ranging between 6 and 8 g per deciliter in low-risk patients if these patients have good cardiovascular reserves or if their anemia is chronic. Hemoglobin levels of high-risk patients are permitted to drop to 6 to 8 g per deciliter temporarily if hypothermia or hemodilution is being used and when blood loss is slower. Patients with higher risk are usually transfused to attain hemoglobin concentrations between 8 and 10 g per deciliter, closer to 10 when the risk is highest. Coronary artery and cerebrovascular disease are the factors that most frequently affect the decision to maintain a higher hemoglobin level, but rapid blood loss and anticipated continuing postoperative blood loss also often necessitate attempts to maintain a hemoglobin of 10 g per deciliter in a bleeding patient. When hypovolemia is suspected in a rapidly bleeding patient, transfusion is indicated even when the hemoglobin is between 10 and 12 g per deciliter. Anemia must be corrected very slowly in normovolemic and hypervolemic patients to avoid congestive heart failure.

perioperative management of sickle cell disease (33). Patients undergoing 604 surgeries were randomized to receive either an aggressive transfusion regimen (exchange transfused to decrease hemoglobin S to <30%) or a conservative regimen (transfused only to maintain the hemoglobin level of about 10 g/dL). These investigators observed that the conservative transfusion regimen was as effective as the aggressive regimen in preventing perioperative complications in patients with sickle cell disease. Furthermore, the conservative approach decreased significantly the incidence of transfusion-associated complications (33).

More recently, Spiess and co-workers reported a multiinstitutional observational study of the effect of hematocrit value after coronary artery bypass graft surgery (CABG) (34). They evaluated the role of hematocrit value on ICU entry on the frequency of Q-wave myocardial infarction (MI) (34). In this study, 2,202 patients undergoing CABG were categorized into three groups according to the hematocrit value on entry into the ICU: high (≥34%), medium (between 33% and 25%) and low (≤24%). Outcomes were compared, and the role of hematocrit on the risk of Q-wave MI was determined. Surprisingly, these researchers found that the higher hematocrit group was associated with an increased rate of MI and death (34). Most would consider patients with a hematocrit of 34% to be overtransfused. These researchers concluded that high hematocrit was deleterious to post-CABG patients because of increased blood viscosity and shear forces between blood and vessels and disturbance in other biochemical mechanisms, including production of free radicals (33).

In conclusion, a hemoglobin level between 7 and 8 g per deciliter seems an appropriate threshold for transfusion in the ICU and the perioperative period (Table 5). In patients at increased risk of myocardial ischemia, however, the threshold may be modified; in these patients, a threshold of 10.0 g per deciliter is commonly used (2). In contrast, prophylactic transfusion of blood is not recommended (2). Furthermore, the use of blood components as volume replacement is strongly discouraged (except in actively bleeding patients), because recent studies indicate that overuse of transfusion may be associated with less favorable outcome (32–34).

FRESH FROZEN PLASMA AND CRYOPRECIPITATE

Fresh frozen plasma (FFP) is prepared by centrifugation and freezing within 8 hours of collection of whole blood from a single donor. It contains all soluble coagulation factors. Because FFP is not heat treated, however, it presents the same infectious risk as do RBCs, whole blood, and platelet concentrates. Few, if any, controlled studies show that FFP improves clinical outcome. There is also a paucity of data as to which patients might benefit from receiving FFP. Therefore, it is likely that a significant portion of the two million units of FFP transfused each year is used inappropriately (2). Several groups have attempted to write guidelines for the use of FFP (Table 6) (2).

Most groups approve the use of FFP for urgent reversal of warfarin therapy because it replaces vitamin-K-dependent coagulation factors more quickly than administration of vitamin K;

TABLE 6. ASA RECOMMENDATIONS FOR FRESH-FROZEN PLASMA

Indications
1. Urgent reversal of warfarin therapy.
2. Correction of known coagulation factor deficiencies for which specific concentrates are unavailable.
3. Correction of microvascular bleeding in the presence of elevated (>1.5 times normal) PT or PTT.
4. Correction of microvascular bleeding secondary to coagulation factor deficiency in massively transfused patients.

Contraindication
FFP is contraindicated for augmentation of plasma volume or albumin concentration

Dose
FFP should be given in doses of 10–15 mL/kg of FFP, except for urgent reversal of warfarin anticoagulation, for which 5–8 mL/kg of FFP usually suffices.

ASA, American Society of Anesthesiologists; FFP, fresh frozen plasma; PT, prothrombin time; PTT, partial thromboplastin time.

5 to 8 mL per kilogram of FFP have been recommended for this indication (2). Other indications include the correction of known coagulation factor deficiencies for which specific concentrates are not available, and the correction of microvascular bleeding in a massively transfused (>1 blood volume) patient with documented coagulopathy by coagulation tests (2). When necessary, large amounts of FFP probably should be used to achieve a minimum of 30% of coagulation factor concentration, which usually requires at least 10 to 15 mL of FFP per kilogram of body weight (2). FFP also can be used in heparin-resistant patients as a source of antithrombin III (AT-III). Because of the associated infectious risks and costs, FFP clearly is not indicated as a volume expander, to promote wound healing, or as a treatment for patients with low serum albumin.

Cryoprecipitate, which contains factor VIII, fibrinogen, fibronectin, and von Willebrand factor, is produced by cold precipitation of the insoluble portion of FFP, which has been thawed at temperatures between 1°C to 6°C. This cold precipitate is isolated and immediately refrozen and can be stored up to 1 year at −18°C. Once thawed for use, cryoprecipitate has a short shelf life of about 6 hours. The major perioperative indication for cryoprecipitate is correction of microvascular bleeding in the setting of a massively transfused patient thought to have fibrinogen deficiency (Table 7). Cryoprecipitate also is indicated in the treatment of von Willebrand factor deficiency (as occurs

TABLE 7. ASA RECOMMENDATIONS FOR CRYOPRECIPITATE

Indications
1. Prophylaxis in nonbleeding perioperative or peripartum patients with congenital fibrinogen deficiencies or von Willebrand disease unresponsive to DDAVP.
2. Bleeding patients with von Willebrand disease and patients with suspected consumptive coagulopathy whose fibrinogen concentration is less than 80–100 mg/dL.
3. Correction of microvascular bleeding in massively transfused patients thought to have fibrinogen deficiency.

ASA, American Society of Anesthesiologists; DDAVP, desmopressin.

in von Willebrand disease) when the patient is unresponsive to desmopressin (DDAVP) (Table 7).

PLATELET CONCENTRATES

Platelet concentrates are produced from platelet-rich plasma obtained by centrifugation of whole blood just after collection. Each unit of platelet concentrate comes from a single donor and contains approximately 5.5×10^{10} platelets in about 50 mL of plasma. One unit of platelets should increase the average adult platelet count by approximately 10×10^9 per liter. By pooling 6 U or more for transfusion, individual donor variation is overcome, and a clinically significant increase in platelet count can be achieved. On the other hand, pooling of different donors' platelets increases the risk of infectious disease transmission, alloimmunization, and platelet refractoriness. Thus, although platelets share the same adverse reactions as RBCs and FFP, the risk is multiplied when multiple-donor units are combined.

Platelets also can be produced by plateletpheresis. Apheresis platelets are obtained from a single donor to produce the equivalent of multiple units of platelet concentrates. A semicontinuous-flow centrifuge is used to return RBCs to the donor after separation of plasma and platelets. More than 3×10^{11} platelets can be collected from a single donor. Donor-recipient matched apheresis platelets are especially helpful in the treatment of refractory patients.

One of the major problems with platelet transfusion is the development of refractoriness. In such patients, platelet concentrate transfusion will not produce the expected increase in platelet count. Many immune and nonimmune factors can cause platelet transfusion refractoriness. Multiply transfused patients often become refractory to platelet transfusion due to the development of human leukocyte antigen (HLA) antibodies. HLA alloimmunization appears to be mediated by leukocytes contained in transfused blood products. Indeed, in a large prospective randomized trial, the use of leukocyte-depleted RBCs and platelet concentrates reduced the incidence of HLA alloimmunization and platelet refractoriness in acute leukemia patients (35–36). Furthermore, when HLA-alloimmunized patients are refractory to platelets, HLA-matched apheresis platelets are required.

More than seven million units of platelet concentrate are transfused each year in the United States. Many are used to protect oncologic patients from the risk of extreme thrombocytopenia induced by chemotherapy. In this setting, guidelines use platelet counts as low as 5×10^9 per liter as triggers for prophylactic transfusion in patients who are not actively bleeding. On the other hand, prophylactic platelet transfusion is not indicated in patients with idiopathic thrombocytopenic purpura (ITP).

In the perioperative setting, platelet transfusion is used to correct thrombocytopenia and platelet dysfunction. It is difficult to determine exactly which level of thrombocytopenia should warrant transfusion of platelet concentrates in the perioperative period; as with RBC transfusion, medical judgment is required. When the problem is dilutional thrombocytopenia with microvascular bleeding, platelet transfusion usually is required when the platelet count is below 50×10^9 per liter and is seldom necessary when the count is above 100×10^9 per liter (Table 8) (2).

TABLE 8. ASA RECOMMENDATIONS FOR PLATELETS

Preoperative
1. Prophylactic platelet transfusion is ineffective when thrombocytopenia is due to increased platelet destruction (e.g., idiopathic thrombocytopenic purpura).
2. Prophylactic platelet transfusion is rarely indicated in surgical patients when the platelet count is greater than 100×10^9/L and is usually indicated when the count is below 50×10^9/L. The determination of whether patients with intermediate platelet counts ($50–100 \times 10^9$/L) require therapy should be based on the risk of bleeding.

Intraoperative
1. Patients with microvascular bleeding usually require platelet transfusion if the platelet count is less than 50×10^9/L and rarely require therapy if it is greater than 100×10^9/L. With intermediate platelet counts ($50–100 \times 10^9$/L), the determination should be based on the patient's risk of developing more significant bleeding.
2. Vaginal deliveries and operative procedures that are ordinarily associated with insignificant blood loss may be undertaken in patients with platelet counts less than 50×10^9/L.
3. Platelet transfusion may be indicated despite an apparently adequate platelet count if there is known platelet dysfunction and microvascular bleeding.

ASA, American Society of Anesthesiologists.

With intermediate platelet counts, the risk of further bleeding should affect the judgment of whether or not to transfuse.

LEUKOCYTE-DEPLETED BLOOD PRODUCTS

As discussed, leukocyte contaminants present in blood products are involved in several adverse reactions to blood component transfusion, including febrile and allergic reactions, TRALI, platelet refractoriness, and CMV transmission. Several clinical trials indicated that leukocyte depletion can reduce the occurrence of these adverse reactions (35–38). Improved technology led to the development of effective blood filters for the production of leukocyte-depleted blood components. Recently, several European countries adopted the so-called prestorage universal leukocyte depletion. In this approach, all (*universal*) blood components produced by the blood bank are passed though a leukocyte filter (*leukocyte depletion*) soon after collection (*prestorage*). It is expected that prestorage universal leukocyte depletion will become the standard for blood component preparation in the United States.

MASSIVE TRANSFUSION

Massive blood transfusion usually is defined as a transfusion equal to or greater than one blood volume. Massive transfusion is encountered frequently in the perioperative period. Problems related to massive transfusion include disturbance of the coagulation system and metabolic complications.

Coagulopathy

The classic teaching is that the mechanism of coagulopathy most often is due to dilutional thrombocytopenia, although

TABLE 9. LABORATORY EVALUATION OF INTRAOPERATIVE COAGULOPATHY

	Dilutional Thrombocytopenia	Clotting Factor Deficiencies	Disseminated Intravascular Coagulation	Platelet Function Disorder	Circulating Heparin
Platelet count	Low	—	Low	—	—
PT, aPTT	—	High	High	—	High
Fibrinogen level	—	Low	Low	—	—
Fibrin split products	—	—	Present	—	—
Thromboelastograph	Low ma	Prolonged r	Prolonged r and low ma	Low ma	Extremely prolonged r

PT, prothrombin time; aPTT, activated partial thromboplastin time.
ma, maximum amplitude; r, reaction time.

clotting-factor dilution, DIC, preoperative coagulation defects, and HTR are also possible. Laboratory studies including platelet count, PT, aPTT, fibrin-split products, and thromboelastogram can assist in defining the mechanism of coagulopathy in the setting of massive transfusion (Table 9).

Prophylactic platelet concentrates early in a massive transfusion are ineffective in preventing coagulopathy (39). In a randomized, prospective study, Reed and colleagues showed that prophylactic infusion of platelets did not affect the incidence of coagulopathy in trauma patients (39). Depending on their initial platelet counts, most patients will not develop dilutional thrombocytopenia until at least 1.5 blood volumes have been transfused. It is appropriate to monitor the platelet count of massively transfused patients and delay platelet therapy until coagulopathy and thrombocytopenia actually coexist. Because RBCs and salvaged autologous blood are virtually depleted of plasma, severe bleeding can occur as a result of dilution of clotting factors during massive transfusion. Prophylactic FFP infusion, however, has not been effective in preventing coagulopathy in massively transfused patients (40). Although neither platelet concentrates nor FFP should be given prophylactically, they can be lifesaving when a coagulopathy actually develops. However, in the setting of severe bleeding and transfusion of more than 2 blood volumes, empiric transfusion of platelets and FFP is standout practice.

Metabolic Complications

Aside from hypothermia, metabolic problems associated with massive transfusion are seldom as serious as coagulation abnormalities. Hypothermia should be prevented by the use of blood warmers. Although all transfusions for adults do not need to be warmed, whenever more than 2 U are infused rapidly, a warmer should be used.

Citrate anticoagulants, which are present in blood products, can accumulate and bind calcium in the recipient blood. Hypocalcemia and hypomagnesemia resulting from citrate binding are rare. Indeed, normothermic adults seldom develop citrate toxicity. This problem is more likely to occur in neonates, in the setting of hypothermia, and in patients with liver disease. Routine prophylactic calcium administration is not recommended in adults unless large volumes of blood products are being transfused rapidly (>50 mL/min) (41) or when severe hepatic failure is present. Patients undergoing liver transplantation are more likely to experience citrate toxicity during massive transfusion. In the setting of hypotension and signs of decreased myocardial contractility, with a prolonged QT interval on the electrocardiogram, calcium should be replaced.

Although stored blood is quite acidic, massively transfused patients become acidotic only when their systemic perfusion is inadequate. Prophylactic bicarbonate administration is not recommended; therapy for acid–base abnormalities should be guided by blood gas measurement. When the infused citrate is metabolized to bicarbonate by the liver, metabolic alkalosis may develop in the setting of massive transfusion. Likewise, the high potassium content of stored RBCs is seldom a problem *in vivo*; electrolyte abnormalities should only be treated when they are actually confirmed by laboratory data.

BLOOD SUBSTITUTES

The term *blood substitutes* has been used broadly to describe oxygen-carrying, volume-expanding solutions. Oxygen-carrying volume expanders have long been attractive to military medical organizations faced with the logistical constraints of the battlefield (42). Concern over fatal blood-borne pathogens, including hepatitis and HIV, also makes oxygen-carrying volume expanders attractive for civilian use (43). Since the blood supply in the United States faces major challenges associated with an aging population and potentially inadequate rates of volunteer donation by healthy citizens (43), blood substitutes may be particularly useful in the near future.

A variety of cell-free substances that transport oxygen and augment intravascular volume are emerging as possible blood substitutes for use in humans. These substances include polymerized or cross-linked hemoglobin solutions, liposome-encapsulated hemoglobin, perfluorocarbons, and possibly recombinant hemoglobin (44,45). None of these compounds replaces coagulation factors, and all have limited circulation half-life. Nevertheless, red cell substitutes may be valuable in specific clinical settings, such as acute normovolemic hemodilution, myocardial and cerebral ischemia, cardiopulmonary bypass extracorporeal circulation, and organ perfusion before transplant.

In conclusion, oxygen-carrying volume-expanding solutions that can sustain life in the absence of RBCs have been developed. Concerns about side effects and ultimate demonstration of efficacy will have to be satisfactorily addressed before physicians routinely administer such solutions. Although blood substitutes will be expensive and still have not been proved clinically safe, their need could become more apparent in the future. It is unlikely, however, that any of these solutions will replace autologous or allogeneic blood in the near future.

USE OF ERYTHROPOIETIN IN CRITICALLY ILL PATIENTS

As discussed, anemia is a common problem in critically ill patients admitted to the ICU (46). It has been reported that about 85% of ICU patients with a length of stay of more than 7 days will be transfused with at least 1 U RBCs (46). Most transfusions in the ICU are not associated with acute blood loss (46).

Critically ill patients appear to have a blunted response to physiologic erythropoietic stimuli (47). Recently, several small trials analyzed the efficacy of recombinant human erythropoietin (rHuEPO) in critically ill patients (48,49). The working hypothesis is that by providing pharmacologic doses of rHuEPO, transfusion requirements for RBCs could be decreased in critically ill patients (48,49). In fact, in a randomized, double-blind, placebo-controlled trial, Corwin and colleagues found that a total of 6 weeks' therapy with pharmacologic doses of rHuEPO resulted in a 45% decrease in the number of units of RBCs transfused (49). In this study, however, a rather high hematocrit level was observed both in the controls and the treated group (49). Furthermore, no significant differences between the two groups either in mortality rates or in the frequency of adverse events was observed (49).

The RBCs that are produced endogenously may be more effective and safer than transfused blood (48,49). Allogeneic blood transfusion is not risk free. It is possible that a combination of conservative blood transfusion strategies (as reported by Hebert and co-workers) with pharmacologic doses of rHuEPO may be a safe and cost-effective way to avoid allogeneic blood transfusion (32, 48,49). Indeed, such strategy may be a possible way to reduce the number of unnecessary blood component transfusions and avoid the expected blood component shortage in the near future (50).

ISCHEMIC OPTIC NEUROPATHY

A number of case reports have described blindness occurring in association with blood loss, anemia, and hypotension. Arteriosclerotic risk factors such as hypertension, diabetes, and smoking are often associated (51). Acute loss of vision is caused by infarctions in one or both optic nerves. Although this syndrome, referred to as *ischemic optic neuropathy* (ION), is more common in older patients, there are case reports of patients as young as 13 years. Reported to occur most frequently after cardiopulmonary bypass, ION also occurs after back and abdominal operations and multiple other procedures as well as after nonsurgical hemorrhage. Katz and colleagues reported the occurrence of ION in four patients who had undergone lumbar laminectomies (aged 41–65 years) and reviewed the literature on other adequately documented cases (52); bilateral eye involvement occurred in 18 of 30 cases (52). The onset sometimes is reported as occurring days after the initial procedure, possibly because initial complaints of blurred vision are ignored immediately postoperatively and an ophthalmoscopic examination is routinely near normal. Although blindness is not always complete, visual acuities were poorer than 20/100 in most cases (52). Although the syndrome of ION is likely to be underdiagnosed and underreported for medicolegal and other reasons, the incidence of this complication is so low that it probably should not affect transfusion practice until its pathophysiologic mechanism is more clearly understood.

SUMMARY

Current transfusion medicine practices have greatly reduced the risks of blood transfusion and make the blood supply as safe as it ever has been. Despite this, various controversies continue in this dynamic field. These include the quest for identification of the optimal hematocrit, appropriate transfusion triggers, and limitation or elimination of deleterious effects when blood is transfused. The major dangers associated with transfusion continue to center around reaction to blood products, catastrophic effects from incompatible blood, transmission of infectious disease, immunomodulation, and the effects of transfusion of aged blood. Research continues in the area of alternatives to blood, augmentation of blood production with erythropoietin, and methods to screen blood products more effectively. Recombinant technologies also remain under investigation. Various approaches, including the treatment of plasma with solvent and detergent, are being broadly advocated as a means to limit transmission of various infectious diseases, particularly enveloped viruses.

The future use of transfusion therapy will continue to evolve, and there are projected shortages of the blood supply as the population ages and donations drop or contraindications to donations increase. Therefore, judicious use of this limited resource and appropriate innovative techniques will have to be applied to optimize the safe use of blood products.

KEY POINTS

Transfusion therapy continues to be refined and has become increasingly safe. This is despite concerns over transfusion reactions, transmission of infectious disease, immune modulation, and the effects of stored blood. Current screening techniques, including nucleic acid testing, have markedly limited the incidence of transmission of viral-mediated diseases. There may be unknown or unanticipated infectious diseases lurking in the blood-borne environment, however.

Blood component therapy still dominates our current approach to transfusion. In addition, various studies have questioned the appropriate level at which we should trigger transfusion and have questioned the efficacy of empirically transfusing individuals or transfusing to a specific endpoint.

Future developments in transfusion medicine will center around refinements in screening blood, techniques to salvage and more judiciously use blood, and finally use of "blood substitutes." Anesthesiologists and critical care physicians continue to be major users of blood products and need to take a leading role in appropriate administration of this limited resource.

REFERENCES

1. Goodnough LT, Brecher ME, Kanter MH, et al. Transfusion medicine (first of two parts): blood transfusion. *N Engl J Med* 1999;340:438–447.
2. American Society of Anesthesiologists Task Force on Blood Component Therapy. Practice guidelines for blood component therapy. *Anesthesiology* 1996;84:732–742.
3. Glynn SA, Kleinman SH, Schreiber GB, et al. Trends in incidence and prevalence of major transfusion-transmissible viral infections in U.S. blood donors. *JAMA* 2000;284:229–235.
4. Ling AE, Robbins KE, Brown TM, et al. Failure of routine HIV-1 tests in a case involving transmission with preseroconversion blood components during the infectious window period. *JAMA* 2000;284:210–214.
5. Klein HG. Will blood transfusion ever be safe enough? *JAMA* 2000;284:238–240.
6. Peterman TA, Ward JW. What's happening to the epidemic of transfusion-associated AIDS? [Editorial] *Transfusion* 1989;29:659–660.
7. Faust RJ. Transfusion medicine. In: Wedel DJ, ed. *Orthopedic anesthesia.* New York: Churchill Livingstone,1993:15–53.
8. Donahue JG, Munoz A, Ness PM, et al. The declining risk of post-transfusion hepatitis C virus infection. *N Engl J Med* 1992;327:369–373.
9. Williams I. Epidemiology of hepatitis C in the United States. *Am J Med* 1999;107:2S–9S.
10. Van der Poel CL. Hepatitis C virus and blood transfusion: past and present. *J Hepatology* 1999;31:101–106.
11. McCullough J. Transfusion-transmitted diseases. In: McCullough J, ed. *Transfusion medicine.* New York: McGraw-Hill, 1998:361–386.
12. Busch M, Chamberland M, Epstein J, et al. Oversight and monitoring of blood safety in the United States. *Vox Sang* 1999;77:67–76.
13. Sazama K. Reports of 355 transfusion-associated deaths: 1976 through 1985. *Transfusion* 1990;30:583–590.
14. Capon SM, Goldfinger D. Acute hemolytic transfusion reaction, a paradigm of the systemic inflammatory response: new insights into pathophysiology and treatment. *Transfusion* 1995;35:513–520.
15. Popovsky MA, Chaplin HC Jr, Moore SB. Transfusion-related acute lung injury: a neglected, serious complication of hemotherapy. *Transfusion* 1992;32:589–592.
16. Silliman CC, Paterson AJ, Dickey WO, et al. The association of bio-chemically active lipids with the development of transfusion-related acute lung injury: retrospective study. *Transfusion* 1997;37:719–726.
17. Klein HG. Immunomodulatory aspects of transfusion: a once and future risk. *Anesthesiology* 1999;91:861–865.
18. National Heart, Lung, and Blood Institute Expert Panel on the Use of Autologous Blood. Transfusion alert: use of autologous blood. *Transfusion* 1995;35:703–711.
19. Klein HG. Transfusion safety: avoiding unnecessary transfusion. [Editorial] *Mayo Clin Proc* 2000;75:5–7.
20. Goodnough LT, Brecher ME, Kanter MH, et al. Transfusion medicine (second of two parts): Blood Conservation. *N Engl J Med* 1999;340:525–533.
21. Spahn DR, Casutt M. Eliminating blood transfusions: new aspects and perspectives. *Anesthesiology* 2000;93:242–255.
22. Nuttal GA, Santrach PJ, Oliver WC, et al. Possible guidelines for auto-logous red blood cell donations before total hip arthroplasty based on the surgical blood order equation. *Mayo Clin Proc* 2000;75:10–17.
23. Napier JA, Bruce M, Chapman J, et al. Guidelines for autologous trans-fusion. II. Perioperative haemodilution and cell salvage. *Br J Anaesth* 1997;78:768–771.
24. Huet C, Salmi LR, Fergusson D, et al. A meta-analysis of the effectiveness of cell salvage to minimize preoperative allogeneic blood transfusion in cardiac and orthopedic surgery. *Anesth Analg* 1999;89:861–869.
25. Linden JV, Tourault MA, Scribner CL. Decrease in frequency of trans-fusion fatalities. *Transfusion* 1997;37:243–244.
26. Hart OJ III, Klimberg IW, Wajsman Z, et al. Intraoperative auto-transfusion in radical cystectomy for carcinoma of the bladder. *Surg Gynecol Obstet* 1989;168:302–306.
27. Umlas J, Foster RR, Dalal SA, et al. Red cell loss following orthopedic surgery: the case against postoperative blood salvage. *Transfusion* 1994;34:402–406.
28. Faust RJ. Perioperative indications for red blood cell transfusion-has the pendulum swung too far? [Editorial] *Mayo Clin Proc* 1993;68:512–514.
29. Fitzgerald RD, Martin CM, Dietz GE, et al. Transfusing red blood cell stored in citrate phosphate dextrose adenine-1 for 28 days fails to improve tissue oxygenation in rats. *Crit Care Med* 1997;25:726–732.
30. Sielenkamper AW, Chin Yee IH, Martin CM, et al. Diaspirin crosslinked hemoglobin improves systemic oxygen uptake in oxygen supply-dependent septic rats. *Am J Respir Crit Care Med* 1997;156:1066–1072.
31. Hebert PC, Schweitzert I, Calder L, et al. Review of the clinical prac-tice literature on allogeneic red blood cell transfusion. *Can Med Assoc J* 1997;156:S9–S26.
32. Hebert PC, Wells G, Blajchman M, et al. A multicentric, random-ized, controlled clinical trial of transfusion requirements in critical care. *N Engl J Med* 1999;340:409–417.
33. Vichinsky EP, Haberkern CM, Neumayr L, et al. A comparison of con-servative and aggressive transfusion regimens in the perioperative man-agement of sickle cell disease. *N Engl J Med* 1995;333:206–213.
34. Spiess BD, Ley C, Body SC, et al. Hematocrit value on intensive care unit entry influences the frequency of Q-wave myocardial infarction after coronary artery bypass grafting. *J Thorac Cardiovasc Surg* 1998;116:460–467.
35. TRAP Trial Study Group. Leukocyte reduction and ultraviolet B irra-diation of platelets to prevent alloimmunization and refractoriness to platelet transfusion. *N Engl J Med* 1997;337:1861–1869.
36. van Marwijk Kooy M, Van Prooijen HC, Moes M, et al. Use of leukocyte-depleted platelet concentrates for the prevention of refractoriness and primary HLA alloimmunization: a prospective, randomized trial. *Blood* 1991;77:201–205.
37. Kao KH, Mickel M, Braine HG, et al. White cell reduction in platelet concentrates and packed red cells by filtration: a multicenter trial. *Transfusion* 1995;35:13–19.
38. Bowden RA, Slichter SJ, Sayers M, et al. A comparision of filtered leukocyte-reduced and cytomegalovirus (CMV) seronegative blood products for the prevention of transfusion-associated CMV infection after marrow transplant. *Blood* 1995;86:3598–3603.
39. Reed RL II, Ciavarella D, Heimbach DM, et al. Prophylactic platelet administration during massive transfusion: a prospective, randomized, double-blind clinical study. *Ann Surg* 1986;203:40–48.
40. Roy RC, Stafford MA, Hudspeth AS, et al. Failure of prophylaxis with fresh frozen plasma after cardiopulmonary bypass. *Anesthesiology* 1988;69:254–257.
41. Denlinger JK, Nahrwold ML, Gibbs PS, et al. Hypocalcemia during rapid blood transfusion in anesthetized man. *Br J Anaesth* 1976;48:995–1000.
42. Webster NR, Ward MJ. Battlefield transfusions. *JAMA* 1994;271:319.
43. Scott MG, Kucik DF, Goodnough LT, et al. Blood substitutes: evolution and future applications. *Clin Chem* 1997;43:1724–1731.
44. Winslow RM. Blood substitutes-a moving target. *Nat Med* 1995;1:1212–1215.
45. Dietz NM, Joyner MJ, Warner MA. Blood substitutes: fluids, drugs, or miracle solutions? *Anesth Analg* 1996;82:390–405.
46. Corwin HC, Parsonnet KC, Gettinger A. RBC transfusion in the ICU: Is there a reason? *Chest* 1995;108:767–771.
47. Rogiers P, Zhang H, Leeman M, et al. Erythropoietin response is blunted in critically ill patients. *Intensive Care Med* 1997;23:159–162.
48. Gabriel A, Kozek S, Chiari A, et al. High-dose recombinant human erythropoietin stimulates reticulocyte production patients with multiple organ dysfunction syndrome. *J Trauma* 1998;44:361–367.
49. Corwin H, Gettinger A, Rodriguez R, et al. Efficacy of recombinant human erythropoietin in the critically ill patient: a randomized, double-blind, placebo-controlled trial. *Crit Care Med* 1999;27:2346–2350.
50. Nucci ML, Abuchowski A. The search for blood substitutes. *Sci Am* 1998;278:72–79.
51. Williams EL, Hart WM Jr, Tempelhoff R. Postoperative ischemic optic neuropathy. *Anesth Analg* 1995;80:1018–1029.
52. Katz DM, Trobe JD, Cornblath WT, et al. Ischemic optic neuropathy after lumbar spine surgery. *Arch Ophthalmol* 1994;112:925–931.

EVALUATION OF FEVER IN THE INTENSIVE CARE UNIT

KENNETH E. WOOD

KEY WORDS

- Infectious fever–catheter infections
- Intraabdominal infection
- Neuroleptic malignant syndrome
- Noninfectious fever—drug fever
- Nosocomial pneumonia
- Postoperative fever
- Transfusion reactions
- Urinary tract infections

Humanity has but three great enemies: fever, famine and war; of these, by far the greatest, by far the most terrible, is fever.

—Sir William Osler

THE FEBRILE RESPONSE

Fever, perhaps more than any other phenomenon, is the thread woven through the fabric of critical illness. It knows no specialty or disease barrier and constantly confronts the critical care practitioner to define its etiology and significance. Despite the incidence of nosocomial complications manifesting as fever in patients requiring critical care, rigid examination of the issue has not been undertaken in the critical care literature. Several investigators have determined, however, that fever occurred in 29% (1) and 36% (2) of patients on general medical inpatient services. Given the acuity of and complications associated with critical illnesses, the incidence of fever in patients in the intensive care unit (ICU) is probably even greater. Previous studies (3,4) have reported a fourfold increase in mortality in patients who developed fever while hospitalized, a factor most likely reflecting the severity of the patients' underlying illnesses and predisposition to fever-provoking events. If fever is a manifestation of an ICU-acquired nosocomial infection, the attributable mortality is approximately 25% (5).

Bearing in mind that some subsets of patients [i.e., older patients; malnourished, azotemic, steroid-dependent, antipyretic-using, leukopenic, and immunosuppressed patients; or those with congestive heart failure (CHF), large burns, or open abdominal wounds] may not mount an effective febrile response to an appropriate stimulus, *fever* is conventionally defined as a core temperature greater than 100.4°F (38°C) (6). The thermistor of a pulmonary artery catheter (PAC) is considered to be the standard for measuring core temperature. Thermistors in indwelling bladder catheters and tympanic membrane temperature by means of infrared ear thermometry are acceptable alternatives. The pattern of the fever is not particularly helpful in defining or establishing the diagnosis (7), nor does the amplitude of the fever or the clinical appearance of the patient correlate with the presence or severity of infection (3,8).

Pathophysiology

Thermoregulation occurs in the anterior hypothalamus and is determined by a balance between heat loss from the periphery and heat production from organs and muscle (Fig. 1). It should be recognized that fever, in contrast to hyperthermia, represents a physiologic upregulation of the hypothalamic set point. Various disease states, including infections, injury, inflammation, neoplasia, and immunologically mediated processes, can stimulate host-cell (monocyte, macrophage) production of pyrogenic cytokines [interleukin (IL)-1, IL-6, tumor necrosis factor (TNF), and others]. These cytokines provoke the synthesis of prostaglandin E_2 (PGE_2) in the anterior hypothalamus and reset the thermoregulatory center to a higher level, initiating processes that favor heat conservation (i.e., vasoconstriction, positional change to minimize the body surface area for heat loss, behavioral changes to seek warm environments, or donning of insulating clothing) and heat production (i.e., muscle contractions with shivering). Because humans produce more heat than is necessary to achieve a core temperature of 37°C, the latter mechanism will be invoked only when the former approach is inadequate to generate and sustain the new higher set point. Cessation of fever will occur when the initiating stimulus is removed and will be accompanied by mechanisms that dissipate heat loss, such as sweating and vasodilation. These phenomena are quite evident, either through personal experience or patient observation, as one witnesses patients curled up in bed, surrounded by blankets with teeth-chattering shakes that eventuate into a profuse sweat with peripheral dilatation. Because temperatures rarely exceed 42°C in humans, endogenous, centrally produced antipyretics (somatostatin, arginine, vasopressin) that limit the fever amplitude are thought to exist. Unknown,

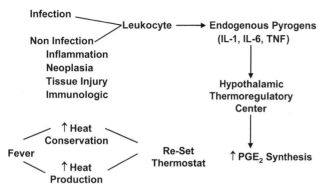

FIGURE 1. Physiology of fever.

however, is whether conventional application of these agents in treating other disease processes blunts temperature production.

Beneficial and Adverse Effects

Fever should not be viewed as an isolated phenomena but as one component of the nonspecific acute-phase response. This response includes changes in the synthesis of liver proteins (i.e., albumin, complement, haptoglobin, fibrinogen, C-reactive protein), an increased number and immaturity of circulating neutrophils, increased gluconeogenesis and muscle proteolysis, depression of serum iron and zinc levels, as well as the clinical findings of lethargy and hypersomnolence. Once might infer that fever and the acute-phase response, taken together, are vital and integral components of the host's defense against infection and malignancy, but firm support of this hypothesis is lacking. Evidence supporting the benefit of fever includes self-potentiation of the local action of IL-1, augmentation of T- and B-cell responses, generation of cytotoxic T-cells, increased B-cell activity, and increased immunoglobulin synthesis. Additionally, certain viral and bacterial replication is impaired at higher temperatures. Although clinical data are limited, it has been reported that an increased temperature is associated with an improved outcome in gram-negative bacteremia (9), spontaneous bacterial peritonitis (10), and children with chickenpox (11). Adverse effects of fever include an increase in oxygen consumption of 13% for each degree over 37°C, the strain on the cardiovascular system to meet this demand, and the changes in mental status that can occur. All effects are particularly pronounced in patients with preexisting cardiac and neurologic disease. Fever and its mediators seemingly have the capacity to potentiate and inhibit resistance to infection.

If one views fever from a species perspective rather than that of an individual, a teleologic viewpoint would explain the salutary effects of fever on mild to moderate infection and the adverse effects of fever on fulminant infection. With preservation of the species (as opposed to survival of the individual) as the ultimate objective, fever and its mediators could have evolved to facilitate survival from localized or moderate systemic infections to achieve species propagation. Fever hastened the demise of fulminantly infected individuals who posed a threat of epidemic disease to the species (12).

Treatment

The decision to treat a fever is predicated on the weighted perception of the beneficial versus adverse effects of fever in an individual patient. Although fever can occur through defective thermoregulation, this type of fever is not hypothalamically mediated, and the topic will not be pursued here. As discussed earlier, temperature elevation with an intact thermoregulatory center essentially defines a new, higher set point as a consequence of cytokine stimulation of hypothalamic PGE$_2$ synthesis. Available therapeutic agents that inhibit brain cyclooxygenase act as central antipyretics. These agents include acetaminophen, which poorly inhibits peripheral cyclooxygenase activity but is oxidized in the brain and effectively lowers temperature; nonsteroidal antiinflammatory agents (e.g., indomethacin, ibuprofen, naproxen), which work similarly; and corticosteroids, which centrally impair PGE$_2$ synthesis and inhibit the transcription of pyrogenic cytokines in the periphery. Cooling blankets are frequently used to reduce temperature in the ICU despite evidence that they are no more effective than central antipyretics and can precipitate large temperature fluctuations with rebound hyperthermia (13). Insofar as the generation of temperature is an appropriate response to a new elevated hypothalamic set point, external cooling can prevent attainment of the set point, thereby inducing hypermetabolism. Active cooling in patients with induced fever is reported to increase oxygen consumption by 35% and also to increase catecholamine levels (14). Cooling blankets should not be used without antipyretic drugs because cold receptors in the skin can cause reflex vasoconstriction and impair further heat loss. Certain drugs, although not advocated for this purpose (phenothiazines interfere with vasoconstriction, and paralytic agents abolish muscle contraction), can minimize the extent of fever. Ultimately, the decision to lower temperature therapeutically is based on the perceived detrimental aspects of high fever in patients with compromised cardiac or neurologic systems.

GENERAL APPROACH AND EVALUATION

The ICU is undoubtedly the ward where one most commonly encounters fever. In addition to having whatever process warranted admission to the ICU, many patients are frequently immunocompromised as well as afflicted with chronic disease, systemic inflammatory response syndrome (SIRS), and multiple-organ dysfunction syndrome (MODS).

Superimposed on these baseline problems are initiation of invasive procedures, transfusion of blood products, and infusion of multiple medications—all factors that add to the complexity of the differential diagnosis. Because nosocomial infections occur most commonly in the ICU (2) and because sepsis or MODS is a leading cause of death among patients in the ICU, it is imperative that the evaluation of fever be undertaken expeditiously, in a thorough and comprehensive manner. It is important to recognize, however, that as many as 10% of septic patients are hypothermic and 35% are normothermic. A significantly worse outcome is reported in septic patients who fail to mount a febrile response (15,16). Therefore, the absence of a temperature should

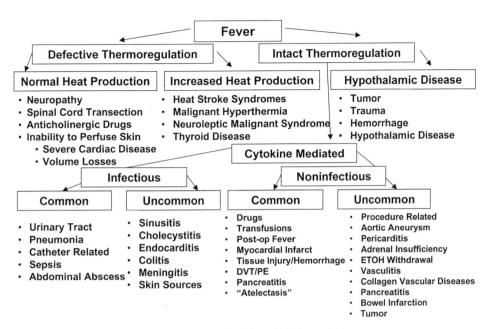

FIGURE 2. Fever–physiology clinical correlates.

not dissuade clinicians from considering sepsis in the differential diagnosis.

In medical patients with a fever and documented infection, the presence of bacteremia, peak respiratory rate, nadir Glasgow Coma Scale score, and peak white blood cell count correlated with the subsequent development of shock (17). As with many problems in critical care medicine, it is reasonable to develop a diagnostic/therapeutic algorithm by proceeding along two conceptual parallels: defining the physiologic abnormality (Fig. 2) and generating a differential diagnosis from the available history, physical, and laboratory data (Fig. 3). This paradigm defines fever as a function of the capacity to thermoregulate. Defective thermoregulation is characterized by the preservation of the normal hypothalamic temperature set point but an inability to dissipate heat, which results in temperature elevation. It is further characterized into instances where heat production is normal but heat cannot be dissipated versus processes where heat production is increased beyond the capacity of the patient to dissipate that heat. Intact thermoregulation reflects an elevation of the hypothalamic set point to a higher level and can occur through pathologic processes in the hypothalamus or through the previously defined cytokine-mediated increases in PGE_2. Infectious as well as most noninfectious causes of fever are mediated by this mechanism.

The clinical evaluation of fever in the ICU begins with a review of the pertinent medical history combined with a physical examination. This evaluation should be performed in a thorough and meticulous manner; given the possible sequelae of sepsis and multiple-system failure, the initial goal should be to confirm or eliminate an infectious cause. After reviewing the patient's admitting problem, ICU course, comorbid processes, and risk factors, the critical care physician attempts to define the clinical context of the fever. The physician also develops a physiologic classification that incorporates pertinent issues (e.g., reason for patient's admission, length of time the indwelling catheter has been in

place, medications taken, use of blood products). A "head-to-toe" physical examination, with careful evaluation of wounds, drains, catheter sites, and dependent areas, should be performed (Fig. 3). The overall clinical assessment should be coupled with diagnostic tests that are reflective of findings in the history and physical. Blood cultures should be drawn from two separate sites by venipuncture using tincture of iodine as a cutaneous antiseptic to reduce contamination. Each blood culture should consist of 20 to 30 mL of blood with 10 to 15 mL inoculated into both aerobic and anaerobic media to significantly improve the yield (18). No more than three blood cultures (10–15 mL each) need to be drawn during the initial 24 hours after onset of a new fever. Judicious use of radiologic studies and ultrasound, as well as additional cultures, should derive from the history and physical assessment.

If an obvious or likely infectious source or process is identified, appropriate therapy should be initiated and necessary confirmatory studies ordered, or the offending agent or process should be withdrawn, if possible. When no obvious source is apparent and the patient is toxic, unstable, or immunocompromised, antibiotics and possibly antifungal or antiviral drugs should be instituted to cover the most commonly encountered pathogens. Consideration should also be given to expanding the diagnostic assessment. For patients who are stable but lack an obvious infectious source, the initial diagnostic studies and the patient's status should be followed carefully and the history and physical examination reassessed. If the patient's clinical condition deteriorates, empiric antimicrobial therapy should be initiated.

INFECTIOUS SOURCES OF FEVER

Infectious sources of fever are common in the ICU. Nosocomial infection is reported to occur in 10% of patients and is related to ICU length of stay (19). In a recent survey of 1,417 European

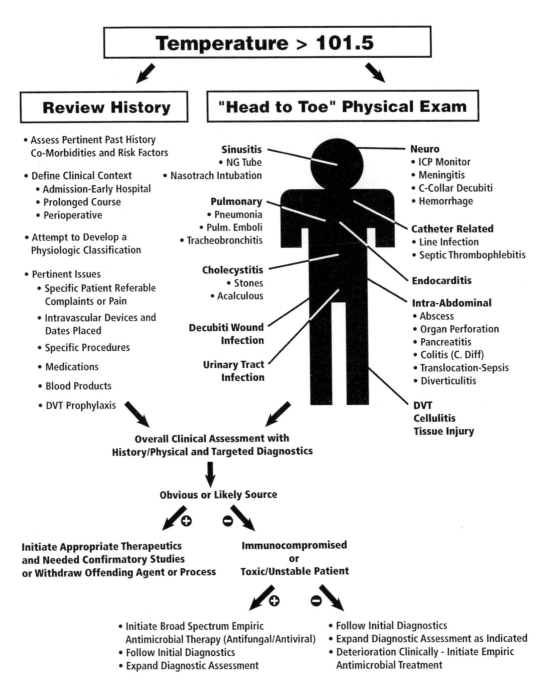

FIGURE 3. General approach to fever.

ICU's involving 10,000 patients, 20% of patients manifested an ICU-acquired infection. Pneumonia (47%) was the most common, followed by urinary tract infection (18%) and bloodstream infection (12%) (20).

Catheter-related Infection

Central venous catheters (CVCs) have become an integral and indispensable component in the care of the critically ill. Their use is associated with a significant infectious risk, however. Although the incidence of secondary bloodstream infections from many areas has declined in the past decade, nosocomial bacteremia has

increased tenfold. This increase is attributed primarily to intravascular catheters, with 80% to 90% of infections arising from CVCs (21,22). It is estimated that 25% of CVCs will become colonized, one-quarter of which will result subsequently in a catheter-related bloodstream infection (23). Thus, the reported 5% to 10% incidence of catheter-related infection (CRI) is responsible for 10% to 20% of ICU nosocomial infections (21,24). With more than five million catheters placed each year, 300,000 CRIs will result, with an estimated attributable mortality of 25%, ranging from 13% for coagulase-negative *Staphylococcus* to 38% for *Candida* infections. The estimated attributable increase in length of stay is 6 to 10 days at a cost of $30,000 per survivor (25,26).

Colonization of the CVC is a prelude to CRI and can occur from the extraluminal or intraluminal route. The former predominates in short-term catheters (≤30 days); molecular DNA subtyping has shown that a vast majority (82%) of CRIs arise from patient skin flora or the catheter hub, whereas 9% originate through hematogenous seeding and 9% are infusion related (27). The following are clinical signs suggestive of CRI: The patient is an unlikely candidate for overt sepsis; the source of sepsis is not apparent; the intravascular device was in place at the onset of sepsis; inflammation or purulence is present at the insertion site; the sepsis had an abrupt shock-associated onset; the sepsis is caused by *Staphylococcus* (coagulase-negative) or high-grade candidemia; the sepsis is refractory to antibiotic treatment; or the patient improves dramatically with catheter removal (23).

From an operational perspective, CRI can be divided into catheter-related bloodstream infections (CRI-BS) and catheter-related localized infections (CRI-LI). Traditionally, a significant semiquantitative culture [≥15 colony forming units (CFU)] will

define a CRI, and CRI-BS and CRI-LI will be differentiated by the presence or absence of blood culture positivity (23). A diagnosis of CRI-BS should require catheter tip-blood culture concordance for the same organism and no other identifiable source of infection. Despite the widespread application of the semiquantitative technique, only the external portion of the CVC is evaluated, and although the sensitivity is excellent, the specificity is less than 50%. Specificity is improved only slightly when the threshold is increased to 100 CFU (28). Therefore, it has been advocated that quantitative catheter cultures be used that are reported to have a sensitivity and specificity greater than 90% for infection when a threshold of 10^3 CFU per milliliter is used (29). Recognizing that only 15% to 25% of CVCs that are removed for suspicion of infection will be proven infected by quantitative catheter-tip culture (30), it is crucial to devise a standardized strategy to define absolute indications for catheter removal and criteria for CRI diagnosis with and without catheter removal. An approach to assessing suspected CRI is presented in Figures 4

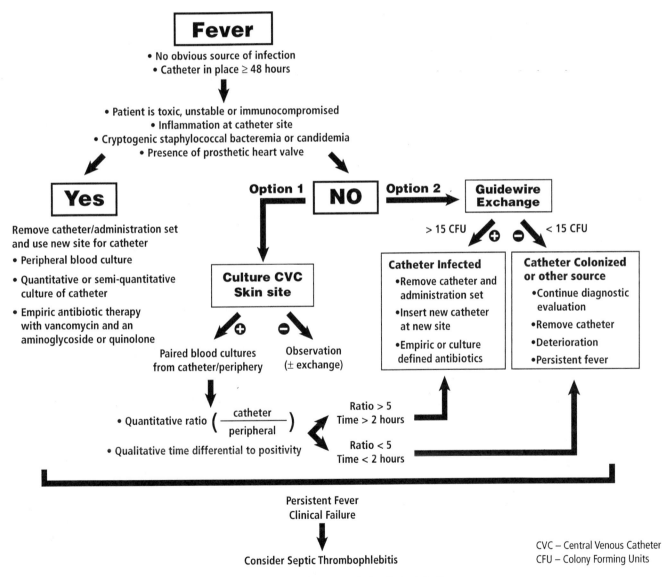

FIGURE 4. Approach to suspected catheter infection.

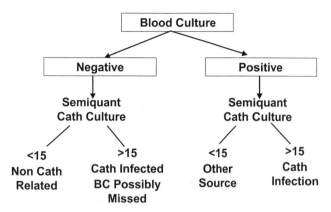

FIGURE 5. Culture interpretation.

and 5. CRI should be considered in febrile patients in whom no source of infection is obvious and the catheter has been in place longer than 48 hours. If the patient is toxic or unstable or the site is inflamed, the catheter should be removed and a new site chosen. Cultures should be performed and empiric therapy instituted to cover the most likely organisms. Deep subcutaneous or tunnel infections are characterized by local purulence with warmth and induration extending more than 2 cm from the insertion site and mandate CVC removal under any circumstance. In the absence of the preceding information, two options are available: (a) a guidewire catheter change and (b) a quantitative culture of the catheter skin site. With the guidewire exchange technique, the presence of 15 CFU or more growth on the removed catheter indicates a CRI. The guidewire exchange catheter that is placed through the newly defined infected site should be removed and a new catheter placed in a new site. Alternatively, one can attempt to define a CRI without removing the catheter. Quantitative cultures of the catheter skin exit site have a high sensitivity and negative predictive value (using a threshold of 15–50 CFU/mL) and are useful in ruling out a suspected CRI. If skin exit-site cultures are positive, CRI is confirmed when simultaneous paired hub-blood and peripheral blood culture ratios show a fivefold to tenfold differential colony ratio or the differential time to culture positivity is longer than 2 hours (30,31). Proven methods of prevention of CRI are depicted in Table 1. Maximal sterile

TABLE 1. PROVEN PREVENTION OF CATHETER-RELATED INFECTIONS

Insertion and maintenance
  Chlorhexidine >10% povidone-iodine >70% alcohol skin
    preparation
  Maximal barrier precautions
  Catheter placement and maintenance by therapy team
  Subclavian approach
  Catheter tunneling
  Antibiotic and iodophor ointments not necessary
  Routine catheter site or guidewire changes not recommended
Catheter material
  Heparin-bonded catheters
  Silicone and hydrophilic polyurethane
  Antiseptic catheters (chlorhexidine and silver sulfadiazine)
  Antibiotic impregnated catheters (minocycline and rifampin)

barrier precautions (skin disinfection, cap, mask, full-length surgical gown, full drapes) reportedly decrease CRI-BS sixfold (32). Impregnation of catheters with antiseptics (chlorhexidine and silver sulfadiazine) and antibiotics (minocycline and rifampin) has been proven to reduce CRIs (33,34). Persistent fever or clinical failure should prompt consideration toward the evaluation of septic thrombophlebitis. CRI with coagulase-negative *Staphylococcus* predominates over *Staphylococcus aureus* and is responsible for 50% or more of all CRIs. Empiric therapy should include vancomycin and gram-negative coverage in the unstable patient. Definitive therapy should be based on culture results, recognizing that *Candida* CRI is becoming exceedingly common.

Abdominal Infection

Although uncommon in the medical ICU (3), intraabdominal infection constitutes 7% to 14% of nosocomial infections in the surgical ICU (35). The diagnosis of intraabdominal sepsis can be quite difficult to make or can be delayed by the variability or masking of physical signs as well as by logistic issues surrounding transport of critically ill patients to the site of diagnostic studies. Abscess formation most likely represents an intermediate position between an overwhelming lethal inoculum of microorganisms and the complete resolution of the inoculum. The abscess represents a barrier to the immune system and antibiotics; hence, there is a mandatory need to drain or evacuate abscesses either surgically or percutaneously. Failure of the inflammatory reaction to contain the microorganisms results in peritonitis. The diagnosis of an abdominal abscess should be entertained whenever the clinician evaluates fever in a patient who has undergone a surgical or invasive abdominal procedure; prompt recognition and drainage of an intraabdominal abscess before SIRS/MODS is established can greatly improve outcome (36).

A diagnostic approach to evaluating patients with a suspected intraabdominal infection is presented in Figure 6. Most patients who develop intraabdominal infection have had previous operations for perforation, enteric injuries, or a complicated elective operation. Infection should be strongly considered in any febrile patient not making reasonable and expected postoperative progress (37). Diagnostic evaluation commences with a thorough physical examination and a two-view abdominal radiographic series, attempting to identify free or bowel air, distention, air–fluid levels, or "thumbprinting" within the bowel wall. Further diagnostic testing is directed by results of the physical examination, although physical assessment of the critically ill, sedated, hemodynamically unstable, or paralyzed patient can be, at best, challenging. Ultrasonography is particularly sensitive in diagnosing cholecystitis and pelvic pathology. Ultrasound findings can direct percutaneous drainage or exploratory operations. Because the abdominal evaluation is frequently limited in the critically ill patient, the computed tomography (CT) scan is a commonly performed diagnostic test for abscess detection. The study by Trynet and colleagues showed that CT scanning is quite sensitive and specific (90%) in the diagnosis of abdominal abscess (38). In this study, all abscesses were detected by CT scan, while negative scans were obtained in 14 of the 16 patients who did not have abscesses. However, other studies suggest that an abdominal CT scan aided or altered management only 55% of the time (39)

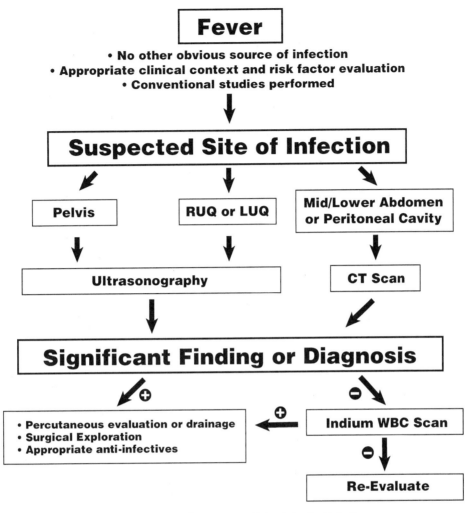

FIGURE 6. Approach to suspected intraabdominal infection.

and provided beneficial interpretation only 23% of the time in patients at risk for developing an intraabdominal abscess (40). Norwood's proposed guidelines (41) to help improve the utilization of CT scans for identifying intraabdominal infection include the following: (a) the scan should not be performed before the eighth postoperative day; (b) the scan should not be done as a final effort to detect a correctable source for sepsis in patients with MODS unless a negative scan would strongly support a decision to withdraw therapy; (c) CT scans should be used sparingly with patients who have an established diagnosis of MODS related to sepsis because useful information is rarely obtained and outcome is not changed; (d) CT scans should be used to search for abdominal abscess only if a reasonable possibility exists that the information will affect treatment decisions; (e) as clinical diagnostic difficulty increases, scan usefulness diminishes.

A labeled leukocyte scan followed by a site-specific imaging study could be used to evaluate patients with a lack of localizing findings, but some clinicians advocate reserving indium scanning for use when imaging studies fail to define a source of infection. Approaches vary, and clinical judgment should be used. *Clostridium difficile* colitis should be a consideration in any patient with a fever and diarrhea, especially in patients receiving broad-spectrum antibiotics. Neutrophilia and fecal leukocytes are common. The tissue culture assay for *C. difficile* toxin is the diagnostic gold standard; however, most laboratories use the enzyme immunoassay for detection of toxin A alone or toxin A and B. Although somewhat less sensitive, the toxin assay can be performed within hours, with a sensitivity of 72% for the first sample. Repeat toxin assay should not be ordered to assess the response to therapy. Direct visualization of pseudomembranes is highly specific (42).

Nosocomial Pneumonia

Ventilator-associated Pneumonia

Ventilator-associated pneumonia (VAP) accounts for 50% of ICU nosocomial infections and is the most common ICU infection. (20) The Canadian Clinical Trials Group reported that 17.5% of patients mechanically ventilated ≥48 hours developed VAP an average of 7 days after ICU admission. Although the overall cumulative incidence was 15 cases per 1,000 ventilator days, the conditional risk diminished over time. VAP rates of 3%, 2%, and 1% per day were reported for the first, second, and third weeks of ventilation, respectively (43). VAP can be defined as either early (≤48 hours) or late (≥48 hours) onset, with the former thought to account for 50% of cases or more. Early onset VAP is associated with common respiratory pathogens or normal oropharyngeal flora (*Streptococcus pneumonia*, *Haemophilus influenza* or *Moraxella catarrhalis*). Late-onset VAP is usually caused by gram-negative bacilli (*Pseudomonas aeruginosa*, *Acinetobacter*, or *Enterobacter*), *S. aureus*, or resistant strains and is heavily influenced by prior antimicrobial therapy (44). VAP is an independent risk factor for mortality with an attributable mortality of 30% and attributable ICU and hospital length of stay durations of 4 and 13 days, respectively (45).

Colonization of the patient's oropharynx with nosocomial pathogens is a prerequisite for the development of VAP. Colonization is multifactorial, heavily influenced by ventilation duration and previous antibiotic pressure (especially third-generation cephalosporins, fluoroquinolones, or imipenem), and occurs in 70% to 90% of ventilated patients (46). Microaspiration of the colonized oropharyngeal contents into the lower respiratory tract, which is facilitated by the supine position and presence of a nasogastric tube, eventually leads to pneumonia. Acute and chronic lung disease, burns, head injury, and manipulation of the ventilator circuit have been identified as independent risk factors for VAP (47,48).

The diagnosis of VAP has remained a contentious topic for debate since Fagan reported that fewer than half of patients with a clinical diagnosis of VAP (fever, leukocytosis, pulmonary infiltrates, and purulent sputum) had positive cultures from specimens obtained by protected catheter brushing (PCB) (49). Literature advocating a clinical (50) versus an invasive approach with PCB or bronchoalveolar lavage (BAL) (51) illustrates the polarity in the diagnosis and therapy of VAP. Unfortunately, there is no gold reference standard to which comparisons can be made; even histopathologic classifications have reported substantial variability (52). Figure 7 illustrates an approach to fever in the ventilated patient with no other obvious source of fever. A chest radiograph should be obtained. If no infiltrate is present, either tracheobronchitis or an alternative diagnosis should be considered. The presence of infiltrates is addressed by a clinical approach or with the aid of specific microbiologic data obtained through BAL or PBC. The latter requires thresholds of 10^4 CFU per milliliter or more and 10^3 CFU per milliliter, respectively. Whatever the approach undertaken, it is crucial to recognize that the early initiation of the appropriate antibiotics is the most important factor affecting outcome (53). Given the predominance of *S. aureus* and gram-negative organisms, empiric coverage should be broad and double cover gram-negative organisms, especially the *Pseudomonas* species. Methods of proven value in diminishing VAP include the following: minimizing ventilator circuit changes, avoiding heated humidifiers, using oral intubation instead of nasal intubation, draining subglottic secretions, and using kinetic bed therapy and semirecumbent position as opposed to full recumbent position (54).

Urinary Tract Infection

Urinary tract infections are probably the most common ICU nosocomial infections (55), and 1% to 3% manifest as bac-

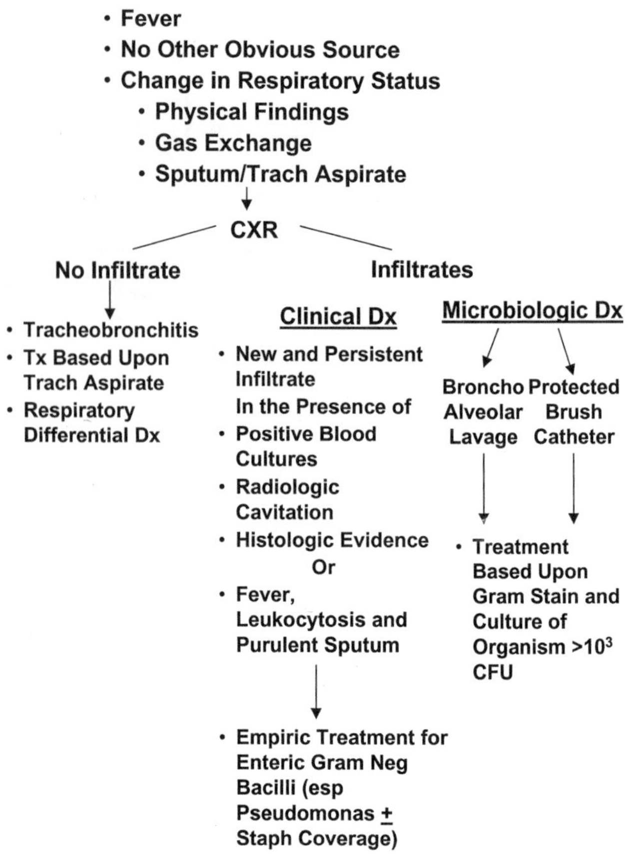

FIGURE 7. Approach to suspected ventilator-associated pneumonia.

teremia (56). Infection most commonly is accompanied by pyuria [>10 white blood cell count (WBC)/mm^2], with a colony count greater than 10^5 to help differentiate infection from colonization. The presence of candiduria should prompt an evaluation for disseminated candidiasis. Empiric therapy should be targeted at gram-negative organisms.

Sinusitis

Maxillary sinusitis is thought to arise from ostial occlusion by nasogastric or nasotracheal tubes, although that concept has been recently challenged (57) in a study which showed no difference in the incidence of sinusitis between the oral and nasal routes. Fever in a nasally instrumented patient should prompt a radiographic sinus series focusing on the maxillary sinuses, with consideration given to the use of CT scan if conventional radiographs are inadequate. Therapy should be directed toward treating gram-negative organisms because these are the most commonly encountered pathogens (58).

NONINFECTIOUS CAUSES OF FEVER

Given the nature of acute and chronic illness, invasive procedures performed, and variety of therapies initiated, patients in the ICU are exposed to a myriad of noninfectious causes of fever. After a thorough evaluation of infectious sources is undertaken and infectious sources are ruled out as the cause of fever, deciphering the cause of noninfectious fever should proceed along the lines of the pathway outlined in Figure 2. A careful history and physical examination and evaluation of appropriate diagnostic tests, in conjunction with the clinical scenario, should provide a point for initiation of further evaluation.

Drug Fever

A diagnosis of drug-induced fever should be suspected when fever coinciding with drug administration occurs in the absence of another cause of the fever (59). Between 2% and 7% of fevers on a general medical service can be ascribed to medications (1,3,4). Such fever is thought to be immunologic and cytokine mediated. The patient's status can be clinically indistinguishable from that accompanying an infectiously mediated temperature elevation (3,59). In contrast to traditional dogma, recent literature suggests that associations with relative bradycardia, rash, or eosinophilia are uncommon. No characteristic drug-induced fever pattern exists. Mackowiak and colleagues noted a variation in the time of onset of the drug-induced fever and that patients without concurrent cardiac disease have a minimal risk with rechallenge of the offending drug (59). If drug fever is suspected, the offending agent should be removed. ICU drugs associated with fever are listed in Table 2.

Transfusion Reactions

When a patient develops a fever during the course of a transfusion, an immediate evaluation should be undertaken because it is difficult to differentiate the cause of the febrile reaction (i.e., the recipient's plasma antibodies reacting to antigens on the transfused leukocyte cell membranes versus an acute hemolytic transfusion reaction caused by the recipient's plasma antibodies reacting to the transfused red blood cells). Allergic reactions to donor plasma and bacterial contamination of blood also can cause fever. Febrile reactions usually begin within 30 minutes of exposure and are generally self-limited. Use of leukocyte-poor products in selected patients can negate a subsequent febrile reaction. Hemolytic reactions are much less common (occurring in approximately 1 in 6,000 U transfused) (60) but are of greater significance. Intravascular hemolysis mediated by IgM or IgG and complement binding can occur quite rapidly after infusion of only several milliliters of blood. The classic symptoms of a hemolytic reaction, such as chest pain, headache, back pain, and dyspnea, may be obscured in the critically ill sedated, paralyzed,

TABLE 2. ICU DRUGS KNOWN TO CAUSE FEVER

Penicillins	Amphotericin B
Cimetidine	Sulfonamides
Hydralazine	Cephalosporins
Phenytoin	Procarbazine
Procainamide	Azathioprine
Quinidine	Dextrans

ICU, intensive care unit.

or unstable patient. Unexplained fever, hypotension, renal failure, and disseminated intravascular coagulopathy may therefore be the initial presenting signs. If any evidence of a transfusion reaction arises, the transfusion should be stopped immediately and a hemolysis evaluation initiated because the severity of the reaction correlates with the number of cells transfused (61).

Neuroleptic Malignant Syndrome and Malignant Hyperthermia

Neuroleptic malignant syndrome is a rare phenomenon that results from an imbalance in central neurotransmitters (decreased dopamine) and usually is due to neuroleptic drug use. This syndrome is characterized by hyperthermia, muscular rigidity, and alterations in consciousness; extrapyramidal signs and catatonia are common. Hyperthermia is thought to arise from the body's inability to dissipate heat produced by muscular contraction and the patient's inability to provide voluntary behavioral heat loss. In contrast to previous reports, recent literature suggests that mortality is quite low (62). Neuroleptic malignant syndrome differs from malignant hyperthermia in that the provocative agents are different, and, in the neuroleptic malignant syndrome, the mechanism of increased temperature is decreased central dopaminergic concentrations rather than abnormal peripheral calcium metabolism. Extrapyramidal signs occur only with neuroleptic malignant syndrome. Treatment consists of withdrawing the offending agent; reducing muscle contraction with dantrolene sodium; and using bromocriptine mesylate, amantadine hydrochloride, or dopamine hydrochloride to increase dopamine concentrations in the central nervous system.

Malignant hyperthermia, a syndrome characterized by a defect in skeletal-muscle calcium metabolism, results in muscle contraction or rigidity. This syndrome, in which net production exceeds the patient's capacity to dissipate that heat (Fig. 2), is associated with the use of halothane and succinylcholine, although multiple other associations have been reported. Injury is attributable to direct thermal damage and consists of rhabdomyolysis, hypercalcemia, cerebral edema, tachycardia, and vascular collapse. Hyperthermia is characteristically a late sign in an acute crisis (63). The differential diagnosis should include thyroid storm and pheochromocytoma. Supportive care combined with dantrolene sodium, which uncouples skeletal muscle contraction, is the treatment of choice.

EVALUATION OF POSTOPERATIVE FEVER

Although fever is common in postoperative patients, it is not common as a manifestation of infection. In one series, 9% of postoperative patients developed fever without a distinguishable origin (64); in another series, fever occurred in 15% of postoperative patients, with infection absent in two-thirds of those febrile patients (65). Noninfectious fever occurs more commonly as a single episode within the first 2 postoperative days and is of shorter duration (64,66). Fever developing after the fourth postoperative day is more likely to be of an infectious nature (65,66).

Given that fever may not represent infection, and that only 50% of infections in postoperative patients may manifest as fever

(66), the evaluation should proceed in a judicious manner using diagnostic studies, as necessary, based on a thorough history and physical examination (41,65). If no physical findings are present, the patient is immunocompetent, and a diagnosis of bacteremia is not suspected, the clinician should follow the patient's condition without further intervention unless the fever recurs. All wounds should be inspected to define a necrotizing process, and the differential diagnosis should include malignant hyperthermia, thromboembolic disease, and adrenal insufficiency.

SUMMARY

Evaluation of the febrile patient in the ICU can be quite difficult and challenging. A comprehensive approach using the history and physical examination is advocated to define a differential diagnosis and subsequent studies. Given the possible development of SIRS or MODS with attendant morbidity and mortality, the initial goal should be to confirm or eliminate an infectious cause of the fever.

KEY POINTS

Evaluation of the febrile response begins with a review of the pertinent medical history combined with a thorough physical examination. Given the sequelae of systemic inflammatory response syndrome (SIRS) and multiple-organ dysfunction syndrome (MODS), the initial focus of the evaluation should be directed toward excluding infectious causes of the fever. Common infectious sources include catheters, nosocomial pneumonia, urinary tract infections, sinusitis, and intraabdominal processes. Noninfectious causes, such as transfusion reactions, drug fever, and neuroleptic malignant syndrome, also need to be considered.

Diagnostic tests should be directed by the findings of the history and physical examination in the clinical context of the patient's presentation, with treatment appropriately targeted at the identified basis of the fever. Empiric antibiotic therapy should be reserved for patients in whom an infectious process has been identified or for patients at great risk for developing SIRS/MODS.

REFERENCES

1. McGowan JE Jr, Rose RC, Jacobs NF, et al. Fever in hospitalized patients: with special reference to the medical service. *Am J Med* 1987;82: 580–586.
2. Donowitz LG, Wenzel RP, Joyt JW. High risk of hospital-acquired infection in the ICU patient. *Crit Care Med* 1982;10:355–357.
3. Filice GA, Weiler MD, Hughes RA, et al. Nosocomial febrile illnesses in patients on an internal medicine service. *Arch Intern Med* 1989;149: 319–324.
4. Bor DH, Makadon HJ, Friedland G, et al. Fever in hospitalized medical patients: characteristics and significance. *J Gen Intern Med* 1988;3: 119–125.
5. Martin MA. Nosocomial infections in intensive care units: an overview of their epidemiology, outcome, and prevention. *New Horizons* 1993;1:162–171.
6. Gleckman R, Hibert D. Afebrile bacteremia: a phenomena in geriatric patients. *JAMA* 1982;248:1478–1481.
7. Musher DM, Fainstein V, Young EJ, et al. Fever patterns: their lack of clinical significance. *Arch Intern Med* 1979;139:1225–1228.
8. Mellors JW, Horwitz RI, Harvey MR, et al. A simple index to identify occult bacterial infection in adults with acute unexplained fever. *Arch Intern Med* 1987;147:666–671.
9. Bryant RE, Hood AF, Hood CE, et al. Factors affecting mortality of gram-negative rod bacteremia. *Arch Intern Med* 1971;127:120– 128.
10. Weinstein MR, Iannini PB, Stratton CW, et al. Spontaneous bacterial peritonitis: a review of 28 cases with emphasis on improved survival and factors influencing prognosis. *Am J Med* 1978;64:592–598.
11. Dorn TF, DeAngelis C, Baumgardner RA, et al. Acetaminophens: more harm than good for chicken-pox? *J Pediatr* 1989;114:1045–1048.
12. Mackowiak PA. Fever: blessing or curse? A unifying hypothesis. *Ann Intern Med* 1994;120:1037–1040.
13. O'Donnel J, Axelrod P, Fisher C, et al. Use of and effectiveness of hypothermia blankets for febrile patients in the intensive care unit. *Clin Infect Dis* 1997;24:1208–1213.
14. Lenhardt R, Negishi C, Sessler DI, et al. The effects of physical treatment on induced fever in humans. *Am J Med* 1999;106:550–555.
15. Clemmer TP, Fischer CJ. Boue RC, et al. Hypothermia in the sepsis syndrome and clinical outcome: the Methylprednisolone Severe Sepsis Study Group. *Crit Care Med* 1992;20:1395–1401.
16. Arons MM, Wheller AP, Bernard GR, et al. Effects of ibuprofen on the physiology and survival of hypothermic sepsis. *Crit Care Med* 1999;27:699–707.
17. Bossink AWJ, Groeneveld ABJ, Koffeman GI, et al. Prediction of shock in febrile medical patients with a clinical infection. *Crit Care Med* 2001;29:25–31.
18. Washington JA II, Illstrup DM. Blood cultures: Issues and controversies. *Rev Infect Dis* 1986;8:792–802.
19. Jarvis WR, Edwards JR, Culver DH, et al. Nosocomial infection rates in adult and pediatric intensive care units in the United States: National Nosocomial Infections Surveillance System. *Am J Med* 1991;91:1855– 1915.
20. Vincent JL, Bihari DJ, Suter PM, et al. The prevalence of nosocomial infection n the intensive care units in Europe: results of the European prevalence of infection in intensive care (EPIC) Study. EPIC International Advisory Committee. *JAMA* 1995;274:639–644.
21. Banerjee SN, Emori TG, Culver DH, et al. Nocturnal Nosocomial Infections Surveillance (NNIS) System: secular trends in primary blood stream infections in the United States. 1980–1989 *Am J Med* 1991;91(Suppl):S86–S89.
22. Richet H, Hubert B, Nitemberg G, et al. Prospective multicenter study of vascular catheter-related complications and risk factors for positive central catheter cultures in intensive care unit patients. *J Clin Microbiol* 1990;28:2520–2525.
23. Maki DG. Infections caused by intravascular devices used for infusion therapy: pathogenesis, prevention and management. In: Bisno AL, Waldvogel FA, eds. *Infections associated with indwelling medical devices*, 2nd ed. Washington, D.C.: American Society for Microbiology; 1994.
24. Sheretz RJ. Surveillance for infections associated with vascular catheters. *Infect Control Hosp Epidemiol* 1996;17:746–752.
25. Heiselman D, Tarora D, Wenzel RP. Nosocomial bloodstream infections in the critically ill. *JAMA* 1994;272:1578–1601.
26. Pittet D, Tarara D, Wenzel RP. Nosocomial bloodstream infections in critically ill patients: excess length of stay, extra costs, and attributable mortality. *JAMA* 1994;271:1598–1601.
27. Maki DG, Stolz SM, Wheeler S, et al. Prevention of central venous

catheter related blood stream infection by use of an anti-septic impregnated catheter: a randomized controlled study. *Ann Intern Med* 1997;127:257–2666.

28. Collignon PJ, Soni N, Pearson IY, et al. Is semiquantitative culture of central vein catheter tips useful in the diagnosis of catheter-associated bacteremia? *J Clin Microbial* 1986;24:532–535.

29. Seigman-Igra Y, Anglim AM, Shapiro DE, et al. Diagnosis of vascular catheter related bloodstream infections: a meta-analysis. *J Clin Microbiol* 1997;35:928–933.

30. Raad II, Bodey GP. Infectious complications of indwelling vascular catheters. *Clin Infect Dis* 1992;15:197–210.

31. Blot F, Nitenberg G, Chachaty E, et al. Diagnosis of catheter related bacterium: a prospective comparison of the time to positivity of central vs. peripheral blood cultures. *Lancet* 1999;354(9184):1071–1077.

32. Raad II, Hohn DC, Gilbreath BJ, et al. Prevention of central venous catheter related infections by using maximal sterile barrier precautions during insertion. *Infect Control Hosp Epidemiol* 1994;15:231–238.

33. Veenstra DL, Saint S, Saha S, et al. Efficiency of antiseptic impregnated central venous catheters in preventing catheter related bloodstream infection: a meta-analysis. *JAMA* 1999;281:261–267.

34. Darouiche R, Raad II, Heard SO, et al. A comparison of two antimicrobial-impregnated central venous catheters. *N Eng J Med* 1999;340:1–8.

35. Brown RB, Hosmer D, Chen HC, et al. A comparison of infections for different ICUs within the same hospital. *Crit Care Med* 1985;13:472–476.

36. Fry DE, Garrison RN, Heitsch RC, et al. Determinants of death in patients with intraabdominal abscess. *Surgery* 1980;88:517–523.

37. Rogers PN, Wright RH. Postoperative intra-abdominal abscess. *Surgery* 1980;88:517–523.

38. Trynet P, Legall JR, Gagwiez PL, et al. Computed tomography and post-laparotomy intra-abdominal abscess. *Intensive Care Med* 1982;8:193–196.

39. Roche J. Effectiveness of computed tomography in the diagnosis of intra-abdominal abscess: a review of 111 patients. *Med J Aust* 1981;2:85–88.

40. Norwood SH, Civetta JM. Abdominal CT scanning in critically ill surgical patients. *Ann Surg* 1985;202:166–175.

41. Norwood SH. An approach to the febrile ICU patient. In: Civetta JM, Taylor RW, Kirby RR, eds. *Critical care*, 2nd ed. Philadelphia: JB Lippincott, 1992:983–994.

42. O'Grady NP, Barie PS, Bartlett J. Practice parameters for evaluating new fever in critically ill adult patients. *Crit Care Med* 1998;26:392–408.

43. Cook DJ, Watter S, Cook RJ, et al. The incidence and risk factors for ventilator associated pneumonia in critically ill patients. *Ann Intern Med* 1998;129:433–440.

44. Rello J, Ausina V, Ricard M, et al. Impact of previous antimicrobial therapy on the etiology and outcome of ventilator-associated pneumonia. *Chest* 1993;104:1230–1235.

45. Heyland DK, Cook DJ, Griffith LE, et al. The attributable morbidity and mortality of ventilator associated pneumonia in the critically ill patient. *Am J Respir Care Med* 1999;159:1249–1256.

46. Trouilette JL, Chastre J, Vuagnat A, et al. Ventilator associated pneu-

monia caused by potentially drug resistant bacteria. *Am Rev Respir Crit Care Med* 1998;157:531–539.

47. Torres A, Aznar R, Garell JM, et al. Incidence, risk and prognosis factors of nosocomial pneumonia in mechanically ventilated patients. *Am Rev Respir Dis* 1990;142:523–528.

48. Kolleff M. Ventilator associated pneumonia: a multivariate analysis. *JAMA* 1992;270:1965–1970.

49. Fagan JY, Chastre J, Hance AJ, et al. Detection of nosocomial lung infection in ventilated patients: use of a protected specimen brush and quantitative culture techniques in 147 Patients. *Am Rev Respir Dis* 1988;138:110–116.

50. Niederman MS, Torres A, Summer W. Invasive diagnostic testing is not needed routinely to manage suspected ventilator-associated pneumonia. *Am J Respir Crit Care Med* 1994;150:565–569.

51. Meduri GU. Ventilator-associated pneumonia in patients with respiratory failure: a diagnostic approach. *Chest* 1990;97:1208–1219.

52. Corley DE, Kirtland SH, Winterbaner RH, et al. Reproducibility of the histologic diagnosis of pneumonia among a panel of four pathologists: analysis of a gold standard. *Chest* 1997;112:458–465.

53. Luna CM, Vajacich P, Niederman MS, et al. Impact of BAL data on the therapy and outcome of ventilation associated pneumonia. *Chest* 1997;111:676–685.

54. Cook DB. Ventilator associated pneumonia. *Curr Opin Crit Care* 1999;5:350–356.

55. Daschner FD, Frey P, Wolff G, et al. Nosocomial infections in intensive care wards: a multicenter prospective trial. *Intensive Care Med* 1982;8:5–9.

56. Turck M, Stamm W. Nosocomial infections of the urinary tract. *Am J Med* 1981;70:651–654.

57. Holzapfel L, Chevret S, Madinier G, et al. Influence of long-term oral or nasotracheal intubation on nosocomial maxillary sinusitis and pneumonia: results of a prospective randomized, clinical trial. *Crit Care Med* 1993;21:1132–1138.

58. Caplan ES, Hoyt NJ. Nosocomial sinusitis. *JAMA* 1982;247:639–641.

59. Mackowiak PA, LeMaistre CF. Drug fever: a critical appraisal of conventional concepts. An analysis of 51 episodes in two Dallas hospitals and 97 episodes reported in the English literature. *Ann Intern Med* 1987;106:728–733.

60. Pineda AA, Brzica SM Jr, Taswell HF. Hemolytic transfusion reaction: recent experience in a large blood bank. *Mayo Clin Proc* 1978;53:378–390.

61. Gregory SA, McKenna R, Sassetti RJ, et al. Hematologic emergencies. *Med Clin North Am* 1986;70:1129–1149.

62. Rosebush P, Stewart T. A prospective analysis of 24 episodes of neuroleptic malignant syndrome. *Am J Psychiatry* 1989;146:717.

63. Garibaldi RA, Brodine S, Matsumiya S, et al. Evidence for non-infectious etiology of early postoperative fever. *Infect Control Hosp Epidemiol* 1985;6:273–277.

64. Freischlag J, Busuttil RW. The value of postoperative fever evaluation. *Surgery* 1983;94:358–363.

65. Galicier C, Richet H. A prospective study of postoperative fever in a general surgery department. *Infect Control* 1985;6:487–490.

66. Steward DJ. Malignant hyperthermia: the acute crisis. *Int Anesthesiol Clin* 1979;17:1–9.

MULTIPLE-ORGAN DYSFUNCTION SYNDROME

STEPHEN O. HEARD
MITCHELL P. FINK

KEY WORDS

- Apoptosis
- Bradykinin
- Complement
- Cytokines
- Leukotrienes
- Multiple-organ dysfunction syndrome
- Multiple-organ failure syndrome
- Nitric oxide
- Oxygen consumption
- Oxygen radicals
- Platelet-activating factor
- Prostaglandins
- Resuscitation
- Sepsis
- Systemic inflammatory response syndrome

INTRODUCTION

Despite vast improvements in critical care medicine, many critically ill patients often suffer progressive deterioration in the function of multiple organs, a phenomenon that has been termed the multiple-organ dysfunction syndrome (MODS) (1). MODS is the primary cause of death for patients in the surgical intensive care unit (ICU). The financial toll is significant: more than 60% of ICU resources are consumed by patients with MODS (2).

Individual organ dysfunction may result from a direct insult, such as pulmonary aspiration of stomach contents or renal contusion (primary MODS), or it can be associated with a systemic process, such as sepsis or pancreatitis (secondary MODS). Although the development of secondary MODS is usually preceded by a period of hemodynamic instability, the precise risk factors for the development of the syndrome are obscure. Alterations in organ function observed during MODS are a continuum rather than sentinel events indicating the failure of a particular organ. There are a number of organ dysfunction scores, each with its own attributes (3) (Table 1). In general, the greater the number of organs that are dysfunctional, the greater the risk of death. The Brussels score can be used to calculate failure-free days (3), a useful feature for clinical trials. Performing daily MOD scores and calculating a maximum MOD score or a "delta" score (by subtracting the maximum score from the baseline score) appears to be more accurate than Acute Physiologic and Chronic Health Evaluation (APACHE) II or the Organ Failure Score (OFS) in predicting outcome (4).

PATHOPHYSIOLOGY

MODS usually occurs in patients who exhibit findings indicative of a generalized inflammatory response that has been defined as the systemic inflammatory response syndrome (SIRS) (1) (Table 2). SIRS commonly occurs as a result of infection, but other conditions, such as necrotizing pancreatitis or severe trauma, can also lead to systemic manifestations of poorly controlled inflammation. SIRS due to infection has been defined as sepsis. For those patients who present with SIRS, a substantial proportion will develop sepsis, septic shock, and MODS (5). Although documented infection is not required for the development of MODS, the entities of SIRS, sepsis, and MODS appear to be closely related entities. As a result, the following review of the pathophysiology of MODS will also include discussions of SIRS and sepsis.

Derangements in Oxygen Delivery and Consumption

In most tissues, oxygen consumption (VO_2) is determined by metabolic demand and is independent of oxygen delivery (DO_2). When DO_2 is reduced, VO_2 is maintained by increased O_2 extraction. If DO_2 is reduced to the point where metabolic needs cannot be met, VO_2 then becomes "supply-dependent" (Fig. 1). The point at which VO_2 becomes supply-dependent is called the critical DO_2. Although one study suggests that the critical DO_2 appears to be approximately 330 mL per minute per M^2 in anesthetized humans (6), another investigation where life support was withdrawn in critically ill patients indicates the value is probably much lower (7).

Many studies from the 1970s and 1980s demonstrated that patients with sepsis or acute respiratory distress syndrome (ARDS) had a systemic VO_2 that was supply-dependent over a wide range of DO_2 values (8,9). Because oxygen consumption is independent of oxygen transport in critically ill patients without sepsis or ARDS, the apparent coupling of these two parameters in

TABLE 1. COMPARISON OF THE PHYSIOLOGIC AND BIOCHEMICAL PARAMETERS USED BY FOUR SCORING SYSTEMS FOR ORGAN DYSFUNCTION AND FAILURE

Organ System	Sequential Organ Failure Assessment (SOFA) (111)	Multiple Organ Dysfunction Score (MODS) (112)	Logistic Organ Dysfunction (LOD) (113)	Brussels (114)
Cardiovascular	Blood pressure and vasopressor use	Blood pressure adjusted heart rate	Blood pressure and heart rate	Blood pressure, fluid responsiveness, and acidosis
Pulmonary	PaO_2/FIO_2 and mechanical ventilation	PaO_2/FIO_2	PaO_2/FIO_2 and mechanical ventilation	PaO_2/FIO_2
Hepatic	Bilirubin	Bilirubin	Bilirubin and prothrombin time	Bilirubin
Hematologic	Platelets	Platelets	Platelets and white blood cell count	Platelets
Renal	Creatinine and urine output	Creatinine	Creatinine, blood urea nitrogen, or urine output	Creatinine
Central nervous system	Glasgow Coma Score (GCS)	GCS	GCS	GCS

Reprinted from Bernard GR. Quantification of organ dysfunction: seeking standardization. *Crit Care Med* 1998;26:1767–1768, with permission.

patients with sepsis or ARDS has been termed pathologic supply dependency (10). The presence of pathologic supply dependency is important as this implies that an oxygen deficit exists at the cellular level and some tissues may be relatively ischemic even when global perfusion is preserved. As a result, inadequate production of adenosine triphosphate (ATP) or other high-energy phosphates at the cellular level may contribute to organ failure in patients with MODS.

TABLE 2. AMERICAN COLLEGE OF CHEST PHYSICIANS/SOCIETY OF CRITICAL CARE MEDICINE DEFINITIONS OF SEPSIS AND ORGAN FAILURE

A. Infection: Microbial phenomenon characterized by an inflammatory response to the presence of the microorganism or the invasion of normally sterile host tissue by those organisms.
B. Bacteremia: The presence of viable bacteria in the blood.
C. Systemic Inflammatory Response Syndrome (SIRS): The systemic inflammatory response to a variety of severe clinical insults, manifested by two or more of the following conditions:
   Temperature >38°C or <36°C
   Heart rate >90 beats/min
   Respiratory rate >20 breaths/min or $PaCO_2$ <32 mm Hg
   WBC >12,000 cells/mm³, <4,000 cells/min³, or >10% immature (band) forms
D. Sepsis: The systemic response to infection. The manifestations are the same as those enumerated for SIRS.
E. Severe Sepsis: Sepsis associated with organ dysfunction, hypoperfusion, or hypotension.
F. Septic Shock: Sepsis with hypotension, despite adequate fluid resuscitation, and perfusion abnormalities, including but not limited to the following:
   Lactic acidosis
   Oliguria
   Acute alteration in mental status
G. Hypotension: A systolic BP <90 torr or a reduction of >40 mm Hg from baseline in the absence of other causes for hypotension.
H. Multiple Organ Dysfunction Syndrome: Presence of altered organ function in an acutely ill patient such that homeostasis cannot be maintained without intervention.

WBC, white blood cells; BP, blood pressure.
Condensed from American College of Chest Physicians/Society of Critical Care Medicine Consensus Conference: Definitions for sepsis and organ failure and guidelines for the use of innovative therapies in sepsis. *Crit Care Med* 1992;20:864–874.

Subsequently, the validity of this concept was challenged, and indeed, this phenomenon may be more artifactual than real. Mathematical coupling of data, pooling of data, and spontaneous changes in metabolic demand can explain many of the findings of these studies. Carefully performed investigations showed that systemic VO_2 is independent of systemic DO_2 in patients with sepsis or ARDS (11,12) and that the critical DO_2 is no higher in patients with sepsis than in critically ill patients without sepsis. Supply dependency may occur in some vascular beds during SIRS or sepsis and there may be a diffusive loss of oxygen at the precapillary level (13), thereby contributing to the development of MODS, but the frequency with which this occurs is unknown.

Functional cellular hypoxia ("cytopathic hypoxia") may occur under certain conditions rendering the cell incapable of using oxygen to produce ATP despite adequate delivery of oxygen (14). Studies using different animal models of sepsis have shown that tissue PO_2 is normal or even increased above normal in many organs despite the presence of systemic or tissue acidosis (15,16). Clinical investigations have shown that skeletal muscle PO_2 is high

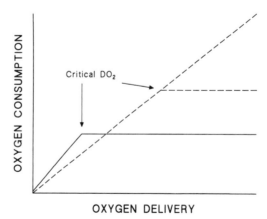

FIGURE 1. The proposed relationship between oxygen consumption and oxygen delivery. The *solid line* depicts the normal relationship; the *dashed line* depicts pathologic supply dependency of oxygen consumption. Some studies have failed to identify a critical DO_2 in septic patients. See text for details.

in septic patients whereas it is low in patients with cardiogenic shock (17,18). These data suggest that oxygen delivery is not deficient in sepsis and the tissue acidosis is due to alterations in cellular function. The mechanism by which cytopathic hypoxia occurs is unclear but may involve a change in the ability of cytochrome a, a$_3$ to donate electrons to oxygen, decreased availability of mitochondrial reduced nicotine adenine dinucleotide (NADH) due to activation of poly (ADP-ribose) polymerase (PARP) (19), or uncoupling of oxidative phosphorylation as a result of the loss of the protonic gradient across the mitochondria or changes in the mitochondrial permeability transition (13). Recent studies using a rat model of endotoxemic shock strongly implicate excessive production of nitric oxide due to increased expression of the enzyme inducible nitric oxide synthase (iNOS) as being important in the development of cytopathic hypoxia (20,21).

Role of Inflammatory and Vasoactive Mediators

Early clinical series describing MODS emphasized the importance of uncontrolled infection in the pathophysiology of MODS (22). Subsequent reports have supported the hypothesis that sepsis is a key risk factor for the development of MODS, but it is important to note that MODS complicates the course of many critically ill patients without documented infections (23). Because of these observations, it has been suggested that either extensive tissue injury (as observed in trauma or pancreatitis) or sepsis can trigger the systemic release of inflammatory mediators that lead to further tissue injury and MODS (24,25).

Complement, Neutrophils, and Reactive Oxygen Metabolites

The complement cascade is activated via two pathways. The classic pathway is triggered by antibody-coated targets or antigen-antibody complexes, while the alternative pathway is activated by aggregated immunoglobulins, products of tissue trauma, lipopolysaccharide (LPS), and other complex polysaccharides (e.g., zymosan). Products of the complement pathway activate neutrophils, which in turn obstruct capillaries and damage endothelium by releasing lysosomal enzymes and toxic oxygen radicals (Table 3). Adhesion molecules, which are expressed on both polymorphonuclear leukocytes (PMNs) and vascular endothelium in response to endotoxin and inflammatory mediators, facilitate the adherence and diapedesis of PMNs through the endothelium.

Complement-mediated activation of neutrophils may be important in the pathophysiology of MODS (26). Activation of both complement and neutrophils occurs in patients with ARDS (an important component of MODS) or thermal injury and in trauma patients who ultimately develop ARDS (26,27). These activated neutrophils accumulate in the lungs of at least some patients with ARDS. In addition, evidence of complement and neutrophil activation can be found in the bronchoalveolar lavage (BAL) fluid from patients with ARDS (28). However, since ARDS can occur in patients with few circulating neutrophils, activated neutrophils are only one of several likely mediators capable of injuring the lung (and presumably other organs) in sepsis and MODS.

TABLE 3. INFLAMMATORY MEDIATORS IMPORTANT IN THE PATHOGENESIS OF SEPSIS AND THE MULTIPLE ORGAN DYSFUNCTION SYNDROME

Complement (C3a, C5a)
Neutrophil products
  Proteases
    Neutral proteases
      Elastase
      Cathepsin G
      Collagenase
    Acid hydrolase
      Cathepsins B and D
      β-glucuronidase
      Glucosaminase
Oxygen radicals
  Superoxide anion
  Hydroxyl radical
  Hydrogen peroxide
  Peroxynitrite
Bradykinin
Lipid mediators
  Prostaglandins
    Thromboxane A$_2$
    Prostaglandin I$_2$
    Prostaglandin E$_2$
Leukotrienes (LTB$_4$, LTC$_4$, LTD$_4$, LTE$_4$)
Platelet-activating factor (PAF)
Cytokines
  Tumor necrosis factor-α (TNF-α)
  Interleukins (IL-1, IL-6, IL-8)
  High-mobility group-1 (HMG-1)
Macrophage migration inhibition factor (MIF)
Nitric oxide

Reactive oxygen species (superoxide anion, hydrogen peroxide, and the hydroxyl radical) are released by activated PMNs and can injure tissues by damaging DNA, crosslinking cellular proteins, and causing peroxidation of membrane lipids (29,30). Lipid peroxidation can alter cellular function by diminishing membrane fluidity and increasing membrane permeability. Clinical data suggest that toxic oxygen metabolites are important mediators in the pathophysiology of ARDS. In humans with ARDS, plasma levels of lipid peroxides are elevated, increased levels of hydrogen peroxide in the expiratory condensate have been measured (31), and analysis of BAL fluid reveals evidence of oxidative damage to proteins (32). Furthermore, patients with ARDS have reduced levels of oxygen radical scavengers in plasma or BAL fluid (33), a sign of "oxidant stress." However, antioxidant therapies thus far have not improved the outcome in humans with ARDS or MODS although such interventions may increase the number of days "free" of acute lung injury (34) and reduce oxidative stress during septic shock (35).

Reactive oxygen species (including peroxynitrite) also cause breaks in DNA, activate PARP, and deplete NADH and ATP in cell culture. PARP catalyzes the cleavage of NADH into ADP-ribose and nicotinamide and helps form a covalent bond between the newly formed ADP-ribose and various proteins. Further cleavage of NADH results in more ADP-ribose attaching to the originally produced ADP-ribose, ultimately forming a large polymer. Since NADH is required for oxidative phosphorylation,

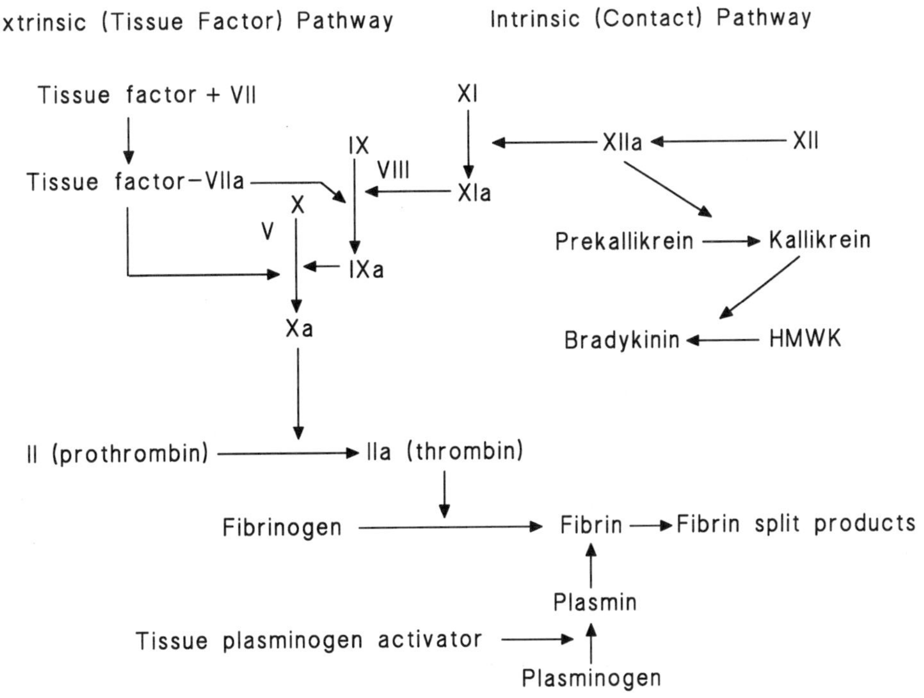

Extrinsic (Tissue Factor) Pathway Intrinsic (Contact) Pathway

FIGURE 2. The coagulation cascade. *HMWK*, high-molecular-weight kininogen.

degradation of NADH can cause cellular energy (ATP) depletion (13).

The Kallikrein-Kinin System

The kallikrein-kinin system is part of the contact system (complement, coagulation, and kallikrein-kinins) (Fig. 2). Bradykinin, the final product of this cascade, is a potent vasodilator and increases vascular permeability. Both experimental and clinical data suggest that the kallikrein-kinin system participates in the pathophysiology of sepsis and MODS. However, a trial of a bradykinin-receptor antagonist (CP-0127) for the adjuvant therapy of sepsis in humans failed to alter 28-day mortality (36). A subset of patients with gram-negative sepsis may benefit from this treatment.

The Coagulation System

Endotoxin and many proinflammatory mediators will activate the coagulation system (Fig. 2). Coagulation in sepsis or inflammatory states is initiated primarily by the extrinsic (tissue-factor dependent) pathway (37) as these mediators (e.g., tumor necrosis factor-α [TNF-α]) induce the expression of tissue factor (TF) on monocytes and endothelial cells. Although these same mediators will cause activation of the fibrinolytic system, subsequent increases in plasminogen activator inhibitor-1 (PAI-1) effectively suppress fibrinolysis. Important inhibitors of coagulation such as antithrombin, tissue factor pathway inhibitor (TFPI), protein C, protein S, and endothelial-bound modulators (heparin sulfate and thrombomodulin) may be downregulated. Thus, the net effect is a procoagulant tendency with the potential for development of disseminated intravascular coagulation (DIC). DIC can result in microvascular thrombosis and organ failure and/or

bleeding from consumption of platelets and clotting factors (38). Inhibition of the coagulation cascade by activated protein C has been shown to reduce the relative risk of death in patients with severe sepsis by over 19% (38a). Other studies evaluating the effectiveness of inhibitors of coagulation in sepsis and septic shock are currently underway (TFPI therapy).

Prostaglandins, Leukotrienes, and Platelet-Activating Factor

Prostaglandins (PGs), leukotrienes (LTs), and platelet-activating factor (PAF) are potent lipid mediators that may be important in the pathophysiology of sepsis and MODS (Table 2). Extensive literature suggests that PGs are important mediators in experimental endotoxicosis, sepsis, and ARDS (39). However, clinical data supporting a predominant role for PGs in the development of MODS and sepsis are weaker. Plasma and urinary concentrations of PGs are elevated in patients with sepsis, septic shock, or ARDS. Plasma phospholipase A2 levels (the enzyme that cleaves the precursor of PG formation, arachidonic acid, from membrane-bound phospholipids) are elevated in patients with septic shock and pancreatitis and correlate with the degree of hypotension (40,41). However, investigations have shown little or no benefit from treating septic or ARDS patients with inhibitors of the enzymes that form PGs or with immunomodulating PGs (42,43).

The role of the LTs as significant mediators in experimental sepsis, other shock states, and ARDS is unclear (44). Clinical studies have implicated LTs in the pathogenesis of ARDS. In a number of investigations, elevated levels of LTs have been found in the BAL fluid or urine of patients with ARDS or at risk for the development of ARDS. In one study, LT levels correlated with the onset of ARDS. The mechanism by which LTs may contribute to the pathogenesis of ARDS is priming of neutrophils for the release of superoxide and elastase (45).

PAF is synthesized and released by platelets, neutrophils, monocytes, macrophages, endothelial cells, and other cell types and has a variety of biologic actions, including aggregation of platelets, activation of neutrophils, bronchoconstriction, and enhancement of microvascular permeability (44). As with the PGs and LTs, results of animal studies indicate an important role for PAF in the pathophysiology of sepsis and MODS; however, clinical data implicating a role for PAF in the development of human sepsis or MODS are somewhat limited. Elevated levels of PAF have been measured in empyema fluid and in plasma from septic patients (46). An association between plasma levels of PAF-acetylhydrolase (the enzyme responsible for PAF degradation) and MODS in trauma patients has been reported (47). Unfortunately, recent randomized, placebo-controlled, double-blind trials evaluating the safety and efficacy of PAF-receptor antagonists used to treat patients with severe sepsis or SIRS failed to demonstrate that these agents were of benefit in reducing mortality (48,49).

Cytokines

Cytokines are small proteins that are secreted by nearly all nucleated cells and exhibit autocrine, paracrine, or endocrine activity (50). These cytokines are generally classified as proinflammatory or antiinflammatory molecules. However, this classification is somewhat arbitrary since an individual cytokine may function either as an antiinflammatory or proinflammatory agent depending on the underlying biologic process. Proinflammatory cytokines (most notably TNF-α and interleukin [IL]-1) can trigger the release of other mediators including PAF, NO, LTs, and PGs. These cytokines also induce the expression of adhesion molecules on neutrophils and endothelial cells, thereby promoting neutrophil recruitment to the site of injury or infection. As mentioned previously, enhanced expression of TF on endothelial cells caused by these cytokines can lead to activation of the extrinsic pathway of coagulation and may result in DIC.

TNF-α plays an important role in the pathogenesis of human sepsis, septic shock, and MODS (51). Small doses of LPS or recombinant human TNF-α, when injected into humans, will reproduce many of the metabolic and cardiovascular changes that are similar to those observed in compensated sepsis (52). Similar findings are observed in animal studies, and administration of anti–TNF-α antibodies will prevent many of the adverse consequences of endotoxic or live gram-negative bacterial shock. However, in studies of critically ill patients, the correlation of plasma TNF-α levels and outcome is variable. These disparate results may be due to timing and method of the TNF-α assay and the acuity and etiology of the patient's illness. Results from multicenter studies of adjuvant therapy of sepsis with either anti–TNF-α antibodies or recombinant-soluble TNF-α receptors have been disappointing: neither the antibodies nor soluble receptors appear to reduce mortality of patients with sepsis. However, in one recent trial where patients were stratified according to initial plasma levels of IL-6, outcome was improved and organ dysfunction ameliorated with the administration of a monoclonal antibody to TNF-α (53).

Recent data suggest that a genetic predisposition for enhanced TNF-α production during inflammation or sepsis may occur in some patients. Individuals who are homozygote for a certain type of TNF-α promoter gene (54) appear to have a higher susceptibility for septic shock and death. Furthermore, trauma patients who are homozygote for a particular TNF-β gene have an increased rate of sepsis and higher levels of TNF-α during sepsis (55). Such patients might be able to be identified early and benefit from anti–TNF-α therapy.

Like TNF-α, IL-1, IL-6, and IL-8 have a wide variety of biologic actions and have been implicated in the pathogenesis of sepsis and MODS (56). In addition, TNF-α and IL-1 often act in a synergistic fashion. Many biologic properties of IL-1 are due to increases in prostaglandin E_2 (PGE_2) as a result of increased transcription of the cyclooxygenase-2 (COX-2) enzyme induced by IL-1 (50). One clinical trial investigating the efficacy of a recombinant IL-1-receptor antagonist for the treatment of sepsis failed to demonstrate an overall survival benefit (57).

Recently, two other cytokines, high-mobility group-1 (HMG-1) and macrophage migration inhibition factor (MIF), have been implicated as causing delayed toxicity due to endotoxemia in experimental animals. Originally described as a T lymphocyte-derived factor that inhibited the random migration of macrophages, MIF is now known to be secreted by the anterior pituitary gland as well as macrophages and T lymphocytes that have been stimulated by glucocorticoids. Once released, MIF overcomes the inhibitory effects of glucocorticoids on TNF-α, IL-1, IL-6, and IL-8 production by LPS-stimulated monocytes *in vitro* and suppresses the protective effects of steroids against lethal endotoxemia *in vivo* (58,59). HMG-1 is a DNA-binding protein that has been known to biochemists and molecular biologists for years, but was just recognized to be a late-acting cytokine that is capable of causing death (60) and acute lung injury (61) in endotoxemic animals. High levels of circulating HMG-1 are detectable in patients with lethal, but not nonlethal sepsis (60).

Nitric Oxide

NO (62) is an inorganic free-radical gas and is derived from one of the terminal guanidino nitrogens of L-arginine, catalyzed by a group of enzymes called NO synthases. Two general classes of NO synthases have been described: constitutive (calcium-dependent) NO synthases (neuronal and endothelial) and inducible (calcium-independent) NO synthase. The production of the latter enzyme is induced by endotoxin, TNF-α, and other inflammatory mediators. NO is released by a variety of cells and tissues, including endothelium, vascular smooth muscle, neutrophils, and mononuclear, glial, mast, hepatic, and adrenal medullary cells. Some of the important physiologic actions of NO include vasorelaxation, neurotransmission, and microbicidal activity. The role that NO plays in the host is a function of the rate and timing of its production and the surrounding environment (62). Normally, it will act as a direct signaling messenger (e.g., vasorelaxation, neurotransmission) and cytoprotective agent (62). Alternatively, it may function as an indirect cytotoxic molecule (Fig. 3).

It appears that NO plays a significant role in the pathophysiology of sepsis and MODS. Increased urinary excretion of two

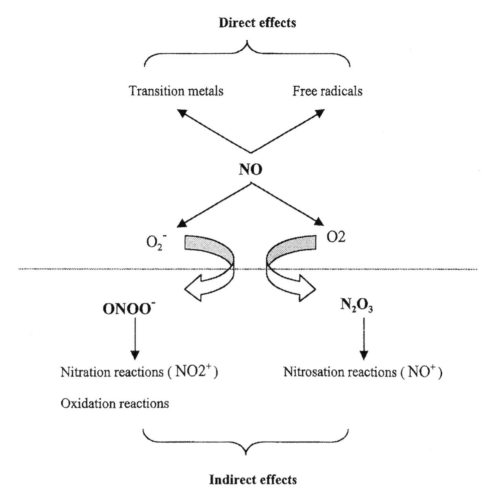

FIGURE 3. The chemistry of nitric oxide. *ONOO⁻*, peroxynitrite. Examples of direct effects include vasodilation, physiologic control of cell respiration, and signal transduction in the nervous system. Examples of indirect effects are inhibition of glycolysis and reduced transcriptional activity. (From Liaudet L, Soriano FG, Szabo C. Biology of nitric oxide signaling. *Crit Care Med* 2000;28:N37–N52, with permission.)

NO metabolites (nitrite and nitrate) has been reported in septic patients and correlates inversely with systemic vascular resistance (SVR) (63). Excretion of nitrate also has been shown to increase dramatically following administration of a cytokine, IL-2, which, when infused in humans, can induce a syndrome similar to MODS (64). In many animal studies, NO reduces myocardial contractility in a concentration-dependent fashion (65). Excess NO in the presence of superoxide anion results in the formation of peroxynitrite, a reactive oxidant that causes lipid peroxidation, inhibits mitochondrial respiration, inactivates glyceraldehyde-3-phosphate dehydrogenase, inhibits membrane sodium/potassium ATP activity, and triggers DNA single-strand breakage. DNA damage activates the nuclear enzyme PARP, which can lead to cellular energy depletion and death (66). In addition, excessive amounts of NO and peroxynitrite can activate the transcription factor, NFκB, thereby increasing the inflammatory response (66).

The efficacy of inhibitors of NO synthase in the treatment of sepsis and MODS is unclear and the use of some inhibitors may actually be detrimental. Although blood pressure rises with the use of nonspecific NO-synthase inhibitors, cardiac performance and perfusion to some vascular beds may be impaired (67). A large randomized, prospective trial evaluating the efficacy of the nonspecific NO-synthase inhibitor, L-N^G-monomethylarginine, in patients with septic shock was terminated early because the experimental agent increased mortality (68). In addition, because NO appears to be an important component in neutrophil function against various pathogens, use of NO-synthase inhibitors for the treatment of septic shock may have an adverse effect on the host response to infection.

Derangements in the Barrier Function of the Intestinal Mucosa

Normally, the mucosa and lymphoid tissue of the gastrointestinal (GI) tract represent an effective barrier that prevents the systemic absorption of intraluminal microbes and microbial products (including LPS). This barrier consists of the tight junctions between mucosal epithelial cells, the mucous layer secreted by the epithelium, secretory immunoglobulin A, and local cell-mediated immune mechanisms. It has been hypothesized that derangements in the barrier function of the intestine permit the systemic absorption of gut-derived microbes (a process termed "translocation") and microbial products, thereby initiating and propagating a septic or generalized inflammatory state. Disruption of this barrier may be due to alterations in oxygen delivery to the tips of the intestinal villi, resulting in ischemia or nutrition factors such as relative deficiencies of glutamine.

The role of altered GI-barrier function in the pathogenesis of MODS in humans remains poorly defined. Gut permeability to nonabsorbable solutes is increased in a number of disease states; however, alterations in gut permeability do not appear to correlate with acuity of illness or survival. Although some investigators have demonstrated a 10% rate of positive mesenteric lymph node cultures in trauma patients (suggesting translocation), it is unclear whether or not this phenomenon is a normal response by gut-associated lymphoid tissue (GALT) or a pathologic event (69).

Apoptosis

Apoptosis is a mode of "active" cell death that is evolutionarily conserved and is energy-dependent (70). It is composed of three phases (Fig. 4). The first phase (initiation) is induced by means of a number of mediators including lipopolysaccharide, TNF-α and Fas ligand (70). These effector molecules stimulate cell surface receptors that activate intermediary signals such as mitogen-activated protein kinase (MAPK). The (second) effector phase involves alterations in mitochondrial membrane per-

meability transition and activation of caspase 3. In the former, a pore opens in the inner mitochondrial membrane and there is a loss of mitochondrial membrane potential and movement of cytochrome c into the cytosol (70). Activation of caspase 3 results in further mitochondrial membrane changes and cleavage of nuclear proteins, causing DNA breakdown. The last phase (or degradative phase) results in the morphologic appearance characteristic of apoptosis.

The exact role of apoptosis in the pathophysiology of MODS remains uncertain. In animal models of infection, lymphocyte, endothelial cell, kidney, lung, and skeletal muscle apoptosis is increased. Neutrophil and hepatocyte apoptosis appears to be delayed (70). Data from clinical studies indicate that upregulation of apoptotic pathways occurs in patients with ARDS (71) and there is widespread apoptosis of splenic and colonic lymphoid populations in patients who die from sepsis and MODS (72). Whether inhibition of these programmed pathways can alter organ injury and death is an area of intense investigation (73).

Complex Nonlinear Systems

The body may be considered as a biologic network that is complex, highly coupled, and nonlinear (74). The behavior of such a system cannot be predicted with great reliability. Nonetheless,

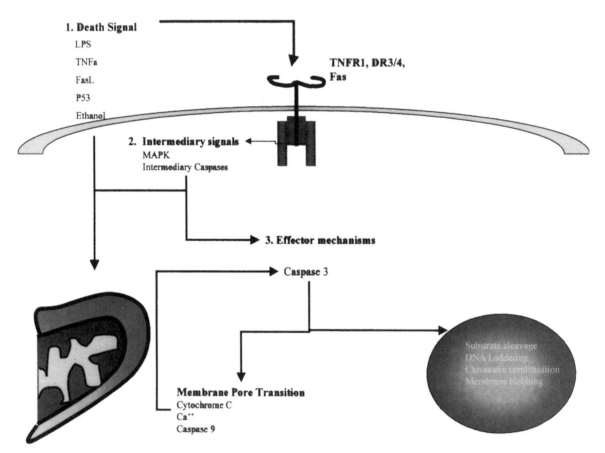

FIGURE 4. Proposed pathway for apoptosis. *LPS*, lipopolysaccharide; *TNFα*, tumor necrosis factor-α; *FasL*, Fas ligand; *TNFR1*, tumor necrosis factor receptor-1; *DR3/4*, death receptor 3/4; *MAPK*, mitogen-activated protein kinase. (From Mahidhara R, Billiar TR. Apoptosis in sepsis. *Crit Care Med* 2000;28:N105–N113, with permission.)

these systems are "attracted" to specific states (75). A large enough perturbation of an organ or cytokine network, for example, can have unexpected and profound results elsewhere, thereby potentially leading to MOD. In the normal, healthy individual, there is a high degree of heart rate (beat-to-beat) variability. Several studies have shown a relationship between loss of heart rate variability and increased mortality in critically ill patients (76). Septic patients or volunteers injected with LPS exhibit loss of heart variability (77). A causal link, however, between this loss of variability and outcome remains elusive. More research into nonlinear dynamics is needed to determine its importance and role in the development of MODS.

PREVENTION AND TREATMENT OF MULTIPLE-ORGAN DYSFUNCTION SYNDROME

Although progress is being made in the study of the pathophysiology of MODS, our knowledge remains very incomplete. As a result, the prevention and treatment of MODS are nonspecific but include the goals of maintaining adequate tissue oxygenation; finding and treating infection; providing adequate nutrition support; and when necessary, providing artificial support (e.g., dialysis or mechanical ventilation) for individual dysfunctional organs. These issues are dealt with in more detail in Chapters 15, 37, 44, and 51.

Resuscitation

An episode of circulatory shock is probably the most common event preceding the development of MODS. Thus, timely restoration of intravascular volume and DO_2 is of great importance in preventing (or ameliorating) MODS in high-risk patients. Controversy continues regarding the correct fluid for resuscitation and the optimal circulating hemoglobin concentration.

Assessing the adequacy of tissue oxygenation can often be difficult. The clinical parameters used most often, including arterial blood pressure, skin color and temperature, urine flow, mixed-venous oxygen saturation, and blood-lactate concentration, may be unreliable. Shoemaker and colleagues (78) report that critically ill patients who maintain a "supranormal" DO_2 (600 mL per minute per M^2), VO_2 (70 mL per minute per M^2), and cardiac index (4.5 L per minute per M^2) have a higher rate of survival than those patients who do not maintain the supranormal levels. As a consequence, Shoemaker and associates reasoned that systemic DO_2, systemic VO_2, and cardiac index should be used as therapeutic endpoints for resuscitation (79). The results of a randomized, prospective study of surgical patients considered to be at high risk for MODS and death showed that survival was significantly improved if the aforementioned levels of resuscitation were maintained after major operations or trauma (80). Other studies using similar therapeutic endpoints in patients undergoing high-risk surgery (81) or suffering from trauma supported such a strategy (82).

Other investigations, however, have failed to show any beneficial effect of resuscitation to predetermined endpoints of oxygen transport. Indeed, one study, which used vigorous fluid replacement and aggressive inotropic and vasopressor support, found

that such a strategy worsened outcome (83). The results of a large European multicenter study also did not support such a strategy (84). More recent data suggest that such aggressive resuscitation in the ICU may be too late. Early (i.e. in the emergency department before hospital admission) goal-directed therapy can reduce mortality and organ dysfunction in patients with severe sepsis and septic shock (85). Practice parameters for the hemodynamic support of the patient with sepsis and septic shock have recently been promulgated (86) and provide useful guidance for the practitioner.

Other largely experimental approaches that may be of value for assessing the adequacy of tissue oxygenation include tonometric determination of subcutaneous-tissue Po_2, monitoring of conjunctival Po_2, use of near-infrared spectroscopy to assess the oxidation state of cerebral cytochrome a, a_3, and tonometric estimation of gastric intramucosal pH (pHi) or Pco_2 (87). The last technique is simple and "minimally invasive." Tonometric evidence of gastric mucosal acidosis has been shown to correlate with both short-term and long-term mortality in critically ill patients and the development of complications after cardiac surgical procedures. In addition, prevention of gastric intramucosal acidosis by using aggressive fluid resuscitation and inotropic therapy may reduce mortality (87). However, more recent data have failed to demonstrate the usefulness of using gastric pHi as a therapeutic endpoint. In addition, the idea that gastric intramucosal acidosis or hypercarbia reflects the hemodynamics in the rest of the splanchnic bed has been cast into doubt (88).

Mechanical Ventilation

The method by which patients are ventilated may contribute to organ dysfunction. Animal and clinical studies indicate that overdistension of the lung through the use of large tidal volumes can cause lung injury and lead to the release of inflammatory mediators, thereby causing derangements in distant organs (89,90). Alveolar collapse and reopening (derecruitment/recruitment) during each tidal volume may also result in lung injury. Recently completed prospective randomized studies of ventilation strategies in patients with acute lung injury (ALI) or ARDS indicate that the use of low tidal volumes (less than 6 mL per kg and limiting plateau pressures to less than 30 cm H_2O) (91) and recruitment strategies (92) reduce mortality and the duration of mechanical ventilation.

Debridement of Dead Tissue and Fracture Stabilization

The presence of dead or devitalized tissue appears to predispose patients to the development of MODS; therefore, aggressive but careful debridement of dead tissue is an important element in the prevention of the syndrome. Timely surgical fixation of major lower extremity fractures will result in a lower incidence of ARDS and pneumonia, and should be considered the standard of care in the management of patients with long-bone fractures.

Infection

Sepsis is an important cause (or correlate) of MODS. It is imperative that the presence of infection is excluded in the critically ill patient with signs of deteriorating organ function. Prophylactic antibiotics should not be used. However, it is often necessary to begin empiric administration of broad-spectrum antibiotics in febrile patients with impending or established MODS while awaiting the results of further diagnostic studies.

Intraabdominal Sepsis

Early and adequate treatment of intraabdominal sepsis is important to prevent the development of MODS. Some surgeons have advocated multiple planned reoperations or open packing for severe cases of intraabdominal sepsis or necrotizing pancreatitis; however, no randomized trial has been undertaken to determine if this approach is optimal. Without clinical or radiologic evidence of intraabdominal infection, "blind" laparotomy in the patient with worsening MODS or frank organ failure does not appear to alter outcome.

Pulmonary Sepsis

Nosocomial pneumonia can play a role in the development and course of MODS and is discussed in greater detail in Chapters 32 and 48. The pathogenesis of pneumonia in intubated patients is controversial. It may be related to the colonization of the proximal GI tract and oropharynx with gram-negative bacteria, with the subsequent aspiration of these organisms around the cuff of the endotracheal tube. Elevating the head of the bed will reduce the risk of silent regurgitation and aspiration of gastric contents (93). Subglottic suctioning may also be effective in preventing nosocomial pneumonia (94).

Early studies indicated that treatment with H2-receptor blockers, antacids, or both, to prevent erosive gastritis promoted the overgrowth of gram-negative bacteria by raising gastric pH. Overgrowth of bacteria may contribute to the development of pneumonia. However, few studies demonstrate that the use of H2-receptor blockers is associated with an increased risk of nosocomial pneumonia (95). It may be the combination of high gastric pH and high gastric volume associated with the use of antacids that is an important factor in the development of nosocomial pneumonia. Sucralfate does not alter gastric pH substantially and is as effective as gastric alkalinization in preventing bleeding from erosive gastritis; thus, use of this agent may lessen the risk of nosocomial pneumonia.

Selective digestive decontamination (SDD) is a technique in which topical nonabsorbable antibacterial and antifungal agents (with or without a concomitant 3- to 5-day course of systemic antibiotic therapy) are applied to the oropharynx and proximal bowel in critically ill patients to reduce the incidence of nosocomial infections and mortality. A metaanalysis of 16 studies investigating SDD showed that the incidence of nosocomial pneumonia and tracheobronchitis is reduced by SDD, but the use of SDD does not improve survival rates (96). Because of expense and fears about selecting multidrug-resistant strains of gram-negative organisms or enterococci, SDD does not enjoy widespread use in the United States.

Immobilization is a risk factor for the development of nosocomial pneumonia. Postural oscillation with a rotating bed (kinetic table) may decrease the incidence of nosocomial lower–respiratory-tract infections in high-risk patients (97).

Catheter-Related Sepsis

Catheter-related sepsis may contribute to the development and propagation of MODS. Strict aseptic technique is required for the insertion of intravascular catheters (personnel inserting central-venous and pulmonary-artery (PA) catheters should wear a cap, gown, gloves and use a large sterile drape to cover the entire patient) (98). Catheters that are placed with suboptimal technique should be removed or replaced as soon as possible. Use of the subclavian insertion site, chlorhexidine/alcohol skin preparations and chlorhexidine impregnated dressing sponges are associated with a lower risk of infection. Routine "prophylactic" catheter changes (either over a guidewire or insertion at a new site) are unnecessary (99,100). Recent strategies to reduce the incidence of catheter-related sepsis include the use of catheters impregnated with minocycline and rifampin or antiseptics (chlorhexidine gluconate/silver sulfadiazine). Both are effective in reducing catheter-related bloodstream infections and appear to be cost-effective (101,102). Their use should be considered in high-risk patients.

Other Sources of Sepsis

Many other less common sources of infection in critically ill patients contribute to the development of MODS. These infections are not always readily apparent. The clinician caring for the patient should remain alert to their presence. Some of these sources of sepsis include purulent sinusitis, suppurative thrombophlebitis, otitis media, perirectal abscess, epididymitis, prostatitis, calculous or acalculous cholecystitis, meningitis or brain abscess (particularly after instrumentation of the central nervous system), prosthetic intravascular graft infection, lower or upper urinary tract infection, and endocarditis. Physical examination and appropriate laboratory and radiographic studies should exclude these conditions.

Nutrition Support

Malnutrition can contribute to the morbidity and mortality of sepsis and MODS (see Chapter 15). Proteolysis is a prominent finding in sepsis, and although it is not suppressed by infusing amino acids, protein anabolism can be achieved by appropriate nutrition support. Early nutrition support may be beneficial in patients at risk for developing MODS (103). The consensus among experts is that if nutrition support is started, enteral feeding is preferable to parental feeding.

Regardless of the route of feeding, overfeeding should be avoided. The excess administration of carbohydrates can alter the respiratory quotient with adverse effects on weaning from mechanical ventilation and can affect hepatic metabolic functions, thereby altering drug clearance (104). Current guidelines for support of hypermetabolic patients with sepsis or MODS include a total nonprotein caloric intake of 20 to 25 kcal per kg per day (2 to 5 g per kg per day of glucose plus 0.5 to 1.0 g per kg per day of fat) and 1.2 to 1.5 g per kg per day of protein (104). The number of calories needed for a given patient can be estimated using the Harris-Benedict equation or indirect calorimetry.

Hyperglycemia can be a difficult problem while feeding patients. A strategy using a continuous infusion of insulin up to doses of 50 units/hr with a serum glucose goal of 80–110 mg/dl can reduce mortality, infection and organ dysfunction (104a). In patients suffering from burns or trauma, severe protein catabolism is evident and is mediated by endogenous catecholamines. Beta-blockade with propranolol in pediatric patients with burns reverses the hypermetabolic response and protein catabolism (104b).

Specialty Formulas

A number of enteral nutritional products are available that provide specific nutrients: glutamine, peptides, arginine, omega-3 fatty acids, nucleic acids, and antioxidants (e.g., vitamins E and C, β-carotene). Arginine is important in NO production, lymphocyte proliferation, and wound healing (104). Omega-3 fatty acids change membrane lipid composition and can alter the inflammatory response (105). Nucleic acids assist in the proliferation of lymphocytes and intestinal crypt cells as well as DNA and RNA synthesis (104). Several proprietary enteral nutrition

formulas are available that include combinations of the aforementioned additives. Some (106–109), but not all (110), studies using these specialty formulas have shown that lymphocyte function may be improved, and postoperative complications, severity of organ dysfunction, hospital length of stay, and/or mortality are reduced.

SUMMARY

Standard therapy for patients with MODS includes adequate cardiovascular resuscitation, identification and treatment of infection, early and aggressive nutrition, and support for dysfunctional or failed organs. Improved outcome may be realized if patients at high risk for developing the syndrome can be identified so that preventive measures can be instituted. Because the pathogenesis of MODS involves numerous mediators, it is doubtful that all patients can be treated adequately with a single agent or mode of therapy. Nonetheless, recent data suggest that certain patients with sepsis or septic shock and organ dysfunction may benefit from anti–TNF-α therapy or modulation of the coagulation cascade. Further research will be needed to better understand the biology and therapy of MODS.

KEY POINTS

Despite significant technologic and therapeutic advances, multiple-organ dysfunction syndrome (MODS) remains the major cause of morbidity and mortality in critically ill patients who require protracted care. The majority of intensive care unit resources are consumed in treating patients with MODS. MODS may be a primary or secondary process. The direct and indirect causes and effects that result in progression to MODS remain incompletely understood, but MODS is most often associated with systemic inflammation. Hemodynamic lability often ensues along with derangements in oxygen delivery, extraction, and utilization.

An imbalance between proinflammatory and antiinflammatory responses via activation and interaction of a plethora of humoral and cellular mediators appears to be the key event that leads to progressive end-organ insult and dysfunction. A host of approaches have been evaluated to ameliorate or retard this deleterious process and ultimate decline. Administration of activated protein C is the only drug thus far which has been shown to reduce mortality in patients with severe sepsis.

Prevention remains the most effective approach to MODS. Preventive measures include very early goal-directed therapy, timely treatment of inadequate resuscitation, reversal of hy-

poperfusion and tissue hypoxia, and infection control. Judiciously timed nutrition using the gastrointestinal tract whenever possible, along with artificial support with noninvasive ventilation, dialytic therapies, and hemodynamic monitoring and support devices are indicated as organ compromise evolves. Pharmacologic therapies are currently mainly supportive in nature and focus on antimicrobials, vasoactive drugs, and prophylactic agents administered to limit stress ulceration and deep venous thrombosis.

Various scoring systems have been applied to define and quantify end-organ disturbance. Although excellent and widely applied for quantifying dysfunction, facilitating research, and providing some prognostic guidance, they have limitations.

Exciting research continues in an attempt to better elucidate risk factors, natural history of systemic inflammation, and progression to MODS. The application of a "lung protective" strategy to limit the deleterious effects of volutrauma and biotrauma is a significant tool in limiting the progression of acute lung injury to MODS. Other forthcoming studies, which modulate the coagulation and inflammatory cascades and reactive oxygen species, are on the horizon.

REFERENCES

1. American College of Chest Physicians/Society of Critical Care Medicine Consensus Conference. Definitions for sepsis and organ failure and guidelines for the use of innovative therapies in sepsis. *Crit Care Med* 1992;20:864–874.

2. Garcia Lizana F, Manzano Alonso JL, Gonzalez Santana B, et al. Survival and quality of life of patients with multiple organ failure one year after leaving an intensive care unit. *Med Clin (Barc)* 2000;114:99–103.

3. Bernard GR. Quantification of organ dysfunction: seeking standardization. *Crit Care Med* 1998;26:1767–1768.

4. Jacobs S, Zuleika M, Mphansa T. The Multiple Organ Dysfunction Score as a descriptor of patient outcome in septic shock compared with two other scoring systems. *Crit Care Med* 1999;27:741–744.

5. Rangel-Frausto MS, Pittet D, Costigan M, et al. The natural history of the systemic inflammatory response syndrome (SIRS). A prospective study. *JAMA* 1995;273:117–123.

6. Komatsu T, Shibutani K, Okamoto K, et al. Critical level of oxygen delivery after cardiopulmonary bypass. *Crit Care Med* 1987;15:194–197.

7. Ronco JJ, Fenwick JC, Tweeddale MG, et al. Identification of the critical oxygen delivery for anaerobic metabolism in critically ill septic and nonseptic humans. *JAMA* 1993;270:1724–1730.

8. Danek SJ, Lynch JP, Weg JG, et al. The dependence of oxygen uptake on oxygen delivery in the adult respiratory distress syndrome. *Am Rev Respir Dis* 1980;122:387–395.

9. Haupt MT, Gilbert EM, Carlson RW. Fluid loading increases oxygen consumption in septic patients with lactic acidosis. *Am Rev Respir Dis* 1985;131:912–916.

10. Nelson DP, Beyer C, Samsel RW, et al. Pathological supply dependence of O2 uptake during bacteremia in dogs. *J Appl Physiol* 1987;63:1487–1492.

11. Ronco JJ, Fenwick JC, Wiggs BR, et al. Oxygen consumption is independent of increases in oxygen delivery by dobutamine in septic patients who have normal or increased plasma lactate. *Am Rev Respir Dis* 1993;147:25–31.

12. Ronco JJ, Phang PT, Walley KR, et al. Oxygen consumption is independent of changes in oxygen delivery in severe adult respiratory distress syndrome. *Am Rev Respir Dis* 1991;143:1267–1273.

13. Sibbald WJ, Messmer K, Fink MP. Roundtable conference on tissue oxygenation in acute medicine, Brussels, Belgium, 14–16 March 1998. *Intensive Care Med* 2000;26:780–791.

14. Fink M. Cytopathic hypoxia in sepsis. *Acta Anaesthesiol Scand Suppl* 1997;110:87–95.

15. VanderMeer TJ, Wang H, Fink MP. Endotoxemia causes ileal mucosal acidosis in the absence of mucosal hypoxia in a normodynamic porcine model of septic shock. *Crit Care Med* 1995;23:1217–1226.

16. Rosser DM, Stidwill RP, Jacobson D, et al. Oxygen tension in the bladder epithelium rises in both high and low cardiac output endotoxemic sepsis. *J Appl Physiol* 1995;79:1878–1882.

17. Boekstegers P, Weidenhofer S, Pilz G, et al. Peripheral oxygen availability within skeletal muscle in sepsis and septic shock: comparison to limited infection and cardiogenic shock. *Infection* 1991;19:317–323.

18. Boekstegers P, Weidenhofer S, Kapsner T, et al. Skeletal muscle partial pressure of oxygen in patients with sepsis. *Crit Care Med* 1994;22:640–650.

19. Kuhnle S, Nicotera P, Wendel A, et al. Prevention of endotoxin-induced lethality, but not of liver apoptosis in poly(ADP-ribose) polymerase-deficient mice. *Biochem Biophys Res Commun* 1999;263:433–438.

20. King CJ, Tytgat S, Delude RL, et al. Ileal mucosal oxygen consumption is decreased in endotoxemic rats but is restored toward normal by treatment with aminoguanidine. *Crit Care Med* 1999;27:2518–2524.

21. Unno N, Wang H, Menconi MJ, et al. Inhibition of inducible nitric oxide synthase ameliorates endotoxin-induced gut mucosal barrier dysfunction in rats. *Gastroenterology* 1997;113:1246–1257.

22. Fry DE, Pearlstein L, Fulton RL, et al. Multiple system organ failure. The role of uncontrolled infection. *Arch Surg* 1980;115:136–140.

23. Rangel-Frausto MS. The epidemiology of bacterial sepsis. *Infect Dis Clin North Am* 1999;13:299–312.

24. Pape HC, Remmers D, Kleemann W, et al. Posttraumatic multiple organ failure—a report on clinical and autopsy findings. *Shock* 1994;2:228–234.

25. Nuytinck HK, Offermans XJ, Kubat K, et al. Whole-body inflammation in trauma patients. An autopsy study. *Arch Surg* 1988;123:1519–1524.

26. Robbins RA, Russ WD, Rasmussen JK, et al. Activation of the complement system in the adult respiratory distress syndrome. *Am Rev Respir Dis* 1987;135:651–658.

27. Fosse E, Pillgram-Larsen J, Svennevig JL, et al. Complement activation in injured patients occurs immediately and is dependent on the severity of the trauma. *Injury* 1998;29:509–514.

28. Fowler AA, Hyers TM, Fisher BJ, et al. The adult respiratory distress syndrome. Cell populations and soluble mediators in the air spaces of patients at high risk. *Am Rev Respir Dis* 1987;136:1225–1231.

29. Lindsay TF, Luo XP, Lehotay DC, et al. Ruptured abdominal aortic aneurysm, a "two-hit" ischemia/reperfusion injury: evidence from an analysis of oxidative products. *J Vasc Surg* 1999;30:219–228.

30. Saikumar P, Dong Z, Weinberg JM, et al. Mechanisms of cell death in hypoxia/reoxygenation injury. *Oncogene* 1998;17:3341–3349.

31. Kietzmann D, Kahl R, Muller M, et al. Hydrogen peroxide in expired breath condensate of patients with acute respiratory failure and with ARDS. *Intensive Care Med* 1993;19:78–81.

32. Lamb NJ, Gutteridge JM, Baker C, et al. Oxidative damage to proteins of bronchoalveolar lavage fluid in patients with acute respiratory distress syndrome: evidence for neutrophil-mediated hydroxylation, nitration, and chlorination. *Crit Care Med* 1999;27:1738–1744.

33. Richard C, Lemonnier F, Thibault M, et al. Vitamin E deficiency and lipoperoxidation during adult respiratory distress syndrome. *Crit Care Med* 1990;18:4–9.

34. Bernard GR, Wheeler AP, Arons MM, et al. A trial of antioxidants N-acetylcysteine and procysteine in ARDS. The Antioxidant in ARDS Study Group. *Chest* 1997;112:164–172.

35. Ortolani O, Conti A, De Gaudio AR, et al. The effect of glutathione and N-acetylcysteine on lipoperoxidative damage in patients with early septic shock. *Am J Respir Crit Care Med* 2000;161:1907–1911.

36. Fein AM, Bernard GR, Criner GJ, et al. Treatment of severe systemic inflammatory response syndrome and sepsis with a novel bradykinin antagonist, deltibant (CP-0127). Results of a randomized, double-blind, placebo-controlled trial. CP-0127 SIRS and Sepsis Study Group. *JAMA* 1997;277:482–487.

37. Levi M, ten Cate H, van der Poll T, et al. Pathogenesis of disseminated intravascular coagulation in sepsis. *JAMA* 1993;270:975–979.

38. van Gorp EC, Suharti C, ten Cate H, et al. Review: infectious diseases and coagulation disorders. *J Infect Dis* 1999;180:176–186.

38a. Bernard GR, Vincent J-L, Laterre P-F, et al.: Efficacy and safety of recombinant human activated protein C for severe sepsis. *New Engl J Med* 2001;344:699–709.

39. Heller A, Koch T, Schmeck J, et al. Lipid mediators in inflammatory disorders. *Drugs* 1998;55:487–496.

40. Vadas P, Pruzanski W, Stefanski E, et al. Pathogenesis of hypotension in septic shock: correlation of circulating phospholipase A2 levels with circulatory collapse. *Crit Care Med* 1988;16:1–7.

41. Bernard GR, Reines HD, Halushka PV, et al. Prostacyclin and thromboxane A2 formation is increased in human sepsis syndrome. Effects of cyclooxygenase inhibition. *Am Rev Respir Dis* 1991;144:1095–1101.

42. Bernard GR, Wheeler AP, Russell JA, et al. The effects of ibuprofen on the physiology and survival of patients with sepsis. The Ibuprofen in Sepsis Study Group. *N Engl J Med* 1997;336:912–918.

43. Abraham E, Baughman R, Fletcher E, et al. Liposomal prostaglandin E1 (TLC C-53) in acute respiratory distress syndrome: a controlled, randomized, double blind, multicenter clinical trial. TLC C-53 ARDS Study Group. *Crit Care Med* 1999;27:1478–1485.

44. Bulger EM, Jurkovich GJ, Gentilello LM, et al. Current clinical options for the treatment and management of acute respiratory distress syndrome. *J Trauma* 2000;48:562–572.

45. Partrick DA, Moore EE, Moore FA, et al. Lipid mediators up-regulate CD11b and prime for concordant superoxide and elastase release in human neutrophils. *J Trauma* 1997;43:297–302.

46. Oda M, Satouchi K, Ikeda I, et al. The presence of platelet-activating factor associated with eosinophil and/or neutrophil accumulations in the pleural fluids. *Am Rev Respir Dis* 1990;141:1469–1473.

47. Partrick DA, Moore EE, Moore FA, et al. Reduced PAF-acetylhydrolase activity is associated with postinjury multiple organ failure. *Shock* 1997;7:170–174.

48. Dhainaut JF, Tenaillon A, Hemmer M, et al. Confirmatory platelet-activating factor receptor antagonist trial in patients with severe gram-negative bacterial sepsis: a phase III, randomized, double-blind,

placebo-controlled, multicenter trial. BN 52021 Sepsis Investigator Group. *Crit Care Med* 1998;26:1963–1971.

49. Froon AM, Greve JW, Buurman WA, et al. Treatment with the platelet-activating factor antagonist TCV-309 in patients with severe systemic inflammatory response syndrome: a prospective, multicenter, double-blind, randomized phase II trial. *Shock* 1996;5:313–319.

50. Dinarello CA. Proinflammatory cytokines. *Chest* 2000;118:503–508.

51. Murphy K, Haudek SB, Thompson M, et al. Molecular biology of septic shock. *New Horizon* 1998;6:181–193.

52. Michie HR, Manogue KR, Spriggs DR, et al. Detection of circulating tumor necrosis factor after endotoxin administration. *N Engl J Med* 1988;318:1481–1486.

53. Panacek E, Marshall J, Fischkoff S, et al. Neutralization of TNF by a monoclonal antibody improves survival and reduces organ dysfunction in human sepsis: results of the MONARCS trial. Presented at: Chest 2000, American College of Chest Physicians; October 2000; San Francisco.

54. Mira JP, Cariou A, Grall F, et al. Association of TNF2, a TNF-alpha promoter polymorphism, with septic shock susceptibility and mortality: a multicenter study. *JAMA* 1999;282:561–568.

55. Majetschak M, Flohe S, Obertacke U, et al. Relation of a TNF gene polymorphism to severe sepsis in trauma patients. *Ann Surg* 1999;230:207–214.

56. Oberholzer A, Oberholzer C, Moldawer LL. Cytokine signaling—regulation of the immune response in normal and critically ill states. *Crit Care Med* 2000;28:N3–N12.

57. Fisher CJ Jr, Dhainaut JF, Opal SM, et al. Recombinant human interleukin 1 receptor antagonist in the treatment of patients with sepsis syndrome. Results from a randomized, double-blind, placebo-controlled trial. Phase III rhIL-1ra Sepsis Syndrome Study Group. *JAMA* 1994;271:1836–1843.

58. Calandra T, Bucala R. Macrophage migration inhibitory factor (MIF): a glucocorticoid counter-regulator within the immune system. *Crit Rev Immunol* 1997;17:77–88.

59. Bozza M, Satoskar AR, Lin G, et al. Targeted disruption of migration inhibitory factor gene reveals its critical role in sepsis. *J Exp Med* 1999;189:341–346.

60. Wang H, Bloom O, Zhang M, et al. HMG-1 as a late mediator of endotoxin lethality in mice. *Science* 1999;285:248–251.

61. Abraham E, Arcaroli J, Carmody A, et al. HMG-1 as a mediator of acute lung inflammation. *J Immunol* 2000;165:2950–2954.

62. Liaudet L, Soriano FG, Szabo C. Biology of nitric oxide signaling. *Crit Care Med* 2000;28:N37–N52.

63. Ochoa JB, Udekwu AO, Billiar TR, et al. Nitrogen oxide levels in patients after trauma and during sepsis. *Ann Surg* 1991;214:621–626.

64. Hibbs JB Jr, Westenfelder C, Taintor R, et al. Evidence for cytokine-inducible nitric oxide synthesis from L-arginine in patients receiving interleukin-2 therapy [published erratum appears in *J Clin Invest* 1992;90:295]. *J Clin Invest* 1992;89:867–877.

65. Horton JW, Maass D, White J, et al. Nitric oxide modulation of TNF-alpha-induced cardiac contractile dysfunction is concentration dependent. *Am J Physiol Heart Circ Physiol* 2000;278:H1955–H1965.

66. Szabo C, Billiar TR. Novel roles of nitric oxide in hemorrhagic shock. *Shock* 1999;12:1–9.

67. Avontuur JA, Biewenga M, Buijk SL, et al. Pulmonary hypertension and reduced cardiac output during inhibition of nitric oxide synthesis in human septic shock. *Shock* 1998;9:451–454.

68. Nasraway SA Jr. Sepsis research: we must change course. *Crit Care Med* 1999;27:427–430.

69. Moore FA. The role of the gastrointestinal tract in postinjury multiple organ failure. *Am J Surg* 1999;178:449–453.

70. Mahidhara R, Billiar TR. Apoptosis in sepsis. *Crit Care Med* 2000;28:N105–N113.

71. Hashimoto S, Kobayashi A, Kooguchi K, et al. Upregulation of two death pathways of perforin/granzyme and FasL/Fas in septic acute respiratory distress syndrome. *Am J Respir Crit Care Med* 2000;161:237–243.

72. Hotchkiss RS, Swanson PE, Freeman BD, et al. Apoptotic cell death in patients with sepsis, shock, and multiple organ dysfunction. *Crit Care Med* 1999;27:1230–1251.

73. Hotchkiss RS, Swanson PE, Knudson CM, et al. Overexpression of Bcl-2 in transgenic mice decreases apoptosis and improves survival in sepsis. *J Immunol* 1999;162:4148–4156.

74. Godin PJ, Buchman TG. Uncoupling of biological oscillators: a complementary hypothesis concerning the pathogenesis of multiple organ dysfunction syndrome. *Crit Care Med* 1996;24:1107–1116.

75. Seely AJ, Christou NV. Multiple organ dysfunction syndrome: exploring the paradigm of complex nonlinear systems. *Crit Care Med* 2000;28:2193–2200.

76. Haji-Michael PG, Vincent JL, Degaute JP, et al. Power spectral analysis of cardiovascular variability in critically ill neurosurgical patients. *Crit Care Med* 2000;28:2578–2583.

77. Godin PJ, Fleisher LA, Eidsath A, et al. Experimental human endotoxemia increases cardiac regularity: results from a prospective, randomized, crossover trial. *Crit Care Med* 1996;24:1117–1124.

78. Shoemaker WC, Chang P, Czer L, et al. Cardiorespiratory monitoring in postoperative patients: I. Prediction of outcome and severity of illness. *Crit Care Med* 1979;7:237–242.

79. Shoemaker WC, Czer LS. Evaluation of the biologic importance of various hemodynamic and oxygen transport variables: which variables should be monitored in postoperative shock? *Crit Care Med* 1979;7:424–431.

80. Shoemaker WC, Appel PL, Kram HB, et al. Prospective trial of supranormal values of survivors as therapeutic goals in high-risk surgical patients. *Chest* 1988;94:1176–1186.

81. Lobo SM, Salgado PF, Castillo VG, et al. Effects of maximizing oxygen delivery on morbidity and mortality in high-risk surgical patients. *Crit Care Med* 2000;28:3396–3404.

82. Boyd O, Grounds RM, Bennett ED. A randomized clinical trial of the effect of deliberate perioperative increase of oxygen delivery on mortality in high-risk surgical patients. *JAMA* 1993;270:2699–2707.

83. Hayes MA, Timmins AC, Yau EH, et al. Elevation of systemic oxygen delivery in the treatment of critically ill patients. *N Engl J Med* 1994;330:1717–1722.

84. Gattinoni L, Brazzi L, Pelosi P, et al. A trial of goal-oriented hemodynamic therapy in critically ill patients. SvO$_2$ Collaborative Group. *N Engl J Med* 1995;333:1025–1032.

85. Rivers E, Nguyen B, Havstad S, et al. Early goal-directed therapy in the treatment of severe sepsis and septic shock. *New Engl J Med* 2001;345:1368–1377.

86. Task Force of the American College of Critical Care Medicine, Society of Critical Care Medicine. Practice parameters for hemodynamic support of sepsis in adult patients in sepsis. *Crit Care Med* 1999;27:639–660.

87. Gutierrez G, Palizas F, Doglio G, et al. Gastric intramucosal pH as a therapeutic index of tissue oxygenation in critically ill patients. *Lancet* 1992;339:195–199.

88. Creteur J, De Backer D, Vincent JL. Does gastric tonometry monitor splanchnic perfusion? *Crit Care Med* 1999;27:2480–2484.

89. Chiumello D, Pristine G, Slutsky AS. Mechanical ventilation affects local and systemic cytokines in an animal model of acute respiratory distress syndrome. *Am J Respir Crit Care Med* 1999;160:109–116.

90. Ranieri VM, Suter PM, Tortorella C, et al. Effect of mechanical ventilation on inflammatory mediators in patients with acute respiratory distress syndrome: a randomized controlled trial. *JAMA* 1999;282:54–61.

91. The Acute Respiratory Distress Syndrome Network. Ventilation with lower tidal volumes as compared with traditional tidal volumes for acute lung injury and the acute respiratory distress syndrome. *N Engl J Med* 2000;342:1301–1308.

92. Amato MB, Barbas CS, Medeiros DM, et al. Effect of a protective-ventilation strategy on mortality in the acute respiratory distress syndrome. *N Engl J Med* 1998;338:347–354.

93. Drakulovic MB, Torres A, Bauer TT, et al. Supine body position as a risk factor for nosocomial pneumonia in mechanically ventilated patients: a randomized trial. *Lancet* 1999;354:1851–1858.

94. Kollef MH, Skubas NJ, Sundt TM. A randomized clinical trial of continuous aspiration of subglottic secretions in cardiac surgery patients. *Chest* 1999;116:1339–1346.

95. Cook D, Guyatt G, Marshall J, et al. A comparison of sucralfate and ranitidine for the prevention of upper gastrointestinal bleeding in patients requiring mechanical ventilation. Canadian Critical Care Trials Group. *N Engl J Med* 1998;338:791–797.

96. Kollef MH. The role of selective digestive tract decontamination on mortality and respiratory tract infections. A meta-analysis. *Chest* 1994;105:1101–1108.

97. Fink MP, Helsmoortel CM, Stein KL, et al. The efficacy of an oscillating bed in the prevention of lower respiratory tract infection in critically ill victims of blunt trauma. A prospective study. *Chest* 1990;97:132–137.

98. Raad, II, Hohn DC, Gilbreath BJ, et al. Prevention of central venous catheter-related infections by using maximal sterile barrier precautions during insertion. *Infect Control Hosp Epidemiol* 1994;15:231–238.

99. Eyer S, Brummitt C, Crossley K, et al. Catheter-related sepsis: prospective, randomized study of three methods of long-term catheter maintenance. *Crit Care Med* 1990;18:1073–1079.

100. Cobb DK, High KP, Sawyer RG, et al. A controlled trial of scheduled replacement of central venous and pulmonary-artery catheters. *N Engl J Med* 1992;327:1062–1068.

101. Veenstra DL, Saint S, Saha S, et al. Efficacy of antiseptic-impregnated central venous catheters in preventing catheter-related bloodstream infection: a meta-analysis. *JAMA* 1999;281:261–267.

102. Darouiche RO, Raad II, Heard SO, et al. A comparison of two antimicrobial-impregnated central venous catheters. Catheter Study Group. *N Engl J Med* 1999;340:1–8.

103. Zaloga GP. Early enteral nutritional support improves outcome: hypothesis or fact? *Crit Care Med* 1999;27:259–261.

104. Cerra FB, Benitez MR, Blackburn GL, et al. Applied nutrition in ICU patients. A consensus statement of the American College of Chest Physicians. *Chest* 1997;111:769–778.

104a. Van den Berghe G, Wouters P, Weekers F, et al. Intensive insulin therapy in critically ill patients. *New Engl J Med* 2001;345:1359–1367.

104b. Herndon DN, Hart DW, Wolf SE, et al. Reversal of catabolism by beta-blockade after severe burns. *New Engl J Med* 2001;345:1223–1229.

105. Endres S, Ghorbani R, Kelley VE, et al. The effect of dietary supplementation with n-3 polyunsaturated fatty acids on the synthesis of interleukin-1 and tumor necrosis factor by mononuclear cells. *N Engl J Med* 1989;320:265–271.

106. Bower RH, Cerra FB, Bershadsky B, et al. Early enteral administration of a formula (Impact) supplemented with arginine, nucleotides, and fish oil in intensive care unit patients: results of a multicenter, prospective, randomized, clinical trial. *Crit Care Med* 1995;23:436–449.

107. Atkinson S, Sieffert E, Bihari D. A prospective, randomized, double-blind, controlled clinical trial of enteral immunonutrition in the critically ill. Guy's Hospital Intensive Care Group. *Crit Care Med* 1998;26:1164–1172.

108. Gadek JE, DeMichele SJ, Karlstad MD, et al. Effect of enteral feeding with eicosapentaenoic acid, gamma-linolenic acid, and antioxidants in patients with acute respiratory distress syndrome. Enteral Nutrition in ARDS Study Group. *Crit Care Med* 1999;27:1409–1420.

109. Galban C, Montejo JC, Mesejo A, et al. An immune-enhancing enteral diet reduces mortality rate and episodes of bacteremia in septic intensive care unit patients. *Crit Care Med* 2000;28:643–648.

110. Mendez C, Jurkovich GJ, Garcia I, et al. Effects of an immune-enhancing diet in critically injured patients. *J Trauma* 1997;42:933–941.

111. Vincent JL, de Mendonca A, Cantraine F, et al. Use of the SOFA score to assess the incidence of organ dysfunction/failure in intensive care units: results of a multicenter, prospective study. Working group on "sepsis-related problems" of the European Society of Intensive Care Medicine. *Crit Care Med* 1998;26:1793–1800.

112. Marshall JC, Cook DJ, Christou NV, et al. Multiple organ dysfunction score: a reliable descriptor of a complex clinical outcome. *Crit Care Med* 1995;23:1638–1652.

113. Le Gall JR, Klar J, Lemeshow S, et al. The Logistic Organ Dysfunction system. A new way to assess organ dysfunction in the intensive care unit. ICU Scoring Group. *JAMA* 1996;276:802–810.

114. Russell JA, Singer J, Bernard GR, et al. Changing pattern of organ dysfunction in early human sepsis is related to mortality. *Crit Care Med* 2000;28:3405–3411.

THE PATIENT WITH SEPSIS OR THE SYSTEMIC INFLAMMATORY RESPONSE SYNDROME

SHARON ORBACH
YORAM G. WEISS
CLIFFORD S. DEUTSCHMAN

KEY WORDS

- Acute respiratory distress syndrome
- Acute-phase response
- Inotropy
- Sepsis
- Stress response
- Systemic inflammatory response syndrome (SIRS)
- Vasodilation

NORMAL RESPONSES TO STRESS AND THE DEFINITIONS OF SEPSIS

Sepsis (also called sepsis syndrome) and the systemic inflammatory response syndrome (SIRS) are often noted complications in surgical patients. At one time the definitions and nomenclature attached to sepsis and SIRS were extremely confusing, involving diverse terms such as infection, septicemia, sepsis, sepsis syndrome, and septic shock (1). To clarify matters, based on the recognition that sepsis and SIRS can occur even in the absence of infection and the need for researchers worldwide to compare results, a series of definitions proposed by Bone and colleagues have been adopted (Table 1) (2). Under these definitions, proposed by the American College of Chest Physicians and the Society for Critical Care Medicine, the term "systemic inflammatory response syndrome" (SIRS) describes the body's response to inflammation regardless of cause (2). Sepsis is defined as the clinical response to the presence of a confirmed infection while severe sepsis and septic shock, representing different aspects of the same disorder, are defined clearly (2). Unfortunately, it has been suggested that these terms are too general and encompass too heterogeneous a population (3). Additional changes in terminology may become necessary.

Sepsis and SIRS are believed to be the most common cause of admission to the surgical intensive care unit (SICU) (2). Indeed, in the United States, there are approximately 400,000 new cases of sepsis or SIRS and 200,000 cases of septic shock per year (1). Sepsis is estimated to lead to 100,000 deaths per year, making it the thirteenth most common cause of death in this country (1). The number of cases is rising; the Centers for Disease Control and Prevention reported a 139% increase in the incidence of sepsis during the 1980s (4). However, it is difficult to estimate the true incidence of this disorder because the septic response represents a continuum of physiologic alterations seen in critically ill patients. Active investigation is currently underway, both in the laboratory and in the ICU, to clarify the elusive point at which an infection elicits sepsis or SIRS. The focus in this chapter will be to (a) define these three states in clinical terms, (b) examine the risk factors and pathogenic processes underlying their development, and (c) discuss the clinical alterations in organ function caused by systemic inflammation (sepsis or sepsis syndrome). The underlying theme is that the transition from infection to sepsis likely results from a fundamental alteration in biologic behavior, while the transition from sepsis to SIRS is probably a matter of degree. Thus, sepsis causes intracellular dysfunction, but compensatory mechanisms or functional reserve render these changes clinically silent, while SIRS involves the loss of the ability to compensate and leads to overt clinical organ dysfunction.

Stress Response or Acute-Phase Response

As detailed in the work of Cuthbertson (5), Moore (6), and others, the response to tissue trauma on any level, including insults as different as operations, an acute myocardial infarction (MI), and respiratory decompensation in chronic obstructive pulmonary disease, is biphasic. The first phase appears to represent activation of mechanisms to ensure short-term survival, which in turn means preservation of substrate delivery to the heart and brain (5). As a result, blood flow to these two organs increases, while flow to all other systems decreases. Substrate is mobilized to a minor degree, but the major change involves maintaining oxygen delivery and intravascular volume by altered ventilation-perfusion (V/Q) matching, renal-fluid retention, and extracellular translocation of intracellular water. Once these mechanisms are activated and short-term survival appears likely, a transition occurs from this "ebb" or "shock" phase into a second, hypermetabolic stage that

TABLE 1. DEFINITIONS OF SEPSIS AND SYSTEMIC INFLAMMATORY RESPONSE SYNDROME

Systemic inflammatory response syndrome (SIRS): The systemic response to a variety of clinical insults. The syndrome manifests by two or more of the following conditions:
 (a) temperature >38°C or <36°C;
 (b) heart rate >90 beats per minute;
 (c) respiratory rate >20 breaths per minute or $Paco_2$ <32 mm Hg;
 (d) white blood cell count >12,000/mm^3 or >10% immature band forms.
Sepsis: The systemic response to infection, manifested by two or more of the following as a result of infection:
 (a) temperature >38°C or <36°C;
 (b) heart rate >90 beats per minute;
 (c) respiratory rate >20 breaths per minute or $Paco_2$ <32 mm Hg;
 (d) white blood cell count >12,000/mm^3 or >10% immature band forms.
Severe sepsis: Sepsis associated with organ dysfunction, hypoperfusion, or hypotension. Hypoperfusion and perfusion abnormalities include, but are not limited to, lactic acidosis, oliguria, or mental status changes.
Sepsis-induced hypotension: Systolic blood pressure <90 mm Hg or reduction of >40 mm Hg in the absence of other causes for hypotension.
Septic shock: Sepsis-induced hypotension in spite of adequate fluid resuscitation plus perfusion abnormalities including, but not limited to, lactic acidosis, oliguria, and mental status changes. Patients who receive vasopressor or inotropic agents to maintain blood pressure are considered to be in septic shock even if they are not hypotensive.

is primarily driven by the demands of damaged tissue (5,6). This demand may arise from a surgical site; a local area of acute inflammation, such as an infarcted or ischemic region of myocardium; or a collection of blood that contains activated white blood cells (WBCs).

WBCs are of key importance; with the initial recruitment of neutrophils into wound tissue and the subsequent migration of macrophages serving to debride and eliminate damaged tissue, these cells provide protection from invading microorganisms and lay down the collagen matrix required for healing (7). A source of energy is required to support these functions. WBCs are obligate glucose or glutamine users, and, thus, the metabolic response is designed to provide these substrates. Relative inhibition of glucose utilization is evident in tissues other than the wound. To support the metabolic requirements of the stress response, glycogen is mobilized from the liver (and if the local damage includes skeletal muscle, from this source as well). Amino acids are released from both skeletal and visceral muscle, as a substrate for hepatic gluconeogenesis, and fat is mobilized to provide an alternate energy source for nonwound tissues. Peripheral vasodilation, fluid retention, decreased intracellular water, and capillary leak facilitate local substrate delivery retention within the area of damage. The vasodilation may be relatively generalized and can lead to a significant increase in cardiac output (CO).

Resting energy expenditure, oxygen consumption, and carbon dioxide production increase in proportion to the magnitude of the injury, reflecting the metabolic demands of the wound and the activities required to support the healing process. Metabolic rate peaks 2 to 3 days following injury and resolves over the next 4 days. The resolution appears to correlate with the process of wound revascularization; as substrate delivery to damaged

tissue improves, the need for gluconeogenesis, high levels of CO, fluid retention, and capillary leak decreases. In the absence of complications, these processes fully resolve 7 days following their onset, with subsequent metabolic alterations directed toward repletion of endogenous resources used to support the response (3). While the time course is relatively fixed, the magnitude of the response is entirely dependent on the magnitude of the injury. The process is modulated by an orchestrated combination of increased activity in the central and autonomic nervous systems; elevations of hormonal secretion; and effects resulting from the release of humoral mediators, such as cytokines, primarily from WBCs (8). It is at the extremes—in patients with severe injuries, highly elevated rates of metabolism, and an increasing contribution by the humoral component of the mediator response—that differentiating the stress response from sepsis becomes difficult.

The Septic Response

There are a number of predisposing conditions and risk factors known to increase the likelihood that a normal stress response will evolve into SIRS/sepsis. These are detailed in Table 2. The hallmark of septic metabolism lies in a biochemical "unbalancing" that results in cellular dysfunction. Organ-system function is acceptable, but evidence shows that this function is inefficient and less than optimal. As an example, during the acute-phase response, the block in glucose oxidation occurs at the peripheral level; in sepsis, the process of gluconeogenesis becomes impaired (9). The delivery of high levels of glucose precursors (alanine, lactate, and pyruvate) to the liver allows hepatic glucose output to remain elevated, but the intrinsic capacity of hepatocytes to engage in gluconeogenesis is decreased (10). Similarly, the capacity of hepatocytes and myocardial cells to use fat is exceeded, perhaps reflecting either saturation of the carnitine carrier that shuttles long-chain fatty acids into mitochondria for β-oxidation or relative carnitine deficiency (11). The result here is deposition of reesterified fat in the bile ducts and within myocardial cells, leading to intrahepatic cholestasis and dysrhythmias. As a final example, the intrinsic ability of cellular processes to respond to neural and hormonal stimulation is altered (12,13). Examples of this phenomenon include the relative inability of catecholamines to stimulate heart rate and myocardial contractility, the inability of alpha-adrenergic agents to cause vasoconstriction,

TABLE 2. RISK FACTORS FOR DEVELOPING SYSTEMIC INFLAMMATORY RESPONSE SYNDROME

Inadequate or delayed resuscitation
Persistent inflammatory or infectious focus
Baseline organ dysfunction
Age >65 years
Immunosuppression
 Steroids
 Chemotherapy/cancer
 Acquired immunodeficiency syndrome
 Transplant patients
 Asplenia
Alcohol abuse
Malnutrition
Invasive instrumentation

or the resistance of gluconeogenesis to modulation by insulin (12,14,15). The net result of this unbalanced milieu is a state that is precariously close to overt organ dysfunction. It is important to note that the clinical picture may differ little from normal, postinjury inflammation and is virtually indistinguishable from SIRS secondary to noninfectious causes. Where the difference lies is in a prolonged time course that is not self-limited. The biochemical etiology of this state remains unknown, but modulation of these responses appears to reflect an overexpression of the effects of the humoral mediators, especially WBC products such as cytokines and perhaps an overexuberant response of the WBCs themselves (8). Neutrophils and macrophages appear to play a particularly important role; some investigators have suggested that the sepsis syndrome really represents a state of disseminated intravascular inflammation, in which WBCs exert their effects in an uncontrolled manner (2).

To compensate, the delivery of substrate to tissues is increased even further than during the stress response. Vasodilation and capillary leak lead to further increases in CO and anasarca, and even greater fluid retention and translocation of intracellular water. These compensatory events can become "discoordinated"; substrates can be depleted, which can aggravate vasodilation and capillary leak that ultimately cannot be compensated by fluid retention, cellular-water translocation, or endogenous catecholamines. This dislocation leads to the state referred to as septic shock. In the absence of shock, however, the clinical manifestations of sepsis may be subtle and will become obvious only with careful scrutiny.

The earliest signs of sepsis are primarily metabolic and include persistent hyperglycemia that is unresponsive to treatment with insulin, and hyperlipidemia or intolerance of exogenously provided long-chain fatty acids. Blood urea nitrogen levels rise reflecting mobilization and deamination of amino acids from skeletal muscle and visceral protein stores. Resting energy expenditure and carbon dioxide production are elevated with a relative lack of a concomitant rise in oxygen extraction and utilization. Physiologic abnormalities, as described in more detail below, follow. The vasculature dilates, the CO rises, fluid in excess of anticipated needs is required, minute ventilation increases to accommodate the increased carbon dioxide production, and urine output decreases as the kidneys attempt to conserve fluid. Fluid transudation into the lungs results in a relative hypoxemia and further reflects the ongoing translocation of fluid from the cellular to the extracellular space.

Weakness, especially of the respiratory muscles, may become apparent as muscle is catabolized. Similar processes in vascular, gastrointestinal (GI), and cardiac muscle result in anastomotic breakdown, loss of the GI mucosal barrier with bacterial and endotoxin translocation, and myocardial dysfunction. At some point the transition to multiple-organ dysfunction syndrome (MODS) occurs.

A number of etiologic agents may provoke the sepsis syndrome. An association with gram-positive, gram-negative, anaerobic, fungal, and viral infection has been noted (16,17). Prior to the 1980s, gram-negative bacteria were the primary reported cause of sepsis (1). Since then, there have been a growing number of infections with gram-positive organisms and fungi. The National Nosocomial Infections Surveillance system reported that between 1992 and 1997 the most common bloodstream pathogen was coagulase-negative staphylococci; there was an increasing incidence of sepsis secondary to enterococci and *Staphylococcus aureus* (1). Because of widespread antibiotic use, the incidence of fungal infection with *Candida* species also increased. However, in 50% of reported cases of sepsis syndrome, no microbiologic etiology can be found. Resolution of large hematomas, as well as noninfectious inflammatory stimuli (such as aspiration pneumonitis, pulmonary contusions, burns, multiple blood transfusions, and pancreatitis) are known to provoke a sepsis-like state. Implicit in these observations is the understanding that the sepsis syndrome is a host-specific response to a number of stimuli, with activation of WBCs and endothelial-cell processes with release of endogenous mediators playing a central role in the development of sepsis and its complications.

Unlike the stress response, the sepsis syndrome does not have a predictable time course. Resolution of the response depends on resolution of the underlying pathology. Thus, drainage of fluid collections, abscesses, eradication of bacteria, and institution of appropriate supportive care are essential in treating sepsis-like processes.

Altered Physiologic Responses and Current Therapy

In defining the pathophysiology of sepsis and determining a useful course of treatment, it is helpful to investigate how recent insights into the nature of the disease have changed our understanding of the pathophysiology and led to a reappraisal of therapy, often resulting in new strategies. Thus, we will examine sepsis in light of "traditional" and "alternative" views of pathophysiology and will attempt to make recommendations regarding treatment.

General Pathophysiology

When sepsis was initially described, microorganisms were believed to be solely responsible for the pathophysiologic state. It was assumed that the patient was an "innocent bystander" whose body was invaded by bacteria. As our understanding has evolved, however, it has become clear that the host's inflammatory response to the infection contributes significantly to the abnormalities observed in sepsis. Because tissue injury from other causes can precipitate a similar inflammatory response, a sepsis-like state can occur even without infection (18). This allows us to discuss the septic state as if it were divided into two stages: initiation and host-mediator response (19).

Initiation

Sepsis, which by definition involves the response to invading microorganisms, can be caused by infiltration of gram-negative or gram-positive bacteria, fungi, viruses, or parasites. Most research has focused on gram-negative bacteria. These organisms possess a cell wall that contains lipopolysaccharide (LPS) in its outer membrane (20). LPS is comprised of an O polysaccharide, a core, and lipid A. The O polysaccharide distinguishes between different types of gram-negative bacteria while lipid A, an endotoxin, is responsible for the compound's toxicity (20). In other diseases specific initiating mediators have not been as well identified.

Host-Mediated Response

The initiating stimulus (whether gram-negative lipid A endotoxin, another infectious stimulus, or a simple inflammatory response) causes activation of the host's defense mechanisms which include molecular (complement and clotting cascades) and cellular components (neutrophils, monocytes, macrophages, and endothelial cells) (17). Cells may elaborate or activate additional mediators such as cytokines, arachidonic acid metabolites, complement, coagulation components, kinins, platelet-activating factor, adhesion markers, and myocardial-depressant factor. Each compound in some way may contribute to the inflammatory response (21). Indeed, all these responses occur after any form of tissue injury. Again, it is the failure of these changes to resolve that distinguishes SIRS/sepsis from the "stress" response.

There is a growing body of evidence implicating cytokines as essential elements in both normal and prolonged inflammatory responses. Cytokines are low-molecular-weight proteins that regulate the amplitude and duration of the body's immune response. These compounds bind to the surface of a target cell and control the release of a number of additional inflammatory mediators. Cytokines may possess both proinflammatory and antiinflammatory properties; in the normal state there is a delicate balance between these two (22). During simple stress and early in sepsis, proinflammatory effects appear to predominate. Tumor necrosis factor, interleukin (IL)-1, IL-6, and IL-8 are proinflammatory mediators that seem to be crucial in the propagation of the inflammatory response in various organ systems (see below). These four cytokines, in turn, stimulate their own production via positive feedback mechanisms and enhance other cells' immune function. Antiinflammatory cytokines, of which IL-10 is the best studied, suppress production of the proinflammatory cytokines (23).

ORGAN DYSFUNCTION

Pulmonary Alterations—Acute Respiratory Distress Syndrome

While low levels of stress result in mild hypoxemia that is easily corrected by provision of elevated concentrations of inspired oxygen, the alterations in pulmonary behavior observed in the sepsis syndrome take the form of acute lung injury (ALI) or the acute respiratory distress syndrome (ARDS).

ALI/ARDS represents the classic pulmonary response to a local or remote inflammatory focus. Studies have shown sepsis to be the precipitator of ALI/ARDS in 32% to 63% of cases (24). Often, the focus is intraabdominal, but the inciting focus may involve direct damage to lung parenchyma, as occurs in pneumonia or aspiration. A number of factors influence the likelihood of developing lung injury as a component of sepsis (Table 3) (25–28).

The initial phase of ALI involves diffuse inflammation and capillary leak. The result is nonhydrostatic pulmonary edema, an increase in lung water and densely congested and consolidated pulmonary parenchyma (29). Traditionally, pathophysiology in the early phase of ALI or ARDS is often defined in terms of V/Q mismatching, resulting in hypoxemia and an increased work of breathing. Thus, patients hyperventilate, in part

TABLE 3. RISK FACTORS FOR SEPSIS-INDUCED ACUTE RESPIRATORY DISTRESS SYNDROME

Increased risk:
   ram-negative sepsis
   Increased severity of sepsis
   Older age
   Chronic alcoholism
Decreased risk:
   Less severe sepsis
   Younger age
   Diabetes

to excrete the carbon dioxide load that results from the increase in global metabolism, and in part to compensate for the greater lung "stiffness" that results from parenchymal edema and consolidation. Ultimately, the combination of carbon dioxide production combined with fatigue due to increased work of breathing affects not just oxygenation but also ventilation, and a need for invasive mechanical support develops. Therapy has traditionally involved the use of supplemental oxygen, mechanical ventilation, and continuous positive airway pressure (CPAP) or positive end-expiratory pressure (PEEP) to normalize blood gases by overcoming the diffusion gradient to oxygen and the mechanical resistance of stiff, edematous lung tissue. The pathogenesis of this early phase of ARDS is inordinately complex, involving interactions between WBCs and endothelial cells, a number of mediators including cytokines, arachidonic acid metabolites, and adhesion molecules (25). However, neutrophils seem to be central players. Tumor necrosis factor, IL-1, and IL-8 activate neutrophils that migrate into the pulmonary vasculature and adhere to the endothelium, increasing surface expression of selectins, integrins, and intracellular adhesion molecules on cell surfaces (25). There is an increase in endothelial permeability with exudative leakage into the interstitium and alveoli (25,28).

While neutrophils may mediate the initial phases of ALI/ARDS, newer data indicate that ARDS is a biphasic disease (30). Initially, the response is as described previously, but secondary injury can develop as a consequence of the barotrauma associated with positive pressure ventilation. Application of even modest elevations of peak airway pressures has been demonstrated to cause direct damage to alveoli. This trauma enhances leakage of proteinaceous fluid into both the interstitium and the alveolar spaces, disrupts the collagen framework of the lungs, leads to alveolar rupture, and causes inflammatory proliferation. This infiltrate ultimately comes to contain not only exudative fluid but cellular elements, most notably white and red blood cells. An eventual decrease in local edema occurs as the infiltrate organizes and eventually becomes fibrotic. Volutrauma likely plays a role in the iatrogenic lung injury caused by mechanical ventilation (31). The key point is that the time course of ARDS is dynamic, with significant temporal variability.

It also is clear that both phases of lung injury involve changes in pulmonary pathophysiology that are spatially heterogeneous, not uniformly distributed throughout the lung parenchyma (32). Infiltrates, especially those associated with the alveoli as seen in the later phases of ARDS, accumulate in the dependent portions of the lung. The weight of these edematous lung segments tends to cause collapse in adjacent regions, which may actually be pathologically uninvolved. Further, the location of these infiltrates is gravity-dependent and will be altered with changes in position. The characteristic alteration in compliance is also not uniform, but seems to reflect a loss of functional lung units in the dependent lung and in adjacent collapsed segments, as opposed to a global, edema-induced reduction in distensibility. The net result is a loss of oxygen-exchanging capacity in consolidated regions of the lung and in other regions that are simply collapsed, while a residual number of lung units are entirely normal. The key point is that the lungs are not necessarily stiff; the low compliance is a manifestation of trying to get a relatively large tidal volume (V_T) into a small amount of relatively normal lung (30).

In summary, then, the several pathologic processes involved in the development and perpetuation of ARDS lead to three distinct populations of alveoli: normal, irreversibly consolidated, and collapsed but recruitable. The result is a reduction in the amount of effective surface for gas exchange. When viewed in this manner, it is clear why standard therapy often fails, since attempting to maximize lung volumes when a portion of the lung is irreversibly consolidated can result in the induction of barotrauma in the normal areas of lung. Similarly, normalization of blood gases, especially $Paco_2$, is likely to be an unattainable goal since the effective ventilatory surface is decreased. A new approach with different therapeutic goals is indicated.

In this new paradigm, based on a clearer understanding of the pathophysiology of ARDS, the goals of therapy become (a) maintaining oxygen exchange; (b) preventing further damage (i.e., barotrauma or volutrauma); and (c) recruiting potentially recruitable alveoli. Recent studies (28,33) indicate that ventilation with small V_Ts, low plateau pressure, and the use of a strategy designed to limit cyclic open and closing of alveoli decreases mortality and improves a number of clinical markers in patients with ARDS (33,34). The approach starts with finding the minimal volume needed to provide adequate exchange in the "normal" lung units. It turns out that this volume, and the ability to maintain oxygenation, is a function of mean airway pressure, although there is significant patient-to-patient variability. Therefore, achievement of the initial goal of therapy, maintenance of oxygen exchange, involves determination of the minimal level of mean airway pressure consistent with adequate oxygen exchange. Increasing PEEP to some "optimal" level is the currently accepted method; PEEP is adjusted to the lowest level that gives acceptable oxygenation and minimizes mean airway pressure. The second goal, prevention of further damage from iatrogenic injury by limiting peak (i.e., end-inspiratory) pressure and the time spent at peak pressure, uses small V_Ts and high rates, an approach that is logical when the lungs in ARDS are viewed as "small." A practical approach is to use pressure-limited ventilation, effectively setting a ceiling on the peak pressure. The third therapeutic goal is to recruit alveoli that are collapsed, but not consolidated. Several methods are useful in trying to accomplish this goal. Optimization of PEEP not only improves oxygenation but, by improving compliance and reducing the work of breathing (the "traditional" reason for its use), may also be effective in recruiting slowly expandable alveoli. Computed tomographic studies of the lung demonstrate that the application of PEEP improves gravity-dependent infiltrates, primarily by recruiting lung units that are not irreversibly consolidated (32). It may also be useful to increase the time spent in inspiration by altering the inspiratory-to-expiratory ratio. This alteration exposes the alveoli to the mean airway pressure for a longer period of time, but may ultimately decrease peak pressures by opening up collapsed airways and reducing resistance. The data on the use of inverse-ratio ventilation are primarily anecdotal and are, therefore, less convincing than those on the use of PEEP, but the theoretical basis is sound. Using a ramp inspiratory mode rather than a square wave may also be useful to limit the time spent at peak pressure and to increase mean pressure. In summary then, the therapeutic strategy is simple: optimization of mean airway pressure, use of PEEP, and limitation of peak pressure, often with the use of pressure-limited or pressure-controlled ventilation with a peak transalveolar (airway-to-pleural) plateau pressure of 30 cm H_2O (30).

New approaches may also result in new complications. Small V_T, longer inspiratory time, and increased mean pressure may lead to air trapping, either because there is insufficient time for expiration or an insufficient pressure gradient for flow. Both circulatory compromise, from an increase in intrathoracic pressure and decreased return to both sides of the heart, and carbon dioxide retention may result. Circulatory problems can be overcome with increased venous return. One approach to dealing with carbon dioxide retention is simply to allow carbon dioxide to rise (permissive hypercarbia). Since mechanisms exist that can correct pH, even in the presence of severe hypercarbia, carbon dioxide retention is not necessarily detrimental. Alternatively, normalization of the pH can be achieved with the use of tracheal insufflation (35). In this method, a catheter is placed through the endotracheal tube to the level of the tracheal carina. $Paco_2$ declines as oxygen flow through the catheter increases. This method effectively reduces dead space; while the total minute volume delivered remains constant, the amount delivered by the ventilator decreases as catheter flow is increased. Tracheal insufflation has proven to be an effective method in patients who are difficult to ventilate.

A final word is required of renewed interest in a therapy that has been tested previously and found wanting—steroids for ARDS. Previous large well-designed prospective, double-blinded, randomized trials had used a large bolus of methylprednisolone (30 mg per kg) over a 48-hour period in early ARDS and sepsis. These studies failed to show a decrease in mortality and actually demonstrated a higher incidence of septic complications (36,37). More recent investigations, focusing on the late, fibroproliferative stage of ARDS, demonstrate that low doses of systemically administered steroids may be beneficial (38–40). One explanation for the difference in outcome is that a lower dose of steroids (120 to 240 mg per day methylprednisolone for 10 to 15 days) is given for a longer time period in the more recent studies with significantly less immunosuppressive effects (41,42).

Cardiac Alterations—Myocardial Depression

Sepsis profoundly alters the behavior of the cardiovascular system. Cerra and colleagues previously characterized cardiovascular physiology in sepsis, noting that the heart initially compensated well but that performance ultimately deteriorated (11). All stress states initially result in tachycardia, an increase in CO, a decrease in systemic vascular resistance (SVR), and a redistribution of blood flow. It is postulated that the transition from the stress response to sepsis involves a change from a balanced hyperdynamic state to clinically silent myocardial depression.

Some investigators, relying mainly on measurements of left ventricular (LV) ejection fraction in both dogs (43) and humans (44), have contended that sepsis-associated increases in CO were dependent on markedly increased filling of a dilated, depressed ventricle (45). The development of radionuclide ventriculography in the 1980s allowed more direct demonstration of myocardial depression in sepsis (46). The decrease in ejection fraction was initially believed to have predictive value, but that claim has not been borne out. However, calculated ejection fraction is both preload- and afterload-dependent and correlation with the intrinsic state of the myocardium has not been well established. Indeed, while ejection fraction has long been the standard by which overt heart failure is characterized, even this concept has been questioned. A second approach to quantify ventricular function in sepsis focuses on a decrease in the maximal ability to increase ventricular pressure over the time of contraction (i.e., dP/dtmax). In studies in endotoxemic sheep, Redl and coworkers demonstrated that progressive endotoxemia reduced the maximal pressure generated in the LV over the course of contraction (47). This pressure is a function of preload and, furthermore, anything that alters LV "stiffness," such as myocardial ischemia, will affect the maximum pressure, independent of sepsis. Sagawa and colleagues have developed an approach based on the construction of pressure-volume loops (Fig. 1) (48). By constructing a series of lines through the origin and tangent to the pressure-volume loops at end-systole, one can come up with a quantifiable measure of contractility. As demonstrated in Fig. 1,

each vertical line in the left-hand panel of the figure (1-C, 2-B, 3-A) represents an isovolumetric contraction, and the corresponding horizontal line (AD, BE, CF) reflects a maximal end-systolic pressure. Reducing outflow impedance (moving from B to A) increases ejection fraction or stroke volume (SV)—indicated by the length of the lines AD, BE, and CF—but contractility is a function of the slope of the line. As the slope of the line is altered, the contractility increases or decreases. As depicted in the right-hand side of Fig. 1, contractility is greater in X than in Y or Z, since at a given pressure or outflow impedance (point 2), the SV (length of line 2-Z versus 2-Y versus 2-X) increases. This approach is valid in isolated ventricles, but its use *in vivo* is unknown. Krosl and associates have proposed an alternative that is designed to allay some of the concerns inherent in other approaches (49). Expressing dP/dtmax as a function of end-diastolic ventricular diameter (EDD) eliminates diameter concerns regarding preload dependence.

When the change in dP/dtmax is plotted as a function of the change in EDD (Fig. 2), four possible alterations can occur. While in two alterations the behavior cannot be classified, when dP/dt increases and EDD decreases, contractility is clearly increased; when dP/dt is decreased, despite an increase in EDD, contractility is decreased. Krosl and associates have tested this model in sheep infused with live *Escherichia coli* over an 8-hour period and validated its use.

Controversy remains regarding the effects of sepsis on LV diastolic function (50–53). Right ventricular (RV) function also is altered in sepsis and septic shock, with a depression of the ejection fraction and increased end-diastolic volume (46).

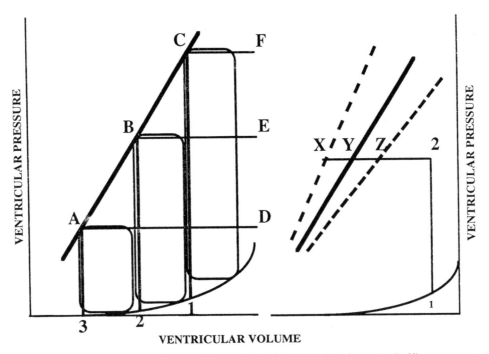

FIGURE 1. Left: Pressure-volume loops at different levels of end-diastolic volume. *Vertical lines* represent changes in pressure during isovolumetric relaxation; *horizontal lines* represent changes in volume during ejection (stroke volume). **Right:** Changes in contractility are represented by a change in the slope of the line connecting the pressure-volume loops at end-systole. See text for details.

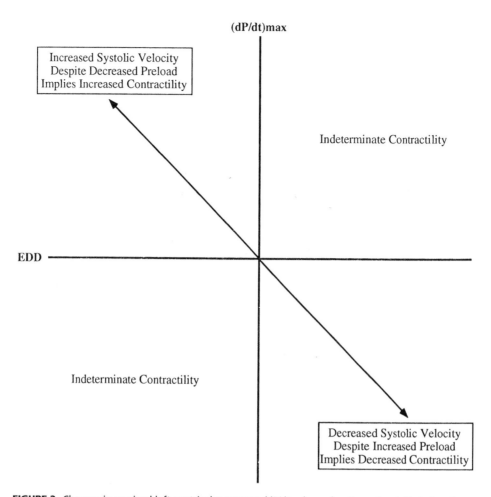

FIGURE 2. Changes in maximal left-ventricular pressure (dP/dt$_{max}$) as a function of end-diastolic volume.

There has been much interest in elucidating the mechanism causing myocardial dysfunction. Two different mechanisms have been suggested (46). The first hypothesis was that global myocardial ischemia caused myocardial dysfunction (46). This theory has been discredited by studies showing normal or increased coronary blood flow (50) and normal myocardial high-energy phosphate levels (54,55). The second theory evokes the production of a circulating myocardial-depressant factor based on studies demonstrating a decrease in extent and velocity of myocardial shortening in isolated rat myocytes treated with serum from septic patients. This did not occur when serum from critically ill nonseptic patients or convalescing former septic patients were applied to myocytes (56). A large, heat-labile polypeptide believed to have myocardial-depressant properties has been isolated from the serum of septic patients. To date, this protein has not been characterized further.

Therefore, it appears that sepsis in some way depresses global cardiac function. What is not clear, however, is where the utility of these findings lies. As in the discussion of ARDS, an alternative approach to the concept of myocardial performance may clarify the clinical situation. Routine measurement of EDD or construction of pressure-volume loops is not clinically feasible. Moreover, CO is inevitably increased in sepsis if venous return is adequate. The information derived from studies on myocardial contractility in sepsis can, however, be used to practically interpret data derived from a pulmonary artery (PA) catheter. The conceptualization involves focusing on the divergent nature of the pulmonary and systemic circulations and examining SV, venous return, and the concept of impedance to ejection. Sepsis is associated with systemic hypotension and pulmonary hypertension. Thus, in septic patients, there is an increase in systemic vascular capacitance, but a decrease in the capacitance of the pulmonary circuit. Venous return to the right heart may be high, reflected in the elevated central venous pressure that accompanies venous pooling, while return to the left heart may be impaired. Similarly, there is little impedance to LV outflow but significant increases in RV-outflow impedance. The pulmonary capillary occlusion pressure may be misleading, since the increase in PA pressure will limit venous return to the left heart despite an apparent increase in LV end-diastolic pressure. If ventricular function (contractility) is only mildly impaired, fluid administration will improve return to the right ventricle, increase right-sided SV, and overcome the resistance in the pulmonary circuit. The result will be an improvement in return to the left ventricle and an increase in the SV calculated from the CO. Should SV fail to improve despite an increase in right-sided filling, the implication is either that pulmonary vasoconstriction is extreme or that ventricular function is depressed. This sort of analysis allows the use of systemic and PA pressures, coupled with determination of SV changes in response to volume infusion, to make qualitative statements regarding the intrinsic contractile state of the myocardium.

The presence of depressed myocardial contractility has direct therapeutic implications. A key lies in optimization of venous return to both sides of the heart, which is best accomplished by fluid administration, with an understanding that the important variable is a change (or lack of change) in SV and that filling pressures may be misleading. Further, intrinsic myocardial depression may require the use of potent inotropes. Breslow and colleagues examined endotoxic shock in dogs whose mean blood pressure decreased from 110 mm Hg to 50 mm Hg and noted that an increase in CO and SV could only be achieved by infusion of norepinephrine (14). Infusions with phenylephrine hydrochloride, dopamine hydrochloride, and dobutamine hydrochloride left CO unchanged. The previous analysis also suggests a role for amrinone lactate, which has pulmonary vasodilatory properties and may also improve RV performance. Finally, this approach underscores the potential use of inhaled nitric oxide (NO). This experimental agent can decrease impedance to RV outflow and improve LV venous return without increasing blood flow to poorly ventilated regions (thus minimizing shunt by avoiding the inhibition of hypoxic pulmonary vasoconstriction) or further decreasing LV outflow impedance (57). A role for selective inotropic support of the RV is also potentially useful.

Vascular Abnormalities—Catechol-Resistant Vasodilation

Vasomotor paralysis is characteristic of sepsis. It has long been understood that sepsis is associated with a decrease in peripheral tone and a redistribution of organ blood flow. The etiology is unclear, but the vasodilation would appear to reflect alterations in metabolism induced by systemic inflammation. Vasodilation may represent a mechanism by which to compensate for impaired oxygen (or some other substrate) use, with the "paralysis" representing the dysfunction that accompanies the transition to organ dysfunction. Recent work has demonstrated that the sepsis-induced alterations in flow and oxygen extraction are not uniform. For example, extraction is low in skeletal muscle, where oxygen consumption is strictly dependent on delivery. In contrast, the splanchnic bed exhibits markedly increased flow, extraction and, presumably, demand. In some organ beds, vasodilation occurs both in the arterial and venous beds. Most recently, studies focusing on the determinants of splanchnic blood flow; the interactions between the mesenteric and portal circulations; and the role of NO, prostacyclin, leukotrienes, tumor necrosis factor, and IL-1 and their importance in mediating sepsis-induced vasodilation, have altered beliefs concerning the peripheral vasculopathy of sepsis in a way that may have therapeutic implications.

The splanchnic circulation is the likely site of increased capacitance in sepsis. Ayuse and coworkers have investigated the relationship between portal and mesenteric blood flow in nonseptic and septic animals (58). Normally, when portal venous pressure increases (and, thus, flow into the liver increases), a reflex arc is activated that constricts the mesenteric circulation. This has been referred to as the venoarterial response. In this study, application of stepwise incremental increases in portal venous pressure under nonseptic conditions resulted in an increase in mesenteric resistance. Sepsis obliterated this response, with the resultant high potential for pooling fluid within the splanchnic bed. Further, given the obligatory capillary leak associated with all inflammatory states, the possibility exists that edema formation in the GI tract might be enhanced.

It is likely that the splanchnic circulation is unresponsive to commonly used therapeutic agents such as natural and synthetic catecholamines. On the other hand, the vasculature that supplies muscle and skin appears to respond to strong alpha-adrenergic agents such as norepinephrine. Data support the theory that norepinephrine may actually increase renal blood flow via a redistribution of flow (59). Thus, it may well be that norepinephrine is the agent of choice to improve the abnormalities of vascular tone and flow distribution in patients with sepsis (60). The use of a potent angiotensin agonist has not been reported, but it is an important area for future investigation since angiotensin II is an important regulator of hepatic perfusion (see below).

Consideration must also be given to sepsis-induced increases in pulmonary resistance. This increased resistance may depress RV function. Agents that decrease pulmonary hypertension, such as epinephrine or dobutamine, may improve RV function but tend to alter V/Q matching by overriding intrinsic pulmonary control mechanisms, such as hypoxic pulmonary vasoconstriction, and may also further compromise systemic pressure. Inhaled NO, which will be selectively directed to open alveoli, has not proven to be as useful as originally hoped.

Altered Aerobic Metabolism (Oxygen Consumption/Delivery)

Tissue hypoxia occurs when there is an imbalance between tissue oxygen demand and tissue oxygen delivery. In normal physiologic conditions, oxygen demand is a major factor in determining the blood flow to the tissues. In sepsis, however, this mechanism appears to fail.

Twenty years ago, Shoemaker and colleagues studied survivors of major surgery and showed that these patients had a significantly higher cardiac index (CI), oxygen delivery (DO_2), and oxygen consumption (VO_2) than nonsurvivors (61). Thereafter, these researchers showed that high-risk surgical patients who were pharmacologically induced to achieve these values also had lower mortality rates, fewer complications, and shorter and less expensive hospital stays. However, this study involved a heterogeneous patient population as well as diverse primary insults (i.e., trauma, perioperative hemodynamic instability, sepsis). In subsequent studies patients with sepsis and septic shock failed to demonstrate similar improvements with interventions designed to increase DO_2 to supranormal values (62). The basis for this failure may be an inability to extract or use oxygen even when delivery is enhanced (63,64). Additional studies indicate that treatment aimed at maximizing oxygen delivery in patients with severe sepsis or septic shock does not reduce mortality or morbidity (65–67). In 1993, a consensus conference on tissue hypoxia evaluated all randomized controlled studies and concluded that "aggressive attempts to increase Do_2 to supranormal values in critically ill patients are unwarranted" (68).

Hepatic Dysfunction

Hepatic blood flow appears to be altered in sepsis. In an important study, Reilly and associates showed that flow across the liver was decreased by vasoconstriction in pigs subjected to cardiogenic shock (69). This decrease is mediated by the angiotensin II pathways but not the alpha-adrenergic or vasopressin pathways. Angiotensin II activity, in turn, is dependent on the renin/angiotensin system and, ultimately, renal perfusion. Additionally, adrenergic agents such as norepinephrine do not markedly alter splanchnic blood flow. However, this pattern may not be applicable in sepsis. Further investigations into splanchnic flow are required.

An altered venoarterial response, as detailed above, indicates that something overrides normal splanchnic venous- and arterial-vasoconstrictive mechanisms in sepsis. Recent studies have implicated NO, which is released by endothelial and inflammatory cells and relaxes vascular smooth muscle via a cyclic-guanosine monophosphate-mediated mechanism. One could postulate that blocking NO might improve the loss of vascular tone. A number of studies in which NO synthase (NOS) was blocked, in both animals and humans, has demonstrated that this is, indeed, the case (70,71). However, the improvement in blood pressure and SVR that followed the use of NOS inhibitors was associated with a worse outcome. These studies, however, employed nonselective NOS inhibition. More recent work, focusing on selective inhibition of inducible NOS, has shown that this isoform of the enzyme has a significant effect on splanchnic flow. However, no studies have been performed in hyperdynamic sepsis.

The clinical hallmark of hepatic failure in sepsis is jaundice that results from intrahepatic cholestasis. Studies in animals indicate that this is likely the result of very early decreases in bilirubin and bile acid transport (72). However, the actual incidence of liver failure in sepsis is unknown because investigators have defined liver failure by different parameters and therefore have reached different conclusions (73).

Hepatic dysfunction is manifest in sepsis in ways other than altered bile acid and bilirubin transport. In animals, hepatic glucose production is initially increased as a result of enhanced substrate delivery and high levels of hormonal tone. This occurs despite a major decrease in the expression and activity of two rate-limiting enzymes, phospho *enol* pyruvate carboxykinase and glucose-6-phosphatase (74,75). Later, glucose production falls as the substrate supply becomes impaired and overt hypoglycemia develops. Similarly, there is an alteration in protein use. The development of a decrease in expression of clotting factors such as fibrinogen and in the use of urea cycle intermediates (76) indicates that somewhere in the course of the transition from the stress response to sepsis-induced organ dysfunction, hepatic protein synthesis becomes selectively and significantly impaired. Failed use of fatty acids results from impaired expression of two rate-limiting enzymes in the beta-oxidative pathway, carnitine palmitoyltransferase and acetyl CoA acyltransferase (77). As a result, intrahepatic steatosis is common in sepsis (79). Drug biotransformation also is altered reflecting decreased activity of

cytochrome P-450 enzymes (77) and decreased bile flow and excretion (78).

These findings have several important therapeutic implications. First, the liver has significant metabolic reserve and can appear to be functioning normally, even in the face of a significant insult. Further, provision of substrate, such as exogenous amino acids or vitamin K, sufficient to maintain hepatic protein synthesis, is imperative. Standard methods of hepatic synthetic function, such as measurement of transport proteins like albumin, cannot be used in sepsis or organ dysfunction because these factors are characteristically depressed in response to any "stress." Finally, clinically evident hepatic dysfunction represents a truly grave situation, with a poor prognosis (8).

Sepsis and the Gastrointestinal Tract

Previously, little importance was attributed to the GI tract and its role in sepsis (80). Recent evidence indicates that the bowel may be important in the propagation and maintenance of sepsis (80).

In the normal physiologic state, the gut acts as a barrier to prevent intestinal bacteria from entering the systemic circulation (80). The intestine provides protection through tight mechanical junctions between intestinal epithelial cells which prevent the exodus of pathogens; chemical substances that recognize and remove foreign antigens; and native bacterial flora that prevent pathogenic overgrowth (80). During sepsis, there is widespread damage to the intestinal mucosa. This damage disrupts tight junctions, potentially permitting access to foreign pathogens, native enteric bacteria, and bacterial breakdown products such as endotoxin (80). General immune impairment, along with local immune failure, further compounds the problem, as does the widespread use of prophylactic antibiotics, which facilitates overgrowth of the endogenous flora with potential pathogens. Additional contributors include ileus and generalized malnutrition with associated stagnation and mucosal atrophy.

Renal Insufficiency—A Pathophysiologic Dilemma

Despite years of interest in and hundreds of studies of the subject, the pathophysiology of renal insufficiency in sepsis remains obscure. Nonetheless, the subject is intensely important. A recent prospective study showed the incidence of acute renal failure to be 19% in sepsis, 23% in severe sepsis, and 51% in septic shock (82,83). The presence of renal failure in sepsis significantly worsens prognosis.

In general, renal dysfunction in sepsis involves the intrinsic renal parenchymal injury known as "acute tubular necrosis" (ATN) or "acute renal failure," a group of disorders generally believed to arise from ischemic (most often resulting from prolonged prerenal azotemia—i.e., functional renal hypoperfusion), nephrotoxic, or nephritic insults (81,84). A detailed examination of the pathogenesis of acute renal failure is beyond the scope of this chapter, but several aspects of the disorder have been the subject of recent controversy and merit discussion. It is important to note that acute renal failure, by definition, involves an intrinsic inability to excrete metabolic waste products (i.e., an inability to clear solute). A further distinction involves the volume of solvent in which the solute is dissolved (i.e., the urine output). While the notion of urine output dominates clinical thinking, it is in a sense spurious with regard to renal dysfunction; the degree of urine output has little correlation with the transition from the stress response to sepsis to organ dysfunction. In fact, urine output as a measure of intrinsic function may actually obscure the underlying problem, a concept that will be returned to in a discussion of the use of dopamine in sepsis. The intrinsic abnormality in renal function is probably present very early (during sepsis), but compensatory mechanisms render the process clinically silent until functional reserve is overwhelmed (during ATN).

The insult most likely to precipitate renal insufficiency in sepsis is prolonged relative hypoperfusion (84). In turn, this insult may on occasion arise as a result of overt shock, either from cardiac failure or unresuscitated vasodilation, but is far more likely to reflect the redistribution of blood flow that is characteristic of sepsis. Blood pooling and vasodilation in the splanchnic bed make the kidneys particularly vulnerable to ischemic insult. Therapeutically, two approaches might be taken: maximization of intravascular volume and the administration of potent adrenergic agonists. The use of these modalities has significance with regard to dysfunction of virtually all organ systems, and will be discussed in more global terms in the section focusing on fluid management ("Fluid and Vasopressor Administration in the Septic Patient—The Common Thread"). A point of note, however, is that recent data focusing on the use of norepinephrine in sepsis indicate that use of this most potent alpha-adrenergic agent is associated with an improvement in renal function, and is not associated with the presumed detrimental effects that have limited its appeal in the past (59). The most reasonable explanation for this phenomenon would appear to lie in an improvement in "central" blood volume, improving perfusion of the kidney at the expense of skeletal muscle.

Similarly, a recent study served to highlight the distinction between solute clearance and solvent losses. Comparing the effects of dopamine and dobutamine on renal function, investigators determined that the former functions as a diuretic, increasing the amount of solvent lost, but not improving creatinine clearance (85). Several explanations, including a dopamine-induced redistribution of blood flow toward the renal medulla, have been advanced. The most likely explanation, however, lies in the identification of D1 receptors on the distal loop of Henle and convoluted tubule, and a vasodilating effect on both flow entering (D1) and leaving (D2) Bowman's capsule. In addition, recent evaluations of renal dysfunction in sepsis have led to a reevaluation of the pathogenic role played by potential nephrotoxins, especially the aminoglycoside antibiotics and radiographic contrast media. Despite the use of pharmacokinetic data and serum levels to direct the dosage regimen of aminoglycosides, the belief remains that the models from which the regimen was developed ineffectively describe the clinical picture associated with sepsis. Newer models (86) have been designed to achieve earlier peak concentration and, thus, minimize the duration of therapy to avoid nephrotoxicity. Similarly, recent studies have highlighted the need for volume loading following a dye load (87,88). Therapeutically then, a limited number of options exist for treating the diagnostic dilemma that is sepsis-associated renal insufficiency.

Maximization of intravascular volume and support of perfusion with strong vasopressors, along with avoiding nephrotoxins, appear to be the keys.

Sepsis and the Nervous System

Septic encephalopathy is the most frequent cause of encephalopathy among intensive care patients (89,90). The incidence of encephalopathy in sepsis is unknown but probably widely underestimated because sedation and neuromuscular blockade, often used to manage ventilation in septic patients, preclude the evaluation of mental status (89). When assessment is possible, septic patients exhibit mental status changes ranging from mild confusion to delirium and coma (91). In addition, sepsis has been associated with a peripheral neuropathy of unclear etiology (89).

Sepsis and Peripheral Metabolism

While the effects of sepsis on hepatic substrate use have been discussed, sepsis also markedly alters metabolism in the periphery. During sepsis, peripheral tissues demonstrate mildly enhanced glucose uptake and peripheral glucose use (92). Glycolysis is increased (93–95). Lactate production is increased as a result of glycolysis (92). However, this increase does not necessarily reflect a deficit in oxygen delivery. Fischer and coworkers (as cited in James, et al.) have shown that increases in epinephrine-induced skeletal muscle metabolism result in stimulation of $Na+/K+$ exchange. This pump is linked to an adenosine triphosphatase that is strictly dependent on the glycolytic pathway, even when oxygen availability is high (96). Thus, one characteristic of septic metabolism is increased aerobic glycolysis. In addition, peripheral responses to insulin are decreased, reflecting a postreceptor defect (97).

Lipolysis is increased in sepsis. This effect of increased hormone-sensitive lipase activity, which increases lipoprotein breakdown and the secretion of fatty acids (92), is accompanied by a cytokine-mediated impairment of lipoprotein lipase. Since lipoprotein lipase is responsible for the uptake and reesterification of free fatty acids in most tissues, the net result is a dramatic rise in circulating levels of free fatty acids (98,99). The excess free fatty acids may contribute to the fatty infiltration of the liver characteristic of sepsis (92,100).

During sepsis, there is net peripheral protein catabolism with consequent increased urea production (92). This catabolism is most pronounced in muscle, gut, and connective tissue (92). The amino-acid metabolites appear to be used by the body as substrate for gluconeogenesis or production of acute phase proteins in the liver (92).

FLUID AND VASOPRESSOR ADMINISTRATION IN THE SEPTIC PATIENT—THE COMMON THREAD

Discussion of the administration of fluid to the septic patient serves to connect the alterations in pulmonary pathophysiology, cardiac function, vascular tone, and hepatic and renal dysfunction that have all been previously detailed in this chapter. Four basic problems make fluid administration in the septic patient a concern:

1. The vasodilation is such that large amounts of exogenous fluid may be required to maintain tissue perfusion.
2. The capillary leak makes maintenance of intravascular volume a challenge; edema, especially in the lung and the gut, compounds the clinical situation.
3. The increase in pulmonary resistance makes adequately estimating volume status a difficult task.
4. Finally, the myocardial depression, splanchnic pooling, and relative renal hypoperfusion make it essential that venous return be maintained.

As previously stated, splanchnic tone appears to be primarily dependent on angiotensin II, which in turn is influenced by renin production. Renin and angiotensin-II levels are further dependent on renal perfusion and hepatic blood flow and function (for the conversion of angiotensin I to angiotensin II). In addition, myocardial depression requires that venous return be maximized for SV to remain acceptable. Maintaining blood flow to the kidney, liver, and heart is therefore essential. However, the obligatory capillary leak results in a constant slow loss of fluid into the "third space," including the pulmonary parenchyma and the splanchnic and somatic beds. These processes make fluid administration a two-edged sword; third-space loss is potentially detrimental to pulmonary function, and may also increase GI dysfunction. Increased lung water, which can be affected by hydrostatic forces, will decrease compliance, altering the ability to ventilate, and may also compromise oxygenation via the collapse of "recruitable" segments of lung. What results is the need to balance oxygenation and edema formation, which mandate a "dry" patient, with the need for renal and hepatic perfusion and increased RV volume to overcome pulmonary hypertension and maintain cardiac performance—goals that are best achieved by keeping the patient "wet."

A recent understanding of several specific pulmonary problems that can impact on fluid administration need to be discussed in more detail. First, the increase in lung water will alter compliance and require that either higher airway pressures or longer ventilator duty cycles be used to ventilate. The higher pressures and longer duty cycles can compromise venous return. Second, hypercapnia by itself is a pulmonary vasodilator and may alter V/Q matching and oxygenation. Third, there is a hydrostatic component to the capillary leak so that increasing preload may also increase the transudation of water into the lungs. Finally, interstitial lung water is in part removed by the lymphatics. In experimental models, lymph flow may either increase or decrease in sepsis; therefore, the actual effects are unknown. Overall, there may be an advantage to minimizing fluid administration in the hypoxemic patient, but this practice will compromise perfusion of other organ systems. Although this view is controversial, ample fluids should be administered while maintaining a PaO_2 above 60 mm Hg or an SaO_2 above about 90%.

In attempting to maintain cardiac function, the goals of fluid therapy are to maximize venous return to both sides of the heart.

However, measurement of venous return can be problematic. For example, altered lung water can increase transpulmonary pressure, which will be reflected in higher PA and wedge pressures. Increased intrathoracic pressure from positive-pressure ventilation can have the same effect. In this setting, pressure may not equal volume, and it is easy to be "misled by the wedge." One possible solution is to use echocardiography to estimate ventricular volume. Finally, while high impedance to ventricular outflow may compromise CO, coronary-artery filling is dependent on diastolic pressure, which needs to be maintained at some minimal level and obviates the use of most vasodilators to reduce pulmonary artery pressure. Inhaled NO will reduce pulmonary artery pressure. However, its use has not proven to reduce mortality or morbidity in sepsis.

Choice of fluid for resuscitation has prompted some of the most vociferous debate in medicine. The controversy surrounds the use of salt solutions (crystalloid), solutions containing large, oncotically active molecule (colloids) and blood or blood products.

Crystalloid solutions are widely available and inexpensive. However, they have a short intravascular half-life (20 to 25 minutes) (101) and a large volume of distribution. Indeed, 1 L of normal saline increases the intravascular volume only by 300 cc after 30 minutes (101). Another putative disadvantage of crystalloid solutions is the lowering of plasma colloid oncotic pressure, which can lead to further tissue extravasation (101). Experimental verification of this widely held belief is lacking.

Proponents for the use of a colloid such as albumin in septic patients argue that the decrease in albumin observed in these patients is accompanied by a significant decrease in colloid osmotic pressure and resultant edema formation. This edema is especially problematic in the lung, where it can alter gas exchange. However, several animal studies suggest that colloid therapy increases interstitial edema (102,103). Investigators also have demonstrated that the decrease in colloid osmotic pressure cannot explain the genesis of pulmonary edema (104). Further, a recent study demonstrated a lack of correlation between mortality and colloid osmotic pressure, further indicated that albumin only contributed 17% of the total colloid osmotic pressure and revealed that survivors of sepsis showed an intrinsic ability to increase serum albumin concentrations, possibly owing to resumption of synthesis (105). Two recent metaanalysis studies have shown that albumin treatment was associated with a higher risk of death than treatment with crystalloid (106,107). The first study included 30 randomized controlled trials, including 1,419 randomized patients. For each patient category (hypovolemia, burns, hypoalbuminemia) the risk of death in the albumin-treated group was higher. These data support the multidisciplinary consensus statement concerning colloid versus crystalloid treatment published in 1995, "... crystalloid is the preferred solution in patients demonstrating septic/SIRS pathophysiology" (108).

The use of blood and component therapy is more complicated and very poorly studied. With the exception of patients with known coronary artery disease, the optimal hemoglobin (Hgb) concentration is unknown. Some early studies showed improved outcome with increased DO_2, prompting a recommendation that

Hgb levels be kept in the 10.0 to 11.5 g per dL range (109). More recent studies, however, dispute this (101), with Dietrich and colleagues demonstrating no improvement in shock when Hgb was increased from 8.2 to 10.5 g per dL by red blood cell transfusion (110) and Hebert and others, in a multicenter prospective trial, demonstrating no difference in outcome when Hgb levels were 7 or 10 g per dL (111,112).

The need to maintain splanchnic flow is the major vascular determinant of fluid administration. The demand for substrate delivery is very high in the septic gut and appears to be directly dependent on flow. Since there is regional variability in flow and demand, and since splanchnic flow cannot be measured directly, one reasonable approach is to keep the intravascular volume high and use agents (alpha-adrenergics such as norepinephrine) that will selectively constrict somatic beds. In addition, a recent study demonstrated a decrease in levels of vasopressin in sepsis (113). The most recent updates in cardiopulmonary resuscitation mandate the use of this agent rather than epinephrine (114). Therefore, use of low doses of vasopressin, although not yet tested in a randomized trial, may be of value in sepsis. Since portal tone is dependent on angiotensin II, which in turn is activated by decreased renal blood flow, it is important to keep renal perfusion at relatively high levels. Finally, it must be remembered that the hepatic venoarterial response may be impaired, and, therefore, there is a gradient for edema formation in the gut. Studies on the use of angiotensin antagonists in sepsis are forthcoming and may be extremely useful in defining the importance of this hormone in determining splanchnic perfusion.

SUMMARY

New information has altered our understanding of the pathophysiology of sepsis and allows for more reasonable decision making in the care of the septic patient. Better comprehension of the pathophysiology of ARDS and the occurrence of secondary injury as a result of viscutrauma, biotrauma, or barotrauma has led us to monitor mean airway pressure, to attempt to minimize peak pressures and decrease V_Ts, and to use increased mean pressure (i.e., optimal PEEP) and increased inspiratory times to recruit alveoli and prevent atelectasis. The use of permissive hypercarbia or tracheal insufflation may be necessary to avoid incurring the risks associated with achieving "normal" blood gases.

Cardiac pathophysiology in sepsis is dominated by intrinsic myocardial depression and impedance to RV outflow (pulmonary hypertension), both of which require that venous return be optimized to achieve an appropriate SV. The use of potent inotropes may be needed, but it may be important to avoid using agents that alter V/Q matching. The management of vascular abnormalities and relative renal hypoperfusion also require optimization of venous volume and the use of potent vasoactive agents such as norepinephrine and perhaps vasopressin. Finally, the use of fluids involves the need to balance the disparate requirements of the heart and vasculature (especially the splanchnic circulation) with the need to maintain adequate oxygenation and limit RV-outflow resistance. A reasonable understanding coupled with a carefully thought out, therapeutic approach potentially can improve the outcome of critically ill septic patients.

KEY POINTS

- Time course of acute respiratory distress syndrome is dynamic with significant temporal variability.
- The lungs are not necessarily stiff; the low compliance is a manifestation of trying to get a relatively large tidal volume into a small amount of relatively normal lung.
- For myocardial contractility, venous return to both sides of the heart is best accomplished by fluid administration.
- The liver has significant metabolic reserve. Provision of substrate, sufficient to maintain hepatic protein synthesis, is imperative. Clinically evident hepatic dysfunction represents a truly grave situation, with a poor prognosis.

- Maximization of intravascular volume and the administration of potent adrenergic agonists.
- The incidence of encephalopathy in sepsis is unknown but probably widely underestimated because sedation and neuromuscular blockade, often used to manage ventilation in septic patients, preclude the evaluation of mental status.
- The increase in lung water will alter compliance and require that either higher airway pressures or longer ventilator duty cycles be used to ventilate. The higher pressures and longer duty cycles can compromise venous return.

REFERENCES

1. Balk RA. Severe sepsis and septic shock definitions, epidemiology and clinical manifestations. *Crit Care Clin* 2000;16(2):179–193.
2. Bone RC, Balk RA, Cerra FB, et al. Definitions for sepsis and organ failure and guidelines for the use of innovative therapies in sepsis. American College of Chest Physicians Society of Critical Care Medicine Consensus Conference Committee. *Chest* 1992;101:1644–1655.
3. Abraham E, Matthay MA, Dinarello CA, et al. Consensus Conference Definitions for Sepsis, Septic Shock, Acute Lung Injury and ARDS: time for a reevaluation. *Crit Care Med* 2000;28(1):232–235.
4. Increase in national hospital discharge survey rates for septicemia—United States 1979–1987. *MMWR* 1992;39:31–34.

5. Cuthbertson D, Tilstone WT. Metabolism during the postinjury period. *Adv Clin Chem* 1969;12:1–55.
6. Moore FD, Olsen KH, McMurrey JD. *The body cell mass and its supporting environment.* Philadelphia: WB Saunders, 1978.
7. Caldwell MD. Importance of cellular metabolism in the inflammatory response to tissue injury. In: Bihari David J, Cerra Frank B, eds. *New horizons: multiple organ failure.* Fullerton, CA: Society of Critical Care Medicine, 1989:37–60.
8. Cerra FB. Hypermetabolism, organ failure and metabolic support. *Surgery* 1987;101:1–14.
9. Deutschman CS, De Maio A, Buchman TG, et al. Sepsis-induced alterations in phospho *enol* pyruvate carboxinase expression: the role of insulin and glucagon. *Circ Shock* 1993;40:295–302.

10. Clemens MG, Chaudry IH, McDermott PH, et al. Regulation of glucose production from lactate in experimental sepsis. *Am J Physiol* 1983;244:R794–R800.

11. Cerra FB, Siegal JB, Border JR, Peters DM, McMenamy RR. Correlations between metabolic and cardiopulmonary measurements in patients after trauma, general surgery, and sepsis. *J Trauma* 1979;19:621–629.

12. Clemens MG, Chaudry IH, Daigneau N, Baue AE. Insulin resistance and depressed gluconeogenic capability during early hyperglycemic sepsis. *J Trauma* 1984;24:701–708.

13. Deutschman CS, De Maio A, Clemens MG. Sepsis-induced attenuation of glucagon and 8Br-cAMP modulation of phospho *enol* pyruvate carboxykinase gene. *Am J Physiol* 1995;269:R584–R591.

14. Breslow MJ, Miller CF, Parker SD, et al. Effect of vasopressors on organ blood flow during endotoxin shock in pigs. *Am J Physiol* 1987;252:H291–300.

15. Ghosh S, Liu MS. Decrease in adenylate cyclase activity in dog livers during endotoxic shock. *Am J Physiol* 1983;245:R737–R742.

16. Wiles JB, Cerra FB, Siegal JH, et al. The systemic sepsis response. Does the organism matter? *Crit Care Med* 1980;8:55–60.

17. Deutschman CS, Konstantinides FN, Tsai M, Simmons RL, Cerra FB. Physiology and metabolism in isolated viral septicemia: further evidence of an organism-independent, host- dependent response. *Arch Surg* 1987;122:21–25.

18. Natanson C. Selected treatment strategies for septic shock based on proposed mechanisms of pathogenesis. *Ann Intern Med* 1994;120(9):771–783.

19. Beal AL, Cerra FB. Multiple organ failure syndrome in the 1990s: systemic inflammatory response and organ dysfunction. *JAMA* 1994;271(3):226–233.

20. Dunn DL. Gram-negative bacterial sepsis and sepsis syndrome. *Surg Clin North Am* 1994;74(3):621–635.

21. Parillo JE. Pathogenetic mechanisms of septic shock. *N Engl J Med* 1993;329:1427–1428.

22. Sheeran P, Hall GM. Cytokines in anaesthesia. *Br J Anaesth* 1997;78:201–219.

23. Parson PE, Moss M. Early detection and markers of sepsis. *Clin Chest Med* 1996;17(2):199–212.

24. Sesslar CN, Bloomfield GL, Fowler AA. Current concepts of sepsis and acute lung injury. *Clin Chest Med* 1996;17(2):213–221.

25. Fein AM, Calalang-Colucci MG. Acute lung injury and acute respiratory distress syndrome in sepsis and septic shock. *Crit Care Clin* 2000;16(2):289–318.

26. Montgomory BA, Stager MA, Carico J, et al. Causes of mortality in patients with acute respiratory distress syndrome. *Am Rev Respir Dis* 1985;132:485–491.

27. Moss M, Guidot D, et al. Diabetic patients have a decreased incidence of ARDS. *Crit Care Med* 2000;28(7):2187–2191.

28. Ware LB, Matthay MA. The acute respiratory distress syndrome. *N Eng J Med* 2000;342:1334–1349.

29. Bernard G, Artigas A, Brigham K, et al. The American European Consensus Conference on ARDS. *Am J Resp Crit Care Med* 1994;149:818–824.

30. Marini JJ. New options for ventilatory management of acute lung injury. *New Horizons* 1993;1:489–503.

31. Corbridge TC, Wood LD, Crawford GP, et al. Adverse effects of large tidal volume and low PEEP in canine acid aspiration. *Am Rev Respir Dis* 1990;142:311–315.

32. Gattinoni L, Presenti A, Bamboni M, et al. Relationships between lung computed tomographic density, gas exchange and PEEP in acute respiratory failure. *Anesthesiology* 1988;69:824–832.

33. Marini JJ, Amato MB. Lung recruitment during ARDS. *Minerva Anesthesiol* 2000;66:314–319.

34. The Acute Respiratory Distress Syndrome Network, Ventilation with lower tidal volumes as compared with traditional tidal volumes for acute lung injury and the acute respiratory distress syndrome network. *N Eng J Med* 2000;342:1301–1308.

35. Nahum A, Ravenscroft SA, Nakos G, et al. Tracheal gas insufflation during pressure-control ventilation. Effect of catheter position, diameter and flow rate. *Am Rev Respir Dis* 1992;146:1411–1416.

36. Luce JM, Montgomery AB, Marks JD, et al. Ineffectiveness of high dose methylprednisolone in preventing parenchymal lung injury and improving mortality in patients with septic shock. *Am Rev Respir Dis* 1988;138:62–68.

37. Bernard GR, Luce JM, Sprung CL. High dose corticosteroids in patients with the adult respiratory distress syndrome. *N Engl J Med* 1987;317:1565–1570.

38. Meduri GU, Tolley EA, Chinn A, et al. Procollagen types I and III aminoterminal peptides levels during acute respiratory distress syndrome and in response to methylprednisolone treatment. *Am J Respir Crit Care Med* 1998;158:1432–1441.

39. Biffl WL, Moore FA, Moore EE, et al. Are corticosteroids salvage therapy for acute respiratory distress syndrome? *Am J Surg* 1995;170:591–595.

40. Meduri GU, Chinn AJ, Leeper KV, et al. Corticosteroids rescue treatment of progressive fibroproliferation in late ARDS. Patterns of response and predictors of outcome. *Chest* 1994;105:1516–1527.

41. Calet J. From mega to more reasonable doses of corticosteroids: a decade to recreate hope. *Crit Care Med* 1999;27:672–674.

42. Auphun NJA, DiDonato C, Roste A, et al. Immunosuppression by glucocorticoids inhibition of NKF-KB activity through induction of INB synthesis. *Science* 1995;270:286–290.

43. Natanson C, Danner RL, Fink MP, et al. Cardiovascular performance with *E. coli* challenges in a canine model of sepsis. *Am J Physiol* 1988;254:H558–H569.

44. Parker MM, Shelhamer JH, Bacharach SL, et al. Profound but reversible myocardial depression in patients with septic shock. *Ann Intern Med* 1984;100:483–490.

45. Parillo JE, Parker MM, Natanson C, et al. Septic shock in humans: advances in the understanding of pathogenesis, cardiovascular dysfunction and therapy. *Ann Intern Med* 1990;113:227–242.

46. Price S, Anning PB, Mitchell JA, et al. Myocardial dysfunction in sepsis: mechanisms and therapeutic implications. *Eur Heart J* 1999;20:715–724.

47. Redl G, Newald J, Schlag G, et al. Cardiac function in an ovine model of endotoxemia. *Circ Shock* 1991;35:31–36.

48. Sagawa K, Maughun L, Suga H, et al. *Cardiac contraction and the pressure volume relationship.* New York: Oxford University Press, 1988.

49. Krosl P, Pretorius J, Redl H, et al. Myocardial function in septic sheep. *Shock* 1994;1:325–334.

50. Kumar A, Haery C, Parillo JE. Myocardial dysfunction in septic shock. *Crit Care Clin* 2000;16(2):251–287.

51. Ellrodt AG, Riedinger MS, Kimchi A, et al. Left ventricular performance in septic shock: reversible segmental and global abnormalities. *Am Heart J* 1985;110:402–409.

52. Jafri SM, Lavine S, Field BE, et al. Left ventricular diastolic dysfunction in sepsis. *Crit Care Med* 1991;18:709–714.

53. Poelaert J, Declerck C, Vogelaers D, et al. Left ventricular systolic and diastolic function in shock. *Intensive Care Med* 1997;23:553–560.

54. Soloman MA, Correa R, Alexander HR, et al. Myocardial energy metabolism and morphology in a canine model of sepsis. *Am J Physiol* 1994;266:H757–H768.

55. Cunnion RE, Parillo JE. Myocardial dysfunction in sepsis. *Crit Care Clin* 1989;5(1):99–117.

56. Parillo JE, Burch C, Shelhamer JH, et al. A circulating myocardial depressant substance is associated with cardiac dysfunction and peripheral hypoperfusion (lactic acidemia) in patients with septic shock. *Chest* 1989;95:1072–1080.

57. Zapol WM, Hurford WE. Inhaled NO in the adult respiratory distress syndrome and other lung diseases. *New Horizons* 1993;1:638–650.

58. Ayuse T, Brienza N, Revelly JP, et al. Alterations in liver hemodynamics in an intact porcine model of endotoxic shock. *Am J Physiol* 1995;268:H1106–H1114.

59. Redl-Wenzl EM, Armbruster C, Edelman G, et al. The effects of norepinephrine on hemodynamics and renal function in severe septic shock states. *Intensive Care Med* 1993;19:151–154.

60. Marik PE, Mohedin M. The contrasting effect of dopamine and norepinephrine on systemic and splanchnic oxygen utilization in hyperdynamic sepsis. *JAMA* 1994;272:1354–1357.

61. Shoemaker WC, Appel PL, Kram HB, et al. Prospective trial of supranormal values of survivors as therapeutic goals in high-risk surgical patients. *Chest* 1988;94:1176–1186.

62. Hayes MA, Timmone AC, Yau ES, et al. Oxygen transport patterns in patients with sepsis syndrome or septic shock: influence of treatment and relationship to outcome. *Crit Care Med* 1997;25:926–936.

63. Pollack MP, Field AI, Ruttiman UE. Distribution of cardiopulmonary variables in pediatric survivors and nonsurvivors of septic shock. *Crit Care Med* 1985;13:454–459.

64. Kreymann G, Grosser S, Buggisch P, et al. Oxygen consumption and resting metabolic rate in sepsis, sepsis syndrome and septic shock. *Crit Care Med* 1993;21:1012–1019.

65. Ronco JJ, Fenwick JC, Wiggs BR, et al. Oxygen consumption is independent of increases in oxygen delivery by dobutamine in septic patients who have normal or increased plasma lactate. *Am Rev Respir Dis* 1993;147:25–31.

66. Ronco JJ, Phang PT, Walley KR, et al. Oxygen consumption is independent of changes in oxygen delivery in severe adult respiratory distress syndrome. *Am Rev Respir Dis* 1991;143:12–67.

67. Alia I, Esteban A, Gordo F, et al. A randomized and controlled trial of the effect of treatment aimed at maximizing oxygen delivery in patients with severe sepsis or septic shock. *Chest* 1999;115:453–461.

68. Caraslet J, Artigas A, Bihari D, et al. Third European consensus conference. Tissue hypoxia: how to detect, how to correct, how to prevent. *Am J Respir Crit Care Med* 1996;154:1573–1578.

69. Reilly PM, MacGoweb S, Miyachi M, et al. Mesenteric vasoconstriction in cardiogenic shock in pigs. *Gastoenterology* 1992;102:1968–1979.

70. Petros A, Bennet D, Vallence P. Effect of NO synthase inhibitors on hypotension in patients with septic shock. *Lancet* 1991;338:1557–1558.

71. Pastor CM, Payen DM. Effect of modifying NO pathway on liver circulation in a rabbit endotoxin shock model. *Shock* 1994;2:196–202.

72. Kim PK, Chen J, Andrejko KM, Deutschman CS. Intrabdominal sepsis downregulates transcription of sodium taurocholate co-transporter and multidrug resistance-associated protein in rats. *Shock* 2000;14:176–181.

73. Pastor C, Sutor P. Hepatic hemodynamics and cell function in human and experimental sepsis. *Anesth Analg* 1999;89:344–352.

74. Deutschman CS, De Maio A, Buchman TG, et al. Sepsis-induced alterations in levels of mRNA coding for phospho *enol* pyruvate carboxykinase: the role of insulin and glucagon 1993;40:295–302.

75. Deutschman CS, Andrejko KM, Haber BA, et al. Sepsis-induced depression of rat glucose-6-phosphotase gene expression and activity. *Am J Physiol* 1997;273:R1709–R1718.

76. Otake Y, Clemes MG. Interrelationship between hepatic ureagenesis and gluconeogenesis in early sepsis. *Am J Physiol* 1991;260:E453–E458.

77. Andrejko KA, Deutschman CS. Altered hepatic gene expression in fecal peritonitis: changes in transcription of gluconeogenic, B oxidative and ureagenic genes. *Shock* 1997;7:164–167.

78. Muller CM, Scierka A, Stiller RL, et al. Nitric oxide mediates hepatic cytochrome P450 dysfunction induced by endotoxin. *Anesthesiology* 1996;84:1435–1442.

79. Moseley RH. Sepsis-associated cholestasis. *Gastroenterology* 1997;112:302–306.

80. Rowland BJ, Soong CV, Gardiner KR. The gastrointestinal tract as a barrier to sepsis. *Br Med J* 1999;55(1):196–211.

81. Camussi G, Ronco C, Montrucchio G, et al. Role of soluble mediators in sepsis and renal failure. *Kidney Int* 1998;53[Suppl 66]:S38–S42.

82. Thijs A, Thijs LG. Pathogenesis of renal failure in sepsis. *Kidney Int* 1998;53[Suppl 66]:S34–S37.

83. Rangel-Frauso MS, Pittet D, Costigman M, et al. The natural history of systemic inflammatory response syndrome (SIRS). A prospective study. *JAMA* 1995;273:117–123.

84. Conger JD, Briner VA, Schrier RW. Acute renal failure: pathogenesis, diagnosis, and management. In: Schrier RW, ed. *Renal and electrolyte disorders.* Boston: Little, Brown and Company, 1992:495–537.

85. Duke GJ, Briedid JH, Weaver RA. Renal support in critically ill patients: low-dose dopamine or low-dose dobutamine? *Crit Care Med* 1994;22:1919–1925.

86. Dorman T, Swoboda S, Zarfeshenfard F, et al. Impact of altered aminoglycoside volume of distribution on the adequacy of a three milligram per kilogram loading dose. *Surgery* 1998;124:73–78.

87. Solomon R, Werner C, Mann D, et al. Effects of saline, mannitol, and furosemide to prevent acute decreases in renal function induced by radiocontrast agents. *N Engl J Med* 1994;331:1416–1420.

88. Tepel M, van der Giet M, Schwarzfeld C, et al. Prevention of radiographic-contrast-agent-induced reductions in renal function by acetylcysteine. *N Engl J Med* 2000;343(3):180–184.

89. Papadopoulus MC, Davies DC, Moss RF, et al. Pathophysiology of septic encephalopathy: a review. *Crit Care Med* 2000;28(8):3019–3023.

90. Bleck TP, Smith MC, Pierre-Louis SJ, et al. Neurologic complications of critical medical illnesses. *Crit Care Med* 1993;21:98–103.

91. Young GB, Bolton CF, Austin TW, et al. The encephalopathy associated with septic illness. *Clin Invest Med* 1990;13:297–304.

92. Mizock BA. Metabolic derangements in sepsis and septic shock. *Crit Care Clin* 2000;16(2):319–335.

93. Meszaros K, Lang CH, Bagby GJ, et al. Tumor necrosis factor increases in vivo glucose utilization of macrophage-rich tissues. *Biochem Biophys Res Commun* 1987;149:1–6.

94. Taylor DJ, Faragher EB, Evanson JM. Inflammatory cytokines stimulate glucose uptake and glycolysis but reduce glucose oxidation in human dermal fibroblasts in vitro. *Circ Shock* 1992;37:105–110.

95. Wolfe RR, Jahoor F, Herndon D, et al. Isotopic evaluation of the metabolism of pyruvate and related substances in normal adult volunteers and severely burned children: effect of dichloroacetate and glucose infusions. *Surgery* 1991;110:54–67.

96. James JH, Wagner KR, King JK, et al. Stimulation of both aerobic glycolysis and Na(+)-K(+)-ATPase activity in skeletal muscle by epinephrine or amylin. *Am J Physiol* 1999;277:E176–E186.

97. Shangraw RE, Jahoor F, Miyoshi H, et al. Differentiation between septic and postburn insulin resistance. *Metabolism* 1989;38:983–989.

98. Hardardottir I, Grunfield C, Feingold KR, et al. Effects of endotoxin and cytokines on lipid metabolism. *Curr Opin Lipid* 1994;5:207–215.

99. Herndon DN, Ngyyen TT, Wolfe RR, et al. Lipolysis in burned patients is stimulated by the beta 2 receptor for catecholamines. *Arch Surg* 1994;129:1301–1304.

100. Aarsland A, Chinkes DL, Wolfe RR. Contributions of de novo synthesis of fatty acids and lipolysis to VLDL secretion during prolonged hyperglycemia and hyperinsulinemia in normal man. *J Clin Invest* 1996;98:2008–2017.

101. Kreimeier U, Peter K. Strategies of volume therapy in sepsis and SIRS. *Kidney Int* 1998;53[Suppl 64]:S75–S79.

102. Wood LD, Prewitt RM. Cardiovascular management in acute hypoxemic respiratory failure. *Am J Cardiol* 1981;47:963–972.

103. Holcroft JW, Trunkey DD. Extravascular lung water following hemorrhagic shock in the baboon: comparison between resuscitation with Ringer's lactate and plasmanate. *Ann Surg* 1974;180:408–417.

104. Stein L, Beraud JJ, Morisetti M, et al. Pulmonary edema during volume infusion. *Circulation* 1975;52:483–489.

105. Blunt MC, Nicholson JP, Park GR. Serum albumin and colloid osmotic pressure in survivors and nonsurvivors of prolonged critical illness. *Anaesthesia* 1998;53:755–761.

106. Cochrane Injuries Group Albumin Reviewers. Human albumin administration in critically ill patients: systemic review of randomized controlled trials. *Br Med J* 1998;317:235–240.

107. Alderson P, Schierhout G, Roberts I, Bunn F. Colloids vs. crystalloids for fluid resuscitation in critically ill patients. *Cochrane Database Syst Rev* 2000;(2):CD000567.

108. Vermeulen LC Jr, Ratko TA, Erstad BL, et al. A paradigm for consensus: The University Hospital Consortium Guidelines for the use of albumin, nonprotein colloid and crystalloid solutions. *Arch Intern Med* 1995;155:373–379.

109. Bryan-Brown CW. Blood flow to organs. Parameters for function and survival in critical illness. *Crit Care Med* 1988;16:170–178.

110. Dietrich KA, Conrad SA, Herbert CA, et al. Cardiovascular and metabolic response to red blood cell transfusion in critically ill volume-resuscitated nonsurgical patients. *Crit Care Med* 1990;18:940–944.

111. Jundal N, Hollenberg SM, Dellinger RP. Pharmacologic issues in the management of septic shock. *Crit Care Clin* 2000;16(2):233–249.

112. Meier-Hellman A, Bredle DL, Specht M, et al. Increasing splanchnic blood flow in critically ill. *Chest* 1995;108:1826.

113. Landry DW, Levin HR, Gallant EM, et al. Vasopressin deficiency contributes to the vasodilation of septic shock. *Circulation* 1997;95:1122–1125.

114. Wenzel V, Ewy GA, Lindner KH. Vasopressin and endothelin during cardiopulmonary resuscitation. *Crit Care Med* 2000;28:N233–235.

MANAGEMENT OF LIFE-THREATENING INFECTION IN THE INTENSIVE CARE UNIT

DENNIS G. MAKI

KEY WORDS

- Abscess
- AIDS
- *Aspergillus*
- Bloodstream infection
- *Candida*
- Catheter-related infection
- Cellulitis
- Cholangitis
- Cytomegalovirus (CMV)
- Endocarditis
- Herpes simplex virus (HSV)
- Malaria
- Meningitis
- Meningoencephalitis
- Methicillin-resistant *Staphylococcus aureus* (MRSA)
- Methicillin-resistant coagulase-negative *Staphylococcus epidermidis* (MRCNS)
- Peritonitis
- Pneumonia
- rhACP
- Rickettsiosis
- Sepsis, septic shock
- Sinusitis
- Soft tissue infection
- Systemic inflammatory response syndrome (SIRS)
- Toxic shock syndrome (TSS)
- VAREC, VRE
- Varicella-zoster virus (VZV)

Life is short, the art is long, opportunity fleeting, experience treacherous, judgment difficult. For extreme illness, extreme treatments are most fitting.

Hippocrates
Aphorisms

INTRODUCTION

Infection shadows the patient in the intensive care unit (ICU) (1–3). Community- or hospital-acquired (nosocomial) infection proves to be a contributory factor to a fatal outcome or the direct cause of death in more than one-half of patients in an ICU (1–4). Over the past two decades there has been a marked increase in resistance to antibiotics of organisms causing life-threatening infection (4,5), especially infections acquired in the ICU (Fig. 1). Infections caused by *Streptococcus pneumoniae* highly resistant to penicillin (6,7); *Staphylococcus aureus* and resistant to methicillin coagulase-negative *Staphylococcus epidermidis* (MRCNS) (and all other beta-lactams) (8,9); enterococci resistant to vancomycin

(VRE), ampicillin, or both (VAREC) (10,11); Enterobacteriaceae and *Pseudomonas aeruginosa* resistant to third-generation cephalosporins and other extended-spectrum beta-lactams (12,13); *Clostridium difficile* (14); and *Candida* (15) are now being encountered by intensivists worldwide on a daily basis, a consequence of the very heavy use of antibiotics in clinical practice (1–5).

Fortunately, major advances have been made in our understanding of patterns of infection in critically ill patients and how to diagnose these infections expeditiously and accurately (16,17). Potent antiinfectives are now available to treat every type of bacterial, rickettsial, or chlamydial infection, nearly all fungal infections, most parasitic infections, and an increasing number of viral infections, especially those caused by the herpes viruses—herpes simplex virus (HSV), varicella-zoster virus (VZV), and cytomegalovirus (CMV). Moreover, we are beginning to achieve a deeper understanding of the pathophysiology of sepsis and septic shock, which has formed the basis for an increasingly evidence-based approach to management and has fostered the first effective novel adjunctive therapies. Finally, perhaps most importantly, the epidemiology of infections occurring in the ICU is now sufficiently understood that preventive measures, designed to block infection by microorganisms acquired from the ICU environment, as well as from a patient's own microflora, can prevent many life-threatening nosocomial infections (1).

DIAGNOSIS

A physician or intensivist can expect to encounter a wide array of infecting pathogens and manifestations of infection because of the extraordinary vulnerability of many hospitalized patients to infection and the increasingly invasive nature of the ICU practice for management of trauma and most forms of critical illness. In order to diagnose life-threatening infections as early as possible, to initiate the most effective therapy, several basic principles of management should be kept foremost in mind.

Prevention

It must be reemphasized that most infections encountered in ICU patients are nosocomial but preventable (1). Successful prevention invariably has a better ICU outcome than the most innovative and effective therapies (as will be discussed below).

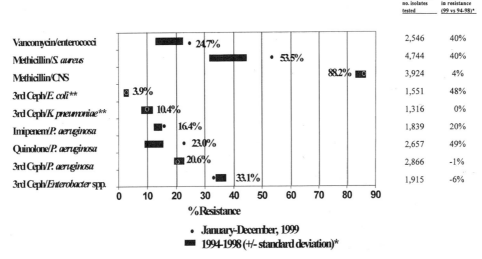

FIGURE 1. Prevalence of selective antimicrobial-resistant pathogens in intensive care units in the United States and comparison of resistance rates from 1994 through 1998, and 1999. (From NNIS System Report. *Am J Infect Control* 2000;28:429–448.)

High Index of Suspicion

A high index of suspicion of infection is essential with an ICU patient who presents with fever or nonspecific signs, such as tachycardia, tachypnea, or hypotension, vis-à-vis, signs of the systemic inflammatory response syndrome (SIRS) (18). Fever reflects infection more than 60% of the time in the ICU patient (19–22) (see Chapter 47). Many patients, particularly those who are profoundly granulocytopenic (23), are older or very debilitated, do not exhibit characteristic findings of local infection on examination.

Patterns of Infection

The spectrum of infectious complications encountered in the ICU patient is influenced powerfully by the alterations in the patient's basic immunity and overall condition. Patients are at risk early in the ICU course, before antiinfective drugs can take effect. There is also potential danger of infection and limitations in establishing a diagnosis of infection, however, later, when surgery or life-support therapy and heavy exposure to antibiotics can themselves cause syndromes that may mimic infection (see Chapters 47 and 48).

The immune defects encountered in critically ill patients are associated with vulnerability to infection by predictable pathogens (Table 1). Multiple myeloma and chronic lymphocytic leukemia produce hypogammaglobulinemia, which predisposes a patient to bacterial pneumonia and bacteremia. Splenectomy increases the risk of overwhelming infection caused by encapsulated bacteria, particularly *S. pneumoniae*. Granulocytopenia (less than 500 per mm³) increases susceptibility to primary staphylococcal and gram-negative bacteremia (source not identified), cellulitis, and pneumonia, as well as invasive infections with *Candida* and filamentous fungi, such as *Aspergillus*. Acquired immunodeficiency syndrome (AIDS) and lymphoreticular malignancies are associated with impaired cell-mediated immunity (CMI) and infection by nocardia, mycobacteria, *Cryptococcus neoformans*,

Pneumocystis carinii, Toxoplasma gondii, CMV, and other herpes viruses. Patients with solid tumors are vulnerable to bacterial infections deriving from tumorous obstruction of vital organs, such as cholangitis with pancreaticobiliary malignancy, urosepsis with obstructive bladder or prostate cancer, and pneumonia or lung abscess distal to obstructing bronchopulmonary neoplasms. Latent infections with *Mycobacterium tuberculosis, Histoplasma capsulatum* or *Coccidioides*, and *T. gondii* are commonly reactivated by AIDS, organ transplantation, or intensive corticosteroid therapy.

Endotracheal intubation, urinary and central venous catheters (CVCs), and surgery—all ubiquitous in ICU patients—are the major causes of ICU-acquired infection brought on by a broad array of nosocomial skin and gastrointestinal microorganisms, especially resistant staphylococci, enterococci, enteric gram-negative bacilli, *P. aeruginosa*, and *Candida* (1–4) (Fig. 2).

These associations are important and helpful when evaluating an immunocompromised ICU patient with fever or other signs that suggest infection.

Noninfectious Syndromes Mimicking Infection

Clinical manifestations of patients' underlying diseases and the various forms of therapy given to the patient, such as blood products, cytotoxic drugs, or enteral feeding, can produce fever, diarrhea, pneumonitis, or systemic erythroderma, mimicking infection.

Drug fever is a relatively common cause of pyrexia in the hospitalized patient (19–22). Contrary to popular dogma, it is not associated in most cases with a rash or eosinophilia, or a history of atopy. The fever can present hours, days, or even weeks after starting the culpable agent, but averages 21 days (24). Most patients will defervesce within 24 to 48 hours after discontinuation of the drug. The agents most commonly implicated in drug fever are the numerous antiinfectives, especially the beta-lactams; all of the antineoplastic agents and anticonvulsants; and, especially, the

TABLE 1. INFECTIONS ASSOCIATED WITH ALTERED HOST IMMUNITY

	Pathogens Encountered at Site of Infection			
Host Defect	Bloodstream or Disseminated	Pulmonary	Central Nervous System	Gastrointestinal
Hypogammaglobulinemia	*Streptococcus pneumoniae* *Haemophilus influenzae* Type B *Neisseria meningitidis*	*S. pneumoniae* *H. influenzae* *Branhamella catarrhalis*	*S. pneumoniae* *H. influenzae*	*Giardia lamblia*
Splenectomy	As above, *plus Bartonella,* malaria, *Babesia*	As above	As above	
Cell-mediated immunity	*Listeria monocytogenes* *Salmonella* *Mycobacterium tuberculosis* *Coccidioides immitis* *Histoplasma capsulatum* *Cryptococcus neoformans* Cytomegalovirus Varicella-zoster virus Herpes simplex virus	*Legionella* *Nocardia* Mycobacteria *C. immitis* *H. capsulatum* *Pneumocystis carinii* Cytomegalovirus	*Listeria* *M. tuberculosis* *C. neoformans* *Toxoplasma gondii* Herpes simplex virus Cytomegalovirus	*Salmonella* *Campylobacter* *Candida* spp. *Cryptosporidium* *Entamoeba histolytica* *Strongyloides stercoralis* Cytomegalovirus Herpes simplex virus

Tumorous obstruction	Cholangitis:
	  Gram-negative bacilli
	  enterococcus
	  Clostridium
	Urosepsis:
	  Gram-negative bacilli
	  enterococcus
	  Candida spp.
	Pneumonia:
	  S. pneumoniae
	  S. aureus
	  Oral anaerobes
		S. pneumoniae
		S. aureus
		Oral anaerobes
				Gram-negative bacilli
				Enterococci
				Clostridium
				Bacteroides fragilis

Granulocytopenia	Gram-negative bacilli, especially: *Pseudomonas aeruginosa* Staphylococci *Fusarium* spp. *Candida* spp.	Gram-negative bacilli Staphylococci *Aspergillus* spp.	*Aspergillus* spp. *Candida* spp.	*Candida* spp. *Clostridium difficile* Other clostridia Herpes simplex virus
Reactivation of latent infections	*H. capsulatum* *C. immitis* Malaria	*M. tuberculosis*	*M. tuberculosis* *H. capsulatum* *C. immitis* *T. gondii*	*S. stercoralis*
Central venous catheter	*Staphylococcus epidermidis* *S. aureus* *Corynebacterium* spp. JK *Mycobacterium* spp. *Bacillus* spp. *Candida* spp. *Fusarium* spp. *Trichosporon* spp.			

lupogenic drugs—isonicotinic acid hydrazide (INH), methyldopa, procainamide, quinidine, hydralazine, and phenytoin.

Diagnostic Studies

The importance of making every effort to diagnose suspected infection cannot be overemphasized. Failure to obtain appropriate cultures before initiating empiric therapy of suspected infection may preclude the physician from determining whether infection was present initially after the patient responds poorly to the antimicrobial regimen. Such an oversight may prove deleterious in the long run. The true diagnosis may be delayed because of empiric therapy, and nonbacterial infection with fungi or viruses might not be recognized sufficiently early enough to institute life-saving therapy. The patient may be subjected also to unnec-

essarily broad-spectrum antimicrobial therapy that increases the risk of drug reactions and superinfection by resistant organisms, such as antibiotic-associated colitis caused by *C. difficile.*

Recent evidence-based guidelines provide the best current information on the evaluation of the ICU patient with fever or other signs of sepsis (16,17). It is indefensible to start antiinfective drugs for suspected or presumed infection in the critically ill ICU patient without first obtaining appropriate cultures, which must always include blood cultures, ideally drawn from peripheral veins by percutaneous venipuncture. Patients in an ICU have a very high incidence of bloodstream infection (BSI) (1–4), particularly patients with organ transplants or profound granulocytopenia (less than 100 per mm^3), patients with peritonitis, cholangitis, or pyohydronephrosis, and all patients with CVCs. Studies have shown that obtaining more than two

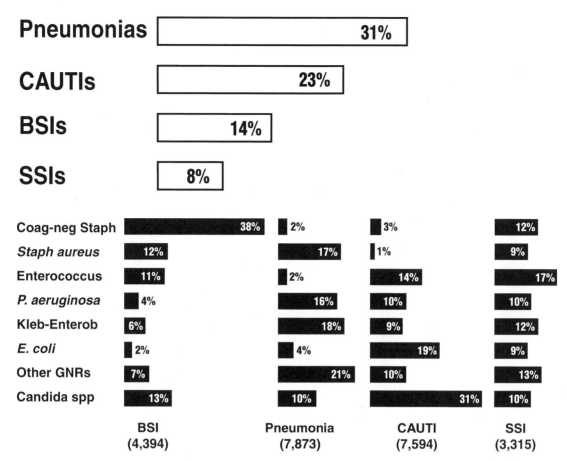

FIGURE 2. Distribution of 129,041 nosocomial infections occurring in 205 medical-surgical intensive care units in the United States from 1992 through 1998, with nosocomial profile of ventilator-associated pneumonias (VAPs), central venous catheter-related bloodstream infections (BSIs), catheter-associated urinary tract infections (CAUTIs), and surgical site infections (SSIs). (From NNIS System Report. *Infect Control Hosp Epidemiol* 2000;21:510–515.)

10- to 15-mL blood cultures provides little additional yield (25), but it is essential in adults that an adequate total volume of blood is cultured, at least 20 mL—ideally 30 mL—to maximize the detection of BSI (25,26).

Standard blood cultures drawn through CVCs provide excellent sensitivity for diagnosis of BSI but are more likely to be contaminated (27,28), resulting in unnecessary or suboptimal antimicrobial therapy; single positive blood cultures drawn through a CVC for coagulase-negative staphylococci reflect contaminants most of the time (28).

The availability of the Isolator blood culture system (Wampole Laboratories, Cranbury, NJ), which provides a quantitative blood culture on solid media, offers improved sensitivity for diagnosis of fungemia (25) and allows diagnosis of infected surgically-implanted cuffed CVCs and subcutaneous central ports without removing the device. With an infected device, the number of organisms per mL of blood drawn through the infected device is tenfold or more higher than in a concomitant blood culture drawn from a peripheral vein (29).

The near universal availability of automated positive blood culture-detection systems in Western hospitals allows the differential time-to-positivity of positive catheter-drawn and peripheral vein–drawn blood cultures to be used to diagnose intravascular device–related BSI without removing the device. If both blood cultures are positive, a delay more than 2 hours in the time for the peripherally drawn blood culture to turn positive indicates that the intravascular device is the source of BSI (28).

Confusion or headache associated with fever or other neurologic signs prompts suspicion of meningitis, especially in a newly admitted patient or a hospitalized patient who has had recent craniofacial or neurologic surgery, which cannot be diagnosed without examination of the cerebrospinal fluid (CSF). Gram stain of an ultracentrifuged CSF specimen shows the infecting organisms 80% to 90% of the time in bacterial meningitis (30). If a hospitalized patient has not had recent surgery on parameningeal structures, nosocomial meningitis is very unlikely and the yield of lumbar puncture is virtually nil (31).

Pneumonia poses the greatest challenge diagnostically. Basing initial therapy of pneumonia on the results of microscopic examination of the expectorated sputum (32) or, better, a tracheal aspirate (33), is reasonable in immunocompetent patients (32–35). However, a large multicenter trial has suggested that with intubated and ventilated patients, proceeding directly to a bronchoscopic examination, with bronchoalveolar lavage or protected brush biopsy, permits more effective therapy, less superinfection, lower mortality, and a shorter ICU length of stay (36). Unfortunately, this could not be confirmed in a smaller trial (37), but the question bears continued study. If a patient with suspected pneumonia is immunocompromised (e.g., with AIDS or an organ transplant), the greatly expanded range of potential pathogens (Table 1) and the physiologic vulnerability of the patient support direct procession to a diagnostic bronchoscopic procedure at the outset (34,35) (see also Chapters 32 and 51). Commercial tests for urinary antigen show 75% to 80% sensitivity and more than 90% specificity for rapid diagnosis of pneumonia caused by *Legionella pneumophila* serogroup I and *S. pneumoniae* (34,35).

Powerful imaging techniques, particularly computerized tomography (CT) and ultrasonography, have greatly facilitated detection of abscesses in the abdomen and pelvis, chest, head, and neck and can aid in the diagnosis of pneumonia and other deep infections in immunocompromised or trauma patients (38–41).

It is important to realize, however, that Foley catheter–associated bacteriuria or candiduria, while extremely common in the ICU (Fig. 2), only rarely causes fever or sepsis (42). Urinary tract infection can be diagnosed with greater than 98% accuracy by a Gram stain of centrifuged urine (43). Pyuria, while very useful for identifying urinary tract infections in noncatheterized patients (44), has much poorer predictive value in patients with urinary catheters (45).

Paranasal sinusitis, a relatively common infection in the intubated ICU patient, cannot be reliably diagnosed by imaging alone, and diagnostic needle aspiration is mandated if fluid is seen within a sinus or sinuses on CT scan of a patient with cryptogenic sepsis (46).

Intense efforts have been made over the past decade to develop a blood test that would permit rapid and reliable diagnosis of bacterial or fungal sepsis, particularly in its early stage (47). The peripheral white blood cell count, erythrocyte sedimentation rate, and C-reactive protein all have too little specificity (47,48). Recent studies suggest that levels of the precursor molecule for calcitonin, procalcitonin, might be the sensitive but specific marker for invasive infection needed to facilitate earlier and more focused therapy of life-threatening infection, minimizing unnecessary empiric antimicrobial therapy (48–52).

Studies have also shown that proactive efforts on the part of the diagnostic laboratory to accelerate the processing of cultures, providing presumptive identification and susceptibility results within 24 hours rather than the usual 48 to 72 hours, improves antiinfective therapy and yields cost savings (53).

Continuous Assessment of the Patient

The decision to initiate antimicrobial therapy is based upon examination of the patient and laboratory studies available at the outset. In many instances, physical examination, imaging studies, or microscopic examinations of sputum and urine, may not identify a definite site of local infection. Empirical antimicrobial therapy must be started on the presumption that the patient has primary BSI or other occult deep infection, however, because the patient is judged to be septic and is highly vulnerable. When empiric antimicrobial therapy has been initiated, the need for continued therapy must be regularly reassessed, particularly if cultures and other diagnostic studies are negative and the patient has not shown significant change. On the other hand, if an infecting pathogen has been identified, the antimicrobial regimen should be adjusted based on the infecting pathogen or pathogens, striving for the most focused and narrow-spectrum therapy possible, which improves the likelihood of therapeutic success and reduces the risk of superinfection and antibiotic-associated colitis.

Patients in an ICU are far more vulnerable than most other hospitalized patients to superinfection caused by resistant bacteria or fungi because the course of the ICU patient is continuously evolving. It is essential to regularly reassess the patient, not simply to confirm a favorable response to the therapy, but also to identify side effects from the treatment, especially superinfection and drug toxicity.

SOURCE CONTROL

Every effort must be made to identify the source of infection and, if possible, to mechanically remove that source from every ICU patient who presents with signs of systemic infection, especially overwhelming infection. Removal techniques include surgically closing an intestinal perforation, draining an intraabdominal abscess (54,55), decompressing an obstructed common bile duct or obstructed ureter; removing an infected intravascular device, even resecting a suppurative vein segment (29), or discontinuing a contaminated intravenous (i.v.) or intraarterial infusion. Such measures are crucial to survival and in many instances supersede antimicrobial therapy.

Antiinfective Therapy

Antiinfectives

Dosing of the different classes of antiinfectives has improved greatly over the past decade. The emerging science of pharmacodynamics attempts to maximize the therapeutic effect and minimize toxicity and the risk of promoting resistance to the agent (56,57).

Beta-Lactams

It has become clear that beta-lactam antibiotics with a short half-life (1 to 2 hours) should be dosed sufficiently often to maintain therapeutic drug levels that exceed the organism's minimum inhibitory concentration (MIC) for at least 50% of dosing interval (56,57). Penicillin, ampicillin, and the antipseudomonal penicillins, ticarcillin (Ticar) and ticarcillin-clavulanate (Timentin), mezlocillin (Mezlin), piperacillin (Pipracil), and piperacillin-tazobactam (Tazocin), should be dosed no less often than every 4 to 6 hours in patients with normal renal function. Accumulating data suggest that continuous infusion of beta-lactams may ultimately prove most effective for a treatment of serious gram-positive infections (58). More extended dosing intervals will not compromise therapeutic goals with beta-lactams, such as cefoperazone (Cefobid), ceftazidime (Fortaz, Tazicef, Tazidime), cefepime (Maxipime), or ceftriaxone (Rocephin), which have longer half-lives.

A number of novel beta-lactam and related antibiotics have become available over the past 20 years. The combination of a beta-lactam with a beta-lactamase inhibitor, ampicillin-sulbactam (Unasyn), ticarcillin-clavulanic acid (Timentin), and piperacillin-tazobactam (Zosyn), are some of the most notable. Others include the potent and very broad-spectrum carbapenems, imipenem-cilastatin (Primaxin); meropenem (Merren); the new, powerful antipseudomonal fourth-generation cephalosporin, cefepime (Maxipime); and the monobactam, aztreonam (Azactam).

Aztreonam is a novel beta-lactam–like drug that has no gram-positive activity, but is highly active against many enteric aerobic gram-negative bacilli—with the exception of many strains of *Serratia, Enterobacter,* and *P. aeruginosa.* It can also be used safely in patients who have had anaphylactic reactions to penicillin (59).

Most of these beta-lactams have an important role in the management of serious infections in critically ill ICU patients, and recommended dosing schedules and indications for their use are provided in Tables 2 and 3.

Aminoglycosides

Aminoglycoside antibiotics are still important drugs for the management of life-threatening gram-negative infections (60), particularly in patients with granulocytopenia (61). Studies suggest that the use of two drugs that show *in vitro* additive effects or, even more desirable, synergy, such as a beta-lactam and an aminoglycoside, improves outcome with gram-negative bacteremia in patients with profound and prolonged granulocytopenia (less than 100 per mm^3) (61,62). Two antibiotics should be used with granulocytopenia and proven gram-negative bacillemia, combining a potent beta-lactam with an aminoglycoside or a fluoroquinolone. It is far less clear that two drugs need to be used or whether synergism translates to an improved therapeutic outcome for patients without granulocytopenia, even with *P. aeruginosa* infections (63).

There are no data showing unequivocal superiority of one aminoglycoside over another—assuming both are effective *in vitro*—especially if the aminoglycoside is combined with a beta-lactam in the initial empiric regimen. However, for *P. aeruginosa* infections, tobramycin is superior *in vitro* to gentamicin and should be the agent of choice. Other than for *P. aeruginosa,* gentamicin is generally more effective than tobramycin *in vitro* against the broad range of enteric gram-negative bacilli. Amikacin is usually effective *in vitro* and would be the aminoglycoside of choice when dealing with gentamicin- or tobramycin-resistant organisms. No data are available, however, to indicate that amikacin is superior therapeutically to gentamicin or tobramycin for infections with organisms susceptible to all of these drugs.

The outcome of treatment of serious gram-negative bacillary infections with aminoglycosides is most heavily influenced by the peak blood level at the outset of therapy because bacterial killing with aminoglycosides is concentration-dependent (56,57). Patients with a subtherapeutic level of gentamicin or tobramycin (less than 5 μg per mL) are far more likely to show therapeutic failure than patients with a peak level greater than 5 μg per mL following the first dose (64,65). Multiple studies have shown that the total daily dose of an aminoglycoside, such as gentamicin (5 to 6 mg per kg), can be given once daily; therapeutic results are comparable to dosing every 8 hours, as was the common practice for many years in patients with normal renal function (66,67). It may be most prudent to begin with doses of 2.5 to 3.0 mg per kg (for a 70-kg patient, 180 to 210 mg) gentamicin or tobramycin every 12 hours with critically ill, hemodynamically unstable patients at high risk for renal failure. Once or twice daily dosing is not associated with an increased risk of ototoxicity or nephrotoxicity, but assures supratherapeutic blood levels at the outset of therapy (10 to 30 μg per mL), when it is most essential. Aminoglycoside levels should be obtained at the outset of therapy (e.g., after the first dose) if once or twice daily dosing is not used in order to confirm that the peak blood level exceeds 5 μg per mL (64).

Macrolides

Erythromycin, one of the oldest antibacterials, remains an excellent and effective alternative to beta-lactams in penicillin-allergic patients in the outpatient setting. In the hospital, its major use is as an adjunct to the treatment of community-acquired pneumonia, usually given with a second- or third-generation cephalosporin (34,35). It is also effective for *Legionella* pneumonia but is being superceded by fluoroquinolones, which are more active *in vitro* (68). Garden-variety erythromycin salts are very irritating to peripheral veins, which limits their use if the patient does not have a central catheter, and produces nausea or vomiting, cramps, and diarrhea in up to 30% of treated patients. More important, erythromycin inhibits the elimination of P450-excreted drugs, such as warfarin, cyclosporine, phenytoin, and theophylline, which can lead to life-threatening toxicity.

The new macrolide, azithromycin (Zithromax) has a long half-life, which permits once-daily dosing, is far better tolerated, including parenterally, has little effect on the pharmacokinetics of other drugs (69), and has largely supplanted erythromycin for parenteral use.

Vancomycin

Vancomycin has come to be used widely throughout the world during the past 20 years, with the marked increase in infections caused by staphylococci resistant to methicillin (Fig. 1) (8,9). Vancomycin exhibits *in vitro* activity against nearly all gram-positive cocci,[1] including methicillin-resistant strains of *S. aureus* and coagulase-negative staphylococci, as well as most enterococci. Vancomycin is the drug of choice for treatment of infections caused by gram-positive organisms resistant to beta-lactam antibiotics, such as methicillin-resistant *Staphylococcus aureus* (MRSA), most coagulase-negative staphylococci, and JK *Corynebacterium* species. It is also the drug of choice for treating serious staphylococcal, streptococcal, and enterococcal infections in patients with penicillin hypersensitivity (71).

The most common side effect of vancomycin is the "red-man syndrome" with diffuse erythroderma and hypotension stemming from nonallergenic release of histamine by peripheral leukocytes, and occasionally associated with urticaria and bronchospasm (72). This syndrome occurs in up to 10% of patients given i.v. vancomycin. The risk of vancomycin-related red-man syndrome and hypotension is heavily influenced by the rate of administration and can be controlled by administration of vancomycin in a solution containing not more than 5 mg per mL, over an interval of

---

[1] Exceptions: *Staphylococcus haemolyticus, Pediococcus,* Leuconostoc, and up to one-half of nosocomial enterococci (10,11) exhibit high-level resistance to vancomycin. Occasional strains of *S. aureus* show reduced or intermediate susceptibility to glycopeptides (GISA) but not yet high-level resistance.

TABLE 2. DOSING OF PARENTERAL ANTIINFECTIVE DRUGS FOR TREATMENT OF LIFE-THREATENING INFECTION[a]

Drug	Total Daily Dose	For 70-kg Adult	Side Effects/Monitoring
Amikacin	15 mg/kg	500 mg q12 h 1 g q24 h	Ototoxicity, nephrotoxicity (3%–5%), neuromuscular blockade (rare)
Ampicillin	100–200 mg/kg	1–2 g q4–6 h	Rashes, diarrhea, *C. difficile* diarrhea or colitis, superinfection
Ampicillin-sulbactam	170 mg/kg	1–3 g q6 h	Similar to ampicillin
Antifungal drugs:			
Amphotericin B	See Table 5	See Table 5	Fever, chills, and phlebitis (frequent); azotemia, renal tubular acidosis with hypokalemia (universal)
Flucytosine	See Table 5	See Table 5	Rash, diarrhea, myelosuppression (common)
Itraconazole	See Table 5	See Table 5	Rash, hepatitis (rare) interactions with P-450 excreted drugs
Fluconazole	See Table 5	See Table 5	Same
Antimalarial drugs:			
Chloroquine	See Table 6	See Table 6	Rash, photosensitivity
Quinine	See Table 6	See Table 6	Cinchonism, hemolysis with G6PD deficiency
Quinidine gluconate	See Table 6	See Table 6	Same + QT prolongation
Atovaquone-proguanil	See Table 6	See Table 6	GI side effects (10%–20%)
Antipneumocystis drugs:			
Pentamidine	4 mg/kg	300 mg/d	Rash, azotemia, hypoglycemia; cardiotoxicity with rapid i.v. administration
Trimethoprim (TMP)-sulfamethoxazole	20 mg/kg of TMP component	4 ampules q6 h	See below
Atovaquone		750 mg q12 h	Rash, diarrhea
Antipseudomonal cephalosporins:			
Cefepime, ceftazidime	50–100 mg/kg	1–2 g q8–12 h	Similar to other third-generation cephalosporins
Antipseudomonal penicillins:			Like ampicillin
Ticarcillin, mezlocillin, piperacillin	250 mg/kg	3–4 g q4–6 h	
Ticarcillin-clavulanate	250 mg/kg	3.1 g q4–6 h	
Piperacillin-tazobactam	200 mg/kg	3.375 g q6 h	
Antiviral drugs:			
Acyclovir	See Table 6	See Table 6	Rash, mental status changes (rare), myelosuppression (rare except in AIDS), azotemia (rare)
Amantadine or rimantadine	See Table 6	See Table 6	Neuropsychiatric, seizures (↑ in older adults)
Cidofovir	See Table 6	See Table 6	Nephrotoxicity (common), myelosuppression, GI
Foscarnet	See Table 6	See Table 6	Nephrotoxicity (common), electrolyte imbalance, seizures
Ganciclovir	See Table 6	See Table 6	Myelosuppression (common)
Ribavirin	See Table 6	See Table 6	Myelosuppression, azotemia
Azithromycin		500 mg day 1, 250 mg/d thereafter	GI (5%), rash
Aztreonam	50–100 mg/kg	1–2 g q6–8 h	Superinfection, rash (however, *no* cross-sensitivity in the patient with pencillin allergy)
Carbapenems			
Imipenem-cilastatin	30–50 mg/kg	0.5–1.0 g q6 h	Like third-generation cephalosporins *plus* seizures (increased risk in renal insufficiency, meningitis, seizure disorder)
Meropenem	50 mg/kg	1 g q8 h	Same but lower incidence of seizures
Cefotaxime, ceftizoxime	100 mg/kg	1–2 g q4–8 h	Rash, diarrhea, *C. difficile* colitis, superinfection with *Candida*, coagulase-negative staphylococci, enterococci
Ceftriaxone	30 mg/kg	1–2 g q24 h	Same
Cefuroxime	30–50 mg/kg	750–1,500 mg q8 h	Similar to ampicillin
Clindamycin	20–35 mg/kg	600–900 mg q8 h	Rash, diarrhea, *C. difficile* colitis
Doxycycline		100 mg q12 h	Rash, diarrhea, photosensitivity, superinfection **Should not be used in children < 8 yrs old**
Erythromycin	30–60 mg/kg	500 mg–1 gm q6 h	GI: nausea, vomiting, diarrhea (25%); interactions with P-450 excreted drugs

(*continued*)

TABLE 2. (*continued*)

Drug	Total Daily Dose	For 70-kg Adult	Side Effects/Monitoring

Fluoroquinolones:
  Ciprofloxacin
		400–600 mg q12 h	Rash, GI, neuropsychiatric
			  (1–2%), photosensitivity
			  Should not be used in children

Levofloxicin, gatifloxicin		500 mg q24 h	Like ciprofloxacin
Gentamicin, tobramycin	5–6 mg/kg	180 mg q12 h 350–500 mg q24 h	Like amikacin
Linezolid		600 mg q12 h	P-450 drug interactions, myelosuppression
Metronidazole	30 mg/kg	500 mg q6–8 h	Rash, nausea, antabuse-like reaction, neutropenia, neuropathy (rare)
Nafcillin or oxacillin	100–200 mg/kg	1–2 g q4 h	Rash, granulocytopenia (common with nafcillin), hepatitis (oxacillin)
Penicillin G	200,000–300,000 U/kg	2–4 million U q4 h	Rashes (1%–5%), anaphylaxis, hypersensitivity nephritis (<1%)

Quinupristin-dalfopristin	15–25 mg/kg	7.5 mg/kg q8–12 h	Rashes, myalgias, or arthralgias
			  (5%–10%), myositis, hepatitis,
			  interactions with P-450 excreted drugs

Trimethoprim-
  sulfamethoxazole
	10–20 mg/kg of
	  TMP component
		2–5 ampules q6 h
		  (5 mL ampule: 80 mg/400 mg)
			Rash (common), Stevens-Johnson
			  syndrome (rare), myelosuppression
			  (rare except in AIDS)

Vancomycin	30–50 mg/kg	0.5–1.0 g q12 h	"Red man syndrome" and hypotension (common),
			  nephrotoxicity and ototoxicity (rare,
			  unless given with aminoglycosides)

GI, gastrointestinal; i.v., intravenous; AIDS, acquired immunodeficiency syndrome.

[a]Assuming normal renal and hepatic function. With renal insufficiency or hepatic failure, *whereas the loading dose is unchanged,* subsequent doses or dosing intervals may need to be modified.

no less than 1 hour (72). Pretreatment with an H1-histamine receptor antagonist, such as diphenhydramine, appears to be highly effective at preventing vancomycin-related hypotension and the red-man syndrome (73). If hypotension occurs during administration of vancomycin, stopping the infusion and giving supplemental i.v. fluids, and if necessary, an alpha-agonist pressor, such as norepinephrine, or higher-dose dopamine (greater than 5 µg per kg per minute), will quickly reverse the hypotension; but the patient should also be treated with diphenhydramine, 50 to 100 mg i.v. Vancomycin can be resumed safely following the occurrence of the red-man syndrome if the patient is pretreated with an H1 antihistamine before each subsequent dose and the concentration of infused drug and rate of administration are carefully controlled (73).

Vancomycin is not particularly hazardous, in terms of ototoxicity or nephrotoxicity (approximately 1% to 2%). When vancomycin is given with an aminoglycoside, such as gentamicin, however, the combination is very toxic (estimate, 25% [74]), especially in older adult patients and those with preexistent renal disease or hearing loss; the combination should be used very cautiously, probably only for enterococcal or staphylococcal endocarditis (75,76).

New Drugs for Multiresistant Gram-Positive Cocci: Quinupristin-Dalfopristin and Linezolid

An alarming increase in nosocomial infections caused by strains of enterococci highly resistant to vancomycin (VRE, VAREC) has occurred worldwide (10,11), and MRSA also exhibiting reduced susceptibility to vancomycin (GISA) are starting to be encountered (70). The older commercial antibiotics, alone or in combinations, have not proven effective for serious infections caused by VRE/VAREC. Two entirely new antibiotics, the novel streptogrammin combination, quinupristin-dalfopristin (Synercid), and the first oxazolidinone, linezolid (Zyvox), are now commercially available for treating infections caused by VRE/VAREC and methicillin-resistant staphylococcal infections in patients unable to tolerate vancomycin or caused by strains exhibiting reduced susceptibility to vancomycin (77–79).

Both agents are active against virtually all gram-positive cocci, with the exception of *Enterococcus faecalis*. Quinupristin-dalfopristin has been associated with myalgias in 5% to 10% of patients, occasionally so severe as to necessitate discontinuation of the drug, but has produced little organ toxicity; however, like macrolides, it also inhibits the excretion of many P450-excreted drugs (77). Linezolid is better tolerated but has been associated with thrombocytopenia or leukopenia in patients treated for longer than a week (79).

Fluoroquinolones

The fluoroquinolone ciprofloxacin (Cipro), exhibits excellent *in vitro* activity against most gram-negative bacilli, including *P. aeruginosa,* and is highly effective clinically (80). Although ciprofloxacin shows *in vitro* activity against many gram-positive cocci, there are reports of therapeutic failure when used as a sole agent for gram-positive infections, and serious gram-positive superinfections, such as pneumococcal meningitis (81), have occurred during ciprofloxacin therapy. Ciprofloxacin should never be the sole therapy for life-threatening gram-positive infections, but rather considered as a valuable drug for treating life-threatening infections caused by aerobic gram-negative bacilli, especially *P. aeruginosa,* and *Legionella* (68).

TABLE 3. RECOMMENDED THERAPY FOR LIFE-THREATENING INFECTION WITH SPECIFIC BACTERIAL PATHOGENS[a]

Pathogen	Syndromes	First Choice(s)	Alternative/Penicillin-Allergic
Streptococcus pneumoniae	Pneumonia	Ceftriaxone or cefotaxime Levofloxicin or gatifloxicin[b]	Vancomycin Levofloxicin or gatifloxicin[b]
	Meningitis	Ceftriaxone, cefotaxime or cefepime *and* vancomycin ± rifampin[c]	
Staphylococcus aureus	Bacteremia/endocarditis Pneumonia Soft-tissue infection	Nafcillin (methicillin-sensitive) Vancomycin (methicillin-resistant) ± gentamicin ± rifampin[d]	Vancomycin Quinupristin-dalfopristin Linezolid
Coagulase-negative staphylococci	Bacteremia Device-related infection	Vancomycin ± gentamicin ± rifampin[d]	Quinupristin-dalfopristin Linezolid
Haemophilus influenzae type b	Bacteremia Meningitis Cellulitis	Ceftriaxone, cefotaxime, or cefepime	Same or ciprofloxacin
Clostridium difficile	Colitis	Metronidazole (oral ± i.v.) Vancomycin (oral *only*)	Same
Listeria monocytogenes	Meningitis Bacteremia	Ampicillin ± gentamicin	Trimethoprim-sulfamethoxazole ± gentamicin
Legionella spp.	Pneumonia	Ciprofloxacin or other fluoroquinolone Macrolide ± rifampin Doxycycline[b]	Same

Pseudomonas aeruginosa	Bacteremia
	Pneumonia
	Soft-tissue infection
		Antipseudomonal beta-lactam[e]
		  and tobramycin or ciprofloxacin[f]
			Aztreonam *and* ciprofloxacin
			  or tobramycin

Enterobacteriaceae	Bacteremia Peritonitis Pneumonia Urosepsis Soft-tissue infection	Third-generation cephalosporin[g] ± ciprofloxacin or gentamicin[f] Carbapenem Ciprofloxacin[b]	Ciprofloxacin[b]
Bacteroides fragilis	Intraabdominal infection	Metronidazole	Clindamycin Ticarcillin-clavulanate Piperacillin-tazobactam Carbapenem
Enterococci	Same	Ampicillin	Vancomycin Quinupristin-dalfopristin
VRE/VAREC	Same	Quinupristin-dalfopristin Linezolid	Same
Stenotrophomonas maltophilia	Pneumonia Bacteremia	Trimethoprim-sulfamethoxazole Ticarcillin-clavulanate Ceftazidime	
Burkholderia cepacia	Pneumonia Bacteremia	Trimethoprim-sulfamethoxazole Ticarcillin-clavulanate Ceftazidime Carbapenem	
Nocardia asteroides	Pneumonia Brain abscess Metastatic infection	Sulfadiazine Trimethoprim-sulfamethoxazole	Imipenem *and* amikacin Minocycline *and* ampicillin

i.v., intravenous; VRE, enterococci resistant to vancomycin; VAREC, enterococci resistant to vancomycin, ampicillin, or both.
[a] These regimens are suggested as initial therapy most likely to be effective, pending the results of susceptibility testing which should guide selection of the final regimen.
[b] Contraindicated in children.
[c] If corticosteroids are also being given.
[d] Add gentamicin and/or rifampin for infection of prosthetic implant or endocarditis.
[e] Antipseudomonal beta-lactams: ticarcillin, ticarcillin-clavulanate, mezlocillin, piperacillin, piperacillin-tazobactam, ceftazidime, cefepime, carbapenem.
[f] Add second drug for *nosocomial* infection.
[g] Cefriaxone, cefotaxime, ceftizoxime, ceftazidime, cefepime.

The newest fluoroquinolones, levofloxacin (Levaquin) and gatifloxacin (Tequin), on the other hand, possess excellent gram-positive activity. These new fluoroquinolones are active against *S. pneumoniae* highly resistant to penicillin (35,82), as well as *Legionella*, *Chlamydia*, and *Mycoplasma*, and have been shown to be excellent drugs for community-acquired pneumonia (83,84).

Dosing of Antibacterials

It is extremely important that drugs used to treat bacterial infections in critically ill patients are dosed adequately (Table 2) (85), especially the aminoglycosides and beta-lactams used to treat *P. aeruginosa* infections. For example, the antipseudomonal

TABLE 4. RECOMMENDED THERAPY FOR LIFE-THREATENING FUNGAL INFECTIONS[a]

Pathogens	Syndrome	First Choice	Alternate Choices/Comments
Candida spp.	Oropharyngeal	Clotrimazole 10 mg troches 5×/d Fluconazole 100 mg/d p.o.	Ketoconazole 200 mg/d p.o. Fluconazole 100 mg/d
	Esophagitis	Fluconazole 100–200 mg/d p.o. or i.v.	Amphotericin 0.3 mg/kg/d i.v.
	Endophthalmitis	Amphotericin B *intravitreal* ± amphotericin B 0.5 mg/kg/d i.v. *plus* flucytosine or fluconazole	Fluconazole 400–800 mg/d i.v. or p.o.
	Cystitis	Fluconazole 100–400 mg/d	Amphotericin B 0.3 mg/kg/d i.v., total dose 1–3 mg/kg
	Candidemia, other deep infections, such as pyelonephritis or peritonitis	Fluconazole, 400 mg/d i.v. or p.o. Amphotericin B IV 0.3–0.7 mg/kg/d, total dose: 5–20 mg/kg; septic thrombosis of great central vein requires total dose >20 mg/kg Lipid-associated amphotericin 2–5 mg/kg/d i.v. Caspofungin 60 mg/d i.v.	Fluconazole 400–800 mg/kg/d i.v. or p.o.
Cryptococcus neoformans	Meningitis	Amphotericin B 0.5–0.7 mg/kg/d i.v. or lipid-associated amphotericin 3–5 mg/kg/d i.v. *and* flucytosine 100–150 mg/kg/d p.o., for 6–8 weeks Intrathecal amphotericin B may be required for refractory meningitis	Fluconazole 400–800 mg/d i.v. or p.o.
Geographic fungi *Histoplasma capsulatum* *Blastomyces dermatitidis* *C. dermitis*	Pulmonary or disseminated, *without* meningitis	Amphotericin B 0.5–0.7 mg/kg/d i.v. (total dose, 1.5–2 g) or lipid-associated amphotericin 5–6 mg/kg/d i.v.	Itraconazole 400 mg/d p.o. or i.v.
Coccidioides immitis	Meningitis	Amphotericin B 0.7–1.0 mg/kg/d i.v., total dose ≥2 g, or lipid-associated amphotericin 5–6 mg/kg/d i.v.	Intrathecal therapy needed in most cases
Aspergillus Zygomycetes *Fusarium* *Trichosporon* *Sporothrix*	Pulmonary or disseminated	Amphotericin B 0.7–1.5 mg/kg/d i.v., total dose ≥2 g Lipid-associated amphotericin 5–6 mg/kg/d i.v. Caspofungin 60 mg/d i.v.	Surgical extirpation or debridement of isolated foci infection (i.e., sinusitis, pulmonary, brain) for aspergillus/zygomycetes infection
Pseudallescheria boydii	Pulmonary or disseminated	Itraconazole 200–400 mg q24 h i.v. or p.o., for 2–4 wks	Fluconazole may also be effective but little published data to guide its use

[a]Adult patients, assuming normal renal and hepatic function; dosing of azoles and flucytosine may need to be modified for renal insufficiency or hepatic failure.

penicillins should be given in a total daily dose not less than 250 mg per kg to assure optimal efficacy in patients with normal renal function. On the other hand, with renal insufficiency, dosing after the first (loading) dose needs to be adjusted with all renally excreted antiinfectives to avert toxicity.

Antifungal Drugs

Amphotericin B deoxycholate (Fungizone), which is given intravenously, is yet another essential drug for the treatment of fungal infections (86–88). Relatively few fungi exhibit primary resistance—the exceptions include *Pseudallescheria boydii*, *Trichosporon* species, *Fusarium* species, occasional strains of *Aspergillus*, and rare strains of *Candida*—and with few exceptions, amphotericin B remains the drug of choice for most life-threatening deep fungal infections (Table 4). The doses of amphotericin deoxycholate necessary to treat various fungal infections vary, but there is no need to adjust the daily dose for renal insufficiency.

Many physicians are reluctant to use amphotericin B because of its formidable toxicity. The side effects of amphotericin B include hyperpyrexic reactions, rigors, nephrotoxicity, and electrolyte imbalance syndromes. These can be reduced greatly by a protocol approach to its use, the most essential features of which are measures to avert dehydration and to counter the effects of the renal tubular acidosis, with renal potassium and magnesium wasting, that invariably occurs. Vigorous hydration and salt loading (1 L of normal saline before, 500 mL after the infusion) and vigorous repletion of potassium and magnesium can substantially reduce nephrotoxicity (86,89). Moreover, pretreatment with diphenhydramine, 50 mg, and acetaminophen, 500 to 625 mg, shortly before each daily dose greatly reduces hyperpyrexic reactions; for patients who continue to experience rigors, despite pretreatment, meperidine, 25 to 50 mg by i.v. bolus immediately prior to beginning the infusion, is usually effective. If pretreatment with acetaminophen and diphenhydramine fail to prevent symptomatic febrile reactions, hydrocortisone, 35 to 50 mg *given as a bolus* immediately prior to beginning the infusion, is usually highly effective (86); hydrocortisone should not be added to the bottle or bag. There is no evidence that addition of heparin or mannitol to the container of amphotericin adds to prevention of side effects.

Recently, lipid-associated forms of i.v. amphotericin B have become available: amphotericin B lipid complex (Abelcet); amphotericin B colloidal suspension (Amphotec); and liposomal amphotericin (AmBisome) (90). In these forms, amphotericin has far less toxicity, and it is usually possible to give very large doses from the outset (e.g., 5 to 10 mg per kg per day) without adverse effects. The results with lipid-associated amphotericin B for treatment of deep *Candida* and especially, life-threatening *Aspergillus* and cryptococcal infections, have been promising (91–93). Unfortunately, the attractiveness of the lipid-associated forms is diminished by its cost, in excess of $500 per day. Expensive lipid-associated forms of amphotericin are restricted to patients with marginal renal function and treatment of invasive *Aspergillus* and other filamentous fungal infections in immunocompromised patients in many centers.

Flucytosine (Ancobon) is an important antifungal drug for the adjunctive therapy of cryptococcal meningitis and selected deep *Candida* infections (94), but is only available in an oral form. Flucytosine should be used with great caution, if at all, in patients with renal insufficiency; fatal bone marrow toxicity has resulted from the use of flucytosine in patients with renal failure. In general, when flucytosine is used for treating deep fungal infections in critically ill patients, serum levels should be monitored, especially if the patient has renal insufficiency or preexistent myelosuppression, to assure levels of 50 to not more than 100 μg per mL.

Three azoles are now available for treatment of systemic fungal infections (87): ketoconazole (Nizoral)—only available orally; the triazolam, fluconazole (Diflucan)—now available in both an oral form and parenterally; and itraconazole (Sporanox)—also available orally and parenterally. They are joined by the newly released first echinocandin, caspofungin (Cancidas) (95)—only available parenterally.

The *in vitro* activity of fluconazole against most yeasts, the excellent results in clinical trials, and its minimal toxicity have made it an attractive alternative to i.v. amphotericin B for the treatment of systemic *Candida* infections in ICU patients. Vascular catheter-related BSIs (96–98) and cryptococcal infection in patients with AIDS (99,100) are the conditions most responsive to fluconazole. Whereas fluconazole is highly active against most yeasts, including *Candida*, it is not active *in vitro* against *Aspergillus* or Zygomycetes, and it should never be relied upon for treating infections potentially caused by *Aspergillus* or other filamentous fungi. The drug has been effective for treating most *Candida* infections although certain species, such as *Candida krusei* and *Candida glabrata,* are characteristically resistant (87,101,102). Intravenous amphotericin B is still the drug of choice for life-threatening deep *Candida* infections, such as high-grade candidemia deriving from catheter-related septic thrombosis of a great central vein (29), especially if it has not been established that the infecting strain is a nonalbicans strain and could be resistant to fluconazole. Studies have also shown that fluconazole is effective prophylactically, for prevention of fungal infection in patients undergoing bone marrow transplantation (102,103).

Itraconazole (Sporanox) is effective for treating infections caused by the geographic fungi, especially *H. capsulatum* and *Blastomyces dermatitidis* (104), unless the patient has meningitis or overwhelming infection, in which event i.v. amphotericin B

is the preferred drug (88). Itraconazole also shows promise for treatment of deep *Aspergillus* infections (105), although full-dose standard i.v. amphotericin B, 0.7 to 1.5 mg per kg per day or lipid-associated amphotericin, 5 to 10 mg per kg per day, remain the drugs of choice for this grave infection (88).

Caspofungin, the newly released echinocandin, is approved for *Aspergillus* infections unresponsive to amphotericin B (95). It may also prove useful for treating fluconazole-resistant *Candida* infections, particularly those caused by the ubiquitous and vexing nosocomial species, *C. glabrata.*

Antiviral Drugs

A number of effective antiviral drugs are now available for treatment of life-threatening viral infections in ICU patients (Table 5). The most important of these drugs are acyclovir (Zovirax) (106), which has excellent efficacy for infections caused by HSV (107, 108) and VZV (109,110); and ganciclovir (Cytovene), for CMV infections (111,112) and possibly Epstein-Barr virus infections as well. Foscarnet (Foscavir) is effective for the treatment of CMV, HSV, and VZV infections, especially ganciclovir- or acyclovir-resistant strains (113,114). Cidofovir (Vistide), a unique, very long half-life nucleotide analog can be used to combat ganciclovir-resistant CMV infections (115). Ribavirin (Virazole) is administered in an aerosol for pneumonias caused by respiratory syncytial virus (116) and, intravenously for severe adenovirus pneumonia and infections with hemorrhagic fever viruses (117, 118), possibly the U.S. Hantavirus (119). Amantadine (Symmetrel, Symadine) and rimantadine (Flumadine) are effective agents for influenza A, while zanamavir (Relenza) and oseltamivir (Tamiflu) can be used to treat both for influenza A and B (120–122). Interferon-alpha (Roferon-A) is administered for hepatitis B (123), and, in combination with ribavirin (Virazole), for hepatitis C (124). Ribavirin in a parenteral form is not yet commercially available but can be obtained for treatment of life-threatening infections, such as with Hantavirus or adenoviruses, on a compassionate basis from the manufacturer, ICN Pharmaceuticals (714-545-0100), usually through the Centers for Disease Control and Prevention (877-232-3322).

Recommended dosing schedules for antiviral drugs are provided in Table 5. These schedules must be followed closely, especially when treating disseminated or central nervous system HSV infections or visceral or disseminated VZV infections with acyclovir, to assure maximal benefit. Ganciclovir, which is used primarily for treating CMV infections, produces myelosuppression and occasionally, hepatotoxicity (111), whereas acyclovir has been associated with minimal toxicity (106). Monitoring for bone marrow toxicity is mandatory with ganciclovir, especially in patients with AIDS or those receiving other potentially myelotoxic drugs. If the patient has renal insufficiency, the doses must be carefully adjusted. Foscarnet, which is now available for treating HSV, VZV, or CMV infections refractory to acyclovir or ganciclovir because of drug resistance, is both nephrotoxic and neurotoxic (113), and treatment must also be monitored closely. Cidofovir, which at this time is only approved for CMV retinitis, is also nephrotoxic (115).

Amantadine, rimantadine, zanamivir, and oseltamivir, which are all well tolerated, are each effective prophylactically for prevention of influenza A in the setting of an epidemic (120,121).

TABLE 5. RECOMMENDED THERAPY FOR LIFE-THREATENING VIRAL INFECTIONS AND MALARIA[a]

Pathogen	Type of Infection	First Choice	Alternate Choice/Comments
Herpes simplex virus (HSV)	Stomatitis	Acyclovir 400 mg t.i.d. p.o. ×7 d	Acyclovir 5 mg/kg q8 h i.v.
	Disseminated or visceral infection	Acyclovir 5 mg/kg q8 h i.v. ×10–14 d	Foscarnet 40 mg/kg q8–12 h i.v. ×7–21 d
	Encephalitis	Acyclovir 10 mg/kg q8 h i.v. ×14–21d	Foscarnet
Varicella-zoster virus (VZV)	Local zoster	Acyclovir 800 mg q4 h p.o. ×10 d or famciclovir 500 mg q8 h p.o. ×7 d or valacyclovir 1 g q8 h p.o. ×7 d	Acyclovir 10 mg/kg q8 h i.v.
	Disseminated or visceral infection	Acyclovir 10 mg/kg q8 h i.v. ×7–14 d	Foscarnet
Cytomegalovirus	Retinitis, colitis, or disseminated infection	Ganciclovir 5 mg/kg i.v. q12 h × 2–3 wks, induction; 5 mg/kg/d, maintenance	Foscarnet Cidofovir 5 mg/kg wk ×2, induction; q2 wk, maintenance
	Pneumonia	Ganciclovir 5 mg/kg i.v. q12 h *and* CMV hyperimmune ISG	Foscarnet Cidofovir
Resistant CMV	All	Foscarnet 40–60 mg/kg q8 h i.v., ×2–3 wks, induction; 90–120 mg/kg/d, maintenance	Cidofovir
Resistant HSV, VZV	All	Foscarnet 40–60 mg/kg, 8–12 h ×7–21 d	Cidofovir
Influenza A	Upper respiratory tract infection or pneumonia	Amantadine or rimantadine 100 mg q12 h p.o. ×7 d Oseltamivir 75 b.i.d. p.o. ×7 d	Amantadine or rimantadine Oseltamivir
Hemorrhagic fever virus: Lassa fever virus Marburg virus Korean Hantaan virus U.S. Hantavirus	Disseminated infection	Ribavirin 33 mg/kg i.v. load, 16 mg/kg q6 h ×4 d, 8mg/kg q8 h ×3 d	None
Malaria Chloroquine-sensitive nonfalciparum spp. or *Plasmodium falciparum*	Disseminated	Chloroquine 1 g p.o. stat, 500 mg 6, 24, and 48 h later *plus* primaquine 15 mg daily ×2 wks	None
Chloroquine-resistant *P. falciparum*		Quinine 600 mg q8 h p.o. *plus* doxycycline 150 mg IV p.o. b.i.d. 3–7 d *or* Quinidine 100 mg/kg i.v. over 2 h, *with ECG monitoring*, then 0.02 mg/kg/min i.v. until can take p.o. quinine *plus* doxycycline	Atovaquone *plus* proguanil (Malarone) 1,000/400 mg/d p.o. ×4 d

CMV, cytomegalovirus; ISG, immune serum globulin; HSV, herpes simplex virus; VZV, varicella-zoster virus; ECG, electrocardiogram.
[a]Adult patients with normal renal and hepatic function; dosing may need to be adjusted for renal insufficiency.
[b]Investigational drug potentially available through ICN Pharmaceuticals (714-545-0100) or the Centers for Disease Control (877-232-3322) on a compassionate protocol.

If given within 24 to 48 hours of the onset of acute influenza A infection, they can also ameliorate the severity of illness in older adult or immunocompromised patients, reducing complications and the need for hospitalization (120,122). Neither amantadine or rimantadine, however, is effective against influenza B, parainfluenza viruses, or any other respiratory viruses than influenza A. Dosing of amantadine and rimantadine must be modified in older adult patients (100 mg per day rather than 200 mg per day) and patients with renal insufficiency to prevent seizures (120).

SELECTION OF ANTIINFECTIVE THERAPY FOR INFECTIOUS DISEASE SYNDROMES

It is essential to emphasize the importance of making every effort at the outset to determine the microbial etiology of an ICU patient's presumed infection, to select initial and guide long-term therapy, and to minimize side effects. In most cases, it is possible to select a specific regimen because the initial evaluation suggests a source of infection, such as bacterial pneumonia (chest radiograph and microscopic examination of sputum, a tracheal aspirate, or bronchoalveolar lavage fluid); urinary tract infection (urinalysis and Gram stain of the urine); or meningitis (Gram stain of sedimented CSF) (17,18). Cultures will ultimately disclose the infecting organism(s). In such circumstances, the clinician chooses an empiric regimen based on the microbial pathogen or pathogens that can predictably be expected to be present at the presumed site of infection (Table 6).

Cryptogenic Sepsis, Without Identified Local Infection

Despite efforts to identify a local infection, patients in an ICU often present with fever, rigors, or even septic shock without a

TABLE 6. INITIAL ANTIINFECTIVE THERAPY FOR LIFE-THREATENING INFECTIOUS DISEASE SYNDROMES

Syndrome	Pathogens	Initial Empiric Regimens
Cryptogenic sepsis *without* identifiable local infection (vis-a-vis, primary bloodstream infection) Community-acquired:		
Immunocompetent	*Staphylococcus aureus* *Neisseria meningitidis* Group A streptococcus	Ceftriaxone or cefotaxime (levofloxicin or gatifloxicin[a]) *plus* vancomycin (*if* MRSA in community-acquired infections or has long-term CVC)
Child, older adult, or immunocompromised individual	Same *plus Streptococcus pneumoniae* (including PRP) *Salmonella* *Listeria*	Ceftriaxone or cefotaxime *plus* ampicillin (vancomycin[a])
Nosocomial	*S. aureus* (including MRSA) Enterococcus (possible VRE) *Pseudomonas aeruginosa* and other resistant Gram-negative bacilli	Cefepime, carbapenem, or antipseudomonal penicillin (aztreonam[a]) *plus* ciprofloxacin or tobramycin *plus* vancomycin (*if* risk MRSA/MRCNS) *plus* drug for VRE *only* if known culture-positive
Granulocytopenic fever	Same	Cefepime or carbapenem *Add* vancomycin (if cellulitis, CVC sepsis, septic shock, or known MRSA-positive) Ciprofloxacin *plus* vancomycin[a]
Acute bacterial endocarditis: Native valve	*S. aureus* Group A streptococcus Gram-negative bacilli *Enterococcus*	Penicillin *plus* nafcillin (vancomycin[a]) *plus* gentamicin
Prosthetic valve	Same *plus* coagulase-negative *Staphylococcus* MRSA Nosocomial Gram-negative bacilli *Candida*	Vancomycin *plus* gentamicin
Suspected i.v. line sepsis	Same	Vancomycin *plus* ciprofloxacin or gentamicin
Presumed bacterial pneumonia Community-acquired	*S. pneumoniae* *S. aureus* Oral anaerobes Enteric Gram-negative bacilli *Legionella* spp. *Chlamydia pneumoniae*	Ceftriaxone or cefotaxime *plus* azithromycin Levofloxicin or gatifloxicin[a]
Nosocomial or severe community-acquired requiring ICU care	Same *plus* *P. aeruginosa* MRSA	Cefepime or piperacillin-tazobactam or carbapenem or (aztreonam[a]) *plus* ciprofloxacin, *plus* vancomycin (*if* risk MRSA)
Sinusitis Community-acquired	*S. pneumoniae* *Haemophilus influenzae* *S. aureus*	Cefotaxime or ceftriaxone Levofloxicin or gatifloxicin[a] *Add* vancomycin (if risk MRSA)
Nosocomial	*S. aureus* (including MRSA) Gram-negative bacilli Fungi	Same as nosocomial pneumonia
Presumed bacterial meningitis Community-acquired	*S. pneumoniae* *H. influenzae* type B *N. meningitidis* *Listeria monocytogenes*	Ceftriaxone, cefotaxime, or cefepime *and* vancomycin, *add* rifampin (if also giving corticosteroids)
Nosocomial	Enteric Gram-negative bacilli *P. aeruginosa* *S. aureus* (including MRSA) coagulase-negative Staphylococcus	Cefepime or piperacillin-tazobactam *plus* ciprofloxacin *plus* vancomycin
Intraabdominal infections Cholangitis	Enteric Gram-negative bacilli Enterococci *Clostridium* spp.	Ciprofloxacin or gentamicin *plus* ampicillin (vancomycin[a]) Third-generation cephalosporin *plus* ampicillin (vancomycin) Carbapenem Aztreonam *plus* vancomycin[a]

(continued)

TABLE 6. (*continued*)

Syndrome	Pathogens	Initial Empiric Regimens
Secondary peritonitis or intraabdominal abscess, granulocytopenic typhlitis	As above *plus Bacteroides fragilis* Other anaerobes	Metronidazole or clindamycin, *plus* gentamicin or ciprofloxacin *plus* ampicillin (vancomycin[a]) Ampicillin-sulbactam *and* gentamicin Piperacillin-tazobactam *and* gentamicin Carbapenem
Spontaneous bacterial peritonitis	Gram-negative bacilli *S. pneumoniae*	Ceftriaxone or cefotaxime Ciprofloxacin *and* vancomycin[a] Levofloxacin or gatifloxacin[a]
Urosepsis[b] Community-acquired	Enteric gram-negative bacilli *Enterococcus*	Ciprofloxacin *and* ampicillin (vancomycin[a]) Gentamicin (tobramycin) *and* ampicillin (vancomycin[a])
Nosocomial	Same *plus P. aeruginosa* VRE	Same Carbapenem Give quinupristin or linezolid *only* for documented VRE
Skin and soft tissue Uncomplicated, without granulocytopenia	*S. aureus* Beta-hemolytic streptococci	Nafcillin *with or without* penicillin (vancomycin[a]) Vancomycin[a] Ceftriaxone or cefotaxime (children)
Granulocytopenia	*S. aureus* Gram-negative bacilli, including *P. aeruginosa*	Cefepime or ticarcillin-claviculate or piperacillin-tazobactam *and* ciprofloxacin or tobramycin *plus* vancomycin
Necrotizing fasciitis	Gram-negative bacilli Clostridia and *B. fragilis* *S. aureus* Group A streptococci *Vibrio vulnificans*	Same as secondary peritonitis Doxycycline Ceftriaxone or cefotaxime
Streptococcal toxic shock syndrome with necrotizing cellulitis	Toxigenic group A streptococci	Penicillin (vancomycin) *plus* clindamycin
Enteric infection Bacterial pathogens	*Salmonella* *Shigella* *Campylobacter* Enteropathogenic *Eschericia coli* *Vibrio* spp.	Ciprofloxacin *orally* Ceftriaxone or cefotaxime i.v.
Antibiotic-associated colitis	*Clostridium difficile*	Metronidazole (mild or moderately severe) Vancomycin (severe), *also* give i.v. metronidazole (if ileus)
Toxic shock syndrome	*S. aureus* Group A streptococci	Nafcillin, vancomycin[a], *and* clindamycin Penicillin G, vancomycin[a], *and* clindamycin
Malaria Nonfalciparum species	*Plasmodium vivax* *P. malariae* *P. ovale*	Chloroquine, followed by primaquine[c]
Falciparum	*P. falciparum*[d]	Quinine p.o. (quinine i.v.) *plus* doxycycline or clindamycin Atovaquone-proguanil Mefloquine[e] Artesunate *plus* mefloquine
Babesiosis	*Babcsica* spp.	Quinine and clindamycin Atovaquone and azithromycin
Rickettsial infections	*Rickettsia rickettsia* *R. typhi* *R. prowazekii* *R. akari* *Coxiella burnetii* *Ehrlichia chaffeensis* and *E. phagocytophilia*	Doxycycline Chloramphenicol

MRSA, methicillin-resistant *Staphylococcus aureus*; CVC, central venious catheters; PRP, penicillin-resistant *Streptococcal pneumoniae*; VRE, enterococci resistant to vancomycin; MRCNS, coagulase-negative staphylococci resistant to methicillin; i.v., intravenous.
[a]For serious penicillin hypersensitivity.
[b]Gram stain of the urine will show organisms and allow determination, with >98% reliability, whether a drug regimen is needed for gram-negative bacilli alone, for gram-positive cocci alone, or both.
[c]Check for G-6-PD deficiency before giving primaquine.
[d]Assume all falciparum infections are caused by chloroquine-resistant strain.
[e]Mefloquine resistance is growing.

clinically identifiable source of infection. Many of these patients, especially those who are granulocytopenic, will have culture-proved bacteremia or even candidemia. It is appropriate, after obtaining diagnostic studies, to treat such patients empirically on the premise that they have a primary BSI. Fever alone, other than in a granulocytic patient (125–127), should not be considered grounds to automatically initiate empiric antimicrobial therapy (16). Fever in association with features of SIRS, however, including tachycardia, tachypnea, hypotension with leukocytosis and a left shift; with severe respiratory alkalosis, cryptogenic metabolic acidosis or lactatemia; and certainly with shock or early multiple-organ failure, all features of severe sepsis (18), comprise firm grounds to begin i.v. antiinfective therapy (16,17).

The selection of the initial antimicrobial regimen in this circumstance is generally influenced by: (a) whether the presumed infection was acquired in the community or is nosocomial; (b) the age of the patient; and (c) whether or not the patient is immunocompromised, especially granulocytopenic (less than 1,000 per mm³).

The regimen must be effective against *S. aureus, Streptococcus pyogenes,* and *Neisseria meningitidis* (Table 6) for the immunocompetent septic adult entering the hospital who does not have granulocytopenia, and can be easily achieved with one drug: a third-generation cephalosporin with activity against penicillin-resistant *S. pneumoniae* (ceftriaxone or cefotaxime). The regimen must also be effective against *S. pneumoniae,* type B *H. influenzae,* and Listeria monocytogenes, which mandate the addition of ampicillin or vancomycin. If the patient is an infant or older adult or is immunocompromised (other than granulocytopenia), vancomycin should be added to the third-generation cephalosporin (Table 6) if the patient enters with a long-term central line, is a hemodialysis patient, or if MRSA is endemic in the community.

If, however, the patient does not have granulocytopenia but has recently been hospitalized or has received recent extensive antimicrobial therapy, or, especially, is known to be colonized by resistant gram-negative bacilli or *P. aeruginosa,* then it is desirable to use two antipseudomonal antibiotics in the initial regimen. Adding an aminoglycoside, such as tobramycin, or a fluoroquinolone, such as ciprofloxacin, to a third-generation cephalosporin with antipseudomonal activity, such as cefepime, and also giving vancomycin, for MRSA (Table 6) is recommended.

For the nonseptic but febrile granulocytopenic patient without an obvious local source of infection, an antipseudomonal penicillin or cephalosporin combined with an aminoglycoside or ciprofloxacin can be given (Table 3). However, monotherapy with ceftazidime (128,129), cefepime (130), or imipenem (128,131) will provide reliable initial coverage, pending the results of cultures; each has been studied in randomized, comparative trials and been shown to provide efficacy comparable to combination regimens including an aminoglycoside. If monotherapy is chosen, it is essential that the regimen be adjusted and tailored if blood cultures identify an infecting organism (e.g., administer two antibiotics effective against the organism if the infecting species is a gram-negative rod) to provide additive—ideally synergistic—activity (61,62) to improve the outcome when the patient has severe granulocytopenia.

There has been considerable controversy regarding the inclusion of vancomycin in the initial empiric regimen for the febrile granulocytopenic patient (125–127), to provide a drug active against methicillin-resistant staphylococci, enterococci, and *Corynebacterium* species. Comparative trials have shown that beginning with empiric vancomycin reduces the frequency of secondary nosocomial BSI with these organisms during therapy (132–134). These studies, however, have also shown that excluding vancomycin from the initial regimen and giving it only when a gram-positive infection is identified is not associated with increased morbidity or mortality; the gram-positive infections can be effectively treated (133,134). Thus, the routine use of vancomycin in the initial antimicrobial regimen for the febrile granulocytopenic patient is not recommended unless:

1. The hospital has a high rate of nosocomial infection with MRSA or the patient is known to have previously been colonized or infected by MRSA.
2. There are reasons to suspect overwhelming alpha-hemolytic viridans streptococcal bacteremia (135) (i.e., shock with respiratory distress).
3. The patient shows evidence of infection at the exit site or tunnel of a CVC (29).
4. The patient is at risk for endocarditis (i.e., has a prosthetic heart valve).

In most cases, vancomycin can be reserved for microbiologically confirmed infections with coagulase-negative staphylococci or other resistant gram-positive organisms.

The increasing effectiveness of antineoplastic therapy and antibacterial drugs have extended the lives of most patients with cancer. Deep fungal infections, however, are encountered more often in most centers, particularly in patients with prolonged granulocytopenia who have received intensive antibiotic therapy (125–127). Studies indicate that addition of i.v. amphotericin B, 0.4 to 0.5 mg per kg per day, to the empiric antibacterial regimen reduces mortality due to deep fungal infections and may have prophylactic value as well (136,137) in patients still febrile after 5 to 7 days of empiric antibacterial therapy. Every effort should be made, however, to identify deep fungal infection in such instances. Methods of identification include biopsies of suspicious skin or pulmonary lesions, use of Isolator fungal blood cultures (25), or contrast-enhanced CT scans of the chest to identify the necrotizing nodular lesions characteristic of invasive *Aspergillus* and other filamentous fungal infection (41).

Acute Infective Endocarditis

Relatively few patients with subacute bacterial endocarditis caused by alpha-hemolytic streptococci, enterococci, or the HACEK (*Haemophilus aphrophilus, Actinobacillus actinomycetemcomitans, Cardiobacterium hominus, Eikenella corrodens,* and *Kingella*) organisms require ICU care, unless they develop congestive heart failure or embolic stroke. Patients with acute bacterial endocarditis, on the other hand, commonly need ICU care because of overwhelming sepsis or cardiac complications. Cardiac pathology includes: acute left ventricular failure precipitated by valve destruction; complete heart block produced by a burrowing ring abscess; embolic infarction of the brain, intestine, spleen, or kidneys; or metastatic infection of these organs or the spine (76). Acute infective endocarditis is most often caused by *S. aureus,* but beta-hemolytic streptococci, enterococci, gram-negative bacilli, and even *Candida* can also be encountered. Blood cultures obtained prior to antimicrobial therapy are almost invariably positive. Echocardiography, particularly transesophageal echocardiography, will show vegetations in nearly all cases (138) and is highly reliable for identifying intracardiac complications, such as valvular disruption or ring abscess (139).

Initial therapy for acute endocarditis may be guided by a Gram stain of material aspirated from an embolic skin lesion or an embolus retrieved at surgery, or by the early results of blood cultures. If not, therapy should have efficacy against *S. aureus*, including MRSA, enterococci, and gram-negative bacilli. Penicillin, vancomycin, and gentamicin should provide reliable initial therapy in most cases (Table 6), pending the results of blood cultures, after which a specific American Heart Association consensus regimen should be used (75).

A cardiologist and cardiovascular surgeon should be consulted at the outset because many patients with endocarditis will require cardiac surgery to replace destroyed valves, to debride burrowing ring or septal abscesses, or to drain the infected pericardial space (140,141). Such surgery is often required emergently and has improved the survival of patients with acute endocarditis in recent years (141).

Line Sepsis

Stable vascular access is essential to the management of the critically ill ICU patient. Most patients will have one or more CVCs and an arterial catheter for hemodynamic monitoring, but an increasing number have permanent, surgically implanted, cuffed CVCs—Hickman, Broviac, or hemodialysis catheters—or subcutaneous central venous ports—the Infusaport or Portacath.

The relative risk of BSI caused by the various devices available ranges widely, depending on the type of device (29,142). The highest risk is with short-term CVCs, in the range of 2% to 4% (two to five cases per 1,000 catheter-days), and is highest (5% to 10%) with noncuffed temporary hemodialysis catheters; surprisingly, arterial catheters pose a risk of BSI comparable to short-term CVCs in the ICU (142). In contrast, the risk of bacteremia with small, peripheral i.v. catheters are now very low, less than 0.2%. Permanent, surgically implanted catheters are also associated with a relatively low risk of bloodstream infection, in the range of one BSI per 1,000 days, with good care. The diagnosis of infection with permanently implanted central devices is more difficult, however, as is the decision whether the device needs to be removed to cure presumed related BSI.

Evaluation of the patient with suspected intravascular device-related sepsis must start with a thorough examination to exclude other sites of infection (29,143). The access site must be carefully examined and any expressible purulence should be Gram stained and cultured. Peripheral percutaneous blood cultures should always be obtained and in patients with surgically implanted catheters or ports, blood cultures from the device and peripherally. Quantitative blood cultures using the Isolator system show improved sensitivity for diagnosis of fungemia and are also very helpful in the diagnosis of central venous device-related sepsis. A marked step-up in the quantitative level of bacteremia or fungemia in a blood culture obtained from the device, compared with that from a percutaneous peripheral venous blood culture, is highly suggestive of infection of the device (29). A differential

time to positivity more than 2 hours between standard BACTEC blood cultures drawn concomitantly from a central venous device and peripheral venipuncture also strongly suggests device-originated BSI (28).

With presumed infection of a temporary noncuffed peripheral, central venous, or arterial catheter, the catheter should be removed and if continued access is necessary, a new catheter inserted at a new site, not over a guidewire at the old site (29,97,143, 144).

Uncomplicated, catheter-related bacteremias that show a clinical and bacteriologic response within 48 to 72 hours of initiating antiinfective therapy without signs of metastatic infection or secondary endocarditis can be treated successfully with 7 to 14 days of antimicrobial therapy. Complicated bacteremias mandate longer treatment of generally 4 or more weeks (143).

Transesophageal echocardiography now permits a more cost-effective way to treat catheter-related *S. aureus* bacteremias. First of all, with *S. aureus* line sepsis, the culpable i.v. device must always be removed; irrespective of whether it is a noncuffed short-term i.v. catheter or is a long-term central device. Thereafter, if the bacteremia appears to have been uncomplicated, a transesophageal echocardiogram which does not show vegetations can be regarded as indicating that it is not necessary to treat the infection for longer than 2 weeks (145).

Most catheter-related candidemias can be treated successfully with a total dose of 3 to 5 mg per kg of conventional i.v. amphotericin B (29,88,101,143). Septic thrombosis of a central vein caused by *Candida*, on the other hand, which is characterized by high-grade candidemia, usually requires a higher daily dose, in the range of 0.7 mg per kg, and a total dose of approximately 20 mg per kg, if not contraindicated (renal failure or neutropenia). Flucytosine should be added to the regimen and if there are no contraindications, the patient should be fully anticoagulated (146). Most intravascular catheter-related candidemias—except those caused by *C. glabrata* or *C. krusei*—can also be treated effectively with i.v. fluconazole, 400 to 800 mg per day (29,96,97,101,143), combined with catheter removal, (97,144); those caused by azole-resistant yeasts, such as *C. glabrata* or *C. krusei*, can be treated with amphotericin or the new antifungal, caspofungin (Table 4).

Most BSIs originating from permanent cuffed CVCs or ports derive from intraluminal contaminants, and many caused by coagulase-negative staphylococci or gram-negative bacilli can be successfully treated without removing the catheter. Effective treatment includes administration of i.v. antibiotics through the presumably infected catheter and locking each lumen with a solution containing heparin plus vancomycin or ciprofloxacin (25 μg per mL) when not in use (143). The cuffed catheter should be removed to prevent unnecessary morbidity if at the outset the infecting pathogen is *S. aureus*, JK *Corynebacterium*, a bacillus species, a mycobacterium, or a fungus, and clinical signs of sepsis do not resolve within 3 days or bacteremia persists despite antimicrobial therapy; if the subcutaneous tunnel is infected at the outset; if there is clinical or echocardiographic evidence of endocarditis, septic thrombosis, or septic emboli; or if the patient is at high risk for endocarditis (29,143).

BSIs originating from an infected subcutaneous central port can be diagnosed by demonstrating large numbers of organisms in quantitative culture of material aspirated from the port. Local cellulitis without BSI can usually be treated successfully with antimicrobial therapy, without removing the port. It is usually desirable to remove the port completely if the patient has bacteremia or candidemia and the causal role of the port has been established by quantitative culture of fluid aspirated from the device, as it is difficult to cure implanted port infections medically (29,143).

Pneumonia

Pneumonia poses the greatest threat to the ICU patient and the greatest challenge to the intensivist. Several points bear emphasis before discussing therapy. First, a clinical picture of pneumonitis may have a noninfectious etiology: many antineoplastic drugs, such as methotrexate, cyclophosphamide, or bleomycin, produce toxic or hypersensitivity pneumonitis, and adult lung injury syndromes, atelectasis, pulmonary emboli, congestive heart failure, pulmonary hemorrhage, neoplastic disease, and radiation therapy can mimic infectious pneumonia. Second, these processes may coexist in the setting of infectious pneumonitis. Finally, in all critically ill or immunocompromised patients, it is especially important to strive to determine the microbial etiology of presumed infectious pneumonia, eschewing empiric therapy without diagnostic studies.

Table 6 lists the major pathogens encountered and suggested drug regimens for the treatment of pneumonia in the ICU patient. Patients with acute pneumonia in which the Gram stain of a good sputum specimen or tracheal aspirate shows large numbers of white blood cells, but no microorganisms, *Legionella*, *Chlamydia*, or *Mycoplasma* infection must be suspected, in addition to viruses or fungi. A macrolide, such as azithromycin, or a fluoroquinolone should be included in the initial empiric regimen (Table 6) (34,35). Recent large studies have shown that a third-generation cephalosporin with activity against resistant *S. pneumoniae* plus a macrolide, or a new fluoroquinolone given alone provided the best results in community-acquired pneumonia requiring hospitalization (147).

Severe, community-acquired pneumonia requiring ICU care is generally best treated with a new fluoroquinolone or an antipseudomonal cephalosporin (cefepime), or penicillin (e.g., piperacillin-tazobactam), or a carbapenem plus a macrolide, such as azithromycin (34,35,82). Nosocomial pneumonia should ideally be guided, to begin, by a Gram stain of tracheal secretions (33): if gram-negative bacilli are seen, multiresistant organisms—especially *P. aeruginosa*—must be assumed, and two drugs with antipseudomonal activity are recommended (Table 6). The only two drugs for which data exist to justify possible monotherapy for the initial empiric regimen for nosocomial pneumonia are imipenem and ciprofloxacin. A multicenter randomized trial in patients with severe pneumonia, most with nosocomial pneumonia, showed that ciprofloxacin was superior to imipenem (148).

Human immunodeficiency virus (HIV) infection must be excluded and studies should also be done to rule out *P. carinii* or CMV infection (34,35) when confronted by diffuse interstitial-alveolar pneumonitis acquired in the community. A wet mount should also be done to rule out overwhelming blastomycosis, histoplasmosis, or coccidioidomycosis (149–151). Hantavirus pneumonia should also be considered, especially if the patient shows hemoconcentration or has had exposure to mice (119).

Sinusitis

Radiographs or a CT scan will allow a diagnosis of sinusitis in most patients: opacification, air fluid levels, or marked mucosal thickening (greater than 10 mm) have been shown to be associated with bacterial sinusitis approximately 90% of the time with community-acquired disease. Whereas most acute sinusitis has a bacterial etiology (Table 6), granulocytopenic patients are vulnerable to fungal sinusitis, especially with Zygomycetes (mucormycosis) or *Aspergillus*. In the critically ill immunocompromised patient, particularly with sinusitis associated with periorbital inflammation, fungal sinusitis must be strongly considered (152) and excluded by endoscopic or open biopsy.

For empiric therapy of presumed severe bacterial sinusitis acquired in the community in the immunocompetent patient without granulocytopenia, a third-generation cephalosporin with activity against *S. pneumoniae* (ceftriaxone or cefotaxime) should prove effective in the vast majority of cases. Therapy should be guided by the results of diagnostic sinus aspiration or biopsy (46) in critically ill patients, especially granulocytopenic patients or ICU patients who have received prolonged, intensive antimicrobial therapy. This allows use of the most specific regimen for infection caused by *S. aureus*, *P. aeruginosa*, or other gram-negative bacilli, or fungi (152–154).

Meningitis

With rare exceptions, treatment of meningitis should be guided by the results of the CSF fluid examination, particularly the Gram stain of ultracentrifuged CSF (30), and if negative, with purulent meningitis, the results of antigen tests for *S. pneumoniae*, *H. influenzae* type b, and *N. meningitidis*. If these studies are inconclusive but the CSF profile strongly suggests bacterial meningitis, vis-à-vis, neutrophilic pleocytosis and hypoglycorrhachia, the initial regimen must provide activity against the three aforementioned pathogens and *L. monocytogenes*, an increasingly important cause of meningitis in infants, older adults, and immunocompromised patients (155). The combination of a third-generation cephalosporin with pneumococcal activity, such as ceftriaxone or cefotaxime (156,157), and ampicillin or vancomycin is recommended (30) (Table 6); with life-threatening penicillin allergy, trimethoprim-sulfamethoxazole or vancomycin can be used in place of the ampicillin. With granulocytopenia, the regimen must also be effective against *P. aeruginosa*, and cefepime or a carbapenem can be used, with ciprofloxacin. These regimens will also provide adequate initial empiric therapy if lumbar puncture is delayed or is contraindicated because of threatened herniation or severe coagulopathy.

Strains of *S. pneumonia* causing bacterial meningitis exhibiting high-level resistance to penicillin (MIC greater than 1 μg per mL) are now widely prevalent in most parts of the world, including the United States (6,7). The combination of ceftriaxone or cefotaxime, *and* vancomycin, with rifampin if corticosteroids are being given, is recommended for the initial therapy of suspected pneumococcal meningitis or suppurative meningitis of unknown etiology, pending the results of cultures (30) (Table 6).

With bacterial meningitis, postexposure prophylaxis must be provided for the household contacts of patients found to have meningococcal or *H. influenzae* type b meningitis, bacteremia, or pneumonia (30).

Viral Meningoencephalitis

Viral meningoencephalitis is extremely common, but in most cases is self-limiting and does not require hospitalization. On the other hand, viral meningoencephalitis caused by some of the arboviruses, lymphocytic choriomeningitis virus, Japanese B encephalitis virus, West Nile encephalitis virus, and HSV can result in severe brain damage or death.

Of the more virulent forms of viral meningoencephalitis, necrotizing encephalitis caused by HSV is perhaps the most common in North America but is also eminently treatable, if therapy is begun sufficiently early (107). In patients with a clinical picture of meningoencephalitis and a compatible CSF profile (lymphocytic pleocytosis with some neutrophils, only modest elevation of protein, little or no hypoglycorrhachia, and a negative Gram stain), who also show focal findings on neurologic examination or focal inflammation on contrast imaging of the brain (CT scan, or better, magnetic resonance imaging [MRI]), especially of the temporal lobes, necrotizing HSV encephalitis must be suspected and treated without delay (158). Detection of HSV DNA in the CSF by polymerase chain reaction (PCR) has obviated the need for brain biopsy in most cases (159). If begun before the patient has progressed to frank coma, acyclovir 10 mg per kg i.v. every 8 hours results in a good outcome in more than 70% of cases (107).

Intraabdominal Infections

Intraabdominal infections fall into three major categories with differing microbial profiles (Table 6): cholangitis, spontaneous bacterial (primary) peritonitis, and secondary peritonitis or intraabdominal abscesses from loss of integrity of the gastrointestinal tract.

Cholangitis

Cholangitis occurs primarily in the setting of biliary tract obstruction, usually by calculi or cancer (160). Suppurative ascending cholangitis with sepsis is an emergency. Shock and death from overwhelming endotoxemia can rapidly occur even in young patients if the obstruction is not promptly relieved endoscopically by percutaneous transhepatic catheter drainage or surgically. Cholangitis with bacteremia occurs occasionally in the absence of obstruction with a surgical choledochojejunostomy or following hepatic transplantation.

Cholangitis is caused predominantly by aerobic gram-negative bacilli, enterococci, and occasionally, *Clostridium* species. *Bacteroides fragilis* and other anaerobic bacteria are rarely encountered in ascending cholangitis, without hepatic abscess (160). Treatment of presumed cholangitis mandates a regimen effective against aerobic gram-negative bacilli and enterococci: gentamicin, ciprofloxacin, an antipseudomonal cephalosporin, such as cefepime, or a carbapenem plus ampicillin (vancomycin, for penicillin-allergic patients) (Table 6).

Spontaneous Bacterial Peritonitis

Spontaneous bacterial (primary) peritonitis is a well-defined syndrome in which enteric gram-negative bacilli—usually *Escherichia coli*—occasionally *S. pneumoniae,* produce unimicrobial peritonitis, associated with bacteremia more than one-half of the time, without identifiable disruption of the integrity of the gastrointestinal tract or cholangitis. Spontaneous bacterial peritonitis is seen almost exclusively in patients with preexistent end-stage liver disease and ascites (161), but also in female children with nephrotic syndrome. Community-acquired spontaneous bacterial peritonitis is effectively treated with a third-generation cephalosporin (ceftriaxone or cefotaxime) or a new fluoroquinolone, such as levofloxacin or gatifloxacin (Table 6) (161,162).

Secondary Peritonitis or Intraabdominal Abscess

Bacteroides fragilis and other anaerobic organisms, together with aerobic gram-negative bacilli and enterococci, are polymicrobial copathogens in most cases of secondary peritonitis due to disruption of the gastrointestinal mucosa and with all types of intraabdominal and pelvic abscesses. Metronidazole or clindamycin, combined with an aminoglycoside or ciprofloxacin, with or without ampicillin; ampicillin-sulbactam and gentamicin; or piperacillin-tazobactam, with or without ampicillin, have all been shown to provide reliable coverage (Table 6) (163,164). For monotherapy, only a carbapenem should be relied upon (165).

Many patients in an ICU with intraabdominal sepsis are immunocompromised or have received prior antimicrobial therapy. Multiresistant nosocomial organisms (166), especially enterococci (167), and yeasts, must always be considered as potential copathogens. The antimicrobial regimen should generally include ampicillin or vancomycin (167). Recovery of *Candida* in a specimen from suppurative intraabdominal infection mandates antifungal therapy with fluconazole or i.v. amphotericin B (164,166,168,169).

Acalculous Cholecystitis

Acalculous cholecystitis is a relatively uncommon and insidious condition seen primarily in patients who have had gastrointestinal surgery, trauma, or other illness that precludes feeding enterally (170). It is often associated with minimal abdominal findings and ultrasound examination or hepatic scintigraphy are most likely to be helpful diagnostically. Surgical exploration is mandated to confirm the diagnosis and drain or, better, resect the necrotic gallbladder in a case of suspected acalculous cholecystitis.

Typhlitis

Patients with prolonged and profound granulocytopenia are uniquely vulnerable to a syndrome characterized by abdominal pain and tenderness, usually in the right lower quadrant, associated with ileus and a clinical picture of systemic sepsis (171,172). Typhlitis appears to represent localized inflammation of the distal small bowel and cecum, and is commonly associated with aerobic gram-negative bacteremia or fungemia. Treatment of typhlitis consists of bowel rest and empiric antimicrobial (and possibly, antifungal) therapy, similar to that which would be used for treatment of secondary peritonitis (Table 6), but with efficacy against *P. aeruginosa*. The role for surgical resection is not clear-cut and remains controversial (171,172)

Gynecologic Infections

Suppurative pelvic infections are usually caused by the same microorganisms encountered in patients with secondary peritonitis due to disruption of the gastrointestinal mucosa: anaerobes, aerobic-enteric gram-negative bacilli, and enterococci (164,173). Thus, the empiric regimen for pelvic infection in ICU patients, many of whom have had recent gynecologic surgery, is similar to that used for the treatment of secondary peritonitis or intraabdominal abscesses.

Urosepsis

Although urinary catheter-associated bacteriuria or candiduria is extremely common in the ICU (1–4) (Fig. 2), it rarely is the cause of nosocomial sepsis (42). Urosepsis is most often encountered in patients admitted from the community with overt pyelonephritis (174). Nosocomial urosepsis, most often seen in urology patients with obstruction or who have undergone recent urinary tract surgery (175), is usually caused by resistant nosocomial organisms, such as *Klebsiella* or *Enterobacter*, *Proteus* species, *P. aeruginosa*, *Serratia*, or enterococci, and not uncommonly, *Candida* (Fig. 2). A Gram stain of infected urine provides highly reliable immediate data pointing at the probable microbial etiology (43). Initial regimens, pending cultures, for nosocomial urosepsis include ampicillin and an aminoglycoside, ciprofloxacin or cefepime, or a carbapenem alone (176). Fluconazole is usually effective for *Candida* urosepsis (101).

It is extremely important with septic shock due to urosepsis that obstruction is promptly excluded by ultrasonography or CT scan. If present, obstruction must be relieved, without delay. Upper tract obstruction must be relieved by percutaneous nephrostomy.

Skin and Soft-Tissue Infections

S. aureus and beta-hemolytic streptococci cause uncomplicated skin and soft-tissue infections in adults almost exclusively. In unimmunized children, type b *H. influenzae* should be considered as well (Table 6). Adults can be treated with nafcillin, with or without penicillin, and children, with ceftriaxone or cefotaxime.

Cellulitis in granulocytopenic patients is often caused by staphylococci or streptococci, but is more often caused by aerobic gram-negative bacilli, especially *P. aeruginosa*. Perianal cellulitis is a syndrome unique to granulocytopenic patients and, contrary to perianal abscesses in nongranulocytopenic patients, is nearly always a unimicrobial, aerobic gram-negative bacillary infection, most often with *P. aeruginosa* (177). Surgical intervention is occasionally justified, but is not routinely recommended unless there is necrotic tissue to debride or a clear-cut abscess to drain.

Patients who have undergone recent gastrointestinal or gynecologic surgery, or with soft-tissue infections complicating decubital ulcers or occurring in the setting of antineoplastic chemotherapy, peripheral vascular disease or, especially, diabetes are vulnerable to life-threatening necrotizing soft-tissue infections—

"necrotizing fasciitis" or "synergistic gangrene"—which may involve underlying muscle (178,179). These infections are usually polymicrobial, caused by aerobic gram-negative bacilli and anaerobic organisms (Table 6), basically, the same pathogens implicated in secondary peritonitis. Bacteremia occurs in up to 40% of cases. Necrotizing group A streptococcal soft-tissue infection with streptococcal toxic shock syndrome must be suspected in patients admitted to the hospital with an acute soft-tissue infection and a picture of septic shock, especially in younger, and previously well patients (180,181) (see below).

Any soft tissue inflammation occurring in a patient at risk for complex cellulitis must be vigorously evaluated diagnostically, at the minimum with Gram stain and culture of percutaneous aspirates or biopsies; in most cases, Gram stain will show the infecting organisms (182). If a grayish hue or frank necrosis is seen or gas is present in the deep tissues on radiographic examination, exploratory surgery and thorough debridement is imperative at the outset (178–181). The case fatality of complex skin and soft tissue infections is exceedingly high unless surgical debridement is employed early in the course.

Uncontrolled data suggest that adjunctive treatment in a hyperbaric oxygen chamber (3 atm), after surgical debridement, may improve survival in patients with necrotizing soft-tissue infections (183).

Enteric Infections

Infants, older adults, and immunocompromised patients of any age are at risk for life-threatening enteric infections with *Campylobacter*, *Salmonella*, *Shigella*, enteropathogenic *E. coli*, or enterocolitis caused by *C. difficile*. With the exception of *C. difficile* enterocolitis, most enteric infections are effectively treated with a fluoroquinolone, such as ciprofloxacin, given orally (184). A third-generation cephalosporin, such as ceftriaxone, will also be effective against the aforementioned pathogens if bacteremia has occurred.

C. difficile enterocolitis (pseudomembranous colitis, antibiotic-associated colitis) is now an extremely common complication of broad-spectrum antimicrobial therapy, especially in the ICU (14). Any patient who has recently received antibiotic therapy and develops watery diarrhea, especially associated with cramps and fever, or who simply develops unexplained ileus, must be suspected of having this syndrome. The diagnosis can be confirmed 80% of the time by flexible sigmoidoscopy, identifying the characteristic pseudomembranes, but tests for the presence of cytotoxin in the stool are equally sensitive diagnostically and highly specific, in the range of 95% (185).

Antibiotic-associated colitis prompts reassessment of the need for continued broad-spectrum antimicrobial therapy. Oral metronidazole appears to be as efficacious therapeutically as oral vancomycin for mild or moderately severe cases (186); for severe antibiotic-related colitis or with unstable patients, vancomycin 125 mg by mouth every 6 hours is considered the regimen of choice (14).

Colectomy is strongly recommended, before catastrophic perforation occurs, if the patient is floridly septic and abdominal radiograph shows severe ileus and progressive or massive colonic dilation (187).

Toxic Shock Syndrome

Most patients who present with septic shock have bacterial infection, often involving the bloodstream, and a local infection, such as pyelonephritis, peritonitis, or pneumonia, is apparent at the outset. One must be suspicious of primary bacteremia when careful history and physical examination do not identify a plausible local source of infection. Cryptogenic (primary) bacteremia caused by gram-negative bacilli, other than rare *Salmonella*, is uncommon in a previously well person without underlying illness. The most frequent causes of primary bacteremia in previously well, younger patients are *N. meningitidis*, *S. aureus*, or group A streptococci (Table 3).

Toxic shock syndrome (TSS) caused by toxigenic strains of *S. aureus* or group A beta-hemolytic streptococci must also be considered with this clinical scenario. TSS caused by *S. aureus* is rarely associated with bacteremia. Staphylococcal TSS usually derives from clinically asymptomatic mucosal colonization, usually of the vagina in association with tampon use in women, of the nasopharynx in small children, or as a complication of surgical nasal packs (188); rarely, it stems from indolent postoperative infection of a surgical wound (189). Ninety percent of *S. aureus* TSS occurs in women during their menses in association with tampon use; with early diagnosis and appropriate treatment, mortality is now very low, less than 1%. On the other hand, postsurgical staphylococcal TSS from a wound infection (189) and TSS caused by group A streptococci (180,181) are far more serious clinically because they originate from a soft tissue infection and, in the case of streptococcal TSS, from primary bacteremia as well; mortality, even in the best hands, is prohibitively high, in the range of 30% to 40%.

TSS is a multisystem syndrome produced by toxigenic strains of *S. aureus* or group A *Streptococcus*. The TSS toxins, enterotoxin F (TSST-1) with *S. aureus* TSS and streptococcal pyrogenic exotoxin A (SPE A) with streptococcal TSS, share greater than 50% DNA homology and do not differ materially in biologic activity. TSST-1 and SPE A are among the most potent biologic toxins known. These toxins act as superantigens inducing large numbers of circulating T-lymphocytes to release massive quantities of cytokines, such as tumor necrosis factor-α (TNF-α), interleukin-1 (IL-1), platelet-activating factor, and other biologic mediators that produce the clinical features of septic shock, as well as TSS. These toxins result in high fever, chills, hypotension, polymyalgias, and headache, with laboratory findings, such as leukocytosis, thrombocytopenia, evidence of disseminated intravascular coagulation, hypoxemia, electrolyte abnormalities, azotemia, and organ failure. TSS might be more accurately termed staphylococcal (or streptococcal) biologic mediator syndrome.

The only natural defense against TSS in a patient who becomes colonized or infected by a toxigenic strain is a preexistent antibody from prior subclinical colonization and exposure to infinitesimally low levels of the toxin sufficient to induce humoral immunity. The use of pooled human immune serum globulin (ISG), which exhibits activity against TSS toxins, can prevent the syndrome, and is also effective for treatment in experimental animal models of TSS (180,181).

TSS should be suspected in any patient with a clinical picture of cryptogenic hypotension and fever without an obvious apparent source of local infection, other than cellulitis. The presence of diffuse, blanchable erythroderma or a scarlatiniform rash should greatly increase suspicion. Such a clinical picture occurring in a woman during her menstrual period who is using tampons should be considered to represent TSS until proven otherwise. Generally, TSS is a diagnosis of exclusion, with other causes of septic shock, such as pyelonephritis, overwhelming pneumonia, or peritonitis, excluded by clinical and laboratory evaluation.

With TSS caused by group A streptococci and originating from a necrotizing cellulitis, the patient typically experiences intractable local pain and tenderness, with a characteristic grayish hue to the skin seen that reflects infarction of underlying tissue (180,181). Gram stain of material aspirated percutaneously will usually show organisms. CT or MRI imaging is helpful diagnostically and usually reveals deep inflammation. Necrotizing infection is confirmed by surgical exploration and treated by surgical debridement of the nonviable tissue.

The Centers for Disease Control and Prevention epidemiologic criteria for diagnosis of TSS require all of the following:

1. Fever $\geq 38.9°C$
2. Rash: diffuse macular erythroderma, with subsequent desquamation
3. Systolic blood pressure ≤ 90 mm Hg
4. Involvement of more than three of the following organ systems:
   Gastrointestinal: vomiting or diarrhea
   Muscular: myalgias or increased creatinine phosphokinase
   Mucous membranes: hyperemia
   Renal: blood urea nitrogen or creatine greater than 2 times the upper limit of normal
   Liver: transaminases greater than 2 times the upper limit of normal
   Blood: thrombocytopenia less than 100,000 per mm^3
   Central nervous system: disorientation without focal signs
5. Negative studies for other infections, such as Rocky Mountain spotted fever, leptospirosis, or measles.

Rigorous confirmation of TSS requires culture of a toxigenic strain of *S. aureus* or group A streptococci and documentation of seroconversion, from no detectable antibody to TSS toxin at the outset of illness to circulating antibody in the convalescent period.

TSS toxin produces profound capillary permeability with transudation of plasma into the interstitial space, resulting in severe hypovolemia. Circulating biologic mediators produce marked vasodilation. The most important measure for treatment of TSS is large-volume fluid resuscitation: 10 to 20 L of normal saline or Ringer lactate solution may be necessary in the first 24 hours. Failure to do so predictably results in multiple-organ failure and, ultimately, death. Inadequate fluid resuscitation with *S. aureus* tampon-related TSS in the early 1980s explains the prohibitive 13% mortality at the time (188), before the syndrome was fully understood in terms of its pathogenesis and needed management.

Antibiotics effective against the infecting or colonizing toxigenic organism should also be given: nafcillin or vancomycin for *S. aureus*, penicillin G (or erythromycin) for group A streptococci. Clindamycin, which unlike penicillin is active against stationary-phase organisms and blocks toxin production independent of its antibacterial activity, is associated with greatly improved survival in animal models (190), and should be included in the initial regimen (Table 6).

One of the most important aspects of management of TSS is "source control," achieved with menstrual-related *S. aureus* TSS by removal of the tampon. Streptococcal TSS, however, as noted, requires surgical debridement of necrotizing soft-tissue infection, if present. Bacteremia, obviously, can be treated only with i.v. antibiotics.

A novel approach to treatment of TSS that is being increasingly used is i.v. immune serum globulin (ISG). Pooled standard human ISG has neutralizing activity against TSS toxins, and if the patient is hemodynamically unstable, a dose of 400 mg per kg of i.v. ISG at the outset may reduce mortality (191). It is likely that a hyperimmune ISG or recombinant monoclonal antitoxin for adjunctive treatment of TSS, to neutralize circulating and possibly even bound TSS toxin, would prove highly beneficial.

Malaria and Babesiosis

Malaria

Malaria is one of the leading causes of mortality due to infection worldwide, accounting for more than 3 million deaths per year (192). Each year, over 30,000 travelers to malarious countries acquire malaria; many die in an ICU, nearly all from unrecognized falciparum malaria that has progressed to an overwhelming stage.

Malaria is easily diagnosed on a peripheral blood smear, especially that caused by *Plasmodium falciparum*: fine, lacy trophozoites with characteristic double chromatin dots, multiply infected erythrocytes, no peripheral schizonts, and characteristic banana-shaped gametocytes. But malaria can be diagnosed and treated expeditiously only if it is considered in the differential diagnosis of fever and sepsis occurring in a patient who has recently returned from a malarious area of the world, regardless of whether they took antimalarial prophylaxis. A new highly sensitive antigen test permits rapid diagnosis, even in the field, and reliable identification of *P. falciparum* infection (193).

Chloroquine resistance in *P. falciparum* is now endemic worldwide, with only selected areas of Central America and the Middle East spared (192). In a critically ill patient with malarial forms seen in the peripheral blood smear, if there is any question whatsoever about the infecting species, particularly if there is high-level parasitemia (greater than 1% to 2%), chloroquine-resistant *P. falciparum* infection must be assumed, and the patient should be given oral quinine 600 mg every 8 hours and doxycycline 100 mg every 12 hours (194). Quinine can be administered through an orogastric tube if the patient is unable to take oral medications, but if the patient has vomiting or ileus, quinidine gluconate, given by continuous i.v. infusion, with doxycycline, is the treatment of choice (195,196). The level of parasitemia should decline rapidly, within 24 hours, of initiating effective therapy.

Exchange transfusion has been successfully used in conjunction with antimalarial drug therapy in the treatment of gravely ill patients with overwhelming falciparum malaria and massive par-

asitemia (30% to 50%) (196). Corticosteroids are not beneficial (197).

Nonfalciparum chloroquine-sensitive malaria is rarely life threatening and is easily treated with the standard 2-day chloroquine regimen (Table 5), followed by 14 days of primiquine to prevent relapse (194).

Babesiosis

Babesia are *Plasmodium* species endemic in the United States. (198), primarily in the North Central and Northeast states, and are acquired from the same ticks that vector Lyme disease—coinfections are well documented. Babesiosis produces a clinical picture similar to malaria but, unfortunately, diagnosis is commonly delayed. In splenic and immunocompromised patients, babesiosis can be rapidly fatal. Babesia infection is treated with oral quinine plus clindamycin, or with atovaquone and azithromycin (199).

Rickettsial Infections

Six rickettsial species are endemic in the United States: the agents of Rocky Mountain spotted fever (*Rickettsia rickettsii*), murine typhus (*Rickettsia typhi*), epidemic typhus (*Rickettsia prowazekii*), rickettsial pox (*Rickettsia akari*), Q fever (*Coxiella burnetii*), and perhaps, most common, erhlichiosis (*Erhlichia chaffeensis* and *Erhlichia phagocytophilia*) (200). Rickettsial infections are the most serious and life-threatening vector-borne infections acquired in the continental U.S. and are characterized by high fever, headache, and profound myalgias, often associated with leukopenia and thrombocytopenia. Patients with Rocky Mountain spotted fever and typhus usually show a nonspecific maculopapular or hemorrhagic rash and those with rickettsial pox, vesicular or pustular skin lesions, whereas the other U.S. rickettsioses are not associated with a rash. Q fever produces atypical pneumonia and hepatitis.

The combination of leukopenia, elevated transaminases, and thrombocytopenia in a septic patient who has had tick exposures should prompt suspicion of rickettsial infection, especially erhlichiosis (200,201). Rickettsial infections can prove fatal if untreated, particularly in older adult or immune-compromised patients. Erhlichiosis can be presumptively diagnosed by identifying morulae in peripheral leukocytes, but the sensitivity of this finding is so low as to not be reliable diagnostically. Rickettsial infections can be diagnosed by demonstrating the microorganisms' DNA in peripheral blood by PCR or by conventional serologic techniques (201,202).

The treatment of choice for all rickettsial infections, including erhlichiosis, is doxycycline, with chloramphenicol reserved for infants or patients unable to tolerate tetracyclines. Beta-lactams are ineffective for treatment of rickettsioses.

Acquired Immunodeficiency Syndrome in the Intensive Care Unit

In recent years, far fewer patients with AIDS chose to enter an ICU during the final stages of their illness. Most AIDS patients

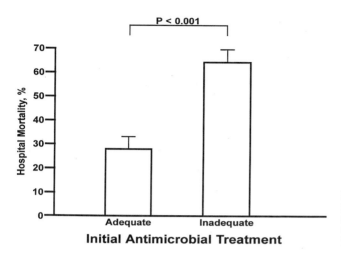

FIGURE 3. Hospital mortality of 492 intensive care unit patients with bloodstream infections between 1997 and 1999, according to the adequacy of initial antimicrobial therapy. (From Ibrahim EH, Sherman G, Ward S, et al. The influence of inadequate antimicrobial treatment of bloodstream infections on patient outcomes in the ICU setting. *Chest* 2000;118:146–155.)

coming to an ICU are admitted for trauma or other conditions unrelated to HIV infection. Many, however, are in the earlier stage of HIV infection and warrant ICU monitoring and care for first episodes of *P. carinii* pneumonia, seizures or coma due to *T. gondii*, cryptococcal meningitis, or tuberculosis mycobacterium infection, or BSI with *S. aureus*, *S. pneumoniae*, or *Salmonella*.

The numerous opportunistic infections are generally easily treated (85). In general, antiretroviral drugs are continued, if enteric administration is possible.

It is essential for ICU personnel to scrupulously adhere to Universal Precautions with all patients, not just those with documented HIV or other chronic bloodborne viral infections, to prevent occupationally acquired infection (203,204). Novel technologies engineered to reduce the risk of catastrophic sharps injuries (e.g., needleless systems) may ultimately provide the greatest protection (205).

Treatment of Antimicrobial-Resistant Infections

There has been a marked increase during the past decade in nosocomial infections caused by MRSA (8,9), VRE/VAREC (10,11), ESBL-positive gram-negative bacilli (12,13), *C. difficile* (14), and *Candida* (15), especially azole-resistant nonalbicans species (Fig. 1). In many areas of the country, community-acquired MRSA is starting to be seen (206), and infections caused by *S. aureus* exhibiting diminished susceptibility to vancomycin (GISA) are beginning to be encountered (70).

It is clear that delay in initiating appropriate antiinfective therapy for BSIs and other serious infections with these microorganisms in ICU patients is associated with greatly increased mortality (Fig. 3) (207). Patients likely to be infected by multiresistant pathogens almost always have characteristic risk factors (208): significant underlying diseases, especially cancer or organ transplantation; recent surgery; nosocomial sepsis, in most cases device-related, especially CVC-related BSI; and, almost universally, history of prior antimicrobial therapy, especially with cephalosporins or other broad-spectrum antibiotics.

The recommended regimens for specific treatment of infections caused by multiresistant organisms are summarized in

Table 7. Infection with a multiresistant organism should be considered and the empiric regimen should take into account the possibility of infection with penicillin-resistant *S. pneumoniae* MRSA or ESBL-positive gram-negative bacilli when critically ill septic patients have one or more risk factors. If a hospitalized patient has received intensive antimicrobial therapy and is known to be colonized by *Candida*, especially in the urinary tract or a surgical wound, or a CVC tip culture has returned positive, empiric therapy with fluconazole or amphotericin B is justified (88,101).

Focused Antiinfective Therapy

The results of cultures and other diagnostic studies identifying the infecting organisms and susceptibility tests form the basis for selection of the definitive antimicrobial regimen for treatment of the patient's infection. In nongranulocytopenic patients, this can allow a change to a less intensive and more focused regimen, particularly if the infecting pathogen is a single gram-positive or aerobic gram-negative bacterium.

With granulocytopenic patients, on the other hand, particularly those with profound granulocytopenia, even if staphylococcal BSI is identified, it is usually desirable to continue the broad-spectrum regimen, such as vancomycin and cefepime. This therapy is based on the premise that the patient is coinfected by other organisms and remains highly vulnerable to superinfection by gram-negative bacilli (125–127,136).

Specific regimens for the treatment of infections caused by the bacterial, rickettsial, chlamydial, fungal, and viral pathogens encountered in ICU patients, and for malaria are summarized in Tables 3 through 7; recommended doses and dosing intervals are provided in Table 2.

SUPPORTIVE THERAPY

Treatment of sepsis, especially associated with shock or early multiple-organ dysfunction (MODS) syndrome, does not stop with source control and antiinfective therapy, but demands the highest skills of the intensivist to keep the patient alive until the infection can be controlled. Recent reviews provide insightful

TABLE 7. RECOMMENDED REGIMENS FOR SPECIFIC TREATMENT OF INFECTIONS CAUSED BY MULTIRESISTANT ORGANISMS

Pathogen	First Choice(s)	Second Choice(s)
Penicillin-resistant *S. pneumoniae* (PRP)	Ceftriaxone, cefotaxime or cefepime Vancomycin	Levofloxacin Gatifloxicin
Methicillin-resistant *S. aureus* (MRSA) or coagulase-negative staphylococci	Vancomycin	Quinupristin-dalfopristin Linezolid
Vancomycin- and ampicillin-resistant enterococci (VRE/ VAREC)	Quinupristin-dalfopristin Linezolid	Ampicillin and imipenem (?)
Third-generation cephalosporin-resistant *Enterobacter, Serratia, Pseudomonas aeruginosa*	Cefepime or carbapenem *and* ciprofloxacin or gentamicin or tobramycin	Amikacin
Extended-spectrum β-lactamase producing gram-negative bacilli	Carbapenem Cefepime	Gentamicin or amikacin Ciprofloxacin
Carbapenem-resistant *P. aeruginosa*	Cefepime Tobramycin Ciprofloxacin	Polymixin B
Fluconazole-resistant *Candida*	Amphotericin B Caspofungin	Flucytosine

Amphotericin-resistant fungi
   Candida (rare)
   Trichosporon
   Fusarium
   Pseudallescheria
	Caspofungin
	
	Itraconazole
		Voriconazole[a]
		
		Fluconazole

Acyclovir-resistant HSV, VZV	Foscarnet	Cidofovir
Ganciclovir-resistant CMV	Foscarnet	Cidofovir

VRE, enterococci resistant to vancomycin; VAREC, enterococci resistant to vancomycin, ampicillin or both; HSV, herpes simplex virus; VZV, varicella zoster virus; CMV, cytomegalovirus.
[a] Experimental drug potentially available on compassionate protocol from Merck & Co., Inc, 1-800-672-6372.

guidelines for the supportive and adjunctive therapy of septic shock (17,209–211).

Circulatory Support

The importance of support of very early and aggressive the circulation in the septic patient with large volumes of i.v. fluids, with or without cardiovascular pressor drugs, cannot be overemphasized (212). The most experienced intensivist cannot by physical examination alone reliably assess a critically ill patient's cardiac performance, vis-à-vis, reliably estimate ventricular filling pressures, or cardiac output (213). Thus, if an infected patient exhibits hypoxemia or hypotension refractory to initial fluid resuscitation, a flow-directed, balloon-tipped, pulmonary-artery catheter can be very helpful to guide fluid therapy and decisions on choice of pressors and inotropic drugs, with the physiologic goal of optimizing oxygen delivery and uptake (214,215). Recent fear, based on retrospective analysis of an unrelated database, that pulmonary-artery catheters increase mortality in critically ill patients (216) has been dispelled by a large, multicenter randomized Canadian trial in older adult postoperative patients showing that pulmonary-artery catheters can be used safely, without increased mortality (217).

There are no data to indicate that colloid solutions, such as albumin, plasma protein fraction, or hydroxyethyl starch (hetastarch), are superior to crystalloids, such as 0.9% normal saline or Ringer lactate, for support of the failing circulation in the patient with septic shock. Three metaanalyses have shown that the use of colloid solutions in the management of critically ill patients is associated with significantly increased hospital mortality

(relative risk, 1.10 to 1.49) (218–220). Crystalloids should be the i.v. fluid of choice for treatment of sepsis and septic shock until an ongoing large, multicenter, randomized international trial resolves the issue. Data from a randomized trial shows that including albumin, 1.5 g per kg, in the initial fluid resuscitation regimen reduces mortality only in patients with end-stage liver disease and spontaneous bacterial peritonitis (221).

With septic shock, the hemodynamic target for volume loading should be a cardiac filling (pulmonary-artery-occlusion) pressure of no more than 12 to 15 mm Hg (222,223). Continued hypotension or a subnormal cardiac output indicates the need for a pressor—dopamine, dobutamine, or even norepinephrine (224–226)—depending on the need for an alpha-agonist as opposed to an inotrope.

Early hopes that pulmonary-artery catheter monitoring, combined with efforts to maximize oxygen delivery mainly by augmenting cardiac output to supranormal levels can improve survival in septic shock (214,215) have not been confirmed in large, multicenter randomized trials (227). Whether bedside monitoring of gastric intramucosal pH, which correlates with tissue oxygenation, can permit more effective use of resuscitation fluids, pressors, and novel therapies sufficient to improve survival remains to be determined (228,229).

Novel Adjunctive Therapies

For nearly 40 years, despite advances in antiinfective therapy and in ICU care, the mortality of septic shock has declined only marginally (230), pointing up the need to modulate the severe SIRS that underlies shock, MODS, and death (231).

Corticosteroids

The long-disputed role of high-dose corticosteroids for adjunctive therapy of septic shock would appear to have been resolved by two large, prospective, randomized double-blind trials: methylprednisolone, 30 mg per kg per day, did not improve survival in either trial (232,233). More recent studies, however, have shown that with acute bacterial meningitis caused by type b *H. influenzae* or *S. pneumoniae*, especially in children, dexamethasone 0.15 mg per kg started immediately before beginning antimicrobial therapy, significantly reduces morbidity (234–236); corticosteroids may even improve survival in adults with pneumococcal meningitis (237). Corticosteroids also appear to be of benefit in tuberculous meningitis (238,239). Prednisone, 50 to 100 mg per day, given to patients with life-threatening typhoid fever—with shock or in coma—also improves survival (240). In patients with AIDS who have *P. carinii* pneumonia and hypoxemia ($PaO_2 < 70$ less than 70 torr or $(A-a)O_2$-greater than 35 torr, on room air), prednisone 20 mg every 6 hours and tapered over 2 weeks also improves survival (241,242).

Patients who have been receiving long-term corticosteroid therapy who develop sepsis must be given supplemental stress doses of corticosteroids, hydrocortisone, 50 to 75 i.v. every 6 hours, to prevent acute adrenal crisis (see Chapter 57). However, there is growing evidence to suggest that these doses of hydrocortisone will improve survival in patients with severe sepsis. Many previously well patients with bacteremic sepsis, especially caused by *N. meningitidis* or other encapsulated bacteria, such as *S. pneumoniae* or type b *H. influenzae*, who develop disseminated intravascular coagulation will show a subnormal response to corticotropin stimulation (243,244). This indicates relative adrenal insufficiency and a beneficial role for stress-level corticosteroid support (245,246). A recent multicenter, double-blind randomized trial in France found that in ICU patients with severe sepsis or septic shock, adjunctive therapy with hydrocortisone, 50 mg i.v. every 6 hours, and fludrocortisone, 5 μg per day orally, reduced mortality 30% (247).

Other Novel Adjunctive Therapies

During the past 20 years, intensive efforts have been made to modulate the systemic inflammatory response syndrome (SIRS) that accounts for the features of sepsis—especially shock—organ failure, and death (231). More than 30 multicenter trials of novel pharmacologic agents for the adjunctive therapy of septic shock have been undertaken following trials demonstrating that high doses of corticosteroids did not improve survival, (17,209,210, 248).

Early trials with hyperimmune immunoglobulins with endotoxin-neutralizing activity showed clear-cut benefit (249–251) but, inexplicably, these products have never been developed and made available commercially. Subsequent trials, most using monoclonal antibodies designed to block the biologic effects of endotoxin or inflammatory cytokines, such as TNF-α, IL-1, or platelet-activating factor, were undertaken, with uniformly disappointing results (248). It has become starkly evident that modulating the immunoinflammatory response to sepsis sufficiently to improve survival but not compromise essential host defense mechanisms is a daunting challenge.

It has long been recognized that most patients with septic shock show evidence of uncontrolled, disseminated intravascular coagulation, with low levels of the most important physiologic anticoagulant, protein C (252). A recent international multicenter trial was undertaken to assess the therapeutic effect of repleting protein C with a recombinant activated form (rhAPC) in patients with severe sepsis, 75% with shock (253). The choice of protein C was also influenced by knowledge of its capacity to modulate inflammation, through inhibition of monocyte production of TNF-α and IL-1b, inhibition of neutrophil activation, and downregulation of endothelial expression molecules, intercellular adhesion molecule (ICAM)-1, E-selectin, and VCAM-1 (254).

In a double-blind trial in 1,640 patients, a continuous infusion of rhAPC 24 μg per kg per minute, begun within 24 hours of the onset of severe sepsis and continued for 96 hours, was associated with a 19% reduction in 28-day all-cause mortality ($P = 0.005$) (253). There was a slight increase in bleeding complications in recipients of rhAPC (serious bleeding, 3.5% versus 2.0%, $P = 0.06$), however, rhAPC was well tolerated, considering the critical illness of most of the recipients. This novel product was recently approved by the Food and Drug Administration and is now available commercially.

Other Issues

Granulocyte transfusions are no longer recommended for most patients with serious infection and profound granulocytopenia. Early studies showed a short-term advantage, but the associated risks of transfusion-related CMV infection, alloimmunization, pulmonary toxicity with concomitant use of amphotericin B, and cost have dampened enthusiasm for the use of granulocyte transfusions as adjunctive therapy in infected granulocytopenic patients (255,256). The major indication for granulocyte transfusion support at the present time is the patient with profound granulocytopenia (less than 100 per mm^3) and overwhelming gram-negative bacillary infection, especially major soft-tissue infection that is unresponsive to antiinfective therapy (256).

The availability of recombinant granulocyte and granulocyte/macrophage–colony-stimulating factors, G-CSF (filgrastim; Neupogen) and GM-CSF (sargramostim; Leukine, Prokine), provides an important adjunctive option for the management of patients with severe but transient granulocytopenia due to cancer chemotherapy, bone marrow transplantation, or drug toxicity (257–259). In general, G-CSF (5 μg per kg per day) and GM-CSF (250 μg per M^2 per day) are used prophylactically to shorten the duration of chemotherapy-related granulocytopenia; their efficacy for treatment of severe bacterial or fungal infections is less well established at this time (260). A new immunomodulator, macrophage–colony-stimulating factor (M-CSF) has shown promise for treatment of severe disseminated fungal infections in granulocytopenic patients (261).

The use of ISG is clearly of value for prevention of infection in many clinical settings (262), but the role of ISG as an adjunct in the treatment of bacterial or fungal sepsis, in the absence of hypogammaglobulinemia, is less secure. In patients with impaired CMI and severe CMV pneumonitis, however, particularly those who have recently undergone bone marrow or organ transplantation, CMV hyperimmunoglobulin, given in conjunction with i.v. ganciclovir, may improve the patient's chance for survival (112).

Finally, beyond all of the therapeutic measures discussed, it is essential to assure that the critically ill patient receives optimal nutritional (263) and transfusion (264) support and protection from thromboembolism (265) and stress-related gastrointestinal hemorrhage (266) (see also Chapters 15, 40, and 44).

PREVENTION OF INFECTION IN THE INTENSIVE CARE UNIT

At least one-half of nosocomial infections in the ICU are preventable (1). It is beyond the scope of this review to consider in detail measures for prevention of infection in the ICU patient; however, important points warrant brief discussion.

Basic Infection Control Practices

It is imperative in the ICU that maximal attention be paid to good aseptic technique. In particular hand washing with an antiseptic-containing agent, such as 2% to 4% chlorhexidine (267–269), or use of a waterless alcohol-containing gel (270), before and after each contact with a patient should be a routine practice. There should be uncompromising compliance with isolation policies (271), including Universal Precautions (203,204); and there should be adherence with consensus infection control guidelines for the management of urinary catheters (272), intravascular devices (29,143,273), and ventilatory support (274).

Technologic Innovations

The promise of novel technology, proven in randomized controlled trials, offers new opportunities to protect the vulnerable ICU patient from serious nosocomial infection. New developments include the use of chlorhexidine rather than povidone-iodine for cutaneous antisepsis for vascular access preparation (275–277), CVCs (278–280), and urinary catheters (281,282) with antiinfective coatings, aspiration-resistant endotracheal tubes (283,284), and immune-enhancing nutritional formulas (285).

Protected Environments

Numerous trials have examined the efficacy of protected environments for granulocytopenic patients: laminar air flow rooms and use of sterile gowns, gloves, masks, and shoe covers for all health care workers entering the patient's room. These studies have shown only marginal benefit, if any, for prevention of infection during the period of profound granulocytopenia (286). As such, few centers routinely use protective isolation for the care of such patients.

A randomized trial, however, has shown that the routine use of simple barrier precautions—nonsterile gloves and a disposable gown—significantly reduces nosocomial colonization by resistant organisms and the incidence of nosocomial infection in high-risk children requiring ventilatory support in an ICU for at least 7 days (287). Moreover, the routine use of nonsterile gloves for all patient contacts has been shown to reduce nosocomial acquisition of

C. difficile (288). To stop the continued spread of resistant nosocomial pathogens, such as MRSA, VRE, resistant gram-negative bacilli, and *C. difficile*, it may be desirable to preemptively use simple barrier precautions routinely for contacts with all ICU and other hospitalized patients who are at high risk of nosocomial infection, especially with resistant organisms (289), as contrasted with screening all high-risk patients and isolating those found to be positive (290).

Patients with prolonged severe granulocytopenia or recipients of liver, heart, or lung transplants are uniquely susceptible to invasive infection by airborne filamentous fungi, especially *Aspergillus fumigatus*, devastating infections that have prohibitively high mortality. Studies have shown that the incidence of filamentous fungal infection during antileukemic therapy or bone marrow transplantation can be greatly reduced by providing spore-free air—accomplished by use of high-efficiency particle (HEPA) filters (291,292). Inexpensive HEPA units for individual patient-care rooms are now available. Spore-free air must be considered a standard of care for the treatment of compromised patients with prolonged and profound granulocytopenia due to acute leukemia or bone marrow transplantation, including during needed care in an ICU. It is probably also warranted for the care of patients undergoing liver, heart, or lung transplants, because of the high risk of airborne filamentous fungal infection in these patients as well.

Immune Serum Globulin

ICU patients with chronic lymphocytic leukemia, multiple myeloma, or lymphoma, or who have recently undergone bone marrow transplantation often have associated hypogammaglobulinemia. Patients with documented hypogammaglobulinemia (IgG level less than 200 mg per dL) or who have experienced recurrent bacterial infections and have subnormal levels of immunoglobulin G, should receive supplemental ISG, 400 mg per kg every 3 weeks (262). In general, immunoglobulin levels should be checked in any compromised patient who develops recurrent bacterial infections of the respiratory tract, especially with encapsulated bacteria. Recent trials suggest that prophylactic use of ISG in unselected critically ill ICU patients may reduce the risk of nosocomial infection, especially pneumonia (293–296).

Antiviral Prophylaxis

Patients who have undergone recent bone marrow or solid organ transplantation are highly susceptible to primary or reactivated infections caused by HSV and CMV. Acyclovir, 5 mg per kg i.v. every 8 hours, markedly reduces the incidence of necrotizing HSV stomatitis and disseminated HSV infection during the period of maximal vulnerability (297,298). In patients who have undergone recent bone marrow or organ transplantation, i.v. ganciclovir 5 mg per kg i.v. every 12 hours, greatly reduces the risk of early posttransplant CMV infection (250,300).

During a hospital influenza A outbreak, susceptible compromised patients who have not been previously immunized should receive amantadine or rimantadine, 200 mg daily (100 mg per day in patients over 60 years of age), or oseltamivir, 75 mg every 12 hours, to prevent severe or even fatal nosocomial influenza A (120,121).

SUMMARY

Life-threatening infection continues to be a major cause of increased morbidity and mortality in the critically ill. Early diagnosis, by comprehensive evaluation, and initiation of the most focused and physiologically based therapy is crucial to survival. When antiinfective therapy is to be initiated, it should be directed against the most likely pathogens and be reevaluated on a daily basis. Renal and hepatic function must be considered in choice of antimicrobial agent or agents, along with proper dosing and monitoring of drug levels. Crystalloid i.v. solutions, such as normal saline or Ringer lactate, should be used, rather than colloids, such as albumin, for support of the failing circulation. Timely surgical intervention is essential to survival with many infections, such as ascending cholangitis or necrotizing soft-tissue infections. Recent trials now show, for the first time, that adjunctive therapy with stress-level hydrocortisone or repletion of protein C with a novel activated recombinant form significantly improves survival in patients with severe sepsis. Finally, consistent application of proven infection control practices can reduce the risk of nosocomial infection, especially the spread of multiple-resistant pathogens.

KEY POINTS

1. Infection, either acquired in the community or, increasingly, in the hospital is the major cause of death of more than one-half of patients dying in an intensive care unit (ICU).

2. Accurate diagnosis of the source of infection is essential to select the most focused and effective antiinfective regimen, and to implement needed source control.

3. Beyond a comprehensive history and physical examination, skilled use of Gram stains, cultures, and other microbiologic studies, and radiologic imaging will identify the source of infection of most patients with life-threatening infection.

4. Toxic shock syndrome caused by *Staphylococcus aureus* or toxigenic strains of group A beta-hemolytic streptococci is a common cause of cryptogenic septic shock and must prompt aggressive studies for the source of toxigenic organisms. This is particularly important in patients with streptococcal toxic shock syndrome that originates from deep necrotizing soft-tissue infections in 50% of cases, and where early surgical debridement is essential if the patient is to survive.

5. More than one-half of nosocomial bloodstream infections acquired in the ICU originate from intravascular devices; a high index of suspicion and the use of microbiologic studies including, where indicated, the use of paired blood cultures, permits the accurate diagnosis of most device-related bloodstream infections.

6. Antibiotic-associated colitis caused by toxigenic strains of *Clostridium difficile* is a common problem in the ICU patient who has received prior antimicrobial therapy and must be excluded with nosocomial diarrhea or unexplained ileus and sepsis.

7. A large number of powerful antiinfectives for treatment of life-threatening bacterial, fungal, and viral infections are now available and, when used properly, greatly improve outcome.

8. With antibiotics in which microbial killing is concentration-dependent, such as fluoroquinolones and aminoglycosides with gram-negative organisms, it is essential that blood and tissue levels be high at the outset. With aminoglycosides, once-daily dosing appears to be as effective as three-times daily dosing. With beta-lactam antibiotics and vancomycin, however, maintaining blood and tissue levels above the minimum inhibitory concentration of the organism for most of the dosing interval enhances effectiveness, indicating that with short half-life beta-lactam antibiotics, frequent dosing is essential, particularly with life-threatening gram-positive infections, such as meningitis or infective endocarditis. Effective antimicrobial therapy also requires knowledge of the patient's renal and hepatic status, and dosing adjustments for organ failure.

9. When antimicrobial therapy has been initiated, the need for continued therapy must be reassessed regularly, particularly if cultures or other diagnostic studies are negative and the patient has not changed. The regimen should be adjusted, based on the organisms identified and drug susceptibilities, if an infecting pathogen or pathogens have been identified.

10. In the ICU patient who presents with signs of systemic infection, especially overwhelming infection or septic shock, every effort must be made to identify the source of infection, and if possible, to mechanically remove that source, if necessary, surgically. Source control is crucial to survival and in many instances supersedes antimicrobial therapy in importance.

11. Circulatory support with intravenous crystalloid fluids, such as normal saline or Ringer lactate solution, is the first and one of the most important therapeutic measures in septic shock, volume loading to a filling pressure of 12 to 15 mm Hg. Other than sepsis from spontaneous bacterial peritonitis with end-stage liver disease, there are no data to support the unmitigated use of colloid solutions, such as albumin or plasma protein fraction; in fact, colloids may increase mortality.

12. For severe sepsis, with organ failure or shock refractory to fluid resuscitation, adjunctive therapy with stress-level corticosteroids or recombinant activated human protein C (rhAPC) significantly improves the likelihood of survival.

REFERENCES

1. Maki DG. Nosocomial infection in the intensive care unit. In: Parrillo JE, Bone RC, eds. *Critical care medicine. Principles diagnosis and management.* St. Louis: Mosby–Year Book, 1995:893–954; 2nd edition, 2001 (*in press*).

2. Vincent J-L, Bihari D, Suter P, et al. The prevalence of nosocomial infection in intensive care units in Europe. Results of the European Prevalence of Infection in Intensive Care (EPIC) Study. EPIC International Advisory Committee. *JAMA* 1995;274:639–644.

3. Pittet D, Tarara D, Wenzel RP. Nosocomial bloodstream infections in critically ill patients. Excess length of stay, extra cost, and attributable mortality. *JAMA* 1994;271:1598–1601.

4. Richards MJ, Edwards JR, Culver DH, Gaynes RP, and the National Nosocomial Infections Surveillance System. Nosocomial infections in combined medical-surgical intensive care units in the United States. *Infect Control Hosp Epidemiol* 2000;21:510–515.

5. Kollef MH, Fraser VJ. Antibiotic resistance in the intensive care unit. *Ann Intern Med* 2001;134:298–314.

6. Whitney CG, Farley MM, Hadler J, et al. Increasing prevalence of multidrug-resistant *Streptococcus pneumoniae* in the United States. *N Engl J Med* 2000;343:1917–1924.

7. Feikin DR, Schuchat A, Kolczak M, et al. Mortality from invasive pneumococcal pneumonia in the era of antibiotic resistance, 1995–1997. *Am J Public Health* 2000;90:223–229.

8. Panlilio AL, Culver DH, Gaynes RP, et al. Methicillin-resistant *Staphylococcus aureus* in U.S. hospitals, 1975–1991. *Infect Control Hosp Epidemiol* 1992;13:582–586.

9. Maranan MC, Moreira B, Boyle-Vavra S, et al. Antimicrobial resistance in staphylococci: epidemiology, molecular mechanisms, and clinical relevance. *Infect Dis Clin North Am* 1997;11:813–849.

10. Centers for Disease Control and Prevention. Nosocomial enterococci resistant to vancomycin—United States, 1989–1993. *MMWR* 1993;42:597–599.

11. Murray BE. Vancomycin-resistant enterococci. *Am J Med* 1997;101:284–293.

12. Jarlier V, Nicholas M-H, Fournier G, et al. Extended broad-spectrum beta-lactamases conferring transferable resistance to newer beta-lactam agents in Enterobacteriaceae: hospital prevalence and susceptibility patterns. *Rev Infect Dis* 1988;10:867–878.

13. Pitout JDD, Sanders CC, Sanders E Jr. Antimicrobial resistance with focus on β-lactam resistance in gram-negative bacilli. *Am J Med* 1997;103:51–59.

14. Johnson S, Gerding DN. *Clostridium difficile*-associated diarrhea. *Clin Infect Dis* 1998;26:1027–1034.

15. Wright WL, Wenzel RP. Nosocomial *Candida*. Epidemiology, transmission, and prevention. *Infect Dis Clin North Am* 1997;11:411–425.

16. O'Grady NP, Barie PS, Bartlett J, et al. Practice parameters for evaluating new fever in critically ill adult patients. *Crit Care Med* 1998;26:392–408.

17. Sprung CL, Bernard GR, Dellinger RP, eds. Guidelines on the management of sepsis and shock. *Intensive Care Med* 2001;27[Suppl 1]:S1–S134.

18. Bone RC, Balk RA, Cerra FB, et al. Definitions for sepsis and organ failure and guidelines for the use of innovative therapies in sepsis. *Chest* 1992;101:1644–1655.

19. Arbo MJ, Fine MJ, Hanusa BH, et al. Fever of nosocomial origin: etiology, risk factors, and outcomes. *Am J Med* 1993;95:505–512.

20. Hall J. Assessment of fever in the intensive care unit. Is the answer just beyond the tip of our nose? *Am J Respir Crit Care Med* 1999;159:695–701.

21. Circiumaru B, Baldock G, Cohen J. A prospective study of fever in the intensive care unit. *Intensive Care Med* 1999;25:668–673.

22. Sehdev PS, Mackowiak PA. Fever in the ICU patient. In: Pankey GA, ed. *Ochsner Clinic reports on serious hospital infections.* New Orleans: Ochsner Clinic, 1999:1–8.

23. Sickles EA, Greene WH, Wiernik PH. Clinical presentation of infection in granulocytopenic patients. *Arch Intern Med* 1975;135:715–719.

24. Mackowiak PA, LeMaistre CF. Drug fever: a critical appraisal of conventional concepts. *Ann Intern Med* 1987;106:728–733.

25. Dunne WM, Nolte FS, Wilson ML, et al. In: Hindler JA, ed. *Blood cultures III.* Washington DC: American Society for Microbiology, 1997.

26. Mermel LA, Maki DG. Detection of bacteremia in adults: consequences of culturing an inadequate volume of blood. *Ann Intern Med* 1993;119:270–272.

27. DesJardin JA, Falagas ME, Ruthazer R, et al. Clinical utility of blood cultures drawn from indwelling central venous catheters in hospitalized patients with cancer. *Ann Intern Med* 1999;131:641–647.

28. Blot F, Nitenberg G, Chachaty E, et al. Diagnosis of catheter-related bacteraemia: a prospective comparison of the time to positivity of hub-blood versus peripheral-blood cultures. *Lancet* 1999;354:1074–1077.

29. Maki DG. Infections caused by intravascular devices used for infusion therapy: pathogenesis, prevention, and management. In: Bisno AL, Waldvogel FA, eds. *Infections associated with indwelling medical devices,* 2nd ed. Washington, DC: American Society for Microbiology, 1994:155–212.

30. Roos KL, Tunkel AR, Scheld WM. Acute bacterial meningitis in children and adults. In: Scheld WM, Whitley RJ, Durack DT, eds. *Infections of the central nervous system,* 2nd ed. Philadelphia: Lippincott–Raven Publishers, 1997:335–401.

31. Metersky ML, Williams A, Rafanan AL. Retrospective analysis: are fever and altered mental status indications for lumbar puncture in a hospitalized patient who has not undergone neurosurgery? *Clin Infect Dis* 1997;25:285–288.

32. Kalin Mats, Lindberg AA, Tunevall G. Etiological diagnosis of bacterial pneumonia by Gram stain and quantitative culture of expectorates. *Scand J Infect Dis* 1983;15:153–160.

33. Salata RA, Lederman MM, Shlaes DM, et al. Diagnosis of nosocomial pneumonia in intubated, intensive care unit patients. *Am Rev Respir Dis* 1987;135:426–432.

34. Bartlett JG, Dowell SF, Mandell LA, et al. Practice guidelines for the management of community-acquired pneumonia in adults. *Clin Infect Dis* 2000;31:347–382.

35. Mandell LA, Marrie TJ, Grossman RF, et al. and the Canadian Community-Acquired Pneumonia Working Group. Canadian guidelines for the initial management of community-acquired pneumonia: an evidence-based update by the Canadian Infectious Diseases Society and the Canadian Thoracic Society. *Clin Infect Dis* 2000;31:383–421.

36. Fagon J-Y, Chastre J, Wolff M, et al. Invasive and noninvasive strategies for management of suspected ventilator-associated pneumonia. *Ann Intern Med* 2000;132:621–630.

37. Luna CM, Vujacich P, Niederman MS, et al. Impact of BAL data on the therapy and outcome of ventilator-associated pneumonia. *Chest* 1997;111:676–685.

38. Moir C, Robins RE. Role of ultrasonography, gallium scanning, and computed tomography in the diagnosis of intraabdominal abscess. *Am J Surg* 1982;143:582–585.

39. Gagliardi PD, Hoffer PB, Rosenfield AT. Correlative imaging in abdominal infection: an algorithmic approach using nuclear medicine, ultrasound, and computed tomography. *Semin Nucl Med* 1988:18:320–334.

40. McDowell RK, Dawson SL. Evaluation of the abdomen in sepsis of unknown origin. *Radiol Clin North Am* 1996;34:177–190.

41. Heussel CP, Kauczor H-U, Heussel G, et al. Early detection of pneumonia in febrile neutropenic patients: use of thin-section CT. *AJR* 1997;169:1347–1353.

42. Tambyah PA, Maki DG. Catheter-associated urinary tract infection is rarely symptomatic: a prospective study of 1497 catheterized patients. *Arch Intern Med* 2000;160:678–682.

43. Kunin CM. The quantitative significance of bacteria visualized in the urinary sediment. *N Engl J Med* 1961;265:89.

44. Stamm WE. Measurement of pyuria and its relation to bacteriuria. *Am J Med* 1983;75[Suppl 1B]:53–58.

45. Tambyah PA, Maki DG. The relationship between pyuria and infection in patients with indwelling urinary catheters. Results of a prospective study of 761 patients. *Arch Intern Med* 2000;160:763–767.

46. Ramadan HH, Owens RM, Tiu C, et al. Role of antral puncture in the treatment of sinusitis in the intensive care unit. *Otolaryngol Head Neck Surg* 1998;119:381–384.

47. Carlet J. Rapid diagnostic methods in the detection of sepsis. *Infect Dis Clin North Am* 1999;13:483–494.

48. Hatherill M, Tibby SM, Sykes K, et al. Diagnostic markers of infection: comparison of procalcitonin with C reactive protein and leucocyte count. *Arch Dis Child* 1999;81:417–421.

49. Viallon A, Zeni F, Lambert C, et al. High sensitivity and specificity of serum procalcitonin levels in adults with bacterial meningitis. *Clin Infect Dis* 1999;28:1313–1316.

50. Enguix A, Rey C, Concha A, et al. Comparison of procalcitonin with C-reactive protein and serum amyloid for the early diagnosis of bacterial sepsis in critically ill neonates and children. *Intensive Care Med* 2001;27:211–215.

51. Müller B, Becker KL, Schächinger H, et al. Calcitonin precursors are reliable markers of sepsis in a medical intensive care unit. *Crit Care Med* 2000;28:977–983.

52. Wanner GA, Keel M, Steckholzer U, et al. Relationship between procalcitonin plasma levels and severity of injury, sepsis, organ failure, and mortality in injured patients. *Crit Care Med* 2000;28:950–957.

53. Trenholme GM, Kaplan RL, Karakusis PH, et al. Clinical impact of rapid identification and susceptibility testing of bacterial blood culture isolates. *J Clin Micro* 1989;27:1342–1345.

54. Glick PH, Pellegrini CA, Stein S, et al. Abdominal abscess. A surgical strategy. *Arch Intern Med* 1983;118:646–650.

55. Olak J, Christou NV, Stein LA, et al. Operative vs. percutaneous drainage of intra-abdominal abscesses. *Arch Surg* 1986;121:141–146.

56. Drusano GL. Human pharmacodynamics of beta-lactams, aminoglycosides and their combination. *Scand J Infect Dis* 1991;74 [Suppl]:235–248.

57. Craig WA. Pharmacokinetic/pharmacodynamic parameters: rationale for antibacterial dosing of mice and men. *Clin Infect Dis* 1998;26:1–12.

58. Craig WA. Continuous infusion of β-lactam antibiotics. *Antimicrob Agents Chemother* 1992;36:2577–2583.

59. Adkinson NF Jr, Saxon A, Spence MR, et al. Cross-allergenicity and immunogenicity of Aztreonam. *Rev Infect Dis* 1985;7[Suppl 4]:S613–S621.

60. Levin S, Karakusis PH. Future trends in aminoglycoside therapy. *Am J Med* 1986;80:190–194.

61. Love LJ, Schimpff SC, Schiffer CA, et al. Improved prognosis of granulocytopenic patients with gram-negative bacteremia. *Am J Med* 1980;68:643–648.

62. DeJongh CA, Joshi JH, Newman KA, et al. Antibiotic synergism and response in gram-negative bacteremia in granulocytopenic cancer patients. *Am J Med* 1986;80[Suppl 5C]:96–100.

63. Vidal F, Mensa J, Almela M, et al. Epidemiology and outcome of *Pseudomonas aeruginosa* bacteremia, with special emphasis on the influence of antibiotic treatment. *Arch Intern Med* 1996;156:2121–2126.

64. Moore RD, Smith CR, Lietman PS. The association of aminoglycoside plasma levels with mortality in patients with gram-negative bacteremia. *J Infect Dis* 1984;149:443–448.

65. Moore RD, Lietman PS, Smith CR. Clinical response to aminoglycoside therapy: importance of the ratio of peak concentration to minimal inhibitory concentration. *J Infect Dis* 1987;155:93–99.

66. Prins JM, Buller HR, Kuijper EJ, et al. Once versus thrice daily gentamicin in patients with serious infections. *Lancet* 1993;341:335–339.

67. Nicolau DP, Freeman CD, Belliveau PP, et al. Experience with a once-daily aminoglycoside program administered to 2,184 adult patients. *Antimicrob Agents Chemother* 1995;39:650–655.

68. Edelstein PH. Antimicrobial chemotherapy for Legionnaires disease: a review. *Clin Infect Dis* 1995;21[Suppl 3]:5265–5276.

69. Piscitelli SC, Danziger LH, Rodvold KA. Clarithromycin and azithromycin: new macrolide antibiotics. *Clin Pharm* 1992;11:137–152.

70. Centers for Disease Control. *Staphylococcus aureus* with reduced susceptibility to vancomycin—United States, 1997. *MMWR* 1997;46(33):765–766.

71. Hospital Infection Control Practices Advisory Committee. Recommendations for preventing the spread of vancomycin resistance. *Infect Control Hosp Epidemiol* 1995;16:105–113.

72. Polk RE, Healy DP, Schwartz LB, et al. Vancomycin and the red-man syndrome: pharmacodynamics of histamine release. *J Infect Dis* 1988;157:502–507.

73. Maki DG, Bohn MJ, Stolz SM, et al. Comparative study of cefazolin, cefamandole, and vancomycin for surgical prophylaxis in cardiac and vascular operations. *J Thorac Cardiovasc Surg* 1992;104:1423–1434.

74. Ryback MJ, Albrecht LM, Boike SC, et al. Nephrotoxicity of vancomycin, alone and with an aminoglycoside. *J Antimicrob Chemother* 1990;25:679–685.

75. Wilson WR, Karchmer AW, Dajani AS, et al. Antibiotic treatment of adults with infective endocarditis due to *Streptococci, Enterococci, Staphylococci,* and HAECK microorganisms. *JAMA* 1995;274:1706–1713.

76. Cunha BA, Gill MV, Lazar JM. Acute infective endocarditis. Diagnostic and therapeutic approach. *Infect Dis Clin North Am* 1996;10:812–834.

77. Winston DJ, Emmanouilides C, Kroeber A, et al. Quinupristin/dalfopristin therapy for infections due to vancomycin-resistant *Enterococcus faecium. Clin Infect Dis* 2000;30:790–797.

78. Drew RH, Perfect JR, Srinath L, et al. Treatment of methicillin-resistant *Staphylococcus aureus* infections with quinupristin-dalfopristin in patients intolerant of or failing prior to therapy. *J Antimicrob Chemother* 2000;46:775–784.

79. Clemett D, Markham A. Linezolid. *Drugs* 2000;59:815–827.

80. Beam TR, Ed. Clinical uses of IV ciprofloxacin. *Infect Med* 1991;8[Suppl C]:1–49.

81. Righter J. Pneumococcal meningitis during intravenous ciprofloxacin therapy. *Am J Med* 1990;88:548.

82. Heffelfinger JD, Dowell SF, Jorgensen JH, et al. Management of community-acquired pneumonia in the era of pneumococcal resistance. *Arch Intern Med* 2000;160:1399–1408.

83. File TM, Segreti J, Dunbar L, et al. A multicenter, randomized study comparing the efficacy and safety of intravenous and/or oral levofloxacin verus ceftriaxone and/or cefuroxime axetil in treatment of adults with community-acquired pneumonia. *Antimicrob Agents Chemother* 1997;41:1965–1972.

84. Sullivan JG, McElroy AD, Honsinger RW, et al. Treating community-acquired pneumonia with once-daily gatifloxacin vs. once-daily levofloxacin. *J Respir Dis* 1999;20:S49–S59.

85. Bartlett JG. *2000 Pocket Book of Infectious Disease Therapy.* Baltimore: Williams & Wilkins, 2000:1–447.

86. Gasslis HA, Drew RH, Pickard WW. Amphotericin B: 30 years of clinical experience. *Rev Infect Dis* 1990;12:308–329.

87. Dismukes WE. Introduction to antifungal drugs. *Clin Infect Dis* 2000;30:653–657.

88. Sobel JD. Practice guidelines for the treatment of fungal infections. *Clin Infect Dis* 2000;30:652–657.

89. Branch RA. Prevention of amphotericin B-induced renal impairment. *Arch Intern Med* 1988;148:2389–2394.

90. Hiemenz JW, Walsh TJ. Lipid formulations of amphotericin B: recent progress and future directions. *Clin Infect Dis* 1996;22[Suppl 2]:S133–S144.

91. Mills W, Chopra R, Linch DC, et al. Liposomal amphotericin B in the treatment of fungal infections in neutropenic patients: a single-centre experience of 133 episodes in 116 patients. *Br J Haemat* 1994;86:754–760.

92. Sharkey PK, Graybill JR, Johnson ES, et al. Amphotericin B lipid complex compared with amphotericin B in the treatment of cryptococcal meningitis in patients with AIDS. *Clin Infect Dis* 1996;22:315–321.

93. Walsh TJ, Finberg TW, Arndt C, et al. Liposomal amphotericin B for empirical therapy in patients with persistent fever and neutropenia. *N Engl J Med* 1999;340:764–771.

94. Bennett JE. Flucytosine. *Ann Intern Med* 1977;86:319–322.

95. Maetens J, Raad I, Sable CA, et al. Multicenter, noncomparative study to evaluate safety and efficacy of caspofungin (CAS) in adults with invasive aspergillosis (IA) refractory (R) or intolerant (I) to amphotericin B (AMB), ABM lipid formulations (lipid AMB), or azoles. In: *Proceedings and abstracts of the 40th Interscience Conference on Antimicrobial Agents and Chemotherapy; Sept 17–20, 2000; Toronto.* Abstract:1103.

96. Rex JH, Bennett JE, Sugar AM, et al. A randomized trial comparing fluconazole with amphotericin B for the treatment of candidemia in patients without neutropenia. *N Engl J Med* 1994;331:1325–1330.

97. Nguyen MH, Peacock JE, Tanner DC, et al. Therapeutic approaches in patients with candidemia. *Arch Intern Med* 1995;155:2429–2435.

98. Annaissie EJ, Darouiche RO, Abi-Said D, et al. Management of invasive candidal infections: results of a prospective, randomized, multicenter study of fluconazole versus amphotericin B and review of the literature. *Clin Infect Dis* 1996;23:964–972.

99. Saag MS, Powderly WG, Cloud GA, et al. Comparison of amphotericin B with fluconazole in the treatment of acute AIDS-associated cryptococcal meningitis. *N Engl J Med* 1992;326:83–89.

100. Powderly WG, SMS, Cloud GA, et al. A controlled trial of fluconazole or amphotericin B to prevent relapse of cryptococcal meningitis in patients with the acquired immunodeficiency syndrome. *N Engl J Med* 1992;326:793–798.

101. Rex JH, Walsh TJ, Sobel JD, et al. Practice guidelines for treatment of candidiasis. *Clin Infect Dis* 2000;30:662–678.

102. Goodman JL, Winston DJ, Greenfield RA, et al. A controlled trial of fluconazole to prevent fungal infections in patients undergoing bone marrow transplantation. *N Engl J Med* 1992;326:845–851.

103. Gubbins PO, Bowman JL, Penzak SR. Antifungal prophylaxis to prevent invasive mycoses among bone marrow transplantation recipients. *Pharmacotherapy* 1998;18:549–564.

104. Dismukes WE, Bradsher Jr RW, Cloud GC, et al., NIAID and the Mycoses Study Group. Itraconazole therapy for blastomycosis and histoplasmosis. *Am J Med* 1992;93:489–497.

105. Jennings TS, Hardin TC. Treatment of aspergillosis with itraconazole. *Ann Pharm* 1993; 27:1206–1211.

106. Whitley RJ, Gnann JW Jr. Acyclovir: a decade later. *N Engl J Med* 1992;327:782–789.

107. Skoldenberg B, Forsgren M, Alestig K, et al. Acyclovir versus vidarabine in herpes simplex encephalitis. *Lancet* 1984;2:707–711.

108. Whitley R, Arvin A, Prober C, et al. A controlled trial comparing vidarabine with acyclovir in neonatal herpes simplex virus infection. *N Engl J Med* 1991;324:444–449.

109. Balfour HH Jr, Bean B, Laskin OL, et al. Acyclovir halts progression of herpes zoster in immunocompromised patients. *N Engl J Med* 1983;308:1448–1453.

110. Nyerges G, Meszner Z, Gyarmati E, et al. Acyclovir prevents dissemination of varicella in immunocompromised children. *J Infect Dis* 1988; 157:309–313.

111. Crumpacker CS. Ganciclovir. *N Engl J Med* 1996;335:721–729.

112. Emanuel D, Cunningham I, Jules-Elysee K, et al. Cytomegalovirus pneumonia after bone marrow transplantation successfully treated with the combination of ganciclovir and high-dose intravenous immune globulin. *Ann Intern Med* 1988;109:777–782.

113. Chrisp P, Clissold SP. Foscarnet. A review of its antiviral activity, pharmacokinetic properties and therapeutic use in immunocompromised patients with cytomegalovirus retinitis. *Drugs* 1991;41:104–129.

114. Hardy WD. Foscarnet treatment of acyclovir-resistant herpes simplex virus infection in patients with acquired immunodeficiency syndrome: preliminary results of a controlled, randomized, regimen-comparative trial. *Am J Med* 1992;92[Suppl 2A]:30S–35S.

115. Hitchcock MJ, Jaffe HS, Martin MC, et al. Cidofovir, a new agent with potent anti-herpesvirus activity. *Antiviral Chem and Chemother* 1996;7:115–127.

116. Smith DW, Frankel LR, Mathers LH, et al. A controlled trial of aerosolized ribavirin in infants receiving mechanical ventilation for severe respiratory syncytial virus infection. *N Engl J Med* 1991;325:24–29.

117. McCormick JB, King JJ, Webb PA, et al. Lassa fever: effective therapy with ribavirin. *N Engl J Med* 1986;314:20–26.

118. Huggins JW, Hsiang CM, Cosgriff TM, et al. Prospective, double-blind, concurrent, placebo-controlled clinical trial of intravenous ribavirin therapy of hemorrhagic fever with renal syndrome. *J Infect Dis* 1991;164:1119–1127.

119. Duchin JS, Koster F, Peters CJ, et al. Hantavirus pulmonary syndrome: clinical description of disease caused by a newly recognized hemorrhagic fever virus in the southwestern United States. *N Engl J Med* 1994;330:949–955.

120. Couch RB. Prevention and treatment of influenza. *N Engl J Med* 2000;343:1778–1785.

121. Hayden FG, Atmar RL, Schilling M, et al. Use of the selective oral neuraminidase inhibitor oseltamivir to prevent influenza. *N Engl J Med* 1999;341:1336–1343.

122. Nicholson KG, Aoki FY, Osterhaus ME, et al. Efficacy and safety of oseltamivir in treatment of acute influenza: a randomised controlled trial. *Lancet* 2000;355:1845–1850.

123. Korenman B, Baker J, Waggoner JE, et al. Long-term remission of chronic hepatitis B after alpha-interferon therapy. *Ann Intern Med* 1991;114:629–634.

124. McHutchison JG, Gordon SC, Schiff ER, et al. Interferon alfa-2b alone or in combination with ribavirin as initial treatment for chronic hepatitis C. *N Engl J Med* 1998;339:1485–1492.

125. Hughes WT, Armstrong D, Bodey GP, et al. Guidelines for use of antimicrobial agents in neutropenic patients with unexplained fever. *J Infect Dis* 1990;161:381–396.

126. Pizzo PA. Management of fever in patients with cancer and treatment-induced neutropenia. *N Engl J Med* 1993;328:1323–1332.

127. Maschmeyer G. Interventional antimicrobial therapy in febrile neutropenic patients. *Diag Microbiol Infect Dis* 1999;34:205–212.

128. Wade JC. Antibiotic therapy for the febrile granulocytopenic cancer patient: combination therapy vs. monotherapy. *Rev Infect Dis* 1989;11(S7):S1572–S1581.

129. Sanders JW, Powe NR, Moore RD. Ceftazidime monotherapy for empiric treatment of febrile neutropenic patients: a meta-analysis. *J Infect Dis* 1991;164:907–916.

130. Yamamura D, Gucalp R, Carlisle P, et al. Open randomized study of cefepime versus piperacillin-gentamicin for treatment of febrile neutropenic cancer patients. *Antimicrob Agents Chemother* 1997;41:1704–1708.

131. Winston DJ, Ho WG, Bruckner DA, et al. Beta-lactam antibiotic therapy in febrile granulocytopenic patients. *Ann Intern Med* 1991;115:849–859.

132. Karp JE, Dick JD, Angelopulos C, et al. Empiric use of vancomycin during prolonged treatment-induced granulocytopenia. *Am J Med* 1986;81:237–242.

133. Rubin M, Hathorn JW, Marshall D, et al. gram-positive infections and the use of vancomycin in 550 episodes of fever and neutropenia. *Ann Intern Med* 1988;108:30–35.

134. European Organization for Research and Treatment of Cancer (EORTC) International Antimicrobial Therapy Cooperative Group and the National Cancer Institute of Canada-Clinical Trials Group. Vancomycin added to empirical combination antibiotic therapy for fever in granulocytopenic cancer patients. *J Infect Dis* 1991;163:951–958.

135. Richard P, Del Valle GA, Moreau P, et al. Viridans streptococcal bacteraemia in patients with neutropenia. *Lancet* 1995;345:1607–1609.

136. Pizzo PA, Robichaud KJ, Gill FA, et al. Empiric antibiotic and antifungal therapy for cancer patients with prolonged fever and granulocytopenia. *Am J Med* 1982;72:101–111.

137. EORTC International Antimicrobial Therapy Cooperative Group. Empiric antifungal therapy in febrile granulocytopenic patients. *Am J Med* 1989;86:668–672.

138. Lowry RW, Zoghbi WA, Baker WB, et al. Clinical impact of transesophageal echocardiography in the diagnosis and management of infective endocarditis. *Am J Cardiol* 1994;73:1089–1091.

139. Daniel WG, Mugge A, Martin RP, et al. Improvement in the diagnosis of abscesses associated with endocarditis by transesophageal echocardiography. *N Engl J Med* 1991;324:795–800.

140. Bogers AJ, van Vreeswijk H, Verbaan CJ, et al. Early surgery for active infective endocarditis improves early and late results. *Thorac Cardiovasc Surg* 1991;39:284–288.

141. Larbalestier RI, Kinchla NM, Aranki SF, et al. Acute bacterial endocarditis. Optimizing surgical results. *Circulation* 1992;86[5 Suppl]:1168–1174.

142. Kluger DM, Maki DG. A meta-analysis of risk factors for catheter-related BSI with percutaneously-inserted central venous catheters (abst). In: *Program and Abstracts of the Fourth Decennial International*

Conference on Nosocomial and Healthcare-Associated Infections, March 5–8, 2000; Atlanta.

143. Mermel LA, Farr BM, Sheretz RJ, et al. Guidelines for the management of intravascular catheter-related infections. *J Intraven Nurs* 2001;24:180–205.

144. Rex JH, Bennett JE, Sugar AM, et al. Intravascular catheter exchange and duration of candidemia. *Clin Infect Dis* 1995;21:994–996.

145. Rosen AB, Fowler VG Jr, Corey GR, et al. Cost-effectiveness of transesophageal echocardiography to determine the duration of therapy for intravascular catheter-associated *Staphylococcus aureus* bacteremia. *Ann Intern Med* 1999;130:810–820.

146. Strinden WD, Helgerson RB, Maki DG. Candida sepsis thrombosis of the great veins associated with central catheters. Clinical features and management. *Ann Surg* 1985;202:653–658.

147. Gleason PP, Meehan TP, Fine JM, et al. Association between initial antimicrobial therapy and medical outcomes for hospitalized elderly patients with pneumonia. *Arch Intern Med* 1999;159:2562–2572.

148. Fink MP, Snydman DR, Niederman MS, et al. Treatment of severe pneumonia in hospitalized patients: results of a multicenter, randomized, double-blind trial comparing intravenous ciprofloxacin with imipenem-cilastatin. *Antimicrob Agents Chemother* 1994;547:57.

149. Wynne JW, Olsen GN. Acute histoplasmosis presenting as the adult respiratory distress syndrome. *Chest* 1974;66:158–161.

150. Deresinski SC, Stevens DA. Coccidioidomycosis in compromised hosts: experience at Stanford University Hospital. *Medicine (Baltimore)* 1975;54:377–395.

151. Meyer KC, McManus EJ, Maki DG. Overwhelming pulmonary blastomycosis associated with the adult respiratory distress syndrome. *N Engl J Med* 1993;329:1231–1236.

152. Blitzer A, Lawson W. Fungal infections of the nose and paranasal sinuses, part 1. *Otolaryngol Clin North Am* 1993;26:1007–1035.

153. George DL, Falk PS, Meduri GU, et al. Nosocomial sinusitis in patients in the medical intensive care unit: a prospective epidemiological study. *Clin Infect Dis* 1998;27:463–470.

154. Kountakis SE, Burke L, Rafie J-J, et al. Sinusitis in the intensive care unit patient. *Otolaryngol Head Neck Surg* 1997;117:362–366.

155. Schuchat A, Robinson K, Wenger JD, et al. Bacterial meningitis in the United States in 1995. *N Engl J Med* 1997;337:970–976.

156. Lebel MH, Hoyt MJ, McCracken GH Jr. Comparative efficacy of ceftriaxone and cefuroxine for treatment of bacterial meningitis. *J Pediatr* 1989;114:1049–1054.

157. Schaad UB, Suter S, Gianella-Borradori A, et al. A comparison of ceftriaxone and cefuroxime for the treatment of bacterial meningitis in children. *N Engl J Med* 1990;322:141–147.

158. Whitley RJ, Soon S-J, Lineman C Jr, et al. Herpes simplex encephalitis: clinical assessment. *JAMA* 1982;247:317–320.

159. Aurelius E, Johansson B, Stoltenberg B, et al. Rapid diagnosis of herpes simplex encephalitis by nested polymerase chain reaction assay of cerebrospinal fluid. *Lancet* 1991;337:189–192.

160. Sinanan MN. Acute cholangitis. *Infect Dis Clin North Am* 1992; 6:571–599.

161. Bhuva M, Ganger D, Jensen D. Spontaneous bacterial peritonitis: an update on evaluation, management, and prevention. *Am J Med* 1994;97:169–175.

162. Felisart J, Rimola A, Arroyo V, et al. Cefotaxime is more effective than is ampicillin-tobramycin in cirrhotics with severe infections. *Hepatology* 1985;5:457–462.

163. Bohnen JMA, Solomkin JS, Dellinger EP, et al. Guidelines for clinical care: anti-infective agents for intra-abdominal infection. A Surgical Infection Society Policy Statement. *Arch Surg* 1992;127:83–89.

164. McClean KL, Sheehan GJ, Harding GKM. Intraabdominal infection: a review. *Clin Infect Dis* 1994;19:100–116.

165. Solomkin JS, Dellinger EP, Christou NY, et al. Results of a multicenter trial comparing imipenem/cilastatin to tobramycin/clindamycin for intra-abdominal infections. *Ann Surg* 1990;212:581–591.

166. Rostein OD, Pruett TL, Simons RL. Microbiologic features and treatment of persistent peritonitis in patients in the intensive care unit. *Can J Surg* 1986;29:247–250.

167. Maki DG, Agger WA. Enterococcal bacteremia: clinical features,

the risk of endocarditis, and management. *Medicine (Baltimore)* 1988;67:248–269.

168. Solomkin JS, Flohr A, Simmons RL. *Candida* infections in surgical patients: dose requirements and toxicity of amphotericin B. *Ann Surg* 1982;195:177–185.

169. Calandra T, Bille J, Schneider R, et al. Clinical significance of *Candida* isolated from peritoneum in surgical patients. *Lancet* 1989;2:1437–1440.

170. Kalliafas S, Ziegler DW, Flancbaum L, et al. Acute acalculous cholecystitis: incidence, risk factors, diagnosis, and outcome. *Am Surg* 1998; 64:471–475.

171. Shaked A, Shinar E, Freund H. Neutropenic typhlitis: a plea for conservatism. *Dis Colon Rectum* 1983;26:351–352.

172. Alt B, Glass NR, Sallinger H. Neutropenic enterocolitis in adults: review of the literature and assessment of surgical intervention. *Am J Surg* 1985;149:405–408.

173. Duff P. Antibiotic selection in obstetric patients. *Infect Dis Clin North Am* 1997;11:1–12.

174. Bryan CS, Reynolds DK. Hospital-acquired bacteremic urinary tract infection: epidemiology and outcome. *J Urol* 1984;132:494–498.

175. Quintiliani R, Klimek J, Cunha BA, et al. Bacteremia after manipulation of the urinary tract: the importance of pre-existing urinary tract disease and compromised host defenses. *Postgrad Med J* 1978;54:668–671.

176. Stamm WE, Hooton TM. Management of urinary tract infections in adults. *N Engl J Med* 1993;329:1328–1334.

177. Barnes SG, Sattler FR, Ballard JO. Perirectal infections in acute leukemia: improved survival after incision and debridement. *Ann Intern Med* 1984;100:515–518.

178. Ahrenholz DH. Necrotizing soft-tissue infections. *Surg Clin North Am* 1988;68:199–214.

179. Bilton BD, Zibari BG, McMillan RW, et al. Aggressive surgical management of necrotizing fasciitis serves to decrease mortality: a retrospective study. *Am Surg* 1998;64:397–400.

180. Cone LA, Woodard DR, Schlievert PM, et al. Clinical and bacteriologic observations of a toxic shock-like syndrome due to *Streptococcus pyogenes*. *N Engl J Med* 1987;317:146–149.

181. Stevens DL. Streptococcal toxic-shock syndrome: spectrum of disease, pathogenesis, and new concepts in treatment. *Emerg Infect Dis* 1995;1:69–78.

182. Stamenkovic I, Lew PD. Early recognition of potentially fatal necrotizing fasciitis: use of frozen-section biopsy. *N Engl Med* 1984; 310:1689.

183. Riseman JA, Zamboni WA, Curtis A, et al. Hyperbaric oxygen therapy for necrotizing fasciitis reduces mortality and the need for debridements. *Surgery* 1990;10:847–850.

184. Dryden MS, Gabb RJE, Wright SK. Empirical treatment of severe acute community-acquired gastroenteritis with ciprofloxacin. *Clin Infect Dis* 1996;22:1019–1025.

185. Doer GV, Coughlin RT, Wu L. Laboratory diagnosis of *Clostridium difficile*-associated gastrointestinal disease: comparison of a monoclonal antibody enzyme immunoassay for toxins A and B with a monoclonal antibody enzyme immunoassay for toxin A only and two cytotoxicity assays. *J Clin Microbiol* 1992;30:2042–2046.

186. Teasley DG, Gerding DN, Olson MM, et al. Prospective randomized trial of metronidazole versus vancomycin for *Clostridium difficile*-associated diarrhoea and colitis. *Lancet* 1983;2:1043–1046.

187. Medich DS, Lee KKW, Simmons RL, et al. Laparotomy for fulminant *Pseudomembranous colitis*. *Arch Surg* 1992;127:847–853.

188. Chesney PJ. Clinical aspects and spectrum of illness of toxic shock syndrome. Overview. *Rev Infect Dis* 1989;11[Suppl 1]:S1–S7.

189. Reingold AL, Hargrett NT, Dann BB, et al. Nonmenstrual toxic shock syndrome. A review of 130 cases. *Ann Intern Med* 1982;96:871–874.

190. Stevens DL, Bryant AE, Hackett AP. Antibiotic effects on bacterial viability, toxin production and host response. *Clin Infect Dis* 1995;20:S1564–S1567.

191. Kaul R, McGeer A, Norrby-Teglund A, et al. Intravenous immunoglobulin therapy for streptococcal toxic shock syndrome: a comparative observational study. *Clin Infect Dis* 1999;28:800–807.

192. Tsai YL, Krogstad DJ. The resurgence of malaria. In: Scheld WM, Craig WA, Hughes JM, eds. *Emerging infections 2*. Washington, DC: American Society for Microbiology 1998:195–212.

193. Palmer CJ, Lindo JF, Klaskala WI, et al. Evaluation of the OptiMAL test for rapid diagnosis of *Plasmodium vivax* and *Plasmodium falciparum* malaria. *J Clin Microbiol* 1998;36:203–206.

194. Anonymous. Drugs for parasitic infections. *Med Lett Drugs Ther* 1998;40:1–12.

195. Centers for Disease Control. Availability and use of parenteral quinidine gluconate for severe or complicated malaria. *MMWR* 2000;49:1138–1140.

196. Miller KD, Greenberg AE, Campbell CC. Treatment of severe malaria in the United States with a continuous infusion of quinidine gluconate and exchange transfusion. *N Engl J Med* 1989;321:65–70.

197. Warrell DA, Looareesuwan S, Warrell MJ, et al. Dexamethasone proves deleterious in cerebral malaria: a double-blind clinical trial in 100 comatose patients. *N Engl J Med* 1982;306:313–318.

198. Gorenflot A, Moubri K, Precigout E, et al. Human babesiosis. *Ann Trop Med Parasitol* 1998;92:489–501.

199. Krause PJ, et al. Atovaquone and azithromycin for the treatment of babesiosis. *N Engl J Med* 2000;16:343:1454–1458.

200. Saah AJ. Introduction to rickettsioses and ehrlichioses. In: Mandell GL, Bennett JE, Dolin R, eds. *Principles and practice of infectious diseases*, 5th ed. New York: Churchill Livingstone, 2000:2033–2035.

201. Fritz CL, Glaser CA. Ehrlichiosis. *Emerg Infect Dis* 1998;12:123–136.

202. Anderson BE, Summer JW, Dawson JE, et al. Detection of the etiologic agent of human ehrlichiosis by polymerase chain reaction. *J Clin Microbiol* 1992;30:775–780.

203. Centers for Disease Control. Update: Universal Precautions for prevention of transmission of human immunodeficiency virus, hepatitis B virus, and other blood-borne pathogens in healthcare settings. *MMWR* 1988;37:377–388.

204. U.S. Department of Labor. Occupational safety and health administration: occupational exposure to blood-borne pathogens: final rule. *Federal Register* 1991;58:5210–5250.

205. McCormick RD, Ircink FG, Maki DG. The epidemiology of sharps injuries in a university hospital. Part III. The impact of 20 years of a multi-faceted control program (abst). In: *Program and Abstracts of the Fourth Decennial International Conference on Nosocomial and Healthcare-Associated Infections*; March 5–8, 2000; Atlanta.

206. Wheeling MSN. Four pediatric deaths from community-acquired methicillin-resistant *Staphylococcus aureus*—Minnesota and North Dakota, 1997–1999. *MMWR* 1999;48(32):707–710.

207. Ibrahim EH, Sherman G, Ward S, et al. The influence of inadequate antimicrobial treatment of bloodstream infections on patient outcomes in the ICU setting. *Chest* 2000;118:146–155.

208. Safdar N, Maki DG. The commonality of risk factors for nosocomial colonization/infection with antimicrobial-resistant *Staphylococcus aureus*, *Enterococcus*, gram-negative bacilli, *Clostridium difficile* and *Candida*. *Ann Intern Med* 2001 (*in press*).

209. Astiz ME, Rackow EC. Septic shock. *Lancet* 1998;351:1501–1505.

210. Wheeler AP, Bernard GR. Treating patients with severe sepsis. *N Engl J Med* 1999;340:207–214.

211. Marini JJ, Wright L. General supportive care of the critically ill patient. *Semin Respir Crit Care Med* 1997;18:3–17.

212. Rivers E, Nguyen B, Havstad S, et al. Early goal-directed therapy in the treatment of severe sepsis and septic shock. *N Engl J Med* 2001;345:1359–1367.

213. Connors AF Jr., McCaffree DR, Gray BA. Evaluation of right heart catheterization in the critically ill patient without acute myocardial infarction. *N Engl J Med* 1983;308:263–267.

214. Shoemaker WC, Appel PL, Kram HB et al. Prospective trial of supranormal values of survivors as therapeutic goals in high-risk surgical patients. *Chest* 1988;94:1176–1186.

215. Tuchschmidt J, Fried J, Astiz M, et al. Elevation of cardiac output and oxygen delivery improves outcome in septic shock. *Chest* 1992;102:216–220.

216. Connors AF, Speroff T, Dawson NV, et al. The effectiveness of right heart catheterization in the initial care of critically ill patients. *JAMA* 1996;276:889–897.

217. Sandham JD, Hull RD, Brant R. A randomized controlled trial of pulmonary artery catheter use in 1994 high-risk geriatric surgical patients. In: *Proceedings and Abstracts of the 97th International Conference of the American Thoracic Society*; May 18–23, 2001; San Francisco. Abstract:16.

218. Schierhout G, Roberts I. Fluid resuscitation with colloid or crystalloid solutions in critically ill patients: a systematic review of randomised trials. *BMJ* 1998;316:961–964.

219. Cochrane Injuries Group Albumin Reviewers. Human albumin administration in critically ill patients: systematic review of randomised controlled trials. *BMJ* 1998;317:235–240.

220. Choi PT, Yip G, Quinonez LG, et al. Crystalloid vs. colloids in fluid resuscitation: a systematic review. *Crit Care Med* 1999;27:200–210.

221. Sort P, Navasa M, Arroyo V, et al. Effect of intravenous albumin on renal impairment and mortality in patients with cirrhosis and spontaneous bacterial peritonitis. *N Engl J Med* 1999;341:403–409.

222. Packman MI, Rackow EC. Optimum left heart filling pressure during fluid resuscitation of patients with hypovolemic and septic shock. *Crit Care Med* 1983;11:165–169.

223. Rackow EC, Kaufman BS, Falk JL, et al. Hemodynamic response to fluid repletion in patients with septic shock: evidence for early depression of cardiac performance. *Circ Shock* 1987;22:11–22.

224. Nataanson C, Hoffman WD, Suffredini AF, et al. Selected treatment strategies for septic shock based on proposed mechanisms of pathogenesis. *Ann Intern Med* 1994;120:771–783.

225. Rudis MI, Basha MA, Zarowitz BJ. Is it time to reposition vasopressors and inotropes in sepsis? *Crit Care Med* 1996;24:525–537.

226. Kumar A, Parrillo JE. Shock: classification, pathophysiology and approach to management. In: Parrillo JE, Bone RC, eds. *Critical care medicine. Principles of diagnosis and management*. St. Louis: Mosby-Year Book, 1995:291–339; 2nd ed, 2001 (*in press*).

227. Gattinoni L, Brazzi L, Pelosi P, et al. A trial of goal-oriented hemodynamic therapy in critically ill patients. *N Engl J Med* 1995;333:1025–1032.

228. Gutierrez G, Palizas F, Doglio G, et al. Gastric intramucosal pH as a therapeutic index of tissue oxygenation in critically ill patients. *Lancet* 1992;339:195–199.

229. Friedman G, Berlot G, Kahn RJ, et al. Combined measurements of blood lactate concentrations and gastric intramucosal pH in patients with severe sepsis. *Crit Care Med* 1995;23:1184–1193.

230. Friedman G, Silva E, Vincent J-L. Has the mortality of septic shock changed in time? *Crit Care Med* 1998;26:2078–2086.

231. Pinsky MR, Vincent J-L, Deviere J, et al. Serum cytokine levels in human septic shock. *Chest* 1993;103:565–575.

232. Veterans Administration Systemic Sepsis Cooperative Study Group. Effect of high-dose glucocorticoid therapy on mortality in patients with clinical signs of systemic sepsis. *N Engl J Med* 1987;317:659–665.

233. Bone RC, Fisher CJ Jr., Clemmer TP, et al. A controlled clinical trial of high-dose methylprednisolone in the treatment of severe sepsis and septic shock. *N Engl J Med* 1987;317:653–658.

234. Lebel MH, Freij BJ, Syrogiannopoulos GA, et al. Dexamethasone therapy for bacterial meningitis: results of two double-blind, placebo-controlled trials. *N Engl J Med* 1988;319:964–971.

235. Odio CM, Faingezicht I, Paris M, et al. The beneficial effects of early dexamethasone administration in infants and children with bacterial meningitis. *N Engl J Med* 1991;324:1525–1531.

236. Schaad UB, Lips U, Gnehm HE, et al. for the Swiss Meningitis Study Group. Dexamethasone therapy for bacterial meningitis in children. *Lancet* 1993;342:457–461.

237. Girgis NI, Farid Z, Kilpatrick ME, et al. Dexamethasone for the treatment of children and adults with bacterial meningitis. *Rev Infect Dis* 1990;12:963–964.

238. Girgis NI, Farid Z, Kilpatrick ME, et al. Dexamethasone adjunctive treatment for tuberculous meningitis. *Pediatr Infect Dis J* 1991;10:179–183.

239. O'Toole RD, Thornton GF, Mukjerjee MK, et al. Dexamethasone in tuberculous meningitis: relationship of cerebrospinal fluid effects to therapeutic efficacy. *Ann Intern Med* 1969;70:39–48.

240. Hoffman SL, Punjabi NH, Kumala S, et al. Reduction of mortality

in chloramphenicol-treated severe typhoid fever by high-dose dexamethasone. *N Engl J Med* 1984;310:82–88.

241. MacFadden DK, Edelson JD, Hyland RH, et al. Corticosteroids as adjunctive therapy in treatment of *Pneumocystis carinii* pneumonia in patients with acquired immunodeficiency syndrome. *Lancet* 1987;1:1477–1479.

242. Gagnon S, Boota AM, Fischl MA, et al. Corticosteroids as adjunctive therapy for severe *Pneumocystis carinii* pneumonia in the acquired immunodeficiency syndrome. *N Engl J Med* 1990;323:1444–1450.

243. Wajchenberg B, Leme CE, Tambascia M, et al. The adrenal response to exogenous adrenocorticotropin in patients with infections due to *Neisseria meningitidis. J Infect Dis* 1978;138:387–391.

244. Annane D, Sébille V, Troché G, et al. A 3-level prognostic classification in septic shock based on cortisol levels and cortisol response to corticotropin. *JAMA* 2000;283:1038–1045.

245. Bollaert PE, Charpentier C, Levy S, et al. Reversal of late septic shock with supraphysiologic doses of hydrocortisone. *Crit Care Med* 1988;26:645–650.

246. Briegel J, Forst H, Haller M, et al. Stress doses of hydrocortisone reverse hyperdynamic septic shock: a prospective, randomized, double-blind single center study. *Crit Care Med* 1999;27:723–732.

247. Annane D. Effects of the combination of hydrocortisone (HC)-Fludro-Cortisone (FC) on mortality in septic shock [Abstract]. In: *Proceedings of the 30th International and Scientific Symposium of the Society of Critical Care Medicine*, 2001; San Francisco. Abstract:63; *Crit Care Med* 2001 (*in press*).

248. Zeni F, Freeman B, Natanson C. Anti-inflammatory therapies to treat sepsis and septic shock: a reassessment. *Crit Care Med* 1997;25:1095–1100.

249. Ziegler EJ, Fisher CJ Jr, Sprung CL, et al. Treatment of gram-negative bacteremia and septic shock with HA-1A human monoclonal antibody against endotoxin: a randomized, double-blind, placebo-controlled trial. *N Engl J Med* 1991;324:429–436.

250. Baumgartner JD, Glauser MP, McCutchan JA, et al. Prevention of gram-negative shock and death in surgical patients by antibody to endotoxin core glycolipid. *Lancet* 1985;2:59–63.

251. Schedel I, Dreikhausen U, Nentwig B, et al. Treatment of gram-negative septic shock with an immunoglobulin preparation: a prospective, randomized clinical trial. *Crit Care Med* 1991;19:1104–1113.

252. Levi M, Cate HT, van der Poll T, et al. Pathogenesis of disseminated intravascular coagulation in sepsis. *JAMA* 1993;270:975–979.

253. Bernard GR, Vincent JL, Laterre P-F, et al. Efficacy and safety of recombinant human activated protein C for severe sepsis. *N Engl J Med* 2001;344:699–709.

254. Esmon C. The protein C pathway. *Crit Care Med* 2000;28 [Suppl]:S44–S48.

255. Strauss RG. Granulocyte transfusion therapy. *Transfusion Med* 1994;8:1159–1166.

256. Lucas KG. Another look at granulocyte transfusions in neutropenic patients with cancer. *Infect Med* 1996;13:79–92.

257. Lieschke GJ, Burgess AW. Granulocyte colony-stimulating factor and granulocyte-macrophage colony-stimulating factor. *N Engl J Med* 1992;327:28–35.

258. Gabrilove JL, Jakubowski A, Scher H, et al. Effect of granulocyte colony-stimulating factor on neutropenia and associated morbidity due to chemotherapy for transitional cell carcinoma or the urothelium. *N Engl J Med* 1988;318:1414–1422.

259. Advani R, Chao NJ, Horning SJ, et al. Granulocyte-macrophage colony-stimulating factor (GM-CSF) as an adjunct to autologous hemopoietic stem cell transplantation for lymphoma. *Ann Intern Med* 1992;116:183–189.

260. Nelson S, Heyder AM, Stone J, et al. A randomized controlled trial of filgrastim for the treatment of hospitalized patients with multilobar pneumonia. *J Infect Dis* 2001;182:970–973.

261. Nemunaitis J, Meyers JD, Bruckner CD, et al. Phase I trial of recombinant human macrophage colony-stimulating factor in patients with invasive fungal infections. *Blood* 1991;78:907–913.

262. Siber GR, Snydman DR. Use of immune globulins in the prevention and treatment of infections. *Curr Clin Top Infect Dis* 1992;12:208–256.

262a. Van den Barghe G, Woutors P, Weekers F, et al. Intensive insulin therapy in critically ill patients. *N Engl J Med* 2001;345:1368–1377.

263. Cerra RB, Benitez MR, Blackburn GL, et al. Applied nutrition in ICU patients: a consensus statement of the American College of Chest Physicians. *Chest* 1997;111:7769–7778.

264. Hebert PC, Wells G, Blajchman MA, et al. A multicenter, randomized, controlled clinical trial of transfusion requirements in critical care. *N Engl J Med* 1999;340:409–417.

265. Jain M, Schmidt GA. Venous thromboembolism: prevention and prophylaxis. *Semin Respir Crit Care Med* 1997;18:79–90.

266. Cook D. Prevention of stress ulcers and ventilator-associated pneumonia: examining the evidence. *Semin Respir Crit Care Med* 1997;18:91–95.

267. Maki DG, Hecht J. Antiseptic-containing handwashing agents reduce nosocomial infections—a prospective study (abst). In: *Proceedings of the Twenty-second Interscience Conference on Antimicrobial Agents and Chemotherapy*; October 1982; Miami Beach, FL.

268. Massanari RM, Hierholzer WJ. A crossover comparison of antiseptic soaps on nosocomial infection rates in intensive care units. *Am J Infect Control* 1984;12:247–248.

269. Doebbeling BN, Stanley GL, Sheetz CT, et al. Comparative efficacy of alternative-handwashing agents in reducing nosocomial infections in intensive care units. *N Engl J Med* 1992;327:88–93.

270. Pittet D, Hugonnet S, Harbarth S, et al. Effectiveness of a hospital-wide programme to improve compliance with hand hygiene. *Lancet* 2000;356:1307–1312.

271. Garner JS and Hospital Infection Control Practices Advisory Committee. Draft guideline for isolation precautions in hospitals. *Infect Control Hosp Epidemiol* 1996;17:53–80.

272. Maki DG, Tambyah PA. Engineering out the risk of infection with urinary catheters. *Emerg Infect Dis* 2001;7:342–347.

273. Hospital Infection Control Practices Advisory Committee. Guideline for prevention of infection in IV therapy. *Federal Register* 2001 (*in press*).

274. Centers for Disease Control and Prevention. Draft guideline for prevention of nosocomial pneumonia. *Federal Register* 1994;59:4980–5022.

275. Maki DG, Ringer M, Alvarado CJ. Prospective randomized trial of povidone-iodine, alcohol and chlorhexidine for prevention of infection associated with central venous and arterial catheters. *Lancet* 1991;338:339–343.

276. Mimoz O, Pieroni L, Lawrence C, et al. Prospective, randomized trial of two antiseptic solutions for prevention of central venous or arterial catheter colonization and infection in intensive care unit patients. *Crit Care Med* 1996;24:1818–1823.

277. Maki DG, Knasinski V, Narans LL, et al. A randomized trial of a novel 1% chlorhexidine-75% alcohol tincture vs. 10% povidone-iodine for cutaneous disinfection with vascular catheters. In: *Eleventh Annual Proceedings and Abstracts of the Eleventh Annual Scientific Meeting of the Society for Healthcare Epidemiology of America*; April 1–3, 2001; Toronto. Abstract:142.

278. Maki DG, Stolz SM, Wheeler S, et al. Prevention of central venous catheter-related bloodstream infection by use of an antiseptic-impregnated catheter. A randomized controlled trial. *Ann Intern Med* 1997;127:257–266.

279. Veenstra DL, Saint S, Saha S, et al. Efficacy of antiseptic-impregnated central venous catheters in preventing catheter-related bloodstream infection: a meta-analysis. *JAMA* 1999;281(3):261–267.

280. Darouiche RO, Raad II, Heard SO, et al. A comparison of two antimicrobial-impregnated central venous catheters. *N Engl J Med* 1999;340:1–8.

281. Maki DG, Knasinski V, Halvorson K, et al. A novel silver hydrogel-impregnated indwelling urinary catheter reduces CAUTIs: a prospective double blind trial (abst). *Infect Control Hosp Epidemiol* 1998;19:682.

282. Bologna RA, Tu LM, Polansky M, et al. Hydrogel/silver ion-coated urinary catheter reduces nosocomial urinary tract infection rates in

intensive care unit patients: a multicenter study. *Urology* 1999;54:982–987.

283. Mahul P, Auboyer C, Jospe R, et al. Prevention of nosocomial pneumonia in intubated patients: respective role of mechanical subglottic secretion drainage and stress ulcer prophylaxis. *Intensive Care Med* 1992;18:20–25.

284. Vallés J, Artigas A, Rello J, et al. Continuous aspiration of subglottic secretions in preventing ventilator-associated pneumonia. *Ann Intern Med* 1995;122:179–186.

285. Beale RJ, Bryg DJ, Bihari DJ. Immunonutrition in the critically ill: a systematic review of clinical outcome. *Crit Care Med* 1999;27:2799–2805.

286. Nauseef WM, Maki DG. A study of the value of simple protective isolation in patients with granulocytopenia. *N Engl J Med* 1981;304:448–453.

287. Klein BS, Perloff WH, Maki DG. Reduction of nosocomial infection during pediatric intensive care by protective isolation. *N Engl J Med* 1989;3210:1714–1721.

288. Johnson S, Gerding DN, Olson MM, et al. Prospective, controlled study of vinyl glove use to interrupt *Clostridium difficile* nosocomial transmission. *Am J Med* 1990:88:137–140.

289. Maki DG, Zilz MA, McCormick R. The effectiveness of using preemptive barrier precautions routinely (protective isolation) in all high-risk patients to prevent nosocomial infection with resistant organisms, especially MRSA, VRE and *C. difficile* (abst). In: *Proceedings and Abstracts of the Thirty-fourth Annual Meeting of the Infectious Disease Society of America*; September 1996; New Orleans. *Clin Infect Dis* 1996;23:43(abst).

290. Ostrowsky BE, Trick WE, Sohn AH, et al. Control of vancomycin-resistant *Enterococcus* in health care facilities in a region. *N Engl J Med* 2001;344:1427–1433.

291. Rhame FS, Streifel AJ, Kersey JH Jr, et al. Extrinsic risk factors for pneumonia in the patient at high risk of infection. *Am J Med* 1984;76[Suppl 5A]:42–52.

292. Sherertz RH, Belani A, Kramer BS, et al. Impact of air filtration on nosocomial *Aspergillus* infections. *Am J Med* 1987;83:709–718.

293. Baker CJ, Melish ME, Hall RT, et al. Intravenous immune globulin for the prevention of nosocomial infection in low–birth-weight neonates. *N Engl J Med* 1992;327:213–219.

294. Silber GR. Immune globulin to prevent nosocomial infections. *N Engl J Med* 1992;327:269–271.

295. The Intravenous Immunoglobulin Collaborative Study Group. Prophylactic intravenous administration of standard immune globulin as compared with core-lipopolysaccharide immune globulin in patients at high risk of postsurgical infection. *N Engl J Med* 1993;327:234–240.

296. Douzinas EE, Pitaridis MT, Louris G, et al. Prevention of infection in multiple trauma patients by high-dose intravenous immunoglobulins. *Crit Care Med* 2000;28:8–15.

297. Seale L, Jones CJ, Kathpalia S, et al. Prevention of herpes virus infections in renal allograft recipients by low-dose oral acyclovir. *JAMA* 1985;254:3435–3438.

298. Saral R, Ambinder RF, Burns WH, et al. Acyclovir prophylaxis against herpes simplex virus infection in patients with leukemia. *Ann Intern Med* 1983;99:773–776.

299. Winston DJ, Ho WG, Bartoni K, et al. Ganciclovir prophylaxis of cytomegalovirus infection and disease in allogeneic bone marrow transplant recipients: results of a placebo-controlled, double-blind trial. *Ann Intern Med* 1993;118:179–184.

299. Deleted in page proofs.

300. Hibberd PL, Tolkoff-Rubin NE, Conti D, et al. Preemptive ganciclovir therapy for preventing cytomegalovirus disease in cytomegalovirus antibody-positive renal transplant recipients: a randomized controlled trial. *Ann Intern Med* 1995;123:18–26.

51

INFECTIONS IN THE IMMUNOCOMPROMISED

ANAND KUMAR
BALA HOTA

KEY WORDS

- Infection
- Immunosuppressed
- Immunocompromised
- Opportunistic infections
- Neutropenia
- Organ transplant
- Bone marrow transplant
- AIDS

INTRODUCTION

Rapid medical, surgical, and pharmaceutical advances in the last 30 years have resulted in a burgeoning population of patients with suppressed immune function. The incidence of infections in this group has risen rapidly as their numbers grow and survival increases. Advances that predispose to such infections include the following:

1. Immunosuppressive chemotherapy of malignancies and various autoimmune diseases
2. Aggressive organ transplantation efforts with concomitant, long-term immunosuppressive drug therapy
3. Supportive therapies such as total parenteral nutrition, dialysis, and advanced intensive care unit (ICU) support, which allow patients with chronic diseases or immune dysfunction to survive for extended periods

The last 20 years also have seen a remarkable increase in those with acquired immunodeficiency resulting from infection with the human immunodeficiency virus (HIV). With advances in medical management of this disease in the United States, longevity of patients continues to increase as disease severity diminishes. Despite a marked decrease in the incidence of opportunistic infections in this population over the last decade as a result of improved antiretroviral therapy, the total number of opportunistic infections in this group remains substantial.

For clinicians and their patients, recognition of the immunocompromised state is imperative. Infections in such patients can involve unusual organisms requiring atypical pharmacologic therapy. In addition to increased susceptibility to common community-acquired and nosocomial pathogens, immunocompromised patients are vulnerable to opportunistic pathogens

(e.g., *Cryptococcus, Candida,* and *Aspergillus* species) and to reactivation of endogenous but latent organisms (e.g., herpesviruses, *Toxoplasma gondii, Pneumocystis carinii*) (Table 1). Infection with these pathogens can present with minimal signs and symptoms or with atypical features in unusual locations. This can considerably delay the diagnosis if the presence of immunocompromise is not appreciated. Although the risk of mortality is high in these patients because of the underlying immunosuppression and the unusual nature of the organisms that may be involved, outcome can be optimized by early diagnosis and aggressive, specific pharmacotherapy.

HOST DEFENSES TO INFECTION

A basic understanding of the elements of host defense and immunity is required to appreciate the probable etiologic basis of infection in any given immunocompromised patient. Both specific (*immune*) and nonspecific (*nonimmune*) host defenses exist. An immunocompromised patient is one in whom any aspect of host defense is deficient. In contrast, immunosuppression occurs when immune defenses are specifically impaired.

Nonspecific defense elements include intact integumentary barriers. Defects of the integument, such as might be seen in burns, severe eczema, or some forms of chemotherapy (cis-platinum leading to gastrointestinal ulceration), effectively denude the body of its primary defense against the normal microbial milieu by both bypassing the anatomic (physical) barriers and also breaching membrane-associated immune defenses. Similarly, invasive intravascular catheters (for infusion, dialysis, or hemodynamic monitoring), intubation, trauma, and operative procedures disrupt the normal barriers to microorganisms. Anatomic defects of host defense typically coexist with concurrent immune deficits because any illness of sufficient severity to result in a major integumentary defect or to necessitate invasive support is likely to be sufficiently severe to result in direct perturbation of immune function.

Other nonspecific elements of host defense include the normal acidity of the stomach; the natural indigenous microbial flora of the skin, mucous membranes, and gut; the physiologic flow of secretions and excretions of various organs; and appropriate

TABLE 1. COMMON CAUSES OF IMMUNOSUPPRESSION AND MAJOR INFECTIONS IN IMMUNOCOMPROMISED PATIENTS

Immunosuppression		Major Infections and Their Causes				
Defect	Cause	Pneumonia	CNS Infection	Mucocutaneous Infection	Disseminated Infection	Septic Shock
Neutropenia	Leukemia Chemotherapy (adriamycin, ARA-C, cyclophosphamide) Total-body radiation Idiopathic drug effect Aplastic anemia	Enteric gram-negative bacilli Pseudomonas aeruginosa Staphylococcus aureus Aspergillus	Enteric gram-negative bacilli Aspergillus spp Mucormycosis spp	HSV VZV	Aspergillus spp Other fungi	Enteric gram-negative bacilli P. aeruginosa Staphylococcus Candida
Cell-mediated	Hodgkin disease Lymphoma Corticosteroid use Chemotherapy (azathioprine, vincristine sulfate, bleomycin sulfate) CMV, EBV, or HIV infection Protein-calorie malnutrition	Pneumocystis carinii Legionella Herpesvirus (CMV, HSV, VZV) Adenovirus Histoplasmosis Coccidiomycosis Cryptococcus neoformans	Cryptococcus neoformans Toxoplasma gondii Listeria monocytogenes	HSV VZV CMV Candida spp	CMV VZV MAI	L. monocytogenes
Humoral	Multiple myeloma Chronic lymphocytic leukemia Chemotherapy (cyclophosphamide, methotrexate, azathioprine) Splenectomy	Streptococcus pneumoniae Hemophilus influenzae Enteric gram-negative bacilli	S. pneumoniae H. influenzae Neisseria meningitidis	—	—	S. pneumoniae H. influenzae N. meningitidis
Complement	Congenital deficiency SLE Multiple myeloma	—	N. meningitidis	—	N. meningitidis Neisseria gonorrhoeae	N. meningitidis

ARA-C, cytosine arabinoside; CMV, cytomegalovirus; CNS, central nervous system; EBV, Epstein–Barr virus; HIV, human immunodeficiency virus; HSV, herpes simplex virus; MAI, Mycobacterium avium-intracellulare; SLE, systemic lupus erythematosus; VZV, varicella zoster virus.

650

nutrition and hormonal factors. Abnormalities of any of these nonspecific elements of host defense can result in an immunocompromised condition. Causative factors may include prolonged antibiotic use, poor nutritional status, a postmenopausal state in women, or surgical or age-related alteration of normal anatomy.

Specific immune defects can be categorized into four clinically relevant groups (Table 1). The first group involves polymorphonuclear leukocytes (PMNs), also called neutrophils or granulocytes, which are responsible for phagocytosis and killing of extracellular microbes. Initially, such microbes are targeted by other immune system components. Specific antibodies and complement bind to the cell walls and membranes of microbes. Subsequently, opsonized organisms can be more easily phagocytosed and eliminated by PMNs. The most common defect of PMN function is related to their absence. Neutropenia due to leukemic bone marrow infiltration, cytotoxic chemotherapy (e.g., adriamycin, cis-platinum, cytosine arabinoside, high-dose cyclophosphamide), aplastic anemia, and idiopathic drug reactions are relatively common and can deplete PMNs to the point of severe immune suppression ($<100/\mu L$). Congenital absence of PMNs is extremely rare, but congenital functional defects of neutrophil chemotaxis and intracellular killing are well described.

The second broad group of immune defects involves cell-mediated immunity. This term encompasses processes by which intracellular pathogens as well as malignant and virus-infected cells are eliminated. Cell-mediated immunity involves monocyte/macrophages and T-lymphocytes. Monocytes are responsible for a variety of functions, including phagocytosis of intracellular pathogens and elimination of malignant cells. T-lymphocytes include CD4 helper lymphocytes that are important in induction of the immune response and CD8 suppressor lymphocytes that appropriately limit the immune response. Natural killer cells and other cytotoxic lymphocytes that eliminate malignant and virus-infected cells as well as maintain immune tolerance to native tissue also are derived from T-lymphocytes. Acquired defects of cell-mediated immunity may be seen in severe malnutrition; lymphoma; HIV infection; following treatment with cyclosporine, tacrolimus, OKT3, antithymocyte globulin or high-dose corticosteroids; and with immunosuppressive chemotherapy using azathioprine, vincristine, bleomycin, fludarabine, or low-dose cyclophosphamide. Congenital defects of cell-mediated immunity are much rarer.

The third clinically relevant category of immune defects includes those involving the humoral arm of the immune system. Humoral immune function involves B-lymphocytes that clonally proliferate to produce appropriate specific antibodies to foreign antigens. Antibodies (along with activating complement) enhance clearance of microorganisms by phagocytes. Multiple myeloma and chronic lymphocytic leukemia are the major acquired conditions in which humoral immunity is impaired. Chemotherapeutic agents such as azathioprine, 6-mercaptopurine, cyclophosphamide, and methotrexate also suppress humoral immunity in addition to their detrimental effects on other elements of the immune system (i.e., neutropenia, mucosal barrier interruption).

The spleen is important for T-cell-independent immune responses and contains a large number of antibody-producing B-lymphocytes. Opsonized immune complexes and bacteria as well as nonopsonized microorganisms are cleared by phagocytes

in the spleen. Anatomic or functional (e.g., sickle cell disease) asplenia results in an immune defect similar to that seen with humoral deficits.

The final category of immune defects involves the complement cascade, which represents one of the major amplification pathways of the normal immune response. Various complement components facilitate phagocytosis by neutrophils, provide chemotactic signals to phagocytes, and can independently mediate the killing of extracellular bacteria. Complement deficiencies (notably systemic lupus erythematosus or multiple myeloma among acquired causes) usually result in infections similar to those associated with direct humoral immune defects. For clinical purposes, complement abnormalities and asplenia can be considered inclusively with defects of humoral immunity.

It is important to realize that immune defects seen in clinical practice do not, as a rule, represent discrete deficiencies of a single element of the immune system. Apart from rare congenital immune defects, immune defects tend to involve multiple arms of the immune system (although one may dominate). The reason is that the components of the immune system are inextricably linked together by molecular signaling mechanisms, such as cytokines, and by other feedback loops. For example, HIV infection–related suppression of cell-mediated immunity also results in humoral immune defects. Chemotherapy-induced granulocytopenia also suppresses T-cell and macrophage function with a resultant defect of cell-mediated immunity. The clinically dominant humoral immune defect in multiple myeloma and chronic lymphocytic leukemia is paralleled by more subtle defects of granulocyte function, cell-mediated immunity, and complement activity. In addition, any injury that is sufficiently severe (e.g. chemotherapy, burns, major trauma) to impair one arm of the immune system is likely to directly impair others.

PRINCIPLES IN ASSESSMENT OF INFECTION

The approach to infections in the immunocompromised patient is straightforward, even though the variety of infections that may be encountered is quite broad. A few basic principles should be used to narrow the initial diagnostic possibilities and target empiric therapy to appropriate etiologic categories (Table 2).

First, the likelihood of a given opportunistic infection is related to the nature of the immune defect. Deficiencies of humoral immune function (including asplenia and complement deficits) predispose to infections with encapsulated bacteria (e.g., *Streptococcus pneumoniae*, *Neisseria meningitidis*). Cellular immune dysfunction, such as seen with HIV infection, lymphoma, and corticosteroid use, predisposes to infection with more unusual organisms. These include atypical bacteria, such as *Listeria* and *Nocardia*; mycobacteria; fungi including *Cryptococcus* and *Candida* species; viruses, particularly herpesviruses including cytomegalovirus (CMV), Epstein-Barr virus (EBV), herpes simplex virus (HSV), and herpes varicella-zoster virus (VZV); and parasites such as *P. carinii*. Neutropenia resulting from acute leukemia, cytotoxic chemotherapy or aplastic anemia, and chronic neutrophil dysfunction such as seen in chronic granulomatous disease is associated with increased infections by pyogenic bacteria (e.g., *Staphylococcus aureus*, enteric gram-negative rods, *Pseudomonas aeruginosa*) and fungi (e.g. *Candida*, *Aspergillus*).

TABLE 2. ANTIMICROBIAL THERAPY IN IMMUNOCOMPROMISED PATIENTS

Antimicrobial Agent	Comments
Antibiotics	
Third-generation cephalosporins	Only ceftazidime and cefoperazone sodium are appropriate for coverage of *P. aeruginosa*. Inappropriate as single agents for organisms capable of producing inducible β-lactamases (e.g., *Enterobacter, Serratia*).
Fourth-generation cephalosporins	Modestly enhanced gram-positive activity and increased gram-negative activity (due to improved stability to inducible β-lactamases)
Extended-spectrum penicillins	Because of the potential for resistance, piperacillin, azlocillin sodium, or mezlocillin sodium should be administered with either an aminoglycoside or a third-generation cephalosporin. Ureidopenicillins (piperacillin, azlocillin, and mezlocillin) have greater enterococcal and anaerobic activity than do carboxypenicillins (carbenicillin and ticarcillin).
Penicillin-β-lactamase inhibitor combinations	Ticarcillin-clavulanate exhibits increased activity against *S. aureus*, anaerobes, and gram-negative bacilli compared with ticarcillin alone. The addition of tazobactam similarly broadens the activity of piperacillin.
Carbapenems	Imipenem-cilastatin and meropenem are the agents with the broadest activity but should be combined with an aminoglycoside if *Pseudomonas* is present.
Aminoglycosides	Preferred agents, in combination with anti-pseudomonal β-lactams for neutropenic fever and sepsis. Recent data suggest that toxicity is decreased and efficacy is preserved with once-daily doses.
Quinolones	Ciprofloxacin may be an effective alternative to aminoglycosides for the treatment of neutropenic fever or sepsis in patients with renal failure. Role of new quinolones with enhanced gram-positive and anaerobic activity is unclear.
Vancomycin hydrochloride	Covers gram-positive cocci, including *Enterococcus* and *Staphylococcus* species. Should be used for treatment of neutropenic fever when a specific risk factor, including a high incidence of MRSA, exists. A major emerging concern is nosocomial infection with ampicillin- and vancomycin-resistant *Enterococcus*.
Antifungals	
Amphotericin B	Most reliably effective treatment for fungal infections; liposomal forms with decreased renal toxicity available *Candida* vascular catheter infections: 0.6 mg $\cdot$ kg^{-1} $\cdot$ d^{-1} to 5 mg/kg total (longer therapy for parenchymal infections) Cryptococcal meningitis in AIDS: 0.5–0.8 mg $\cdot$ kg^{-1} $\cdot$ d^{-1} for 4–6 wk (follow with lifelong fluconazole) *Aspergillus* (invasive): 1.0–1.5 mg $\cdot$ kg^{-1} $\cdot$ d^{-1} to 20–40 mg/kg total dose Mucomycosis (invasive): 1.5 mg $\cdot$ kg^{-1} $\cdot$ d^{-1} to 30–40 mg/kg total dose (rhinocerebral infection frequently requires surgical debridement)
Fluconazole	Effective for thrush and *Candida* esophagitis; some evidence supports the use for *Candida* infection of intravascular catheters; maintenance therapy for cryptococcal meningitis
Itraconazole	Broader activity than fluconazole; possibly particular utility in *Candida* infection of biliary system. Now available in intravenous form
Caspofungin	Novel parenteral echinocandin, wide spectrum of activity including P. carinii but ineffective for cryptococcus
Antivirals	
Acyclovir	Mucocutaneous herpes[a] 5 mg $\cdot$ kg^{-1} $\cdot$ d^{-1} every 8 h for 7 to 14 d Dermatomal herpes zoster[a] 10–12 mg $\cdot$ kg^{-1} $\cdot$ d^{-1} every 8 h for 7 to 10 d Disseminated herpes zoster or primary varicella[a]: 10–12 mg/kg every 8 h for 7 to 14 d
Ganciclovir	CMV retinitis and other infections in HIV-infected patients: 5 mg $\cdot$ kg^{-1} $\cdot$ d^{-1} for 21 d (utility of treatment of pulmonary CMV isolate from AIDS patients with other pulmonary pathogens unclear) CMV pneumonitis in bone marrow transplant and other solid organ transplant recipients: 7.5–10 mg $\cdot$ kg^{-1} $\cdot$ d^{-1} for 10 to 20 d May have utility for other herpes viruses (simplex or zoster)
Antiparasitics	
Trimethoprim-sulfamethoxazole (TMP-SMX)	Optimal therapy for *Pneumocystis carinii*: 15–20 mg $\cdot$ kg^{-1} $\cdot$ d^{-1} in four divided doses for 21 d (if PaO$_2$ < 70 mm Hg on room air, corticosteroid therapy should be instituted)
Pentamidine	Alternative treatment of *P. carinii* pneumonia; more side effects than TMP-SMX
Sulfadiazine + pyrethamine + folinic acid	Optimal therapy of cerebral toxoplasmosis; chronic suppressive therapy should follow. Use corticosteroids (dexamethasone, 4 mg every 6 h) if significant brain edema or mass effect.

AIDS, acquired immunodeficiency syndrome; CMV, cytomegalovirus; HIV, human immunodeficiency virus; MRSA, methicillin-resistant *S. aureus*; PaO$_2$, partial pressure of oxygen in arterial blood.
[a]For patients who are immunosuppressed.
Adapted from Pizzo PA. Management of fever in patients with cancer and treatment-induced neutropenia. *N Engl J Med* 1993;328:1323–1332, with permission.

Second, the probable cause of infection is linked to the severity of the immune defect. Infection caused by neutrophil depletion following chemotherapy is unusual with an absolute neutrophil count (ANC) greater than 500 per microliter but is almost predictable as ANC falls below 100 per microliter. Similarly, although prednisone can broadly suppress the immune system, *P. carinii* infections are rare unless doses greater than 80 mg daily are taken for prolonged periods. Opportunistic infections in HIV-infected patients are uncommon when the CD4 count

exceeds 800 per microliter. Various opportunistic infections, including *Candida, P. carinii* and *Mycobacterium avium* intracellulare (MAI) become sequentially more common as the CD4 count falls to less than 100 cells per microliter.

Finally, the duration of the immune deficit helps to define the probable infecting agents. As a classic example, bacterial infection is common early in the neutropenic period, whereas fungal infections become increasingly important after the first week(s) of neutropenia. In organ-transplant patients, prolonged immunosuppression leads to a predictable evolution of infection risk. Within the first month posttransplant, patients are at risk for the same early postoperative infectious complications seen in immunocompetent patients with similarly extensive surgery. Between 1 and 6 months' posttransplant, infections with various fungi (e.g., *Cryptococcus, Candida, Aspergillus*), protozoa (e.g., *P. carinii*) and viruses (e.g., CMV, EBV, VZV dissemination, non-A, non-B hepatitis) dominate. After 6 months, the risk of opportunistic infections declines as immunosuppressive regimens are tapered. Despite decreased immunosuppression, however, some chronic risk of infection with atypical organisms, notably CMV (chorioretinitis), *Listeria* (meningitis, bacteremia) and *Cryptococcus* (meningitis) remains. Similar data exist for infection risk in bone marrow transplant patients.

CLINICAL APPROACH TO THE INFECTED, IMMUNOCOMPROMISED PATIENT

The general approach to the potentially infected, immunocompromised patient involves early assessment, careful evaluation of subtle clinical findings, aggressive diagnostic tests, empiric broad-spectrum antimicrobial therapy, anticipation of potential complications and coinfections, monitoring of clinical response and side effects, and, whenever possible, reduction of immunosuppression.

Patients must undergo a detailed history, physical examination, and laboratory evaluations. Based on these data, rapid implementation of a rational empiric therapeutic regimen tailored to the probable etiologic agents is required.

The history should evaluate the nature, severity, and duration (or expected duration) of the immunosuppressed state. In addition, localizing symptoms, if present, can narrow the field of potential pathogens. Knowledge of prior treatment can help to differentiate between therapy-induced disease and infection (e.g., bleomycin- or radiation-induced pulmonary fibrosis versus atypical pneumonia). Previous infections can point to the possibility of recurrence (particularly with defects of cell-mediated immunity). Prior antibiotic use can alter endogenous flora changing the identity of probable pathogens. Use of prophylactic regimens can influence the differential diagnosis of infection in critically ill patients. It also can lower the likelihood of certain diagnoses [e.g., *P. carinii* infection in HIV-infected patients receiving trimethoprim–sulfamethoxazole (TMP-SMX)] or increase the chance of others (e.g., α-hemolytic streptococcal or resistant gram-negative bacteremia in neutropenic patients receiving ciprofloxacin or TMP-SMX).

The physical examination should be complete and include specific areas often underappreciated in routine examinations. Fundoscopic examination may show evidence of *Candida endophthalmitis, Toxoplasma gondii* chorioretinitis, or CMV chorioretinitis. The skin may show herpetic vesicles, ecthyma gangrenosum associated with *Pseudomonas* or, less commonly, *Aeromonas* infection or lesions typical of disseminated *Candida* or *Aspergillus*. In the oropharynx, subtle evidence of odontogenic abscesses, *Candida* esophagitis/pharyngitis, and herpetic mucositis may exist. Intertriginous areas may conceal *Candida* or bacterial abscesses. Examination of the anus and surrounding tissue is necessary to rule out perirectal abscesses and cellulitis. A close neurologic examination may reveal subtle findings consistent with

cryptococcal meningitis or cerebral toxoplasmosis (e.g., nuchal rigidity, focal deficits).

Laboratory examination of specimens from the potentially infected immunocompromised patient can be extremely useful. Relatively trivial laboratory abnormalities may be indicative of significant disease. The initial workup should include a complete blood count with a manual differential white blood cell count (WBC). Severe neutropenia (ANC $<100/\mu L$) indicates a marked propensity to develop life-threatening bacterial and fungal infections (potentially in the absence of focal signs and symptoms). The leukocyte differential count may be useful in immunosuppressed patients who are unable to mount a substantial leukocytosis. A shift of the leukocyte population to immature neutrophil forms along with toxic granulation and Döhle bodies suggests overwhelming marrow stress, as seen in bacterial and fungal sepsis. Predominance of lymphocytes or monocytes is consistent with viral or mycobacterial infection, respectively. Thrombocytopenia with schistocytes suggests sepsis-associated disseminated intravascular coagulation (DIC). MAI and CMV infection can directly involve bone marrow resulting in pancytopenia. Electrolyte abnormalities associated with adrenal insufficiency (decreased serum Na^+, increased serum K^+) may indicate meningococcal, tuberculous, or fungal adrenalitis. Alterations of transaminases, bilirubin, amylase, and other routine blood tests can be useful in identifying potential sites of infection when clinical signs and symptoms are blunted or equivocal. Because many infected, immunocompromised patients have decreased creatinine clearance, assessment of renal function may be useful for dose adjustment of antimicrobials.

Examination of available body fluids and tissues is of key importance in the evaluation of the immunocompromised patient suspected of harboring infection. The selection of necessary tests and assessment of results are dependent on understanding the underlying immune deficit. If sputum is obtainable, a Gram stain and routine culture are required, even if pulmonary symptoms are relatively minor. Direct immunofluorescence for *Legionella* also is indicated for both community- and hospital-acquired disease. A number of institutions have documented nosocomially acquired *Legionella* infections. Neutropenic patients may exhibit marked symptoms of pulmonary origin in the absence of significant infiltrates and sputum production. Gram stain may show a paucity of neutrophils, but pathogenic bacteria or fungi may be visible. In patients with cell-mediated immune deficits, special stains, such as a Ziehl-Nielson (acid-fast stain) for mycobacteria (e.g., *M. tuberculosis*, MAI) or *Nocardia* and toluidine blue stain for *P. carinii* and fungi are required. Polymerase chain reaction (PCR) techniques also can be used (i.e., on acid-fast smear-positive specimens for species identification or on smear-negative sputum specimens); sensitivity and specificity are approximately 50% and greater than 95%, respectively, for acid-fast smear-negative sputum specimens (1). If sputum cannot be obtained noninvasively and clinical suspicion is high [e.g., chest x-ray (CXR) infiltrates], bronchoscopy with bronchoalveolar lavage (BAL) with or without biopsy may be indicated (Fig. 1).

The presence of gastrointestinal symptoms is an indication for stool examination and culture. Acid-fast stains and direct examination for mycobacteria, *Isospora*, and *Cryptosporidium* are particularly indicated for those with cell-mediated immune defects (particularly HIV infection). Patients with humoral deficits

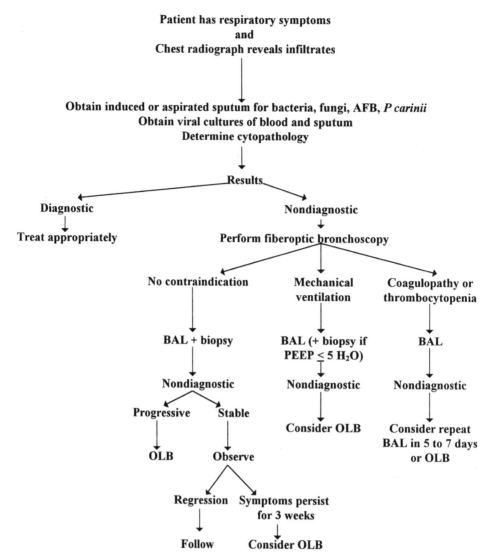

FIGURE 1. Diagnostic approach to pulmonary infiltrates in the immunosuppressed. CXR, chest x-ray; AFB, acid-fast bacilli; BAL, bronchoalveolar lavage; OLB, open-lung biopsy; PEEP, positive end-expiratory pressure.

have increased risk for *Giardia, Cryptosporidium,* and rotavirus infections.

Urine examination and culture may be similarly useful. The genitourinary tract is a potential source for sepsis in all patients. *M. tuberculosis* and CMV can be isolated in the urine from patients with disseminated disease.

Bacterial culture of the blood is routinely performed. Patients with clearance defects (neutropenia, immunoglobulin deficiency, complement deficiency, asplenia) are susceptible to rapidly progressive, fulminant, bacterial septic shock. In immunosuppressed patients, particularly those with severe neutropenia, bacteremia can be present with minimal symptoms initially. In these patients, multiple blood cultures should be obtained. Those with cell-mediated immune deficits should, in addition, have blood cultured for CMV. HIV-seropositive patients with persistent fever should have mycobacterial blood cultures for MAI. Persistent fever despite empiric antibiotics during prolonged neutropenia can indicate fungal infection. Although most fungi grow on regular blood culture media, the yield can be increased with fungal media. On occasion, in the appropriate clinical context, stain and culture of invasively obtained body fluids or tissue may be useful [e.g., cerebrospinal fluid (CSF) for tuberculous or cryptococcal meningitis, bone marrow for disseminated MAI].

Ancillary diagnostic tests may include serum cryptococcal antigen and urine for *Legionella* and *Histoplasma* antigen. Serology is rarely of use for acute management but can help in the later diagnosis of various viral and fungal infections.

The lung is the single most frequently infected organ in immunocompromised patients. Not surprisingly, a high-quality CXR (posteroanterior and lateral) is the most useful initial radiologic test and is mandatory in all immunocompromised patients suspected of serious infection. A computerized axial tomogram (CT) occasionally can detect otherwise occult lesions (normal CXR) or further delineate suspected pathologies. In the presence of neurologic findings, a cranial CT or magnetic resonance imaging (MRI) scan may reveal infectious (e.g., *Toxoplasma gondii*) or noninfectious (e.g., lymphoma) sources of fever in the immuno-compromised host. In general, MRI provides a higher diagnostic yield of brain parenchyma than does CT scan. CT examination of the abdomen has potential utility if an intraabdominal, intra-hepatic, or splenic abscess is suspected. Nuclear imaging techniques also occasionally can be useful [e.g., gallium scanning for *P. carinii* pneumonia (PCP), indium-labeled WBC scanning for occult abdominal abscesses]; however, the immune defects of this patient group (particularly neutropenia) can limit the utility of such leukocyte-dependent studies. Newer modalities, such as indium-labeled immunoglobulin G may prove of greater utility in the immunocompromised patient.

Despite the need for an aggressive search for infection in immunocompromised patients, the potential for noninfectious causes of fever resulting from underlying or unrelated diseases must be considered. Among malignancies, lymphoma and hyper-nephroma frequently are associated with fever. Allograft rejection may be the most common cause of fever in organ-transplant re-cipients. Antibiotics, among the myriad of medications given im-munocompromised patients, are well known to cause drug fever. Postsurgical hematoma, pulmonary embolism, and myocardial infarction are other potential causes of fever in immunocompro-mised patients.

INFECTION IN THE NEUTROPENIC PATIENT

Most patients become neutropenic as a consequence of leukemia or the treatment of malignancy with chemotherapy or bone mar-row transplantation (2). Occasional patients have aplastic anemia or neutropenia secondary to idiosyncratic responses to drugs.

Although overt focal processes may be seen, fever is the typi-cal presenting feature in most patients with infection and severe neutropenia (<100 PMN/μL). Unfortunately, a definitive fever source cannot be determined in the majority (60%–70%) of these cases. An organism is identified in only 30% (2). Because of these problems, neutropenic patients with fever ($>38.3°$C) in the absence of a defined cause must be assumed to have in-fection. In cases where an anatomic source of infection can be identified, 85% are localized to periodontium, oropharynx, lung, distal esophagus, colon, perianal area, or skin. Bacterial and fungal pathogens dominate in all patients with neutropenia regardless of the etiology. Patients with neutropenia secondary to untreated leukemia/lymphoma or aplastic anemia are also at increased risk of reactivation of herpes viruses resulting in severe HSV mucosi-tis, disseminated varicella-zoster, and CMV infection. In the past, viral hepatitis B and C as a consequence of multiple blood product transfusions were problems, but the incidence of primary infec-tion has declined dramatically with the development of screening tests; however, reactivation of chronic viral hepatitis (B or C) re-mains a recognized complication of induction chemotherapy.

Several factors have an impact on the risk of infection during neutropenia. One such factor is the underlying cause of neutrope-nia. Conditions that are associated with concurrent abnormalities of other components of the immune system during neutropenia result in a marked increase in the risk of infectious complica-tions. Neutropenia resulting from drug reactions, aplastic ane-mia, or congenital cyclic neutropenia involves a relatively isolated

immune defect without mucosal injury. In contrast, cytotoxic chemotherapy impairs mucosal integrity (breaching the anatomic barrier to endogenous organisms). It also impairs the phagocytic function of surviving neutrophils and adversely affects both hu-moral and cell-mediated immunity. As a consequence, the risk of infection during cytotoxic chemotherapy-induced neutropenia is far higher than for other groups.

The dominant predictor of risk of infection during neutrope-nia resulting from chemotherapy is the degree and duration of the neutropenia (2,3). The risk of bacterial infection is signifi-cantly increased when the ANC falls below 500 per microliter. A marked increase in risk is seen with counts below 100 per micro-liter. Most severe infections and bacteremias are seen with ANC counts below this level. It is well recognized, however, that brief periods of even total neutropenia infrequently result in signifi-cant infectious complications. In addition, the rate of neutrophil decline influences the risk of infection; the likelihood of infection increases with more rapid declines in PMN counts.

Along with degree of neutropenia, duration of neutropenia is critically important in the development of infection. Within a week after the administration of chemotherapy, over 50% of patients with neutropenia develop fever. In patients given chemo-therapy, the nadir of neutrophil count and peak severity of mu-cositis occur about 10 days after chemotherapy is started. If fever and infection does occur in the first few days (<1 week) of neu-tropenia, gram positive cocci are frequently responsible. In those with more prolonged neutropenia, gram negative bacilli become problematic in the second and third weeks. After 3 weeks of neutropenia, there is an increase in the incidence of opportunis-tic fungal infections, particularly with *Candida* and *Aspergillus* species.

Typically, infections in patients with neutropenia are due to endogenous bacteria (although half may be hospital acquired). Nosocomial acquisition may have occurred from physical con-tact (gram-negative rods, gram-positive cocci), water sources (e.g., *Legionella*) or air (e.g., *Aspergillus*). Potential sources for infection with endogenous organisms include the skin (e.g., *Staphylococcus* species, *Corynebacterium* species [especially *C. jeikeium*], *Bacillus* species, gram-negative rods, and *Candida* organisms), and gut (e.g., gram-negative rods and *Candida* species). Insertion of inva-sive lines can allow introduction of staphylococci, gram-negative rods, and *Candida* organisms.

Traditionally, early infections in neutropenic patients had been related to gram-negative rods such as *Escherichia coli*, *Klebsiella* species, and *P. aeruginosa*, although staphylococcal and strepto-coccal species occasionally were seen; the last decade has seen a shift away from gram-negative infections toward staphylococcal species (including *S. aureus* and coagulase-negative staphylococci) and nonenterococcal, nonpneumococcal, α-hemolytic strepto-coccal species ("strep viridans"). These α-hemolytic streptococci, in particular, have been associated with a severe syndrome of sepsis and acute respiratory distress syndrome (ARDS) in this patient population. The last decade also has seen the emergence of new early pathogens in infections such as necrotizing fasci-itis (*Aeromonas hydrophila*), pneumonia (*Stenotrophomonas mal-tophilia*), and line sepsis (*Burkholderia* [formerly *Pseudomonas*], *cepacia*, or *S. maltophilia*). Other emerging pathogens unique to the neutropenic host are *Leuconostoc* species (line sepsis, dental

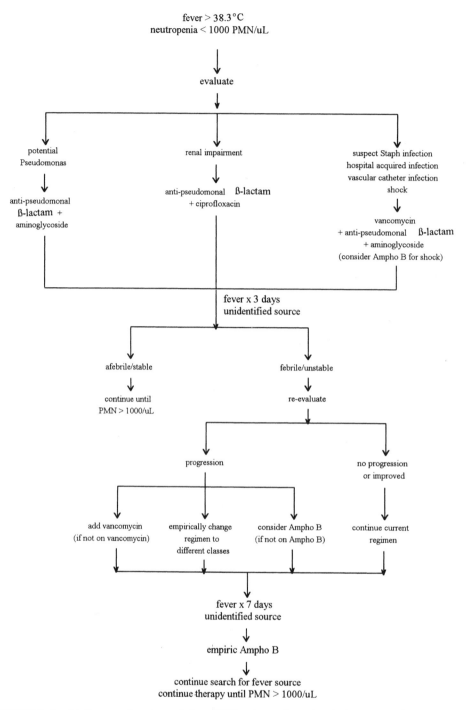

fever > 38.3 °C
neutropenia < 1000 PMN/uL

↓

evaluate

↓

potential	renal impairment	suspect Staph infection
Pseudomonas		hospital acquired infection
		vascular catheter infection
		shock

potential Pseudomonas
↓
anti-pseudomonal ß-lactam + aminoglycoside

renal impairment
↓
anti-pseudomonal ß-lactam + ciprofloxacin

suspect Staph infection / hospital acquired infection / vascular catheter infection / shock
↓
vancomycin + anti-pseudomonal ß-lactam + aminoglycoside (consider Ampho B for shock)

fever x 3 days
unidentified source

afebrile/stable
↓
continue until PMN > 1000/uL

febrile/unstable
↓
re-evaluate

progression

no progression or improved
↓
continue current regimen

add vancomycin (if not on vancomycin)

empirically change regimen to different classes

consider Ampho B (if not on Ampho B)

fever x 7 days
unidentified source
↓
empiric Ampho B
↓
continue search for fever source
continue therapy until PMN > 1000/uL

FIGURE 2. Empiric therapy of neutropenic fever. PMN, polymorphonuclear leukocyte; Ampho B, amphotericin B.

abscess, and meningitis), *Corynebacteria* (pneumonia, line sepsis, and skin infection), *Bacillus* species (line sepsis and pneumonia), *Capnocytophaga* (sepsis), and *Rhodococcus equi* (necrotizing pneumonia). This shift has occurred for a variety of reasons, including the use of prophylactic antibiotics and chemotherapeutic regimens causing greater mucositis.

As noted, fungal infections predominate after 3 weeks of neutropenia. Traditional later-onset pathogens have included *Candida albicans, Aspergillus,* and *Mucor* species. Partially as a result of the widespread application of fluconazole prophylaxis,

these traditional late pathogens have been supplemented in recent years by emerging pathogens, such as *Torulopsis glabrata* (line sepsis and pneumonia), *C. tropicalis* (line sepsis and soft-tissue infections), *Trichosporon* species (soft-tissue infections and pneumonia), and *Fusaria* species (line sepsis).

A number of principles, developed in the 1960s and 1970s, continue to be relevant to the management of fever from an undefined source in the neutropenic host (Fig. 2). Many of these principles are also applicable for fever from a defined source. The primary principle is based on the observation that, despite the difficulty in defining a site of infection at the time of fever onset, empiric therapy with antibiotics clearly decreases mortality during neutropenic fever. Therefore, neutropenic patients (PMN count <500 cells/μL) with fever (temperature >38.5°C on one occasion or >38°C on two occasions) should be started on empiric antibiotic therapy.

Second, as a rule, broad empiric combinations of antibiotics should be used, particularly in the ICU. With narrow regimens (even when a specific organism is identified), there is an unacceptably high risk of a secondary bacterial infection. This high risk may be due to the fact that most neutropenic infection occurs in patients who have received cytotoxic chemotherapy for leukemia and bone marrow transplantation. Such cytotoxic chemotherapy results in gastrointestinal mucosal injury, which allows invasion by multiple organisms.

Third, broad-spectrum antibiotics should be continued for the duration of the neutropenia or for 10 to 14 days if the ANC recovers to more than 500 per microliter (whichever is longer). Failure to continue antibiotics for the duration of neutropenia has been associated with relapse and/or recurrence of fever and infection.

Fourth, the specific choice of the initial antibiotic regimen is dependent on the microbial flora of the local environment. This includes both sensitivity patterns of likely endogenous flora present on the individual and sensitivity patterns of pathogens known to circulate in the local nosocomial environment. It is important to note that standard antibiotic regimens evolve over time as a result of changing nosocomial pathogens and susceptibility patterns. Historically, standard regimens have included a broad-spectrum antipseudomonal β-lactam and an aminoglycoside (e.g., ceftazidime and tobramycin, piperacillin and amikacin). In recent years, most institutions have favored the cephalosporin/aminoglycoside combinations. Although acceptable in most patients, monotherapy with carbapenems (imipenem-cilastin or meropenem are currently marketed) or antipseudomonal cephalosporins should be avoided in patients sufficiently ill to require ICU care. In addition, monotherapy with third-generation cephalosporins should be avoided in institutions with a high incidence of infections with *Enterobacter, Citrobacter,* and *Serratia* species because these organisms may harbor inducible β-lactamases that can rapidly render these organisms resistant. Monotherapy with β-lactamase stable fourth-generation cephalosporins or carbapenems are acceptable in noncritically ill patients in such institutions. Although evidence supports the use of a double β-lactam combination as an alternative to a cephalosporin and aminoglycoside in renal failure, the combination of an antipseudomonal cephalosporin with ciprofloxacin may be preferable (ciprofloxacin still has the greatest *Pseudomonas* activity of the available quinolones). Despite the increasing incidence of gram-positive infections, it is not necessary routinely to add vancomycin to the initial empiric regimen unless a specific suspicion for a gram-positive infection is present (line infection, high incidence of hospital-acquired methicillin-resistant *S. aureus* or *S. mitis* infection).

Finally, it is a well-accepted principle of therapy that if fever persists or recurs in a neutropenic patient after 4 to 7 days of broad-spectrum antibacterial therapy, empiric antifungal therapy with intravenous amphotericin B (0.5–1.0 mg/kg daily) should be initiated. Antifungal therapy can be initiated earlier if clinical deterioration is present. Documented fungal infection, particularly hepatic candidiasis, requires prolonged amphotericin B treatment. Currently, the major role of imidazoles (e.g., fluconazole, itraconazole) in the management of the neutropenic patient is as either primary or secondary prophylaxis. For the most part, patients with neutropenic fever in whom a potential fungal infection is suspected should not receive such drugs as primary therapy. The only exception may be hemodynamically stable patients with a high suspicion of *C. albicans* sepsis. Recent data suggest that treatment with intravenous fluconazole may be effective in this circumstance. Newer azoles in development, such as voriconazole may offer excellent microbiologic and clinical activity against fungal pathogens, including *Aspergillus.* Similarly, the newly released echinocandin, caspofungin, is also effective for a variety of invasive fungal infections. For the moment, however, life-threatening fungal infections in neutropenic patients should continue to be treated with amphotericin B.

A myriad of other clinical findings either can alter the initial empiric regimen for neutropenic fever or cause later modifications of that initial regimen. Therapy of neutropenic fever can be tailored according to specific findings as listed in Table 3.

In contrast to immunocompetent patients, intravascular catheter-associated bacteremia (particularly if caused by coagulase negative staphylococci) can be treated without catheter removal in most neutropenic patients. For multilumen vascular access catheters, the antibiotic infusion ports should be alternated, and it may be useful to leave antibiotic containing flush in lumens when they are not being used. Blood isolation of certain organisms (*Bacillus, C. jeikium, Candida*), tunnel infections, and failure to eliminate fever with antimicrobial therapy necessitates catheter removal (in addition to antibiotic therapy). In addition, catheter infection with other bacteria (*S. aureus, P. aeruginosa*) may be relatively resistant to therapy without catheter removal.

A new therapeutic modality now seeing extensive use involves the various leukocyte growth factors. Both granulocyte colony stimulating factor (G-CSF) and granulocyte-macrophage colony stimulating factor (GM-CSF) can abbreviate the duration of chemotherapy-related neutropenia and also decrease the incidence of infections in high-risk patients. They probably should be reserved for patients in whom a relatively prolonged duration of neutropenia (>10 days) is anticipated. In contrast, various antiendotoxins and anticytokines (monoclonal antibodies, receptor antagonists) have not been shown to have utility in treating any form of clinical infection. Protrecogin-alfa (activated), a recombinant form of activated protein C, has recently been approved for use in sepsis with organ failure, (severe sepsis) and septic shock. This therapy is likely to see substantial use in neutropenic and other immunocompromised patients.

INFECTIONS IN SOLID-ORGAN TRANSPLANT RECIPIENTS

Since 1980, solid-organ transplantation success rates have risen dramatically. One-year survival for renal, hepatic, and cardiac allografts now exceeds 80%. This improvement has been due largely to the introduction of effective immunosuppressive compounds such as cyclosporine and to advances in surgical technique. The last 15 years have been notable for the substantial

TABLE 3. COMMON MODIFICATIONS OR ADDITIONS TO INITIAL EMPIRIC ANTIBIOTIC THERAPY IN PATIENTS WITH NEUTROPENIA AND FEVER

Status or Symptoms	Modifications of Primary Regimen
Fever	
Persistent for >1 wk	Add empiric antifungal therapy.
Recurrence after 1 wk or later in patient with persistent neutropenia	Add empiric antifungal therapy.
Persistent or recurrent fever at time of recovery from neutropenia	Evaluate liver and spleen by CT, ultrasonography, or MRI for hepatosplenic candidiasis and evaluate need for antifungal therapy.
Bloodstream	
Cultures before antibiotic therapy	
Gram-positive organism	Add vancomycin hydrochloride pending further identification.
Gram-negative organism	Maintain regimen if patient is stable and isolate is sensitive. If *P. aeruginosa*, *Enterobacter*, or *Citrobacter* is isolated, add an aminoglycoside; if potential inducible β-lactamase producer (*Enterobacter, Citrobacter, Serratia*), ensure primary agent has enhanced β-lactamase stability (carbapenem or 4th generation cephalosporin).
Organism isolated during antibiotic therapy	
Gram-positive organism	Add vancomycin
Gram-negative organism	Broaden gram-negative coverage (e.g. ceftazidime + tobramycin → carbapenem or fourth generation cephalosporin + amikacin). Use inducible β-lactamase stable agent (carbapenem or fourth generation cephalosporin) if potential inducible β-lactamase producers (*Enterobacter, Citrobacter, Serratia*). Consider possibility of a central venous catheter infection.
Shock	Add vancomycin. Consider using amphotericin B. If no other site identified and shock not resolving, remove central venous catheters.
Head, eyes, ears, nose, throat	
Necrotizing gingivitis	Change antibiotics to increase antianaerobic activity (e.g., piperacillin → piperacillin/tazobactam, ceftazidime → imipenem-cilastin or meropenem) or add specific antianaerobic agents (e.g., metronidazole, clindamycin).
Vesicular or ulcerative lesions	Suspect herpes simplex infection. Culture and begin acyclovir therapy.
Sinus tenderness or nasal ulcerative lesions	Suspect fungal infection with *Aspergillus* or *Mucor* spp.
Gastrointestinal tract	
Retrosternal burning pain	Suspect *Candida*, herpes simplex, or both. Add fluconazole or amphotericin B and, if no response, acyclovir. Bacterial esophagitis is also a possibility. For patients who do not respond within 48 h, endoscopy should be considered.
Acute abdominal pain	Suspect typhlitis, as well as appendicitis if pain in right lower quadrant. Change antibiotics to increase antianaerobic activity (e.g., ceftazidime → imipenem-cilastin or meropenem) or add specific antianaerobic agents (e.g., metronidazole, clindamycin). Monitor closely for need for surgical intervention.
Perianal tenderness	Change antibiotics to increase antianaerobic activity (e.g., ceftazidime → imipenem-cilastin or meropenem) or add specific antianaerobic agents (e.g., metronidazole). Monitor need for surgical intervention, especially when patient is recovering from neutropenia.
Respiratory tract	
New focal lesion in patient recovering from neutropenia	Observe carefully because this lesion may be a consequence of inflammatory response in concert with neutrophil recovery.
New focal lesion in patient with continuing neutropenia	*Aspergillus* is the chief concern. Perform appropriate cultures and consider biopsy. If patient is not a candidate for procedure, administer high-dose amphotericin B ($1.5 \text{ mg} \cdot \text{kg}^{-1} \cdot \text{d}^{-1}$).
New interstitial pneumonitis	Attempt diagnosis by examination of induced sputum or bronchoalveolar lavage. If not feasible, begin empiric treatment with trimethoprim-sulfamethoxazole or pentamidine. Consider noninfectious causes and the need for open lung biopsy if condition has not improved after 4 d of therapy.
Central venous catheters	
Positive culture for organisms other than *Bacillus* species or *Candida*	Attempt to treat. Rotate antibiotic administration with multiple lumen into different lumens of central venous catheters.
Positive culture for *Bacillus* species or *Candida*	Remove catheter and treat.
Exit-site infection with *Mycobacterium* or *Aspergillus*	Remove catheter and treat.
Tunnel infection	Remove catheter and treat.

CT, computed tomography; MRI, magnetic resonance imaging.
Adapted from Pizzo PA. Management of fever in patients with cancer and treatment-induced neutropenia. *N Engl J Med* 1993;328:1323–1332, with permission.

increase in the number of heart and kidney transplants along with the emergence of heart–lung, lung, liver, pancreas, kidney–pancreas and, most recently, small bowel transplantation.

Along with HIV infection and lymphoreticular malignancies, immunosuppressed organ-transplant recipients probably represent the majority of individuals with major deficits of cell-mediated immunity in the developed world. Immunosuppression in these patients primarily reflects iatrogenic pharmacologically induced depression of cell-mediated immunity (cellular immune function) for purposes of graft retention. Pharmaceutical agents that induce defects of cell-mediated immunity include high-dose steroids (>60 mg prednisone equivalent daily), azathioprine, low-dose cyclophosphamide, vincristine, bleomycin, OKT3, antilymphocyte or thymocyte globulin, and, to a lesser extent, cyclosporine and tacrolimus. In contrast to the industrialized world, the dominant causes of cell-mediated immune defects in developing nations are malnutrition and HIV infection.

As with other forms of immune suppression, impaired cell-mediated immunity predisposes to infection with a variety of organisms (endogenous, community-acquired, or nosocomial in origin). These infections can manifest with clinically attenuated or otherwise unusual presentations. Although this section deals with organ-transplant patients, most patients with defects of cell-mediated immunity will exhibit a similar variety of infections. In transplant patients, fever without a defined focus and pneumonia are the most common infectious manifestations after the first month posttransplant (when surgical infections predominate).

The risk of infection and the most likely cause are related to a number of factors (4–7). These include the nature of the immune defect, the degree and duration of the postoperative immunosuppression, the time since the transplant, and the organ transplanted.

The nature of the immune defect defines the spectrum of likely infections. Unlike PMNs, which are required to clear extracellular organisms and bacteria, cell-mediated immunity (deficient in posttransplant patients) is responsible for defense against intracellular pathogens, including most viruses. For this reason, pharmacologically immunosuppressed organ-transplant recipients (as well as patients with lymphoreticular malignancies) are at substantial risk for systemic infections involving reactivation of latent viruses of the herpes group (HSV, CMV, EBV, VZV). In addition, they are at increased risk for papovavirus, adenovirus, and hepatitis B and C infections. They also have increased susceptibility to specific bacterial (e.g., *Listeria, Nocardia*), mycobacterial (e.g., *M. tuberculosis*), fungal (e.g., *Aspergillus, Cryptococcus*) and parasitic (e.g., *P. carinii, T. gondii*) infections. The specific immunosuppressive chemotherapy affects the etiology of infections. Prolonged high-dose corticosteroids (>80–120 mg prednisone equivalent daily) specifically increases risk for fungal and *P. carinii* infections. Azathioprine, cyclophosphamide, and OKT3 are associated with high risk for CMV reactivation. The relatively narrow T-cell immunosuppressive agents, cyclosporine and tacrolimus, appear to have relatively little impact on risk of opportunistic infection.

The level of risk and the probable causes of infection in transplant recipients also are related to the duration of time since the transplantation (Fig. 3). This phenomenon is explained by the multiple and sequential nature of the insults sustained by the transplant recipient and by the decreasing need for pharma-

cologic immunosuppression over time. Although the severity and clinical impact of infections may differ, the pattern of infections is similar for all forms of solid organ transplants.

Posttransplantation infections are divided into three major categories based on the postsurgical period. In the first period, the first month posttransplant, most infections are similar to those in any postsurgical patient. In the second period, the period from the second until the sixth month posttransplant, opportunistic infections predominate. The third period, 6 months or longer posttransplant, is characterized by infections similar to those in an immunocompetent person. Certain chronic herpesvirus infections (CMV and EBV) as well as augmentation of immunosuppression because of episodes of rejection alter this time course of susceptibility.

In the first month posttransplantation, recipients are at increased risk for developing infections resulting from preoperative illness and surgical insult. Solid-organ transplant recipients undergo an operative insult to implant the graft, resulting in the potential for wound or perigraft infection. Many of these patients have severe medical illnesses (uncompensated liver, cardiac, or respiratory failure), which can nonspecifically impair host defenses, impair wound healing, and predispose patients to develop severe infections. The invasive hemodynamic catheters, orotracheal intubation, and blood transfusions that most organ-transplant recipients receive perioperatively all increase their risk of developing early infection. Acute rejection also increases infection risk in the early postoperative phase.

Most early postoperative infections (90%–95%) in solid-organ transplant recipients are similar to those occurring in nonimmunosuppressed patients undergoing comparably extensive operations, although the infections in transplant recipients may be more severe. Surgical wound and intravenous catheter infections, urinary tract infections (UTI), and pneumonia are typical. Early postoperative infections represent a particular problem in major-organ transplants (e.g., heart–lung and liver transplants) because these patients frequently are substantially debilitated prior to surgery. Pathogens responsible for these infections generally are nosocomial in origin and will carry resistance patterns endemic to ICU organisms.

Most remaining early posttransplant infections are caused by reactivation of latent or subclinical infections that were present in the recipient before transplantation. Reactivation is triggered by perioperative nonspecific insults and intense immunosuppression. Typical organisms include HSV, *M. tuberculosis*, geographically restricted mycoses, and occasionally *Strongyloides*. Early postoperative infections due to hepatitis B, hepatitis C, or CMV carried by the allograft or perioperatively administered blood products have been common in the past; however, modern screening technologies have resulted in a sharp decline in such infections.

It is important to note that opportunistic pathogens normally do not present in this early postoperative period because they require a prolonged period of immunosuppression to manifest. The occurrence of such opportunistic pathogens implies either an excessive environmental exposure (*Aspergillus, Nocardia, Legionella*) or failure to appreciate latent or subclinical disease (tuberculosis, *Strongyloides*, geographically restricted mycoses).

HSV antibodies are present in three-quarters of adult solid-organ transplant recipients; HSV reactivation occur in the first

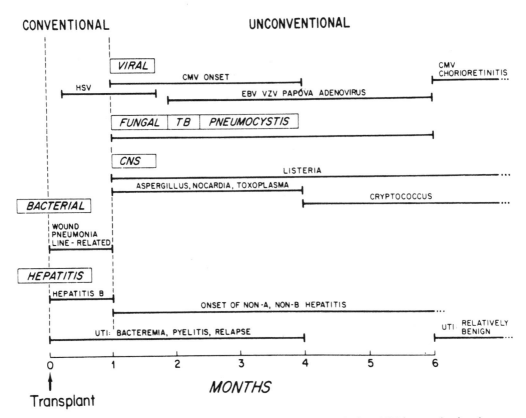

FIGURE 3. Infection in the renal transplant patient. CMV, cytomegalovirus; HSV, herpes simplex virus; EBV, Epstein–Barr virus; VZV, varicella-zoster virus; CNS, central nervous system; UTI, urinary tract infection. (From Rubin RH, Wolfson JS, Cosimi AB, et al. Infection in the renal transplant recipient. *Am J Med* 1981;70:405–411, with permission.)

month posttransplantation in about one-third of adults and 8% of pediatric cases (due to a lower rate of latent infection) (7). Clinically, these patients will have oral or genital mucocutaneous lesions but occasionally have either target-organ disease (pneumonitis, tracheobronchitis, esophagitis, or hepatitis) or disseminated disease. Aggressive treatment with high-dose acyclovir is required in this circumstance.

Of the geographically restricted mycoses, *Histoplasma capsulatum* (central United States) and *Coccidiodes immitis* (Southwestern United States, New Mexico, and Central America) disseminate or reactivate more frequently in organ-transplant patients, whereas there appears to be no increase in risk of *Blastomyces dermatiditis*. *M. tuberculosis* also has an increased risk of reactivation and has been reported in outbreaks among transplantation populations. Clinically, most patients have fever. Tuberculin skin tests are positive in 25% to 33% of cases, but patients may be highly infectious. Diagnosis should proceed with sputum smears and cultures for acid-fast organisms; bronchoscopy with lavage, transbronchial biopsy, or open lung biopsy may be necessary to evaluate patients with negative smears in whom the diagnosis is suspected.

Following the first month posttransplantation, defects of cellular immunity due to pharmacologic intervention begin to have a greater impact on the etiology of infections. All allograft recipients require pharmacologic immunosuppression to ensure graft survival. Solid-organ transplantation recipients typically have decreasing immunosuppressive requirements over time as immunotolerance to the allograft develops. The risk for infections due to pharmacologically induced depression of cellular immunity is maximal between 1 and 6 months. The immunomodulating viruses (CMV, EBV, and HIV) are one of the major infectious concerns during this period. Infection with these viruses can further increase the patient's risk of developing opportunistic infections caused by *P. carinii*, *Listeria monocytogenes*, *Aspergillus*, *Nocardia*, *T. gondii*, *S. stercoralis*, and *Cryptococcus* species. The maximum period of risk for serious life-threatening infections appears to be at about 3 to 4 months after transplantation. During this period, all risk factors (surgery, graft dysfunction, and immunosuppression) overlap.

With regard to parasitic infections, these generally are not associated with unique clinical syndromes that require a change of approach in transplant populations. Exceptions are disease caused by *T. gondii*, *P. carinii*, and *S. stercoralis*.

Strongyloides stercoralis is endemic in rural Puerto Rico and the southeastern United States (Louisiana, Tennessee, and Kentucky). In most patients, symptoms develop in the first 6 months posttransplantation. Some patients are asymptomatic. Most have predominantly gastrointestinal symptoms (e.g., diarrhea, abdominal pain, nausea, emesis, ileus, or bowel obstruction). These patients can have an autoinfection cycle in which larvae both infect colon and invade intestinal mucosa or perianal skin. This can progress to systemic disease as larvae disseminate throughout the body [heart, lungs, central nervous system (CNS), and skin]. As larvae migrate from the gastrointestinal tract, enteric gram-negative organisms can migrate as well, and active disease may be associated with gram-negative bacteremia or, less commonly, meningitis. Immunosuppressive therapy, especially with corticosteroids, can lead to increased autoinfection and tissue invasion and the hyperinfection syndrome. Dissemination can occur years after the primary infection. With aggressive tissue invasion and disseminated disease, the mortality rate can reach 71% (7,8). The diagnosis is made by examination of stool specimens for larvae; to improve yield, several stool samples should be examined. Duodenal fluid also can be examined for the organism; other sites that can be examined include urine, ascitic fluid, wounds, sputum, and jejunal biopsy. Peripheral blood can be examined for eosinophilia, although this feature may not be present; serologic tests also exist. Therapy is traditionally with thiabendazole; ivermectin and albendazole are promising. In addition, reduction of immunosuppression should be attempted, if possible, and therapy of associated gram-negative infections treated, if present.

Normally, at 6 months posttransplantation, pharmacologic immunosuppression is minimized and graft function is optimal. At this point, the risk and etiology of infections for most graft recipients (75%) begin to approximate those of immunocompetent individuals. Twenty-five percent continue to have difficulties, and 10% have chronic viral infections (CMV, EBV, and hepatitis), leading to graft failure or malignancy (hepatocellular carcinoma due to hepatitis B or C or posttransplant lymphoproliferative disorder due to EBV). About 15% of transplant recipients continue to have chronic rejection, which necessitates sustained use of high-level pharmacologic immunosuppression with the attendant increased susceptibility to developing opportunistic pathogens.

Although the extent of time following the transplant is crucially important in determining the range of infections for which the patient is at risk, the risk of infection is also related to the actual organ transplanted, especially during the first 3 months. Because of surgical anastomoses and surgical denervation of the graft, recurrent and severe infections tend to occur in the transplanted organ. For example, lung-transplant recipients tend to exhibit recurrent pneumonias, involving both standard bacterial pathogens and opportunistic organisms; CMV pneumonitis is particularly severe in these patients. Liver transplant recipients exhibit biliary sepsis with increased frequency. CMV hepatitis, which is typically mild in most transplant recipients, can be fulminant in liver allograft recipients. Renal transplants often are complicated by recurrent urinary tract infection.

The most common syndrome in organ-transplant infections is fever without a defined source. The clinical approach is similar for any immunocompromised patient; however, the focus should be on pathogens for which the patient is known to be high risk. The assessment includes a close review of the patient's history (including serologic status); a physical examination, with a view toward localizing signs; and laboratory examination, including chest radiograph and culture (including viral studies) of available body fluids and tissues. Pathogens that can present with fever without a defined clinical focus include CMV, EBV, toxoplasmosis, and disseminated candidiasis. PCP can present with only fever, nonspecific pulmonary symptoms, and a normal chest radiograph. Graft rejection and drug reactions are other potential causes of fever in this patient group.

Cytomegalovirus infection is the most common infection-related cause of fever without a defined source in allograft recipi-

ents. It occurs in 44% to 85% of kidney, heart, and liver transplant patients. Typically, the infection occurs through reactivation of latent virus in a seropositive transplant recipient. Most adults have antibodies that demonstrate prior infection with CMV. Primary acquisition of infection from the graft itself or perioperative blood products occurs occasionally. Seronegative recipients who receive CMV seropositive organs carry a higher risk of clinical disease due to CMV infection; in such cases, the clinical course of the infection may be especially severe. Although the initial presentation may involve fever and malaise alone in mild cases, hypotension, pneumonitis, hepatitis, glomerulonephritis, encephalitis, and enterocolitis are not uncommon in patients admitted to ICU. Cell-count abnormalities such as leukopenia or thrombocytopenia are frequently present. Involvement of the transplanted organ always should be suspected: hepatitis in liver transplant patients, pancreatitis in pancreas transplant patients, pneumonitis in lung and heart–lung transplant patients, and glomerulopathy in renal transplant patients. CMV infection also has been associated with graft rejection and viral-induced immunosuppression beyond the first 6 months posttransplant resulting in prolonged susceptibility to other opportunistic infections.

The diagnosis of CMV disease can be difficult. Viral cultures using the tube culture (7–14 days of incubation) method or the shell vial method (16 hours of incubation) of tissue or blood are useful when positive. Viral blood cultures are insensitive, but when they are positive indicate CMV viremia. Typical intranuclear inclusions in biopsied tissues or, less reliably, a positive nonhematologic fluid culture (urine or BAL) in a patient with a likely clinical presentation may also indicate disease. Serology is rarely clinically useful except in primary infections in which seroconversion may be noted.

Both DNA hybridization techniques and immunohistochemistry are gaining in importance in the diagnosis of CMV disease. These techniques can detect CMV in biopsy tissues and provide greater sensitivity than culture. Rapid detection of CMV in blood by using PCR techniques is as or more sensitive than culture methods. Data are forthcoming regarding the correlation of target-organ disease and CMV viremia.

Clinical information on a variety of opportunistic pathogens has grown rapidly over the last 15 years. In many cases, this is due to the increased incidence of formerly rare infections in the HIV-positive population. Data derived from HIV-positive patients may not, however, be directly applicable to the organ-transplant population because significant differences exist in the clinical presentation of disease and the utility of diagnostic techniques between the two groups. Compared with organ-transplant recipients, CMV disease in HIV-positive persons is less common as a cause of fever and rarely causes specific organ dysfunction. In contrast, disseminated MAI infection is relatively common and contributes substantially to morbidity in HIV-positive patients but is uncommon in organ-transplant recipients. Similarly, PCP tends to be a much more virulent illness with a higher mortality rate in transplant (and oncology) patients than in those who are HIV seropositive. In addition, standard diagnostic techniques, such as examination of induced sputum and BAL fluid, are less effective for the diagnosis of PCP in transplant (and oncology) patients than HIV patients. Open-lung biopsy (OLB) still is required occasionally to make a definitive diagnosis in such patients but is rarely required in patients with HIV infection.

Although the treatment of infections is generally similar for these groups, organ-transplant recipients have at least one major consideration unique to them. Several antibiotics and antimicrobial chemotherapies interact with cyclosporine and tacrolimus, antirejection agents commonly used for transplant patients. Clearance of these compounds involves the hepatic enzyme, cytochrome P450. Rifampin and isoniazid upregulate cytochrome P450 activity and result in increased clearance of cyclosporine (potentially leading to rejection). In contrast, macrolides (erythromycin, azithromycin, and clarithromycin) and azoles (ketoconazole, fluconazole, and itraconazole) inhibit activity of the enzyme and can result in cyclosporine toxicity. Use of any of these drugs necessitates close cyclosporine monitoring. Similar problems exist with the use of tacrolimus, although limited data are available because it was introduced to the market more recently. Synergistic nephrotoxicity with other compounds is also a major clinical concern with both drugs. The potential for nephrotoxicity and renal failure is enhanced by coadministration with amphotericin, aminoglycosides, vancomycin, high-dose TMP-SMX, pentamidine isethionate, and itraconazole.

INFECTION IN BONE MARROW TRANSPLANT RECIPIENTS

Bone marrow transplant (BMT) recipients incur the combined early risks of ablative chemotherapy resulting in profound leukope-

nia, and the later risks of depression of cell-mediated and humoral immunity secondary to cytotoxic injury and ongoing immunosuppressive therapy (Fig. 4) (9–11). Although granulocytopenia usually resolves by 20 to 30 days if engraftment is successful, phagocytic function may remain depressed for prolonged periods. Similarly, cell-mediated immunity as measured by T-cell number is grossly normal by 2 months posttransplant, but specialized tests show functional abnormalities for years following transplantation. Likewise, CD8 suppressor cell numbers may be increased for the first year, and CD4 helper-cell numbers remain depressed for up to 2 years. Immunoglobulin production also may be suppressed for a year or longer following transplantation.

Three broad periods corresponding to the nature of infectious risk have been defined for BMT recipients; as with solid-organ transplantation, these general designations vary from patient to patient based on additional factors such as concurrent CMV infection and degree of iatrogenic immunosuppression from medications.

The first period, the preengraftment period, occurs from bone marrow ablation until 30 days posttransplant. Infections in this period relate primarily to the severe neutropenia and mucositis caused by the cytotoxic conditioning regimen given for the transplant. Clinical disease and treatment are therefore similar to those of other febrile neutropenic patients. Relatively prolonged neutropenia, however, should be anticipated.

Various prophylactic regimens to prevent infectious complications may be given in this period, and these may influence

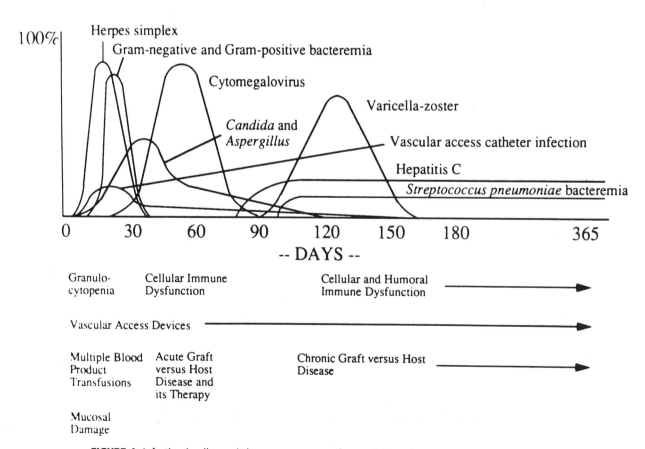

FIGURE 4. Infection in allogeneic bone marrow transplant recipients. (From Schimpff SC. Infection in bone marrow transplantation: a model for examining predisposing factors to infection in cancer patients. *Recent Results Cancer Res* 1993;132:15–34, with permission.)

predominant pathogens, shifting bacterial species to more re-sistant gram-negatives, increasing the incidence of *C. difficile* diarrhea, or increasing the incidence of colonization with flu-conazole resistant *Candida* species. HSV infections reactivate in up to 80% of HSV-seropositive patients who do not receive acy-clovir prophylaxis.

The postengraftment period lasts from 30 to 100 days post-transplant. For the most part, infection risk in this period occurs as a consequence of the defect of cell-mediated immunity caused by the antirejection immunosuppressive regimen. Immune dys-function caused by the bone marrow ablating conditioning reg-imen (as described previously) as well as graft-versus-host dis-ease and the augmented immunosuppression required by this complication may contribute. Since allogeneic transplants re-quire greater immunosuppression, they tend to have higher rates of infection than autologous transplants. Because cell-mediated immunity is predominantly affected, infections in this period involve pathogens similar to those seen in organ-transplant re-cipients. The dominant concerns are CMV infection, *P. carinii*, and nonspecific interstitial pneumonia. All have similar presenta-tions, with fever, nonproductive cough, dyspnea, hypoxemia, and diffuse interstitial infiltrates. The approach to diagnosis is simi-lar to that for other immunosuppressed patients with pulmonary infiltrates (Fig. 1). CMV pneumonitis is of particular concern in patients who are CMV seropositive prior to BMT and in CMV-seronegative patients who receive granulocytes or bone marrow from CMV-seropositive donors. Patients receiving total-body ir-radiation are also at increased risk for developing CMV infections. CMV pneumonia is most reliably diagnosed by the demonstra-tion of typical intranuclear inclusions in lung biopsies. If the pa-tient's clinical status precludes transbronchial biopsy, BAL (and occasionally sputum or tracheal aspirate) cytology demonstration of typical inclusions is also diagnostic although probably less sen-sitive. Shell vial CMV-positive blood cultures provide supportive evidence of an active infection. Recently developed antigen de-tection assays and PCR techniques may be useful. *P. carinii*, less common than CMV in this setting, sometimes can be diagnosed by BAL, although OLB may be necessary. Prophylaxis with TMP-SMX decreases the likelihood of *P. carinii* infection. Nonspecific interstitial pneumonitis occurs in a considerable number of pa-tients, but can be reliably diagnosed only by OLB.

Invasive *Aspergillus* is also a concern in these patients. Flucona-zole prophylaxis for *Candida* infections has resulted in *Aspergillus* accounting for most fungal infections found in BMT patients postmortem. The incidence is approximately 8%, and infection can occur either early or late post transplant. Early disease is associated with neutropenia, whereas late disease is associated with corticosteroid use. Disease often occurs in the lung, but hematogenous spread is not uncommon; blood cultures are usu-ally negative. High-dose amphotericin B (1.0–1.5 mg/kg daily) is required for therapy.

Other potential pathogens in the postengraftment period in-clude HSV and VZV (usually reactivation), fungal infections with *Candida* species, and occasionally parasitic disease caused by *T. gondii* or *Cryptosporidium*. Venoocclusive disease, a syn-drome of fever, hepatomegaly, and liver function abnormality, is a noninfectious cause of fever that typically occurs in the early postengraftment period and should be considered in the differ-ential diagnosis of fever in this setting.

During the late posttransplantation period, beginning 100 days posttransplant, VZV reactivation and viral respiratory in-fections become more common. About 40% of patients will de-velop a significant VZV infection (either zoster or varicella-like syndrome) during their posttransplant course. One third of pa-tients experience dissemination, with a mortality rate of 30% to 35%. In contrast, aggravation of chronic carriage of hepatitis B and C is uncommon and these infections do not preclude marrow transplantation. Potential causes of viral respiratory tract infec-tions in the late posttransplant period include respiratory syncy-tial virus (RSV) and parainfluenza. These are the most common causes of viral pneumonia in this population, and they carry a high mortality rate. Diagnosis is made by nasopharyngeal swab sent for viral culture by conventional and shell vial methods and by direct immunofluorescent (DFA) assay. Therapy with antiviral agents is available (ribavirin and IVIG for RSV; amantadine or rimantadine for parainfluenza or influenza); therapy appears to be more effective earlier in the course of disease. Humoral immu-nity defects with decreased production of opsonizing antibodies also persist for years, resulting in increased risk of infection with encapsulated bacteria. Pneumococcal and *S. aureus* pneumonia are most common. Chronic graft-versus-host disease substantially increases the risk for all these infections.

INFECTIONS IN ACQUIRED IMMUNE DEFICIENCY SYNDROME

First reported in 1981, acquired immunodeficiency syndrome (AIDS) is defined by the occurrence of specific opportunistic infections and immunosuppression-related malignancies in per-sons infected with HIV. Since 1993, the diagnosis of AIDS has required evidence of a defined spectrum of clinical disease (spe-cific opportunistic infections, specified malignancies, or primary HIV-related phenomenon) (Table 4) or marked depletion of CD4 cell counts (<200 cells/μL or <14% total) with direct evidence of HIV infection (12).

In recent years, the therapy for HIV has undergone a revolu-tion. The advent of highly active antiretroviral therapy in which multiple antiviral drugs used in combination almost completely suppress viral replication has had a dramatic impact. With these new therapies, the incidence of opportunistic infections has fallen as patients have experienced stabilization and reconstitution of their immune systems and suppression of viral proliferation. As deaths related to new HIV-related infections and malignancies has fallen, the number of persons living with HIV/AIDS has risen. Current estimates suggest between one and two million HIV-infected persons live in the United States. By the end of 1999, more than 700,000 cases of AIDS in the United States had been reported to the Centers for Disease Control and Prevention in Atlanta, Georgia (13).

Although HIV infections and AIDS cases in North Amer-ica are centered primarily in urban centers, it is likely that every intensivist in the country has dealt with the disease. As noted, the last decade has seen an improvement in the mortality and the severity of illness as well as a decrease in the incidence of opportunistic infections. The prototypical patient in the early years of the epidemic was a white male homosexual or intra-venous drug abuser between the age of 20 and 50. As a result of

TABLE 4. CONDITIONS INCLUDED IN THE 1993 AIDS SURVEILLANCE DEFINITION

Candidiasis of bronchi, trachea, or lungs
Candidiasis, esophageal
Cervical cancer, invasive
Coccidioidomycosis, disseminated or extrapulmonary
Cryptococcosis, extrapulmonary
Cryptosporidiosis, chronic intestinal (>1-mo duration)
Cytomegalovirus disease (other than liver, spleen, or nodes)
Cytomegalovirus retinitis (with loss of vision)
Encephalopathy, HIV-related
Herpes simplex: chronic ulcer(s) (>1-mo duration); or
    bronchitis, pneumonitis, or esophagitis
Histoplasmosis, disseminated or extrapulmonary
Isosporiasis, chronic intestinal (>1-mo duration)
Kaposi sarcoma
Lymphoma, Burkitt (or equivalent term)
Lymphoma, immunoblastic (or equivalent term)
Lymphoma, primary, of brain
Mycobacterium avium complex of *M. kansasii*, disseminated or
    extrapulmonary
Mycobacterium tuberculosis, any site (pulmonary or extrapulmonary)
Mycobacterium, other species or unidentified species, disseminated or
    extrapulmonary
Pneumocystis carinii pneumonia
Pneumonia, recurrent
Progressive multifocal leukoencephalopathy
Salmonella septicemia, recurrent
Toxoplasmosis of brain
Wasting syndrome due to HIV

AIDS, acquired immunodeficiency syndrome; HIV, human immunodeficiency virus.

heterosexual transmission and continued dissemination among intravenous drug abusers, substantial increases in the rate of new cases of HIV infection have been noted among women and minorities. As of December 1999, 82% of HIV-infected persons were men, 18% were women; 43% were white, 37% were black, and 18% Hispanic. Of new cases of HIV infection, 47% occur in homosexual males, 25% in intravenous drug users, and 10% are acquired through heterosexual contact. AIDS patients are still relatively young, with more than 40% of cases occurring between ages 30 and 39 and about 80% occurring between ages 20 and 45.

The epidemic is more severe in developing nations and in areas where resources are poor, including some areas of the former Soviet Union, Southeast Asia (India, Thailand, Myanmar, Malaysia, and southern China), the Caribbean (including Haiti and the Dominican Republic), and Africa (including the eastern and southern African countries of Botswana, Zimbabwe, Namibia, and Swaziland). In some of these regions, one in four adults may be infected. As of 1998, the worldwide burden was thought to be 33 million people, with a cumulative number of deaths from HIV/AIDS at almost 14 million (14).

Infection occurs through exchange of body fluids during sexual intercourse, infusion of contaminated blood products, needle sharing between intravenous drug users, and vertical perinatal transmission. Transmission through needle-stick injuries to health care professionals is extremely rare; the frequency is reduced by the rigorous application of universal precautions. Guidelines have been developed for postexposure prophylaxis for health care workers; these guidelines assess the infectious risk

of a given exposure and recommend regimens of antiretroviral agents based on this assessment.

The four major causes of disease in HIV infection are as follows: (a) direct HIV-mediated injury of individual organs (e.g., encephalitis, myelitis, cardiomyopathy, nephropathy); (b) immune-mediated phenomena (e.g., glomerulonephritis and immune thrombocytopenic purpura); (c) immunosuppression-related malignancies (e.g., Kaposi sarcoma and lymphoma); and (d) immunosuppression-related infections (e.g., PCP, tuberculosis, *Candida* esophagitis, cryptococcal meningitis, *Cryptosporidium* or *Isospora* enteritis, disseminated MAI disease, disseminated CMV with chorioretinitis, and *T. gondii* brain abscess) (15).

The role of the intensivist in the care of the HIV patient has undergone a substantial evolution in the last decade. In the initial phases of the epidemic, many intensivists believed that AIDS represented a terminal condition for which ICU support was inappropriate. This view was supported by early studies that documented mortality in excess of 80% to 90% for AIDS patients requiring ICU admission. The life expectancy of HIV-infected and AIDS patients has improved significantly over the last ten years, however. This is related to improved supportive care (nutrition, general medical care), specific antiretroviral therapy [including combination therapy, e.g., azidothymidine (AZT or zidovudine), didanosine (ddI), dideoxycytidine (zalcitabine or ddC)], and prophylaxis for opportunistic infections (TMP-SMX or inhaled pentamidine for *P. carinii*, rifabutin for MAI). Recent data demonstrate >50% survival of AIDS patients admitted to the ICU. These data suggest that intensivists must determine appropriateness of ICU support for HIV-positive patients on an individual basis.

As when caring for other immunosuppressed patients, the clinician should have an idea of likely pathogens to help delineate a diagnostic strategy and determine empiric therapy. In the absence of antiretroviral therapy, immunodeficiency progresses during the course of HIV infection. An untreated patient in the early phase of HIV infection is likely to be less immunosuppressed than a patient who has harbored HIV for a longer period. There is, however, naturally an exceptional amount of intraindividual variation in this phenomenon. In addition, the advent of effective antiretroviral therapy has substantially confounded the association of duration of infection with degree of immunosuppression. An accurate way to define a patient's risk status is through the CD4 (T4 helper cell) count (15,16) (Fig. 5). These lymphocytes, which are responsible for controlling cell-mediated immune functions, are directly infected by HIV. Depletion leads to the classic opportunistic infections of AIDS.

A CD4 count of greater than 800 cells per microliter (close to normal range) is associated with essentially normal immune function. Infections in such patients generally reflect standard community-acquired pathogens. HIV-related malignancies and tuberculosis are among the HIV-associated conditions that may present at modest levels of CD4 depletion (500–800 cells/μL). In fact, tuberculosis can occur at any CD4 count and provides synergistic suppression of cell-mediated immunity with active disease. With higher CD4 counts, upper lobe disease and cavitation are typical. As CD4 counts decline, miliary disease, adenopathy, and lower-lobe infiltrates become more frequent. With CD4 counts of 500 cells per microliter or less, classic opportunistic

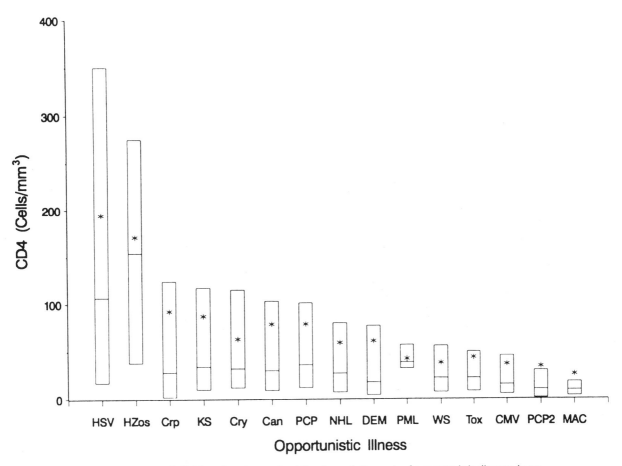

FIGURE 5. Range of CD4 lymphocyte counts at the time of diagnosis of opportunistic diseases in patients with human immunodeficiency virus (HIV) infection. Boxes represent the 25th to 75th percentiles, bars represent medians, and asterisks represent means. Can, *Candida* esophagitis; CMV, cytomegalovirus; Crp, cryptosporidiosis; Cry, cryptococcosis; Enc, HIV encephalopathy; HSV, herpes simplex virus; Hzos, herpes zoster; KS, Kaposi sarcoma; MAC, *Mycobacterium avium* complex; NHL, non-Hodgkin lymphoma; PCP, first episodes of *Pneumocystis carinii* pneumonia; PCP2, recurrent *P.carinii* pneumonia; PML, progressive multifocal leukoencephalopathy; Tox, toxoplasmosis; WS, wasting syndrome. (From Moore RD, Chaisson RE. Natural history of opportunistic disease in an HIV-infected urban cohort. *Ann Intern Med* 1996;124:633–642, with permission.)

infections begin to appear. At this CD4 count, HIV-infected patients become susceptible to esophageal candidiasis as well as reactivation of herpes simplex and varicella zoster. Low-grade fevers and unexplained weight loss also may be noted. Significant risk for PCP begins at CD4 counts under 200 to 300 cells per microliter. Disseminated disease resulting from reactivation of histoplasmosis or coccidioidomycosis in patients with a history of habitation or travel in an endemic area also occurs in this range. Below 100 cells per microliter, infection with *T. gondii* (encephalitis), *Cryptococcus neoformans* (meningitis), and disseminated *M. tuberculosis* can be anticipated. Below 50 cells per microliter, pathogens such as *Cryptosporidia* (enteritis), *Microsporidia* (enteritis), *Isospora* (enteritis), MAI, CMV, and JC virus (progressive multifocal leukoencephalopathy) begin to present. CNS lymphoma also presents at these low CD4 counts. Concurrent with defects of cell-mediated immunity, HIV infection also may result in humoral immune defects by reducing immunoglobulin production by B-lymphocytes. This leads to a susceptibility to infections by encapsulated bacteria, such as *S. pneumoniae* and *H. influenza*. Less commonly used clinically, the HIV viral load is also predictive of the degree of immunosuppression and the range of opportunistic infections to which a given patient is susceptible.

With the advent of highly effective combination antiretroviral therapy, the CD4 count of a patient may rise over time, with reconstitution of clones of CD4 cells and immune recovery. Immune recovery, however, may be incomplete, with specific defects within the immune system remaining despite overall recovery of the CD4 level. Despite these potential defects in specific CD4 clones, several studies have shown low rates of new infections with *P. carinii* or MAI when prophylaxis was stopped after CD4 count rises above the threshold for prophylaxis. Immune recovery also can result in so-called immune-reconstitution syndromes, in which immunity presumably is regained to pathogens infecting a patient, resulting in acute onset of inflammation and immune response to infected sites. Such responses have been described in patients with infections with CMV, MAI, and hepatitis C.

Respiratory failure with fever, hypoxemia, and diffuse pulmonary infiltrates is the most common syndrome in HIV-positive

ICU patients. As noted, the probable pathogen is dependent on the degree of immunosuppression, as reflected by the CD4 count. Standard community-acquired pulmonary pathogens are seen in patients with normal CD4 counts. Fungal pulmonary infections and PCP become more common as CD4 counts fall. CMV pneumonitis is infrequent in patients with CD4 counts greater than 50 cells per microliter. Geographic locale also affects the prevalence of specific pulmonary infections in HIV-positive patients. Tuberculosis is a serious concern in urban centers. In the Ohio River Valley, pulmonary histoplasmosis may be seen as frequently as is PCP. Similarly, in the southwest United States, pulmonary coccidioidomycosis becomes a significant concern.

The diagnostic approach to respiratory failure in HIV-seropositive patients with diffuse pulmonary infiltrates involves an aggressive assessment (Fig. 1). Definitive diagnosis depends on demonstration of the organism. Induced sputum has a 70% to 90% sensitivity for *P. carinii* (less if the patient is receiving inhaled pentamidine prophylaxis) and is also very useful for the diagnosis of bacterial, mycobacterial, and fungal pneumonias. If such samples do not yield a diagnosis, BAL (with or without transbronchial biopsy) is indicated. The sensitivity of BAL for the diagnosis of PCP in HIV-positive patients approaches 100%. BAL is also highly effective in the diagnosis of bacterial, mycobacterial, and fungal pneumonias; OLB is rarely required. Ancillary diagnostic tests include serum for *Cryptococcus* antigen and urine for *Histoplasma* antigen. Serum lactate dehydrogenase has been proposed as a marker for PCP, but it is also known to be elevated in other pulmonary processes that can produce diffuse infiltrates, including other forms of pneumonia, pulmonary embolism with infarction, and lymphoma.

The most common cause of pneumonia (and the most common opportunistic infection) in HIV-seropositive patients with significant CD4 depletion is *P. carinii* (17). Historically, as many as 80% of HIV-positive patients have eventually developed PCP. In contrast to its presentation in other immunosuppressed patients, in whom the onset may be relatively rapid, PCP in HIV-positive patients typically presents with gradually progressive fever, nonproductive cough, and shortness of breath over a period of weeks. The chest radiograph typically shows diffuse interstitial infiltrates without effusions, but these can appear early in the course. On rare occasions, atypical patterns, including lobar involvement or nodules, can be found.

Cytomegalovirus also can be frequently isolated from the lungs of HIV-positive patients who are ill enough to undergo BAL; however, CMV can be isolated from the body fluids of most CMV-seropositive patients with CD4 counts below 100 cells per microliter. A diagnosis of CMV pneumonia requires either cytologic evidence of cytopathic effect with intranuclear viral inclusions or concurrent CMV disease in other organs (e.g., CMV chorioretinitis). *M. tuberculosis* also can cause a diffuse pneumonitis. Although MAI is common in AIDS patients, it typically presents in disseminated form, causing fever and weight loss but rarely pneumonitis. *Cryptococcus* typically presents with indolent meningitis but can cause diffuse pneumonia. Blastomycosis, histoplasmosis, and coccidioidomycosis are relevant in specific geographic areas. Nonspecific interstitial pneumonitis, pulmonary Kaposi sarcoma, and pulmonary lymphoma also can cause respiratory failure with diffuse infiltrates but usually do not present with fever.

Any HIV-positive patient with pneumonitis who requires ICU support should have an urgent, aggressive diagnostic assessment, with BAL if necessary. Pending the results, empiric broad-spectrum antibiotic therapy based on the CD4 count and geographic locale is appropriate. Patients with CD4 counts greater than 200 to 300 cells per microliter should be treated with standard regimens to cover typical and atypical community-acquired pneumonia. If the CD4 count is below that level, TMP-SMX should be added to the standard regimen to ensure coverage of *P. carinii*. Depending on the geographic locale, a low index of suspicion can be used to initiate antifungal therapy. Treatment can be narrowed once a firm diagnosis is made.

If *P. carinii* is confirmed and the patient's partial pressure of oxygen in arterial blood (PaO_2) is less than 70 mm Hg on room air, then 40 mg of prednisone or an equivalent should be given twice daily for 5 days, followed by 40 mg once daily of a prednisone equivalent for 5 days, and then 20 mg daily for 11 days (total of 21 days). This regimen has been shown to improve the mortality rate for patients with severe PCP. If the patient's condition fails to improve after 5 to 10 days, the clinician should reevaluate the diagnosis and, if necessary, repeat the BAL. Concurrent CMV pneumonitis and bacterial superinfection should be considered. If PCP without coinfection or superinfection is confirmed, some authorities advocate switching to intravenously administered pentamidine. Continued failure to respond after 2 weeks is associated with a poor outcome.

Apart from pneumonia, the other frequent cause of ICU admission in HIV-positive patients is CNS dysfunction (Fig. 6) (18). Fever and headache in an HIV-positive patient necessitate an urgent evaluation. Unless the history and physical examination are entirely benign (no evidence of altered level of consciousness, focal neurologic deficits, or seizures), the patient should undergo an enhanced CT scan or MRI. Evidence of cerebral toxoplasmosis; CNS lymphoma; brain abscesses caused by bacteria, *Nocardia*, or *M. tuberculosis*; or encephalitis due to herpes, CMV, or primary HIV infection may be visualized. Although progressive multifocal leukoencephalopathy, caused by the JC virus, can cause CNS lesions in HIV-infected individuals, fever is uncommon. In the absence of an intracranial lesion or mass effect, a lumbar puncture should be performed. The CSF should be examined and cultured for bacteria, mycobacteria, fungi, and viruses. The CSF can be used to diagnose meningitis resulting from standard bacterial pathogens and opportunistic infections, including meningitis due to *Cryptococcus* and *M. tuberculosis*. Detection of p24 HIV antigen or HIV DNA by PCR may indicate primary HIV meningitis. In the appropriate clinical context, PCR also may be useful in defining HSV encephalitis or meningitis. Serum and CSF cryptococcal antigen may be useful in diagnosing cryptococcal meningitis. If an intracranial lesion or lesions are noted, the absence of serum *T. gondii* antibody can rule out cerebral toxoplasmosis.

Initially, management should focus on airway protection and aggressive therapy of seizures. If the presentation involves altered mental status with focal neurologic signs or seizures in a patient with a CD4 count of less than 100 cells per microliter who has not been receiving prophylaxis with TMP-SMX, cerebral toxoplasmosis should be suspected. Cerebral toxoplasmosis is seen in 4% of American but in 25% of French AIDS patients during the course of their illness. The incidence is probably related to

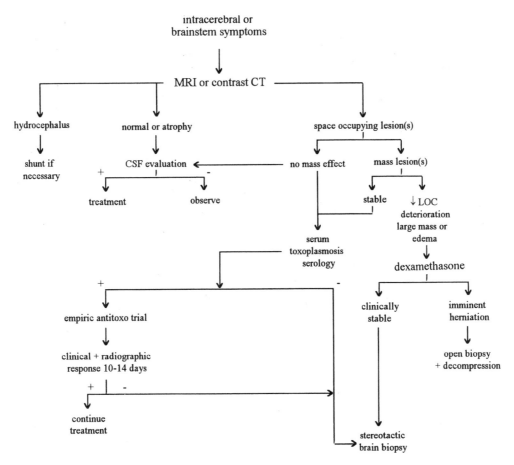

FIGURE 6. Diagnostic approach to central nervous system (CNS) abnormalities in human immunodeficiency virus (HIV) infection. MRI, magnetic resonance imaging; CT, computerized axial tomography; CSF, cerebrospinal fluid; LOC, level of consciousness. (Adapted from Levi RM, Berger JR. Neurologic critical care in patients with human immunodeficiency virus infection. *Crit Care Clin* 1993;9:49–72, with permission.)

T. gondii seroprevalence in the at-risk population (20%–60% in the United States; 80%–90% in France). The CT scan usually shows a ring-enhancing lesion or lesions. Empiric therapy with sulfadiazine and pyrimethamine is appropriate in such cases, even though bacterial or mycobacterial brain abscesses also can exhibit ring enhancement. Corticosteroids may be useful to decrease cerebral edema. If the patient's condition fails to improve within 7 to 10 days, a stereotactic biopsy may be necessary to confirm the diagnosis (18). Therapy for cryptococcal meningitis in HIV patients requires intravenously administered amphotericin B plus flucytosine followed by fluconazole for a minimum of 10 weeks. Chronic suppression is accomplished with lifelong oral fluconazole (19).

As a final note, medication side effects should be considered in the differential diagnosis of the critically ill HIV patient. Many of these pharmacologic complications may be confused with infectious syndromes, including hepatitis, pneumonia, and sepsis with lactic acidosis. Pancreatitis has been well described with pentamidine, TMP-SMX, or steroids (used for *P. carinii*). Cytopenias (like leukopenia or granulocytopenia) may occur with ganciclovir, TMP-SMX, and pentamidine. Antiretroviral medications themselves have complications: Pancreatitis has been described with ddI, ddC, and 3TC and cytopenias with AZT. The drug abacavir can cause an idiosyncratic hypersensitivity reaction, which can present with headache, rash, malaise, or respiratory complaints;

after onset of symptoms, rechallenge with the drug can cause death. Nucleoside reverse transcriptase inhibitors (e.g., stavudine) may rarely cause a type B lactic acidosis. This syndrome occurs mainly in patients with prior exposure to the drug, may have an increased association with d4T use, and is theorized to occur due to mitochondrial toxicity; therapy is with supportive care. Nonnucleoside reverse transcriptase inhibitors (e.g., nevirapine) have been reported to cause liver failure as an idiosyncratic drug reaction.

INFECTIONS IN PATIENTS WITH HUMORAL IMMUNE DEFECTS, ASPLENIA, OR COMPLEMENT DEFICIENCY

Defects of humoral immunity, complement deficiencies, and functional or anatomic asplenia impair clearance of extracellular bacteria. This results in a predisposition to bacteremia and shock as a result of encapsulated organisms.

Multiple myeloma and chronic lymphocytic leukemia represent the most common causes of a dominant defect of humoral immune function (20). Multiple myeloma causes a decrease in synthesis and an increase in the degradation of normal immunoglobulins. As the tumor burden increases, normal B-lymphocytes and plasma cells are suppressed, resulting in a decrease of normal antibodies to encapsulated bacteria. Although the humoral defect is clinically dominant, elements of functional complement deficiency, cellular immune impairment, and granulocyte dysfunction are present as the disease advances. In the late stages, as marrow is replaced by malignant cells, neutropenia may develop.

Pneumococcal infections, including pneumonia, meningitis, and septic shock, are the leading concern in this group of patients. *H. influenzae* (pneumonia, septic shock) and *N. meningitidis* (meningitis, septic shock) are the next leading pathogens. *Klebsiella* (pneumonia) and *E. coli* (pyelonephritis) infections are also common. Appropriate management requires an awareness that infections in these patients may progress rapidly into fulminant septic shock. Culture and gram stain of appropriate body fluids should be rapidly followed by the empiric administration of broad-spectrum antibiotics, including a β-lactam.

Anatomic (surgical excision for trauma, chronic lymphocytic leukemia, Hodgkin disease) and functional (sickle cell disease) asplenia leads to impairment of clearance of nonopsonized bacteria and, to a lesser extent, opsonized bacteria (20,21). Asplenia also is associated with deficiencies of specific complement factors (such as properdin), defective neutrophil phagocytosis (the spleen synthesizes tuftsin, a basic peptide that enhances granulocyte function), and impaired humoral immune function (the primary immunoglobulin response occurs in the spleen). All splenectomized patients should receive pneumococcal and meningococcal vaccination. Regular revaccination is required to maintain protective antibody titers. Children also should receive *H. influenzae* vaccination.

Overwhelming septicemia occurs in about 5% of patients splenectomized as adults for staging of hematologic malignancy or treatment of hematologic disorders. The risk is lower for otherwise healthy patients with splenectomy due to trauma. Septic shock with purpura fulminans caused by *S. pneumoniae* is a well-reported phenomenon (22). Occasional cases have been associated with *N. meningitidis* and *H. influenzae*. Mortality is extremely high (approaching 80%) and severe morbidity with multiple amputations is typical among survivors.

Fever in an asplenic patient requires immediate treatment with antipneumococcal antibiotics. Sepsis in these patients is a medical emergency in which imminent pneumococcal septic shock must be considered. Such patients should receive high-dose parenteral antipneumococcal antibiotics and an aggressive diagnostic assessment that includes culture of blood and sputum, sinus and chest radiographs, and, if indicated, a lumbar puncture for CSF examination. Given the increasing incidence of penicillin-resistant pneumococci in many parts of the country (>15%–20%), the optimal regimen combines high dose ceftriaxone (or cefotaxime) with vancomycin. If the clinical suspicion of meningeal involvement is high or CSF is shown to harbor organisms, rifampin may be useful because vancomycin does not penetrate the blood–brain barrier well. Once sensitivities of the organism are established, therapy can be narrowed. For an asplenic patient with pneumococcal septicemia, the best chance of survival lies in rapid, empiric initiation of appropriate antibiotic therapy along with supportive care. Asplenic patients are also at risk for fulminant infections with intraerythrocyte protozoa such as *Plasmodium malariae* and *Babesia*.

Patients with congenital deficiencies of functional complement components are rare (20). Such patients tend to be susceptible to severe and potentially overwhelming infections with encapsulated bacteria such as *N. meningitidis*, *S. pneumoniae*, and less commonly, *N. gonorrhoeae* or *H. influenzae*. Culture of blood, CSF, and joint fluid may be required. Empiric therapy with a nonantipseudomonal third-generation cephalosporin is usually sufficient. The most common cause of a relatively isolated hypocomplementemia is systemic lupus erythematosus (SLE). Hypocomplementemia may be partially responsible for the predisposition of patients with SLE to overwhelming pneumococcal infections.

NONSPECIFIC IMMUNODEFICIENCY STATES AND INFECTION

A number of diseases and other conditions that do not specifically impair immune function can cause immunocompromise secondarily. Each results in a predisposition to severe, potentially life-threatening infections. Such conditions include protein–calorie malnutrition, diabetes, renal failure, and hepatic failure.

There is a bidirectional relationship between nutrition and infection. A deficient nutritional state predisposes toward infection while infection increases the metabolic rate and nutritional requirements. Malnutrition is both a risk factor and an aggravating factor for infection (20,23). Although the leading cause of immunodeficiency on a worldwide level, malnutrition has not been well appreciated as a cause of immunosuppression related infections. It results in a myriad of immune function abnormalities that involve T-cell, B-cell, neutrophil, and complement function. These include thymic and lymph node atrophy, impaired T-cell-dependent B-lymphocyte responses, reductions in CD4 count, and impaired neutrophil chemotaxis/bactericidal activity. In addition, vitamin and mineral deficiency (zinc, copper, vitamin A, vitamin B6, folate, biotin, thiamine, riboflavin) in chronic malnutrition can impair leukocyte function. Defects of cell-mediated immunity are most important clinically. In the first half of this century, before the advent of pharmacologic immunosuppression and HIV infection, PCP, the classic opportunistic infection of cellular immune depression, was primarily known as a disease of malnourished infants. Rare cases are still reported. Malnutrition also results in increased susceptibility to and severity of measles infections in the developing world. In addition, the risk of progressive tuberculosis and herpes virus infections is also elevated. Finally, malnutrition also is associated with impaired wound healing and increased wound infections. The important role of nutrition in ensuring an appropriate immune response is reflected in recent efforts to optimize the nutritional status of critically ill patients.

Diabetes, in contrast to malnutrition, is well known to be associated with increased risk of infection (20). The cause is not entirely clear. Possibilities include the direct consequences of diabetic vasculopathy or neuropathy as well as the indirect consequences of diabetic hyperglycemia that impair neutrophil chemotaxis, adherence, and phagocytosis. Increased glucose concentration in urine and mucosal secretions leading to increased colonization with bacteria and *Candida* species also may contribute. As a consequence of these factors, diabetics have an increased risk for a variety of life-threatening infections, including bacterial pyelonephritis, pulmonary tuberculosis, and necrotizing polymicrobial cellulitis.

Two life-threatening conditions almost unique to diabetics deserve special mention (24). Invasive ("malignant") external otitis is a necrotizing infection of the external auditory canal and surrounding tissues. The condition presents with severe ear pain, otitis externa, and radiographic evidence of erosion through the auditory canal. Patients may appear toxic. Cultures of blood and otic discharge or tissue should be obtained because, although *P. aeruginosa* is almost universally the cause, rare cases have been caused by *S. aureus*, *Klebsiella oxytoca*, *Actinomyces*, and *Aspergillus*. Prompt treatment with a combination of two antipseudomonal drugs should be implemented immediately and continued for 4 to 8 weeks. Optimal therapy also demands rigorous control of blood sugars and avoidance of ketoacidosis. Surgical debridement is occasionally required. Despite aggressive treatment, the mortality rate remains at 10% to 20% (60% in the face of cranial nerve abnormalities).

Rhinocerebral mucormycosis (*zygomycosis*) is a devastating necrotizing fungal infection seen in diabetics (most frequently in association with diabetic ketoacidosis) and in patients with severe granulocytopenia. The infection, acquired by inhaling spores that are ubiquitous in the environment, begins in the nasal passage and extends to the paranasal sinuses. The infection may spread to the orbit or directly to the frontal lobe of the brain. The presentation is typically fulminant. Clinical signs include lethargy, palatine or nasal necrotic lesions, and evidence of ocular and periocular involvement. Cranial nerve palsies and thrombosis of the cavernous sinus, carotid artery, and jugular vein may occur. Although a CT or MRI may help to delineate the extent of disease, a biopsy is required for a definitive diagnosis. Treatment requires a combination of rigorous control of blood sugars with avoidance of ketoacidosis, high-dose amphotericin B (1–1.5 mg/kg daily to a total of 2–3 g typically) and aggressive surgical debridement. Some suggest the addition of rifampin for synergy with amphotericin B. Despite aggressive management, mortality is substantial.

Renal failure and its management are associated with defects of both specific and nonspecific elements of host defenses (20,25). Defects of nonspecific defenses include vascular and peritoneal access devices for dialysis. Specific immune defense elements are impaired by exposure of blood to hemodialysis membranes (complement depletion, leukocyte dysfunction) and by the direct effects of uremia, which cause cellular immune deficits (thymic atrophy, lymphopenia, decreased interferon production, and impaired delayed hypersensitivity responses). Splenic clearance of opsonized and nonopsonized pathogens also appears to be defective as does neutrophil chemotaxis and phagocytosis. The result is a propensity to infections associated with breaches of integumentary barriers (intravenous catheter related infections, peritonitis in peritoneal dialysis patients, urinary tract infections, wound infections) and with specific immune deficits (PCP, esophageal candidiasis, chronic viral hepatitis, bacterial pneumonia, and bacteremia). Infection is the leading cause of death (30%–70%) in patients with acute renal failure.

Finally, hepatic failure and end-stage cirrhosis represent an immunocompromised state (20,26). Serious infections develop in as many as 80% of patients with fulminant hepatic failure. Approximately a quarter will demonstrate bacteremia. At least three factors will place such patients at increased risk of infection. First, in hepatic failure, the Kupffer cells of the liver fail to clear the many enteric bacteria normally found in the portal venous flow, resulting in systemic bacteremia. Second, the liver synthesizes 90% of the complement components and is the major organ through which opsonized pathogens (primarily bacteria) are removed. Hepatic failure severely impairs this function both by reducing opsonizing complement and by damaging the liver's ability to clear opsonized (and nonopsonized) organisms. Finally, patients with fulminant hepatic failure and end-stage cirrhosis require supportive care (endotracheal intubation, intravascular devices, urinary catheterization), which breaches normal mucocutaneous barriers to infection. Most also require substantial coagulation support with pooled blood products, which can carry a variety of infections.

Hepatic failure is associated with a marked increase in a broad range of bacterial infections. The primary sites of involvement are respiratory, urinary, and peritoneal. Staphylococcal species (intravascular catheter infections) and gram-negative rods (pneumonia, urinary tract infection) are common isolates. Bacteremia with enteric organisms is frequent as a consequence of the damaged liver's inability to clear enteric bacteria in the portal circulation. These organisms may seed to the peritoneum where, in the presence of ascites, spontaneous bacterial peritonitis may result. Because of the impairment of the inflammatory response (complement depletion) and frequent encephalopathy, clinical findings such as fever, peritoneal signs, and abdominal pain may be equivocal or absent. The diagnosis is best made by the presence of an ascitic leukocyte count over 250 per microliter or isolation of a single organism from ascitic fluid inoculated directly into blood culture bottles. Pneumococci and enteric gram-negative rods (*E. coli* and *Klebsiella*) account for more than 75% of cases. Surgical peritonitis is indicated by a leukocyte count greater than 10,000 per microliter or polymicrobial or anaerobic organisms. Treatment of spontaneous bacterial peritonitis is with a non-antipseudomonal third-generation cephalosporin such as cefotaxime or ceftriaxone. Patients with hepatic failure are also susceptible to fungal infections, mostly with *Candida* species. These may be seen in 25% to 33% of patients, particularly those with renal failure and prolonged antibiotic therapy.

SUMMARY

With the increasing ability of medicine to support aggressively patients with chronic or previously fatal illnesses (including AIDS and malignancy) through ICU supportive care, organ transplantation, and chemotherapy, the population of patients with ongoing risk for severe infections is exploding. The approach to infection in these immunocompromised patients is similar to that in other critically ill patients, although the spectrum of causative organisms may be broader, leading to differences in the diagnostic approach and therapeutic management. Fundamental to the approach to infection in immunocompromised patients is the concept that the probable etiologic organisms are predictable based primarily on awareness of the immunologic defect and its duration. With a rational assessment of each patient's specific risks, timely initiation of appropriate empiric therapy, and an application of an aggressive diagnostic algorithm, outcome for each individual can be optimized.

KEY POINTS

Immunocompromised patients are vulnerable to an exceptionally broad variety of infections, including those caused by newly acquired opportunistic pathogens, reactivation of latent organisms, and typical community or nosocomial pathogens. The most likely pathogens at any given point are predictable in immunocompromised patients.

The keys to determining probable etiologies of infection include knowledge of the nature of the immune defect (humoral, cell-mediated, neutrophil) and the duration and severity of the defects. Severely neutropenic (<100 PMN/μL) patients are susceptible to bacterial infections within the first weeks of severe neutropenia and fungal infections thereafter; recovery typically ensues as PMN levels climb over 500 per microliter. In solid-organ transplant recipients, standard perioperative infections are common during the early perioperative period, with opportunistic pathogens dominating between 1 and 6 months; successful engraftment is associated with a relatively normal infection profile after 6 months. In bone marrow transplant recipients, neutropenia-associated bacterial and fungal infections are common during the first 20 to 30 days, whereas cytomegalovirus (CMV) and *Pneumocystis carinii* pneumonia (PCP) dominate from 30 to 100 days posttransplant; varicella-zoster virus (VZV) and viral respiratory infections are problematic after 100 days.

In human immunodeficiency virus (HIV)-positive patients, CD4 helper lymphocyte counts define the risk for specific infections: counts above 500 are associated with a normal pattern of infectious risk; 250 to 500 with *Candida* esophagitis; below 300 with PCP; below 100 with *T. gondii* central nervous system disease or cryptococcal meningitis; and below 50 with CMV disease, *Mycobacterium avium* intracellulare (MAI) infection, or enteritis due to *Cryptosporidium*, *Microsporidia*, or *Isospora*. Humoral or complement defects and asplenia predispose to bacterial infections and septic shock, particularly with encapsulated organisms.

Early assessment, careful evaluation of subtle clinical findings, aggressive diagnostic testing (including invasive procedures where necessary), empiric broad-spectrum antimicrobial therapy, and reduction of immunosuppression where possible are key to the successful management of infections.

The future will see an increase in the overall incidence of infections in immunocompromised patients as a result of an increasingly aged and chronically ill population. Concurrently, emerging pathogens such as methicillin-resistant *S. aureus*, vancomycin-resistant enterococci, multidrug-resistant tuberculosis, HIV, and CMV will continue to alter the infectious disease landscape.

These changes will be matched by the advances in both diagnosis and therapy of disease in the immunocompromised host. In the past decade, diagnostic advances have included lysis-centrifugation blood cultures for bacteria and yeasts, shell-vial cultures for CMV, and immunofluorescent and enzyme-linked immunoassays for detection of cryptococcal, *Legionella* and various bacterial antigens. Polymerase chain reaction has begun to emerge as a broad-based diagnostic tool. Future developments may include improvements in nuclear imaging (e.g., indium-111-labelled immunoglobulin G and magnetic resonance imaging). Advances in therapy over the last decade include antivirals such as acyclovir, ribavirin, ganciclovir, zidovudine, dideoxyinosine, nevirapine, and interferon-α; antibacterials such as the new quinolones (levofloxacin, gatifloxacin), new carbapenems (meropenem), and fourth-generation cephalosporins (cefepime) with enhanced gram-positive, gram-negative, or anaerobic activity as well as streptogramins (quinupristin/dalfopristin) and oxazolidinones (linezolid) for methicillin-resistant *S. aureus* and vancomycin-resistant enterococci; antifungals, such as liposomal amphotericin B, echinocandins (caspofungin), and the new triazoles (itraconazole, voriconazole); and various antiparasitics such as atovaquone for PCP. Nearing release or late in development are a variety of new agents including new glycylcylcines, ketolides, and everninomycines for gram-positive infections, other echinocandins/pneumocandins for *P. carinii* and fungal infections, and novel protease inhibitors for HIV infection.

Despite continued diagnostic and therapeutic advances, management of infections in the immunocompromised will remain problematic. Outcome will remain dependent on a high index of suspicion resulting in an early diagnosis and specific pharmacotherapy.

REFERENCES

1. Anonymous. Rapid diagnostic tests for tuberculosis: what is the appropriate use? American Thoracic Society Workshop. *Am J Respir Crit Care Med* 1997;155:1497–1498.
2. Pizzo PA. Management of fever in patients with cancer and treatment-induced neutropenia. *N Engl J Med* 1993;328:1323–1332.
3. Hughes WT, Armstrong D, Bodey GP, et al. The Infectious Disease Society of America. Use of antimicrobial agents in neutropenic patients with unexplained fever. *Clin Infect Dis* 1997;25:551–573.
4. Rubin RH. Infection in the organ transplant recipient. In: Rubin RH, Young LS, eds. *Clinical approach to infection in the compromised host.* New York: Plenum, 1994;629–707.
5. Rubin RH, Wolfson JS, Cosimi AB, et al. Infection in the renal transplant recipient. *Am J Med* 1981;70:405–411.
6. Winston DJ, Emmanouilides C, Busuttil RW. Infections in liver transplant patients. *Clin Infect Dis* 1995;21:1077–1091.
7. Patel R, Paya C. Infections in solid organ transplant recipients. *Clin Microbiol Rev* 1997;10:86–124.
8. Mahmoud A. Strongyloidiasis. *Clin Invest Dis* 1996;23:949–953.
9. Bowden RA, Meyers JD. Infection complicating bone marrow transplantation. In: Rubin RH, Young LS, eds. *Clinical approach to infection in the compromised host.* New York: Plenum, 1994:601–628.
10. Schimpff SC. Infection in bone marrow transplantation: a model for examining predisposing factors to infection in cancer patients. *Recent Results Cancer Res* 1993;132:15–34.

11. Van Burik J, Weisdorf D. Infections in recipients of blood and marrow transplantation. In: Mandell GL, Bennett JE, Dolin R, eds. *Principles and practice of infectious diseases*, 5th ed. Philadelphia: Churchill Livingstone, 2000:3136–3147.

12. Centers for Disease Control and Prevention. 1993 Revised classification system for HIV infection and expanded surveillance case definitions for AIDS among adolescents and adults. *MMWR Morb Mortal Wkly Rep* 1992;41:1–19.

13. UNAIDS and WHO. *AIDS epidemic update, 1998*. Geneva: UNAIDS, 1998.

14. Chaisson RE, Sterling TR, Gallant JE. General clinical manifestations of human immunodeficiency virus infection. In: Mandell GL, Bennett JE, Dolin R, eds. *Principles and practice of infectious diseases*, 5th ed. Philadelphia: Churchill Livingstone. 2000:1398–1415.

15. Powderly WG. Prophylaxis for opportunistic infections in an era of effective antiretroviral therapy. *Clin Infect Dis* 2000;31:597–601.

16. Moore RD, Chaisson RE. Natural history of opportunistic disease in an HIV-infected urban cohort. *Ann Intern Med* 1996;124:633–642.

17. Bartlett MS, Smith JW. *Pneumocystis carinii*, an opportunist in immunocompromised patients. *Clin Microbiol Rev* 1991;4:137–149.

18. Levy RM, Berger JR. Neurologic critical care in patients with human immunodeficiency virus infection. *Crit Care Clin* 1993;9:49–72.

19. Saag MS, Graybill RJ, Larson RA, et al. The Infectious Diseases Society of America. Practice guidelines for the management of cryptococcal disease. *Clin Infect Dis* 2000;30:710–718.

20. Van der Meer JW. Defects in host defense mechanisms. In: Rubin RH, Young LS, eds. *Clinical approach to infection in the compromised host*. New York: Plenum, 1994:33–66.

21. Fabri PJ. Postsplenectomy infections. In: Fry DE, ed. *Surgical infections*. Boston: Little, Brown, 1995:565–568.

22. Schwartz PE, Sterioff S, Mucha P, et al. Post-splenectomy sepsis and mortality in adults. *JAMA* 284;1982:2279–2283.

23. Chandra RK. Nutrition and immunity. In: Lackham PJ, Peters K, Rosen FS, et al., eds. *Clinical aspects of immunology*. London: Blackwell Scientific, 1993:1325–1328.

24. Tiemey MR, Baker AS. Infections of the head and neck in diabetes mellitus. *Infect Dis Clin North Am* 1995;9:195–216.

25. Montgomerie JZ, Kalmanson OM, Guze LB. Renal failure and infection. *Medicine (Baltimore)* 1968;47:1–32.

26. Wilcox CM, Dismukes WE. Spontaneous bacterial peritonitis. A review of pathogenesis, diagnosis, and treatment. *Medicine (Baltimore)* 1987;66:447–456.

THE USE OF ANTIMICROBIALS IN THE INTENSIVE CARE UNIT

EUGENE Y. CHENG
CYNTHIA R. HENNEN

KEY WORDS

- Antibacterial agents
- Antifungal agents
- Antimicrobial use
- Antiviral agents
- Bacterial resistance

INTRODUCTION

Antimicrobial agents account for approximately one-third of a hospital's formulary budget. Antimicrobials are used for patients on various hospital wards, but nowhere are they used more frequently and in more combinations than in the intensive care unit (ICU). Patients admitted to the ICU with overwhelming community-acquired or nosocomial infections often require the use of a wide variety and different combinations of antibiotic medications because of the resistant and virulent nature of the infecting organism. Patient history and clinical findings are key in selecting antimicrobial agents for empiric therapy. Positive culture results with antibiotic sensitivities are helpful in ensuring effective antimicrobial therapy. Appropriate selection, dosage, and timing of antibiotic administration decrease morbidity and mortality and help reduce drug toxicity and cost.

PRINCIPLES OF THERAPY

Diagnosis

Before initiating antimicrobial therapy, the clinician should be fairly certain that the systemic inflammatory reaction is secondary to infection and should collect specimens for Gram stain and culture. Microscopic examination of the Gram-stained specimen can provide the earliest information about the microbial pathogen; cultures of blood, urine, or sputum may be positive as soon as 18 to 24 hours after incubation. Unfortunately, more often than not, the infecting organism is not detected through routine cultures of blood and other body fluids. New culturing techniques, such as adding resins to the blood-culture medium, may increase the yield in the presence of antimicrobial therapy. DNA probes, antigen assays, and fluorescent antibody staining can help iden-tify the infecting organism in cases in which cultures have been persistently negative. Consideration of epidemiologic and host factors is important in guiding further testing in the patient with an illness that is difficult to diagnose. Computed tomography scan, magnetic resonance imaging, or tissue biopsy of areas likely to be infected (as indicated by host factors) may significantly increase the probability of detecting the infective organism in the patient with a prolonged undiagnosed febrile illness.

Antibiotic Selection

In clinical situations in which the infecting pathogen is known, *in vitro* testing is usually performed to determine the minimum concentrations of an antibiotic necessary to inhibit the growth of most bacteria (MIC). The concentration of antibiotics needed to kill bacteria (MBC) also can be obtained but usually is not needed except for specific circumstances, such as in patients with endocarditis or in those who are neutropenic.

Two common methods of susceptibility testing are in use today: the broth-dilution method and the disk (agar)-diffusion, or Kirby-Bauer, method. In the broth-dilution method, the bacteria are inoculated onto liquid media containing graduated concentrations of the test antimicrobial agents. The bacteria are allowed to grow under controlled conditions for the direct determination of MIC. Although less labor intensive and less expensive than broth dilution, the disk-diffusion method is also less accurate because it does not provide MIC values. This method entails inoculating the test bacteria onto an agar plate, after which a disk containing a standardized amount of antibiotic is placed on the plate. The test bacteria are allowed to grow under controlled conditions while the antimicrobial agent diffuses out into the agar. The distance of no bacterial growth around the disk is measured. The diameter of growth inhibition determines whether the organism is very susceptible, moderately sensitive, or resistant to the tested antibiotics. Disk diffusions are sufficient for determining the susceptibility of many organisms, particularly if susceptibility or resistance to the antibiotic is clear. With intermediate results, however, it is unclear whether a specific antibiotic at its usually achievable tissue concentration will be effective. In these circumstances, determining the specific *in vitro* antibiotic concentration (breakpoint) that is ineffective or effective in bacterial growth

TABLE 1. ANTIBIOTIC SELECTION FOR COMMON BACTERIA ENCOUNTERED IN THE INTENSIVE CARE UNIT

Antibiotic	*Streptococcus*	*Staphylococcus*	Gram-Negative β-Lactamase (Negative)	Gram-Negative β-Lactamase (Positive)	*Pseudomonas*	*Bacteroides Fragilis*
Penicillins						
Penicillin G	1	0	2	0	0	0
Ampicillin	1	0	1	0	0	0
Penicillinase-resistant penicillins						
Penicillin-β-lactamase inhibitor combinations	2	2	1	1	2	2
Antipseudomonal penicillins	1	0	1	1	2	0
Cephalosporins						
1st generation	1[a]	2	2	2	0	0
2nd generation	1[a]	2	2	2	0	0
3rd generation	2[a]	2	1	1	2[b]	0
Ceftazidime	2[a]	0	1	1	1	0
4th generation	1[a]	1	1	1	1	
Macrolides	1[a]	0	2	0	0	0
Tetracyclines	2	0	2	2	0	0
Vancomycin	1	1	0	0	0	0
Trimethoprim-sulfamethoxazole	1[a]	2	1	1	0	0
Chloramphenicol	2[a]	0	2	2	0	0
Aminoglycosides	2	2	1	1	1	0
Clindamycin	2[a]	2	1	1	1	0
Metronidazole	0	0	0	0	0	1
Aztreonam	0	0	1	1	2	0
Imipenem	1	1	1	1	2	1
Ciprofloxacin	2	2	1	1	1	0
Oxizolidinones	1	1	0	0	0	0
Streptogramins	1	1	0	0	0	0

1 = first line; 2 = second line; 0 = minimal activity in vivo.
[a] Except against enterococci, for which activity is zero.
[b] Cefoperazone = 2.

inhibition can be done with serial broth dilution. As with all *in vitro* testing, the results will suggest the potential efficacy of the tested antimicrobial agent. Many factors, however, can affect actual *in vivo* activity, such as the ability of the antibiotic to penetrate into infected tissues or fluid collections, to cross the blood–brain barrier, and to penetrate cellular membranes to reach intracellular organisms.

Empiric therapy may be necessary because the patient's condition mitigates against waiting for culture results or the clinical presentation suggests infection despite the inability to identify a pathogen (Table 1). In choosing an antibiotic or antibiotic combination for empiric therapy, one should consider several important factors: site of the infection as determined by clinical presentation (e.g., meningitis, cellulitis, or pneumonia); regional or hospital-specific bacterial sensitivities; host factors such as immunocompetency, hepatic and renal function, prior antibiotic exposure, and drug allergies; and pharmacokinetics (achieved tissue levels).

ANTIBACTERIAL AGENTS

β-Lactam Antibiotics

The largest group of antimicrobial agents, the β-lactams, is so named because they contain the four-sided β-lactam ring. These antimicrobial agents work primarily by inhibiting the synthesis of and promoting the lysis of bacterial cell walls. The agents included in this category are penicillins, cephalosporins, carbapenems, and monobactams. The β-lactam agents are usually bactericidal, but they may be only bacteriostatic if MIC levels are not reached. Many of these agents can be used effectively against gram-positive and gram-negative organisms.

Penicillins

Penicillins are bactericidal antibiotics that destroy bacteria by causing lysis of the bacterial cell wall. The bactericidal "activity" of a particular penicillin is related to the ability of the penicillin to penetrate the outer wall of a bacterium and the interaction with specific penicillin-binding proteins, which lead to inhibition of cell-wall synthesis or activation of autolytic enzymes. Without intact cell walls, the bacteria either rupture or fail to reproduce.

Penicillins share a basic structure that consists of a thiazolidine ring connected to a β-lactam ring with an attached side chain. The pharmacologic and antibacterial properties of penicillin are modified by altering the side chain. This change in structure results in several groups of penicillin compounds that are effective against a wide variety of bacterial organisms.

The first generation or the naturally occurring penicillins are represented by penicillin G (benzylpenicillin) and penicillin V (phenoxymethyl penicillin). Naturally occurring penicillins are useful for the treatment of gram-positive organisms such as *Streptococcus, Clostridium tetani* and *perfringens,* gram-negative organisms such as *Neisseria meningitides* and *Pasteurella multocida,* and spiral organisms *Leptospira* species and *Treponema pallidum.* The increasing number of organisms that produce penicillinase makes this group of antibiotics less useful than previously. Therefore, subsequent generations of penicillin have been developed.

The next generations of penicillins are based on semisynthetic penicillins. Semisynthetic penicillinase-resistant penicillins were the start of the next three generations. Methicillin, oxacillin, nafcillin, cloxacillin, and dicloxacillin are representatives of this group, which has improved activity against gram-positive organisms, especially penicillin-resistant streptococcus and *Staphylococcus aureus.* The next generation, extended-spectrum penicillins (ampicillin, amoxicillin, bacampicillin), provided increased activity against some of the gram-negative bacilli but are not resistant to the action of penicillinase unless a β-lactamase inhibitor, such as sulbactam is added (Unasyn). In addition to better gram-negative activity, this group of penicillins, particularly ampicillin, has the greatest activity against enterococci. The latest extended-spectrum penicillins, also referred to as the *fourth-generation* or *antipseudomonal* penicillins, provided a wider coverage of gram-negative organisms. These penicillins (mezlocillin, azlocillin, piperacillin), because of their unique structure that allows for greater cell wall penetration and selected affinities for penicillin-binding proteins, produce enhanced gram-negative activity.

β-Lactamase Inhibitors

Clavulanic acid, sulbactam sodium, and tazobactam sodium are based on the β-lactam structure. They have poor intrinsic antimicrobial activity but bind irreversibly to β-lactamases produced by a wide range of gram-negative and gram-positive organisms. The β-lactamases are secreted extracellularly by gram-positive bacteria, but are "cell bound" in the periphery of gram-negative bacteria and present a barrier to the diffusion of penicillins and cephalosporins in microorganisms of the latter group. Antibiotics that are usually substrates for these enzymes can be spared as a result of enzyme inactivation with β-lactamase inhibitors. Thus far, the penicillins are the only group of β-lactams combined with these β-lactamase inhibitors. The addition of these inhibitors to penicillins can extend the penicillins' activity against most β-lactamase-producing strains of bacteria. The β-lactamase enzymes of *Enterobacter* and *Pseudomonas* species are intrinsically resistant to all available inhibitors.

Cephalosporins

Cephalosporins are structurally similar to penicillins and inhibit bacterial cell-wall synthesis in much the same manner as do penicillins. Cephalosporins are divided into "generations," with increasing generations representing broadening of the antibiotic spectrum. First-generation cephalosporins are most active against gram-positive organisms, such as the staphylococci and streptococci. They are not effective against methicillin-resistant strains of staphylococci and have little or no activity against enterococci. They also are not effective against anaerobes and many gram-negative organisms, with the exceptions of *Escherichia coli, Klebsiella,* and *Proteus mirabilis.*

First-generation cephalosporins (cefazolin, cephalexin, and cephalothin) are the most frequently used antibiotics for antimicrobial prophylaxis during operations. Critically ill patients are usually more susceptible to infection because of their immunosuppressed condition and the presence of indwelling catheters. The usual antimicrobial surgical prophylaxis does not need to be changed, however, unless an endemic problem with antibiotic-resistant organisms is present in the ICU. Prophylactic antibiotic therapy should be modified to cover any known resistant organisms. While retaining much of the original gram-positive activity, second-generation cephalosporins also possess greater gram-negative activity than do the first-generation agents. Two second-generation cephalosporins, cefoxitin sodium and cefotetan disodium, also have significant activity against anaerobes. Compared with the second-generation agents, the extended-spectrum or third-generation cephalosporins offer improved gram-negative activity. In general, third-generation cephalosporins (ceffriaxone, cefotaxime, ceftazidime, ceftizoxime) are relatively resistant to β-lactamases and often are reserved for use in patients who have a documented or suspected high risk of being infected with gram-negative organisms.

Fourth-generation cephalosporin antibiotics provide good gram-negative and gram-positive coverage. Currently, cefepime is the only clinically available fourth-generation cephalosporin (1). It has good β-lactamase stability, antipseudomonal activity similar to ceftazidime, and gram-positive activity similar to first-generation cephalosporins. In addition, the drug has been shown to inhibit various *Enterobacteriaceae* resistant to cefotaxime and ceftazidime. Cefepime is similar to other second- and third-generation cephalosporins in that it is not useful against methicillin-resistant staphylococcus or enterococcal species.

Carbapenems

Carbapenems are β-lactam antibiotics that are resistant to most commonly produced β-lactamases and have the broadest activity of any β-lactam agent. Imipenem is prepared in combination with cilastatin. Cilastatin is included to inhibit a renal-tubular enzyme, hydropeptidase, which metabolizes imipenem and produces nephrotoxic metabolites. This drug combination is usually reserved for use against multiple–antibiotic-resistant gram-negative organisms or as an alternative antimicrobial agent against enterococci. It can be used as a single agent, but usually it is combined with an aminoglycoside for improved coverage against either gram-negative organisms or enterococci. Resistance to imipenem occurs with most strains of methicillin-resistant *S. aureus,* non-aeruginosa strains of *Pseudomonas,* and *Stenotrophomonas maltophilia.* Another carbapenem, meropenem, has a mechanism of action and indications for use similar to imipenem. Meropenem provides better activity against *Enterobacteriaceae* and some *Pseudomonas* species. Meropenem may be less likely to cause seizures when dosed at higher concentrations. Nephrotoxicity with meropenem is negligible even without a cilastatin component.

Monobactams

Aztreonam, the only monobactam approved for clinical use, is a synthetic β-lactam antibiotic that is structurally different from cephalosporins and penicillins. Its basic structure consists of a monocyclic β-lactam ring. Aztreonam provides selective therapy for gram-negative infections but has no anaerobic or gram-positive coverage. Aztreonam is often considered a nonnephrotoxic substitute for aminoglycosides. It is thought that this narrow spectrum of coverage may decrease disruptions in normal flora, as are seen with the use of broader-spectrum agents.

Distribution and Elimination

Penicillins penetrate well into most areas of the body. Therapeutic concentrations are also achieved in sinus, peritoneal, pleural, pericardial, biliary, and synovial fluids as well as in abscesses. In cerebrospinal fluid (CSF), concentrations are usually less than 17% of plasma values. With the presence of meningeal inflammation, CSF concentration levels may rise to within 5% of plasma concentrations. Distribution to prostatic fluid is low, whereas urinary concentrations are generally high. Most penicillins are excreted in the urine unchanged. Adjustment of dosage is necessary in the presence of severe renal dysfunction, especially if creatinine clearance is less than 30 mL per minute.

Therapeutic cephalosporin levels can be found in most body sites, including bile, pericardial fluid, and synovial fluid. Only third-generation agents and cefepime penetrate the CSF in sufficient concentrations to treat meningitis. Depending on the specific cephalosporin, elimination may be by the renal or hepatic route. All the cephalosporins, including those eliminated primarily by hepatic mechanisms (cephalothin sodium, cefaclor, cefotaxime sodium), provide urine concentrations high enough to treat urinary tract infections. Accumulation of the agents depends on the status of renal clearance mechanisms because of varying degrees of tubular secretion and glomerular filtration. Significant renal or hepatic disease requires dosage adjustments (Table 2).

Imipenem and meropenem are widely distributed to all tissues but enter the CSF in therapeutic levels only in the presence of inflammation. The serum half-life of imipenem increases as creatinine clearance falls, and doses should be modified in patients with impaired renal function. Meropenem does not have to be adjusted for decreased creatinine clearance.

Aztreonam is widely distributed to all body sites and compartments, including the CSF. The drug is removed from the body by glomerular filtration and tubular secretion. The half-life may increase up to 6 hours when creatinine clearance falls below 10 mL per minute.

Adverse Reactions

Adverse reactions with penicillins, fortunately, are few. The most common adverse reactions are minor allergies to antimicrobials in the ICU (Table 3). Minor allergic reactions are manifested by

TABLE 2. ANTIBIOTIC MANAGEMENT FOR PATIENTS WITH RENAL AND HEPATIC DYSFUNCTION

	Requires Dose Adjustment for Renal Dysfunction (CrCl < 30 mL/min)	Requires Dose Adjustment for Hepatic Failure	Serum Concentration Altered by Hemodialysis	Serum Concentration Altered by Peritoneal Dialysis
Penicillins				
Penicillin G	Yes	No	No	No
Ampicillin	Yes	No	Yes	No
Piperacillin	Yes[a]	No	Yes	Yes
Nafcillin	Yes[a]	No	No	No
Cephalosporins				
Cefazolin	Yes	No	Yes	No
Cefotetan	Yes	No	Yes	[b]
Cefuroxime	Yes	No	Yes	No
Cefotaxime	Yes[a]	No	No	No
Ceftazidime	Yes	No	Yes	Yes
Ceftriaxone	Yes[a]	No	No	No
Cefepime	Yes	No	Yes	Yes
Carbapenems	Yes	No	Yes	[b]
Aztreonam	Yes	No	Yes	Yes
Aminoglycosides	Yes	No	Yes	Yes
Quinolones	No	No	No	No
Trimethoprim-sulfamethoxazole	Yes	No	Yes	Yes
Erythromycin	No	Yes	No	No
Clindamycin	No	Yes	No	No
Metronidazole	Yes[a]	No	Yes	[b]
Vancomycin	Yes	No	No	Yes
Chloramphenicol	Yes[a]	Yes	No	No
Linezolid	Yes[a]	No	Yes	Yes
Quinopristim/dalfopristin	Yes	No	No	No

[a]CrCl < 10 mL/min.
[b]No information.

TABLE 3. COMMON ADVERSE REACTIONS TO ANTIBACTERIAL THERAPY

Cutaneous reactions	Morbilliform eruptions
	Urticaria
	Purpura
	Erythema multiforme
	Erythema nodosum
	Exfoliative dermatitis
Generalized hypersensitivity reactions	Fever
	Angioedema
	Serum sickness
	Anaphylactic shock
Mucosal reactions	Dryness, burning, soreness, and itching of the mouth and tongue
GI reactions	Nausea
	Vomiting
	Diarrhea
	Pseudomembranous colitis
	Liver damage
	Fungal overgrowth
	Steatorrhea
Urinary tract complications	Hematuria
	Crystalluria
	Nephrotoxicity
Neurologic reactions	Peripheral neuritis
	Paresthesias
	8th nerve damage
	Sleep disturbance or mood change
	Psychosis or convulsions
	Respiratory paralysis
Hematologic complications	Hemolytic anemia
	Eosinophilia
	Aplastic anemia
	Thrombocytopenia
	Leukopenia
Electrolyte disturbances	Hyperkalemia
	Hypernatremia
	Hypokalemic alkalosis

maculopapular rash, urticaria, and fever, which occur in about 5% of patients taking penicillins. Anaphylaxis occurs in approximately 0.01% of patients who have no previous history of penicillin allergy. Hepatic function abnormalities, such as elevations of serum transaminase or alkaline phosphatase concentrations, often follow the use of high-dose antistaphylococcal penicillins or extended-spectrum antipseudomonal agents. In general, hepatic function rapidly returns to normal when these agents are discontinued.

Allergic reactions to cephalosporins are less common than are reactions to penicillin. Fewer than 5% of individuals who have an anaphylactic reaction to a penicillin will have an anaphylactic reaction to a cephalosporin. Patients who have had minor reactions to penicillin have a minimal risk of developing a cross-reaction with cephalosporins (2). Therefore, a cephalosporin may be given safely to patients who have had only a minor reaction to penicillin. A history of an anaphylactic reaction to a penicillin, however, is a contraindication for the use of cephalosporins.

Carbapenems can cause allergic reactions similar to those produced by penicillins and should not be administered to patients who have had anaphylactic reactions to cephalosporins or peni-

cillins. Seizures resulting from central nervous system (CNS) stimulation from high imipenem levels occur most often in patients with decreased renal function or in patients with an underlying seizure focus. Dose adjustment for patients with renal disease usually prevent imipenem-induced seizures.

Aztreonam is from the monobactam family of β-lactams and does not cross-react with antibodies directed against penicillin and penicillin derivatives. Because of the structural difference, aztreonam can be given safely to patients with a history of anaphylaxis to other β-lactams.

Aminoglycosides

The aminoglycosides are a group of natural and semisynthetic compounds that exert bactericidal action by entering the bacterial cell, binding to 30S ribosomal sites, and inhibiting protein synthesis. Gentamicin sulfate, tobramycin sulfate, and amikacin sulfate are the most frequently used aminoglycosides. Other clinically available aminoglycosides are netilmicin sulfate, kanamycin sulfate, neomycin sulfate, and streptomycin sulfate. Aminoglycosides are frequently used in combination with other antibiotics for empiric therapy in the septic patient.

These drugs are highly effective against gram-negative bacilli but have no activity against anaerobic organisms and only limited activity against aerobic gram-positive cocci. Aminoglycosides with β-lactams or glycopeptides have synergistic activity against enterococcal, staphylococcal, and some streptococcal infections. When aminoglycosides are combined with β-lactams, synergistic activity is seen against most *Enterobacter* and *Pseudomonas* species and against multiresistant strains of many other gram-negative bacilli (3).

Aminoglycosides also have a postantibiotic effect with most gram-negative bacteria. This increased duration of action for a period less than the MIC of the bacterium being treated allows extended-interval dosing when patients achieve adequate peak levels with each dose of aminoglycoside (4).

Distribution and Elimination

Aminoglycosides are distributed into interstitial fluid with a volume of distribution essentially equal to that of extracellular fluid. Aminoglycoside concentrations are highest in the renal cortex, where the drug concentrates in the proximal renal tubular cells. Levels are low in most tissues and do not reliably penetrate into the CSF. Aminoglycosides are eliminated unchanged by glomerular filtration. A small amount undergoes reabsorption into proximal renal tubular cells. Dose adjustments must be made in patients with reduced renal capacity.

Measuring peak serum levels helps the clinician to ensure that therapeutic levels of drug are achieved. Following trough levels determines the rate of drug elimination and helps in calculating dosing intervals.

Adverse Reactions

Aminoglycosides can cause severe renal, vestibular, and cochlear damage. Irreversible ototoxicity usually occurs gradually and is seen most often in patients receiving long-term therapy.

Nephrotoxicity, which can occur after only a few days of therapy, has an initial presentation of proteinuria and renal casts, followed by a reduction in glomerular filtration rate and a rise in the serum creatinine level. Coadministration of aminoglycosides with vancomycin hydrochloride, amphotericin B, cis-platinum, and cyclosporin A, especially in the volume-depleted patient, is associated with increased renal toxicity. Renal function often returns to normal if the aminoglycosides are discontinued before severe renal failure occurs.

Neuromuscular paralysis is a rarely seen adverse reaction associated with aminoglycoside use. Aminoglycosides inhibit the influx of calcium at the presynaptic nerve terminal, preventing the release of acetylcholine in the neuromuscular junction. Prolonged paralysis after the use of neuromuscular blocking agents can be due to the concomitant use of aminoglycosides.

Macrolide and Azalide Antibiotics

Erythromycin is either bactericidal or bacteriostatic, depending on the serum concentration and the sensitivity of the infecting microorganism. Erythromycin binds to the 50S subunit of bacterial ribosomes, disrupting protein synthesis. Erythromycin is primarily active against gram-positive species, such as staphylococci and streptococci, but it also inhibits the growth of some enterococci and gram-negative bacilli. Also useful against *Mycoplasma pneumoniae*, *Legionella pneumophila*, *Moraxella catarrhalis*, and *Chlamydia*, erythromycin is primarily used in the ICU for the treatment of *Legionella* or *Mycoplasma* pneumonias. Because of its variable activity against *S. aureus*, *S. pneumoniae*, and *Haemophilus influenzae*, this drug is considered an alternative to penicillin derivatives. Erythromycin can be used as prophylaxis for bacterial endocarditis in penicillin-allergic patients.

Clarithromycin and azithromycin are macrolide congeners (azalides) that have longer clinical activity and fewer gastrointestinal side effects than does erythromycin. Their spectrum of activity is similar to that of erythromycin, but additionally, both drugs have activity against *Mycobacterium avium* complex, *Cryptosporidium*, and *Toxoplasma gondii*. These two drugs are available for enteral use, but only azithromycin has an intravenous preparation.

Distribution and Elimination

Macrolides penetrate into most tissues and produce therapeutic concentrations in middle-ear fluid, lung, liver, and bile but do not diffuse well into the CSF. The main route of elimination is urinary excretion after demethylation by the liver. Only a small percentage of the drug (approximately 15%) is excreted unchanged in the urine. The half-lives of macrolides are prolonged by severe liver disease.

Adverse Reactions

Macrolide-associated side effects usually are limited to nausea, vomiting, and diarrhea, particularly with the use of the oral preparation of erythromycin. Intravenously administered erythromycin frequently causes phlebitis. Azithromycin causes little, if any, phlebitis and other adverse effects intravenously. Erythromycin at high doses can cause reversible deafness. Hepatotoxicity most often occurs with the oral estolate salt preparation of erythromycin. Clarithromycin, azithromycin, and intravenously administered erythromycin are rarely associated with hepatic toxicity. Fever, eosinophilia, and rash occasionally occur. Macrolides, especially erythromycin, will inhibit cytochrome P-450 enzymes and alter drug metabolism, which can increase the risk of drug toxicity. Renal toxicity as a result of high cyclosporine levels after starting a macrolide in transplant patients is a well-known complication.

Lincosamides

Clindamycin phosphate, a lincosamide derivative, is a ribosomally active bacteriostatic antibiotic against most gram-positive cocci and many anaerobes. This drug is frequently used with an aminoglycoside or third-generation cephalosporin for the treatment of severe polymicrobial infections. Considered an alternative agent to broad-spectrum penicillins for the treatment of aspiration pneumonia, clindamycin should not be considered first-line treatment for *S. aureus*, nor is it active against enterococci. Clindamycin alone or in combination with primaquine phosphate is effective for the treatment of CNS *T. gondii*.

Distribution and Elimination

Clindamycin penetrates most body tissues and can achieve adequate concentrations in lung, liver, bone, and abscesses. Although it does not reliably enter the CSF and concentrations are inadequate to treat bacterial meningitis, clindamycin can be used to treat CNS toxoplasmosis. Only 10% of the dose is eliminated as unmetabolized drug in urine. The half-life of clindamycin is prolonged with severe liver disease.

Adverse Reactions

When copious amounts of bloody diarrhea are associated with clindamycin use, a diagnosis of pseudomembranous colitis should be suspected. The use of most other antibiotics also may be associated with pseudomembranous colitis, secondary to overgrowth of *Clostridium difficile*. Treatment consists of stopping clindamycin and administering oral metronidazole or vancomycin.

Glycopeptides

Vancomycin, a bacterial cell-wall inhibitor, is structurally and functionally different from all other antimicrobial compounds. Vancomycin is bactericidal against *Staphylococcus epidermidis*, *S. aureus*, most streptococci, and *Corynebacterium*, *S. haemolyticus*, and coagulase-negative *Staphylococcus*; *Enterococcus* may have variable resistance to vancomycin. No gram-negative organisms and only a few anaerobes are susceptible to vancomycin. Vancomycin is the drug of choice for the treatment of infections caused by methicillin-resistant *S. aureus* and provides an alternative to penicillin for patients with life-threatening penicillin allergies who have infections from gram-positive organisms (5). Vancomycin is the preferred antibiotic for surgical prophylaxis against *S. aureus* and *S. epidermidis* in patients allergic to penicillin who have permanently implanted foreign bodies, such as pacemakers, prosthetic valves, and intravascular catheters.

Teicoplanin is a glycopeptide antibiotic recently made available for clinical use. Teicoplanin differs chemically from vancomycin, having different carbohydrate moieties, dihydroxyphenylglycines in place of the aspartic acid and N-methylleucine side chains, and additional fatty-acid moieties. Teicoplanin has an antibacterial spectrum and mechanism of action similar to those of vancomycin. Although teicoplanin has greater inhibitory activity against enterococci than does vancomycin, it too is rarely bactericidal for this species. Teicoplanin and vancomycin exhibit similar bactericidal synergism in combination with aminoglycosides or rifampin against staphylococci, enterococci, other streptococci, and *Listeria* organisms (6,7).

Vancomycin-resistant staphylococci and enterococci also are usually resistant to teicoplanin (8). Teicoplanin, potentially an effective alternative to vancomycin, may be most useful in patients who have had neutropenic or allergic reactions to vancomycin.

Distribution and Elimination

Because vancomycin is not absorbed orally, it should be administered intravenously except when treating *C. difficile* colitis. Vancomycin penetrates into bile, pleural, peritoneal, and synovial fluids and only crosses the meninges during inflammation. About 90% of the drug is eliminated unchanged in the urine through glomerular filtration. Because of its large molecular size, vancomycin is not removed by hemodialysis but is removed by peritoneal dialysis. The dosage is usually adjusted based on creatinine clearance and vancomycin serum concentrations for renal-compromised patients.

With its greater tissue and cellular penetration (due to its fatty-acid moieties), teicoplanin is far more lipophilic than is vancomycin (7). Teicoplanin also exhibits a much higher protein-binding capacity than does vancomycin. Because of the difference in protein binding and the larger volume of distribution, teicoplanin has a much lower clearance rate. The elimination half-life for teicoplanin is approximately 40 hours, compared with 6 hours for vancomycin. Because of this long half-life, it can be given intramuscularly or intravenously once per day. In patients with renal impairment, dosage adjustments must be made. Teicoplanin is not removed by hemodialysis. No information is available regarding the clearance of teicoplanin with peritoneal dialysis.

Adverse Effects

Ototoxicity and nephrotoxicity previously were a significant problem associated with vancomycin use. Because of improved commercial preparation (with removal of toxic impurities), ototoxicity and nephrotoxicity now are rarely encountered. Clinicians frequently monitor trough concentrations and attempt to keep levels below 10 micrograms per milliliter to minimize toxicity. Peak serum levels usually are not measured unless high levels (25–35 μg/mL) are needed to help ensure good bactericidal tissue concentrations for serious *S. aureus* infections.

Vancomycin, when used concurrently with aminoglycosides or amphotericin, will increase the risk of renal toxicity. The risk of ototoxicity is not known to be increased when vancomycin is used concomitantly with other ototoxic drugs (9). Hypersensitivity reactions may occur with the infusion of vancomycin. Much more commonly, a diffuse macular skin rash about the neck, upper extremities, and upper torso is seen, with or without hypotension. This reaction, which results from infusing a therapeutic dose of vancomycin over less than 1 hour, is due to histamine release and has been referred to as "red-man" or "red-neck" syndrome.

Significant adverse effects with teicoplanin use are uncommon. The red-man or red-neck syndrome is not seen with teicoplanin administration.

Quinolones

The quinolones are derivatives of nalidixic acid and exhibit bactericidal activity by inhibiting an important bacterial replication enzyme, DNA gyrase. The quinolone antibiotics have a wide spectrum of antibacterial activity, including activity against *Chlamydia, Mycoplasma, Legionella,* and some mycobacteria. An intrinsic reduced activity against *S. aureus, S. pneumoniae,* and *P. aeruginosa* appears to be worsening, possibly from overuse. This group of drugs has no activity against anaerobes. Quinolones are nonnephrotoxic alternative agents against most pathogenic gram-negative organisms.

Like the cephalosporins, the quinolones can be placed in different generations according to their coverage for important pathogens (Table 4). Nalidixic acid was the first oral quinolone that gained significant use. Because of its reliable activity against most Enterobacteriaceae, it became a popular choice for the treatment of uncomplicated urinary tract infections. In fact, it was often referred to as an oral form of kanamycin. Unfortunately, its serum and tissue concentrations were so low that it could not be used for infections in other body sites. Several other similar quinolones (i.e., oxolinic acid, cinoxacin) were developed that were essentially identical to nalidixic acid but could be given less frequently. None of these first-generation quinolones has any activity against *P. aeruginosa,* anaerobes, or gram-positive bacteria.

The next or second-generation expanded the bacterial coverage to *P. aeruginosa.* This change was the result of the discovery that the placement of a fluorine into the 6-position of the 4-quinolone molecule and the replacement of the methyl side-chain of nalidixic acid with a piperazine group markedly enhanced

TABLE 4. QUINOLONE ANTIBIOTICS

Generation	Quinolone	Sensitive Organisms
First	Naladixic acid Oxolinic acid Cinoxacin	Enterobacteriaceae
Second	Norfloxacin Lomafloxacin Enoxacin	Enterobacteriaceae and *P. aeruginosa*
Third	Ciprofloxacin Ofloxacin	Enterobacteriaceae and *P. aeruginosa*
Fourth	Levofloxacin Grepafloxacin Gatifloxacin Moxifloxacin	Enterobacteriaceae, *P. aeruginosa,* and streptococci

the microbiologic activity. As a result of this observation, all the newer agents in this class are referred to as *fluoroquinolones*. These new quinolones have microbiologic activity closely similar to that of the aminoglycosides but still are not able to reach clinically effective levels in body tissues other than in the urinary tract.

The third-generation quinolones, ciprofloxacin and ofloxacin, expanded the clinical utility beyond that of the first- and second-generation agents. These quinolones, as a class, achieve high enough serum and tissue concentrations to allow for the treatment of infection in body sites other than the urinary tract. Moreover, third-generation quinolones exhibit high intracellular penetration, allowing the therapy of atypical organisms, like *Chlamydia*, *Mycoplasma*, and *Legionella* species, which are susceptible to these agents. These agents are available in both intravenous and oral formulations.

Unfortunately, none of these third-generation quinolones exhibited adequate activity against streptococci. Temofloxacin, a third-generation fluoroquinolone, had streptococcal activity, but it had to be withdrawn from the market because of serious adverse reactions. The creation of fourth-generation quinolones, although still active against gram-negative organisms, provided coverage of gram-positive bacteria. These new agents allow single-agent therapy in community-acquired lung infections becaise they provide coverage for the leading bacterial and atypical microorganisms. Levofloxacin, gatifloxacin, and moxifloxacin are fourth-generation agents that are available in both intravenous and oral formulations. A fifth-generation quinolone, trova-floxacin, which exhibited good antipseudomonal, antianaerobic, and antistreptococcal activity, was available for a short time before being removed from clinical use because of adverse effects.

Distribution and Elimination

Fluoroquinolones are widely distributed in the body, entering all compartments, including the eye, CSF, bronchial epithelium, and bile. These drugs are removed by glomerular filtration and tubular secretion, with 30% of a dose recovered unchanged in the urine. Dosage adjustment is not needed for hepatic or renal dysfunction. Quinolones that are currently under investigation have anaerobic coverage and greater activity against *P. aeruginosa*.

Adverse Effects

All quinolones can cause gastrointestinal reactions such as nausea, vomiting, and abdominal pain. Seizures have been a rare problem, with dizziness, headache, depression, and insomnia more frequent side effects. Quinolones damage cartilage in immature animals and therefore are not recommended for use in children less than 14 years old (10). Allergic reactions are uncommon, but urticaria, rashes, photosensitivity, and interstitial nephritis have occurred.

Sulfonamides and Trimethoprim

The sulfonamides and trimethoprim are members of the first chemotherapeutic agents used to treat bacterial infections in humans. The bactericidal combination of trimethoprim-sulfamethoxazole prevents the ability of bacteria to use folic acid. This combination has a wide antimicrobial spectrum that includes gram-positive cocci (including methicillin-resistant *S. aureus* when sensitive *in vitro* but usually not *Enterococcus*), gram-negative rods (except *P. aeruginosa*), *Chlamydia*, *Neisseria*, *Toxoplasma*, *Plasmodium*, *Pneumocystis carinii*, *Nocardia*, *Aeromonas*, *M. catarrhalis*, and *Yersinia enterocolitica*. Occasionally, the antimicrobial activity of this drug combination is not as effective as predicted by *in vitro* testing (e.g., methicillin-resistant *S. aureus*). This may be due to less than optimal *in vivo* drug concentration for each drug, thus not achieving a synergistic drug ratio that is seen in the *in vitro* testing.

Distribution and Elimination

The sulfonamides and trimethoprim are widely distributed through most body compartments and will cross the blood–brain barrier. Most sulfonamides and trimethoprim are metabolized by the liver, with renal excretion of the metabolites. Several sulfonamide derivatives may have varying amounts of the drug excreted unchanged in the urine.

Adverse Effects

As a group, the sulfonamides cause a large number of adverse reactions. Hypersensitivity reactions, which occur in approximately 2% to 3% of patients, can be life threatening. Rashes may be urticarial; maculopapular; or, rarely, exfoliative, as in Stevens–Johnson syndrome. A serum sickness–like illness, with fever, joint pain, and rash, can be seen. Sulfonamide use produces several hematologic toxicities, including aplastic anemia, hemolytic anemia, thrombocytopenia, and agranulocytosis; agranulocytosis occurs in fewer than 0.1% of patients. Hepatotoxicity is rarely seen with sulfonamide use. Trimethoprim use alone has little intrinsic toxicity but is known to cause nausea, vomiting, and diarrhea.

Metronidazole

Metronidazole, a synthetic nitroimidazole, is active against most anaerobes, but a few gram-positive anaerobic bacilli are resistant. The bactericidal activity of metronidazole occurs through the reductive activation of its nitro group and interaction of the metabolite with the organism's DNA or other macromolecules. Metronidazole is the drug of choice for the treatment of protozoan infections, including amoebae, *Giardia*, and *Trichomonas*. It is commonly used as part of a multidrug regimen for the treatment of *H. pylori* and suspected polymicrobial infections. Oral metronidazole is as effective as and less expensive than oral vancomycin for treating antibiotic-associated colitis caused by *C. difficile*.

Distribution and Elimination

The absence of significant protein binding and the small size of the metronidazole molecule favor good distribution throughout body tissues and fluids. Metronidazole penetrates well into CSF. In patients with normal meninges, the spinal fluid levels are approximately half the simultaneously measured serum concentrations. Most of the administered metronidazole is metabolized in the liver and excreted with the unmetabolized form in urine.

Adverse Effects

The incidence of untoward effects associated with metronidazole use is low. The drug is generally well tolerated, with exceptions being nausea, vomiting, urticaria, and an unpleasant metallic taste. Rare neurologic side effects have included seizures, ataxia, and encephalopathy. Although rare, reversible neutropenia has been reported with metronidazole use.

Tetracyclines

Tetracyclines are similar to the aminoglycoside class of antibiotics in that they act by binding to ribosomes and interrupting bacterial peptide-chain synthesis. Tetracyclines are broad-spectrum agents that are primarily bacteriostatic, inhibiting a wide variety of aerobic and anaerobic gram-positive and gram-negative bacteria and other microorganisms, such as *Mycoplasma, Chlamydia,* and *Rickettsia.* Unlike aminoglycosides, the tetracyclines are only weakly bound to ribosomal proteins, rendering them poorly active *in vivo* despite indicating good activity *in vitro.* The tetracyclines previously had many clinical uses, but increasing bacterial resistance and the development of newer, more effective agents have decreased their use.

As mentioned, resistance has moved tetracyclines to the area of "alternative agents" for many of their previous indications. They remain the preferred agent for treating rickettsial diseases, however, such as Rocky Mountain spotted fever, typhus, and Q fever, as well as *Borrelia*-related infections, such as Lyme disease and relapsing fever. They are also frequently used for treating sexually transmitted chlamydial infections.

Distribution and Elimination

Tetracyclines are distributed to all body compartments. They are metabolized hepatically, but significant amounts are excreted unchanged in the urine and bile. Only doxycycline does not accumulate in the presence of decreased renal function.

Adverse Effects

Phototoxicity is a common problem. Dental staining and interference with dental and bone growth are particular problems for patients aged less than 8 years. Fatty liver changes and renal insufficiency have been seen with the use of tetracyclines.

Chloramphenicol

Chloramphenicol is an antibiotic produced by *Streptomyces venezuelae.* Like erythromycin and clindamycin, chloramphenicol binds to the same site or sites on the ribosomal 50S subunit, preventing the formation of peptide bonds and protein synthesis. Chloramphenicol can be useful for treating infections in critically ill patients because this drug has a broad antibacterial spectrum; it is bacteriostatic for a wide variety of gram-positive and gram-negative organisms, including *Neisseria meningitidis,* nonenterococcal streptococci, most anaerobes, *H. influenzae,* and many enteric gram-negative bacilli. This drug, however, has been used with decreasing frequency because of bone marrow toxicity and the availability of less toxic alternatives.

Distribution and Elimination

Chloramphenicol penetrates into all body tissues, including the CSF. About 90% of the drug is metabolized in the liver. The plasma half-life of the drug correlates with plasma bilirubin concentrations, and the dosage should be adjusted for patients for hepatic insufficiency. No dosage adjustments are needed for patients with decreased renal function.

Adverse Effects

Aplastic anemia, the most common type of bone marrow toxicity, occurs once per 25,000 treated patients and almost exclusively in young women with previous exposure to the drug. A dose-related hematologic toxicity of thrombocytopenia and leukopenia is most often seen with serum levels greater than 25 μg per milliliter. This selective bone marrow suppression, unlike drug-induced aplastic anemia, is reversible when chloramphenicol is discontinued.

Oxazolidinediones

The oxazolidinediones are inhibitors of protein synthesis and are bacteriostatic against different bacteria. These agents bind to the 50S subunit of bacterial ribosomes, which blocks a step in early protein synthesis. Linezolid, the only oxazolidinedione approved for clinical use, possesses activity against gram-positive organisms, including methicillin-resistant strains of *S. aureus,* coagulase-negative staphylococci, vancomycin-resistant strains of *Enterococcus* species, and penicillin-resistant strains of *S. pneumoniae* [11]. Most gram-positive cocci are inhibited by linezolid in concentrations of 4 micrograms per milliliter or less. Linezolid is especially useful for the treatment of vancomycin-resistant enterococcal infections and methicillin-resistant *S. aureus* (MRSA).

Distribution and Elimination

Linezolid readily distributes to well-perfused tissues. Linezolid is not metabolized by, nor is it an inducer of, cytochrome P-450. Renal excretion is responsible for elimination of 80% to 85% of linezolid and its metabolites. About 30% is excreted in the urine unchanged. Linezolid and both major metabolites are removed by hemodialysis.

Adverse Effects

Predominant adverse effects have included nausea, diarrhea, and headache. Pseudomembranous colitis or superinfection may occur. Patients should be monitored for thrombocytopenia. Linezolid inhibits monoamine oxidase, so patients should avoid consumption of high-tyramine content foods or concomitant administration of drugs that modulate CNS levels of dopamine or serotonin.

Quinupristin/Dalfopristin

Quinupristin/dalfopristin is a streptogramin antibacterial agent indicated for the treatment of patients with serious or life-threatening infections associated with vancomycin-resistant *Enterococcus faecium* (VREF) bacteremia. Quinupristin/dalfopristin also has demonstrated bactericidal activity against methicillin-sensitive or -resistant gram-positive organisms as well as some gram-negative organisms and anaerobes (12). Quinupristin/dalfopristin exerts its antimicrobial activity through inhibition of protein synthesis by binding to different sites on the 50S ribosome, resulting in a stable ternary drug-ribosome complex.

Distribution and Elimination

The total protein binding of quinupristin/dalfopristin is moderate: quinupristin 23% to 32% and dalfopristin 50% to 56%. There is good penetration to all tissue sites. Quinupristin/dalfopristin is extensively metabolized in both blood and liver by drug hydrolysis. Less than 5% of unmetabolized quinupristin/dalfopristin is excreted in the urine. The elimination half-life of quinupristin/dalfopristin is 1.3 to 1.5 hours, with no apparent dose-dependency metabolism. The clearance of quinupristin, dalfopristin, and their respective metabolites is negligibly affected by peritoneal dialysis and is unlikely to be affected by hemodialysis.

Adverse Effects

Quinupristin/dalfopristin has been well tolerated in clinical studies. Local reactions at the infusion site (muscle pain, erythema) are the predominant adverse effects. Headache, gastrointestinal disturbances, nonlocal skin reactions, and liver enzyme elevations also have been reported. Quinupristin/dalfopristin does not appear to induce histamine release.

Mupirocin

Mupirocin, a topical agent derived from *Pseudomonas fluorescens*, may become an important prophylactic antibiotic in ICUs and transplant units. Mupirocin inhibits bacterial RNA and protein synthesis by binding to tRNA synthetase. Mupirocin is active against many gram-positive and gram-negative bacteria and may be useful to decrease the carrier state when applied to areas that are frequently colonized with *S. aureus* or methicillin-resistant *S. aureus*. Mupirocin is inactive *in vitro* against *P. aeruginosa*, *Enterobacteriaceae*, and anaerobes.

FACTORS INFLUENCING ANTIBACTERIAL ACTIVITY

Antagonism

Antagonism occurs when one antibiotic diminishes the antibacterial effectiveness of another antibiotic. This is an *in vitro* phenomenon that can be seen between bactericidal and bacteriostatic drugs (13). Significant antagonism is seen with the use of erythromycin, chloramphenicol, and tetracycline (bacteriostatic agents) with penicillins, cephalosporins, or aminoglycosides (bactericidal agents), which require bacterial multiplication (e.g., protein or cell-wall synthesis) for optimal killing effect. Significant antagonism is seen most often when near subtherapeutic amounts of a bacteriostatic drug are added to low therapeutic concentrations of bactericidal drug. When antimicrobials are antagonistic,

the activity of the combination is fourfold less than the sum of the independent agents (14).

Synergy

Synergistic or additive drug combinations are popular approaches for treating bacterial infections (13). Synergy arises with the use of two antibiotics when one drug enhances the antibacterial activity of the other against a specific microorganism. Synergy frequently is defined as a fourfold or greater reduction in the MIC or MBC for either agent. One of the best established synergistic combinations is a penicillin or glycopeptide and an aminoglycoside for the treatment of *Enterococcus* endocarditis. The MBC of ampicillin against *Enterococcus* is 64 micrograms per milliliter, and the MBC of gentamicin is 4 micrograms per milliliter. In combination, the MBCs are 4 and 0.5 micrograms per milliliter, respectively. The combination results in increased bacterial uptake of aminoglycoside, resulting from cell-wall damage induced by penicillin or vancomycin (15). Extended-spectrum penicillins plus aminoglycosides for treating *Pseudomonas* infections, nafcillin sodium plus an aminoglycoside for *S. aureus*, and flucytosine plus amphotericin B for *Cryptococcus* are other synergistic antibacterial combinations.

Drug combinations are also used to reduce the dose required of each antibacterial agent, resulting in a decreased incidence or intensity of adverse reactions to the individual agents and preventing the emergence of resistance because of improved bacterial killing capabilities. The treatment of *M. tuberculosis* with isoniazid, ethambutol hydrochloride, and rifampin is an example of combining antibiotics to decrease individual drug toxicity while improving therapeutic outcome.

Resistance

Antibiotic resistance appears to be an inevitable problem, with antibiotics exerting pressure on bacteria, resulting in the selective survival of resistant strains. The more frequently bacterial populations are exposed to antibiotics, the more resistance emerges. The Centers for Disease Control and Prevention (CDC) estimated that approximately 50% of all antibiotics are prescribed unnecessarily (16). Most of these prescriptions are for ambulatory respiratory infections. Other factors affecting antibiotic resistance include older age, prolonged hospital stays, admission to the ICU, indwelling catheters and tubes, prior or prolonged antibiotic therapy, and exposure to patients with MRSA. The cost of treating infections from resistant organisms has been estimated at $30 billion.

Mechanisms of bacterial resistance (Table 5) include altered antibiotic penetration into bacterial cells, mutated antibiotic target sites within the bacterial cell, and production of antibiotic-inactivating enzymes by bacteria (17). Bacterial resistance is either plasmid or chromosomally mediated. Plasmid-mediated resistance to an antibiotic agent can be passed from one species to another and can render resistance to one or more antibiotics. Genes that encode bacterial resistance via chromosomes are not passed between species or between members of different species. This type of resistance is more stable but can result in outbreaks of infection, especially in crowded patient care areas. Patients in

TABLE 5. ANTIBIOTICS AND BACTERIAL RESISTANCE

Antibiotics	Mechanism of Resistance	Problematic Inducible Strains
β-Lactams	ESBL Penicillins Cephalosporins	*Enterobacter* spp Enterococcus *Serratia* spp *Morganella morganii* *Citrobacter freundii* *Pseudomonas* spp
Glycopeptides Aminoglycosides	Changes in PBPs Cell-wall permeability	Enterococcus *Pseudomonas* spp *Enterobacter* spp Enterococcus *S. aureus*
Quinolones	Cell-wall permeability DNA gyrase modifications	*Enterobacter* spp *Pseudomonas* spp *S. aureus*

ESBL, extended spectrum β-lactamases; PBPs, penicillin-binding proteins.

ICUs can acquire resistant organisms in both ways from exposure to hospital flora. Substantial antibiotic pressure on these patients can also select out endogenous flora that have multiple antibiotic resistance (18).

Current methods used to minimize microbial resistance are through strengthening infection-control practices, limiting the use of antibiotics, rotating antibiotics, limiting the formulary to select antibiotics, requiring antibiotic order sheets requiring documentation of need, and permitting the pharmacy to intervene and modify the dose of selected therapy or even change the antibiotic therapy.

β-Lactam Resistance

In gram-positive bacteria, peptidoglycan is a major component of the cell wall. Binding of β-lactam antibiotics to the penicillin-binding proteins (PBPs) found on the inner membrane of the bacterial cell wall inhibits peptidoglycan cross-linking and enhances intrinsic autolysis, resulting in breakdown of the bacterial cell wall and eventually cell death (19). Bacterial β-lactamase acylates the β-lactam ring, which inactivates the antibiotic. β-Lactamase resistance with gram-positive bacteria occurs primarily through the spread of plasmid-mediated β-lactamases. The gram-positive bacteria with a broad-based β-lactam resistance is *S. aureus*. Methicillin-resistant strains of *S. aureus* are not inhibited by any of the currently available β-lactams because of the presence of β-lactamase and low-affinity PBPs. Other gram-positive organisms with increased resistance caused by PBP alterations include additional species of staphylococci, enterococci, pneumococci, *Neisseria, Listeria monocytogenes*, and *H. influenzae*.

In gram-negative bacteria, the presence of β-lactamases and failure of the drug to reach PBPs are the common causes of resistance, but alteration of the antibiotic target site also can occur. Gram-negative bacteria produce a wider variety of β-lactamases than do gram-positive bacteria, and these β-lactamases can be either plasmid or chromosomally mediated.

Numerous gram-negative organisms have inducible β-lactamase, in which the bacteria produce only small amounts of enzyme until the organisms are challenged by an inducer (β-lactams), after which large amounts of enzyme are synthe-sized. The chromosomally inherited β-lactamases of *Enterobacter, Citrobacter*, indole-positive *Proteus, Providencia, Serratia, Morganella*, and *P. aeruginosa* are inducible. Antibiotics that are capable of strongly inducing β-lactamase production include third-generation cephalosporins and carbapenems. This type of resistance can occur in up to 25% of patients treated with β-lactams, resulting in clinical failures and longer duration of antibiotic therapy (20). This is one of the reasons that narrow-spectrum antibiotics should be used and only identified infections should be treated whenever possible.

Quinolone Resistance

Bacterial cell walls have protein channels that extend from the outer to the inner membrane. These water-filled channels, called *porins*, allow oxygen-dependent semiselective diffusion of various hydrophilic solutes, such as antibiotics. A number of bacteria produce more than one type of porin, depending on nutritional needs and surrounding environment pressures. Alterations in porins have been found to be responsible for acquired resistance during quinolone therapy. The altered porins prevent quinolones from gaining access to the bacterial cytoplasm to inactivate DNA gyrase (21). Also, acquired changes in the DNA gyrase make it less sensitive to quinolones. Bacteria resistant to quinolones have been found in patients who were then treated for urinary tract infections with antibiotics other than quinolones; this resistance occurs particularly in cystic fibrosis patients infected with *Pseudomonas* and methicillin-resistant staphylococci.

Aminoglycoside Resistance

Changes in the permeability of porin channels (reducing the intracellular penetration of aminoglycosides) and alterations in bacterial ribosomes (limiting the avidity of ribosomes for aminoglycosides) are probably not significant factors in increasing bacterial resistance. Plasmid-mediated encoding of aminoglycoside-modifying enzymes is the primary mechanism of bacterial resistance to this group of antibiotics. These enzymes alter the structure of specific aminoglycosides by phosphorylation, acetylation, adenylation, or other enzymatic modifications, which either prevent ribosomal binding or interfere with intracellular drug accumulation. Anaerobic bacteria are inherently resistant to aminoglycosides because intracellular transport and accumulation of aminoglycosides through porins are oxygen dependent. The wide variability in aminoglycoside resistance depends on location and usage patterns. Prediction of resistance to a particular aminoglycoside is not feasible at present, and little evidence supports the theory that restricting the use of a particular aminoglycoside will prevent the development of resistance (22).

Vancomycin Resistance

The increasing prevalence of methicillin-resistant staphylococci has resulted from a major increase in vancomycin use. This drug also has become the mainstay of parenteral therapy for treating other gram-positive bacteria that are resistant to ß-lactam antibiotics and for patients with serious β-lactam allergies. Unfortunately, the liberal use of vancomycin for patients who do not meet these indications has caused a high level of resistance among

TABLE 6. *IN VITRO* ANTIFUNGAL ACTIVITY

Organism	Fluconazole[a]	Ketoconazole[a]	Itraconazole[a]	Amphotericin B[b]	Flucytosine[c]	Triazoles
Candida albicans[d]	+	+	+	+	+	+
Candida glabrata	+[e]	−	+	+	+	+
Candida tropicalis	+	−	+	+	+	+
Candida krusei	−	+	+	+	+	−
Cryptococcus	+	+	+	+	+	+
Aspergillis	−	−	+	+	+	+
Pseudallescheria	±	+	±	−	−	+
Fuserium	±	±	±	+	−	±
Coccidioides	+	+	+	+	−	+
Blastomyces	±	+	+	+	−	±
Histoplasma	+	+	+	+	−	+
Sporothis	+	+	+	+	−	+
Torulopsis	+	−	+	+	−	+
Paracoccidioides	+	+	+	+	−	+
Mucormycosis	−	−	−	+	−	−

+, active; −, inactive; ±, uncertain or unknown.
[a]Azoles most frequently used for less severe infections.
[b]Amphotericin B is the drug of choice for life-threatening fungal infection.
[c]Used only as a synergistic combination with amphotericin B.
[d]Intravenous fluconazole i.v. is as effective as amphotericin B for life-threatening *C. albicans* infection.
[e]High doses only.

coagulase-negative staphylococci and enterococci. The recent induction of high resistance levels, which makes these organisms impervious to almost all antibiotics, is mandating the reduction of vancomycin use to decrease antibiotic induction pressure. Resistance to vancomycin occurs primarily through plasmid transference of genetic material that induces the production of a protein that interferes with the bacterial binding of vancomycin.

Pharmacodynamics and Dosing

The integrated roles of host bacterial susceptibility and pharmacokinetics have been established for prescribing antimicrobial agents. Individual variability, however, can make precise prediction of pharmacodynamic response difficult.

In general, the strategy for concentration-independent antibiotics is low-level exposure at some concentration above the bacterial MIC. For concentration-dependent antibiotics, high-peak concentrations for short periods may be optimal. "Single-daily-dose" therapy (high-dose extended-interval therapy) has been suggested as a more beneficial method of administering aminoglycosides (23). Continuous infusion of β-lactam antibiotics to specific bacterial MIC levels has been suggested as a method to improve clinical outcome for patients receiving this group of agents (24). These tailored dosing strategies may have advantages, such as decreased cost of antimicrobials, reduced incidence of adverse drug reactions and improved or at least equal clinical efficacy.

Antifungal Therapy

Fungal infections occur less frequently than do bacterial and viral infections, and many that do exist are superficial and respond to topical therapy. Systemic life-threatening fungal infections usually are seen in patients with immunodeficiency problems. Fungi have different cell-wall components and ribosomes than do bacteria and have a nuclear membrane, which is not seen with bacteria. These structural differences make bacterial antibiotics ineffective against fungi. The available antifungal agents are few (Table 6), and drug susceptibility testing is not readily available or standardized, as it is for antibacterial agents. Frequently, empiric therapy is started and continued because rapid diagnosis of fungal infections is difficult and because of the severe nature of the patients' infective process.

Amphotericin B

Amphotericin is from the polyene antibiotic family, which is fungistatic or fungicidal for a wide variety of fungi but has no activity against bacteria or viruses (25). Polyenes act by binding to sterols (preferentially to ergosterol) in the cell membrane and forming channels, allowing potassium ions and magnesium molecules to leak out of the cell. Compromised cell-wall integrity and the inability to maintain intracellular ionic balance lead to cell death.

Amphotericin B is the drug of choice to treat most serious fungal infections. Resistance has been observed in some *Candida* species, such as *C. lusitaniae* and *guilliermondi*; *Pseudallescheria boydii* should be considered resistant. When given in the standard dose (0.4–1.0 mg/kg), therapeutic serum concentrations of amphotericin are reached in the approximate range of 1.5 to 2.1 microgram per milliliter. These serum levels exceed the MIC of most of the commonly encountered fungal infections (*Candida albicans, tropicalis, parapsilosis, immitis,* and *neoformans; Aspergillus; H. capsulatum; Blastomyces dermatitidis; Sporothrix schenckii;* and *Zygomycetes*) (26). This agent also is used as empiric therapy in febrile neutropenic patients who have not responded to antibacterial agents.

Distribution and Elimination

The pharmacokinetics of amphotericin B are complex, with several distribution and elimination phases. Therefore, clinical efficacy may not correlate with a given daily dose. The daily and total doses of amphotericin B depend on the severity of infection and the type of fungus as well as the patient's response. Although some clinicians suggest gradual increases in dose until therapeutic doses are reached over several days, no increase in toxicity has been seen with initiating the daily dose at 0.6 mg per kilogram. Once the fungal disease is under control, it may be possible to change to alternate-day therapy to decrease the adverse effects of the drug.

Amphotericin B generally has good tissue uptake except in the CNS and vitreous humor of the eye. It also does not cross epithelial surfaces well; therefore, systemic amphotericin B does not penetrate into the gastrointestinal tract. The principal pathway for amphotericin B disposition is not known. Only 3% of a dose is eliminated in the urine. A small amount of amphotericin B is eliminated by the biliary route. Renal dysfunction or hemodialysis does not affect plasma concentrations of the drug.

Adverse Effects

Amphotericin B must be administered by slow intravenous infusion. Because of serious hypersensitivity effects, a test dose is given (approximately 1 mg over the first 30–60 minutes) at the start of therapy, with the remainder of the therapeutic dose given over 4 to 6 hours. Further test dosing is not needed unless a hyperacute reaction is seen. Other less severe acute infusion-related reactions, such as fever, chills, rigors, nausea, hypotension, and tachycardia, commonly occur. The cause of these symptoms may be the amphotericin-induced release of tumor necrosis factor and interleukin-1 from macrophages and monocytes. If these reactions limit the amount of drug that can be infused, patients may benefit from premedication. Acetaminophen, 650 mg; diphenhydramine hydrochloride, 25 to 50 mg; or intravenously administered hydrocortisone, 25 to 50 mg, can decrease the incidence and severity of fever, nausea, hypotension, and fever. Intravenously administered meperidine hydrochloride, 25 to 50 mg, is useful for treating rigors and chills.

Renal toxicity, a common side effect of amphotericin-B therapy, is manifested by an early decrease in the glomerular filtration rate resulting from vasoconstriction of afferent arterioles. Using prehydration and avoiding simultaneous administration of other nephrotoxic drugs can reduce the incidence of acute renal failure. One pilot study suggested that the use of pentoxifylline may reduce nephrotoxicity in humans (27). Limiting the daily dose to 1 mg per kilogram of amphotericin and limiting the total dose to less than 3 g will help minimize renal toxicity. If the serum creatinine concentration increases above 3.5 mg per deciliter, amphotericin should be discontinued for a few days. Administration of amphotericin B may be resumed at 50% to 75% of the original dose or may be given every other day when the serum creatinine level falls below 3 mg per deciliter.

Reversible renal tubular loss of potassium, magnesium, and bicarbonate is seen with chronic amphotericin administration. Replacement electrolyte therapy is commonly needed throughout amphotericin therapy. Other unusual adverse side effects seen with amphotericin use are neurotoxicity, cardiac arrhythmias, and pulmonary infiltrates.

Liposomal Amphotericin

The encapsulation of amphotericin B in liposomes represents a promising addition for antifungal therapy. Use of liposomal amphotericin B reduces infusion-related symptoms and the incidence of renal toxicity compared with the use of amphotericin B. It is possible that encapsulation of amphotericin B in phospholipids results in decreased interaction with mammalian cellular membranes compared with fungal membranes owing to different cellular binding affinities for the amphotericin B-lipid complex. Although clinically attainable serum levels of amphotericin B are fungistatic, it has concentration-dependent fungicidal activity. Previously, it has not been possible to take advantage of this pharmacodynamic property because of the dose-limiting nephrotoxicity. Optimal dosing of liposomal formulations based on pharmacodynamic principles has yet to be elucidated; however, liposomal amphotericin B has an improved therapeutic index compared with amphotericin B, and long-term (22 weeks) high total dose (30 g) therapy has been reported in the literature without toxicity attributable to the drug (28). Direct comparative studies between liposomal formulations of amphotericin B are lacking; however, structural differences suggest efficacy and tolerability may differ among the liposomal formulations

Flucytosine

Flucytosine (5-fluorocytosine) is a fluorinated pyrimidine, which is an antimetabolite that undergoes intracellular metabolism to an active form that leads to inhibition of DNA synthesis. Flucytosine is active against *Cryptococcus neoformans*, many *Candida* species, blastomycosis, and chromomycosis. Approximately 30% of cryptococci develop resistance during therapy. Resistance also has occurred during therapy for *Candida* infection. Because of this variability in the susceptibility of these organisms, flucytosine's role as a single agent is limited to the treatment of chronic blastomycosis. Its primary use is in combination with amphotericin B for the treatment of cryptococcal infections and disseminated *Candida* infections (29). Flucytosine is not effective against *Aspergillus*, *Sporothrix*, *Histoplasma*, or *Coccidioides immitis*.

Distribution and Elimination

Flucytosine is widely distributed in body tissues, including CSF, bronchial secretions, saliva, and bone. Approximately 85% to 95% is excreted unchanged by glomerular filtration. Flucytosine has a half-life of 3 to 6 hours, with a marked increase with renal dysfunction. The drug can be removed by hemodialysis and peritoneal dialysis.

Adverse Effects

High levels of flucytosine are associated with anemia, leukopenia, and thrombocytopenia. These hematologic effects can occur because a small fraction of flucytosine is converted by intestinal bacteria to 5-fluorouracil, a known cytotoxic agent. Serum concentrations should be monitored and maintained between 30 and 80 micrograms per milliliter, especially in patients with renal dysfunction, to reduce the risk of bone marrow suppression. Patients occasionally experience nausea, vomiting, and diarrhea with the use of flucytosine. Transient episodes of hepatotoxicity also have been reported.

Azoles

Azoles or imidazole derivatives inhibit cytochrome P-450–dependent enzymes and block ergosterol synthesis, which are essential for maintaining the integrity of fungal cell membranes. Ketoconazole, the first oral azole, is capable of inhibiting many of the common infecting fungi, except *Aspergillus* organisms and *Mucor* species; however, ketoconazole has been replaced for most indications by newer triazoles (N-substitution of imidazole) that are better absorbed, cause fewer gastrointestinal disturbances, and do not suppress testosterone or corticosteroid synthesis. Ketoconazole is still commonly used topically for the treatment of mucosal candidiasis and tinea versicolor.

Fluconazole is a bistriazole that is effective against most *Candida* species except *C. glabrata* and *krusei,* which are resistant (30). Fluconazole also does not appear to have good clinical activity against *Aspergillus* species. The drug is available in both oral and intravenous forms. After oral administration, serum concentrations are almost identical to those achieved with intravenous administration. Administered intravenously, fluconazole is effective therapy for many of the same indications as is amphotericin B, but because of the associated slower response time, earlier deaths may occur in seriously ill patients. In addition to its use as a primary antifungal therapy, fluconazole is used as chronic suppressive therapy for cryptococcosis and candidiasis in immunodeficient patients.

Itraconazole, another triazole, is available in oral and intravenous preparations. Itraconazole is as effective as amphotericin B for the treatment of less serious infections of blastomycosis, histoplasmosis, chromomycosis, sporotrichosis, and aspergillosis. This azole derivative is the only one that has substantial activity against *Aspergillus* species (30). Itraconazole is not significantly active against *Candida* or *Cryptococcus* organisms (31).

Voriconazole, an investigational triazole, has been shown to be effective in treating acute and chronic invasive aspergillosis in patients failing on other antifungals. Most clinically important fungal pathogens are inhibited by voriconazole levels of 0.5 micrograms per milliliter or less (32).

Distribution and Elimination

Ketoconazole and itraconazole absorption is significantly reduced with the use of antacids or H_2-receptor blockers. Acidic gastric pH augments enteral absorption of itraconazole. Both drugs are distributed into skin, bone, saliva, and peritoneal and aqueous humor fluids, but penetration into the CSF is poor and therapeutic concentrations are not achieved.

Ketoconazole and itraconazole are extensively metabolized by the liver. Very little free drug is excreted in urine, and renal insufficiency does cause significant drug accumulation. Decreased hepatic function requires an adjustment in doses for both drugs.

Fluconazole is distributed into all body tissues, including the vitreous and aqueous humor of the eye and the CNS. The drug is excreted mainly in the urine, with minimal hepatic metabolism. The half-life of fluconazole is approximately 30 hours and is greatly prolonged in patients with renal insufficiency. Because hemodialysis and peritoneal dialysis significantly reduce serum concentrations, the maintenance dose should be given after each course of dialysis.

Adverse Effects

Adverse effects associated with the use of all azole derivatives include nausea, vomiting, headache, diarrhea, hypokalemia, and, rarely, exfoliative dermatitis and hepatocellular inflammation. Transient abnormalities of liver function have been observed in approximately 3% of patients receiving fluconazole. Serum cyclosporin-A concentrations rise in patients receiving ketoconazole and possibly in patients receiving fluconazole or itraconazole. Measurement of cyclosporin-A and serum creatinine levels, to check for cyclosporin-A renal toxicity, is advisable when these antifungal agents are used. Fluconazole is known to inhibit the metabolism of phenytoin, oral hypoglycemic agents, and warfarin. Ketoconazole and itraconazole may decrease the metabolism of the antihistamines terfenadine and astemizole and cause life-threatening arrhythmias.

ANTIVIRAL THERAPY

Viruses are responsible for a large portion of the infectious morbidity and mortality seen worldwide. Fortunately, most viral infections do not result in overwhelming infection and inflammation. The availability of antiviral therapy is much more limited than that of antibacterial drugs; however, considerable progress has been made in the development of treatment for several significant viral groups (Table 7). Antiviral drugs work through a variety of mechanisms, including interference with viral nucleic acid synthesis, prevention of viral uncoating, and inhibition of the function of viral replicative enzymes.

TABLE 7. ANTIVIRAL THERAPY

Antiviral Agent	HSV I & II	VZV	CMV	HPV	Inf A	RSV	Hepatitis B & C
Acyclovir	++	++	+	−	−	−	−
Ganciclovir	+	+	++	−	−	−	−
Oseltamivir	−	−	−	−	++	−	−
Amantadine	−	−	−	−	++	−	−
Ribavirin	−	−	−	−	+	+	−

−, no activity; +, moderate activity; ++, good activity; CMV, cytomegalovirus; HPV, human papillomavirus; HSV, herpes simplex virus; Inf A, influenza A; RSV, respiratory syncytial virus; VZV, varicella-zoster virus.

Guanine Nucleoside Analogs

Acyclovir (acycloguanosine), a synthetic guanosine analog, undergoes monophosphorylation by viral thymidine kinase. Further intracellular phosphorylation occurs, and acyclovir triphosphate is formed. Acyclovir triphosphate binds to viral DNA polymerase, acting as a DNA chain terminator. Acyclovir is the drug of choice for the treatment of herpes simplex (HSV) and varicella-zoster (VZV) viruses; however, the development of thymidine kinase–deficient viral mutants is causing a significant resistance problem in patients who have undergone prolonged or repeated therapy with acyclovir. These mutants are susceptible to alternative agents, such as vidarabine and foscarnet sodium. Acyclovir is available for intravenous, oral, or topical use. Acyclovir is not effective in treating cytomegalovirus (CMV) pneumonia or visceral disease, even though early studies showed some efficacy.

Ganciclovir is an acyclic nucleoside analog of acyclovir. Compared with acyclovir, ganciclovir has greater *in vitro* activity against all herpes viruses, particularly CMV. Like acyclovir, ganciclovir depends on activation by viral thymidine kinase. Because of the dose-related bone marrow toxicity of ganciclovir, its use is limited primarily to the treatment of CMV. CMV infection is a common problem for the immunocompromised patient. A 10- to 14-day course of ganciclovir is effective in the treatment of CMV retinitis, pneumonia, or gastroenteritis. Relapse is frequent with CMV infections, and maintenance therapy with ganciclovir may be necessary. Ganciclovir-resistant strains of CMV can emerge during chronic treatment. Ganciclovir is currently available in both intravenous and oral forms.

Distribution and Elimination

Acyclovir and ganciclovir have good penetration to all body compartments. Both guanine derivatives are dependent on renal excretion. Sixty percent to 90% of acyclovir is excreted unchanged in the urine through glomerular filtration and tubular secretion. Because of the large amounts that are processed through the kidneys, acyclovir may interfere with the renal excretion of drugs that are dependent on renal tubular excretion. This problem is not apparent with ganciclovir use. Dosage adjustments are necessary for both drugs in patients with renal insufficiency.

Adverse Effects

The major adverse effect is alteration of renal function. Large bolus injections of acyclovir can cause crystallization in renal tubules, resulting in elevation of serum creatinine or acute tubular necrosis. Up to 50% of patients receiving high-dose acyclovir for treatment of herpes zoster have some elevation in serum creatinine levels (33).

Dose-related leukopenia, neutropenia, and thrombocytopenia are frequent problems with ganciclovir use. Lowering the dose or stopping therapy for a short time will frequently allow the bone marrow to recover; however, irreversible leukopenia has occurred. Coadministration of any other myelotoxic drug markedly increases the risk of bone marrow suppression.

Neuraminidase Inhibitors

Oseltamivir, an inhibitor of influenza A and B virus neuraminidase, is indicated for the treatment of uncomplicated acute illness due to influenza. Oseltamivir must be started within 2 days of onset of influenza symptoms and continued for a total of 5 days. It has shown some benefit as a prophylactic agent; however, the influenza vaccine remains the prophylaxis of choice. Dosage adjustments are required for creatinine clearance below 30 milliliter per minute.

Distribution and Elimination

Oseltamivir is an ethyl ester prodrug; it is converted to its active form, oseltamivir carboxylate, via hepatic esterase hydrolysis. The prodrug, oseltamivir, is readily absorbed and extensively hydrolyzed. It is neither a substrate for, nor an inhibitor of, cytochrome P-450 isoforms. Oseltamivir carboxylate is entirely eliminated by renal excretion.

Adverse Effects

Most frequent adverse effects were mild to moderate nausea and vomiting.

Tricyclic Amines

Amantadine, a tricyclic amine, was the first antiviral agent approved for sale in the United States. Its mechanism of action is unclear but may be related to the prevention of viral uncoating or inhibition of virus assembly. Amantadine, used for the treatment and prophylaxis of influenza A infections, is not effective against influenza B, which lacks the protein to which amantadine binds in influenza A. Amantadine is most effective when given before exposure or within 48 hours after the development of symptoms. Clinical effectiveness has been estimated at 50% protection against infection and 60% to 70% protection against illness. The protective effect is lost approximately 48 hours after stopping treatment. Amantadine therapy would benefit unvaccinated persons exposed to influenza who have underlying cardiopulmonary, renal, metabolic, neuromuscular, or immunodeficiency diseases. Ramantadine is a structural analog of amantadine and has the same spectrum of activity, mechanism of action, and clinical indications.

Distribution and Elimination

Amantadine and ramantadine achieve good tissue levels for the treatment of influenza A. Both are eliminated by kidney glomerular filtration and tubular secretion, with more than 90% excreted unchanged in the urine. Dosage adjustment must be made for older patients or those with renal dysfunction.

Adverse Effects

Side effects related to amantadine and ramantadine use are few and usually mild. CNS side effects are most common and include confusion, anxiety, insomnia, and hallucinations. These side effects resolve rapidly with discontinuation of therapy.

Purine Nucleoside Analog

Ribavirin is a synthetic purine nucleoside analog that is active *in vitro* against a number of viruses. The specific mechanism of action is not known but may be related to its ability to alter nucleotides used in the synthesis of mRNA. At this time, ribavirin is approved only for the treatment of severe respiratory syncytial virus (RSV) infections. Aerosolized ribavirin for RSV improves oxygenation, decreases viral shedding, and improves the symptoms of pneumonia. Ribavirin, administered orally or intravenously, is the therapy of choice for Lassa fever, an otherwise fatal disease, but is not yet approved by the U.S. Food and Drug Administration. It is also being used intravenously to treat patients with the Hantavirus pulmonary syndrome, recently seen in the western United States (34). Ribavirin is not known to be effective against the Ebola virus. Treatment of Junin, Machupo, and Congo–Crimean hemorrhagic fever (CCHF) viral infections with ribavirin is currently under investigation.

Distribution and Elimination

Ribavirin, given intravenously, has good tissue penetration. At steady state, CSF levels are approximately 70% of plasma levels (35). It undergoes extensive metabolism, but up to 40% of ribavirin is excreted in the urine unchanged.

Adverse Effects

Deterioration of pulmonary function has been reported with aerosol therapy. Precipitation of the drug within the ventilatory apparatus can cause significant mechanical damage. Reticulocytosis, rash, and conjunctivitis also have been seen with the use of aerosolized ribavirin. Oral or intravenously administered ribavirin may cause a transient increase of serum bilirubin and anemia. Ribavirin may be absorbed passively by employees working with patients receiving aerosolized therapy. Although no human data are available, pregnant women should not be exposed to the aerosol because of the teratogenic and embryolethal effects found in animal models treated with ribavirin.

Antiretroviral Drugs

At present, three classes of antiretroviral drugs are available: nucleoside analog reverse transcriptase inhibitors (NRTIs), nonnucleoside analogue reverse transcriptase inhibitors (NNRTIs), and protease inhibitors (PIs) (Table 8). Selecting an appropriate antiretroviral therapeutic regimen involves addressing multiple interdependent issues, including patient adherence, pharmacokinetic properties of the drugs (including food effects and drug–drug interactions), drug resistance, and overlapping adverse effects (36,37).

The NRTIs were the first agents to be developed as antiretrovirals. These agents are structurally similar to the building blocks of nucleic acids (RNA, DNA) but differ from their natural analogs by the replacement of the hydroxy group in the 3' position. NRTIs block reverse transcriptase (viral DNA polymerase) activity by competing with the natural substrates and incorporating into viral DNA to act as chain terminators in the synthesis of proviral DNA. To exert their antiviral activity, NRTIs must

TABLE 8. ANTIRETROVIRAL THERAPY

Nucleoside Reverse Transcriptase Inhibitors (NRTIs)	Nonnucleoside Reverse Transcriptase Inhibitors (NNRTIs)	Protease Inhibitors (PIs)
Zidovudine (Retrovir, AZT)	Nevirapine (Viramune) Delavirdine (Rescriptor)	Saquinavir (Fortovase) Ritonavir (Norvir)
Lamivudine (epivir, 3TC)	Efavirenz (Sustiva)	Indinavir (Crixivan)
Didanosine (Videx, ddI)		Nelfinavir (Viracept) Amprenavir (Agenerase)
Zalcitabine (Hivid, ddC)		Lopinavir/ritonavir (Kaletra)
Stavudine (Zerit, d4T)		
Abacavir (Ziagen)		

first be intracellularly phosphorylated to their active 5' triphosphate forms by cellular kinases. Different nucleoside analogs may require separate metabolic pathways for their anabolic phosphorylation. Based on their phosphorylation profiles, NRTIs can be classified into two groups: (a) those that have greater activity in replicating cells—that is, those that are preferentially phosphorylated in replicating cells—and (b) those that are cell-activation independent and have greater activity in resting cells. Zidovudine and stavudine belong to the first group, whereas didanosine, zalcitabine, and lamivudine belong to the latter.

The NNRTIs bind directly and noncompetitively to the enzyme reverse transcriptase. Although the drugs differ chemically from each other, they all bind to the same site, a site distinct from the substrate binding site. They block DNA polymerase activity by causing conformational change and disrupting the catalytic site of the enzyme. Unlike nucleoside analogues, NNRTIs do not need phosphorylation to become active, and they are not incorporated into viral DNA. In addition, they have no activity against human immunodeficiency virus-2 (HIV-2). When NNRTIs are administered as a single agent or as a part of an inadequately suppressive treatment regimen, resistance emerges rapidly. Mutations conferring resistance to one drug in this class generally confer cross-resistance to most other NNRTIs.

Protease inhibitors exert their antiviral effect by inhibiting HIV-1 protease. HIV-1 protease is a member of the aspartyl class of protease enzymes, composed of two identical halves (symmetric dimer) with an active site located at the base of the cleft created by the dimerization process. This process occurs in the final stages of the HIV life cycle. Inhibition of the protease enzyme results in the release of structurally disorganized and noninfectious viral particles. PIs have antiviral activity in both acutely and chronically infected cells. PIs are metabolized by the cytochrome P-450 system and are themselves, to varying degrees, inhibitors of this system. This leads to a substantial number of interactions with drugs that are inducers, inhibitors, or substrates of this system.

The inhibitory effect of PIs on each other's metabolism has led to the evaluation of specific combinations that may delay or prevent the onset of resistance and may facilitate dose reductions, more convenient dosing regimens, and less toxicity for this class of drugs. Currently, the ritonavir–saquinavir combination is the one for which the most data is available, and it is the only combination recommended by the Department of Health and Human Services. Other PI combinations, including ritonavir–indinavir, indinavir–nelfinavir, ritonavir–nelfinavir, nelfinavir–saquinavir, and amprenavir-based regimens are currently being evaluated. The long-term safety and efficacy of these combinations are unknown.

Triple combination therapy is known as *highly active antiretroviral treatment* (HAART). By using HAART, HIV in the blood is often lowered to undetectable levels for extended periods. The number of new HIV infections has not dropped in recent years; however, the number of AIDS-related deaths has dropped dramatically because of the use of HAART and other treatments. AIDS-related deaths between 1996 and 1997 dropped by 42%. Between 1997 and 1998, AIDS-related deaths decreased by another 20%. Changes in HAART occur frequently enough that timely reviews of the literature are needed to find the most up-to-date guidelines (36).

SUMMARY

Antimicrobial agents are essential for the treatment of life-threatening infections. Today's antibiotics often have a wide spectrum of activity against several classes of organisms; however, even as more potent antimicrobial agents are being developed, organisms are also mutating and developing resistance to these newer agents as well as to many of the older antimicrobials. Appropriate antibiotic selection is extremely important in minimizing the morbidity and mortality rates associated with sepsis. Knowledge of the probable source of infection, the patient's underlying medical problems, and the hospital's microbial sensitivities to antibiotics are key in starting empiric therapy. Identifying the infecting organism is important in guiding further antimicrobial therapy. Narrowing the spectrum of antibiotic therapy to the specific infecting organism or organisms will help decrease the emergence of resistant organisms. In addition, major cost savings may be realized if fewer antibiotics can be used and if sensitivity patterns show that an older drug (often available in generic form) may be therapeutically equivalent to a more recently developed antimicrobial agent.

Most antibiotic dosages must be adjusted for patients with renal or hepatic dysfunction. In many instances, adjustments can be made by using readily available dosing algorithms and tables. Monitoring drug levels for the more toxic antibiotics, such as aminoglycosides and vancomycin, may help avoid the complications of nephrotoxicity or ototoxicity. In the near future, many new antibiotics will be approved for clinical use. These antibiotics may be derivatives of current antibiotics or based on new molecular entities. Some of the new antibiotics will be in the form of ketolides, glycopeptides, everninomicins, streptogramins, oxazolidinones, fluoroquinolones, and β-lactams.

Despite the administration of appropriate antimicrobial agents, morbidity and mortality rates from infection-induced systemic inflammatory response syndrome and multiple-organ dysfunction remain high. Research is continuing on improving the current methods of antimicrobial treatment. Significant improvements in the treatment of infection may come from other modes of therapy. Most of the new therapy is based on genetic cloning technology. Active investigation of ways to suppress the release of systemic mediators of sepsis, such as tumor necrosis factor or interleukins, may help to improve outcome. Development of monoclonal antibodies against specific humoral mediators of sepsis may also ameliorate some of the adverse systemic reactions. The use of cloned granulocyte or macrophage colony-stimulating factors can decrease neutropenic days and possibly improve recovery in the neutropenic patient. Unfortunately, many of these new modalities of therapy are still early in their developmental phase or are so expensive that the costs far outweigh any potential benefit from their use. Additional studies are needed to define which patient populations may benefit from the new biotechnology and how the biotechnology can be incorporated into current antimicrobial therapy.

KEY POINTS

Antimicrobials, which include antibiotics, antifungals, antivirals, and antiparasitic agents, are crucial tools in the armamentarium used daily to control infection and support critically ill patients. Although it is most appropriate to obtain cultures with sensitivities to guide proper selection of antimicrobial therapy, empiric treatment is common in those with critical illness and life threatening infection. The choice of drug(s) must be based on careful review of the patient's history; the physical examination; integration of laboratory data and diagnostic studies; and consideration of potential synergistic, antagonistic, or additive drug interactions. Drug selection must take into account the location of infection, the immune state of the patient, hospital and community-wide sensitivities of the suspected offending organism, hepatic and renal function of the patient, recent antibiotic exposure, history of drug allergies, and pharmacodynamic and pharmacokinetic properties of the drug.

Although fungal infections are less common than bacterial illnesses, they continue to be on the increase. Newer antifungal agents with less toxicity and greater efficacy are under investigation.

Viral illnesses are ubiquitous and may be life threatening, particularly in immunocompromised patients. Antiviral efficacy and number are limited but hopefully will expand in the near future. Clearly, for certain viral pathologies such as human immunodeficiency virus, cytomegalovirus, and herpes simplex, life-sparing agents have been produced.

In the dynamic ICU setting, increasing resistance to antimicrobials continues to occur at an alarming rate. Judicious selection and use of antiinfectives, along with standard infection control measures, must be applied to limit this development. Antimicrobial use should be limited when possible, and drugs should be given in proper amounts for appropriate periods. Some advocate rotating antibiotics to limit microbial exposure, restricting the ICU formulary to select agents, implementing standard antimicrobial order forms to document indications, and allowing the pharmacy to restrict use of specific drugs or substitute more appropriate drugs.

REFERENCES

1. Sanders CC. Cefepime: the next generation? *Clin Infect Dis* 1993;17: 369–379.
2. Anderson JA, Adkinson NF Jr. Allergic reactions to drugs and biologic agents. *JAMA* 1987;258:2891–2899.
3. Eliopoulos GM, Moellering RC Jr. Azlocillin, mezlocillin, and piperacillin: new broad-spectrum penicillins. *Ann Intern Med* 1982;97: 755–760.
4. Fantin B, Ebert S, Leggett J, et al. Factors affecting duration of in-vivo postantibiotic effect for aminoglycosides against gram-negative bacilli. *J Antimicrob Chemother* 1991;27:829–836.
5. Cook FV, Farrar WE Jr. Vancomycin revisited. *Ann Intern Med* 1978; 88:813–818.
6. Van der Auwera P, Klastersky J. Bactericidal activity and killing rate of serum in volunteers receiving vancomycin or teicoplanin with and without amikacin given intravenously. *J Antimicrob Chemother* 1987;19:623–635.
7. Tuazon CU, Washburn D. Teicoplanin and rifampicin singly and in combination in the treatment of experimental *Staphylococcus epidermidis* endocarditis in the rabbit model. *J Antimicrob Chemother* 1987;20:233–237.
8. Fekety R. Vancomycin and teicoplanin. In: Mandell GL, Bennett JE, Dolin R, eds. *Principles and practice of infectious diseases*, 4th ed. New York: Churchill Livingstone, 1995:346–354.
9. Rybak MJ, Albrecht LM, Boike SC, et al. Nephrotoxicity of vancomycin, alone, and with an aminoglycoside. *J Antimicrob Chemother* 1990;25:679–687.
10. Sanford JP, Gilbert DN, Sande ME. The Sanford guide to antimicrobial therapy, 1995. Dallas: Antimicrobial Therapy, Inc., 2000.
11. Eliopoulos GM, Wennersten CB, Gold HS, et al. *In vitro* activities of new oxazolidinone antimicrobial agents against enterococci. *Antimicrob Agents Chemother* 1996;40:1745–1747.
12. Chant C, Rybak MJ. Quinupristin/dalfopristin (RP 59500): a new streptogramin antibiotic. *Ann Pharmacother* 1995;29:1022–1027.
13. Rahal JJ Jr. Antibiotic combinations: the clinical relevance of synergy and antagonism. *Medicine* 1978;57:179–195.
14. Moellering RC Jr. Use and abuse of antibiotic combinations. *R I Med J* 1972;55:341–345.
15. Moellering RC Jr, Weinberg AN. Studies on antibiotic synergism against enterococci. II. Effect of various antibiotics on the uptake of C-14 labeled streptomycin by enterococci. *J Clin Invest* 1971;50:2580–2584.
16. Centers for Disease Control and Prevention, Division of Bacterial and Mycotic Diseases. Antibiotic resistance. 2000 http://www.cdc.gov/ncidod/dbmd/antibioticresistance/. Accessed October 26, 2001.
17. Reed RL II. Antibiotic choices in surgical intensive care unit patients. *Surg Clin North Am* 1991;71:765–789.
18. Jenkins SG. Mechanism of bacterial antibiotic resistance. *New Horizons* 1996;4:321–332.
19. Weinstein L, Dalton AC. Host determinants of response to antimicrobial agents. *N Engl J Med* 1968;279:524–531.
20. McCraney S, Rapp RP. Antibiotic agents in critical care. *Crit Care Nurs Clin North Am* 1993;5:313–323.
21. Dever LA, Dermody TS. Mechanisms of bacterial resistance to antibiotics. *Arch Intern Med* 1991;151:886–895.
22. Bryan LE. Aminoglycoside resistance. In: Bryan LE, ed. *Antimicrobial drug resistance.* Orlando: Academic Press, 1984:241–277.
23. Gilbert DN. Once-daily aminoglycoside therapy. *Antimicrob Agents Chemother* 1991;35:399–405.
24. Craig WA, Ebert SC. Continuous infusion of beta-lactam antibiotics. *Antimicrob Agents Chemother* 1992;36:2577–2583.
25. Bennett JE. Antifungal agents. In: Mandell GL, Bennett JE, Dolin R, eds. *Principles and practice of infectious diseases*, 4th ed. New York: Churchill Livingstone, 1995;401–410.
26. Winn RE. Antifungal therapy in critical care. *Probl Crit Care* 1992;6: 107–131.
27. Bianco JA, Almgren J, Kern DL, et al. Evidence that oral pentoxifylline reverses acute renal dysfunction in bone marrow transplant recipients receiving amphotericin B and cyclosporine. Results of a pilot study. *Transplantation* 1991;51:925–927.
28. Anaisse E, Solomkin JS. Fungal infections: approach to the surgical patient at risk for candidiasis. In: Wilmore DW, Brennan MF, Harken AH, et al., eds. *American College of Surgeons: care of the surgical patient.* New York, Scientific American, 1994, 2:2.
29. Bennett JE, Dismukes WE, Duma RJ, et al. A comparison of amphotericin B alone and combined with flucytosine in the treatment of cryptococcal meningitis. *N Engl J Med* 1979;301:126–131.
30. Bodey GP. Azole antifungal agents. *Clin Infect Dis* 1992;14:S161–S169.
31. Wong-Beringer A, Jacobs RA, Guglielmo BJ. Treatment of funguria. *JAMA* 1992;267:2780–2785.
32. Radford SA, Johnson EM, Warnock DW. *In vitro* studies of activity of voriconazole (UK-109,496), a new triazole antifungal agent, against emerging and less-common mold pathogens. *Antimicrob Agents Chemother* 1997;41:841–843.
33. Bean B, Aeppli D. Adverse effects of high-dose intravenous acyclovir in ambulatory patients with acute herpes zoster. *J Infect Dis* 1985;151: 362–365.
34. Huggins JW, Hsiang CM, Cosgriff TM, et al. Prospective, double-blind, concurrent, placebo-controlled clinical trial of intravenous ribavirin therapy of hemorrhagic fever with renal syndrome. *J Infect Dis* 1991;164:1119–1127.
35. Connor E, Morrison S, Lane J, et al. Safety, tolerance, and pharmacokinetics of systemic ribavirin in children with human immunodeficiency virus infection. *Antimicrob Agents Chemother* 1993;37:532–539.
36. Carpenter CC, Fischl MA, Hammer SM, et al. Antiretroviral therapy for HIV infection in 1998. *JAMA* 1998;280:78–86.
37. Wei X, Ghosh SK, Taylor ME, et al. Viral dynamics in HIV-1 infection. *Nature* 1995;373:117–122.

53

THE BIOLOGY OF TRANSPLANTATION

L. THOMAS CHIN
STUART J. KNECHTLE

KEY WORDS

- Antimetabolites
- Corticosteroids
- Immune defense
- Immune tolerance
- Immunosuppression
- Macrolide antibiotics
- Monoclonal antibody
- Rejection
- T-cell and B-cell function
- Transplant biology

INTRODUCTION

Immunologic rejection of organ transplants is a complex and incompletely understood process involving mechanisms that include those used for natural host defense and that may include unique mechanisms that exist only when the artificial situation of tissue transplantation takes place. The biologic basis of rejection is becoming better understood, thus permitting the development of biologic strategies for tolerance induction. Nevertheless, the backbone of successful organ transplantation continues to be generalized pharmacologic immunosuppression, using agents that have proven to be efficacious and relatively safe. Most immunosuppressive agents currently in use target the T-lymphocyte and only indirectly inhibit B-lymphocytes by suppressing T-helper (T_H) cells. Despite the relative safety of immunosuppressants in current clinical use, transplant patients continue to have a high rate of infection and malignancy resulting from immunosuppression.

INDUCTION OF IMMUNOLOGIC TOLERANCE

Self-tolerance is the normal state of unresponsiveness of an individual's immune system to self-peptides bound to molecules of self-MHC (major histocompatibility complex). In 1953, Billingham and colleagues (1) demonstrated that tolerance could be acquired during lymphocyte development. Tolerance is acquired by at least three possible mechanisms. First, immature T cells during development may undergo clonal deletion in the thymus if they are capable of binding self-antigen with a high affinity. Second, the cells could be functionally inactivated in the periphery (outside the thymus), a process known as *clonal anergy*. Third, potentially autoreactive cells could be inhibited by other cells by an active process called *suppression*. Clonal deletion occurs centrally in the thymus during T-cell development, whereas anergy or functional inactivation of matured T cells occurs principally in the periphery, that is, extrathymically.

T cells recognize foreign antigens that are associated with MHC molecules, a concept termed *MHC restriction*, which originally was described by Zinkernagel and Doherty in 1974 (2). T cells are somewhat analogous to a social "snob" who, when a stranger tries to approach, ignores the stranger, but if the stranger is introduced by an old friend, the snob cordially greets the stranger. For T_H cells, the stranger is a foreign peptide and the old friend is an MHC class II molecule. For cytotoxic T cells, the familiar friend is an MHC class I molecule. The process of MHC restriction applies in T-cell development and maturation in the thymus and helps to orchestrate the processes known as *positive* and *negative selection*. Positive selection refers to the requirement that for T cells to survive the selection process in the thymus, they must express receptors capable of recognizing self-MHC. The cells undergo further negative selection, meaning that cells with a high affinity for self will also be destroyed by a process of apoptosis. Only about 2% of immature T-cell precursors reaching the thymus ever leave the thymus as mature functional T cells.

Biologic approaches to transplantation tolerance are varied. Thymic tolerance refers to an approach that tries to mimic the normal development process of central tolerance, in which T cells that are responsive to self are eliminated. This approach depends on having a functional thymus gland and includes inoculation of the recipient thymus gland with donor cells that express the MHC antigen. Simultaneously, an antilymphocyte preparation, either an antibody or irradiation, is administered. Recipients are rendered tolerant to islet cells (injected into the thymus) or to a subsequent organ transplant. Questions that remain to be answered are whether thymic tolerance can be reproduced reliably in humans and whether adults can develop thymic tolerance.

Other approaches to transplantation tolerance seek to inactivate the ability of peripheral lymphocytes to respond to donor antigen. Recent attention focused on a potential role for chimerism in promoting immunologic tolerance to the donor. *Chimera* refers to an individual who contains cells from two or more genetically distinct individuals. Because organ transplants and, obviously, bone marrow transplants transfer leukocytes from the donor to the recipient, if the recipient is treated so that his or her immune system will not destroy the donor cells, lymphocytes from the donor can develop within the recipient, rendering him or her chimeric. Radiation and pharmacologic immuno-suppression may permit the development of chimerism, but the question remains whether chimerism is a result of tolerance or is functionally involved in promoting tolerance. If stable chimerism of hematopoietic cells develops, this state may confer an advantage for the development of specific immunologic tolerance to an organ transplant. If, however, the donor leukocytes become the dominant immunologic force, they may attack the host. Graft-versus-host reaction occurs if the donor leukocytes mount an immune response toward the recipient. This phenomenon generally occurs when the recipient is unable to reject the transplant, but the "transplanted" lymphocytes reject the host. Tolerance therefore requires a balance between host-versus-graft reaction and graft-versus-host reaction.

IMMUNOBIOLOGY

Rejection Mediated by T-Lymphocytes

Acute allograft rejection refers to immunologic rejection occurring within days to weeks of an organ transplant and is characterized histologically by a dense lymphocytic infiltrate in the transplanted organ. Although clinical parameters are useful for suggesting the diagnosis of rejection, needle biopsy has become the standard of diagnosis for organ-transplant rejection. Hematoxylin and eosin staining of tissue specimens during acute allograft rejection demonstrates a lymphocytic infiltrate with eosinophils as well. The effector cell for acute rejection is the cytotoxic T cell, which expresses a CD8 cell-surface marker. Such infiltrates also will contain numerous T_H cells (CD4+) which, as their name implies, are regulatory cells that assist other cells of the immune system to differentiate into effector cells. A third subset of T cells, called *suppressor cells*, is thought to inhibit T-lymphocytes from attacking an allograft; however, it is not clear whether these cells are a distinct subset. Nevertheless, the T-lymphocytes as a whole are the cells most responsible for orchestrating acute allograft rejection. An unmodified immune response typically results in immunologic destruction of an allograft in 7 to 14 days, depending on the degree of MHC disparity between donor and recipient. The goal of pharmacologic immunosuppression is either to kill T-lymphocytes or to prevent their activation or effector mechanisms.

In the 1960s, Gowans and Knight (3) identified lymphocytes as the cells responsible for generating an immune response. They also demonstrated the ability of lymphocytes to circulate through the blood and lymphoid tissues. T-lymphocytes originate in the bone marrow but mature in the thymus, where they differentiate into the subtypes mentioned earlier. The process of clonal selection of lymphocytes during maturation leads to antigen-specific immune responses because any particular lymphocyte expresses only one receptor, conferring specificity of the immune response. Any lymphocyte capable of binding to a particular antigen will respond to that antigen, but not to unrelated antigens. The activation of lymphocytes and their differentiation require not only binding of a particular antigen but also delivery of a second signal, usually delivered by another cell. Typically, this second signal can be provided only by antigen-presenting cells (APCs), which include B-lymphocytes, macrophages, and dendritic cells.

In addition to presenting antigens to T cells, APCs deliver a costimulatory signal, which permits proliferation and differentiation of T cells to their effector function.

Rejection Mediated by Antibody

Allograft rejection mediated by antibody occurs within minutes to hours and is termed *hyperacute rejection*. These antibodies are typically immunoglobulin M (IgM) and immunoglobulin G (IgG), which are capable of binding complement and activating the complement cascade and a full-blown inflammatory response. Hyperacute rejection is characterized histologically by microvascular thrombosis; hemorrhage into the parenchyma; severe edema of the tissue with a massive neutrophil infiltrate; and, ultimately, ischemia and necrosis of the organ. Hyperacute rejection mediated by antidonor antibody is currently an untreatable type of rejection, hence the development of screening techniques for prevention. The cross-match test consists of reacting recipient serum, potentially containing antidonor IgM and IgG, with donor lymphocytes to screen for potential lymphocytotoxic antibodies. In the event of a positive cross-match test between donor and recipient, the transplantation would be contraindicated.

Another example of antibody-mediated or humoral rejection occurs in the setting of ABO-incompatible organ transplantation. The ABO blood group antigens are ubiquitously expressed glycoproteins, and persons who do not express either the A or the B blood group antigens express natural antibody to these antigens. *Natural antibody* refers to antibody that is produced toward antigens even in the absence of previous exposure to them. Hyperacute rejection is predictable in ABO-incompatible organ transplants, except in the case of liver transplants, which are less susceptible to hyperacute rejection but nevertheless have a poorer prognosis in the setting of ABO incompatibility.

The cellular basis for the immunoglobulin response to an allograft is the B-lymphocyte, which displays on its surface immunoglobulin molecules of a predetermined specificity that serve as its antigen receptors. When B-lymphocytes encounter antigen, they undergo clonal expansion and differentiation to plasma cells, which secrete antibody of the same specificity—initially IgM isotype with later elaboration of IgG isotype. To undergo clonal expansion and differentiation, B-lymphocytes also require the assistance of T_H cells.

Role of Cytokines in Rejection and Graft Injury

Cells of the immune system secrete and respond to soluble factors, called *cytokines*, that exert diverse effects on the immune system. Many cytokines are produced by T cells and macrophages, but other cells secrete them as well. Cytokines currently include ten interleukins (ILs), the interferons (IFN), tumor necrosis factor (TNF), and colony-stimulating factors. The names of these cytokines are not necessarily a useful guide to their properties. In humans, some cytokine genes are located on the long arm of chromosome 5, and others are located on chromosome 6 within the MHC locus.

Cytokines act through specific cell-surface receptors. Despite the structural diversity of cytokines themselves, cytokine receptors

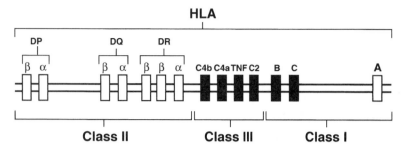

FIGURE 1. Gene map of the HLA (human leukocyte antigen) region located on chromosome 6.

fall into three distinct families: (a) members of the immunoglobulin supergene family, (b) the hematopoietin receptor family, and (c) the TNF receptor family. Different cytokines may produce similar effects because of the ability of cytokine receptors to cross-react with more than one cytokine.

T cells and macrophages are the major sources of cytokines. T_H cells can be divided into two subpopulations based on the cytokines they produce: T_{H1} cells elaborate IL-2, lymphotoxin, and IFN-γ; T_{H2} cells elaborate IL-4, IL-5, IL-6, and IL-10. In addition, IFN-γ made by T_{H1} cells inhibits cytokine production by T_{H2} cells, and IL-10 made by T_{H2} cells inhibits cytokine production by T_{H1} cells. Another example of antagonism between different cytokines is transforming growth factor-beta (TGF-β), which inhibits the production of IL-2 by T_{H1} cells.

The importance of cytokines in the immune response is exemplified by CD4+ T cells, which respond to recognition of MHC class II antigen and IL-1 elaborated by the APC. Similarly, CD8+ T-cell responses are enhanced by IL-1 and IL-6. IFN-γ increases MHC class II expression by macrophages and nonlymphoid cells capable of MHC class II induction. These cytokines play a key role in activation of the immune system, but they also may play an important role in tolerance induction. For instance, the T_{H2}-type immune response generally is associated with unresponsiveness to tissue transplants, and a T_{H2} response is associated with IL-4, IL-5, IL-6, and IL-10. These same cytokines are associated with B-cell activation, proliferation, and differentiation.

Activation of CD4 and CD8 T cells depends on the production of IL-2 and IL-2 receptors. The major source of IL-2 for both cell types is the CD4+ T cell. Binding of antigen to the T-cell receptor activates resting T cells in the G_0, or resting phase of the cell cycle, to proceed to G_1. In G_1, T cells become responsive to IL-1 and other cytokines and begin to synthesize cytokines themselves. The number of T cells that pass from G_1 to S phase of the cell cycle and therefore are committed to division depends on the number of IL-2 receptors occupied by IL-2. The proliferative response of T cells thus depends directly on the number of receptors, the IL-2 concentration, and the length of the IL-2/IL-2 receptor interaction.

The principal cytokines involved in B-cell activation and differentiation are IL-4, IL-5, and IL-6. Cytokines also are involved in the regulation of isotype expression by B cells. Finally, macrophage activation is mediated substantially by IFN-γ, which upregulates MHC class I and class II expression and stimulates macrophages to become more active. The contribution of cytokines to the immune response toward organ transplants is an area of intensive research.

Chronic rejection of organ transplants refers to a gradual process of organ injury occurring months to years after transplantation and resulting in parenchymal fibrosis and ischemic changes. Chronic rejection may be mediated largely by cytokines.

The Role of MHC in Rejection

The principal antigens involved in immunologic rejection of organ transplants were identified in the mouse by Snell (4) and are called *histocompatibility antigens*. The analogous system in the human is called the HLA system (human leukocyte antigen) (5–7). The HLA genes are located on the short arm of chromosome 6 and can be divided into class I, class II, and class III genes (Fig. 1). MHC class I molecules are the principal target for cytotoxic T-cells and antibody and are, therefore, the principal target for the effector arm of the immune response. MHC class II molecules are recognized by T_H cells and are involved in antigen presentation to the immune system. MHC class III molecules include some of the complement proteins involved in the complement cascade and some cytokine genes.

The major MHC class I molecules in the human are the HLA-A and HLA-B antigens and are expressed on all nucleated cells. Both these loci are highly polymorphic. The MHC class I molecule consists of a heavy chain with α-1, α-2, and α-3 domains; a transmembrane domain and cytoplasmic tail; and a noncovalently bound light chain called β_2-microglobulin. An approximately 10–amino acid peptide is bound to the peptide-binding groove in the MHC class I molecule during transport to the cell surface and aids in proper conformation and, therefore, function. MHC class I molecules are recognized by CD8+ T-cells, either during activation or by effector cytotoxic cells during allograft rejection.

The MHC class II molecules are expressed only on B-lymphocytes, monocytes, macrophages, and vascular endothelial cells. Their expression is inducible on some other cell types, and the degree of expression is upregulated in response to IFN-γ. The MHC class II molecules consist of α and β chains, each containing two domains. The variable portion of the molecule is located in the β chain. Class II-bearing APCs present peptide that is associated with their MHC class II molecule to CD4+ T-cells (Fig. 2), a process called *indirect antigen presentation*, and thus initiate CD4-mediated immune responses (Fig. 3).

The HLA typing of organ donors and recipients developed as a serologic test that is dependent on serologic definition of HLA class I and class II loci. More recently, it has become possible to perform DNA typing of the MHC. For practical reasons, organ donors and recipients typically are typed at the two major HLA class I loci (A and B) and at the principal HLA class II locus (DR). Because each person expresses two codominant alleles at each locus, it follows that donors and recipients can match

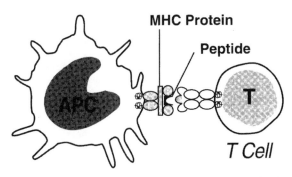

FIGURE 2. Major histocompatibility complex (MHC) molecules on antigen-presenting cells associate with peptide and present the foreign peptide to T cells, initiating the immune response.

a maximum of six antigens. The more HLA antigens that are matched between donor and recipient, the weaker the biologic force promoting rejection.

Because of the central importance of the HLA system in the immunobiology of transplantation and because of the possibility of selecting well-matched donors and recipients for kidney transplantation, all donors and all potential renal transplant recipients undergo serologic HLA typing based on lymphocytotoxicity testing. Because of the availability of sequence information for many of the HLA molecules, DNA typing using allele-specific oligonucleotide methods eventually will replace serologic and cellular typing methods.

To prevent immediate or hyperacute rejection of organ transplants, a cross-match test is routinely performed on potential kidney transplant recipients to identify their preformed antidonor antibodies. Cross-matching uses a lymphocytotoxicity test in which recipient serum is tested for its ability to lyse donor lymphocytes when complement is added. A positive reaction generally indicates antibodies to MHC class I antigens and would indicate a high risk of hyperacute rejection. Such a positive cross-match would exclude the potential recipient from receiving a kidney transplant from that donor because the risk of hyperacute rejection would be greater than 85%.

PHARMACOLOGIC IMMUNOSUPPRESSION

Because specific tolerance of the organ transplant recipient to the donor organ cannot yet be reliably achieved in humans, the long-term success of organ transplantation depends on the chronic use of nonspecific immunosuppressive agents to suppress the alloimmune response. Unfortunately, no reliable means exists of evaluating the alloimmune response to the donor organ after transplantation; despite substantial efforts, immunologic monitoring of organ transplant recipients is imprecise, and no reliable tests are currently available. Because of the redundancy of the immune system, immunosuppression using a combination of agents that work by different mechanisms tends to provide more successful immunosuppression. Although 10 years ago only a handful of immunosuppressive agents were in use, the number and variety of agents are proliferating rapidly, requiring the transplant physician to be familiar with an ever-expanding pharmacopeia (Table 1).

Corticosteroids

Corticosteroids have been used in transplantation longer than any other drug. In combination with other agents, relatively low

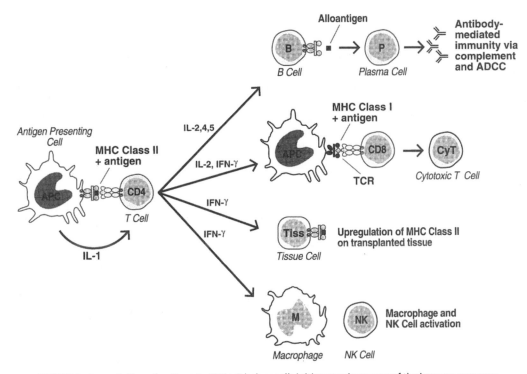

FIGURE 3. Presentation of antigen to CD4+ T-helper cells initiates various arms of the immune response. Direct presentation of antigen to CD8+ cytotoxic T cells also plays an important role. IL, interleukin; MHC, major histocompatibility complex; TCR, thymocyte receptor; NK, natural killer cells.

TABLE 1. CURRENT AGENTS FOR CLINICAL TRANSPLANTATION

Drug	Classification	Major Side Effects	Mechanism of Action
Corticosteroid	Adrenal glucocorticoid	See Table 2	Inhibits T-lymphocyte cytokine production; causes lymphocytes to migrate from blood to lymphoid tissue
Azathioprine	Antimetabolite	Bone marrow suppression	Inhibits purine synthesis
Cyclophosphamide	Antimetabolite	Bone marrow suppression; GI disturbance	Inhibits nucleic acid
Mycophenolate mofetil	Antimetabolite	GI disturbance	Inhibits purine synthesis
Cyclosporine	Macrolide antibiotic	Nephrotoxic, neurotoxic	Inhibits cytokine gene transcription by lymphocytes
Tacrolimus	Macrolide antibiotic	Nephrotoxic, neurotoxic, should not be used with cyclosporine, must wait at least 24 h before initiating therapy with cyclosporine. Must monitor potassium levels	Inhibits cytokine gene transcription by lymphocytes
Rapamycin	Macrolide antibiotic	Elevated cholesterol/triglycerides	Inhibits response of T cell to IL-2
ALG (antilymphocyte globulin)	Polyclonal antibody	Serum sickness	Kills lymphocytes
OKT3	Monoclonal antibody	Cytokine release syndrome	Eliminates CD3+ lymphocytes

GI, gastrointestinal; IL-2, interleukin 2.

doses are used for maintenance of immunosuppression. Higher doses, sometimes called *pulse-steroid therapy*, are used to treat acute cellular rejection.

The side effects of corticosteroid use are multiple and dose related, with higher doses and longer treatment resulting in a higher frequency of side effects (Table 2). The mechanism of action of steroids is complex and incompletely understood, but steroids are known to inhibit antigen-stimulated T-lymphocyte proliferation by a variety of mechanisms. Steroids block IL-1 synthesis by macrophages and inhibit the induction of MHC class II antigens required for antigen presentation. They block IFN-γ production, neutrophil migration, and lysosomal enzyme release by polymorphonucleocytes; they indirectly inhibit IL-2 synthesis. Steroids inhibit the actions of vasodilators, such as histamine and prostacyclin, and blunt the response of leukocytes to chemotaxins, agents that increase vascular permeability. Despite their profound effect on lymphocytes, neutrophils, eosinophils, and monocytes, steroids do not have a significant impact on antibody-mediated rejection.

Steroids induce a profound redistribution of leukocytes, as reflected in the peripheral blood leukocyte count. Lymphocyte, monocyte, eosinophil, and basophil counts decrease and neutrophil counts increase within hours of administration of a pulse

TABLE 2. SIDE EFFECTS ASSOCIATED WITH STEROID USE

Acute
  Fluid retention
  Psychosis
  Peptic ulcers
  Diabetes
  Delayed wound healing
Chronic
  Cataracts
  Osteoporosis
  Myopathy
  Growth retardation (prepuberty)

dose of steroids. The increase in peripheral neutrophils occurs because of demargination of the cells from capillary endothelium and reduced migration out of the circulation. Lymphocytes, on the other hand, tend to leave the circulation and migrate to the lymphoid tissue in response to steroids.

One of the goals of clinical transplantation is to minimize the dose of steroids used and therefore reduce the incidence of side effects by adding other immunosuppressive agents. Subsets of patients—such as HLA-identical living-related kidney transplant recipients, some haploidentical living-related kidney transplant recipients, and some liver transplant recipients—may require no maintenance steroid therapy at all.

Azathioprine

Schwartz and Damashek (8) discovered that 6-mercaptopurine (6-MP) prevents antibody formation in rabbits injected with human serum albumin. To increase the therapeutic index of 6-MP, Hitchings and colleagues (9) synthesized an analog, azathioprine (Imuran). Elion (10) found that azathioprine had a greater immunosuppressive effect. Azathioprine is converted to 6-MP in vivo and inhibits purine nucleotide synthesis by altering DNA structure. The drug therefore acts nonspecifically on proliferating lymphocytes and polymorphonuclear leukocytes at the level of DNA and RNA synthesis. Calne and Murray (11) reported on its use in a canine renal transplant model. Azathioprine has been used clinically since 1963 for maintenance immunosuppression (usually at a dose of 2–3 mg/kg daily), but, unlike steroids, it has no value in treating ongoing rejection. Its principal toxicity is related to bone marrow suppression, and an excessive dose may result in leukopenia. The leukopenia generally reverses when the dose is lowered or the drug is stopped. This drug should not be used in combination with allopurinol because this combination may result in profound leukopenia. Although the finding is controversial, some reports have indicated that azathioprine is hepatotoxic. Patients with significant liver dysfunction should not receive azathioprine.

Mycophenolate Mofetil

Mycophenolate mofetil (MMF) is a morpholinoethyl ester of the fungal antibiotic mycophenolic acid. This molecule inhibits the synthesis of lymphocyte guanosine monophosphate. Because of this inhibition, the drug blocks the proliferative response of lymphocytes. Its selective effect on lymphocytes occurs because lymphocytes rely on *de novo* purine synthesis, whereas other cell types use the salvage pathway for purine synthesis. Although mycophenolic acid is poorly absorbed after oral administration, MMF has improved bioavailability.

In vitro, mycophenolic acid suppresses antibody formation, inhibits cytotoxic T-cell generation, and reduces the expression of adhesion molecules on lymphocytes. In preclinical studies in a variety of animal models of organ transplantation, MMF, in combination with cyclosporine or other immunosuppressants, is effective in preventing rejection and treating ongoing rejection (12–14). MMF also may exert a preventive effect on the development of proliferative arteriopathy, a critical lesion in the development of chronic rejection.

Multicenter double-blinded placebo controlled trials showed a 40% to 50% reduction in the incidence of acute rejection in patients treated with MMF compared with patients treated with either placebo or azathioprine without a concomitant increase in adverse events. A recent retrospective analysis of the U.S. Renal Data System (USRDS) registry showed that MMF decreases the risk of graft loss secondary to chronic allograft nephropathy by reducing acute rejection. In addition, MMF appears to have an independent protective effect against graft loss from chronic allograft nephropathy because a decreased incidence of chronic allograft failure was found in patients without a history of rejection (15).

In 1995, MMF was approved for clinical use. In most transplant centers, MMF has essentially replaced azathioprine. The current recommended dose is 2 g daily. MMF is generally well tolerated. The most common adverse effects are on the gastrointestinal tract: diarrhea in approximately 30% of the patients, esophagitis and gastritis in approximately 5%, and gastrointestinal hemorrhage in 4%. Most of these symptoms respond to a reduction in drug dosage. Leukopenia and anemia occur with a similar frequency to that seen with azathioprine.

Cyclosporine

Borel (16) demonstrated the potent immunosuppressive properties of cyclosporine, a cyclic endecapeptide isolated from the fungus *Tolypocladium inflatum gams*. Clinical studies were initiated in the late 1970s, and in 1983, the drug was approved for use in the United States. This drug had the most profound impact on immunologic rejection of organ transplants of any drug introduced in the past 30 years. The use of cyclosporine permitted establishment of clinically acceptable results in cardiac and hepatic transplantation. Results of cadaveric renal transplantation improved about 25% and continue to improve with increasing experience.

Cyclosporine is a cyclic polypeptide that is soluble in lipids and organic solvents but insoluble in aqueous solutions. This insolubility has made the preparation of reliable pharmaceutical formulations difficult. A microemulsification of the drug is currently being used; it is better absorbed, bile independent, and gives more consistent blood levels. Cyclosporine is metabolized by the hepatic cytochrome P-450 enzymes; therefore, blood levels of the drug are increased by inhibitors of cytochrome P-450 (ketoconazole, erythromycin, some calcium-channel blockers) and are decreased by cytochrome P-450 inducers (rifampin, phenobarbital, phenytoin). Ninety percent of the metabolites of cyclosporine are cleared in the bile; therefore, the dose of cyclosporine should be lowered in patients with liver failure. Metabolites of cyclosporine are less immunosuppressive and less toxic than is the parent compound. Renal failure does not significantly alter cyclosporine clearance. Response to the drug is variable among individuals, and the dose should be guided by blood levels. Numerous assays are commercially available to measure cyclosporine levels, but the current state-of-the-art method uses measurement of only the parent compound, with either high-pressure liquid chromatography or an immunoassay. If given intravenously, cyclosporine should be administered slowly over 12 to 24 hours because of the associated risk of seizures. The typical side effects of cyclosporine include nephrotoxicity resulting from its vasoconstrictive effect on the afferent arterioles in the kidney; neurotoxicity, manifested by tremors; and, occasionally, seizures, hypertension, hyperlipidemia, gingival hypertrophy, and hirsutism.

Cyclosporine acts intracellularly in the lymphocyte by binding to calcineurin, a calcium- and calmodulin-dependent protein phosphatase. The cyclosporine–calcineurin complex blocks the nuclear translocation of nuclear factor of activated T-cells (NFAT-1) and thus prevents activation of the transcription of IL-2. Cyclosporine, like tacrolimus and rapamycin, depends for its activity on its ability to complex with endogenous intracellular proteins, called immunophilins (cyclophilin). Although cyclophilin is a systranspeptidal prolyl isomerase (rodamase), the immunosuppressive action of cyclosporine is unrelated to the isomerase activity of the immunophilin. Instead, the complex of cyclosporine and cyclophilin permits binding of the complex to calcineurin.

Cyclosporine nephrotoxicity can be difficult to diagnose and can be manifested in both acute and chronic forms. Acute cyclosporine toxicity generally responds to withholding the drug, is diagnosed histologically by striped fibrosis seen on renal transplant biopsy, and is a reversible phenomenon. Chronic cyclosporine toxicity, on the other hand, is manifested by vascular sclerosis, interstitial fibrosis, and thickening of the renal tubular and glomerular basement membranes. These changes are often irreversible despite discontinuance of cyclosporine.

Cyclosporine remains the backbone of immunosuppression therapy for most organ transplant recipients in the United States, and its interesting pharmacologic properties have spawned a vast amount of research into its mechanisms of action and side effects. Cyclosporine has interactions with many other drugs (Table 3).

Tacrolimus

Similar to cyclosporine, tacrolimus (formerly FK506) is a macrolide antibiotic derived from a soil fungus; however, tacrolimus is about 100 times more potent than cyclosporine. Its mechanism of action is analogous to that of cyclosporine. Specifically, tacrolimus binds to FK-binding protein, and this complex binds

TABLE 3. DRUGS THAT INTERACT WITH CYCLOSPORINE[a]

Drugs that increase cyclosporine levels by decreasing its metabolism
  Calcium channel blockers
    Diltiazem hydrochloride
    Verapamil hydrochloride
    Nicardipine hydrochloride
  Erythromycin
  Clarithromycin
  Ketoconazole
  Methylprednisolone
  Danazol
  Bromocriptine mesylate
  Metoclopramide hydrochloride
  Fluconazole
  Itraconazole

Drugs that decrease cyclosporine levels by increasing its metabolism
  Phenytoin
  Phenobarbital
  Rifampin
  Carbamazepine

[a]For detailed list of interactions, contact Novartis Pharmaceuticals, East Hanover, NJ, U.S.A.

calcineurin and blocks nuclear translocation of the cytosolic subunit of NFAT, thus preventing the activation of genes, including the gene encoding for IL-2. In short, both drugs work by inhibiting IL-2 gene transcription and, hence, IL-2 production. Inhibition of IL-2 blocks antigen-driven T-cell proliferation and differentiation.

Tacrolimus is absorbed from the gastrointestinal tract more easily than is cyclosporine, and its absorption is not bile dependent. This factor is advantageous for liver transplant recipients whose bile is drained initially by a T-tube. Tacrolimus is cleared by the hepatic cytochrome P-450 system, and, therefore, like cyclosporine, it is dramatically affected by enzymes that either induce or inhibit the cytochrome P-450 system. Monitoring of plasma levels of tacrolimus is necessary to guide therapy, and a manual microtiter plate enzyme immunoassay is currently used. This immunoassay relies on a monoclonal antibody and enzyme-labeled tacrolimus to measure plasma or whole-blood levels.

Tacrolimus was developed primarily at the University of Pittsburgh beginning in 1989. In a multicenter, randomized trial that compared tacrolimus with cyclosporine in human liver transplant recipients (17), tacrolimus resulted in fewer rejection episodes and a lower incidence of steroid-resistant rejection. Nevertheless, tacrolimus is associated with a higher incidence of side effects, particularly neurotoxicity and nephrotoxicity. It has been used successfully in small bowel transplantation to prevent rejection. Its side-effect profile is similar to that of cyclosporine and includes nephrotoxicity, neurotoxicity, diabetes, and diarrhea.

Sirolimus

Sirolimus (the U.S. approved name for rapamycin) was released by the U.S. Food and Drug Administration for clinical use in 1999. It is a macrolide antibiotic that is structurally related to tacrolimus but has a different mechanism of action. Activation of T cells occurs in three phases. The first phase causes transcriptional activation of immediate and early genes (i.e., IL-2 receptor)

that allow T cells to progress from a quiescent (G_0) to a competent (G_1) state. In the second phase, T cells transduce the signal triggered by cytokines, leading to entry into the cell cycle with resultant clonal expansion and acquisition of effector function (third phase). Whereas cyclosporine and tacrolimus inhibit the first phase by inhibiting IL-2 production, sirolimus inhibits the second phase by inhibiting the response to IL-2. Both sirolimus and tacrolimus bind to the same family of immunophilins, the intracellular FK-binding proteins (FKBP). Once complexed with FKBP, sirolimus binds to and modulates the activity of a protein called the mammalian target of rapamycin (TOR), which results in cell cycle arrest at the G_1-S interface. Specifically, the sirolimus–FKBP–TOR complex blocks the IL-2-stimulated phosphorylation activation of $p70^{S6K}$, which prevents the phosphorylation of the 70s ribosomal protein S6. This blocks the synthesis of ribosomal and elongation factor proteins required for the accelerated rate of protein synthesis necessary for progression of T cells into S phase. The sirolimus–FKBP–TOR complex also appears to inhibit the activity of cyclin-dependent kinase complexes and the activation of the retinoblastoma protein, which are essential steps for the transition from G_1 to S. In addition to inhibiting T-cells, sirolimus blocks stimulation of B-cell proliferation and immunoglobulin synthesis. Sirolimus also appears to inhibit growth factor–induced cell proliferation of fibroblasts, endothelial cells, hepatocytes, and smooth-muscle cells. Because sirolimus occupies the same binding protein as tacrolimus, it was initially thought that sirolimus would act as a competitive inhibitor of tacrolimus. Whereas this was shown *in vitro*, immunosuppressive concentrations of tacrolimus *in vivo* are not sufficient for these drugs to be antagonistic. In fact, it has been demonstrated that the combined use of sirolimus and tacrolimus (as well as cyclosporine) is synergistic.

Sirolimus has demonstrated potent antirejection activity, as well as the ability to prolong allograft survival in a number of animal models of organ transplantation. Two phase 3 multicenter, randomized, double-blind studies evaluating the efficacy of sirolimus in preventing acute allograft rejection after transplantation have been performed. The Rapamune U.S. Multicenter Study compared three groups: sirolimus 2 mg daily, sirolimus 5 mg daily, and azathioprine 2 to 3 mg per kilogram of body weight daily. Immunosuppression also consisted of cyclosporine and prednisone. Both sirolimus regimens were significantly more effective than azathioprine in reducing the incidence of acute rejection. Moreover, the sirolimus groups required less antibody therapy for the treatment of steroid-resistant rejection. Six- and 12-month graft survival did not differ among treatment groups. The Rapamune Global Study Group was similar to the U.S. study, but it compared the two sirolimus groups with a placebo group. The results mirrored those of the U.S. study, with the sirolimus groups being significantly more effective than placebo in preventing acute rejection. Whereas previous studies showed no effect of sirolimus on renal function, a surprising finding of both phase 3 studies is that a dose-related elevation in serum creatinine was seen in sirolimus-treated patients. At 6 and 12 months, the mean serum creatinine levels were approximately 10% higher in the sirolimus-treated groups. No effect on renal function was noted in the monotherapy trials of sirolimus. The elevation in serum creatinine may represent enhanced cyclosporine-associated renal effects. The major side effects of sirolimus are thrombocytopenia, leukopenia, and hyperlipidemia. In general, these effects can be controlled by dose reduction or adding lipid-lowering agents (18). Clinical experience with sirolimus remains limited and the ultimate role of sirolimus in maintenance immunosuppression remains to be determined.

Antilymphocyte Globulin

Antilymphocyte globulin is a polyclonal serum preparation made by inoculating horses, rabbits, or goats with human lymphocytes; collecting the plasma; and purifying the IgG fraction. Alternatively, thymocytes may be used, resulting in antithymocyte globulin (ATG). ATGAM (Upjohn, Kalamazoo, MI, U.S.A.) was introduced in 1972 and is produced in the horse. In 1999 SangStat (Fremont, CA, U.S.A.) introduced an antithymocyte globulin prepared in rabbits and marketed as Thymoglobulin. Both preparations include antibodies to multiple antigenic determinants and are a polyclonal preparation of antibodies. Some of the antibodies are lymphocytotoxic, and the preparation acted through opsonization of lymphocytes and through the reticuloendothelial system to clear the lymphocytes.

OKT3

The technology of monoclonal antibodies stems from the hybridoma work of Kohler and Milstein in the late 1970s. The only commercially available preparation of monoclonal antibodies for use in organ transplantation is the murine monoclonal antibody to the CD3 determinant on human T-lymphocytes, Muromonab-CD3 (Orthoclone OKT3; Ortho Pharmaceuticals, Raritan, NJ, U.S.A.). OKT3 is the product of a hybridoma formed by fusing a myeloma cell line with a murine lymphocyte specific for CD3. The hybridoma is cultured in mouse ascites, and OKT3 is purified from the ascites.

The CD3 determinant is located on all mature human T-lymphocytes and is closely associated with the T-cell receptor complex. This complex is responsible for transmitting the intracellular message once the T-cell receptor has engaged its antigen target. By binding to the CD3 determinant, OKT3 prevents antigen recognition and, ultimately, the generation of cytotoxic T cells. Additionally, OKT3 results in rapid opsonization and clearance of T cells by the reticuloendothelial system. There is a decrease not only in CD3+ T cells but also in the CD4+ and CD8+ T-cells. Another mechanism of action of OKT3 is through modulation of the T3 surface protein. T-lymphocytes that do not express CD3 are incapable of participating in allograft rejection. Finally, in addition to interfering with the generation of cytotoxic T cells and modulating their cell-surface proteins, OKT3 blocks the cytotoxic activity of already formed cytotoxic T-cells.

The most common side effects associated with the use of OKT3 include fever, headache, and severe malaise. Pretreatment with at least 250 mg of methylprednisolone prior to the first dose can blunt the side effects. The side effects are most prominent with the first and second doses of OKT3 and gradually decline in severity with continued use. The most common severe side effect of OKT3 use is pulmonary edema, which is typically seen in patients with preexisting fluid overload. Hypertension resulting from cytokine release can be serious in patients with severe underlying cardiovascular disease. The central nervous system side effects of OKT3 are, again, most severe in patients with underlying cerebrovascular disease, old age, and diabetes. Nevertheless, most older patients tolerate OKT3 without significant difficulty.

Initially, OKT3 was used to treat acute renal allograft rejection. Cyclosporine should be withheld during treatment, and steroid therapy can be minimized except to blunt OKT3 side effects. In renal transplant recipients, the serum creatinine level often increases after the first dose of OKT3 but declines thereafter. To prevent a rebound of T-cell clones involved in rejection, at least 7 days of therapy are recommended, and, in general, a maximum of 14 days of therapy is recommended. More than 14 days of therapy can be used, but the risk of lymphoproliferative disorders increases after more than 2 weeks of consecutive doses of OKT3.

In addition, OKT3 is used in induction immunotherapy. Typically, a 7- to 14-day course is started on the day of the transplantation, with the goal of preventing acute allograft rejection. The efficacy of OKT3 induction protocols has not been clearly established, although the drug is commonly used for this purpose. As with the treatment of acute allograft rejection, administration of OKT3 should be accompanied by monitoring of CD3 levels to ascertain the drug's efficacy in a given patient. CD3+ cells should represent fewer than 10% of peripheral T cells to achieve therapeutic efficacy. Because OKT3 is a xenogeneic antibody, xenoantibodies may be produced in the murine portion of the molecule and may prevent the efficacy of OKT3. The presence of xenogeneic antibodies can be measured by a commercially available assay, and use of this assay should be considered in patients with previous exposure to OKT3 or in those who lack a reduction of CD3 levels during treatment.

The use of OKT3 has been associated with a high reactivation rate of cytomegalovirus and with Epstein–Barr viral infections, leading to lymphoproliferative disorders. For this reason, prophylaxis with ganciclovir is recommended to minimize the risk of cytomegalovirus reactivation.

Anti–IL-2 Receptor-α (CD25)

Monoclonal antibodies against the IL-2α receptor (CD25) were introduced in 1997 by Roche (daclizumab) and in 1998 by Novartis (basiliximab). Resting lymphocytes express only the intermediate affinity IL-2 receptor, the IL-2Rβ/γ complex. On T-cell activation, increased expression of IL-2Rβ/γ parallels *de novo* expression of IL-2Rα chains. This results in the expression of a high affinity IL-2 receptor complex, IL-2R$\alpha/\beta/\gamma$. The expression of such an activation-induced cell-surface protein provides a convenient target for the selective destruction of activated lymphocytes. Both daclizumab and basiliximab have been genetically engineered to contain most of the human immunoglobulin sequence while retaining the original specificity of the original antibody. This allows reduced immunogenicity of the antibody and allows the antibody to participate in antibody-directed cell-mediated cytotoxicity and complement-directed cytotoxicity. As a result, both preparations have minimal side effects. Both can reduce acute rejection episodes significantly during the first six posttransplant months. Most transplant centers that used monoclonal or polyclonal antibodies as part of early posttransplant immunosuppression have switched to one of the anti-IL-2Rα receptor monoclonals.

SUMMARY

The trends in the clinical use of immunosuppressive agents for organ transplantation over the past 2 years have included (a) developing steroid-free approaches and discontinuing steroids after a period of months to years; (b) reduced use of OKT3 because, in combination with calcineurin inhibitors, the risk of PTLD increases; (c) an increased interest in rapamycin-based strategies to decrease reliance on steroids and decrease the dose of a calcineurin inhibitor; (d) increased use of tacrolimus; and (e) increased use of anti-CD25 monoclonal antibody. Experimental protocols being evaluated currently include protocols aimed at tolerance induction, typically through the use of a T-cell-depleting antibody in combination with rapamycin or mycophenolate mofetil. A clinical trial of anti-CD154 with initial promising results in nonhuman primates was disappointing in clinical application. Other targets of costimulation blockade such as B7 or use of the agent CTLA4-Ig are currently being investigated. Many other immunosuppressive drugs are in clinical trials using a broad variety of drug classes. Testing of new strategies ultimately should benefit patients by increasing the success of organ transplantation and decreasing the side effects of immunosuppressive therapy.

KEY POINTS

Successful organ transplantation has evolved through an improved understanding of immune function combined with an expanded drug armamentarium and directed immunosuppression.

Despite advances in immunosuppression, transplant patients have an increased incidence of infection and malignancy.

At present, immunosuppressive therapy targets the T-lymphocyte and indirectly inhibits B-lymphocytes by suppressing T-helper cells.

Current immunosuppressive regimens use a three- or four-drug approach. These drugs usually consist of low-dose corticosteroids, an antimetabolite (e.g., azathioprine or mycophenolate), and a macrolide antibiotic (e.g., cyclosporine A or tacrolimus).

High-dose pulse steroids and T-cell specific monoclonal antibody therapy (e.g., ALG, and OKT3) are used most commonly to control acute rejection.

Genetic modification of donor organs will be required to modify the xenograft response if the prospect of xenotransplantation is ever to be realized.

Exciting research is under way to alter the genetic makeup of transplanted organs, to store and clone native tissue, and to develop more specific immunotherapy to prevent complications such as post-transplantation infection or malignancy.

REFERENCES

1. Billingham RE, Brent L, Medawar PB. "Actively acquired tolerance" of foreign cells. *Nature* 1953;172:603–606.
2. Zinkernagel RM, Doherty PC. Restriction of *in vitro* T cell-mediated cytotoxicity in lymphocytic choriomeningitis within a syngeneic or semi-allogeneic system. *Nature* 1974;248:701–702.
3. Gowans JL, Knight EJ. The route of re-circulation of lymphocytes in the rat. *Proc R Soc Lond [Biol]* 1964;159:257–282.
4. Snell GS. T-cells, T cell recognition structures, and the major histocompatibility complex. *Immunol Rev* 1978;38:63–69.
5. Dausset J, Ivanyi P, Ivanyi D. Tissue alloantigens in humans: identification of a complex system (Hu-1). In: Balner H, Cleton FJ, Eernisse JG, eds. *Histocompatibility testing 1965*. Copenhagen: Munksgaard, 1965:51.
6. van Rood JJ, van Leeuwen A. Leukocyte grouping: a method and its application. *J Clin Invest* 1963;42:1382.
7. Amos DB. Human histocompatibility locus HL-A. *Science* 1968; 159:659–660.
8. Schwartz R, Damashek W. Drug-induced immunological tolerance. *Nature* 1959;183:1682–1683.
9. Hitchings GH, Elion GB, Falco EA, et al. Antagonists of nucleic acid derivatives. I. The *Lactobacillus casei* model. *J Biol Chem* 1950;183:1–9.
10. Elion GB. The comparative metabolism of Imuran and 6-MP in man. *Proceedings of the Annual Meeting of the American Association for Cancer Research* 1969;10:21.
11. Calne RY, Murray JE. Inhibition of the rejection of renal homografts in dogs by Burroughs-Wellcome 322. *Surg Forum* 1961;12:118–120.
12. Morris RE, Hoyt EG, Eugui EM, et al. Prolongation of rat heart allograft survival by RS 61443. *Surg Forum* 1989;40:337–338.
13. Platz KP, Sollinger HW, Hullett DA, et al. RS-61443–a new, potent immunosuppressive agent. *Transplantation* 1991;51:27–31.
14. Sollinger HW, Belzer FO, Deierhoi MH, et al. RS-61443 (mycophenolate mofetil): a multicenter study for refractory kidney transplant rejection. *Ann Surg* 1992;216:513–519.
15. Ojo AO, Meier-Kriesche HU, Hanson JA, et al. Mycophenolate mofetil reduces late renal allograft loss independent of acute rejection. *Transplantation* 2000;69:2405–2409.
16. Borel JF. Cyclosporine-A—present experimental status. *Transplant Proc* 1981;13:344–348.
17. The U.S. Multicenter FK506 Liver Study Group. A comparison of tacrolimus (FK506) and cyclosporine for immunosuppression in liver transplantation. *N Engl J Med* 1994;331:1110–1115.
18. Kelly PA, Gruber SA, Behbod F, et al. Sirolimus, a new, potent immunosuppressive agent. *Pharmacotherapy* 1997;17:1148–1156.

CARDIOPULMONARY TRANSPLANTATION

BYRON P. UNGER

KEY WORDS

- ABO
- Accelerated atherosclerosis
- Acute bronchiolitis
- Acute rejection
- Allograft
- Antithymocyte globulin (ATG)
- Autonomic
- Azathioprine
- Bilateral sequential
- Bronchiolitis obliterans
- Cadaveric
- Cardiac
- Cardiac allograft vasculopathy (CAV)
- Cardiomyopathy
- Cardioplegia
- Chronic bronchiolitis
- Chronic rejection
- Coronary artery disease
- Cyclosporine
- Denervation
- Donor
- Double-lung
- FK-506
- Heart
- Heart failure
- Heart-lung
- HLA (human leukocyte antigen)
- Hyperacute rejection
- Immunosuppressant
- International Society for Heart and Lung Transplantation (ISHLT), Registry of
- Ischemic time
- Living-related
- Lung
- Methylprednisolone preservation solution
- Mycophenolate mofetil (MMF)
- OKT3
- Orthotopic heart
- Panel of reactive antibodies (PRA)
- Pulmonary hypertension
- Rejection
- Single-lung
- T-cell
- Tacrolimus (FK-506)
- Transesophageal echocardiography (TEE)
- Transplant
- University of Wisconsin (UW) solution
- Xenotransplantation

ORTHOTOPIC HEART TRANSPLANTATION

Christian Barnard performed the first successful human heart transplant in 1967 in South Africa (1). This followed Lower and Shumway's successful canine cardiac transplant in 1960 (2) and the first human heart transplant attempt by Hardy and colleagues in 1964 using the heart of a chimpanzee (3). Despite dismal initial outcomes, there were significant advances in donor and recipient management and substantially increased knowledge of all aspects of transplantation. The discovery of the immunosuppressive qualities of cyclosporine by Borel in 1976, and its introduction to clinical practice in the early 1980s (4) led to a renewed interest in heart and heart-lung transplants in the 1980s. Exponential growth occurred in the number of these procedures performed over the past two decades, and these have now become relatively common procedures for end-stage cardiopulmonary disease. A total of 55,359 orthotopic heart transplants (OHTs) and 2,698 heart-lung transplants worldwide have been reported to the Registry of the International Society for Heart and Lung Transplantation (ISHLT) as of March 2000 (5). The majority of recipients are men between 40 and 65 years of age primarily for either cardiomyopathy or coronary artery disease. The number of OHTs performed worldwide plateaued in 1991 at approximately 4,000 annually, largely due to a shortage of compatible donor organs (Fig. 1). In fact, worldwide heart transplantation volume over the past few years has clearly declined such that the number performed in 1999 was the lowest in over a decade (5). This has occurred despite the practice of using less stringent donor and recipient selection criteria.

Indications for Heart Transplantation

Patients with end-stage cardiac disease that have New York Heart Association (NYHA) class IV symptoms and a poor prognosis despite maximal medical and surgical therapy are considered potential candidates for heart transplantation (6). However, American College of Cardiology consensus guidelines for the selection of cardiac transplant recipients have suggested that an ejection fraction of 20% or NYHA class IV symptoms alone may be insufficient indications for transplantation. Transplantation is indicated if either of these two factors is associated with refractory ventricular arrhythmias, a maximal oxygen consumption (VO_{2max}) of less than 14 mL per kg per minute, or unstable coronary ischemia that is not amenable to angioplasty or surgery (7,8).

Coronary artery disease and primary cardiomyopathy (most commonly idiopathic dilated cardiomyopathy) are the most common indications for adult heart transplantation, accounting for over 90% of all transplants (Fig. 2) (5). Miscellaneous causes (4.9%) include etiologies such as cardiac tumors, restrictive

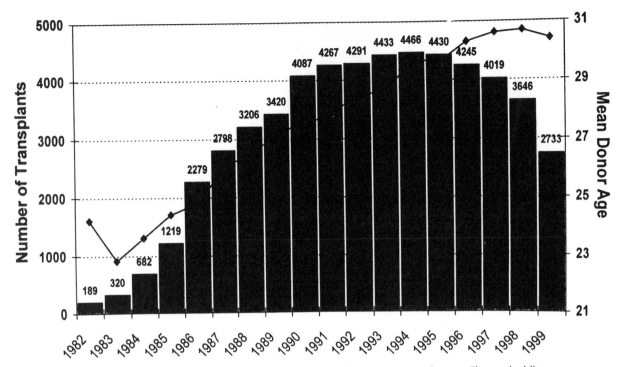

FIGURE 1. Worldwide heart transplantation volumes and mean donor age by year. The *marked line* indicates the mean age of heart donors. (From Hosenpud JD, Bennet LE, Keck BM, et al. The Registry of the International Society for Heart and Lung Transplantation: Seventeenth Official Report—2000. *J Heart Lung Transpl* 2000;19:909–931, with permission.)

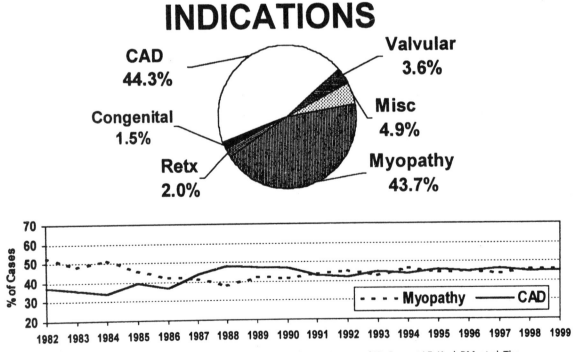

FIGURE 2. Indications for adult heart transplantation. (From Hosenpud JD, Bennet LE, Keck BM, et al. The Registry of the International Society for Heart and Lung Transplantation: Seventeenth Official Report—2000. *J Heart Lung Transpl* 2000;19:909–931, with permission.)

TABLE 1. GENERAL CONTRAINDICATIONS TO ORGAN TRANSPLANTATION

Age > 60–65 yrs
Incurable malignancy
Systemic or incurable infection
Severe pulmonary disease or recent pulmonary embolism/infarction
Diabetes with poor control or severe end-organ complications
Irreversible renal or hepatic dysfunction
Severe cerebral or peripheral vascular disease
Morbid obesity
Alcohol, tobacco, or drug abuse
Emotional instability or major psychiatric disorder
Noncompliance with medical therapy
Unsupportive social environment

cardiomyopathy due to sarcoidosis or amyloidosis, and dilated cardiomyopathy secondary to doxorubicin toxicity or infection (such as coxsackie B virus or *Trypanosoma cruzi*).

Contraindications to Heart Transplantation

Contraindications to heart transplantation include general contraindications to any organ transplant (Table 1) in addition to those that are specific to OHT. Controversy exists regarding which factors constitute general contraindications to transplantation, such as the appropriate maximum recipient age, and the presence of diabetes or malignancy. Although physiologic age is more important than chronologic age, it is clear that 1-year, and particularly 5-year mortality rates, are higher following OHT in recipients over the age of 65 (5). Diabetes has been shown to be compatible with successful heart transplantation since the steroid component of immunosuppression can be tapered or discontinued in many patients, allowing better glucose control. However, transplantation remains contraindicated in diabetics with associated end-organ damage or poor glucose control, as well as in those experiencing severe or irreversible dysfunction in other organ systems (Table 2) secondary to end-stage heart disease. On the other hand, malignancies such as Hodgkin lymphoma that have been cured are no longer grounds for disqualification, and even patients with selected systemic diseases, such as

TABLE 2. MULTISYSTEM PATHOPHYSIOLOGIC CONSEQUENCES OF END-STAGE HEART DISEASE

Organ System	Consequence
Central nervous system	Confusion
Pulmonary	Interstitial edema
	Pulmonary venous hypertension
	Increased alveolar-arterial oxygen gradient
Renal	Prerenal azotemia
	Oliguria
Hepatic	Chronic venous congestion
	Synthetic and metabolic dysfunction
	Ascites
	Hepatomegaly
Endocrine	Elevated serum renin/angiotensin/ aldosterone
	Elevated serum catecholamines

amyloidosis, have successfully undergone heart transplantation (9).

One absolute contraindication to isolated OHT is refractory pulmonary hypertension, since the donor right ventricle (RV) rapidly fails when contracting against an elevated, fixed pulmonary vascular resistance (PVR). Maximum tolerable levels are generally accepted to be a transpulmonary gradient (mean pulmonary artery [PA] pressure minus mean left atrial [LA] pressure) of greater than 15 mm Hg or an irreversible PVR of greater than 6 Wood units (480 dynes $\cdot$ sec $\cdot$ cm^{-5}) (10). The PVR index (PVR normalized for body surface area) may be a more useful predictor of RV failure after OHT than PVR itself (11).

Mechanical support devices, such as left-ventricular assist devices (LVAD), implantable cardioverter defibrillators (ICD), or intraaortic balloon pumps (IABP) were once considered absolute contraindications to heart transplantation, but are now often used preoperatively in patients who go on to have successful outcomes following OHT (12–15).

Recipient Selection

General evaluation includes a detailed history, physical examination, and laboratory investigations such as a complete blood count (CBC), serum electrolytes, glucose, blood urea nitrogen (BUN), creatinine, creatinine clearance, urinalysis, liver enzyme and function tests, thyroid function tests, serum lipoprotein profile, and coagulation studies. Infectious diseases should be ruled out. Investigation of pulmonary status includes an arterial blood gas, chest x-ray (CXR), pulmonary function tests (PFT), and occasionally ventilation-perfusion (V/Q) scanning or pulmonary angiography as clinically indicated. Finally, immunologic evaluation includes an ABO blood type, antibody screen, and human leukocyte antigen (HLA) type. A panel of reactive antibodies (PRA) screen is used to detect the presence of preformed antibodies in the recipient's serum that may be directed against donor HLAs. Such preformed antibodies usually exist as a result of a prior blood transfusion or pregnancy in the recipient and can lead to hyperacute rejection and fulminant graft failure following transplantation (16). A prospective crossmatch between donor cells and recipient serum is generally only performed if the PRA screen is positive.

Cardiovascular assessment of heart transplant candidates includes an electrocardiogram (ECG), CXR, echocardiogram, right- and left-heart catheterization, exercise testing with measurement of VO$_{2max}$, and often a myocardial biopsy. Ventricular ejection fraction should be accurately measured, the presence of reversible coronary lesions should be ruled out, and PA hypertension with a fixed PVR must be excluded. PA vasodilators used to assess the reversibility of PVR include prostaglandin E$_1$ (PGE$_1$), prostacyclin, nitroglycerin, sodium nitroprusside, inhaled nitric oxide (NO), phosphodiesterase-III inhibitors (amrinone and milrinone), dobutamine, and isoproterenol. Knowledge of which PA vasodilators are effective in an individual patient is valuable for the management of PA hypertension, which may be present after separation from cardiopulmonary bypass (CPB), and in the early period in the intensive care unit (ICU) (17). Pulmonary hypertension and an elevated PVR must be aggressively treated to prevent acute RV failure.

Priority Status Level

Once contraindications to transplantation are ruled out and transplant candidates have been thoroughly evaluated, they are placed on a waiting list and assigned a priority status level as defined by the United Network for Organ Sharing (UNOS). Three UNOS categories now exist for heart transplant candidates. UNOS status 1A candidates are those with the most immediate need for transplantation. These candidates generally require support with inotropic agents and possibly mechanical ventilation in the ICU. Their survival may be dependent on mechanical devices, such as an LVAD or IABP. UNOS status 2 patients are more stable and are not necessarily even hospitalized while on the waiting list.

Donor Selection

Donor hearts must be carefully selected to ensure compatibility and prolonged survival in the recipient, despite the fact that a shortage of donor organs dramatically limits the number of transplants that could be performed annually. However, less stringent donor selection criteria have been used during the past several years in an effort to expand the pool of donor organs. The donor selection process begins with the diagnosis of brain death in a patient and obtaining consent for organ donation. Evaluation of the donor then includes consideration of the patient's age, gender, heart size, ABO blood group, hemodynamic stability, history of current and past medical problems and surgery, and a review of the circumstances leading to brain death. Although some centers have accepted hearts from donors over the age of 50, donor age over 35 years is associated with increased 1-year and 5-year recipient mortality rates following transplantation (5). Similarly, patients receiving a heart from a female donor have an increased risk of mortality. The absence of major thoracic trauma, previous cardiac surgery, hypoxia, and significant infection in the donor is also important. Although the majority of brain-dead organ donors have some degree of hemodynamic instability, the heart may be acceptable for transplantation provided that excessive inotropic support (greater than 10 μg per kg per minute of dopamine or dobutamine) is not required to maintain a mean arterial pressure (MAP) between 70 and 90 mm Hg, following volume resuscitation to a central venous pressure (CVP) of at least 5 to 10 mm Hg. There should also be no history of prolonged hypotension or excessive cardiopulmonary resuscitation.

Thorough cardiac evaluation of the donor is essential. Ideally, there should be an absence of risk factors for coronary artery disease, such as a strong family history, hypertension, hyperlipidemia, diabetes mellitus, and significant smoking history. The donor ECG should show no evidence of ischemia or prior infarction; however, ST segment changes or T-wave abnormalities that are commonly seen with brain death may make it difficult to rule out myocardial ischemia with an ECG alone. Echocardiography is used to rule out significant regional wall motion abnormalities, valvular dysfunction, anatomic abnormalities such as a patent foramen ovale, and to assess global ventricular function and ejection fraction. If suspicion of coronary artery disease remains following this evaluation, coronary angiography should be performed. Perhaps the most important evaluation of the donor heart is at the time of organ harvesting. Visual inspection is used to assess size and contractility of the heart, and to rule out a significant myocardial contusion. The coronary arteries are palpated to detect any evidence of atherosclerosis, and the PA and CVPs are estimated either by palpation or by transducing the pressure via a needle placed directly into the PA or central veins. A palpable thrill may indicate the presence of valvular abnormalities.

Donor-Recipient Matching

Recipients and donors are matched primarily on the basis of ABO blood type, heart size, UNOS status, geographic location, and time that the recipient has been on the waiting list. ABO compatibility is mandatory since mismatch results in hyperacute rejection, due to the presence of preformed recipient antibodies reacting against donor tissue antigens. Recipients with blood type AB generally have the shortest waiting times for organs, whereas those with type O blood wait the longest. The HLA antibody screen (PRA screen) is used to detect the presence of preformed antibodies in the recipient's serum directed against a panel of HLAs. If the PRA screen yields greater than 10% reactivity, then a negative prospective crossmatch between donor cells and recipient serum is required prior to transplantation (18). The relatively short safe ischemic time for hearts precludes routine prospective HLA crossmatching prior to transplantation.

The "safe" ischemic time for hearts, defined as the time from donor aortic cross-clamping during harvest to recipient cross-clamp removal and reperfusion following transplantation, is 4 to 6 hours. Mortality risk is increased when an ischemic time of 4 hours is exceeded (5,19). The limited time is one reason for considering geographic location in the allocation of donor organs. Finally, donor body weight should be within 20% of that of the recipient. Somewhat oversized donor hearts may be desirable for recipients with pulmonary hypertension.

Donor Heart Procurement

Donor cardiectomy is usually the initial procedure in multi-organ procurement. However, since this may follow hours of surgical dissection of the heart and other organs, hypovolemia and hypothermia must be prevented prior to cardiectomy. Premature cardiac arrest may also occur, secondary to absorption of potassium-containing organ preservation solutions used for *in situ* perfusion of abdominal organs being harvested. Excessive use of inotropes and vasopressors to support systemic perfusion prior to cardiectomy may also jeopardize the donor heart.

The donor heart is inspected following median sternotomy and pericardiotomy, the epicardial coronary arteries are palpated for atherosclerotic plaques, then the aorta and both vena cavae are dissected. Many hearts are found to be unacceptable for transplantation at this stage, but may still be used for homograft valve procurement. If the heart is suitable for transplantation, the donor is heparinized, a cardioplegia cannula is inserted into the aortic root, the superior vena cava (SVC) is ligated, and the inferior vena cava (IVC) and right inferior pulmonary vein are transected. The heart is then decompressed and 1 to 3 L of University of Wisconsin (UW) solution or cardioplegia (typically a crystalloid solution consisting of sodium, chloride, bicarbonate, dextrose, mannitol, and a high concentration of potassium) is delivered into the aortic root, perfusing the coronaries to arrest and preserve the heart. Topical cooling with iced saline slush and coronary perfusion with cold preservative solutions are used to produce hypothermic arrest, significantly extending the safe ischemic time (20). The aorta is cross-clamped when the heart ceases to eject. The SVC, pulmonary veins, PA, and aorta are then transected. Following excision, the heart is examined for subtle valve lesions or other anatomic abnormalities. If no abnormalities are found, the heart is placed in a sterile bag, which is then placed inside a second sterile bag containing cold saline, and then stored inside an insulated cooler at 4 to 6°C for transportation.

Recipient Preoperative Management

The recipient transplant anesthesiologist and team are often informed of the available organ only a few hours prior to the transplant operation. Fortunately, extensive evaluation is generally not required immediately preceding transplantation, as most candidates have already been thoroughly evaluated. Exceptions are patients that deteriorate suddenly. The etiology and type of heart failure, current medical management, allergies, and NPO status should be reviewed preoperatively. Hemodynamic parameters and reversibility of elevated PVR should be noted, and volume status assessed.

Patients are usually maintained on multidrug regimens that may include inotropes, vasodilators, antiarrhythmics, and diuretics, which should be continued preoperatively if the patient has been optimized on a particular drug combination. All oral anticoagulants should be stopped and coagulation status may need to be restored with fresh frozen plasma (FFP) preoperatively. Minimal or no sedative premedication should be given. The time of last oral intake should be ascertained, as aspiration prophylaxis is often required. Drug side effects, such as hypokalemia and hypovolemia from diuretics or multisystem effects of amiodarone, must be evaluated and corrected if possible. Preoperative management requires knowledge of mechanical devices, such as LVADs and IABPs, that are often used to support patients awaiting OHT.

Intraoperative Management

To minimize donor organ ischemia time, it is crucial that the recipient is cannulated and ready for CPB just as the allograft arrives in the operating room. The anesthesiologist, operating room nurses, surgeons, and perfusionist must be present at the time of anesthetic induction as patients are critically ill and may require emergency surgical intervention.

The recipient is transferred to the operating room breathing supplemental oxygen. Routine intraoperative monitors are placed. External defibrillator/pacing pads should be placed prior to induction since there is a relatively high incidence of life-threatening arrhythmias in these patients. Large-bore peripheral intravenous (i.v.) access is obtained. Invasive hemodynamic monitors are then placed prior to induction, including an arterial catheter and central venous ± PA catheter. All invasive monitors are placed with meticulous attention to aseptic technique, since these patients are at increased risk for postoperative infection secondary to therapeutic immunosuppression. During placement of invasive monitors, PA pressure elevation secondary to Trendelenburg positioning or hypoxia and hypercarbia following i.v. sedation may be poorly tolerated. PA catheter placement in heart transplant recipients may be difficult, has associated risks, and its

benefit is controversial. Difficulty is often encountered placing a PA catheter, as RV dilation is often present and low cardiac output or severe tricuspid regurgitation limits forward blood flow floating the balloon. Placing a PA catheter also introduces potential risks, such as infection and PA rupture in patients with elevated PA pressures. Finally, the pulmonary capillary occlusion pressure (PCOP) often may not accurately reflect LA and left ventricle (LV) end-diastolic volume status in the presence of elevated PA pressures. Newer PA catheters capable of continuously monitoring cardiac output or mixed venous oxygen saturation may be helpful during OHT. If this monitor is to be used, PA catheterization is most often performed via the right internal jugular vein. It has been shown that intraoperative use of the right internal jugular vein for invasive monitoring does not jeopardize future endomyocardial biopsies via this same route (16,21). The catheter should be withdrawn into its sheath prior to snaring the SVC cannula and cardiectomy, keeping the catheter sterile so that it may be advanced into the donor heart after separation from CPB. Finally, intraoperative transesophageal echocardiography (TEE) is now routinely employed in most centers performing heart transplants (22). TEE may be used intraoperatively to assess contractility, ventricular volume, aortic atherosclerosis, and valvular function. Specific to OHT, TEE may be used to detect the presence of cardiac thrombi prior to recipient cardiectomy, and to assess atrial or caval suture lines, pulmonary venous flow, and intracardiac air in the allograft heart.

Transplants are emergency procedures and patients should be considered to have a "full stomach." Ideally, a "rapid-sequence" induction would be used; however, the need for a rapid induction and intubation to prevent aspiration is tempered by the need for a controlled induction to avoid myocardial depression and maintain hemodynamic stability. A combination of etomidate (0.1 to 0.3 mg per kg), fentanyl (up to 10 μg per kg), and succinylcholine (1.5 mg per kg) has been suggested as one way to achieve these goals on induction (23). Prolonged circulation time and a reduced volume of distribution associated with a low cardiac output state should be anticipated, and drug dosage should be carefully titrated. Maintenance of anesthesia relies heavily on opiates, such as fentanyl (10 to 30 μg per kg) or sufentanil (1 to 5 μg per kg), in addition to low-dose volatile anesthetics, benzodiazepines, and neuromuscular blocking drugs. This "balanced" anesthetic technique generally maintains hemodynamic stability and still allows for tracheal extubation within 12 to 18 hours postoperatively. Nitrous oxide is avoided because it may increase PVR, reduce the inspired oxygen concentration, and expand intracardiac air bubbles. Following induction, even small changes in preload and afterload critically affect ventricular performance and may result in systemic arterial hypotension. Treatment of hypotension prior to CPB should rely on inotropes and vasopressors rather than fluid loading, unless significant hypovolemia exists, since excess fluid contributes to pulmonary hypertension and right heart failure.

Antibiotics are given at the time of anesthetic induction and immunosuppressive therapy is initiated perioperatively. Although immunosuppression protocols vary between transplant centers, the induction phase of therapy is most commonly a triple-drug regimen, consisting of cyclosporine or tacrolimus (FK-506), azathioprine, and corticosteroids (5). Azathioprine is often the first immunosuppressant to be administered, typically given either

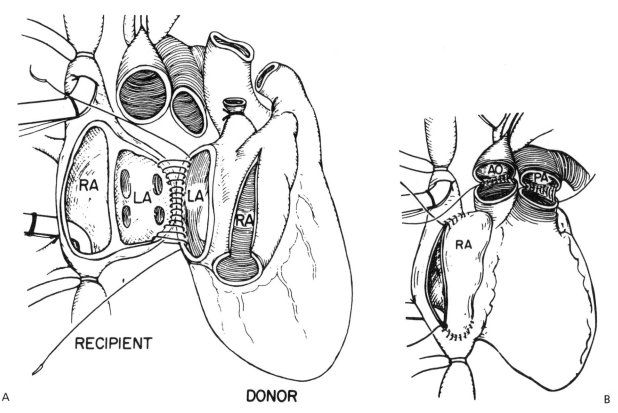

FIGURE 3. Traditional biatrial anastomotic technique for orthotopic heart transplantation. **A:** The initial sutures of the donor and recipient left atrial anastomosis. A segment of the recipient right atrium has been resected and the donor right atrium incised in preparation for right atrial anastomosis. **B:** The right atrial, aortic, and pulmonary artery anastomoses near completion. (From Bolman RM. Cardiac transplantation: the operative technique. In: Thompson ME, ed. *Cardiac transplantation.* Philadelphia: FA Davis Co, 1990:136–144, with permission.)

orally in the preoperative period, or infused intravenously following the induction of anesthesia. Methylprednisolone 500–1000 mg is also given following anesthetic induction or immediately prior to release of the aortic cross-clamp during the latter stages of CPB, whereas cyclosporine is most commonly first administered in the ICU following transplantation. Some centers also use antithymocyte globulin (ATG) as part of the perioperative immunosuppression induction.

Prior to CPB, manipulation of the heart should be minimized since intracardiac thrombi may be present (a diagnosis typically made by intraoperative TEE). Following systemic heparinization (300 to 400 IU per kg), both vena cavae and the aorta are cannulated, CPB is initiated, and the patient is cooled to 28° to 30°C. During recipient heart excision an LA cuff containing the pulmonary veins, and adequate lengths of the recipient aorta and PA are left *in situ* for anastomosis to the donor left atrium and great vessels. In the past, a right atrial (RA) cuff containing the vena cavae was left *in situ* for anastomosis to the donor right atrium (Fig. 3). Anastomosis of donor and recipient right atria created large atrial cavities with abnormal geometry ("snowman" enlargement of the left atrium), impaired atrial function because of asynchronous donor and recipient atrial contraction, sinus node injury, and an increased risk of atrial septal aneurysm and thrombus formation. More recently, a bicaval reimplantation technique has commonly been employed, in which the recipient right atrium has been excised with the remainder of the recipient

heart, leaving only the IVC and SVC for anastomosis to the donor vena cavae (Fig. 4) (24). The bicaval technique has been shown to better preserve RA function, lower RA pressure, improve cardiac output, and reduce the incidence of atrial arrhythmias, tricuspid regurgitation, atrial thrombus formation, and the development of atrial septal aneurysms (25–27). Perhaps most important, the bicaval technique allows the return of sinus rhythm in nearly all cardiac transplant recipients; in contrast, conduction abnormalities require permanent pacemaker implantation in 5% to 10% of patients using the traditional biatrial anastomotic technique (26,28). The bicaval anastomotic technique is safe, technically no more difficult than anastomosis of the donor and recipient atria, and does not prolong CPB or graft ischemic time. Following anastomosis of the donor and recipient IVC and SVC or right atria, the left atria (including pulmonary veins) are anastomosed, the heart is then filled with cold saline to displace intracardiac air, and the aorta and pulmonary arteries are attached. The heart is then de-aired and the aortic cross-clamp is removed, allowing reperfusion of the donor heart and ending the ischemic time. Electromechanical activity of the heart generally resumes spontaneously following reperfusion but pacing may be required, particularly if the bicaval anastomosis technique was not used (28,29).

Prior to weaning from CPB, the "water-tightness" of all anastomoses is verified, the heart is filled with blood, adequacy of de-airing is confirmed by TEE, epicardial pacing wires are placed, the lungs are ventilated, the PA catheter is advanced, and serum

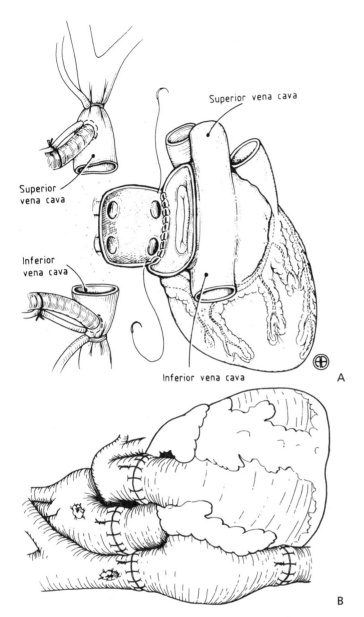

FIGURE 4. Bicaval anastomotic technique for orthotopic heart transplantation. **A:** The recipient inferior vena cava (IVC) and superior vena cava (SVC) remnants, in addition to the left atrial cuff containing four pulmonary veins *in situ*. The allograft left atrium is partially anastomosed to the recipient left atrial cuff. **B:** The completed IVC, SVC, pulmonary artery, and aortic suture lines following anastomosis using the bicaval technique. (**A:** From Deleuze PH, Benvenuti C, Mazzucotelli JP, et al. Orthotopic cardiac transplantation with direct caval anastomosis: is it the optimal procedure? *J Thorac Cardiovasc Surg* 1995;109:731–737, with permission; **B:** From Gamel AE, Yonan NA, Grant S, et al. Orthotopic cardiac transplantation: comparison of standard and bicaval Wythenshawe techniques. *J Thorac Cardiovasc Surg* 1995;109:721–730, with permission.)

ionized calcium is restored to normal. Patients with excessive blood volume should be ultrafiltrated and hemoconcentrated prior to separation from CPB. If the heart rate (HR) is less than 70 to 90 beats per minute (bpm), despite chronotropic drug infusions, epicardial pacing is initiated to maintain a HR of at least 90 to 110 bpm.

Weaning from CPB is almost always achieved with the infusion of catecholamines, since even well-preserved allograft hearts

may have somewhat impaired contractility and transient bradyarrhythmias. In addition, allograft hearts often have comparatively noncompliant ventricles that deliver a relatively fixed stroke volume and are dependant on adequate preload and a HR of 90 to 110 bpm to produce an adequate cardiac output. Many centers consider isoproterenol (0.03 to 0.15 μg per kg per minute) the drug of choice to improve contractility and increase HR in this setting, while others prefer to use dobutamine or dopamine. Aggressive treatment of pulmonary hypertension and the use of other drug infusions may be required to treat RV dysfunction. The management of RV dysfunction is reviewed in the following section on postoperative cardiovascular support.

Successful weaning from CPB is followed by ongoing support of cardiovascular and respiratory function. Bleeding is more common following OHT than other cardiac procedures because of an increased number of anastomoses that have the potential to leak, and a relatively high incidence of coagulopathy in these patients. Coagulopathy may be secondary to prolonged CPB, hypothermia, dilution of coagulation factors, preoperative aspirin or oral anticoagulant therapy, and liver dysfunction due to congestive heart failure. Once all heparin is completely reversed with protamine, transfusion of packed red blood cells, FFP, platelets, and cryoprecipitate is often required to ensure an adequate hemoglobin and achieve hemostasis. Transfusion of blood products should be selective and guided by laboratory results and assessment of clinical bleeding. Only CMV-free blood products should be transfused to seronegative recipients, since CMV sepsis is life threatening in immunosuppressed recipients. Drugs, such as aprotinin, tranexamic acid, and epsilon-aminocaproic acid, are helpful in reducing blood transfusion requirements during these procedures and may be infused intraoperatively and in the early postoperative period. Finally, hemodynamics and drug infusion rates should be stabilized and volume status optimized (often with the aid of TEE monitoring) prior to transferring the patient to the ICU.

Acute Postoperative Management

Cardiovascular Support

Allograft heart function may be affected by ischemia, insufficient cardioplegia, reperfusion injury, surgical trauma to conducting tissue, hyperacute rejection, and autonomic denervation. Functional changes in myocardial performance, particularly diastolic dysfunction, are often apparent, despite the effectiveness of cardioplegia in protecting against ischemia and reperfusion injury. Thus, most transplant centers will use catecholamine infusions for inotropic and chronotropic support from the time just before weaning the patient off CPB and into the postoperative period.

Transient RV dysfunction is particularly common following OHT for all of the reasons already noted, and is exacerbated by increased RV afterload due to elevated recipient PVR. Medical therapy of RV dysfunction involves optimizing volume status and HR, improving myocardial contractility, and reducing PVR, as outlined in Table 3. Volume infusion to increase preload is often required to treat low cardiac output associated with RV dysfunction, but excess volume infusion may exacerbate RV dysfunction if PVR is high and RV distension or increased wall

TABLE 3. TREATMENT OF RIGHT VENTRICULAR DYSFUNCTION FOLLOWING CARDIAC TRANSPLANTATION

1. Optimize volume status:
   Increased preload is usually required if PVR is normal
   Avoid volume overload if PVR is increased

2. Increase myocardial contractility and/or heart rate:
   Treat myocardial ischemia/maintain RV coronary perfusion pressure
   Isoproterenol (0.03–0.25 μg/kg/min)
   Dobutamine (2–20 μg/kg/min)
   Epinephrine (0.05–0.5 μg/kg/min) or norepinephrine
     (0.05–0.5 μg/kg/min)
   Phosphodiesterase III inhibitors (milrinone 0.25–0.75 μg/kg/min)
   Epicardial pacing
   RV assist device

3. Decrease PVR:
   Ensure adequate oxygenation (reduce hypoxic pulmonary
     vasoconstriction)
   Hyperventilation
   Decrease peak airway pressures (minimize PEEP and tidal volumes)
   Correct acidosis
   Avoid hypothermia
   Inhaled nitric oxide (0.5–40 ppm)
   Prostaglandin E₁ (PGE₁) (0.05–0.4 μg/kg/min)
   Nitroglycerin (0.1–5 μg/kg/min) or nitroprusside (0.1–5 μg/kg/min)
   Isoproterenol (0.03–0.25 μg/kg/min)
   Phosphodiesterase III inhibitors (milrinone 0.25–0.75 μg/kg/min)

PVR, pulmonary vascular resistance; RV, right ventricular; PEEP, positive end-expiratory pressure.

tension result. Drugs that increase myocardial contractility and simultaneously lower PVR, such as isoproterenol, dobutamine, and milrinone, are ideal drugs for the treatment of RV dysfunction. Of the drugs used to lower PVR, only inhaled NO selectively causes pulmonary vasodilation without associated systemic hypotension. Inhaled NO effectively treats pulmonary hypertension and primary graft failure following OHT (30,31). Anatomic factors contributing to RV dysfunction, such as kinking of a redundant PA at the site of anastomosis, must be ruled out following OHT. As a last resort, mechanical RV-assist devices (RVADs) have been successfully used to support RV function following transplantation (32).

Other cardiovascular problems in the early postoperative period include LV dysfunction (primarily due to prolonged donor heart ischemia or inadequate preservation), low systemic vascular resistance (SVR), and bradyarrhythmias. Low SVR, as seen in patients who have been on long-term amiodarone therapy prior to transplantation, may require very high-dose catecholamine infusions for correction. Transplant recipients who were previously in severe heart failure also have reduced sensitivity to stimulation with alpha₁-adrenergic agonists. Consequently, infusion of vasopressors, such as phenylephrine and norepinephrine, that are commonly used to support SVR postoperatively, may need to be increased accordingly (33). Temporary epicardial pacing is commonly required for transient bradyarrhythmias following OHT, and permanent pacing is necessary in 5% to 10% of recipients who have had the donor heart implanted by the traditional RA anastomotic technique (26,28,29). The need for pacing is somewhat unexpected because vagal denervation, which occurs during heart transplantation, removes the vagal influence on the sinus node and should result in an atrial rate that is higher in the trans-

planted heart than in the native atria. However, bradyarrhythmias are quite common following OHT and may result from surgical trauma to conducting tissue, allograft ischemia, and inadequate preservation. They are rarely due to hyperacute rejection.

Cardiac allograft denervation occurs during transplantation because the donor heart's cardiac plexus (which resides on the anterior surface of the great arteries) is transected during donor cardiectomy. All afferent and efferent sympathetic and parasympathetic innervation is lost. Posttransplantation cardiac denervation is generally thought to be permanent in humans. However, the fact that some patients perceive angina and that norepinephrine may be released in response to a tyramine challenge following transplantation suggest that partial afferent reinnervation may rarely occur (34–36). Several clinically important physiologic consequences accompany cardiac autonomic denervation. Although intrinsic mechanisms, such as spontaneous pacemaker depolarization and the Frank-Starling mechanism, can sustain the circulation under resting conditions, the response of the denervated heart is very different from usual when demands for increased cardiac output are seen during exercise or physiologic stress. Immediate increases in cardiac output (CO) are mediated by elevation in HR, with little change in stroke volume (SV) in the normal heart. In contrast, the denervated heart responds to increased demand by acutely augmenting SV rather than HR. This partly explains why heart transplant recipients are considered to be "preload dependent" and rely on adequate volume status postoperatively. Nevertheless, the denervated heart is capable of increasing HR at times of heightened demand, but does so more slowly than normal and in response to the direct effects of catecholamines. HR is slow to return to baseline values when demand is decreased, because vagal innervation is absent. Evidence of late improvement in exercise capacity following OHT has not been found, further substantiating the belief that reinnervation does not occur (37). Autonomic denervation of the heart also results in silent myocardial ischemia and abnormal responses to drugs that rely on autonomic activity for their action (Table 4).

Heart transplant recipients that have had the traditional biatrial anastomosis during transplantation will have both donor RA tissue and remnants of their native right atrium present. These patients often have two P-waves that are dissociated from each other on the ECG. Vagotonic stimuli (Valsalva maneuver, respiration, cholinesterase-inhibiting drugs) will continue to influence the intact native recipient sinus node tissue, but this atrial activity and P-wave are dissociated from the donor heart's R-wave.

TABLE 4. ABNORMAL CARDIOACTIVE DRUG RESPONSES IN THE DENERVATED (TRANSPLANTED) HEART

Drug	Abnormal Response
Adenosine	Increased sensitivity
Anticholinesterases	Vagotonic effect absent
Atropine sulfate	Vagolytic effect absent
Digoxin	Vagotonic effect absent
Ephedrine	Cardiostimulatory effect reduced
Norepinephrine bitartrate	Chronotropic (β) effect unmasked
Pancuronium bromide	Vagolytic effect absent
Vasodilators	Reflex tachycardia initially absent

In contrast, the donor atrial tissue is denervated, resulting in a donor P-wave that is independent of vagotonic stimuli, but that is associated with conduction to the ventricle and the observed R-wave. Recipients that have had the newer bicaval anastomosis during OHT will have a single P-wave that is associated with the R-wave, because only donor RA tissue is present.

Respiratory Support

The trachea should be extubated as soon as possible to minimize the risk of nosocomial pulmonary infection, the most common site of infection in immunosuppressed patients following OHT. Criteria for weaning from mechanical ventilation following other types of cardiac surgery and in other ICU patients are described elsewhere in this text and apply to OHT recipients as well. Traditional high-dose opioid (particularly fentanyl) anesthetics may depress respiratory drive and delay extubation until well into the first postoperative day. The use of opioids that have a shorter duration of action, such as sufentanil (1 to 3 μg per kg), and the use of inhalational anesthetics to reduce total opioid dose intraoperatively may allow earlier extubation in the ICU. Other intraoperative events that may delay extubation in the ICU include damage to the vagus, recurrent laryngeal, or phrenic nerves as a result of surgical dissection or injury from the ice-cold saline slush used for allograft preservation during implantation.

Significant concurrent pulmonary disease that is irreversible must be excluded when candidates for OHT are evaluated preoperatively and should not complicate the immediate postoperative management of transplant recipients. Nonetheless, many candidates (particularly those with coronary artery disease and ischemic cardiomyopathy necessitating transplantation) have a significant history of cigarette smoking and may have some degree of obstructive pulmonary disease that impedes weaning from mechanical ventilation following OHT. Pulmonary edema and small pleural effusions present preoperatively, as a result of congestive heart failure, and generally resolve within a few days following transplantation.

Hemostasis and Blood Coagulation

OHT is associated with considerable intraoperative and postoperative blood loss due to the number of anastomoses and a relatively high incidence of coagulopathy. Prolonged CPB, hypothermia, dilution of coagulation factors, preoperative aspirin or oral anticoagulant therapy, and liver dysfunction due to congestive heart failure may all contribute to coagulopathy following OHT. Extensive mediastinal collateral vessels in patients with end-stage congenital heart disease may also lead to profuse postoperative bleeding. Excessive postoperative bleeding that is not adequately drained by mediastinal chest tubes may result in hemodynamic compromise due to mediastinal tamponade.

Following separation from CPB, heparin is completely reversed with protamine, coagulopathy is treated, and blood products are transfused as necessary. Shed blood is commonly reinfused via closed scavenging systems intraoperatively and in the initial period in the ICU if significant nonsurgical bleeding continues. Perioperative infusions of aprotinin, epsilon-aminoca-

proic acid, or tranexamic acid may also decrease postoperative bleeding. However, transfusion of banked blood products, such as packed red blood cells, FFP, platelets, and cryoprecipitate, is often still necessary to ensure an adequate hemoglobin level and achieve hemostasis. It is critical that CMV-seronegative patients are transfused only with blood products that are free of CMV, since CMV sepsis is potentially fatal in immunosuppressed transplant recipients.

Immunosuppression

Pharmacologic immunosuppression usually begins during or immediately prior to the OHT procedure and is continued throughout the remainder of the recipient's life. Although immunosuppression protocols vary between transplant centers, most have traditionally employed "triple therapy" consisting of cyclosporine, azathioprine, and corticosteroids (5). Azathioprine is often the first immunosuppressant to be administered, typically given either orally in the preoperative period, or infused intravenously (2 to 4 mg per kg) following the induction of anesthesia. Methylprednisolone 500 to 1,000 mg is also given following anesthetic induction or immediately prior to release of the aortic cross-clamp during the latter stages of CPB, whereas cyclosporine is most commonly initiated within 1 to 4 hours of arrival in the ICU following transplantation. Cyclosporine may be replaced with alternative immunosuppressants, such as OKT3, initially in patients with postoperative renal dysfunction (38). In an effort to reduce complications, most centers decrease steroids as soon as possible and many recipients have steroid therapy discontinued for prolonged periods of time; however, over 70% of patients remain on corticosteroids at 5 years following OHT (5).

An increasing number of patients are being treated with newer immunosuppressive drugs, such as tacrolimus (FK-506), mycophenolate mofetil (MMF), and polyclonal antisera, that may supplement or replace one or more of the traditional "triple therapy" drugs (5,39). These newer agents may also be used intermittently to induce remission during episodes of acute rejection (40). MMF is an antimetabolite that inhibits T- and B-lymphocyte proliferation and activity by depleting nucleotides required for DNA synthesis, a mechanism of action similar to azathioprine (41). ATG and antilymphocyte globulin (ALG) are both polyclonal antibodies, derived from rabbit or horse serum, that result in potent immunosuppression by causing complement-dependant depletion of T-cells. Investigational immunosuppressive drugs that have the potential to enter clinical use in the future include rapamycin (sirolimus), leflunomide, deoxyspergualin, class I–derived peptides, and a variety of monoclonal antibodies directed against various components of the immune response that cause allograft rejection.

Mechanisms of action and the chemical structures of various immunosuppressants are summarized elsewhere in this text (see Chapter 53). Most immunosuppressants increase the risk of infection and many increase the risk of developing a malignancy (42). Fortunately, a certain degree of graft tolerance develops over time, allowing immunosuppressive therapy to be progressively tapered, with a resultant decrease in infections and other complications. Drug interactions with immunosuppressants are

TABLE 5. DRUGS KNOWN TO AFFECT CYCLOSPORINE SERUM LEVELS

Increased Cyclosporine Levels	Decreased Cyclosporine Levels
Amiodarone	Anticonvulsants:
Antifungals:	Carbamazepine
Fluconazole	Phenobarbital
Itraconazole	Phenytoin
Ketoconazole	Isoniazid
Calcium channel blockers	Nafcillin
Cimetidine	Octreotide
Fluoroquinolones (ciprofloxacin)	Rifampin
Macrolide antibiotics	Sulfamethoxzole
(erythromycin)	
Metoclopramide	
Oral contraceptives	
Tacrolimus (FK506)	

TABLE 6. STANDARDIZED GRADING SYSTEM OF CELLULAR REJECTION BASED ON ENDOMYOCARDIAL BIOPSY SPECIMENS

Grade	Current Nomenclature	Former Nomenclature
0	No rejection	No rejection
IA	Focal perivascular or interstitial infiltrate without necrosis	Mild rejection
IB	Diffuse but sparse infiltrate without necrosis	
II	One focus only with aggressive infiltration, focal myocyte damage, or both	Focal moderate rejection
IIIA	Multifocal aggressive infiltrates, myocyte damage, or both	Low to moderate rejection
IIIB	Diffuse inflammatory process with necrosis	Borderline severe rejection
IV	Diffuse aggressive polymorphous infiltrate, edema, hemorrhage, or vasculitis, with necrosis	Severe acute rejection

Adapted from Billingham ME, Cary NR, Hammond ME. A working formulation for the standardization of nomenclature in the diagnosis of heart and lung rejection: Heart Rejection Study Group. *J Heart Transplant* 1991;9:587–592, with permission.

also common. Immunosuppressants may affect the actions and blood levels of drugs commonly administered postoperatively; conversely, many drugs can affect blood levels of immunosuppressants, particularly cyclosporine (Table 5). Drugs that inhibit hepatic cytochrome P450 isoenzymes can increase cyclosporine's plasma concentration to a toxic level. In contrast, drugs such as barbiturates and phenytoin induce cytochrome P450 isoenzymes and may result in a decrease of cyclosporine plasma levels, leading to allograft rejection.

Nonpharmacologic approaches to immunosuppression, such as total lymphoid irradiation and photophoresis, have also been used following OHT, particularly for the treatment of rejection episodes (43). Total lymphoid irradiation appears to be moderately effective as "salvage therapy" for the treatment of recurrent cardiac rejection and has minimal side effects. Extracorporeal photochemotherapy is a more recently developed immunomodulatory treatment, primarily used for recurrent or refractory episodes of allograft rejection. The recipient's mononuclear cells in the blood are irradiated with ultraviolet light in the presence of 8-methoxypsoralen and are then reinfused. Episodes of rejection that could not be reversed with pharmacologic immunosuppression alone have been safely controlled with photochemotherapy. However, the cost and inconvenience of this mode of therapy will likely limit its future use.

Rejection Complications

Hyperacute (humoral) rejection results from preformed cytotoxic antibodies directed against allograft antigens. It is a very rare complication following OHT, provided the donor and recipient are ABO-matched and there is low reactivity on the PRA. It is characterized by rapid development of intravascular thrombosis within the first few hours of reperfusing the donor heart, resulting in a cyanotic allograft that ceases to function. Aggressive treatment of hyperacute rejection with modalities such as high-dose corticosteroids, tacrolimus, lymphocytotoxic therapy, and plasmapheresis to reduce the level of circulating preformed antibodies has limited efficacy. Death often results unless the patient is supported mechanically until retransplanted.

Unlike hyperacute rejection, acute and chronic rejection are cell-mediated and take longer to develop; however, the tendency toward rejection diminishes over time. Acute cellular rejection may develop at any time, most commonly in the first 6 months following transplantation, and is diagnosed by both clinical and histologic criteria. Unfortunately, clinical symptoms and signs of acute rejection (such as fever, new onset of arrhythmias, exercise intolerance, and evidence of congestive heart failure) are often nonspecific or not present in the early stages of rejection, and may be irreversible in the later stages (6,38). Consequently, transvenous endomyocardial biopsy remains the "gold standard" method for diagnosing acute rejection. The ISHLT developed a standardized nomenclature in 1991 for the grading of acute rejection severity, based on histologic findings of allograft RV tissue obtained by endomyocardial biopsy (Table 6) (44). The degree of cellular infiltration has significance for both treatment and prognosis. In the absence of clinical evidence of acute rejection, the frequency of endomyocardial biopsies for surveillance of acute rejection varies between transplant centers, but typically consists of weekly biopsies for the first month or until discharged from hospital, followed by every other week for another month, then monthly until 6 months following surgery, and finally every 3 months until the end of the first postoperative year. Chronic rejection, another form of cellular rejection, is characterized by premature coronary artery disease.

Therapy for rejection depends on clinical status and histologic grade of the endomyocardial biopsy specimen. The mainstay of rejection therapy remains augmented doses of corticosteroids, often as "pulse" doses of methylprednisolone (500 to 1,000 mg per day), generally administered intravenously for a few days and then followed by tapering doses of oral corticosteroids. Substitution of tacrolimus for cyclosporine may also expedite the resolution of acute rejection. The adjunctive use of total lymphoid irradiation, photophoresis, methotrexate, mycophenolate mofetil, and lympholytic therapy with ATG or OKT3 may induce remission in refractory, steroid-resistant rejection (6).

Infectious Complications

Infection remains one of the most common causes of morbidity and mortality following OHT. It is the leading cause of death between 1 month and 1 year following transplantation, and is second only to primary graft failure as the most common cause of death in the first 30 days. Infection may occur anywhere, but is most commonly found in the lung. Early (within the first 30 days) infections following OHT are most commonly nosocomial bacterial infections caused by *Staphylococcus aureus*, *Pseudomonas aeruginosa*, Enterobacteriaceae, and enterococci. Mucocutaneous herpes simplex and *Candida* infections are also common in the early period, in part related to the use of broad-spectrum antibiotics. Despite an increased risk of nosocomial infection, the incidence of mediastinitis following OHT is comparable to that following other emergency cardiac operations. Late infectious complications, occurring between the first month and first year following transplantation, most commonly involve opportunistic organisms that are associated with therapeutic immunosuppression. Such organisms include cytomegalovirus [CMV], *Pneumocystis carinii*, *Legionella* species, *Toxoplasma gondii*, and fungi, such as *Aspergillus*, *Histoplasma*, and *Cryptococcus*.

Broad-spectrum antibacterial prophylaxis, typically a second-generation cephalosporin and vancomycin hydrochloride, is initiated immediately prior to transplantation and continued for 1 to 3 days postoperatively. In the absence of signs of infection, prophylactic antibiotics are discontinued following tracheal extubation and the removal of intravascular catheters. Only a few regimens for infection prophylaxis have been shown to be effective in transplant recipients, including prophylaxis against *P. carinii* with trimethoprim and sulfamethoxazole, and the use of ganciclovir or CMV hyperimmunoglobulin in CMV-seronegative recipients of a seropositive donor's heart (6). However, the use of prophylactic ganciclovir to prevent reactivation of CMV and its use in asymptomatic CMV-seronegative recipients of a CMV-seropositive donor heart remains controversial. *T. gondii*–seronegative recipients who are transplanted with a seropositive donor heart are at high risk of developing potentially fatal meningoencephalitis or myocarditis and should receive at least a 6-week course of pyrimethamine, sulfadiazine, and folinic acid (leucovorin) prophylaxis. Other antibiotics are not used unless symptoms or signs of infection develop. When signs of infection emerge, a prompt and aggressive search for the source is essential for patient survival. This may include cultures of catheter tips and of samples of sputum, urine, blood, and wound drainage, and serial CXRs, as clinically indicated. If pathogens are revealed on culture, the choice of antibiotics should be guided by culture and sensitivity reports.

Neurologic Complications

Although neurologic complications are relatively infrequent after OHT, a thorough preoperative neurologic examination should be documented for all cardiac transplant candidates because these patients are at increased risk of such an event. Cardiac transplant recipients are particularly vulnerable to both ischemic and hemorrhagic cerebrovascular complications perioperatively. Ischemic strokes may result from reduced cerebral blood flow associated with low cardiac output, prior episodes of cardiac arrest, and polycythemia secondary to congenital heart disease. Embolic sources of ischemic neurologic injury include thromboemboli from a ventricular aneurysm or mechanical circulatory support device, air emboli from inadequate de-airing prior to weaning from CPB, and cholesterol or other particulate emboli generated from aortic transection and reanastomosis. Hemorrhagic strokes are associated with long-term use of anticoagulants and perioperative coagulopathy.

Other Noncardiac Surgical Complications

Cardiac allograft recipients require noncardiac surgical procedures reasonably often in the months and years following OHT. General surgical intervention is required for intraabdominal complications in up to 20% of OHT recipients (45). Immunocompromise is likely a key factor in the development of intraabdominal abscesses and diverticulitis, whereas both immunosuppression and antibiotic therapy predispose patients to *Clostridium difficile* pseudomembranous colitis. Corticosteroid use could account for an increased incidence of pancreatitis and gastrointestinal (GI) ulceration, with associated GI bleeding and viscus perforation. A high index of suspicion is required to diagnose intraabdominal pathology in these patients because corticosteroids may mask common symptoms and signs of complications, such as a perforated viscus. Chronic corticosteroid use also leads to osteoporosis and joint complications, which may require orthopedic surgical intervention.

Long-Term Complications

Cardiovascular Complications

The major factor limiting long-term success of OHT is the development of accelerated atherosclerosis in the allograft coronary arteries, termed cardiac allograft vasculopathy (CAV). It is a unique and unusually accelerated form of coronary artery disease, affecting both intramural and epicardial coronary arteries and veins, with an incidence of 5% to 10% per year (46,47). Transplant atherosclerosis is believed to represent a form of chronic rejection that is characterized by diffuse, uniform, concentric narrowing of the coronary vessels by a proliferative, fibrocellular intima (48). The diffuse nature of CAV may result in a gross underestimate of its severity on angiography, since angiography only outlines the lumen of a vessel, and has led to the use of intravascular ultrasound as a sensitive modality for detecting and following the progression of CAV (6,49). Although CAV is believed to be primarily immune-mediated, vascular endothelial damage from ischemia-reperfusion injury, viral infection (particularly CMV), immunosuppressive drugs, and classic risk factors for atherosclerosis, such as hypertension, hyperlipidemia, and diabetes, may all be involved in its pathogenesis (47,50). It is thought to progress through repetitive endothelial injury, followed by a repair response involving endothelial cells, smooth muscle cells, and inflammatory cells.

CAV is difficult to treat and ultimately limits the useful life of cardiac allografts. No currently available treatment prevents CAV, but factors that may limit its progression include calcium channel blocker therapy and control of hypertension and hyper-lipidemia. Although early focal coronary lesions are often initially amenable to angioplasty, coronary revascularization procedures have a limited role in treating this condition because of the diffuse involvement of distal vessels. Transmyocardial laser revascularization has recently been shown to improve both symptoms and myocardial perfusion in some cases of CAV (51). Nonetheless, repeat transplantation currently provides the only definitive treatment in patients who are severely affected (48,52). However, retransplantation is associated with significantly worse outcome than initial transplantation and there is considerable ethical controversy regarding the use of scarce donor organs for retransplantation (5).

Transient conduction abnormalities are common in the initial period following OHT, particularly if donor and recipient right atria were anastomosed instead of using the newer bicaval technique, but the majority of these resolve. However, some recipients will have chronic atrial and ventricular arrhythmias and conduction abnormalities (most commonly a right bundle-branch block); 5% to 10% of patients who have had a traditional biatrial anastomosis will require permanent pacing (26,28,29,53).

Autonomic denervation of the transplanted heart is another long-term complication that seems to be permanent in humans (34). As a result, myocardial ischemia is typically silent following OHT and may present with atypical symptoms and signs, such as paroxysmal dyspnea due to LV dysfunction, ventricular arrhythmias, or sudden death, rendering clinical diagnosis difficult. In addition, abnormal chronotropic and hemodynamic responses to exercise and cardioactive drugs persist (37).

Other Long-Term Complications

Other long-term complications following OHT are commonly related to immunosuppressive therapy. Opportunistic infections, malignancy, and immunosuppressant drug side effects and toxicities unfortunately occur quite often over the years following OHT. CMV, *P. carinii*, and *Aspergillus* are common opportunistic infections. The development of malignancy in immunosuppressed recipients is also not uncommon: 3.7% of all recipients are found to have a malignancy at 1-year follow-up and this increases to 9.6% at 5-year follow-up (5). The pathogenesis of posttransplant malignancy is multifactorial, but there is convincing evidence that most posttransplant lymphoproliferative disease is related to either primary or reactivation Epstein-Barr virus infection (6,54). Nearly one-third of malignancies present at 1-year posttransplantation are lymphoid malignancies, but an unexpectedly high percentage of malignancies are of nonlymphoid origin in later years. At 5-year follow-up only 15.2% of all malignancies are of lymphoid origin, whereas skin cancer increases to over half of all diagnosed malignancies. Surprisingly, between 4 and 5 years following OHT the second most common cause of death becomes malignancy (predominantly nonlymphoid), following CAV by only a small margin. Finally, common immunosuppressive drug side effects and toxicities include the following incidences of complications, even at 1 year after OHT: hypertension, 67.1%; renal dysfunction or failure 20.2%; hyperlipidemia 39.3%; and diabetes 19.9% (5).

Outcome Following Orthotopic Heart Transplant

Mortality rates declined significantly following the introduction of cyclosporine into clinical practice in the early 1980s. Recent worldwide survival rates at 1 and 3 years following OHT were 85.6% and 79.5%, respectively (5). However, survival rates for carefully selected subgroups of patients transplanted at the most experienced centers may exceed 90% at 1 year. The highest mortality rate is in the first year posttransplantation, followed by a constant mortality rate of approximately 4% per year beyond the first year. Factors associated with an increased risk of mortality include repeat transplantation, dependence on a ventilator or ventricular-assist device preoperatively, transplantation for diagnoses other than coronary artery disease or idiopathic-dilated cardiomyopathy, a female donor heart, advanced recipient or donor age, preoperative amiodarone treatment for more than 4 weeks, transplantation in a center with low procedure volume, elevated recipient PVR, and an allograft ischemic time exceeding 3 hours.

In addition to traditional measures of outcome, factors such as the recipient's perceived well being, exercise tolerance, and return to work status are important in evaluating overall outcome following OHT. Quality of life is generally reported to be markedly improved by most recipients, the majority return to NYHA functional class I, and exercise capacity is only slightly less than that of the age-matched general population. Despite this, only slightly more than 40% of recipients return to work by 5 years posttransplantation.

HETEROTOPIC HEART TRANSPLANTATION

Heterotopic heart transplantation is a rarely used technique, performed at a limited number of centers for highly selected patients. The native recipient heart remains *in situ* and the donor heart is placed in the right hemithorax. The two hearts are then joined to form a parallel circulation, with side-to-side anastomoses between the donor and native atria and end-to-side anastomoses between the donor and native pulmonary arteries and aortas. A conduit made of either Dacron or pericardium usually joins the pulmonary arteries. The ventricles are not anastomosed primarily, but both LVs provide cardiac output into the native aortic trunk and both RVs empty into the native PA. Although ventricular compliance partly determines the relative contribution of the native and donor LV, most of the cardiac output is usually delivered by the donor LV. However, contribution of the native LV to cardiac output is increased in the initial period following transplantation and during episodes of allograft rejection. Since the donor heart is denervated and the native heart retains its innervation, the two hearts often do not have the same rhythm and asynchronous LV ejection results, but total cardiac output is generally not compromised despite this.

Indications for use of the heterotopic technique may include significant donor and recipient heart size mismatch, and recipient pulmonary hypertension that is severe and irreversible, and when donor heart function is marginal. In the future, porcine xenotransplantation may lead to renewed interest in the technique of heterotopic heart transplantation as a bridge to potential native heart recovery or allotransplantation in selected patients (55). The primary disadvantage of heterotopic OHT is that survival

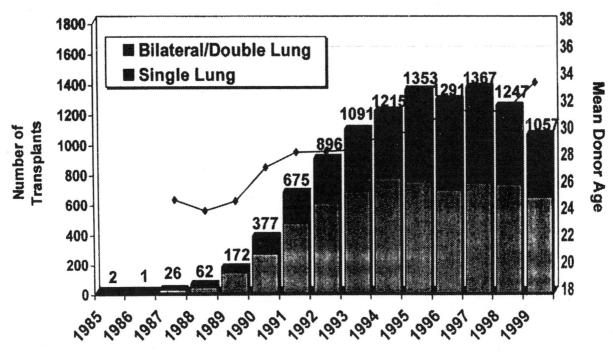

FIGURE 5. Lung transplant volume and donor age by year. (From Hosenpud JD, Bennet LE, Keck BM, et al. The Registry of the International Society for Heart and Lung Transplantation: Seventeenth Official Report—2000. *J Heart Lung Transpl* 2000;19:909–931, with permission.)

rates are significantly lower compared to the orthotopic procedure (56).

ISOLATED LUNG TRANSPLANTATION

End-stage lung disease is among the five leading causes of death and disablement among adults in North America. Pulmonary transplantation, including single- and double-lung operations, has gained widespread acceptance as a therapeutic option for severe parenchymal lung disease and pulmonary vascular disease. The first human lung transplant was reported by Hardy and coworkers in 1963 (57). Over the next 20 years, a total of 40 lung transplants were performed, but only one recipient survived greater than one month (58). High postoperative mortality rates prior to the early 1980s were predominantly due to primary allograft failure, rejection, infection, and dehiscence of the bronchial anastomosis. The introduction of cyclosporine in the early 1980s significantly improved outcomes. During the same time period, Dr. Joel Cooper and colleagues at the University of Toronto demonstrated that wrapping the bronchial anastomosis with omentum improved bronchial healing and neovascularization. In 1983, Cooper performed the landmark single-lung transplant (SLT) on a patient with pulmonary fibrosis that went on to become the first long-term lung transplant survivor (58,59). Following this success, exponential growth occurred in the number of lung transplants being performed during the 1980s to early 1990s and these have now become relatively common procedures for the treatment of end-stage pulmonary disease. A total of 6,514 SLTs and 4,634 bilateral sequential single-lung transplants (BSSLTs) and *en bloc* double-lung transplants (DLTs) worldwide

have been reported to the ISHLT as of March 2000 (5). Largely due to a shortage of compatible donor organs, the number of lung transplants being performed worldwide plateaued in 1994 at approximately 1,200 to 1,300 annually (Fig. 5) (5). Despite use of less stringent donor and recipient selection criteria and similar to OHT, worldwide lung transplantation volume has decreased over the past several years (5).

Indications and Selection Criteria for Lung Transplantation

Indications for adult lung transplantation include various etiologies of end-stage pulmonary vascular disease and obstructive, restrictive, and septic parenchymal lung disease (Table 7). General

TABLE 7. ADULT LUNG TRANSPLANT DISTRIBUTION BY INDICATION

Indication	SLT (%)	DLT/BSSLT (%)
Emphysema	42.6	17.5
Idiopathic pulmonary fibrosis	19.5	7.1
Alpha$_1$-antitrypsin deficiency	10.6	9.6
Primary pulmonary hypertension	3.9	9.2
Cystic fibrosis	2.4	31.5
Repeat transplantation	2.3	2.2
Miscellaneous	18.1	22.9

SLT, single-lung transplant; DLT/BSSLT, double-lung transplant/bilateral sequential single-lung transplant.
Adapted from Hosenpud JD, Bennet LE, Keck BM, et al. The Registry of the International Society for Heart and Lung Transplantation: Seventeenth Official Report—2000. *J Heart Lung Transpl* 2000;19:909–931, with permission.

selection criteria include the presence of deteriorating end-stage pulmonary disease for which no further medical or surgical therapy exists. Progressive exercise intolerance, increasing oxygen requirements, carbon-dioxide retention, deteriorating right heart function, and social debilitation are often present. When compared to the natural history of the patient's pulmonary disease, lung transplantation generally confers a survival advantage in candidates that have a pretransplant life expectancy of 1 to 2 years despite maximal medical therapy. The optimal time for transplantation varies significantly between patients. An ideal candidate is one who deteriorates after all reasonable medical and surgical therapies have been exhausted, but who remains ambulatory and is not so critically ill that surviving the transplant procedure is improbable. Preoperative ambulatory status is an objective measurement useful in predicting both survival prior to transplantation and outcome following lung transplantation. Candidates who are unable to walk at least 300 to 400 M during a 6-minute walk have a significantly increased risk of death prior to transplantation (60). An increased risk of death following transplantation is associated with a candidate's inability to walk at least 200 M in 6 minutes prior to the procedure (61). The rate of functional deterioration and the ability of the RV to tolerate progression of pulmonary hypertension also influence the timing of transplantation. Finally, no contraindications to transplantation should exist, candidates must abstain from tobacco for at least 6 months, and should be under 65 years of age for an SLT or under 60 years of age to be considered for a BSSLT/DLT.

Specific criteria exist for each major pulmonary disease necessitating lung transplantation (62) and are reviewed in a recent article (63). Specific diseases requiring lung transplantation (Table 7) also influence the choice of surgical procedure, either SLT or BSSLT/DLT.

Contraindications to Lung Transplantation

Contraindications specific to isolated lung transplantation include advanced RV failure, LV dysfunction (ejection fraction less than 35%), significant coronary artery disease, and factors that may complicate surgical dissection or impair postoperative ventilation, such as pleural or neuromuscular disease and musculoskeletal disorders.

Several factors previously considered to be absolute contraindications to lung transplantation are now controversial. Infection with multidrug-resistant *Pseudomonas* and the persistence of *Aspergillus* in the sputum of cystic fibrosis (CF) patients were once considered contraindications to lung transplantation. Recent evidence suggests that these factors may not negatively impact survival following lung transplantation (64,65). Adequately treated *Mycobacterium tuberculosis* and colonization with fungi or atypical mycobacteria are not absolute contraindications to lung transplantation (63). Preoperative mechanical ventilator dependence for more than several days was considered an absolute contraindication to lung transplantation because airway colonization with bacteria may lead to nosocomial infection, and respiratory muscle deconditioning may necessitate prolonged postoperative ventilatory support. These concerns do not seem to be clinically significant if the period of preoperative mechanical ventilation is less than 2 weeks (66,67). Patients on any dose of corticosteroids were also once refused lung transplantation, based on concerns that bronchial anastomotic healing would be impeded and the risk of infection increased. Most transplant centers now accept candidates for lung transplantation provided the preoperative dose of prednisone is less than 0.3 mg per kg per day (63,64,68). Prior thoracic surgery was traditionally considered a contraindication, since pleural adhesions are associated with increased bleeding and technical difficulty during lung transplantation. Prior open lung biopsy, chest tube drainage of a pneumothorax, lung lobectomy, and palliative procedures, such as thoracoscopic bullectomy and lung volume-reduction surgery, are common and do not preclude future lung transplantation in carefully selected patients (69). Finally, controversy surrounds the use of BSSLT for treatment of bronchoalveolar lung carcinoma. There are reports of long-term survival following lung transplantation for bronchoalveolar lung carcinoma, however, recurrence of this tumor in lung allografts has also been reported. Other forms of active malignancy are an absolute contraindication to transplantation.

Choice of Lung Transplant Procedure

Lung transplantation comprises four distinct surgical procedures: SLT, BSSLT, heart-lung transplantation (HLT), and transplantation of a lung lobe from a living-related donor (LRDT). The distribution of adult single- and bilateral-lung transplants for common indications is outlined in Table 7.

SLT is the most common lung transplant procedure. Although pulmonary function would improve more in most patients if both lungs were transplanted, SLT provides excellent functional outcomes in many patients. It also optimizes the use of scarce donor lungs, involves a technically less demanding surgical procedure, leaves carinal innervation and the cough reflex intact, and is associated with less postoperative morbidity. The most common indications for SLT are emphysema (due to smoking or alpha$_1$-antitrypsin deficiency) and pulmonary fibrosis (5,70). The first successful SLT was performed in a patient with pulmonary fibrosis, which remains perhaps the ideal indication for SLT physiologically, since most pulmonary blood flow and ventilation go to the transplanted lung in these patients (71). Conversely, patients with emphysema were initially thought to be physiologically unsuitable for SLT. Ventilation/perfusion (V/Q) mismatching would result from the majority of pulmonary blood flow going to the transplanted lung, while the more compliant native lung would be preferentially ventilated. V/Q mismatching and overdistension of the native lung does occur following SLT in these recipients, but is generally only a concern during positive-pressure ventilation in the early postoperative period. Independent lung ventilation resolves this problem prior to extubation. Recently, lung volume-reduction surgery has been performed on the remaining native lung, either during the SLT procedure or postoperatively as a separate procedure, in an effort to avoid native lung overdistension (64,72,73). Despite the above concerns, emphysema accounts for the majority of SLTs performed. It is associated with the lowest mortality rates of all lung transplant indications (5). Finally, SLT is seldom used for lung diseases, such as CF or bronchiectasis that are associated with chronic pulmonary infection, since an SLT would rapidly become infected by the remaining diseased lung.

If lung pathology is more advanced on one side than the other, or if a prior thoracic surgical procedure has been performed on one side only, the lung transplanted preferentially is the most diseased lung or the side with the least intrathoracic adhesions, respectively. If the native lungs are equally impaired and pleural scarring is absent, the left lung is preferable because the left hemithorax can more easily accommodate an oversized donor lung, the native right pulmonary veins are less accessible than those on the left, and the recipient's left bronchus is longer. The right lung may be transplanted preferentially in patients with emphysema and severe hyperinflation, however, as the left hemidiaphragm is able to descend more freely than the right. This minimizes mediastinal shift and inhibits the hyperinflated native lung from compressing the transplanted lung (71).

No consensus exists regarding which lung transplant procedure is the most appropriate for patients with primary pulmonary hypertension (PPH). End-stage pulmonary vascular disease (primary and secondary) is treated by both SLT and DLT, provided RV compromise is deemed reversible. HLT is reserved for cases where cor pulmonale is irreversible. Advantages of SLT for the treatment of PPH are that the surgical technique is simpler than BSSLT, donor lungs are conserved, CPB time is shortened, PVR declines rapidly following transplantation, RV function is substantially improved, and recent studies have shown that functional status is the same following SLT or BSSLT for the treatment of PPH (74). The primary disadvantage of SLT in recipients with PPH is that at least 85% to 90% of the pulmonary blood flow goes to the allograft lung because of persistently elevated PVR in the recipient's native lung (58,74,75). Allograft dysfunction or rejection is poorly tolerated in these patients because of the resultant V/Q mismatch. Excessive pulmonary blood flow to the allograft lung also increases the incidence of reperfusion pulmonary edema. Some studies suggest that a higher incidence of bronchiolitis obliterans develops in recipients with PPH who have been treated with SLT, but this is debatable. Patients with PPH are the only group of SLT patients who routinely require CPB during transplantation, since RV failure often results when the PA of the lung to be transplanted is clamped and the entire cardiac output must flow through one diseased branch PA.

Over twice as many BSSLT/DLTs than SLTs have been performed for PPH as of March 2000. The primary advantages of BSSLT for the treatment of PPH are less reperfusion edema and V/Q mismatch result, since pulmonary blood flow is more evenly distributed to two lungs following BSSLT. Rejection episodes are better tolerated as a result. Although controversial, a small survival advantage may exist for BSSLT versus SLT in the treatment of PPH, even though both procedures effectively lower PVR and improve RV function (5,58,74,75). The disadvantages of BSSLT are that two lungs are used per patient, ischemic time of the second lung and CPB time are prolonged, and the procedure is technically more difficult than a SLT.

HLT was previously the transplant procedure of choice for treatment of PPH. However, in the absence of significant coexisting cardiac disease, HLT is now rarely required for the treatment of PPH, since early and persistent normalization of PVR and RV ejection fraction follow lung transplantation alone (76,77).

Bilateral sequential single-lung transplantation has replaced traditional en bloc DLT as the procedure of choice for patients who require replacement of both lungs. BSSLT involves sequential transplantation of single-lung grafts in a single recipient, rather than a complete double-lung block that remains attached to the donor trachea. Bibronchial anastomoses used in the BSSLT technique heal with significantly fewer complications than does the tracheal anastomosis required by the en bloc DLT procedure. In addition, full systemic heparinization and CPB are often avoided with use of the BSSLT technique. Indications for BSSLT include severe bilateral bullous emphysema, selected patients with PPH, and end-stage bilateral lung disease associated with infection, such as CF and bronchiectasis.

HLT is performed rarely for either end-stage lung disease or cardiac disease. The three main indications for HLT include congenital heart disease, PPH, and CF. HLT is discussed later in this chapter.

Due to a shortage of donor organs, LRDT of lung lobes is the most recently developed lung transplant procedure. LRDT involves implantation of bilateral lower lobes from two separate compatible living donors. To avoid infection, the native recipient lungs must be excised, particularly in patients with CF. Although the indications have broadened in recent years, children and young adults with CF account for the majority of recipients (75,78,79). These patients generally have smaller chest cavities and are good candidates for this procedure, since, ideally, the donor lobes are large enough to fill each recipient hemithorax. Postoperative management, complications, and immunosuppression are the same as for other techniques of lung transplantation. It remains to be seen whether adequate lobar tissue is transplanted to provide sufficient gas exchange and vascular surfaces for long-term survival, whether obliterative bronchiolitis develops at the same rate as is observed after cadaveric donation, and whether the incidences of reperfusion injury and rejection will be comparable. A recent series of 60 LRDTs documented an encouraging 1-year survival rate of 71.7% in recipients and no donor mortality (78). No significant difference in survival rates existed between the CF versus non-CF groups. Donation of a lower lung lobe decreased average donor forced vital capacity (FVC) by 15%, forced expiratory volume (FEV_1) by 14%, and total lung capacity (TLC) by 16% at 1 year following lobectomy (78) and did not result in long-term limitation of donor activity.

Donor Lung Selection

Healthy donor lungs are in exceedingly short supply. Pulmonary contusion, massive fluid resuscitation, neurogenic pulmonary edema, aspiration, ventilator-associated pneumonia or oxygen toxicity, and possibly chronic cigarette smoking often damage donor lungs, since most organ donors are the victims of trauma or cerebral aneurysm rupture. Consequently, fewer than 20% of cadaveric donors have lungs suitable for transplantation (64,80).

Ideal donors should be less than 55 years of age and have no history of lung or pleural disease, chronic smoking, malignancy, systemic or pulmonary infection, chest tube or tracheostomy placement, or prior cardiothoracic surgery. The donor should be on a ventilator for less than 1 week and have a Pao_2 of at least 100 mm Hg on 40% oxygen or a Pao_2 greater than 300 mm Hg on 100% oxygen, with a positive end-expiratory pressure (PEEP) of 5 cm H_2O, and a tidal volume of 12 mL per kg

(58,71). The CXR should be clear and the sputum examination negative for infection within 2 hours of harvesting. Small infiltrates on CXR are not an absolute contraindication to transplantation, provided they are not associated with the presence of purulent sputum on bronchoscopy. Since sputum culture results typically are not available at the time of organ harvesting, the assessment of infection is based on the quantity and Gram stain of airway secretions obtained by bronchoscopy. The presence of moderate polymorphonuclear cells and mixed gram-positive and possibly gram-negative organisms is acceptable as long as secretions are moderate in volume, nonpurulent, and uniformly distributed. No fungal growth should be present in the sputum. Donor size should be matched to within 10% to 20% of the recipient's body surface area and within 8 to 9 cm of the recipient's chest circumference at the nipple line. Vertical and horizontal lung dimensions are also reviewed on CXR to confirm that the vertical dimension of the donor's lungs is within 75% of the recipient's. However, size matching by CXR measurements may be less reliable than matching by comparison of predicted lung volumes (TLC and FVC) of the donor and recipient calculated by established formulas based on height, age, and gender (71). ABO compatibility must be present to avoid hyperacute rejection. Although the value of HLA matching for lung transplants is controversial, recent evidence shows a strong influence of HLA matching on graft survival and the development of acute rejection (81,82). Suitable donor lungs have a maximum tolerable ischemic time of 6 to 8 hours, even when UW solution is used for lung preservation. Mortality rates and the future development of bronchiolitis obliterans increases when lung ischemic time exceeds 4 hours.

Donor Lung Procurement

Lung donor management focuses on lung preservation and maintenance of hemodynamic stability. Inotropes and vasopressors may be required to maintain a MAP above 70 mm Hg, as fluid resuscitation should be limited to keep CVP less than 8 to 10 mm Hg and PCOP below 10 to 12 mm Hg, to minimize posttransplant pulmonary edema (83). Inspired oxygen concentration (F_{IO_2}) should be limited to the lowest concentration that maintains donor Pa_{O_2} greater than 100 mm Hg, to decrease oxygen toxicity. Donor ventilator settings usually include PEEP of 5 mm Hg. Pulmonary suctioning is done as little as possible and performed with strict aseptic technique, to avoid lung contamination.

Lungs are procured through a median sternotomy. Two grams of methylprednisolone is generally administered to the donor prior to lung procurement. Following dissection of the lungs and heart, the patient is heparinized (300 U per kg), PGE_1 (500 μg) or prostacyclin is infused into the PA, the vena cavae are ligated and transected, the LA appendage is incised, and the aorta is cross-clamped. The lungs are then flushed with a cold (4°C) preservative solution delivered into the PA, while the lungs are ventilated with 100% oxygen. PGE_1 or prostacyclin are infused into the PA prior to the preservative solution to prevent reflex pulmonary vasoconstriction and ensure uniform cooling and distribution of the preservative solution. These drugs may also have beneficial antiinflammatory effects. Crystalloid preservative solutions commonly used to flush the lungs include UW, modified Euro-Collins, and low-potassium dextran solutions. The lungs are often topically cooled with iced-saline slush. The left atrium is then divided between insertion of the left and right pulmonary veins, providing a cuff of LA tissue for each harvested lung. The airway is then stapled and the lungs are removed partially inflated.

Preoperative Preparation

Lung transplants are performed as emergency procedures, to minimize donor lung ischemia time. This limits preoperative evaluation and preparation of recipients. However, the vast majority of candidates have had a thorough, multidisciplinary medical and surgical evaluation before a donor organ becomes available. Preoperative evaluation is focused on a review of the candidate's medical history and indication for transplantation, significant changes in the interval since the most recent evaluation, allergies, current medical therapy and oxygen requirements, anesthetic history, and time of last oral intake. No sedative premedication is given; many of these patients have limited reserve and chronically border on respiratory arrest. Pulmonary vasodilators, bronchodilators, antiarrhythmics, and similar medical therapy must be continued preoperatively, with the exception of anticoagulants (common treatment in candidates with PPH). Since many patients have had oral intake in less than 8 hours preceding surgery, aspiration prophylaxis with antacids or gastric propulsant medication is given. Chest physiotherapy and suctioning of copious airway secretions are continued until immediately prior to surgery, especially in CF patients.

Epidural analgesia provides effective pain control following lung transplantation, and may aid in weaning patients from mechanical ventilation in the postoperative period. Some centers routinely place thoracic epidural catheters in recipients preoperatively, but this should be avoided if CPB will be necessary during transplantation. High-dose heparinization required for CPB increases the risk of epidural hematoma formation and associated neurologic injury following epidural catheter placement. Most transplant centers place an epidural catheter postoperatively, once coagulation has been restored.

Intraoperative Management

Organ procurement and recipient transplant teams must be well coordinated to minimize donor lung ischemia time. It is crucial to synchronize the insertion of invasive monitors, induction of anesthesia, and start of operation so that the recipient is ready for pneumonectomy and immediate transplantation as soon as the donor lung arrives. The patient is given 100% oxygen to breathe while routine and invasive (arterial and PA catheters) monitors are placed and large-bore i.v. access is obtained. Central venous access and PA catheter placement may be deferred until after induction in patients who are too dyspneic to tolerate supine or Trendelenburg positioning for placement. All invasive monitors must be placed with strict aseptic technique. PA placement may be difficult prior to lung transplantation. The PCOP may not accurately reflect left-sided heart pressures in the presence of PA hypertension, or when the patient is in the lateral decubitus position for SLT if the PA catheter tip is in the nondependent PA. The PA catheter must be enveloped in a long, sterile sheath so that it may be withdrawn during PA anastomosis and subsequently readvanced.

All intraoperative transplant team members must be present at the time of anesthetic induction, since these critically ill patients may require emergency surgical intervention following induction. As in OHT, use of a rapid-sequence induction to prevent aspiration is tempered by the need to provide a controlled, hemodynamically stable induction. Drugs not associated with myocardial depression or histamine release are preferred. Opioids are the principal drugs used for anesthetic induction and maintenance, supplemented by low-dose inhaled anesthetics, benzodiazepines, and neuromuscular blockers. Nitrous oxide is avoided, since it dilutes the F_{IO_2}, increases PVR (in adults), and may expand lung bullae, pneumothoraces, and entrained air bubbles in the heart or circulation.

Lung transplant candidates must be intubated rapidly; desaturation and hypercarbia promptly ensue following induction of anesthesia. A left-endobronchial double-lumen endotracheal tube, of the largest size that will fit easily, is placed so that the lungs may be independently ventilated or deflated during the procedure. Double-lumen endotracheal tube positioning is always confirmed with the aid of a fiberoptic bronchoscope. Thorough suctioning prior to one-lung ventilation is essential if copious amounts of viscous pulmonary secretions are present, particularly in patients with CF. Adequate ventilation must be provided between suctioning attempts to maintain oxygenation and avoid hypercarbia-induced PA hypertension and RV failure.

Fundamental differences exist between recommended ventilator settings for patients with emphysema versus those with CF and restrictive lung disease. Prior to allograft lung implantation, patients with emphysema are ventilated with tidal volumes of 8 to 10 mL per kg, a slightly increased respiratory rate, but prolonged expiratory time (inspiratory to expiratory [I:E] ratio of 1:3 to 1:5) in an effort to prevent air trapping (dynamic hyperinflation) and "pulmonary tamponade" during positive-pressure ventilation. If this occurs, cardiovascular collapse must be prevented through judicious volume infusion, immediate disconnection of the expiratory limb of the ventilator circuit, to allow lung deflation, and initiation of inotropes and vasopressors as necessary (84). Permissive hypoventilation and limitation of airway pressures may be required. In patients with chronic carbon dioxide retention, pH reflects the adequacy of ventilation more accurately than $Paco_2$ during permissive hypoventilation. Minimizing peak airway pressure decreases the risk of emphysematous bullae rupture and pneumothorax.

In contrast, patients with CF and restrictive lung disease are ventilated with a slow respiratory rate, I:E ratios of 1:1, and peak airway pressures that often exceed 50 cm H_2O. Peak inspiratory pressures of 75 cm H_2O have been described for ventilating patients with CF (85). Chronic, recurrent pneumonia and pleural inflammation in patients with CF result in pleural adhesions that significantly reduce the risk of pneumothorax, despite high airway pressures. Finally, the primary goal of ventilation in patients with PPH is to minimize PVR by avoiding hypoxia, hypercarbia, and either lung distension or atelectasis.

One-lung ventilation (OLV) is required during lung transplantation to allow deflation and removal of the diseased lung and implantation of the donor lung. It may also be necessary following transplantation to allow delivery of different modes of mechanical ventilation to each lung. Lungs are generally isolated from each other with a double-lumen endotracheal tube. Other methods of lung separation include the use of a Univent endotracheal tube or a standard single-lumen endotracheal tube accompanied by a bronchial blocker (usually a Fogarty catheter). Acute deterioration in gas exchange or hemodynamics occurs with deflation of the operative lung and initiation of OLV. Strategies for improving oxygenation during OLV include the use of 100% oxygen, continuous positive airway pressure (CPAP) in the nondependent (operative) lung, PEEP in the dependent lung, ligation of the operative lung PA (to decrease V/Q mismatch), and return to two-lung ventilation. CPB may be required if severe hypoxia or RV failure occurs during OLV, particularly if the native lung has already been removed but the allograft lung anastomoses have not yet been completed.

TEE probe placement follows intubation and initiation of mechanical ventilation. TEE is used prior to lung implantation to assess RV volume and function, rule out right-to-left shunting across a patent foramen ovale or atrial septal defect (ASD) (particularly in patients with PPH), approximate PA pressures when patients are in the lateral position (when the PA catheter may be inaccurate), and identify proximal PA thrombi (22,71,86). Transient bacteremia is associated with the use of intraoperative TEE, but is not clinically significant.

For SLT, the patient is placed in the lateral decubitus position for a thoracotomy incision at the fourth or fifth intercostal space. The patient may be placed somewhat more supine and the femoral vessels exposed for cannulation if CPB is required. Following dissection of the mainstem bronchus, PA, and pulmonary veins entering the left atrium, the branch PA is clamped for several minutes and the operative lung is deflated to assess oxygenation, ventilation, and RV function. CPB is required to complete the transplant procedure if oxygenation or ventilation are inadequate with one-lung ventilation or if RV failure occurs as a result of increased afterload with one branch PA clamped. If the patient remains stable, the mainstem bronchus, branch PA, and a segment of the left atrium are transected and the native lung is excised. If CPB is required, 300 U per kg heparin is given, otherwise only 30 to 100 U per kg is given during SLT. The donor lung is implanted, with anastomoses between the donor and recipient pulmonary arteries and mainstem bronchi, and a cuff of donor left atrium containing the pulmonary veins is joined to the recipient left atrium (Fig. 6). The donor bronchus is entirely dependent on PA collaterals for perfusion since the donor lung's bronchial blood supply is lost when the lung is harvested. Consequently, limiting donor bronchial length is associated with improved bronchial healing. The donor mainstem bronchus is excised within two bronchial rings of the upper lobe bronchus and anastomosed to the recipient mainstem bronchus.

The earliest successful lung transplants were performed in Toronto. Dr. Joel Cooper and colleagues used a segment of omentum "wrapped" around the bronchial anastomosis to improve its vascularity and maintain airway integrity if a partial dehiscence of the bronchial anastomosis occurred. With improved surgical technique and medical management in recent years, it is unnecessary to wrap the bronchial anastomoses with omentum. The bronchi are now commonly joined with a "telescoping"

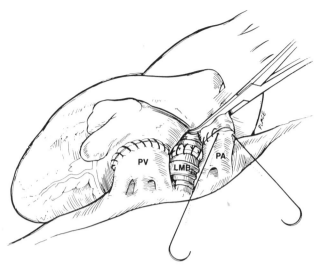

FIGURE 6. Left lung transplant anatomy. Anastomoses of the donor pulmonary veins (with a left atrial cuff) to recipient left atrium, and between the donor and recipient pulmonary arteries and left mainstem bronchi are shown. (From Calhoon JH, Grover FL, Gibbons WJ, et al. Single lung transplantation. Alternative indications and technique. *J Thorac Cardiovasc Surg* 1991;101:816–825, with permission.)

anastomosis; a short segment of the smaller bronchus is intussuscepted inside the larger bronchus and anastomosed. Direct end-to-end bronchial anastomoses are also performed safely. Following implantation, the allograft lung is suctioned and gently reinflated with an FIO_2 of 0.5, peak inspiratory pressure of 10 to 25 cm H_2O, and PEEP of up to 5 cm H_2O prior to reperfusion. Solumedrol 500 to 1000 mg is given i.v. The PA cross-clamp is slowly removed over several minutes, allowing rewarming and reperfusion of the lung, and the lung is de-aired by allowing the blood and preservative solution to drain out the incomplete LA anastomosis. Once de-aired, the atrial clamp is removed and the LA anastomosis completed.

Patients requiring BSSLT remain in the supine position and a bilateral anterolateral thoracotomy with transverse sternotomy ("clam shell") incision is made (Fig. 7). Following implantation

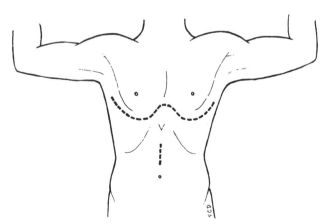

FIGURE 7. The "clam shell" incision used for bilateral sequential single-lung transplant (*dotted line*). (From Egan TM, Detterbeck FC. Technique and results of double lung transplantation. *Chest Surg Clin North Am* 1993;3:89–111, with permission.)

of the first donor lung the allograft lung is ventilated and perfused while the second donor lung is implanted with the same technique used for SLT. The recipient lung removed and transplanted first is the most diseased lung or the lung with the least blood flow, as identified by preoperative V/Q scan. The lung transplanted first is at risk for developing pulmonary edema, reperfusion injury, PA hypertension, and primary graft failure during implantation of the second lung. Severe hypoxia or RV failure may result, necessitating CPB for implantation of the second lung.

The first DLTs were performed en bloc, involving implantation of both donor lungs attached to the donor trachea as one unit. The DLT technique has been replaced with the BSSLT procedure for several reasons. DLT required a median sternotomy, full systemic heparinization, cardioplegic arrest, CPB, tracheal anastomosis, large atrial anastomoses, and extensive retrocardiac dissection that resulted in cardiac denervation and excessive postoperative bleeding. Tracheal anastomosis is associated with a much higher complication rate than bibronchial anastomosis used in the BSSLT technique, and carinal denervation during the DLT procedure results in loss of the cough reflex. Overall perioperative morbidity and mortality were greater following DLT than BSSLT.

CPB is required for HLTs and lung transplants combined with cardiac repair, but it is not required for many isolated lung transplants performed by either the SLT or BSSLT technique. It is generally used only when there is inadequate oxygenation or ventilation, and hemodynamic instability resulting from PA clamping and RV failure. The need for CPB during single-lung transplantation is difficult to predict. The presence of severe hypoxia, poor RV function, or pulmonary hypertension in the preoperative period increases the likelihood that CPB will be required (87,88). Since PA pressure increases dramatically when the operative lung's branch PA is clamped in patients with pulmonary hypertension, pulmonary edema of the first transplanted lung or RV failure may develop if CPB is not used in these patients. Transplantation of lung lobes also generally requires CPB to avoid perfusion of one lung lobe with the entire cardiac output during implantation of the second lobe. Since bronchial blood flow is absent in the donor lung, blood flow to the lung itself and the bronchial anastomosis depends on collaterals from the PA. If CPB is used during BSSLT, flow rates must be lowered, no cardioplegia is given, the patient is not actively cooled, and the heart is allowed to eject blood into the PA to ensure perfusion of the first allograft lung during implantation of the second lung. Limiting CPB flow to one-half to three-fourths of normal also minimizes reperfusion injury and pulmonary edema in the first lung. Gentle mechanical ventilation of the first lung is continued while on CPB. Whether there are deleterious effects of CPB on early allograft function and whether these influence outcome following lung transplantation remains controversial. Conflicting results have been reported in comparison studies of CPB versus non-CPB for lung transplantation in identifying differences in oxygenation, hemodynamic stability, pulmonary vasomotor dysfunction, severity of pulmonary infiltrates, duration of postoperative ventilation, and ICU stay (71,83,87,89). It is clear, however, that perioperative blood loss is increased when CPB is used, particularly in patients with CF that require extensive dissection and lysis of dense pleural adhesions to resect the native lung. The systemic inflammatory response associated with CPB may also play a role in the development of reperfusion injury in the allograft lung. In contrast, CPB may limit reperfusion pulmonary edema and improve function in the first transplanted lung in patients with PPH undergoing BSSLT, since PA pressure and the amount of blood flow in the first lung can be controlled while the second lung is implanted.

Several factors contribute to the development of pulmonary edema following lung transplantation. Although most interstitial fluid in alveoli is absorbed through alveolar epithelial cells, the remainder is normally cleared by the lymphatic system. Since lymphatic drainage of the allograft lung is interrupted at the time of lung dissection and removal from the donor, excessive intraoperative fluid administration may increase postoperative pulmonary edema. Consequently, crystalloid infusion should be limited during lung transplantation, in an effort to minimize allograft pulmonary edema. The use of colloids in place of crystalloids is not beneficial. Vasopressors should be used to treat episodes of hypotension instead of fluids. Low-dose norepinephrine is often infused intraoperatively to minimize fluid administration during episodes of hypotension associated with obstruction of venous return and heart retraction during dissection of the hilum and left atrium.

TEE is used to assess the anastomosis between donor pulmonary veins and recipient left atrium for stenosis or obstruction, rule out the presence of a pulmonary vein thrombus, quantify intracardiac air, and evaluate RV and LV filling volumes and function near completion of the lung transplant procedure. The patient is moved to the supine position and the double-lumen endotracheal tube is replaced with a single-lumen tube, unless postoperative independent lung ("split-lung") ventilation is required following donor lung implantation and chest closure. Bronchoscopy is then performed to suction secretions and blood from the airways and confirm patency of the airway anastomosis.

Acute Postoperative Management

Respiratory Management

Adequate oxygenation (Pa_{O_2} of 60 to 100 mm Hg) should be achieved with the lowest F_{IO_2} possible to reduce the risk of oxygen toxicity. Tidal volume and both peak and plateau airway pressures should be limited to avoid bronchial anastomotic damage, volutrauma, and barotrauma. Mechanical ventilation is usually delivered through a single-lumen endotracheal tube with the addition of 5 to 10 mm Hg PEEP. Patients with emphysema that have undergone SLT may require differential (independent) ventilation with a double-lumen endotracheal tube and a separate ventilator for each lung to deliver low tidal volumes with a prolonged expiratory time and no PEEP applied to the native lung to avoid hyperinflation. Native lung hyperinflation may result in V/Q mismatch, mediastinal shift, compression of the transplanted lung, and hemodynamic instability. Differential ventilation of the two lungs does not need to be synchronous. Patient positioning can also improve V/Q matching after SLT, or following BSSLT when function of one lung is worse than the other (83). Patients with PPH may have improved ventilation and perfusion matching when the transplanted lung is in the nondependent position, since ventilation is improved in the transplanted lung that receives

most of the pulmonary blood flow. Conversely, patients with restrictive lung disease may improve with the transplanted lung dependent, because the lungs will be ventilated more uniformly.

Early postoperative respiratory insufficiency following lung transplantation results from primary graft failure, inadequate donor lung preservation, ischemic lung injury, rejection, and pulmonary edema due to reperfusion injury, interruption of lung lymphatics, excessive fluid administration, prolonged CPB (when used), pulmonary venous obstruction or thrombosis, and surgical trauma. General causes of postoperative respiratory insufficiency, such as atelectasis, aspiration, pneumothorax, and pulmonary infection, must be considered. Reperfusion injury is characterized by impaired oxygenation, noncardiogenic pulmonary edema, and poor lung compliance (64,90). Initial management is supportive; it includes increased F_{IO_2} and PEEP as necessary, alternate modes of mechanical ventilation, diuresis, and avoidance of fluid overload. Differential ventilation may be beneficial if one lung is affected more than the other. Severe, life-threatening hypoxia and occasionally pulmonary hypertension resulting from reperfusion injury may require treatment with inhaled NO, PGE_1 infusion, or extracorporeal membrane oxygenation (ECMO) (90).

Lung transplant patients are extubated as soon as possible postoperatively to minimize the risk of pulmonary infection. Reperfusion pulmonary edema, however, may necessitate mechanical ventilation with PEEP until resolution. Injury to the recurrent laryngeal and phrenic nerves may also delay extubation. Epidural analgesia provides effective postoperative pain relief and often aids in weaning patients from mechanical ventilation.

Vagal denervation of the transplanted lung and airway alter recipient pulmonary physiology. The denervated lung exhibits resting bronchodilation, a less effective cough reflex, and decreased clearance of secretions, response to hypercapnia, and sensitivity to foreign bodies (71,83). The ability of the lung to bronchoconstrict in response to hypocapnia is unchanged. Phrenic nerve injury also alters pulmonary physiology, secondary to diaphragmatic dysfunction.

Airway Complications

Airway complications were a frequent cause of morbidity and mortality following early lung transplants, but now occur in less than 15% of patients (64,91). The most common airway complications are anastomotic dehiscence or stenosis, and bronchomalacia. Complete dehiscence is the most serious airway complication, but is rare since the abandonment of tracheal anastomoses and the introduction of the telescoping technique of bronchial anastomosis. Dehiscence is generally the result of airway ischemia and is associated with a high mortality rate. Immediate surgical intervention is required to repair the anastomosis and prevent mediastinitis. Partial airway dehiscence is managed conservatively, with tube thoracostomy drainage of the associated pneumothorax and reduction in the dose of steroids (64). The most frequent airway complication is anastomotic stenosis resulting from granulation tissue, concentric scarring, or bronchomalacia. Stenosis typically presents with wheezing, dyspnea, and recurrent lower respiratory tract infections several weeks to months following lung transplantation. Fiberoptic bronchoscopy confirms the diagnosis along with spirometry, which reveals variable or fixed intrathoracic airway obstruction. Progressive airway narrowing that compromises more than 50% of the lumen area is treated with dilation or placement of an expandable airway stent (91,92). Airway stenosis from granulation tissue has also been treated with laser ablation.

Cardiovascular Management

Minimal cardiovascular support is generally required following lung transplantation, particularly if CPB was not necessary during the procedure. Transient hypotension is common in the first 24 to 48 hours following lung transplantation, as a result of low SVR. Vasopressors, such as low-dose norepinephrine, are administered to minimize fluid resuscitation and prevent pulmonary edema. Fluid replacement is used only to maintain euvolemia, with a CVP less than 10 and PCOP less than 14, a MAP greater than 65 to 70, and adequate urine output. PVR will decrease and RV function gradually improves in patients with preoperative pulmonary hypertension. Postoperative pulmonary hypertension must be avoided in patients who have undergone SLT for PPH, since the transplanted lung receives more than 85% to 90% of the pulmonary blood flow and is prone to pulmonary edema when PA pressures increase.

Hematologic Management

Perioperative blood loss depends on the procedure and indication for transplantation. SLT commonly requires transfusion of 1 to 2 U of packed red blood cells; 2 to 5 U may be necessary for BSSLT. Transfusion requirements are increased if CPB is used during the procedure, if dense pleural adhesions are dissected (common in patients with CF), and in patients with congenital heart disease or Eisenmenger syndrome who have extensive mediastinal collateral vessels. The former en bloc DLT procedure was also associated with greater blood loss than either SLT or BSSLT. Blood loss is decreased with the use of antifibrinolytic agents, such as aprotinin, tranexamic acid, and epsilon-aminocaproic acid, particularly in patients undergoing repeat transplantation or requiring CPB. Use of closed red cell scavenging devices to reinfuse shed blood will also decrease homologous blood transfusion rates. It is essential that CMV-seronegative patients are transfused only with blood products that are free of CMV, since CMV sepsis is potentially fatal in immunosuppressed transplant recipients.

Therapeutic anticoagulation with low-dose heparin or dextran is often initiated in the ICU following lung transplantation, once postoperative bleeding has ceased. Anticoagulation may improve microcirculatory flow to the bronchial anastomosis that is dependent on PA collateral perfusion, and prevent both pulmonary venous thrombosis and deep venous thrombosis (DVT). Prevention of DVT is essential, since an associated pulmonary embolism may result in ischemia or infarction of a larger segment of the lung than usual because the transplanted lung is devoid of bronchial blood flow which normally perfuses and maintains viability of the lung itself.

Immunosuppression

Allograft lungs necessitate the most aggressive immunosuppression and have the highest incidence of acute and chronic rejection of any solid organ transplant (43). Although immunosuppression protocols vary between different transplant centers, traditional "triple therapy" consisting of cyclosporine, azathioprine, and corticosteroids remains the most common regimen (5,43). As with OHT, some recipients may be weaned off corticosteroids when the risk of rejection is reduced following lung transplantation and newer agents are being administered (5,39,43) (see "Orthotopic Heart Transplant" earlier in the chapter). Dacliximab and basiliximab are two new antiinterleukin-2 receptor antibodies that have minimal toxicity, are clinically available, and may replace older cytolytic immunosuppressants following lung transplantation if future studies confirm their benefit.

Hyperacute and Acute Rejection

Hyperacute (humoral) rejection is the result of preformed cytotoxic antibodies directed against allograft antigens and is very rare following lung transplantation provided the donor and recipient are ABO matched and there is low reactivity on the PRA. It is characterized by rapid development of intravascular thrombosis within the first few hours of reperfusing the donor lung, resulting in a cyanotic allograft that ceases to function. High-dose corticosteroids, tacrolimus, lymphocytotoxic therapy, and plasmapheresis to reduce the level of circulating preformed antibodies have been used to treat hyperacute rejection, but are of limited efficacy. Death often results unless the patient is retransplanted, particularly in DLTs.

Acute rejection is cell-mediated and takes longer to develop. Although it may occur at any time, the majority of lung transplant recipients will have at least one episode of acute rejection within the first 6 months following transplantation, and the incidence declines thereafter. Clinical presentation is often nonspecific and includes dyspnea, nonproductive cough, hypoxia, malaise, low-grade fever, and leukocytosis (93). Mild rejection may be present in completely asymptomatic patients. CXR may reveal interstitial or alveolar opacification and pleural effusions, but is often unremarkable during rejection episodes that occur after 1 month following transplantation (64). Since clinical presentation and CXR may not identify patients with acute rejection, some centers recommend surveillance with home spirometry. Greater than a 10% decline in spirometric values suggests the presence of acute rejection, but does not rule out etiologies such as pulmonary infection or variability in native-lung mechanics in patients who have had only one lung transplanted (64). Histologic confirmation is mandatory given the unreliability of clinical presentation, CXR, and spirometry in the diagnosis of acute rejection. Biopsy specimens obtained by bronchoscopy with transbronchial biopsy and bronchoalveolar lavage remain the "gold standard" for diagnosis and demonstrate histologic evidence of minimal-to-mild grade acute rejection in nearly 40% of asymptomatic patients (64,93,94).

Acute rejection usually responds promptly and completely to treatment with a short course of high-dose corticosteroids (750 to 1,000 mg i.v. methylprednisolone daily for 3 days), in addition to transiently increased doses of cyclosporine and azathioprine. Tacrolimus and MMF have also been used to treat acute rejection. Histologic evidence of acute rejection often persists after clinical, spirometric, and CXR abnormalities have resolved, necessitating follow-up transbronchial biopsies. It is essential to differentiate rejection from other causes of impaired respiratory function to avoid an unnecessary increase of immunosuppressive drugs and delayed treatment of etiologies other than rejection.

Infectious Complications

Infection remains one of the leading causes of morbidity and mortality following lung transplantation. The lung is uniquely predisposed to infection because it is the only transplanted organ that is exposed to the external environment. Other factors that contribute to an increased risk of infection include therapeutic immunosuppression, a depressed cough reflex and impaired ciliary clearance of secretions due to lung denervation, disruption of pulmonary lymphatics, preexisting infection of the donor lung, airway anastomosis ischemia, the presence of sutures in the airway, and unresolved upper airway or sinus infection in recipients transplanted for septic lung diseases. Pneumonia is common in the early postoperative period, primarily due to nosocomial gram-negative bacteria, such as *P. aeruginosa*, *Klebsiella*, and *Haemophilus influenzae*. Pulmonary or systemic infection with organisms, such as CMV, fungi (most commonly *Candida albicans* and *Aspergillus*), and *P. carinii*, typically occurs beyond the first postoperative month. Clinical presentation of pulmonary infection shares several features with rejection, such as fever, cough, leukocytosis, and impaired oxygenation. Unlike rejection, pulmonary infiltrates on CXR tend to be more localized and sputum is more often purulent with infection. Confirmation of the diagnosis via bronchoscopy with transbronchial biopsy, bronchoalveolar lavage, and examination of specimen histology, culture and sensitivity, and Gram stain is necessary to differentiate infection from rejection and to identify the specific infectious agent.

Prevention and prompt, specific treatment of infection is essential for survival. Lung donors and recipients are routinely given preoperative cefotaxime or cefuroxime, and all recipients are started on prophylactic antibiotics in the immediate postoperative period to prevent bacterial infection. A combination of clindamycin and a third-generation cephalosporin, such as ceftazidime, is commonly used for prophylaxis postoperatively. Antibiotic therapy is often modified in response to final bacterial culture and sensitivity reports of specimens obtained preoperatively from the donor and recipient airways. Antibiotics are continued at least until the patient is extubated, culture results from the donor are known, and evidence of infection is absent.

Viruses, fungi, and *P. carinii* are other common etiologies of infection following lung transplantation. Although not a problem in the immediate postoperative period, CMV is a potentially devastating viral infection that occurs most often in the first few months following transplantation. Prophylaxis against CMV is commonly initiated by the end of the first postoperative week. Recipients at greatest risk for severe, primary CMV infection are CMV-seronegative preoperatively and transplanted with a CMV-positive donor organ. Such patients are treated with ganciclovir for up to 3 months. Ganciclovir prophylaxis is also given for 3 weeks to recipients who were CMV-positive prior to transplantation and received a CMV-positive lung, since these patients may experience reactivation of latent CMV infection or become infected with a new strain of virus from a CMV-positive donor. Ganciclovir effectively treats active CMV infection and reduces CMV-related mortality, but the use of prophylactic ganciclovir in the absence of active CMV infection and in recipients who were CMV-positive prior to transplantation is controversial and seems to only modestly reduce the incidence of active CMV infection (64,83,95,96). Some centers supplement ganciclovir therapy with CMV hyperimmunoglobulin, primarily in recipients at risk for primary CMV infection. Foscarnet is used to treat ganciclovir-resistant CMV, but is more toxic than ganciclovir. Patients not receiving ganciclovir are maintained on acyclovir prophylaxis against herpes simplex and herpes zoster, two common viral infections following lung transplantation. Fungal infections are also common following lung transplantation, most commonly caused by *C. albicans* and *Aspergillus*. Fluconazole is often used to treat *Candida* infection. *Aspergillus* is treated with itraconazole. Both of these fungi respond to inhaled or i.v. amphotericin B. *P. carinii* infection occurs in nearly all lung recipients in the absence of preventive therapy. Consequently, prophylaxis with trimethoprim-sulfamethoxazole is universal.

Long-Term Complications

Bronchiolitis obliterans (BO) is the major factor limiting long-term survival following lung transplantation. It generally occurs beyond 6 months following transplantation and has a reported prevalence of 32% to over 50% by 5 years posttransplantation (5,64,97–99). The term BO refers to histologic abnormalities within the allograft lung including inflammation, submucosal fibrosis, and luminal obliteration of the small airways, and is thought to represent chronic rejection (97,98). Unlike acute rejection, which requires histologic confirmation of the diagnosis, chronic rejection is identified by clinical criteria without pathologic evidence (Table 8). Consequently, the term bronchiolitis obliterans syndrome (BOS) is commonly used to describe chronic rejection following lung transplantation. This clinical syndrome is characterized by increasing dyspnea, airflow limitation on PFTs, and impaired gas exchange, as a result of irreversible, progressive airway obstruction. Onset of chronic rejection is often insidious and may present with vague symptoms, such as malaise or a mild nonproductive cough. Use of home spirometry and pulse oximetry, with resting and exercise saturations daily, may lead to earlier diagnosis of chronic rejection. Any consistent decrease of at least 10% to 20% in FEV_1 and FVC that persists for more than a few days on home spirometry should be reported and

TABLE 8. CLINICAL CLASSIFICATION OF BRONCHIOLITIS OBLITERANS SYNDROME[a]

Stage 0:	FEV_1 >80% of baseline
Stage 1:	Mild BOS FEV_1 66%–80% of baseline
Stage 2:	Moderate BOS FEV_1 51%–65% of baseline
Stage 3:	Severe BOS FEV_1 50% of baseline

FEV_1, forced expiratory volume in 1 second; BOS, bronchiolitis obliterans syndrome.
[a]Each stage is subclassified as "a", without histologic confirmation; or "b", with histologic confirmation.
Adapted from Cooper JD, Billingham M, Egan T, et al. A working formulation for the standardization of nomenclature and for clinical staging of chronic dysfunction in lung allografts. *J Heart Lung Transpl*, 1993;12:713–716, with permission.

confirmed with formal PFTs in a qualified laboratory. Maximal forced expiratory flow rate at 25% to 75% of FVC ($FEF_{25\%-75\%}$) is a less effort-dependent PFT that indicates airflow limitation in the small airways when decreased. A decline in $FEF_{25\%-75\%}$ may be more useful than other PFTs in diagnosing chronic rejection early, since it generally precedes the fall in FEV_1 and FVC (64,100). CXRs are often normal until late in the disease, whereas high-resolution computed tomography of the chest may reveal peripheral lucency, decreased peripheral vascular markings, bronchiectasis, and air trapping, especially on expiratory images (101). Although bronchoscopy and transbronchial biopsies are not sensitive methods of diagnosing chronic rejection, they are often still performed to rule out acute rejection and infection.

The etiology and pathogenesis of BO are not fully understood. Predisposing factors for the development of BO include HLA mismatching, ischemia-reperfusion injury, CMV pneumonitis, and an increased number and severity of acute rejection episodes in the early posttransplant period (64,97–99). No effective prevention for BO exists, but prevention and early treatment of acute rejection episodes and CMV infection may delay its onset and severity. BO has a variable course, ranging from slow progression over several years to a rapid decline in function, resulting in death within a few months from the time of onset. Treatment of chronic rejection includes high-dose corticosteroids, augmentation of other immunosuppressants, and occasionally the addition of lymphocytotoxic therapy with ALG, ATG, or OKT3. However, medical treatment is generally ineffective and only slows or temporarily inhibits the progression of BO. Retransplantation is the only definitive treatment available, but is associated with worse outcome than primary transplantation and remains ethically controversial.

Other long-term complications following lung transplantation are predominantly related to immunosuppressive therapy, and are similar to the long-term problems seen after OHT. These include opportunistic infections, malignancy (especially lymphoproliferative disorders), and immunosuppressant drug side effects and toxicities, such as hypertension, renal dysfunction, hyperlipidemia, and diabetes (5).

Outcome Following Lung Transplantation

Lung transplant recipients generally have a significantly improved quality of life, increased exercise tolerance, normalization of PA pressures, and restoration of RV function. Over 80% of survivors report no limitation of activity at 1 and 5 years following transplantation (5). Survival rates following lung transplantation have consistently improved over the past decade. Although the greatest improvement has been since 1992, a smaller, but still statistically significant improvement in survival has occurred since 1996 (5). Nonetheless, survival rates following lung transplantation are the lowest of any solid organ transplant, primarily because no available therapy consistently halts or reverses the progression of chronic rejection in the allograft lung. Since 1996, actuarial survival of all lung recipients (adult and pediatric) is approximately 76% at 1 year and slightly over 60% at 3 years following transplantation (5). Survival rates in the pediatric population are lower than in adults. No statistically significant difference exists in the survival rates between SLT and BSSLT. Risk factors for

1- and 5-year mortality following lung transplantation include preoperative ventilator support, repeat transplantation, diagnosis other than emphysema, year of transplantation prior to 1996, female donor lung, and advanced recipient age. The leading cause of death in the first 30 days is primary graft failure, whereas infection is the predominant cause overall in the first year. Survival beyond the first year is primarily limited by BO.

HEART-LUNG TRANSPLANTATION

The first successful human HLT was performed at Stanford University in 1981 (102). This procedure was increasingly performed worldwide during the 1980s, but plateaued in the early to mid-1990s. Subsequently, the number of HLTs has sharply declined in recent years. Only 91 of these procedures worldwide were reported to the ISHLT in 1999. Several factors account for the decline in HLT numbers. Isolated heart or lung transplant procedures have replaced HLT for some pathologic processes, such as PPH, that were traditionally considered indications for heart-lung transplantation. Even secondary pulmonary vascular destruction and irreversible pulmonary hypertension (Eisenmenger syndrome) associated with end-stage congenital heart disease is now commonly treated with an isolated SLT or BSSLT and primary cardiac repair, instead of HLT (75). Eisenmenger syndrome, one of the first and most common indications for HLT, is also less prevalent now, since early repair of congenital cardiac defects is common and prevents secondary pulmonary vascular damage. Similarly, patients with end-stage lung disease and associated moderate RV dysfunction are now known to have good outcomes and improvement in RV function following SLT or BSSLT alone, obviating the need for HLT. Other reasons for the declining use of HLT include an extreme shortage of suitable donor heart-lung blocs, and ethical concerns regarding the use of two lungs and a heart for one recipient. Primary indications for the limited number of HLTs currently performed include congenital heart disease (30.6%), PPH (28.1%), and CF (8.5%) (5,70).

Preoperative evaluation and care, intraoperative monitoring, and anesthetic management for HLT candidates is similar to that for patients presenting for isolated heart or lung transplantation. Intracardiac shunting and severe polycythemia in some patients with congenital heart disease present additional challenges when these patients undergo HLT. Surgical technique has historically involved implantation of the heart and lungs as a single unit, using a tracheal airway anastomosis. As in the DLT procedure, a tracheal anastomosis used for HLT requires extensive retrocardiac dissection and is associated with higher rates of airway dehiscence and stenosis postoperatively. Consequently, the bibronchial anastomotic technique used for BSSLT is now employed for lung implantation during HLT. Other surgical concerns include the presence of pleural adhesions and extensive mediastinal vascular collaterals that often complicate surgical dissection and contribute to excessive perioperative blood loss. It is also difficult to uniformly cool and preserve the heart-lung bloc during transportation and implantation because of its large size.

Postoperative management of HLT recipients is similar to that described for isolated heart or lung transplantation. Actuarial survival rates for HLT are the lowest of any form of cardiopulmonary transplantation. The 1-year survival is approximately 63%, whereas 12-year survival is 23% (5).

SUMMARY

Heart and lung transplantation evolved from experimental procedures of last resort to therapies of choice for selected patients with end-stage cardiopulmonary disease during the last two decades. Improved organ preservation and surgical technique, a better understanding of heart and lung transplant physiology and immunology, the development of donor and recipient selection criteria, improved immunologic surveillance and therapeutic immunosuppression, and early diagnosis and treatment of common postoperative problems, such as rejection and infection, resulted in this success. Properly selected patients often enjoy an active, productive life and long-term survival following transplantation.

KEY POINTS

Although the number of cardiopulmonary transplants performed worldwide has declined in recent years due to a shortage of donor organs, heart and lung transplantations remain relatively common procedures for the treatment of end-stage cardiopulmonary disease. The success of these procedures is related to effective immunosuppressants, enhanced organ preservation, and improved operative techniques developed over the past two decades.

Coronary artery disease and idiopathic-dilated cardiomyopathy are the primary indications for cardiac transplants. The most common indications for lung transplantation vary according to the type of procedure performed, but include emphysema, idiopathic pulmonary fibrosis, cystic fibrosis, and primary pulmonary hypertension.

Orthotopic heart transplant nearly always employs the orthotopic technique. Combined heart-lung transplantation is now rarely performed. Lung transplantation is currently comprised of four distinct surgical procedures: single-lung transplant (SLT), bilateral sequential single-lung transplant (BSSLT), heart-lung transplant (HLT), and living-related donor transplant (LRDT). The most common lung transplant procedure performed worldwide is SLT.

The diagnosis of acute and chronic cardiac allograft rejection require histologic confirmation. Cardiac tissue specimens are obtained from transvenous endomyocardial biopsy. The diagnosis of acute rejection following lung transplantation requires histologic confirmation, whereas the diagnosis of chronic rejection in the allograft lung does not. Transbronchial biopsies and bronchoalveolar lavage are used to collect histologic specimens from the allograft lung. Bronchiolitis obliterans and cardiac allograft vasculopathy are the result of chronic rejection in transplanted lungs and hearts, respectively. These complications ultimately limit the longevity of the allograft organs.

Corticosteroids, azathioprine, and cyclosporine are the most commonly used drugs for triple-therapy immunosuppression following cardiopulmonary transplantation. The use of newer agents, such as mycophenolate mofetil and tacrolimus, is becoming increasingly common.

REFERENCES

1. Barnard CN. A human cardiac transplant: an interim report of a successful operation performed at Groote Schuur Hospital, Cape Town. *S Afr Med J* 1967;41:1271–1274.
2. Lower RR, Shumway NE. Studies on orthotopic hemotransplantation of the canine heart. *Surg Forum* 1960;11:18–19.
3. Hardy JD, Chavez CM, Kurrus FD, et al. Heart transplantation in man. *JAMA* 1964;188:114–118.
4. Borel J. Comparative study of in vitro and in vivo drug effects on cell-mediated cytotoxicity. *Immunology* 1976;31:631–641.
5. Hosenpud JD, Bennet LE, Keck BM, et al. The Registry of the International Society for Heart and Lung Transplantation: Seventeenth Official Report—2000. *J Heart Lung Transpl* 2000;19:909–931.
6. Hunt SA. Current status of cardiac transplantation. *JAMA* 1998;280:1692–1698.
7. Mudge GH, Goldstein S, Addonizio LJ, et al. Task Force 3: recipient guidelines/prioritization. *J Am Coll Cardiol* 1993;22:21–30.
8. Mancini DM, Eisen H, Kussmaul W, et al. Value of peak exercise oxygen consumption for optimal timing of cardiac transplantation in ambulatory patients with heart failure. *Circulation* 1991;83:778.
9. Barbers RG. Role of transplantation (lung, liver, and heart) in sarcoidosis. *Clin Chest Med* 1997;18:865–874.
10. Murali S, Kormos RL, Uretsky BF, et al. Preoperative pulmonary hemodynamics and early mortality after orthotopic cardiac transplantation: the Pittsburgh experience. *Am Heart J* 1993;126:896–904.
11. Addonizio LJ, Gersony WM, Robbins RC, et al. Elevated pulmonary vascular resistance and cardiac transplantation. *Circulation* 1987;76[Suppl V]:V52–V55.
12. Scherr K, Jensen L, Koshal A. Mechanical circulatory support as a bridge to cardiac transplantation: toward the 21st century. *Am J Crit Care* 1999;8:324–337.
13. Schmidinger H. The implantable cardioverter defibrillator as a "bridge to transplant": a viable clinical strategy? *Am J Cardiol* 1999;83:151D–157D.
14. Goldstein DJ, Oz MC, Rose EA. Implantable left ventricular assist devices. *N Engl J Med* 1998;339:1522–1533.
15. Hunt SA, Frazier OH. Mechanical circulatory support and cardiac transplantation. *Circulation* 1998;97:2079.
16. Jhaveri R, Davis RD, Tardiff B, Leone B. Heart and heart-lung transplantation. In: Sharpe MD, Gelb AW, eds. *Anesthesia and transplantation.* Woburn, MA: Butterworth-Heinemann, 1999:113–141.
17. Murali S, Uretsky BF, Reddy PS, et al. Reversibility of pulmonary hypertension in congestive heart failure patients evaluated for cardiac transplantation: comparative effects of various pharmacologic agents. *Am Heart J* 1991;122:1375–1381.
18. O'Connell JB, Bourge RC, Costanzo-Nordin MR, et al. Cardiac transplantation: recipient selection, donor procurement, and medical follow-up. A statement for health professionals from the Committee on Cardiac Transplantation of the Council on Clinical Cardiology, American Health Association. *Circulation* 1992:86:1061–1079.
19. Young JB, Nafter DC, Bourge RC, et al. Matching the heart donor and

heart transplant recipient—clues for successful expansion of the donor pool: a multivariate, multiinstitutional report. *J Heart Lung Transplant* 1994;13:353–365.

20. Jahania MS, Sanchez JA, Narayan P, et al. Heart preservation for transplantation: principles and strategies. *Ann Thorac Surg* 1999;68:1983–1987.

21. Firestone L. Heart transplantation. *Intl Anesth Clin* 1991;29:41–58.

22. Suriani RJ. Transesophageal echocardiography during organ transplantation. *J Cardiothorac Vasc Anesth* 1998;12:686–694.

23. Waterman PM, Bjerke R. Rapid-sequence induction technique in patients with severe ventricular dysfunction. *J Cardiothorac Anesth* 1988;2:602–606.

24. Sarsam MA, Campbell CS, Yonan NA, et al. An alternative surgical technique in orthotopic cardiac transplantation. *J Card Surg* 1993;8:344–349.

25. El Gamel A, Yonan NA, Grant S, et al. Orthotopic cardiac transplantation: comparison of standard and bicaval Wythenshawe techniques. *J Thorac Cardiovasc Surg* 1995;109:721–730.

26. Deleuze PH, Benvenuti C, Mazzucotelli JP, et al. Orthotopic cardiac transplantation with direct caval anastomosis: is it the optimal procedure? *J Thorac Cardiovasc Surg* 1995;109:731–737.

27. El Gamel A, Deiraniya AK, Rahman AN, et al. Orthotopic heart transplantation hemodynamics: does atrial preservation improve cardiac output after transplantation? *J Heart Lung Transplant* 1996;15:564–571.

28. Melton IC, Gilligan DM, Wood MA, et al. Optimal cardiac pacing after heart transplantation. *Pacing Clin Electrophysiol* 1999;22:1510–1527.

29. Miyamoto Y, Curtiss EI, Kormos RL, et al. Bradyarrhythmia after heart transplantation. Incidence, time course, and outcome. *Circulation* 1990;82:IV313–IV317.

30. Carrier M, Blaise G, Belisle S, et al. Nitric oxide inhalation in the treatment of primary graft failure following heart transplantation. *J Heart Lung Transplant* 1999;18:664–667.

31. Cannon PJ. The role of nitric oxide in cardiac transplantation. *Coronary Artery Dis* 1999;10:309–314.

32. Fonger JD, Borkon AM, Baumgartner WA, et al. Acute ventricular heart failure following heart transplantation: improvement with prostaglandin E1 and right ventricular assist. *J Heart Transpl* 1986;5:317–321.

33. Borow KM, Neumann A, Arensman FW, et al. Cardiac and peripheral vascular responses to adrenoceptor stimulation and blockade after cardiac transplantation. *J Am Coll Cardiol* 1989;14:1229–1238.

34. Mancini D. Surgically denervated cardiac transplant: rewired or permanently unplugged? *Circulation* 1997;96:6–8.

35. Wilson RF, Christensen BV, Olivari MT, et al. Evidence for structural sympathetic reinnervation after orthotopic cardiac transplantation in humans. *Circulation* 1991;83:1210–1220.

36. Stark RP, McGinn AL, Wilson RF. Chest pain in cardiac-transplant recipients. Evidence of sensory reinnervation after cardiac transplantation. *N Engl J Med* 1991;324:1791–1794.

37. Givertz MM, Harley H, Colucci WS. Long-term sequential changes in exercise capacity and chronotropic responsiveness after cardiac transplantation. *Circulation* 1997;96:232–237.

38. Spann JC, Van Meter C. Cardiac transplantation. *Surg Clin North Am* 1998 Oct;78:679–690.

39. Kobashigawa JA. Advances in immunosuppression for heart transplantation. *Adv Card Surg* 1998;10:155–174.

40. Spencer CM, Goa KL, Gillis JC. Tacrolimus. An update of its pharmacology and clinical efficacy in the management of organ transplantation. *Drugs* 1997;54:925–975.

41. Mele TS, Halloran PF. The use of mycophenolate mofetil in transplant recipients. *Immunopharmacology* 2000;47:215–245.

42. Hullett DA, Little DM, Sollinger HW. Biology of immunosuppression and immunosuppressive agents. In: Sharpe MD, Gelb AW, eds. *Anesthesia and transplantation*. Woburn, MA: Butterworth-Heinemann, 1999:389–403.

43. Hausen B, Morris RE. Review of immunosuppression for lung transplantation. Novel drugs, new uses for conventional immunosuppressants, and alternative strategies. *Clin Chest Med* 1997;18:353–366.

44. Billingham ME, Cary NR, Hammond ME. A working formulation for the standardization of nomenclature in the diagnosis of heart and lung rejection: Heart Rejection Study Group. *J Heart Transplant* 1991;9:587–592.

45. Augustine SM, Yeo CJ, Buchman TG, et al. Gastrointestinal complications in heart and heart-lung transplant patients. *J Heart Lung Transplant* 1991;10:877–887.

46. Conraads V, Lahaye I, Rademakers F. Cardiac graft vasculopathy: aetiologic factors and therapeutic approaches. *Acta Cardiol* 1998;53:37–43.

47. Weis M, von Scheidt W. Cardiac allograft vasculopathy: a review. *Circulation* 1997;96:2069–2077.

48. Atkinson JB. Accelerated arteriosclerosis after transplantation: the possible role of calcium channel blockers. *Intl J Cardiol* 1997;62[Suppl 2]:S125–S134.

49. St Goar FG, Pinto FJ, Alderman EL, et al. Intracoronary ultrasound in cardiac transplant recipients: in vivo evidence of "angiographically silent" intimal thickening. *Circulation* 1992;85:979–987.

50. Hosenpud JD. Coronary artery disease after heart transplantation and its relation to cytomegalovirus. *Am Heart J* 1999;138:S469–S472.

51. McFadden PM, Robbins RJ, Ochsner JL, et al. Transmyocardial laser revascularization for cardiac allograft vasculopathy. *J Thorac Cardiovasc Surg* 1998;115:1385.

52. Weis M, von Scheidt W. Coronary artery disease in the transplanted heart. *Annu Rev Med* 2000;51:81–100.

53. Little RE, Kay GN, Epstein AE, et al. Arrhythmias after orthotopic cardiac transplantation. Prevalence and determinants during initial hospitalization and late follow-up. *Circulation* 1989;80[Suppl III]:140–146.

54. Hanto DW. Classification of Epstein-Barr virus-associated posttransplant lymphoproliferative diseases: implications for understanding their pathogenesis and developing rational treatment strategies. *Annu Rev Med* 1995;46:381–394.

55. Kadner A, Chen RH, Adams DH. Heterotopic heart transplantation: experimental development and clinical experience. *Eur J Cardiothorac Surg* 2000;17:474–481.

56. Martich GD, Boujoukos AJ. Adult cardiac transplantation. *J Intensive Care Med* 1996;11:79–89.

57. Hardy JD, Webb WR, Dalton ML Jr, et al. Lung homotransplantation in man: report of the initial case. *JAMA* 1963;186:1065–1074.

58. Grover FL, Fullerton DA, Zamora MR, et al. The past, present, and future of lung transplantation. *Am J Surg* 1997;173:523–533.

59. Toronto Lung Transplant Group. Unilateral lung transplantation for pulmonary fibrosis. *N Engl J Med* 1986;314:1140–1145.

60. Kadikar A, Maurer J, Keston S. The six-minute walk test: a guide to assessment for lung transplantation. *J Heart Lung Transplant* 1997;16:313–319.

61. Manzetti JD, Hoffman LA, Sereika SM, et al. Exercise, education, and quality of life in lung transplant candidates. *J Heart Lung Transplant* 1994;13:297–305.

62. Edelman JD, Kotloff RM. Lung transplantation. A disease-specific approach. *Clin Chest Med* 1997;18:627–644.

63. Maurer JR, Frost AE, Estenne M, et al. International guidelines for the selection of lung transplant candidates. *J Heart Lung Transplant* 1998;17:703–709.

64. Arcasoy SM, Kotloff RM. Lung transplantation. *N Engl J Med* 1999;340:1081–1091.

65. Aris RM, Gilligan PH, Neuringer IP, et al. The effects of panresistant bacteria in cystic fibrosis patients on lung transplant outcome. *Am J Respir Crit Care Med* 1997;155:1699–1704.

66. Flume PA, Egan TM, Westerman JH, et al. Lung transplantation for mechanically ventilated patients. *J Heart Lung Transplant* 1994;13:15–21.

67. Low DE, Trulock EP, Kaiser LR, et al. Lung transplantation of ventilator-dependent patients. *Chest* 1992;101:8–11.

68. Schafers HJ, Wagner TOF, Demertzis S, et al. Preoperative corticosteroids: a contraindication to lung transplantation? *Chest* 1992;102:1522–1525.

69. Dusmet M, Winton TL, Keston S, Maurer J. Previous intrapleural procedures do not adversely affect lung transplantation. *J Heart Lung Transplant* 1996;15:249–254.

70. Patterson GA. Indications. Unilateral, bilateral, heart-lung, and lobar transplant procedures. *Clin Chest Med* 1997;18:225–230.
71. Singh HJ, Bossard RF. Perioperative anesthetic considerations for patients undergoing lung transplantation. *Can J Anaesth* 1997;44:284–299.
72. Anderson MB, Kriett JM, Kapelanski DP, et al. Volume reduction surgery in the native lung after single lung transplantation for emphysema. *J Heart Lung Transplant* 1997;16:752–757.
73. Todd TR, Perron J, Winton T, et al. Simultaneous single lung transplantation and lung volume reduction. *Ann Thorac Surg* 1997;63:1468–1470.
74. Gammie JS, Keenan RJ, Pham SM, et al. Single- versus double-lung transplantation for pulmonary hypertension. *J Thorac Cardiovasc Surg* 1998;115:397–403.
75. Gridelli B, Remuzzi G. Strategies for making more organs available for transplantation. *N Engl J Med* 2000;343:404–410.
76. Kramer MR, Valantine HA, Marshall SE. Recovery of the right ventricle after single-lung transplantation in pulmonary hypertension. *Am J Cardiol* 1994;73:494–500.
77. Pasque MK, Trulock EP, Cooper JD, et al. Single lung transplantation for pulmonary hypertension: single institution experience in 34 patients. *Circulation* 1995;92:2252–2258.
78. Barr ML, Schenkel FA, Cohen RG, et al. Recipient and donor outcomes in living related and unrelated lobar transplantation. *Transplant Proc* 1998;30:2261–2263.
79. Starnes VA, Barr ML, Schenkel FA, et al. Experience with living-donor lobar transplantation for indications other than cystic fibrosis. *J Thorac Cardiovasc Surg* 1997;114:917–922.
80. Winton TL, Miller JD, Scavuzzo M, et al. Donor selection for pulmonary transplantation. *Transplant Proc* 1991;23:2472–2474.
81. Schulman LL, Weinberg AD, McGregor C, et al. Mismatches at the HLA-DR and HLA-B loci are risk factors for acute rejection after lung transplantation. *Am J Respir Crit Care Med* 1998;157:1833–1837.
82. Wisser W, Wekerle T, Zlabinger G, et al. Influence of human leukocyte antigen matching on long-term outcome after lung transplantation. *J Heart Lung Transplant* 1996;15:1209–1216.
83. Bracken CA, Gurkowski MA, Naples JJ. Lung transplantation: historical perspectives, current concepts, and anesthetic considerations. *J Cardiothorac Vasc Anesth* 1997;11:220–241.
84. Myles PS, Ryder IG, Weeks AM, et al. Diagnosis and management of dynamic hyperinflation during lung transplantation. *J Cardiothorac Vasc Anesth* 1997;11:100–104.
85. Robinson RJS, Shennib H, Noirclerc M. Slow-rate, high-pressure ventilation: a method of management of difficult transplant recipients during sequential double lung transplantation for cystic fibrosis. *J Heart Lung Transplant* 1994;13:779–784.
86. Gorscan J III, Edwaards TD, Ziady GM, et al. Transesophageal echocardiography to evaluate patients with severe pulmonary hypertension for lung transplantation. *Ann Thorac Surg* 1995;59:717–722.
87. Triantafillou AN, Paque MK, Huddleston CB, et al. Predictors, frequency, and indications for cardiopulmonary bypass during lung transplantation in adults. *Ann Thorac Surg* 1994;57:1248–1251.
88. de Hoyas A, Demajo W, Snell G, et al. Preoperative prediction for the use of cardiopulmonary bypass in lung transplantation. *J Thorac Cardiovasc Surg* 1993;106:787–795.
89. Aeba R, Griffith BP, Kormos RL, et al. Effect of cardiopulmonary bypass on early graft dysfunction in clinical lung transplantation. *Ann Thorac Surg* 1994;57:715–772.
90. Christie JD, Bavaria JE, Palevsky HI, et al. Primary graft failure following lung transplantation. *Chest* 1998;114:51–60.
91. Kshettry VR, Kroshus TJ, Hertz MI, et al. Early and late airway complications after lung transplantation: incidence and management. *Ann Thorac Surg* 1997;63:1576–1583.
92. Susanto I, Peters JI, Levine SM, et al. Use of balloon-expandable metallic stents in the management of bronchial stenosis and bronchomalacia after lung transplantation. *Chest* 1998;114:1330–1335.
93. King-Biggs MB. Acute pulmonary allograft rejection: mechanisms, diagnosis, and management. *Clin Chest Med* 1997;18:301–310.
94. Guilinger RA, Paradis IL, Dauber JH, et al. The importance of bronchoscopy with transbronchial biopsy and bronchoalveolar lavage in the management of lung transplant recipients. *Am J Respir Crit Care Med* 1995;152:2037–2043.
95. Soghikian MV, Valentine VG, Berry GJ, et al. Impact of ganciclovir prophylaxis on heart-lung and lung transplant recipients. *J Heart Lung Transplant* 1996;15:881–887.
96. Gutierrez CA, Chaparro C, Krajden M, et al. Cytomegalovirus viremia in lung transplant recipients receiving ganciclovir and immune globulin. *Chest* 1998;113:924–932.
97. Boehler A, Keston S, Weder W, et al. Bronchiolitis obliterans after lung transplantation: a review. *Chest* 1998;114:1411–1426.
98. Schlesinger C, Meyer CA, Veeraraghavan S, et al. Constrictive (obliterative) bronchiolitis: diagnosis, etiology, and a critical review of the literature. *Ann Diagn Pathol* 1998;2:321–334.
99. Heng D, Sharples LD, McNeil K, et al. Bronchiolitis obliterans syndrome: incidence, natural history, prognosis, and risk factors. *J Heart Lung Transpl* 1998;17:1255–1263.
100. Patterson GM, Wilson S, Whang JL, et al. Physiologic definitions of obliterative bronchiolitis in heart-lung and double lung transplantation: a comparison of the forced expiratory flow between 25% and 75% of the forced vital capacity and forced expiratory volume in one second. *J Heart Lung Transpl* 1996;15:175–181.
101. Leung AN, Fisher KL, Valentine V, et al. Bronchiolitis obliterans after lung transplantation: detection using expiratory HRCT. *Chest* 1998;113:365–370.
102. Reitz BA, Wallwork JL, Hunt SA, et al. Heart-lung transplantation: successful therapy for patients with pulmonary vascular disease. *N Engl J Med* 1982;306:557–564.

LIVER, KIDNEY, PANCREAS
TRANSPLANTATION

WOLF H. STAPELFELDT

KEY WORDS

- Orthotopic liver transplantation
- Kidney transplantation
- Pancreas transplantation
- Preoperative evaluation
- Routine postoperative management
- Immunosuppression
- Postoperative complications

INTRODUCTION

Human organ transplantation has assumed a firmly established role in the cornucopia of contemporary medical therapy, offering unprecedented options in treating advanced disease. With success and ensuing societal acceptance, transplantation has progressively been inculcated into the American health care consciousness, generating increasing demand for procedures that promise return to a quality of life not attained by conventional therapies. The field has been revolutionized by successful introduction of the novel immunosuppressive agents cyclosporine, discovered by J.F. Borel in 1972 and approved for commercial use in 1983; and tacrolimus, a discovery by researchers for the Fujisawa Company in 1984 and made commercially available in 1994. In the United States alone more than 4,000 liver, 10,000 kidney, and 1,000 pancreas transplants are now being performed annually in steadily rising numbers, thereby creating a new and essential role for critical care before and after transplantation.

LIVER TRANSPLANTATION

Orthotopic liver transplantation (OLT) has emerged from its more than three-decade history as a commonly sought, effective treatment available to patients who would otherwise succumb to end-stage hepatic disease. Since its inception with T.E. Starzl's first successful OLT in 1967, the field has progressed markedly, particularly during the past 20 years as benefits were realized from scientific advances in immunosuppressive therapies, organ procurement procedures (University of Wisconsin [UW] solution), surgical techniques (venovenous bypass, piggyback technique),

new and rediscovered technologies (rapid infusion system, thromboelastography), and refined perioperative management by anesthesiologists and intensivists.

In 1983 the National Institutes of Health (NIH) Consensus Development Conference concluded that OLT was no longer experimental, but "a therapeutic modality for end-stage liver disease that deserves broader application," largely due to the improvement in outcome incurred with the use of cyclosporine. By the 1990s tacrolimus (FK506, Prograf) became the principal immunosuppressive agent of choice offering the significant advantage of fewer episodes of steroid-refractory organ rejection (1). One-year graft survival rates began to exceed 80%, and more than two-thirds of patients began to survive for longer than 5 years with relatively acceptable side effects, notably renal insufficiency and hypertension (2).

Success gave impetus to growing demand for the procedure reflected in an evolution of patient candidacy, fewer and revised contraindications, tangible societal support (Medicare reimbursement approval extended in 1991), and an ever exacerbating disequilibrium between recipient need and supply of available organs, compounded by the recently emerging epidemiologic trend of a greater prevalence of hepatitis C.

Patient candidacy evolved with the acknowledgment of a wider range of indications for OLT. Changes in contraindications included more favorable views of hepatic malignancy, substance abuse, and viral etiology of liver disease. OLT is being offered to patients with the following:

fulminant hepatic failure from viral hepatitis (A, B, C, D),

chemically induced hepatic necrosis (mushrooms, acetaminophen, halothane),

chronic liver disease (postnecrotic cirrhosis from chronic viral hepatitis, alcoholism, autoimmune disease, or cholestatic disease [primary biliary cirrhosis, primary sclerosing cholangitis]),

vascular disease (Budd-Chiari syndrome, venoocclusive disease),

congenital disease (biliary atresia, congenital hepatic fibrosis),

metabolic disease (steatohepatitis, Wilson disease, hemochromatosis, α_1-antitrypsin deficiency),

certain neoplasms confined to the liver (hepatoma, cholangiocarcinoma, hemangioendothelioma, hepatic metastases of endocrine malignancies, polycystic liver disease),

TABLE 1. CONTRAINDICATIONS TO ORTHOTOPIC LIVER TRANSPLANTATION

Absolute	Relative
Extrahepatic malignancy	Cholangiocarcinoma
Extrahepatic infection	HIV
Brain death	Severe comorbidities (coronary artery
Replicative hepatitis B	disease, severe hepatopulmonary
Failure to comply with	syndrome, portopulmonary
treatment regimens	hypertension)
Multifocal hepatocellular	Progressive encephalopathy with
carcinoma	sustained intracranial hypertension
Cardiovascular instability	
Severe ARDS	
Active pancreatitis	

ARDS, acute respiratory distress syndrome; HIV, human immunodeficiency virus.

inborn errors of metabolism (hemophilia A and B, primary hyperoxaluria type I, tyrosinemia, glycogen storage disease, primary amyloidosis, hyperlipidemia type II), and/or

hepatic cirrhosis and failure of no detectable underlying etiology (cryptogenic cirrhosis).

Advanced chronologic age is no longer considered an absolute contraindication, with patients in over 70 years of age beginning to be accepted not only for organ donation but also as recipients. Currently recognized contraindications are listed in Table 1.

Epidemiologic trends further contributed to rising need as noncholestatic etiologies grew in proportion from about 45% to over 60%, with hepatitis C virus (HCV) now responsible for more than 40% of chronic liver disease and more than half the transplants performed in many centers (3). With the prevalence

of HCV being highest in Americans between the ages of 30 and 49 (4), OLT for HCV alone is expected to nearly triple over the next decade. Related is a predictable need for late retransplantation in up to 5% of previous transplant recipients, at a higher morbidity and mortality compared with initial OLT (3).

These developments continue to accelerate demand for OLT. In 1988, there were 1,713 transplants in the U.S. By 1999, this figure had more than doubled to 4,698 (Fig. 1). However, an even larger number of new patient registrations has continued to be added to the transplant list annually for the past 10 years (Fig. 1). Consequently, the median waiting period expanded from 1 month in 1988 to more than 1 year by 1997, patient registrations on the waiting list soared to nearly 17,000 in 2001, and the number of patients dying while awaiting transplantation is approaching 2,000 yearly (Fig. 1).

A widening gap between available and needed organs creates a major challenge that has yet to be effectively addressed. Continually more OLTs will be necessitated through improved organ utilization including an expansion of the donor pool (nonheartbeating donors) and wider implementation of living-related, split-liver, and domino transplant procedures.

Some of the liver transplant recipients have survived for nearly 30 years. As a result, a cumulative number of recipients are in need of intermittent care for procedures unrelated to yet complicated by their posttransplant state as well as related medical problems, including retransplantation. Thus, increasingly complex intensive care will likely be required for more patients in advanced disease states having to wait longer, deteriorate further, and being more difficult to manage until their priority status matches graft availability. In due course the intensivist's expertise in caring for this evolving segment of critically ill patients will become vitally important.

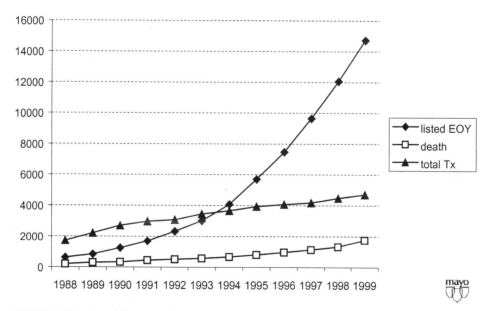

FIGURE 1. Number of liver transplant registrations between 1988 and 1999. *listed EOY*, number of patients on the transplant list at the end of the year; *death*, number of patients on the list who died during the year; *total Tx*, number of patients transplanted during the year. (Data from the United Network for Organ Sharing. Available at: http://www.unos.org. Accessed October 17, 2001.

Preoperative Care

Intensivists may participate in various aspects of patient preparation for transplantation, and an awareness of those conditions that preclude transplantation is essential. While a majority of transplant candidates in the past have not routinely required preoperative intensive care unit (ICU) care, approximately 20% of patients have done so, including—by definition—all patients with fulminant hepatic failure listed under United Network for Organ Sharing (UNOS) status I and those with complications from chronic liver disease listed under UNOS II A. Such patients are at an increased risk for multiorgan system failure and death dependent on their number of comorbid conditions (5–7), and are admitted to the ICU mainly for the purpose of invasive monitoring, vasoactive drug administration, and respiratory support. Common indications for ICU admission include:

infection (pneumonia, subacute bacterial peritonitis),
gastrointestinal (GI) bleeding (from gastroesophageal varices, portal hypertensive gastropathy, gastroduodenal ulcerations) or hepatic encephalopathy precipitated by acute hepatic failure, infected ascites,
sedative/analgesic medication,
a protein overload such as seen with GI bleeding, or
increased portosystemic shunting following a transjugular intrahepatic portosystemic shunting procedure.

Because of the high mortality of recipient sepsis, antimicrobial coverage needs to be instituted and cardiovascular stability restored in any candidate presenting with fever, hypotension, and dependence on vasopressors before OLT can proceed.

Chest infections (aspiration pneumonia), pulmonary edema, pleural effusions, massive ascites, anemia (hemoglobin less than 8 g per dL), and/or electrolyte abnormalities (K^+ greater than 5.5 mEq per L, K^+ less than 3.0 mEq per L, Na^+ less than 120 mEq per L) need to be treated and corrected prior to surgery.

Every effort must be made to prevent or minimize renal failure secondary to acute tubular necrosis (ATN) or a worsening of hepatorenal syndrome for which these patients are at a progressive risk, particularly in the presence of a diminished baseline glomerular filtration rate (GFR) (8). Precipitation of renal failure for any reason carries a high mortality before or after liver transplantation due largely to an increased risk of bacterial or fungal infection (6,7). This is prevented or minimized primarily through meticulous preservation of an adequate cardiac output and intravascular volume status (9).

Cerebral edema and elevated intracerebral pressure (ICP) may occur in patients with fulminant hepatic failure (10), primary graft nonfunction, or much less commonly decompensating chronic liver disease (11). It may develop in as many as 60% of patients with hepatic failure progressing to grade III hepatic encephalopathy (12). Suggestive new patient symptoms include decerebrate or decorticate posturing, seizures, anisocoria, disconjugate gaze, sluggish pupillary reflexes, and/or absent corneal or cold caloric reflexes. If confirmed by computed tomography (CT) or magnetic resonance imaging (MRI), ICP monitoring may be indicated in otherwise acceptable candidates to allow the timely

initiation of treatment prior to a progression to coma and thereby minimize the likelihood of poor outcome (10). Therapeutic options include head elevation (10 to 20 degrees), hyperventilation, mannitol administration, and induction of pentobarbital coma to lower the ICP to less than 20 mm Hg while maintaining adequate systemic blood (mean arterial pressure greater than 60 mm Hg) and cerebral perfusion (greater than 50 mm Hg) pressures. In refractory cases, instituting moderate perioperative hypothermia to $32°$ to $33°C$ may be successful (13), albeit at the cost of increased intraoperative transfusion requirements and an independently increased risk for postoperative cytomegalovirus (CMV) infection (14). If available, extracorporeal liver assist devices may help bridge time to transplantation at the earliest opportunity (15).

In addition to such acute, direct complications from hepatic failure the intensivist may encounter other, frequently asymptomatic conditions that may preclude the patient's candidacy for transplantation. Significant coronary artery disease (CAD) may be detected during dobutamine stress echocardiography in 5% to 10% of candidates (Fig. 2), giving rise to a greater than 50% 3-year mortality (16,17). Severe hepatopulmonary syndrome may be manifested by platypnea, nail clubbing, or orthodeoxia caused by intrapulmonary vascular dilations best documented by contrast echocardiography and quantified by technetium-99-labeled macroaggregated albumin scanning. This syndrome is associated with a prohibitive 30% mortality within 3 months of transplantation if the patient's room air Po_2 is less than 50 mm Hg, but is more likely to improve long-term posttransplant if the Po_2 is greater than 50 mm Hg (18). Severe portopulmonary hypertension may be present in 2% to 5%, often without causing any clinical symptoms (19), but occasionally presenting with a loud pulmonary valve closure (S2) on physical examination, right ventricular strain or right bundle-branch block on the electrocardiogram, or prominent pulmonary vessels on the chest radiograph. It is most commonly suspected following routine transthoracic echocardiography (Fig. 2), which demonstrates a prevalence of estimated right ventricular systolic pressures greater than 50 mm Hg in approximately 10% of transplant candidates (16). These patients need to be further examined by right heart catheterization. Any confirmed pulmonary artery pressure greater than 50 mm Hg, or mean greater than 35 mm Hg coinciding with a pulmonary vascular resistance (PVR) greater than 250 dynes $\cdot$ sec $\cdot$ cm^{-5}, especially if proven refractory to vasodilator treatment, precludes transplantation because of hospital survival rates less than 50% (20).

Transplantation should only proceed after each one of these conditions has been carefully ruled out by following a preoperative evaluation algorithm as shown in Fig. 2.

Postoperative Care

Transplant recipients may require ICU care immediately following transplantation or may be (re-)admitted for early (days to weeks) or late (months to years) complications. Routine ICU care may not be necessary in as many as 50% of liver transplant recipients who can be successfully "ultra-fast-tracked" (defined as a form of perioperative and intraoperative anesthetic management aimed at extubation in the operating room, recovery

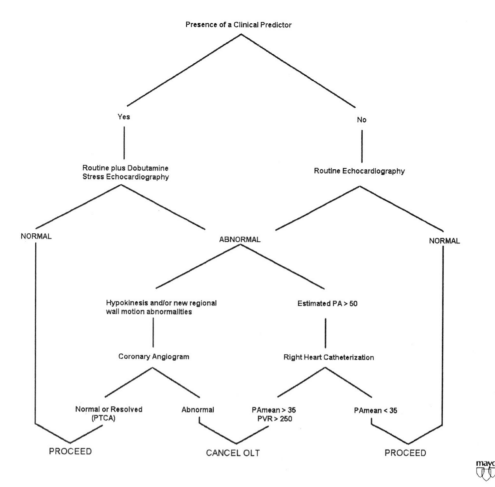

FIGURE 2. Algorithm for the evaluation of candidacy for liver transplantation. Clinical predictors include: advanced age; limited functional capacity; abnormal electrocardiogram (ST-T abnormalities, conduction abnormalities [left bundle-branch block], rhythm other than sinus, dysrhythmias); history of angina, myocardial infarction, congestive heart failure, or stroke; uncontrolled hypertension; diabetes mellitus; smoking history; hypercholesterolemia; or a positive family history for coronary artery disease. *PA*, estimated right ventricular systolic pressure; *PAmean*, measured mean pulmonary artery pressure; *PVR*, measured pulmonary vascular resistance in dynes · sec · cm^{-5}; *OLT*, orthotopic liver transplantation.

in the postanesthesia care unit, and transfer to the ward, circumventing routine ICU admission—W.H. Stapelfeldt, unpublished data). However, it is advisable in many cases, particularly when caring for patients who are at an increased risk such as older adult recipients (more than 65 years), repeat transplants (3), and patients with renal failure or any other medical condition that indicates pretransplant ICU admission. These patients are at a greater risk for bacterial and fungal infections, need for renal support, and overall mortality (6). Other considerations include the condition of the donor organ (age of the donor, extent of fatty infiltration, cold and warm ischemia times, and duration of donor hypotension) (21), and details of the intraoperative anesthetic course (hemodynamic stability, transfusion requirements). While any of these factors alone or in combination may give rise to concern and warrant ICU admission, stable patients with well-preserved extrahepatic organ function who undergo an uneventful transplantation with good postoperative graft function may be successfully extubated within less than 4 hours of surgery, either bypass completely ("ultra-fast-track") or leave the ICU within less

than 24 hours, and be discharged from the hospital within less than 1 week (22).

On the intensivist's initial assessment of the cardiorespiratory and neurologic status, satisfactory allograft function is likely if the patient is hemodynamically stable and appropriately responsive, with adequate breath sounds and satisfactory oxygenation at a fraction of inspired oxygen (F$_{IO_2}$) less than 50%, and without evidence of active bleeding. Initial measures include a determination of the patient's:

arterial blood gases,
electrolytes (including ionized calcium and magnesium),
glucose,
complete blood count,
coagulation status (prothrombin time [PT], activated partial thromboplastin time [aPTT],
fibrinogen, factor V, fibrin split products, thromboelastogram [TEG]),
12-lead electrocardiogram, and
chest radiograph.

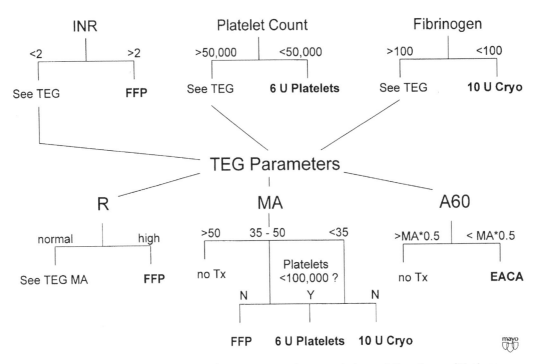

FIGURE 3. Algorithm for the perioperative assessment and treatment of coagulation abnormalities in patients undergoing orthotopic liver transplantation. *FFP*, fresh frozen plasma; *Cryo*, cryoprecipitate; *TEG*, thromboelastogram; *R*, TEG reaction time; *MA*, TEG maximal amplitude; *A60*, TEG amplitude 60 minutes after the time of MA; *Tx*, treatment; *EACA*, ε-aminocaproic acid.

Graft function is monitored by the serial assessment of liver enzymes and coagulation status. Aspartate aminotransferase (AST) and alanine aminotransferase (ALT) typically peak within the first 3 days, reflective of the extent of hepatocellular injury. Canalicular enzymes rise to 4 to 5 times normal values and then return to normal over the first few postoperative weeks. PT should be less than 25 seconds and gradually normalize over the course of the first week while the celite-activated TEG should be within an acceptable range when the patient first arrives from the operating room (i.e., the maximal amplitude [MA] should be greater than 50 mm, Fig. 3). To assure adequate vascular anastomoses and flow, duplex ultrasonography is performed within the first 24 hours, confirming the patency of the hepatic arterial branches and that of the portal and hepatic venous systems.

Most patients maintain a characteristic hyperdynamic circulatory state that improves only gradually. Resolution may be delayed by graft dysfunction or sepsis. The goal of the hemodynamic management is to maintain cardiac output and mean arterial pressure while minimizing intravenous (i.v.) fluid administration to keep the central venous pressure less than 12 cm H_2O, maximize pressure-limited graft perfusion (arteriovenous pressure gradient), and avoid hepatic venous congestion. If necessary, colloid (5% albumin) is preferred for the treatment of hypovolemia-induced hypoperfusion. It is also important to avoid hypertension (greater than 160/95 mm Hg) because of the risk of anastomotic bleeding or central nervous system (CNS) hemorrhage. New onset hypertension may reflect inadequate analgesia, hypoglycemia, impaired gas exchange, volume overload, renal failure, or the toxic effect of immunosuppressants. Once these possible etiologies are ruled out or corrected, antihypertensive therapy may be indicated.

Complications Requiring Prolonged Stay or Readmission to the Intensive Care Unit

Hemodynamic

Up to 15% of patients require reoperation for bleeding (23). Causes include hemorrhage from a vascular anastomosis, a ruptured intraabdominal varix, the adrenal bed, cystic artery, skin closure site, drain site, liver laceration, or gallbladder bed. Bleeding may also be an indication of poor graft function. In the case of active bleeding it is important to maintain blood pressure and restore intravascular volume and coagulation states acceptable for a return to the operating room by administering coagulation products according to the patient's particular needs (Fig. 3).

While the majority of patients maintain a hyperdynamic circulation for several weeks there is evidence for early postoperative mortality associated with myocardial depression in some patients (24). This condition may be reversible with careful management through optimization of ventricular filling pressures by cardiac output or stroke work indices combined with judicious use of inotropes (25). Marked or worsening peripheral vasodilation, particularly in the face of otherwise improving graft function, should prompt an evaluation for a focus of inflammation, infection, pancreatitis, or beginning rejection. Hypotension must be avoided to prevent precipitation of graft failure.

Pulmonary

The role of early resumption of spontaneous ventilation in hemodynamically stable patients remains unclear. Positive intrapleural pressure impairs venous return as indicated by pancardiac cycle tricuspid regurgitation into the hepatic veins during lung inflation, even in the presence of only mild baseline tricuspid regurgitation and normal peak airway pressure (26). A majority of patients readily achieve adequate airway competency and spontaneous minute ventilation, and can be successfully extubated within less than 4 hours without an increased incidence of aspiration or need for reintubation (22). Most early pulmonary complications are noninfectious: right-sided or bilateral pleural effusions that occur in many patients during the first week after transplantation (27) rarely cause respiratory compromise, and tend to resolve during the first postoperative month. More significant problems include V-Q mismatch, impaired hypoxic pulmonary vasoconstriction, intrapulmonary or intrapleural arteriovenous shunts, atelectasis from ascites, fluid overload, pulmonary edema, or aspiration pneumonia. Factors favoring prolonged ventilatory support include severe malnutrition, persistent hepatic failure (hepatic encephalopathy), or neurologic complications such as profound muscle weakness, phrenic nerve injury, or immunosuppressant neurotoxicity.

Pulmonary infiltrates are commonly encountered during the postoperative period, often due to episodes of cardiogenic or noncardiogenic pulmonary edema, which occur in between 15% to upwards of more than 50% of transplant recipients (27–29). Occasionally, early infiltrates are caused by bacterial pneumonia secondary to the tracheal aspiration of gastric content. New infiltrates and fever appearing after the fourth postoperative week are most likely caused by CMV, *Pneumocystis carinii*, or fungal infections (27). A bronchoalveolar lavage specimen with or without protected brush may be needed to identify the causative mechanism. If prolonged tracheal intubation and mechanical ventilation are required, airway pressure and positive end-expiratory pressure should be minimized and the FIO_2 increased if necessary. Weaning and extubation may be attempted after the infiltrates have cleared in the face of adequate and improving liver function. The presence of renal failure (creatinine greater than 1.5 mg per dL) independently predicts poor outcome in patients with refractory pulmonary infiltrates (29).

Neurologic

Neurologic function is a sensitive marker of hepatic graft function. Initial alterations in the level of cognition and alertness in postoperative transplant patients are usually due to a combination of hepatic insufficiency, electrolyte and metabolic derangements, residual drug effects (anesthetics, sedatives), and/or medication neurotoxicity. Several CNS complications can occur at any time postoperatively including seizures, hepatic encephalopathy, cerebral edema, central pontine myelinolysis, leukoencephalopathy, stroke, intracranial hemorrhage, or (fungal) abscesses (30,31).

Seizures are encountered in up to approximately 4% of patients (32). These may be generalized tonic-clonic, complex partial, or akinetic, and may include x-ray findings of reversible white matter demyelination (leukoencephalopathy) (33). They are caused most commonly by immunosuppressant toxicity (cyclosporine, tacrolimus, OKT-3) (34), or, less often, by electrolyte disturbances including hyponatremia, hypomagnesemia, hypocalcemia, hypoglycemia, or mass lesions (stroke, hemorrhage, abscesses). Hypomagnesemia, hypocholesterolemia (33), and an

i.v. route of administration increase the likelihood of immunosuppressant toxicity. Treatment is symptomatic with correction of the underlying cause such as adjustment of immunosuppressant dosage. The likelihood of significant drug interaction with the anticonvulsant medication needs to be taken into consideration. Long-term anticonvulsant treatment is generally unwarranted (32).

In patients with postoperative hepatic encephalopathy, flumazenil may be temporarily effective in improving mental status. Refractory or worsening encephalopathy unresponsive to selective bowel decontamination with lactulose and neomycin demands a high level of suspicion regarding any focal neurologic signs and warrants radiographic examination (CT/MRI) to search for the possibility of cerebral edema or structural lesions such as central pontine myelinolysis (31).

After the first week, leukodystrophy, vascular events (hemorrhage, infarct, subdural hematoma), infections (meningitis, fungal abscesses), or malignant lesions (posttransplantation lymphoproliferative disease) need to be considered as cause for CNS symptoms (31,35). The risk of intracerebral hemorrhage is diminished by the prevention of hypertension, correction of severe hypocoagulability, and aggressive treatment of infections. Established infectious and malignant CNS lesions carry a greater than 70% mortality (31).

Peripheral nerve injuries (cranial nerve lesions, distal lower extremity neuropathy, brachial plexopathy, polyneuropathy, or mononeuropathy such as phrenic nerve injury) have also been reported in some patients following transplantation.

Graft Function

Successful engraftment is by and large evident within the first 48 to 72 hours, indicated by the production of dark bile, improved coagulation with a PT of less than 25 seconds, a modest increase in liver enzymes with peak AST and ALT levels less than 2,000 IU per L followed by a steady decline, and gradual development of metabolic alkalosis. Graft failure (initial poor function or primary nonfunction) occurs in up to 5% to 10% of cases, heralded by hyperkalemia, acidosis, persistent coagulopathy, bleeding, poor biliary output, markedly elevated liver enzymes, hypoglycemia, progressive renal dysfunction, obtunded mental status, and acute respiratory distress syndrome. Until an improvement in graft function or retransplantation occurs, the care for these patients is challenging and aimed at preventing and treating complications including infections, cerebral edema, hemodynamic instability, pulmonary insufficiency, renal failure, acid-base disturbances, or coagulopathy. Occasionally, isolated marked enzyme elevations without hepatic dysfunction may be the result of localized hepatic infarction and tolerated well without any consequence. When graft function is uncertain, bedside duplex ultrasonography is used to examine the vessels supplying the transplanted liver. Concern about the adequacy of flow should prompt an immediate angiographic evaluation.

Hepatic arterial thrombosis occurs in approximately 5% of transplant patients and requires immediate diagnosis and reexploration in an effort to save the graft (23). Portal venous thrombosis is uncommon (at least in adults) and may cause recurrent symptoms of portal hypertension, ascites, and GI hemorrhage from gastroesophageal varices or hypertensive gastropathy. It may be treated with anticoagulation, open thrombectomy, or retransplantation. Graft edema (from venous congestion or plasma hypoosmolarity), hypercoagulability, and hemoconcentration (overtransfusion) must be avoided to minimize the risk of portal venous thrombosis. Stenosis of the suprahepatic caval anastomosis occurs rarely and may present with hepatic congestion, portal hypertension, lower extremity edema, and renal failure. Infrahepatic anastomotic stricture may cause lower extremity edema and renal failure. Any upper GI bleeding during the early postoperative period requires immediate evaluation for the possibility of recurrent portal hypertension for any of these reasons. In contrast to acute hepatic arterial thrombosis, delayed hepatic artery thrombosis is often less dramatic, gradually producing multiple intrahepatic strictures, bilomas, and intrahepatic abscesses. A disproportionate rise of bilirubin and recurrent bacteremia may occasionally be the only indication.

Biliary strictures/leaks are reported in up to 10% of patients, usually after the first week, and may be caused by delayed hepatic artery thrombosis, ductopenic rejection, CMV infection, or graft ischemia time exceeding 12 hours. Small bile leaks may be asymptomatic and may be discovered on a routine postoperative cholangiogram. Symptomatic leaks causing recurrent enteric bacteremia, peritonitis with fever, leukocytosis, and/or right upper quadrant tenderness require surgical reexploration, and in most instances, permanent conversion to a Roux-en-Y choledochojejunostomy.

Occasionally, persistent graft dysfunction for reasons other than acute rejection may be difficult to diagnose and evidenced only by the patient's continued failure to thrive.

Hyperglycemia is common in the immediate postoperative period, posing a problem only if in excess of 500 mg per dL or causing symptoms of hyperosmolarity. It is important to serially check glucose and electrolytes, avoid precipitous increases in Na^+ by more than 12 mEq per L within 24 hours to diminish the risk of central pontine myelinolysis, and replace potassium to prevent hypokalemic metabolic alkalosis induced by improving graft function (23).

Coagulation

Coagulopathy in the immediate postoperative period should be treated with transfusion of coagulation factors to maintain adequate surgical hemostasis (Fig. 3). Subsequently, PT should be corrected to less than 25 seconds and otherwise be allowed to normalize on its own within 1 week. A platelet count nadir occurs typically 3 to 4 days after transplantation and remains abnormal for several weeks requiring platelet transfusions in case of hemorrhage, a platelet count of less than 20,000, or poorly controlled hypertension. It is advisable to avoid overtransfusion (Fig. 3) and correct any evidence of hypercoagulability or hemoconcentration, aiming for a hematocrit of 30% to 35% to maximize oxygen transport while minimizing the risk of hepatic arterial or portal venous thrombosis.

Infection

Infection is by far the most common problem and principal cause for mortality in transplant recipients. Two-thirds of recipients experience at least one episode of serious infection (mostly during the first 2 months) (2). Most of the infections are bacterial, 20% to 40% viral, 5% to 15% fungal, and less than 10% caused by *P. carinii* or *Toxoplasma gondii*. The likelihood of postoperative sepsis and death caused by secondary multiorgan failure is increased in relation to several factors including increased preoperative Acute Physiologic and Chronic Health Evaluation (APACHE II) and Child-Turcotte-Pugh scores (5), the duration of transplant surgery (more than 12 hours), the extent of the preoperative bilirubin elevation (greater than 12 mg per dL), the need for extended (more than 5 days) antibiotic therapy pretransplant or posttransplant (fungal infections), increased intraoperative transfusion requirements (greater than 25 U red blood cells, greater than 30 U fresh frozen plasma), the total number of abdominal surgeries (including retransplantation), and the extent of renal dysfunction (6).

Prophylactic coverage with broad-spectrum antibiotics for 24 to 72 hours is routine practice as is prophylaxis for *P. carinii* with either trimethoprim-sulfamethoxazole or inhaled pentamidine, and antifungal prophylaxis with nystatin. While oral small bowel decontamination has been suggested by some investigators to moderately decrease the postoperative risk of infection at key sites (abdominal, wound, pulmonary) (36) its role in liver transplantation remains unclear, and it is not routinely administered by most liver transplant programs. Routine surveillance cultures for bacteria and fungi are obtained from the throat, trachea, rectum, urine, and bile on the first postoperative day and twice weekly thereafter. Blood cultures are obtained weekly while patients are in the ICU.

Sites of infections are most often intraabdominal (surgical wound, peritonitis, cholangitis, hepatic/extrahepatic abscesses); they are less often pulmonary or within the CNS. During the first month infections are commonly found in patients with biliary obstruction or poor liver function. Thereafter they are encountered in connection with vascular ischemia or chronic rejection. The most common microorganisms include Gram-positive bacteria (*Staphylococcus aureus*, coagulase-negative staphylococci, group D streptococcus) and aerobic Gram-negative bacteria (Enterobacteriaceae, *Pseudomonas aeruginosa*). Less common pathogens are *Nocardia*, *Listeria*, *Legionella*, *Candida* species, herpes simplex virus (HSV) reactivation (during the first 3 weeks), CMV infection (with a peak during the latter part of the first month to 6 weeks posttransplant), *P. carinii*, *Cryptococcus*, or Epstein-Barr virus (causing primary infection or reactivation during the first 6 months posttransplant). Development of pneumonia is usually the result of the tracheal aspiration of orogastric or pulmonary secretions. An urgent identification of the pathogen is critical in any case because of a high mortality of up to 40%. Bacterial pneumonitis is particularly common in patients with fulminant hepatic failure. CNS infections are least frequent and predominantly of nonbacterial (HSV, fungal) etiology.

CMV infection occurs in between 5% and 60% of recipients (with the highest risk in CMV-seronegative patients receiving grafts from CMV-seropositive donors). Risk factors include intraoperative hypothermia (14), rejection, and antilymphocyte immunoglobulin (OKT-3) treatment. Clinical expression varies from asymptomatic seroconversion to disseminated disease resulting in multiorgan system failure and death at a peak incidence during the fifth week posttransplant. Symptoms include fever and neutropenia with hepatitis as the most common organ manifestation (in 50% of recipients). Other affected sites include pneumonitis (in 30% of recipients), GI ulceration, or retinitis. Patients with CMV disease are at an increased risk for bacterial, fungal, and/or *P. carinii* superinfection. The first choice of pharmacologic agent for the preemptive treatment in high-risk patients (in CMV-seronegative patients receiving CMV-seropositive donor grafts) is oral ganciclovir for 3 months. Active CMV disease with or without mucosal involvement is treated with i.v. ganciclovir. An alternative is foscarnet in case of ganciclovir-resistant infection or uncontrollable leukopenia. In patients not receiving ganciclovir, acyclovir is administered for routine antiviral prophylaxis.

Similarly to bacterial infection, most fungal infections occur during the first month. *Candida* is responsible for 75% of fungal infections, *Aspergillus* for approximately 20%. The remainder are represented by sporadic infections with *Mucor*, *Cryptococcus*, and *Trichosporon*. Invasive fungal infections carry a mortality of 50% to 80%. While aspergillosis is predominantly pulmonary in origin, CNS manifestations are not uncommon, usually fatal, and often diagnosed complicating acute hepatic failure (10). Patients deemed to be at particularly high risk for invasive fungal infection (patients with hepatic or graft failure, retransplants, or renal failure) may benefit from preemptive antifungal treatment with microsomal amphotericin B, an issue that is unclear and under active investigation.

Hepatitis C virus (HCV)-related graft disease develops over a period of 5 years in the majority of recipients transplanted for HCV disease. The graft disease shows variable histologic expression ranging from minimal changes to recurrent cirrhosis. HCV recurrence has been reported to account for nearly half of all late (more than 6 months) retransplants performed in one recent study (3).

In eligible transplant candidates with nonreplicative hepatitis B treatment with lamivudine and administration of antihepatitis B immunoglobulin are being evaluated for their effectiveness in preventing graft reinfection.

Nutrition/Gastrointestinal Function

Transplant patients have increased postoperative caloric requirements (37). Enteric feeding via a feeding tube or immediate advancement to an oral clear liquid diet is usually well tolerated following the return of bowel sounds within 24 hours in uncomplicated cases (38). Rarely, pancreatitis may present with unexplained fever and/or an isolated left-sided pleural effusion. GI bleeding may be an indication of recurrent portal hypertension (portal or hepatic venous thrombosis), stress ulceration, or, during the later postoperative course, CMV enteritis, fungal esophagitis, *Clostridium difficile* enterocolitis, posttransplant lymphoproliferative disease, or hemorrhage from a vascular enteric fistula. In unstable patients the diagnosis and detection of the source of bleeding may require emergent endoscopy, radionuclide scanning, and/or selective arteriography.

Renal Function

Adequate renal function is of paramount importance in transplantation because of its dramatic effect on long-term outcome, which is worse in oliguric patients regardless of whether renal failure occurs preoperatively or postoperatively (7). The 1-year mortality is greater than 50% in those patients who require continuous renal replacement therapy or maintenance hemodialysis (39). Renal failure may be caused by ATN or (exacerbation of) hepatorenal syndrome, particularly in patients with preoperative renal dysfunction (6,8,39).

ATN may result from intravascular fluid shifts, hypotensive episodes, an array of nephrotoxic drugs (cyclosporine A, tacrolimus, amphotericin B), hemolysis, postoperative hemorrhage with resulting abdominal distension, or sepsis.

Hepatorenal syndrome (HRS) is encountered in approximately 10% of transplant candidates (40). Its only definitive treatment is liver transplantation upon which patients with HRS enjoy a long-term prognosis similar to that of patients without HRS albeit after typically longer ICU stays (8,40). Up to 20% of patients with HRS may require temporary postoperative dialysis, and up to 10% may develop end-stage renal failure but less than 1% require long-term maintenance hemodialysis. In any patient with poor initial allograft function or primary nonfunction who subsequently develops hepatorenal failure, recovery of renal function is dependent on a resolution of the graft dysfunction—the single most important predictor of the requirement for dialysis—or, in hemodynamically less stable patients, continuous arteriovenous hemofiltration in the postoperative period (39).

Minimization of the risk of renal failure requires an early detection and correction of intravascular hypovolemia, low cardiac output, and/or hypotension through volume expansion and renal dopamine, adjustment of immunosuppressive drug dosing, and aggressive treatment of septicemia. Albumin is the preferred volume expander, particularly if the plasma level is less than 2.5 mg per dL. It is administered in a 5% solution or in a 25% solution if intended to mobilize extravascular free water (9). Patients requiring hemodialysis for prolonged periods of time are more likely to develop ischemic or infectious CNS lesions (31), and a creatinine of greater than 1.5 mg per dL independently predicts increased mortality in patients with pulmonary infiltrates in the ICU (29).

Following the initiation of treatment with cyclosporine or tacrolimus there is a predictable, gradual 30% to 50% decline in GFR over the course of the first postoperative year, the most common toxic side effect of both agents (1,2).

Rejection

Rejection of the liver graft can occur at any time after transplantation and by a variety of mechanisms. It is rare during the first week after surgery but may occur in patients with preexisting antibodies who received an ABO-incompatible donor graft or exhibited a strongly positive cytotoxic crossmatch, usually resulting in irreversible graft failure. Late onset acute rejection after the second week is more common and most often caused by subtherapeutic T-cell suppression. A highly variable clinical presentation may include fever, leukocytosis, thrombocytopenia, and/or extrahepatic organ dysfunction. Liver biopsy is diagnostic, demonstrating inflammation and mononuclear infiltration of the portal triads. It is usually reversible with antirejection therapy. Chronic rejection typically occurs after the fourth postoperative week, is characterized by a progressive graft dysfunction (ductopenic rejection), and often requires retransplantation.

Immunosuppression

Tacrolimus is the mainstay in immunosuppressive therapy. It is a macrolide that binds to cytoplasmic immunophilins to cause inhibition of T-cell receptor-triggered cytokine gene expression, leading to decreased interleukin (IL)-2 release (41). Tacrolimus affords better rejection prophylaxis, fewer cases of steroid-resistant rejection, and less need for OKT-3 (1) than cyclosporine. However, similar to cyclosporine, it is subject to a multitude of important drug interactions (Table 2) (41) and toxic side effects for which liver transplant patients are more susceptible than other solid organ recipients. Neurotoxic side effects may be found in as many as 25% to 40% of patients ranging from minor complications such as headache, lethargy, confusion, insomnia, tremor, or dysesthesias to major complications (in up to 8%) such as seizures, cortical blindness, visual hallucinations, aphasia, neuropathy, delirium, psychosis, obtundation, or coma. These symptoms typically reverse with dose reduction.

Another relatively recent immunosuppressant is mycophenolate mofetil (CellCept), the morpholinoethylester of mycophenolic acid which acts at a late stage in lymphocyte proliferation by selectively inhibiting inosine monophosphate dehydrogenase, an important enzyme in the de novo synthesis of guanine nucleotides (41). While it causes more GI side effects (diarrhea or vomiting) it is less bone marrow toxic and preferred over azathioprine, effectively replacing it as an adjunct agent which may allow dose reduction in patients exhibiting tacrolimus toxicity.

Tapered doses of steroids (prednisone) remain a common component of most (triple) immunosuppressant agent combinations. A steroid bolus (methylprednisolone 1 g i.v. every other day, 3 doses) is also commonly used as the initial drug of choice to treat biopsy-proven acute rejection, and is usually effective in reversing this condition.

OKT-3 (Muromonab CD3) is a therapeutic option in case of steroid-resistant rejection. It is a mouse monoclonal antibody that binds to the CD3 antigen on T-lymphocytes, causing immunologic inactivation of CD3+ cells (41). Complications include a cytokine release syndrome manifested by hyperpyrexia, rigors, bronchospasm, pulmonary edema, seizures (in uremic

TABLE 2. AGENTS POTENTIALLY ALTERING TACROLIMUS METABOLISM AND BLOOD LEVELS

Drugs Causing a Potential Increase in Tacrolimus Blood Levels	Drugs Causing a Potential Decrease in Blood Tacrolimus Levels

Calcium channel blockers
  Diltiazem
  Verapamil
  Nifedipine
  Nicardipine
	Anticonvulsant agents
	  Carbamazepine
	  Phenobarbital
	  Phenytoin

Gastrointestinal prokinetic agents
  Metoclopramide
  Cisapride
	Antibiotics
	  Rifabutin
	  Rifampin

Antifungal agents
  Clotrimazole
  Fluconazole
  Itraconazole
  Ketoconazole	

Macrolide antibiotics
  Erythromycin
  Clarithromycin
  Troleandomycin	

Miscellaneous drugs
  Bromocriptine
  Cimetidine
  Cyclosporine
  Danazol
  Methyprednisolone
  Protease inhibitors	

From Fujisawa Healthcare, Inc. Available at: http://www.fujisawa.com /medinfo/mono/mono_page_pg.htm. Accessed October 24, 2001.

patients), and aseptic meningitis (34). Its use requires judicious fluid management; pretreatment with steroids, antihistamine, and acetaminophen; and prophylaxis against subsequent CMV infection with the concomitant administration of intravenous, followed by oral, ganciclovir for a total of 3 months.

Most transplant centers typically develop their own, unique agent combinations and modifications to immunosuppressive treatment schedules based on their experiences and preferences, including the investigational use of yet more recently released, novel agents such as sirolimus (rapamycin) or inolimomab which are being evaluated in liver transplantation. A very basic immunosuppressive schedule is depicted in Table 3.

TABLE 3. BASIC IMMUNOSUPPRESSION FOR ORTHOTOPIC LIVER TRANSPLANT RECIPIENTS

Agent	Dose	Timing
Methylprednisolone	1 g i.v. 200 mg/d, taper to 20 mg/d over 6 d 1 g i.v. q.o.d.	At the beginning of surgery Daily, i.v. or p.o. Three doses for rejection
Tacrolimus	0.05 mg/kg i.v. 0.05 mg/kg p.o. b.i.d.	Starting on day 2, continuous infusion[a] until taken p.o. Twice daily p.o. doses[a]
Cyclosporine	3 mg/kg i.v. 5 mg/kg p.o. b.i.d.	If intolerant to tacrolimus, continue, i.v.[a] until taken p.o. Twice daily p.o. doses,[a] if intolerant to tacrolimus
Mycophenolate	1 g q.d. p.o. b.i.d.	Twice daily, as an adjunct

[a]Titrated to the desired target blood levels; oral route of administration is preferred.

KIDNEY TRANSPLANTATION

The era of human organ transplantation was conceived with the advent of the first successful kidney transplant by J.E. Murray in 1954. During the intervening years renal transplantation has developed progressive societal support (marked by Medicare reimbursement approval at 80% coverage initiated in 1973), accompanied by heightened demand as graft survival rates continued to improve. Superior immunosuppressive therapies (cyclosporine, tacrolimus, genetically engineered T-cell antibodies) contributed immensely to improved outcome, as did advances in perioperative care.

Living-related transplantation has reemerged as the most successful technique, gaining acceptance by patients and their families. Historically, this technique originally mandated by rejection prevention has progressed from 20% in 1988 to nearly 50% in 1999, with 1-year graft survival rates exceeding 90% and 4-year rates topping 80%. In the U.S. alone, more than 185,000 cadaveric and living-related transplants were performed between 1979 and 1999; and more than 10,000 such transplants annually for each of the last 10 years. Even more extensive numbers may be predicted for this decade, as the patient waiting list exceeded 47,000 in January 2001, with a median waiting time beyond 3 years.

Indications for transplantation include diabetic nephropathy, glomerular diseases, polycystic kidneys, hypertensive nephrosclerosis, renovascular diseases, congenital and metabolic diseases, tubular and interstitial diseases, neoplasms, and graft failure. Contraindications are active infection, human immunodeficiency virus (HIV), active substance abuse, disseminated malignancy, preformed cytotoxic antibodies, and thrombosis of the vena cava or iliac veins. In suitable candidates, transplantation is the preferred, definitive treatment modality offering patients a profoundly enhanced quality of life and long-term medical solution for recipients of functional grafts at only 30% the cost of hemodialysis.

Preoperative Care

Patients with end-stage renal disease constitute a high-risk patient population due to an increased prevalence of cardiovascular disease, hypertension, fluid and electrolyte abnormalities, hematologic abnormalities, bacterial infections, neurologic disorders, and GI bleeding. While the intensivist's involvement in the preoperative care is not routine, it may be required to treat acute electrolyte disturbances, hypervolemia, acidosis (pH less than 7.25), coronary ischemia, congestive heart failure, hypertension, uremic pericarditis, uremic encephalopathy, or diabetic ketoacidosis, and to assist the transplant nephrologist in optimizing the patient's cardiac and pulmonary status for transplantation.

Preoperative diagnosis and treatment of ischemic heart disease are of utmost importance. Asymptomatic ischemic heart disease occurs in 35% to 55% of patients on maintenance hemodialysis, especially in diabetics, and is the cause of death in 50% of patients with end-stage renal failure. Two-year survival of patients with unrevascularized coronary stenoses is less than 50%. Patient age is a major predictor for significant CAD in diabetic patients with end-stage renal failure (42). While CAD is prevalent in nearly 90% of renal failure patients 45 years of age or older, it is also en-countered in a significant number of patients less than 45 years old who present with an abnormal electrocardiogram (ST-changes), a positive smoking history (for more than 5 years), or duration of diabetes for more than 25 years (42). Such patients are subjected to a coronary stress test or coronary angiography. Angiography is indicated for a definitive assessment following a positive stress test or in cases of strong clinical suspicion. Dobutamine stress echocardiography may be suited to noninvasively identify those patients in definite need of angiography by detecting CAD with a sensitivity of 95% (92% for one-vessel, 100% for two-vessel or more extensive disease) and a specificity of 86% (43), and may allow potentially harmful angiography to be avoided in patients with a negative stress test. Confirmed significant coronary stenoses greater than 50% should be corrected either surgically or angiographically before considering transplantation.

Postoperative Care

While kidney transplant recipients do not routinely require intensive care, admission to the ICU may be mandated either immediately after surgery or for late complications. Possible indications for immediate ICU admission include fluid overload, electrolyte disturbances, or (an increased risk of) cardiac complications (dysrhythmias, ischemia, myocardial infarction, congestive heart failure), particularly in patients with a history of cardiac disease and episodes of intraoperative hypotension (44). Hyperkalemia may develop secondary to tissue trauma, protein catabolism, excessive bleeding (transfusions), the use of β-blockers for hypertension, and/or institution of immunosuppressive therapy (cyclosporine, tacrolimus), especially in the presence of delayed graft function or ATN. Hypokalemia and/or hypomagnesemia may result from polyuric graft failure. With supportive care (symptomatic treatment, replacement therapy) and careful monitoring most of the patients presenting with these types of problems eventually fare well with a survival rate better than predicted by their APACHE II scores (44). In contrast, patients admitted to the ICU at a later time and for reasons other than immediate postoperative monitoring have twice the mortality of general surgical ICU patients, mainly because of infection in the presence of immunosuppression (44).

Other than treating complications or monitoring vital signs to rule out the possibility of myocardial ischemia or infarction, patient management is primarily concerned with assessing and maintaining adequate graft function. This is accomplished through an hourly measurement of urine output, blood pressure, and central venous pressure, as well as laboratory determination of the patient's electrolytes, ionized calcium, magnesium, bicarbonate, glucose, blood urea nitrogen, creatinine, and complete blood count. In order to optimize conditions for normal graft function it is of critical importance to maintain normal volume status, an adequate hemoglobin, oxygen saturation, and perfusion pressure by keeping the systolic blood pressure greater than 120 mm Hg and mean blood pressure greater than 70 mm Hg (in previously normotensive patients, higher in patients with inadequately controlled hypertension). Hypertension (systolic blood pressure greater than 160 mm Hg) and volume overload need to be avoided because of the increased risk of anastomotic bleeding, coronary ischemia, or pulmonary edema. Normovolemia is

TABLE 4. FLUID MANAGEMENT IN RENAL TRANSPLANT RECIPIENTS

Hourly Urine Output (mL/kg)	Treatment

>1	Maintenance i.v.: DSW 0.45% normal saline at 75 mL/h
	Hourly urine replacement with 0.45% normal saline
	  0–200 mL urine/h: replace 1 mL for each mL
	  200–400 mL urine/h: replace 0.5 mL for each mL
	  >400 mL urine/h: replace 0.25 mL for each mL
	Change to maintenance i.v., and stop replacement after 24 h if urine output <200 mL/h
	If K$^+$ < 3.2 mEq/L, supplement as needed, consider changing fluids to lactated Ringer solution

<1	Check urinary catheter patency Check central venous pressure (CVP) Bolus with normal saline or 5% albumin as needed to maintain 5 < CVP < 15 cm H$_2$O Give diuretic (furosemide, 1 mg/kg) *if* CVP and urinary catheter okay If no response after 2 hours, contact surgical team
0	Maintenance D5W at 20 mL/h Do not bolus or give diuretics after the diagnosis of acute tubular necrosis has been established Minimize other fluids if CVP > 12

D5W, 5% dextrose in water.

dependent upon meticulous adherence to a fluid management schedule like that depicted in Table 4.

ATN is the primary reason for delayed graft function or oliguria in the postoperative period. Other differential causes include low cardiac output, hypotension, hypovolemia, ureteric obstruction, nephrotoxic drugs (immunosuppressants), renal artery stenosis, arterial thrombosis, venous thrombosis, infection (sepsis), or rejection. In diagnosing the cause of oliguria the following steps are helpful. Initially, it is most important to assess and rectify the patient's volume and hemodynamic status by regularly reviewing fluid balance, weight, central venous pressure, cardiac output (if available), and blood pressure data. If these are adequate it is crucial to rule out benign mechanical problems such as blood clots at the ureter/bladder anastomosis, a kink in the urinary catheter, or a urine leak by flushing and irrigating the urinary catheter as a second step. If this does not solve the problem or provide a satisfactory explanation one must rule out serious vascular complications in need of immediate surgical correction such as arterial or venous graft thrombosis. This is accomplished by performing a bedside duplex ultrasound examination of the blood vessels supplying the renal graft. Finally, if prerenal or postrenal causes are ruled out it is appropriate to assume and search for a parenchymal etiology such as toxicity (antibiotics, immunosuppressants), rejection, or most commonly ATN. Acute drug toxicity is typically reversible with dose reduction. ATN also gradually improves in most instances over the course of several days to weeks with supportive care and avoidance of aggravating factors (hypotension, hypovolemia, low cardiac output, nephrotoxic drugs, or sepsis). Maintenance of adequate volume status is especially important in the event of a nonoliguric stage to minimize the risk of secondary ATN or thrombosis (from hypovolemia and/or hemoconcentration).

If rejection is suspected either clinically or on the basis of suggestive sonographic findings an ultrasound-guided percutaneous graft biopsy is performed to arrive at a definitive diagnosis. Confirmed rejection is treated with a steroid bolus or an antilymphocytic induction drug such as thymoglobulin (ATG) or OKT-3 (discussed later in the chapter).

Other management issues include glucose monitoring and adjustment of insulin dosing in diabetic patients who did not receive a simultaneous pancreas transplant, especially during the rapid postoperative advancement to a regular diet. Postoperative patients are at an increased risk of GI bleeding (from gastroduodenal ulceration, CMV enteritis), pancreatitis, and neurotoxic symptoms (obtundation, seizures), which may result from accumulation of active metabolites of drugs used for postoperative pain control such as morphine or meperidine, or immunosuppressant toxicity. (For a list of symptoms list refer to "Liver Transplantation" at the beginning of this chapter). Other causes for neurologic complications and symptoms include metabolic or hypertensive encephalopathy, cerebrovascular events, or CNS infections most commonly caused by *Listeria, Cryptococcus, Nocardia, Aspergillus, Mucor, Toxoplasma, Coccidia,* CMV, or HSV.

Prophylactic drug regimens include gastric ulcer prophylaxis; perioperative antibiotics; treatment with trimethoprim-sulfamethoxazole or pentamidine (via nebulizer or intravenously in sulfaallergic patients) for *P. carinii* prophylaxis; treatment with oral nystatin or fluconazole for antifungal prophylaxis (initially after transplantation and following any antilymphocyte treatment); and routine antiviral prophylaxis with acyclovir. When patients receive antilymphocyte treatment, concomitant CMV prophylaxis with intravenous ganciclovir (adjusted to serum creatinine) followed by oral ganciclovir is indicated for a total duration of 3 months. Mismatched CMV-seronegative recipients are prophylactically treated with oral ganciclovir for 3 months.

Immunosuppression

Principal immunosuppressant agents are steroids, tacrolimus (which allows the eventual elimination of steroids in many patients and tends to produce slightly less long-term hypertension or hypercholesterinemia than cyclosporine but a slightly higher incidence of diabetes), mycophenolate, and daclizumab (Zenapax).

Daclizumab is a novel, genetically engineered human immunoglobulin-1 antibody containing those regions of the parent murine monoclonal antibody that bind specifically to the α-chain of the IL-2 receptor of alloantigen-reactive T-lymphocytes. It causes a decreased frequency of acute rejection in kidney transplant recipients, an increased time to a first episode of rejection, and a decreased number of episodes of rejection per patient, resulting in increased graft survival without any concomitant increase in infection or malignancies (45). A basic immunosuppressive regimen is shown in Table 5.

Rejection

Rejection may occur over different time frames and via different mechanisms. Hyperacute rejection may occur shortly after reperfusion because of preformed antibodies present in the recipient, resulting in irreversible graft failure. Accelerated acute rejection may develop during the first 2 days and may be successfully managed by intense immunosuppression. Both forms are rare with current crossmatch techniques. Acute rejection may

TABLE 5. BASIC IMMUNOSUPPRESSION FOR KIDNEY OR PANCREAS TRANSPLANT RECIPIENTS

Agent	Dose	Timing
Methylprednisolone	500 mg i.v.	At the beginning of surgery
	250 mg/d taper to 30 mg/d over 6 d	Daily, i.v. or p.o.
	500 mg i.v. q.d.	For 3 days for rejection
Tacrolimus	0.075 mg/kg p.o. b.i.d.	Starting as soon as serum creatinine is ≤50% baseline or on day 5 in patients with delayed graft function[a]
Cyclosporine	5 mg/kg p.o. b.i.d.	Twice daily p.o. doses[a] if intolerant to tacrolimus
Mycophenolate	1 g q.d. p.o. b.i.d.	Twice daily, as an adjunct, first dose before surgery; continued unless dose reduction necessary due to leukopenia or gastrointestinal side effects
Daclizumab[b]	2 mg/kg i.v.	Immediately prior to surgery
	1 mg/kg i.v.	Second postoperative week (postoperative day 10–14)

[a]Titrated to the desired target blood levels.
[b]Kidney transplants only.

occur within 1 to 2 weeks or any time thereafter as a result of T-lymphocyte activation. It is characterized by a rising creatinine in the presence of abnormal ultrasonic findings (increased renal volume, loss of corticomedullary junction, enlargement of the medullary pyramids). Following its histopathologic confirmation via ultrasound-guided core biopsy, antirejection treatment is required to save the graft.

Antirejection treatment options include a steroid bolus (500 mg methylprednisolone daily for 3 days) and, if signs of rejection are not clinically resolved within 3 days of steroid bolus therapy, antilymphocyte treatment with ATG or OKT-3 for 10 to 14 days. These agents are used in some centers for routine induction of immunosuppression ("quadruple therapy").

Following premedication with methylprednisolone (500 mg), acetaminophen, and diphenhydramine prior to each of the first three applications, ATG is administered at a daily dose of 15 mg per kg over 4 to 6 hours via a central venous line. The dose should be reduced or held in case of severe leukocytopenia or thrombocytopenia. The therapeutic effectiveness is monitored by a daily creatinine and differential WBC count, aiming at a lymphocyte count of less than 200 per mm^3.

Treatment with OKT-3 requires a careful assessment and optimization of the patient's volume status by reviewing the patient's fluid balance and ruling out signs of edema upon physical examination, lung auscultation, and chest radiography. If the patient is fluid-overloaded (by more than 3% above dry weight for the previous 7 days) or shows signs of peripheral or pulmonary edema, it may be necessary to induce aggressive diuresis or dialyze the patient prior to the initiation of OKT-3 therapy. For the treatment to be effective the CD3 count must be maintained at less than 25 cells per mm^3. Nonspecific symptoms such as fever and chills are common during the first 3 to 4 days of OKT-3 therapy and should not invariably trigger the usual workup (blood cultures). Symptomatic treatment with acetaminophen and a cooling blanket may be indicated in some cases. Screening for anti-OKT-3 antibodies should be performed 4 weeks after the end of therapy and before the initiation of any subsequent therapeutic course with OKT-3 because OKT-3 is not effective in sensitized patients with an elevated anti-OKT-3 antibody titer. Elevated titers may require the consideration of an alternative therapy such as ATG if indicated. CMV prophylaxis with ganciclovir is indicated similarly as described previously for OLT.

After ATN and rejection, which may under the most adverse circumstances lead to graft loss and return to hemodialysis, infections are the most common, serious, and potentially lethal complications in the early postoperative period (44). They may occasionally mandate the difficult decision to intentionally withhold immunosuppressive drugs in order to save a patient's life at the cost of sacrificing the transplanted organ.

PANCREAS TRANSPLANTATION

Pancreas transplantation entered the human transplantation arena during the 1960s, with the introduction of the field's first successful procedures: simultaneous pancreas kidney (SPK) by W.D. Kelly and R.C. Lillehei in 1966; and isolated pancreas (PTA) by Lillehei in 1968. The ensuing three decades found the progressive course of the field hindered by unsatisfactory graft survival rates. This dramatically changed in the 1990s as greater graft survival was realized following the introduction of the new immunosuppressive agents tacrolimus and mycophenolate (46). Since 1996 more than 1,000 pancreas transplants have been performed each year in the U.S., in more than 75% as SPK, the most successful approach with 1-, 2-, and 3-year survival rates of 94%, 92%, and 91% for patients; 83%, 80%, and 77% for pancreas grafts; and 90%, 88%, and 85% for kidney grafts, respectively. For pancreas after kidney transplants (PAK) these figures are 95%, 92%, and 88% for patients; and 71%, 61%, and 55% for pancreas grafts. PTA remains the least promising approach with 64%, 58%, and 50% graft survival rates, respectively. Consequently, SPK and PAK, but not PTA received approval for Medicare reimbursement effective July 1, 1999.

Candidates for pancreas transplantation are type-I diabetics with or without uremia. Eighty percent have end-stage renal disease and are thus candidates for SPK. Justification for pancreas transplantation includes a significantly improved quality of life, prevention of life-threatening complications from diabetes, and, as a result, increased long-term (greater than 5-year) life expectancy of pancreas transplant recipients. Complications from long-standing diabetes occur in up to 50% of patients who have been insulin-dependent for more than 20 years including an increased incidence of cardiovascular disease (CAD, cardiomyopathy, peripheral vascular disease, hypertension), diabetic glomerulosclerosis, and neuropathologic changes. In comparison to isolated kidney transplantation alone, SPK reduces by 75% the 10-year mortality rate of 80%, which is due largely to cardiac causes (47). Pancreas transplantation may not only prevent a progression of diabetic complications such as glomerulosclerosis in transplanted kidneys but may also contribute to an eventual histologic improvement of nephropathy after a period of 5 years in those patients who do not receive combined kidney transplants (48). In an analogous fashion it may also improve diabetic neuropathy over the long term (49) and thus contribute to a decrease in the risk for sudden cardiac death from autonomic neuropathy.

PTA without kidney transplantation may be indicated in patients with extremely labile diabetes mellitus, poor quality of life, and a risk of diabetic complications deemed to exceed that of side effects of immunosuppression. Those patients considered candidates for pancreas and kidney transplantation are recommended to receive SPK since PAK carries an increased risk of graft loss secondary to either thrombosis or rejection attributable to the introduction of different human leukocyte antigen types of kidney and pancreas grafts (50).

Preoperative Care

Diabetic transplant candidates pose a particular challenge because of complications from long-standing diabetes in conjunction with a greatly increased general risk of infection. Preoperative care includes a comprehensive assessment and management of:

> comorbid conditions, notably ischemic heart disease (42),
> renal insufficiency,
> hypertension,
> diabetic neuropathy (extent of motor, sensory, and/or autonomic neuropathy as manifested by loss of beat-to-beat variability in heart rate, orthostasis, or silent ischemia),
> gastroparesis, and
> the possibility of a difficult airway secondary to stiff joint syndrome which may be found in more than 10% of diabetics.

Additionally, the patient's metabolic (plasma glucose, acid-base status, electrolytes) and volume status need to be corrected prior to transplantation to minimize the risk of osmotic, acid-base, electrolyte, or fluid derangements during transplantation. While not routinely indicated in every pancreas transplant candidate, preoperative ICU care may be necessary for the preparation of severely decompensated patients (presenting with diabetic ketoacidosis, congestive heart failure, or severe electrolyte abnormalities) or the procurement of vascular access prior to transplantation.

Postoperative Care

Patients undergoing pancreas transplantation (PTA, PKA, or SPK) are usually extubated postoperatively either in the operating room or in the postanesthesia care unit, recovered from the effects of general anesthesia, and transferred either to the ICU or the hospital ward. Reasons to admit patients to the ICU include:

> concerns about an increased risk of cardiac ischemia in patients with a history of CAD,

> a history of myocardial infarction or congestive heart failure,
> an episode of severe intraoperative bleeding or hypotension,
> manifestation of perioperative electrocardiographic changes (ST-changes, dysrhythmias), or
> a history of autonomic neuropathy which may blunt the patient's reflex responses to hypovolemia or hypoxia and thus increase and prolong the need for postoperative monitoring.

Routine monitoring includes:

> hemodynamics (via arterial and central venous or pulmonary artery catheters if indicated),
> urine output,
> hourly glucose for 12 hours,
> electrolytes,
> acid-base status,
> complete blood count,
> PT,
> aPTT,
> creatinine,
> pulse oximetry,
> a postoperative chest radiograph,
> serial electrocardiograms,
> cardiac isoenzymes (CK-MB, troponin),
> daily amylase and lipase levels, and
> urine amylase (a 25% to 50% decrease alone typically precedes any rise in plasma glucose during pancreas graft dysfunction).

While most patients require insulin administration to prevent or correct intraoperative hyperglycemia there is generally no persistent need for continued insulin supplementation in the absence of a significant postoperative problem with the graft. If insulin supplementation is required it may be infused according to a schedule like the one shown in Table 6 while the underlying cause for hyperglycemia is sought and the possibility of graft malfunction is explored (discussed subsequently). Following SPK, in addition to these specific issues, the same monitoring and management considerations apply as discussed previously under "Kidney Transplantation," except that sodium bicarbonate may need to be added to the i.v. maintenance fluid regimen in order to inhibit the development of progressive hyperchloremic metabolic acidosis for which 20% of bladder-drained pancreas graft recipients are at an increased risk.

A number of possible complications threaten the graft in the postoperative period and may require re-laparotomy in up to

TABLE 6. INSULIN INFUSION PROTOCOL IN DIABETIC TRANSPLANT RECIPIENTS

Plasma Glucose (mg/dL)	Insulin Infusion Rate (IU/h)
>250	3.0
200–249	2.5
150–199	2.0
120–149	1.5
100–119	1.0
70–99	0.5[a]
<70	0.0[a,b]

[a]Dextrose should be continually infused (50 mg/kg/h) to prevent iatrogenic hypoglycemia.
[b]Dextrose should be bolused (0.25 g/kg) to correct hypoglycemia.

one-fourth of transplant recipients. One percent of patients experience hemorrhage resulting either from incomplete surgical hemostasis or at a later time, an arterial fistula. Another principal problem in 5% to 10% of cases is acute arterial graft thrombosis (50). It is characterized by an indolent sudden and sharp rise in plasma glucose in association with a decrease in serum and urine amylase levels. Risk factors for thrombosis include donor age over 45 years, preservation time longer than 24 hours, and cerebrovascular disease as the cause of donor death (50). Upon duplex ultrasonographic confirmation this diagnosis nearly always requires transplant graft pancreatectomy. Venous thrombosis is a differential diagnosis for a sudden rise in plasma glucose associated with an increased amylase level, a tender swelling of the graft, and occasionally, bleeding from the bladder-drained graft (blood-stained urine), especially during the first 48 hours. Its occurrence is minimized by routine prophylactic anticoagulant treatment with acetylsalicylic acid.

Within the first 2 weeks graft pancreatitis may occur and present as a febrile tenderness of the graft associated with elevated serum amylase levels, yet typically normal plasma glucose levels due to usually sufficient endocrine function. This condition may result from the surgical handling of the graft, prolonged graft ischemic time, or urinary reflux from the bladder. It is treated conservatively with i.v. fluids, bowel rest, analgesics, and somatostatin. A pancreatic fistula may present with the discharge of amylase-containing fluid from a reddened skin lesion. Later complications include anastomotic leaks, and intraabdominal or intrapancreatic abscesses which may present with fever, tenderness, and amylase and glucose elevations reflecting the extent of graft involvement. While anastomotic leaks are successfully treated either conservatively or with a surgical conversion to a Roux-en-Y enterostomy, infections represent the most serious postoperative complication, causing the majority of graft failures and deaths, similar to those following kidney or liver transplantation. Risk factors for infection include donor age over 45 years, preservation time longer than 24 hours, and recipient age over 50 years (50).

Finally, episodes of acute rejection are reported in more than three out of four of transplant recipients, and are responsible for approximately 30% of graft losses during the first year after transplantation. Thus, the incidence of graft loss due to rejections remains higher than that found following kidney or liver transplantation. Rejection is heralded by biochemical changes (hyperglycemia, hypoamylasemia), often preceded by renal deterioration in SPK patients (in 90%), and confirmed via core biopsy of the kidney (SPK) or fine needle biopsy of the pancreas graft. Most episodes of rejection are successfully reversed using agents and protocols analogous to those described for kidney transplantation. Anti–T-cell treatment-refractory rejection may require graft pancreatectomy to prevent sepsis.

The need for re-laparotomy for any of the reasons given is associated with a decrease in 1-year patient survival rate from more than 90% to less than 80%, and a decrease in graft survival rate from greater than 70% to less than 30%. Thus, every effort needs to be made by the attending staff to diligently observe the infectious prophylaxis and immunosuppressive protocols that are being established for these procedures, and carefully monitor transplant recipients for the earliest detection of emerging signs of complications that may arise at any time during the immediate perioperative period and beyond.

SUMMARY

Transplantation has benefited immensely from improvements in immunosuppressive therapy, refined surgical techniques, and highly developed perioperative care. Severe limitations remain in the form of relatively low therapeutic indices and propensity for significant toxicity exhibited by most of today's immunosuppressants. Future trends will likely include the genetic engineering of more specific immunosuppressive probes with fewer side effects. Liver transplantation will undergo an implementation of strategies aimed at maximizing the impact of available organ grafts through expansion of the donor pool, refinement of split-liver transplantation, and increased use of living-related transplant procedures; the development of therapeutic strategies designed to prevent HCV disease recurrence in grafts; and the perfection and more widespread use of bioartificial assist devices to bridge time to transplantation. Further exploration of hepatic and renal xenotransplantation will be facilitated by novel gene manipulation techniques (knock-outs, knock-ins). Such imminent developments will fundamentally transform the challenges and tasks faced by the intensivist caring for transplant patients as the twenty-first century begins to take shape.

Acknowledgments. I would like to acknowledge the many people who have in so numerous ways helped to create the field of transplantation and continually contribute to reshaping it every day. In particular, I wish to thank my colleagues at the Mayo Clinic and the Thomas Starzl Transplantation Institute for shared experiences, triumphs, and losses. My specials thanks are extended to the clinician teachers who first stimulated my interest in transplantation, Drs. Steven Rettke and David Plevak. I also want to thank Dr. Jeffery Steers for reviewing this manuscript, and N. Marlena Jones for providing expert editorial assistance.

KEY POINTS

Transplantation of the liver, kidney, and pancreas are well-established, cost-effective treatment modalities for growing numbers of patients with advanced organ disease. Refinements in organ procurement, surgical technique, anesthetic management, and perioperative care (including recipient selection) have rendered previously experimental procedures more predictively successful. Advances in immunosuppression have provided the basis for greatly improved long-term graft and patient survival following transplantation of all three organs. The development of tacrolimus and introduction into routine clinical use have played a central role in this continued progress since the pivotal discovery of cyclosporine. However, the intensivist needs to remain aware of toxicity and propensity for multiple drug interactions.

Improved success rates have placed transplantation in steadily rising demand, exceeding organ availability. New and improved organ procurement procedures (split liver, living-related donor grafts) have begun to play an increasingly important role in an effort to meet these needs.

Meticulous attention to detail remains essential in the perioperative, intensive care for transplant recipients threatened by rejection, side effects of immunosuppression, and/or infection in addition to organ-specific medical problems and technical complications affecting graft viability and function. With growing lists of patients either awaiting transplantation, being treated for immediate or delayed posttransplant complications, or requiring subsequent care for unrelated medical or surgical problems posttransplantation, more intensivists and their staffs can expect to be called upon for their expertise in dealing with these vitally important challenges.

REFERENCES

1. Anonymous. Comparison of tacrolimus (FK 506) and cyclosporine for immunosuppression in liver transplantation. The U.S. Multicenter FK506 Liver Study Group. *N Engl J Med* 1994;331:1110–1115.
2. Sheiner PA, Magliocca JF, Bodian CA, et al. Long-term medical complications in patients surviving > or = 5 years after liver transplant. *Transplantation* 2000;69:781–789.
3. Facciuto M, Heidt D, Guarrera J, et al. Retransplantation for late liver graft failure: predictors of mortality. *Liver Transpl* 2000;6:174–179.
4. Williams I. Epidemiology of hepatitis C in the United States. *Am J Med* 1999;107:2S–9S.
5. Spanier TB, Klein RD, Nasraway SA, et al. Multiple organ failure after liver transplantation. *Crit Care Med* 1995;23:466–473.
6. Baliga P, Merion RM, Turcotte JG, et al. Preoperative risk factor assessment in liver transplantation. *Surgery* 1992;112:704–710.
7. Fraley DS, Burr R, Bernardini J, et al. Impact of acute renal failure on mortality in end-stage liver disease with or without transplantation. *Kidney Int* 1998;54:518–524.
8. Gines A, Escorsell A, Gines P, et al. Incidence, predictive factors, and prognosis of the hepatorenal syndrome in cirrhosis with ascites. *Gastroenterology* 1993;105:229–236.
9. Sort P, Navasa M, Arroyo V, et al. Effect of intravenous albumin on renal impairment and mortality in patients with cirrhosis and spontaneous bacterial peritonitis. *N Engl J Med* 1999;341:403–409.
10. Daas M, Plevak DJ, Wijdicks EF, et al. Acute liver failure: results of a 5-year clinical protocol. *Liver Transpl Surg* 1995;1:210–219.
11. Donovan JP, Schafer DF, Shaw BW Jr, et al. Cerebral oedema and increased intracranial pressure in chronic liver disease. *Lancet* 1998;351:719–721.
12. Cordoba J, Blei AT. Brain edema and hepatic encephalopathy. *Semin Liver Dis* 1996;16:271–280.
13. Jalan R, Damink SW, Deutz NE, et al. Moderate hypothermia for uncontrolled intracranial hypertension in acute liver failure. *Lancet* 1999;354:1164–1168.
14. Paterson DL, Stapelfeldt WH, Wagener MM, et al. Intraoperative hypothermia is an independent risk factor for early cytomegalovirus infection in liver transplant recipients. *Transplantation* 1999;67:1151–1155.
15. Watanabe FD, Mullon CJ, Hewitt WR, et al. Clinical experience with a bioartificial liver in the treatment of severe liver failure. A phase I clinical trial. *Ann Surg* 1997;225:484–491.
16. Donovan CL, Marcovitz PA, Punch JD, et al. Two-dimensional and dobutamine stress echocardiography in the preoperative assessment of patients with end-stage liver disease prior to orthotopic liver transplantation. *Transplantation* 1996;61:1180–1188.
17. Plotkin JS, Scott VL, Pinna A, et al. Morbidity and mortality in patients with coronary artery disease undergoing orthotopic liver transplantation. *Liver Transpl Surg* 1996;2:426–430.
18. Krowka MJ, Porayko MK, Plevak DJ, et al. Hepatopulmonary syndrome with progressive hypoxemia as an indication for liver transplantation: case reports and literature review. *Mayo Clin Proc* 1997;72:44–53.
19. Hadengue A, Benhayoun MK, Lebrec D, et al. Pulmonary hypertension complicating portal hypertension: prevalence and relation to splanchnic hemodynamics. *Gastroenterology* 1991;100:520–528.
20. Krowka MJ, Plevak DJ, Findlay JY, et al. Pulmonary hemodynamics and perioperative cardiopulmonary-related mortality in patients with portopulmonary hypertension undergoing liver transplantation. *Liver Transpl* 2000;6:443–450.
21. Strasberg SM, Howard TK, Molmenti EP, et al. Selecting the donor liver: risk factors for poor function after orthotopic liver transplantation. *Hepatology* 1994;20:829–838.
22. Stapelfeldt WH, Willingham D, Sitzman T, et al. Early extubation following liver transplantation. *Liver Transpl* 1999;5(4):C2.
23. Plevak DJ, Southorn PA, Narr BJ, et al. Intensive-care unit experience in the Mayo Liver Transplantation Program: the first 100 cases. *Mayo Clin Proc* 1989;64:433–445.
24. Nasraway SA, Klein RD, Spanier TB, et al. Hemodynamic correlates of outcome in patients undergoing orthotopic liver transplantation. Evidence for early postoperative myocardial depression. *Chest* 1995;107:218–224.
25. Sampathkumar P, Lerman A, Kim BY, et al. Post-liver transplantation myocardial dysfunction. *Liver Transpl Surg* 1998;4:399–403.
26. Jullien T, Valtier B, Hongnat JM, et al. Incidence of tricuspid regurgitation and vena caval backward flow in mechanically ventilated patients. A color Doppler and contrast echocardiographic study. *Chest* 1995;107:488–493.
27. Afessa B, Gay PC, Plevak DJ, et al. Pulmonary complications of orthotopic liver transplantation. *Mayo Clin Proc* 1993;68:427–434.
28. Snowden CP, Hughes T, Rose J, et al. Pulmonary edema in patients after liver transplantation. *Liver Transpl* 2000;6:466–470.
29. Singh N, Gayowski T, Wagener MM, et al. Pulmonary infiltrates in liver transplant recipients in the intensive care unit. *Transplantation* 1999;67:1138–1144.
30. Menegaux F, Keeffe EB, Andrews BT, et al. Neurological complications of liver transplantation in adult versus pediatric patients. *Transplantation* 1994;58:447–450.
31. Bonham CA, Dominguez EA, Fukui MB, et al. Central nervous system lesions in liver transplant recipients: prospective assessment of indications for biopsy and implications for management. *Transplantation* 1998;66:1596–1604.
32. Wijdicks EF, Plevak DJ, Wiesner RH, et al. Causes and outcome of seizures in liver transplant recipients. *Neurology* 1996;47:1523–1525.
33. de Groen PC, Aksamit AJ, Rakela J, et al. Central nervous system toxicity after liver transplantation. The role of cyclosporine and cholesterol. *N Engl J Med* 1987;317:861–866.
34. Thistlethwaite JR Jr, Stuart JK, Mayes JT, et al. Complications and monitoring of OKT3 therapy. *Am J Kidney Dis* 1988;11:112–119.
35. Wijdicks EF, de Groen PC, Wiesner RH, et al. Intracerebral hemorrhage in liver transplant recipients. *Mayo Clin Proc* 1995;70:443–446.
36. Arnow PM, Carandang GC, Zabner R, et al. Randomized controlled trial of selective bowel decontamination for prevention of infections following liver transplantation. *Clin Infect Dis* 1996;22:997–1003.
37. Plevak DJ, DiCecco SR, Wiesner RH, et al. Nutritional support for liver

transplantation: identifying caloric and protein requirements. *Mayo Clin Proc* 1994;69:225–230.

38. Hasse JM, Blue LS, Liepa GU, et al. Early enteral nutrition support in patients undergoing liver transplantation. *J Parenter Enteral Nutr* 1995;19:437–443.

39. Bilbao I, Charco R, Balsells J, et al. Risk factors for acute renal failure requiring dialysis after liver transplantation. *Clin Transplant* 1998;12:123–129.

40. Gonwa TA, Morris CA, Goldstein RM, et al. Long-term survival and renal function following liver transplantation in patients with and without hepatorenal syndrome—experience in 300 patients. *Transplantation* 1991;51:428–430.

41. Mignat C. Clinically significant drug interactions with new immunosuppressive agents. *Drug Saf* 1997;16:267–278.

42. Manske CL, Thomas W, Wang Y, et al. Screening diabetic transplant candidates for coronary artery disease: identification of a low risk subgroup. *Kidney Int* 1993;44:617–621.

43. Reis G, Marcovitz PA, Leichtman AB, et al. Usefulness of dobutamine stress echocardiography in detecting coronary artery disease in end-stage renal disease. *Am J Cardiol* 1995;75:707–710.

44. Sadaghdar H, Chelluri L, Bowles SA, et al. Outcome of renal transplant recipients in the ICU. *Chest* 1995;107:1402–1405.

45. Vincenti F, Kirkman R, Light S, et al. Interleukin-2-receptor blockade with daclizumab to prevent acute rejection in renal transplantation. Daclizumab Triple Therapy Study Group. *N Engl J Med* 1998;338:161–165.

46. Gruessner AC, Sutherland DE. Analysis of United States (US) and non-US pancreas transplants as reported to the International Pancreas Transplant Registry (IPTR) and to the United Network for Organ Sharing (UNOS). *Clin Transpl* 1998;53–73.

47. Tyden G, Bolinder J, Solders G, et al. Improved survival in patients with insulin-dependent diabetes mellitus and end-stage diabetic nephropathy 10 years after combined pancreas and kidney transplantation. *Transplantation* 1999;67:645–648.

48. Fioretto P, Steffes MW, Sutherland DE, et al. Reversal of lesions of diabetic nephropathy after pancreas transplantation. *N Engl J Med* 1998;339:69–75.

49. Navarro X, Sutherland DE, Kennedy WR. Long-term effects of pancreatic transplantation on diabetic neuropathy. *Ann Neurol* 1997;42:727–736.

50. Troppmann C, Gruessner AC, Benedetti E, et al. Vascular graft thrombosis after pancreatic transplantation: univariate and multivariate operative and nonoperative risk factor analysis. *J Am Coll Surg* 1996;182:285–316.

HEMATOPOIETIC STEM CELL TRANSPLANTATION

BABAK KHARRAZI
NORMAN W. RIZK

KEY WORDS

- Hematopoietic stem cell transplantation
- Bone marrow transplantation
- Graft-versus-host disease
- Idiopathic pneumonia syndrome
- Diffuse alveolar hemorrhage
- Hepatic venoocclusive disease
- Bone marrow transplant nephropathy
- *Aspergillus*
- Cytomegalovirus

INTRODUCTION

Following discovery of the human leukocyte antigen (HLA) system by Jean Dausset in 1958, the stage was set for living-related hematopoietic stem cell transplants (HSCT). The initial success with transplantation of hematopoietic stem cells occurred in 1968, when two children with immunodeficiency states received grafts from living-related siblings. This was followed in 1973 by the first unrelated allogeneic transplant for severe combined immunodeficiency, performed at Memorial Sloan-Kettering Cancer Center in New York with marrow from a Danish donor. Since then autologous and allogeneic transplants have been used in the treatment of more than 100,000 patients worldwide for a variety of malignant and nonmalignant diseases; many of the latter are congenital in nature, although marrow aplasia and even inflammatory disorders are on the list of indications (1). Currently, between 40,000 and 50,000 transplants are estimated to occur each year, and the rate of increase is averaging 15% to 20% per year.

AUTOLOGOUS TRANSPLANTATION

In the 1970s and early 1980s it was known that hematopoietic stem cells circulate in small numbers in peripheral blood, but not until 1986 were the first peripheral blood stem cell (PBSC) transplants performed in humans. By 1990, PBSC had become the most common form of HSCT. Since it does not require a donor, autologous PBSC transplantation was widely adopted, chiefly to achieve dose intensification of chemotherapy for solid tumors and hematologic malignancies. Autotransplants are associated with lower mortality, are not complicated by graft-versus-host disease (GVHD) and its attendant requirement of immunosuppression, and are characterized by faster marrow recovery and shorter periods of neutropenia.

Harvesting mobilized stem cells is substantially easier than collecting bone marrow. Since 1988 it has been recognized that pretreatment with granulocyte or granulocyte-macrophage colony stimulating factor for 5 to 7 days enhances mobilization of stem cells to the extent that one to three sessions of continuous apheresis can yield an adequate number of cells to reconstitute the marrow. Standards employing the count of cells expressing CD34 antigen are widely used to determine the adequacy of collected cells; about 2.5 to 5×10^6 CD34+ cells per kg of recipient weight constitutes an adequate dose. The harvested cells are cryopreserved at $-80°C$ or colder while the patient undergoes high-dose chemotherapy. A real concern is that mobilized stem cells are accompanied by circulating tumor cells, so that autotransplants may reintroduce malignant cells to the patient. Because of this concern, manipulation or treatment of the harvested cells to purge or kill tumor cells is commonly attempted.

ALLOGENEIC TRANSPLANTATION

In the early experience with HSCT, allogeneic transplants were mainly applied in far-advanced active hematologic malignancies, as desperate attempts at salvage after failed conventional therapy. With more experience and technical advances in this modality, allotransplants are increasingly used successfully in early-stage disease in patients with good functional status. Since only about 20% to 25% of patients have a suitable sibling donor, the availability of marrow sources for HLA-matched transplants from unrelated donors was greatly improved after development of volunteer marrow registries of HLA-typed donors. As of August 2000, there were roughly 6 million donors worldwide, with approximately 4 million in the Minnesota-based National Marrow Donor Program in the United States. Because of HLA polymorphism across ethnic groups, access to suitable donor marrow is easier for Caucasian patients than it is for patients from other racial groups; Caucasians have an approximately 70% chance of finding a suitable donor in the registries. HSCT from unrelated donors is associated with a higher morbidity and mortality than is living-related transplantation, but at the same time, it extends the therapy to many patients who would otherwise have no appropriate donor source.

The actual donation is achieved by aspirating a volume of approximately 10 to 15 mL per kg from the anterior and posterior iliac crests of the donor, who is most often under general anesthesia. Bony spicules and fat are filtered out by 0.2- to 0.3-mm screens through which the heparinized aspirate passes. Typically less than 1% of donors experience a serious complication, and fatal complications are extremely rare. Reinfusion of the marrow to the recipient is similarly well tolerated, except for occasional fever, cough, or dyspnea.

Alternative potential sources of marrow stem cells include PBSC and umbilical cord blood. PBSCs, as in autologous PBSC transplants, are collected by continuous flow apheresis from donors primed with hematopoietic growth factors. These grafts have a higher percentage of mature T-lymphocytes, as compared to bone marrow aspirates, and consequently increase the risk of GVHD in the recipient. However, they also induce a more rapid hematopoietic recovery and are easier to obtain and less traumatic for donors. Cord blood donations from neonates have other advantages. They can be harvested at delivery and frozen and stored indefinitely in cord blood banks; there were five such banks collaborating with the National Marrow Donor Program as of 1999. This technology also carries promise for ameliorating the deficiency of marrow sources for non-Caucasian patients. Cord blood transplantation has been most widely used in children, since the stem cell dose required for early and successful engraftment in adults sometimes exceeds the dose available through neonatal sources. Nonetheless, searches for unrelated donors in the National Marrow Donor Program now automatically identify cord units that are compatible for both children and adults. PBSC and cord blood transplantation have engendered substantial excitement and are expanding as programs, but the large majority of allogeneic transplants still arise from living-related donors.

INDICATIONS

Indications for HSCT continue to evolve, reflecting improving technology, the shift from allogeneic to autologous transplants, and greater use of PBSC methodologies. Autologous transplants are now most commonly used for Hodgkin and non-Hodgkin lymphomas, multiple myeloma, and a minority of acute and chronic leukemias. Previously the most common indication was breast cancer, but adequate trials with long-term follow-up indicate that the improvement in survival conferred by the procedure is small, if there is any survival advantage at all. Allogeneic transplants are most often given as therapy for the acute and chronic leukemias, aplastic anemias, myelodysplasia, and some solid tumors. These are summarized in Table 1.

TABLE 1. INDICATIONS FOR HEMATOPOIETIC STEM CELL TRANSPLANTATION

Allogeneic Transplants	Autologous Transplants
Severe aplastic anemia	Acute lymphoblastic leukemia (certain subtypes)
Chronic myeloid leukemia	
Acute myeloid leukemia	Hodgkin disease
Myelodysplasia	Non-Hodgkin lymphoma
Acute lymphoblastic leukemia	Multiple myeloma
Severe congenital immunodeficiency	Certain solid tumors such as neuroblastoma and ovarian cancer
Thalassemia	Autoimmune disorders such as systemic sclerosis
Multiple myeloma	Chronic lymphocytic leukemia
Sickle cell anemia	Chronic myeloid leukemia
Inherited metabolic disorders	
Hodgkin disease	
Non-Hodgkin lymphoma	

PREPARATIVE REGIMENS

Prior to transplantation, a preparative regimen is administered both to eliminate malignant or abnormal cells and to clear the marrow of immunocompetent cells, so that disease recurrence and graft rejection do not ensue. Agents whose limiting toxicity is myelosuppression are desirable, since this problem is corrected by the transplant. Total body irradiation, alkylating agents, and cytotoxic drugs are the most commonly employed.

ENGRAFTMENT

Until engraftment occurs, patients are particularly vulnerable to infection and bleeding; rapid engraftment, therefore, is crucial in minimizing morbidity and mortality of the procedure. The rate of engraftment depends upon the source of stem cells, extent of colony stimulating factor use, and the use of immunosuppressive and myelosuppressive agents. PBSC grafts achieve adequate cell production most rapidly but are less responsive to growth factors. By day 12 to 14 posttransplantation, granulocyte counts usually exceed 500 per mm^3, and platelet recovery follows shortly thereafter. Marrow and cord blood transplants usually take 14 to 20 days to achieve similar granulocyte counts.

HEMATOPOIETIC STEM CELL TRANSPLANT OUTCOMES

Disease-free survival rates are determined by the mortality and complications of the specific transplant procedure, age and functional status of the patient, disease entity, and the marrow source of the therapy selected. For most malignant diseases treated by HSCT, the most common cause of death posttransplant is disease recurrence. Timing is also key in determining outcome; for example acute myelogenous leukemia is cured with HSCT in only about 15% to 20% of patients who fail induction therapy but in up to 60% of patients in first remission with HLA-matched

TABLE 2. FOUR-YEAR SURVIVAL RATES FOR COMMON DISEASES TREATED WITH STEM CELL TRANSPLANTATION

Acute Leukemias		Chronic Myelogenous Leukemia (CML)		Other Diseases	
AML, first remission	25%	CML, first chronic phase	39%	Severe aplastic anemia	36%
AML, second remission	28%	CML, second chronic phase and accelerated phase	20%	Myelodysplastic and related syndromes	26%
AML, third or greater remission or relapse	9%	CML blast phase	5%	Non-Hodgkin lymphoma	24%
ALL, first remission	34%			Nonmalignant diseases	43%
ALL, second remission	32%				
ALL, third or greater remission	24%				
ALL relapse	6%				

AML, acute myeloid leukemia; ALL, acute lymphoblastic leukemia.
From disease outcome data as of June 1999 provided by the National Marrow Donor Program. Available at: http://www.marrow.org/MEDICAL/disease_outcome_data.html. Accessed October 24, 2001.

siblings. Average 4-year survival rates for common indications are provided in Table 2. HSCT outcomes continue to improve with better therapy and posttransplant support services.

COMPLICATIONS OF HEMATOPOIETIC STEM CELL TRANSPLANTS

HSCT as a therapy is associated with substantial morbidity and mortality. Complications tend to be relatively stereotypic and organ-specific and often occur in a characteristic time frame posttransplant. Most complications reflect either toxicity from the preparative regimen or infectious or immunologic sequelae of cytopenia and altered immunologic status.

PULMONARY COMPLICATIONS

Pulmonary complications occur in approximately half of patients who undergo HSCT; the exact incidence depends upon marrow source, patient age and functional status, preparative regimen employed, and any underlying lung disease. In the first 2 to 3 weeks following the conditioning regimen and transplantation, virtually all patients develop mucositis, with loss of integrity of oral and pharyngeal epithelial lining cells; the mucositis predisposes to both infection and aspiration. The requirement for narcotic analgesia exacerbates the aspiration in many cases.

Specific chemotherapeutic agents cause characteristic clinical and radiographic syndromes of toxicity, reflected in underlying histopathology (2). Carmustine (BCNU), for example, is associated with bilateral airspace consolidation occurring at a median of 45 days following administration. Histologically this resembles nonspecific interstitial pneumonia (NSIP) or diffuse alveolar damage (DAD). Patients typically have fever, cough, and hypoxemia; if the syndrome is recognized and treated, over 90% respond to corticosteroid therapy and are left without sequelae. Bleomycin, busulfan, carmustine, and alkylating agents commonly cause a cytotoxic effect evident as DAD on biopsy. These patients rarely have fever, but bilateral radiographic opacities, dyspnea, and cough are the rule. Sometimes this progresses to diffuse opacification and frank respiratory failure. An exudative and a proliferative stage are recognized; pulmonary fibrosis with honeycombing sometimes ensues. Whether corticosteroids are of value, particularly during the proliferative phase, is debated. For

some of these agents, toxicity is dose-related. The incidence of carmustine toxicity is typically 20% to 30% in treated patients but rises to almost 50% in patients receiving over 1.5 g per m². Bleomycin toxicity affects 2% to 5% of patients but is far more common when a cumulative dose of over 450 mg per m² is given.

NSIP and DAD are the most common histopathologic patterns of regimen-related toxicity, but even more often, noninfectious lung injury occurs outside of a single identifiable etiology. The term "idiopathic pneumonia syndrome" has been applied to this group of conditions. This form of lung injury is presumably multifactorial in causation, with drug toxicity, cytokines from recovering marrow elements, sepsis, alloreactivity, hemorrhage, and edema all contributing. The syndrome presents with fever, dyspnea, hypoxemia, and bilateral opacities on chest radiography, with onset typically about 3 weeks following HSCT. It is clinically indistinguishable from common infectious disorders occurring in this setting and should only be considered after infectious and intravascular volume-overloaded states have been excluded by diagnostic measures. In a large series from Seattle, idiopathic pneumonia syndrome was diagnosed in 7% of marrow recipients, both autologous and allogeneic, and was associated with a 62% mortality rate from progressive respiratory failure (3). Some groups have reported a more favorable outcome with use of systemic corticosteroid therapy but not everyone accepts its value in the absence of large controlled trials.

A subgroup of idiopathic pneumonia syndrome cases include features of diffuse alveolar hemorrhage (DAH) (Fig.1). Initially described in autologous HSCT recipients, it is now recognized commonly in their allogeneic counterparts. The diagnosis rests on the observation of progressively bloodier return of lavage fluid during bronchoscopy in patients with otherwise fairly typical idiopathic pneumonia syndrome. Among autologous transplant patients in some centers, DAH had an incidence as high as 21%, but this frequency is now rarely observed. DAH is important to recognize since its in-hospital mortality ranges between 50% and 80% and early treatment with corticosteroids may improve prognosis.

In the original report, DAH was associated with age older than 40, solid malignancies, high fevers, severe mucositis, renal insufficiency, total body irradiation, and white blood cell recovery (4). This syndrome develops a median time of 12 days after transplantation (range 7 to 40 days). Its etiology remains unclear, but hypothesized causes include body irradiation, transplant preparative regimens, infection, and neutrophil influx. On pathology, affected lungs show diffuse alveolar damage.

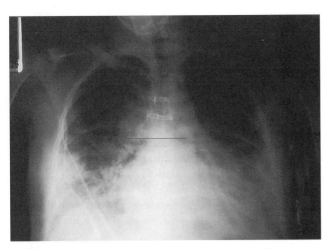

FIGURE 1. The most common radiographic finding in diffuse alveolar hemorrhage is a bilateral alveolar-filling process that involves the middle and lower lung zones.

Corticosteroids are the major therapeutic option in DAH. In a retrospective analysis of 63 patients with DAH, those who received greater than 30 mg of methylprednisolone per day had a significantly lower mortality than those who received less methylprednisolone or none at all (67% versus 91%) (5). Two other case series, each with four patients, also demonstrated possible benefit of corticosteroid use: in one, all four patients were discharged home (6), and in the other, all four demonstrated an immediate clinical response (7). In the absence of a randomized controlled trial, these results have made high-dose corticosteroids the accepted treatment for DAH. A typical regimen is 0.5 to 1.0 g of methylprednisolone per day for 3 to 5 days with subsequent tapering over 2 to 4 weeks. Despite prompt treatment with high doses of corticosteroids, approximately 50% of the patients in these series required mechanical ventilatory support.

Another common confounding entity following transplantation is pulmonary edema, due to both cardiogenic and increased vascular permeability causes. Hepatic venoocclusive disease, acute GVHD, sepsis syndromes, and high-dose chemotherapy have all been implicated in abnormal vascular permeability. Coexisting renal insufficiency often further impairs fluid and sodium excretion. Pragmatically, separating pulmonary edema from other forms of idiopathic pneumonia syndrome can only be achieved by attention to weight gains, echocardiography, or even pulmonary artery catheterization. Because pulmonary edema is so common following HSCT, bilateral pleural effusions, interstitial edema, or other clinical signs suggestive of volume-overloaded states should prompt empiric diuresis and fluid restriction, assuming the patient has adequate renal function.

In addition to airspace-filling diseases, HSCT in allogeneic transplant recipients is sometimes complicated by chronic airflow obstruction. As many as 10% of patients with chronic GVHD develop progressive bronchiolitis obliterans, similar to the disorder seen in patients with lung or heart-lung transplants (8). Presumably a function of alloreactivity, it usually appears after the first 90 to 100 days, presenting as cough, dyspnea, and hyperinflation on chest radiography. Spirometry first shows impairment of flow in midlung volumes, then reduced expiratory volume in the first

second of a maximal maneuver (FEV$_1$). Progression may be slow or rapid; immunosuppression with corticosteroids, azathioprine, or cyclosporine has been used with mixed success. Many of these patients pursue a relentless downhill course to death despite attempts to control the small airway injury. Airflow obstruction severe enough to warrant intensive care unit (ICU) care portends a poor prognosis, as does early posttransplant onset and rapid initial progression.

DIAGNOSIS OF PULMONARY COMPLICATIONS

Since the pulmonary complications associated with HSCT are few in number, a consensus approach to diagnosis has evolved at most centers. The disorders can most easily be classified according to whether they exhibit radiographically focal or diffuse opacity. Diffuse opacities are most often due to volume overload, ventricular dysfunction, hemorrhage, other forms of idiopathic pneumonia, and viral or protozoal pneumonias. Pulmonary edema often manifests as reticular opacities and pleural effusions on chest radiography and is dependent in distribution on computed tomography (CT). Distinguishing the other entities by imaging is not reliable; therefore diagnostic bronchoalveolar lavage (BAL) is the next step. Simple inspection during BAL is definitive for alveolar hemorrhage; analysis of cultures, cytology, and special stains of the BAL fluid are necessary for diagnosis of infectious entities. Idiopathic pneumonia syndrome is a diagnosis of exclusion and neither requires nor benefits from histologic confirmation. Video-assisted thoracoscopy is usually unnecessary and also has significant bleeding hazards, given its limited operative field and

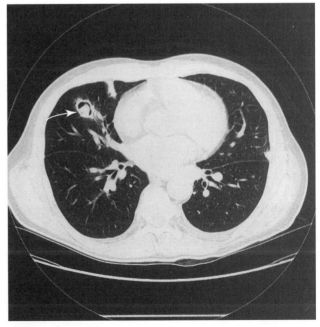

FIGURE 2. Chest computed tomography of a patient with invasive pulmonary aspergillosis of the right upper lobe revealing a cavitary mass with a crescentic "halo" (*arrow*). The "halo" sign is highly distinctive for invasive fungal disease (usually caused by *Aspergillus*) and represents infarcted lung tissue full of hyphae that extend beyond the area of infarction.

the usual concomitant thrombocytopenia. Open lung biopsy has largely been abandoned.

Focal opacities may be attributed to recurrent malignancy or pneumonia that is fungal or bacterial in origin. An opacity larger than a lung segment can be reliably sampled by BAL, whereas subsegmental lesions require the more directed approach of CT-guided fine needle aspiration. Many subsegmental lesions are due to fungal disease, particularly invasive aspergillosis. This observation is especially true when the lesions are nodular or mass-like and are surrounded by a halo of density consistent with blood on CT (Fig. 2). Cavitary necrotizing lesions are usually infectious in origin and essentially never due to simple alveolar hemorrhage or pulmonary edema. Focal areas of consolidation that are segmental or larger most often are bacterial in origin.

HEPATIC VENOOCCLUSIVE DISEASE

Venoocclusive disease (VOD) of the liver is the most common life-threatening toxicity of the HSCT conditioning regimen, occurring in 10% to 60% of patients. The syndrome consists of painful hepatomegaly, fluid retention, and an elevated serum bilirubin following cytoreductive therapy. High-dose cytoreductive therapy presumably produces an endothelial injury to sinusoids and small hepatic venules, leading to thrombosis and hepatic venous outflow obstruction (9). With time, this leads to fibrosis of centrilobular sinusoids and portal hypertension.

The diagnosis of VOD should be entertained when painful hepatomegaly along with fluid retention occurs in the first 20 days after HSCT. Jaundice usually ensues in a few days. The differential diagnosis includes GVHD, hepatic vein obstruction, sepsis, heart failure, renal failure, and pancreatic disease (10). Confirmatory laboratory data for VOD include hyperbilirubinemia and elevated transaminases. Thrombocytopenia and refractoriness to platelet transfusions may also be early signs associated with severe VOD. Ultrasound and CT can demonstrate hepatomegaly and ascites. Doppler studies can display diminished hepatic venous flow, a finding with insufficient sensitivity in the early stages of VOD. In instances where other causes of cholestasis coexist and the presence of VOD is unclear, transjugular liver biopsy with simultaneous intrahepatic pressure measurements may be useful. A hepatic venous pressure gradient of greater than 10 mm Hg using the occlusive balloon technique is greater than 90% specific for this entity.

The clinical course of hepatic VOD is difficult to predict. In one study, the amount of weight gain and the concentration of bilirubin best correlated with the outcome (11). The majority of patients have mild to moderate disease that reverses with supportive care. Severe VOD is defined as irreversible despite therapy, and its associated 100-day mortality approaches 100% (10). Overall, the mortality of VOD is 20% to 50% (9), and death is usually due to renal or cardiopulmonary failure and rarely the result of liver dysfunction.

In mild and moderate cases of hepatic VOD, the goals of treatment are maintaining intravascular volume and renal perfusion and avoiding extravascular fluid accumulation by judicious use of diuretics. Paracentesis can be performed for tense ascites. Hepatotoxic and nephrotoxic drugs should be avoided if possible.

For severe VOD, several studies have used recombinant tissue plasminogen activator (rtPA) to resolve hepatic venular occlusion. Variable efficacy with rtPA, often combined with infusion of heparin, has been shown. The response rate in one large series was 29%, but 24% of patients experienced a severe bleeding episode (12). A typical dosing regimen is 20 mg of rtPA over 4 hours for 4 consecutive days plus a continuous infusion of heparin at 150 U per kg per day. It is important to recognize that rtPA has never been studied in a randomized controlled fashion for hepatic VOD and that the optimal dose and duration of this agent are not established for this indication.

More recently, defibrotide has shown promise for the treatment of hepatic VOD. Defibrotide is an adenosine receptor agonist extracted from mammalian organs and has antithrombotic and thrombolytic activities without systemic anticoagulant effects. Its exact mechanism of action is unclear but probably includes decreasing plasminogen activator inhibitor levels, increasing rtPA function, and stimulating thrombomodulin synthesis. In one series of 19 patients with severe VOD who either failed rtPA or were not candidates for thrombolytics, 42% had a complete response to a 14-day course of defibrotide (13). No significant drug toxicity was reported; the initial dose used was 10 mg per kg per day divided into 4 doses with the dose increased by 10 mg per kg every 1 to 2 days to a maximum of 60 mg per kg per day.

RENAL FAILURE

Renal insufficiency is a common complication of HSCT, affecting as many as 50% of transplant recipients. Its numerous causes in this setting can be categorized as early or late, in relation to transplantation. Whereas the majority of early cases are the result of nephrotoxic drugs, late impairment of renal function in HSCT is predominantly due to damage from irradiation (14).

The preparative regimens for HSCT often contain antineoplastic drugs that are potentially nephrotoxic. Commonly used cytoreductive drugs with this effect include high-dose methotrexate, ifosfamide, cisplatin, and carboplatin. In addition, given a large tumor cell burden, cancer cytotoxic treatment may result in tumor lysis syndrome, with release of massive amounts of intracellular material causing renal failure by renal tubular deposition of uric acid and phosphate. Preventive and treatment measures for tumor lysis syndrome consist of intravenous hydration, urinary alkalinization, and allopurinol therapy. The use of cyclophosphamide and ifosfamide uncommonly leads to hemorrhagic cystitis, where a large clot burden in the bladder results in urinary outlet obstruction and acute renal failure (15). Infections and consequent sepsis syndrome often occur after HSCT, especially before marrow engraftment. The hypoperfusion of kidneys in septic shock, compounded by the nephrotoxic drugs often used for treatment of infections, can lead to significant renal insufficiency. Table 3 lists several nephrotoxic antimicrobial agents commonly used in the peritransplantation period.

Hepatic VOD in the first month after HSCT often produces a functional renal abnormality no different than the hepatorenal syndrome (HRS) associated with other causes of cirrhosis. HRS is diagnosed in liver disease when other common causes of renal failure such as intravascular hypovolemia, urinary obstruction,

TABLE 3. COMMON ANTIMICROBIAL AGENTS WITH NEPHROTOXIC EFFECTS

Amphotericin B
Aminoglycosides
Vancomycin
Teicoplanin
Acyclovir
Ganciclovir
Foscarnet

and intrinsic renal disease are eliminated (16). Clinically, the syndrome is typified by avid sodium retention, edema and ascites formation, low urinary sodium levels, and azotemia. The pathophysiology of HRS is poorly understood; no specific treatment has proved effective, and the prognosis is dismal. Therapy of this syndrome is comprised of attempts to reverse the underlying liver pathology while the kidneys are supported with dialysis as needed.

The syndrome called "bone marrow transplant nephropathy" (BMTN) usually occurs months after transplantation. It is characterized by azotemia, hypertension, and a disproportionate degree of anemia. Its histologic changes are very similar to those of radiation nephritis (17). Despite this similarity, other factors likely play a significant role in its development: several chemotherapy agents such as busulfan, cisplatinum, and BCNU can enhance renal radiation damage in a rat model, and more important, the syndrome has been described in the absence of total body irradiation (TBI) (17). In short, BMTN is likely the manifestation of renal injury from HSCT preparative regimens sometimes potentiated by TBI. Treatment of BMTN is largely supportive and includes blood pressure control, erythropoietin and red cell transfusions for anemia, and renal replacement therapy if needed. Angiotensin-converting enzyme inhibitors may prove to be useful. A subset of patients with BMTN shows features of hemolytic-uremic syndrome (HUS) and thrombotic thrombocytopenic purpura as discussed below.

Because cyclosporine (CSP) is often administered for GVHD in the first 6 to 12 months, it can be a cause of both early and delayed renal insufficiency after allogeneic stem cell transplantation. CSP nephrotoxicity is amplified with larger doses, longer exposure times, higher trough levels, and TBI conditioning (14). Despite its high incidence, CSP nephropathy rarely progresses to end-stage renal disease since awareness of its toxicity usually leads to prompt dose reduction.

CARDIAC INSUFFICIENCY

Cardiac sequelae of antineoplastic agents include cardiac insufficiency, pericardial disease, arrhythmias, and infectious complications that involve the heart. Cardiac insufficiency, which is the most common and clinically significant of these complications, often stems from the transplant conditioning regimen and/or prior exposure to anthracyclines or mediastinal irradiation.

Cyclophosphamide (CY) is largely responsible for the majority of the cardiotoxic effects of conditioning regimens. This complication usually presents within 3 weeks of CY administration (18) and results from CY directly damaging the endothelium, causing capillary microthromboses and capillary leak within the heart,

in a dose-dependent fashion. With doses of less than 120 mg per kg, electrocardiogram (ECG) abnormalities (ST and T segment changes and loss of QRS voltage) and mild impairment in ventricular function are common and often transient. The majority of the fatal cases of CY cardiotoxicity, on the other hand, have occurred with doses exceeding 180 mg per kg. It has been suggested that dosing may be more appropriately based on body surface area for less toxicity (19). Pretransplantation evaluation of ventricular function has not been shown to reliably predict CY-induced cardiomyopathy.

Anthracyclines are commonly used antineoplastic agents with significant associated cardiotoxicity. In long-term follow-up, up to 7% of exposed patients develop overt heart failure. The pathogenesis of this disease is hypothesized to involve free-radical–mediated injury, myocyte damage from calcium overload, and cellular toxicity from anthracycline metabolites. The different syndromes of anthracycline-induced cardiac disease are classified based on time of presentation in relation to anthracycline exposure. The most common and clinically significant of these syndromes is chronic anthracycline-induced cardiomyopathy which presents within 1 year of treatment (20), and is dependent on the cumulative dose of the drug. The incidence of heart failure is 0.14% when total anthracycline dose is less than 400 mg per M^2 body surface area, and it increases to 7% at a dose of 550 mg per M^2 (21). Noninvasive methods to detect cardiotoxicity (echocardiography and radionuclide angiocardiography) are of limited value in that they detect systolic dysfunction only when a significant amount of the myocardium has been injured. Evaluation for diastolic abnormalities may be able to detect cardiotoxicity at an earlier stage (20). Recently, dexrazoxane, an iron chelator, has been approved for prevention of anthracycline-induced myocardial damage (22).

Radiation therapy that involves the mediastinum can also result in cardiac injury. This complication is a direct function of the amount of radiation delivered to the heart and can consequently be diminished by using techniques such as equally weighted anterior and posterior fields and subcarinal blocks. The most clinically relevant aspects of this complication in the setting of HSCT are the delayed pericarditis that typically occurs within 12 months after therapy and the pancarditis that results in myocardial and endocardial fibrosis. The delayed pericarditis, in addition to the usual fever, pleuritic chest pain, and ECG abnormalities, can be accompanied by a large pericardial effusion. Up to half of these patients have some degree of tamponade and require pericardiocentesis (23). Constrictive pericarditis can also occur in these patients. Radiation-induced injury involving the myocardium and endocardium occurs less often and results in a restrictive cardiomyopathy. In the presence of pericardial disease, differentiating constrictive pericarditis from restrictive cardiomyopathy can be difficult, and the two may coexist.

The treatment of cardiac complications that occur in the setting of HSCT are extrapolated from treating heart dysfunction in other, more common circumstances. Therapy of systolic dysfunction involves the use of diuretics, digitalis, vasodilators (e.g., angiotensin-converting enzyme inhibitors), and β-blockers. Diuretics are the mainstay of management in restrictive cardiomyopathies. When pericardial disease predominates, pericardiocentesis may be useful if effusions with tamponade exist,

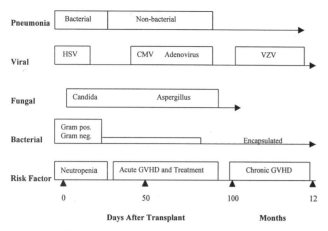

FIGURE 3. Infectious syndromes at different times after hematopoietic stem cell transplantation. (Redrawn with permission from Meyers JF. Infections in marrow recipients. In: Mandell GL, Douglas RG, Bennett JE, eds. *Principles and practice of infectious diseases*, 2nd ed. New York: John Wiley and Sons, 1985:1674–1676.)

and pericardiectomy may be indicated if constrictive pericarditis is present.

INFECTIONS IN HEMATOPOIETIC STEM CELL TRANSPLANTATION RECIPIENTS

The HSCT recipient is susceptible to different infectious syndromes at different times after transplantation. Which infections predominate depends on a complex interaction between the host's immune status and the infectious agents to which it is exposed. Immune recovery occurs first in granulocytes and later in elements of cellular and humoral immunity. Immune status is also altered in allogeneic transplants when additional immunosuppressive agents are administered for the prevention or treatment of GVHD. Exposure to pathogens can be treatment-related (e.g., introduction of gut flora into the bloodstream in the setting of mucositis), environmental (e.g., nosocomial bacteria, *Aspergillus*), or due to reactivation of prior infections (e.g., cytomegalovirus, herpes simplex virus). Figure 3 depicts the typical timeline for infectious complications after HSCT.

BACTERIAL INFECTIONS

Bacterial infections are a particularly frequent complication in the first 30 days after HSCT. The frequency of infections and the organisms involved vary immensely and depend on factors such as time elapsed from transplantation, type of transplantation (autologous versus allogeneic), the degree of HLA match between donor and recipient, presence of GVHD, severity of mucositis, presence of central vascular catheters or other medical devices, type of bacteria colonizing the patient, and the use of prophylactic antibiotics. Traditionally, these infections have been categorized into three time periods: (a) preengraftment (neutropenic); (b) early postengraftment (up to 3 months); and (c) late recovery (after 3 months). In this section, we will discuss each susceptibility period and its associated risk factors and bacteriology.

TABLE 4. COMMON PATHOGENIC BACTERIA IN THE PREENGRAFTMENT PERIOD

Gram-Positives	Gram-Negatives
Coagulase-negative *Staphylococcus*	*Escherichia coli*
Streptococcus viridans	*Klebsiella* spp.
Enterococcus spp.	*Enterobacter* spp.
Staphylococcus aureus	*Citrobacter* spp.
Corynebacterium spp.	*Acinetobacter* spp.
	Pseudomonas spp.

Bacteria cause more than 90% of infections during the neutropenic period. Important risk factors during this time include mucositis and presence of central venous catheters, both of which introduce defects into the physical barriers of the immune system. Mucositis of the oropharynx allows mouth flora such as *Streptococcus viridans* access to the bloodstream, whereas gastrointestinal involvement usually results in infection with enteric gram-negative organisms. A particularly devastating preengraftment infection is necrotizing enterocolitis, in which gastrointestinal mucositis results in invasion of the bowel wall with enteric organisms. The extraluminal surface and hub of central venous catheters (CVC) often become colonized with skin flora (gram-positive cocci and *Candida* species) and, in hospitalized patients, with gram-negative organisms. Colonization can lead to bacteremia or exit site infection. Table 4 lists common pathogenic organisms during the preengraftment period. In centers where prophylactic antibiotics against gram-negative organisms are used, there is an increased incidence of infection with *Clostridium difficile*, coagulase-negative staphylococci, less common gram-negative organisms, and *S. viridans* (24).

Fever in the neutropenic phase is often bacterial in origin and requires prompt empiric broad-spectrum antibiotic treatment. The choice of antibiotics varies between centers but should cover gram-positive skin flora and gram-negative organisms including *Pseudomonas* species. In the critically ill neutropenic patient, a reasonable choice would be the combination of vancomycin plus an antipseudomonal β-lactam, imipenem, or a fluoroquinolone (25). An aminoglycoside can be added for double coverage of gram-negative organisms.

Despite engraftment and neutrophil recovery, humoral and cellular immune deficiencies usually persist. Risk factors for bacterial infections during the postengraftment period include allogeneic transplantation, donor-recipient HLA mismatches, T-cell depleted stem cells, immunosuppressive therapy for GVHD, and the presence of viral infections (e.g., cytomegalovirus). Common bacterial infections in this time period are sinusitis, CVC-related infections, and gram-negative bacteremia due to mucositis of GVHD.

The bacterial infections of the late recovery period (after 3 months) mostly occur in patients with chronic GVHD. The functional asplenia and immunoglobulin deficiency present in chronic GVHD make these patients particularly susceptible to infections with encapsulated organisms such as pneumococcus, *Haemophilus influenzae*, meningococcus, *Staphylococcus aureus*, *Escherichia coli*, and *Pseudomonas* species. Since chronic GVHD often leads to a pulmonary sicca syndrome and sinusitis, these infections often occur in the lungs and sinuses.

FUNGAL INFECTIONS

Fungal infections occur in 10% to 20% of patients after stem cell transplantation, and the vast majority of these infections are caused by *Candida* or *Aspergillus* species. Many factors predispose transplant patients to develop fungal infections; important among these are GVHD and chemotherapeutic agents that damage mucosal barriers, neutropenia which debilitates the immune system, and antibiotic use which permits fungal overgrowth. Based on these risk factors, allogeneic transplant recipients are much more susceptible than their autologous counterparts: allogeneic transplant patients are neutropenic for a longer period and are susceptible to GVHD which is treated with further immunosuppressive agents. With the advent of fluconazole prophylaxis during the neutropenic phase after transplantation, the number of *Candida albicans* and *Candida tropicalis* infections is decreasing while *Aspergillus* and nonalbicans *Candida* infections are on the rise (26,27). The clinical presentation of fungal infections is often subtle, and the diagnosis is often delayed until microbial burden is overwhelming. As a result, the mortality rate of invasive fungal infections in the setting of HSCT is 75% to 95%.

The spectrum of *Candida* infections ranges from mucosal disease to fungemia with or without visceral organ involvement. The liver and spleen are the organs most commonly involved because the microbes enter the portal circulation from the gut due to mucositis. The most common presentation of invasive candidiasis is neutropenic fevers that do not abate with antibacterial agents (28). Fevers and an elevated alkaline phosphatase should suggest hepatosplenic involvement. Diagnostic tools for invasive candidiasis are suboptimal. Blood cultures are negative in 50% of cases of visceral disease. Radiologic imaging may demonstrate abscess(es) accessible to needle aspiration for cytologic and microbiologic analysis (Fig. 4). Polymerase chain reaction (PCR) and antigen detection for diagnosis are still being investigated.

Aspergillus is acquired by inhalation of airborne conidia, making the lungs and sinuses the most common sites of infection. *Aspergillus* species are angioinvasive; infection therefore may lead to pulmonary infarction and hemorrhage. Fevers, pleuritic chest

pain, and hemoptysis may be part of the presenting signs. Involvement of the heart and central nervous system (CNS) can follow pulmonary vascular invasion and dissemination. Aspergillosis is the most common cause of CNS disease in HSCT. Visceral organ involvement occurs late in the disease. As with *Candida* infections, definitive diagnosis can be difficult: blood cultures are rarely positive and culture results from bronchoalveolar lavage are negative in up to 50% of cases. In one autopsy series, 23% of cases were diagnosed postmortem (29).

Several preventive measures decrease the incidence of fungal infections post-HSCT. Prophylactic fluconazole, at a dose of 400 mg per day, in the neutropenic phase of transplantation has significantly decreased the incidence of *Candida* infections, mostly those due to *C. albicans* and *C. tropicalis* species (30,31). Low-dose intravenous amphotericin B (AmB) may be as effective, but its use is limited by significant toxicity. Rooms with laminar airflow or high-efficiency particle air (HEPA) filtration systems can minimize *Aspergillus* exposure. Patients with a history of prior invasive fungal infection require secondary prophylaxis with AmB and may benefit from surgical resection of previous disease (e.g., unilobar pulmonary aspergillosis). Fungal therapy should be empirically started when neutropenic fevers persist despite antibacterial therapy. AmB is the treatment of choice, with doses of 0.5 mg per kg per day for suspected *Candida* and 1 to 1.5 mg per kg per day for suspected *Aspergillus* infections. For documented *Candida* infections, AmB at doses of 0.5 to 1.0 mg per kg per day is first-line therapy; 5-fluorocytosine may be added in unstable patients or those with deep-organ infections. Sensitive species in stable patients can be as effectively treated with fluconazole 400 to 800 mg per day. A recent consensus statement strongly suggests that removal or changing of all intravascular catheters be considered (32). The treatment of choice for documented aspergillosis is AmB at a dose of 1.0 to 1.5 mg per kg per day. Surgical resection of solitary lung nodules and drainage of sinuses may have a role in certain patients. Lipid formulations of AmB are likely as effective as standard AmB for all of the above-stated indications, and they produce significantly less nephrotoxicity (33–35). The duration of treatment of fungal disease in HSCT is poorly studied and is often guided by clinical response.

CYTOMEGALOVIRUS

Table 5 lists several of the viruses and their associated diseases that affect the HSCT population; of these viruses, cytomegalovirus (CMV) is clinically the most significant. CMV infection is defined as the isolation of the virus from any tissue or body fluid using any culture technique, histochemical stain, or antigen or DNA assay; CMV disease is defined as organ damage caused by the virus. After HSCT, the majority of cases of CMV infection are due to reactivation, which occur in a seropositive recipient or in a seronegative recipient who receives a seropositive organ. Primary infection in the CMV-seronegative recipient has been reduced to less than 3% with the use of CMV-negative or leukocyte-filtered blood products for transfusions (36). With the advent of preemptive antiviral therapy in the last decade, mostly with ganciclovir (GCV), rates of antigenemia and disease among HSCT recipients have been reduced to less than 40% and 5%, respectively

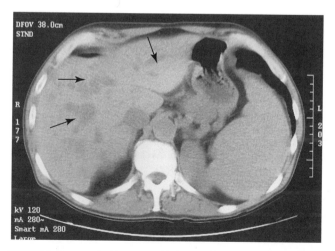

FIGURE 4. A computed tomographic image demonstrating hypodense lesions (*arrows*) throughout the liver typical of hepatic candidiasis in the setting of hematopoietic stem cell transplantation.

TABLE 5. COMMON VIRAL INFECTIONS AFTER HEMATOPOIETIC CELL TRANSPLANTATION

Virus	Peak Susceptibility Period	Common Manifestation(s)
Herpes simplex virus	1–2 wks	Oropharyngeal, esophageal, and/or perianal involvement
Respiratory viruses	2–5 wks	Upper and lower respiratory tract infections
Respiratory syncitial virus		
Parainfluenza virus		
Influenza virus		
Rhinovirus		
Adenovirus	4–8 wks	Hemorrhagic cystitis; infection of lung, liver, or kidneys
Cytomegalovirus	7–15 wks	Pneumonitis, enteritis, retinitis
Varicella-zoster virus	12–52 wks	Localized (skin) or disseminated (visceral organ involvement)
Epstein-Barr virus	—	Posttransplant lymphoproliferative disorder
Human herpesvirus-6	—	Bone marrow suppression, meningoencephalitis, pneumonia

(37). With the use of GCV prophylactically, the median time to CMV disease has also been delayed from 50 days to past day 100 after transplantation.

Success of preemptive therapy depends on recognizing infection and starting treatment early to prevent end-organ damage. Amplification of CMV DNA in peripheral blood leukocytes using PCR is the most sensitive screening method available. Antigenemia assays, using monoclonal antibodies to detect pp65, a viral matrix protein, are also useful, and are superior in sensitivity to culture-based assays such as shell vial technique. It is important to recognize that CMV antigen assays are not valid in neutropenic patients since the assay relies on circulating leukocytes. CMV blood infection strongly correlates with disease development; as a result, once the stem cells have engrafted, many centers begin scheduled weekly blood monitoring for CMV using PCR, antigen assays, or shell vial culture. At first evidence of CMV infection, intravenous GCV therapy is begun at 5 mg per kg every 12 hours for 10 to 14 days and then 5 mg per kg once daily for several weeks beyond negative screening results or until day 100 posttransplant. Use of preemptive GCV regimens have been shown to significantly reduce CMV disease and mortality (38,39). Foscarnet may also have a role in preventing CMV disease. Indications for its use include refractory neutropenia due to GCV and GCV-resistant CMV, usually manifested as a persistently positive CMV assay or development of disease while on preemptive therapy.

Despite prophylactic measures, up to 5% of marrow recipients develop end-organ damage from CMV disease. Common manifestations, in order of decreasing incidence, are pneumonitis, enteritis, and retinitis. Other presentations include fevers, pancytopenia, hepatitis, encephalitis, arthritis, and oral involvement. CMV pneumonitis usually presents with hypoxemia, fevers, and bilateral interstitial infiltrates (Fig. 5). Bronchoalveolar lavage is the preferred diagnostic test, with the fluid sample demonstrating CMV by culture, antigen presence, or histology. A positive PCR assay of the lavage fluid is not diagnostic due to its lack of specificity. Without therapy, CMV pneumonitis has an 85% mortality rate. With the use of GCV and immunoglobulin (IVIG), its mortality has halved. A typical treatment regimen is GCV 5 mg per kg every 12 hours + IVIG 500 mg per kg every other day for 21 days, followed by GCV 5 mg per kg every day, 5 times per week + IVIG 500 mg per kg once weekly for an extended time based on the patient's immunosuppression. CMV-specific IVIG does not improve outcome compared with standard IVIG. Some experts recommend switching GCV to foscarnet if absolute neutrophil count is lower than 1,000 per μL on 2 consecutive days (40). Hypoxemia and fevers usually abate with 1 week of treatment; if not, alternate diagnoses or GCV-resistance should be suspected.

CMV-associated enteritis typically presents with pain, nausea, vomiting, and/or diarrhea. Mucosal pathology such as inflammation or ulcerations may be seen anywhere in the gastrointestinal tract. Diagnosis is based on showing inclusion bodies or antigen in biopsied tissue. The optimal treatment regimen is not known but is based on experience with CMV pneumonitis.

THROMBOTIC MICROANGIOPATHY OF STEM CELL TRANSPLANTATION

The thrombotic microangiopathy (TM) that occurs after HSCT is the hematologic complication most likely to require critical care support. This clinical syndrome ranges from isolated mechanical hemolysis of RBCs to hemolysis concomitant with varying degrees of organ dysfunction. The underlying pathology in TM is endothelial damage (41). Factors that have been implicated in causing endothelial damage include chemotherapeutic agents

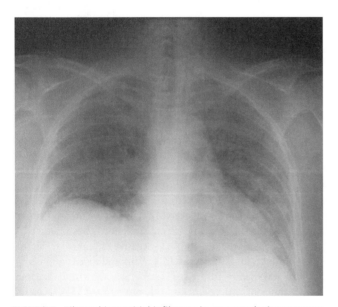

FIGURE 5. Bilateral interstitial infiltrates in cytomegalovirus pneumonitis.

(cyclophosphamide, nitrosoureas, platinum-based compounds), body irradiation, CSP, FK 506, and various cytokines that are expressed in the setting of GVHD and infections. Endothelial damage likely leads to thrombus formation in the small arterioles and capillaries. Thrombosis in the microcirculation consequently causes a mechanical hemolysis and impairs blood flow to different organs, explaining the clinical presentation of TM. The overall incidence of HSCT-TM is approximately 7%, with allograft recipients having twice the risk compared with their autograft counterparts (42).

TM of HSCT typically appears 3 to 6 months after transplantation. Diagnosis is based on the presence of nonimmune-mediated hemolytic anemia, thrombocytopenia, and evidence of organ dysfunction. Organ systems commonly involved include the kidneys, causing an HUS-like syndrome, and the nervous system, presenting similar to thrombotic thrombocytopenic purpura (TTP). Zeigler and colleagues in their case series demonstrated that the degree of hemolysis correlated with the clinical severity and outcome of the disease (43). Milder cases had less than 5% of red blood cells (RBCs) fragmented and median survival was greater than 400 days, whereas moderate and severe cases, with greater than 5% fragmentation of RBCs, had median survivals of only 60 days. Schriber and Herzig retrospectively identified three risk factors associated with a higher 3-month mortality: (a) presentation within 120 days of transplantation, (b) treatment with CSP or FK 506 for GVHD, and (c) presence of neurologic symptoms from the onset (41).

Clinical entities that can obscure the diagnosis of HSCT-TM include disseminated intravascular coagulation (DIC) and CSP and FK 506 toxicity. Compared to DIC, the thrombocytopenia of TM is more profound, and fibrinogen and factor VIII in TM are not consumed. CSP and FK 506 may both result in RBC hemolysis and renal insufficiency, and CSP can also cause neurologic symptoms. These drug effects, however, usually resolve with decreasing the dose or stopping the offending agent.

The treatment of HSCT-TM has never been studied in a prospective, controlled manner. Mild cases are generally treated with supportive care such as control of hypertension, judicious use of diuretics for fluid-overload states, and discontinuation of exacerbating drugs such as CSP and FK 506. Therapy of moderate and severe cases is fashioned after the treatment of classic TTP with plasma exchange. Whereas TTP is more than 90% responsive to plasma exchange therapy, at best 50% of HSCT-TM cases respond. There may be a better response rate when cryosupernatant, which is deficient in factor VIII multimers, is used instead of fresh frozen plasma. The role of other adjunctive treatment modalities such as corticosteroids, vincristine, splenectomy, IVIG, and protein A immune absorption are still being investigated.

PROGNOSIS OF CRITICALLY ILL HEMATOPOIETIC STEM CELL TRANSPLANTATION RECIPIENTS

Critical care support of the HSCT patient is a controversial topic. Admission to an ICU depends not only on the patient's clinical condition, but in many instances on the availability of ICU beds and the level of care that can be provided outside the ICU.

Many studies, therefore, have concentrated specifically on respiratory failure and the need for mechanical ventilation to assess the prognosis of critically ill transplant recipients.

Overall, 10% to 20% of HSCT recipients require ventilatory support. Studies published up to the mid-1990s cited hospital survival rates of less than 10%, with long-term survival (greater than 6 months) of only 3%. Based on these high mortality rates, the limited availability of resources, and the burden of critical care on the patients and their families, some have questioned the utility of providing intensive care to these patients. Over the last two decades, numerous studies have attempted to identify variables that predict survival after intensive care support. Unfortunately, many studies report conflicting results, and none have succeeded in predicting mortality with 100% accuracy. In the largest cohort analyzed to date, Rubenfeld and colleagues found no survivors among the 398 HSCT patients who had lung injury (F_{IO_2} greater than 0.6 or positive end-expiratory pressure greater than 5 after the first 24 hours of mechanical ventilation) and received more than 4 hours of vasopressor therapy or had sustained hepatic and renal failure (creatinine greater than 2 mg per dL and bilirubin greater than 4 mg per dL) (44). Other reports, however, have described patients who survived in spite of meeting the above criteria (45,46). Inconsistencies arise because patients in different cohorts vary in their underlying diseases, the conditioning regimens they have received, the type of transplant they underwent, and the severity of their illness at presentation to the ICU. In addition, several conditions requiring ventilatory support are more easily reversible, and the proportion of these diseases among different cohorts varies. Easily treatable processes include hydrostatic pulmonary edema, airway obstruction from mucositis, corticosteroid-responsive DAH, and engraftment syndrome. More recent studies also indicate that the survival of bone marrow transplant recipients with respiratory failure has improved over time (44,45,47,48). This improvement can probably be attributed to less toxic preparative regimens, better prophylaxis of infections, more sensitive diagnostic techniques, and more transplants using peripheral blood stem cells.

Despite conflicting reports with respect to ICU outcomes, several trends have persisted throughout most studies involving HSCT recipients: the majority of ICU admissions are due to respiratory insufficiency; mortality significantly increases when mechanical ventilation is required and as the number of organs with dysfunction increases; and severity of illness scores such as the Acute Physiologic and Chronic Health Evaluation (APACHE) II often underestimate mortality.

Transplant recipients should be informed of the incidence and outcome of critical care support, and their preferences ought to be established in the pretransplant period. When the patient's wishes are not known, and since outcomes often cannot be accurately predicted, it is reasonable to provide life support for a limited period of time during which the prognosis can become more clear. Progression to multiorgan failure is associated with a hospital mortality approaching 100% (44,49,50).

SUMMARY

HSCT is now offered worldwide to approximately 40,000 patients per year, primarily as treatment for malignancies and genetic conditions. The number of transplants is increasing by 15% to 20% per year as indications for HSCT expand and as marrow sources increase due to volunteer marrow registries and umbilical cord blood availability. Over the last two decades conventional bone marrow transplantation is gradually being supplanted by PBSC transplants. Complications of HSCT are relatively stereotypic and derive predictably from the kind of transplant, time elapsed since transplantation, and the conditioning regimens used. Organ-specific complications often result from endothelial damage caused by the preparative regimens; idiopathic pneumonia syndrome, hepatic VOD, and thrombotic microangiopathy of HSCT are a few examples of this phenomenon. Infectious complications are also prevalent in the setting of HSCT due to neutropenia and alterations in the cellular and humoral immunity.

Protocol-driven prophylactic and therapeutic regimens are widely used to diminish the morbidity and mortality of infectious complications; nevertheless, bacterial, fungal, and viral infections remain important determinants of outcome following transplantation. Pulmonary complications remain the most common cause of admission to an ICU. HSCT recipients have a poor prognosis once mechanical ventilation, hemodialysis, or hemodynamic support is required because of multiple-organ system failure; there is not yet a consensus, however, regarding the best predictors of outcome in patients requiring critical care support services in this population.

Acknowledgments. We would like to thank Dr. Frandics P. Chan for providing Fig. 2 and Dr. Keith Stockerl-Goldstein for providing Fig. 4.

KEY POINTS

- Each year more than 40,000 hematopoietic stem cell transplants are performed worldwide for a variety of malignant and nonmalignant conditions, and this number is increasing by 15% to 20% per year.
- Advances that facilitate this growth include the use of colony-stimulating factors and peripheral blood stem cells, development of volunteer marrow registries, and application of protocol-driven regimens to diminish complications.
- Complications of this therapy usually result from infections,

toxicity of the preparative regimen, or graft-versus-host disease.
- The nature of these complications is often predictable based on type of transplant, time elapsed since transplantation, and the conditioning regimen used.
- Respiratory failure is the most common complication requiring admission to an intensive care unit.
- Outcome of critically ill transplant recipients significantly worsens when mechanical ventilation is required and as the number of organs with dysfunction increases.

REFERENCES

1. Lennard A, Jackson G. Stem cell transplantation. *BMJ* 2000;321:433–437.
2. Rossi S, Erasmus J, McAdams P, et al. Pulmonary drug toxicity: radiologic and pathologic manifestations. *Radiographics* 2000;20:1245–1259.
3. Kantrow S, Hackman R, Boeckh M, et al. Idiopathic pneumonia syndrome: changing spectrum of lung injury after marrow transplantation. *Transplantation* 1997;63:1079–1086.
4. Robbins R, Linder J, Stahl M, et al. Diffuse alveolar hemorrhage in autologous bone marrow transplant recipients. *Am J Med* 1989;87:511–518.
5. Metcalf J, Rennard S, Reed E, et al. Corticosteroids as adjunctive therapy for diffuse alveolar hemorrhage associated with bone marrow transplantation. *Am J Med* 1993;96:327–334.
6. Chao N, Duncan S, Long G, et al. Corticosteroid therapy for diffuse alveolar hemorrhage in autologous bone marrow transplant recipients. *Ann Intern Med* 1991;114:145–146.
7. Raptis A, Mavroudis D, Suffredini A, et al. High-dose corticosteroid therapy for diffuse alveolar hemorrhage in allogeneic bone marrow stem cell transplant recipients. *Bone Marrow Transpl* 1999;24:879–883.
8. Philit F, Weisendanger T, Achibaud E, et al. Post transplant obstructive lung disease ("bronchiolitis obliterans"): a clinical comparative study of bone marrow and lung transplant patients. *Eur Respir J* 1995;8:551–558.
9. Carreras E. Veno-occlusive disease of the liver after hemopoietic cell transplantation. *Eur J Haematol* 2000;64:281–291.
10. Ribaud P, Gluckman E. Hepatic veno-occlusive disease. In: Atkinson K, ed. *Clinical bone marrow and blood stem cell transplantation*, 2nd ed. Cambridge: Cambridge University Press, 2000;783–790.
11. Bearman S, Anderson G, Mori M, et al. Veno-occlusive disease of the liver: development of a model for predicting fatal outcome after marrow transplantation. *J Clin Oncol* 1993;11:1729–1736.
12. Bearman S, Lee J, Baron A, et al. Treatment of hepatic venoocclusive disease with recombinant human tissue plasminogen activator and heparin in 42 marrow transplantation patients. *Blood* 1997;89:1501–1506.
13. Richardson P, Elias A, Krishnan A, et al. Treatment of severe venoocclusive disease with defibrotide: compassionate use results in response without significant toxicity in a high-risk population. *Blood* 1998;92:737–744.
14. Savdie E. Renal complications. In: Atkinson K, ed. *Clinical bone marrow and blood stem cell transplantation*, 2nd ed. Cambridge: Cambridge University Press, 2000:930–942.
15. Kapeluchnik J, Verstandig A, Or R. Hydronephrosis in children after bone marrow transplantation: case reports. *Bone Marrow Transpl* 1996;17:873–875.
16. Bataller R, Gines P, Guevara M, et al. Hepatorenal syndrome. *Semin Liver Dis* 1997;17:233–247.
17. Cruz D, Perazella M, Mahnensmith R. Bone marrow transplant nephropathy: a case report and review of the literature. *J Am Soc Nephrol* 1997;8:166–173.
18. Bearman S, Petersen F, Schor R, et al. Radionuclide ejection fractions in the evaluation of patients being considered for bone marrow transplantation: risk for cardiac toxicity. *Bone Marrow Transpl* 1990;5:173–177.
19. Goldberg M, Antin J, Giunan E, et al. Cyclophosphamide cardiotoxicity: an analysis of dosing as a risk factor. *Blood* 1986;68:1114–1118.
20. Shan K, Lincoff A, Young J. Anthracycline-induced cardiotoxicity. *Ann Intern Med* 1996;125:47–58.
21. Von Hoff D, Layard M, Basa P, et al. Risk factors for doxorubicin-induced congestive heart failure. *Ann Intern Med* 1979;91:710–717.

22. Hellman K. Preventing the cardiotoxicity of anthracyclines by dexrazoxane: a real breakthrough. *BMJ* 1999;319:1085–1086.
23. Benoff L, Schweitzer P. Radiation therapy-induced cardiac injury. *Am Heart J* 1995;129:1193–1196.
24. van Burik J, Weisdorf D. Infections in recipients of blood and marrow transplantation. *Hematol Oncol Clin North Am* 1999;13:1065–1089.
25. Hughes W, Armstrong D, Bodey G, et al. 1997 guidelines for the use of antimicrobial agents in neutropenic patients with unexplained fever. Infectious Diseases Society of America. *Clin Infect Dis* 1997;25:551–573.
26. Wingard J, Merz W, Rinaldi M, et al. Increase in *Candida krusei* infection among patients with bone marrow transplantation and neutropenia treated prophylactically with fluconazole. *N Engl J Med* 1991;325:1274–1277.
27. van Burik J, Leisenring W, Myerson D, et al. The effect of prophylactic fluconazole on the clinical spectrum of fungal diseases in bone marrow transplant recipients with special attention to hepatic candidiasis: an autopsy study of 355 patients. *Medicine* 1998;77:246–254.
28. Wingard J. Fungal infections after bone marrow transplant. *Biol Blood Marrow Transpl* 1999;5:55–68.
29. Wald A, Leisenring W, van Burik J, et al. Epidemiology of *Aspergillus* infections in a large cohort of patients undergoing bone marrow transplantation. *J Infect Dis* 1997;175:1459–1466.
30. Slavin M, Osborne B, Adams R, et al. Efficacy and safety of fluconazole prophylaxis for fungal infections after marrow transplantation—a prospective, randomized, double-blind study. *J Infect Dis* 1995;171:1545–1552.
31. Goodman J, Winston D, Greenfield R, et al. A controlled trial of fluconazole to prevent fungal infections in patients undergoing bone marrow transplantation. *N Engl J Med* 1992;326:845–851.
32. Edwards JE, Bodey GP, Bowden RA, et al. International conference for the development of a consensus on the management and prevention of severe candidal infections. National Institute of Allergy and Infectious Diseases Mycoses Study Group. *Clin Infect Dis* 1997;25:43–59.
33. White M, Anaissie E, Kusne S. Amphotericin B colloidal dispersion vs. amphotericin B as therapy for invasive aspergillosis. *Clin Infect Dis* 1997;24:635–642.
34. Wingard J. Efficacy of amphotericin B lipid complex injection (ABLC) in bone marrow transplant recipients with life-threatening systemic mycoses. *Bone Marrow Transpl* 1997;19:343–347.
35. Walsh T, Finberg R, Arndt C, et al. Liposomal amphotericin B for empirical therapy in patients with persistent fever and neutropenia. National Institute of Allergy and Infectious Diseases Mycoses Study Group. *N Engl J Med* 1999;340:764–771.
36. Bowden R, Slichter S, Sayers M. A comparison of filtered leukocyte-reduced and cytomegalovirus seronegative blood products for the prevention of transfusion-associated CMV infection after marrow transplant. *Blood* 1995;86:3598–3603.
37. van Burik J, Weisdorf D. Infections in recipients of blood and marrow transplantation. In: Mandell G, Bennett J, Dolin R, eds. *Principles and practice of infectious diseases*, 5th ed. Philadelphia: Churchill Livingstone, 2000;3137–3147.
38. Einsele B, Ehninger G, Hebart H. Polymerase chain reaction monitoring reduces the incidence of cytomegalovirus disease and the duration and side effects of antiviral therapy after bone marrow transplantation. *Blood* 1995;86:2815–2820.
39. Schmidt G, Horak D, Niland JC. A randomized, controlled trial of prophylactic ganciclovir for cytomegalovirus pulmonary infection in recipients of allogeneic marrow transplant. *N Engl J Med* 1991;324:105–111.
40. Zaia J. Cytomegalovirus infections. In: Thomas E, Blume K, Forman S, eds. *Hematopoietic cell transplantation*, 2nd ed. Malden, MA: Blackwell Science, 1999;560–583.
41. Schriber J, Herzig G. Transplantation-associated thrombotic thrombocytopenic purpura and hemolytic uremic syndrome. *Semin Hematol* 1997;34:126–133.
42. Pettitt A, Clark R. Thrombotic microangiopathy following bone marrow transplantation. *Bone Marrow Transpl* 1994;14:495–504.
43. Zeigler Z, Shadduck R, Nemunaitis J, et al. Bone marrow transplant-associated thrombotic microangiopathy: a case series. *Bone Marrow Transpl* 1995;15:247–253.
44. Rubenfeld G, Crawford S. Withdrawing life support from mechanically ventilated recipients of bone marrow transplants: a case for evidence-based guidelines. *Ann Intern Med* 1996;125:625–633.
45. Shorr A, Moores L, Edenfield W, et al. Mechanical ventilation in hematopoietic stem cell transplantation: can we effectively predict outcome? *Chest* 1999;116:1012–1018.
46. Marin D, Berrade J, Ferra C, et al. Engraftment syndrome and survival after respiratory failure post-bone marrow transplantation. *Intensive Care Med* 1998;24:732–735.
47. Jackson S, Tweeddale M, Barnett M, et al. Admission of bone marrow transplant recipients to the intensive care unit: outcome, survival, and prognostic factors. *Bone Marrow Transpl* 1998;21:697–704.
48. Price K, Thall P, Kish S, et al. Prognostic indicators for blood and marrow transplant patients admitted to an intensive care unit. *Am J Respir Crit Care Med* 1998;158:876–884.
49. Torecilla C, Cortes J, Chamorro C, et al. Prognostic assessment of the acute complications of bone marrow transplantation requiring intensive therapy. *Intensive Care Med* 1988;14:393–398.
50. Afessa B, Tefferi A, Hoagland H, et al. Outcome of recipients of bone marrow transplants who require intensive-care unit support. *Mayo Clin Proc* 1992;67:117–122.

CARE OF THE PATIENT
WITH ENDOCRINE EMERGENCIES

GARY P. ZALOGA

KEY WORDS

- Diabetes insipidus
- Hypoparathyroidism
- Hypocalcemia
- Hyperparathyroidism
- Hypercalcemia
- Hypothyroidism
- Hyperthyroidism

- Adrenal insufficiency
- Pheochromocytoma
- Carcinoid syndrome
- Hyperglycemia
- Diabetic ketoacidosis
- Hyperglycemic hyperosmolar syndrome

INTRODUCTION

The endocrine glands secrete a variety of hormones that regulate cellular activity. Oversecretion or undersecretion of hormones can impair cell and organ function, the net result being increased morbidity and mortality. Undersecretion or oversecretion of some hormones (e.g., estrogens, testosterone, follicle-stimulating hormone, prolactin) alters selected cellular functions but does not result in life-threatening emergencies. In this chapter, we discuss the clinical presentation, diagnosis, and treatment of endocrine emergencies that are likely to present in the perioperative period. We concentrate on acute management of these disorders and cover alterations in hormonal production by the pituitary gland (diabetes insipidus), parathyroid glands (hypoparathyroidism, hyperparathyroidism), thyroid gland (hypothyroidism, hyperthyroidism), adrenal glands (adrenal insufficiency, pheochromocytoma), carcinoid tissue, and pancreas (diabetic ketoacidosis and hyperglycemic hyperosmolar syndrome).

PITUITARY: DIABETES INSIPIDUS

Diabetes insipidus (1–3) results from deficient secretion or action of antidiuretic hormone (ADH). The syndrome is characterized by hypotonic polyuria (the inability to conserve water by the kidneys), hypernatremia, hyperosmolality, dehydration, intravascular volume depletion, and ultimately hypovolemic shock.

Diabetes insipidus results from decreased hypothalamic-pituitary secretion of ADH (central diabetes insipidus) or renal resistance to ADH (nephrogenic diabetes insipidus). Central diabetes insipidus occurs in patients with destructive lesions within the hypothalamic-pituitary area (e.g., tumors, head trauma, thrombosis with infarction, surgery, infiltrative disease). Diabetes insipidus may occur in a triphasic pattern after trauma or brain surgery (1). The initial diabetes insipidus (first phase) is due to axon shock and lack of function of the damaged neurons. This phase lasts several hours to days and is followed by an antidiuretic phase (second phase) due to release of vasopressin from the disconnected posterior pituitary or remaining severed neurons. Overly aggressive fluid administration during this phase can lead to hyponatremia and volume overload. The antidiuresis can last 2 to 14 days, after which diabetes insipidus (third phase) may return. Diabetes insipidus occurs in approximately 50% of patients receiving frontal craniotomies for lesions in the hypothalamic-pituitary gland area (approximately 20% to 30% are permanent). Diabetes insipidus is less common in patients undergoing transphenoidal surgery (approximately 15%) and is usually transient. Nephrogenic diabetes insipidus occurs in patients with a variety of renal disorders (i.e., renal insufficiency, hypercalcemia) and following a variety of drugs (e.g., amphotericin B).

Patients with diabetes insipidus present with hypotonic polyuria, which left untreated results in water loss, hypernatremia, hyperosmolality, cellular dehydration, and volume depletion. It is important to rule out other causes of polyuria in these patients. Urinary osmolality and serum sodium are very helpful in the differential diagnosis of the polyuria. The most frequent reason for hypotonic polyuria is postresuscitation diuresis (in which there is physiologic suppression of ADH). It is important to note that patients with postresuscitation diuresis are appropriately excreting fluid and do not become hypernatremic or hypotensive. Patients with diabetes insipidus continue to excrete fluid despite development of hypernatremia and hypotension. At times, it may be difficult to distinguish between partial central diabetes insipidus and normal function. In general, if a patient fails to concentrate urine maximally (usually greater than 600 mOsm per kg H_2O) in the presence of hypernatremia or hypotension, he or she should be treated as though they have partial diabetes insipidus. Definitive diagnosis can await recovery from the acute condition. Of course, treatment will depend upon the degree of water loss.

Hypertonic polyuria may be caused by hyperglycemia, mannitol administration, use of radiocontrast dye, or ingestion/injection of other osmolar agents.

The emergency treatment of diabetes insipidus is aimed at volume and water repletion. Intravascular volume should be replaced rapidly using isotonic fluids. Water can be replaced with intravenous (i.v.) fluids (e.g., 5% dextrose in water, 0.5 normal saline) or enteral water (orally or via orogastric or nasogastric tube). The total body water deficit can be estimated as [(0.6) (weight in kg) (plasma sodium in mEq/L per $140 - 1$)]. Blood pressure, heart rate, and plasma sodium concentration should be monitored at frequent intervals.

When polyuria is excessive (i.e., greater than 300 mL per hour), we favor administration of the ADH analog desmopressin (DDAVP) along with fluid administration. Desmopressin is devoid of significant vasopressor activity and should be used in place of vasopressin (which has both vasopressor and antidiuretic activities). Desmopressin may be administered i.v. (1 to 4 μg every 12 to 24 hours), subcutaneously (s.c.) (1 to 4 μg every 12 to 24 hours), or intranasally (5 to 20 μg once to twice daily). The onset of action of desmopressin is rapid after parenteral or nasal administration (i.e., 1 hour) and the duration of effect is 12 to 24 hours. Desmopressin is also available in tablet form for chronic nonemergent oral treatment of central diabetes insipidus. The usual starting dose is 0.05 to 0.1 mg twice daily. The major side effects of desmopressin administration are water retention and volume overload. However, with careful monitoring of the patient (i.e., urinary volume, fluid input and output, urinary osmolality, serum sodium, intravascular volume status) these effects are rarely clinically significant. The patient should be allowed to escape from the effects of previous medication before administering the next dose. Alternatively, one may administer aqueous L-arginine vasopressin (duration of action 2 to 8 hours) s.c. at a dose of 5 to 10 U every 6 to 12 hours.

The management of nephrogenic diabetes insipidus is more difficult since these patients do not respond to ADH. Emergency management is based upon intravenous/enteral water and electrolyte administration. Volume depletion is treated with isotonic fluids.

All patients with the acute onset of central diabetes insipidus require an evaluation for possible anterior pituitary insufficiency. The patient should be given stress doses of hydrocortisone (initially 100 mg every 8 hours i.v.) until anterior pituitary function (especially adrenal and thyroid status) can be definitively evaluated.

Serum electrolytes (especially potassium) must be monitored closely and replaced as indicated by monitoring since they are lost in the urine along with water. If hypernatremia is chronic (i.e., greater than 2 days), it should be corrected slowly to avoid neurologic sequelae, such as seizures and cerebral edema. The plasma sodium concentration should be reduced approximately 1 to 2 mEq per L per hour. If changes in plasma sodium are acute, they can be corrected over a shorter period of time. If a patient is having ongoing seizures, serum sodium should be reduced rapidly until seizures stop (usually reducing the plasma sodium to 160 to 170 mEq per L is sufficient to stop seizures).

PARATHYROID DISEASE

The parathyroid glands secrete parathyroid hormone (PTH), which, along with vitamin D (1,25-dihydroxyvitamin D) is responsible for regulating circulating ionized calcium levels within narrow limits (1.0 to 1.3 mmol per L). Loss of PTH secretion results in hypocalcemia (hypoparathyroidism) while excess PTH secretion causes hypercalcemia (hyperparathyroidism) (4–8).

Hypoparathyroidism (ionized hypocalcemia) may occur in the perioperative period following parathyroidectomy (usually for hyperparathyroidism) and rarely after nonparathyroid neck surgery. Hypoparathyroidism is also occasionally seen as an acquired disorder in patients with severe hypomagnesemia, hypermagnesemia, and sepsis.

Hyperparathyroidism (ionized hypercalcemia) is the most common cause of hypercalcemia in the outpatient setting. Many of these patients are asymptomatic and the hypercalcemia is detected when the patient presents for medical attention for other problems, such as infection, trauma, or elective surgery. Some patients present with renal calculi. Other causes of hypercalcemia include malignancies (especially metastatic disease, multiple myeloma), granulomatous disease (e.g., sarcoidosis), and vitamin A and D intoxication (4).

The diagnoses of hypoparathyroidism and hyperparathyroidism are based upon measurement of circulating ionized calcium and PTH levels. Although one may suspect the diagnosis based upon total serum calcium levels, this test lacks specificity (for detecting hypocalcemia) and lacks sensitivity (for detecting hypercalcemia). Calcium circulates in the blood in ionized (approximately 50%), albumin bound (approximately 40%), and chelated (approximately 10%) forms (4). It is the ionized form that is physiologically active. Total serum calcium levels are affected by albumin level, percent of calcium bound to albumin, acid-base status, and chelators (4). Most critically ill patients will have low albumin levels and low total serum calcium levels despite the presence of normal ionized calcium levels. Patients with elevated ionized calcium levels may have normal total serum calcium levels, partially as a result of low albumin levels. Thus, we recommend ionized calcium assessment (which can be performed on most blood gas analyzers) when evaluating calcium status (4,9).

The clinical features of ionized hypocalcemia and hypercalcemia relate to the degree of calcium decrease or elevation and the acuteness of the change in calcium level. The organs most affected by calcium alterations are the cardiovascular, gastrointestinal, and central nervous systems (Table 1).

Mild to moderate ionized hypocalcemia rarely requires treatment. Ionized hypocalcemia is part of the acute phase response to stress and illness and is believed to be protective to cells. It rarely causes cardiovascular or other organ compromise. Intracellular calcium levels are usually elevated during states of shock and critical illness. Administration of calcium may further increase these detrimental levels. Thus, we do not recommend calcium repletion until ionized calcium concentrations decrease below 0.7 to 0.8 mmol per L (normal levels 1.0 to 1.3 mmol/L).

It is always important to evaluate and treat the underlying disease responsible for changes in calcium levels (e.g., shock, sepsis, cancer, drugs). Patients with ionized hypocalcemia

TABLE 1. CLINICAL FEATURES OF IONIZED HYPOCALCEMIA AND HYPERCALCEMIA

Organ System	Hypocalcemia	Hypercalcemia
Cardiovascular	Hypotension Heart failure Bradycardia Heart block Arrhythmias Cardiac arrest Insensitivity to digitalis QT and ST prolongation	Hypertension Cardiac arrhythmias Heart block Heart failure Digitalis sensitivity Catecholamine resistance QT shortening
Neuromuscular	Tetany Spasm Hyperreflexia Paresthesias Weakness Chvostek sign Trousseau sign Seizures Papilledema	Weakness Hypotonia Hyporeflexia Seizures Headache
Psychiatric	Anxiety Irritability Psychosis Confusion Dementia Depression	Lethargy Depression Obtundation Coma Memory impairment Confusion Disorientation Psychosis
Respiratory	Laryngeal spasm Bronchospasm Apnea	
Gastrointestinal	Irritable bowel Abdominal pain	Peptic ulcer Pancreatitis Constipation Anorexia Nausea, vomiting
Urinary tract		Polyuria (nephrogenic diabetes insipidus) Tubular dysfunction Nephrocalcinosis Nephrolithiasis Glomerular dysfunction Interstitial nephritis
Miscellaneous	Cataracts Dry skin Brittle nails Coarse hair	Osteopenia Fractures Skin necrosis Pruritis Conjunctivitis Hypomagnesemia Ectopic calcification Vasculitis

must have levels of phosphorus and magnesium measured (4). Hyperphosphatemic hypocalcemia (i.e., rhabdomyolysis, tumor lysis syndrome) is best treated by lowering phosphorus levels (i.e., with diuresis, phosphorus binders, dialysis). Administration of calcium to these patients may cause calcium precipitation, organ injury, and death. Severe hypomagnesemia and hypermagnesemia inhibit parathyroid gland function and/or PTH action. Normalization of the magnesium level in these patients usually corrects the circulating calcium concentration. In patients with severe (ionized calcium less than 0.7 mmol per L) or symptomatic ion-

ized hypocalcemia, we recommend administration of i.v. calcium (100 mg elemental calcium over 5 minutes, followed by an infusion of calcium at 0.5 to 1.0 mg per kg per hour) (4). We usually administer calcium as the chloride salt and closely monitor ionized calcium levels during calcium infusion. The rate of calcium administration is adjusted to maintain ionized calcium levels between 0.8 to 1.0 mmol per L. It is important to administer calcium as an infusion since bolus doses produce only a transient elevation because calcium is eliminated in the urine and diffuses into the tissues. When stable, patients who continue to require calcium can be switched to oral calcium with or without vitamin D (4,6).

Ionized hypercalcemia also requires evaluation and treatment of the underlying disease. Hyperparathyroidism is best treated by surgical removal of adenomatous or hyperplastic parathyroid tissue although asymptomatic patients with mild hypercalcemia may be followed without treatment (5,8). Treatment of hypercalcemia of malignancy usually requires chemotherapy, radiotherapy, or surgery. General supportive measures for hypercalcemic patients (4,7) include removal of drugs which may elevate calcium (e.g., thiazide diuretics, lithium, vitamin D, calcium supplements) and correction of concomitant electrolyte disorders. Mobilization is helpful to minimize bone resorption. Intravascular volume should be repleted. Many hypercalcemic patients are volume-depleted secondary to calcium-induced nephrogenic diabetes insipidus. Normal saline is the fluid of choice since sodium excretion by the kidney inhibits calcium reabsorption. Once intravascular volume and renal perfusion are restored, calcium excretion by the kidneys can be further augmented with a loop diuretic such as furosemide. It is essential to maintain intravascular volume during diuresis. Calcium excretion can also be augmented by dialysis in patients with renal failure. The next step in treatment of hypercalcemic patients is to decrease bone resorption (the source of calcium in most hypercalcemic patients). Bisphosphonates (e.g., pamidronate 30 to 90 mg in 250 mL saline i.v. over 4 to 24 hours) are the drugs of choice. Onset of action is typically 24 to 48 hours and duration of action can last several weeks. Injection of calcitonin (4 to 8 IU per kg every 6 to 12 hours i.v., s.c., or intramuscularly [i.m.]) may also be useful. Glucocorticoids are beneficial in the treatment of hypercalcemia in patients with granulomatous disease (such as sarcoidosis), vitamin A and D toxicity, and some malignancies. Rarely, phosphates can be used to acutely lower calcium levels. However, phosphates may precipitate with calcium, especially when administered i.v., and cause organ injury.

THYROID DISEASE

The thyroid gland secretes primarily thyroxine (T_4) along with smaller amounts of triiodothyronine (T_3). T_3 is the active form of thyroid hormone and regulates gene expression. T_4 is converted to T_3 (5'-deiodinase enzyme) or reverse T_3 (rT_3; inactive hormone) in various tissues. Thus, the primary control of cellular metabolism lies in the tissues themselves. Synthesis and secretion of thyroid hormone by the thyroid gland is stimulated by pituitary-derived thyroid stimulating hormone (TSH), which in turn is stimulated by thyrotropin-releasing hormone (TRH) from the hypothalamus. The secretion of TRH and TSH is regulated by T_3 through a negative feedback mechanism. Thus, circulating T_4 levels are a measure of thyroid gland function while circulating T_3 assesses peripheral conversion of T_4 to T_3 (5′-deiodinase function). TSH is a measure of pituitary function. Low TSH levels indicate failure of the pituitary gland (i.e., secondary hypothyroidism), hyperthyroidism (via negative feedback) or depressed pituitary function (euthyroid sick syndromes). Elevated TSH levels usually indicate decreased negative feedback due to low T_4/T_3 levels (primary hypothyroidism).

Hypothyroidism (Myxedema)

Primary hypothyroidism results from the loss of thyroid tissue (10–13). The most common etiologies are Hashimoto thyroiditis (autoimmune), thyroidectomy, radioiodine treatment, iodide deficiency, infectious thyroiditis, and drug use (e.g., amiodarone, lithium, iodide excess, propylthiouracil, methimazole, aminoglutethimide). Secondary hypothyroidism results from hypothalamic pituitary failure and may result from tumors, thrombosis, infarction, hemochromatosis, and sarcoidosis. The diagnosis of hypothyroidism (Table 2) is established by measuring circulating levels of TSH and thyroid hormone (usually free T_4 or total T_4).

Thyroid hormone deficiency results in decreased metabolic activity of all organ systems. There is a generalized slowing of metabolic functions. Symptoms include fatigue, lethargy, weakness, headache, weight gain, cold intolerance, menstrual irregularities, infertility, galactorrhea, dry skin, hair loss, constipation, decreased sweating, paresthesias, neuropathy, myalgias, confusion, and memory impairment. Clinical signs include goiter, bradycardia, heart failure, pericardial effusions, hypertension, slow mentation, apathy, slow relaxation of the reflexes, obtundation, coma, slow movements, edema, dry scaly skin, coarse hair, brittle nails, hypothermia, facial edema, diminished ventilatory response to hypoxia and hypercarbia, macroglossia, muscle weakness, failure to wean from mechanical ventilation, pleural effusions, ascites, hoarseness, and failure to grow or thrive. Laboratory findings include elevated cholesterol and triglycerides, elevated prolactin, increased P_{CO_2}, hyponatremia, anemia, hypoglycemia, and decreased voltage and bradycardia on electrocardiogram. There may also be an increase in hepatic transaminases, lactic dehydrogenase, and creatine phosphokinase (CPK). CPK-MB may be elevated.

The initial management of hypothyroidism is supportive (10–13): maintain intravascular volume, support ventilation, maintain body temperature, and provide nutritional support. Electrolyte levels should be checked and corrected. Hyponatremia usually results from the syndrome of excess ADH secretion and is treated with free water restriction and/or saline plus furosemide. It is important to make an appropriate diagnosis of the cause of hypothyroidism. Secondary hypothyroidism may indicate hypothalamic-pituitary disease, which requires specific workup and treatment. Pituitary failure resulting in hypothyroidism is usually associated with other endocrine abnormalities (such as adrenal insufficiency). It is important to treat precipitating disease such as infection, trauma, heart failure, and stroke. The actions of many drugs are altered in hypothyroid patients due to altered metabolism (clearance) or cellular action. Thus, drug therapy must be followed closely during repletion with thyroid hormone.

The definitive treatment of hypothyroidism is thyroid hormone replacement (10–13). Thyroid hormone may be administered as T_4 or T_3. Thyroid extract (a combination of T_4 and T_3) is rarely used today. The most common agent used to treat hypothyroidism is T_4. The agent may be administered orally or intravenously. The intravenous dose is 50% to 75% of the oral dose (to account for absorption). The amount of T_4 administered to a patient depends upon their age, length of hypothyroidism, and underlying cardiac disease. Treatment of patients who are older, have underlying cardiac disease, or long-standing untreated hypothyroidism is best initiated with low doses of T_4. Begin with 0.025 to 0.05 mg per day and increase the dose every 2 to 4 weeks by 0.025 to 0.05 mg per day until the maintenance dose is reached (usually 0.1 to 0.15 mg per day). Treatment of young adults can be initiated with 0.1 mg per day of T_4. The dose can be increased by 0.025 to 0.05 mg per day every 2 to 4 weeks. T_4 has a long half-life (approximately 10 days) and steady state is not achieved for approximately 25 to 30 days. T_3 is seldom used to treat hypothyroidism. It is short-acting and may precipitate cardiac arrhythmias. The usual replacement dose is 25 μg every 8 hours. It is important to follow clinical status, T_4, and TSH levels during treatment. T_4 dosage should be adjusted to suppress TSH into the normal range.

Myxedema coma (13–15) represents acute life-threatening metabolic decompensation in a patient with underlying untreated hypothyroidism. Patients develop failure of multiple-organ systems, evidenced by stupor, coma, hypoventilation, hypothermia, hypotension, bradycardia, hyponatremia, and hypoglycemia, in addition to other features of hypothyroidism (see previous discussion). The mortality rate is reported to be 20% to 50%. The patient should be supported with mechanical ventilation, appropriate fluids based upon volume status and serum sodium concentrations, glucose, and body warming (as required by the clinical state). The clinician should look for and treat precipitating causes

TABLE 2. DIAGNOSIS OF THYROID ABNORMALITIES

Disorder	T_4	Free T_4	T_3	Free T_3	rT_3	TSH	RT_3U
Normal	4–12 μg/dL	0.8–2.7 ng/dL	75–195 ng/dL	0.25–0.65 ng/dL	2.6–18.9 ng/dL	0.5–5 μU/mL	0.8–1.2
Primary hypothyroidism	Low	Low	Low	Low	Low	High	Low
Secondary hypothyroidism	Low	Low	Low	Low	Low	Very low	Low
Hyperthyroidism	High	High	High	High	High	Suppressed	High
Sick-euthyroid	Low	Normal	Low	Low	High	Normal or low	High

T_4, thyroxine; T_3, triiodothyronine; rT_3, reverse T_3; TSH, thyroid stimulating hormone; RT_3U, T_3 resin uptake.

such as pneumonia, sepsis, hypothermia, stroke, gastrointestinal bleeding, surgery, trauma, and use of sedatives and hypnotic agents. Blood is sent for analysis of thyroid hormones, TSH, and cortisol. Treatment is begun with thyroid hormone immediately while awaiting laboratory confirmation. A loading dose of T_4 (0.3 to 0.4 mg) is administered and followed with a maintenance dose of 0.1 mg per day. Many experts also recommend a dose of T_3 (10 μg over 5 minutes). The presence of adrenal insufficiency should be considered and hydrocortisone administered (100 mg i.v. every 8 hours) while awaiting results. Administration of thyroid hormone to patients with untreated adrenal insufficiency may precipitate addisonian crisis.

Hyperthyroidism

Hyperthyroidism results from overactivity of the thyroid gland, functioning thyroid carcinoma, or excess administration of thyroid hormone. It is convenient to divide the etiologies of hyperthyroidism into those associated with increased uptake of radioiodine and those associated with decreased uptake (Table 3). Graves disease is an autoimmune disease caused by the production of thyroid-stimulating antibodies and is the most common cause of hyperthyroidism. A number of other autoantibodies are also produced in patients with Graves disease. The net result includes a number of autoimmune abnormalities such as ophthalmopathy and dermopathy.

Hyperthyroidism (10,16–18) is characterized by increased metabolism and function of multiple organs. Symptoms include restlessness, irritability, agitation, emotional lability, diminished mentation, poor sleep, fatigue, muscle weakness, increased appetite, weight loss, palpitations, heat intolerance, increased sweating, increased bowel movements, dyspnea, periodic paralysis (very rare), oligomenorrhea, and angina pectoris. Signs of hyperthyroidism include goiter, lid lag, tachycardia, heart failure (high output), hypertension, atrial fibrillation, wide pulse pressure, tremor, hyperreflexia, muscle wasting, onycholysis, warm moist skin, increased sweating, fine hair, exophthalmos, pretibial myxedema, and weight loss. Cardiovascular demands may cause myocardial ischemia, infarction, and cardiac arrhythmias, and result in shock. Oxygen consumption is increased and the demand upon the cardiovascular system is high. Laboratory findings include an elevated alkaline phosphatase (from bone), hypercalcemia, hypokalemia, hyperglycemia, rarely hypoglycemia, anemia, and an increased heart rate and arrhythmias.

TABLE 3. ETIOLOGIES OF HYPERTHYROIDISM

Increased Radioiodine Uptake	Decreased Radioiodine Uptake
1. Graves disease (diffuse enlargement)	1. Subacute thyroiditis
2. Toxic multinodular goiter	2. Exogenous thyroid hormone
3. Toxic adenoma	3. Metastatic thyroid carcinoma
4. Functioning thyroid carcinoma (in thyroid)	4. Thyroiditis
5. TSH-secreting tumor (rare)	
6. Struma ovarii (hCG secretion)	

TSH, thyroid stimulating hormone; hCG = human chorionic gonadotropin.

The diagnosis of hyperthyroidism is confirmed by measuring thyroid hormone and TSH circulating levels (Table 2). T_4 and T_3 levels are usually elevated and TSH is suppressed below normal levels. An occasional patient may present with a normal T_4 but elevated T_3 (T_3 toxicosis). In addition, critical illness decreases levels of T_4 and T_3 and may mask the diagnosis of hyperthyroidism. TSH is suppressed in these patients and suggests the presence of the hyperthyroid state.

The primary aim of treatment is to decrease the hypermetabolic state by inhibiting the secretion and action of thyroid hormone. Treatment is aimed at inhibiting the thyroid gland with propylthiouracil (PTU; initially 300 mg every 6 hours for severe hyperthyroidism) or methimazole (initially 15 to 30 mg every 6 hours for severe hyperthyroidism). Surgery is rarely indicated for initial therapy since it may precipitate thyroid storm and has a high morbidity and mortality in patients with uncontrolled hyperthyroidism. Radioiodine takes weeks to months to produce a significant clinical effect. It is used to destroy the thyroid gland following control of the hyperthyroidism with medications. High-dose iodine produces a blocking effect on the thyroid gland. It may be used following administration of PTU or methimazole (i.e., Lugol solution 10 drops every 8 hours; potassium iodide 3 drops every 8 hours; sodium iodine 1 g every 24 hours; or ipodate 500 mg orally daily). Iodine must be given after PTU or methimazole so as to prevent its use in the synthesis of additional thyroid hormone. One may also block the conversion of T_4 to T_3 in the peripheral organs with glucocorticoids (hydrocortisone 100 mg i.v. every 8 hours), PTU, or ipodate. Glucocorticoids are beneficial because they reduce conversion of T_4 to T_3, reduce levels of thyroid receptor antibodies, and treat the patient for possible underlying adrenal insufficiency. Drugs that decrease hyperadrenergic manifestations include beta-adrenergic blockers such as propranolol (40 to 60 mg orally every 6 hours or 0.5 to 1 mg i.v. every 5 to 10 minutes) or esmolol (50 to 200 μg per kg per minute). Most patients benefit from use of an antiadrenergic drug since thyroid hormone facilitates the action of the adrenergic system in target tissues (which leads to increased cardiac stimulation and increased tissue oxygen consumption). Beta-adrenergic blockers are tapered to control the heart rate (i.e., 80 to 100 beats per minute).

It is also important to provide supportive care (fluids, electrolytes, nutrition, control of body temperature) and treat underlying diseases (especially hypotension, heart failure, cardiac arrhythmias, sepsis, stroke, trauma). Elevated temperatures should not be treated with aspirin, which displaces thyroid hormone from its binding proteins. Centrally acting agents (prostaglandin inhibitors) are marginally effective in controlling fever because the increased temperature results from hypermetabolism in peripheral organs.

Thyroid storm (17,18) represents a life-threatening hypermetabolic crisis in a patient with underlying decompensated hyperthyroidism. It is characterized by end-organ dysfunction that includes fever, profuse sweating, psychosis, delirium, coma, heart failure, tachycardia, and ventricular arrhythmias. Vomiting, profuse diarrhea, and hepatomegaly with jaundice may occur. The clinical features of hyperthyroidism are worsened and cardiovascular collapse may result. It is often precipitated by underlying illnesses such as infection, myocardial infarction, stroke, diabetic ketoacidosis, surgery, or trauma. Treatment is multifactorial. Patients are usually given a combination of PTU (600 mg orally or by nasogastric tube, then 200 mg every 4 hours), iodine after PTU (Lugol solution 10 drops orally every 8 hours; potassium iodide 3 drops orally every 8 hours; sodium iodine 1 g i.v. every 24 hours; or ipodate 500–1000 mg orally every 24 hours), glucocorticoid (hydrocortisone 100 mg i.v. every 8 hours), and beta-adrenergic blocker (e.g., propranolol 40 to 80 mg orally every 4 to 6 hours; propranolol 0.5 to 1.0 mg i.v. every 5 to 10 minutes; or esmolol 50 to 200 μg per kg per minute i.v.). Fluid administration is often required to support intravascular volume and cooling may be required to control fever.

Rarely, one encounters patients in thyroid storm who cannot be treated with PTU or methimazole (e.g., due to a prior history of agranulocytosis). Surgery is precluded due to the high risk of worsening thyroid storm. In these patients, direct removal of thyroid hormone from the blood with plasmapheresis, charcoal plasma perfusion, or peritoneal dialysis can be beneficial (19,20). In patients with iodine allergies, lithium carbonate (300 mg every 6 hours) may be used to inhibit thyroid hormone release (21).

Iodine should not be used in patients with iodine-overload-induced hyperthyroidism or thyroid storm such as may be seen after radiocontrast dye administration or amiodarone. In such patients, antithyroid drugs should be used (as described above) in combination with potassium perchlorate, which blocks iodine uptake into thyroid cells (0.5 g daily). Many patients with asthma will not tolerate beta-adrenergic antagonists. Hyperadrenergic symptoms in these patients can be inhibited with reserpine (2.5 mg orally every 4 hours) or guanethidine (30 mg orally every 6 hours). Diltiazem has also been effective in controlling heart rate in hyperthyroid patients.

Some critically ill and older adult patients manifest what is termed apathetic hyperthyroidism. This is a form of hyperthyroidism in which symptoms and signs are localized to one or a few organ systems. Typical features may include one or more of the following: atrial fibrillation, weight loss, diarrhea, or poor sleep.

ADRENAL INSUFFICIENCY

The adrenal glands produce glucocorticoids, mineralocorticoids, sex hormones, and catecholamines. This discussion will focus upon the adrenal cortex and disease processes that alter the synthesis of the glucocorticoids (e.g., cortisol). Cortisol is required for function of all cells in the body. It is required for carbohydrate-protein-lipid metabolism, immune function, synthesis and action of catecholamines and adrenergic receptors, cardiac contractility, vascular tone, endothelial integrity, and numerous other functions. Deficiency of cortisol is associated with increased morbidity and mortality during critical illness. Absence of cortisol results in death of the organism.

Adrenal insufficiency (22) may result from destruction of the adrenal cortex (primary adrenal insufficiency), impairment of the hypothalamic-pituitary-adrenal (HPA) axis (secondary adrenal insufficiency), or tissue resistance to cortisol (Table 4). Primary

TABLE 4. CAUSES OF ADRENAL INSUFFICIENCY

I. Primary
  A. Infectious
    Human immunodeficiency virus (HIV)
    Bacterial sepsis
    Tuberculosis
    Meningococcemia
    Cytomegalovirus
    Fungal
  B. Thrombosis
    Heparin-induced
    Antiphospholipid syndrome
  C. Hemorrhage
    Coagulopathy
    Disseminated intravascular coagulation
    Anticoagulant use
  D. Cancer
  E. Autoimmune adrenalitis
  F. Drugs
    Ketoconazole
    Etomidate
    Megestrol acetate
II. Secondary
  A. Previous use of glucocorticoids
  B. Sepsis
  C. HIV
  D. Hypothalamic disease
    Cancer
    Infiltrative disease
      Sarcoidosis
      Histiocytosis
      Lymphoma
  E. Pituitary disease
    Tumors
    Surgery
    Irradiation
    Necrosis infarction
      Postpartum
    Head trauma
III. Tissue Glucocorticoid Resistance
  A. Sepsis
  B. Multiple-organ failure

adrenal insufficiency is associated with deficiency of both glucocorticoids and mineralocorticoids while secondary adrenal insufficiency involves primarily glucocorticoids (mineralocorticoid secretion remains intact).

The most common causes of primary adrenal insufficiency are infections. Gram-negative sepsis and human immunodeficiency virus (HIV) infection (23) are the most common infections associated with primary adrenal insufficiency in critically ill patients. Other infections causing primary adrenal insufficiency include meningococcal infections, fungal infection, and tuberculosis. Although it was once thought that direct organism invasion of the adrenal glands caused most cases of primary adrenal insufficiency, current evidence indicates that most critically ill patients develop a reversible form of adrenal insufficiency, which likely results from release of inflammatory mediators during infection and other cell injuries (24). These substances (e.g., tumor necrosis factor, corticostatin) impair adrenal gland synthesis of cortisol or inhibit corticotropin (e.g., adrenocorticotropic hormone [ACTH]) action on the adrenal glands (25–27). We have recently found that a significant number of patients with septic shock who develop adrenal insufficiency have ACTH resistance. Patients may also develop primary adrenal insufficiency as a result of thrombosis (e.g., disseminated intravascular coagulation, hypercoagulable states) or hemorrhage into the adrenal glands. Autoimmune adrenalitis and cancer are less common causes of primary adrenal insufficiency. Primary adrenal insufficiency may also result from the use of drugs such as etomidate and ketoconazole.

The most common etiology of secondary adrenal insufficiency is previous glucocorticoid use (Table 4). The second most common etiology is septic shock, in which impairment of the HPA axis is caused by substances (e.g., cytokines, peptides) released during sepsis. These substances suppress release of corticotropin-releasing hormone (CRH) and/or corticotropin. Gram-negative sepsis and HIV infection are commonly associated with septic shock-induced secondary adrenal insufficiency. Less common causes of secondary adrenal insufficiency involve destructive processes in the hypothalamus and pituitary regions (i.e., cancer, infiltrative diseases, sarcoidosis, hemochromatosis, surgery). Pituitary infarction (e.g., following trauma, thrombosis, or pregnancy) may also cause secondary adrenal insufficiency.

A third form of adrenal insufficiency results from tissue resistance to cortisol. This form of adrenal insufficiency is difficult to diagnose because patients may have high levels of circulating cortisol. However, cortisol fails to enter the cells. This form of adrenal insufficiency partially explains the high mortality associated with very high circulating cortisol levels. Adrenal insufficiency in these patients is diagnosed by demonstrating decreased clearance of cortisol from the circulation. Experimental models implicate an acquired defect in the glucocorticoid receptor for binding of cortisol. It is unclear whether this form of adrenal insufficiency improves with exogenous glucocorticoids.

Tissue deficiency of glucocorticoids affects all cells in the body. Unfortunately, most signs and symptoms of adrenal insufficiency are nonspecific and common in critically ill patients. Thus, a high index of suspicion is essential to the diagnosis. Cardiovascular insufficiency (i.e., hypotension, low systemic vascular resistance, impaired cardiac contractility) is common in critically ill patients with adrenal insufficiency (28) and usually improves with glucocorticoid treatment. Patients who remain hypotensive despite fluids and vasopressors have a high likelihood of having adrenal insufficiency. Other manifestations of adrenal insufficiency are weakness, anorexia, lethargy, mental depression, failure to wean from mechanical ventilation, abdominal pain, nausea, vomiting, diarrhea, and impaired wound healing. Laboratory findings include hyponatremia, hyperkalemia, salt wasting in the urine, hypoglycemia, and eosinophilia. One must always consider adrenal insufficiency in patients with underlying hypothalamic-pituitary disease or injury (i.e., head trauma, central nervous system surgery, gonadal dysfunction, optic nerve defects).

The diagnosis of adrenal insufficiency (29) has been hampered by a low index of suspicion of adrenal insufficiency on the part of the clinician and a failure to fully understand normal responses of the HPA axis to critical illness. An important issue relates to the normal circulating cortisol response to critical illness (an index of adrenal function). Hypotension, cardiac arrest, hypoglycemia, hypoxemia, multiple trauma with tissue injury, and major surgery are potent stimuli for cortisol secretion and test the integrity of the entire central nervous system–hypothalamic-pituitary-adrenal axis (CNS-HPA). Since the HPA axis evolved to respond to endogenous stresses, these stimuli are the "gold standards" for evaluating adrenal function. Thus, to define the normal cortisol response to critical illness one needs to examine levels of cortisol that are obtained during these endogenous stresses and not the response to biochemical stimuli (i.e., ACTH, CRH). When these responses (especially hypotension) have been used as the "gold standard" for stress, the vast majority of patients achieve circulating cortisol levels in excess of 25 to 30 μg per dL. Thus, this is the level that should be used when assessing adrenal gland function. Patients who fail to achieve a circulating stress cortisol in excess of 25 μg per dL should be considered to have adrenal insufficiency. It is important to note that stress (i.e., critical illness) tests the function of the entire CNS-HPA axis. It requires appropriate sensing of the stress by the CNS. Once sensed, there must be release of CRH from the hypothalamus and ACTH from the pituitary. The adrenal gland must also be capable of responding to corticotropin and synthesizing and releasing cortisol.

At times the level of stress is low or uncertain and a baseline cortisol is less than 25 μg per dL. To determine if the adrenal glands can respond appropriately to stress, dynamic testing is best. Induction of hypoglycemia (e.g., insulin tolerance test) may not be desirable. In these instances, one usually performs a corticotropin stimulation test. This test bypasses the CNS-HPA and stimulates the adrenal glands directly. Thus, it fails to evaluate the integrity of a large part of the CNS-HPA axis. Failure to respond to corticotropin with an elevation in circulating cortisol above 25 to 30 μg per dL at 30 to 60 minutes following corticotropin administration indicates the presence of adrenal insufficiency (primary or secondary). On the other hand, a normal response does not rule out adrenal insufficiency. Patients with acute-onset secondary adrenal insufficiency may continue to respond to the standard corticotropin stimulation test (250 μg corticotropin) for 10 to 14 days following CNS-hypothalamic-pituitary failure. Patients with partial secondary adrenal insufficiency (i.e., deficiency of CRH or ACTH) may respond normally to the standard corticotropin stimulation test but be unable to increase cortisol appropriately during stress. Patients with adrenal corticotropin resistance may also respond normally to the standard corticotropin stimulation test. The standard corticotropin stimulation test uses 250 μg corticotropin, which is 200-fold greater than stress ACTH levels. Thus, this high dose can override ACTH resistance. As a result, many metabolism experts now use the low-dose corticotropin stimulation test (1 to 2 μg) which uses stress levels of corticotropin (30–32). This test is more sensitive for diagnosing adrenal insufficiency. We recommend the low-dose corticotropin stimulation test when testing for adrenal insufficiency. In a recent study of patients with septic shock, we found that the standard corticotropin stimulation test had a 42% sensitivity for detecting adrenal insufficiency while the low-dose corticotropin stimulation test had a sensitivity of 76% (29). Some have advocated the use of the CRH stimulation test for diagnosing adrenal insufficiency in the intensive care unit (ICU) since it tests the integrity of both the pituitary and adrenal glands. However, experience with this test in the ICU is lacking.

We advocate treating all patients with suspected adrenal insufficiency with stress doses of hydrocortisone (100 mg every 8 hours) until results of testing (i.e., stress cortisol or low-dose corticotropin stimulation test) are available. If the stress cortisol is greater than 25 to 30 μg per dL, hydrocortisone can usually be discontinued. However, if the patient deteriorates following discontinuation of the hydrocortisone, it should be restarted and slowly tapered based upon clinical response.

The available data indicate that treatment of adrenal insufficiency with hydrocortisone improves outcome. Adrenalectomy in animals subjected to shock increases mortality, an effect reversed by corticosteroids. McKee and Finlay (33) randomized 18 critically ill patients with adrenal insufficiency to glucocorticoids or placebo. Steroid-treated patients had a 13% mortality versus 90% in placebo-treated patients. Use of etomidate, which causes adrenal insufficiency, increased mortality from 27% to 44% in multiple-trauma patients (34). We found that hydrocortisone treatment of septic shock patients with adrenal insufficiency improved survival from 35% to 68% (29). In addition, two recent prospective randomized studies of hydrocortisone treatment (100 mg every 8 hours) of patients with septic shock revealed improved outcome with hydrocortisone treatment. Bollaert and colleagues (35) randomized 41 critically ill septic patients to hydrocortisone or placebo and reported that glucocorticoid-treated patients had greater reversal of shock and lower mortality. Briegel and colleagues (36) randomized 40 septic patients to hydrocortisone or placebo. Hydrocortisone treatment was associated with improved shock reversal, decreased ventilator time, earlier resolution of organ dysfunction, and shorter ICU stay. A large multicenter prospective randomized trial of hydrocortisone versus placebo in patients with sepsis is underway. However, to date the results suggest that physiologic stress doses of hydrocortisone (100 mg every 8 hours for many days) improve outcome in patients with sepsis. These positive studies contrast with previous negative studies of steroids in sepsis, which used pharmacologic doses of steroids (e.g., 30 mg per kg methylprednisolone) for short periods (i.e., 1 to 2 doses).

PHEOCHROMOCYTOMA

Pheochromocytomas are tumors that arise from enterochromaffin tissue (37–40). Ninety percent arise from the adrenal medullae (10% bilateral) and 10% from extraadrenal loci (anywhere from the carotid bodies to the urinary bladder). Pheochromocytomas may occur along with other endocrine tumors (e.g., thyroid tumors, parathyroid hyperplasia) as part of the multiple-endocrine neoplasia syndromes. Most of these tumors are endocrinologically active and secrete a variety of hormones such as norepinephrine, epinephrine, and dopamine.

The signs and symptoms in patients with pheochromocytomas are usually the result of catecholamine excess. The most common sign (present in 90% of patients) is hypertension (0.1% of all hypertensive patients). Of the hypertensive patients, approximately 50% have sustained hypertension while the remaining half have paroxysmal blood pressure elevations that may reach life-threatening levels. Paroxysmal hypertension is often precipitated by acute physical stress such as trauma, surgery, and

induction of anesthesia. Hypertension may be precipitated by drugs that acutely lower blood pressure such as apresoline or saralasin; opiates such as morphine or fentanyl; glucagon; dopamine antagonists such as metoclopramide or droperidol; intraarterial injection of radiocontrast dye; atracurium or pancuronium; and cocaine, tricyclic antidepressants, and monoamine oxidase inhibitors. An important clue to the diagnosis of pheochromocytoma is that the hypertension is poorly responsive to standard antihypertensive agents. Complications of the hypertension include headache, congestive heart failure, myocardial infarction, renal failure, and cerebrovascular accidents. Clinical features of catecholamine excess also include sweating, cutaneous flushing, anxiety, panic attacks, peripheral vasoconstriction, skin pallor, tachycardia, palpitations, cardiac arrhythmias, angina pectoris, tremulousness, nausea, vomiting, decreased gastrointestinal motility, and acute abdominal pain. Occasionally, patients may present with orthostatic hypotension, severe fever, encephalopathy, seizures, and organ failure. Hypermetabolism resembling hyperthyroidism may occur. Fever and weight loss are not uncommon. The association of headache, sweating, and palpitations with hypertension has high sensitivity (91%) and specificity (93%) for the presence of pheochromocytomas. Glucose intolerance and hyperglycemia are common. Hypercalcemia is a rare manifestation.

The diagnosis of pheochromocytoma is confirmed using biochemical tests that assess catecholamines and their metabolic products. Classically, 24-hour urine collections for vanillylmandelic acid (VMA), metanephrine, normetanephrine, and free catecholamines are used to screen patients for the presence of pheochromocytoma. The diagnosis can be further confirmed using plasma catecholamine levels and suppression testing with clonidine (if initial results are equivocal). At times it may be difficult to separate the patient with critical illness from the patient with a pheochromocytoma. Definitive diagnosis in these patients may have to await recovery from illness. In the intervening period, treatment of the patient for pheochromocytoma should be initiated. Following biochemical confirmation of the presence of a pheochromocytoma, localization studies are essential to direct surgical removal of the tumor. A variety of procedures are available and include computerized tomography, magnetic resonance imaging, radioiodinated metaiodobenzylguanidine (MIBG) scanning, and vena caval sampling for catecholamines.

Definitive treatment of pheochromocytoma involves surgical removal of the functioning tumor. However, prior to surgery and in some patients in whom surgery is not possible, medical management is required (37–40). Medical management is geared toward control of hypertension and associated cardiovascular symptoms. Phenoxybenzamine (initial dose 10 mg twice daily), a noncompetitive alpha-adrenergic receptor blocker, is the drug of choice to control blood pressure when treatment is not emergent. The drug allows for reexpansion of intravascular volume (which usually takes 1 to 2 weeks). Other alpha-adrenergic agents that can be used include prazosin hydrochloride (begin at 1 mg every 6 hours; may increase to 5 mg every 6 hours), terazosin (2 to 5 mg twice daily), and doxazosin (2 to 8 mg daily). Intravenous phentolamine (2 to 5 mg i.v. bolus followed by 1 mg per minute infusion) can be used to manage hypertensive crises when immediate blood pressure lowering effects are required. Intravenous sodium nitroprusside (0.5 to 1.5 μg per kg per minute) has also been used with success. In addition, calcium channel blockers (e.g., nicardipine, diltiazem) are effective for the control of blood pressure in most patients with pheochromocytoma. Combination of an alpha-adrenergic antagonist with a calcium channel blocker is useful in refractory hypertensive cases. Beta-adrenergic antagonists are contraindicated in the absence of alpha$_1$-adrenergic blockade because of exacerbation of vasoconstriction and precipitation of hypertensive crisis. Although labetalol (a beta- and alpha-adrenergic antagonist) has been used successfully in some cases, there are reports of it worsening hypertension in some patients (which may relate to the drug's predominant beta-blocking activity). Beta-adrenergic blockers are added to control tachycardia and cardiac arrhythmias, once blood pressure is controlled with an alpha-adrenergic antagonist. Esmolol (500 μg per kg loading dose followed by 50 to 200 μg per kg per minute), a selective beta$_1$-adrenergic antagonist with a short duration of action, should be used in unstable patients or when a short duration of beta-blockade is desired. Catecholamine-induced arrhythmias usually respond to i.v. lidocaine. Some patients (especially patients with unresectable tumors) may benefit from treatment with alpha-methyl-L-tyrosine (metyrosine), an inhibitor of tyrosine hydroxylase (the rate-limiting step in catecholamine synthesis). Combination therapy of metyrosine with an alpha-adrenergic antagonist is also useful for patients undergoing surgical resection of pheochromocytomas (41).

Patients with pheochromocytoma have high fluid requirements (before and after surgery). Postoperative patients are at risk for bleeding and may require blood as well as fluids to maintain blood pressure and oxygen-carrying capacity. Hypoglycemia is common after removal of tumors. Causes include depletion of glycogen stores and rebound hyperinsulinemia.

CARCINOID SYNDROME

Carcinoid tumors (42,43) arise from serotonin-producing enterochromaffin cells and most occur in the gut (40% in the appendix). Most carcinoids are nonfunctioning and of no clinical consequence. However, because these tumors occur throughout the gastrointestinal tract and may metastasize and produce the carcinoid syndrome, it is important to be knowledgeable of the emergency management of this syndrome.

The major manifestations of the carcinoid syndrome that require therapy are flushing and diarrhea (present in most cases), cardiac disease (25%), bronchospasm (10%), and hepatic enlargement and pain. Cardiac disease includes congestive failure, fibrotic valvular lesions, and metastatic involvement of the myocardium or pericardium. Hypotension and shock may occur in a severe carcinoid crisis. Minor features of the syndrome include peptic ulcer disease, severe hypoalbuminemia, pellagra, muscle wasting, myopathy, arthropathy, retroperitoneal fibrosis, brawny edema, and hyperglycemia. Rarely, one may encounter inferior or superior venacaval obstruction, intestinal obstruction, or gastrointestinal bleeding.

Carcinoids vary in the quantity of peptides produced (e.g., serotonin, bradykinin, prostaglandin E$_2$, substance P, neurotensin, motilin, histamine, and endorphins). Unless the tumor arises in an area that drains directly into the central circulation, large deposits of carcinoid metastases are needed in the liver before manifestations of the syndrome are apparent. Diagnosis of the disease can be made by measuring levels of indole metabolites in the urine or serotonin and chromogranin-A in the blood. Once the syndrome is clinically present, cure by surgical resection is usually not possible.

Adrenergic agonists, such as epinephrine, and stress can precipitate the carcinoid syndrome. Importantly, hypotension and shock should be treated with the direct acting vasoconstrictor, methoxamine, to avoid exacerbation of hypotension, bronchospasm, and shock. Monoamine oxidase inhibitors (e.g., found in some antidepressants) should be avoided since they prolong the action of serotonin and other amines.

Therapy is aimed at control of clinical features and palliation of the tumors (42,43). Palliation of tumor may be accomplished with chemotherapy and hepatic artery embolization and chemotherapy injection (42). Initial treatment is directed at preventing or reducing the tumor's chemical production, inhibiting release of these substances, and blocking the effects on target tissues. Octreotide, the most useful and specific drug available for treating carcinoid syndrome, is effective in most cases for control of diarrhea, flushing, bronchospasm, and hypotension. It is usually administered by s.c. injection (0.05 to 0.5 mg) every 8 to 12 hours. Other drugs that may be useful in treating symptoms (especially diarrhea and flushing) include diphenoxylate plus atropine, loperamide, cyproheptadine (antiserotonin), methysergide (antiserotonin), propantheline (anticholinergic), combined histamine-1 and histamine-2 receptor antagonists, clonidine, and ondansetron (5-hydroxytryptamine-3 receptor antagonist). Most patients with secretory diarrhea are depleted of fluids and electrolytes and malnourished (vitamin deficiencies and protein deficiency). Niacin synthesis is deficient because of conversion of its precursor tryptophan to serotonin and should be replaced. Patients with the carcinoid syndrome tolerate anesthesia and surgery poorly and should be premedicated with octreotide (0.1 to 0.5 mg s.c. prior to the procedure), an antiserotonin drug such as ondansetron or methotrimeprazine, an antikinin agent such as aprotinin, and hydrocortisone (inhibits prostaglandin and kinin production; 100 mg i.v.). Additional octreotide (50 μg i.v. followed by an infusion) may be given during the procedure to treat symptoms. If hypotension develops and fails to respond to octreotide, i.v. methoxamine is the agent of choice for treating the hypotension. In the rare patient who develops hypertension that does not respond to the above treatments, nitroprusside can be used to lower blood pressure.

HYPERGLYCEMIC EMERGENCIES (DIABETES MELLITUS)

Hyperglycemic emergencies usually result from insulin deficiency (absolute or relative) in patients with diabetes mellitus. Insulin deficiency may result from lack of insulin secretion to meet metabolic demands, insulin receptor defects, postreceptor defects, or circulating insulin antibodies. There is also often an elevation in insulin-antagonistic hormones (e.g., epinephrine, norepinephrine, glucagon, cortisol, growth hormone), which contributes to an insulin-deficient state. The net effect of insulin deficiency is hyperglycemia and/or ketosis. Hyperglycemia results from increased liver gluconeogenesis (from amino acids), increased liver glycogenolysis, and decreased tissue utilization of glucose. Ketosis results from increased lipolysis, increased fatty acid oxidation, decreased liver synthesis of very low-density lipoprotein, and decreased peripheral use of fatty acids and ketones. However, it is important to realize that insulin deficiency also alters protein-carbohydrate-lipid metabolism, accelerates atherosclerosis, causes neuropathy and retinopathy, and causes renal and other end-organ disease.

Patients with diabetes mellitus fall into three major categories. Patients may require insulin to prevent diabetic ketoacidosis (DKA) or hyperglycemic hyperosmolar nonketotic syndrome (HHNS). These patients are "insulin-dependent" and have type I diabetes mellitus. Most acquire their diabetes while young and have near total destruction of their islet cells. The second group of patients require insulin to maintain "normal" blood glucose levels. These patients have type II or "insulin-requiring" diabetes mellitus. Most of these patients have elevated insulin levels and a receptor or postreceptor defect. The third group of patients have hyperglycemia that can be controlled with diet or oral hypoglycemic agents. They are a subgroup of type II diabetes mellitus.

Acute metabolic decompensation in a diabetic patient may result in DKA or HHNS (44–48). Decompensation may be associated with cessation of insulin therapy, stress (increased counterregulatory hormones), drug use (antagonizes insulin action), or excess intake of carbohydrates.

The clinical features of DKA and HHNS relate primarily to hyperglycemia (both DKA and HHNS) and ketosis (DKA). Hyperglycemia results in an osmotic diuresis, fluid and electrolyte losses, hyperosmolality, dehydration, and volume depletion. Reduction in the filtered load of glucose by the kidney aggravates the hyperglycemia. Vomiting and decreased oral intake adds to the state of volume depletion. Ketosis causes a metabolic acidosis and contributes to an osmotic diuresis. Clinical manifestations of the syndromes include malaise, weakness, dehydration, polyuria, polydipsia, muscle aches, depressed mental status, drowsiness, stupor, coma, headache, tachycardia, arrhythmias, hypotension, heart failure, anorexia, nausea/vomiting, gastric stasis, abdominal pain, ileus, hyperpnea, Kussmaul breathing (DKA only), and fruity odor on the breath (DKA only).

The laboratory features of DKA and HHNS include hyperglycemia, ketosis (DKA only), hyperosmolality (estimated as $P_{osm} = [2 \times Na$ mEq per L] + glucose [mg per dL]/18 + blood urea nitrogen [mg per dL]/2.8), glucosuria, ketonuria, acidosis (DKA only, anion gap), altered electrolyte levels (Na^+, K^+, Mg^+, PO_4^-), leukocytosis, azotemia, and elevated enzymes (amylase, CPK, hepatic transaminases). Patients may also develop lactic acidosis when tissue perfusion is poor. Hyperkalemia may occur during the initial presentation due to insulinopenia, accelerated loss of intracellular potassium (catabolism), acidosis, and solvent drag. Levels of potassium decrease rapidly during treatment.

The diagnosis of DKA or HHNS should be suspected in patients presenting with altered mental status, dehydration, hypotension, hyperpnea, vomiting, acetone on the breath, polyuria, and polydipsia. The diagnosis can be easily confirmed at the bedside using a blood glucose analyzer and urine ketone test.

Serum ketones are assessed using the nitroprusside reaction. This test reacts primarily with acetoacetate (AcAc) and not beta-hydroxybutyrate (BOHB). Thus, ketone levels may appear low when most of the ketones are in the form of BOHB. In addition, BOHB is metabolized to AcAc during recovery from DKA. Measured ketone levels may increase as the patient is improving. Thus, we do not advocate following serum ketones closely during therapy. We test them initially when making the diagnosis. We follow the anion gap and blood pH during treatment with fluids and insulin. We only test the ketones again at the end of therapy to be sure that the ketosis has resolved.

The goals for the treatment of DKA and HHNS are to restore fluid status and electrolytes to normal, provide insulin, and identify and treat underlying disease. Isotonic glucose-free crystalloids should be given to restore intravascular volume and urinary output to normal. Once restored, additional fluid administration

TABLE 5. ELECTROLYTE ALTERATIONS DURING DIABETIC KETOACIDOSIS

Electrolyte	Average Body Deficit	Recommended Treatment
Sodium	Slightly negative	1. Hyponatremia: reflects dilution due to elevated glucose and retention of water; partially results from elevated ADH and intake of hypotonic fluids; improves with lowering of glucose; restrict free water, may occasionally require saline + furosemide 2. Hypernatremia: usually indicates dehydration
Potassium	3–10 mEq/kg	1. Hypokalemia: give K 20–40 mEq/h (10 mEq/h if oliguric), follow K level 2. Normal K level: give K 20 mEq/h, follow K level 3. Hyperkalemic: no K until K level normalizes *Note:* K levels will decrease during therapy due to dilution from fluids, K loss in urine, and intracellular shift from insulin
Magnesium	Low total body levels	1. Hypomagnesemia: give Mg 2. Normal or elevated Mg: follow levels; will decrease during therapy
Phosphorus	1 mmol/kg	1. Hypophosphatemia: give PO_4 (250 mg every 6 h orally or give K_2PO_4 5–8 mmol/6 h i.v.) 2. Normal or elevated PO_4: follow levels, will decrease during therapy
Bicarbonate	Low serum levels reflect HCO_3 loss in urine and underlying metabolic acidosis	Give HCO_3 if pH < 6.9 or HCO_3 < 5–7 mEq/L

ADH, antidiuretic hormone; K, potassium; Mg, magnesium; PO_4, phosphate; i.v., intravenous.

is guided by the serum sodium level and clinical response. The average volume deficit in patients presenting with DKA/HHNS averages between 6 to 10 L. We usually give an initial bolus of 1 L 0.9% saline, followed by 1 L in the next hour and another L over the next 2 hours. This is followed by a maintenance infusion of 250 to 500 mL per hour of 0.9% or 0.45% saline. Fluid losses in both DKA and HHNS are largely hypotonic and hypotonic fluids are required to rehydrate cells. Thus, once intravascular volume is replaced, we usually switch to hypotonic fluids. When blood glucose decreases below 250 mg per dL, we consider adding dextrose to the infusion.

We monitor blood pressure, heart rate, respiratory rate, urinary output, blood glucose, blood pH, anion gap, and serum/blood electrolytes during therapy. Rarely do we require central hemodynamic monitoring with a pulmonary arterial catheter. The most common electrolyte disorders encountered in patients with DKA/HHNS involve sodium, potassium, phosphorus, and magnesium (Table 5). Levels of electrolytes (especially potassium) change rapidly during initial treatment and must be monitored at frequent intervals (i.e., every 4 to 6 hours) to avoid complications such as cardiac arrhythmias and respiratory failure. Serum potassium decreases during therapy due to dilution with i.v. fluids, increased renal clearance, and insulin action. Most patients require 10 to 40 mEq of potassium per hour to maintain normal levels.

Bicarbonate is rarely required and should be reserved for the few patients with severe metabolic acidosis (i.e., pH less than 6.9 or bicarbonate less than 5 to 7 mEq per L) or severe hyperkalemia. Bicarbonate should only be administered to raise pH to 7.1 and bicarbonate to 10 mEq per L. Ketoacidosis will resolve during treatment as ketones are metabolized to bicarbonate. Administration of exogenous bicarbonate prolongs the ketotic state and causes rebound alkalosis (49,50). Hyperchloremic acidosis may develop during treatment secondary to loss of ketones (bicarbonate precursors) and use of high-chloride–containing fluids. Hyperchloremic acidosis usually resolves with a decrease in chloride intake (i.e., use of 0.45% saline).

Following restoration of intravascular volume, insulin should be administered (44–48,50) (Table 6). Insulin, administered before volume resuscitation, can lead to further reductions in circulating volume as a result of glucose (and water) movement into cells. Insulin may be administered i.v., i.m., or s.c. The preferred route for initial treatment of DKA or HHNS is the i.v. route. Regular insulin is the only form approved for i.v. administration. Human insulin is the preferred type. It is not essential that one administer a loading dose of insulin (due to its short half-life). However, some prefer a loading dose of 5 to 10 U i.v. regular insulin. We usually begin i.v. infusion of insulin at 5 to 10 U regular insulin per hour. Glucose is monitored at the bedside and the dose adjusted to provide for a decrease in glucose of approximately 100 mg per dL per hour. When the glucose level

TABLE 6. INSULIN CHARACTERISTICS

Type of Insulin	Route	Peak	Duration
Regular	i.v.	1–5 min	1–2 h
	i.m.	5–10 min	2–4 h
	s.c.	1–3 h	4–6 h
Intermediate-acting insulin (NPH)	s.c.	6–8 h	12–18 h

reaches 250 mg per dL, dextrose-containing fluids are added, the insulin infusion is decreased to 1 to 4 U per hour, and the infusion is continued until acidosis and ketosis resolve. The patient is then switched to s.c. intermediate-acting insulin (NPH). Half the total infusion dose is given s.c. every 12 hours and the patient supplemented with regular insulin by sliding scale. If the i.v. route is not available, one may administer regular insulin i.m. (begin with 5 to 10 U every 2 to 4 hours). In patients with refractory hyperglycemia, administration of octreotide (decreases glucagon levels) or addition of an oral hypoglycemic agent (50) may improve glucose control.

It is also important to treat the underlying precipitating cause of the DKA or HHNS. Common precipitating causes include infection (e.g., pneumonia, urinary tract infection, meningitis, sinusitis), surgery, trauma, burns, myocardial infarction, stroke, pancreatitis, gastrointestinal bleed, failure to take insulin, and drugs (e.g., steroids, thiazides, phenytoin). Most patients who reach the hospital do not die from DKA or HHNS. Mortality usually relates to the underlying disease that caused metabolic decompensation. However, patients may occasionally die or suffer injury from complications of their diabetic treatment. Such complications include shock, hypoglycemia, hypokalemia (with arrhythmias), hypophosphatemia, hypomagnesemia, fluid overload (e.g., pulmonary edema, heart failure), myocardial infarction, cerebral edema (especially when glucose is lowered rapidly), thrombosis, and disseminated intravascular coagulation.

SUMMARY

Overproduction or underproduction of hormones from endocrine glands impairs cell and organ function. Altered production of some hormones does not cause significant organ dysfunction and does not result in life-threatening conditions. However, altered production of ADH, PTH, thyroid hormone, cortisol, catecholamines, serotonin, and insulin can impair organ function and if left untreated result in life-threatening emergencies. The presentation and acute management of these conditions has been discussed in this chapter. Optimal outcome requires that all physicians be familiar with the emergency management of these endocrine syndromes.

KEY POINTS

■ Diabetes insipidus, if untreated, results in water loss, hypernatremia, hyperosmolality, cellular dehydration, and volume depletion.

■ Most critically ill patients have low albumin levels and low total serum calcium levels despite normal ionized calcium levels.

- The treatment of thyroid storm includes propylthiouracil, iodine (after propylthiouracil), glucocorticoids, and beta-adrenergic blockers.
- Patients subjected to the stress of critical illness usually have serum cortisol levels in excess of 25 to 30 μg per dL; if the level is lower in a stressed patient, the corticotropin stimulation test can be used to determine if the adrenal glands can respond appropriately to stress.
- The pharmacologic management of pheochromocytoma, pending definitive surgical treatment, consists of phenoxybenzamine (or other alpha-adrenergic blockers), sometimes calcium entry blockers (in refractory hypertension), and beta-adrenergic blockers (require preceding alpha-1 blockage).
- The goals for the treatment of diabetic ketoacidosis and hyperglycemic hyperosmolar nonketotic syndrome include restoring fluid status and electrolytes to normal and identifying and treating the underlying disease.

REFERENCES

1. Robinson AG, Verbalis JG. Diabetes insipidus. In: Bardin CW, ed. *Current therapy in endocrinology and metabolism*, 6th ed. St. Louis: Mosby, 1997:1–7.
2. Ober KP. Diabetes insipidus. *Crit Care Clin* 1991;7:109–125.
3. Buonocore CM, Robinson AG. The diagnosis and management of diabetes insipidus during medical emergencies. *Endocrinol Metab Clin North Am* 1993;22:411–423.
4. Zaloga GP, Roberts PR. Calcium, magnesium and phosphorus disorders. In: Grenvik A, Ayres SM, Holbrook PR, eds. *Textbook of critical care*, 4th ed. Philadelphia: WB Saunders, 2000:862–875.
5. Marx SJ. Hyperparathyroid and hypoparathyroid disorders. *N Engl J Med* 2000;343:1863–1875.
6. Rude RK. Hypocalcemia and hypoparathyroidism. In: Bardin CW, ed. *Current therapy in endocrinology and metabolism*, 6th ed. St. Louis: Mosby, 1997:546–551.
7. Jan de Beur SM, Levine MA. Hypercalcemia. In: Bardin CW, ed. *Current therapy in endocrinology and metabolism*, 6th ed. St. Louis: Mosby, 1997:551–556.
8. Attie JN. Primary hyperparathyroidism. In Bardin CW, ed. *Current therapy in endocrinology and metabolism*, 6th ed. St. Louis: Mosby, 1997:557–565.
9. Zaloga GP, Chernow B, Cook D, et al. Assessment of calcium homeostasis in the critically ill surgical patient. The diagnostic pitfalls of the McClean-Hastings nomogram. *Ann Surg* 1985;202:587–594.
10. Singer PA, Cooper DS, Levy EG, et al. Treatment guidelines for patients with hyperthyroidism and hypothyroidism. *JAMA* 1995;273:808–812.
11. Ringel MD. Management of hypothyroidism and hyperthyroidism in the intensive care unit. *Crit Care Clin* 2001;17:59–74.
12. Gaitan E, Cooper DS. Primary hypothyroidism. In: Bardin CW, ed. *Current therapy in endocrinology and metabolism*, 6th ed. St. Louis: Mosby, 1997:94–98.
13. Pittman CS, Zayed AA. Myxedema coma. In: Bardin CW, ed. *Current therapy in endocrinology and metabolism*, 6th ed. St. Louis: Mosby, 1997:98–101.
14. Jordan RM. Myxedema coma–pathophysiology, therapy and factors affecting prognosis. *Med Clin North Am* 1995;79:185–194.
15. Nicoloff JT, Lopresti JS. Myxedema coma–a form of decompensated hypothyroidism. *Endocrinol Metab Clin North Am* 1993;22:279–290.
16. Hashizume K, Suzuki S. Hyperthyroidism. In: Bardin CW, ed. *Current therapy in endocrinology and metabolism*, 6th ed. St. Louis: Mosby, 1997:71–76.
17. Dillmann WH. Thyroid storm. In: Bardin CW, ed. *Current therapy in endocrinology and metabolism*, 6th ed. St. Louis: Mosby, 1997:81–85.
18. Burch HB, Wartofsky L. Life-threatening thyrotoxicosis: thyroid storm. *Endocrinol Metab Clin North Am* 1993;22:263–277.
19. Candrina R, DiStefano O, Spandrio S, et al. Treatment of thyrotoxic storm by charcoal plasmaperfusion. *J Endocrinol Invest* 1989; 12: 133–134.
20. Tajiri J, Katsuya H, Kiyokayo T. Successful treatment of thyrotoxic crisis with plasma exchange. *Crit Care Med* 1984; 12: 536–537.
21. Lazarus JH, Richards AR, Addission GH, et al. Treatment of thyrotoxicosis with lithium carbonate. *Lancet* 1974;2:1160–1163.
22. Oelkers W. Adrenal insufficiency. *N Engl J Med* 1996;335:1206.
23. Membreno L, Irony I, Dere W, et al. Adrenocortical function in the acquired immune deficiency syndrome. *J Clin Endocrinol Metab* 1987;65:482.
24. Soni A, Pepper GM, Wyrwinski PM, et al. Adrenal insufficiency occurring during septic shock: incidence, outcome, and relationship to peripheral cytokine levels. *Am J Med* 1995;98:266.
25. Gaillard RC, Turnill D, Sappino P, et al. Tumor necrosis factor alpha inhibits the hormonal response of the pituitary gland to hypothalamic releasing factors. *Endocrinology* 1990;127:101.
26. Zhu Q, Solomon S. Isolation and mode of action of rabbit corticostatin (antiadrenocorticotropin) peptides. *Endocrinology* 1992;130:1413.
27. Jaattela M, Ilvesmaki V, Voutilainen R, et al. Tumor necrosis factor as a potent inhibitor of adrenocorticotropin-induced cortisol production and steroidogenic P450 enzyme gene expression in cultured human fetal adrenal cells. *Endocrinology* 1991;128:623.
28. Lamberts SWJ, Bruining HA, deJong FH. Corticosteroid therapy in severe illness. *N Engl J Med* 1997;337:1285.
29. Zaloga GP, Marik P. Hypothalamic-pituitary-adrenal insufficiency. *Crit Care Clin* 2001;17:25–41.
30. Richards ML, Caplan RH, Wickus GG, et al. The rapid low dose (1 μg) cosyntropin test in the immediate postoperative period: results in elderly subjects after major abdominal surgery. *Surgery* 1999;125:431.
31. Tordjman K, Jaffe A, Grazas N, et al. The role of the low dose (1 μg) adrenocorticotropin test in the evaluation of patients with pituitary disease. *J Clin Endocrinol Metab* 1995;80:1301.
32. Rasmuson S, Olsson T, Hagg E. A low dose ACTH test to assess the function of the hypothalamic-pituitary-adrenal axis. *Clin Endocrinol* 1996;44:151.
33. McKee JI, Finlay WEI. Cortisol replacement in severely stressed patients. *Lancet* 1983;1:484.
34. Ledingham IM, Watt I. Influence of sedation on mortality in critically ill multiple trauma patients. *Lancet* 1983;1:1270.
35. Bollaert PE, Charpentier C, Levy B, et al. Reversal of late septic shock with supraphysiologic doses of hydrocortisone. *Crit Care Med* 1998;26:645.
36. Briegel J, Forst H, Haller M, et al. Stress doses of hydrocortisone reverse hyperdynamic septic-shock: a prospective randomized double-blind single-center study. *Crit Care Med* 1999;27:723.
37. Bravo EL. Pheochromocytoma. In: Bardin CW, ed. *Current therapy in endocrinology and metabolism*, 6th ed. St. Louis: Mosby, 1997:195–197.
38. Boutros AR, Bravo EL, Zanettin G, et al. Perioperative management of 63 patients with pheochromocytoma. *Clev Clin J Med* 1990;57:613–617.
39. Bravo EL. Evolving concepts in the pathophysiology, diagnosis and treatment of pheochromocytoma. *Endocrinol Rev* 1994;15:356–368.
40. Mueller GL. Pheochromocytoma. *Problems Crit Care* 1990;4:372–381.
41. Perry RR, Keiser HR, Norton JA, et al. Surgical management of

pheochromocytoma with the use of metyrosine. *Ann Surg* 1990;212:
621–628.

42. Warner RRP. Gut neuroendocrine tumors. In: Bardin CW, ed. *Current therapy in endocrinology and metabolism*, 6th ed. St. Louis: Mosby, 1997:606–614.

43. Arnold R, Kloppel G, Rothmond M. Carcinoid tumors. *Digestion* 1994;55[Suppl 3]:1–115.

44. Magee MF, Bhatt BA. Management of decompensated diabetes–diabetic ketoacidosis and hyperglycemia hyperosmolar syndrome. *Crit Care Clin* 2001;17:75–106.

45. Kitabchi AE, Wall BM. Diabetic ketoacidosis. *Med Clin North Am* 1995;79:9.

46. Genuth SM. Diabetic ketoacidosis and hyperglycemic hyperosmolar

coma. In: Bardin CW, ed. *Current therapy in endocrinology and metabolism*, 6th ed. St. Louis: Mosby, 1997:438–447.

47. DeFronzo RA, Matsuda M, Barrett EJ. Diabetic ketoacidosis: a combined metabolic-nephrologic approach to therapy. *Diabetes Metab Rev* 1994;2:209–238.

48. Fleckman AM. Diabetic ketoacidosis. *Endocrinol Metab Clin North Am* 1993;22:181–207.

49. Okuda Y, Adrogue HJ, Field JB, et al. Counterproductive effects of sodium bicarbonate in diabetic ketoacidosis. *J Clin Endocrinol Metab* 1996;81:314.

50. Zaloga GP, Chernow B. Insulin and oral hypoglycemics. In: Chernow B, ed. *The pharmacologic approach to the critically ill patient*, 3rd ed. Baltimore: Williams & Wilkins, 1994:758–776.

CARE OF CRITICALLY ILL OBSTETRIC PATIENTS

JAMES W. VAN HOOK
RAKESH B. VADHERA

KEY WORDS
■ Amniotic fluid embolism   ■ Monitoring, fetal heart rate
■ Beat-to-beat variability   ■ Preeclampsia
■ Late deceleration   ■ Variable deceleration

INTRODUCTION

Intensive care of the pregnant or recently postpartum patient is simultaneously similar to and different from general intensive care of the nonpregnant adult. Changes in maternal physiology, fetal considerations, and the presence of disease states unique to pregnancy are all challenges to successful critical care of the pregnant woman facing critical illness. This chapter highlights the similarities and differences of obstetric critical care and discusses specific topics germane to the diagnosis and treatment of the critically ill mother and fetus.

NORMAL AND ABNORMAL PREGNANCY

Pregnancy normally is characterized by a gestation of 260 to 294 days (37–42 weeks) from the last normal menstrual period (arbitrarily determined to be 2 weeks before actual fertilization). Delivery before 37 weeks' gestation is described as *preterm*. In the United States, most persistent morbidity and mortality from prematurity occur in infants born before 32 weeks' gestation. The imprecise phrase *fetal viability* usually is defined as the gestational age at which 50% survival is expected. In the United States, fetal viability (serious morbidity notwithstanding) is between 24 and 26 weeks' gestation (1). Birth weight and fetal condition at birth also profoundly influence fetal outcome. The management of critically ill pregnant patients always includes consideration of neonatal outcome if delivery is accomplished. Treatment of pathophysiology initiated or aggravated by pregnancy always includes risk-to-benefit evaluations for both mother and fetus. The relative maternal and fetal risks may change as the fetus grows and develops. Therefore, appropriate treatment or pregnancy

intervention may differ, depending on the gestational age of the pregnancy.

PHYSIOLOGIC CHANGES SECONDARY TO PREGNANCY

During pregnancy, many important physiologic adaptations contribute to successful outcome. These adaptations strongly influence the treatment of critically ill obstetric patients. The following physiologic changes are relevant to intensive care.

Blood Volume

By late pregnancy, maternal plasma volume increases by as much as 50% above prepregnancy levels. Red cell mass also increases, but to a lesser extent, resulting in a mild, relative "anemia" (2). The maternal red cell 2,3-diphosphoglycerate concentration is increased during pregnancy, helping to facilitate maternal-to-fetal oxygen transport (3).

Hemodynamics

Mean arterial blood pressure decreases by midpregnancy and then gradually rises toward prepregnancy values near term. Cardiac output increases by 30% to 50%, accompanied by a reciprocal decrease in total peripheral resistance, with most changes occurring by 28 to 32 weeks' gestation (4). Although the precise etiology is not known, these changes may result from altered ventricular filling as blood volume increases and a transplacental arteriovenous (A-V) shunt develops as a result of low-resistance choriodecidual vessels. Hyperreninism and aldosterone-mediated volume expansion, coupled with relatively reduced responsiveness of vascular smooth muscle, could account for the hemodynamic effects present during normal pregnancy. Clark and colleagues (5) measured hemodynamic changes during normal late pregnancy by serial placement of pulmonary arterial (PA) catheters in normal parturients (Table 1). It is important to note that the decrease in plasma colloid osmotic pressure as pregnancy progresses to term may predispose the gravid woman to pulmonary edema.

TABLE 1. HEMODYNAMICS OF LATE PREGNANCY AND THE POSTPARTUM PERIOD IN NORMAL WOMEN[a]

Parameter	Late Pregnancy	Postpartum	Change[b] (%)
Cardiac output (L/min)	6.2 ± 1	4.3 ± 1	+43
Mean arterial pressure (mm Hg)	90 ± 6	86 ± 8	NS
Heart rate (beats/min)	83 ± 10	71 ± 10	+17
Systemic vascular resistance (dyne·sec·cm^{-5})	$1,210 \pm 266$	$1,530 \pm 520$	−21
Central venous pressure (mm Hg)	4 ± 3	4 ± 3	NS
Pulmonary artery wedge pressure (mm Hg)	8 ± 2	6 ± 2	NS
Pulmonary vascular resistance (dyne·sec·cm^{-5})	78 ± 22	119 ± 47	−34
Colloid osmotic pressure (mm Hg)	18 ± 1.5	0.8 ± 1	−14
Left ventricular stroke work index (g·m·m^{-2})	49 ± 6	41 ± 8	NS

NS, not significant at $P, < 0.05$.
[a]All measurements are mean ± standard deviation.
[b]In comparison with postpartum levels, assumed to be comparable to nonpregnant levels.
Adapted from Clark SL, Cotton DB, Lee W, et al. Central hemodynamic assessment of normal term pregnancy. *Am J Obstet Gynecol* 1989;161:1439–1442, with permission.

Gas Exchange and Acid–Base Changes

In the second half of pregnancy, several important changes in lung volumes and capacities occur (6,7). Total lung capacity remains unchanged during pregnancy. Tidal volume (V_T) increases by approximately 200 mL, thus decreasing expiratory reserve volume and functional residual capacity (FRC). Under normal circumstances, these changes place critical closing capacity (CC) very near the FRC. Under situations in which FRC is further decreased (mechanical ventilation, supine positioning, and obesity) or CC is increased (small airway disease), airway closure may occur during tidal breathing.

Total airway resistance is probably unchanged during pregnancy, perhaps as a result of the offsetting effects of small airway vascular congestion and large airway bronchodilation. One-second forced expiratory volume is not altered during pregnancy. Total minute exhaled volume (V_E) and alveolar ventilation (V_A) both increase by 40% to 50% during pregnancy (being mediated predominantly by the increase in V_T). The increase in V_A occurs despite increased dead space from bronchodilation.

Because of pregnancy-associated increases in V_A, the partial pressure of carbon dioxide in arterial blood ($Paco_2$) is decreased by 5 to 10 mm Hg compared with the nonpregnant state. A compensated respiratory alkalosis with reduced serum bicarbonate is therefore normal. The net effects of chronic compensated respiratory alkalosis reduce serum buffering capacity (by decreasing bicarbonate) and increase the partial pressure of oxygen in alveolar gas (Pao_2) at any given fractional concentration of oxygen in inspired gas. Nonetheless, under normal circumstances, the partial pressure of oxygen in arterial blood (Pao_2) changes little during normal pregnancy (7). Intrapulmonary shunt (Qs/Qt) is somewhat increased during pregnancy. In healthy, pregnant patients, position change does not appear to appreciably affect intrapulmonary shunt (8).

Metabolic Alterations

To detail all the metabolic changes that occur during pregnancy is beyond the scope of this chapter; however, several particularly important adaptations occur. Basal metabolic energy expenditure increases during pregnancy. By late pregnancy, the fetoplacental

unit requires approximately an additional 1,260 kJ daily. Maternal fasting hypoglycemia is evident early in gestation. Fasting blood glucose is reduced by 5 to 10 mg per deciliter by 10 to 15 weeks of pregnancy. Hence, pregnancy is a condition of "accelerated starvation" (9) Conversely, in the second half of pregnancy, relative insulin resistance in response to the fed state is apparent. This decreased tolerance to carbohydrates occurs despite exaggerated insulin release in response to a given carbohydrate load. Late in pregnancy, gravid patients are therefore predisposed to primary glucose intolerance [gestational diabetes mellitus (GDM)] as well as to secondary alterations in glucose homeostasis from starvation or medical therapies that are diabetogenic (corticosteroid or β-sympathomimetic therapy). The diminished bicarbonate buffering, mentioned earlier, places pregnant diabetics at increased risk of diabetic ketoacidosis (DKA) (10).

Renal blood flow increases by up to 80% during pregnancy. The glomerular filtration rate increases by 30% to 50%. The filtration fraction decreases somewhat in early pregnancy but subsequently rises slightly by the third trimester. Serum creatinine levels above 80 μmol per liter generally should be considered abnormal in pregnancy. Tubular reabsorption of amino acids and glucose is less effective during pregnancy. Anatomically, the renal collecting system shows pronounced dilatation. Both direct obstruction from the growing uterus and progesterone-mediated smooth-muscle relaxation may contribute to this phenomenon. Asymptomatic bacteriuria and pyelonephritis occur more frequently in gravid women (11).

The cardiac, respiratory, acid–base, and metabolic adaptations make the gravid state unique. As will be seen in subsequent sections, these adaptations can be advantageous or detrimental in conjunction with the pathophysiologic processes found in critically ill pregnant or immediately postpartum patients.

MATERNAL–FETAL INTERACTIONS DURING PREGNANCY

By term, up to 30% of maternal cardiac output flows through the uterine arteries: a high-flow, low-resistance circuit that supplies the metabolic needs of the uterus, placenta, and fetus. In many ways, the fetoplacental unit is poorly understood; many complex interactions between the fetal and the maternal compartments are necessary for proper fetal growth and survival. How these interactions occur, how they are altered by critical illness, and how the fetoplacental compartment can be monitored are questions that must be considered in the care of critically ill pregnant patients.

Placental Function

The human placenta is hemochorioendothelial. Maternal blood bathes frond-like trophoblasts that reside in the intervillous space. Fetal blood cells traverse embryonic capillaries inside each trophoblast, with gas and nutrient transfer through the trophoblastic tissues (12). Oxygen tension is much lower in the fetal than in the maternal compartment. The oxyhemoglobin dissociation curve of fetal hemoglobin is displaced to the left compared with maternal hemoglobin (Fig. 1). Therefore, oxygen transfer to the fetal compartment is facilitated. Because maternal–fetal transfer occurs from the maternal venous compartment (*intervillous sinuses*), changes in maternal venous oxygen content influence the oxygen that is available for transplacental passage to the fetus. Small shifts in maternal venous (*intervillous*) content are therefore likely to produce larger changes in fetal oxygen content (13). Because of the demands for cardiac output placed by the fetoplacental unit on the pregnant patient, the fetus and placenta are sensitive to what are otherwise clinically unimportant changes in intravascular volume and perfusion.

Fetal heart rate monitoring (FHRM) is commonly used to monitor fetal status. The clinical principles behind the applicability of FHRM are based on the supposition that the hypoxic fetus will progressively display a pattern of heart rate (HR) abnormalities in the presence and absence of uterine contractions (14). The fetus normally displays a resting HR of 120 to 160 beats per minute. Beat-to-beat variability (BTBV) in the R-R interval between successive heartbeats is normally found in healthy fetuses. "Reactivity" (acceleration of the fetal HR) also typically is present during the latter stages of pregnancy in the healthy fetus. Applied to pregnancies at gestational ages that are viable (>24 weeks' gestation), interpretation of FHRM improves as gestational age advances beyond 32 weeks' gestation. The positive predictive value of FHRM for impending fetal death or the

diagnosis of perinatal asphyxia is poor. Conversely, provided the maternal–fetal unit is in a steady state, the negative predictive value of FHRM is generally quite good (15).

Fetal heart rate monitoring usually is accomplished by external (Doppler) continuous monitoring or direct fetal ECG monitoring via internal fetal scalp electrode placement. The presence of BTBV is detectable only with scalp electrode placement. Uterine activity usually is measured concurrently.

Fetal HR changes are thought predominantly to reflect underlying parasympathetic stimulation. BTBV and reactivity are probably due to alterations in the phase rates of parasympathetic and less influential sympathetic stimuli. Alterations in fetal HR during pathologic conditions are a result of alterations in the phase rates of baroreceptor or chemoreceptor influences or of direct hypoxic effects on the fetal myocardium. Selective shunting of fetal blood flow to the brain also may occur acutely and chronically. Adaptation of fetal cardiac circulation to *in utero* life includes the presence of two sites of intracardiac right-to-left shunts (ductus arteriosus and foramen ovale) and one site of direct umbilical vein–central venous mixture (ductus venosus). The anatomic relationship of the ductus arteriosus facilitates a relative mismatch of oxygen content of postductal blood sent cephalically to the fetal brain and head (relatively oxygenated, predominantly from umbilical–placental circulation) compared with that sent caudally to the lower fetal trunk and extremities. During chronic placental underperfusion, this mismatch between upper- and lower-body oxygen delivery is accentuated, presumably as a teleologic adaptation of the fetus for central nervous system sparing (16).

Acute hypoxia usually causes a predictable series of changes in the fetal HR, including an absence of reactivity, loss of BTBV, fetal tachycardia, and ultimately fetal HR decelerations after uterine contractions (late decelerations), followed by bradycardia if hypoxia persists (17). Continuous FHRM may be useful in monitoring the effects of a given maternal intervention or therapy. Figure 2 illustrates such a case.

Ultrasound is another useful tool in the evaluation of pregnancy. Early in gestation, ultrasound may confirm the location and viability of the pregnancy. Later, ultrasound may serve as an adjunct to gestational age determination, or it may be used in evaluation of the intrauterine environment. Ultrasound or FHRM can be applied periodically to measure the intrauterine environment. Fetal biophysical profile testing (15,18) (ultrasound and FHRM) or nonstress testing (14,15,17) (FHRM alone) are two techniques of antepartum fetal surveillance used to evaluate the unborn fetus systematically. Antepartum fetal surveillance is generally accurate in the late second and third trimesters of pregnancy and is useful for the day-to-day (or week-to-week) monitoring of an at-risk fetus, provided the mother and the fetus are in steady state.

NONOBSTETRIC DISEASES IN CRITICALLY ILL OBSTETRIC PATIENTS

An extensive review of all medical or surgical conditions that could require intensive care for pregnant patients is beyond the scope of this text; however, a review of several commonly found

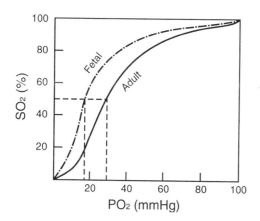

FIGURE 1. Fetal and maternal oxyhemoglobin dissociation curves.

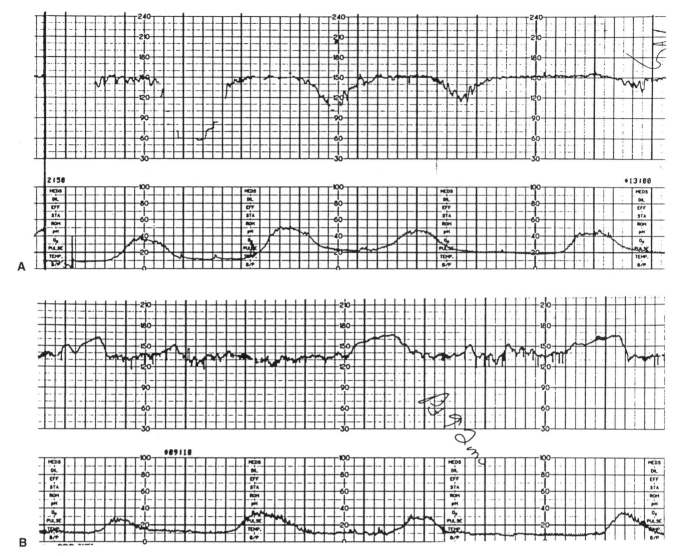

FIGURE 2. Fetal monitoring as affected by maternal pharmacotherapy. **A:** Before pharmacotherapy (nonreassuring pattern and late heart rate decelerations). **B:** After pharmacotherapy (reassuring fetal heart pattern).

conditions will underscore the important similarities and differences in various pathophysiologic states during pregnancy.

Cardiac Disease

Predicting outcome in pregnant patients with structural cardiac disease is based on clinical classification of functional status. Several excellent sources are available for review (19,20). Generally speaking, conditions characterized by pulmonary hypertension, right-to-left intracardiac shunting, or left-sided valvular stenosis are not tolerated as well as other cardiac conditions. Increasing cardiac demand peaks at approximately 28 to 32 weeks' gestation. Intrapartum, an additional 25% to 50% increase in cardiac output, coupled with obligate parturitional blood loss, poses a particular set of cardiac demands on the structurally altered heart (20). This problem can be worsened in the immediate postpartum period, when the cardiac output rises by 80%.

Mitral stenosis (MS), the most common rheumatic valvular lesion of pregnancy, may pose a particular problem during the labor and delivery of the affected patient. Critical MS (valvular area <1.0 cm²) often produces intrapartum and postpartum pulmonary edema secondary to an increase in pulmonary arterial occlusion pressure (PAOP). The PAOP increases up to 16 mm Hg immediately postpartum (21). If the left atrium cannot empty normally, the increase in left atrial pressure frequently increases pulmonary capillary hydrostatic pressure sufficiently above colloid osmotic pressure to produce edema. Tachycardia from intrapartum pain or postpartum blood loss aggravates the adverse effects of increasing blood flow velocity on the transvalvular mitral gradient. Pregnancy also may predispose parturients with MS to atrial fibrillation. Definitive correction of MS by valvulotomy or valvuloplasty usually is delayed until after delivery. For treatment of intractable heart failure during pregnancy, some investigators recommend balloon valvuloplasty. Nonetheless, the precise role of balloon valvuloplasty during pregnancy remains uncertain (21).

Antepartum medical treatment of critical MS involves rate control with β-blockers and avoidance or treatment of atrial fibrillation. Rate control is essential. Intrapartum, the use of intrathecal opioids provides excellent pain relief in early labor while maintaining hemodynamic stability. As labor progresses, a slowly implemented conduction block with low concentrations of local anesthetics can be used for analgesia. Pulmonary arterial catheterization facilitates titration of left atrial filling to a level that produces an acceptable compromise between systemic cardiac output and pulmonary capillary hydrostatic pressure and may improve outcome in pregnant patients with critical MS (22).

Severe aortic stenosis (AS) is generally somewhat better tolerated during pregnancy than is MS. Nonetheless, the "fixed output" characteristics of severe AS make the patient sensitive to obstetric blood loss, sympathetic blockade from rapidly initiated conduction anesthesia, or diminished filling from uterine compression of the abdominal vena cava. Patients with transvalvular gradients exceeding 100 mm Hg are at particular risk. Maintaining adequate ventricular preload is the preferred strategy in the intrapartum care of the pregnant patient with AS (23). Intrathecal opioids are optimal for early labor. Conduction anesthesia requires patience and caution. Maintenance of adequate preload and afterload and early anticipation of blood loss are important management goals.

Pulmonary hypertension as a result of congenital structural cardiac disease portends a particularly poor prognosis during pregnancy. Reported maternal mortality during pregnancy in patients with Eisenmenger syndrome is as high as 50%, although at least one recent series reports lower maternal mortality (20,24). Apparently, peripartum changes in pulmonary vascular tone, when accompanied by hypoxic pulmonary vasoconstriction, can cause a potentially irreversible process of progressive right-to-left intracardiac shunting and intractable hypoxemia.

Treatment is based on either prevention (pregnancy termination) or expectant hemodynamic management (25,26). Limited experience with the use of epoprostenol suggests that the agent may be safe during pregnancy. Epoprostenol has been chronically administered in a limited number of pregnant patients with noncardiac etiologies of pulmonary hypertension (27,28). Efficacy during acute administration is limited by the relative nonresponsiveness of fixed pulmonary vasculature to vasodilators. Although not described during pregnancy, long-term administration of epoprostenol for pulmonary vascular remodeling may be an interesting option for treatment. The risk of catastrophic deterioration can be reduced by ensuring adequate preload to maintain ventricular filling, aggressively replacing blood loss, and avoiding dramatic reduction in afterload by the use of regional anesthesia and attenuating hypoxic pulmonary vasoconstriction by administration of oxygen. Anticoagulation with heparin also is advocated (26).

Marfan syndrome is an autosomal dominant trait with a variable expression that affects elastic connective tissue. Cardiovascular manifestations of Marfan syndrome include aortic insufficiency, mitral insufficiency, and cystic medial necrosis manifested by aortic aneurysms along the aortic root or distal aorta. The increased vascular blood flow velocity and the adjusted increase in the rate of pressure change in the aorta (D_p/D_t) seen during pregnancy and delivery place the pregnant patient with Marfan syndrome at increased risk of acute aneurysm dissection (29). Risk of dissection during pregnancy is appreciably increased if

aortic root diameter exceeds 40 mm (30). As with Eisenmenger syndrome, the patient with Marfan syndrome who is contemplating pregnancy should be carefully informed of the particular risks of pregnancy on maternal outcome; generally, pregnancy should be discouraged. Intrapartum management of the patient with Marfan syndrome is similar to that of nonpregnant patients who have cerebral or peripheral vascular aneurysms: β-blockade (e.g., with intravenous esmolol) should be used to reduce D_p/D_t. Maneuvers and manipulations that result in reflex tachycardia (hypovolemia, suboptimal pain control, antihypertensive treatment with vasodilators, β-agonist treatment or sympathetic blockade) should be limited or avoided if possible (31). Despite the potential for reflex tachycardia, carefully titrated epidural anesthesia has been used successfully in the care of patients with Marfan syndrome (32).

Myocardial infarction (MI) during pregnancy or just before delivery is associated with a 35% mortality rate (33,34). MI occurs more frequently in the third trimester. Mortality is significantly higher when MI presents in late pregnancy. Delivery should be delayed, if possible, for about 2 weeks. Nitrates, calcium-channel blocking agents, β-blockers, and heparin must be used with caution. Thrombolytics are contraindicated in the delivered or soon-to-be-delivered patient. Limited experience has been reported concerning the successful use of thrombolytics in the non-laboring gravida (35).

Pulmonary Disease

The physiologic alterations associated with pregnancy complicate the care of the pregnant patient who is undergoing mechanical ventilation and also complicate medical treatment of acute pulmonary disease.

Asthma commonly complicates pregnancy. Generally, pregnancy does not appreciably alter the natural course of the disease. Compared with the nonpregnant state, management of status asthmaticus is not appreciably different (12), but assessment of the necessity for mechanical ventilation is somewhat altered. The baseline respiratory alkalosis normally present in pregnancy influences blood gas analysis and interpretation. Given that $Paco_2$ normally is decreased in pregnancy, a measurement of $Paco_2$ in or near the normal nonpregnant range may be indicative of impending ventilatory failure. Pharmacologic therapy of asthma is essentially unchanged in pregnancy (36), although subcutaneous epinephrine probably should be avoided during pregnancy because of epinephrine's possible adverse effects on uterine blood flow and contractility. Although carrying at least theoretical fetal risks early in pregnancy and a possibly increased risk of preeclampsia in late pregnancy, corticosteroids are recommended by most authorities during acute management of asthmatic decompensation during pregnancy as they are for the treatment of nonpregnant individuals. Semiselective β-sympathomimetics and magnesium sulfate, frequently given during pregnancy to treat preterm labor, are not contraindicated. Available data suggest that the use of ipratropium, aminophylline, and cromolyn is safe during pregnancy as indicated. Data are less clear regarding leukotriene modifier agents (37).

Pulmonary embolism (PE), including amniotic fluid embolism (AFE) (discussed subsequently), is the most common cause of maternal mortality. Deep venous thrombosis (DVT) occurs five times more frequently during pregnancy than in the nonpregnant state. The risk of DVT (and of PE) is probably highest immediately postpartum. The antepartum risk of PE is arguably highest in the third trimester. The diagnosis of DVT in pregnant women is more difficult because the site of thrombosis is often in the pelvic venous system rather than in the lower extremities and because radioactive fibrinogen testing is contraindicated during pregnancy. Contrast venography, Doppler studies for lower-extremity venous thrombosis, and magnetic resonance imaging (MRI) for pelvic-vessel imaging are appropriate. The diagnosis of PE is unaltered in the pregnant patient (38). Ventilation/perfusion scanning, which presents only minimal radiation exposure to the fetus, is not contraindicated when necessary. Pulmonary angiography also is acceptable. Treatment of the pregnant patient with PE is altered by the fact that warfarin derivatives are contraindicated during pregnancy. Heparin is acceptable and does not cross the placenta. Thrombolytics have not been well studied but are probably at least as safe as emergency surgical embolectomy (35,39).

Limited published findings are available regarding mechanical ventilation during pregnancy. In our experience, pregnancy does not alter initiation of mechanical ventilation, weaning, and extubation of the patient. Relevant considerations include the potential for hypoxemia (because of FRC alterations), the risk of aspiration, and the possibility of supine vena cava compression (from the gravid uterus). If possible, maternal PaO_2 should be maintained at 75 to 85 mm Hg to maximize fetal oxygen delivery (by optimization of maternal venous oxygen content) (6,10). As needed, opioids, anxiolytics, and nondepolarizing muscle relaxants (with the possible exception of gallamine) are acceptable during pregnancy. Avoiding hypotension and using fetal monitoring are helpful in the care of critically ill pregnant patients undergoing mechanical ventilation.

Acute respiratory distress syndrome (ARDS) occurs in pregnant patients in response to a wide variety of circumstances. A surprising number of pregnant patients with bacterial pyelonephritis develop ARDS (40). This syndrome is also a complication of severe preeclampsia (discussed subsequently); a similar process that arguably is related to the development of pregnancy-associated, β-sympathomimetic drug-induced "pulmonary edema." These associations emphasize that during pregnancy ARDS often is initiated by potentially reversible or self-limiting disease processes. Therefore, ARDS during pregnancy potentially carries a greater chance for resolution of the underlying disease and perhaps a greater chance for recovery from ARDS (41).

Few trials have compared management strategies in pregnant patients with ARDS. Our group's experience with ARDS during pregnancy suggests that pregnant patients, if cared for appropriately, generally respond favorably because of the reversibility of underlying disease. No published data describe a large experience with barotrauma-limiting strategies of mechanical ventilation in pregnant patients with ARDS. We have used low-tidal-volume, volume-cycled ventilation; pressure-controlled, inverse-ratio ventilation; and extracorporeal membrane oxygenation in pregnant and recently postpartum patients. Use of permissive hypercapnia theoretically should be avoided during pregnancy because of the potentially deleterious maternal effects of superimposing acute respiratory acidosis on hypobicarbonatemia and the unknown

effects of prolonged hypercapnia on uteroplacental blood flow or fetal acid–base homeostasis (42).

Mechanical ventilation during pregnancy should include consideration of the physiologic alterations normally present during pregnancy. Two frequently overlooked circumstances are uterine compression of the maternal vena cava while the mother is in the supine position and the somewhat increased nutritional requirements of the pregnant woman. Careful positioning will avoid supine hypotension. Recognition of maternal caloric requirements and possible use of indirect calorimetry may help to facilitate adequate nutrition of the pregnant patient undergoing prolonged intensive care.

Cardiopulmonary Resuscitation

Cardiopulmonary arrest during pregnancy carries the additional burden of fetal well-being and survival. Several important tenets regarding cardiopulmonary resuscitation (CPR) during pregnancy follow (Fig. 3).

1. Anticipation of potential cardiopulmonary arrest is vital in a pregnant patient with a viable fetus. A cogent multidisciplinary plan for management of the critically ill pregnant patient should be formulated in advance of urgent situations.
2. During arrest, aortocaval compression may severely limit the effectiveness of CPR (43). Lateral positioning of the patient or manual displacement of the uterus must be performed immediately in pregnant patients at risk for aortocaval compression (i.e., those >24 weeks' gestation) who develop arrest. Lateral position limits the effectiveness of chest compressions. Aortocaval compression generally does not exist until at least 20 weeks' gestation and is not common before to 24 to 26 weeks.
3. Despite lateral displacement, the already marginal efficacy of external cardiac compression may be dangerously degraded.

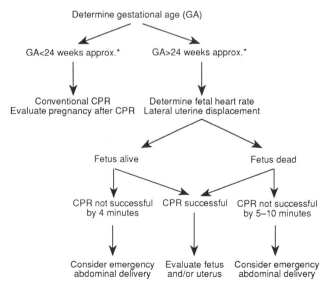

FIGURE 3. Cardiopulmonary resuscitation during pregnancy by clinical dating or history, immediate ultrasound, or fundal height measurement (uterine fundus palpable to 2 to 4 cm above maternal fundus).

Therefore, cesarean section may be lifesaving for the pregnant patient undergoing CPR. Bedside, emergent uterine evacuation is suggested for maternal indications after 5 to 10 minutes of unsuccessful CPR (44).

4. Intact fetal survival is not, surprisingly, directly proportional to the duration of maternal resuscitation. Therefore, if the fetus is alive and at or exceeding a gestational age associated with fetal viability (see first part of this chapter), fetal outcome is optimized by emergent bedside delivery after 5 minutes of unsuccessful CPR (44). Early delivery of a viable fetus may produce good fetal outcome as well as improve maternal survival.

5. No medication, therapy, or treatment is absolutely contraindicated during resuscitation of the pregnant patient if the alternative is maternal death. Femoral venous injection of medications should be avoided. Thrombolytics should be administered with care in the patient who will be delivered subsequently because of the almost certain complication of massive bleeding.

OBSTETRIC DISEASES IN CRITICALLY ILL OBSTETRIC PATIENTS

This section reviews several circumstances unique to pregnancy that may be encountered in intensive care of the critically ill parturient. Pregnancy-induced hypertension (*preeclampsia*), amniotic fluid embolism, the manifestations of diabetes during pregnancy, the consumptive coagulopathy of fetal death, postpartum hemorrhage, and acute fatty liver will be reviewed.

Severe Preeclampsia

Preeclampsia (edema–proteinuria–hypertension, or EPH) is defined as a pregnancy-generated disorder that produces new-onset hypertension and proteinuria, with or without pathologic edema. In pregnant women, blood pressures of 140/90 mm Hg or higher may indicate EPH. By definition, EPH presents after 20 weeks' gestation. Preeclampsia can be mild or severe, the latter often including multiple-organ system involvement. Seizure activity thought to be produced by EPH is defined as *eclampsia*. Preeclampsia frequently complicates underlying chronic hypertension, renal disease, diabetes mellitus, and multiple gestation (12).

The cause of EPH is unknown. Endothelial injury (not unlike the systemic inflammatory response syndrome) is central to multisystem organ involvement in patients with EPH. Furthermore, evidence suggests that severe preeclampsia is associated with a fixed oxygen-extraction state (45). Table 2 outlines the criteria for severe EPH. Seizures notwithstanding, one of the most seriously ill cohorts of patients with severe EPH consists of those with microangiopathic hemolytic anemia, elevated liver function studies, and thrombocytopenia (HELLP syndrome).

The only definitive cure for EPH is delivery. In the severe EPH patient at or near term (>32–34 weeks' gestation), delivery usually is undertaken. At gestational ages less than 32 weeks, limited attempts at expectant management are sometimes tried—although delivery is dictated by unrelenting maternal disease (cerebropreeclampsia, hepatic involvement, thrombocytopenia,

TABLE 2. SIGNS AND SYMPTOMS OF SEVERE PREECLAMPSIA

Hypertension	> 160/110 mm Hg
Proteinuria	> 5 g/24 h
Fetal	Intrauterine growth delay
Oliguria	< 500 mL/24 h
Central nervous system (CNS)	Visual disturbances or other CNS symptoms
Pulmonary	Pulmonary edema or cyanosis
Hepatic	Epigastric pain or diminished liver function
Hematologic	Thrombocytopenia

or uncontrollable hypertension). For the fetus, the main benefit of expectant management is additional time in which maternal corticosteroid administration can promote fetal pulmonary maturation. Severe EPH generally resolves within 24 to 48 hours postpartum, although some patients (particularly those with HELLP syndrome) show persistence of severe EPH for several days postdelivery. Parenteral corticosteroid administration has been shown to be beneficial in severe, refractory postpartum EPH (46,47).

Inexplicably, control of hypertension per se does not reverse the natural course of EPH. Treatment generally is undertaken to avoid the maternal complications associated with hypertensive crises. Obstetricians frequently use older antihypertensive agents such as α-methyldopa and hydralazine to treat hypertension in severe EPH. Experience is being gained gradually with the use of β-adrenergic blocking agents, calcium-channel blocking agents, and intravenous nitrates. Sodium nitroprusside is used occasionally but carries the additional risk of fetal cyanide toxicity. Angiotensin-converting enzyme inhibitors are contraindicated. Most authorities recommend avoiding overaggressive antihypertensive therapy in patients who present with hypertension. This philosophy is suggested in the hope of avoiding uteroplacental hypoperfusion secondary to excessive reduction of blood pressure. The target blood pressure in the treatment of hypertension in severe EPH is controversial. Persistent blood pressure values greater than 160/110 mm Hg usually dictate the use of antihypertensive pharmacotherapy (48).

The cause of seizure activity in eclampsia is unclear but may be the loss of global cerebral autoregulation or focal ischemia from vasogenic cerebral vasospasm and edema (49,50). Obstetricians use magnesium sulfate for both the prevention and treatment of seizure activity, and large clinical trials attest to its efficacy (51). The action mechanism of magnesium sulfate in the prevention or treatment of seizure activity in severe EPH and eclampsia is uncertain, but existing evidence suggests that magnesium functions to prevent or attenuate cerebral vasospasm (52). Intractable seizures resistant to magnesium sulfate may be treated with conventional antiseizure regimens. In such patients, it is necessary to rule out secondary causes of seizures (e.g., intracerebral hemorrhage, metabolic derangements, uncontrolled hypertension, acute cerebral edema). Fortunately, elevated intracranial pressure and clinically significant cerebral edema are not common complications in eclampsia. Treatment is conventional. It is not known whether the underlying respiratory alkalosis of pregnancy alters cerebral blood flow responses to deliberate hyperventilation in pregnant patients compared with nonpregnant patients.

The hemodynamics of severe preeclampsia vary among patients. Most oliguric EPH patients who receive PA catheters have low ventricular filling pressures, increased systemic vascular resistance, and hyperdynamic ventricular function coupled with contracted plasma volume (53). Monitoring with the PA catheter is nonetheless believed to be helpful in severe EPH in cases of pulmonary edema, refractory oliguria, or unremitting hypertension requiring continuous infusion of antihypertensive agents.

Amniotic Fluid Embolism

Amniotic fluid embolism (AFE) is a rare but often catastrophic complication of labor or delivery. Thought to be due to either direct embolism of the pulmonary vasculature or (more likely) anaphylactoid reaction with activation of endothelial mediator cascades from some direct effect of a constituent of amniotic fluid, AFE produces a syndrome of hypoxemia, myocardial pump failure, and (frequently) consumptive coagulopathy. Myocardial dysfunction in AFE—long thought to be a result of right heart failure—more recently was attributed to left-sided heart failure and ischemia from direct myocardial depression (54). Therefore, treatment generally should consist of treatment of left-sided heart failure and coagulopathy, if present. A prompt diagnosis and aggressive resuscitation and treatment (possibly guided by echocardiography or pulmonary artery catheterization) in the early stage are of paramount importance in patient survival. Recovery can occur if a patient survives the initial insult and the immediate hemodynamic depression (46). Nonetheless, AFE remains a highly lethal condition.

Diabetes Mellitus (DM) in Pregnancy

As stated earlier, normal glucose homeostasis is altered by several physiologic responses to pregnancy, including fasting blood sugar, insulin resistance, and diminished buffering capacity (9,10).

The National Diabetes Data Group of the National Institutes of Health has classified DM in pregnancy (55). The nomenclature includes type I (ketosis-prone, insulin-deficient), type II (non-insulin-dependent), and type IV (secondary diabetes), subtypes familiar to the nonobstetric provider. An additional subtype, type III or GDM, complicates approximately 3.5% of pregnancies (56); insulin is required in 1 of every 200 pregnancies (57). Types I and II DM are generally aggravated by the accelerated starvation and relative insulin resistance of pregnancy. The insulin resistance of pregnancy is probably similar to the postreceptor impairment of glucose handling in type II DM. Gestational diabetes mellitus appears to result from impaired secretion of insulin in response to a given metabolic challenge (58).

Issues germane to the intensivist regarding DM during pregnancy include the relative frequency with which glucose intolerance occurs in pregnancy, the propensity of the pregnant patient to develop secondary (type IV) DM, the increased possibility of DKA at relatively lower blood glucose levels, and the altered management philosophy for DM during pregnancy.

Preexisting DM is managed aggressively during (and preferably immediately before) pregnancy. Treatment goals during pregnancy are to keep fasting serum glucose less than 105 mg% and 2-hour postprandial serum glucose less than 120 mg% (59).

Hypoglycemia is most common early in pregnancy and immediately postpartum. Otherwise, once midpregnancy is reached, progressive insulin resistance develops, necessitating a progressive increase in insulin requirements as the pregnancy progresses (59). Maternal outcome, the risk of congenital malformations, and fetal mortality rates are improved by fastidious glucose control (57,60,61). Diabetic glomerulopathy is not permanently worsened by pregnancy (62). Diabetic retinopathy may worsen with pregnancy (63). In all patients, the risk of superimposed pregnancy-associated hypertension (preeclampsia) is increased.

Pregnant women with type I DM are at increased risk of developing DKA (58). Although serum glucose is often lower in pregnant patients with DKA than in nonpregnant patients, serum glucose is generally greater than 330 mg per deciliter. The acceleration of lipolysis and ketogenesis evident during pregnancy probably precipitates the manifestation of insulin resistance. Diminished buffering capacity predisposes the diabetic parturient to acidemia. Treatment of DKA in pregnancy is similar to treatment in nonpregnant patients. A key difference lies in the fact that fetal mortality is as great as 50% in the presence of maternal DKA. Ideally, maternal treatment will effectively resuscitate the fetus compromised by DKA (58,64).

All pregnant patients are screened for GDM. Unless other factors suggest the need to screen earlier, most clinicians screen for GDM at 24 to 28 weeks' gestation (58). Most patients with GDM are treated with diet alone; a smaller percentage require insulin (9,10,58,65), often in association with previously undiagnosed type II DM. In the absence of preexisting DM, most patients do not require treatment postpartum, although postpartum screening is recommended. Other complications are commonly associated with GDM, including fetal macrosomia and maternal hypertension, but there is no evidence to suggest that congenital malformation occurs more frequently in the offspring of patients with GDM (58).

Patients with GDM usually do not present with DKA. In the presence of other factors or treatments, however, the gestational (and type II) diabetic can develop DKA. Both β-sympathomimetics and glucocorticoids, frequently used in the management of preterm labor, may impair glucose tolerance or aggravate preexisting glucose intolerance (66).

During labor, patients with insulin-requiring DM usually are treated with low-dose insulin and glucose infusions (61). Postpartum dose reductions are recommended. During pregnancy, insulin usually is provided as multiple injections of intermediate and regular insulin. Refractory and resistant patients often are treated with long-acting insulin for basal control, with regular insulin used to treat glycemic excursions (9,58,61). Occasionally, the disease is controlled with programmable insulin pumps (67). There is no place for oral hypoglycemic agents in the treatment of DM during pregnancy (58).

Hematologic Manifestations of Fetal Death

Fetal loss is often an inevitable consequence of critical illness during pregnancy. An important issue for the intensivist caring for the pregnant patient with fetal death is the potential for alterations of coagulation as the result of two related processes. Placental abruption can produce acute or subacute changes in intravascular coagulation. Coagulopathy from delay in delivery of an intrauterine fetal demise can incite a chronic consumptive coagulopathy. As a general rule, the latter does not occur in gestations of less than 16 to 20 weeks.

Abruption occurs as a consequence of hypertension, trauma, hypotension, uterine hyperstimulation, and a host of other conditions. Clinically significant coagulopathy complicates approximately 10% of abruptions. Fetal death increases the risk. The induction of coagulopathy from placental abruption probably occurs through entry of placental thromboplastins into the maternal circulation. Extrinsic pathway activation is self-perpetuating until the placenta is delivered. Progressive consumptive hypofibrinogenemia results. It should be remembered that in pregnancy serum fibrinogen is normally increased by 25% to 50%. Consequently, a serum fibrinogen level in the "low normal" range may indicate significant consumption (68). End-organ infarction often is not evident from concomitant activation of the fibrinolytic system. Fibrin degradation products are markedly elevated. The coagulopathy of placental abruption is usually disproportionate to the degree of intravascular volume depletion from the abruption itself (69).

The coagulopathy of undelivered fetal loss is thought to occur through a similar mechanism. Hypofibrinogenemia is often the primary manifestation of fetal death with delayed delivery. In the absence of other complicating factors, clinically important coagulopathy is usually not evident for at least 4 weeks after fetal death (69).

Delivery is the definitive treatment for consumptive coagulopathy caused by fetal death or abruption. Vaginal delivery is preferred over cesarean section. Factor replacement occasionally is necessary to accomplish delivery. In cases of coagulopathy from delayed delivery of a dead fetus, heparin may allow an increase in maternal fibrinogen before uterine evacuation (12).

Obstetric Peripartum Hemorrhagic Shock

Obstetric hemorrhage is one of the leading causes of maternal mortality. It may present as a complication of vaginal or cesarean delivery. Hemorrhage may occur as a result of bleeding in the placental site or as a consequence of uterine or lower genital tract lacerations occurring during childbirth. Postpartum hemorrhage secondary to uterine atony is a common cause of obstetric hemorrhage. Increase in maternal plasma and red cell volume evident during pregnancy increase the tolerance of the immediately postpartum patient for moderate blood loss. Normal vaginal or cesarean delivery typically results in 500 or 1,000 mL of blood loss, respectively (12). The ability of the postpartum gravida to tolerate some degree of blood loss under normal circumstances, plus the fact that pregnant patients are often young and otherwise healthy, makes the diagnosis of hypovolemic postpartum shock much more elusive than in the nonpregnant patient. In the complicated antepartum or postpartum patient, unrecognized intraabdominal hemorrhage may be easily confused with severe preeclampsia, intraabdominal sepsis, or a variety of other conditions. Bleeding visualized during C-section or complications that result in vaginal bleeding are more easily appreciated. Nonetheless, the amount of vaginal bleeding may be easily underestimated and frequently inadequately replaced.

A detailed description of the treatment of obstetric hemorrhage is beyond the scope of this text. Several issues are important to the intensivist who may be involved in the care of the postpartum patient with hemorrhagic shock, however. Severe intrapartum hemorrhage invariably affects the fetus, thus necessitating delivery, whereas postpartum hemorrhage is likely to require pharmacologic or surgical prevention. Uterine atony is the diagnosis of exclusion in postpartum vaginal bleeding. Other causes of obvious vaginal bleeding include vaginal wall and cervical lacerations, vaginal hematoma, uterine rupture, and preexisting or acquired hemostatic disorder. Inspection of the vagina and cervix serves as a screening test for lacerations with the exception of uterine rupture. Uterine atony may be palpated manually. Pharmacologic treatment with oxytocin, intramuscular ergonovine, or prostaglandin preparations is generally used in most cases of suspected uterine atony. The management of bleeding and hemorrhagic shock from uterine rupture or cesarean section site bleeding is generally surgical. Uterine artery ligation, hypogastric artery ligation, simple repair, and hysterectomy are all management options. Radiographic embolization is another choice for persistent refractory bleeding. The use of radiographic embolization is generally much less effective in patients who previously received hypogastric artery ligations. Intractable postpartum intraabdominal hemorrhage may be treated with abdominal packing or (temporarily) with inflatable military antishock trousers (MAST)—albeit with limited effectiveness. Despite appropriate and varied options available for management, obstetric hemorrhage may result in catastrophic maternal consequences (1,70,71).

Acute Fatty Liver of Pregnancy

Idiopathic acute fatty liver of pregnancy (AFLP) is a rare but serious disorder unique to pregnancy (72). It is characterized by microvesicular fatty infiltration leading to massive hepatic necrosis and failure, encephalopathy, disseminated intravascular coagulopathy, and death. Acute fatty liver of pregnancy occurs approximately once in 10,000 deliveries, and the maternal mortality from AFLP has improved to approximately 25%. The etiology of AFLP is unclear. *Microvesicular* steatosis (unlike in Reye syndrome) is panlobular, with sparing of periportal areas.

Acute fatty liver of pregnancy usually presents in the late second or third trimester. A noticeable overlap with preeclampsia (at least 30%) suggests a relation between the disease processes; however, hepatic failure from severe preeclampsia also can occur without steatosis. The hepatorenal syndrome with the early presence of hypoglycemia characterizes AFLP. Deranged coagulation with prolonged partial thromboplastin time, increased international normalized ratio (INR), and microangiopathic hemolytic anemia are all consistent with the diagnosis. Maternal and fetal outcomes do not correlate with transaminase levels; many cases of massive necrosis are characterized by normalization of transaminase levels. The diagnosis is clinical, with computed tomographic scanning or MRI irregularly showing low hepatic attenuation (73).

Delivery and supportive measures appear to be the only effective treatments for AFLP. Standard supportive therapy includes maintenance of blood glucose level, correction of coagulopathy, use of lactulose to limit effects of intestinal bacteria, administration of vitamin K, and renal support. Hepatic rupture, hepatic encephalopathy, and refractory hypoglycemia complicate severe cases. Some patients with AFLP gradually recover normal or near-normal hepatic function after delivery. Others will progress to inexorable hepatic failure. Successful hepatic transplantation has been reported in patients with refractory AFLP. In patients with spontaneous recovery, the disease might recur with subsequent pregnancies, and a relationship between AFLP and deficiency in long-chain 3-hydroxyacyl-CoA dehydrogenase suggests a direct genetic link in some cases of AFLP (74).

SUMMARY

Pregnancy encompasses a unique set of circumstances that may have important ramifications in the treatment of the pregnant or recently delivered critically ill obstetric patient. Multidisciplinary care, meticulous attention to the physiologic alterations normally present during pregnancy, and concomitant recognition of both the fetus and the mother will optimize the recovery of that special pair of patients: the parturient and her unborn child.

KEY POINTS

By late pregnancy, blood volume is increased by as much as 50%, cardiac output is increased by 30% to 50%, systemic vascular resistance is proportionately decreased, and renal blood flow is increased by as much as 80%.

By late pregnancy, functional residual capacity is reduced, airway resistance is unchanged, and $PaCO_2$ is decreased.

The positive predictive value of fetal heart rate monitoring for impending fetal death or perinatal asphyxia is poor; however, the negative predictive value is generally quite good.

Cardiac diseases that may decompensate secondary to the increased cardiac demands of pregnancy and labor include mitral stenosis, severe aortic stenosis, and Eisenmenger complex.

Mechanical ventilation of pregnant patients is similar to mechanical ventilation of nonpregnant patients.

During cardiopulmonary resuscitation of pregnant patients, aortocaval compression by the gravid uterus may severely limit the effectiveness of manual cardiac compression.

Severe preeclampsia cannot be treated medically; treatment requires delivery, although medical management may be attempted at gestational ages less than 32 weeks.

During labor, patients with insulin-requiring diabetes mellitus usually are treated with low-dose insulin and glucose infusions.

REFERENCES

1. The American College of Obstetricians and Gynecologists. *Committee opinion: perinatal care at the threshold of viability.* Washington, DC: American College of Obstetricians and Gynecologists, 1995, no. 163.
2. Pritchard JA. Changes in the blood volume during pregnancy and delivery. *Anesthesiology* 1965;26:393–399.
3. Tsai CH, de Leeuw NK. Changes in 2,3-diphosphoglycerate during pregnancy and puerperium in normal women and in beta-thalassemia heterozygous women. *Am J Obstet Gynecol* 1982;142:520–523.
4. Lee W, Cotton DB. Cardiorespiratory changes during pregnancy. In: Clark SL, Cotton DB, Hankins GD, et al., eds. *Critical care obstetrics,* 2nd ed. Boston: Blackwell Scientific, 1991:2–34.
5. Clark SL, Cotton DB, Lee W, et al. Central hemodynamic assessment of normal term pregnancy. *Am J Obstet Gynecol* 1989;161:1439–1442.
6. de Sweit M. The respiratory system. In: Hytten F, Chamberlain G, eds. *Clinical physiology in obstetrics,* 2nd ed. London: Blackwell Scientific, 1991:83–100.
7. Myers SA, Gleicher N. Physiologic changes in normal pregnancy. In: Gleicher N, Elkayam U, Galbraith RM, et al., eds. *Principles and practice of medical therapy in pregnancy,* 2nd ed. Norwalk, CT: Appleton & Lange, 1992:35–52.
8. Hankins GDV, Harvey CJ, Clark SL, et al. The effects of maternal position and cardiac output on intrapulmonary shunt in normal and third-trimester pregnancy. *Obstet Gynecol* 1996;88:1–4.
9. Freinkel N, Dooley SL, Metzger BE. Care of the pregnant woman with insulin-dependent diabetes mellitus. *N Engl J Med* 1985;313:96–101.
10. Bender HS, Chickering WR. Pregnancy and diabetes: the maternal response. *Life Sci* 1985;37:1–9.
11. Lindheimer MD, Davison JM. Renal disorders. In: Barron WM, Lindheimer MD, eds. *Medical disorders during pregnancy.* St Louis: Mosby–Year Book, 1991:42–72.
12. Cunningham FG, MacDonald PC, Gant NF, et al. *Williams obstetrics,* 20th ed. Stamford, CT: Appleton & Lange, 1997.

13. Bauer C, Ludwig M, Ludwig I, et al. Factors governing the oxygen affinity of human adult and fetal blood. *Respir Physiol* 1969;7:271–277.
14. Parer JT. Fetal heart rate. In: Creasy RK, Resnik R, eds. *Maternal–fetal medicine: principles and practice,* 3rd ed. Philadelphia: WB Saunders, 1994:298–325.
15. The American College of Obstetricians and Gynecologists. *Practice bulletin: antepartum fetal surveillance.* Washington, DC: American College of Obstetricians and Gynecologists, 1999, no. 9.
16. Clyman RI, Heymann MA. Fetal cardiovascular physiology. In: Creasy RK, Resnik R, eds. *Maternal fetal medicine,* 4th ed. Philadelphia: WB Saunders, 1999:249–259.
17. Parer JT. Fetal heart rate. In: Creasy RK, Resnik R, eds. *Maternal fetal medicine,* 4th ed. Philadelphia: WB Saunders, 1999:271–299.
18. Manning FA, Morrison I, Lange IR. Fetal assessment based on fetal biophysical profile scoring: experience in 12,620 referred high-risk pregnancies. *Am J Obstet Gynecol* 1985;151:343–345.
19. Clark SL, Cotton DB, Hankins GD, Phelan JP, eds. *Critical care obstetrics,* 3rd ed. Boston: Blackwell Scientific, 1997.
20. Shabetai R. Cardiac diseases. In: Creasy RK, Resnik R, eds. *Maternal fetal medicine,* 4th ed. Philadelphia: WB Saunders, 1999:249–259.
21. Glantz JC, Pomerantz RM, Cunningham MJ, et al. Percutaneous balloon valvuloplasty for severe mitral stenosis during pregnancy: a review of therapeutic options. *Obstet Gynecol Surv* 1993;7:503–508.
22. Clark SL, Phelan JP, Greenspoon J, et al. Labor and delivery in the presence of mitral stenosis: central hemodynamic observations. *Am J Obstet Gynecol* 1985;152:984–988.
23. Easterling TR, Chadwick HS, Otto CM, et al. Aortic stenosis in pregnancy. *Obstet Gynecol* 1988;72:113–118.
24. Avila WS, Grinberg M, Snitcowsky, R, et al. Maternal and fetal outcome in pregnant women with Eisenmenger's syndrome. *Eur Heart J* 1995;16:460.
25. Gleicher N, Midwall J, Hochberger D, et al. Eisenmenger's syndrome and pregnancy. *Obstet Gynecol Surv* 1979;34:721–741.
26. Wess BM, Hess OM. Pulmonary vascular disease and pregnancy: current controversies, management strategies, and perspectives. *Eur Heart J* 2000;21:104–115.

27. Badalian SS, Silverman RK, Aubry RH, et al. Twin pregnancy in a woman on long-term epoprostenol therapy for primary pulmonary hypertension: a case report. *J Reprod Med* 2000;45:149–152.

28. Easterling TR, Ralph DD, Schmucker BC. Pulmonary hypertension in pregnancy: treatment with pulmonary vasodilators. *Obstet Gynecol* 1999;93:494–498.

29. Rossiter JP, Repke JT, Morales AJ, et al. A prospective longitudinal evaluation of pregnancy in the Marfan syndrome. *Am J Obstet Gynecol* 1995;173:1599.

30. Pyeritz RE. Maternal and fetal complications of pregnancy in Marfan's syndrome. *Am J Med* 1984;71:784.

31. Wells DG. Anaesthesia and Marfan's syndrome: a case report. *Can J Anaesth* 1987;34:311.

32. Mor-Yosef S, Younis J, Granat M, et al. Marfan's syndrome in pregnancy. *Obstet Gynecol Surv* 1988;43:382.

33. Mabie WC, Freire MV. Sudden chest pain and cardiac emergencies in the obstetric patient. *Obstet Gynecol Clin North Am* 1995;22:19–37.

34. Hankins GD, Wendel GD Jr, Leveno KJ, et al. Myocardial infarction during pregnancy: a review. *Obstet Gynecol* 1985;65:139–146.

35. Schumacher B, Belfort MA, Card RJ. Successful treatment of acute myocardial infarction during pregnancy with tissue plasminogen activator. *Am J Obstet Gynecol* 1997;176:716.

36. Greenberger PA. Pregnancy and asthma. *Chest* 1985;7:855–875.

37. The American College of Obstetricians and Gynecologists and the American College of Allergy, Asthma, and Immunology. Position statement: the use of newer asthma and allergy medications during pregnancy. *Ann Allergy Asthma Immunol* 2000;84:475–480.

38. Rutherford SE, Phelan JP. Clinical management of thromboembolic disorders in pregnancy. *Crit Care Clin* 1991;7:809–828.

39. Mazeika PK, Oakley CM. Massive pulmonary embolism in pregnancy treated with streptokinase and percutaneous catheter fragmentation. *Eur Heart J* 1994;15:1281–1283.

40. Towers GV, Kaminskas CM, Garite CJ, et al. Pulmonary injury associated with antepartum pyelonephritis: can patients at risk be identified? *Am J Obstet Gynecol* 1991;164:974–978.

41. Van Hook JW. Acute respiratory distress syndrome in pregnancy. *Semin Perinatol* 1997;21:320–327.

42. Catanzarite VA, Willms D. Adult respiratory distress syndrome in pregnancy: report of three cases and review of the literature. *Obstet Gynecol Surv* 1997;52:381–392.

43. Rees GA, Willis BA. Resuscitation in late pregnancy. *Anesthesia* 1988;43:347–349.

44. Katz VL, Dotters DJ, Droegemueller W. Perimortem cesarean delivery. *Obstet Gynecol* 1986;68:571–576.

45. Belfort MA, Anthony J, Saade GR, et al. The oxygen consumption/oxygen delivery curve in severe preeclampsia: evidence for a fixed oxygen extraction state. *Am J Obstet Gynecol* 1993;169:1448–1555.

46. Van Hook JW. Management of complicated preeclampsia. *Semin Perinatol* 1999;23:79–90.

47. Martin JN, Perry KG Jr, Blake PG, et al. Better maternal outcomes are achieved with dexamethasone therapy for postpartum HELLP (hemolysis, elevate liver enzymes, and thrombocytopenia) syndrome. *Am J Obstet Gynecol* 1997;177:1011.

48. Roberts JM. Pregnancy-related hypertension. In: Creasy RK, Resnik R, eds. *Maternal fetal medicine.* 4th ed. Philadelphia: WB Saunders, 1999:833–872.

49. Lucas MJ, Levenao KJ, Cunningham FG. A comparison of magnesium sulfate with phenytoin for the prevention of eclampsia. *N Engl J Med* 1995;333:201.

50. Williams KP, Wilson S. Persistence of cerebral hemodynamic changes in patients with eclampsia: A report of three cases. *Am J Obstet Gynecol* 1999;181:1162–1165.

51. Eclampsia Trial Collaborative Group. Which anticonvulsant for women with eclampsia? Evidence from the collaborative eclampsia trial. *Lancet* 1995;345:1445.

52. Belfort MA, Moise KJ. Effect of magnesium sulfate on maternal brain blood flow in preeclampsia: a randomized placebo-controlled study. *Am J Obstet Gynecol* 1992;167:661–666.

53. Clark SL, Cotton DB. Clinical indications for pulmonary artery catheterization in the patient with severe preeclampsia. *Am J Obstet Gynecol* 1988;158:453–458.

54. Hankins GD, Snyder RR, Clark SL, et al. Acute hemodynamic and respiratory effects of amniotic fluid embolism in the pregnant goat model. *Am J Obstet Gynecol* 1993;168:1113–1129.

55. National Diabetes Data Group. Classification and diagnosis of diabetes mellitus and other categories of glucose intolerance. *Diabetes* 1979;23:1039–1057.

56. Dooley SL, Metzger BE, Cho N, et al. The influence of demographic and phenotypic heterogeneity on the prevalence of gestational diabetes mellitus. *Int J Gynaecol Obstet* 1991;25:13–18.

57. Cousins L. Pregnancy complications among diabetic women: review. *Obstet Gynecol Surv* 1987;42:140–149.

58. Moore TR. Diabetes in pregnancy. In: Creasy RK, Resnick R, eds. *Maternal-fetal medicine: principles and practice,* 3rd ed. Philadelphia: WB Saunders, 1994:934–978.

59. The American College of Obstetricians and Gynecologists. Technical Bulletin. *Diabetes and pregnancy.* Washington, DC: American College of Obstetricians and Gynecologists, 1995:200.

60. Landon MB, Gabbe SG, Piana R, et al. Neonatal morbidity in pregnancy complicated by diabetes mellitus: predictive value of maternal glycemic profiles. *Am J Obstet Gynecol* 1987;156:1089–1095.

61. Jovanovic L, Peterson CM. Management of the pregnant, insulin-dependent diabetic woman. *Diabetes Care* 1980;3:63–68.

62. Reece EA, Coustan DR, Hayslett JP, et al. Diabetic nephropathy: pregnancy performance and fetomaternal outcome. *Am J Obstet Gynecol* 1988;159:56–66.

63. Klein BE, Moss SE, Klein R. Effect of pregnancy on progression of diabetic retinopathy. *Diabetes Care* 1990;13:34–40.

64. Hughes AB. Fetal heart rate changes during diabetic ketosis. *Acta Obstet Gynecol Scand* 1987;66:71–73.

65. Dornhorst A, Nicholls JS, Probst F, et al. Calorie restriction for treatment of gestational diabetes. *Diabetes* 1991;40(Suppl 2):161–164.

66. Rodgers BD, Rodgers DE. Clinical variables associated with diabetic ketoacidosis during pregnancy. *J Reprod Med* 1991;36:797–800.

67. Coustan DR, Reece EA, Sherwin RS, et al. A randomized clinical trial of the insulin pump vs intensive conventional therapy in diabetic pregnancies. *JAMA* 1986;255:631–666.

68. Green JR. Placenta previa and abruptio placentae. In: Creasy RK, Resnik R, eds. *Maternal–fetal medicine: principles and practice,* 3rd ed. Philadelphia: WB Saunders, 1994:602–19.

69. Pritchard JA. Haematological problems associated with delivery, placental abruption, retained dead fetus, and amniotic fluid embolism. *Clin Haematol* 1973;2:563–586.

70. Cunningham FG, MacDonald PC, Gant NF, et al. Obstetrical hemorrhage. In: *Williams obstetrics,* 19th ed. Norwalk, CT: Appleton & Lange, 1993:819–851.

71. Hankins GDV, Clark SL, Cunningham FG, Gilstrap LC, eds. *Operative obstetrics.* Norwalk, CT: Appleton & Lange, 1995.

72. Purdie JM, Walters BN. Acute fatty liver of pregnancy: clinical features and diagnosis. *Aust NZ J Obstet Gynaecol* 1988;28:62–67.

73. Rolfes DB, Ishak KG. Acute fatty liver of pregnancy: a clinicopathologic study of 35 cases. *Hepatology* 1985;5:1149–1158.

74. Schoeman MN, Batey RG, Wilcken B. Recurrent acute fatty liver of pregnancy associated with a fatty acid oxidation defect in the offspring. *Gastroenterology* 1991;100:544.

PEDIATRIC CRITICAL CARE: SELECTED ASPECTS OF PERIOPERATIVE MANAGEMENT OF INFANTS AND CHILDREN

SHEKHAR T. VENKATARAMAN
JOSEPH A. CARCILLO
MARK W. HALL
RANDALL A. RUPPEL
PATRICK M. KOCHANEK

KEY WORDS

- Acute respiratory distress syndrome
- Airway
- Congenital heart disease: preoperative assessment, critical care
- Development
- Disseminated intravascular coagulation
- Extracorporeal membrane oxygenation
- Fluid therapy
- Heart failure
- Immunosuppressants
- Infection; immunocompromise, postoperative, posttransplantation

- Inotropes
- Metabolism
- Multiple-organ failure
- Nutrition
- Pancreatitis
- Pediatric critical care
- Pediatric intensive care unit
- Pediatric transplantation: heart, kidney, liver, lungs, multivisceral, rejection
- Respiratory failure
- Pain management
- Sedation
- Shock: hemorrhagic, septic

INTRODUCTION

Numerous chapters and textbooks have been written in the field of pediatric critical care medicine on the unique spectrum of disease processes encountered in the pediatric intensive care unit (PICU) (1–4). Likewise, numerous chapters have been written describing the fundamental developmental differences in the biology, pathophysiology, and management of critically ill infants and children compared with adults (5). Few chapters, however, have been devoted to contemporary perioperative management of infants and children in the PICU. In this chapter, six areas

of perioperative care are addressed. PICU-related aspects of the management of infants and children after general, neurologic, and cardiothoracic surgery are discussed. PICU-related management of infants and children after solid-organ transplantation and management of hemorrhagic shock and subsequent multiple-organ failure (MOF) also are addressed. Each area focuses on key developmental issues and selected issues in diagnosis and management. Conditions that represent extremely common postoperative admissions to the PICU also are discussed. Finally, the unique features of the MOF syndrome in infants and children are discussed. Pediatric aspects of this important syndrome often are not addressed even in classic and contemporary textbooks in the field (6,7). The focus in each area is on management issues that are most germane to pediatric intensivists or anesthesiologists working in collaboration with their colleagues in either general pediatric surgery or one of the pediatric surgical subspecialties.

GENERAL ISSUES FOR THE PERIOPERATIVE PATIENT

General pediatric surgical care encompasses a wide variety of pediatric problems, including correction of congenital anomalies, gastrointestinal diseases, and other conditions. Many key differences between adults and children are pertinent to all general pediatric perioperative care in the PICU.

Airway

Infants and toddlers have a prominent occiput and a large head-to-body ratio that combine to result in flexion of the neck when the patient is in the supine position. Optimal patient positioning may include the use of a shoulder roll to provide head extension and open the airway. Children frequently have generous tonsillar and adenoidal tissue that, combined with a relatively large tongue and small oral cavity, may result in upper airway obstruction. A nasal or oral airway can aid in relieving this obstruction, particularly in the somnolent child.

When intubation of the airway is indicated, additional anatomic differences between adults and children come into play. The position of the larynx in the child is typically much more anterior and cephalad than that of the adult. In neonates, the larynx can be found at the level of C1 and descends throughout childhood to reach the level of C4 to C7 by adolescence. Additionally, the epiglottis often lacks rigidity in infants and toddlers. The use of a straight blade is therefore often desirable to lift the epiglottis when visualizing the airway. When choosing the appropriate endotracheal tube for a pediatric airway, it is important to remember that well into school age the narrowest part of the pediatric airway occurs at the cricoid ring rather than at the vocal cords. Typically, uncuffed tubes are used in children aged younger than 8 years because the cricoid ring acts as a natural cuff. Cuffed endotracheal tubes may be indicated even in infancy in cases where high airway pressures are required. The cuff should be inflated to a pressure just sufficient to prevent clinically significant air leak. Cuffs should be inspected frequently to ensure that they are not overinflated, adding to the risk for development of subglottic stenosis. Estimation of appropriate endotracheal tube size can be made by the following formula: (age in years + 16)/4. Right mainstem bronchus intubation is a common complication of pediatric intubations, especially in infants and toddlers, given the short length of the trachea. Auscultation of breath sounds in both lung fields can be deceiving given the easy transmission of sound through a small chest. Radiographic confirmation of tube position is therefore an important part of the intubation process.

Breathing

There is considerable age-related variation in respiratory rate in children. Neonates typically breathe 40 to 60 times per minute with the normal respiratory rate decreasing to 20 to 30 in toddlers, 18 to 22 in school-aged children, and 16 to 20 in adolescents (8). Tachypnea, with nasal flaring, grunting, and use of accessory respiratory musculature, are the hallmark signs of respiratory distress in infants and young children. Early intervention with supplemental oxygen, airway positioning, airway adjuncts, and mechanical ventilation can be lifesaving. Bronchospasm is a common pediatric problem and can complicate perioperative management. The presence of respiratory distress in the face of wheezing or a prolonged expiratory phase of respiration identifies patients who may benefit from a trial of inhaled bronchodilator therapy. Another problem common to small infants is that of airway malacia. This condition, characterized by a lack of airway tone that may exist from the larynx to the distal airways, can present with stridor or monophonic wheezing. Infants with malacia often improve when placed in the prone position. Bronchodilators may exacerbate malacia by further decreasing airway tone. Recognition and treatment of these conditions may help to prevent the need for intubation or facilitate extubation.

If mechanical ventilation is necessary, volume ventilation with effective tidal volumes of 8 to 10 cc per kilogram measured at the endotracheal tube, a respiratory rate of 15 to 20 breaths per minute, and positive end-expiratory pressure (PEEP) of 3 to 5 cm H_2O is appropriate for most children with normal lung compliance. If lung compliance worsens, the increase in airway pressure required to deliver a given tidal volume may necessitate a change in the approach to ventilation. In this setting, pressure-control ventilation with peak pressures adjusted to produce effective tidal volumes of 6 to 8 cc per kilogram, with a concomitant increase in respiratory rate, may maintain the same minute ventilation using lower peak pressures. Increased PEEP may be necessary to maintain functional residual capacity, but it is important to remember that PEEP of 10 cm H_2O or greater may impede venous return and can result in a relatively hypovolemic state as well as increased intracranial pressure.

The process of weaning from mechanical ventilation in the postoperative period can be optimized in the following ways. First, sedation and pain control should be titrated in such a way that the patient is arousable and has good spontaneous respiratory effort with an absence of splinting due to thoracic or abdominal pain. Next, mechanical impediments to airflow should be minimized by trimming unnecessary dead space from the endotracheal tube. A continuous flow ventilator circuit or a low-sensitivity trigger for delivery of augmented breaths may be important for weaning small infants from the ventilator. The use of pressure support ventilation may allow weaning of mandatory breaths while continuing to provide ventilatory support. A pressure support level of more than 5 to 10 cm of H_2O, however, may represent a significant amount of ventilation and itself may require weaning before extubation. Nutritional status and strength also must be taken into consideration, particularly for children with prolonged intubations. These patients may benefit from graduated trials of continuous positive airway pressure (CPAP) or T-piece ventilation while strength and nutrition are optimized. Although uniformly accepted parameters for extubation readiness in children are lacking, our practice is to consider a patient for extubation if he or she has a Glasgow Coma Scale (GCS) score greater than 8, intact cough and gag reflexes, an oxygen requirement below 0.4 fraction of inspired oxygen (Fio_2), peak inspiratory pressure below 30 cm H_2O, PEEP 3 to 5 cm H_2O, and a spontaneous tidal volume of 5 to 7 cc per kilogram on CPAP (9).

Circulation

Just as normal values for respiratory rate vary with age within the pediatric population, so do heart rate and blood pressure (Table 1). The lower normal limit for systolic blood pressure

TABLE 1. THRESHOLD HEART RATES AND PERFUSION PRESSURE (MAP-CVP OR MAP-IAP) FOR AGE

	Heart Rate (b.p.m.)	MAP-CVP (cm H_2O)
Term newborn	120–180 b.p.m.	55
Up to 1 year	120–180 b.p.m.	60
Up to 2 years	120–160 b.p.m.	65
Up to 7 years	100–140 b.p.m.	65
Up to 15 years	90–140 b.p.m.	65

b.p.m., beats per minute; MAP, mean arterial pressure; CVP, central venous pressure.
Modified from Krovetz JL, Goldbloom S. Hemodynamics in normal children, *Johns Hopkins Med J* 1971;130:187–195; and Anonymous. Report of the second taskforce on blood pressure control in children. *Pediatrics* 1987;79:1.

can be estimated with the following formula: systolic blood pressure (mm Hg) = 70 + (2 × age in years). Children have a remarkable ability to preserve blood pressure during hypovolemia through autoregulation of systemic vascular resistance and heart rate. Hypotension may not become evident until more than 30% of a child's blood volume has been lost. Signs of autoregulation should be used as cues to early treatment of shock rather than hypotension. Because stroke volume is relatively fixed in childhood, tachycardia is an early sign of compensated shock. Unfortunately, tachycardia is nonspecific and can be seen with fever, anxiety, and pain. Other signs of compensated shock include delayed capillary refill longer than 2 seconds, cool extremities, decreased urine output (<1 mL/kg per hour), tachypnea, and depressed mental status. These topics are discussed later.

Whereas controversy exists regarding the use of albumin as the optimal resuscitative fluid (10), it is appropriate to use any isotonic fluid (normal saline, lactated Ringer solution, 5% albumin) for initial fluid resuscitation. In the setting of hypovolemia, fluid should be administered serially in 20 mL per kilogram boluses until signs of tissue perfusion normalize. If signs of hypovolemia persist after a total of 60 mL per kilogram of fluid, the addition of a catecholamine infusion such as dopamine or epinephrine should be considered. If shock persists, or if there is a history of recent steroid use, stress dose hydrocortisone (50 mg/m^2) followed by an infusion at 50 mg/m^2 daily should be strongly considered.

After the acute resuscitative phase, many children will develop significant soft-tissue edema, particularly following extensive abdominal exploration or sepsis. Whereas treatment with supplemental albumin remains controversial, it is clear that patients can become intravascularly depleted as a result of third spacing. Careful titration of fluids to maintain normal perfusion and central venous pressure during the acute phase followed by a period of diuresis after the capillary leak has resolved will serve to optimize organ function and minimize respiratory insufficiency.

Fluids, Nutrition, and Metabolism

Maintenance fluids for children are calculated by weight according to Table 2. A 5% dextrose solution with 0.25 normal saline and 20 mEq KCl per liter is appropriate for most infants and toddlers, whereas 0.5 normal saline in 5% dextrose with 20 mEq KCl per liter will suffice for most children and adolescents. Changes in maintenance fluid composition should be guided by serum electrolyte assessment. The volume and content of ongoing losses such as nasogastric or ostomy output also must be considered.

Caloric requirements vary with age and clinical situation. In general, baseline caloric needs are between 90 and 120 kcal for infants, 75 and 90 kcal for toddlers, 60 and 75 kcal day for children, and 30 and 60 kcal per kilogram of body weight daily for adolescents. In patients with sepsis, major surgery, trauma, and burns, these requirements may increase by 30% to 60% (11). Indirect calorimetry with volumetric spirometry as well as measurement of urinary nitrogen can provide an accurate measurement of caloric needs in intubated patients. When enteral nutrition is not feasible, parenteral nutrition should be initiated. Baseline protein requirements are greatest for infants, at 2 to 3 g per kilogram of body weight daily and then decrease to between 1.5 and 2 g per kilogram of body weight daily in childhood. Protein calories should not account for more than 25% of total calories. Fats in the form of 20% intralipids should be started at 0.5 g per kilogram daily and advanced by increments of 0.5 to 1 g per kilogram daily to a maximum of 3 g per kilogram daily. Carbohydrate in the form of dextrose is typically begun with 10% to 15% solutions, advancing up to 30% as tolerated. A 12.5% dextrose solution is typically the highest concentration tolerated in a peripheral vein. Essential vitamins, minerals, and trace elements should be added according to institutional protocol. Albumin, prealbumin, or transferrin, as well as triglyceride levels, should be assessed. A weight gain of 20 to 30 g daily should be anticipated for infants and 0.5% of total body weight per day in children (12).

Enteral nutrition is preferable to intravenous nutrition whenever possible. There is mounting evidence that even small-volume enteral feedings can have beneficial effects on intestinal immunity (13). In cases of severe gastroesophageal reflux or gastroparesis, a transpyloric feeding tube often will allow safe and effective advancement of enteral feedings.

Children are at risk for hypothermia because of their large ratio of surface area to body mass. Hypothermia itself increases peripheral vascular resistance, making cardiovascular assessment more difficult. Prompt measurement of the child's temperature and maintenance of normothermia with a warm ambient temperature and warmed intravenous fluids are important, particularly in the early postoperative period. Optimal temperature during and after shock remains controversial. Children have high metabolic demands with limited glycogen stores. Monitoring of plasma glucose is important.

PERIOPERATIVE MANAGEMENT OF INFANTS AND CHILDREN AFTER NEUROLOGIC SURGERY

Neurosurgical procedures in infants and children include elective and emergent operations in all ages of children for a variety of conditions. Although a number of general principles apply to the care of pediatric patients in the postoperative period, several management considerations are specific to the care of a neurosurgical patient.

Diagnoses

The need for admission to the PICU is largely determined by the potential complications associated with the specific surgical procedure. The most common postoperative complications that require intensive monitoring following neurologic surgery include

TABLE 2. PEDIATRIC MAINTENANCE FLUID CALCULATION

Weight	Daily Fluid Volume
1–10 kg	100 mL/kg/day
10–20 kg	1,000 mL/day plus 50 mL/kg/day for each kg between 10 and 20 kg
>20 kg	1,500 mL/day plus 20 mL/kg/day for each kg over 20 kg

hydrocephalus, airway compromise, bleeding, vascular complications, fluid and electrolyte abnormalities, and seizures.

Intracranial hypertension is a concern in patients undergoing procedures to treat hydrocephalus with shunting, ventriculostomy, or a decompressive procedure. Patients with congenital hydrocephalus require intensive monitoring, depending largely on their preoperative status. A child with slowly progressive hydrocephalus with few clinical symptoms may not require admission to the PICU, whereas preoperative symptoms that raise a concern of potential herniation will require close observation and monitoring. Patients with Chiari malformations, tumors impinging on cerebrospinal fluid (CSF) drainage, or intraventricular hemorrhage all carry a significant risk of developing postoperative hydrocephalus.

Airway compromise is a potentially life-threatening complication that is of particular concern after neurosurgical procedures involving the brainstem because vocal cord paralysis or cranial nerve damage is possible. Patients with congenital anomalies that include facial abnormalities are also at particular risk for respiratory compromise (Table 3). Neurosurgical procedures requiring prone positioning during surgery also may increase risk for postoperative airway compromise because facial swelling can result.

Although the potential for bleeding is always a concern after surgical procedures, certain conditions carry more than the typical risk for postoperative hemorrhage. Surgical resection of a vascular malformation is of concern for bleeding if complete resection is impossible.

Surgical procedures near major arteries can be associated with vasospasm and resultant cerebral ischemia or infarction. Also, subarachnoid hemorrhage from aneurysmal or vascular

malformation rupture is a well-known cause of vasospasm. Carotid vasospasm occurs frequently during resection of craniopharyngioma; however, this is rarely associated with cerebral infarct unless combined with hypovolemia (14).

Electrolyte abnormalities can result from three disturbances in normal regulatory mechanisms: diabetes insipidus, syndrome of inappropriate antidiuretic hormone (SIADH) secretion, and cerebral salt wasting. Management of these problems is described below. Other complications that are unique to neurosurgical procedures include CSF leak, aseptic meningitis, and pseudo-meningocoele.

Monitoring

All patients in the PICU should have cardiorespiratory monitoring. Monitoring strategies should address all the potential complications described above. Therefore, respiratory monitoring should be designed to warn of impending airway compromise, including measurement of respiratory rate, pulse oximetry, and repeated examinations evaluating the work of breathing, air entry, and evidence of stridor.

Hemodynamic monitoring is useful for evaluating both cardiovascular and neurologic status. Increases in heart rate and blood pressure can be an indication of pain or of seizure activity. Systemic hypertension accompanied by bradycardia (*Cushing response*) can be associated with intracranial hypertension and impending herniation. Tachycardia with hypotension or delayed capillary refill may indicate excessive fluid losses, either from bleeding, third-space losses, or excessive urine output. Tachycardia and hypotension also can result from loss of vasomotor tone, either from infection or medications, or after spinal surgery. Invasive blood pressure monitoring is necessary when patients are at high risk for any of the preceding complications.

Strict measurement of fluid intake and output is essential to monitor fluid balance, evaluate overall perfusion, and detect disturbances in fluid and electrolyte regulation. In surgical procedures carrying a high risk for disturbances in fluid regulation, such as resection of a craniopharyngioma, serum and urine electrolytes, should be assessed every 4 to 6 hours, along with continuous urine measurement and possibly central venous pressure monitoring.

Temperature control is extremely important after neurosurgical procedures; therefore, it should be monitored closely. Normothermia and mild hypothermia are safe, whereas aggressive measures to prevent hyperthermia are warranted because neurologic injury is exacerbated by high brain temperature.

Physical Examination

As with all postoperative patients, the immediate examination should include an evaluation of airway, breathing, and circulation. Specific to neurosurgical patients, however, a rapid neurologic examination is important to evaluate for baseline deficits following surgery. This is essential for evaluation of changes in neurologic status. For example, unequal pupillary size may be a result of surgical intervention and would therefore be present immediately after the surgery. Delayed development of unequal pupils in a patient may be the first sign of impending herniation.

TABLE 3. SYNDROMES ASSOCIATED WITH POTENTIAL AIRWAY PROBLEMS

Micrognathia
    Aniridia–Wilms Tumor Association
    Cerebro-oculo-facio-skeletal syndrome
    Cornelia de Lange syndrome
    Craniofacial dysostosis
    Dubowitz syndrome
    Goldenhar syndrome
    Miller–Dieker syndrome
    Noonan's syndrome
    Pierre–Robin sequence
    Russell–Silver syndrome
    Seckel syndrome
    Smith–Lemli–Opitz syndrome
    Treacher Collins syndrome
    Turner syndrome
    William syndrome
Airway abnormalities
    Hemihypertrophy
    Klippel–Feil syndrome
    Sturge–Weber syndrome
Atlantoaxial instability
    Down syndrome
    Osteogenesis imperfecta
Macroglossia
    Beckwith–Wiedemann syndrome
    Down syndrome
    Hurler syndrome

The initial neurologic examination should include a gross evaluation of mental status. Patients routinely have a depressed level of consciousness after anesthesia, but repeated examinations are necessary to ensure that mental status continues to improve. Measurement of the GCS score is one means of objectively quantifying a child's level of consciousness. A cranial nerve examination is limited by the child's ability to cooperate but should include pupillary response (cranial nerve II), observation of extraocular movements (cranial nerves III, IV, and VI), jaw deviation during sucking in an infant (cranial nerve V), facial asymmetry while crying or laughing (cranial nerve VII), gag reflex (cranial nerves IX and X), and shoulder droop (cranial nerve XI). The initial motor examination relies heavily on careful observation of movements because few patients are able to cooperate with a formal examination immediately after surgery. Similarly, the sensory examination involves observing gross responses to stimuli. A full evaluation of deep tendon reflexes is usually possible, however. Neurologic evaluation should be repeated frequently during the first 24 hours, evaluating for new neurologic deficits or progression of existing problems.

Fluid Management

Fluid management for the postoperative neurosurgical patient differs from that for other postoperative patients in a few key ways. Although maintenance of circulating volume is important, it is important to avoid fluid overload to prevent exacerbating cerebral edema. In general, neurosurgical procedures do not result in the large third-space losses seen with other surgeries. Once adequate volume status is achieved to maintain perfusion, fluid requirements usually will be met with a maintenance fluid rate. Euglycemia is important following neurologic surgery because both hypoglycemia and hyperglycemia can exacerbate neurologic injury. Initial intravenous fluids in older children should contain little or no dextrose, but serum glucose levels must be monitored closely. Infants, on the other hand, do not have the same capacity for maintaining serum glucose levels and will quickly become hypoglycemic if maintained with no source of carbohydrate intake.

Hyponatremia is of particular concern in neurosurgical patients because the blood–brain barrier is highly impermeable to sodium, and osmotic effects thus can increase cerebral edema. Normal saline is preferable to avoid this complication. When hyponatremia occurs in conjunction with a decreasing urine output and an increased urinary specific gravity and sodium concentration, it is likely a result of SIADH. In this case, fluid restriction is indicated. Neurosurgical patients also have two unique possible sources for excessive sodium loss: CSF losses from extraventricular drainage and urine losses from cerebral salt wasting. Both require replacement of sodium losses.

Mild hypernatremia is not generally detrimental and usually results from excessive sodium intake or osmotic diuresis. A progressively increasing serum sodium concentration in the face of increasing volume of hypo-osmolar urine, however, is suggestive of diabetes insipidus. This complication is seen after surgeries with potential for pituitary injury. Management of diabetes insipidus requires careful titration of fluids with a maintenance rate to equal insensible losses (300 mL/m^2 daily) plus total replacement of urine output with a fluid that matches the urinary

electrolyte levels. Vasopressin or desmopressin (DDAVP) may be required to control the free water loss that results from this problem.

Medications

Several general medications should be considered in all neurosurgical patients. Antiemetics are important to prevent postanesthesia nausea and vomiting because vomiting can cause a dramatic increase in intracranial pressure. Ondansetron and droperidol are good choices for antiemetic therapy because they are minimally sedating (15). Anticonvulsants should be considered in all patients at risk for postoperative seizures. Phenytoin is the least sedating drug for seizure prophylaxis in patients who did not require preoperative seizure therapy. Patients on chronic medications for seizures should have their usual regimen started as soon as possible after surgery. Dexamethasone is commonly used to reduce cerebral edema around tumors (16). The use of steroids is controversial in most other settings. Patients who received steroids preoperatively may require stress-dose steroids during the postoperative period. Prophylaxis with H$_2$ blockers reduces gastrointestinal hemorrhage in critically ill patients (17) but also may increase the risk of nosocomial infections (18). Gastrointestinal bleeding is more common following resection of a posterior fossa tumor, and the use of prophylaxis has been advocated in these patients (19).

Emergency Procedures

The postoperative problem that causes the most concern and sometimes is the most difficult to evaluate in children is an altered mental status. Anesthetics or narcotics can cause an altered sensorium, but emergent evaluation is indicated if reversal of these medications does not yield a reassuring examination. If the patient's GCS score is less than 8, intubation should be performed before any transport or testing. If an extraventricular drain is in place, it should be opened to facilitate CSF drainage. Hyperventilation should be initiated for signs of impending herniation, and mannitol and other neuroprotective measures, such as thiopental or pentobarbital, should be administered. Emergent head computed tomography (CT) examination then should be performed as soon as the patient is stabilized. Further action will be guided by the CT findings.

PERIOPERATIVE CARE OF INFANTS AND CHILDREN WITH CONGENITAL HEART DISEASE

Infants and children with congenital heart disease may require critical care both before and after cardiac surgery. About one-third of all children born with congenital heart defects become critically ill during the first year of life. A thorough understanding of the anatomy and physiology of congenital heart defects is essential in the perioperative management of these infants and children. A multidisciplinary approach involving the pediatric cardiac surgeons, pediatric intensivists, and pediatric cardiologists is optimal in the management of these patients. A detailed review of this topic is beyond the scope of this chapter, and the reader is referred to several excellent texts and reviews on this

TABLE 4. GOALS OF PERIOPERATIVE CARE OF INFANTS AND CHILDREN WITH CONGENITAL HEART DEFECTS

Preoperative goals
  Initial stabilization
    Airway control and mechanical ventilation
    Maintenance of a patent ductus arteriosus in duct-dependent lesions
    Support of circulatory system
  Accurate diagnosis of the congenital heart defect
    Noninvasive echocardiography
    Cardiac catheterization
  Preoperative preparation
    Correction of metabolic and acid-base imbalances
    Support of respiratory and circulatory systems
    Maintenance of secondary organ function
  Prevention of secondary insults to the myocardium and to other organs
Postoperative goals
  Minimize the myocardial workload
    Airway control and mechanical ventilation
    Temperature homeostasis
    Optimize preload and afterload
  Maintain adequate tissue perfusion
    Optimize preload and afterload
    Support and maintain contractility
    Maintain metabolic and acid-base balance
  Prevention of secondary insults to the myocardium and to other organs
  Withdrawal of external cardiopulmonary support

subject (1–3,20). We briefly review the guiding principles for the perioperative care of infants and children after surgery for congenital heart disease. The general goals of perioperative management are given in Table 4.

Initial Postoperative Assessment and Critical Care Management

Postoperative assessment in the PICU must be performed soon after the patient's arrival. The components of the initial postoperative assessment include the following: (a) a review of the preoperative anatomy, physiology, and interventions; (b) a review of the intraoperative events and the current postoperative anatomy; (c) a thorough evaluation of the cardiac and respiratory systems; (d) review of laboratory analyses (chest radiography, electrocardiography, blood gas analysis, complete blood count, serum electrolytes including ionized calcium, serum glucose, and coagulation profile, if necessary); and (e) critical evaluation of the cardioactive agents being used.

Developmental Issues

There are important differences between the immature and the adult myocardium. The immature myocardium exhibits a decreased oxidative capacity, increased glycogen stores, and increased glycolytic flux (21). Hypoglycemia is an important cause of myocardial dysfunction in the neonate. Infants increase their cardiac output largely by increasing heart rate rather than stroke volume (22). Thus, tachycardia is tolerated better in infants than adults. The immature myocardium is quite sensitive to norepinephrine because it is poorly tolerant of increases in afterload. The immature myocardium is also highly dependent on

extracellular sources of calcium and therefore does not tolerate hypocalcemia (23). In contrast, restitution of contractility after an extrasystole is rapid in the immature myocardium; therefore, extrasystoles are better tolerated without loss of cardiac output in infants, in contrast to adults. The immature myocardium has considerable ability to withstand hypoxemia. Levels of adenosine monophosphate (AMP) are higher in infants compared with adults during hypoxemia because of the deficiency of 5′-nucleotidase in the immature myocardium, and the immature myocardium may be able to recover from ischemia more successfully than the adult myocardium (24).

Physiology

Heart rate, preload, contractility, and afterload determine cardiac output. Adequate filling is important. The determinants of diastolic filling of the heart are heart rate, venous return, distensibility of the ventricles, pericardial restraint, and the presence or absence of synchronized atrioventricular contraction. Inadequate venous return is manifested by low filling pressures. Decreased ventricular distensibility is manifested by the presence of high filling pressures coupled with a small heart as noted on a chest x-ray or by echocardiograph. Decreased ventricular distensibility may be due to a stiff myocardium, poor ventricular relaxation, or encroachment by the opposite ventricle through the ventricular septum. Decreased ventricular filling may result from pericardial fluid, most commonly due to bleeding, postoperatively. Atrioventricular dissociation results in asynchronous contraction of the atria and ventricles with the loss of the "atrial kick," which normally accounts for a 20% to 25% of diastolic filling. Systolic dysfunction is due to decreased contractility. After cardiopulmonary bypass, there is often decreased oxidative phosphorylation and increased glycolysis in a dysfunctional heart. Intrinsic myocardial metabolic demands take precedence over external work. Coronary blood flow is affected by diastolic pressure, diastolic time, increased filling pressure, increased wall tension, and myocardial edema.

Postoperative Issues in Common Cardiac Lesions

Although a comprehensive discussion of the individual perioperative diagnostic and management issues in each of the common cardiac lesions is beyond the scope of this chapter, Table 5 summarizes key anatomic, functional, and management issues. General issues are addressed in the following sections.

Treatment of Postoperative Cardiovascular Failure

Volume replacement should be directed toward maintaining adequate central and left atrial pressures. It is more important to assess the impact of volume loading on the changes in filling pressures than to select an absolute pressure value. For example, after repair of tetralogy of Fallot, a child with diastolic dysfunction may have central venous pressures of 10 to 15 mm Hg. A 5 mL per kilogram fluid bolus increases central venous pressure from 12 to 20 mm Hg, suggesting that the ventricle is stiff and at the high end of its compliance curve. Further volume loading would be unlikely to improve cardiac output and may

TABLE 5. PERIOPERATIVE ISSUES IN COMMON CARDIAC LESIONS AND MANAGEMENT STRATEGIES

Lesion	Postperative Issues	Manifestations	Management Strategies
Systemic to pulmonary shunts	Excessive shunt flow Inadequate shunt flow	Pulmonary edema High oxygen saturation Congestive heart failure Cyanosis/low SpO_2	Afterload reduction of the systemic ventricle Inotropic support of the volume loaded ventricle Revision of the shunt Increasing systemic vascular resistance with vasopressors Prostaglandin-E_1 (temporarily) until the shunt is revised Thrombolytic therapy if there is clotting of the shunt
Bidirectional cavopulmonary anastomosis	Inadequate pulmonary blood flow	Cyanosis	Volume loading Decrease pulmonary vascular resistance Minimize mean airway pressure if mechanically ventilated
Coarctation of aorta	Systemic hypertension Congestive heart failure	Pulmonary edema Hepatomegaly Poor perfusion	Nitroprusside ACE-inhibitors β-blockers Inotropic support Diuretics
Closure of atrial and ventricular septal defects	Myocardial dysfunction Dysrhythmias Pulmonary hypertension	Poor perfusion Low cardiac output Junctional ectopic tachycardia A-V dissociation Low cardiac output Decreased oxygenation	Inotropic support Adequate preload Afterload reduction Cooling A-V sequential pacing Hyperoxygenation Hyperventilation Inhaled nitric oxide
Fontan operation	Inadequate pulmonary blood flow	Low cardiac output	Volume loading Minimal mean airway pressure—sometimes early extubation and encouragement of spontaneous breathing
Repair of right ventricular outflow tract obstruction (including repair of tetralogy of Fallot)	Right ventricular dysfunction Dysrhythmias	High CVP Low cardiac output Ventricular	Judicious volume loading Inotropic support Afterload reduction for both ventricles Aggressively keep normal potassium levels Early treatment of ventricular arrythmias
Norwood procedure and other operations with single-ventricle physiology	Inadequate systemic output Inadequate pulmonary blood flow	Poor perfusion coupled with increased oxygen saturation Good peripheral perfusion coupled with decreased oxygen saturation	Decrease pulmonary blood flow by increased inspired carbon dioxide or nitrogen Inotropic support Volume loading Increased FiO_2 Volume loading
Arterial switch procedure	Myocardial dysfunction	Poor perfusion	Inotropic support Afterload reduction

SpO_2, arterial oxyhemoglobin saturation; ACE, angiotensin converting enzyme; A-V, arterioventricular; FiO_2, fraction of inspired oxygen.

exacerbate edema and pleural effusions. Conversely, a minimal change in central venous pressure after fluid challenge suggests a more compliant ventricle and the likelihood of improvement in cardiac output.

Common inotropes used to improve contractility are dobutamine, dopamine, and epinephrine. Phosphodiesterase inhibitors such as milrinone have both inotropic and vasodilator properties [25]. Milrinone is also thought to have beneficial effects on ventricular relaxation. All adrenergic inotropes increase myocardial oxygen demand. One undesirable side effect of inotropes is tachycardia. Hypocalcemia is common after surgery for congenital heart disease, especially after cardiopulmonary bypass or in infants with DiGeorge syndrome (congenital hypoplasia of the thymus). Hypocalcemia impairs contractility. Maintaining an ionized calcium level greater than 1.0 mg per deciliter improves cardiac contractility. Afterload reduction is another important component of cardiac support. Nitrosovasodilators are the most common agents used to decrease afterload. Increasingly, milrinone is supplanting nitrosovasodialtors to reduce afterload [26]. Cardiac pacing is sometimes necessary to maintain cardiac output. Indications for cardiac pacing are complete heart block, atrioventricular dissociation with low cardiac output, junctional escape rhythm with a low ventricular rate, and a sinus rate that is insufficient to maintain cardiac output.

When cardiac function cannot be supported using pharmacologic agents, mechanical support of the heart may become necessary [27]. Extracorporeal membrane oxygenation (ECMO) is sometimes necessary for severe postoperative myocardial dysfunction. Adequate left atrial drainage with an atrial septectomy is occasionally needed for ECMO. Aortic counterpulsation, when feasible, is an option in some older children and adolescents (28).

Pulmonary Dysfunction after Cardiothoracic Surgery

The respiratory system is compromised by cardiovascular dysfunction because of a decrease in respiratory reserve, an increase in respiratory work, and impaired gas exchange. Respiratory failure results when the cardiovascular system fails to meet the increased metabolic demands imposed by the respiratory muscles. Positive pressure ventilation, by unloading the respiratory muscle work, can decrease the metabolic demands and myocardial work. Thus, moderate to severe cardiovascular dysfunction is a major indication for mechanical ventilation both before and after cardiac surgery. Mechanical ventilation is required to recruit the lung after cardiopulmonary bypass and to reduce the workload on the respiratory muscles and myocardium. PEEP is often necessary to recruit the alveoli. Increased intrathoracic pressure has diverse cardiovascular effects, some beneficial and some detrimental. Ventilator settings should be carefully titrated to optimize the beneficial effects while minimizing the negative effects of positive pressure breathing. In patients after the Fontan procedure, early extubation, and encouragement of spontaneous breathing are desirable because positive-pressure breathing may decrease venous return and pulmonary blood flow (29). On the other hand, patients with left ventricular dysfunction may experience an improvement in cardiac output with positive-pressure breathing.

Perioperative Pain, Sedation, Metabolism, and Nutrition

Adequate pain control decreases the stress response after cardiac surgery (30). Pain increases ventricular afterload and imposes a burden on myocardial oxygen demand. Adequate sedation is sometimes necessary to decrease patient–ventilator asynchrony, which is common in neonates and infants after cardiac surgery. Older children and adolescents may benefit from patient-controlled analgesia. Electrolyte imbalances are common after cardiac surgery, particularly with the preoperative and postoperative use of diuretics. It is important to maintain normal glucose, potassium, acid–base, calcium, and magnesium balance. Metabolic demands are increased after cardiac surgery. Fever increases myocardial metabolic demands and should be aggressively controlled. Adequate nutrition is important in the postoperative management. As soon as it is feasible, enteral feedings should be encouraged. Caution is advised with lesions associated with compromise of enteric blood flow, such as coarctation of the aorta or low-output states.

PEDIATRIC TRANSPLANTATION

Pediatric transplantation has evolved into an accepted therapy for numerous congenital and acquired diseases. With development of multidrug immunosuppressive regimens, along with improved surgical and anesthetic techniques and PICU management, short-term survival approaches 80% for pediatric liver, kidney, and heart transplants (31–34) and nearly 70% for multivisceral and lung transplant (35,36). Whereas many problems are specific to the individual organ being transplanted, there are a number of PICU issues that are shared by all transplant patients. These include an appropriate preoperative evaluation, immunosuppressive medications, and posttransplant rejection and infection.

Preoperative Concerns

Patients undergoing a transplant evaluation must have immunologic screening to identify human leukocyte antigen (HLA) A, B, and DR genotypes. A panel reactive antibody screen also may help to identify patients at risk for developing acute rejection. Serologies against varicella, cytomegalovirus (CMV), toxoplasmosis, measles (if patient has been vaccinated), Epstein–Barr virus (EBV), and herpes simplex virus (HSV) should be obtained to provide a baseline for interpreting posttransplant titers and assessing the need for chemoprophylaxis. Preoperative and intraoperative cultures aid in selecting appropriate anti-microbial therapy for patients with unique infectious disease issues [e.g., patients with cystic fibrosis (CF)].

The general health of the patient in the pretransplant phase will impact on the postoperative course. Whereas some patients are critically ill at the time of transplantation, it is important that all patients have careful attention paid to optimization of nutrition, minimizing toxic medications, and avoidance of nosocomial infections. Equally important is the cultivation of a supportive environment for the patient and family. A multidisciplinary team—including physicians, nurses, social workers, and mental health professionals—is invaluable.

Immunosuppressive Medications

Immunosuppressive regimens consisted primarily of azathioprine and corticosteroids until the introduction of cyclosporine in 1980. Since then, combination induction therapy using steroids and either cyclosporine or tacrolimus has become the mainstay of most centers. Although regimens differ somewhat from center to center, these drugs represent the core of antirejection therapy (Table 6).

Posttransplant Rejection

Hyperacute (humoral) rejection mediated by preformed antibodies against donor antigen manifests in the first hours to days after transplant. The combination of pretransplant screening and early, aggressive immunosuppression makes this a rare event. Acute cellular rejection is lymphocyte-mediated and may manifest during the initial postoperative PICU stay but usually takes days to weeks to develop. The signs and symptoms of rejection vary according to the organ system involved, but organ dysfunction and fever are typically seen. Intravenous steroid pulses and increased cyclosporine/tacrolimus doses are usually the first-line treatment for rejection. Mycophenolate or azathioprine often are added (if not already present) during acute rejection. Antilymphocyte

TABLE 6. PEDIATRIC IMMUNOSUPPRESSIVE AGENTS[a]

Drug	Class	Mechanism of Action	Adverse Effects	Route
Methylprednisolone (Solu-Medrol) Prednisone	Corticosteroid	Inhibition of T-cell proliferation via decreased transcription of genes encoding proinflammatory cytokines	Infection, hypertension, hyperglycemia, weakness, impaired wound healing, growth delay Interactions: phenytoin, phenobarbital, rifampin	i.v., oral
Tacrolimus (formerly FK506) (Prograf)	Macrolide antibiotic	Calcineurin inhibition	Infection, nephrotoxicity, neurotoxicity: seizure, tremor, headache, gastrointestinal toxicity, hypertension, hyperglycemia, electrolyte disturbances Interactions: phenytoin, phenobarbital, TMP/SMX, rifampin, amphotericin B, macrolides, azole antifungals, aminophylline	i.v., oral Unreliable pharmacokinetics typically necessitate use of i.v. form immediately posttransplant; follow whole blood levels
Sirolimus (Rapamycin) (Rapamune)	Macrolide antibiotic	Complex T- and B-cell inhibition	Infection, hypercholesterolemia, hypertension, nephrotoxicity, gastrointestinal toxicity, rash, thrombocytopenia, leukopenia Interactions: cyclosporine	Oral, poor bioavailability; follow blood levels
Cyclosporine (Sandimmune, Neoral)	Cyclic polypeptide	Calcineurin inhibition	Infection, nephrotoxicity, neurotoxicity, hypertension, gastrointestinal toxicity, hirsutism, gingival hyperplasia Interactions: phenytoin, phenobarbital, TMP-SMX, rifampin, amphotericin B, macrolides, azole antifungals, aminophylline	i.v., oral; erratic enteral absorption, but i.v. formulation has higher incidence of adverse effects; follow blood levels
Azathioprine (Imuran)	Purine antimetabolite	Purine synthesis inhibition	Infection, bone marrow suppression, gastrointestinal toxicity, cholestasis Interactions: allopurinol, nondepolarizing NMBs	i.v., oral; titrate to degree of leukopenia
Mycophenolate mofetil (Cellcept)	Inosine monophosphate dehydrogenase inhibitor	Purine synthesis inhibition	Infection, bone marrow suppression, gastrointestinal toxicity, hypertension Interactions: Aluminum and magnesium containing antacids, cholestyramine, probenecid	Oral
Antithymocyte globulin (ATGAM)	Animal antiserum	Direct binding and inhibition of circulating T-cells	Infection, fever, serum sickness, anaphylaxis, rash	i.v.
Muromonab-CD3 (OKT3)	Murine monoclonal antibody	Blockade of CD3-related T-cell antigen recognition complex	Infection, fever, anaphylaxis, seizure, encephalopathy Interactions: Azathioprine, cyclosporine, tacrolimus	i.v.

i.v., intravenous; TMP-SMX, trimethoprim-sulfamethoxazole; NMB, neuromuscular blockage.
[a]Doses and target levels vary significantly between clinical scenarios and practitioners.

immunotherapy with OKT3 or antithymocyte globulin can be used for refractory rejection.

Posttransplant Infection

Profound immunosuppression places the transplant patient at high risk for the development of nosocomial and opportunistic infections. Chemoprophylaxis with trimethoprim-sulfamethoxazole for the immediate posttransplant period effectively

prevents pneumonia with *Pneumocystis carinii*. Patients who are seronegative for CMV who receive a CMV-positive organ generally receive some form of CMV prophylaxis as well. Ganciclovir and CMV immune globulin have been used with good results (37). Similarly, patients with pretransplant HSV seropositivity usually receive antiviral prophylaxis with either acyclovir or ganciclovir during the early posttransplant period. Lastly, empiric antibacterial and antifungal therapies should be tailored to cover the patient's known flora and adjusted based on culture results.

Oral nystatin typically is used in all patients four times daily to reduce fungal carriage. Although it is important to provide early and aggressive antimicrobial therapy in the immunosuppressed patient, care must be taken to monitor drug levels and avoid adverse drug interactions.

Pediatric Liver Transplantation

Liver transplantation has become an effective treatment for cholestatic disease (e.g., biliary atresia), fulminant hepatic failure (e.g., viral, toxins), autoimmune hepatitis, hepatic malignancies, and a myriad of metabolic diseases. The development of reduced-size grafts and split-liver techniques has increased the number of organs available to pediatric patients. Before transplantation, children may suffer from profound coagulopathy, encephalopathy, and pulmonary and renal dysfunction as well. The coagulopathy often stems from a combination of clotting factor deficiency and thrombocytopenia (usually as a result of splenic sequestration). Variceal bleeding is common and presents a significant risk of exsanguination or aspiration or both. This can be managed by improving clotting times and platelet counts with blood product transfusion. Patients may require continuous fresh frozen plasma (FFP) and platelet infusions to improve clotting function. Regular plasma exchange can be helpful in managing this refractory coagulopathy without leading to fluid overload. Endoscopy with sclerotherapy or banding of varices is an important palliative therapy in the event of recurrent or ongoing bleeding.

The encephalopathy associated with hepatic failure can be initially treated with enteral lactulose; however, hemodialysis or intracranial pressure monitoring may be necessary if hyperammonemia and mental status changes progress. Metabolism of both endogenous and exogenous sedatives can be unpredictable in this patient population. Iatrogenic oversedation can interfere with the evaluation of encephalopathy both pretransplant and posttransplant, and so care should be taken to individualize sedation regimens.

Patients with end-stage liver disease are, in general, susceptible to capillary leak and pulmonary edema. Some patients suffer from an additional pulmonary insult. Hepatopulmonary syndrome occurs in patients with long-standing liver dysfunction and is characterized by the development of intrapulmonary arteriovenous fistulae. These fistulae often represent significant shunt, which can lead to hypoxia unresponsive to positive pressure or supplemental oxygen. It is important to recognize this phenomenon preoperatively so that postoperative blood gases can be interpreted with the proper expectations. Hepatopulmonary syndrome tends to resolve over several months after transplantation.

Renal function often is compromised before transplantation. A combination of increased intraabdominal pressure (leading to decreased renal perfusion pressure), exposure to nephrotoxic medications, and a poorly characterized interaction between the failing liver and the kidney often leave patients with some degree of renal insufficiency. Hepatorenal syndrome may require the removal of ascitic fluid or the addition of volume or vasopressors to improve the transglomerular pressure gradient. Drug doses and intervals should be adjusted according to measured creatinine clearance. Hepatorenal syndrome typically improves after transplantation, but if severe, its presence may preclude transplantation.

Immediately after surgery, fluid balance is of primary concern. The transplant procedure typically involves a long operating time with significant fluid shifts and insensible losses. Patients may require repeated doses of fluid during the initial postoperative phase, titrating to maintain a normal central venous pressure, perfusion, heart rate, and urine output. Older children usually can be extubated within 1 or 2 days after transplantation. Infants who were ventilated before transplantation or have restriction of diaphragmatic movement because of a large abdomen often require a more prolonged ventilator wean.

Graft failure early after transplantation usually is related to one of four phenomena: prolonged ischemic time, hyperacute rejection, primary nonfunction, or vascular thrombosis. Of these, vascular thrombosis is the most common cause of early allograft loss. Hepatic artery thrombosis occurs three to four times more commonly in children than in adults, likely secondary to smaller vessel size (31). Hepatic artery thrombosis can present in any of the following ways: (a) massive ischemic necrosis resulting in rapid graft failure; (b) biliary leak, often with accompanying sepsis; (c) relapsing bacteremia without hepatic dysfunction; or (d) late biliary strictures with cholestasis (38,39). Vascular thrombosis can be treated prophylactically with aspirin, Dipyramidole, dextran, or heparin infusions in young patients. Daily Doppler ultrasound studies of the hepatic vessels in the initial posttransplant period can screen for hepatic artery and, less commonly, portal vein thrombosis. If thrombosis is suspected, either open exploration or angiography can be performed. If the diagnosis of hepatic artery thrombosis is confirmed within 24 hours of either transplantation or a previously normal ultrasound, urgent operative revascularization is typically attempted (40). Whereas planned explorations of asymptomatic liver transplant recipients have been advocated by some authorities (41), this is not standard care in most centers.

Pediatric Kidney Transplantation

Since the late 1980s, about 300 living related and 300 cadaveric kidney pediatric transplants have been performed in North America each year (32,33). Few of these patients are critically ill before surgery, but many suffer from electrolyte disturbances, growth failure, and hypertension as a result of chronic renal insufficiency. Most kidney recipients are extubated in the operating room, and the immediate posttransplant care is directed toward the allograft function. Graft thrombosis is particularly common in infants, occurring in 3.5% of living related transplant recipients aged younger than 2 years and 9% of infant cadaveric transplant recipients (compared with 2% in adolescents) (42). Risk factors for graft thrombosis include young age of recipient or donor, absence of prophylactic antilymphocyte therapy, prolonged cold ischemia time, and prior renal transplantation (43). To avoid this complication, an approach combining early and aggressive immunosuppression with vigorous hydration is typically adopted. Polyuria is common in the early postoperative period, and if urinary losses are not adequately replaced, patients can become hemoconcentrated, increasing the risk of thrombosis. Also, large bicarbonate losses in the urine are common, necessitating replacement with an appropriate bicarbonate-containing solution. Multidrug immunosuppression is begun early, with about half of pediatric patients receiving prophylactic antilymphocyte therapy before transplantation (32,33). Serum electrolyte and creatinine concentrations and urine output, as well as renal ultrasound, are used to monitor for thrombosis.

Pediatric Heart Transplantation

Transplantation has become an accepted therapy for the treatment of end-stage cardiomyopathy and some forms of surgically uncorrectable congenital heart disease. Some degree of hepatic and renal dysfunction is common because of a chronic low-output state in patients awaiting heart transplantation. Optimization of cardiac function with infusions of dobutamine or milrinone with meticulous fluid management is the mainstay of care. ECMO and ventricular assist devices also have been used as bridges to transplantation. The nature of the postoperative course depends largely on the interaction between the donor heart and the native vasculature. If the heart has a long ischemic time or significant preharvest dysfunction, a longer period of postoperative inotropic support or afterload reduction may be required. The right ventricle of the allograft may be sensitive to the higher pulmonary artery pressures often seen in heart transplant recipients. A trial of a pulmonary artery vasodilator such as inhaled nitric oxide may be indicated until the ventricle becomes conditioned. In ideal circumstances, patients can be extubated and weaned from inotropic support within 2 days of transplantation. A multidrug immunosuppression regimen consisting of tacrolimus, steroids, and azathioprine typically is instituted after transplantation (34).

Pediatric Lung Transplantation

Pediatric lung and heart–lung transplantation are performed in selected centers for the treatment of cystic fibrosis (CF), primary pulmonary hypertension, congenital heart disease, obliterative bronchiolitis, surfactant protein B deficiency, and other rare pulmonary parenchymal diseases (36,44). Single-lung and living donor lobar transplants have evolved to address the shortage of available organs (45). Patients with CF constitute the largest group of patients, and their unique set of perioperative issues deserves special mention. At transplantation, virtually all patients with CF are chronically infected with pseudomonal species or other nosocomially acquired gram-negative bacteria. The prevalence of multidrug resistance among these bacteria and the problem of concomitant fungal infection make chronic immunosuppression an unattractive option, and strategies for containing infection have been developed. These include preoperative and postoperative treatment with an antibacterial and antifungal regimen tailored to the sensitivities of the patient's flora and procedures such as sinus debridement designed to eliminate other foci of infection. Patients with CF also frequently have glucose intolerance, malnutrition, hepatic dysfunction, and renal insufficiency, which complicate the posttransplant course.

Immediately after surgery, most lung transplant recipients exhibit some degree of reduced pulmonary compliance. These problems are proportional to the degree of anatomic size mismatch and the ischemic time and preharvest condition of the lungs. Most patients are mechanically ventilated for 24 to 72 hours or until clinical and radiographic evidence of reperfusion injury is waning. After extubation, pain management and pulmonary toilet are important and often mutually exclusive problems. Patient-controlled analgesia and thoracic epidural catheters are helpful adjuncts. Chest physiotherapy, noninvasive positive pressure delivered by facial bilevel positive airway pressure or intermittent positive-pressure breaths also can help to mobilize mucous plugs, improve atelectasis, and maintain lung volumes.

The airway anastomosis is of particular concern because of the high incidence of stenosis, 18% to 27% in children versus 10% in adults (36). Whereas this may not manifest in the initial postoperative period, it is common to observe edema at the anastomotic site, which, coupled to the malacia frequently seen in pediatric airways, can cause fixed obstruction to airflow. If such an obstruction is clinically apparent and bronchoscopy fails to identify a lesion amenable to surgical repair, an inspired helium/oxygen mixture may allow for adequate ventilation until perioperative edema resolves.

A multidrug immunosuppression regimen is typical of postoperative lung transplant management. Immunosuppressive drug levels, however, are generally maintained at higher ranges than after hepatic, renal, or cardiac transplantation as a result of the inherent immunogenicity of the lung.

Pediatric Multivisceral Transplantation

Multivisceral abdominal organ transplantation has evolved over the last 15 years as a rescue therapy for patients suffering from short gut and chronic malabsorptive syndromes with associated parenteral nutrition-related hepatotoxicity. Many of the perioperative issues are identical to those of the isolated liver transplant patient; however, the potent immunogenicity of the transplanted bowel necessitates a significant escalation in immunosuppression, often exceeding that required even after lung transplantation. Although the transplanted bowel often requires delayed abdominal closure as a result of edema and size discrepancies, the ostomy provides an easily accessible site for frequent biopsy and graft monitoring.

Although technical and pharmacologic advances have greatly improved outcomes in pediatric solid-organ transplantation, many challenges remain. Infection, rejection, and the toxicities of the immunosuppressive medications remain as major obstacles to recovery. Careful attention to nutrition, drug interactions and toxicities, fluid balance, and the psychosocial needs of the patient and family will help improve and shorten the PICU course.

HEMORRHAGIC SHOCK AND MULTIORGAN FAILURE

Children at Risk for Postoperative Hemorrhage

Early recognition and treatment of hemorrhage are important. Timely identification and appropriate response to blood loss prevent the development of uncompensated hemorrhagic shock and result in a nearly 100% favorable outcome in children after surgery. Many conditions predispose children to ongoing blood loss. Severe blunt trauma with splenic or hepatic laceration is managed in children with blood transfusion; the intact native capsule gives tamponade-mediated hemostasis. Two common pediatric surgeries, fronto-orbital advancement, and anterior–posterior spinal fusion are associated with ongoing bleeding from the subgaleal veins and broken vertebral facets, respectively. Bleeding diatheses also contribute to hemorrhage. Risk of postoperative bleeding is increased in liver transplantation as a result of underlying liver dysfunction. Severely ill children with disseminated intravascular coagulation (DIC) associated with tissue injury or hemodilution are also susceptible to bleeding.

Early Recognition and Treatment of Hemorrhage

Hemoglobin concentration may not accurately reflect blood loss in the perioperative period. Therefore, the clinician must recognize the signs of the early physiologic compensatory response to blood loss. As previously discussed, children have a robust neurohormonal response that maintains cardiac output and then blood pressure. Two important equations symbolize this response. First, cardiac output = heart rate × stroke volume (CO = HR × SV); second, mean arterial pressure − central venous pressure = cardiac output × systemic vascular resistance (MAP − CVP = CO × SVR). The first compensatory neurohormonal response is an increase in heart rate, which maintains cardiac output despite the hemorrhage-associated decrease in preload and stroke volume. Patients retain perfusion and blood pressure by increasing heart rate. Unfortunately, tachycardia can be a misleading sign because it is a nonspecific response that also can be associated with pain, anxiety, or fever. If blood loss is ongoing and tachycardia is no longer able to maintain cardiac output, a second compensatory neurohormonal response is needed. Systemic vascular resistance increases to maintain blood pressure, despite decreasing cardiac output. Children in this stage of compensated shock have a narrow pulse pressure with somewhat weaker peripheral pulses (radial, dorsalis pedis) compared with central pulses (axillary, femoral). Children continue to maintain mentation and adequate urine output despite a decreasing cardiac output because perfusion of the brain and kidney is dependent on perfusion pressure (MAP–CVP). This stage of shock is thought to occur with less than 10% blood volume loss. The estimated blood volume of a child is 80 to 90 mL per kilogram of body weight; so this represents a blood loss of about 10 mL per kilogram of body weight. Children can be resuscitated at this stage of shock with one to two boluses of lactated Ringer's, 20 mL per kilogram of body weight. A decrease in heart rate, an increase in pulse pressure, and an equalization of proximal and distal pulses represent a good response. Return of signs of shock strongly suggests ongoing hemorrhage, a requirement for blood replacement and a need for assessment by the surgeon.

Late Recognition and Treatment of Hemorrhagic Shock

If the early physiologic signs of compensation are unrecognized, shock will progress. Eventually, pulses become weak and thready; the child becomes lethargic, irritable, and confused; the skin becomes cool and clammy; and urine output begins to decrease. There is also a slight decrease in systolic pressure that can go unrecognized as systemic vasoconstriction becomes maximal. These signs are thought to occur with a blood loss of less than 25%

(20 mL/kg). If these signs continue to be unrecognized, then the child no longer responds appropriately to pain; capillary refill increases to longer than 3 seconds; and urine output is minimal. Ongoing, untreated hemorrhage (45% blood volume loss or 40 mL/kg) causes hypotension, coma, anuria, and preterminal bradycardia. Therapy during these late stages of compensated and uncompensated shock frequently requires airway and breathing management as well as resuscitation with both volume and blood. After 40 mL per kilogram of lactated Ringer's, whole blood or packed red blood cells should be administered as a rapid push until restoration of normal heart rate, pulses, blood pressure, pulse pressure, mental status, and urine output is attained. If hypotension is not promptly treated, then intractable shock may develop despite successful control of hemorrhage. Children with prolonged hypotension who recover from intractable shock still can develop MOF.

Multiple Organ Failure Syndrome in Children during the Perioperative Period

There is a paucity of literature on MOF associated with perioperative hemorrhage in children versus adults (46), in part because it usually can be avoided by early recognition and appropriate fluid/blood therapy during the compensated phase of hemorrhagic shock. MOF usually occurs in the perioperative setting as a result of one or more of the following causes: (a) prolonged shock or ongoing ischemia, (b) DIC, (c) primary organ failure, (e.g., liver failure), (d) a persistent nidus of inflammation or infection, (e) trauma, and (f) toxin or drug toxicity.

Ongoing ischemia after resuscitation can be underdiagnosed. Although fluid and blood resuscitation are the mainstays of therapy of hemorrhagic shock and third-space fluid loss, cardiovascular failure can also be important. Adequate perfusion pressure (MAP-CVP) must be provided to prevent renal failure. It is important to maintain urine output greater than 1 mL per kilogram of body weight per hour and to maintain a normal creatinine clearance for age. Creatinine clearance can be measured in a 1-hour urine collection. Hemorrhagic shock also can produce endotoxemia secondary to bowel ischemia (47). Ongoing shock can be caused by cardiac dysfunction. When fluid refractory shock persists, dopamine can be used as a first-line inotrope. Children are relatively unresponsive to dopamine or dobutamine compared with adults; so epinephrine infusion may be required for fluid-refractory shock. As suggested, adrenal insufficiency also should be evaluated in this group of patients and, if present, hydrocortisone therapy is warranted.

Disseminated intravascular coagulopathy causes MOF. Microvascular thrombi lead to inadequate perfusion of organs (48). Numerous forms of DIC exist. First, dilutional DIC occurs because blood replacement therapy does not keep up with platelet and coagulation factor requirements. Administering platelets, FFP, and cryoprecipitate as directed by platelet count, prothrombin time (PT), and partial thromboplastin time (PTT) can correct this problem. This condition also can be prevented by including platelet and FFP transfusion with packed red blood cell replacement during resuscitation (1 U platelets for each 5 U packed red blood cells and 1 U FFP for each 3 U packed red blood cells). Second, tissue disruption can lead to release of tissue factor and resultant DIC with a bleeding diathesis (49). Optimal treatment of these patients includes platelets, cryoprecipitate, and FFP according to platelet count and PT and PTT. Third, bleeding diathesis, particularly in newborns, can result from a relative deficiency or dysfunction in von Willebrand factor. These patients respond to therapy with DDAVP. Fourth, a "hypercoagulable" form of DIC is caused by systemic bacterial or fungal infection. Consumption of the anticoagulants antithrombin III and protein C and increased plasminogen activator inhibitor type 1 activity leads to a hypercoagulable and hypofibrinolytic state that is associated with microvascular thrombosis and little evidence of bleeding (50). These patients can be treated with antithrombin III or protein C according to measured levels (51). When concentrates are not available, FFP replacement is indicated according to PT and PTT.

Patients with liver failure have a remarkable degree of MOF with cerebral edema, hyperammonemia, acute respiratory distress syndrome (ARDS), bleeding diathesis, hypoglycemia, hypoalbuminemia, and hepatorenal syndrome. Supportive therapies include intracranial pressure monitoring, when possible, and management, ammonia scavengers and binders, FFP and cryoprecipitate replacement, high glucose infusions, replacement of albumin, and attention to abdominal compartment syndrome. Intraabdominal pressure can be increased from ascites. If abdominal pressure increases relative to mean arterial pressure, then renal perfusion pressure and renal function are compromised. These children can require volume or pressors to maintain adequate perfusion pressures.

Ongoing infection from a persistent nidus is the most common cause of MOF in children (52). Numerous mediators associated with hypercoagulation, hypofibrinolysis, and immune paralysis lead to MOF. The mainstay of therapy includes removal of the nidus and eradication of infection. Children can commonly be infected with opportunistic organisms, including *Candida* and *Aspergillus*. Antifungal therapy is often required. If the nidus of infection is removed, outcomes are favorable.

Multiple-organ failure associated with trauma is rare and usually is associated with crush injury in children (53). ARDS and pulmonary contusion are common with multitrauma victims. Use of PEEP to maintain functional residual capacity and low tidal volumes to prevent iatrogenic lung injury are indicated. Methyl prednisolone can be used in patients with ARDS that is not resolving by 7 days if bronchoalveolar lavage shows no evidence of pneumonia. Rhabdomyolysis and hyperuricemia cause renal failure. Myoglobinuria should be rapidly treated with mannitol and urine alkalinization to prevent renal failure (54). Renal failure is not an ominous condition in children. Dialysis is rarely needed after 6 weeks to 3 months because renal function uniformly returns. Pancreatitis is another common cause of MOF. Supportive therapy remains the mainstay. Prognosis with severe pancreatitis is also generally good in children.

Drug toxicity must be investigated in any child with MOF. Adverse drug reactions and drug interactions can occur in a subtle fashion. Renally excreted drugs should be dosed according to creatinine clearance. Hepatically metabolized drugs should be avoided in children with liver dysfunction. Drug holidays should be considered for any nonessential medication. Drugs should be carefully administered using a pediatric dosing handbook. Toxins also should be considered in children with an osmolar gap.

SUMMARY

Key developmental, physiologic, diagnostic, and management issues have been discussed for infants and children in the PICU before and after general, neurologic, and cardiothoracic surgery or solid-organ transplantation. Although there are a number of guiding principles, the unique nature of each surgical condition mandates both specific expertise and careful titration of care at the bedside. Finally, related to its importance in perioperative management, a contemporary assessment of the area of hemorrhagic shock and MOF in infants and children was provided. Both the complexity of this important PICU problem and the need for aggressive and carefully titrated multimodal therapies delivered by a highly trained and cooperative team were readily identified. Critical care expertise is essential to optimize the outcome of our most seriously ill infants and children with surgical conditions.

KEY POINTS

There are crucial developmental, physiologic, diagnostic, and medical and surgical management priorities and differences between caring for infants and children compared with adults. Guiding principles about the unique nature of the infant's or child's airway, fluid requirements, cardiopulmonary reserve, metabolic rate, and nutritional needs must be factored into the perioperative assessment and critical care of children undergoing general surgical, neurosurgical, cardiac, or transplant procedures. Congenital anomalies and metabolic abnormalities must be fully delineated and addressed to optimize perioperative care.

For the child undergoing neurologic surgery, common postoperative complications that require intensive monitoring include hydrocephalus, airway compromise, bleeding, vascular complications, fluid and electrolyte abnormalities, and seizures. Airway and respiratory compromise are particular concerns in patients after major maxillofacial reconstruction, in patients who have undergone procedures involving the brainstem (because respiratory center dysfunction, vocal cord paralysis, or cranial nerve damage is possible) and in patients who have undergone procedures that required prolonged prone positioning.

Approximately a third of infants with congenital heart disease require critical care within the first year of life. A multidisciplinary approach with pediatric cardiologists, intensivists, surgeons, and other subspecialists is the optimal approach to the care of these children perioperatively. Neonates and infants are dependent on maintaining and increasing heart rate to preserve cardiac output and cardiovascular function. Hypoglycemia and hypocalcemia must be recognized and treated in a timely fashion to avoid cardiac depression. Inotropic and vasoactive drugs must be used judiciously to limit excessive tachycardia, afterload increase, and myocardial work. Appropriate respiratory support is important to limit the work of breathing in children with cardiac failure. Finally, extracorporeal circulatory support is beneficial in selected patients with severe or refractory cardiopulmonary dysfunction.

Pediatric transplantation is an accepted treatment for children with various congenital and acquired pathologies and is associated with very favorable outcomes with the continued refinement of patient selection, surgical techniques, critical care, and modern immunosuppression. These patients are at risk for bleeding, infectious, and immune complications in the perioperative and postoperative periods.

Timely identification and intervention in the treatment of shock are important to improving outcome for pediatric patients. Bleeding may be secondary to traumatic or surgical insult, disseminated intravascular coagulopathy (DIC), dilutional coagulopathy, hypothermia, or hypocalcemia, among others. Children are able to maintain cardiac output and blood pressure despite significant blood loss. In addition, the hemoglobin may not accurately reflect the degree of hemorrhage. Therefore, the early physiologic response (tachycardia, narrow pulse pressure) to bleeding or volume depletion must be sought, recognized, and treated.

Multiple-organ failure (MOF) occurs most frequently in the perioperative setting secondary to one or more of the following causes: (a) prolonged shock or ongoing ischemia, (b) DIC, (c) primary organ failure (e.g., liver failure or pancreatitis), (d) a persistent nidus of inflammation or infection, (e) trauma, or (f) toxin or drug toxicity. Prevention and supportive care remain key to limiting the development of MOF.

REFERENCES

1. Rogers MC, ed. *Textbook of pediatric intensive care.* Baltimore: Williams & Wilkins, 1987:1–752.
2. Fuhrman BP, Zimmerman JJ, eds. *Pediatric critical care.* Baltimore: Mosby, 1998:1–1438.
3. Singh NC, ed. *Manual of pediatric critical care.* Philadelphia: WB Saunders, 1997:1–430.
4. Rogers MC, Helfaer MA, eds. *Case studies in pediatric intensive care.* Baltimore: Williams & Wilkins, 1993:1–362.
5. Shoemaker WC, Thompson WL, Holbrook PR, et al., eds. *The Society of Critical Care Medicine textbook of critical care.* Philadelphia: WB Saunders, 1984:1–1063.
6. Cowley RA, Trump BF, eds. *Pathophysiology of shock, anoxia, and ischemia.* Baltimore: Williams & Wilkins, 1982:1–710.
7. Schlag G, Redl H, eds. *Pathophysiology of shock, sepsis, and organ failure.* Berlin: Springer-Verlag, 1993:1–1165.
8. Iliff A, Lee VA. Pulse rate, respiratory rate, and body temperature of children between two months and eighteen years of age. *Child Dev* 1952;23:237–245.
9. Venkataraman ST, Khan N, Brown A. Validation of predictors of extubation success and failure in mechanically ventilated infants and children. *Crit Care Med* 2000;28:2991–2996.
10. Ferguson ND, Stewart TE, Etchells EE. Human albumin administration in critically ill patients. *Intensive Care Med* 1999;25:323–325.
11. Wesley JR, Coran AG. Intravenous nutrition for the pediatric patient. *Semin Pediatr Surg* 1992;1:212–230.
12. Moront ML, Eichelberger MR. Intensive care management of the injured child. In: Grenvik A, ed. *Textbook of critical care,* 4th ed. Philadelphia: WB Saunders, 2000:352–365.
13. Okada Y, Klein N, van Saene HK, et al. Small volumes of enteral feedings normalize immune function in infants receiving parenteral nutrition. *J Pediatr Surg* 1998;33:16–19.
14. Hoffman HJ, DeSilva M, Humphreys RP, et al. Aggressive surgical management of craniopharyngiomas in children. *J Neurosurg* 1992; 76:47–52.
15. Fabling JM, Gan TJ, El-Moalem HE, et al. A randomized, double-blinded comparison of ondansetron, droperidol, and placebo for prevention of postoperative nausea and vomiting after supratentorial craniotomy. *Anesth Analg* 2000;91:358–361.
16. Gutin PH. Corticosteroid therapy in patients with brain tumors. *J Natl Cancer Inst Monogr* 1977;46:151–156.
17. Levine B, Sirinek K, Mcleod C. The role of cimetidine in the prevention of stress induced gastric mucosal injury. *Surg Gynecol Obstet* 1979;148:399–402.
18. MacLean L. Prophylactic treatment of stress ulcers: first do no harm. *Can J Surg* 1988;31:76–77.
19. Ross AJ, Siegel KR, Bell W, et al. Massive gastrointestinal hemorrhage in children with posterior fossa tumors. *J Pediatr Surg* 1987;22:633–636.
20. Bengur AR, Meliones JN. Cardiogenic shock. *New Horizons* 1998; 6:139–149.
21. Schroedl NA, Hartzell CR, Ross PD, McCarl RL. Glucose metabolism, insulin effects, and developmental age of cultured neonatal rat heart cells. *J Cell Physiol* 1982;113:231–239.
22. Friedman WF. The intrinsic physiologic properties of the developing heart. *Prog Cardiovasc Dis* 1972;15:87–111.
23. Klitzner TS. Maturational changes in excitation-contraction coupling in mammalian myocardium. *J Am Coll Cardiol* 1991;17:218–225.
24. Grosso MA, Banerjee A, St Cyr JA, et al. Cardiac 5′-nucleotidase activity increases with age and inversely relates to recovery from ischemia. *J Thorac Cardiovasc Surg* 1992;103:206–209.
25. Colucci WS. Cardiovascular effects of milrinone. *Am Heart J* 1991; 121:1945–1947.
26. Barton P, Garcia J, Kouatli A, et al. Hemodynamic effects of i.v. milrinone lactate in pediatric patients with septic shock. A prospective, double-blinded, randomized, placebo-controlled, interventional study. *Chest* 1996;109:1302–1312.
27. Dalton HJ, Siewers RD, Fuhrman BP, et al. Extracorporeal membrane oxygenation for cardiac rescue in children with severe myocardial dysfunction. *Crit Care Med* 1993;1020–1028.
28. Akomea-Agyin C, Kejriwal NK, Franks R, et al. Intra-aortic balloon pumping in children. *Ann Thorac Surg* 1999;67:1415–1420.
29. Shekerdemian LS, Bush A, Shore DF, et al. Cardiopulmonary interactions after Fontan operations: augmentation of cardiac output using negative pressure ventilation. *Circulation* 1997;96:3934–3942.
30. Anand KJ, Hickey PR. Halothane-morphine compared with high-dose sufentanil for anesthesia and postoperative analgesia in neonatal cardiac surgery. *N Engl J Med* 1992;326:1–9.
31. Alonso M, Ryckman F. Current concepts in pediatric liver transplant. *Semin Liver Dis* 1998;18:295–307.
32. McDonald R, Donaldson L, Emmett L, et al. A decade of living donor transplantation in North American children: the 1998 Annual Report of the North American Pediatric Renal Transplant Cooperative Study (NAPRTCS). *Pediatr Transplant* 2000;4:221–234.
33. Elshihabi I, Chavers B, Donaldson L, et al. Continuing improvement in cadaver donor graft survival in North American children: the 1998 Annual Report of the North American Pediatric Renal Transplant Cooperative Study (NAPRTCS). *Pediatr Transplant* 2000;4:235–246.
34. Webber S. 15 years of pediatric heart transplantation at the University of Pittsburgh: lessons learned and future prospects. *Pediatr Transplant* 1997;1:8–21.

35. Grant D. Intestinal transplantation: 1997 report of the international registry. *Transplantation* 1999;67:1061–1064.

36. Stillwell P, Mallory G. Pediatric lung transplantation. *Clin Chest Med* 1997;18:405–414.

37. Gajarski RJ, Rosenblatt HM, Denfield SW, et al. Outcomes among pediatric heart transplant recipients after dual-therapy cytomegalovirus prophylaxis. *Tex Heart Inst J* 1997;24:97–104.

38. McDiarmid S. Liver transplantation in children. In: Ginns L, ed. *Transplantation*, 1st ed. Malden, Massachusetts: Blackwell Science, 1999:374–394.

39. Tzakis A, Gordon R, Shaw B. Clinical presentation of hepatic artery thrombosis after liver transplantation in the cyclosporine era. *Transplantation* 1985;40:667–671.

40. Mazariegos GV, O'Toole K, Mieles LA, et al. Hyperbaric oxygen therapy for hepatic artery thrombosis after liver transplantation in children. *Liver Transplant Surg* 1999;5:429–436.

41. Renz JF, Rosenthal P, Roberts JP, et al. Planned exploration of pediatric liver transplant recipients reduces post-transplant morbidity and lowers length of hospitalization. *Arch Surg* 1997;132:950–955.

42. Harmon W. Pediatric organ transplantation. *Transplant Proc* 1998; 30:1952–1955.

43. Singh A, Stablein D, Tejani A. Risk factors for vascular thrombosis in pediatric renal transplantation. *Transplantation* 1997;63:1263–1267.

44. Huddleston CB, Sweet SC, Mallory GB, et al. Lung transplantation in very young infants. *J Thorac Cardiovasc Surg* 1999;118:796–803.

45. Woo M, MacLaughlin E, Horn MV, et al. Living donor lobar lung transplantation: the pediatric experience. *Pediatr Transplant* 1998;2: 185–190.

46. Regel G, Grotz M, Weltner T, et al. Pattern of organ failure following severe trauma. *World J Surg* 1996;20:422–429.

47. Charpentier C, Audibert G, Dousset B, et al. Is endotoxin and cytokine release related to a decrease in gastric intramucosal pH after hemorrhagic shock? *Intensive Care Med* 1997;23:1040–1048.

48. Kreuz W, Veldmann A, Fischer D, et al. Neonatal sepsis: a challenge in hemostaseology. *Semin Thromb Hemost* 1999;25:531–535.

49. Abraham E. Tissue factor inhibition and clinical trial results of tissue factor pathway inhibitor in sepsis. *Crit Care Med* 2000;28(9 Suppl): S31–S33.

50. Smith OP, White B, Vaughan D, et al. Use of protein-C concentrate, heparin, and haemodiafiltration in meningococcus-induced purpura fulminans. *Lancet* 1997;350:1590–1593.

51. Kreuz WD, Schneider W, Nowak-Gottl U. Treatment of consumption coagulopathy with antithrombin concentrate in children with acquired antithrombin deficiency—a feasibility pilot study. *Eur J Pediatr* 1999;158(Suppl 3):S187–S191.

52. Hall MW, Volk HD, Reinke P, et al. Validation of monocyte HLA-DR expression less than 30% as a marker of immune paralysis in children with multiple organ dysfunction. *Crit Care Med* 2000;27:A36.

53. Tattersall JE, Richards NT, McCann M, et al. Acute haemodialysis during the Armenian earthquake disaster. *Injury* 1990;21:25–28.

54. Wang AY, Li PK, Lui SF, et al. Renal failure and heatstroke. *Ren Fail* 1995;17:171–179.

CARE OF THE PATIENT WITH MULTIPLE TRAUMA

KIMBERLY K. NAGY
CATHERINE CAGIANNOS
KIMBERLY T. JOSEPH

KEY WORDS

- Abdominal compartment syndrome
- Acute renal failure; acute tubular necrosis
- Acute respiratory distress syndrome
- Blunt cardiac injury
- Cerebral blood flow
- Cerebral perfusion pressure
- Coagulopathy; dilutional, platelets, plasma
- Closed head injury
- Hypothermia
- Immune modulation
- Immune suppression
- Inflammation; systemic,

- antiinflammation, proinflammation
- Inflammatory mediators; cytokines, tumor necrosis factor, interleukins, interferon, adhesion molecules
- Intracranial pressure; monitoring, treatment
- Nutrition support; enteral, parenteral, monitoring, lipids, carbohydrates, protein
- Pulmonary contusion
- Resuscitation
- Starvation
- Transfusion; plasma, platelets, red cells

INTRODUCTION

In the United States, trauma is a major factor in health care. Injury constitutes the third leading cause of death and remains the leading cause of death in children, adolescents, and young adults (1). In 1998, more than 146,000 people died as a result of trauma. An additional 2.5 million were hospitalized for treatment of their injuries (2). Many of these people will require either short- or long-term intensive care management of their injuries.

This chapter summarizes some of the many aspects of the care of the trauma patient, from the basics of resuscitation and management, to the immune response to trauma, to consideration of some specific injuries and their specialized care. It is not the goal of this chapter to review the initial diagnostic and therapeutic procedures that occur in the trauma patient because much of that is completed before the patient is admitted to the intensive care unit (ICU).

RESUSCITATION OF THE TRAUMA PATIENT

Trauma patients frequently come to the ICU requiring ongoing resuscitation. It is important to determine the degree of resuscitation that is still needed both to continue resuscitation as well as to avoid over-resuscitating the patient. If the patient remains under-resuscitated, there is a risk of extension of the injury zone. This is especially important in head injured patients who are subject to ongoing cerebral damage from ischemia (3). On the other hand, overaggressive resuscitation can result in complications such as pulmonary edema and abdominal compartment syndrome (4).

The most widely used method of monitoring in the ICU is measurement of volume status, most commonly preload. In the severely injured patient, this requires the placement of a pulmonary artery catheter (5). Whereas preload can be estimated by measuring central venous pressure (CVP) and pulmonary artery occlusion pressure (PAOP), patients with elevated airway pressures or intrapleural pressures may have a falsely elevated CVP and PAOP. This occurs in patients with increased levels of positive end-expiratory pressure (PEEP) as well (6). In such patients, the measurement of right and left ventricular end diastolic volumes (RVEDVI and LVEDVI) may give a more accurate estimation of preload (7).

Oximetric calculations are useful in determining the patient's degree of resuscitation. Continuous measurement of the mixed venous oxygen saturation (SvO$_2$) will alert the clinician to a drop in the patient's oxygen delivery or an increase in their oxygen consumption, either of which should be addressed (5).

Yu (8) recommends striving to achieve the following "oxygen-delivery goals": an adequate blood pressure, urine output greater than 30 to 50 mL per hour, SvO$_2$ greater than 65%, and oxygen delivery greater than 600 mL per minute per m^2. Older patients also may require maintenance of a hemoglobin level greater than 12 g per deciliter (9). The first line of therapy to improve perfusion in these patients is usually through optimization of their preload status. This may be accomplished by bolus of either crystalloids or colloids. If the patient has a concomitant low hemoglobin level, blood is an ideal choice (8). Once the patient has been determined to have an adequate preload and the oxygen delivery is still low, inotropes may be judiciously added (10). Most trauma patients do not require, and indeed may not tolerate, afterload reduction (8).

Hypoperfusion results in metabolic acidosis, which is reflected in a number of laboratory values that may be followed as measures of end-organ perfusion as well. Measurement of the base deficit is easy, rapid, and widely available. A persistently elevated base deficit is an indication of impaired oxygen utilization, which in these patients indicates inadequate perfusion (11). The best treatment for metabolic acidosis resulting from hypoperfusion is to improve cardiac output and oxygen delivery. The administration of sodium bicarbonate is contraindicated in these patients because of associated rebound alkalemia (12).

Another widely available laboratory marker of perfusion is serum lactate. Because an elevated lactate indicates that anaerobic metabolism is occurring, the patient's lactate measurements can be used to document improvement in the oxygen debt by demonstrating a decrease in serum lactate (13). If the patient has sustained an ischemia/reperfusion insult, there may be an initial increase in the serum lactate, the so-called washout phenomenon, but this lactate should clear as the patient becomes adequately resuscitated (10).

Several relatively new methods of determining specific end-organ perfusion are being evaluated. Perhaps the most promising of these is the gastric tonometer. The tonometer measures the actual mucosal perfusion of the gastrointestinal tract (stomach). Patients with a persistent intramucosal acidosis [i.e., intramucosal pH (pHi) < 7.32 after 24 hours] have been shown to have an increased incidence of multiple-organ failure (MOF) and death compared with patients who have been resuscitated to a normal pHi (14).

VENTILATORY SUPPORT OF THE TRAUMA PATIENT

Not infrequently, the severely injured trauma patient requires ventilatory support. Many of these patients are at risk for the development of acute respiratory distress syndrome (ARDS). In the trauma patient, ARDS may be of either a direct or an indirect etiology (15). *Direct* etiologies result from pulmonary injuries such as pulmonary contusions; severe penetrating lung injuries; smoke inhalation; and, later during the hospitalization, pneumonia. *Indirect* causes of ARDS in trauma patients are shock; massive soft-tissue injury; and, later, sepsis. Direct ARDS is characterized by normal chest-wall compliance with a consolidation of lung parenchyma and is less responsive to alveolar recruitment measures, such as application of PEEP or prone positioning. Barotrauma is more likely to occur in patients with direct ARDS resulting from regional hyperperfusion. Indirect ARDS has abnormal chest-wall and lung compliance and is characterized more by pulmonary edema and alveolar collapse. These patients respond better to PEEP and prone positioning but are more likely to have hemodynamic abnormalities. Many trauma patients may have a combination of both direct and indirect ARDS.

Treatment of patients at risk for ARDS is started by attempts to maintain arterial oxygen saturation (SaO_2) above 90% on inspired oxygen concentrations (FiO_2) less than 0.6 (8). Increased levels of PEEP may be required in these patients. The optimal PEEP for most patients with early ARDS is between 10 and 18 cm H_2O. This level will aid in oxygenation while still limiting overdistension of the alveoli and subsequent barotrauma (16).

A "lung-protective strategy" (17,18) may be used in an attempt to prevent further injury. This involves the use of lower tidal-volume settings (6–8 mL/kg) in an effort to minimize overdistension of the alveoli (19). This lower tidal volume may result in a hypercarbia and respiratory acidosis. This so-called permissive hypercarbia is not harmful, and the pH may be allowed to go as low as 7.20 (20). An acid buffer such as *Tris* (hydroxymethyl)-aminomethane (THAM) may be considered if the pH drops lower than 7.10. Pressure-control mode of ventilation is often necessary to limit the peak inspiratory pressure to 35 to 40 cm H_2O, also reducing the risk of barotrauma (21).

The late phase of ARDS (i.e., after 10–14 days) is characterized by a brittle fibrotic lung. The patient requires a higher minute ventilation and is at greater risk for barotrauma from elevated levels of PEEP (22). There is some evidence that systemic steroids given at the beginning of this stage may be helpful in minimizing fibrosis (21).

RENAL DYSFUNCTION IN TRAUMA

Acute renal failure (ARF) is defined as an abrupt reduction in glomerular filtration rate (GFR) caused by intrinsic parenchymal disease or diminished renal hemodynamics. The trauma patient may develop ARF because of (a) hypovolemia from acute blood loss or postoperative third spacing; (b) direct organ injury to the kidney, ureter, or bladder leading to hydronephrosis; (c) increased filtration of toxic pigments as seen in rhabdomyolysis; (d) use of nephrotoxic agents; and (e) sepsis. Acute tubular necrosis (ATN) accounts for 80% of cases of ARF in the critical care setting. Aminoglycoside antibiotics and radiographic contrast agents are common toxins causing ATN. Ischemic etiologies for ATN include prolonged hypotension, necessity for suprarenal aortic clamping, and sepsis. The renal tubular cells at the corticomedullary junction are particularly susceptible to ischemia.

The mortality rate from ARF remains 50% on average (23); however, mortality rate for ARF associated with ventilatory failure, sepsis, or burns approaches 70% to 80%. Mortality rate approaches 100% if three or more organ systems have failed concomitantly.

Tubular cell injury and cast formation in the tubular lumen from sloughed cellular material increase tubular pressures and decrease GFR. The S3 segment of the proximal tubule and the thick ascending limb of the loop of Henle are susceptible to injury because they normally exist in a state of relative hypoxia (24). Any added ischemic insult promotes tubular injury secondary to accumulation of intracellular calcium, depletion of adenosine triphosphate (ATP), generation of oxidants, and apoptosis (25). There is impaired distribution of integrin receptors on the basolateral membrane of tubular cells with the resultant aberrant adhesion to the adjacent matrix facilitating the sloughing of cells into the tubular lumen (26). Integrin receptors translocate onto the luminal membrane and can contribute to intratubular obstruction by promoting adhesion between tubular cells and sloughed cellular debris. Redistribution of Na^+-K^+-ATPase pumps from the basolateral membrane to the luminal membrane of tubular cells may interfere with the normal sodium transport into tubular cells (27). Endotoxin release may play an important role in ARF associated with sepsis and trauma. Neutrophils primed by endotoxin to release tumor necrosis factor-α (TNF-α), elastases, and oxygen free radicals can result in renal vasoconstriction and direct tubular cell damage (28,29).

Treatment of ARF is supportive, with hydration being paramount. Although "renal dose" dopamine increases sodium excretion, renal blood flow, and GFR in patients with ARF, most studies have not shown an improved outcome (30). Loop diuretics can minimize renal injury by potentially washing out cellular casts and decreasing oxygen requirements in the proximal tubule (31). Mannitol may preserve mitochondrial function by osmotically minimizing the degree of post-ischemic cell swelling (32). It is unknown, however, whether converting a patient from oliguric to nonoliguric ARF using diuretics influences patient survival. Responders may simply have had less severe disease with a greater number of functioning nephrons irrespective of the diuretic. As the pathophysiology of ARF has been elucidated, various agents involved in different aspects of tubular injury have been used as interventions. Use of these agents in animals has met with some success; however, use in humans has not resulted in consistent results. The administration of anti-intracellular adhesion molecule 1 (anti-ICAM-1) antibodies and synthetic Arg-Gly-Asp (RGD) proteins that inhibit integrins has been shown to lessen duration of ATN (26,33). Atrial natriuretic peptide (ANP) increases renal blood flow, improves glomerular blood flow, and decreases endothelin release in animal models of ARF; however, ANP did not improve survival or decrease the need for dialysis in patients with ARF (34). Animal evidence suggests that use of insulin-like growth factor (IGF) and epidermal growth factor may improve renal function, decrease histologic injury, and reduce mortality (35); however, a recent trial with IGF-1 in humans was disappointing (36).

Although dialysis is lifesaving when hypervolemia, hyperkalemia, acidosis, or uremia develop, there are concerns that institution of dialysis may have detrimental effects on renal function by induction of hypotension, activation of complement, upregulation of adhesion receptors, and stimulation of neutrophil infiltration into the kidney (37,38). Continuous renal replacement therapy (CRRT), such as continuous arteriovenous hemofiltration (CAVH), has several advantages over hemodialysis in critically ill patients. CRRT is better tolerated hemodynamically and is as efficient in removing solutes as hemodialysis over a 24-hour period. Preliminary human evidence suggests that the porous membranes used in CAVH may be more efficient at removing endotoxin, interleukin 1 (IL-1), platelet activating factor (PAF), and TNF-α in septic or catabolic patients and may thus act in an immunomodulatory fashion (39). These studies are uncontrolled, and to date there has not been consistent evidence showing improved outcomes in septic patients who have had removal of inflammatory mediators by CRRT (40).

Infection remains the most common cause of death in trauma patients with ARF. Although renal recovery is clinically complete, as many as 50% of patients have functional derangements with defects in GFR, decreased concentrating ability, and defects in

urinary acidification. Thirty percent of ICU patients who survive ARF with dialysis will require long-term renal replacement therapy.

HYPOTHERMIA AND COAGULOPATHY IN THE TRAUMA PATIENT

Trauma patients are at risk for the development of hypothermia for several reasons (41). Patients with severe closed head injury or those undergoing general anesthesia lose the ability to autoregulate their body temperature. They lose heat rapidly because of blood loss as well as increased surface area during laparotomy or thoracotomy. In addition, most resuscitative fluid is given at temperatures lower than body temperature, especially fluids given in the prehospital setting. There is an inverse correlation between body temperature and mortality, even when controlling for injury severity (41). Patients with persistent core temperatures below 92°F have a 100% mortality.

The major physiologic derangement that results from hypothermia is coagulopathy. The coagulation cascade is not functional in the severely hypothermic patient (42). This is difficult to measure, however, because laboratory measurements of coagulation—such as prothrombin time (PT) and partial thromboplastin time (PTT)—are performed after heating the blood sample to body temperature. In addition, there is decreased platelet aggregation and prolonged bleeding time in the hypothermic patient (43). All these hypothermia-induced coagulation abnormalities are reversible on rewarming of the patient (42).

Hypothermia is not the only cause of coagulopathy in the trauma patient. The most common cause is actually hemodilution after hemorrhage and massive transfusion (44). Persistent acidosis contributes to coagulation dysfunction, and there may be a consumptive coagulopathy as well in these patients (45). Thrombocytopenia is the prime culprit in nonsurgical bleeding in the massively transfused patient (46). In patients with severe closed head injury, the injured brain tissue will release a thromboplastin-like substance, which further contributes to the coagulopathy (47).

Correction of coagulopathy in the trauma patient requires correction of its many causative factors. It is imperative that these patients are rewarmed and perfusion restored (48). If the patient remains hypothermic and acidotic, replacement of factors and platelets will be futile (49).

These unstable patients require intense ongoing care. They are best treated with two nurses and a physician at the bedside providing ongoing fluid resuscitation, aggressive rewarming, and transfusion. Aggressive rewarming is carried out by increasing the ambient temperature in the room, warming the ventilator mist, placing convection heating blankets, and warming all intravenous fluids and blood products (48). The small blood-warmer devices are not sufficient for ongoing massive resuscitation. A rapid infusion device, such as the Level I fluid warmer is required to heat fluid and blood to 40°C while infusing it rapidly into the patient.

As the patient is being rewarmed, blood products may be transfused based on actual laboratory values. Cookbook-type formulas that dictate a certain number of units of fresh frozen plasma (FFP) or platelets per units of blood are inaccurate and should not be followed (48). Blood is transfused based on the patient's hemoglobin. FFP is given based on the patient's PT and PTT, and platelets are given when the patient's platelet count is less than 50,000. Cryoprecipitate may be given if the patient has a concomitant consumptive coagulopathy demonstrated by a decreased fibrinogen level (49). These patients also may require replacement of calcium to aid in coagulation function. Calcium replacement is guided by serum-ionized calcium because the bound calcium will be low secondary to dilutional hypoalbuminemia.

IMMUNE DYSFUNCTION IN TRAUMA

There is a relationship between trauma, shock, systemic inflammatory response syndrome (SIRS), and sepsis. Studies have shown that trauma and hemorrhagic shock can induce SIRS or downregulate immune function (50). Trauma is associated with tissue necrosis and bacterial translocation, which can induce the release of superoxide radicals and cytokines as well as alter the expression of adhesion molecules and cell-associated cytokine receptors. Cytokines are proteins and glycoproteins that are released by macrophages and lymphocytes in response to tissue necrosis or foreign-antigen presentation. Cytokines mediate and regulate immune and inflammatory responses (51). Understanding and modifying the proinflammatory and antiinflammatory cytokine milieu may help to regulate the immune response to trauma.

Typically, after severe trauma, an early proinflammatory response is followed by a more sustained antiinflammatory response. The former proinflammatory response is known as SIRS, whereas the latter response, which involves increased expression of antiinflammatory cytokines, is known as *compensatory antiinflammatory response syndrome* (CARS) (52). Homeostasis is achieved if a balance between the proinflammatory and antiinflammatory mediators can be reached; alternatively, MOF or sepsis develops if SIRS or CARS predominates.

Cytokine Levels after Trauma

Trauma, ischemia–reperfusion, and shock induce the release of mediators from monocytes and macrophages. Monocytes activated by trauma synthesize a series of proinflammatory (TNF-α, IL-1, IL-6, IL-8) and anti-inflammatory mediators (IL-4, IL-10, IL-11, IL-13 and transforming growth factor-β). Within minutes of severe trauma, Schinkel and colleagues found increases in chemotactic cytokines such as IL-8 and soluble selectin adhesion molecules (53). Human studies demonstrate early release of TNF-α, IL-1, and IL-6. Studies confirmed increased IL-6, C-reactive protein, and TNF-α levels in trauma patients with MOF and an association between these mediators and poor prognosis.

Usually a balance exists between the activity of proinflammatory and antiinflammatory mediators, but a significant depression of cell-mediated and humoral immunity has been observed in patients following soft tissue trauma, bone fractures, and hemorrhagic shock. After trauma, the synthesis of IL-1, IL-2, IL-2 receptors, IL-3, gamma-interferon (IFN-γ), and mixed histocompatibility complex (MHC) class II antigens on and by macrophages and monocytes is downregulated (50). Decreased levels of IFN-γ may impair macrophage activation (54) as well as decrease natural killer (NK) cell activity, decrease T- and B-cell proliferation and differentiation, and decrease granulocyte chemotaxis and phagocytosis. In addition, activated macrophages elaborate a powerful endogenous immunosuppressant, prostaglandin E_2 (PGE$_2$), which induces T-helper cells to synthesize immunosuppressive cytokines, such as IL-4 and IL-10 (55). Patients with trauma and major burns have increased production of IL-4 and IL-10 as well as decreased levels of IL-12, thus producing a relative anergic state (56). IL-10 suppresses IL-2 synthesis and T-cell proliferation. In CARS, neutrophils are induced to undergo apoptosis by IL-10, thus resulting in reduced antigen presentation to T cells and decreased production of proinflammatory cytokines (57). Failure of neutrophil apoptosis is postulated to mediate tissue injury and precipitate SIRS (58).

Immunomodulatory Therapies

The goals of immunomodulation are (a) to avoid the excessive stimulation of macrophages and T cells, which leads to SIRS and MOF, and (b) to prevent the suppression of cell-mediated immunity, which leads to sepsis. Trauma causes impaired gut perfusion. During ischemia and reperfusion, translocation of bacteria and endotoxin from the gut into the systemic circulation is hypothesized to result in release of proinflammatory mediators from activated cells. Investigators have attempted to improve gut perfusion and reduce the intensity of endotoxin-mediated inflammation by a variety of methods. Hypertonic saline reduces blood viscosity, reduces regional vasoconstriction (59), reduces endothelial adhesion-molecule expression (60), and reduces neutrophil oxidative burst (61). Behrman et al. demonstrated improved perfusion in renal and jejunal mucosa following resuscitation with hypertonic saline (62). Using a rat model of controlled hemorrhage, Coimbra and colleagues reported reductions in lung injury and bacterial translocation following resuscitation with pentoxifylline and hypertonic saline (63). Using pentoxifylline in severe sepsis, Staubach and co-workers observed an improved multiple-organ dysfunction syndrome (MODS) score and PaO$_2$ to FiO$_2$ ratios (64). IL-12 induces the production of IFN-γ, which in turn potentiates macrophage activation, release of TNF-α, and induction of cytotoxic T-cell function. O'Sullivan and colleagues demonstrated that administration of IL-12 restored resistance to infection (65). Attempts to decrease susceptibility to infection and mortality from septic complications by using IFN-γ (66) and anti-TNF-α monoclonal antibodies (67) or soluble TNF receptors (68) have been unsuccessful.

To date, the most efficacious immunomodulatory therapy for trauma patients is the use of enteral feeds. Enteral feeding restores gut barrier function. Use of enteral feeds supplemented with glutamine, arginine, and omega-3 polyunsaturated fatty acids resulted in fewer infectious complications and lower MOF scores (69).

NUTRITIONAL SUPPORT OF THE TRAUMA PATIENT

In 1930, Cuthbertson described the metabolic response to stress in terms of the *ebb* and *flow* phases, terms still in use today (70). The *ebb* phase is characterized by circulatory compromise or insufficiency and a normal or depressed metabolic state. The *flow* phase, which follows this, is notable for increases in energy expenditure, nitrogen excretion, and protein catabolism. Although initially the ebb phase was described as lasting 2 to 48 hours, this phase can vary widely depending on the patient and the clinical situation. The flow phase, in fact, can begin mere hours after the initial trauma or stress. In the last 30 years, enhanced understanding of these processes and advances in technology have allowed for improvements in care for patients experiencing severe metabolic challenge. Although nutrition support is recognized as an important component in the management of such patients, controversy remains regarding the type, timing, composition, and degree of nutritional intervention necessary to achieve an optimal outcome.

Stress Versus Starvation

In the starved patient, there is a decrease in the basal energy expenditure with limited use of glucose and an adaptive increase in the use of fatty acids and ketones for energy; ultimately, at least partial sparing of the skeletal muscle/lean body mass is found, except in extreme cases (71). Furthermore, the body remains very responsive to exogenous fuels if they are provided (71,72). In contrast, the stress state (once in the flow phase) is characterized by increases in substrate flow but poor utilization of these same substrates. For example, although the cellular uptake of glucose peripherally remains somewhat constant, insulin resistance is commonly observed. There is a decrease in ketone production and utilization despite an increase in lipolysis. It is when one considers protein catabolism, however, that the differences between the stressed and starved patient become most dramatic. In the stressed patient, the body's need for protein (to provide for coagulation, wound healing, and host defense, and so on) increases, and a resulting increase in hepatic protein synthesis does occur; however, this is *far* outweighed by the increase in protein catabolism (71,72). Skeletal muscle is broken down to allow use of the branched-chain amino acids (leucine, isoleucine, and valine) as substrates for gluconeogenesis, but this is an inefficient source of energy relative to fat. Because protein is being used preferentially, wasting occurs. The body is also less responsive to administration of exogenous fuels, including protein (72). In severe stress states, progressing to multisystem-organ dysfunction, substrate utilization only worsens; hypertriglyceridemia (due to increased lipolysis), decreased hepatic protein synthesis, increased ureagenesis, and hypoglycemia (caused by the failure of gluconeogenesis) all may be observed (73).

Nutritional Assessment and Estimation of Nutritional Requirements

Because the metabolic processes of the stressed patient are so deranged, traditional methods of nutritional assessment may be less reliable. Fluid shifts and rapid wasting may render anthropometric measurements of little use in these circumstances. Furthermore, frequent changes in a critically ill patient's metabolic status require equally frequent reassessments and careful monitoring. The temptation to provide excessively large amounts of calories based on the misconception that the stress state warrants it should be avoided; it must be remembered that despite increased demands, the body's overall utilization is markedly less efficient.

Hepatic transport protein measurements (transferrin, thyroid-binding protein prealbumin, and retinol-binding protein) have been used to estimate the adequacy of protein synthesis in the liver; however, serum levels of these proteins may be affected by changes in a patient's volume status. In addition, the liver shifts production in favor of acute phase proteins in times of stress (74). C-reactive protein may be detectable in serum in the early inflammatory phase (71) and has been suggested as an alternative to measuring transport proteins. A decline in C-reactive protein accompanied by an increase in prealbumin may indicate a positive response to nutrition support; however, it simply may reflect resolution of the inflammatory process not related to the patient's nutritional status per se. Traditional measurements of urinary nitrogen excretion also may be useful; however, their use must be tempered with the knowledge that the measurements may be inaccurate in the face of renal insufficiency. Also, patients with diarrhea or fistulas may experience significant nitrogen losses via the gastrointestinal tract that also must be taken into account. Measurements of cell-mediated immunity are generally not reliable as indicators of the adequacy of nutrition support in the stressed patient. Anergy is associated with metabolic stress in and of itself and may not represent malnutrition.

Estimates of caloric needs in these patients also may be difficult and may need frequent revision. In general, requirements range from 25 to 35 kcal per kilogram daily of total caloric support. The use of formulas to estimate basal energy requirements, such as the Harris-Benedict equation, may be used with the appropriate stress factor added as a starting point. More precise measurements, such as those obtained using indirect calorimetry, are widely recommended; however, they require the use of specialized and sometimes expensive equipment. Protein requirements in hypermetabolic patients usually range between 1.5 to 2 g per kilogram daily with a suggested nonprotein calorie to nitrogen ratio of 100:1 or less. Literature demonstrates that this lower ratio appears to promote nitrogen retention, increases plasma transferrin, and lowers the respiratory quotient (75). Fat calories should not exceed 40% of the total daily intake and may have to be adjusted in the face of hypertriglyceridemia. Carbohydrate should be provided at a minimum of 100 g daily. The glucose administered should be such that the oxidative rate does not exceed 5 mg per kilogram per minute. Excessive glucose infusion can lead to hepatic fatty infiltration or difficulties in ventilator weaning (71).

In recent years, specific "immune-enhancing" nutrients have received much attention. Glutamine, normally a nonessential amino acid, appears to be conditionally essential in the stress state. It is the preferred fuel source of enterocytes (76) and also may reduce protein degradation in skeletal muscle as well as enhance protein synthesis in the liver (77). One of the hypothetical models of nosocomial infection following trauma involves bacterial translocation due to a loss of gut mucosal integrity. Kouznetsova and colleagues demonstrated rapid reduction of protein kinase C-mediated hyperpermeability of intestinal cells grown in culture when exposed to glutamine (78). Although Kouznetsova and co-workers' work suggests that direct (i.e., enteral) exposure of the intestine to glutamine may be more efficient and result in a better outcome, Hwang and colleagues demonstrated some preservation of small-bowel mucosa integrity when glutamine was delivered by the parenteral route (79). Sheltinga and co-workers (80) also reported lower rates of clinical infection in patients receiving glutamine-enhanced parenteral nutrition. In the United States, parenteral glutamine-enhanced formulas are not yet available; however, several exist for delivery by the enteral route. In some situations, glutamine may be detrimental. Because the end product of glutamine metabolism is ammonia, concern has been expressed about the use of glutamine-rich diets in patients with renal failure, head injuries, and hepatic encephalopathy (71). Arginine, a nitric oxide precursor, also is considered by many to be a conditionally essential amino acid in stressed patients; it may augment immune function and thus improve outcome. Nitric oxide is a vasodilator and may play a role in sepsis-induced myocardial depression. Patients on arginine-enhanced diets should be monitored with this in mind (71). Controversy also exists regarding the use of omega-3 ("fish oil") versus omega-6 polyunsaturated fatty acids. The release of TNF and IL-1 by the macrophage appears to be influenced by the omega-3 to omega-6 *ratio* in the cell membrane, not merely the total content (71,77,81). Medium-chain triglycerides (MCTs) delivered enterally or parenterally appear to have protein-sparing characteristics and are enterally better absorbed than their long-chain counterparts (82); however, pure MCT formulations have been associated with metabolic acidosis and essential fatty acid deficiency. Structured lipid formulas, consisting of a mixture of medium- and long-chain fatty acids on a glycerol backbone, appear to provide the advantages of MCTs without the side effects (82,83); however, there are only a few such formulas available in the United States, and they are all enteral. Antioxidant therapy with high doses of vitamins A, C, and E is advocated by some practitioners, but studies done to date have not been conclusive (81,84).

Combining the preceding elements, the relatively new concept of "immunonutrition" has emerged in recent years. Studies of immune-enhanced formulas suggested that they may be useful in select patient populations, including critically-ill patients (85). A recent study by Gianotti amd colleagues (86) suggests that perioperative use of immunonutrition may result in cost savings by decreasing the incidence of postoperative complications and length of stay. Further work is needed to ascertain what specific formulation given at what time and in what dose is optimal in critical illness.

The Case for Early Enteral Nutrition

Although introduction of total parenteral nutrition revolutionized the field of nutrition support, few would disagree that the intestine, if functional, should be used in the critically ill patient. In the ebb phase of stress, the priority should be on maintenance of fluid balance and initiation of control of the inciting trauma (hemorrhage, infection, thermal injury, and so on). Attempting enteral feeding during this period actually may result in an unreasonable metabolic demand on the gut. Once the flow phase begins (keep in mind that, temporally, this may be only hours after the actual trauma or stress), nutrition support should be initiated; if possible, it should be provided via the gut. The use of early enteral feeding in posttraumatic patients has been demonstrated to preserve intestinal brush border integrity and function as well as to help maintain immunologic function and reduce infectious complications (87–89). Work by Kiyama and colleagues in rats (90) suggests that the route of nutrition may play a role in

wound healing in its early phase. Enteral nutrition appeared to provide superior results in terms of wound breaking strength and wound collagen accumulation. Whether or not enteral feeding should be supplied via the gastric or postpyloric route remains an area of argument. Some practitioners have concerns regarding aspiration in patients who are fed directly into the stomach; some studies have shown, however, that postpyloric feeding may not, in fact, reduce this risk (91,92). Heyland and co-workers suggest that gastric feeding in the critically ill patient is well tolerated if appropriate protocols are followed (93).

In patients in whom the gut cannot be used, parenteral nutrition, of course, should be initiated. Combined parenteral and enteral regimens may be useful in patients who have limited enteral feeding tolerance or in patients who require a more prolonged period to achieve their caloric goals via the enteral route (94).

CARE OF THE HEAD INJURED PATIENT

The multiply injured patient with a severe closed-head injury presents additional challenges for the intensive care physician. In 1995, the Brain Trauma Foundation published a comprehensive series of guidelines on the care of the head-injured patient. These guidelines (95) are based on all available literature and provide the basis for this section of the chapter.

Many patients with a Glasgow Coma Score below 9 will have an intracranial monitor placed. This is the decision of the neurosurgeon based on patient status, neurologic examination, and findings on computed tomogram of the head. Regardless of whether the monitor is placed intraventricular, intraparenchymal, subdural, or epidural, the resultant reading is managed in the same way.

In general, the intracranial pressure (ICP) should be maintained less than 20 mm Hg and the cerebral perfusion pressure (CPP) should be kept above 70 mm Hg. The CPP is the difference between the mean arterial pressure (MAP) and the ICP. The CPP is a reflection of the cerebral blood flow (CBF). By increasing the CPP, we can minimize local and global ischemic insults to the injured brain. An increase in MAP will increase the CPP by a similar amount but has little effect on the ICP. Maintenance of an adequate CPP may require the use of pressors once the patient has been fluid resuscitated.

The mainstay of treatment of elevated ICP is the use of mannitol. Mannitol is given as a bolus of 0.25 to 1.0 g per kilogram and may be repeated every 4 to 6 hours. It works by immediately increasing the plasma volume, thus increasing the CPP. It also functions as an osmotic diuretic to help draw fluid from the injured brain tissue. Mannitol should not be given unless the patient has been fluid resuscitated. It is also important to avoid hypovolemia and hyperosmollemia when using mannitol.

Hyperventilation is no longer used as the mainstay of decreasing ICP. Occasionally, it may be useful for acute treatment of neurologic deterioration, although it should be avoided in the initial 24 hours posttrauma because it may actually decrease the CBF and worsen the outcome of the patient.

In the occasional patient who is refractory to increasing the CPP and use of mannitol, barbiturate coma may be used. This involves giving high-dose pentobarbital to suppress cerebral metabolism and is monitored by burst suppression on the electroencephalogram. Decompressive craniotomy is another rarely used, but occasionally necessary, technique to lower the ICP.

CARE OF THE PATIENT WITH BLUNT CARDIAC INJURY

Patients who sustain severe blunt chest trauma are at risk for a blunt cardiac injury ("cardiac contusion"). Patients with cardiogenic shock or abnormal electrocardiogram (ECG) findings such as dysrhythmias, interventricular or bundle branch blocks, or ischemic changes are at risk for development of complications from a blunt cardiac injury (96). These patients should be placed on a cardiac monitor for 24 to 48 hours because about 15% will develop a complication during that time frame (97). These complications may take the form of a dysrhythmia, such as atrial or ventricular fibrillation or development of pulmonary edema resulting from heart failure. Such complications are treated as they arise. All are self-limiting and usually will resolve within 72 hours (97).

Cardiogenic shock may require the placement of a pulmonary artery catheter and institution of inotropic support or even the placement of an intraaortic balloon pump to support the patient through the acute injury phase (98). It is important to rule out a concomitant source of hemorrhagic shock before ascribing hypotension to the blunt cardiac injury (98). Echocardiography may be helpful in determining the degree of myocardial hypokinesia from the injury (96).

It is safe for the patient with a blunt cardiac injury to undergo general anesthesia if needed for repair of other injuries (96,97). Invasive monitoring in the form of a central venous catheter or pulmonary artery catheter may be useful in guiding fluid replacement and inotropic therapy if the patient is hemodynamically unstable (98).

CARE OF THE PATIENT WITH INCREASED ABDOMINAL PRESSURE

Not infrequently, the multiply injured patient has undergone a damage-control laparotomy to address the immediately life-threatening injuries. Bleeding and intestinal spillage are controlled, but definitive repair of injuries has not been accomplished because of patient instability, hypothermia, acidosis, and coagulopathy. Injuries may be packed to control nonsurgical blood loss. Such patients then are brought to the ICU for continued resuscitation. The goals are to restore perfusion, warm the patient, correct the acidosis, and reverse the coagulopathy (99).

Patients who have undergone a damage-control laparotomy are at risk for development of abdominal compartment syndrome (ACS). Other patients at risk for ACS are those who have had a massive resuscitation (for nonabdominal injuries and burns as well) and those with retroperitoneal hematomata from posterior pelvic fractures. These patients have either massively edematous viscera or hematomata that are causing an increased intraabdominal pressure (IAP) (4).

For patients at risk of developing ACS, the IAP may be measured. The easiest technique is by measurement of the intravesicular pressure (4). The Foley catheter is connected to a pressure transducer. The bladder is filled with 50 mL of sterile saline, and the Foley is clamped distal to the transducer, which is held at the level of the pubic symphysis. This measurement should be repeated every 2 to 4 hours in patients at risk for development of ACS.

The normal IAP is less than 10 mm Hg. As the IAP increases, it affects many systemic functions (4,100). It will cause an increase in peak inspiratory pressure and a decrease in pulmonary compliance through upward displacement of the diaphragm. The cardiac output will decrease, although the PAOP may be falsely elevated. The urine output will decrease, and the serum creatinine will increase as a result of a decrease in the creatinine clearance. As the IAP increases to over 20 mm Hg, the clinical picture is one of oliguria and elevated pulmonary pressures in a patient with a tense distended abdomen (100).

The initial treatment of a patient with ACS is to start fluid resuscitation (4). Unfortunately, the volume status of these patients may be difficult to assess because of the effect of the ACS on preload measurements and urine output. If the IAP is greater than 40 mm Hg, then abdominal decompression is mandatory (4). If the patient is extremely unstable, this may be done in the ICU to avoid transporting the patient to the operating room. The abdomen is opened and intraperitoneal hematoma is evacuated. Any obvious source of bleeding may be controlled. Immediately on relieving the ACS, the airway pressures will decrease, the hemodynamics will stabilize, and the patient should begin to make urine again (100).

Reclosure of the abdomen may result in return of ACS; therefore, a temporary closure method using a prosthetic closure such as GORE-TEX (W.L. Gore & Assoc., Flagstaff, AZ) is suggested (101). When a temporary prosthetic closure is used, the patient will have increased insensible fluid losses from their abdomen, which must be taken into consideration when evaluating the patient's fluid status.

SUMMARY

In summary, intensive care of the multiply traumatized patient involves attainment of a careful balance in the treatment of all systems. Fluid resuscitation must be judiciously performed to optimize perfusion without causing fluid overload. Attempts should be made to avoid further injury to the lungs or the kidneys through lung protective strategies of ventilatory management and intense efforts to avoid ATN.

A carefully designed and monitored nutritional support plan can play an important role in the overall management of the critically ill patient. Care should be taken not to overfeed such patients, and attention should be given to tailor the components of the nutritional support formulation(s) to the patients' needs as they change over time. Whenever possible, the enteral route is the preferred route of delivery of nutritional support in these patients.

Certain injuries, such as blunt cardiac injury and severe closed-head injury, require modifications in management or special attention. Awareness of the possibility of development of ACS should allow prompt diagnosis and treatment of this often unrecognized syndrome in the trauma patient.

With the proper care and attention to details required of these complex patients with multiple systemic derangements, outcomes are improved.

KEY POINTS

Despite tremendous advances in patient transport and triage, resuscitation, and intervention at specialized centers, trauma remains a major public health problem. It is the third leading cause of death in the United States. Timely and appropriate, ongoing resuscitation remains a backbone of trauma management in the emergency department, operating room, and ICU. Under-resuscitation results in hypoperfusion and hypoxia of vital end organs and may be particularly devastating in the victim of head trauma. Over-resuscitation also may be deleterious with excessive tissue edema, altered gas exchange, increased intraabdominal pressure, and other complications. Clinical judgment combined with hemodynamic monitoring is the current state of the practice in resuscitation. Newer techniques, such as gastric tonometry and identification of cellular metabolic markers, may be more widely used in the future to guide the adequacy of tissue perfusion.

Hypothermia and coagulopathy are common complications in injured patients. Aggressive warming of the environment, fluids, and inhaled gases can limit or reverse hypothermia. Hypothermia is frequently a cause of coagulation abnormalities, as is dilutional effect after large-volume resuscitation. Because blood coagulation is compromised during hypothermia, cold patients should be actively rewarmed.

Inflammation and the balance between antiinflammatory and proinflammatory forces are associated with homeostatic and pathologic response to traumatic insult. Inflammatory imbalance is associated with altered immune function, excess catabolism, organ dysfunction, and ultimately morbidity and death. Immune and nutritional modulation after trauma continues to be a major focus of ongoing research.

Appropriate ventilatory, hemodynamic, and nutrition support measures are important interventions in severely injured patients to limit such severe complications as acute respiratory distress syndrome, acute renal failure, or starvation. A lung-protective strategy, which limits peak airway pressure and barotrauma, is currently advocated for patients at risk for or with evolving acute lung injury. Enteral feeding is the preferred route of nutrition support. The role of specialized diets, such as those enriched with glutamate or special fatty acids, remains under investigation.

The closed-head injured patient has specialized needs, and care of such a patient has been well reviewed by the Brain Trauma Foundation. Intracranial pressure monitoring to identify intracranial hypertension is used in many of the more severely head-injured patients (Glasgow Coma Scale <9) on a case-by-case basis. It allows timely intervention to maintain cerebral perfusion pressure. Mannitol is a mainstay of treatment, and routine hyperventilation is no longer recommended.

REFERENCES

1. Magnitude and costs. In: Fulco CE, Bonnie RJ, Liverman CT, eds. *Reducing the burden of injury: advancing prevention and treatment.* Washington, DC: National Academy Press, 1999:41–49.

2. National Center for Health Statistics. *Injuries 2000.* Internet Communication. http://www.cdc.gov/nchs.

3. Suntharalingam G, Evans TW. Current trends in the management of acute respiratory distress syndrome. *Curr Opin Crit Care* 1999;5:1–8.

4. Fulda G. Intra-abdominal hypertension. *Crit Care Report* 1990;1:336–343.

5. Nelson LD. Continuous venous oximetry in surgical patients. *Ann Surg* 1986;203:329–333.

6. Diebel LN, Myers T, Dulchavsky S. Effects of increasing airway pressure and PEEP on the assessment of cardiac preload. *J Trauma* 1997;42:585–590.

7. Chang MC, Blinman P, Rutherford EJ. Preload assessment in trauma patients during large volume resuscitation. *Arch Surg* 1996;131:728–731.

8. Yu M. Oxygen transport optimization. *New Horizons* 1999;7:46–53.

9. Horst HM, Obeid FN, Sorensen VJ. Factors influencing survival of elderly trauma patients. *Crit Care Med* 1986;14:681–684.

10. Moore EE, Burch JM, Franciose RJ, et al. Staged physiologic restoration and damage control surgery. *World J Surg* 1998;22:1184–1191.

11. Kincaid EH, Miller PR, Meredith JW. Elevated arterial base deficit in trauma patients: a marker of impaired oxygen utilization. *J Am Coll Surg* 1998;187:384–392.

12. Cooper DJ, Walley KR, Wiggs BR. Bicarbonate does not improve hemodynamics in critically ill patients who have lactic acidosis. *Ann Intern Med* 1990;112:492–498.

13. Chernow B, Aduen J, Bernstein WK. Lactate: the ultimate blood test in critical care? In: Parker MM, Shapiro MJ, Porembka DT, eds. *Critical care: state of the art.* Vol 15. Anaheim, CA: Society of Critical Care Medicine, 1995:253–268.

14. Chang MC, Cheatham ML, Nelson LD. Gastric tonometry supplements information provided by the systemic indicators of oxygen transport. *JAMA* 1994;37:488–494.

15. Gattinoni L, Pelosi P, Suter P. Acute respiratory distress syndrome caused by pulmonary and extrapulmonary disease. *Am J Respir Crit Care Med* 1998;158:3–11.

16. Levy P, Similowski T, Corbeil C. A method for studying the static pressure-volume curves of the respiratory system during mechanical ventilation. *J Crit Care* 1989;4:83–89.

17. ARDS Network. Ventilation with lower tidal volume as compared with the traditional tidal volume for acute lung injury and the acute respiratory distress syndrome. *N Engl J Med* 2000;342:1301–1308.

18. Roupie E, Dambrosio M, Servillo G. Titration of tidal volume and induced hypercapnia in acute respiratory distress syndrome. *Am J Respir Crit Care Med* 1995;152:121–128.

19. Slutsky AS. Consensus conference on mechanical ventilation. *Intensive Care Med* 1994;20:64–79.

20. Hickling KG. Low volume ventilation with permissive hypercapnia in the adult respiratory distress syndrome. *Clin Intensive Care* 1992;3:67–78.

21. Suntharalingam G, Evans TW. Current trends in the management of acute respiratory distress syndrome. *Curr Opin Crit Care* 1999;5:1–8.

22. Gattinoni L, Bombino M, Pelosi P. Lung structure and function in different stages of severe adult respiratory distress syndrome. *JAMA* 1994;271:1772–1779.

23. Star R. Treatment of acute renal failure. *Kidney Int* 1998;54:1817–1831.

24. Bonventre J, Lieberthal W, Nigam SK. Acute renal failure. I. Relative

importance of proximal vs. distal tubular injury. *Am J Physiol* 1998; 275:F623–F631.

25. Kelly K, Molitoris B. Acute renal failure in the new millenium: Time to consider combination therapy. *Semin Nephrol* 2000;20:4–19.

26. Noiri E, Romanov V, Forest T, et al. Pathophysiology of renal tubular obstruction: Therapeutic role of synthetic RGD peptides in acute renal failure. *Kidney Int* 1995;48:1375–1380.

27. Fish E, Molitoris B. Mechanisms of disease: alterations in epithelial polarity and the pathogenesis of disease states. *N Engl J Med* 1994;330:1580–1592.

28. Linas S, Whittenburg D, Repine J. Role of neutrophil derived oxidants and elastase in lipopolysaccharide-mediated renal injury. *Kidney Int* 1991;39:618–624.

29. Khan R, Badr K. Endotoxin and renal function: perspectives to the understanding of septic acute renal failure and toxic shock. *Nephrol Dial Transplant* 1999;14:814–820.

30. Power D, Duggan J, Brady H. Renal-dose (low-dose) dopamine for the treatment of sepsis-related and other forms of acute renal failure: Ineffective and probably dangerous. *Clin Exp Pharmacol Physiol Suppl* 1999;26:S23–S28.

31. Hanley M, Davidson K. Prior mannitol and furosemide infusion in a model of ischemic acute renal failure. *Am J Physiol* 1981;241:F556.

32. Schrier RW, Arnold PE, Gordon JA, et al. Protection of mitochondrial function by mannitol in ischemic acute renal failure. *Am J Physiol* 1984;247:F365–F369.

33. Kelly KJ, Williams WW Jr, Colvin RB, et al. Intercellular adhesion molecule-1-deficient mice are protected against ischemic renal injury. *J Clin Invest* 1996;97:1056–1063.

34. Allgren RL, Marbury TC, Rahman SN, et al. Anaritide in acute tubular necrosis. *N Engl J Med* 1997;336:828–834.

35. Hammerman M. Growth factors and apoptosis in acute renal injury. *Curr Opin Nephrol Hypertens* 1998;7:419–424.

36. Hirschberg R, Kopple J, Lipsett P, et al. Multicenter clinical trial of recombinant human insulin-like growth factor I in patients with acute renal failure. *Kidney Int* 1999;55:2423–2432.

37. Schulman G, Fogo A, Gung A, et al. Complement activation retards resolution of acute ischemic renal failure in the rat. *Kidney Int* 1991; 40:1069–1074.

38. Hakim R, Wingard R, Parker R. Effect of dialysis membrane in the treatment of patients with acute renal failure. *N Engl J Med* 1994;331:1343–1346.

39. Hoffman JN, Hartl WH, Deppish R, et al. Hemofiltration in human sepsis: Evidence for elimination of immunomodulatory substances. *Kidney Int* 1995;48:1563–1570.

40. De Vriese AS, Vanholder RC, DeSutter JH, et al. Continuous renal replacement therapies in sepsis: where are the data? *Nephrol Dial Transplant* 1998;13:1362–1364.

41. Luna GK, Maier RV, Pavlin EG, et al. Incidence and effect of hypothermia in seriously injured patients. *J Trauma* 1987;27:1014–1018.

42. Valeri CR, Cassidy G, Khuri S, et al. Hypothermia-induced reversible platelet dysfunction. *Ann Surg* 1987;205:175–181.

43. Harrigan C, Lucas CE, Ledgerwood AM, Walz DA. Serial changes in primary hemostasis after massive transfusion. *Surgery* 1985;98:836–843.

44. Hewson JR, Kumar N, Neame PB. Coagulopathy related to dilution and hypotension during massive transfusion. *Crit Care Med* 1985; 13:387–391.

45. Harrigan C, Lucas CE, Ledgerwood AM. The effect of hemorrhagic shock on the clotting cascade in injured patients. *J Trauma* 1989; 29:1416–1421.

46. Reed LR, Ciaverella D, Heimbach D. Prophylactic platelet administration during massive transfusion. *Ann Surg* 1986;203:40–48.

47. Hulka F, Mullins RJ, Frank EH. Blunt brain injury activates the coagulation process. *Arch Surg* 1996;131:923–928.

48. Ku J, Brasel KJ, Baker CC, Rutherford EJ. Triangle of death: hypothermia, acidosis, and coagulopathy. *New Horizons* 1999;7:61–72.

49. Gubler KD, Gentilello LM, Hassantash SA. The impact of hypothermia on dilutional coagulopathy. *J Trauma* 1994;36:847–851.

50. Napolitano LM, Faist E, Wichmann MW, et al. Immune dysfunction in trauma. *Surg Clin North Am* 1999;79:1385–1416.

51. Bone R. The pathogenesis of sepsis. *Ann Intern Med* 1991;115:457–469.

52. Oberholzer A, Oberholzer C, Moldawer LL, et al. Cytokine signaling—regulation of the immune response in normal and critically ill states. *Crit Care Med* 2000;28(4 Suppl):N3–N12.

53. Schinkel C, Faust E, Zimmer S, et al. Kinetics of circulating adhesion molecules and chemokines after mechanical trauma and burns. *Eur J Surg* 1996;162:763–768.

54. Faist E, Mewes A, Strasser T, et al. Alteration of monocyte function following major injury. *Arch Surg* 1988;123:287–292.

55. Faist E, Schinkel C, Zimmer S. Update on the mechanisms of immune suppression of injury and immune modulation. *World J Surg* 1996;20:454–459.

56. O'Sullivan ST, Lederer JA, Horgan AF, et al. Major injury leads to predominance of the T helper-2 lymphocyte phenotype and diminished interleukin-12 production associated with decreased resistance to infection. *Ann Surg* 1995;222:482–490.

57. Keel M, Ungethum U, Steckholzer U, et al. Interleukin-10 counter-regulates proinflammatory cytokine-induced inhibition of neutrophil apoptosis during severe sepsis. *Blood* 1997;90:3356–3363.

58. Jimenez MF, Watson RW, Parodo J, et al. Dysregulated expression of neutrophil apoptosis in the systemic inflammatory response syndrome. *Arch Surg* 1997;132:1263–1269.

59. Scalia S, Burton H, Van Wylen D, et al. Persistent arteriolar constriction in the microcirculation of the terminal ileum following moderate hemorrhagic hypovolemia and volume restoration. *J Trauma* 1990;30:713–718.

60. Angle N, Hoyt DB, Cabello-Passini R, et al. Hypertonic saline resuscitation reduces neutrophil margination by suppressing neutrophil L selectin expression. *J Trauma* 1998;45:7–13.

61. Junger WG, Hoyt DB, Davis RE, et al. Hypertonicity regulates the function of human neutrophils by modulating chemoattractant receptor signaling and activating mitogen-activated protein kinase. *J Clin Invest* 1998;101:2768–2779.

62. Behrman SW, Fabian TC, Kudsk KA, et al. Microcirculatory flow changes after initial resuscitation of hemorrhagic shock with 7.5% hypertonic saline/6% dextran 70. *J Trauma* 1991;31:599–600.

63. Coimbra R, Yada MM, Rocha-e-Silva M, et al. Hypertonic saline and pentoxifylline resuscitation reduce bacterial translocation and lung injury following hemorrhagic shock: lactated Ringers does not. In: *Proceedings of the 75th Annual Meeting of the American Association for the Surgery of Trauma*, 1997.

64. Staubach KH, Schroder J, Stuber F, et al. Effect of pentoxifylline in severe sepsis: Results of a randomized, double-blind, placebo-controlled study. *Arch Surg* 1998;133:94–100.

65. O'Sullivan ST, Lederer JA, Horgan HF, et al. Major injury leads to predominance of the T helper-2 lymphocyte phenotype and diminished interleukin-12 production associated with decreased resistance to infection. *Ann Surg* 1995;222:482–492.

66. Wasserman D, Ioannovich JD, Hinzmann RD, et al. Interferon-gamma in the prevention of severe burn-related infections: a European phase III multicenter trial. *Crit Care Med* 1998;26:434–439.

67. Abraham E, Anzueto A, Gutierrez G, et al. Double-blind randomised controlled trial of monoclonal antibody to human tumor necrosis factor in treatment of septic shock. *Lancet* 1998;351:929–933.

68. Abraham E, Glauser MP, Butler T, et al. P55 tumor necrosis factor receptor fusion protein in the treatment of patients with severe sepsis and septic shock. Ro45-2081 Study Group. *JAMA* 1997;277:1531–1538.

69. Weimann A, Bastian L, Bischoff WE, et al. Influence of arginine, omega-3 fatty acids and nucleotide-supplemented enteral support on systemic inflammatory response syndrome and multiple organ failure in patients after severe trauma. *Nutrition* 1998;14:165–172.

70. Cuthbertson CP. The disturbance of metabolism produced by bony and non-bony injuries, with notes on certain abnormal conditions of bone. *Biochem J* 1930;24:1245–1263.

71. Hutchins AM, Shronts EP. Metabolic stress and immune function. In: Skipper A, ed. *Dietician's handbook of enteral and parenteral nutrition.* Gaithersburg, MD: Aspen Publishers, 1998:353–379.

72. Fish J, Shronts EP. A case for nitrogen balance vs. caloric balance in critically ill patients. *Nutr Immunol Digest* 1993;2:1–5.

73. Kinney JM. Metabolic response to starvation, injury and sepsis. In: Payne-James J, Grimble G, Silk D, eds. Artificial nutrition support in clinical practice. London: Edward Arnold/Hodder-Headline Group, 1995:1–11.

74. Shronts EP. Nutritional assessment of adults with end-stage hepatic failure. *Nutr Clin Pract* 1988;3:133–199.

75. Cerra FB, Shronts EP, Raup S, et al. Enteral nutrition in hypermetabolic surgical patients. *Crit Care Med* 1989;17:619–622.

76. Pastores SM, Kvetan V, Katz DP. Immunomodulatory effect and therapeutic potential of glutamine in the critically ill surgical patient. *Nutrition* 1994;10:385–391.

77. Takala J, Pitkanen O. Nutritional support in trauma and sepsis. In: Payne-James J, Grimble G, Silk D, eds. *Artificial nutrition support in clinical practice.* London: Edward Arnold/Hodder-Headline Group, 1995:403–413.

78. Kouznetsova L, Bijlsma PB, van Leeuwen PAM, et al. Glutamine reduces phorbol-12, 13-dibutyrate-induced macromolecular hyperpermeability in HT-29Cl.19A intestinal cells. *JPEN J Parenter Enteral Nutr* 1999;23:136–146.

79. Hwang TL, O'Dwyer ST, Smith RJ, et al. Preservation of small bowel mucosa using glutamine enriched parenteral nutrition. *Surg Forum* 1987;38:56.

80. Scheltinga MR, Young LS, Benfell K, et al. Glutamine-enriched intravenous feedings attenuate extracellular fluid expansion after a standard stress. *Ann Surg* 1991;214:385–395.

81. Barton RG. Nutrition support in critical illness. *Nutr Clin Pract* 1994;9:127–139.

82. Hyltander A, Sandstrom R, Lundholm K. Metabolic effects of structural triglycerides in humans. *Nutr Clin Pract* 1995;10:91–97.

83. Dahn MS. Structural lipids: an alternative energy source [Editorial]. *Nutr Clin Pract* 1995;10:89–90.

84. Elia M. Changing concepts of nutrient requirements in disease: implications for artificial nutritional support. *Lancet* 1995;345:1279–1284.

85. Barton RG. Immune-enhancing enteral formulas: are they beneficial in critically ill patients? *Nutr Clin Pract* 1997;12:51–62.

86. Gianotti L, Braga M, Frei A, et al. Health care resources consumed to treat postoperative infections: cost savings by perioperative immunonutrition. *Shock* 2000;14:325–330.

87. Kudsk KA, Croce MA, Fabian TC, et al. Enteral vs. parenteral feeding: Effects on septic morbidity after blunt and penetrating abdominal trauma. *Ann Surg* 1992;215:503–513.

88. Kudsk KA, Minard G, Wojtysiak SL, et al. Visceral protein response to enteral versus parenteral nutrition and sepsis in patients with trauma. *Surgery* 1994;116:516–523.

89. Moore EE, Moore FA. Immediate enteral nutrition following multisystem trauma: a decade perspective. *J Am Coll Nutr* 1991;10:633–648.

90. Kiyama T, Witte MB, Thornton FJ, et al. The route of nutrition support affects the early phase of wound healing. *JPEN J Parenter Enteral Nutri* 1998;22:276–285.

91. Strong RM, Condon SC, Solinger MR, et al. Equal aspiration rates from post-pylorus and intragastric-placed feeding tubes: a randomized, prospective study. *JPEN* 1992;16:59–63.

92. Montecalvo MA, Steger KA, Farber HW, et al. Nutritional outlook and pneumonia in critical care patients randomized to gastric versus jejunal tube feedings. *Crit Care Med* 1992;20:1377–1387.

93. Heyland DK, Konopad E, Alberda C, et al. How well do critically ill patients tolerate early intragastric enteral feeding? Results of a prospective, multicenter trial. *Nutr Clin Pract* 1999;14:23–28.

94. Wagner DR, Elmore MF, Tate JT. Combined parenteral and enteral nutrition in severe trauma. *Nutr Clin Pract* 1992;7:113–116.

95. Brain Trauma Foundation. *Guidelines for the management of severe head injury.* 2000. Ref Type: Internet Communication. http://www.braintrauma.org.

96. Pasquale MD, Nagy KK, Clarke JR. Practice management guidelines for trauma from the eastern association for the surgery of trauma: practice management guidelines for screening of blunt cardiac injury. *J Trauma* 1998;44:941–945.

97. Nagy KK, Krosner SM, Roberts RR, et al. Determining which patients require evaluation for blunt cardiac injury following blunt chest trauma. *World J Surg.* 2001;25.

98. Newman PG, Feliciano DV. Blunt cardiac injury. *New Horizons* 1999;7:26–34.

99. Brasel KJ, Ku J, Baker CC, Rutherford EJ. Damage control in the critically ill and injured patient. *New Horizons* 1999;7:73–86.

100. Schein M, Wittmann DH, Aprahamian CC, et al. The abdominal compartment syndrome: The physiological and clinical consequences of elevated intra-abdominal pressure. *J Am Coll Surg* 1995;180:745–753.

101. Nagy KK, Fildes JJ, Mahr C, et al. Experience with three prosthetic materials in temporary abdominal wall closure. *Am Surg* 1996;62:331–335.

ACUTE CARE OF BURNS

R. E. BARROW
D. N. HERNDON

KEY WORDS

- Burn wound
- "Rule of nines"
- Fluid management
- Hypermetabolic response
- Infection, burn wound
- Antimicrobial agents, topical
- Excision, burn wound
- Skin graft, cadaver allograft
- Inhalation injury
- Burns, chemical
- Burns, electrical

INTRODUCTION

The number of burn injuries in the United States ranges from 1.4 to 2 million per year (1,2). In 1998, 3,813 burn deaths occurred, for a crude death rate of 1.4 per 100,00 population or an age-adjusted rate of 1.2 per 100,000 population (2). House fires are responsible for nearly 75% of all burn deaths, with nearly 80,000 persons each year requiring in-hospital care for burns in the United States alone (7). Scald burns are the most common form of thermal injury, with more than 100,000 patients treated in hospital emergency departments each year (8). Hot-liquid spills are the primary cause of burns in children (9). In New York State, 45% of admissions for scalds were in children aged younger than 5 years (10,11). New and innovative advances in burn care have focused on improved survival and long-term quality of life. Over the last few decades, advances in burn care that have contributed to a decrease in the mortality rate from burns include new fluid resuscitation formulas (12–15), nutritional support regimens (16,17), the use of topical antimicrobials (18), early surgical excision of eschar to reduce the occurrence of sepsis (19–22), and management of the life-threatening hypermetabolic response to large burns (23–34). With new therapies for treating the burn wounds, pulmonary failure now has been identified as one of the leading causes of death in the burn patient and has been implicated in nearly 40% to 60% of the mortalities associated with severe thermal injuries (35). Clinical research on the pathophysiology of inhalation injury has provided new therapies that have decreased burn-related pulmonary edema and pneumonia (36–41); however, acute respiratory distress syndrome (ARDS) associated with inhalation injury and concomitant thermal injury remains a serious complicating problem (42,43).

BURN-WOUND PATHOLOGY

The pathologic processes at the skin level differ according to the degree of burn injury. In *first-degree burns*, only the epidermis is involved; tissue injury is minimal. Pain, the usual symptom, generally resolves within 36 to 72 hours. The protective barrier of the skin is preserved. In most cases, the damaged tissue peels about 1 week after injury. Exposure to the sun is the major cause of first-degree burns.

Second-degree burns, which involve the epidermis and all or part of the dermis, are classified as either superficial or deep. Superficial burns usually are associated with blister formation and involve all the epidermis and the upper third of the dermis. Pain is a major problem because viable nerve endings are exposed. Second-degree burns generally heal between 7 and 14 days after the burn, with minimal scarring, as the epithelial cells that line hair follicles and sweat glands stimulate healing (44–46).

In *deep second-degree burns*, pain is not as severe as in superficial second-degree burns because most nerve endings are destroyed by the injury. There are few epithelial cells, so repopulation of the skin takes longer than in superficial burns.

In *third-degree burns*, the epidermis and the entire dermis are destroyed (46). In many cases, the underlying fat layer and blood vessels are destroyed. Most pain fibers are destroyed by the injury; so patients will generally not be in as much pain as are those with second-degree burns. In this injury, reepithelialization does not occur and treatment generally requires homo-skin grafting.

AMERICAN BURN ASSOCIATION CRITERIA FOR BURNS REFERRAL

Superficial minor burns in adults involving less than 10% total body-surface area (TBSA) rarely require hospitalization. In children, hospitalization may be necessary if abuse is suspected. Moderate burns greater than 10% TBSA require only brief hospitalization. Patients with moderate to major burns always should be referred to a burn center. The American Burn Association (ABA) has established specific criteria for burn referrals (Table 1).

TABLE 1. CRITERIA FOR BURN CENTER REFERRAL[a]

Burns involving face, hands, feet, genitalia, perineum, and major joints
Third-degree burns in any age group
Partial thickness burn covering more than 10% of the total body
  surface area
Electrical burns
Chemical burns
Inhalation injury
Burned patients with complicating preexisting medical disorders
Burns with a concomitant trauma in which burn injury poses the
  greatest risk of morbidity or mortality
Burned children in hospitals without qualified personnel or equipment
Burn injury in patients requiring special social, emotional, or long-term
  intervention

[a]Established by the ABA.
ABA, American Burn Association.

MANAGEMENT OF THE PATIENT

Treatment of burn injury is directed toward replacement of skin function. These include (a) conservation of body fluids, (b) temperature regulation, (c) protection from infection, and (d) the protective functional properties of the external body surface with contributions to joint mobility, appearance, and sensation.

When patients first arrive at an emergency department, providers should assess the time, type, size, depth, and degree of burn injury and evaluate associated injuries. Because children have a greater ratio of body surface area to weight, their burn size is calculated differently from that in adults (Fig. 1). These calculations are important because they lay the foundation for the initial resuscitation.

The initial treatment of thermal trauma begins with the establishment of an adequate airway and maintenance of intravascular volume. Thermal injuries cause massive fluid shifts into normal as well as burned tissues. A marked increase in capillary permeability, which allows both large and small molecules to escape the capillary bed, is observed within the first 24 hours in burns involving more than 20% of the total body surface. Several replacement formulas advanced over the last 40 years are predicated on the size of the patient and the size of the burn injury. Lund and Browder charts, relating changes in body surface with age, are used to predict the extent of the burn injury (47). Less precise estimates of burn size can be derived from the "rule of nines" in adult patients, in which the head and each upper extremity are counted as 9%, the anterior trunk and posterior trunk, 18% each, and the legs, 18% each (Table 2). With adults the neck is counter as 1%.

The cardiovascular status should be evaluated, and fluid resuscitation should be initiated as rapidly as possible. A recent study showed that delay of reliable venous access of more than two hours was significantly associated with an increase in mortality (14). The patient should be evaluated rapidly and associated injuries noted. Life-threatening injuries, such as tension pneumothorax or cardiac tamponade, should be dealt with as soon as identified (48). Extremities with circumferential burns should be evaluated for the presence of distal pulses. The absence of peripheral pulses requires escharotomy, which can be performed at the bedside using a scalpel or electrocautery unit. Escharotomies should be performed along the lateral and medial aspects of the extremities through the entire expansion of eschar to release the constriction leading to compromised circulation (49).

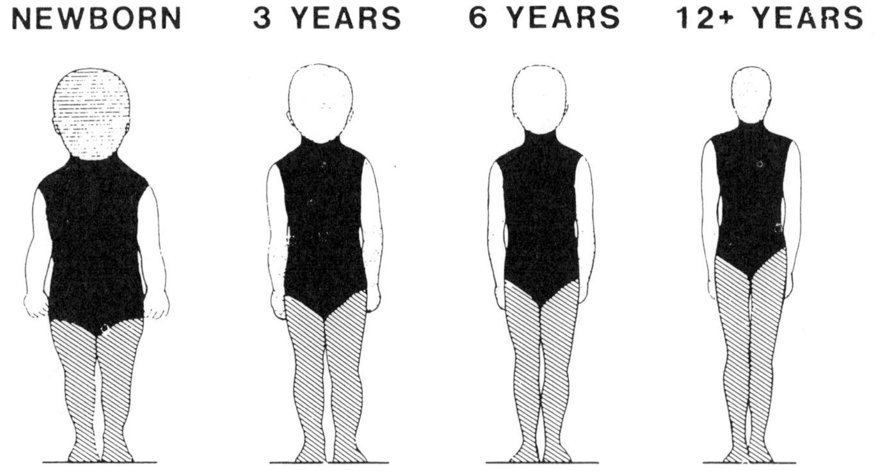

	NEWBORN	3 YEARS	6 YEARS	12+ YEARS
	%	%	%	%
HEAD	19	15	13	10
TRUNK	32	32	32	36
ARMS	9 1/2	9 1/2	9 1/2	9
LEGS	15	17	18	18

FIGURE 1. Influence of age on body surface area. Note the large proportion of body surface area represented by the head and face in the infant and child. (From Vassallo SA, Martyn JAJ. Pathophysiology and anesthetic management of burn injury. *Semin Anesth* 1989;8:275–284, with permission).

TABLE 2. "RULE OF NINES" FOR CALCULATING PERCENTAGE OF BODY SURFACE AREA BURNED

Area	Children	Adults
Head/neck	18	9
Arm	9	9
Anterior trunk	18	18
Posterior trunk	18	18
Leg (groin to toe)	14	18

Chest and neck escharotomines are rare except when lung volumes are restricted.

The Parkland formula (50–52) is the most commonly administered resuscitation regimen in the United States. This formula requires 4 mL of lactated Ringer solution per kilogram of body weight per percentage of TBSA burn administered in the first 24 hours after injury. One-half the amount is given in the first 8 hours after injury, and the remainder is administered over the subsequent 16 hours postburn. This formula is based on a regression analysis of the amount of lactated Ringer solution required in major burns to maintain urinary output of 30 to 70 mL per hour. Other advocated formulas contain various amounts of colloid or hypertonic saline. The argument against colloid administration in the first 12 hours postburn is that there is a diffuse postburn capillary leak that allows colloids to extravasate through endothelial junctions, thereby not producing any demonstrable oncotic benefit over administration of crystalloid. Hypertonic saline resuscitation lowers the amount of fluid that must be given to selected patients but can cause severe hypernatremia and should be used only by highly experienced investigators (53).

Patients with smoke inhalation injury typically require 2 mL per kilogram of percentage of burn more fluid than similar sized burns without an inhalation injury to resuscitate to normal urinary output. All resuscitation formulas are considered approximations, and the patient's blood pressure and urine output must be monitored every hour as a minimum precaution. Resuscitation fluids should be titrated to maintain a stable and adequate blood pressure, with a urinary output of 0.5 mL per kilogram per hour in adults and 1.0 mL per kilogram per hour in children. All burns greater than 20% to 30% TBSA should have indwelling Foley catheters for monitoring urinary output. This is the single best indicator of resuscitation for patients with previously normal renal function who have not sustained periods of shock and do not have congestive heart failure or pulmonary dysfunction. Central venous catheters and pulmonary arterial catheters are not routinely inserted; however, in patients with risk factors or certain electrical injuries, or when the response to resuscitation is not proceeding as predicted, there should be no hesitation in using pulmonary arterial catheters.

The time after injury at which capillary integrity is restored varies from individual to individual. We believe that capillary integrity usually is restored between 12 and 24 hours after the injury. Our practice is to administer colloids thereafter to restore albumin levels to 2.0 to 3.0 mg per deciliter. Whereas controversy exists about which type of colloid should be administered, no real comparative data on this subject exist. Some burn centers use salt-poor albumin, and others use fresh frozen plasma.

We use albumin because the purported advantages of other constituents of fresh frozen plasma do not seem to outweigh the risks of hepatitis or jaundice from multiple transfusions with fresh blood products.

Massive evaporative water loss replacement is the other major consideration in fluid management after the first 24-hour period after the injury occurs. The primary solution given is D5W, the goal being to maintain sodium concentration near 140 mEq per liter. After the first 24 hours, the formula we use to predict the daily rate of infusion that will meet this goal is 1,500 mL per m^2 TBSA + 3,750 mL per m^2 BSA burned. The patient's TBSA is calculated using standard nomograms. Additional evaporative water loss may be as much as 250 mL daily per degree Centigrade of body temperature above normal. Support of fluid needs is switched as quickly as possible from intravenous fluid to continuous enteral feeding. Milk has a normal osmolarity and provides 0.6 calories per milliliter. A 70-kg man can meet his caloric and fluid needs with one carton (240 mL) of milk per hour.

Most resuscitation formulas based on adult patients are not applicable to pediatric patients and therefore are used with great variability. In small children with small burns, resuscitation requirements that are defined by the Parkland formula fall below basic-maintenance fluid requirements. In children with large burns, the commonly used Parkland formula will grossly overpredict the amount of fluid required. For example, a 12-kg child with a 24% TBSA having a BSA of 0.5 m^2 would receive via the Parkland formula: (4 mL) × (12 kg) × 24% TBSA burn = 1,152 mL for the first 24 hours. The same child's maintenance requirements would be 100 mL per kilogram for the first 10 kg of weight per 24 hours and 50 mL per kilogram for the next 2 kg in weight for 24 hours, for a total of 1,100 mL. The Parkland formula administers no extra fluid for the extravasated fluid loss due to increased microvascular permeability from the injury or from increased evaporative water loss. Individualization of resuscitation in children is critical, and caution must be observed when using weight-based formulas in this age group. The most commonly used fluid resuscitation regimens are shown in Table 3. Delay in resuscitation rather than the type of fluid given in the first 2 hours postinjury may be the most significant contributor to mortality from burns (14). Such patients arrive at the hospital hyperosmolar and acidemic with hemolysis and often develop renal failure

TABLE 3. FLUID RESUSCITATION REQUIREMENTS

Adults	
Parkland	Ringer Lactate; 4 mL/kg/% burn, 1/2 during first 8 h postburn, the other 1/2 over next 16 h
Brooke	Ringer Lactate; 1.5 mL/kg/% burn; colloid 5; 0.5 mL/kg D5W; 2,000 mL
Modified Brooke	Ringer Lactate; 2 mL/kg/% burn in first 24 h
Hypertonic (Monafo)	250 mEq/L Na—in volume to maintain urinary output at 30 mL/h
Children	
SBH Galveston	Ringer Lactate; 5,000 mL/m^2 BSA burn + 2,000 mL/m^2 BSA, 1/2 in the first 8 h postburn, the other 1/2 over next 16 h

SBH, Shriners Burn Hospital; BSA, body surface area.

(54). They typically require 2 mL more fluid per kilogram of body weight per the percentage of TBSA burn to resuscitate to normal urine output than do patients of similar burn size who were resuscitated more quickly.

Support of the Hypermetabolic Response to Thermal Injury

A second priority in burn treatment is maintenance of body temperature. Hypermetabolism, increased glucose flux, and severe protein and fat wasting are characteristic of the response to major trauma and infection. In no other disease state is this response as severe as it is following thermal injury. Patients with peritonitis have an increased metabolic rate from 5% to 25% above normal; multiple trauma and respirator-dependent patients can have metabolic requirements 30% to 75% above normal. The metabolic rate of patients with burns covering more than 40% TBSA is often twice normal (55,56). In patients with major thermal injury, tissue breakdown liberates as much as 30 g per day of nitrogen (57), approaching lethality from the depletion of essential protein stores within 3 to 4 weeks following injury. Resting metabolic rates increase in a curvilinear fashion, with rates ranging from near normal for burns less than 10% TBSA to 1.5 times normal for 25% TBSA burns (maximum twice normal).

The hypermetabolic response is temperature sensitive but not temperature dependent; that is, it may be decreased but not abolished by environmental heating. At room temperatures greater than skin temperatures, the metabolic rate is twice normal in patients with greater than 40% TBSA burned. Individuals with large burns strive to maintain core and skin temperatures approximately 1° to 2°C above normal (58,59). Ambient temperatures must be kept at 28° to 33°C to minimize the metabolic expenditure needed to maintain adequate core temperatures and maximize comfort. When patients are allowed to select their own environmental temperature, their choice will be in this range. Metabolic rate and catecholamine release increase with pain and anxiety. Burn-care procedures (debridement, range-of-motion exercises, dressing changes, and application of certain antimicrobials) increase the nearly unbearable pain. Maximum utilization of narcotics and sedatives and supportive psychology help reduce these effects. The need for uninterrupted sleeping intervals, so frequently overlooked, is of critical importance.

Glucose kinetics in the hypermetabolic burn patient are always abnormal. Glucose tolerance curves obtained during the shock phase of resuscitation resemble those of diabetic patients, with elevations in fasting glucose levels and prolonged or decreased rates of disappearance. The total glucose space in adequately resuscitated patients is increased and total glucose flow to peripheral tissues is slightly elevated. During the flow phase of the hypermetabolic response, between the seventh postburn day and the time of wound closure, the integrity of the extracellular fluid compartment is reestablished, and the rate of glucose disappearance returns to normal, with total glucose flow increasing markedly. Normal glucose flow is approximately 3.3 mg per minute, whereas that of the 50% TBSA burn patient is 10.0 mg per minute at the 16th postburn day (60). Increased lactate production suggests that glucose utilization in burned patients is almost entirely through relatively inefficient anaerobic metabolism (16,48,61),

which may account for the increased glucose consumption. Further analysis indicated that most glucose consumption occurs within the burn wound. This is supported by the fact that the major constituents of granulation tissue are anaerobic cells (i.e., fibroblasts, leukocytes, and epithelial cells).

In the absence of dietary glucose, new glucose is formed from breakdown of protein to alanine, which can combine with the carbon atoms from lactate formed in the burn wound. Three-carbon amino acids, principally alanine, are released, primarily from peripheral muscle degradation but also by systemic enzyme degradation. Increases in urinary nitrogen excretion are paralleled by increases in the excretion of sulfur, phosphorous, magnesium, zinc, creatinine, and the muscle protein metabolite 3-methyl histidine. Daily nitrogen losses from 30% to 35% TBSA burns have been shown to be 20 to 25 g per m^2 BSA daily at the peak of the hypermetabolic response between the postburn day 7 and 17 (57). Although the three-carbon fragments utilized in making new glucose in the liver are derived from muscle protein and lactate produced in the wound, the energy that drives this gluconeogenesis is from fat metabolism.

Increased oxygen consumption, metabolic rate, urinary nitrogen excretion, fat breakdown, and steady erosion of body mass are directly related to burn size and continue for up to 1 year after the injury (34). Patients with greater than 40% TBSA burns who are treated with the most vigorous possible oral alimentation have been shown to lose 25% of their preadmission weight by 3 weeks after injury (62). This approaches lethality from body weight loss alone. Only recently, using enteral hyperalimentation, has it been possible to deliver sufficient exogenous energy to prevent postburn weight loss. Even when body weight is maintained, body composition is markedly altered with loss of lean body mass and increase in central fat.

Abston and colleagues demonstrated that with hourly administration of milk, one third of severely burned children could actually gain weight, one third maintained a stable weight, and the remaining third lost less than 10% of their preadmission weight (63).

The precise energy requirements needed to reach weight and nitrogen balance and energy equilibrium have been calculated from linear regression analysis of weight change versus predicted dietary intake in a small number of adults with large burns (64). This requirement is approximately 25 kcal per kilogram of body weight plus 40 calories per percentage BSA burn per 24 hours. In some cases, this caloric load can reach more than 5,000 kcal daily. Approximately 50 g per day of nitrogen is needed in addition to some polyunsaturated fats to prevent essential fatty acid deficiency. Multivitamins and increased amounts of vitamin C, potassium, zinc, and magnesium also are required.

A burn patient's appetite seldom exceeds the level before the burn occurred, and voluntary eating from the hospital tray almost never meets protein, fat, and caloric requirements in any but patients with small burns. Between meals, high caloric liquid supplements may be sufficient in moderate burns, but large burns require constant interval feedings through feeding tubes. With around-the-clock administration, caloric loads as high as 5,000 kcal daily can be easily tolerated. Blended or commercially prepared solutions are available that give from 1 kcal per milliliter to 2 kcal per milliliter with protein supplements. Milk, at

0.6 kcal per milliliter, is the least expensive and best tolerated of all feedings. Diarrhea is the most frequent problem encountered with enteral feedings with solutions of higher osmolarity. We currently use an iso-osmolar elemental diet with a low-fat content. Constant drip or hourly bolus infusion into the stomach with hourly monitoring of gastric residuals and gastric pH is performed. Gastric residuals are replaced up to 100 mL in volume to simplify electrolyte management. If milk is used, antacids are rarely required. Maalox in itself can cause severe diarrhea.

Infrequently, gastric retention, which we believe is due to the development of duodenitis, requires placement of duodenal tubes via fluoroscopy. This technique also is recommended for patients at high risk for aspiration or when more calories are needed for equilibrium. Often there is weight loss despite adequate caloric loads. If prolonged paralytic ileus is present, parenteral hyperalimentation, usually through the central venous route, may be required. In some instances, peripherally administered isotonic mixtures of amino acids, glucose, vitamins, and fat may suffice.

When peripheral or central parenteral hyperalimentation is required, absolute aseptic technique for catheter insertion and alternation of intravenous sites every 3 days is essential to prevent septic thrombophlebitis in surface-contaminated patients. Insulin supplementation usually is required when sufficient caloric loads are administered. Insulin, 250 U or more, may be required per day. Frequent serum and regular urinary glucose determinations are obligatory, as are serial liver function tests to monitor for the possible development of cholestasis or fatty infiltration. Potassium supplementation is needed to maintain serum electrolytes.

During the initial burn period, 8% to 19% of the circulating red blood cell mass may have been destroyed, and additional blood loss is slow and constant as debridement proceeds. One unit of blood is lost every 3 to 4 days in adults with burns exceeding 40% TBSA. Frequent transfusions and maintenance of blood volume will significantly decrease catecholamine output and diminish catabolic stress.

Failure to maintain the large caloric loads required for weight maintenance, nitrogen balance, and energy equilibrium results in delayed and abnormal wound healing, with defects in fibroblast and white cell metabolic rates. Isolated leukocytes from patients 7 to 15 days postburn with 40% to 50% TBSA burns consume one-half to one-third the amount of oxygen that normal leukocytes consume. Decreases in leukocyte chemotaxis and phagocytosis also have been demonstrated, and active transport across the cell membrane is reversibly inhibited (65).

Most early investigators believed that postburn hypermetabolism represented a physiologic response that generated energy to offset heat losses from obligatory evaporative water loss through the water-permeable eschar. Evaporative water loss can be as high as 200 mL per m² of BSA burn per hour (66,67). The heat of vaporization of water is 0.576 kcal per milliliter; thus, when skin temperature is less than environmental temperature, the patient must supply this energy or become hypothermic. Severely burned patients remain hypermetabolic even at high environmental temperatures (33°C) at which the energy of vaporization is derived from the environment and not from the patient (68). The metabolic rate of adult rats with 30–50% of their total body

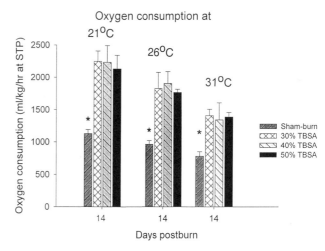

FIGURE 2. Oxygen consumption at STP for sham, 30% and 50% TBSA burns on the 14th day postburn at 21°C (room temperature), 26°C and 31°C. All burned rats showed an increase in oxygen consumption compared with sham-burned animals. There was no significant difference between the 30%, 40% and 50% TBSA burns within each temperature tested. *Significant difference between sham vs. 30%, 40% and 50% TBSA burns at $p < 0.05$.

surface area burned is consistently elevated at ambient temperatures from 21°C to 31°C when compared to unburned rats (69) (Fig. 2). This confirms that a severe burn causes a temperature reset in which burn patients are striving for a core temperature over 2°C higher than controls. Environmental heating does not change the increase in metabolic rate over controls. It does, however, decrease the metabolic rate of any individual, as would be expected.

Environmental heating should eliminate the response if hypermetabolism is simply a response to evaporative cooling. When evaporation is completely eliminated as a driving force, burn patients remain hypermetabolic (70). Postburn hypermetabolism is a manifestation of a true central-temperature control reset, and burned patients have an elevated core temperature. This reset, like other physiologic central resets such as cold acclimatization, is believed to be mediated by the hypothalamus.

Central-temperature reset, increased hypothalamus activity, fat mobilization, glycogenolysis, increased gluconeogenesis, and elevated glucose flow, which characterize postburn hypermetabolism, are mediated by complex changes in hormonal milieu. Thyroid hormone, prostaglandins, and catecholamines have been implicated as primary mediators of the response. Thyroid hormone, the critical controller of basal metabolic rate, has been suspected as an effector of this response, but serial T4 analyses in burn patients failed to reveal any elevations. Catecholamines have been implicated in humans as a primary efferent mediator (71) with urinary excretion of catecholamines elevated in proportion to increases in metabolic rate subsequent to increasing burn size. Hypermetabolic responses can be partially blocked in burn patients with combined α- and β-adrenergic blockade (72). Elevated prostaglandin levels were found in burn-wound exudate and burn-wound lymph draining from thermally injured tissues (73).

Increased catecholamine output stimulates an increase in glucagon secretion; cortisol levels are elevated to normal. These hormones all promote hepatic gluconeogenesis and ureagenesis when increased relative to insulin. During the postburn "ebb" or "resuscitation" phase, insulin levels are low, and, in the uncomplicated fed patient, return to normal but are never elevated (60). Insulin seems central to the regulation of skeletal muscle uptake and release and stimulates both amino acid and lactic acid efflux from muscle and fat breakdown and release from lipocytes. Glucose and insulin, growth hormone IGF-1/IGFBP-3, and propranolol support in burn patients does not decrease hypermetabolism but does preserve body mass, reverses nitrogen losses, and retains energy stores (16,73).

MANAGEMENT OF THE WOUND

Control of Infection by Conservative Methods

The third major function of viable skin is to prevent infection. Colonization with fungi and bacteria of nonviable, frequently necrotic burn-wound eschar and granulating surfaces presents a constant potential reservoir of microbes and their by-products. Burn-wound surfaces provide a warm, moist, protein-laden growth medium for microorganisms. The general consensus is that it is not realistic to try to maintain the burn wound sterile by environmental techniques or by the application of topical prophylactic antibiotics because any contaminating organism, whether exogenous or endogenous (specifically from the patient's own gut), will quickly grow and spread throughout this type of wound (74). Control of the microbial flora is, however, realistic and obtainable, and many prophylactic topical agents are currently used.

Prophylactic topical agents used from the time of admission to a burn ward include 0.5% silver nitrate (75), mafenide acetate (18), nitrofurazone (76), povidone iodine (77), silver sulfadiazine (78), gentamicin (79), and nystatin (80). The effectiveness of any of these topical agents must be related to their ability to inhibit bacterial growth *in vitro* and reduce *in vivo* colony counts in the burn. It is important to realize that no single agent is totally effective against all burn-wound microbes; thus, treatment therapy should be guided by *in vitro* testing or *in vivo* results (81). We perform quantitative and qualitative eschar and granulating wound biopsies three times weekly on all patients with open wounds (82). Samples are obtained from all patients with deep second-degree and third-degree burns and granulating wounds, one or two samples per every 18% TBSA burn. Identification of organisms and antibiotic sensitivities can be available within 48 hours after sampling. A Gram stain and rapid histologic biopsy are obtained at times of clinical suspicion of burn-wound sepsis if the possibly contaminated wound has not been cultured.

Wounds in which quantitative culture counts remain below 102 organisms per gram of tissue may remain dressed in the primary topical agent until wound closure can be managed. Wounds that demonstrate a tenfold increase or greater in bacterial count should be treated differently.

Silver sulfadiazine is the primary topical agent of choice on admission (83). The most common adverse reaction to silver

sulfadiazine is transient leukopenia (84,85), and serial complete blood counts (CBCs) should be monitored and the agent replaced with other agents if the white blood cell (WBC) count falls below 3,000 WBC per mm³. Silver sulfadiazine may be reinstituted when the WBC count comes back to a normal range, arbitrarily defined as 4,000 to 5,000 WBC per mm³.

When colony counts increase, we empirically change to mafenide acetate cream, which is an effective broad-spectrum bacteriostatic agent (86). Mafenide acetate is the only topical agent that has been shown definitely to diffuse through third-degree eschar to the burn wound–blood margin; this occurs within 3 hours after application (87,88). Twice-daily application maintains an inhibitory concentration within the necrotic tissue. Acid–base changes may occur in patients being treated with mafenide acetate as the drug enters the bloodstream (89,90). Mafenide acetate, a potent carbonic anhydrase inhibitor in the blood, is broken down rapidly into an inactive acid salt that is excreted in the urine. This produces metabolic acidosis, initially compensated for by hyperventilation. The amount of acid–base change that occurs and the renal and pulmonary complications are related to the surface area being treated. The oral administration of Bicitra or intravenous sodium bicarbonate usually corrects the metabolic acidosis. When less than 20% of the TBSA burn is treated with mafenide acetate at any one time, the effect on acid–base equilibrium and pulmonary function are usually minor. Sequential serial applications of mafenide acetate to different sites of full-thickness wounds, each less than 20% TBSA, for a duration of approximately 2 to 3 hours is relatively safe. After this period, the residual carrier cream is removed and the wound is covered with the primary treatment agent. A rotation schedule can be established so that all burn areas are treated with mafenide acetate twice daily. We refer to this as *pulse therapy*. Wound colony counts of more than 105 organisms per gram of tissue can be reduced to fewer than 102 organisms per gram of tissue with a two- to nine-day pulse treatment period with mafenide acetate. We have observed that about 10% of the patients treated with pulse mafenide acetate therapy had overgrowth of yeast, requiring nystatin to be added in a 1:1 proportion to their primary agent, silver sulfadiazine. The yeast counts were reduced to below 102 within less than 7 days after initiation of nystatin therapy in all of these patients. Routine cultures to detect fungal overgrowth must be obtained from any patient receiving mafenide acetate (91).

Maintaining wounds at low contamination levels reduces the number and duration of septic episodes caused by wound flora (92). This in turn reduces the caloric and fluid demands placed on the patient with each septic episode. The burn unit as a whole benefits from thus limiting the sources of cross-contamination. Longer skin-graft survival has been shown on wounds with low bacterial colony counts (93). Skin-graft survival was 94% in wounds with fewer than 105 bacteria per gram of tissue present but only 19% in wounds with a bacteria count greater than 105 present per gram of tissue. Scarring over areas as a result of graft loss over areas may be reduced to a cosmetically acceptable and functionally superior wound (94).

It is our practice to use systemic antimicrobial agents for patients with evidence of systemic infection. The clinical signs monitored are obtundation, changing mental signs, hyperventilation, hyperglycemia, thrombocytopenia, and hypothermia. Whenever these signs supervene and colony counts in the wound are greater than 105 bacteria present per gram of tissue, systemic antimicrobial therapy specific for the burn-wound culture is instituted. At all times, and most importantly, when the burn wound appears clean, other sources of sepsis such as the lungs, the genitourinary tract, or thrombophlebitis should be suspected. If no specific bacteriologic data are available from these sources, and Gram stains and histologic sections are not directive, presumptive antimicrobial therapy must be initiated based on unit-specific epidemiologic data. Our presumptive antimicrobial coverage is usually vancomycin. This choice will vary from unit to unit depending on predominant organism sensitivity patterns. Prophylactic systemic antimicrobial therapy is not advocated in an inpatient setting (95). The increased incidence of methicillin-resistant strains of *Staphylococcus* and the increasing prevalence of *Candida* and fungus in burn wards has become particularly troublesome. The administration of penicillin as prophylaxis is somewhat controversial, and our policy is to await the development of a cellulitis before administration of antibiotics in hospitalized patients. Inpatients usually are treated with vancomycin due to the high incidence of colonization of wounds in hospitalized patients with methicillin-resistant *Staphylococcus*; however, we still tend to give penicillin to outpatients. Tetanus toxoid prophylaxis is given to all patients who have not received tetanus toxoid within 6 months of the injury. If the patient never has received tetanus toxoid or has not received it within 10 years, both tetanus toxoid and human tetanus hyperimmune globulin (250 U) are administered. Vancomycin, levofloxacin, and imipenem are administered preoperatively and for approximately 48 hours postoperatively with subsequent administration of oral rifampin and levofloxacin for 5 days. It is our belief that this polyantibiotic therapy serves to protect burn patients from the seeding that accompanies wound manipulation (96).

Alternatives to Topical Antimicrobial Agents: Biologic Dressings

The application of topical antimicrobial agents in all cases inhibits the rate of wound epithelialization and may cause increased metabolic rate and alterations in the internal milieu, such as sodium leaching by silver nitrate and acid–base abnormalities with mafenide acetate (97). A major effort has been made to develop biologic dressings (pigskin, heterograft, human skin allograft) that, when applied to debrided, relatively uncontaminated wounds, adhere to the wound surface (98), reduce the wound colony count (99), limit fluid and protein loss (100), reduce pain, and increase the rate of epithelialization over that obtained with application of topical antimicrobial agents. Pigskin heterograft evolved as a substitute for human skin allograft in certain situations because it is cheaper and more readily available than human skin (101). Pigskin serves in all functions equally as well as human skin except when used following burn-wound excisions. Pigskin, currently in use in the United States, is not living and will not undergo vascularization (102). Some

Chinese surgeons use fresh frozen pigskin and claim that it is in every way the equivalent of fresh cadaver skin. Current indications for the use of biologic dressings or Biobrane are (a) immediate coverage of superficial fully debrided, second-degree burn wounds; (b) coverage of granulating excised wounds while autograft donor sites are healing; (c) as a test graft prior to autograft applications; and (d) debridement of granulating wounds with patches of necrotic tissue still adherent to the wound surface (103).

Application of pigskin or Biobrane to fresh (within 16 hours after injury) second-degree wounds (104) provides a physiologic environment for reepithelialization. Second-degree wounds treated with biologic dressings, Biobrane, or Opsite heal at a faster rate than wounds treated with mafenide acetate or silver sulfadiazine (105,106). When graft or Biobrane is allowed to adhere to the burn wound, epithelial cells proliferate and spread under the graft. The pigskin then will detach as keratinization occurs, leaving a normal epidermal covering. The vast majority of burns are second degree and can be treated by immediate Biobrane application, thereby decreasing pain and time to heal relative to application of topical antibiotics. The success of this technique depends on the adherence of the graft to the wound bed. Remaining necrotic tissue or accumulation of serum under the graft will create a closed fluid loculation that can become infected and destroy remaining epidermal components, converting the partial-thickness injury to a full-thickness wound. Application of heterografts and synthetic skin substitutes to second-degree burn wounds must be carried out with the same diligence as an autograft procedure. All grafted areas must be protected from shear forces and inspected frequently for development of subgraft fluid or infection.

Pigskin and Biobrane application to granulating and excised wounds is not recommended for long-term coverage (107). Cadaver skin allograft is a more suitable substitute when the wound cannot be readily closed with autograft. If allograft is not available and pigskin is used, it must be changed every 3 to 4 days to prevent suppuration in a potentially contaminated wound. Heterograft or synthetic material application to fully debrided, bacterially clean, granulating wounds before autografting may be used as a test to indicate the potential of success for the autograft. Human allograft also may be used in this situation. The successful "take" of these grafts assures eventual survival of autografts (93).

Debridement of untidy granulating wounds with serial applications of biologic dressings is practiced in many burn units; however, this procedure is not recommended. When the bacterial counts in necrotic tissue remaining under the dressing increase, suppuration of nonviable tissue occurs (103). Frequently, the biologic dressings themselves are dissolved (108). Any evidence of hyperpyrexia in this process should stimulate removal of the graft. Use of closed dressings for debridement results in high wound colony counts, which then must be reduced prior to autograft application if the autografts are to survive (102). Clearly, human skin allograft should not be used in any treatment modality unless graft "take" is an expected result. The use of skin allograft as biologic dressing, rather than as a true transplant, is expensive and wasteful of a valuable resource.

Excision of the Burn Wound

The ultimate protection of the body from burn-wound pathogens is obtained by covering the burn wound with viable autologous skin. This is also the ultimate solution to the restoration of the other functions of the skin. Controversies remain on how, in whom, and when to excise. If normal skin does not regenerate within a matter of a few weeks through healing of partial-thickness injury and through closure of the wound, morbidity and scarring will be severe. Excision of all deep components of the burn wound, whether deep second-degree wounds taking more than a few weeks to heal or full-thickness, third-degree wounds, becomes the treatment of choice if the patient can stand the stress of operation physiologically (109). Superficial second-degree burns that will heal within 3 weeks usually can be accurately recognized on a clinical basis. The physiologic and functional consequences of deep second-degree burns are not dissimilar from those of third-degree burns; so their distinction becomes somewhat academic. For example, a deep second-degree burn on the back of the hand will cause severe burn scar hypertrophy and deformity across any joint in much the same way as a third-degree wound allowed to go on to spontaneous eschar separation and grafting.

Excision of as much of the burn wound as possible should be carried out whenever a patient is hemodynamically stable and the risks of the operation would not increase the mortality that would be expected from traditional treatment. In patients with associated injuries such as inhalation injury or patients at the extremes of age or with cardiac conditions that make operative risks quite high, extraordinary surgical judgment is required in making the decision to excise. Sequential layered tangential excision to viable bleeding points, even to fat, while minimizing the loss of viable tissue, is the generally accepted technique. Excision of burn wounds to fascia is reserved for large third-degree burns over 60% TBSA where the risks of massive blood loss and possibility of skin slough from less vascularized grafts on fat may lead to higher mortality. The timing of excision is an area of controversy. It is recommended that all third-degree wounds be excised within 72 hours of the time of injury. Recently, it became apparent that early excision of scald injuries may not be appropriate because more wound than necessary may be excised because of difficulty in accurately determining the depth of injury. Our overwhelming prejudice is that burn wounds should be excised before high bacterial counts occur in the wound, which generally occurs within 5 days of the injury. After that time, the incidence of sepsis and graft failure increases to unacceptable levels.

Expanded meshed autografts are used to cover wounds if sufficient donor sites are available. The expansion ratio of graft-to-wound area cover ranges from 1:1.5 to 1:9 (110). Wounds with an expansion ratio greater than 1:3 heal in a suboptimal manner, leading to contractures and thin, easily injured skin.

The Use of Cadaver Allograft

Donor sites for autografts in smaller burns, that is, less than 40% TBSA, are seldom a problem unless the patient is at risk of surgical complication resulting from age, cardiopulmonary problems,

TABLE 4. INDICATORS FOR USE OF CADAVER ALLOGRAFT

Patients with burns >40% TBSA, who are at risk from preexisting illnesses or who have hemodynamic complication during excision of the burn wound where blood loss and anesthesia times are critical factors

Patients with large burns >40% TBSA, who have complications associated with blood loss, anesthesia time, or lack of available autograft donor sites

In massive thermal injuries >60% TBSA third-degree burn size

TBSA, total body-surface area.

or coagulopathy. Patients with greater than 40% TBSA burn have a scarcity of available donor sites because about 30% of the body surface, including the face, neck, and hands, is unsuitable. Large surface-area donor sites add to the morbidity and mortality of burn injury through blood loss as they are being harvested and in subsequent fluid and heat loss, with increased metabolic demands, while healing. Artifical skin replacement (111–113) and pigskin heterograft have been used as temporary wound coverage (101,102) with limited success.

We use viable cadaver skin allograft obtained within 18 hours after death as a physiologic temporary transplant (114,115). The allograft decreases the size of an open wound until autograft becomes available as the partial-thickness burn area is healed or previously harvested donor sites heal (21 days) (115). This temporary covering helps to control wound infection, preserves deeper tissues, eliminates fluid and heat loss, maintains function, prevents wound contracture, and relieves pain (99,103,114–116). Primary indications for the use of skin allograft are summarized in Table 4. Skin donors must be free of any disease that could be transmitted to the recipient (117).

Most burn wounds (<30% TBSA), whether deep second-degree or third-degree, can and probably should be excised within the early postburn period and replaced with autograft. Larger burns in hemodynamically stable individuals who are physiologically good risks should undergo massive excision with allograft replacement (118). Current research is directed toward the development of human autografts grown in tissue culture that can expand a patient's skin 40 times within 2 weeks (119). Development of collagen artificial dermis for application of this autograft will simplify this procedure greatly (120).

INHALATION INJURY

The single most important associated injury that contributes to burn mortality is inhalation injury. In 25% of all hospitalized burn patients, some pulmonary complication will develop, with an attendant mortality of approximately 50% (121). Mortality from major burns has decreased in the past 20 years. Burn shock, which accounted for almost 20% of burn deaths from 1939 to 1947, has been nearly eliminated as a major cause of death by widespread understanding of the need for early vigorous fluid resuscitation (122). Topical antimicrobial therapy with mafenide acetate as well as aggressive debridement has led to gains in the

TABLE 5. INCIDENCE AND MORTALITY RELATED TO AGE AND PRESENCE OF INHALATION INJURY

Age (yr)	No. of Patients	% With Inhalation Injury (n)	Mortality	
			% Without Inhalation Injury (n)	% With Inhalation Injury (n)
≤4	317	5 (16)	2 (5)	44[a] (7)
5–14	195	7 (13)	1 (2)	38[a] (5)
15–44	394	9 (35)	5 (17)	54[a] (19)
45–59	67	18 (12)	15 (8)	58[a] (7)
≥59	45	27 (12)	24 (8)	92[a] (11)

[a]Significant difference at $P < 0.01$.

control of burn-wound sepsis. Advances have been made in monitoring and supporting the body's hemodynamic and metabolic response to trauma. Improvements in patient care in these areas have decreased contribution to mortality, and today respiratory complications have emerged as the predominant cause of death of persons with major thermal injury. Pulmonary pathology, primarily as a result of inhalation injury, now accounts for 20% to 84% of burn mortality (122–127).

In patients with thermal burns, mortality increases with the severity of burn injury, advancing age, and the presence of inhalation injury. A retrospective audit of records of 1,018 patients admitted to our service over a 3-year period yielded 88 patients with inhalation injury (8.6% incidence) (128). The mortality rate in these 88 patients was 56%. In patients with burns exceeding 20% TBSA, the incidence of inhalation injury was 20%, and 58% of those patients died. Tables 5 and 6 show the incidence and mortality rates related to age and TBSA burned with and without lung injury. From these data, we concluded that inhalation injury alone is one of the most significant determinants of mortality inpatients with thermal injury, regardless of age and TBSA burned.

Lung injury resulting from smoke inhalation is commonly associated with increased pulmonary capillary permeability and pulmonary edema. Studies using laboratory rats show progressive increases in lung permeability during the first 6 hours following acute thermal injury to the skin (129). During the first hour, no significant difference from controls was noted; however, 2 hours later, significant increases in lung permeability were evident from radio-tagged albumin leaking into the extravascular compartment.

In a review of the literature, using indirect clinical criteria such as facial burns, singed nasal vibrissae, and a history of closed-space injury for diagnosis, 3% to 15% of thermally injured patients admitted to burn units were found to have inhalation injury. The use of other methods of examination, such as bronchoscopy and xenon-133 (^{133}Xe scanning), led to the recognition of inhalation injury in patients previously not suspected to have such injuries. New methods have increased the identification of inhalation injury to as high as 33% in all major burns (130,131), with a mortality between 38% and 58% (Tables 5 and 6) (123,132,133).

For major advances to be made in the care of patients with inhalation injury, it is imperative that methods of early detection be improved. Traditionally, the diagnosis has been based on a series of indirect observations, the presence of each of which was believed to increase the likelihood of an injury being present. Physical findings of facial burns, singed nasal vibrissae, bronchorrhea, and sooty sputum, as well as auscultatory findings of wheezing and rales, are complemented by a history of exposure to smoke in a closed space, particularly in patients who are stuporous or unconscious. Laboratory findings of hypoxemia or elevated levels of carbon monoxide may be present. The incidence of each clinical sign depends on the criteria used to make the final diagnosis of inhalation injury. There is a high incidence of false-positive values for each finding. For example, although facial burns are present in 70% of patients with inhalation injury, 70% of those with facial burns do not have significant respiratory tract damage (134). Hypoxemia, which is significant if present, may be absent acutely in 80% of patients who subsequently demonstrate pulmonary damage. Early findings of adventitious breath sounds (e.g., rales, rhonchi, wheezing), although unusual, may be indicative of severe lung injury (132). The strongest correlation with eventual pulmonary failure occurs with a history of closed-space injury of patients who are stuporous or unconscious, usually from drug

TABLE 6. INCIDENCE AND MORTALITY RELATED TO TOTAL BODY SURFACE AREA (TBSA) BURN AND PRESENCE OF INHALATION INJURY

% TBSA Burn	No. of Patients	% With Inhalation Injury (n)	Mortality	
			% Without Inhalation Injury (n)	% With Inhalation Injury (n)
0–20	627	2 (11)	1 (6)	36[a] (4)
21–40	200	11 (21)	2 (4)	38[a] (8)
41–60	102	20 (20)	18 (15)	50[a] (10)
61–80	56	32 (18)	24 (9)	67[a] (12)
81–100	33	55 (18)	47 (7)	83[a] (15)

[a]Significant difference at $P < 0.01$.

or alcohol intoxication. A drug screen and blood alcohol level determination should be done for any unconscious or stuporous burn patient.

The presence of an elevated carbon monoxide level [carboxyhemoglobin (COHb) >10%] is significant, but high levels will be detected only if measurements are made soon after exposure. The time for serum COHb levels to fall by one-half is 4 hours if the subject is breathing room air and less than 1 hour when breathing 100% oxygen (135). In a series of 22 patients who developed severe pulmonary complications from smoke inhalation, only two had greater than 15% COHb on admission (136).

Standard chest x-ray films are an insensitive measure of inhalation injury. Although Putman and colleagues reported that 12 of 21 patients with inhalation injury eventually had abnormal chest roentgenograms (six with focal infiltrates, four with diffuse patchy infiltrates, and three with pulmonary edema), admission studies are seldom abnormal and may remain normal as long as 7 days after injury (137,138).

Fiberoptic bronchoscopy, now the standard technique for diagnosis of inhalation injury, is performed routinely on admission at most burn centers. Positive findings are airway edema and inflammation, mucosal necrosis, and the presence of soot and charring in the airway (139). The technique identifies approximately twice as many victims of true inhalation injury as do the indirect previously described criteria. A significant number of false-positive results based on indirect criteria alone can be identified. Bronchoscopy directly evaluates the upper airway injury only. Introduced to define parenchymal injury in 1972, ^{133}Xe lung scanning involves intravenous injection of radioactive xenon gas followed by serial chest scintiphotography. The technique, which is safe and rapid and does not require patients' cooperation (140), identifies areas of air trapping from small-airway partial or total obstruction by demonstrating areas of decreased alveolar gas washout. The principal sites of damage after inhalation injury are depicted in Table 7. Inequalities in the ventilation pattern can be missed in patients who are hyperventilating and rapidly clearing the radioactive gas from the lungs. An abnormal admission chest roentgenogram (not usually attributable to the injury) or a history of preexisting pulmonary disease or heavy cigarette smoking will confound the specificity of an abnormal scan. Delay in performing the scan to day 4 after the burn or later is another potential source of false-negative tests because clearance returns to normal in 80% of patients by postburn day 4 (126). Unfortunately, the equipment and personnel needed to complete this useful test are rarely available to burn units, or the condition of the patients prohibits their transfer to the nuclear medicine laboratory.

Pulmonary function tests, especially measurements of lung compliance and airway resistance, are altered by inhalation injury.

Aub and Pitman reported in 1943 that, 1 week postburn, the vital capacities of 19 survivors of the Coconut Grove fire were reduced to an average of 73% of their predicted values (141). Garzon and colleagues showed that respiratory resistance can be as high as four times normal and that pulmonary compliance can be reduced by more than 50% (142). Based on the results of pulmonary function tests performed in the first 72 hours postburn, there were increased pulmonary resistance and decreased flow in those with abnormal ^{133}Xe scans (143). An obvious limitation to this type of examination is the need for patient cooperation.

Traditional indirect clinical diagnostic criteria, such as facial burns, singed nasal vibrissae, and a history of closed-space injury now are being complemented by fiberoptic bronchoscopy, ^{133}Xe lung scanning, and lung water determinations to provide an accurate assessment of injury to the small airways and pulmonary parenchyma. Pulmonary function tests described previously are probably most useful in providing information regarding the extent of disease rather than from initial diagnosis (134).

In the most severely injured, the first 36 hours are characterized by acute pulmonary insufficiency with several contributing components. During a fire, most of the available oxygen in a closed space may be consumed, with resultant asphyxia. If carbon monoxide is produced by the fire, death from carbon monoxide poisoning is the next immediate threat to the burn victim (144). Tracheobronchitis, bronchospasm, and cough related to the irritating effect of incomplete products of combustion contribute further to hypoxia (123). Another component of early pulmonary insufficiency is atelectasis, which often appears within seconds of smoke insult (145). The patient with normal oxygenating capability is threatened by laryngeal and upper-airway edema in the first 12 to 36 hours postburn. Tracheobronchial swelling, compounded by the necessary resuscitative efforts, is usually resolved by day 3 or 4. Early severe pulmonary insufficiency not relieved by endotracheal intubation or tracheostomy is almost universally fatal (133,146). The second stage, that of pulmonary edema, occurs in 5% to 30% of patients, usually from 6 to 72 hours postburn, and is associated with a mortality of 60% to 70% (147–150).

Bronchopneumonia appears in 15% to 60% of these patients and has a reported mortality of 50% to 86% (132,136,146,149). Bronchopneumonia, typically occurring 3 to 10 days postburn, often is associated with the expectoration of large mucus casts formed in the tracheobronchial tree. Those pneumonias appearing in the first few days are usually due to penicillin-resistant *Staphylococcus* species, whereas, after 3 to 4 days, the changing flora of the burn wound is reflected in the appearance in the lung of gram-negative organisms, especially *Pseudomonas* species.

In patients with inhalation injury who have survived, the long-term pulmonary sequelae are few. Bronchiectasis (diagnosed

TABLE 7. CHARACTERISTICS OF THE THREE MAJOR SITES OF INHALATION INJURY

Injury	Time of Onset	Duration	Complications	Therapy
Supraglottic	0–24 h	48–72 h	Airway obstruction	Tracheal intubation
Upper airway	0–24 h	2–7 d	Airway debris; secondary infection with tracheobronchitis	Airway access and toilet with suctioning
Lower airway	4–7 d	Weeks	Pulmonary edema; bronchopneumonia	Mechanical ventilatory assistance

by bronchography) developed in two patients in one series of 28 inhalation injury survivors. Subglottic stenosis requiring tracheostomy occurred in two of 38 survivors among 84 patients who required nasotracheal intubation at the time of injury (129, 140). It should be emphasized that the more severely injured patients die during the acute phase of injury. As survival of severely injured patients improves, long-term problems will surface.

The lung lesions evident clinically in thermally injured patients are multifactorial in cause. Pulmonary edema, airway infection, and airway obstruction occur with thermal injury to the skin, inhalation injury, and sepsis (150).

Lung lesions associated with pure thermal damage to the dermis involve an increase in lung lymph flow and edema formation (151–154). The quality of the fluid formed suggests that systemic hypoproteinemia and reduced oncotic pressure develop secondary to increased microvascular permeability in the cutaneous burn area, which promotes protein and fluid leakage into the interstitial space (152). During the resuscitation phase, fluid losses usually are replaced by crystalloid solutions with little or no colloid content; thus, as the volume status of the individual is restored, he or she becomes functionally hypoproteinemic. In addition, after resuscitation, burned patients have an elevated metabolic rate, a corresponding increase in cardiac output, and consequently increased pulmonary blood flow. This increased perfusion of the pulmonary capillary areas concomitant with hypoproteinemia increases edema formation (152–155). Permeability edema involving the margination of polymorphonuclear cells in the pulmonary microcirculation, with release of oxygen-free radicals, also has been proposed (156) and has been demonstrated in other forms of multiple trauma and severe hypovolemia (157). Lung edema associated with pure epidermal injury seldom manifests itself in the clinical setting, but these microvascular changes make the lung more sensitive to fluid overload, septic insults, and smoke inhalation.

Inhalation injury may involve the oropharyngeal, tracheobronchial, or parenchymal areas. Edema formation in the upper airway is a direct result of thermal injury; however, the mechanisms of damage to the lower airway are considerably different. Direct thermal damage to the lung is seldom seen except as a result of high-pressure steam, which has 4,000 times the heat-carrying capacity of dry air. Laryngeal reflexes and the efficiency of heat dissipation in the upper airways prevent heat damage to the lung parenchyma (158).

The carbonaceous material generated in smoke has not been shown in and of itself to be damaging (159). The primary pathogenic substances seem to be aldehydes. Oxides of sulphur and nitrogen combine with water in the lung to yield corrosive acids and nascent oxygen radicals. Thermal degradation of polyvinyl chloride (PVC) results in the formation of at least 75 known toxic compounds, including carbon monoxide and hydrochloric acid (HCl). At 15 parts per million (ppm), HCl is an irritant to the mucous membranes of the eyes and respiratory tract and at concentrations greater than 100 ppm, causes pulmonary edema and laryngeal spasm. Because of its solubility, the irritating action of HCl in the gas phase is limited to the upper airways. When HCl is reversibly absorbed to soot particles smaller than 5 μm in diameter, it can reach the bronchioles and alveoli in damaging concentrations.

Carbon monoxide, an odorless, colorless gas, has an affinity for hemoglobin approximately 200 times that of oxygen. Breathing 0.1% of carbon monoxide in room air (21% O_2) results in equal quantities of oxygenated and deoxygenated hemoglobin. The shift to the left of the oxyhemoglobin dissociation curve by carbon monoxide increases tissue hypoxia (160). Even at COHb levels below 10%, CO interferes with oxidation-reduction reactions in metabolically active alveolar type II cells, causing fragmentation of lamellar bodies and dilation of smooth endoplasmic reticulum in these cells. Complete inhibition of *in vitro* oxygen consumption has been shown in mouse pulmonary parenchymal cells (160). Rabbits exposed to high levels of carbon monoxide show increased alveolar epithelial membrane permeability. Much of the damage from COHb is due to altered O_2 transport and is not a direct result of histotoxicity (161,162).

Aldehydes and other chemicals can directly damage the epithelial alveolar macrophage and pneumocyte cell lines with a release of chemotactic substances such as histamine, serotonin, and kallikreins. Leukocytes are then recruited into the airways and parenchyma. During the first 24 hours after injury, bronchoscopic evaluation reveals edematous tracheobronchial mucosa. During this time, there may be mucosal shedding with areas of almost complete deepithelialization, along with formation of an exudate containing large quantities of polymorphonuclear cells and β-glucuronidase, both of which contribute to progressive pulmonary damage (163,164). As the lesions progress, a castlike material composed of insoluble fibrin and cells can cause partial or complete obstruction of large and small airways, resulting in patchy areas of atelectasis and emphysema (123,165). The protein content of the exudate formed indicates that it is a filtrate of plasma. There is a large concentration of low-molecular-weight substances, indicating that the permeability changes responsible for this protein leakage are selective (133,166,167). After inhalation injury, the formation of lung lymph and interstitial edema increases, which correlates with an elevation in extravascular lung water (133,163,168–175). An examination of lung lymph shows, in contrast to the hydrostatic edema of congestive heart failure, an elevated ratio of lymph to plasma protein concentration. Cardiac output and left atrial pressure, however, are either normal or reduced, indicating a change in microvascular permeability (163,170,176).

Chemical by-products of combustion stimulate pulmonary macrophages that secrete chemotactic substances, causing sequestration of leukocytes in the pulmonary microvasculature, lung lymph, and endotracheal exudate (172,177–179). A similar injury has been produced by aerosolized chemoattractants (180). The sequestered leukocytes cause increased release of proteolytic enzymes, as indicated by increased levels of β-glucuronidase and decreased levels of trypsin and elastase inhibitory capacity in the lung. The release of proteolytic enzymes and free radicals of oxygen by leukocytes may contribute to the progressive permeability changes of inhalation injury.

Interstitial edema may be produced by the bronchial or pulmonary microvascular beds. Both areas can be injured by smoke. A marked redistribution of bronchial blood flow occurs following inhalation injury, with more than a ten-fold increase in tracheobronchial blood, which contributes to the formation of exudate and interstitial edema. The mediators responsible for the increase in blood flow are yet to be identified but probably come from the release of vasoactive polypeptides and/or histamine. An examination of the chemical composition of the exudate formed after inhalation injury reveals large quantities of thromboxane B2, which is the stable metabolite of the potent vasoconstrictor thromboxane A2 170. Perhaps of greatest importance to the survival of a patient with inhalation injury is the marked decline in lung compliance.

Treatment

Treatment of inhalation injury must begin even before the diagnosis is confirmed. Oxygen should be administered by face mask or nasal cannula, starting at the site of the accident. This helps counteract the effects of carbon monoxide and aids in its clearance, as 100% oxygen lowers the half-time for carbon monoxide elimination from 250 to less than 50 minutes (149). Intravenous bronchodilators can provide dramatic relief from the acute irritating effects of combustion by-products on the tracheobronchial mucosa.

Control of the upper airway should be achieved by endotracheal intubation or tracheostomy at the first sign of impending airway obstruction. Other widely accepted criteria for early intubation are as follows: smoke inhalation associated with coma or respiratory depression (many subjects of inhalation injury have concomitantly high blood levels of alcohol and other central nervous system depressing drugs), posterior pharyngeal swelling, nasolabial full-thickness burns, or circumferential neck burns (181). Other researchers have more liberal criteria for early intubation and intubate prophylactically all patients with a clinical diagnosis of inhalation injury for humidification, pulmonary toilet, and positive pressure ventilation (166).

It is not yet clear whether long-term nasotracheal intubation or early tracheostomy is the treatment of choice. The advantages of tracheostomy include ease of pulmonary toilet, comfort to the patient, and ease of oral alimentation. The advantages of nasotracheal intubation include nonoperative placement, an ability to remove the tube easily if no longer necessary, a longer and less direct route for bacterial contamination of the lungs, and the obvious value of not interfering with care of neck burns. Reported complications of nasotracheal intubation are infrequent but include subglottic stenosis, vocal cord damage, and necrosis of nasal cartilage. A randomized prospective study comparing the two methods has not yet been performed, but the trend appears to favor long-term nasotracheal intubation (132,133,182,183).

The onset of severe, noncardiac pulmonary edema within minutes of tracheostomy or endotracheal intubation has been associated with a mortality rate as high as 25%. Mathru and colleagues reported that these patients developed bilateral fluffy infiltrates on chest roentgenograms but had normal-sized hearts and no clinical evidence of heart failure (166). Ratios of edema to plasma protein averaging 0.81 indicate the noncardiac nature of this pulmonary edema. Many researchers have commented on the lifesaving effects of continuous positive airway pressure (CPAP) in treating this syndrome and postulate that it restores the glottic mechanism of maintaining greater than atmospheric intrapulmonary pressures, which is eliminated by tracheal intubation (132,166,182,184).

Traditionally, fluid resuscitation has been kept to a minimum in patients with inhalation injury in an attempt to minimize or prevent pulmonary edema. This was first described in 1943 when Cope and Runinelander, using serial hematocrits as a guide to fluid status, maintained Coconut Grove fire victims who evidenced respiratory distress in a slightly dehydrated state (185). This practice has been questioned because animal studies have shown that fluid resuscitation appropriate for the patient's other needs (that is, to maintain pulmonary capillary wedge pressure and cardiac output) results in decreased formation of lung water, has no adverse effect on pulmonary histology, and actually improves survival (163,186,187). This may relate to the status of pulmonary blood flow in relationship to sequestration of neutrophils in the lung because these cells seem so intimately related to lung injury (188). Fluid administration in excess of requirements for resuscitation and the concomitant formation of hydrostatic edema also must be carefully avoided.

Humidification of inspired air had been used for decades, when steam kettles and steam from room heaters resulted in improvements in comfort and breathing for patients (127). Humidification is a possible contributor to fluid overload, but it aids in preventing drying of secretions and clearing thick casts (182). Antibiotics are clearly indicated in instances of documented infection. Empiric choices for treatment of pneumonias prior to culture results should include coverage of penicillin-resistant *Staphylococcus aureus* in the first few days postburn and of gram-negative organisms (especially *Pseudomonas* species) in subsequent days. Prophylactic use of antibiotics is of no benefit.

Other treatment modalities include endotracheal suction and lavage as needed. Shook and colleagues described the use of several agents administered by nebulizer (125). Heparin, presumably by its mucolytic and antiinflammatory effects, caused expectoration of large amounts of proteinaceous material followed by symptomatic and radiographic improvement. There is anecdotal evidence of rapid improvement in clinical signs of respiratory insufficiency from smoke inhalation following hyperbaric oxygen therapy (189).

BURNS OF A SPECIAL NATURE

Other special forms of burn injury that require specialized treatment include electrical injury that may be characterized by relatively small thermal injury with deep tissue damage. It is estimated that in the United States alone, nearly 52,000 trauma admissions each year are due to electrical injuries. Electricity is conducted most rapidly along nerves and arteries. Damage is most severe to muscles closest to bone, which offer the greatest resistance to electrical transmission and therefore generate the most heat during conduction (190). Resuscitation in these instances cannot be governed by the size of the surface injury but must be given massively to maintain high urinary output to prevent pigment deposits in the renal tubules and tubular necrosis. When urinary output cannot be supported by fluid resuscitation alone, osmotic diuretics (e.g., mannitol) may be considered. This is the one instance in burn therapy in which osmotic diuretics may be considered. Low-dose administration of sodium bicarbonate to prevent pigment deposits in the tubules is also advised. When osmotic diuretics must be administered, a central venous catheter or pulmonary arterial catheter should be considered to ensure the maintenance of adequate intravascular volume. Early operative exploration with visualization of muscles close to bone in the involved extremities is obligatory in high-voltage injuries. With high-voltage electrical injury, muscle damage may be progressive. Repeated explorations at 24- to 48-hour intervals after the injury are required. Complications may be numerous and involve all body systems. Immediate death from myocardial infarction is well described. Central nervous system complications, such as transverse myelitis, and late ophthalmic complications, such as cataracts, are examples of widespread effects (191).

Acid and alkali burns, although infrequent, require special treatment. A strong acid can cause coagulation necrosis of the skin. With a few exceptions, mineral acid burns are not as destructive as alkali burns. Mineral acids commonly used in industry include nitric acid, which is highly corrosive and produces a yellow eschar; hydrochloric acid, which produces a white or grayish-brown eschar; and sulfuric acid, which is a strong dehydrating agent and produces a dry black or brown eschar. The sulfuric acid burn often extends through the skin into subcutaneous tissue. The primary treatment for these acid burns is lavage with large amounts of water and debridement of all loose nonviable tissue.

Specific agents such as hydrofluoric acid require special antidotes. This highly corrosive acid is toxic not only because hydrogen ions produce tissue destruction but also because the free fluoride ions deeply penetrate to form calcium and magnesium salts (192–195). Tendons and bones can be damaged by direct contact with the fluoride ion, and life-threatening hypocalcemia may develop with prolonged contact. Systemic application of calcium gluconate is the most effective remedy for attenuating invasive tissue damage and persistent hypocalcemia. Without treatment, a hydrofluoric acid burn will lead to full-thickness skin loss and decalcification of underlying bone.

Phosphorus burns require aspiration of blebs prior to excision and irrigation with 1% copper sulfate. White phosphorus spontaneously ignites in air and, in contact with skin, causes a burn wound that is yellowish and has a characteristic smell of garlic (196,197). Carbolic acid or phenol and its cresol derivatives are highly corrosive acids that cause extensive coagulation necrosis leaving a light gray or light brown eschar (198). Phenols are highly lipid soluble and penetrate deeply into adjacent tissue. Standard water irrigation is not recommended unless a high-volume source is used. Phenol, however, is highly soluble in a 50% polyethylene glycol 50% solution. This solution should be removed by copious amounts of water irrigation.

Strong alkali, generally hydroxides of alkali and alkaline earth metals, form alkaline proteins, saponify fats, and cause cellular dehydration. Edema is characteristic of an alkali burn during the shock phase, resulting in extensive fluid loss and hypovolemia. Attempts to neutralize the alkali are not recommended; however, until the agent is removed, it will continue to destroy tissue. Ocular damage is common in an alkali injury because a very small amount can cause extensive damage. As with strong acid burns, irrigation with copious amounts of water, along with debridement of all loose, nonviable tissue, is effective.

KEY POINTS

Burn wounds are classified as first-degree (involving only the epidermis), second-degree (involving all or part of the dermis), and third-degree (entire dermis is destroyed and underlying fat and blood vessels may be destroyed) burns.

The Parkland formula, the most common formula for burn resuscitation in the United States, requires 4 mL of lactated Ringer solution per kilogram of body weight per percent total body surface area burn in the first 24 hours, half within 8 hours and the remainder over the subsequent 16 hours.

Prophylactic topical agents used from the time of admission to a burn unit are chosen from silver sulfadiazine (the agent of choice on admission), mafenide acetate (usually used when colony counts increase), 0.5% silver nitrate, nitrofura-zone, povidone iodine, gentamicin, and nystatin. The choice after admission is based on quantitative and qualitative eschar and granulating wound biopsies and cultures.

Inhalation injury is the single most important associated injury that contributes to burn mortality.

The treatment of inhalation injury includes oxygen, endotracheal intubation for impending airway obstruction or severe respiratory insufficiency, fluid resuscitation appropriate to restore systemic perfusion, humidification of inspired air, and antibiotics (for documented infection).

Electrical burns most severely damage muscle closest to bone because bone offers the greatest resistance to conduction, therefore generating the greatest heat.

REFERENCES AND SUGGESTED READINGS

1. Baker SP, O'Neill B, Ginsberg NJ, et al. Fire, burns and lightening. In: *The injury fact book*, 2nd ed. New York: Oxford University Press, 1992:161–173.
2. United States fire/burn deaths and rates per 100,000. *National Center for Health Statistics mortality data tapes for number of deaths*. Atlanta: Division of Unintentional Injury Prevention, National Center for Injury Prevention and Control, Centers for Disease Control and Prevention, 1991.
3. Karter MJ. 1991 U.S. fire loss. *NFPA Journal* 1992;Sept-Oct:30–43.
4. U.S. Department of Health. *Injury mortality: national summary of injury mortality data: 1984–1990*. Washington, DC: U.S. Department of Health and Human Resources, 1993.
5. U.S. Department of Health and Human Services: *Detailed diagnoses and surgical procedures for patients from short-stay hospitals: United States, 1979*. Washington, DC: DHHS publication no. (PHS) 82-1274-11, Washington, DC, 1985.
6. Hight DW, Bakalar HR, Lloyd JR. Inflicted burns in children: recognition and treatment. *JAMA* 1979;242:517.
7. Burns causes and costs. *A Burn Foundation report*. Philadelphia: Burn Foundation, 1989.

8. Graitcer PL, Sniezek JE. Hospitalization due to tap water scalds 1978–1985. *MMWR Morb Mortal Wkly Rep* 1988;37:35–38.

9. Milo Y, Robinpour M, Glicksman A, et al. Epidemiology of burns in the Tel Aviv area. *Burns* 1993:19:352–357.

10. Baptiste MS, Feck G. Preventing tap water burns. *Am J Public Health* 1980;70:727–729.

11. Lindblad BE, Mikkelsen SS, Larsent TK, et al. A comparative analysis of burn injuries at two burn centers in Denmark. *Burns* 1994;20:173–175.

12. Wolf SE, Rose JK, Desai MH, et al. Mortality determinants in massive pediatric burns: an analysis of 103 children with 80% TBSA burns (70% full-thickness). *Ann Surg* 1997;225:554–569.

13. Baxter CR, Marvin JA, Aurreri PW. Fluid and electrolyte therapy of burn shock. *Heart Lung* 1973;2:707–713.

14. Barrow RE, Jeschke MG, Herndon DN. Early fluid resuscitation improves extended outcomes in thermally injured children. *Resuscitation* 2000;45:91–96.

15. Tadros T, Traber DL, Herndon DN. Hepatic blood flow and oxygen consumption after burn and sepsis. *J Trauma* 2000;49:101–108.

16. Hart DW, Wolf SE, Shinkes DL, et al. Determinants of skeletal muscle catabolism after severe burn. *Ann Surg* 2000;232:455–465.

17. Hildreth MA, Herndon DN, Desai MH, et al. Reassessing caloric requirements in pediatric burn patients. *J Burn Care Rehabil* 1988;9:616–618.

18. Moncrief JA, Lindberg RB, Switzer WE, et al. Use of topical antibacterial therapy in treatment of the burn wound. *Arch Surg* 1966;92:558.

19. Burke JF, Bandoc CC, Quinby WC. Primary burn excision and immediate grafting: a method for shortening illness. *J Trauma* 1974;14:389–395.

20. Engrav LH, Heimbach DM, Resus JL, et al. Early excision and grafting vs. nonoperative treatment of burns of indeterminate depth: a randomized prospective study. *J Trauma* 1983;23:1001–1004.

21. Herndon DN, Barrow RE, Rutan RL, et al. A comparison of conservative versus early excision therapies in severely burned patients. *Ann Surg* 1989;209:547–553.

22. Desai MH, Herndon DN, Broemling L, et al. Early burn wound excision significantly reduces blood loss. *Ann Surg* 1990;211:753–762.

23. Herndon DN, Nguyen TT, Wolfe RR, et al. Lipolysis in burned patients is stimulated by the B2-receptor for catecholamines. *Arch Surg* 1994;129:1301–1305.

24. Wilmore DW, Long JM, Mason AD Jr, et al. Catecholamines: mediator of the hypermetabolic response to thermal injury. *Ann Surg* 1974;180:653–669.

25. Sakurai Y, Aarsland A, Herndon DN, et al. Stimulation of muscle protein synthesis by long-term insulin infusion in severely burned patients. *Ann Surg* 1995;222:283–297.

26. Aarsland A, Chinkes D, Wolfe RR, et al. Beta-blockade lowers peripheral lipolysis in burn patients receiving growth hormone. *Ann Surg* 1996;223:777–789.

27. Ferrando AA, Chinkes D, Wolfe SE, et al. Acute dichloroacetate administration increases skeletal muscle free glutamine concentrations after burn injury. *Ann Surg* 1998;228:249–256.

28. Aarsland A, Chinkes DL, Sakurai Y, et al. Insulin therapy in burn patients does not contribute to hepatic triglyceride production. *J Clin Invest* 1998;101:2233–2239.

29. Ferrando AA, Chinkes DL, Wolf SE, et al. A submaximal dose of insulin promotes net skeletal muscle protein synthesis in patients with severe burns. *Ann Surg* 1999;229:11–18.

30. Herndon DN, Ramzy PI, DebRoy MA, et al. Muscle protein catabolism after severe burn: effects of IGF-1/IGFBP-3 treatment. *Ann Surg* 1999;229:713–720.

31. Jeschke MG, Barrow RE, Perez-Polo JR, et al. Attenuation of the acute-phase response in thermally injured rats by cholesterol-containing cationic liposomes used as a delivery system for gene therapy. *Arch Surg* 1999;134:1098–1102.

32. Hart DW, Wolf SE, Chinkes DL, et al. Anti-catabolic synergism between growth hormone and propranolol after burn. *Surg Forum* 2000;51:196–197.

33. DebRoy MA, Wolf SE, Zhang XJ, et al. Anabolic effects of insulin-like growth factor in combination with insulin-like growth factor binding protein-3 in severely burned adults. *J Trauma* 1999;47:904–911.

34. Hart DW, Wolf SE, Mlcak R, et al. Persistence of muscle catabolism after severe burn. *Surgery* 2000;128:312–319.

35. Thompson PD, Herndon DN, Traber DL, et al. Effect on mortality of inhalation injury. *J Trauma* 1986;26:163–165.

36. Shirani KZ, Pruitt BA Jr, Mason AD Jr. The influence of inhalation injury and pneumonia on burn mortality. *Ann Surg* 1987;205:82–87.

37. Herndon DN, Barrow RE, Linares HA, et al. Inhalation injury in burned patients: effects and treatment. *Burns* 1988;14:349–356.

38. Cioffi WG Jr, Rue LW III, Graves TA, et al. Prophylactic use of high-frequency percussive ventilation in patients with inhalation injury. *Ann Surg* 1991;13:575–582.

39. Pierre EJ, Zaiwchenberger JB, Angel C, et al. Extracorporeal membrane oxygenation in the treatment of respiratory failure in pediatric patients with burns. *J Burn Care Rehabil* 1998;19:131–134.

40. Desai MH, Mlcak R, Richardson J, et al. Reduction in mortality in pediatric patients with inhalation injury with aerosolized heparin/N-acetyl cystine therapy. *J Burn Care Rehabil* 1998;19:210–212.

41. Cortiella J, Mlcak R, Herndon DN. High frequency percussive ventilation in pediatric patients with inhalation injury. *J Burn Care Rehabil* 1999;20:232–235.

42. Mlcak R, Cortiella J, Desai M, et al. Lung compliance, airway resistance, and work of breathing in children after inhalation injury. *J Burn Care Rehabil* 1997;18:531–534.

43. Mlcak R, Desai MH, Robinson E, et al. Lung function following thermal injury in children: an 8-year follow up. *Burns* 1998;24:213–216.

44. Tredget EE, Yu MY. Thermometabolic effects of thermal injury. *World J Surg* 1992;16:68–79.

45. Curreri PW, Luterman A. Burns. In: Schwartz SI, Shires GT, Spencer FC, et al., eds. *Principles of surgery*. New York: McGraw-Hill Book Company, 1984.

46. Herndon DN. *Total burn care.* London: WB Saunders, 1995:68–69.

47. Lund CC, Browder NC. The estimate of areas of burns. *Surg Gynecol Obstet J* 1944;79:352–358.

48. Wolf SE, Herndon DN. Burns. In: Townsend CM, ed. *Sabiston's textbook of surgery*. New York: WB Saunders, 2001:20,245.

49. American Burn Association. *Advanced burn life support course provider's manual*, revised ed. Chicago: American Burn Association, 2000.

50. Baxter CR. Fluid and electrolyte changes of the early postburn period. *Clin Plast Surg* 1974;1:693.

51. Deitch EA. The management of burns. *N Engl J Med* 1990;323:1249–1253.

52. Baxter CR. Guidelines for fluid resuscitation. *J Trauma* 1981;21:687–689.

53. Milner SM, Kinsky MP, Guha SC, et al. A comparison of two different 2400 mOsm solutions for resuscitation of major burns. *J Burn Care Rehabil* 1997;18:109–115.

54. Jeschke MG, Barrow RE, Wolf SE, et al. Mortality in burned children with acute renal failure. *Arch Surg* 1998;133:752–756.

55. Kenney JM, Long CL, Grump FE, et al. Tissue composition of weight loss in surgical patients: I. Elective operations. *Ann Surg* 1968;168:459.

56. Long CL, Spencer JL, Kinney JM, et al. Carbohydrate metabolism in man: effectiveness of elective operations and major injury. *J Appl Physiol* 1971;31:110.

57. Soroff HS, Pearson E, Artz CP. An estimation of nitrogen requirements for equilibrium in burn patients. *Surg Gynecol Obstet* 1961;112:159.

58. Wilmore DW, Long JM, Skreen RW, et al. Studies of the effect of variation of temperature and humidity on energy demands of the burned solider in a controlled metabolic room. *Fort Sam Houston, U.S. Army Institution of Surgical Research, annual report*. Report Control Symbol MEDDH-288 (R1), 1973.

59. Herndon DN, Wilmore DW, Mason AD Jr, et al. Development and analysis of a small animal model simulating the human postburn hypermetabolic response. *J Surg Res* 1978;25:394.

60. Wilmore DW, Mason AD Jr, Pruitt BA Jr. Insulin response to glucose in hypermetabolic burn patients. *Ann Surg* 1976;186:314.

61. Wilmore DW, Aulick LH, Pruitt BA Jr. Influence of the burn wound on local and systemic response to injury. *Ann Surg* 1977;186:314.

62. Newsoms TW, Mason AD Jr, Pruitt BA Jr. Weight loss following thermal injury. *Ann Surg* 1973;178:215.

63. Abston S, Maxwell RR, Larson DL. Nutritional management of the acutely burned child. In: Matter P, Barclay TL, Zonickeva Z, eds. *Research in burns*. Bern, Switzerland: Hans Huber, 1970.

64. Currieri PW, Richmond D, Marvin JA. Dietary requirements of patients with major burns. *J Am Diet Assoc* 1974;65:415.

65. Currieri PW, Wilmore DW, Mason AD Jr, et al. Intracellular action alterations following major trauma: effect of superabnormal caloric intake. *J Trauma* 1971;11:390.

66. Barr PO, Birke G, Liljedahl SO, et al. Oxygen consumption and water loss during treatment of burns with warm dry air. *Lancet* 1968;1:164.

67. Caldwell FT Jr. Metabolic response to thermal trauma: two nutritional studies with rats at two environmental temperatures. *Ann Surg* 1962;115:119.

68. Wilmore DW, Mason AD Jr, Johnson DW, et al. Effect of ambient temperature of heat production and heat loss in burn patients. *J Appl Physiol* 1975;38:593.

69. Barrow RE, Meyer NA, Jeschke MG. Effect of varying burns size and ambient temperature on the hypermetabolic rate in thermally injured rats. *J Surg Res* 2001;29:253–257.

70. Zawacki BE, Spitzer KW, Mason AD Jr, et al. Does increased evaporative water loss cause hypermetabolism in burn patients? *Ann Surg* 1970;171:236.

71. Goodall MC, Stone C, Haynes BW Jr. Urinary output of adrenaline in severe thermal burns. *Ann Surg* 1957;145:479.

72. Wilmore DW, Long JM, Mason AD Jr, et al. Catecholamines: mediator of the hypermetabolic response to thermal injury. *Ann Surg* 1974;180:653.

73. Arturson G. Prostaglandins in human burn wound secretions. *Burns* 1977;3:112.

74. Moncrief JA. Topical antibacterial treatment of the burn wound. In: Art CP, Moncrief JA, Pruitt BA Jr, eds. *Burns, a team approach*. Philadelphia: WB Saunders, 1979.

75. Moyer CA, Brentano L, Gravens DL, et al. Treatment of large human burns with 0.5% silver nitrate solution. *Arch Surg* 1956;90:812.

76. Georgiade N, Lucas M, Georgiade R, et al. The use of new potent topical antibacterial agent for the control of infection in the burn wound. *Plast Reconstr Surg* 1967;39:349.

77. Robson MC, Schaerf RHM, Zrizek TJ. Evaluation of topical povidone iodine ointment in experimental burn would sepsis. *Plast Reconstr Surg* 1974;54:328.

78. Fox JCL, Rappole BW, Stanford W. Control of *Pseudomonas* infection in burns by silver sulfadiazine. *Surg Gynecol Obstet* 1969;128:1021.

79. MacMillan BG. Ecology of bacteria colonizing the burned patient given topical and systemic gentamicin therapy: a five year study. *J Infect Dis* 1971;124:5278.

80. Stone HH, Kolb LD, Currie CA, et al. *Candida* sepsis: pathogenesis and principles of treatment. *Ann Surg* 1974;179:697.

81. Nathan P, Law EJ, Murphy DF, et al. A laboratory method for the selection of topical 71: antimicrobial agents to treat infected burn wounds. *Burns* 1978;4:177.

82. Loebl E, Marvin JA, Heck EL, et al. The use of quantitative biopsy cultures in bacteriologic monitoring of burn patients. *J Surg Res* 1974;16:1.

83. Baxter CR. Topical use of 1.0% silver sulfadiazine. In: Polk HC Jr, Stone HH, eds. *Contemporary burn management*. Boston, Little Brown and Company, 1971.

84. Jarrett F, Ellerbee S, Demling R. Acute leukopenia during topical burn therapy with silver sulfadiazine. *Am J Surg* 1978;135:818.

85. Chan CK, Jarret F, Moylan JA. Acute leukopenia as an allergic reaction to silver sulfadiazine in burn patients. *J Trauma* 1976;16:395.

86. Holder IA, Schwab M, Jackson L. Eighteen months of routine topical antimicrobial susceptibility testing of isolates from burn patients: results and conclusions. *J Antimicrob Chemother* 1979;5:455.

87. Harrison HN, Bales H, Jacoby F. The behavior of mafenide acetate as a basis for its clinical use. *Arch Surg* 1971;103:449.

88. Harrison HN, Blackmore WP, Bales HW, et al. The absorption of C-14 labeled Sulfamylon acetate through burned skin: I. Experimental methods and initial observations. *J Trauma* 1972;12:986.

89. Schaner P, Shuck JM, Richey CR. A possible ventilatory effect of carbonic anhydrase inhibition following topical sulfamylon in burn patients. *Anesthesia* 1968;29:207.

90. White NG, Asch MJ. Acid base effects of topical mafenide acetate in the burn patient. *N Engl J Med* 1971;284:1281.

91. Bruck HM, Nash G, Stein JM, et al. Studies on the occurrence and significance of yeast and fungi in the burn wound. *Ann Surg* 1972;108:176.

92. Teplitz C. The pathology of burns and the fundamental of burn wound sepsis. In: Artz CP, Moncrief JA, Pruitt BA Jr, eds. *Burns, a team approach*. Philadelphia: WB Saunders Company, 1979.

93. Robson MC, Krizek TS. Predicting skin graft survival. *J Trauma* 1973;13:213.

94. Bryant WM. *Wound Healing Clinical Symposia*. Sarasota, FL: Ciba Pharmaceutical Company, 1977.

95. Larkin JM, Moylan JA. The role of prophylactic antibiotics in burn care. *Am Surg* 1976;42:247.

96. Sasaki TM, Welch GW, Herndon DN, et al. Burn wound manipulation induced bactermia. *J Trauma* 1979;19:46.

97. Herndon DN, Wilmore DW, Mason AD Jr, et al. Increases in postburn hypermetabolism caused by application of topical ointment. *Surg Forum* 1978;29:49.

98. Burleson R, Eiseman B. Nature of the bond between partial-thickness skin and wound granulations. *Surgery* 1972;72:315.

99. Burleson R, Eiseman B. Mechanism of antibacterial effect of biologic dressings. *Ann Surg* 1973;177:181.

100. Lamke LO, Nilsson GE, Reithne HS. The evaporative water loss from burns and the water-vapor permeability of grafts and artificial membranes used in the treatment of burns. *Burns* 1978;3:159.

101. Bromberg BE, Song IC, Mohn MP. The use of pigskin as a temproary biologic dressing. *Plast Reconstr Surg* 1965;36:80.

102. Shuck JM. The use of heteroplastic grafts. *Burns* 1977;2:47.

103. Pruitt BA Jr, Currieri PW. The use of homograft and heterograft skin. In: Polk HC, Stone H, eds. *Contemporary burn management*. Boston: Little Brown and Company, 1971.

104. Zawacki BE. Reversal of capillary stasis and prevention of necrosis in burns. *Ann Surg* 1974;180:98.

105. Burleson R, Eiseman E. Effect of skin dressings and topical antibiotic on healing of partial thickness skin wounds in rats. *Surg Gynecol Obstet* 1973;136:158.

106. Lal S, Barrow RE, Wolf SE, et al. Biobrane improves wound healing in burned children without increased risk of infection. *Shock* 2000;14:314–319.

107. Luterman A, Kraft E, Bookless S. Biological dressing: an appraisal of current practices. *J Burn Care Rehabil* 1980;1:18.

108. Kraft E, Luterman A, Currieri PW. What type of pigskin should I use? Presented at the 12th Annual Meeting of the American Burn Association, San Antonio, Texas, March 27–29, 1980.

109. Burke JF, Quimby WC, Bondoc CC. Primary excision and prompt grafting as routine therapy for the treatment of thermal burns in children. *Surg Clin North Am* 1976;56:477.

110. Synder WH, Bowles BM, MacMillan BG. The use of expansion meshed grafts in the acute and reconstructive management of thermal injury: a clinical evaluation. *J Trauma* 1970;10:740.

111. Oluwaganmi J, Chvapil M. A comparative study of four materials in local burn care in rabbit model. *J Trauma* 1976;16:348.

112. Saymen DG, Nathan P, Holder IA, et al. Control of surface wound infection: skin versus synthetic grafts. *Appl Microb* 1973;25:921.

113. Guldalian BS, Jelenko C, Callaway D, et al. Comparative study of synthetic and biological materials for wound dressing. *J Trauma* 1973;13:32.

114. Berggren RB, LehrHB. Clinical use of a viable frozen skin bank. *JAMA* 1962;194:149.

115. MacMillan BG. Homograft skin: a valuable adjunct to treatment of thermal burns. *J Trauma* 1962;2:130.

116. Bondoc CC, Burke JF. Clinical experience with viable frozen skin and frozen skin bank. *Ann Surg* 1971;174:371.

117. Guidelines for banking of skin tissue: report of the Standards Committee of the Skin Council of the American Association of Tissue Banks. *American Association Tissue Banks Newsletter* 1979;3:5.

118. Rose JK, Desai MH, Mlakar JM, et al. Allograft is superior to topical antimicrobial therapy in the treatment of partial-thickness scald burns in children. *J Burn Care Rehabil* 1997;18:338–341.

119. Eisinger M, Moden M, Raaf JH, et al. Wound coverage by a sheet of epidermal cells grown in vitro from dispersed single cell preparations. *Surgery* 1980;88:287.

120. Bell E, Ehrlich PH, Sher S, et al. Development and use of a living skin equivalent. *Plastic Reconstr Surg* 1981;67:386.

121. Pruitt BA Jr, Flemma RJ, DiVincenti FC, et al. Pulmonary complications in burn patients, a comparative study of 697 patients. *J Thorac Cardiovasc Surg* 1970;59:7.

122. Phillips AW, Cope O. Burn therapy: II. The revelation of respiratory tract damage as a principal killer of the burned patients. *Ann Surg* 1962;155:1.

123. DiVincenti FC, Pruitt BA Jr, Reckler JM. Inhalation injuries. *J Trauma* 1971;11:109.

124. Foley FD, Moncrief JA, Mason AD Jr. Pathology of the lung in fatally burned patients. *Ann Surg* 1968;167:251.

125. Shook CD, MacMillan BG, Altermeir WA. Pulmonary complications of the burn patient. *Arch Surg* 1968;97:215.

126. Silverstein P, Dressler DP. Effect of current therapy on burn mortality. *Ann Surg* 1970;171:124.

127. Skornik WA, Dressler DP. Lung bacterial clearance in the burned rat. *Ann Surg* 1970;172:837.

128. Thompson PB, Herndon DN, Abston S. Effect on mortality of inhalation injury. *J Trauma* 1986;26:163.

129. Till GO, Beauchamp C, Menapace D, et al. Oxygen radical dependent lung damage following thermal injury of rat skin. *J Trauma* 1983;23:269.

130. Moylan JA, Alexander G Jr. Diagnosis and treatment of inhalation injury. *World J Surg* 1978;2:185.

131. Moylan JA, Chan CK. Inhalation injury: an increasing problem. *Surgery* 1978;188:34.

132. Stone HH, Rhame DW, Corbitt JD, et al. Respiratory burns: a correlation of clinical and laboratory results. *Ann Surg* 1967;165:157.

133. Venus A, Matsuda T, Copiozo JB, et al. Prophylactic intubation and continuous positive airway pressure in the management of inhalation injury in burn victims. *Crit Care Med* 1981;9:519.

134. Moylan JA. Inhalation injury: a primary determinant of survival. *J Burn Care Rehabil* 1981;3:78.

135. Mellins RB, Park S. Medical progress: respiratory complications of smoke inhalation in victims of fires. *J Pediatr* 1975;87:1.

136. Achauer BM, Allyn PA, Furnas DW, et al. Pulmonary complications of burns: the major threat to the burn patient. *Ann Surg* 1973;177:311.

137. Putman CE, Loke J, Matthay RA, et al. Radiographic manifestations of acute smoke inhalation. *AJR Am J Roentegenol* 1977;129:865.

138. Zikria BA, Budd DC, Floch F, et al. What is clinical smoke poisoning? *Ann Surg* 1975;181:151.

139. Moylan JA, Adib K, Birnbaum M. Fiberoptic bronchoscopy following thermal injury. *Surg Gynecol Obstet* 1975;140:541.

140. Nider A. The effects of low levels of carbon monoxide on the fine structures of terminal airways. *Am Rev Respir Dis* 1971;103:898.

141. Aub JC, Pittman H. The pulmonary complications: a clinical description. *Ann Surg* 1943;117:834.

142. Garzon AA, Seltzer B, Song IC, et al. Respiratory mechanics in patients with inhalation burns. *J Trauma* 1970;10:57.

143. Petroff PA, Hander EW, Clayton WH, et al. Pulmonary function studies after smoke inhalation. *Am J Surg* 1976;132:346.

144. Zikria BA, Weston GC, Chodoff M, et al. Smoke and carbon monoxide poisoning in fire victims. *J Trauma* 1972;12:641.

145. Nieman GF, Clark WR, Wax SD, et al. The effect of smoke inhalation on pulmonary surfactant. *Ann Surg* 1980;191:171.

146. Wooton R, Hodgson E. Physiotherapy in treatment of burns with inhalation involvement. *Physiotherapy* 1977;63:153.

147. Wroblewski DA, Bower GC. The significance of facial burns in acute smoke inhalation. *Crit Care Med* 1979;7:335.

148. Zawacki BE, Jung RC, Joyce J, et al. Smoke, burns, and natural history of inhalation injury in fire victims. *Ann Surg* 1977;185:100.

149. Fein A, Leff A, Hopewell PC. Pathophysiology and management of the complications resulting from fire and the inhaled products of combustion: review of the literature. *Crit Care Med* 1980;8:94.

150. Traber DL. Pulmonary microvascular dysfunction during shock. In: Barnes J, eds. *Cardiovascular shock: basic and clinical implications.* New York: Academic Press, 1984.

151. Demling RH. The pathogenesis of respiratory failure after trauma and sepsis. *Surg Clin North Am* 1980;60:1373.

152. Demling RH. Burn edema: I. Pathogenesis. *J Burn Care Rehabil* 1982;3:138.

153. Traber DL, Bohs CT, Carvajal HF, et al. Early cardiopulmonary and renal function in thermally injured sheep. *Surg Gynecol Obstet* 1979;148:753.

154. Traber DL, Bohs CT, Carvajal HF, et al. Nicotinic acid-mannitol supplement in post-burn resuscitation: a double-blind study in sheep. *Burns* 1979;5:299.

155. Herndon DL, Traber DL, Brown M, et al. Lung microvascular lesions with and without inhalation injury in thermally injured sheep. *Prog Clin Biol Res* 1988;264:403–408.

156. Till GO, Johnson KJ, Kunkel R, et al. Intravascular activation of complement and acute lung injury. *J Clin Invest* 1982;69:1126.

157. Redl H, Schlag G, Griswold W, et al. Early morphological changes of the lung in shock demonstrated in the light (LM), transmission electron (TEM) and scanning electron microscopy (SEM). *Scanning Electron Microsc* 1978;2:555.

158. Moritz AR, Henriques FC Jr, McLean R. The effects of inhaled heat on the air passages and lungs: an experimental investigation. *Am J Pathol* 1945;21:311.

159. Zikria BA, Ferrer JM, Loch HF. The chemical factors contributing to pulmonary damage. *Surgery* 1972;71:704.

160. Rhodes ML. The effect of carbon monoxide on mitochondrial respiratory enzymes in pulmonary tissue. *Am Rev Respir Dis* 1971;103:906.

161. Fein A, Grossman RF, Jones JG, et al. Carbon monoxide effect on alveolar epithelial permeability. *Chest* 1980;78:726.

162. Fisher AB, Hyde RW, Baue AE, et al. Effect of carbon monoxide on function and structure of the lung. *J Appl Physiol* 1969;26:4.

163. Herndon DN, Traber DL, Niehaus GD, et al. The pathophysiology of smoke inhalation injury in a sheep model. *J Trauma* 1984;24:1043.

164. Henriques FC Jr. Studies of thermal injury: V. The predictability and the significance of thermally induced rate process leading to irreversible epidermal injury. *Arch Pathol* 1947;43:489.

165. Walker HL, McLeod CG, McManus WL. Experimental inhalation injury in the goat. *J Trauma* 1981;21:804.

166. Mathru M, Venus B, Rao TLK, et al. Noncardiac pulmonary edema precipitated by tracheal intubation in patients with inhalation injury. *Crit Care Med* 1983;11:804.

167. Stone HH, Martin JD Jr. Pulmonary injury associated with thermal burns. *Surg Gynecol Obstet* 1969;129:1242.

168. Davies LK, Pulton TJ, Modell JH. Continuous positive airway pressure is beneficial in treatment of smoke inhalation. *Crit Care Med* 1983;11:726.

169. Esrig BC, Stephenson SF, Fulton RL. Role of pulmonary infection in the pathogenesis of smoke inhalation. *Surg Forum* 1975;26:204.

170. Herndon DN, Traber DL, Linares HA, et al. Etiology of the pulmonary pathophysiology associated with inhalation injury. *Resuscitation* 1986;14:43–59.

171. Herndon DN, Traber DL, Traber LD, et al. Mediators of tracheobronchial fluid formation and pulmonary destruction following smoke inhalation, abstracted. *Physiologist* 1983;26:55.

172. Morgan A, Knight D, O'Connor N. Lung water changes after thermal burns. *Ann Surg* 1977;187:288.

173. Traber DL, Schlag G, Redl H, et al. The mechanism of the pulmonary edema of smoke inhalation, abstracted. *Circ Shock* 1984;13:77.

174. Herndon DN, Barrow RE, Traber DL, et al. Extravascular lung water changes following smoke inhalation and massive burn injury. *Surgery* 1987;42:665–674.

175. Tranbaugh RF, Lewis FR, Christensen JM, et al. Lung water changes after thermal injury. *Ann Surg* 1980;192:479.

176. Head JM. Inhalation injury in burns. *Am J Surg* 1980;129:508.

177. Bringham KL, Meyrick B. Interaction of granulocytes with the lungs. *Circ Res* 1984;54:623.

178. Staub NC, Schultz EL, Albertine KH. Leukocytes and pulmonary microvascular injury. *Ann NY Acad Sci* 1982;384:332.

179. Stein MD. Boyden chamber analysis of sheep neutrophil chemotaxis. *Circ Shock* 1984;13:77.

180. Johnson KJ, Ward PA. Acute and progressive lung injury after contact with phorbol myristate acetate. *Am J Pathol* 1982;107:29.

181. Bartlett RH, Niccole M, Tavis MJ, et al. Acute management of the upper airway in facial burns. *Arch Surg* 1976;111:774.

182. Lloyd E, MacRae WR. Respiratory tract damage in burns. *Br J Anesth* 1971;43:365.

183. Trunkey DD. Inhalation injury. *Surg Clin North Am* 1978;8:1133.

184. Reed GF, Camp HL. Upper airway problems in severely burned patients. *Ann Otol* 1972;78:472.

185. Cope O, Runinelander FW. The problem of burn shock complicated by pulmonary damage. *Ann Surg* 1943;117:915.

186. Fineberg C, Mille BJ, Allbritten FF Jr. Thermal burns of the respiratory tract. *Surg Gynecol Obstet* 1954;98:318.

187. Stephenson SF, Esrig BC, Polk HC Jr, et al. The pathophysiology of smoke inhalation Injury. *Ann Surg* 1975;182:652.

188. Thommasen HV, Martin BA, Wiggs BR, et al. Effect of pulmonary blood flow on leukocyte uptake and release by dog lung. *J Appl Physiol* 1984;56:966.

189. Gorman JF, Rejent MM. Treatment of pulmonary complications of smoke inhalation. *Clin Pediatr* 1965;4:577.

190. Rai J, Jschke MG, Barrow RE, et al. Electrical injuries: a 30-year review. *J Trauma* 1999;46:1–4.

191. Baxter CR. Present concepts in the management of major electrical injury. *Surg Clin North Am* 1970;50:1401.

192. Mistry D, Wainwright D. Hydrofluoric acid burns. *Am Fam Physician* 1992;45:1748–1754.

193. McIvor M. Delayed fatal hyperkalemia in a patient with acute fluoride intoxication. *Ann Emerg Med* 1987;16:118–120.

194. Klauder JV, Shelanski L, Gavriel K. Industrial uses of compounds of fluoride and oxalic acid. *Archives of Industrial Health* 1955;12:412–419.

195. Division of Industrial Hygiene, National Institutes of Health. Hydrofluoric acid burns. *Industrial Medicine* 1943;12:412–419.

196. Summerlin WT, Walder AI, Moncrief JA. White phosphorous burns and massive haemolysis. *J Trauma* 1967;7:476–484.

197. Cioffi GC, Rue LW, Buescher TM, et al. A brief history and the pathophysiology of burns. In: Zaitchuk R, ed. *Textbook of military medicine.* Washington, DC: Office of the Surgeon General, Department of the Army, 1989.

198. Saunders A, Geddes L, Elliott P. Are phenolic disinfectants toxic to staff members? *Aust Nurses J* 1988;17:25.

CARE OF THE POISONED PATIENT

BRIAN S. KAUFMAN
ROBERT S. HOFFMAN

KEY WORDS

- Antidotes
- Cathartics
- Activated charcoal
- Gastric emptying
- Hemodialysis
- Hemoperfusion
- Overdose
- Poisoning
- Whole-bowel irrigation

INTRODUCTION

Poisoning continues to represent a significant sociomedical problem in the United States, both in terms of direct medical costs as well as indirect costs from lost labor and wages. Since oral ingestions account for 75% of human poison exposures and 76% of fatalities, we will focus our discussion on this route of exposure (1). This chapter's purpose is to briefly review the epidemiology of poisoning, discuss diagnostic and general supportive management principles, review the various decontamination techniques available, and discuss the appropriate use of antidotes. A brief summary of the diagnosis and treatment of specific, commonly encountered poisonings is also included.

EPIDEMIOLOGY

The American Association of Poison Control Centers (AAPCC) through its Toxic Exposure Surveillance System (TESS) has annually reported data regarding calls to participating poison control centers in the United States (1). The data obtained from these centers represent an estimated 95.7% of the human poison exposures that precipitated poison center contacts in 1999. Extrapolating from the 2.2 million human poison exposures reported in this database, 2.3 million human poison exposures are estimated to have been reported to all U.S. poison centers in 1999. Ninety-two percent of exposures occurred at a residence, most often involving unintentional oral exposure to a single toxin in a child younger than 6 years. In direct contrast, in clinical series of overdoses in adults, ingestion of two or more drugs (particularly ethanol) occurred in approximately 50% to 60% of cases (2). A male predominance was found among poison exposure victims younger than 13 years of age, but the gender distribution was reversed in teenagers and adults.

The majority of cases reported to poison centers were managed in a nonhealth care facility (78%), usually at the patient's own home (1). Of cases managed in a health care facility, 57.1% were treated and released without admission, 13% were admitted to an intensive care unit (ICU), and 7% were admitted to a medical or psychiatric unit. There were 873 reported fatalities in the 1999 database. Fatalities differed from the total exposure population in several ways. Although the majority of exposures occurred in children under the age of 6, this group comprised only 2.7% of the fatalities. The majority of fatalities (61%) occurred in patients aged 20 to 49. Although a single substance was implicated in 92.4% of exposures, 45% of the fatal cases occurred in individuals with ingestions of two or more toxins. Analgesics, antidepressants (most often tricyclics), cardiovascular drugs, and stimulant and street drugs were the primary substances involved in 64% of the fatalities with 71% of the analgesic related deaths occurring with ingestion of acetaminophen, aspirin, or other salicylates.

In general, poisonings follow one of two patterns. Children usually ingest small quantities of poison unintentionally and suffer minimal morbidity or mortality related to their ingestion. In contrast, adolescents and adults tend to intentionally ingest larger quantities and, as a result, suffer substantially more morbidity and mortality. Although the overall risk of mortality in the 1999 AAPCC report was 0.04%, it must be recognized that data generated by poison control centers are inherently flawed. This is because the data collected and disseminated by these centers are on exposures and many exposures are of no consequence because of the properties of the substance involved, the magnitude or duration of the exposure, or confusion about whether an actual exposure has occurred. Statistics generated by poison control centers may grossly underestimate the number of poisoning deaths as documented by the medical examiner system (3). Nonetheless, the vast majority of poisoned patients, given appropriate care, will have a satisfactory outcome.

DIAGNOSIS OF POISONING

The principal objectives in the diagnosis and evaluation of a patient exposed to a poison are: (a) to recognize the presence of a poisoning; (b) to identify the involved poison or poisons; (c) to estimate the potential toxicity of the poison; and (d) to assess the severity of the poisoning. Although an accurate diagnostic evaluation is a prerequisite for optimal patient management, arriving at the correct diagnosis of a poisoning is often difficult due to multiple confounding variables, including unreliable history, mixed toxin ingestions, concomitant traumatic injury, underlying medical conditions and their treatment, and unpredictable pharmacology of the (often unknown) ingested agent or agents. Thus, it is important that the clinician maintains a high index of suspicion for poisonings in all patients who present with multisystem organ dysfunction of unknown etiology.

Historical information on drug intake has been reported to be inaccurate or unavailable in 75% of toxicologic emergencies (4). Unreliable data regarding the amounts and time of ingestion are a particular problem in patients with intentional self-poisoning. Attempts should be made to elicit data regarding the specific toxin ingested, quantity, time of ingestion, decontamination techniques initiated prior to hospital arrival, nature and progression of symptoms occurring since ingestion, medical history, psychiatric history (including suicide gestures or attempts), current medications used by the patient or others living with the patient, and any history of incidental trauma related to the toxin exposure. A worst case scenario should always be assumed. When pill bottles are brought in with the patient, all missing or not clearly accounted for pills should be considered to have been ingested. For known ingestants, the potential toxicity can then be predicted from existing toxicodynamic data. When patients are unwilling or unable to provide historical information, attempts should be made to obtain data from ambulance personnel, police, family, friends, personal physician, local pharmacies, and previous medical records. These resources can also be used to confirm historical information obtained from the "cooperative" patient. Poison control centers, computer-based information systems (*Poisondex*, Micromedex, Inc., Greenwood Village, CO), and standard toxicology textbooks can prove quite useful for both the routine and puzzling case.

The assessment of the severity of a poisoning is primarily determined by the findings on physical examination. A complete physical examination should be performed in all patients, but the examination should be initially focused on the assessment of respiratory function (including the presence of airway protective reflexes), cardiovascular stability, and the patient's neurologic status.

Cardiopulmonary stabilization should be provided while the rest of the physical examination is completed. The accurate measurement of vital signs is essential and must include measurement of core temperature to exclude hypothermia or hyperthermia. Such temperature disturbances may be due to ingested toxin (e.g., salicylates, stimulants, and anticholinergics) rather than to environmental exposure. Identification of central nervous system (CNS) dysfunction (particularly mental status depression or seizures) should prompt immediate consideration of pharmacologic therapy (for seizures) as well as an evaluation for the possibilities of head and cervical spine injury while the cervical spine is protected until injury can either be excluded or diagnosed and treated. The physical examination should be completed by searching carefully for any signs of head, neck, chest and abdominal trauma, incidental fractures, or occult hemorrhage. Stigmata of substance abuse such as puncture wounds and needle "tracks" should be sought. Focal neurologic findings, abnormal pupillary responses, unusual breath or skin odors, abnormal respiratory breathing pattern and abnormal respiratory, cardiac, and abdominal sounds should be documented.

With some toxins, a characteristic constellation of signs and symptoms consistently develops. Mofenson and Greensher coined the term "toxidrome" from toxic syndromes to describe these typical grouped clinical findings (5). The most typical toxic syndromes are described in Table 1. These autonomic syndromes are best described by a combination of the vital signs and clinically obvious end-organ manifestations. The organ system signs that prove most clinically useful for toxin identification include the CNS (mental status), ophthalmologic (pupil size and reactivity), gastrointestinal (peristalsis), skin (dryness versus diaphoresis), mucous membranes (salivation versus dryness), and genitourinary system (urinary retention). Table 2 reviews many of the commonly encountered toxins and their typical clinical findings. The clinical manifestations of an ingestion are often however much more variable than the signs, symptoms, and clinical findings described in Table 2.

The number and type of laboratory testing required to assess metabolic and organ function should be determined primarily by the clinical severity of the poisoning and secondarily by the history. Measurement of serum chemistries, hematologic studies,

TABLE 1. TOXIC SYNDROMES

Group	BP	P	RR	T	Mental Status	Pupil Size	Peristalsis	Diaphoresis	Other
Adrenergic agonists	↑	↑	↑	↑	Altered	↑	↑	↑	Flush
Anticholinergic agents	±	↑	±	↑	Altered	↑	↓	↓	Dry mucous membranes, flush, urinary retention
Cholinergic agents (muscarinic, nicotinic)	±	±	−	−	Altered	±	↑	↑	Salivation, lacrimation, urination, bronchorrhea, fasciculations
Opioids	↓	↓	↓	↓	Altered	↓	↓	↓	Hyporeflexia
Withdrawal of opioids	↑	↑	—	—	Normal	↑	↑	Present	Nausea, vomiting, hyperactivity, rhinorrhea, piloerection
Sedative-hypnotics or ethanol	↓	↓	↓	↓	Altered	±	↓	↓	Hyporeflexia
Withdrawal of sedative-hypnotics or ethanol	↑	↑	↑	↑	Altered	↑	Normal to ↑	Present	Nausea, tremor, seizures

BP, blood pressure; P, pulse; RR, respiratory rate; T, temperature.
From Goldfrank LR, et al. Vital signs and toxic syndromes. In: Goldfrank LR, et al., eds. *Goldfrank's toxicologic emergencies*, 6th ed. Stamford, CT: Appelton & Lange, 1998, with permission.

TABLE 2. SPECIFIC DRUGS OR TOXINS AND THEIR TOXIC SYNDROMES

Toxin	Vital Signs	Mental Status	Signs and Symptoms	Clinical Findings
Acetaminophen	Normal (early)	Normal	Anorexia, nausea, vomiting	Right upper quadrant tenderness, jaundice (late)
Amphetamines	Hypertension, tachycardia, tachypnea, hyperthermia	Hyperactive, agitated, toxic psychosis	Hyperalertness, panic, anxiety, diaphoresis	Mydriasis, hyperactive peristalsis, diaphoresis
Antihistamines	Hypotension, hypertension, tachycardia, hyperthermia	Altered (agitation, lethargy to coma) hallucinations	Blurred vision, dry mouth, inability to urinate	Dry mucous membranes, mydriasis, flush, ↓ peristalsis, urinary retention
Barbiturates	Hypotension, bradypnea, hypothermia	Altered (lethargy to coma)	Slurred speech, ataxia	Dysconjugate gaze, bullae, hyporeflexia
Beta-adrenergic antagonists	Hypotension, bradycardia	Altered (lethargy to coma)	Dizziness	Cyanosis, seizures
Carbon monoxide	Often normal	Altered (lethargy to coma)	Headache, dizziness, nausea, vomiting	Seizures
Clonidine	Hypotension, hypertension, bradycardia, bradypnea	Altered (lethargy to coma)	Dizziness, confusion	Miosis
Cocaine	Hypertension, tachycardia, tachypnea, hyperthermia	Altered (anxiety, agitation, delirium)	Hallucinations, paranoia, panic, anxiety, restlessness	Mydriasis, nystagmus
Cyclic antidepressants	Hypotension, tachycardia	Altered (lethargy to coma)	Confusion, dizziness, dry mouth, inability to urinate	Mydriasis, dry mucous membranes, distended bladder, flush, seizures
Digitalis	Hypotension, bradycardia	Normal to altered, visual distortion	Nausea, vomiting, anorexia, visual disturbances	None
Ethylene glycol	Tachypnea	Altered (lethargy to coma)	Abdominal pain	Slurred speech, ataxia
Isoniazid	Often normal	Normal or altered (lethargy to coma)	Nausea, vomiting	Seizures
Lead	Hypertension	Altered (lethargy to coma)	Irritability, abdominal pain (colic), nausea, vomiting, constipation	Peripheral neuropathy, seizures, gingival pigmentation
Lithium	Hypotension (late)	Altered (lethargy to coma)	Diarrhea, tremor, nausea	Weakness, tremor, ataxia, myoclonus, seizures
Methanol	Hypotension, tachypnea	Altered (lethargy to coma)	Blurred vision, blindness, abdominal pain	Hyperemic discs, mydriasis
Opioids	Hypotension, bradycardia, bradypnea, hypothermia	Altered (lethargy to coma)	Slurred speech, ataxia	Miosis, ↓ peristalsis
Phencyclidine	Hypertension, tachycardia, hyperthermia	Altered (agitation, lethargy to coma)	Hallucinations	Miosis, diaphoresis, myoclonus, blank stare, nystagmus, seizures
Phenothiazines	Hypotension, tachycardia, hypothermia, or hyperthermia	Altered (lethargy to coma)	Dizziness, dry mouth, inability to urinate	Miosis or mydriasis, decreased bowel sounds, dystonia
Salicylates	Hypotension, tachycardia, tachypnea, hyperthermia	Altered (agitation, lethargy to coma)	Tinnitus, nausea, vomiting	Diaphoresis, tender abdomen, pulmonary edema
Sedatives-hypnotics	Hypotension, bradypnea, hypothermia	Altered (lethargy to coma)	Slurred speech, ataxia	Hyporeflexia, bullae
Theophylline	Hypotension, tachycardia, tachypnea, hyperthermia	Altered (agitation)	Nausea, vomiting, diaphoresis, anxiety	Diaphoresis, tremor, seizures, arrhythmias

From Goldfrank LR, et al. Vital signs and toxic syndromes. In: Goldfrank LR, et al., eds. *Goldfrank's toxicologic emergencies.* 6th ed. Stamford, CT: Appelton & Lange, 1998, with permission.

arterial blood gases, and electrocardiography, are infrequently helpful in the diagnosis of acute poisoning. Asymptomatic or potentially poisoned patients, should have blood and urine samples obtained on emergency room presentation. These samples should be saved and if there is a subsequent clinical deterioration, laboratory analysis should be completed to document baseline values (6,7). Symptomatic or suicidal patients should have blood samples sent for a complete blood count, serum chemistries (including calcium and magnesium measurements if indicated), urinalysis, and a 12-lead electrocardiogram (ECG). An arterial blood gas may be indicated early after hospital arrival to assess ventilation, oxygenation, detect carboxyhemoglobin or methemoglobin (by cooximetry), and for patients with altered mental status to confirm or exclude some toxic-metabolic etiologies

(e.g., a wide anion gap metabolic acidosis). A more extensive laboratory evaluation should be performed in patients with respiratory symptoms (chest radiograph), and clinical indications of severe stimulant or depressant poisoning (coagulation studies, amylase, creatine phosphokinase, hepatic enzyme levels). The decision whether to perform neurodiagnostic studies for the patient with altered mental status must be individualized.

Although many hospitals can perform "toxicology screens," these tests often provide delayed results that rarely impact on patient management. In one study of 209 overdoses, toxicology screen results changed therapy in only three cases, with no apparent impact on outcome (8). In contrast to screening tests, quantitative analysis for specific chemical concentrations in the serum, blood, or urine can sometimes help in assessing the severity of poisoning and aid with management decisions. For a quantitative chemical measurement to be clinically useful, the measurement must be able to be made rapidly so that the critical time for specific intervention (e.g., an antidote) is not exceeded. Additionally, there must be a predictable relationship between the concentration of the poison and its toxicologic effects, so that management decisions can be made based on the measurement. Less than two dozen substances have demonstrated reliable correlations between body fluid concentration and toxic effects (acetaminophen, acetone, alcohols, antiarrhythmics, antiepileptics, barbiturates, carbon monoxide, calcium, digoxin, ethylene glycol, heavy metals, lithium, magnesium, salicylates, theophylline). Tests for one or more of these specific drugs or toxins should be performed when their ingestion is suggested by history, physical examination, or bedside diagnostic tests. An acetaminophen level should be requested for all potentially suicidal patients. The use of invasive, expensive, potentially dangerous, or poison-specific therapies is difficult to justify without laboratory documentation of toxic levels of these toxins. For the vast majority of intoxications, assay for other chemicals is not indicated; if present it will only confirm the clinical impression and will not change supportive management.

GENERAL MANAGEMENT

Emergency Stabilization and Supportive Care

Because most calls to poison control centers are for nontoxic or minimally toxic ingestions, rapid reference to a list of nontoxic products may obviate the need for any further medical intervention (Table 3) (1). When medical intervention is necessary, the vast majority of poisoned or overdosed patients will benefit from aggressive institution of an organized, clinical management plan.

The initial management of patients with toxic or potentially toxic overdoses begins with attention to the ABCs: *a*irway compromise, *b*reathing difficulties, and *c*irculatory problems. Establishing and maintaining the patency of the upper airway is the first priority. When airway patency is in question, maneuvers to establish and protect the airway are of prime importance. This may often simply involve repositioning the chin, jaw, or head, or suctioning secretions or vomitus from the airway. However, insertion of an oral or nasopharyngeal airway, endotracheal intubation, or cricothyroidotomy may all be required as clinically indicated. Pulmonary aspiration of gastric contents is a relatively common complication of poisoning and of its treatment (e.g., gastrointestinal decontamination techniques). The airway should be secured by emergent tracheal intubation in all obtunded patients who lack protective gag and cough reflexes. An absent gag reflex is not an indication by itself for intubation, as many normal individuals lack this reflex. Prophylactic intubation is indicated in situations in which progressive mental status deterioration with loss of protective airway reflexes is anticipated based on the history, physical examination, and pharmacology of the ingested agent(s). Use of an endotracheal tube with a high-volume, low-pressure cuff, however, does not provide complete protection from aspiration. In one study, activated charcoal was recovered from the airway of 25% of patients who were given it by nasogastric tube despite prior intubation (9). Intubation may also be required for patients

TABLE 3. HOUSEHOLD ITEMS GENERALLY REGARDED AS NONTOXIC

Personal-use items	Medications
Bath oils	Antacids
Body conditioners	Antibiotics (with some exceptions)
Bubble bath	Birth control pills
Cologne (low alcohol content)	Calamine lotion
Cosmetics	Corticosteroids
Deodorant	Hydrogen peroxide 3%
Eye makeup	Mineral oil
Hair spray and tonic	Zinc oxide
Hand lotions	Zirconium oxide
Lipstick	
Petroleum jelly	**Miscellaneous**
Rouge	Book matches (one book)
Shampoo (small amounts)	Candles
Shaving cream	Cigarettes
Suntan lotion	Grease, motor oil
Thermometer (elemental	Incense
mercury not toxic if ingested)	Latex paint
Toothpaste	Lubricating oil
	Newspaper
Art supplies	Putty
Ballpoint pen ink	Silica gel
Chalk	Spackle
Charcoal	
Clay	**Cleaning products**
Crayons (marked A.P., C.P.)	Fabric softener
Felt-tip pens (water base)	Household bleach 2%–5%
Pencils (graphite)	Laundry detergent
Watercolors	
White glue, paste	
Toys	
Bathtub toys	
Caps (for toy guns)	
Etch A Sketch	
Play-Doh	
Silly Putty	
Teething rings	
Toy cosmetics	

From Weisman RS. Identifying the nontoxic exposure. In: Goldfrank LR, et al., eds. *Goldfrank's toxicologic emergencies*, 6th ed. Stamford, CT: Appelton & Lange, 1998, with permission.

with extreme behavioral or physiologic stimulation who require aggressive pharmacologic therapy with sedatives, antipsychotics, anticonvulsants, or neuromuscular blockers. Cervical spine precautions should be undertaken before airway manipulation in all situations in which coexisting trauma is possible. Given the uncertain nature of most poisonings, patients at low risk for requiring intubation based on clinical criteria (drowsy but easily arousable, intact protective airway reflexes, etc.) should be placed in "aspiration-preventive positioning" (head-down, left lateral decubitus) to protect against aspiration should unanticipated deterioration occur.

Once the airway is secured (if necessary) high-flow supplemental oxygen should be provided and the depth, rate, and rhythm of respirations evaluated. Pulse oximetry is indicated in all patients, recognizing that such readings may be spuriously high with carbon monoxide exposure, and spuriously high or low if toxin-induced methemoglobinemia is present. Hypoventilation resulting from an inadequate respiratory rate or tidal volume leads to hypoxia and ventilatory failure. The symptoms of hypoxia and hypercarbia are nonspecific and resemble toxicity from many agents; therefore in patients who present with drug overdose and possible ventilatory failure, arterial blood gas analysis (with cooximetry) must be used early in the evaluation.

Efforts should next be directed to establishing circulatory stability. Intravenous (i.v.) access with a large-bore cannula and cardiac monitoring should be instituted rapidly. Hemodynamically significant cardiac dysrhythmias should, in general, be treated following Advanced Cardiac Life Support guidelines, with appropriate modification for specific toxins (such as avoidance of class I-A antiarrhythmic agents with ventricular dysrhythmias from QT-interval prolongation in tricyclic overdoses). Hypotension should be treated initially using an i.v. bolus of isotonic crystalloid, with the cautious use of vasopressors restricted to patients who do not respond to judicious fluid therapy. Exaggerated responses to these sympathomimetic vasoconstrictors can occur in overdoses such as cocaine and tricyclic antidepressants, and with monoamine oxidase inhibitors. Symptomatic hypertension should be treated using vasodilators, β-blockers, calcium channel blockers, or α-blockers as appropriate. The clinician should generally resist the urge to acutely treat asymptomatic hypertension in patients at low risk for permanent end-organ dysfunction, given the ill-defined cause and occasionally short-lived nature of the disturbance; however, we aggressively treat hypertension induced by monoamine oxidase inhibitor–food/drug interactions because of a high risk for end-organ damage.

After assessment and stabilization of the airway, breathing, and circulation, a trial of naloxone, hypertonic dextrose, and thiamine (coma cocktail), may be indicated for patients with altered mental status, clonic seizures, and/or respiratory compromise. Since opioid overdose and hypoglycemia are rapidly reversible, potential causes of respiratory failure, these diagnoses should be addressed before most other interventions are considered. However, more recently, this once routine practice has become somewhat controversial (10). Toxin-induced CNS depression and even coma are usually well tolerated and arousal does not necessarily improve prognosis. Former ingredients of the coma cocktail (e.g., doxapram, physostigmine) increased arousal but were abandoned because of adverse effects. Analysis favors empiric administration of hypertonic dextrose (0.5 to 1.0 g per kg dextrose i.v.), accompanied by thiamine (100 mg i.v. or intramuscular in adults) to prevent the development of Wernicke encephalopathy. In a setting in which focal cerebral ischemia is possible (trauma, intracerebral hemorrhage, etc.) rapid reagent strip measurement of blood glucose should also precede i.v. dextrose because of the possible adverse impact of hyperglycemia on this condition. These reagent strips are not infallible, and they fail to recognize clinical hypoglycemia that may occur without numeric hypoglycemia (10). Although critical review offers little evidence to support the empiric use of thiamine in patients with altered mental status, its routine use in the coma cocktail is probably still warranted, as its use is safe, inexpensive, and will prevent the possibility of delayed deterioration secondary to nutritional deficiency.

A trial of naloxone (0.4 to 2.0 mg) should be reserved for patients with clear signs and symptoms of opioid intoxication (CNS and respiratory depression). Its use has been associated with life-threatening complications, but most of these case reports occurred with use in the postoperative setting. Yealy and associates demonstrated that the rate of adverse reactions in 813

patients who received naloxone in the prehospital setting was less than 1%, and all reactions were believed to be inconsequential (11). Opioid withdrawal is commonly associated with naloxone administration. The effects of opioid withdrawal in adults are not considered life threatening; however, significant clinical events can occur when naloxone is administered to patients with polydrug intoxication. Naloxone can be administered without demonstrable risk in patients who present with CNS and/or respiratory depression and have a low likelihood of opioid addiction and polydrug intoxication (small children). For all others naloxone can be administered selectively to patients with a high clinical suspicion for opioid presence (e.g., respiratory rate less than 12), or at decreased dosage (0.1 to 0.2 mg) in potentially dependent patients (10).

Flumazenil is a pure, competitive benzodiazepine antagonist. The use of flumazenil in the treatment of poisoning is very controversial. (10) Proponents cite both the diagnostic and therapeutic value of benzodiazepine reversal and the avoidance of the need for intensive care support and expensive diagnostic testing. Others have cautioned against the routine use of flumazenil in patients with mixed or unknown overdoses because of the risk of serious side effects, including withdrawal, seizures, and dysrhythmias in patients taking cyclic antidepressants and other potential proconvulsant or proarrhythmic agents. Fatalities from benzodiazepine intoxication are rare and are usually associated with respiratory depression and aspiration. Benzodiazepine-induced respiratory depression responds poorly and unpredictably to flumazenil, therefore current recommendations advise airway protection prior to administration if there is evidence of hypoxia or hypoventilation (12,13). Once airway protection has been accomplished, reversal of the depressant effects of benzodiazepines seems unnecessary as the threat to life has been removed. If respiratory depression is not present, the safety and value of reversal is questionable, as acute withdrawal may be precipitated and can include prolonged seizure activity that may be refractory to therapy because of the presence of the benzodiazepine antagonist.

The use of flumazenil in patients with acute overdosage may be justified when there is a reliable history of ingestion corroborated by clinical manifestations consistent with benzodiazepine intoxication and the likelihood of a significant proconvulsant or proarrhythmic coingestion or benzodiazepine dependency is small. Since the half-life of flumazenil (0.7 to 1.3 hours) is much shorter than almost all currently used benzodiazepines, patients will still need to be closely monitored for recurrent sedation after its use. Appropriate regimens for continuous infusion have not been well established. Currently recommended initial dose is 0.2 mg for adults (10 μg per kg to a maximum dose of 0.2 mg for children) infused over 30 seconds, to be followed 30 seconds later by 0.3 mg if the patient does not respond. Subsequent doses of 0.5 mg may also be given. Most patients respond to total doses of less than 1 mg (10).

DECONTAMINATION TECHNIQUES
Evacuation of Unabsorbed Toxin

Limiting ongoing absorption of toxic compounds is one of the core principles of care for poisoned patients. Although gastrointestinal decontamination has been a critical and familiar part of therapy of the poisoned patient for some time, no other area of medical toxicology has generated as much recent and continuing controversy. The controversy has arisen because the results of clinically relevant studies of gastric emptying, activated charcoal, and cathartics have challenged many of the assumptions on which previous therapy was based. Studies of gastric emptying have failed to show benefit or found benefit only in limited circumstances. Activated charcoal appears to be more effective than gastric emptying in many cases and often may enhance drug elimination in addition to decreasing absorption.

The decision to use or forego gastric emptying should be based on whether it is reasonable to expect that a clinically beneficial amount of drug removal can be safely accomplished. Several factors must be considered: (a) the risk of potential harm to the patient caused by the ingestion; (b) the likelihood that gastric emptying will remove a clinically significant amount of the ingestion; (c) the benefits of removing that amount of agent; (d) the risks of gastric emptying; and (e) the availability and use of alternative methods to limit absorption.

An assessment of the risk to the patient includes a consideration of the amount and type of agent ingested and the clinical course since ingestion. If the clinician is confident that the ingestion was of a nontoxic agent or a nontoxic amount of a potentially toxic agent, then gastric emptying is not indicated. If the history obtained suggests a toxic ingestion but the clinical course excludes toxicity, then gastric emptying is again not appropriate. Such an approach is appropriate when other ingestants can be excluded. Another exception should be made for ingestions of extraordinary high potential risk. Although the benefit of gastric emptying remains unproved, in this subset of patients the available data are very limited and some data suggest benefit. The safest course therefore at this time is to perform gastric emptying on patients with unknown potentially lethal ingestions, or known very high-risk ingestions (e.g., cyanide, colchicine, chloroquine, aspirin, tricyclic antidepressants, verapamil); sometimes this may be indicated even if the patient is asymptomatic beyond the time the onset of toxicity would be expected by history.

The likelihood that gastric emptying will effectively remove a clinically significant amount of ingestant depends on both whether any toxin remains in the stomach and whether gastric emptying will successfully remove it. Absorption of many toxins is so rapid that essentially no toxin remains in the stomach after a few hours and gastric emptying is therefore not indicated. Even for the many toxins that are more slowly absorbed, the yield of delayed gastric emptying is often unimpressive. Uncontrolled clinical studies have suggested that other than for drugs that slow gastrointestinal motility such as anticholinergics, sedative-hypnotics, and opioids, that a drug is unlikely to be recoverable by gastric emptying more than 2 to 4 hours after ingestion (14,15). These studies fail to resolve the question of benefit to the subset of individuals at very high risk.

Drugs with or without the ability to slow gastrointestinal motility can also remain in the stomach if they tend to form adherent masses. These drugs include enteric-coated aspirin, iron, meprobamate, and phenobarbital. Drugs such as aspirin that may cause pylorospasm also cause prolonged gastric retention. Clinical anecdotes clearly show that in some cases large amounts of drug can remain in the stomach for hours to days. These observations continue to stimulate the use of delayed gastric emptying despite the lack of proven clinical efficacy.

The occurrence of antecedent spontaneous vomiting is often considered another determinant of whether or not a significant amount of an agent remains in the stomach. Although some drug may remain in the stomach after repeated episodes of spontaneous vomiting, it is unlikely that a significant amount can be subsequently removed by either lavage or emesis. How much antecedent vomiting is sufficient to obviate gastric emptying is speculative and a matter of clinical judgment.

Volunteer studies and observations made in poisoned patients demonstrate that gastric emptying can result in removal of drug but clinical benefit has not been proven. New guidelines have emphasized clinical studies that describe no benefit and concluded that gastric emptying should be entirely abandoned or used only in extraordinary situations (16,17). While these studies do demonstrate that the majority of patients can be treated effectively with activated charcoal alone, they clearly do not prove that delayed gastric emptying is ineffective in all cases. In fact, Kulig and coworkers' 1985 study proved that there is benefit for ill patients lavaged within 1 hour of ingestion (2).

The decision to perform gastric emptying should be largely based on speculation that the ingestion may lead to a clinically unstable life-threatening condition for which even a small decrease in toxic exposure may be critical. The impact of gastric emptying on the clinical outcome of patients with the most dangerous exposures is therefore of greatest interest. Studies thus far include patients with a wide variety of overdoses and possible overdoses, the vast majority of whom could be expected to do well with supportive care alone. Clearly it is difficult to show any therapeutic benefit in such cases and study of such patients does not resolve the question in the most important subset. Understandably, no controlled study to date has included enough patients with confirmed life-threatening ingestions to adequately compare outcome with and without gastric emptying. A case-by-case analysis considering the factors that make gastric emptying more or less logical is appropriate (Table 4). Until these issues are resolved, the value of gastric emptying will remain controversial. Studies clearly support the use of a selective approach and the more limited use of gastric emptying has resulted in decreased patient discomfort, complications, and cost.

The underlying principle behind these modes of therapy is to empty the stomach of any residual toxin before it can pass the pylorus and be absorbed by the small-bowel mucosa. This is typically accomplished either by inducing emesis with syrup of ipecac or by instituting orogastric lavage. Comparisons of the efficacy of these two techniques for evacuation of unabsorbed toxin are difficult to interpret as there is a wide range of results, largely due to differences in study design.

Syrup of ipecac is prepared from the dried rhizome and roots of the *Cephaelis acuminata* or *Cephaelis ipecacuanha* plants. Syrup of ipecac has two main pharmacologically active components: the alkaloids emetine and cephaeline, which induce vomiting through both peripheral and central mechanisms (18). The emetic alkaloids stimulate gastric mucosal sensory receptors which activate the vomiting center in the brain. They also directly stimulate the central chemoreceptor trigger zone in the brainstem.

TABLE 4. FACTORS THAT CUMULATIVELY INCREASE THE APPROPRIATENESS OF GASTRIC EMPTYING

- Substantial risk of consequential toxicity: e.g., ingestion of aspirin, chloroquine, colchicine, cyclic antidepressants, calcium channel blockers
- Evidence of consequential toxicity: e.g., repeated seizures, hypotension, cardiac dysrhythmias, apnea, acid-base or other metabolic disturbances
- Antidotal or adjunctive therapy ineffective or nonexistent: e.g., calcium channel blockers, colchicine, iron, paraquat
- Recent ingestion (<1–2 h)
- Ingestion exceeds adsorptive capacity of initial activated charcoal dosing: e.g., >100 mg/kg of large pills such as aspirin, sustained-release verapamil, sustained-release theophylline
- Ingested agent not adsorbed by activated charcoal: e.g., iron, lithium
- Ingested agent likely to form durable mass after overdose: e.g., large amounts of aspirin, enteric-coated agents, iron, meprobamate
- Ingestions of extended- or sustained-release formulations: e.g., calcium channel blockers, theophylline
- No antecedent vomiting
- No contraindications to gastric emptying

From Smilkstein MJ. Techniques used to prevent gastrointestinal absorption of toxic compounds. In: Goldfrank LR, et al., eds. *Goldfrank's toxicologic emergencies*, 6th ed. Stamford, CT: Appelton & Lange, 1998, with permission.

Syrup of ipecac is available as a nonprescription drug at pharmacies in many countries and may be administered at home shortly after an ingestion. The United States Pharmacopeia (USP DI, 1997) recommends the following oral dose regimen for ipecac syrup, USP: children 6 to 12 months of age, 5 to 10 mL preceded or followed by 120 to 240 mL of water; children 1 to 12 years of age, 15 mL preceded or followed by 120 to 240 mL of water; adolescents or adults, 15 to 30 mL preceded or followed by 240 mL of water. Water ingestion is not essential for success. Emesis occurs in the vast majority of patients within 20 to 30 minutes and typically subsides in 30 to 60 minutes (although effects may persist for 2 hours or more in some patients). The dose may be repeated in all age groups if emesis does not occur in 20 to 30 minutes. When used at home, patients should be warned that persistent vomiting for more than 2 hours may indicate toxicity from the primary substances ingested rather than persistent effects of the ipecac and at that point medical evaluation may be necessary.

Rationale for the use of syrup of ipecac include: (a) it effectively produces emesis in the vast majority of patients within 20 to 30 minutes; (b) it is noninvasive; (c) it uses a physiologic mechanism; and (c) it consumes little staff time.

Although syrup of ipecac has a long history of safety, potential complications of its therapeutic use are well documented and on occasion produce serious sequelae. The most common complications or adverse consequences of using syrup of ipecac are diarrhea, lethargy, drowsiness, and prolonged (greater than 1 hour) vomiting. Less frequent complications include irritability, hyperactivity, fever, and diaphoresis. Rare but more serious complications include Mallory-Weiss tears, aspiration pneumonia, and pneumomediastinum. Fatalities have been described secondary to traumatic diaphragmatic hernia with gastric entry into the chest, gastric rupture, and intracranial hemorrhage.

There are many contraindications for inducing emesis with syrup of ipecac: (a) the presence of compromised airway protective reflexes; (b) ingestion of a substance that is expected to depress mental status and compromise airway protective reflexes; (c) age less than 6 months; (d) ingestion of substances in which the hazard of vomiting and aspiration of the ingested substance (e.g., hydrocarbons) outweighs the risk associated with systemic absorption; (e) ingestion of corrosive substances such as acids or alkali; (f) patients with medical conditions that may be further compromised by the induction of emesis (including debilitated, older adult patients); (g) patients with significant prior vomiting, and (h) a well-documented nontoxic ingestion.

Despite the widespread use of therapeutic doses of syrup of ipecac for induction of emesis (an estimated 3 million doses during the 14-year period of 1983–1996), there is no evidence from clinical studies that syrup of ipecac-induced emesis improves the outcome of poisoned patients (2,19,20). Experimental studies in dogs evaluating the ability of syrup of ipecac to reduce marker absorption demonstrate a highly variable (17.5% to 62.0%) mean recovery of ingested material, with greater efficacy with decreased time interval between dosing and onset of emesis, and with a shorter time interval between marker ingestion and syrup of ipecac dosing (16).

Ten studies conducted in volunteers have examined the value of syrup of ipecac in preventing the absorption of marker substances (16). The results of these studies are similar to the animal data, again demonstrating a high variability in the amount of marker recovered with emesis and better recovery with earlier use of syrup of ipecac and faster onset of emesis. However, the clinical value of these studies seems very limited given that they involved the use of nontoxic amounts of drugs, and in clinically significant poisonings, much greater amounts of drugs may be ingested, which can influence dissolution, absorption, and gastric emptying rates.

Clinical studies usually exclude the use of syrup of ipecac in life-threatening poisonings; therefore, the benefit of ipecac in the more severely intoxicated patient is uncertain. Two clinical studies showed no beneficial patient outcome effects (number of hospital admissions, number of patients who were considered to have suffered clinical deterioration after presentation to the emergency department) with the use of syrup of ipecac followed by activated charcoal versus activated charcoal alone (2,20). Clinical studies have also demonstrated that the use of syrup of ipecac delays the administration of activated charcoal and may prolong the length of stay in the emergency department (2). However, a study in overdose patients suggests that when activated charcoal is given 10 minutes after syrup of ipecac, vomiting still occurs in the majority of cases, probably because the syrup of ipecac is absorbed so quickly (21).

The American Academy of Clinical Toxicology/European Association of Poisons Centre and Clinical Toxicologists' position statement on the use of syrup of ipecac points out that clinical studies have not confirmed the benefit of syrup of ipecac even when it was administered less than 60 minutes after poison ingestion. However, since there is insufficient data to support or exclude syrup of ipecac administration soon after poison ingestion, it should be considered only for alert patients who have ingested a potentially toxic amount of a poison and if it can be administered within 60 minutes of ingestion (16). Syrup of ipecac was administered in 1% of more than 2 million cases reported to the American Association of Poison Control Centers in 1999 (1).

TABLE 5. DECONTAMINATION TRENDS

Year	Ipecac Administered (% of Exposures)	Activated Charcoal (% of Exposures)
1990	6.1	6.7
1991	5.2	7.0
1992	4.3	7.3
1993	3.7	7.3
1994	2.7	6.8
1995	2.3	7.7
1996	1.8	7.3
1997	1.5	7.1
1998	1.2	6.8
1999	1.0	6.6

Data adapted from Litovitz TL, Klein-Schwartz W, White S, et al. 1999 Annual Report of the American Association of Poison Control Centers Toxic Exposure Surveillance System. *Am J Emerg Med* 2000;18:517–574.

Syrup of ipecac was used most often in children under 6 years of age (83.4% of all syrup of ipecac use). There has been a continuing decline in the use of syrup of ipecac-induced emesis in the treatment of poisoning (Table 5).

Orogastric lavage involves the passage of an orogastric tube and the sequential administration and aspiration of small volumes of liquid with the intent of removing toxic substances present in the stomach. Orogastric lavage has been employed widely for more than 180 years to facilitate the removal of poisons from the stomach. However, although the procedure is physiologically appealing, the routine use of orogastric lavage is no longer recommended for the management of the poisoned patient for the following reasons:

1. Most experimental animal studies fail to demonstrate that orogastric lavage is of significant benefit even when undertaken within 60 minutes of toxin dosing, and most poisoned patients arrive at a treatment facility more than 60 minutes after overdose (an average of 3.3 hours for adults in one large series) (2).

2. Data from volunteer studies are difficult to extrapolate to poisoned patients because the amounts ingested in poisoned patients may influence drug dissolution and absorption. Radiotracer studies in volunteers have shown that gastric emptying techniques recover less than approximately 50% of an oral marker, even when used within 1 hour of ingestion (22,23). Orogastric lavage performed 60 minutes after administration of 1.5-g aspirin as twenty 75-mg tablets to twelve volunteers did not produce a clinically important reduction in the absorption of aspirin as judged by salicylate recovery in the urine (24). An endoscopic study performed in 17 poisoned patients demonstrated that after lavage, most patients (88%) still had residual tablet or food debris in the stomach; 12 of 17 patients had tablet debris (25). Newer drug formulations are often too big to fit up orogastric lavage tubes.

3. Orogastric lavage may also cause gastric contents to be propelled into the small bowel, thereby potentially increasing the amount of drug available for absorption or allowing for continued absorption of drug after lavage is completed (26). In addition, drug concretions may be found in the stomach even after orogastric lavage.

4. Complications of lavage may outweigh any benefits. Allan evaluated the value of orogastric lavage in 68 patients poisoned with barbiturates (27). In most cases only small quantities of ingested barbiturates were removed. In the 53 patients who were unconscious on admission, nine developed laryngospasm during intubation attempts (for airway protection during lavage) and five had evidence of gastric aspiration. Allan concluded that routine lavage of unconscious patients should be regarded as potentially dangerous in all cases and of no value in most. Currently, the risk of laryngospasm should be minimal with the widespread use of neuromuscular blockers for intubation of severely poisoned patients.

5. The time required to implement gastric emptying necessarily delays activated charcoal administration. In a prospective, randomized controlled trial involving 876 patients over the age of 13 with an ingested overdose within the previous 12 hours, Pond and coworkers compared orogastric lavage followed by activated charcoal and sorbitol with activated charcoal and sorbitol without orogastric lavage (20). The group of patients who underwent orogastric lavage received their activated charcoal a mean of 36 minutes later than the group of patients who did not receive orogastric lavage.

6. Several large randomized trials comparing gastric evacuation plus activated charcoal with activated charcoal alone report no significant difference in outcome (including the study by Pond and colleagues). Merigan and associates prospectively evaluated the efficacy of gastric emptying in symptomatic patients (19). One group of patients received activated charcoal alone whereas two other study groups had their stomachs evacuated by either orogastric lavage or syrup of ipecac-induced emesis followed by activated charcoal. Gastric emptying did not shorten emergency room length of stay, mean duration of intubation, or mean length of stay in the ICU. The use of orogastric lavage and syrup of ipecac were associated with a significantly higher incidence of aspiration pneumonia and need for ICU admission. However, these studies were poorly designed with strong biases against gastric emptying (e.g., exclusion of toxins known to be poorly adsorbed to activated charcoal, and sustained-release drug formulations).

Since experimental studies demonstrate that the amount of marker removed by orogastric lavage diminishes with time and clinical studies have not confirmed the benefit of orogastric lavage even when it was performed within 60 minutes after poison ingestion, orogastric lavage should no longer be routinely employed for the management of the poisoned patient. However, since anecdotal reports exist in which orogastric lavage was associated with impressive drug recovery, orogastric lavage is still used selectively. Orogastric lavage should only be considered if the patient has ingested a potentially life-threatening amount of a poison and the procedure can be undertaken when it is likely that a clinically significant amount of toxin remains within the stomach. With these guidelines the majority of poisoned patients will not be subjected to the risks of gastric evacuation.

Orogastric lavage is usually safe but can cause significant morbidity. Complications are very rare and most are preventable by appropriate patient selection and the use of appropriate techniques. In addition to the usual complications of orogastric tube placement, orogastric lavage can cause nasal, oral, and pharyngeal injury and/or pyriform sinus, esophageal, or gastric perforation and aspiration. Attempts at gastric emptying may also propel ingested material beyond the pylorus where many drugs are more readily absorbed. In the combative patient who resists attempts at lavage, alternatives should be considered. Almost always the risks of sedation, intubation, and paralysis to allow lavage safely far outweigh the benefits of gastric emptying.

Contraindications to orogastric lavage include any situation when it is unnecessary or ineffective or potentially dangerous (e.g., following ingestion of alkaline caustics, which cause consequential local injury but carry little risk from systemic absorption). Patients who are unresponsive or with depressed airway reflexes should be intubated prior to placement of an orogastric lavage tube. The patient should be placed in the left lateral decubitus/head down (20 degrees) position to minimize transpyloric passage of toxin. The length of tube to be inserted should be measured and marked before insertion. A large bore 36 to 40 F- (adults) or 24 to 28 F-gauge (children) tube should be used. Once appropriate positioning is confirmed by air insufflation or fluid aspiration, residual gastric contents are evacuated by aspiration. Lavage is then carried out by using small aliquots of liquid. In the adult, 200 to 300 mL of preferably warm (38°C) fluid, such as normal saline or tap water are repeatedly instilled and evacuated until the recovered lavage fluid is clear of particulate matter. In a child, a total volume of 10 mL per kg body weight of warm saline should be given in 50 to 100 mL aliquots. Tap water should be avoided in young children because of the risk of inducing hyponatremia. Warming the fluid avoids the risk of hypothermia in the very young and very old and those receiving large volumes of lavage fluid. Small volumes are used to minimize the risk of enhancing toxin entry into the small intestine. Studies suggest that continuing lavage for an extra 1,000 mL after the effluent is clear may evacuate as much as 40% additional toxin, with approximately 90% of the total recoverable toxin being found in the first 5 L (22,28). Upon completion of lavage, appropriate doses of activated charcoal and a cathartic should be instilled through the tube, and the tube should be either replaced with an appropriately sized nasogastric tube or removed as clinically indicated.

Endoscopic or surgical removal of ingested toxin is rarely of practical value. Endoscopic removal might be appropriate for severe or life-threatening ingestions of toxins that remain in the stomach after other less invasive means of removal have been unsuccessful; however, clinical data regarding the benefits of this technique are unavailable. Gastric endoscopy with the use of baskets or snares can be used to remove potentially toxic foreign bodies (e.g., button batteries that fail to pass beyond the pylorus), gastric pill bezoars, or drug concretions (29–31), but drug masses due to iron, enteric aspirin, meprobamate, and others, despite their solid appearance on radiographs, cannot be effectively grasped through an endoscope. Endoscopy should not be used for the removal of drug packets in body packers and body stuffers since the packets may rupture during attempted removal (32,33).

A few indications exist for surgical gastrointestinal decontamination. Immediate surgery is indicated if patients develop signs of significant toxicity due to presumed packet rupture, following the ingestion of packets containing cocaine (32). Ruptured packets

of cocaine can also produce bowel ischemia requiring surgical intervention (34). When the ruptured packets contain a nonlethal drug (e.g., marijuana) or a drug for which an effective antidote is available (i.e., naloxone for opioids), medical management is sufficient. Surgical intervention is also necessary when packets produce mechanical bowel obstruction. Surgery (i.e., gastrotomy, enterotomy) should also be considered in the same situations as endoscopy, when the latter is unsuccessful or impossible due to the location of the toxin or foreign body (35,36).

Adsorption of Unabsorbed Toxin

Activated charcoal, a fine, black, odorless, and tasteless powder has long been recognized to be an effective adsorbent of many substances. Activated charcoal can prevent the absorption of ingested toxins by binding them within the gut lumen, and since activated charcoal is neither absorbed or metabolized, the toxin bound to activated charcoal is normally eliminated with stool.

Activated charcoal is produced in a two-step process: (a) controlled pyrolysis of various carbonaceous materials such as coconut shells, peat, coal, wood pulp, or petroleum, producing charcoal followed by; (b) activation, by heating the charcoal at temperatures of 600 to 900°C in the presence of various activating (oxidizing) agents such as steam or carbon dioxide. Activation increases the charcoal's adsorptive capacity through the formation of an internal network of pores with a huge surface area and small particle size. The adsorptive capacity of the resultant product depends on both its external pore size and its internal surface area with most commercially available forms having surface areas of 1,000 to 2,000 M^2/g. *In vitro* experiments have demonstrated several factors that can influence adsorption by activated charcoal including pore size of activated charcoal, particle size of activated charcoal, surface area of activated charcoal, temperature, solubility of the poison, ionization state of the poison, pH, and the presence of food or other gastric contents. In the clinical setting, most of these factors are uncontrolled; therefore, the actual amount of drug that will be adsorbed to a given dose of activated charcoal will be unpredictable.

Activated charcoal has been studied with hundreds of substances *in vitro*, in animals, in volunteers, and in clinical overdose. However, there are no satisfactorily designed, controlled clinical studies assessing benefit from single-dose activated charcoal. Volunteer studies of single-dose activated charcoal have demonstrated that when administered within 30 minutes of drug ingestion, drug bioavailability was significantly reduced compared to activated charcoal administration 60 minutes after ingestion (37).

There are two distinct potential benefits for the use of activated charcoal in the poisoned patient: (a) preventing the absorption of toxic agents from the gastrointestinal tract and (b) enhancing the elimination of agents already absorbed. Activated charcoal is most likely to be efficacious if a toxin has been ingested that will adsorb to it, and a significant amount of the toxin remains in the gastrointestinal tract at the time of activated charcoal administration. The sooner activated charcoal is administered after ingestion, the more efficacious the intervention. Rapid instillation is most important for toxins that are rapidly absorbed from the gastrointestinal tract.

There is no single correct dose of activated charcoal in poisoned patients. Available data imply a dose-response relationship that favors larger doses. *In vitro* studies have demonstrated that the ideal activated charcoal-to-toxin ratio varies widely, but a ratio of 10:1 is a representative optimal value for many typical drugs. The maximum amount of activated charcoal that can be given safely is unknown. The type and amount of agent ingested (if known) along with the age and size of the patient should influence the dose selected. The optimal activated charcoal dose theoretically would be the minimum dose that would completely adsorb the ingested toxic agent and maximize enhanced elimination, but this optimal dose cannot be known in individual patients where factors such as the physical properties of the drug formulation ingested, gastric volume, food content, and pH will all influence activated charcoal activity. The United States Pharmacopeia (USP DI, 1997) recommends the following oral dose regimen: children up to 1 year of age, 1 g per kg; children 1 to 12 years of age, 25 to 50 g; adolescents and adults, 25 to 100 g. In adults, a dose of 1 to 2 g per kg administered enterally, mixed in a relatively unpalatable slurry with water or a cathartic (such as 70% sorbitol), is commonly recommended.

Achieving a high activated charcoal-to-toxin ratio is easily accomplished for drugs dispensed in small formulation such as digoxin (0.25 mg) but impossible for drugs such as sustained-release theophylline (200 to 400 mg). Maximal initial dosing (e.g., 1.5 to 2 g per kg) should be used for massive potentially life-threatening ingestions of substances that are well adsorbed to activated charcoal (e.g., aspirin, theophylline, sustained-release verapamil).

Although activated charcoal is efficacious in binding most inorganic and organic materials, it is relatively ineffective in adsorbing low-molecular-weight substances such as heavy metals, caustics, lithium, iron, cyanide, and the alcohols. Typical ingestions of ethanol, iron, and lithium involve several grams of drug and given their minimal adsorption to activated charcoal, it is not surprising that activated charcoal is completely ineffective here. However, regardless of the ingestion history, administration of activated charcoal may be appropriate due to the frequency of inaccurate history regarding the nature of the ingestant and unrecognized coingestion of agents that are well adsorbed.

Activated charcoal is generally safe and there are few contraindications to its use. Patients who have ingested caustics and who require endoscopic evaluation should not receive activated charcoal as the activated charcoal does not adsorb most caustics, and the endoscopist's view will be obscured. It is also contraindicated in patients who have ingested hydrocarbons or other agents that are not well adsorbed to activated charcoal and have a high aspiration potential. Relative contraindications to activated charcoal administration include conditions such as paralytic ileus and bowel obstruction. Patients should have an intact or protected airway prior to the administration of the activated charcoal.

Minor adverse reactions to activated charcoal use include nausea, vomiting, and constipation. Cases of bowel obstruction requiring surgical intervention and pseudoobstruction have been described following multidose activated charcoal use (38). Given the inherent constipating nature of activated charcoal, a single cathartic dose is usually given with the initial dose of activated charcoal. If subsequent doses of activated charcoal are given, the cathartic should be eliminated to avoid complications of cathartic use. Aspiration is the most serious complication and this can lead to death. When clinically significant aspiration has occurred it usually was a result of a failure to secure the airway prior to activated charcoal use, or direct instillation of activated charcoal into the trachea after improper enteral tube placement (39). Unintentional spillage of activated charcoal into the eyes can cause transient corneal abrasions (37).

Single-dose activated charcoal should not be administered routinely in the management of the poisoned patient. It should be considered if a patient has recently ingested a potentially toxic amount of a poison (known to be adsorbed to activated charcoal). There are insufficient data to support or exclude its use after 1 hour of ingestion (37). There is no evidence that the administration of activated charcoal improves clinical outcome.

Additionally, certain poisonings exhibit favorable pharmacokinetics for potential benefit from repeated doses of activated charcoal. Multidose activated charcoal might be indicated in several circumstances in which a significant amount of the agent is likely to remain within the gastrointestinal tract: (a) massive drug overdoses where a standard initial dose of activated charcoal is unlikely to achieve a 10:1 activated charcoal-to-drug ratio; (b) drug bezoars or concretions; (c) enteric-coated or sustained-release formulations; and (d) drugs that slow gastrointestinal motility. All of these circumstances favor the persistence of undissociated luminal toxin and ongoing toxin absorption from the small intestine. Multidose activated charcoal also might be useful when drug reabsorption can be prevented (enterohepatic circulation of active drug, active metabolites, or conjugated drug hydrolyzed by gut bacteria to active drug). Multidose activated charcoal is much more controversial as a method to enhance elimination of toxic substances that are already absorbed into the body. It should be most useful when free drug in the plasma is substantial enough to permit an enteroenteric effect. Drugs with a small volume of distribution, low or saturable plasma protein binding, and a long elimination phase are theoretically most accessible.

Drugs can diffuse from the circulation into the gut lumen by passive diffusion provided that the concentration of the drug within the gut lumen is lower than that in the blood. The amount of drug that will diffuse depends upon the concentration gradient, intestinal surface area, permeability, and splanchnic blood flow. The activated charcoal adsorbs the drug as it continuously diffuses into the gut lumen creating an "infinite sink," and this maintains the concentration gradient. This process has been called "gastrointestinal dialysis" (40). To enhance elimination of a given drug, the substance must either undergo enterohepatic recirculation or, more often, be present to a significant extent in circulating blood and be well adsorbed to activated charcoal. For some substances such as theophylline, carbamazepine, dapsone, phenobarbital, and quinine, there is evidence from experimental and clinical studies that multidose activated charcoal substantially limits absorption and enhances elimination and its use should be considered if a patient has ingested a life-threatening amount of the drug (39). Minimal clinical data are available for other drugs (e.g., digoxin, phenytoin, disopyramide) in which enhanced elimination has been demonstrated in volunteer studies, and because of the paucity of data, the role for multidose activated charcoal is uncertain. However, despite documented pharmacokinetic effects, multidose activated charcoal has not been demonstrated to improve clinical outcome, and for most toxins possibly affected by this treatment, better alternative treatments are available or patients do well with supportive care alone.

Clinical experience suggests that, after an initial dose of 50 to 100 g given to an adult, activated charcoal may be administered hourly, every 2 hours, or every 4 hours at a dose equivalent to 12.5 g per hour (39). In some cases, continuous nasogastric administration of activated charcoal can be employed, especially when vomiting is a problem. Activated charcoal should be continued until the patient's condition and laboratory parameters including plasma drug concentrations are improving.

Enhanced Fecal Elimination

Cathartics were often given to poisoned patients in the belief that these agents will reduce the absorption of the poison by decreasing the amount of time the poison or poison-activated charcoal complex remains within the gut. Cathartics are now used much less often. Data are limited regarding the mechanism of action of cathartics. Postulated mechanisms include a direct effect of the cathartic in the lumen of the intestines which either promotes osmotic retention of fluid or extracts water from the intestinal circulation. Cathartics are relatively nonabsorbable and create a hyperosmolar state within the intestinal lumen. Water is drawn into the bowel. The resulting increase in intraluminal contents activates gastrointestinal motility reflexes which enhance the expulsion of the intraluminal contents. A decrease in gastrointestinal transit time theoretically minimizes systemic toxin absorption, and augments enteral toxin elimination from the body. Cathartics may also counteract the constipating effects of activated charcoal.

Although cathartics are still used for the treatment of the poisoned patient, their efficacy remains unproved. Clinical benefit has not been demonstrated from the use of cathartics alone and there are some data suggesting that their use could be deleterious secondary to increased drug dissolution. In a simulated theophylline overdose model, the administration of theophylline with a cathartic resulted in both a higher maximal serum concentration, and a shorter time to maximal serum concentration compared with the administration of theophylline alone (41). When combined with activated charcoal, occasional benefit in terms of decreased drug levels has been demonstrated, but clinical benefit has never been demonstrated and cathartics may reduce the efficacy of activated charcoal (42).

Several animal studies have evaluated the effects of cathartics on bioavailability, peak drug concentrations, and survival but the clinical relevance of these studies is limited as all of these studies used doses of cathartics that exceeded therapeutic recommendations and none used intervals between the ingestion and administration of cathartics that are common in the treatment of poisoned patients (42). The same limitations apply to animal studies in which cathartics were given simultaneously with activated charcoal. In most of these studies, the addition of cathartics to activated charcoal results in minimal or no decrease in toxin absorption compared with activated charcoal alone (41,43).

Several volunteer studies demonstrated that cathartics alone did not enhance drug elimination (42). When combined with

activated charcoal, the use of cathartics reduces the transit time of stool through the gut but this decrease in transit time has not been associated with significantly reduced drug absorption (42).

Two general types of osmotic cathartics are used in poisoned patients: (a) saccharide cathartics (70% sorbitol); and (b) saline cathartics (magnesium citrate, magnesium sulfate, sodium sulfate). Some studies have suggested that sorbitol is the more effective cathartic and its use predominates in the United States.

Cathartic dosage is largely empiric. An initial dose of sorbitol of 1 g per kg in adults is reasonable. A 100 mL dose of 70% sorbitol contains 89.95 g of sorbitol. Typical recommended dosage for 6% magnesium citrate is 4 mL per kg up to a maximum of 300 mL.

When used in appropriate dosage and when contraindications to their use are excluded, there is no evidence that a single dose of cathartic is harmful. Therapeutic doses can produce nausea, vomiting, and abdominal cramping. More serious adverse reactions including dehydration, hypotension, hypermagnesemia, and hypernatremia may occur in patients receiving multiple doses or inadvertent overdosage of saline cathartics. Dehydration secondary to water loss in the stool can result from any of the cathartics.

Contraindications to cathartic use include paralytic ileus, intestinal obstruction, bowel perforation, recent bowel surgery, hypovolemia, significant electrolyte imbalance, or ingestion of a corrosive. There is no need to use it in patients with diarrhea. Magnesium-containing cathartics should not be used in patients with renal insufficiency.

The 1997 position statement published by the American Academy of Clinical Toxicology/European Association of Poisons Centres and Clinical Toxicologists states: "The administration of a cathartic alone has no role in the management of the poisoned patient and is not recommended as a method of gut decontamination. Experimental data are conflicting regarding the use of cathartics in combination with activated charcoal. No clinical studies have been published to investigate the ability of a cathartic, with or without activated charcoal, to reduce the bioavailability of drugs, or to improve the outcome of poisoned patients. Based on available data, the routine use of a cathartic in combination with activated charcoal is not endorsed. If a cathartic is used, it should be limited to a single dose in order to minimize adverse effects" (42).

Because repeated dosage of cathartics risks creation of serious fluid and electrolyte disturbances, other methods of gastrointestinal decontamination have recently been considered. Whole-bowel irrigation is a variant of catharsis in which large quantities of isosmotic polyethylene glycol electrolyte solutions (PEG-ES) such as Colyte or Golytely are administered enterally until liquid stool is produced with the physical appearance of the infusate. The duration of treatment however can be extended if there is corroborative evidence (e.g., radiographs) of continued presence of drug in the gastrointestinal tract. These solutions, originally introduced for preoperative bowel preparation, are nonabsorbable, and because they are isotonic, significant changes in water and electrolyte balance do not occur. Rather than inducing diarrhea by drawing water into the stool or by directly stimulating gut motility, whole-bowel irrigation washes bowel contents through the gastrointestinal tract mechanically by the use of large volumes of fluid. Whole-bowel irrigation has the potential to reduce drug absorption by physically expelling intraluminal contents.

Animal and volunteer studies have demonstrated that whole-bowel irrigation reduces absorption of some ingested drugs (e.g., lithium, enteric-coated salicylates) (44). Case reports have provided visually impressive radiographic and bedside evidence of gastrointestinal passage of iron, arsenic, lead, and sustained-release calcium channel blockers, but without control groups, the clinical benefits of the procedure are uncertain (44). No controlled clinical studies using whole-bowel irrigation have been performed.

Concerns exist regarding the potential of PEG-ES to enhance drug dissolution and also for its potential to bind to activated charcoal and thereby limit its adsorptive capacity. *In vitro* studies have demonstrated that the binding of salicylates, theophylline, and cocaine to activated charcoal is decreased in the presence of PEG-ES (44). The results of these studies suggest that activated charcoal should not be mixed with PEG-ES. Whether the magnitude of benefit from whole-bowel irrigation outweighs the risk from slightly decreased activated charcoal absorption is uncertain. Whole-bowel irrigation will likely have a role in life-threatening overdoses of drugs that are minimally adsorbed to activated charcoal (e.g., iron, lithium, lead); or with ingested foreign bodies (e.g., body packers, miniature disc batteries, drug bezoars) when the foreign bodies cannot be removed safely or effectively by other methods. In cases where there has been a massive ingestion of sustained release drugs such as verapamil and theophylline, multidose activated charcoal is essential, and the detrimental effects of PEG-ES on activated charcoal is an important clinical consideration when a decision regarding use of PEG-ES is being made. Whole-bowel irrigation should not be substituted or added to activated charcoal in overdoses for which activated charcoal has proven efficacy.

Whole-bowel irrigation is usually performed through a nasogastric tube. Once gastric placement of the tube is confirmed, the proximal end of the tube is attached to an elevated reservoir bag filled with PEG-ES. The patient should be seated or the head of the bed should be elevated to at least 45 degrees. The PEG-ES should be given at a rate of 500 mL per hour for children 9 months to 6 years; 1,000 mL per hour for children 6 to 12 years; and 1,500 to 2,000 mL per hour for adolescents and adults. A commode is used to collect the effluent. Whole-bowel irrigation is contraindicated in patients with ileus, bowel obstruction, bowel perforation, intractable vomiting, hemodynamic instability, or patients with an unprotected and compromised airway. Side effects of PEG-ES when used for bowel preparation include nausea, vomiting, abdominal cramps, and bloating. Little clinical data are available regarding side effects in poisoned patients, however there were no complications attributed to whole-bowel irrigation in the published case reports in this patient population. We usually add a promotility, antiemetic like metoclopramide to decrease side effects and improve tolerance of whole-bowel irrigation.

At the present time, there is no established indication for the use of whole-bowel irrigation. Whole-bowel irrigation can reduce absorption and augment removal of toxic agents in the gastrointestinal tract although the clinical benefit that results is unproven. It should not be used routinely in the management of the poisoned patient. Based on volunteer studies it may be considered for potentially toxic ingestions of sustained-release or enteric-coated drugs. It is also an option for potentially toxic ingestions of iron, lead, zinc, lithium, and packets of illicit drugs.

Enhanced Renal Elimination

Small, water-soluble toxins with a low volume of distribution, a low endogenous clearance rate, and relatively high-plasma concentrations of their free, uncharged form have the potential for augmented elimination using "ion-trapping" combined with forced diuresis or the application of an extracorporeal technique such as hemodialysis (6). Agents with these characteristics should be freely filtered at the glomerulus, resulting in ultrafiltrate toxin levels comparable to those in plasma. Subsequent conversion of the neutral toxin into its ionized form by pH manipulation "traps" the toxin in the urine, preventing passive toxin reabsorption by the renal tubules. Forced diuresis using large quantities of isotonic crystalloids plus a loop diuretic should augment toxin elimination in the urine by bulk flow and generally acts synergistically with manipulation of the urinary pH. Complications of this therapy primarily involve iatrogenic changes in the patient's intravascular volume and systemic acid-base status. Although alkalinization with bicarbonate for weak acids (barbiturates, chlorpropamide, salicylates) is still used (particularly for salicylates), acidification with ammonium chloride for weak bases (amphetamines, phencyclidine) is no longer used and "ion-trapping" is currently an infrequently used modality for treatment of intoxicated patients.

Certain toxins can be removed through an extracorporeal technique such as hemodialysis, hemoperfusion, continuous arteriovenous hemofiltration (CAVH), continuous arteriovenous hemofiltration with dialysis (CAVHD), and continuous venovenous hemofiltration with dialysis (CVVHD). Pharmacokinetic factors that favor the use of hemodialysis using a standard semipermeable membrane include toxins with: (a) molecular weight less than 500 daltons; (b) high water solubility; and (c) low plasma protein binding. Hemoperfusion with a charcoal-impregnated semipermeable membrane would be favored for toxins that bind effectively to charcoal. One of the hemofiltration techniques (usually performed continuously) would be favored for toxins with molecular weight between 10,000 to 40,000 daltons that have a slow redistribution from a second compartment to the plasma.

No randomized, controlled, clinical trials have been performed to document the clinical efficacy of extracorporeal toxin removal. Beneficial effects are expected theoretically for certain toxins and on the basis of case reports for others. These invasive techniques should be considered for intoxications with substances with appropriate pharmacokinetic characteristics, when the patient remains unstable despite maximal supportive care and decontamination, when the endogenous route of toxin elimination is impaired, or when the patient is at high risk for serious morbidity or mortality. Complications of these techniques include infection, bleeding, and hypotension. Charcoal hemoperfusion can also induce thrombocytopenia, leukopenia, hypocalcemia, and rarely, charcoal embolism.

Agents amenable to removal by hemodialysis include ethylene glycol, methanol, lithium, salicylate, and theophylline (if charcoal hemoperfusion is not available). Ethanol and isopropanol can also be removed by hemodialysis but this is rarely necessary.

TABLE 6. THERAPY PROVIDED IN HUMAN EXPOSURE CASES

Therapy	%
Decontamination	
Dilution/irrigation	51.0
Activated charcoal, single dose	6.2
Cathartic	3.1
Gastric lavage	1.7
Ipecac syrup	1.0
Activated charcoal, multidose	0.4
Whole bowel irrigation	0.1
Measures to enhance elimination	
Alkalinization	0.28
Extracorporeal technique	0.05

Data adapted from Litovitz TL, Klein-Schwartz W, White S, et al. 1999 Annual Report of the American Association of Poison Control Centers Toxic Exposure Surveillance System. *Am J Emerg Med* 2000;18:517–574.

Hemoperfusion can remove drugs that are more highly protein bound and may be useful for theophylline, and if initiated very early for *Amanita phalloides* toxin (mushroom) and paraquat. The various hemofiltration techniques (CAVH, CAVHD, CVVHD) can remove lithium and procainamide. The invasiveness, cost, equipment demands, and personnel required to implement urgent dialysis therapy necessarily limit its clinical application. In the 1999 American Association of Poison Control Centers summary, extracorporeal techniques were used in only 0.05% of the reported patients (1). Table 6 summarizes the 1999 data reported to poison control centers regarding therapy provided in human exposure cases.

Antidotes

Table 7 highlights the antidotes most commonly administered early in the care of poisoned adults. It is meant to serve as a useful

TABLE 7. ANTIDOTES USED EARLY IN THE TREATMENT OF A PATIENT WITH AN OVERDOSE

Opiates	Naloxone	Starting dose 0.1 mg. Increase to 0.4 mg then 2 mg and finally 10 mg. If respiratory depression recurs, start continuous infusion at a dose per h = 2/3 of the total naloxone dose that resulted in reversal.
Methanol, ethylene glycol	Ethanol	Loading dose = 0.8 g/kg of a 10% solution = 8 mL/kg, administered i.v. over 20 to 60 min as tolerated. Maintenance dose = 0.15 mL/kg/h. Double maintenance dose during dialysis. Titrate to a blood ethanol level of at least 22 mmol/L (100 mg/dL).
	4-Methylpyrazole (fomepizole)	Loading dose 15 mg/kg i.v. over 30 min, followed in 12 h by 10 mg/kg every 12 h for 4 doses, and then increased to 15 mg/kg every 12 h as long as necessary. Give additional dose if patient is dialyzed.
Anticholinergic agents	Physostigmine	1–2 mg i.v. over 5 min. Use only for severe delirium. May be useful to treat seizures or tachyarrhythmias, but strong clinical evidence is lacking and substantial risks exist.
Organophosphate or carbamate insecticides	Atropine	Test dose 2 mg i.v. Repeat in larger increments until drying of pulmonary secretions occurs.
Isoniazid	Pyridoxine (vitamin B$_6$)	Give 1 g of pyridoxine for each g of isoniazid ingested, to a maximum of 5 g when the history is uncertain. For a patient who is actively seizing, give by slow i.v. infusion at 0.5 g/min until the seizures stop or the maximum dose is reached. Once the seizures stop, the remainder of the dose should be infused over 4 to 6 h. An overdose of pyridoxine may cause neuropathy.
Beta-blockers	Glucagon	Initial i.v. bolus of 50 μg/kg infused ovr 1 min. Higher doses may be necessary if the initial dose is ineffective, and up to 10 mg may be tried in an adult. Titrate to response (normalization of vital signs). Maintenance dose of 2 to 5 mg/h may be used.
Cyclic antidepressants	Bicarbonate	1 to 2 mEq/kg i.v. bolus over 1 to 2 min, for substantial cardiac conduction delay or ventricular arrhythmias. Titrate to response and pH. Try to achieve a blood pH of 7.50 to 7.55. Continuous infusion usually required after the i.v. bolus.
Digitalis glycosides	Digoxin-specific Fab antibodies	Equimolar to ingestion: the number of mg of digoxin ingested ÷ 0.6 = required number of vials. If amount ingested is unknown and the patient has life-threatening arrhythmias, give 10–20 vials i.v. Each vial contains 38 mg of digoxin-specific antibody fragments. If serum digoxin concentration is known, the number of vials to administer = (concentration [in ng/mL] × 5.6 × weight in kg) ÷ 600. Give as an i.v. bolus in unstable clinical situations. Otherwise administer over 30 min.
Benzodiazepines	Flumazenil	0.2 mg i.v. over 30 s. If no response after 30 s, give 0.3 mg over 30 s. If no response after 30 sec, give 0.5 mg over 30 sec at 1-min intervals up to a total dose of 3 mg. Risk of precipitating acute withdrawal limited when total dose < 1 mg. Relative contraindications: serious overdose from coingestion of cyclic antidepressants or benzodiazepine use for control of seizures.
Acetaminophen	N-acetylcysteine	Most effective if given within 8 h of ingestion. Give if history suggests an ingestion of 150 mg/kg close to 8 h earlier or if plasma acetaminophen level falls on or above the nomogram (acute overdose). 140 mg/kg oral loading dose, then 70 mg/kg every 4 h for an additional 17 doses. Dilute to a 5% solution with a soft drink.
Calcium channel blockers, fluorides	Calcium	1 g calcium chloride, or 3 g calcium gluconate given over 10 min by i.v. infusion with continuous cardiac monitoring. Faster infusion rate for patients in extremis. Dose may be repeated every 10 to 20 min for 3 to 4 additional doses.

Adapted from data from Howland MA. Antidotes in depth. In: Goldfrank LR, et al., eds. *Goldfrank's toxicologic emergencies*, 6th ed. Stamford, CT: Appelton & Lange, 1998, with permission.

framework for integration with supportive care and decontamination techniques in the majority of poisonings. Further details on certain antidotes have been discussed in the text. Readers are referred to their regional poison control center or reference texts for information on less commonly used antidotes (see "Bibliography" at the end of this chapter).

EVALUATION AND MANAGEMENT OF SPECIFIC INTOXICATIONS

Digoxin

Digoxin is used to slow the ventricular rate in patients with atrial fibrillation, atrial flutter, and supraventricular tachycardia. It is also used to increase ventricular contractility in patients with congestive heart failure. There are many other naturally occurring cardiac glycosides besides digoxin, and their toxicities are similar. With oral ingestion, digoxin is approximately 75% bioavailable. Between 60% and 80% of the drug is renally eliminated, with the remainder being eliminated by the liver. Therapeutic serum levels are 0.8 to 2.0 ng per mL. Digoxin inhibits the cardiac Na^+/K^+ adenosine triphosphatase (ATPase) exchange pump. This increases intracellular sodium and extracellular potassium. The increased intracellular sodium decreases calcium excretion and produces increased intracellular calcium concentration which enhances cardiac contractility and increases automaticity, which predisposes toward the development of tachydysrhythmias. Digoxin also increases vagal tone, decreases atrioventricular node conduction velocity, and increases atrioventricular node refractoriness.

Early signs of toxicity are nonspecific and include nausea, vomiting, and malaise. CNS symptoms include headaches, visual disturbances (halos, blurring, color aberrations), confusion, delirium, and rarely seizures. Hyperkalemia may occur secondary to blockade of Na^+/K^+ ATPase. The potassium level is an accurate predictor of outcome in adult patients with acute digoxin overdose. Cardiac effects may include sinus bradycardia, atrioventricular block, paroxysmal atrial tachycardia with block, intraventricular conduction delays, and ventricular dysrhythmias. Digoxin toxicity should be suspected in patients with unexplained bradycardia, nonspecific gastrointestinal or neurologic complaints, evidence of "digoxin effect" on ECG, or hyperkalemia of unclear etiology. It is important to note that serum digoxin levels are only interpretable after the end of redistribution from the central compartment (i.e., more than 4 to 6 hours after ingestion). Therefore, a digoxin level taken earlier after ingestion only confirms the presence of the drug.

Death from massive overdose in adults results from ventricular dysrhythmias (65% of deaths), conduction impairment or asystole (25% of deaths), or pump failure secondary to negative inotropic effects, increased sympathetic tone-induced vasoconstriction, and bradycardia (10% of deaths). Fatal mesenteric infarction may also occur, particularly in older adults (45).

Supportive treatment should include the use of activated charcoal. Bradydysrhythmias can be treated with atropine and with electric pacing, although caution against internal pacing is advised as a retrospective study found increased mortality in patients treated with internal pacing. (46) Ventricular tachydysrhythmias

should be treated with lidocaine, with phenytoin as an alternate agent. Potassium or magnesium replacement may be effective if the respective serum levels are low. In the setting of digoxin toxicity, cardioversion may precipitate refractory ventricular tachycardia, ventricular fibrillation, or asystole. When necessary, one should start with very low-energy levels (10 to 25 J).

Hyperkalemia when present is usually not clinically significant other than as a marker for digoxin intoxication. A level of greater than 5 mEq per L in an acute overdose is an absolute indication for Digibind. Calcium is contraindicated in digoxin toxicity except after the use of Digibind (see below). Hypokalemia predisposes patients on digoxin to toxicity and should be corrected if present.

Digoxin-Specific Antibody Fragments (Digibind) provides definitive treatment for severe digoxin toxicity (47). These antibody fragments are derived from sheep immunized with a digoxin-albumin conjugate. The digoxin-specific antibodies are cleaved to smaller and less immunogenic Fab fragments. Digibind binds digoxin in the serum creating a concentration gradient that helps dissociate digoxin from the heart. The antibody-digoxin complex is then renally eliminated. Indications for Digibind include: (a) ventricular dysrhythmias and symptomatic bradydysrhythmias not responsive to atropine; (b) serum potassium level greater than 5 mEq per L in an acute ingestion in an otherwise healthy patient; (c) serum digoxin level of 10 to 15 ng per mL in an acute ingestion; and (d) a digoxin ingestion of greater than 10 mg (4 mg in a child). Digibind may be effective even during cardiac arrest of short duration. A simplified formula for Digibind dosing is:

$$dose \ (vials) = (digoxin \ level \ in \ ng/mL) \times (wt \ in \ kg)/100$$

For patients with suspected digoxin overdose and an unknown digoxin level, overdosing with Digibind is preferable to underdosing. An empiric dosing regimen would be 10 to 20 vials for an acute overdose in adults or children, 5 vials for a chronic overdose in adults, and 2 vials for a chronic overdose in children.

The full dose of Digibind may be given intravenously over 30 minutes or as a bolus if cardiac arrest is imminent. Allergic reactions to Digibind treatment are extremely rare. Morbidity may result from acute withdrawal of digoxin effect (e.g., exacerbation of congestive heart failure, increased ventricular response in patients with atrial fibrillation). Digoxin levels are meaningless following Digibind therapy as both free and bound digoxin are measured by most laboratories.

Lithium

Lithium is an alkali metal approved for oral use in the treatment of bipolar affective disorders. It is also occasionally used to treat other psychiatric disorders and as prophylaxis for cluster headaches. The typical adult dose is 900 to 1,200 mg per day. The mechanisms of action for lithium's antimanic effects are undefined; its antidepressive effects may be secondary to increased synthesis and turnover of serotonin. Lithium is rapidly absorbed from the gastrointestinal tract. Peak levels usually occur 2 to 4 hours after ingestion but may be delayed to more than 8 hours with sustained-release products. Lithium is 95% renally cleared, with 80% of the lithium filtered by the kidneys being reabsorbed in the proximal tubule (like sodium) and 20% excreted in the urine unchanged. These percentages are influenced by the sodium avidity of the kidney which is affected by the patient's intravascular volume status. The therapeutic serum concentration for treatment of acute mania is 0.7 to 1.2 mEq per L, while the goal for maintenance therapy is 0.5 to 0.8 mEq per L. Lithium demonstrates a narrow therapeutic-toxic ratio and can induce severe complications if slight changes in dosing or elimination occur.

Acute intoxication is usually intentional. Toxic effects after acute overdose are typically dose-dependent. Chronic intoxication often occurs and is usually precipitated by an intercurrent illness or introduction of a new therapeutic drug. Patients on chronic lithium therapy may also become intoxicated if clinical events occur that either enhance renal resorption of sodium (e.g., dehydration, sodium depletion, or drug interactions), or decrease renal function. Drugs that decrease lithium excretion include diuretics, nonsteroidal antiinflammatory drugs, angiotensin-converting enzyme inhibitors, and metronidazole.

The mechanism of lithium toxicity is poorly understood. Initial evaluation should include attempts to determine if the intoxication is acute, chronic, or acute on chronic. The severity of acute intoxication does not correlate well with the serum level as toxicity does not occur until lithium distributes into cells. The patient with acute intoxication will have higher serum levels with less symptoms compared to the patient with chronic overdose. Acute overdose usually causes nausea, vomiting, and diarrhea, followed by CNS effects, whereas with chronic overdose, CNS effects predominate. CNS toxic effects include apathy, lethargy, tremor, hyperreflexia, slurred speech, ataxia, and confusion, which may develop over hours to days. Severe toxicity can cause seizures, coma, dysrhythmias, cardiovascular collapse, and acute respiratory distress syndrome (ARDS). Permanent neurologic sequelae may occur, including ataxia, cerebellar atrophy, basal ganglia degeneration, and altered mental status (48).

Treatment of lithium overdose should focus on decontamination, rehydration, and initiation of hemodialysis if indicated. Gastric lavage should be performed for adults presenting within 1 hour of a large ingestion or if serious effects are present. Activated charcoal should only be used if a coingestion is suspected as activated charcoal does not bind to lithium. Whole-bowel irrigation should be initiated if it has been more than 2 to 4 hours since the ingestion or if a sustained release preparation has been ingested. Serum electrolytes should be measured. If the patient is not in renal failure, hydration should be initiated with normal saline at twice the estimated maintenance rate as this will increase the renal elimination of lithium. A serum lithium level should be measured and repeated every 2 to 4 hours until levels decline and symptoms improve. Hemodialysis increases lithium clearance and is an effective treatment for acute ingestions where it may prevent further lithium distribution into the CNS. Hemodialysis is recommended for patients with: (a) acute ingestion and lithium levels greater than 4.0 mEq per L even in the absence of symptoms; (b) acute-on-chronic or chronic toxicity when the lithium level is greater than 2.5 mEq per L; (c) elevated lithium levels and neurologic symptoms of moderate to severe toxicity; (d) renal failure (unable to clear lithium); and (e) for patients who are poor candidates for aggressive hydration secondary to underlying medical conditions (49).

Lithium levels often rebound after completion of hemodialysis as intracellular lithium redistributes back into the intravascular compartment. A repeat lithium level should be measured immediately postdialysis and 6 hours later. Hemodialysis should be repeated if either of these levels are elevated and severe symptoms persist.

Salicylates

Salicylates are widely used analgesic, antipyretic, antiinflammatory and anti-platelet agents. They are available in a variety of forms for oral and topical use. Salicylates are often present in mixed pharmaceutical preparations (e.g., Percodan, Fiorinal, Pepto-Bismol). Topical liniments may contain up to 30% methyl salicylate while oil of wintergreen is 100% methyl salicylate. The rate of absorption following oral ingestion is dependent upon the amount and formulation of the drug. Absorption of a liquid such as methyl salicylate begins within minutes while enteric-coated tablets may require hours. Therapeutic doses of acetylsalicylic acid (ASA) are absorbed quickly after ingestion (peak serum levels in 1 to 2 hours), but with large ingestions the rate of absorption is decreased secondary to formation of clumps of ASA tablets (concretions) and a direct inhibitory effect of ASA on gastric emptying (peak levels greater than 4 hours after ingestion). After absorption ASA is hydrolyzed to salicylic acid (salicylate), which is responsible for both its therapeutic and toxic effects. Salicylate is a weak acid ($pKa = 3.5$); almost all salicylate molecules are ionized at physiologic pH which delays distribution of the drug into tissues. Metabolic or respiratory acidosis shifts the equilibrium to formation of nonionized molecules which can penetrate tissues more rapidly. Salicylate is hepatically metabolized but the responsible enzymes are saturable, and therefore with overdose, elimination is prolonged.

Salicylates stimulate the medullary respiratory center, producing an increased rate and depth of breathing and an initial respiratory alkalosis. Respiratory alkalosis rarely occurs in infants or small children who lack the inspiratory reserve volume. Salicylates also uncouple cellular oxidative phosphorylation, resulting in increased oxygen consumption, increased heat production, and fever with simultaneous decreased ATP production. At higher salicylate concentrations, dehydrogenase enzymes in the Krebs cycle are inhibited and this contributes to the development of lactic acidosis. Ketoacidosis may develop secondary to increased fatty acid metabolism. As metabolic acidosis progresses, a viscious cycle is created as more nonionized salicylate is formed, which further worsens the clinical status.

Salicylates affect both central and peripheral glucose homeostasis. Profound decreases in CNS glucose concentrations may occur despite normal serum glucose levels. Therefore the supply of glucose to the brain in salicylate poisoning may be inadequate even though the serum glucose level is normal (50).

The earliest signs and symptoms of acute salicylate toxicity include nausea, vomiting, diaphoresis, and tinnitus or hearing impairment. CNS effects may progress to signs of hyperactivity including hyperventilation, agitation, delirium, hallucinations, and seizures. At higher salicylate levels, lethargy, stupor, and rarely coma may occur. Hyperthermia due to uncoupling of oxidative phosphorylation is a sign of severe toxicity and is often a preterminal finding. Chronic intoxication often presents insidiously with a change in mental status in an older adult patient. Chronic intoxication is often misdiagnosed as dementia, acute psychosis, encephalopathy of undetermined origin, sepsis, respiratory failure, or congestive heart failure. In one study of chronic intoxication, 30% of patients were misdiagnosed for up to 72 hours after admission and the mortality was 25% (51). ARDS often occurs in chronic salicylate intoxication and is secondary to alterations in pulmonary capillary permeability.

The presence of salicylates can be confirmed by performing a ferric chloride test on urine. This test is very sensitive for small amounts of salicylate. If positive, a stat salicylate level should be obtained. The therapeutic salicylate level is 15 to 30 mg per dL. With acute ingestions, signs or symptoms are usually present when the level is greater than 30 mg per dL. Patients with levels greater than 100 mg per dL tend to be critically ill and require hemodialysis. Salicylate levels have limited use in chronic intoxications. Patients may be critically ill with salicylate levels of 50 mg per dL. The patient's acid-base status will also influence the severity of toxicity. For example, if acetazolamide instead of sodium bicarbonate is used to create an alkaline diuresis, a metabolic acidosis may develop which can increase the concentration of freely diffusible nonionized salicylate molecules and thereby enhance CNS penetrance. Severe toxicity in this setting may be seen with low salicylate levels.

The patient's clinical condition and early course should guide management decisions rather than the salicylate level alone. Serum salicylate levels should be followed until at least two consecutive measurements demonstrate a significant decline. Gastrointestinal decontamination through orogastric lavage should be performed in patients who present early following a large ingestion, or if serious clinical effects occur. Sustained release preparations and drug concretions may be too large to be removed through lavage. ASA is effectively adsorbed to activated charcoal; multiple doses may be important for serious ingestions because large ASA ingestions tend to form concretions. Dehydration secondary to hyperthermia, diaphoresis, hyperpnea, and vomiting is often present, requiring careful fluid resuscitation. A glucose-containing fluid should be infused in most cases to help prevent cerebral hypoglycemia. Intubation may be required for airway protection in patients with altered mental status, for treatment of severe hypoxemia, if ARDS has developed, or for an increasing $PaCO_2$, as respiratory acidosis increases the nonionized fraction of salicylate which more easily crosses cell membranes. Alkalinization should be considered for patients with signs and symptoms consistent with salicylate toxicity, or with a salicylate level greater than 40 mg per dL. Alkalinization can be accomplished by an i.v. infusion of a 1 to 2 mEq per kg bolus of sodium bicarbonate followed by an isotonic bicarbonate drip with a goal of a urinary pH of 7.5 to 8.0 and a blood pH of 7.45 to 7.55. Alkalinization of the blood will maintain more salicylate in the ionized form and decrease entry into tissues. Urinary alkalinization increases the amount of ionized salicylate in the ultrafiltrate, decreasing salicylate reabsorption in the proximal tubule. Adding aggressive hydration to alkalinization (forced alkaline diuresis), or aggressive hydration alone (forced diuresis) increases the risk for complications such as ARDS. Hypokalemia, if present, should be corrected as it impairs the ability to alkalinize the urine.

Hemodialysis and charcoal hemoperfusion are both effective methods for the extracorporeal removal of salicylates. Although charcoal hemoperfusion removes more salicylate from serum than hemodialysis, the latter is considered to be the method of choice because in addition to effective salicylate removal, this technique provides the ability to correct severe acid-base disturbances and electrolyte abnormalities. Reasonable indications for initiation of hemodialysis include: (a) clinical deterioration despite adequate supportive care (including urinary alkalinization); (b) manifestations of salicylism in vital end-organs (e.g., mental status alteration, ARDS, coagulopathy, persistent acidemia); (c) renal failure in the presence of toxicity; and (d) serum level of more than 100 mg per dL with acute toxicity or 60 mg per dL (relative indication) with chronic intoxication.

Acetaminophen

Acetaminophen (N-acetyl-p-aminophenol [APAP]) is the most commonly reported pharmaceutical ingestion in both adults and children, with over 100,000 annual calls to United States poison control centers. It is also the leading cause of hospitalization and fatality reported to result from a pharmaceutical agent. APAP is used for relief of mild to moderate pain and for temperature reduction in febrile patients. APAP is available alone, in combination with other analgesics, or as a component of cough and cold preparations. All formulations of APAP are readily absorbed with peak plasma concentrations occurring 30 minutes to 2 hours after a therapeutic dose of 10 to 15 mg per kg. With overdose, peak levels occur within 2 to 4 hours. Over 90% of APAP is metabolized in the liver to inactive and nontoxic sulfate and glucuronide conjugates which are subsequently excreted in the urine. Approximately 5% of APAP is excreted unchanged in the urine and the remainder is metabolized by the P450 mixed-function oxidase system to N-acetyl-para-benzoquinoneimine (NAPQI), a highly reactive and toxic intermediate. With therapeutic APAP dosing, the glutathione supply far exceeds the amount needed to detoxify NAPQI, and the small amount of NAPQI that is formed is reduced by glutathione into a nontoxic mercaptate conjugate which is then eliminated in the urine.

Overdose leads to saturation of the sulfation and glucuronidation pathways with subsequent shunting of more APAP down the P450 pathway with increased production of NAPQI. The increase in NAPQI depletes hepatic glutathione stores and the NAPQI binds nonspecifically to intracellular proteins, particularly those with sulfhydryl groups, producing cell dysfunction and death. Clinical conditions that produce an increase in the metabolism of the CYP2E1 or CYP1A2 subfamilies of the P450 mixed-function oxidase system, decreased glutathione availability, or decreased hepatic capacity for sulfation or glucuronidation, may predispose to hepatic toxicity.

Early recognition and treatment of APAP poisoning is essential for prevention of morbidity and mortality. The clinical presentation occurs in four stages (52). Stage I develops 0.5 to 24 hours after ingestion. Hepatic injury has not yet occurred and patients may be completely asymptomatic or complain of nausea, vomiting, anorexia, and malaise. Laboratory studies are normal. Stage II develops 24 to 48 hours after ingestion and begins when liver function abnormalities become evident. If present, stage I symptoms resolve while right upper quadrant pain and tenderness develop along with elevation of hepatic enzymes and prothrombin time. Stage III is defined as the time of maximal hepatotoxicity and usually occurs between 72 to 96 hours after ingestion. The symptoms and signs are dependent upon the degree of maximal liver injury and, with cases of fulminant hepatic failure, may include hepatic encephalopathy, coma, hypoglycemia, bleeding, anuric renal failure, and cerebral edema. Patients who survive this period reach stage IV in which hepatic dysfunction resolves, with eventual return of normal liver function without development of cirrhosis.

Renal dysfunction occurs in up to 25% of cases with documented hepatotoxicity and may be secondary to direct toxic effects of NAPQI on the kidney or to the hepatorenal syndrome in patients with fulminant hepatic failure. Serious organ toxicity other than that of the hepatic and renal organs is rare, but can include pancreatitis and cardiac toxicity.

Evaluation of the patient with acute APAP poisoning should initially focus on predicting the risk of toxicity and assessing the degree of hepatic injury. At present, the clinician must rely upon the ingestion history (time and amount of ingestion) and measurement of APAP plasma concentration to predict the risk of toxicity. When reliable information is available regarding the ingested dose, patients with ingestions of less than 150 mg per kg in children or 7.5 g in adults may not require further evaluation for APAP toxicity. These amounts are debated and are probably too low. When the history is likely to be unreliable (e.g., suicide attempts, or in poisonings with uncertain agents), a plasma APAP concentration should be measured. The APAP level should be measured 4 hours after ingestion or as soon as possible thereafter. At 4 hours after ingestion, absorption is usually complete and there is no improvement in the efficacy of N-acetylcysteine (NAC) therapy when started earlier than 4 hours after the overdose. The APAP level versus time after acetaminophen ingestion is used to determine the potential for toxicity through use of the acetaminophen toxicity nomogram (Fig. 1). (53) Overtreatment with NAC is preferred to undertreatment as the treatment is well tolerated and APAP toxicity has significant morbidity and mortality.

If a toxic APAP level is present, the aspartate aminotransferase (AST) level should be measured. AST is a sensitive marker for the presence of hepatic injury but has no prognostic implications. If AST elevation is noted, then serial determinations of AST, alanine aminotransferase (ALT), prothrombin time, bilirubin, electrolytes, and glucose, are appropriate.

Gastric emptying is rarely a consideration for patients with isolated APAP overdose because of the very rapid gastrointestinal absorption of APAP and the availability of NAC. Gastric emptying should be considered to reduce the toxicity of coingestants. There has been some controversy regarding the use of activated charcoal as NAC binds to the activated charcoal. Since most patients are treated with a large excess of NAC, any loss due to binding to activated charcoal is clinically insignificant. There is no value to activated charcoal greater than 4 hours after ingestion as absorption is complete.

NAC acts in several ways to prevent APAP toxicity: (a) it is converted to cysteine, which in turn is converted to glutathione to increase glutathione supply; (b) it directly reduces NAPQI to a nontoxic cysteine conjugate; (c) it can supply substrate for sulfation, increasing the capacity for nontoxic metabolism; and (d) it can directly reduce NAPQI to APAP. These effects of NAC will help prevent the covalent binding of NAPQI to hepatocytes, prior to the onset of hepatotoxicity. NAC may also have beneficial effects through alternative mechanisms of action even after hepatic toxicity is established (54). In a prospective, randomized trial, initiation of i.v. NAC even after fulminant hepatic failure was evident diminished the need for vasopressors and decreased the incidence of cerebral edema and death (55).

The Food and Drug Administration has only approved NAC for oral dosing in the United States. The patient should be given a loading dose of 140 mg per kg followed by a maintenance dose of 70 mg per kg every 4 hours for 17 additional doses. This provides a total dose of 1,330 mg per kg over 72 hours. NAC is poorly tolerated orally and over 50% of patients vomit after NAC administration. To improve tolerance, the NAC should be diluted to a 5% solution with a sweet juice, and antiemetics such as metoclopramide should be used liberally. If any dose is vomited within 1 hour of administration, it should be repeated. Intravenous dosing is used in Europe, Canada, and experimentally in the United States. Intravenous NAC is associated with more significant side effects including anaphylaxis compared to oral therapy. The two routes of treatment are equally effective if treatment is initiated within 8 hours of ingestion. The i.v. formulation was used in all the studies that demonstrated the benefit of NAC in established hepatic failure. Prolonging the use of NAC beyond the standard 18 doses is a potentially useful but incompletely studied option for patients with liver damage.

The success of liver transplantation for APAP-induced liver failure has created an unmet need for early identification of patients with a poor prognosis with medical therapy alone. The presence of a pH less than 7.30 after fluid and hemodynamic resuscitation, or the combination of prothrombin time greater than 100 seconds, creatinine greater than 3.3 mg per dL, and grade III or IV encephalopathy is highly predictive of a patient who will die without transplantation (56). A liver transplant service should be contacted for patients who meet these criteria.

Cyclic Antidepressants

Cyclic antidepressants (CAs) are one of the leading causes of death from prescription drug overdose. Representative agents include doxepin, amitriptyline, imipramine, nortriptyline, and desipramine. Poisoning occurs commonly due to the narrow therapeutic/toxicity ratio and the use of these agents in patients with an increased risk for suicide. CAs are rapidly absorbed from the small intestine with peak serum concentrations occurring 2 to 8 hours after a therapeutic dose. Peak serum concentration, however, is often more delayed when an overdose has been ingested due to the anticholinergic effects of these drugs on gastric emptying. Most of the drug is protein bound at physiologic pH and is pharmacologically inactive. Increased free drug is found in patients with acidosis. These drugs have an extremely large volume of distribution due to extensive tissue distribution of the CAs and their active metabolites. This explains the long elimination half-life and the lack of efficacy of treatment with extracorporeal techniques.

CAs block the reuptake of norepinephrine, dopamine, and serotonin at the central presynaptic terminals. The subsequent

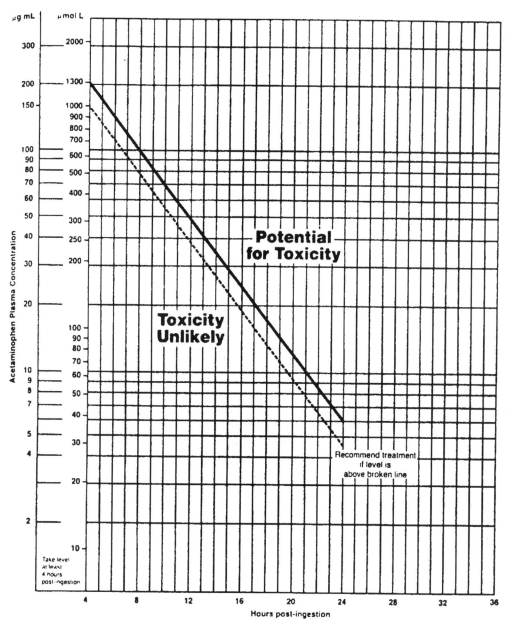

FIGURE 1. Acetaminophen toxicity nomogram: plasma or serum acetaminophen concentration versus time after acetaminophen ingestion. (Reprinted with permission from Management of Acetaminophen Overdose. McNeil Consumer Products Co., 1986.)

accumulation of aminergic transmitters in the CNS may partially account for their antidepressant effects. Central and peripheral anticholinergic effects may be present with therapeutic dosing but are markedly accentuated with overdose. The earliest toxic symptoms are usually anticholinergic and excitatory and may include tachycardia, hyperthermia, dry flushed skin, dilated pupils, decreased gastrointestinal motility, urinary retention, agitation, hallucinations, ataxia, and seizures. Coma is the most common presenting symptom in eventually fatal ingestions.

CAs are highly concentrated within the myocardium where they produce sodium channel blockade and create type IA "quinidinelike" membrane depressant effects on the myocardial conduction system. This prolongs phase 0 depolarization with resulting QRS widening. Hypotension occurs secondary to: (a) direct

myocardial depression resulting from inhibition of the fast sodium channel; (b) blockade of alpha-adrenergic neurotransmitters at postsynaptic sympathetic neurons with resulting vasodilation; and (c) inhibition of norepinephrine reuptake leading to norepinephrine depletion. Hypotension is a manifestation of severe toxicity. Hypoventilation and ARDS are also associated with clinically significant CA overdose.

The diagnosis of CA toxicity is clinical and measuring drug levels is not helpful as a relatively poor correlation has been found between plasma levels and symptoms of serious poisoning. Patients at risk for serious complications of CA overdose manifest signs and symptoms of toxicity early in their course, and life-threatening complications are most likely to occur within 6 hours of presentation. The ECG is a useful screening tool as the QRS duration is a better predictor of toxicity than serum drug levels. When the QRS duration is less than 100 msec, significant toxicity is unlikely to occur. Patients with QRS duration of greater than 100 msec are at high risk for seizures, and those with QRS duration greater than 160 msec are at high risk for ventricular dysrhythmias (57). Other laboratory tests recommended include an arterial blood gas to identify metabolic and respiratory acidosis (both of which increase CA toxicity), serum electrolytes, blood urea nitrogen, creatinine, and creatinine phosphokinase to assess other causes of hypotension, rhabdomyolysis and dysrhythmias, acetaminophen and aspirin levels to exclude coingestion, and CNS diagnostic testing to assess other causes of confusion, coma, or seizures.

Management of CA overdose is largely supportive. Initial goals are to protect the airway and provide respiratory and cardiac support as necessary. Orogastric lavage should be employed if it can be initiated on a timely basis. The anticholinergic-mediated delay in gastric emptying may permit removal of CAs for several hours after ingestion. Syrup of ipecac is contraindicated because rapid deterioration of mental status often occurs, predisposing the patient to emesis-induced aspiration. Activated charcoal is routinely recommended for treatment of CA overdose, with a second dose given 2 to 4 hours after the first dose to decrease enterohepatic recirculation in patients with severe toxicity.

Seizures should be treated with diazepam or lorazepam. Long-acting anticonvulsant therapy is generally not necessary. Phenytoin is contraindicated because its cardiac effects may lead to an increased incidence of ventricular dysrhythmias and is an ineffective anticonvulsant in animals. Patients with possible mixed CA and benzodiazepam overdose should not receive flumazenil as its use may unmask seizures and dysrhythmias. Physostigmine is no longer recommended to treat the anticholinergic manifestations of severe CA overdose, as its use has been associated with serious complications including seizures, vomiting, bradycardia, asystole, and death (58).

Most deaths from CA overdose are due to cardiovascular toxicity. Inducing a systemic alkalosis either through infusion of sodium bicarbonate or by hyperventilation reverses the cardiac toxicity, presumably by decreasing CA binding to the myocardium. Hypertonic saline is also beneficial which suggests that some of the beneficial effects of sodium bicarbonate are secondary to the sodium-loading, reversing CA-induced sodium channel blockade. Sodium bicarbonate should be given if ventricular dysrhythmias occur, or if the QRS duration is greater than 100 msec. A 1 to 2 mEq per kg bolus should be given, followed by either a bicarbonate infusion or repeat boluses as needed. The goal is to maintain the arterial pH between 7.45 and 7.55. Narrowing of the QRS duration indicates a beneficial response.

Sinus tachycardia alone usually does not require treatment. Lidocaine should be used to treat ventricular dysrhythmias if systemic alkalinization fails. If cardiac arrest occurs, the standard advanced cardiac life support protocol should be followed but: (a) sodium bicarbonate should be infused early to achieve systemic alkalinization; (b) type IA and IC antidysrhythmic drugs should be avoided; and (c) resuscitation efforts should be prolonged.

Hypotension should be initially treated with volume administration. If volume repletion (guided by central monitoring if appropriate) is ineffective in restoring systemic blood pressure, catecholamines should be infused. Norepinephrine may be preferable to dopamine as CAs are believed to directly inhibit dopamine-induced release of norepinephrine (59).

Theophylline

Theophylline is a methylxanthine derivative that is used as a bronchodilator for the treatment of asthma and chronic obstructive pulmonary disease. It has a narrow therapeutic index. Multiple theophylline formulations exist, including liquids, tablets, sustained-release preparations, and i.v. (aminophylline). Theophylline is well absorbed orally with levels rising rapidly within 30 minutes to 1 hour following ingestion. Sustained release products result in delayed absorption. Theophylline is metabolized in the liver by the CYP1A2 isozyme of the cytochrome P450 mixed function oxidase enzymes. Many interactions affect the kinetics of theophylline. Several drugs including cimetidine, ciprofloxacin, diltiazem, erythromycin, and norfloxacin, inhibit the CYP1A2 isozyme, raising plasma theophylline levels and increasing the risk for toxicity. Hepatic clearance of theophylline is decreased by factors that lead to diminished hepatic blood flow such as congestive heart failure or by preexisting liver disease. Cigarette smoking, phenobarbital, and phenytoin enhance metabolism of theophylline by as much as 50%.

The mechanism of action of theophylline is uncertain. It appears to act as an adenosine receptor antagonist, inhibits bronchoconstricting prostaglandins and causes adrenal release of epinephrine. At toxic levels, it also inhibits phosphodiesterase. The net effect is bronchodilation, CNS stimulation, increased diaphragmatic contractility, tachydysrhythmias, and vomiting.

Acute theophylline overdose presents with gastrointestinal, cardiovascular, CNS, and metabolic manifestations. Gastrointestinal symptoms include nausea and protracted vomiting secondary to direct CNS stimulation of the chemoreceptor trigger zone as well as increased acid secretion and relaxation of lower esophageal sphincter tone. Cardiovascular manifestations of toxicity may include atrial and ventricular tachydysrhythmias secondary to excessive catecholamine stimulation of the myocardium, a widened pulse pressure due to simultaneous increase in peripheral beta-2 adrenergic receptor mediated vasodilation and beta-1 adrenergic receptor induced inotropy. With more severe toxicity the vasodilatory effects predominate leading to hypotension, which will be exacerbated by vomiting-induced volume depletion. Cardiovascular toxicity may be enhanced by the metabolic effects of theophylline, which lead to development of hypokalemia and lactic acidosis. Other metabolic effects include hyperglycemia, hypophosphatemia, and hypomagnesemia. Tremor, agitation, and psychosis are due to catecholamine release. The exact cause of seizures remains unclear but loss of CNS adenosine anticonvulsant activity probably plays a major role along with cerebral vasoconstriction. Acute toxicity follows acute overdose and presents with the complete spectrum of CNS, gastrointestinal, cardiovascular, and metabolic effects. Chronic toxicity is usually secondary to changes in clearance or unintentional overmedication. Toxicity may occur at lower serum concentrations in patients chronically receiving theophylline than in patients with acute overdoses. Chronic toxicity often presents with nonspecific gastrointestinal distress or tremor, but seizures and life-threatening dysrhythmias may occur without warning. Metabolic changes occur infrequently. Older age markedly increases the risk for CNS or cardiovascular complications with chronic poisoning (60).

The diagnosis of theophylline toxicity is made clinically by the common presentation of protracted vomiting, CNS excitation, and tachydysrhythmias. Theophylline levels should be obtained when the diagnosis is first suspected and then every 1 to 2 hours until the theophylline level decreases into the therapeutic range. Onset of toxicity usually occurs within 1 to 2 hours following acute oral ingestion but can be delayed for greater than 6 hours if sustained release preparations have been ingested. Serum concentrations greater than 90 μg per mL with acute overdose are generally predictive of life-threatening complications, particularly seizures. Serum concentrations are less predictive of serious complications in the chronic overdose setting but levels greater than 40 μg per kg should be considered potentially life threatening.

Treatment decisions regarding gastrointestinal decontamination will depend on the theophylline dosage form, when the ingestion occurred, and the patient's clinical condition. Syrup of ipecac is usually avoided because the protracted vomiting that results from its use limits the ability to use activated charcoal which is highly effective in absorbing theophylline. Orogastric lavage should be performed in patients with potentially toxic theophylline ingestions where the administration of activated charcoal requires placement of a gastric tube. Many preparations of theophylline do not fit through a large bore orogastric tube. Activated charcoal should be given to all patients with a toxic theophylline ingestion because of its ability to absorb drug remaining in the gastrointestinal tract as well as to decrease serum concentrations through "gut dialysis." Multiple doses increase clearance, and multidose activated charcoal is the cornerstone of therapy for theophylline toxicity. Activated charcoal is efficacious even when aminophylline is administered intravenously (61). One to two g per kg of activated charcoal should be given every 2 to 4 hours to a maximum of 5 to 7 doses. Antiemetics may be necessary for successful use of multidose activated charcoal in this setting. Metoclopramide and ondansetron may theoretically be more beneficial than the phenothiazine antiemetics because they do not lower the seizure threshold. Whole-bowel irrigation may be useful to enhance the evacuation of sustained-release theophylline products.

Extracorporeal removal of theophylline should be considered for patients with acute overdose with serum concentrations of greater than 90 μg per mL or with levels greater than 40 μg per mL when seizures, hypotension refractory to fluid resuscitation, life-threatening ventricular dysrhythmias, or protracted vomiting unresponsive to antiemetics are present. For patients with acute on chronic toxicity, extracorporeal techniques should be considered if the theophylline level is greater than 70 μg per mL 4 hours after ingestion of a sustained release form. With chronic ingestions, significant toxicity may occur at lower serum theophylline concentrations. The indications for extracorporeal removal are much more controversial in chronic toxicity. It should be considered in patients with a theophylline level greater than 60 μg per mL and for levels between 40 to 60 μg per mL in patients greater than 60 years old. Charcoal hemoperfusion is the optimal extracorporeal technique due to the high affinity of activated charcoal for theophylline. If this technique is not available then hemodialysis should be used (62).

Cocaine

The National Institute of Drug Abuse estimated that in 1990 over 25 million Americans had tried cocaine at least once and 5 million admitted to using cocaine at least once a month (63). Any dosage is potentially toxic. Fatality has been associated with use of a dose as low as 20 mg. Cocaine is an ester-type local anesthetic. The onset of action depends on the dose and route of administration. With nasal insufflation the onset of action is within 1 to 3 minutes with peak effect in 20 to 30 minutes. When used intravenously or when smoked the onset of action occurs within seconds to minutes. Cocaine has two primary mechanisms of action: (a) it blocks presynaptic re-uptake of biogenic amine neurotransmitters (norepinephrine, dopamine, serotonin) and (b) it produces a local anesthetic effect due to blockade of sodium channels. Cocaine is metabolized by liver esterases and plasma cholinesterase to largely inactive metabolites. Its biologic half-life is 0.5 to 1.5 hours.

The most prominent effect of cocaine use is CNS stimulation. The cortex is initially stimulated which may result in euphoria, hyperactivity, and agitation. Hyperthermia may be present secondary to the increase in psychomotor activity which increases heat production and systemic vasoconstriction which decreases heat dissipation. Subsequently, stimulation of lower motor centers can produce tonic-clonic seizures, probably mediated through excitatory amino acids. Neurologic findings may also occur from hypertensive complications such as intracerebral bleeding secondary to a ruptured aneurysm, or cerebral infarction secondary to vasospasm and hypercoagulability. Cardiovascular effects include tachycardia, hypertension, coronary artery vasoconstriction with subsequent myocardial ischemia or infarction, and dysrhythmias (64). Other complications that may occur include aortic dissection, ARDS, barotrauma, rhabdomyolysis, intestinal ischemia, and placental abruption in the second or third trimester of pregnancy.

Only benzodiazepines and cooling measures have been repeatedly demonstrated to decrease mortality from cocaine intoxication in animal studies; therefore external cooling with an ice water bath and reduction in psychomotor agitation with benzodiazepines are critical early therapeutic maneuvers. Intravenous doses of benzodiazepines should be used until sedation is achieved. Gastric decontamination is of limited value except for body packers. Laboratory tests that may be useful include an ECG looking for evidence of ischemia or infarction, chest x-ray and arterial blood gas, head computed tomography scan followed by a lumbar puncture in patients with altered mental status or agitation, and urinalysis to detect rhabdomyolysis-induced myoglobinuria.

Chest pain usually resolves when the patient is adequately sedated. When an acute coronary ischemic syndrome is suspected, the patient should be given aspirin (325 mg), sublingual nitroglycerin, small doses of morphine to relieve chest pain, and a heparin bolus and infusion. If the response is inadequate, phentolamine, 1 mg i.v. at a time should be used. Cardiac consultation is also appropriate at this stage to determine if acute cardiac catheterization or thrombolytic therapy is indicated. Unresolving hypertension can be treated with nitroglycerin, nitroprusside, or phentolamine. Beta-blockers are contraindicated in acutely toxic patients as unopposed alpha-adrenergic activity may occur. Ventricular dysrhythmias that develop rapidly following cocaine use should be presumed to occur from the local anesthetic effects of cocaine on the myocardium. In some animal models, cocaine-induced, wide-complex ventricular dysrhythmias respond to the administration of sodium bicarbonate (65). If patients present several hours after cocaine use with ventricular dysrhythmias, these are likely ischemic in origin and standard management including the use of lidocaine is appropriate. Seizures should be treated with benzodiazepines. Agitated patients should be given glucose and thiamine. Extracorporeal techniques for cocaine removal are not useful. Body packers should be treated with multi-dose activated charcoal and whole-bowel irrigation; if the patient is toxic and has evidence of abdominal obstruction, surgical removal should be considered.

POISONING-INDUCED HIGH-ANION GAP METABOLIC ACIDOSIS

Metabolic acidosis with a large anion gap may develop secondary to poisoning with various agents or may be secondary to uremia, hypoperfusion-related lactic acidosis, or ketoacidosis (alcoholic or diabetic). Lactic acidosis may be the etiology for the increased anion gap with carbon monoxide, cyanide, and salicylate poisoning. The lactic acidosis associated with isoniazid (INH) intoxication is secondary to seizures. Lactic acidosis secondary to seizures may also develop with theophylline overdose. Iron intoxication produces lactic acidosis secondary to hypotension and disruption of oxidative phosphorylation. Metformin toxicity often presents as lactic acidosis. This toxicity should be suspected in diabetics on this drug who have had a deterioration in renal function.

Methanol and ethylene glycol ingestion are associated with the development of a high-anion gap metabolic acidosis. Typically the acidosis develops from 1 hour to 24 hours after methanol ingestion and 1 hour to 4 to 6 hours after ingestion of ethylene glycol. The acidosis is secondary to the metabolism of methanol to formic acid and of ethylene glycol to glycolic acid. Paraldehyde has been associated with the development of a high-anion gap metabolic acidosis, but this drug has been withdrawn from the market in the United States.

SUMMARY

Poisoning is a common cause of morbidity and mortality. Despite difficulties in establishing which specific toxin may be present in many patients, most patients still do well with early institution of supportive care. The value of decontamination techniques other than single-dose activated charcoal remain unproved, but are likely beneficial for selected patients. Only in a few patients are specific antidotes required or useful.

Acknowledgments. Jeffrey S. Kelly, MD, contributed to this chapter in a previous edition.

KEY POINTS

Poisoning is a heterogeneous disease state whose presentation is affected by such variables as the patient's age, amount, and type of toxin ingested, time since toxin exposure, preexisting medical and psychiatric conditions, and concomitant trauma. The patient's history is often unobtainable or unreliable and therefore other resources (friends, family, etc.) should be used to try to identify the toxin. A thorough physical examination is mandatory to assess for the presence of traumatic injuries, stigmata of substance abuse, or "toxidromes." Laboratory studies are rarely diagnostic in the setting of acute overdose, and appropriate therapy should not be withheld pending their results. Tests for specific toxins for which antidotes are available should be performed when their ingestion is suggested by history, physical examination, or bedside diagnostic tests. The cornerstone of overdose management is aggressive institution of supportive care and stabilization of vital-organ function. Early use of antidotes may also be required to stabilize the patient or prevent delayed life-threatening organ dysfunction. The value of decontamination techniques other than single-dose activated charcoal remains unproven. Dialysis treatment of overdoses is usually limited to patients who remain unstable from dialyzable toxins despite maximal supportive care. Despite the complexities inherent in most clinical overdoses, the outcome from poisoning is usually satisfactory when promptly diagnosed and appropriately treated.

REFERENCES

1. Litovitz TL, Klein-Schwartz W, White S, et al. 1999 annual report of the American Association of Poison Control Centers Toxic Exposure Surveillance System. *Am J Emerg Med* 2000;18:517–574.
2. Kulig K, Bar-Or D, Cantrill SV, et al. Management of acutely poisoned patients without gastric emptying. *Ann Emerg Med* 1985;14:562–567.
3. Linakis JG, Frederick KA. Poisoning deaths not reported to the regional poison center. *Ann Emerg Med* 1993;22:1822–1828.
4. Osterloh JD. Utility and reliability of emergency toxicologic testing. *Emerg Med Clin North Am* 1990;8:693–723.
5. Mofenson HC, Greensher J. The nontoxic ingestion. *Pediatr Clin North Am* 1970;17:583–590.
6. Collee GG, Hanson GC. The management of acute poisoning. *Br J Anaesth* 1993;70:562–573.
7. Kulig K. Initial management of ingestions of toxic substances. *N Engl J Med* 1992;326:1677–1681.
8. Brett AS. Implications of discordance between clinical impression and

toxicology analysis in drug overdose. *Arch Intern Med* 1988;148:437–441.

9. Roy TM, Ossorio MA, Dipolla LM, et al. Pulmonary complications after tricyclic antidepressant overdose. *Chest* 1989;96:852–856.

10. Hoffman RS, Goldfrank LR. The poisoned patient with altered consciousness: controversies in the use of a "coma cocktail." *JAMA* 1995;274:562–569.

11. Yealy DM, Paris PM, Kaplan RM, et al. The safety of prehospital naloxone administration by paramedics. *Ann Emerg Med* 1990;19:902–905.

12. Mordel A, Winkler E, Almog S, et al. Seizures after flumazenil administration in a case of combined benzodiazepine and tricyclic antidepressant overdose. *Crit Care Med* 1992;20:1733–1734.

13. Geller E, Cromae P, Schaller MD, et al. Risks and benefits of therapy with flumazenil (anexate) in mixed drug intoxications. *Eur Neurol* 1991;31:241–250.

14. Comstock EG, Faulkner TP, Boisaubin EV, et al. Studies on the efficacy of gastric emptying as practiced in a large metropolitan hospital. *Clin Toxicol* 1981;18:581–597.

15. Comstock EG, Boisaubin EV, Comstock BS, et al. Assessment of the efficacy of activated charcoal following gastric lavage in acute drug emergencies. *Clin Toxicol* 1982;19:149–165.

16. American Academy of Clinical Toxicology; European Association of Poisons Centres and Clinical Toxicologists. Position statement: ipecac syrup. *Clin Toxicol* 1997;35:699–709.

17. American Academy of Clinical Toxicology; European Association of Poisons Centres and Clinical Toxicologists. Position statement: gastric lavage. *Clin Toxicol* 1997;35:711–719.

18. Manno B, Manno J. Toxicology of ipecac. *Clin Toxicol* 1977;10:221–242.

19. Merigian KS, Woodard M, Hedges JR, et al. Prospective evaluation of gastric emptying in the self poisoned patient. *Am J Emerg Med* 1990;8:479–483.

20. Pond SM, Lewis-Driver DJ, Williams GM, et al. Gastric emptying in acute overdose: a prospective randomised controlled trial. *Med J Aust* 1995;163:345–349.

21. Freedman G, Pasternak S, Krenzelok E. A clinical trial using syrup of ipecac and activated charcoal concurrently. *Ann Emerg Med* 1987;16:164–166.

22. Young WF Jr, Bivins HG. Evaluation of gastric emptying using radionuclides: gastric lavage versus ipecac-induced emesis. *Ann Emerg Med* 1993;22:1423–1427.

23. Vasquez TE, Evans DG, Ashburn WL. Efficacy of syrup of ipecac-induced emesis for emptying gastric contents. *Clin Nucl Med* 1988;13:638–639.

24. Danel V, Henry JA, Glucksman E. Activated charcoal, emesis, and gastric lavage in aspirin overdose. *BMJ* 1988;296:1507.

25. Saetta JP, Quinton DN. Residual gastric content after gastric lavage and ipecacuanha-induced emesis in self-poisoned patients: an endoscopic study. *J Roy Soc Med* 1991;84:35–38.

26. Saetta JP, March S, Gaunt ME, et al. Gastric emptying procedures in the self-poisoned patient: are we forcing gastric content beyond the pylorus? *J Roy Soc Med* 1991;84:274–276.

27. Allan BC. The role of gastric lavage in the treatment of patients suffering from barbiturate overdose. *Med J Aust* 1961;2:513–514.

28. Watson WA, Leighton J, Guy J, et al. Recovery of cyclic antidepressants with gastric lavage. *J Emerg Med* 1989;7:373–377.

29. Marsteller HJ, Gugler R. Endoscopic management of toxic masses in the stomach. *N Engl J Med* 1977;296:1003–1004.

30. Bartecchi CE. Removal of gastric drug masses. *N Engl J Med* 1977;296:282–283.

31. Litovitz TL. Button battery ingestions: a review of 56 cases. *JAMA* 1983;249:2495–2500.

32. Trent M, Kim U. Cocaine packet ingestion: surgical or medical management. *Arch Surg* 1987;122:1179–1181.

33. Hoffman RS, Smilkstein MJ, Goldfrank LR. Whole bowel irrigation and the cocaine body packer. *Am J Emerg Med* 1990;8:523–527.

34. Nalbandian H, Sheth N, Dietrich R, et al. Intestinal ischemia caused by cocaine ingestion: report of two cases. *Surgery* 1985;97:374–376.

35. Schwartz HS. Acute meprobamate poisoning with gastrotomy and removal of a drug-containing mass. *N Engl J Med* 1976;295:1177–1178.

36. Landsman J, Bricker J, Reid BS, et al. Emergency gastrostomy: treatment of choice for iron bezoar. *J Pediatr Surg* 1987;22:184–185.

37. American Academy of Clinical Toxicology; European Association of Poisons Centres and Clinical Toxicologists. Position statement: single-dose activated charcoal. *Clin Toxicol* 1997;35:721–741.

38. Atkinson SW, Young Y, Trotter GA. Treatment with activated charcoal complicated by gastrointestinal obstruction requiring surgery. *Br Med J* 1992;305:563–564.

39. American Academy of Clinical Toxicology; European Association of Poisons Centres and Clinical Toxicology. Position statement and practice guidelines on the use of multi-dose activated charcoal in the treatment of poisoning. *Clin Toxicol* 1999;37:731–751.

40. Levy G. Gastrointestinal clearance of drugs with activated charcoal. *N Engl J Med* 1982;307:676–678.

41. Al-Shareef AH, Buss DC, Allen EM, et al. The effects of charcoal and sorbitol (alone and in combination) on plasma theophylline concentrations after a sustained-release formulation. *Hum Exp Toxicol* 1990;9:179–182.

42. American Academy of Clinical Toxicology; European Association of Poisons Centres and Clinical Toxicologists. Position statement: cathartics. *Clin Toxicol* 1997;35:743–752.

43. Keller RE, Schwab RA, Krenzelok EP. Contribution of sorbitol combined with activated charcoal in prevention of salicylate absorption. *Ann Emerg Med* 1990;19:654–656.

44. American Academy of Clinical Toxicology; European Association of Poisons Centres and Clinical Toxicologists. Position statement: whole bowel irrigation. *Clin Toxicol* 1997;35:753–762.

45. Taboulet P, Baud FJ, Bismuth C. Clinical features and management of digitalis poisoning—rationale for immunotherapy. *Clin Toxicol* 1993;31:247–260.

46. Taboulet P, Baud FJ, Bismuth C, Vicaut E. Acute digitalis intoxication—is pacing still appropriate? *Clin Toxicol* 1993;31:261–271.

47. Antman EM, Wenger TL, Butler VP, et al. Treatment of 150 cases of life-threatening digitalis intoxication with digoxin-specific Fab antibody fragments: final report of a multicenter study. *Circulation* 1990;81:1744–1752.

48. Schou M. Long-lasting neurologic sequelae after lithium intoxication. *Acta Psychiatr Scand* 1984;70:594–602.

49. Jaeger A, Sauder P, Kopeferschmitt J, et al. When should dialysis be performed in lithium poisoning? A kinetic study in 14 cases of lithium poisoning. *J Toxicol Clin Toxicol* 1993;31:429–447.

50. Thurstin JH, Pollock PG, Warren SK, et al. Reduced brain glucose with normal plasma glucose in salicylate poisoning. *Clin Invest* 1970;49:2139–2145.

51. Anderson RJ, Potts DE, Gabow PA, et al. Unrecognized adult salicylate intoxication. *Ann Intern Med* 1976;85:745–748.

52. Linden CH, Rumack BH. Acetaminophen overdose. *Emerg Med Clin North Am* 1984;2:103–119.

53. Rumack BH, Peterson RC, Koch GG, et al. Acetaminophen overdose: 662 cases with evaluation of oral acetylcysteine treatment. *Arch Intern Med* 1981;141:380–385.

54. Harrison PM, Wenson JA, Gimson AES, et al. Improvement by acetylcysteine of hemodynamics and oxygen transport in fulminant hepatic failure. *N Engl J Med* 1991;324:1852–1857.

55. Keays R, Harrison PM, Wendon JA, et al. Intravenous acetylcysteine in paracetamol induced fulminant hepatic failure: a prospective controlled trial. *Br Med J* 1991;303:1026–1029.

56. O'Grady JG, Alexander GJM, Hayllar KM, et al. Early indicators of prognosis in fulminant hepatic failure. *Gastroenterology* 1989;97:439–445.

57. Boehnert MT, Lovejoy FH. Value of the QRS duration versus the serum drug level in predicting seizures and ventricular arrhythmias after an acute overdose of tricyclic antidepressants. *N Engl J Med* 1985;313:474–479.

58. Pentel P, Peterson CD. Asystole complicating physostigmine treatment of tricyclic antidepressant overdose. *Ann Emerg Med* 1980;9:588–590.

59. Teba L, Schiebel F, Dedhia HV, et al. Beneficial effect of norepinephrine in the treatment of circulatory shock caused by tricyclic antidepressant overdose. *Am J Emerg Med* 1988;6:566–568.

60. Shannon M, Lovejoy FH. The influence of age versus serum concentration on life-threatening events after chronic theophylline intoxication. *Arch Intern Med* 1990;50:2045–2048.

61. Radomski L, Park GD, Goldberg MJ, et al. Model for theophylline overdose treatment with oral activated charcoal. *Clin Pharmacol Ther* 1984;35:402–408.

62. Ahlmen C, Heath A, Herlitz H, et al. Treatment of oral theophylline poisoning. *Acta Med Scand* 1984;216:423–426.

63. National Institute of Drug Abuse. National household survey on drug abuse. Population estimates, 1991. DHHS number (ADM) 92-1887, Rockville, MD: Department of Health and Human Services, 1992.

64. Beckerman KJ, Parker RB, Hariman RJ, et al. Hemodynamic and electrophysiologic actions of cocaine: effects of sodium bicarbonate as an antidote in dogs. *Circulation* 1991;83:1799–1807.

65. Amin M, Gabelman G, Karpel J, et al. Acute myocardial infarction and chest pain: syndromes after cocaine use. *Am J Cardiol* 1990;66:1434–1437.

BIBLIOGRAPHY

Goldfrank LR, Flomenbaum NE, Lewin NA, et al, eds. *Goldfrank's toxicologic emergencies*, 6th ed. Stamford, CT: Appleton & Lange, 1998.

Haddad LM, Shannon MW, Winchester JF, eds. *Clinical management of poisoning and drug overdose*, 3rd ed. Philadelphia: WB Saunders, 1998.

Klaassen CD, ed. *Casarett & Doull's toxicology: the basic science of poisons*, 5th ed. New York: McGraw-Hill, 1995.

ADVANCED IMAGING IN THE INTENSIVE CARE UNIT

JANET E. KUHLMAN

KEY WORDS

- Imaging: body, head, spine, chest, abdomen, critical care
- Ultrasound: chest, abdomen
- Computerized tomography: head, spine, chest, abdomen, contrast, noncontrast, spiral, multidetector
- Magnetic resonance imaging: brain, spinal cord, body
- Angiography
- Radiographic intervention

INTRODUCTION

Radiologic imaging is an important part of critical care medicine that involves the integration of clinical and radiologic information on a daily, hourly, and sometimes minute-by-minute basis. As the severity, complexity, and variety of conditions managed in intensive care units (ICUs) increases and our ability to prolong life with technologic advances improves, the intensivist is confronted with a vast array of diagnostic considerations and therapeutic options. At the same time, clinical findings and physiologic data, such as fever, sepsis, hemodynamic instability, change in mental status, or respiratory decompensation, that indicate potentially life-threatening alterations are by their very nature nonspecific as to their etiology. The results of radiologic imaging often are pivotal both in determining a cause by narrowing the differential diagnosis and in choosing an appropriate course of action or change in therapy or intervention.

Portable radiographs of the chest and abdomen are the most frequently ordered radiologic examinations in ICU patients. They provide important information regarding the cardiopulmonary status of critically ill patients and document proper placement of central lines, tubes, and other life-support hardware. The use of plain films in the evaluation of ICU patients has been extensively reviewed in the literature and will not be reiterated here. Readers may wish to consult an excellent and comprehensive text on this topic edited by Goodman and Putman entitled *Critical Care Imaging* (1).

Although essential to the daily management of critical care patients, portable films have severe limitations in terms of qua-

lity and diagnostic accuracy (2). When portable radiographs fail to provide the needed information, advanced imaging often is required. The use of advanced imaging in the ICU is the primary focus of this chapter, including an overview of recent developments in spiral and multidetector computerized tomography (CT) technology. The chapter includes a review of the major indications for advanced imaging of the chest, abdomen, and central nervous system (CNS) as well as a discussion of image-guided interventional procedures in the ICU patient.

Advanced imaging technologies such as CT, ultrasound, and magnetic resonance imaging (MRI) have several distinct advantages over conventional radiography in the assessment of critically ill patients. In the ICU setting, conventional radiographs are usually portable, supine, and often of poor image quality because of patient factors and equipment limitations. Advanced imaging technologies are cross-sectional in format and thus allow evaluation of the internal organs unencumbered by superimposed structures.

Recent advances in CT technology in particular have produced a quantum leap in the speed of such examinations. Utilizing high-speed spiral and multidetector CT scanners, the rate-limiting factor in evaluating critical care patients is no longer scanning time. The newest multidetector CT technology represents a several-fold increase in speed over traditional CT scanners. In practical terms, this means that once an ICU patient is on the CT table, scanning can be done literally from head to toe in a matter of seconds rather than minutes. Obstacles to CT scanning remain significant, however, and the primary ones are those related to patient preparation and stabilization and assuring safe transport of the patient with adequate monitoring en route to the CT unit. The risks involved in moving a critically ill patient from the carefully monitored and controlled environment of the ICU never should be underestimated or minimized (2). Certain patients cannot be moved because of indwelling devices, such as intraaortic balloon pumps. In addition, the nurse, physician, and other medical personnel required to transport the patient safely to the CT suite deplete the staff remaining to care for other critically ill patients (2). Nevertheless, with proper use of portable monitoring and life-support equipment and availability of adequate ICU staff to accompany the patient, transport to the CT scanning suite can be accomplished safely and efficiently when required. To expedite the process, communication and coordination between ICU, CT, and transport personnel are crucial.

As a result of faster exposure times, state-of-the-art multidetector CT scanners also minimize artifacts from respiratory and patient motion. Most examinations of the chest and abdomen done in ICU patients can be completed without additional sedation. Highly agitated patients, however, may require additional sedation to achieve a diagnostic examination. Multidetector CT scanners employ a bank of detectors rather than a single row of x-ray detectors. This configuration allows acquisition of more images with thinner, overlapping slices and better resolution in less time. Such scanners make possible the acquisition of enough CT data to computer-generate angiographic images of the vascular tree that are comparable to conventional angiograms but are achieved in a noninvasive manner. CT angiography obtained with the new multidetector scanners can be acquired 24 hours a day without the need for an angiographic suite and its specialized personnel and can be done with the speed of a CT examination. New and emerging applications of CT angiography in the ICU setting include the evaluation of aortic vascular disorders, such as aortic trauma, aortic dissection, and leaking aneurysms as well as evaluation of thromboembolic disease and pulmonary embolism.

For the critical care patient, magnetic resonance imaging (MRI) examination remains less practical than CT in most cases and a much more cumbersome modality. Not only do most MRI examinations require study times exceeding one-half hour or more but, in addition, any patient motion can significantly degrade MRI quality and usefulness. Additional sedation is often required, and careful attention must be paid to MRI-specific safety factors. Only non-ferromagnetic materials can enter the MRI scanner area. Meticulous screening of all external and internal monitoring and support devices for compatibility with the powerful magnets used for MRI is mandatory. Nevertheless, MRI does have an important and indispensable role in the management of certain conditions in select ICU patients, particularly those with disorders involving the CNS and spinal canal.

Ultrasound is the one advanced imaging modality that is highly portable. Although it has limited applications in the brain, it does have several useful applications in the chest and many in the abdomen, including a role in image-guided drainage and interventional procedures. Ultrasound, however, is not particularly useful for evaluating the lungs. In addition, the abdomens of many ICU and postoperative patients are difficult to evaluate with ultrasound because of overlying matter, drains, and surgical incisions. Ultrasound also suffers from being operator dependent and does not give the global, multiorgan visualization that CT provides. Often, CT must be resorted to when ultrasound does not result in a diagnosis or the diagnosis is equivocal or when a definitive answer is needed. Of note, there is at least one model on the market of a portable CT unit that has been in use since 1997 (Tomoscan, Philips Medical Systems, Shelton, CT, U.S.A.). This mobile CT scanner does not require that the patient be moved from the ICU (2).

THORACIC COMPUTED TOMOGRAPHY

The portable chest radiograph remains the primary tool for the daily imaging assessment of critical care patients. Readily available and relatively inexpensive, the portable chest film provides invaluable information regarding the cardiopulmonary status of ICU patients as well as a reliable means for checking the proper positioning of various support catheters and devices. Although the portable chest x-ray may clearly show the presence of pneumonia, pulmonary edema, pleural effusions, pneumothorax, or other complications, the limited diagnostic accuracy of portable chest films in ICU patients is well known (2). Chest films in ICU patients are obtained using portable units that can generate only limited amounts of kilovoltage. Coupled with the fact that only one frontal view is obtained, often in the supine position, this means that image quality is less than optimal. Variable techniques and difficulties in properly positioning critically ill patients often contribute to inadequate examinations. In one study, the diagnostic accuracy of the portable chest films for pneumonia in ICU patients was reported to be only 52% (3).

Chest CT may play a clinically useful role in the ICU patient when the portable chest film is nondiagnostic or equivocal (2,4–8). Particularly when the chest film is complicated and both pleural and parenchymal processes are present, CT is often more definitive regarding the presence or absence of such findings as loculated collections, pleural effusions, pneumothorax, cavitation, empyema, pneumonia, atelectasis, barotrauma-related pneumatoceles, and bronchopleural fistula (BPF). In addition, CT is superior to plain films in detecting and diagnosing mediastinal, vascular, and chest-wall complications, such as abscesses, and bleeding from trauma, surgery, and invasive procedures (2,4,5). Miller and colleagues reported that 30% of 108 consecutive chest CT examinations of ICU patients detected at least one new and clinically important finding that was not seen on the portable chest film (4). Clinically significant findings included abscesses or postoperative fluid collections, malignancies, unsuspected pneumonia, or pleural effusions. According to these researchers, the results of the CT scan changed clinical management 22% of the time (4).

How can chest CT help in the ICU patient? (a) CT may detect new findings not appreciated on the plain films or detect abnormalities earlier than the plain film can detect them. (b) CT may confirm a suspected or possible diagnosis based on a nonspecific or equivocal plain film finding. (c) CT can be used to exclude more definitively than plain films the presence of significant disease, for example, in ruling out a chest source of fever or sepsis such as a fluid collection, abscess, or empyema. Other chest diagnoses that may need to be excluded with CT include the presence of malignancy, loculated pleural effusions, interstitial lung disease, pulmonary emboli, constrictive pericarditis, pneumothorax, aortic injury, aortic dissection, sternal wound infection, and mediastinitis (4). (d) CT can further evaluate and elucidate the complex or confusing chest film. (e) CT also can assist in planning invasive procedures, including bronchoscopy, biopsy, thoracoscopy, and operative interventions as well as image-guided interventional procedures such as drainages and pleural tube placements.

Most ICU requests for chest CT fall into one of the following general categories (4): (a) to search for a source of infection; (b) to evaluate for postoperative complications (e.g., breakdown of surgical anastomoses, bleeding complications for cardiac and thoracic surgery); (c) to determine the presence, size, location, or loculation of a pleural effusion, fluid collection, air collection, or pneumothorax; (d) to establish the presence or absence of a neoplastic process; (e) to seek a reason for failure to wean.

In addition to these general categories, other requests for chest CT are for more specific problems, such as evaluating a refractory pneumothorax, a persistent air leak, or an enlarging pleural collection despite adequate chest tube drainage or to rule out specific entities such as pericardial tamponade. When the problem or likely pathology involves the mediastinum or deep chest wall, chest CT is also indicated given the relatively limited information that portable plain films provide regarding these anatomic structures (4).

Other emerging CT applications in the ICU patient include the role of spiral and multidetector scanning in (a) the detection of pulmonary embolus, (b) the evaluation of thoracic complications of chest trauma, and (c) the use of CT for image-guided interventional procedures to manage complex pleural, chest wall, mediastinal, or lung collections.

SPECIFIC CHEST APPLICATIONS FOR ADVANCED IMAGING

Searching for a Source of Infection, Sepsis, or Fever

What can CT tell us about the ICU patient that plain films cannot? When the plain film is nondiagnostic, equivocal, or complex, CT may demonstrate definitive findings, such as the presence of a lung abscess, empyema, septic emboli, or fungal infection (9,10). Particularly in the immunocompromised patient, the transplant recipient, or the debilitated ICU patient who is at risk for opportunistic infection, CT can play a role in the early detection of such infections. As experience with CT has accumulated, recognizable patterns and signs of specific lung diseases have emerged. CT helps to evaluate more fully nonspecific lung infiltrates seen on plain films. Patterns of involvement, distribution, and specific signs demonstrable on CT help to narrow the differential diagnosis (9–11).

Indications for chest CT examination that we find helpful include the following: (a) early detection of occult pulmonary infection and (b) characterization of the nature and extent of lung disease initially identified on chest radiographs. Chest CT is a rapid, expeditious method for determining the presence or absence of occult lung infection, particularly in cases where the chest radiograph is equivocal. Once the presence of lung disease has been established, CT patterns of parenchymal lung involvement and associated CT findings help to narrow the differential diagnosis. Although many CT patterns of parenchymal lung involvement are nonspecific, given the appropriate clinical setting, certain patterns are more suggestive of some pathologic processes than others.

Septic Emboli

An increasing number of ICU patients are at risk for developing septic emboli, including immunocompromised patients; organ-transplant recipients; and patients with indwelling catheters, prosthetic valves, or other internal devices. Early detection, along with prompt administration of broad-spectrum antibiotics, is an im-

portant factor in the prognosis of the patient with septic emboli. Unfortunately, the initial clinical diagnosis is often difficult; a heart murmur may or may not be present, and blood cultures may remain negative early during the course of infection. Characteristic chest radiographic findings of septic emboli may not be present or may be obscured by limited portable chest-film techniques available in the ICU. A significant number of patients will have nonspecific or equivocal infiltrates that are not definitive for septic emboli.

On CT, septic emboli have a characteristic appearance of multiple peripheral nodules or wedge-shaped opacities abutting the pleura. The nodules often demonstrate differing degrees or stages of cavitation and may show a feeding vessel leading to them (9) (Fig. 1). Because CT is more sensitive than plain films in detecting pulmonary nodules, such infected foci will be demonstrable earlier and more definitively with CT than by conventional radiographs. CT findings of septic emboli also may be the first indication of endocarditis or other intravascular source of infection in unsuspected cases (9,11).

Pneumocystis carinii Pneumonia

Computed tomography is not used routinely to diagnose *Pneumocystis carinii* pneumonia (PCP) in the ICU patient; rather, bronchoscopy with lavage is used. In unsuspected cases, however, the patient may be referred to CT for evaluation of unexplained fevers or pulmonary symptoms, and some of these patients will have evidence of unsuspected *Pneumocystis* infection. In the hope of finding a treatable complication or evidence of a mixed infection, CT evaluation also may be requested in cases of known or suspected PCP when the patient fails to respond to appropriate therapy. For these reasons, it is important to be aware of the spectrum of CT findings in PCP.

Computed tomography patterns of PCP are varied, but the most common pattern is one of diffuse or patchy ground-glass infiltrates that do not obscure bronchovascular margins (11,13). The resultant CT pattern is often dramatic and has a geometric or mosaic appearance. Increased interstitial markings can be seen in patients who have had repeated PCP infections because of the fibrosis. There is also a cystic form of the infection characterized on CT by the presence of one or more thin-walled cysts or cavities (14–18). This cystic form of PCP can be associated with CT manifestations of disseminated infection, such as calcifications in the liver, spleen, kidneys, and enlarged lymph nodes (14–18).

Spontaneous pneumothorax is a known complication of PCP infection and can be difficult to manage, particularly in the ICU patient who requires mechanical ventilation (19–21). Such pneumothoraces may be refractory to simple chest-tube evacuation, and persistent air leaks may require invasive procedures such as pleurodesis, lung stapling, or pleurectomy.

Mycobacterium Infection

Plain film findings and CT manifestations of tuberculosis in the ICU patient will depend on the patient's immune status. In the patient with normal immunity, classic manifestations of tuberculosis include cavities and bronchogenic spread of infection. Bronchogenic spread of infection has a characteristic CT appearance of "tree-in-bud opacities." These small opacities represent

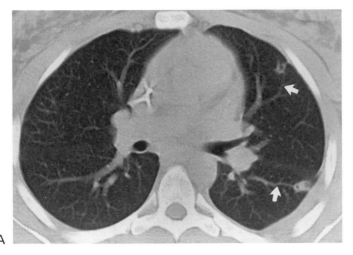

A   B

FIGURE 1. A,B: Computed tomography findings of septic emboli showing multiple peripheral nodules in varying stages of cavitation. A feeding vessel is seen leading to some of the nodules (arrows). This 22-year-old woman presented with an acute febrile syndrome, acute renal insufficiency, peritonitis, and positive blood culture for *Fusobacterium*.

inflamed bronchials that contain inspissated caseous debris that has been expelled from tuberculosis cavities.

In the immunocompromised host, tuberculosis may be atypical and more aggressive in its manifestations. It may resemble primary tuberculosis, primary progressive tuberculosis, or miliary tuberculosis. Cavities may not be present; rather, multiple pulmonary nodules or masses may be seen. In addition, mediastinal and hilar adenopathy may be present, and dissemination beyond the lungs to extrapulmonary sites may be demonstrated on CT.

Cytomegalovirus

Cytomegalovirus (CMV) is ubiquitous in acquired immunodeficiency syndrome (AIDS) patients and is a common infectious complication of organ transplantation, particularly lung transplantation (22). Clinically, CMV can cause pulmonary infiltrates and severe esophagitis. The CT findings of CMV pulmonary infection are nonspecific and mimic those of PCP. Often, both infections are identified together in the symptomatic patient.

Fungal Infections and Invasive Pulmonary Aspergillosis

Fungal infections are increasing in ICU patients. When they involve the lungs, fungal infections usually present as multiple nodules or cavities. Other nonpulmonary manifestations of fungal disease also may be detected on CT, including CT findings of esophagitis or focal lesions in the liver or spleen, indicating a disseminated infection (11). Numerous fungal species can cause pulmonary infection in the ICU patient, depending on the patient's immune status, the type of immune defect, and the underlying disease process. Considerations include infections with *Candida albicans, Coccidioides immitis, Histoplasma capsulatum, Cryptococcus neoformans,* and *Aspergillus* organisms.

The ICU patient with acute leukemia, prolonged neutropenia, and new or refractory fever despite broad-spectrum antibiotics represents a clinical scenario in which early CT examination

can be very helpful in providing a specific diagnosis. Invasive pulmonary aspergillosis (IPA) is the primary concern in this setting, and early infections have a characteristic appearance on CT: one or more pulmonary nodules or masses surrounded by a ring of ground-glass opacity called the *CT halo sign* (10) (Fig. 2). A similar appearance of IPA can be seen in other susceptible hosts, such as bone marrow and other organ-transplant recipients who are receiving immunosuppressant agents.

Blunt Thoracic Trauma

Blunt trauma from high-speed motor-vehicle accidents accounts for a significant number of ICU admissions. Head injuries,

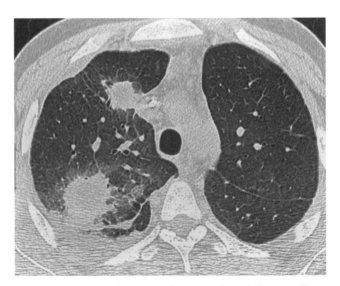

FIGURE 2. Characteristic computed tomography (CT) features of invasive pulmonary aspergillosis include the CT halo sign—a pulmonary mass surrounded by a ring of ground-glass opacity. The CT shows two masses with surrounding halos resulting from invasive fungal infection. This 22-year-old man with acute lymphocytic leukemia and pancytopenia following chemotherapy presented with fever and tachycardia.

extremity trauma, and abdominal and chest injuries are often present in isolation or in combination (23,24). With the advent of fast scanning capabilities, many institutions are screening trauma patients for such injuries using spiral and multidetector CT. In particular, trauma victims with suspected or possible aortic injuries are being evaluated increasingly with chest CT. Most of these patients have normal aortas, but many also have other serious injuries identified coincidentally on chest CT. Unsuspected injuries that can be detected by chest CT in addition to aortic transection include tracheobronchial tears; diaphragmatic rupture; esophageal tears; thoracic spine injuries; chest-wall and seat-belt injuries; lung lacerations; cardiac injuries; occult pneumothorax, pneumomediastinum, pneumopericardium, and hemothorax; and malpositioned trauma chest tubes.

Aortic Transections

The role of CT in screening patients for aortic injury is becoming less and less controversial. A negative chest CT scan obviates the need for invasive aortography in a significant number of trauma patients and has potential cost savings as a triage technique (23,25–27).

Computed tomography findings of aortic injury include mediastinal blood; aortic contour irregularities; intimal flaps; intraaortic thrombus; pseudoaneurysms; abrupt changes in caliber of the descending aorta compared with the ascending aorta ("pseudocoarctation"); and, rarely, extravascular leakage of intravenous contrast (25,28) (Fig. 3).

With spiral and multidetector CT, the aorta can be scanned rapidly using very thin, overlapping slices. This has improved our ability to evaluate the aorta directly rather than to rely on

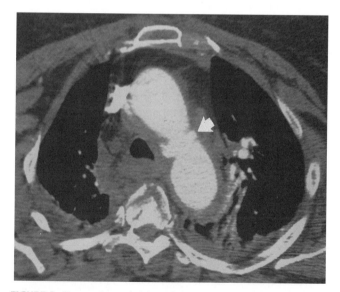

FIGURE 3. Traumatic aortic injury demonstrated with the use of multidetector computed tomography (CT) scanning. Numerous CT slices measuring 2.5 mm in thickness were obtained throughout the entire course of the aorta in less than 15 seconds. They demonstrate a focal irregularity and outpouching of the contrast column in the aortic arch compatible with a pseudoaneurysm resulting from acute aortic injury (arrow). Mediastinal blood is present, and there is also a burst fracture of the T4 vertebral body. This patient was a 70-year-old woman who fell from a mule she was riding on a farm.

indirect, less specific signs of aortic injury such as mediastinal hematoma. Gavant and colleagues, using spiral CT in 1,518 patients with blunt chest trauma, reported a sensitivity of 100% and a specificity of 81.7% for the detection of aortic injury (26).

Tracheobronchial Tears

Tracheobronchial tears frequently are missed on initial trauma evaluation, and delayed diagnosis is common. Most bronchial fractures occur within 2.5 cm of the carina (29,30). CT findings of bronchial fractures include persistent pneumothorax despite adequate placement of one or more chest tubes; massive pneumomediastinum and subcutaneous emphysema; focal peribronchial collections of air; discontinuity or irregularity of the bronchial wall; and a drooping or collapsed lung (30). When a tracheal tear is present, CT may demonstrate eccentric positioning of the endotracheal tube or projection of the tip of the endotracheal tube beyond the tracheal wall (30). Suspected tracheobronchial tears are confirmed with bronchoscopy. Long-term sequelae of unrecognized tracheobronchial tears include airway strictures or bronchomalacia that predispose the patient to recurrent atelectasis or pneumonia in the affected lobe.

Diaphragmatic Rupture

Although the chest film is usually abnormal in patients with diaphragmatic rupture, the diagnosis, nevertheless, is still frequently missed on initial trauma evaluation. Mortality in unrecognized cases is significant (30%), with bowel strangulation being one of the dire consequences (31). Early recognition and repair of diaphragmatic injuries are imperative and improve overall prognosis (32).

In cases of diaphragmatic rupture, the portable chest film may show one or more of the following: an elevated irregular diaphragm, an abnormal course of the nasogastric tube, mediastinal shift to the opposite side of the diaphragmatic injury, or bowel or abdominal contents within the chest (33–35). When the plain film is equivocal, further imaging may be required. In the acute setting, spiral or multidetector CT scanning is the method of choice. Using these fast CT scanners, thin overlapping CT slices through the diaphragm are acquired during a single breath-hold. The CT data then are used to computer-generate reconstructions in the sagittal and coronal plane. These multiplanar reconstructions are particularly helpful for detecting discontinuities in the diaphragm. Not all diaphragmatic discontinuities detected by CT are due to trauma, however. Some are related to congenital Bochdalek hernias, whereas others appear as part of the normal aging process (31–36).

Thoracic Spine Injury

Fractures of the thoracic spine occur in 3% of blunt trauma cases, and many of these fractures will cause significant spinal cord injury (29,37). Most T-spine fractures occur at the thoracoabdominal junction involving the T9–11 vertebral bodies (29,37). Sternal fractures are often associated with T-spine fractures.

Initial trauma films may fail to identify significant T-spine injuries, and many of the plain film findings are nonspecific, such as mediastinal widening, apical capping and deviation of the nasogastric tube (38). As many as 69% of patients with thoracic spine fractures will have chest film findings that suggest an aortic injury (38). By contrast, T-spine fractures are readily identifiable on CT, particularly when bone windows are used to view the images. CT data also can be used to produce sagittal and coronal images of the spinal column, which are often useful in evaluating vertebral body fractures. The extent of soft-tissue injury to the spinal cord, however, is best displayed using MRI.

Chest-wall Trauma and Rib Fractures

Rib fractures occur in 60% of blunt trauma cases, but only about 20% of rib fractures are detectable on initial trauma chest films (8,9). By contrast, rib fractures are readily apparent on trauma chest CT when the images are viewed using a bone algorithm. Fractures of the first rib usually indicate that the patient has sustained a severe impact, and they may be associated with aortic injuries, bronchial tears, or lacerations of the subclavian vessels (29,37). When five or more rib fractures in a row or three or more segmental rib fractures (two fractures in one rib) occur, a flail chest may be present. Paradoxic movement of the flail segment of the rib cage can be a cause of respiratory failure (29,37).

Lung Parenchymal Injury: Contusions, Lacerations, Hematomas, and Pneumatoceles

Pulmonary contusions occur as the result of bleeding into the alveoli from trauma. They appear quickly after trauma as focal infiltrates on both chest films and CT, and typically these infiltrates clear relatively quickly within days to weeks (37,39). Pulmonary lacerations are tears in the lung parenchyma. They may go on to form hematomas or air-filled pneumatoceles (37,39). CT is more sensitive than plain films for detection of contusions and lacerations (39).

Other common causes for lung infiltrates in trauma patients include aspiration pneumonia, atelectasis due to splinting or mucous plugs, cardiogenic and noncardiogenic pulmonary edema, and acute respiratory distress syndrome (ARDS). Fat embolization is another consideration, particularly in patients with long-bone fractures (37).

Pneumothorax and Hemothorax

Chest CT will frequently identify pneumothoraces that have gone undetected on the plain film. CT is also more specific than plain films in characterizing pleural effusions that occur in the setting of trauma. A rapidly accumulating pleural effusion is most often due to a hemothorax, but occasionally it is due to a chylothorax. With CT, the density of the fluid can be measured.

Malpositioned Chest Tubes

Chest tubes that are placed emergently in the setting of trauma can be inadvertently positioned in abnormal locations: extrathoracic, intraparenchymal, mediastinal, and within the fissures (40–42). Misdirected chest tubes also can cause lacerations of the intercostal artery, liver, spleen, and diaphragm. CT is more accurate than portable chest films in detecting malpositioned chest

tubes (41,42). A study by Mirvis and colleagues of ICU trauma patients undergoing CT identified abnormalities such as malpositioned or occluded chest tubes in 15% of their trauma patients (5).

Thoracic Vascular Disease

The number of vascular applications of spiral and multidetector CT in ICU patients continues to grow. Both types of scanners allow fast acquisition of multiple thinly collimated and overlapping slices through the vasculature during the peak phase of contrast enhancement. The CT data that are acquired can be reviewed using traditional axial images, or the data can be reformatted in other planes. In addition, the same CT data can be used to computer-generate angiographic-like images that have replaced conventional angiograms in many cases. Applications of spiral and multidetector CT in the chest include evaluation of the thoracic aorta for dissections, aneurysms, leaks, and injury (43–46). Because of the improved detailing of the pulmonary arteries, spiral and multidetector CT are being used increasingly to evaluate patients for pulmonary embolism (47–51). CT angiography also is playing a role as a substitute for conventional angiography in the evaluation of congenital vascular anomalies, vascular shunts, and pulmonary arteriovenous malformations (48).

Pulmonary Embolism

The role of CT in the evaluation of suspected pulmonary emboli is evolving rapidly. Spiral CT has a reported sensitivity for detecting central pulmonary emboli of 85% to 90% and specificity of greater than 90% (45,47–51). The accuracy of spiral CT for detecting isolated small peripheral, subsegmental emboli is still in question and appears to be lower (45,48,50,51). The risk of subsequent pulmonary embolism after a negative spiral CT is low, however: an estimated 1% in one study by Goodman and colleagues compared with 3.1% for a negative ventilation-perfusion (V/Q) scan (50). Multidetector CT represents additional technologic improvements over spiral CT, both in terms of speed and in the number of ultrathin slices that can be obtained rapidly through the pulmonary arteries. Because of these improvements, when a patient is referred to CT for suspected pulmonary embolus at our institution, we scan all such patients using a multidetector scanner.

The CT findings of acute pulmonary emboli include intravascular filling defects within contrast-enhanced pulmonary arteries (43,47) (Fig. 4). CT also can demonstrate ancillary findings, such as wedge-shaped lung opacities abutting the pleura that are due to pulmonary infarcts. In chronic thromboembolic disease, a particular pattern of mixed CT attenuation also can be seen in the lung and is called *mosaic attenuation*. Chronic thrombi tend to become adherent to the walls of the pulmonary arteries, where they form crescentic filling defects that line the walls of the vessels (43,47). These chronic clots are particularly difficult to image with conventional angiography. Spiral CT and multidetector CT, therefore, have become important alternative modalities for evaluating patients with pulmonary hypertension and suspected chronic thromboembolism (48).

What role should spiral and multidetector CT play in the evaluation of ICU patients with suspected acute pulmonary emboli?

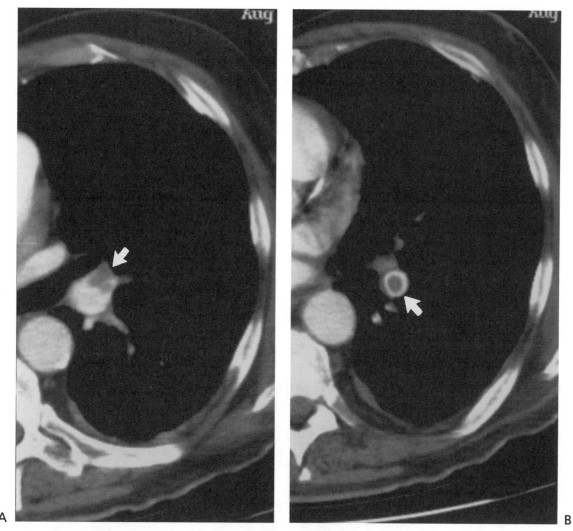

FIGURE 4. A,B: Multidetector computed tomography demonstration of acute pulmonary embolus. Fast scanning allows acquisition of multiple thin slices through the pulmonary arteries during peak contrast enhancement. A filling defect is seen in the pulmonary artery to the left lower lobe (arrow). This 62-year-old man developed acute onset of shortness of breath while gardening.

The definitive answer is likely to be determined by prospective studies that include a multicenter comparative imaging trial (48). In the meantime, several approaches can be considered. Because many, if not most, patients with suspected or possible pulmonary emboli in the ICU have abnormal chest x-rays with infiltrates and effusions, many of these patients will likely have V/Q scans that are intermediate or indeterminate in probability. Spiral and multidetector CT offer reasonable alternatives for establishing the diagnosis of significant pulmonary embolus. Spiral or multidetector CT also can be considered an alternative to angiography in patients with suspected pulmonary emboli who require verification of a high probability or indeterminate V/Q scan when there is a contraindication to anticoagulation or filter placement (48).

Part of the workup for thromboembolic disease involves a search for the most common sources of embolism. This usually requires evaluating the lower extremities for deep venous thrombosis (DVT). Doppler ultrasound is an effective noninvasive method for diagnosing DVT that does not involve radiation

exposure. The disadvantage of Doppler ultrasound is that it does not evaluate the deep pelvic veins or inferior vena cava (IVC) as effectively as the thigh veins. CT venography is an alternative method for looking for clot that does not have this disadvantage. CT venography involves scanning the lower extremities from the knees up through the pelvis and up to the IVC if necessary. The study can be performed immediately after a multidetector CT study of the chest to rule out pulmonary embolism and therefore uses just one dose of intravenous contrast. The disadvantage of CT venography is that it increases the gonadal radiation dose significantly.

EVALUATING COMPLEX PLEURAL DISEASE IN THE ICU PATIENT

Pleural processes are often complex in the ICU patient and difficult to diagnose based solely on clinical grounds and portable chest films. Commonly asked questions in the ICU include the following: (a) Is the opacity on portable chest x-ray due to a large pleural effusion, empyema, or hemothorax? (b) Is the focal air-fluid level seen on chest x-ray due to a lung abscess or empyema? (c) Is this a malignant pleural effusion? (d) Why is this pleural effusion refractory to thoracentesis or chest tube drainage, and is it loculated? (e) Can the interventional radiologist drain this effusion (empyema, malignant effusion, and refractory pneumothorax)? CT evaluation frequently provides important additional information over the plain films that help to answer these questions.

Pleural Space Infection: Does the Patient Have an Empyema?

Computed tomography features of empyema or complicated parapneumonic effusion include thickening of the visceral and parietal pleura that enhances with intravenous contrast (52,53). Pleural fluid trapped between the thickened, enhancing pleurae forms the "split-pleura sign" (52,53) (Fig. 5). Any type of exudative effusion can produce the split-pleura sign, but in the patient with fever or sepsis, it is most often due to infection (52,54,55). CT demonstration of gas bubbles in pleural fluid collections usually indicates one of three things: (a) a recent thoracentesis or invasive procedure has been performed and introduced air into the pleural space; (b) a bronchopleural fistula has developed; or (c) a gas-forming organism is present.

Is This Air-Fluid Level Due to a Lung Abscess or Empyema?

Distinguishing a lung abscess from empyema based on portable ICU chest film may be difficult, and CT can help (52–54,56). On CT, empyemas usually are oblong shaped, and the collection compresses and displaces the adjacent lung and airways. The inner walls of empyemas are smooth and demonstrate the split-pleura sign. Lung abscesses are usually round with irregular inner margins of the cavity. Rather than compress adjacent lung, abscesses destroy lung to form a cavity. A lung abscess often forms an acute angle with the pleural surface (52–54,56).

Is This A Malignant Pleural Effusion?

Computed tomography often is requested in the setting of a new, unexplained pleural effusion to rule out malignancy. On CT, malignant pleural effusions demonstrate irregular pleural

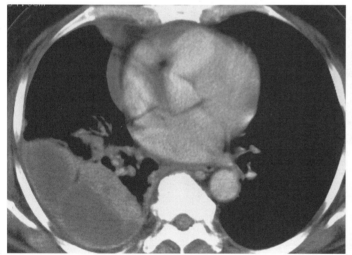

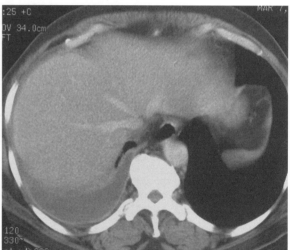

FIGURE 5. Computed tomography (CT)-assisted management of purulent fluid collection. A 63-year-old man with right lower-lobe pneumonia and persistent pleural effusion. **A,B:** CT demonstrates a loculated right pleural fluid collection with enhancing visceral and parietal pleura: the "split pleura sign." Thoracentesis revealed purulent fluid with a pH of 6.6, low glucose level, high lactate dehydrogenase level, and elevated white blood cell count. **C:** An image-guided percutaneous pigtail catheter was placed, and a repeat CT showed marked drainage of the pleural collection. (B,C: Reproduced from Kuhman JE. Complex disease of the pleural space: the 10 questions most frequently asked of the radiologist—new approaches to their answers with CT and MR imaging. *Radiographics* 1997;17:1043–1050, with permission.)

thickening, often with nodules in the pleural space that enhance with intravenous contrast. Malignancy usually involves all pleural surfaces, including the mediastinal pleural surfaces; and it often causes marked pleural thickening exceeding a 1-cm depth (52,54,57–60). CT also may show evidence of other metastatic disease to the lung; bones or lymph nodes and CT can be used to look in the lung, breast tissue, or thymus for a primary tumor (58).

Refractory Pleural Effusions or Pneumothoraces: Why Will This Collection not Drain?

Pleural collections of air or fluid may fail to drain with thoracentesis or chest tube placement. Reasons include the following: (a) improperly positioned or malfunctioning chest tubes; (b) the pleural collections are loculated; (c) the pleural fluid is thick and viscous, as can occur with some chronic empyemas, malignant effusions, or hemothoraces; and (d) a persistent pneumothorax or hydropneumothorax may be due to a bronchopleural fistula.

A bronchopleural fistula (BPF) is a communication between the airways or lung parenchyma and the pleural space (61). A BPF can form in the setting of necrotizing pneumonia, bronchiectasis, tumor, trauma, surgery, barotrauma, and complicated emphysema. CT findings can establish the diagnosis of BPF and sometimes will indicate the underlying cause (61,62). CT may show air and fluid in the pleural space as well as the presence of a communicating tract to the pleural space (61).

Thoracic Interventional Procedures: Can the Interventional Radiologist Drain This Collection (Empyema, Malignant Effusion, Refractory Pneumothorax, or Pneumocele)?

With the aid of image guidance, the answer is often yes. The use of image-guided interventional procedures in the chest and elsewhere in the body has increased dramatically in recent years (63–74). New approaches to management of complex pleural processes include the following: (a) using CT to assess chest-tube positioning and effectiveness of drainage; (b) using image guidance to direct thoracenteses, pleural biopsies, and small-bore catheter drainage; (c) using CT to provide localization for thoracoscopy (54,65,66,69,70).

The loculated or refractory empyema or pneumothorax that fails to drain with conventional chest-tube placement often can be evacuated using small-bore, flexible drainage catheters that are positioned under CT, fluoroscopic, or ultrasound guidance (4,52,63,68,75). Ultrasound, because it is portable to the ICU, is often the first technique used to guide pleural drainage procedures; however, loculated pleural collections may be difficult to locate with ultrasound and often require CT image guidance (2). Image-guided catheter placement can be used with fibrinolytic agents such as streptokinase or urokinase to treat loculated empyemas or hemothoraces, and this approach may obviate the need for operative decortication (57,63,71–73,76). Malignant pleural effusions also can be managed palliatively using small-bore, flexible drainage catheters placed under image guidance. Once adequate drainage has been achieved, a sclerosing agent can be

instilled through the same catheter for sclerotherapy (63,64,77–79).

Image-guided percutaneous catheter drainage is also an effective treatment option for refractory pneumatoceles and lung abscesses, particularly in mechanically ventilated patients who have ARDS (75). Percutaneous catheter drainage of these collections does not appear to increase the risk of BPF or pneumothorax (75). Persistent pneumothoraces and large barotrauma-related pneumatoceles may be causes of failure to wean or cardiopulmonary deterioration in patients with severe respiratory failure (Fig. 6). Many of these refractory air collections are loculated and relatively inaccessible to conventional chest tubes placed blindly at the bedside (75). With image guidance, small-bore drainage catheters can be placed directly into loculated air collections, and because they are flexible, patients better tolerate these small-bore catheters (75).

Central Venous Catheter Complications

Indwelling catheters, particularly central venous catheters, and other devices are used extensively in the ICU patient. Such catheters are often indispensable for providing essential drugs, blood products, and hyperalimentation; however, they are associated with significant complications. Pneumothorax is the most common immediate complication following catheter placement, and postcatheter-placement chest films are mandatory. Central catheters also may become a nidus for clot formation or infection that can lead to pulmonary infarcts and septic emboli. Spiral or multidetector CT scans performed with intravenous contrast can detect not only evidence of pulmonary infarcts or septic emboli, as discussed in previous sections, but also may identify evidence of clot around the distal ends of central catheters. CT also may show that the catheter has caused more extensive thrombosis of an innominate, subclavian, or jugular vein.

Hickman catheters and other operatively placed catheters sometimes become infected around their entrance site in the chest wall. Severe chest-wall infections can result, particularly when invasive *Aspergillus* organisms are the culprit, and may require extensive chest-wall debridement. When an intravenous catheter is improperly positioned, it can erode outside the vessel lumen into the pleural space or the mediastinum. Rapidly enlarged pleural effusions, hematomas, or mediastinitis may result. Broken-off catheters can migrate through the venous system, eventually lodging in the heart or pulmonary arteries. Such sheared off catheter fragments are sometimes difficult to recognize on limited portable ICU films, but they are readily identified on noncontrast CT scans as high-density tubular structures in the vascular system. Embolized catheter fragments often can be removed by interventional radiologists using retrieval baskets and other catheter devices. Accurate localization of the catheter fragment with CT facilitates such attempts at retrieval (80).

ABDOMINAL IMAGING IN THE ICU

The ICU patient with sepsis or an acute abdomen represents a difficult and complex clinical problem. Many of these patients are

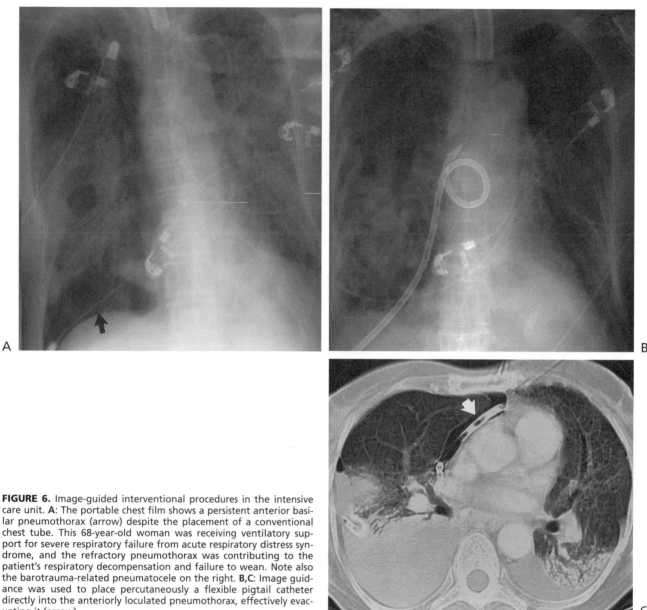

FIGURE 6. Image-guided interventional procedures in the intensive care unit. **A:** The portable chest film shows a persistent anterior basilar pneumothorax (arrow) despite the placement of a conventional chest tube. This 68-year-old woman was receiving ventilatory support for severe respiratory failure from acute respiratory distress syndrome, and the refractory pneumothorax was contributing to the patient's respiratory decompensation and failure to wean. Note also the barotrauma-related pneumatocele on the right. **B,C:** Image guidance was used to place percutaneously a flexible pigtail catheter directly into the anteriorly loculated pneumothorax, effectively evacuating it (arrow).

critically ill with multisystem failure and require urgent medical or surgical attention. Patient obtundation or sedation may hamper clinical assessment. Underlying immunodeficiency, recent surgery, ongoing pain medications, and use of corticosteroids frequently mask common signs and symptoms and dampen the host's normal response to serious abdominal illness. An accurate diagnosis must be arrived at expeditiously, preferably through the use of noninvasive techniques. The presence of multiple coexisting disorders further compounds the problem. Signs and symptoms may be similar for a wide variety of conditions involving any number of abdominal organ systems (81).

Computed tomography remains the most versatile and clinically useful of the advanced imaging techniques in this setting. The ability to evaluate multiple anatomic sites and structures rapidly and accurately with CT, including the bowel, solid organs, retroperitoneum, peritoneal cavity, and vasculature, is un-

paralleled. Ultrasound, because it is portable and can be done at the bedside, also has many important and useful applications in the critically ill ICU patient (82). Particularly in the abdomen, many conditions can be accurately diagnosed with this imaging technique without having to transport the patient. As a technique, however, ultrasound has significant limitations in many ICU patients, particularly with regard to the postoperative patient who has abdominal wound incisions and complicating drains and hardware that interfere with an effective ultrasound examination (81). In addition, the ultrasound examination, by its very nature, is less global and comprehensive, and it is considerably operator dependent (81). CT, therefore, remains the most powerful tool at the clinician's and radiologist's disposal for pinpointing the probable site and cause of acute abdominal disorders in ICU patients. CT findings may help to triage the ICU patient between surgical and medical management by narrowing the list of diagnostic possibilities and directing further workup to those organ systems most likely to be involved. In the setting of major trauma, CT examination of the abdomen and pelvis has become routine in the exclusion of major abdominal organ injury.

When evaluating the ICU patient with acute abdominal symptoms, a survey examination of the entire abdomen and pelvis is usually required. Administration of oral and intravenous contrast media is ideal but not always possible. Adequate amounts of oral contrast are essential to opacify the bowel. Because bowel perforation is often occult in these patents, a water-soluble oral contrast material is used. Intravenous contrast administration is critical for evaluating the patency of vessels and is very helpful in demonstrating renal, liver, splenic, and solid-organ pathology. Administration of intravenous contrast may not always be possible, however, when there is a history of severe contrast reaction or in the setting of impending or profound renal insufficiency. A recent study, however, has suggested the protective effect of pretreatment with oral N-acetyl-cysteine in patients with renal insufficiency who undergo intravenous contrast CT studies (83).

Right Upper-Quadrant Conditions and Considerations

Nausea, vomiting, and right upper-quadrant tenderness may indicate a right upper-quadrant cause for sepsis or acute abdomen. Diseases that affect the liver, biliary tract, gastric antrum or duodenum, pancreas, or right kidney may be involved. Entities as diverse as hepatitis, liver abscess, biloma, cholangitis, cholecystitis peptic ulcer disease, pancreatitis, renal abscess, infarct, or bleed are diagnostic considerations.

Liver and Biliary Tract

Several disease processes affect the liver and biliary tract in ICU patients and produce right upper-quadrant pain, fever, and elevated liver function tests (82). The differential diagnosis includes infection, hepatitis, liver abscess, cholangitis, and cholecystitis. Postoperative complications include abscess, biloma, and hematoma as well as vascular complications due to portal vein thrombosis and, less commonly, hepatic infarcts.

Demonstration by CT of multiple, round, low-density liver lesions may be the first indication of a disseminated bacterial, viral, or fungal infection in the ICU patient with fever of unknown origin. In the postoperative patient, particularly those receiving liver transplants, complications include anastomotic leak, liver abscess, biloma, hematoma, and vascular complications due to thrombosis or anastomotic strictures. CT findings in the liver can be used to direct further diagnostic and therapeutic maneuvers, such as liver biopsy, aspiration, and drainage.

Fatty infiltration of the liver, hepatitis, and cirrhosis cause diffuse parenchymal liver changes on CT and ultrasound examinations and are commonly found abnormalities in ICU patients. Hepatic infarcts can be seen in the setting of sepsis, systemic vasculitis, and as a complication of some liver surgeries. On CT, hepatic infarcts appear as geographic and wedge-shaped areas that demonstrate less intravenous contrast enhancement compared to the rest of the liver.

Cholecystitis and cholangitis are additional diagnostic considerations. When acute cholecystitis is suspected, ultrasound is usually the first imaging modality used to establish the diagnosis (82). Both ultrasound and CT can demonstrate findings indicative of acute cholecystitis, including the presence of a dilated gallbladder with a thickened edematous wall, surrounding pericholecystic inflammation or fluid, and the presence of gallstones (82). Air in the wall of the gallbladder indicates emphysematous cholecystitis.

Biliary duct dilation is another important finding that may indicate the presence of bile duct obstruction or cholangitis. Finding air in the biliary tree on CT or ultrasound usually indicates one of the following: biliary tract infection; a recent or previous surgical or gastrointestinal procedure, such as endoscopic retrograde cholangiopancreatography (ERCP) with sphincterotomy; or the presence of an enteric–biliary communication, such as a fistula or surgically created communication.

Pancreas

Pancreatitis, pancreatic pseudocyst, and phlegmon are most reliably identified by CT (82) (Fig. 7). The presence of pancreatic necrosis also can be evaluated using CT by assessing the degree and uniformity of gland enhancement after rapid bolus administration of intravenous contrast (82). CT also plays an important role in monitoring patients with severe pancreatitis for the development of complications such as abscesses, pseudoaneurysms, and enlarging peripancreatic fluid collections. Many peripancreatic fluid collections, including pseudocysts and abscesses, can be effectively drained using image-guided percutaneous techniques, often obviating the need for more invasive open surgical procedures.

In most cases, CT or ultrasound initially will be used in the evaluation of pancreatic, biliary, and liver disease. In the special setting of biliary or pancreatic duct obstruction, however, when ultrasound and CT do not provide an answer regarding the cause of the obstruction, MRI may play an adjunctive role. A special

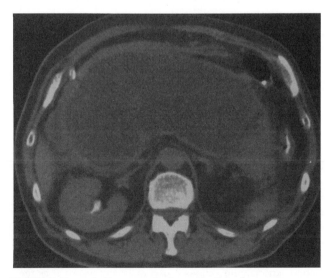

FIGURE 7. Computed tomography demonstration of a massive pancreatic pseudocyst that has replaced most of the pancreas. Such a collection would be amenable to image-guided percutaneous catheter drainage.

type of MRI examination called an MRCP (magnetic resonance cholangiopancreatography) uses heavily T2-weighted sequences. The data from this special MRI examination can be manipulated to produce cholangiographic-like images of the biliary tree, common bile duct, and pancreatic duct, similar to those obtained from ERCP or percutaneous cholangiography. Such images have been used to diagnose the cause of biliary tract obstruction, such as biliary calculi, masses, and strictures, in an entirely noninvasive way.

Left Upper-Quadrant Considerations

Left upper-quadrant pathology encountered in ICU patients includes gastritis, pancreatitis, and diseases involving the left kidney and spleen, such as septic infarction. Septic emboli to the spleen or the kidneys appear on CT and ultrasound as focal, often wedged-shaped lesions that show poor contrast enhancement. Splenic and kidney infarcts can be the result of both bland infarcts and septic arterial emboli.

Renal and Retroperitoneal Considerations

A wide array of renal conditions, including pyelonephritis, renal abscess, renal infarction, and traumatic renal injuries and lacerations, are effectively diagnosed using CT (84). Perinephric collections surrounding native kidneys or renal transplants are also readily identified using CT or ultrasound, including perinephric seromas, hematomas, urinomas, lymphoceles, and abscesses. Such collections may be a source of fever and infection or, if large enough, can cause renal failure secondary to obstruction. CT findings serve as an indispensable guide for planning diagnostic or therapeutic drainage procedures on such collections.

Computed tomography can be used to diagnose hydronephrosis rapidly and to search for the cause of ureteral obstruction. Considerations include ureteral calculi, tumor masses, and adenopathy, retroperitoneal fibrosis, and fungus balls. To detect renal and ureteral calculi, a non-contrast CT scan should be performed before the administration of intravenous contrast (84).

Spontaneous retroperitoneal or perinephric bleeds are important causes of unexplained blood loss and may occur in the setting of sepsis and disseminated intravascular coagulopathy, overanticoagulation, or coagulopathies. Acute bleeds are easily evaluated and quantified on CT (Fig. 8).

Renal infarction may be secondary to bland or septic arterial emboli, vasculitis, trauma, or arterial or venous thrombosis. Renal infarcts due to segmental arterial occlusion have a characteristic appearance on CT, appearing as wedge-shaped, poorly enhancing defects in the renal parenchyma when intravenous contrast is administered. With the advent of spiral and multidetector CT scanning, computer generation of angiographic-like images (CT angiography) of the renal vascular anatomy is now routinely possible. Such CT-generated images facilitate detection of both arterial and venous causes of infarction, such as renal artery thrombosis or occlusion, renal vascular pedicle injuries, and renal vein thrombosis.

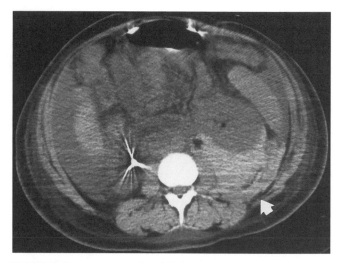

FIGURE 8. Spontaneous perinephric hematoma. A computed tomography (CT) scan was requested to investigate an unexplained drop in hematocrit in this patient in the intensive care unit with sepsis and disseminated intravascular coagulopathy. CT demonstrates a large left perinephric fluid collection with high CT attenuation resulting from acute blood (arrow). (Reprinted from Kuhlman JE. Renal and urinary tract complications. In: Kuhlman JE, ed. *CT of the immunocompromised host.* New York: Churchill Livingstone, 1991:101, with permission.)

Acute Renal Failure due to Acute Tubular Necrosis

Numerous renal insults can precipitate renal failure and the development of acute tubular necrosis (ATN), including sepsis and prolonged hypotension, dehydration, and exposure to nephrotoxic drugs, such as aminoglycoside and amphotericin B. Often the cause is multifactorial (84). Intravenous contrast can cause or contribute to the development of ATN and should be avoided, if possible, in patients with new or impending renal failure.

Gastrointestinal Tract

In the ICU setting, evaluation of the gastrointestinal tract is particularly difficult using conventional techniques such as barium studies (85–87). Although CT does not provide mucosal detail of the bowel, it does allow rapid survey of the gastrointestinal tract for important findings, such as focal bowel-wall thickening, pneumatosis, pneumoperitoneum, and interloop abscesses. Often, the likely site of bowel involvement can be identified with CT, whether it is the esophagus, stomach, duodenum, proximal, or distal small bowel, cecum, or rectosigmoid colon. Once a suspicious area has been identified on CT, endoscopy or colonoscopy can be directed more specifically toward these affected areas for further evaluation and biopsy, if necessary. In addition, CT is superior to conventional gastrointestinal studies in detecting the presence and extent of extraluminal disease, such as peritonitis, ascites, mesenteritis, carcinomatosis, abscesses, adenopathy, and masses. CT also may demonstrate important findings that indicate the presence of bowel ischemia and, if adequate amounts of intravenous contrast are used, CT can assess the patency of proximal major vessels, such as the celiac axis and the superior mesenteric artery and vein.

Right Lower-Quadrant Considerations

Causes of right lower-quadrant pathology in the ICU patient include such diverse entities as acute appendicitis, Meckel diverticulum, infectious or ischemic colitis or ileitis, neutropenic colitis (typhlitis), graft-versus-host disease, inflammatory bowel disease, pseudomembranous colitis, right-sided diverticulitis, and perforated colon cancer. Emergent CT examination of patients with right lower-quadrant pain often identifies the cause of symptoms and effectively triages patients between surgical and medical management.

An increasingly common complication seen in ICU patients is the development of pseudomembranous colitis (85). Pseudomembranous colitis is caused by an overgrowth of *Clostridium difficile* that occurs when antibiotic use alters the normal colonic flora (85,86). *C. difficile* produces a toxin that incites inflammation, ulceration, and sloughing of the colonic mucosa. Severe cases may progress to toxic megacolon and perforation. When pseudomembranous colitis is suspected, the diagnosis can be established by isolating *C. difficile* toxin within the stool or demonstrating pseudomembranes at colonoscopy (85,86). Particularly in the critically ill ICU patient, however, pseudomembranous colitis may not be suspected initially because of atypical presentations or because characteristic signs and symptoms are masked by concurrent problems. CT findings may be the first clue to the correct diagnosis (85). Although many of the CT findings of pseudomembranous colitis are nonspecific, such as colonic wall thickening and edema and overlap with entities such as CMV colitis and ischemic colitis, the pattern of distribution is often quite characteristic. The findings in pseudomembranous colitis are striking in the marked degree of colonic wall thickening, and typically, although not always, the colon is uniformly affected from cecum to anus (85) (Fig. 9).

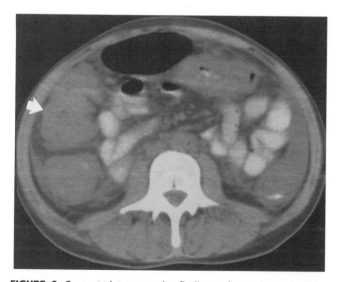

FIGURE 9. Computed tomography findings of pseudomembranous colitis showing marked colonic wall thickening involving the entire colon with the most severe changes noted in the cecum and right colon (arrow).

Typhlitis

Typhlitis, also known as neutropenic colitis, is a severe inflammatory process that targets the cecum, but it also may involve the terminal ileum and appendix. The inflammation can lead to mural ischemia, ulceration, and perforation. It is a condition seen primarily in patients with leukemia and severe neutropenia, but it also has been seen in other severely immunocompromised patients. CT typically shows marked bowel-wall thickening of the cecum, ulcerations, and pericolonic edema. Findings may be similar to those seen with CMV colitis/ileitis.

Left Lower-Quadrant Considerations

Computed tomography is a noninvasive and accurate way to detect causes of left lower-quadrant pain, including acute diverticulitis and its complications of perforation and peridiverticular abscess (87,88). It can be performed without special patient preparation, without delay, and it avoids the potential risks of perforation that conventional barium enema studies pose in this setting.

Gastrointestinal Perforation

When gastrointestinal perforation occurs in the ICU patient, the presentation may be obvious and catastrophic (86,87). In other instances, however, perforation initially may go unrecognized because its presentation can be remarkably occult and the cause equally obscure. Signs and symptoms of perforation may be masked by medications, antibiotics, and altered mental status, and they frequently overlap with other nonsurgical disorders such as pancreatitis. Even tiny amounts of free air that may go undetected with portable abdominal radiographs are readily identifiable on CT. The presence of pneumoperitoneum indicates the presence of bowel perforation unless some other cause of free air can be established, for example, recent intraabdominal surgery, invasive procedures, or extension of pneumomediastinum into the abdomen. The likely site of perforation often can be established with CT by searching for ancillary findings, such as ulcers, focal areas of abnormal bowel wall thickening, or localized fluid collections that occur in the vicinity of the perforated bowel segment (86,87).

Gastrointestinal Obstruction

Symptoms or signs of partial or complete bowel obstruction are other indications for CT evaluation of the ICU patient. In the setting of bowel obstruction, CT aids in identifying the level of the obstruction, its cause, and other associated complications such as ischemic compromise, perforation, or abscess formation.

Ischemic Bowel

Bowel ischemia in critically ill patients may be due to many different causes, including prolonged hypotension, systemic vasculitis, arterial embolism, and traumatic and nontraumatic causes of vascular compromise (81). CT findings of ischemic bowel include thumbprinting and thickening of the bowel wall. These findings are nonspecific, however, and can be seen in inflammatory bowel disease, such as Crohn disease, and with bleeding into the bowel wall. Nonspecific bowel dilatation also may be seen, and abnormal enhancement of the bowel may be present. When there has been infarction and necrosis of the bowel, CT may demonstrate air in the bowel wall or pneumatosis intestinalis. Air also may be detected in the mesenteric veins, portal vein, and within the intrahepatic portal venous branches (86).

Occult Sites of Infection or Bleeding

There are numerous sites in the abdomen and pelvis where occult abscesses and hematomas may collect; these sites include the retroperitoneum and the iliopsoas, paraspinal, and gluteal muscles. Occult osteomyelitis may affect the lumbar spine, the sacrum, and pelvic bones. Hematomas forming in the retroperitoneum and other occult sites can become massive and can account for significant blood loss (Fig. 8). They may be postsurgical as a result of bleeding diathesis or anticoagulant therapy or secondary to trauma. Bleeding complications are, in fact, common in ICU patients and can occur at any site: in the brain, in the lung, in the bowel wall, in solid abdominal organs, in soft tissues or muscles, and within the pericardium. Acute and subacute bleeds and hematomas are easily recognized on CT by their high CT attenuation. Many hematomas have mixed CT attenuation with high- and low-density components reflecting different stages of clot formation or lysis. Often, a serum hematocrit level can be identified on CT (89).

IMAGING OF THE CENTRAL NERVOUS SYSTEM

Evaluating the CNS in the ICU patient poses particular challenges for the intensivist. Clinical history and physical examination are rarely straightforward. The ICU patient may be obtunded, sedated, or have altered mental status secondary to drugs, sepsis, postoperative state, or pain medications. Even relatively minor deficits found on physical examination may indicate that serious CNS abnormalities are present (90,91). Probably nowhere else in the ICU does advanced imaging with CT and MRI play a more crucial role in the evaluation process. Although CT remains the initial imaging modality of choice in most instances of acute neurologic disorders and in the setting of acute trauma, MRI is being used increasingly to follow the progress of many CNS insults. MRI also has a special role in the evaluation of spinal cord pathology. Whereas CT depicts acute hemorrhage and skeletal fractures better than MRI, the soft-tissue differentiation of MRI is superior (91).

Brain Infarction

Stroke may be due to thrombosis; embolism; hypotension; or vascular spasm, compression, or obstruction (91). One of the primary objectives of emergency imaging of the acute stroke patient is to detect any evidence of CNS hemorrhage, thus differentiating between a hemorrhagic stroke and a bland infarct (Fig. 10). Noncontrast head CT remains the imaging modality of choice for this task. It is important to be aware, however, that within the first 24 hours of a stroke, the CT findings of acute infarct may be difficult to discern and a follow-up CT is often required to

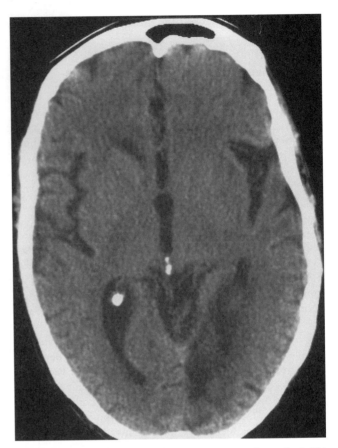

FIGURE 10. Acute stroke occurring in a postoperative patient. This 81-year-old man developed changes in mental status following repair of a ruptured abdominal aortic aneurysm. Computed tomography demonstrates a large, nonhemorrhagic infarct involving the posterior left hemisphere in the distribution of the posterior left cerebral artery.

detect focal abnormalities that indicate the location and extent of the infarct (91).

Acute Intracerebral Hemorrhage

Bleeding into the brain parenchyma may be due to a hemorrhagic stroke or secondary to head trauma; it may result from a bleeding aneurysm or AVM; or it may occur because of bleeding into a neoplasm or bland infarct. Parenchymal blood is high density on CT compared with normal brain tissue and is readily identifiable (91).

Subarachnoid Hemorrhage

Because acute and subacute blood appear high density compared with normal brain tissue and cerebrospinal fluid on CT, head CT is the test of choice for diagnosing subarachnoid bleeds (Fig. 11). The density of active, ongoing bleeding, however, may be similar to that of the brain tissue. Causes of subarachnoid bleeding include head trauma, bleeding aneurysms, arteriovenous malformations, and dural fistulas. Subarachnoid hemorrhage may cause herniation due to mass effect, secondary hydrocephalus, and vasospasm severe enough to produce brain infarction (91).

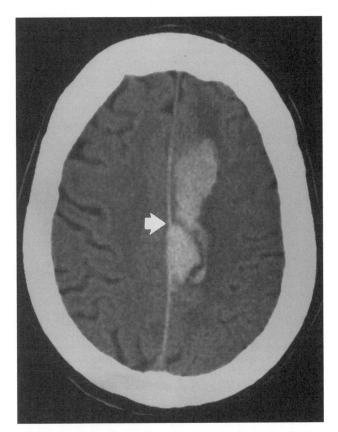

FIGURE 11. An 86-year-old woman fell and hit her head after developing third-degree heart block. Computed tomography shows subarachnoid hemorrhage (arrow) and an adjacent intraparenchymal hematoma on the left. Acute and subacute blood are high density compared with normal brain tissue and normal cerebrospinal fluid.

CNS Infection

As the complexity of diseases treated in the ICU and the degree to which ICU patients are immunocompromised increase, the number and variety of CNS infections have increased. All manner of organisms may cause meningitis; encephalitis; ventriculitis; and epidural, subdural, and brain abscesses, including bacteria, fungi, and viral agents (90). The most common bacterial culprits include *Pseudomonas*, *Staphylococcus aureus*, and *Streptococcus pneumoniae* (90,91). In the organ-transplant recipient, the patient with lymphoma or leukemia, or the patient with AIDS, however, other unusual CNS pathogens must be considered, including CMV, herpes virus, *Listeria*, *Toxoplasma gondii*, *Aspergillus*, mucormycosis, *Cryptococcus*, *Candida*, *Nocardia*, and *Mycobacterium* (90).

Central nervous system infections may result from infections in the adjacent sinuses, mastoid air cells, or skull bones that extend into the CNS; or they may result as a complication of surgery, trauma, or invasive procedures. The CNS also may be seeded hematogenously by blood-borne pathogens arising from infected heart valves and other intravascular foci of infection. In addition, patients with pulmonary AVMs and right-to-left cardiac shunts are at risk of developing brain abscesses (90,91).

The CT findings in cases of infectious meningitis include the presence of hydrocephalus, atrophy, and meningeal enhancement when intravenous contrast is administered. CT findings of brain abscess include focal, round, low CT attenuation lesions that often demonstrate a distinct ring of contrast enhancement surrounding them. If ventriculitis is also present, the ependyma will abnormally enhance as well. In many instances, MRI may display more dramatically the presence and extent of CNS infections, particularly brain abscesses, because of its superior soft-tissue differentiation (90,91).

Central Nervous System Trauma

Computed tomography remains the imaging modality of first resort in the setting of acute head trauma (91). CT is highly sensitive for detecting fractures, acute intracerebral hemorrhage, and acute subarachnoid, epidural, and subdural hematomas. MRI is more time consuming and less versatile in the acutely injured and unstable trauma patient. It requires the use of completely nonferromagnetic stabilization and monitoring devices (91). In addition, MRI demonstrates fractures and some stages of acute blood less well than CT; however, MRI is increasingly used in the follow-up of head trauma patients, after stabilization and initial management. Particularly in the later stages of head injury, MRI may more accurately display the extent of brain injury and its complications (91).

Head injuries can be divided into extraaxial and intraaxial injuries (91). Subdural and epidural hematomas and subarachnoid bleeds are examples of extraaxial injuries, whereas sheer injuries, contusions, intracerebral bleeds, and brainstem transections represent intraaxial injuries. Head injuries can be complicated by herniation, hydrocephalus, infarction, hemorrhage, and cerebrospinal leaks (91).

Spinal cord injuries in the acutely traumatized patient are usually due to fractures, subluxations, and dislocations of the bony structures of the spinal canal. Initial emergency room evaluation of the spine relies on screening radiographs, but these are immediately supplemented with emergent CT evaluation for more accurate and detailed examination of the spine when required. Both CT and MRI may play an important role in evaluating spinal cord injuries (91). Whereas CT displays bone injuries better, including the location of small bone fragments, MRI provides better visualization of spinal cord tissue (91). MRI may be crucial for determining the extent of spinal cord injury secondary to edema, hematoma, or compression by disc herniation, bone fragments, or subluxation (91). MRI is also the imaging modality of choice for the evaluation of nontraumatic spine disorders, such as acute cord compression, which may be due to extradural or intradural lesions often from metastatic disease (91).

SUMMARY

Advanced imaging plays an increasingly important role in the management of today's complex ICU patient. CT, ultrasound, and MRI supplement the portable bedside x-ray and often provide additional information that is critical for the prompt evaluation of thoracic, abdominal, and neurologic conditions that affect ICU patients. Indications for advanced imaging in the ICU can be summarized as in the Key Points.

KEY POINTS

Early detection and diagnosis: In the ICU patient with non-specific symptoms, fever of unknown origin, unexplained sepsis, or altered mental status, further evaluation with advanced imaging may be critical for documenting the presence or absence of significant disease, particularly when routine plain films fail to provide a definitive answer.

Confirmation and characterization of plain film findings: In cases where the portable chest or abdominal film is complex, confusing, or equivocal, advanced imaging with CT or ultrasound may help to characterize further the nature and extent of the abnormality in a more precise cross-sectional format and narrow the differential diagnosis.

Search for possible or suspected complications: When ICU patients fail to respond to appropriate therapy or their condi-

tion inexplicably worsens, complications must be considered. Advanced imaging is often the most expeditious method for conducting such a search and identifying complications.

Plan invasive diagnostic or therapeutic procedures: Advanced imaging provides important anatomic information that serves as a road map for planning many invasive procedures, such as bronchoscopy, thoracoscopy, open surgical procedures, and image-guided therapeutic maneuvers such as percutaneous biopsy and catheter drainage.

Monitor disease progress: In many ICU settings, advanced imaging is more accurate than plain films for documenting the response to therapy, for determining the adequacy of drainage, or for identifying changes in the nature of disease that might suggest a new process has developed.

REFERENCES

1. Goodman LR, Putman CE, eds. *Critical care imaging*, 3rd ed. Philadelphia: WB Saunders, 1992.
2. White CS, Meyer CA, Wu J, et al. Portable CT: assessing thoracic disease in the intensive care unit. *AJR Am J Roentgenol* 1999;173:1351–1356.
3. Winer-Muram HT, Tubin SA, Ellis JV, et al. Pneumonia and ARDS in patients receiving mechanical ventilation: diagnostic accuracy of chest radiography. *Radiology* 1993;288:479–485.
4. Miller WT, Tino G, Friedburg JS. Thoracic CT in the intensive care unit: assessment of clinical usefulness. *Radiology* 1998;209:491–498.
5. Mirvis SE, Tobin KD, Kostrubiak I, et al. Thoracic CT in detecting occult disease in critically ill patients. *AJR Am J Roentgenol* 1987;148:685–689.
6. Golding RP, Knape P, Strack RJM, et al. Computed tomography as an adjunct to chest x-rays of intensive care unit patients. *Crit Care Med* 1988;16:211–216.
7. Snow N, Bergin KT, Horrigan TP. Thoracic CT scanning in critically ill patients: information obtained frequently alters management. *Chest* 1990;97:1467–1470.
8. Peruzzi W, Garner W, Bools J, et al. Portable chest roentgenography and computed tomography in critically ill patients. *Chest* 1988;93:722–726.
9. Kuhlman JE, Fishman EK, Teigen C. Pulmonary septic emboli: diagnosis with CT. *Radiology* 1990;174:211–213.
10. Kuhlman JE, Fishman EK, Siegleman SS. Invasive pulmonary aspergillosis in acute leukemia: characteristic findings on CT, the CT halo sign, and the role of CT in early diagnosis. *Radiology* 1985;157:611–614.
11. Kuhlman JE, Fishman EK, Hruban RH, et al. Diseases of the chest in AIDS: CT diagnosis. *Radiographics* 1989;9:827–857.
12. Deleted in page proofs.
13. Kuhlman JE, Kavuru M, Fishman EK, et al. *Pneumocystis carinii* pneumonia: spectrum of parenchymal CT findings: *Radiology* 1990;175:711–714.
14. Kuhlman JE, Knowles MC, Fishman EK, et al. Premature bullous damage in AIDS: CT diagnosis. *Radiology* 1989;173:23–26.
15. Panicek DM. Cystic pulmonary lesions in patients with AIDS. *Radiology* 1989;173:12–14.
16. Gurney JW, Bates FT. Pulmonary cystic disease: comparison of *Pneumocystis carinii* pneumatoceles and bullous emphysema due to intravenous drug abuse. *Radiology* 1989;173:27–31.
17. Sandhu J, Goodman PC. Pulmonary cysts associated with *Pneumocystis carinii* pneumonia in patients with AIDS. *Radiology* 1989;173:33–35.
18. Radin DR, Baker EL, Klatt EC, et al. Visceral and nodal calcification in patients with AIDS-related *Pneumocystis carinii* infection. *AJR Am J Roentgenol* 1990;154:27–31.
19. Joe L, Gordin F, Parker RH. Spontaneous pneumothorax in *Pneumocystis carinii* infection. *Arch Intern Med* 1986;146:1816–1817.
20. Goodman PC, Daley C, Minagi H. Spontaneous pneumothorax in AIDS patients with *Pneumocystis carinii* pneumonia. *AJR Am J Roentgenol* 1986;147:29–31.
21. Fleisher AG, McElvaney G, Lawson L, et al. Surgical management of spontaneous pneumothorax in patients with acquired immunodeficiency syndrome. *Ann Thorac Surg* 1988;45:21–23.
22. Dee P. AIDS and other forms of immunocompromise. In: Armstrong P, Wilson AG, Dee P, et al., eds. *Imaging of diseases of the chest*, 2nd ed. St. Louis: Mosby, 1995:253.
23. Hunink MGM, Bos JJ. Triage of patients to angiography for detection of aortic rupture after blunt chest trauma: cost-effectiveness analysis of using CT. *AJR Am J Roentgenol* 1995;165:27–36.
24. Stern EJ, Frank MS. Acute traumatic hemopericardium. *AJR Am J Roentgenol* 1994;162:1305–1306.
25. Mirvis SE, Shanmuganathan K, Miller BH, et al. Traumatic aortic injury: diagnosis with contrast-enhanced thoracic CT: five-year experience at a major trauma center. *Radiology* 1996;200:413–422.
26. Gavant ML, Menke PG, Fabian T, et al. Blunt traumatic aortic rupture: detection with helical CT of the chest. *Radiology* 1995;197:125–133.
27. Ben-Menachem Y. Exploratory and interventional angiography in severe trauma: present and future procedure of choice. *Radiographics* 1996;16:963–970.
28. Gavant ML, Flick P, Mendke P, et al. CT aortography of thoracic aortic rupture. *AJR Am J Roentgenol* 1996;166:955–961.
29. Gurney JW. ABCs of blunt chest trauma. In: *Thoracic imaging 1996*. Society of Thoracic Radiology Syllabus. Oak Brook, IL: Society of Thoracic Radiology, 1996:349–352.
30. Unger JM, Schuchmann GG, Grossman JE, et al. Tears of the trachea and main bronchi caused by blunt trauma: radiologic findings. *AJR Am J Roentgenol* 1989;153:1175–1180.
31. Murray JG, Caoili E, Gruden JF, et al. Acute rupture of the diaphragm due to blunt trauma: diagnostic sensitivity and specificity. *AJR Am J Roentgenol* 1996;166:1035–1039.
32. Israel RS, McDaniel PA, Primack SL, et al. Diagnosis of diaphragmatic trauma with helical CT in a swine model. *AJR Am J Roentgenol* 1996;167:637–641.
33. Worthy SA, Kang EY, Hartman TE, et al. Diaphragmatic rupture: CT findings in 11 patients. *Radiology* 1995;194:885–888.
34. Shanmuganathan K, Mirvis SE, White CS, et al. MR imaging evaluation of hemidiaphragms in acute blunt trauma: experience with 16 patients. *AJR Am J Roentgenol* 1996;167:397–402.
35. Gelman R, Mirvis SE, Gens D. Diaphragmatic rupture due to blunt trauma: sensitivity of plain chest radiographs. *AJR Am J Roentgenol* 1991;156:51–57.

36. Caskey CI, Zerhouni EA, Fishman EK, et al. Aging of the diaphragm: a CT study. *Radiology* 1989;171:385–389.

37. Mirvis ST, Young JWR. *Imaging in trauma and critical care.* Baltimore: Williams & Wilkins, 1992.

38. Dennis LN, Rogers LF. Superior mediastinal widening from spine fractures mimicking aortic rupture on chest radiographs. *AJR Am J Roentgenol* 1989;152:27–30.

39. Wagner RB, Crawford WO, Schimpf PP. Classification of parenchymal injuries of the lung. *Radiology* 1988;167:77–82.

40. Curtin JJ, Goodman LR, Quebbeman EJ, et al. Complications after emergency tube thoracostomy: assessment with CT. *Radiology* 1996; 198:19.

41. Baldt MM, Bankier AA, Germann PS, et al. Complications after emergency tube thoracostomy: assessment with CT [Reply]. *Radiology* 1996;198:20.

42. Baldt MM, Bankier AA, Germann PS, et al. Complications after emergency tube thoracostomy: assessment with CT. *Radiology* 1995: 195:539–543.

43. Costello P. Thoracic helical CT. *Radiographics* 1994;14:913–918.

44. Costello P, Dupuy DE, Ecker CP, et al. Spiral CT of the thorax with reduced volume of contrast materials: A comparative study. *Radiology* 1992;183:663–666.

45. Gefter WB, Davis SD, Gurney JW, et al. RSNA '95 meeting notes: thoracic radiology. *Radiology* 1996;198:926–931.

46. Costello P, Ecker CP, Tello R, et al. Assessment of the thoracic aorta by spiral CT. *AJR Am J Roentgenol* 1992;158:1127–1130.

47. Remy-Jardin M, Remy J, Wattinne L, et al. Central pulmonary thromboembolism: diagnosis with spiral volumetric CT with the single breath hold technique—comparison with pulmonary angiography. *Radiology* 1992;185:381–387.

48. Zeman RK, Sliverman PM, Vieco PT, et al. CT angiography *AJR Am J Roentgenol* 1995;165:1079–1088.

49. Remy-Jardin M, Remy J, Cauvain O, et al. Diagnosis of central pulmonary embolism with helical CT: role of two-dimensional multiplanar reformations. *AJR Am J Roentgenol* 1995;165:1131–1138.

50. Goodman LR, Lipchik RJ, Kuzo RS, et al. Subsequent pulmonary embolism: risk after a negative helical CT pulmonary angiogram—prospective comparison with scintigraphy. *Radiology* 2000;215:535–542.

51. Goodman LR, Curtin JJ, Mewissen MW, et al. Detection of pulmonary embolism in patients with unresolved clinical and scintigraphic diagnosis: helical CT versus angiography. *AJR Am J Roentgenol* 1995;164:1369–1374.

52. McLoud TC, Flower CDR. Imaging the pleura: sonography, CT, and MR imaging. *AJR Am J Roentgenol* 1991;145:1145–1153.

53. Stark D, Federle MP, Goodman PC, et al. Differentiating lung abscess and empyema: radiography and computed tomography. *AJR Am J Roentgenol* 1983;141:163–167.

54. Muller NL. Imaging of the pleura. *Radiology* 1993;186:297–309.

55. Aquino SL, Webb WR, Gushiken BJ. Pleural exudates and transudates: diagnosis with contrast-enhanced CT. *Radiology* 1994;192: 803–808.

56. Godwin JD, ed. *Computed tomography of the chest.* Philadelphia: JB Lippincott, 1984:130–137.

57. Dynes MC, White EM, Fry WA, et al. Imaging manifestation of pleural tumors. *Radiographics* 1992;12:1191–1201.

58. O'Donovan PB, Eng P. Pleural changes in malignant pleural effusions: appearance on computed tomography. *Cleve Clin J Med* 1994;61:127–131.

59. Kawashima A, Libshitz HI. Malignant pleural mesothelioma: CT manifestations in 50 cases. *AJR Am J Roentgenol* 1990;155:965–969.

60. Leung AN, Muller NL, Miller RR. CT in differential diagnosis of diffuse pleural disease. *AJR Am J Roentgenol* 1990;154:487–492.

61. Westcott JL, Volpe JP. Peripheral bronchopleural fistula: CT evaluation in 20 patients with pneumonia, empyema, or postoperative air leak. *Radiology* 1995;196:175–181.

62. Samuels LE, Shaw PM, Blaum LC. Percutaneous technique for management of persistent air space with prolonged air leak using fibrin glue. *Chest* 1996;109:1653–1655.

63. Klein JS, Schultz S, Heffner JE. Interventional radiology of the chest: image-guided percutaneous drainage of pleural effusions, lung abscess, and pneumothorax. *AJR Am J Rjoentgenol* 1995;164:581–588.

64. Seaton KG, Patz EF Jr, Goodman PC. Palliative treatment of malignant pleural effusions: value of small-bore catheter thoracostomy and doxycycline sclerotherapy. *AJR Am J Roentgenol* 1995;164:589–591.

65. Baldt MM, Bankier AA, Germann PS, et al. Complications after emergency tube thoracostomy: assessment with CT. *Radiology* 1995; 195:539–543.

66. Curtin JJ, Goodman LR, Quebbeman EJ, et al. Thoracostomy tubes after acute chest injury: relationship between location in a pleural fissure and function. *AJR Am J Roentgenol* 1994;163:1339–1342.

67. Noppen MMP, De Mey J, Meysman M, et al. Percutaneous needle biopsy of localized pulmonary, mediastinal, and pleural diseased tissue with an automatic disposable guillotine soft-tissue needle. *Chest* 1995; 107:1615–1620.

68. Westcott JL. Percutaneous catheter drainage of pleural effusion and empyema. *AJR Am J Roentgenol* 1985;144:1189–1193.

69. Scott EM, Marshall TJ, Flower CD, et al. Diffuse pleural thickening: percutaneous CT-guided cutting needle biopsy. *Radiology* 1995;194:867–870.

70. Lenglinger FX, Schwarz CD, Artmann W. Localization of pulmonary nodules before thoracoscopic surgery: value of percutaneous staining with methylene blue. *AJR Am J Roentgenol* 1994;163:297–300.

71. Taylor RFH, Rubens MB, Pearson MC, et al. Intrapleural streptokinase in the management of empyema. *Thorax* 1994;49:856–859.

72. Bouros D, Schiza S, Panagou P, et al. Role of streptokinase in the treatment of acute loculated parapneumonic pleural effusions and empyema. *Thorax* 1994;49:852–855.

73. Robinson LA, Moulton AL, Fleming WH, et al. Intrapleural fibrinolytic treatment of multiloculated thoracic empyemas. *Ann Thorac Surg* 1994;57:803–814.

74. Klein JS, Schultz S, Heffner JE. Interventional radiology of the chest: image-guided percutaneous drainage of pleural effusions, lung abscess, and pneumothorax. *AJR Am J Roentgenol* 1995;164:581–588.

75. Chon KS, vanSonnenberg E, D'Agostino HB, et al. CT-guided catheter drainage of loculated thoracic air collections in mechanically ventilated patients with acute respiratory distress syndrome. *AJR Am J Roentgenol* 1999;173:1345–1350.

76. Jerjes-Sanchez C, Ramirez-Rivera A, Delgado R, et al. Intrapleural fibrinolysis with streptokinase as an adjunctive treatment in hemothorax and empyema. *Chest* 1996;109:1514–1519.

77. Sahn SA. Chemical pleurodesis for malignant effusions: what is the best agent? *Pulmonary Perspectives* 1996;13:1–3.

78. Seaton KG, Patz EF, Goodman PC. Palliative treatment of malignant pleural effusions: value of small-bore catheter thoracostomy and doxycycline sclerotherapy. *AJR Am J Roentgenol* 1995;164:589–591.

79. Patz EF, McAdams HP, Goodman PC, et al. Ambulatory sclerotherapy for malignant pleural effusions. *Radiology* 1996;199:133–135.

80. Kuhlman JE. Case no. 3: atypical chest pain: CT of the immunocompromised host. In: Kuhlman JE, ed. *Contemporary issues in computed tomography.* New York: Churchill Livingstone, 1991:177–178.

81. Teplick SK, Brandon JC, Shah HR, et al. Acute gastrointestinal disorders. In: Goodman LR, Putman CE, eds. *Critical care imaging*, 3rd ed. Philadelphia: WB Saunders, 1992:313–353.

82. Jeffrey RB Jr. Acute hepatobiliary and pancreatic disease. In: Goodman LR, Putnam CE, eds. *Critical care imaging*, 3rd ed. Philadelphia: WB Saunders, 1992:355–372.

83. Tepel M, van der Giet M, Schwarzfeld C, et al. Prevention of radiographic-contrast-agent–induced reductions in renal function by acetylcysteine. *N Engl J Med* 2000;343:180–184.

84. Kuhlman JE. Renal and urinary complications: CT of the immunocompromised host. In: Kuhlman JE, ed. *Contemporary issues in computed tomography.* New York: Churchill Livingstone, 1992.

85. Fishman EK, Kavuru M, Jones B, et al. CT of pseudomembranous colitis: CT evaluation of 26 cases. *Radiology* 1991;180:57–60.

86. Nemcek AA. CT of acute gastrointestinal disorders. *Radiol Clin North Am* 1989;27:773–786.

87. Jeffrey RB, Federle MP, Wall S. Value of computed tomography in detecting occult gastrointestinal perforation. *J Comput Assist Tomogr* 1983;7:226–229.

88. Kuhlman JE, Fishman EK, Jones B, et al. Computed tomography in the evaluation of diverticular disease: a review. *Revista Interamericana de Radiologia* 1987;10:197–206.

89. Scott WW Jr, Fishman EK, Siegelman SS. Evaluation of abdominal pain in the anticoagulated patient: The role of computed tomography. *JAMA* 1984;252:2053.

90. Yousem DM, Cranial CT in the immunocompromised host. CT of the immunocompromised host. In: Kuhlman JE, ed. *Contemporary issues in computed tomography*. New York: Churchill Livingstone, 1991: 139–167.

91. Graves VB, Partington CR. Imaging evaluation of acute neurologic disease. In: Goodman LR, Putnam CE, eds. *Critical care imaging*, 3rd ed. Philadelphia: WB Saunders, 1992:391–409.

SUBJECT INDEX

Page numbers in *italic* followed by *f* indicate figures; page numbers in *italic* followed by *t* indicate tabular material.

A

AACN. *See* American Association of Critical Care Nurses
AAG. *See* α-1-acid glycoprotein
AAPCC. *See* American Association of Poison Control Centers
AARC. *See* American Association for Respiratory Care
ABA. *See* American Burn Association
Abciximab
  for acute coronary syndromes, *314t*
  effect on coagulation, 313
Abdomen. *See also* Abdominal compartment syndrome; Gastrointestinal hemorrhage
  acute cholecystitis, 478–479, *479t*
  acute conditions in the perioperative intensive care unit patient, 474–484
  anatomy and physiology, 474–475
  common surgeries and associated abdominal complications, *476t*
  diarrhea and, 475–476
  etiology, 475, *476t*
  ileus, 476–477
  imaging in the intensive care unit, 849–854
  infection as source of fever, 582–583, *583f*
  intraabdominal sepsis, 596
  key points, 483
  mechanical obstruction, 477–478
  mesenteric ischemia, 480
  open, following surgery, 172–173
  pancreatitis, 479–480
  pressure, 797
  as source of occult infection, 481–482
Abdominal compartment syndrome (ACS). *See also* Abdomen
  acute, 480–481, *481t*
  care of the patient with multiple trauma and, 797
  causes of intraabdominal hypertension, *171t*
  clinical manifestations, *171t*
  following surgery, 171–172, *171t, 172t*
  physiologic consequences and treatment, *481t*
  transvescial measurement of intraabdominal pressure, *172t*
Abdominal pressure, care of the patient with increased, 797
ABG. *See* Arterial blood gas analysis

Abscess
  brain, recommended therapy for life-threatening, *624t*
  intraabdominal/secondary peritonitis, 633
Acalculous cholecystitis, 633
ACC. *See* American College of Cardiology
Accelerography, 159
Accessory pathways, supraventricular tachyarrhythmias and, 325–327, *326f, 327f*
Accolate (zafirlukast), for asthma, 379
ACCP. *See* American College of Chest Physicians
ACD-CPR. *See* Active compression-decompression CPR
ACE-I. *See* Angiotensin-converting enzyme inhibitors
Acetaminophen
  antidotes for overdose, *830t*
  with antifungal drugs, 625
  as cause of fulminant hepatic failure, 495
  evaluation and management for intoxication of, 833–834, *835f*
  for fever, 578
  in the intensive care unit, 151–152
  toxic syndromes, *820t*
Acetate, administration in the critically ill patient, 182
Acid-base abnormalities
  calcium, 218–219
    hypercalcemia, 219
    hypocalcemia, 218, *219t*
  in critically ill obstetric patients, 766
  diagnosis and management, 206–224
  equilibrium overview, 206
  interpretation, 210–211, *210t, 211t*
  key points, 222–223
  magnesium, 219–221
    hypermagnesemia, 221
    hypomagnesemia, 220–221, *221t*
  metabolic acidosis, 207–208, *208t, 209t*
  metabolic alkalosis, 207, *207f, 207t, 208t*
  phosphate, 221–222
    hyperphosphatemia, 222
    hypophosphatemia, 221–222
  potassium, 215–217
    hyperkalemia, 216–217, *217f, 217t*
    hypokalemia, 215–216
  respiratory acidosis, 209–210
  respiratory alkalosis, 209, *209t*
  sodium, 211–215

hypernatremia, 214–215, *214f, 214t, 215f*
    hyponatremia, 211–214, *212f, 213f*
Acid burns, 813
α-1-acid glycoprotein (AAG), 189
Acinetobacter, 391
ACLS. *See* Advanced cardiac life support
Acquired immunodeficiency syndrome (AIDS)
  bland-aerosol therapy and, 439
  blood donations and, 566
  causes, 664
  conditions included in the 1993 definition, *664t*
  infections in, 663–667, *664t, 665f, 667f*
  in the intensive care unit, 636–637
  patterns of infection and, 617
ACS. *See* Abdominal compartment syndrome
ACT. *See* Activated clotting time
Actinobacter, fever and, 584
Activated charcoal
  combined with cathartics, 828
  dose, 827–828
  for overdose of digoxin, 831
  for poisoning, 826–827
Activated clotting time (ACT), in perioperative hemostasis and coagulopathy, 552
Activated partial thromboplastin time (aPTT), for pulmonary embolism, 540
Active compression-decompression CPR (ACD-CPR), 366
Acuity systems, as quality assessment tools, 23–24
Acute care medicine. *See* Critical care medicine
Acute cholecystitis
  following surgery, 173
  in the perioperative intensive care unit patient, 478–479, *479t*
Acute fatty liver, in critically ill obstetric patients, 773–774
Acute infective endocarditis, 630–631
Acute intermittent peritoneal dialysis (AIPD), for renal replacement therapy, 526–527
Acute intracerebral hemorrhage, evaluation with computed tomography in the intensive care unit, 854

Acute lung injury/acute respiratory distress
syndrome (ALI/ARDS), 408–416
clinical presentation, 408–409, *409f*
definition, 408, *409f*
key points, 415
mechanical ventilation and, 412–413
pathology and pathogenesis, 409–411,
410f
cytokines, 410–411
fibrosing alveolitis, 411
neutrophil-dependent lung injury, 410
ventilator-induced lung injury, 411
predisposing factors, 409, *409t*
resolution, 411–414, *412f*
respiratory care and, 429
sepsis and, 604
treatment, 412–414
acceleration of resolution, 414
fluid and hemodynamic management,
413
glucocorticoids and other
antiinflammatory strategies, 414
inhaled nitric oxide and other
vasodilators, 414
mechanical ventilation, 412–413
surfactant therapy, 413–414
Acute mitral regurgitation, cardiogenic shock
and, 294
Acute myopathy of intensive care (AMIC),
162–163, *163t*
Acute normovolemic hemodilution, 570
Acute Physiology and Chronic Health
Evaluation (APACHE), 11, *11t*,
23–24, 60–61, 352, 479, 521, 730
Acute renal failure (ARF)
in the cardiac surgical patient, 352–353,
353t
care of the patient with multiple trauma
and, 792
complications of acute dialytic therapies,
527–528
air embolism, 528
dialysis disequilibrium syndrome, 527
fever during dialysis, 527–528
first-use syndrome, 527
hemorrhage, 528
hypotension, 527
hypoxemia, 527
sudden death during dialysis, 527
continuous removal of cytokines in the
systemic inflammatory response
syndrome (SIRS), 529–530
controversies of renal replacement therapy
in the critically ill patient, 528-530
dialyzer membrane biocompatibility,
529
initiation and adequacy in the intensive
care unit, 529
mode of renal replacement therapy, 528
in the critically ill patient, 521–532
indications for renal replacement therapy,
524, *524t*
key points, 530
mortality, 792
patterns of postoperative, *507f*
perioperative renal protection, 503–520

prevention and general medical
management of, 522–524
anemia, 524
fluid and electrolyte management, 524
loop diuretics and mannitol, 523
maintenance of renal perfusion pressure,
522
nephrotoxicity avoidance, 523, *523t*
nutritional support, 524
renal dose dopamine and fenoldopam,
522–523
treatment options, *522t*
principles of water and solute removal by
dialysis, 524–525
research, 70
techniques of renal replacement therapy,
525–527
acute intermittent peritoneal dialysis
(AIPD), 526–527
continuous arteriovenous
hemodiafiltration (CAVHDF),
526
continuous arteriovenous hemodialysis
(CAVHD), 526
continuous arteriovenous hemofiltration
(CAVH), 526
continuous renal replacement therapy
(CRRT), 525, *526t*
continuous venovenous
hemodiafiltration (CVVHDF),
526
continuous venovenous hemodialysis
(CVVHD), 526
continuous venovenous hemofiltration
(CVVH), 525–526
intermittent hemodialysis, 525
slow continuous ultrafiltration (SCUF),
526
sustained low-efficiency daily dialysis
(SLED), 526
treatment, 793
treatment options, *522t*
Acute respiratory distress syndrome (ARDS)
cardiogenic shock and, 296
care of the patient with multiple trauma
and, 792
in critically ill obstetric patients, 770
mechanical ventilation and, 403
nitric oxide and, 298
perioperative evaluation, 375
research, 70
sepsis and, 604–605, *604t*
shock and, 193
tracheal intubation and, 89
Acute tubular necrosis (ATN)
evaluation with computed tomography in
the intensive care unit, 852
hemodynamics, 504
initiation of injury, 504
perpetuation of injury, 504
management, 521
oxygen supply–demand paradigm,
504–505
pancreatitis and, 479
pathogenesis, 504–506
research, 70

vasomotor nephropathy, 505
acute renal failure, 505
liver failure (hepatorenal syndrome),
505
nephrotoxic (drug-induced) vasomotor
nephropathy, 505–506
septic shock, 505
Acyclovir (Zovirax)
adverse effects, 686
as antiviral prophylaxis, 640
distribution and elimination, 686
dosing, *622t*
in immunocompromised patients, *652t*
nephrotoxic effects, *745t*
for viral infections, 626
Adenosine
abnormal cardioactive response in the
denervated heart, 706–707, *706t*
in animal studies for acute renal failure,
522t
for cardiogenic shock, 299, *299t*
for paroxysmal supraventricular
tachycardia, 322
for perioperative myocardial ischemia, 315
renal ischemic preconditioning and, 516
Adenovirus, as complication of hematopoietic
stem cell transplantation, 747–748,
748t
ADH. *See* Antidiuretic hormone
Adolescents. *See* Pediatric care
Adrenal insufficiency, 757–759, *757t*
causes, 757, *757t*
diagnosis, 758
treatment, 759
Adrenergic agents
cardioselectivity, 340
for hypertension in the intensive care unit,
340–342, *341t*
intrinsic sympathetic activity, 340
mechanism of action, 340
membrane stabilizing effect, 340
β-adrenergic receptor blockers
for acute myocardial ischemia, 311, *312t*
adverse reactions, 341
antidotes for overdose, *830t*
as antihypertensive drugs, 340
cardioselectivity, 340
as cause of qualitative platelet disorders,
555t
contraindications, 313
inhaled, *441t*
for myocardial ischemia, 312–313
parenteral blockers, 340–341
for pheochromocytoma, 760
for rate control in atrial flutter or atrial
fibrillation, 322–323
selection, 341
toxic syndromes, *820t*
Adrenocortical suppression, preoperative
assessment, 9, *10t*
Adult polycystic kidney disease, hypertension
and, 336
Adult T-cell leukemia (ATL), blood
transfusions and, 567
Advanced cardiac life support (ACLS)
airway management, 89

in the cardiac surgical patient, 352
in cardiopulmonary resuscitation, 363
poisoning and, 822
Advance directives, 47–48
AECG. *See* Ambulatory electrocardiography
Aeromonas hydrophila, 655
Aeromonas spp., 653
Aerosol therapy, 439–443
  aerosolized medications, 439–440
  aerosol mask and T-piece, 432–433
  bland-aerosol therapy, 439
  continuous positive airway pressure,
    442–443, *443f*
  small-volume nebulizers, metered-dose,
    and dry-powder inhalers, 440–442,
    441t, *442f*
AFE. *See* Amniotic fluid embolism
Aflatoxin, as cause of fulminant hepatic
    failure, 495
AFLP. *See* Idiopathic acute fatty liver of
    pregnancy
Afterload, 288, *289f*, *290f*
Age. *See also* Elderly; Pediatric care
  influence on body surface area in burn
    patients, 802, *802f*
  mechanical ventilation in older patients,
    467–468, *468f*
  as risk factor for perioperative pulmonary
    complications, 394
Agency for Health Care Policy and Research,
    23
Agitation, assessment algorithm, *40f*
α-2 agonists
  in the intensive care unit, *151t*
  as neuroprotectants, *233t*
AIDS. *See* Acquired immunodeficiency
    syndrome
AIPD. *See* Acute intermittent peritoneal
    dialysis
Air
  embolism in dialysis for acute renal failure,
    528
  leakage in perioperative care of thoracic
    surgical patients, 421–422
Airway management
  in cardiopulmonary resuscitation,
    363–364, *364f*
  clearance techniques, 433–439
    alternative techniques, 435
    bronchoscopy, 436–439, *437f*, *438t*
    chest physical therapy, 434
    contraindications, 435
    humidification, 433–434
    incentive spirometry, 434
    indications, 435
    intermittent positive-pressure breathing,
      435–436
    percussion and vibration, 435
    postural drainage, 434, *434f*
    prophylactic versus therapeutic, 433
    suctioning, 436
  in infants and children, 776–777
  in lung transplantation, 717–718
  neuromuscular blocking agents and, 92
  syndromes associated with potential airway
    problems, *779t*

tracheal intubation in a difficult patient,
    96–97, *97f*
Airway obstruction
  in perioperative care of thoracic surgical
    patients, 418–419, 421
  in postoperative care of thoracic surgical
    patients, 421
AKBR. *See* Arterial ketone body ratio
Akinetic mutism, definition, 244
Albuterol, *441t*
Aldehydes, thermal damage to the lungs and,
    811
ALG. *See* Antilymphocyte globulin
ALI/ARDS. *See* Acute lung injury/acute
    respiratory distress syndrome
Alkali burns, 813
Alleles, definition, 63
Allergic reactions
  anaphylactic, 569
  to blood transfusions, 568, *568t*
  hemolytic transfusion reaction, 568–569
  immunomodulation, 569
Allografts. *See also* Cardiac allograft
    vasculopathy
  for burn patients, 808
  cadaver, in acute care of burns, 808,
    808t
  indicators for use of cadaver allograft in
    burn patients, 808, *808t*
  in orthotopic heart transplantation, 705
  rejection, 691
Allopurinol
  as neuroprotectant, 232
  for tumor lysis syndrome, 744
Alveolar oxygen tension, 428, *429f*
  inspiratory flow pattern and
    inspiratory–expiratory time
    manipulations, 451-452
  positive end-expiratory pressure, 450–451,
    452f
  recruitment and gas exchange, 450–452
Amanita phalloides
  as cause of fulminant hepatic failure, 495
  hemoperfusion for, 830
Amantadine (Symmetrel, Symadine)
  adverse effects, 686
  as antiviral prophylaxis, 640
  distribution and elimination, 686
  dosing, *622t*
  for viral infections, 626
Ambulatory electrocardiography (AECG), for
    myocardial ischemia, 307
American Academy of Clinical
    Toxicology/European Association
    of Poisons Centre and Clinical
    Toxicologists, 824, 828
American Association for Respiratory Care
    (AARC), 463
American Association of Critical Care Nurses
    (AACN), 22
American Association of Poison Control
    Centers (AAPCC), 818, 824–825,
    830
American Burn Association (ABA), 801–802,
    802t
American College of Cardiology (ACC), 699

American College of Chest Physicians
    (ACCP), 463
  definitions of sepsis and organ failure,
    589t
American College of Physician Guidelines, 6
American–European Consensus Conference,
    408, *409f*
American Heart Association/American
    College of Cardiology Task Force
    on Perioperative Evaluation of the
    Cardiac Patient undergoing
    Noncardiac Surgery, 4, *4t*, *5t*
  algorithms for testing for noncardiac
    surgical procedures, *6t*
American National Red Cross, 566
American Society of Anesthesiologists (ASA),
    3, *4t*, 21, 32, 48, 133, 357, *357t*,
    394, 566
  difficult airway algorithm, 90–91, *91f*,
    96–97, *97f*
  recommendations for cryoprecipitate,
    572t
  recommendations for fresh-frozen plasma,
    572t
  recommendations for platelets, *573t*
  recommendations for red blood cells,
    571t
American Society of Echocardiography (ASE),
    133
American Thoracic Society, 391
AMIC. *See* Acute myopathy of intensive care
Amikacin
  dosage adjustments in the intensive care
    unit, *523t*
  dosing, *622t*
Amikacin sulfate, 676
Amino acid receptor antagonists, as
    neuroprotectants, 232
Aminoglycosides
  adverse reactions, 676–677
  antibiotic management of renal and hepatic
    dysfunction in the intensive care
    unit, *675t*
  for bacteria in the intensive care unit, *673t*
  distribution and elimination, 676
  in immunocompromised patients, *652t*
  infection and, 621
  nephrotoxic effects, *745t*
  resistance, 681–682, 682, *682t*
Aminosteroids, for intensive care unit use,
    155t
Amiodarone
  acquired prolonged repolarization
    syndromes and, *329t*
  for atrial fibrillation, 323
  in cardiopulmonary resuscitation, 369–370
  drug interactions in critically ill patients,
    189t
  for rate control in atrial flutter or atrial
    fibrillation, 322–323
  for supraventricular tachyarrhythmias, 322
Amitriptyline, acquired prolonged
    repolarization syndromes and, *329t*
Amniotic fluid embolism (AFE), in critically
    ill obstetric patients, 772
Amphetamines, toxic syndromes, *820t*

Amphotericin, *683t*
  for bronchoconstriction, 439–440
  in the intensive care unit, 684
Amphotericin B
  adverse effects, 684
  as cause of fever, *585t*
  distribution and elimination, 683–684
  dosing, *622t*
  in immunocompromised patients, *652t*
  nephrotoxic effects, *745t*
  toxicity, 625
Amphotericin B deoxycholate (Fungizone),
      625
Ampicillin, 620
  antibiotic management of renal and hepatic
      dysfunction in the intensive care
      unit, *675t*
  for bacteria in the intensive care unit, *673t*
  dosing, *622t*
Ampicillin-sulbactam (Unasyn), 620
  dosing, *622t*
Amrinone
  for cardiogenic shock, 293
  for shock, *201t*
Analgesics. *See also* individual drug names
  administration during life-sustaining
      treatment, 48–49
  alternate drugs and routes of administration
      in the intensive care unit, *151t*
  epidural, 425–426
  in the intensive care unit, 150–152, *151t*
  intercostal, 425
  interpleural, 425
  nonsteroidal antiinflammatory drugs
      (NSAIDS), 150–151
  opioids, 151–152, *151t*
  postthoracotomy, 424
  systemic, 425–426
Anaphylactic reaction, to blood transfusion,
      569
Anastomosis, vascular, *476t*
Anastomotic techniques, for orthotopic heart
      transplantation
  biatrial, 704, *704f*
  bicaval, 704, *705f*
Anatomic shunting, 428–429
Ancobon (flucytosine), 626, *683t*
  adverse effects, 684–685
  distribution and elimination, 684
  dosing, *622t*
Ancrod, for cerebral ischemia, 260
Anemia
  in the critically ill patient, 177
  postoperative, 316
  prevention and general medical
      management in acute renal failure,
      524
  shock and, 196
Anesthesia
  as cause of fulminant hepatic failure, 495
  choice, 400
  considerations for perioperative pulmonary
      complications, 396–397
  critical care medicine orders, *35f*
  epidural, 382–383
  general, 383

guidelines for preoperative testing, 32, *34f*
  hematologic influences, 10
  in high-risk patients, 382–383
  inhaled, in the intensive care unit, 150
  local, 382
      as cause of qualitative platelet disorders,
          555t
  management in organ donors, 282
  minimal anesthetic concentration, 32–33
  as neuroprotectants, 232–234, *233t*
  perioperative management, 32, *32t*
  in perioperative management of pulmonary
      diseases, 382–383
  in perioperative myocardial ischemia,
      314–316, *315f, 316f*
  pulmonary diseases and, 382–383
  standardized approach to preoperative
      testing, 32–33, *33t, 34f*
  for tracheal intubation, 91–92, 95
Anesthesiologist
  compensation, 32
  primary function, 29–30
  as provider of acute care medicine, 29
  recruiting and training, 38, 42
Aneurysms
  classification systems, 266, *266t*
  diagnosis, 265–266
  giant, 269–270
  operative management, 268–270
  pathophysiology, 265
  postoperative care, 255–256, *255t*
  postoperative management in the intensive
      care unit, 272
  surgical alternatives, 270
Angiography, for determination of brain
      death, 278
Angioplasty. *See also* Percutaneous
      transluminal coronary angioplasty
  for vasospasm, 256
Angiotensin-converting enzyme inhibitors
      (ACE-I)
  acute tubular necrosis and, 505
  for cardiac insufficiency as complication of
      hematopoietic stem cell
      transplantation, 745
  for hypertension in the intensive care unit,
      343
  for myocardial ischemia, 314
  for preoperative antihypertensive
      medication, 339
  for prevention and treatment of renal
      injury, 515
  for renal failure, 336
  for shock, 203
Aniridia–Wilms tumor, *779t*
ANP. *See* Atrial natriuretic peptide
Antagonism, 681
Anthracyclines, as complication of
      hematopoietic stem cell
      transplantation, 745
Antibacterial therapy, 624–625, 673–
      681
  common adverse reactions to, *676t*
Antibiotics
  beta-lactam, 620–621, *622t–623t, 624t*
  bronchoscopy and, 439

as cause of qualitative platelet disorders,
      555t
  effect of renal failure on drug disposition,
      188
  following kidney transplantation, 734
  following liver transplantation, 730
  in immunocompromised patients,
      652t
  for infection following surgery, 170
  for intraoperative management of heart
      transplantation, 703–704
  in patients with neutropenia and fever,
      658t
  resistance to, 681–682, *682t*
Antibodies
  natural, 691
  in transplantation, 691
Anticholinergic drugs
  antidotes for overdose, *830t*
  inhaled, *441t*
Anticholinesterases, abnormal cardioactive
      response in the denervated heart,
      706–707, *706t*
Anticonvulsant therapy
  in the intensive care unit, *151t*
  perioperative management of infants and
      children, 780
  for subarachnoid hemorrhage, 270–271
Antidepressants. *See also* individual drug
      names
  antidotes for overdose, *830t*
  evaluation and management for
      intoxication of, 834–836
  in the intensive care unit, *151t*
  toxic syndromes, *820t*
Antidiuretic hormone (ADH), 138–139
  acid-base abnormalities and, 212
  in diabetes insipidus, 752
Antidotes, for care of the poisoned patient,
      830–831, *830t*
Antifibrinolytic therapy, for postoperative
      bleeding, 357
Antifungal drugs, *683t*
  in immunocompromised patients, *652t*
  for infection, 625–626, *625t*
  in the intensive care unit, 683, *683t*
Antihistamines
  acquired prolonged repolarization
      syndromes and, *329t*
  as cause of qualitative platelet disorders,
      555t
  toxic syndromes, *820t*
Anti-IL-2 receptor-α (CD25), in
      transplantation, 697–698
Antiinfective therapy
  for infections, 620–627. *See also* individual
      drug names
  for infectious disease syndromes, 627–637,
      628t–629t, 637f, 638t
Antiinflammatory agents. *See also* individual
      drug names
  for vasospasm, 271
Antilymphocyte globulin (ALG)
  for postoperative management of heart
      transplantation, 707
  in transplantation, *694t*, 697

Antimicrobial therapy
amphotericin B, 683–684
adverse effects, 684
distribution and elimination, 683–684
antibacterial agents, 673–681
aminoglycosides, 676–677
adverse reactions, 676–677
distribution and elimination, 676
carbapenems, 674
cephalosporins, 674
chloramphenicol, 680
adverse effects, 680
distribution and elimination, 680
glycopeptides, 677–678
adverse effects, 678
distribution and elimination,
678
β-Lactam antibiotics, 673
β-Lactamase inhibitors, 674
lincosamides, 677
adverse reactions, 677
distribution and elimination, 677
macrolide and azalide antibiotics,
677
adverse reactions, 677
distribution and elimination, 677
metronidazole, 679–680
adverse effects, 680
distribution and elimination,
679–680
monobactams, 675–676
adverse reactions, 675–676, *676t*
distribution and elimination, 675,
675t
mupirocin, 681
oxazolidinediones, 680
adverse effects, 680
distribution and elimination, 680
penicillins, 673–674
quinolones, 678–679, *678t*
adverse effects, 679
distribution and elimination, 679
quinupristin/dalfopristin, 680–681
adverse effects, 681
distribution and elimination, 681
sulfonamides and trimethoprim, 679
adverse effects, 679
distribution and elimination, 679
tetracyclines, 680
adverse effects, 680
distribution and elimination, 680
antifungal therapy, 683, *683t*
antiviral therapy, 685–688, *685t*
antiretroviral drugs, 687–688, *687t*
guanine nucleoside analogs, 686
adverse effects, 686
distribution and elimination, 686
neuraminidase inhibitors, 686
adverse effects, 686
distribution and elimination, 686
purine nucleoside analogs, 687
adverse effects, 687
distribution and elimination, 687
tricyclic amines, 686
adverse effects, 686
distribution and elimination, 686

azoles, 685
adverse effects, 685
distribution and elimination, 685
versus biological dressings in acute care of
burns, 807–808
factors influencing antibacterial activity,
681–685
aminoglycoside resistance, 682
antagonism, 681
β-lactam resistance, 682
pharmacodynamics and dosing, 683
quinolone resistance, 682
resistance, 681–682, *682t*
synergy, 681
vancomycin resistance, 682–683
flucytosine, 684–685
adverse effects, 684–685
distribution and elimination, 684
in immunocompromised patients, *652t*
in the intensive care unit, 672–689
key points, 688–689
liposomal amphotericin, 684
principles of therapy, 672–673
antibiotic selection, 672–673, *673t*
diagnosis, 672
treatment of resistant bacteria, 637, *637f,*
638t
Antioxidant agents, for vasospasm, 271
Antiparasitic drugs, in immunocompromised
patients, *652t*
Antipseudomonal penicillins, 674
Antiretroviral drugs, in the intensive care unit,
687–688, *687t*
Antithymocyte globulin (ATG), in pediatric
transplantation, *784t*
Antiviral drugs
dosing, *622t*
in immunocompromised patients,
652t
for infections, 626–627, *627t*
in the intensive care unit, 685–688
Antiviral prophylaxis, in the intensive care
unit, 640
Anxiety, assessment algorithm, *40f*
Aortic dissection
clinical features, 336
hypertension and, 335–336
management, 336
pathophysiology, 336
Aortic stenosis (AS), in critically ill obstetric
patients, 769
Aortic transections, computed tomography
for, 845, *845f*
Aortoenteric fistulas
diagnosis, 491
hemorrhage in the critically ill, 491
pathogenesis, 491
treatment, 491
APACHE. *See* Acute Physiology and Chronic
Health Evaluation
Apnea, in comatose patients, *249t*
Apneustic respiration, in comatose patients,
249t
Apoptosis
in acute lung injury/acute respiratory
distress syndrome, 411–412

in multiple organ dysfunction syndrome,
594, *594f*
Aprotinin, in post-cardiopulmonary bypass,
560
aPTT. *See* Activated partial thromboplastin
time
Arboviruses, 633
ARDS. *See* Acute respiratory distress
syndrome
Arduan (pipecuronium), for intensive care
unit use, *155t*
ARF. *See* Acute renal failure
Arginine, in immune-enhancing diets, 182
Arginine vasopressin (AVP)
for cardiogenic shock, 293–294, *293t*
for prevention and treatment of renal
injury, 516–517
Arousal, definition, 244
Arrhythmias, airway management and, 99
Arterial blood gas (ABG) analysis
for perioperative evaluation of pulmonary
disease, 380–381
Arterial cannulation
complications of arterial line placement,
105, *105t*
in the intensive care unit, 102–105, *103f,*
104f, 105f, 105t
sources for contamination of intravascular
access, 105, *105f*
Arterial ketone body ratio (AKBR), in
management of organ donors, 280
Arteriography, for vasospasm after
subarachnoid hemorrhage, 256
Arteriovenous malformations (AVMs)
classification systems, 266–267, *267t*
diagnosis, 266
epidemiology, 264–265
operative management, 269
pathophysiology, 265
postoperative care, 259
postoperative management in the intensive
care unit, 272–273
surgical alternatives, 270
Arthroplasty, total hip, 569–570
AS. *See* Aortic stenosis
ASA. *See* American Society of
Anesthesiologists
ASCOT. *See* A Severity Characterization of
Trauma
ASE. *See* American Society of
Echocardiography
A Severity Characterization of Trauma
(ASCOT), 11
Aspergillosis, as complication of
hematopoietic stem cell
transplantation, 743–744, *743f*
Aspergillus spp., 617, 625, 649, 655, 656, 660
as complication of hematopoietic stem cell
transplantation, 747
evaluation with computed tomography in
the intensive care unit, 844
following kidney transplantation, 734
fulminant hepatic failure, 498
in pediatric transplantation, 788
in postoperative management of heart
transplantation, 709, 719

Aspergillus spp. (*contd.*)
  in postoperative management of lung
    transplantation, 719
  recommended therapy for life-threatening,
    625t
Aspiration
  airway management and, 99
  tracheal intubation and, 90
Aspirin
  for acute coronary syndromes, *314t*
  acute tubular necrosis and, 505
  as cause of qualitative platelet disorders,
    555t
  effect on coagulation, 313
  in the intensive care unit, 151–152
  platelet counts and, 555
  for poisoning, 823
Asplenia, infection and, 667–668
Association of Medical Colleges, 73
Asthma
  antiasthmatic drugs, *441t*
  in critically ill obstetric patients, 769
  perioperative evaluation, 378–379, *378t*
  preoperative assessment of patient, 8–9
  treatment, 378–379
AT877, for vasospasm, 257
Atelectasis
  oxygen absorption, 433, *433f*
  in perioperative care of thoracic surgical
    patients, 420
  pulmonary diseases and, 383
Atenolol
  for acute myocardial ischemia, 311, *312t*
  as antihypertensive drug, 341, *341t*
  for malignant hypertension, 335
  for myocardial ischemia, 306, *307f*
ATG. *See* Antithymocyte globulin
Atherosclerosis, risk for coronary artery
    disease, 5
ATL. *See* Adult T-cell leukemia
ATN. *See* Acute tubular necrosis
Atovaquone
  for babesiosis, 636
  dosing, *622t*
Atovaquone-proguanil, dosing, *622t*
Atracurium (tracrium), for intensive care unit
    use, *155t*, 157, 164
Atrial natriuretic peptide (ANP), 138–139
  for acute renal failure, 793
  for prevention and treatment of renal
    injury, 515–516
Atrial tachycardia, 324, *324f*
Atropine
  for bradyarrhythmias, 320
  in cardiopulmonary resuscitation, 369
  for overdose of organophosphate or
    carbamate insecticides, *830t*
Atropine sulfate, *441t*
  abnormal cardioactive response in the
    denervated heart, 706–707, *706t*
Authority-based medicine. *See* Evidence-based
    medicine
Autohaler, 440
Autoimmune thrombocytopenia purpura. *See*
    Idiopathic thrombocytopenic
    purpura

Autonomic hyperreflexia
  hypertension and, 337
  spinal cord injuries and, 242
Autopsy studies, of patients with
    ventilator-associated pneumonia,
    390
Autosomal dominance, 64
Autosomal recessive inheritance, 64
AVMs. *See* Arteriovenous malformations
AVP. *See* Arginine vasopressin
Axillary artery, in arterial cannulation, 104
Azactam (azlocillin, aztreonam). *See*
    Aztreonam
Azalide antibiotics
  adverse reactions, 677
  distribution and elimination, 677
Azathioprine (Imuran)
  for autoimmune thrombocytopenia
    purpura, 562–563
  as cause of fever, *585t*
  for intraoperative management of heart
    transplantation, 703–704
  for myasthenia gravis, 420
  in pediatric transplantation, 783, *784t*
  for postoperative management of heart
    transplantation, 707
  in transplantation, 694, *694t*
Azithromycin (Zithromax), 621
  for babesiosis, 636
  dosing, *622t*
Azlocillin. *See* Aztreonam
Azoles
  adverse effects, 685
  distribution and elimination, 685
  in the intensive care unit, 685
Aztreonam (azactam, azlocillin), 620, 621,
    675, 676
  antibiotic management of renal and hepatic
    dysfunction in the intensive care
    unit, *675t*
  for bacteria in the intensive care unit, *673t*
  dosing, *622t*
  for pneumonia, 389

B
Babesia, 636
Babesiosis, 636
Bacillus, 655
Bacteremia, recommended therapy for
    life-threatening, *624t*
Bacteria
  antiinfective therapy for life-threatening
    infectious disease syndromes,
    628t–629t
  drugs for multiresistant gram-positive
    cocci, 623
  in immunocompromised patients, 655
  infections and, *618t*
    with hematopoietic stem cell
      transplantation, 746, *746t*
    in liver transplantation, 730–731
    in the preengraftment period in
      hematopoietic stem cell
      transplantation, 746, *746t*
  recommended therapy, *624t*
  resistance, 681–682, *682t*

  treatment of antimicrobial-resistant, 637,
    637f, 638t
Bacterial endocarditis, initial therapy for
    life-threatening, *628t*
Bacteroides fragilis, 633
  antibiotic selection in the intensive care
    unit, *673t*
  recommended therapy, *624t*
BAEPs. *See* Brainstem auditory evoked
    potentials
BAL. *See* Bronchoalveolar lavage
Balloon tamponade, for portal hypertension,
    490
Barbiturates
  coma and, 239
  in the intensive care unit, 149–150
  as neuroprotectant, 233, *233t*
  toxic syndromes, *820t*
Barnard, Christian, 699
Barrier function, derangements in multiple
    organ dysfunction syndrome,
    593–594
Baylor Bleeding Score, 486
BCNU. *See* Carmustine
Beat-to-beat variability (BTBV), in critically
    ill obstetric patients, 767
Beckwith–Wiedemann syndrome, *779t*
Beclomethasone acetonide, *441t*
Behavior, information-seeking, 86
Benchmarking, databases, 84
Beneficence, 45
Benzocaine, for tracheal intubation, 92
Benzodiazepines
  antidotes for overdose, *830t*
  in the intensive care unit, 147–148
  as neuroprotectants, *233t*, 234
Benzylisoquinolinium drugs, for intensive
    care unit use, *155t*
Bepridil, acquired prolonged repolarization
    syndromes and, *329t*
Biatrial anastomotic technique, for orthotopic
    heart transplantation, 704, *704f*
Bicarbonate, for overdose of cyclic
    antidepressants, *830t*
Bicaval anastomotic technique, for orthotopic
    heart transplantation, 704, *705f*
Bilateral sequential single-lung transplant
    (BSSLT), 711
Biliary sepsis, following surgery, 173
Biliary strictures, in liver transplantation, 730
Biliary tract
  evaluation with computed tomography in
    the intensive care unit, 851
  surgery for perioperative renal protection,
    508
Biobrane, for burn patients, 807
Biochemistry, for nutrition support in the
    critically ill patient, 178
Biologic causation, experimental evidence for
    genomics, 66–67
BiPAP. *See* Biphasic-airway-pressure therapy
Biphasic-airway-pressure (BiPAP) therapy,
    443
Bisoprolol, effect on perioperative mortality,
    29
Bitolterol, *441t*

Bland-aerosol therapy, 439
Blastomyces dermatitidis, 626, 660
    recommended therapy for life-threatening,
        625t
β-blocker therapy, effect on perioperative
        mortality, 29
Blood
    infections associated with, *618t*
    leukocyte-depleted products, 573
    substitutes in transfusion, 574
Blood donation
    advantages and disadvantages of
        preoperative, *569t*
    preoperative, 569–570
Blood flow
    in cardiopulmonary resuscitation, 365
    for cerebroprotective intervention, 230
Blood gas studies, perioperative evaluation,
        380–381
Blood pressure
    classification, *334t*
    control in postoperative neurosurgical
        patients, 261
    hemodynamics, 333
    in postoperative management of
        aneurysms, 272
Blood salvage
    intraoperative, 570
    postoperative, 570
Blood transfusion, 566–576
    algorithm, 347, *347t*
    allergic reactions to, 565, 568, *568t*
    anaphylactic reaction to, 569
    autologous, 569–570
        acute normovolemic hemodilution, 570
        advantages and disadvantages of
            preoperative blood donation, *569t*
        intraoperative blood salvage, 570
        postoperative salvage, 570
        preoperative blood donation, 569–570
    blood substitutes, 574
    in the cardiac surgical patient, 357–358,
        357t
    complications, 357
    Creutzfeld–Jakob disease and, 567
    cytomegalovirus and, 567
    evaluation of reactions, *568t*
    exchange, for malaria, 636
    fever as reaction to, 585
    fresh frozen plasma and cryoprecipitate,
        572–573
        ASA recommendations for
            cryoprecipitate, *572t*
        ASA recommendations for fresh-frozen
            plasma, *572t*
    hepatitis and, 566–567
    HIV and, 566
    immunomodulation and, 569
    infectious disease transmission and,
        566–567, *568t*
    ischemic optic neuropathy (ION), 575
    key points, 575
    leukocyte-depleted blood products, 573
    massive, 561, 573–574
        coagulopathy, 573–574, *574t*
        metabolic complications, 574

with perioperative hemostasis and
        coagulopathy, 561
    platelet concentrates, *573t*
        ASA recommendations for, *573t*
    posttransfusion purpura, 563
    red blood cells, 570–572
        guidelines for RBC transfusion,
            571–572, *571f, 571t*
    refusal by Jehovah's Witness patient, 46
    risks, 566–569, *567t*
        allergic and febrile reactions, 568, *568t*
        anaphylactic reaction, 569
        hemolytic transfusion reaction (HTR),
            568–569
        immunomodulation, 569
        transfusion-related lung injury, 569
        of transmission of infectious diseases,
            566–567, *568t*
    septic reactions to, 567–568, *568t*
    shock and, 568
    T-cell keukemia and, 567
    use of erythropoietin in critically ill
        patients, 575
Blood volume, in critically ill obstetric
        patients, 765
Blunt cardiac injury, 797
Blunt thoracic trauma, computed tomography
        for detection of, 844–845
BMT. *See* Bone marrow transplant
BMTN. *See* Bone marrow transplant
        nephropathy
BN80933, as neuroprotectant, 232
BO. *See* Bronchiolitis obliterans
Bone marrow transplant (BMT). *See also*
        Hematopoietic stem cell
        transplantation
    infections in recipients, 662–663, *662f*
Bone marrow transplant nephropathy
        (BMTN), 746
Bowel
    decontamination in fulminant hepatic
        failure, 499, 500
    obstruction, 476–477
Brachial artery, in arterial cannulation, 104
Bradyarrhythmias, acute therapy in patients
        with, 320–321, *321f*
Bradycardia
    acquired prolonged repolarization
        syndromes and, *329t*
    airway management and, 99
    symptomatic, *321f*
Brain
    death criteria, 250
    determination and diagnosis of brain
        death, 276–277, *276t*
    edema, 238–239
    electrocardiogram changes in brain death,
        279f
    herniation syndromes, 247–249
    injuries, 236–239
    parenchyma reduction, 238–239
    reticular formation, 244
    testing for brain death, 277–278, *277t*
    tissue volume, 261
    traumatic injuries. *See* Traumatic brain
        injury

Brain abscess, recommended therapy for
        life-threatening, *624t*
Brain infarction, evaluation with computed
        tomography in the intensive care
        unit, 854, *854f*
Brainstem
    death, 277
    decreased level of consciousness and,
        259
Brainstem auditory evoked potentials
        (BAEPs), 278
Breathing
    breath cycling, 455
    perioperative management of infants and
        children, 777
    postoperative, 401
    ventilator breath triggering, 453
Bretylium, in cardiopulmonary resuscitation,
        369–370
Bronchiectasis, perioperative evaluation, 377,
        377t
Bronchiolitis obliterans (BO)
    classification, *719t*
    in postoperative management of lung
        transplantation, 719–720
Bronchoalveolar lavage (BAL), 437–438
Bronchodilators, *441t*
Bronchopleural fistula, in perioperative care
        of thoracic surgical patients, 422
Bronchopneumonia, from smoke inhalation,
        810
Bronchoscopy
    for airway management, 436–439, *437f,
        438t*
    laser, 417
    in perioperative care of thoracic surgical
        patients, 417–418
    in postoperative care of thoracic surgical
        patients, 421
    pulmonary resection, 417–418
    rigid, 417
Bronchospasm
    adverse reaction to β-blockers, 341
    preoperative assessment of patient, 8
Brown-Séquard syndrome, 240
BSSLT. *See* Bilateral sequential single-lung
        transplant
BTBV. *See* Beat-to-beat variability
Budesonide, *441t*
Bumetanide, as antihypertensive drug,
        339–340
Burkholderia cepacia, 655
    recommended therapy, *624t*
Burns, 801–817
    acid and alkali burns, 813
    burn-wound pathology, 801
    criteria for burns referral, 801–802,
        802t
    deep second-degree, 801
    electrical injury, 812–813
    first-degree, 801
    hypovolemic shock and, 197
    inhalation injury, 808–812
        characteristics of sites of, 810, *810t*
        incidence and mortality related to age
            and presence of, 809, *809t*

Burns, inhalation injury (*contd.*)
incidence and mortality related to total body surface area burn and presence of, 809, *809t*
treatment, 812
key points, 813
nutrition and, 805
patient management, 802–806
calculating percentage of body surface area burned, 802, *803t*
escharotomy incisions, 802, *803f*
fluid resuscitation requirements, 804, *804t*
influence of age on body surface area, 802, *802f*
support of the hypermetabolic response to thermal injury, 804–806
second-degree, 801
third-degree, 801
wound management, 806–808
biological dressings as alternatives to topical antimicrobial agents, 807–808
control of infection by conservative methods, 806–807
debridement, 807–808
excision of the burn wound, 808
use of cadaver allograft, 808, *808t*
Butyrophenone, in the intensive care unit, 149–150

C

CABG. *See* Coronary artery bypass graft
Cachexia, effect of renal failure on drug disposition, 188
CAD. *See* Coronary artery disease
Cadaver allografts, 808, *808t*
Calcitriol, calcium abnormalities and, 218
Calcium
diagnosis and management of abnormalities, 218–219
monitoring in the critically ill patient, 182
for overdose of calcium channel blockers, *830t*
Calcium channel antagonists
for acute myocardial ischemia, 311, *312t*
adverse reactions, 343
for angina, 313
in animal studies for acute renal failure, *522t*
antidotes for overdose, *830t*
for hypertension in the intensive care unit, 342–343, *342t*
for myocardial ischemia, 313
as neuroprotectants, 231–232
for pheochromocytoma, 760
for prevention and treatment of renal injury, 514–515
for Prinzmetal angina, 313
for rate control in atrial flutter or atrial fibrillation, 322–323
for renal failure, 336
selection, 343
for vasospasm, 257
Calcium entry blockers, for cerebral ischemia, 260

Calcium salts, in cardiopulmonary resuscitation, 370
California Administrative Code, 23
Calories. *See also* Nutrition
chronic deficiency, 177
cAMP. *See* Cyclic adenosine monophosphate
Campylobacter spp., 634
Cancidas (caspofungin), 626
Candida albicans, 491
evaluation with computed tomography in the intensive care unit, 844
fulminant hepatic failure and, 498
in postoperative management of lung transplantation, 719
Candida endophthalmitis, 653
Candida glabrata, 631
Candida guilliermondi, 683
Candida krusei, 631
Candida lusitaniae, 683
Candida spp., 616, 617, *619f,* 625, 626, 631–632, 633, 634, 637, 649, 651, 684
in burn patients, 807
in central venous catheterization, 107
as complication of hematopoietic stem cell transplantation, 747, *747f*
fever and, 580, 582
following liver transplantation, 730
genomic identification, 64
nutrition in the critically ill patient and, 178
in pediatric transplantation, 788
in postoperative management of heart transplantation, 709
in postoperative management of lung transplantation, 719
recommended regimens for treatment of multiresistant, *638t*
recommended therapy for life-threatening, *625t*
secondary to sepsis, 603
Candida tropicalis, 656
Cannulation, central venous, 126
CAP. *See* Community-acquired pneumonia
Capacitance (volume reservoir), definition, 534
Capnocytophaga, 656
Capnometry, 380–381
Captopril, acute tubular necrosis and, 505
Carbamate insecticides, antidotes for overdose, *830t*
Carbamazepine, drug interactions in critically ill patients, *189t*
Carbapenems
allergic reactions to, 676
antibiotic management of renal and hepatic dysfunction in the intensive care unit, *675t*
in immunocompromised patients, *652t*
in the intensive care unit, 674
Carbon monoxide
thermal damage to the lungs and, 811
toxic syndromes, *820t*
Carbon tetrachloride, as cause of fulminant hepatic failure, 495
Carboplatin, for renal failure, 744

Carcinoid syndrome, 760
Cardiac allograft vasculopathy (CAV), in postoperative management of heart transplantation, 709–710
Cardiac Anesthesia Risk Evaluation (CARE), 3, *4t*
Cardiac arrest, pulmonary embolism and, 544–545
Cardiac arrhythmias
acute therapy in patients with, 320–332
bradyarrhythmias, 320–321, *321f*
tachyarrhythmias, 321–331
role of lidocaine in treatment, 330–331
supraventricular, 321–327, *323f, 324f, 325f, 326f, 327f*
ventricular, 327–328, *327f, 328f, 329f, 329t, 330t*
wide-complex, 328–330, *330f, 331f*
Cardiac disease
aortic stenosis in critically ill obstetric patients, 769
cardiac risk stratification for noncardiac surgical procedures, *5t*
cardiac surgery specific risk indices, 3, *4t*
clinical evaluation in patients undergoing noncardiac surgery, 3–8, *4t, 5t, 6t, 7f*
clinical predictors of increased perioperative cardiovascular risk, *4t*
in critically ill obstetric patients, 767–771
end-stage, 701, *701t*
mechanical support devices, 701
mitral stenosis in critically ill obstetric patients, 768–769
myocardial depression with sepsis, 605–606
myocardial infarction in critically ill obstetric patients, 769
noncardiac risk indices, 2–3
patients at risk for coronary artery disease (CAD), 5
preoperative assessment, 2–8
Cardiac herniation, in postoperative care of thoracic surgical patients, 423
Cardiac injury, blunt, 797
Cardiac insufficiency, with hematopoietic stem cell transplantation, 745–746
Cardiac output
arterial pressure wave to determine, 130
continuous, 130
definition, 534
following surgery in the intensive care unit, 169
hypertension and, 333–334
lithium dilution to determine, 130
partial CO_2 rebreathing to determine, 130–131
principles of thermodilution measurement, 127–128
shock and, 193
thoracic impedance cardiography to determine, 130
Cardiac surgery
perioperative cardiac evaluation decision analysis form, 29, *30f–31f*
perioperative management in infants and children, 781, *782t*

perioperative renal protection, 506–507
specific risk indices, 3, *4t*
Cardiac surgical patient, perioperative management, 346–362
  assessment and management, 346–349
    admission, 346–347, *347t*
    postextubation phase, 349
    rehabilitation phase, 349
    stabilization phase, 347–348, *348t*
    weaning phase, 348–349, *348t*
  key points, 358–359
  management of perioperative complications, 349–355
    accelerated recovery from cardiac surgery, 354–355
    dysrhythmias, 351–352
    electrocardiogram changes, 350–351
    hypotension, 349–350
    infection, 352
    neurocognitive deficits, 353–354, *353t*
    oliguria, 352–353, *353t*
    ventricular dysrhythmias, 352
    weaning from ventilation, 354
  minimally invasive cardiac surgery, 355–357, *356t*
    direct coronary artery bypass, 355
    off-pump coronary artery bypass, 355–356
    port-access surgery, 355
    transmyocardial laser revascularization, 356–357
  risk stratification, 358
  transfusion, 357–358, *357t*
Cardiac tamponade, cardiogenic shock and, 295
Cardiogenic shock, 196–197, *197f*, 287–302. *See also* Heart
  cardiac function, 287–289
    afterload, 288, *289f*, *290f*
    contractility, 289
    heart rate, 287
    preload, 287–288, *288f*
  care of the patient with multiple trauma and, 797
  causes, 196–197
  definition, 287
  interrelationship with hyperdynamic and hypovolemic shock, 192–193, *192f*
  key points, 300
  management, 291–294, *291t*
    amrinone and milrinone, 293
    arginine vasopressin, 293–294, *293t*
    combination therapy, 294
    phosphodiesterase fraction III inhibitors, 292
    thyroid hormone, 293
  mechanical complications, 294–295
    acute mitral regurgitation, 294
    cardiac tamponade, 295
    free-wall rupture, 295
    ventricular septal rupture, 294–295
  myocardial infarction, 289–290
    clinical presentation, 290, *291t*
    evolution of pump failure, 290
    pathophysiology of acute, 289–290
  right ventricular dysfunction, 295–300

management of right ventricular failure, 296–298, *297f*, *297t*, *298t*
    nitrous oxide with phenylephrine, 298
    phosphodiesterase inhibition, 298–300, *299t*
    right ventricular infarction, 295–296, *296f*
  risk factors, 196
Cardiopulmonary bypass (CPB)
  in orthotopic heart transplantation, 703–705
  with perioperative hemostasis and coagulopathy, 560–561
  shock and, 196–197
Cardiopulmonary resuscitation (CPR), 363–373
  airway management, 93, 363–364, *364f*
  circulation, 364–367
    adequacy of, 367
    alternative methods of circulatory support, 366, *366f*
    distribution of blood flow, 365
    gas transport, 365
    physiology during closed chest compressions, 364–365
    technique of closed chest compression, 365–366
  closed chest compressions, 364–365
  in critically ill obstetric patients, 770–771, *770f*
  defibrillation, 367–368
    defibrillators, 367–368
    duration and electric pattern, 367
    energy requirements and adverse effects, 368
  drug therapy, 368–370, *368t*
    amiodarone, 369
    atropine, 369
    bretylium, 369–370
    calcium salts, 370
    catecholamines and vasopressors, 368–369
    lidocaine, 369
    routes of administration, 370
    sodium bicarbonate, 370
  key points, 371–372
  postresuscitation care, 370–371
  prognosis, 371
  return of spontaneous circulation, 369
  ventilation, 364
    physiology, 364
    technique of rescue breathing, 364
  withholding, 47
Cardiopulmonary status (CPS), in the critically ill patient, 533
Cardiopulmonary transplantation, 699–723
  heart-lung transplant, 720–721
  heterotopic transplant, 710–711
  isolated lung transplant, 711–720
  orthotopic heart transplant, 351, 699–710
Cardiothoracic surgery
  perioperative management in infants and children, 781, *782t*
  pulmonary dysfunction in infants and children after, 783

Cardiovascular system
  effect on organ donors, 278–280, *279f*
  fulminant hepatic failure and, 496–497
  long-term complications in orthotopic heart transplantation, 709–710
  management in lung transplantation, 718
  as risk factor for perioperative pulmonary complications, 394
  spinal cord injuries and, 241–242
  support in orthotopic heart transplantation, 705–707, *706t*
  treatment of infants and children after cardiovascular failure, 781–783
Cardioversion, for supraventricular tachyarrhythmias, 322
CARE. *See* Cardiac Anesthesia Risk Evaluation
CareSuite, 82
Carmustine (BCNU), as complication of hematopoietic stem cell transplantation, 742
Carotid endarterectomy, postoperative care, 253–254
CARS. *See* Compensatory antiinflammatory response syndrome
CAs. *See* Cyclic antidepressants
Caspofungin (Cancidas), 626
CASS. *See* Coronary artery surgery study
Catabolic index (CI), 179
Catalase, as neuroprotectant, 232
Catecholamines
  for cardiogenic shock, 292
  in cardiopulmonary resuscitation, 368–369
  during catabolic phase of response to injury, 176
  hypertension and, 337
Catechol-resistant vasodilation, sepsis and, 608
Cathartics
  combined with activated charcoal, 828
  contraindications, 828
  for poisoning, 828–829
  repeated dosages, 828–829
Catheters
  "dampened" tracings, 123
  "fling" tracings, 123
  mixed-venous oxygen-saturated, 128–129, *128f*, *129f*
  passage, 126–127
  presence in pulmonary artery, 127
  sepsis in multiple organ dysfunction syndrome, 596
  as source of infection, 580–582, *581f*, *582f*, *582t*
Causal mutation, 65
CAV. *See* Cardiac allograft vasculopathy
CAVH. *See* Continuous arteriovenous hemofiltration
CAVHD. *See* Continuous arteriovenous hemodialysis
CAVHDF. *See* Continuous arteriovenous hemodiafiltration
CBC. *See* Complete blood count
CBF. *See* Cerebral blood flow
CBV. *See* Cerebral blood volume
CCM. *See* Critical care medicine

CCO. *See* Continuous cardiac output
CCTR. *See* Cochrane Controlled Trials Register
CDC. *See* Centers for Disease Control and Prevention
CDSR. *See* Cochrane Database of Systematic Reviews
Cefazolin, antibiotic management of renal and hepatic dysfunction in the intensive care unit, *675t*
Cefepime (Maxipime), 620, 621, 674
  antibiotic management of renal and hepatic dysfunction in the intensive care unit, *675t*
  dosing, *622t*
Cefobid (cefoperazone), 620
  for pneumonia, 389
Cefoperazone (Cefobid), 620
  for pneumonia, 389
Cefotaxime
  dosage adjustments in the intensive care unit, *523t*
  dosing, *622t*
Cefotetan, antibiotic management of renal and hepatic dysfunction in the intensive care unit, *675t*
Ceftazidime
  antibiotic management of renal and hepatic dysfunction in the intensive care unit, *675t*
  dosage adjustments in the intensive care unit, *523t*
  dosing, *622t*
  for pneumonia, 389
Ceftazidime (Fortaz, Tazicef, Tazidime), 620
Ceftizoxime, dosing, *622t*
Ceftriaxone
  antibiotic management of renal and hepatic dysfunction in the intensive care unit, *675t*
  dosage adjustments in the intensive care unit, *523t*
  dosing, *622t*
Ceftriaxone (Rocephin), 620
Cefuroxime
  antibiotic management of renal and hepatic dysfunction in the intensive care unit, *675t*
  dosing, *622t*
Cell-mediated immunity (CMI)
  infections associated with, *618t*
  patterns of infection and, 617
Cellular mechanisms, of cerebral injury, 228–229
Cellulitis, recommended therapy for life-threatening, *624t*
Centers for Disease Control and Prevention (CDC), 192, 387, 601, 626
  definitions for nosocomial pneumonia, *387t*
  epidemiologic criteria for diagnosis of toxic shock syndrome, 635
Central cord syndrome, 240
Central nervous system (CNS), *163t*
  in the cardiac surgical patient, 353–354, *353t*

diagnostic approach to abnormalities, 666, *667f*
dialysis disequilibrium syndrome and, 527
dysfunction, *248t*
evaluation infections with computed tomography in the intensive care unit, 855
evaluation trauma with computed tomography in the intensive care unit, 855
evaluation with computed tomography in the intensive care unit, 854–855
in immunocompromised patients, 649, *650t*
infections associated with, *618t*
neuromuscular blocking agents and, 164
sepsis and, 610
Central neurogenic hyperventilation. *See* Central reflex hyperpnea
Central reflex hyperpnea (CRH), in comatose patients, *249t*
Central venous cannulation, 126
  evaluation with computed tomography, 849
  infections associated with, *618t*
Central venous catheterization
  complications, 108–109
  equipment for, *109t*
  indications for, *106t*
  in the intensive care unit, 105–106, *106t*
  site-specific complications, *106t*
Central venous pressure (CVP) catheter
  in an intensive care unit, 46
  shock and, 195
Cephalosporins
  allergic reactions to, 676
  antibiotic management of renal and hepatic dysfunction in the intensive care unit, *675t*
  for bacteria in the intensive care unit, *673t*
  as cause of fever, *585t*
  as cause of qualitative platelet disorders, *555t*
  dosing, *622t*
  in immunocompromised patients, *652t*
  in the intensive care unit, 674
Cerebral aneurysm, epidemiology, 264
Cerebral blood flow (CBF)
  carotid endarterectomy and, 253
  cerebroprotection and, 227–228
  changes in, *227f*
  in traumatic brain injury, 236
Cerebral blood volume (CBV), reduction in, 238
Cerebral death, 277
Cerebral edema, as complication of subarachnoid hemorrhage, 270
Cerebral hyperperfusion syndrome, 253–254
Cerebral injury, pathophysiology of, 228–230
Cerebral ischemia
  cerebral injury and, 228
  postoperative care, 260
Cerebral perfusion pressure (CPP), 225
  in traumatic brain injury, 237
Cerebral reperfusion, cerebral injury and, 228
Cerebral vascular lesions
  postoperative care, 255–258

Cerebro-oculo-facio-skeletal syndrome, *779t*
Cerebroprotection, 225–235
  cerebral blood flow, 227–228
  key points, 234
  nonpharmacologic cerebroprotective interventions, 230–231
    hyperventilation, 230–231
    hypothermia, 231
    promotion of blood flow and oxygen delivery, 230
  pathophysiology of cerebral injury, 228–230
    cellular and molecular mechanisms, 228–229
    cerebral ischemia/reperfusion, 228
    excitotoxicity, 229
    inflammation, 230
    nitric oxide toxicity and oxidant injury, 229–230
    programmed cell death (PCD), 230
    traumatic brain injury (TBI), 228
  pharmacologic neuroprotectants, 231–234
    anesthetic agents, 232–234, *233t*
    calcium channel antagonists, 231–232
    excitatory amino acid receptor antagonists, 232
    hormonal neuroprotection, 232
    nitric oxide synthase inhibitors, 232
    osmotherapy, 231
    radical scavengers, 232
  regulation of function, 225–227, *226f*, *227f*, *227t*
Cerebrospinal fluid
  analysis for consciousness, 251
  drainage, 238
Cerebrovascular accident
  acquired prolonged repolarization syndromes and, *329t*
  subarachnoid hemorrhage and, 264–274
Certification process, 21
Cervicoocular reflex (COR), 247–248
CF. *See* Cystic fibrosis
Charcoal
  dose, 827–828
  for poisoning, 826–827
Chemicals, thermal damage to the lungs and, 811
Chemotherapeutic agents
  for autoimmune thrombocytopenia purpura, 562–563
  as cause of qualitative platelet disorders, *555t*
Chest physical therapy, for airway management, 434
Chest radiograph, for perioperative evaluation of pulmonary disease, 380
Chest wall, computed tomography for detection of trauma to, 846
Cheyne-Stokes respiration, in comatose patients, *249t*
CHF. *See* Congestive heart failure
Children. *See* Pediatric care
Child-Turcotte-Pugh scores, following liver transplantation, 730
Chimera, 690

Chlamydia, 385, 677, 680
Chloramphenicol
 adverse effects, 680
 antibiotic management of renal and hepatic dysfunction in the intensive care unit, *675t*
 for bacteria in the intensive care unit, *673t*
 distribution and elimination, 680
 for rickettsial infections, 636
Chlorhexidine, for cutaneous antisepsis, 640
Chloride, administration in the critically ill patient, 182
Chloroquine
 dosing, *622t*
 resistance to malaria, 636
Chlorpromazine, acquired prolonged repolarization syndromes and, *329t*
Cholangitis, 633
 evaluation with computed tomography in the intensive care unit, 851
 initial therapy for life-threatening, *628t*
Cholecystitis
 acalculous, 633
 evaluation with computed tomography in the intensive care unit, 851
 following surgery, 173
Chromium, daily requirements in total parenteral nutrition, *182t*
Chronic bronchitis
 perioperative evaluation, 376, *376t*
 preoperative assessment of patient, 8
Chronic lymphocytic leukemia, in immunocompromised patients, 668
Chronic obstructive pulmonary disease (COPD). *See also* Pulmonary diseases
 mechanical ventilation and, 465–466, *466f, 466t*
 preoperative assessment, 8, *8t*
 pulmonary pathology, 375
 research, 73
 risk of perioperative pulmonary complications and, 395
 tracheal intubation and, 89
Chronic pyelonephritis, hypertension and, 336
Chronotropic agents, shock and, 201
CI. *See* Catabolic index
Cidofovir (Vistide)
 dosing, *622t*
 for viral infections, 626
CIIS. *See* Computerized Intensity Intervention Score
Cilastatin, 674
Cimetidine
 as cause of fever, *585t*
 drug interactions in critically ill patients, *189t*
CIP. *See* Critical illness polyneuropathy
Cipro (ciprofloxacin). *See* Ciprofloxacin
Ciprofloxacin (Cipro), 623, 679
 for bacteria in the intensive care unit, *673t*
 dosage adjustments in the intensive care unit, *523t*
 dosing, *623t*
 for pneumonia, 389

Circulation
 in cardiopulmonary resuscitation, 364–367
 hydraulic model of, 534, *535f, 535t*
 perioperative management of infants and children, 777–778, *777t*
 support in the intensive care unit, 638
 support methods, 364–367
CIS. *See* Clinicomp International Clinical Information System
Cisapride, acquired prolonged repolarization syndromes and, *329t*
Cisatracurium (nimbex), for intensive care unit use, *155t,* 157, 164
Cisplatin, for renal failure, 744
Citrate phosphate dextrose adenine (CPDA-1), 570
CJD. *See* Creutzfeld–Jakob disease
Clarithromycin, 677
Clavulanic acid, 674
Clearance (Cl), 187, 190
Clindamycin
 antibiotic management of renal and hepatic dysfunction in the intensive care unit, *675t*
 for babesiosis, 636
 for bacteria in the intensive care unit, *673t*
 dosing, *622t*
 for infection following surgery, 170
 for pneumonia, 389
 for toxic shock syndrome, 635–636
Clindamycin phosphate
 adverse reactions, 677
 distribution and elimination, 677
Clinical trials, 57
 for acute respiratory distress syndrome in critically ill obstetric patients, 770
 ARDS network, 403
 for barrier precautions, 640
 definition, 73
 for efficacy of protected environments, 640
 for hydrocortisone, 639
 milrinone, 299
 for mycophenolate mofetil (MMF), 695
 organizational chart, *75f*
 for orogastric lavage for poisoning, 825–826
 outcome of thrombolysis versus heparin in, 543–544, *544t*
 research, 73–74
 spontaneous breathing, 463
 Urokinase Pulmonary Embolism Trial (UPET), 537–538
 Urokinase-Streptokinase Pulmonary Embolism Trials (USPET), 537–538
 weaning from mechanical ventilatory support, 460–465
Clinicomp International Clinical Information System (CIS), 82
Clonal anergy, 690
Clonidine (Duraclon)
 as antihypertensive drug, 342
 for preoperative antihypertensive medication, 338–339
 toxic syndromes, *820t*
Clopidigrel

for acute coronary syndromes, *314t*
 effect on coagulation, 313
Clorgyline, for hypertension, 337
Closed chest compressions, in cardiopulmonary resuscitation, 364–365
Closed head trauma, mechanical ventilation and, 466–467, *467f*
Clostridium difficile, 476, 616, 618, 634, 677
 following liver transplantation, 731
 recommended therapy, *624t*
Clostridium perfringens, 674
 following surgery in the intensive care unit, 170
Clostridium spp., 633
Clostridium tetani, 674
Cluster (Biot) breathing, in comatose patients, *249t*
CMI. *See* Cell-mediated immunity
CMV. *See* Cytomegalovirus
CNS. *See* Central nervous system
Coagulase-negative staphylococci, recommended therapy, *624t*
Coagulation disorders
 anticoagulant drugs in acute coronary syndromes, *314t*
 effect of aspirin on, 313
 effect of heparin on, 313
 fulminant hepatic failure and, 497, *497f, 498f*
 laboratory assessment, 553–554
 in multiple organ dysfunction syndrome, 591
 preoperative assessment, 10
 regulation in liver transplantation, 730
 regulation in organ donors, 282
Coagulopathy
 care of the patient with multiple trauma and, 793–794
 hemostasis and, 549–565
 in management of organ donors, 282
 nasotracheal intubation and, 90
Cocaine
 evaluation and management for intoxication of, 837–838
 hypertension and, 337
 toxic syndromes, *820t*
Coccidia spp., following kidney transplantation, 734
Coccidiodes immitis, 660
 recommended therapy for life-threatening, *625t*
Coccidioides immitis, evaluation with computed tomography in the intensive care unit, 844
Coccidioides spp., 617
Cochrane, Archie, 57
Cochrane Collaboration, 57
Cochrane Controlled Trials Register (CCTR), 57
Cochrane Database of Systematic Reviews (CDSR), 57
Coding, diagnosis-related group, 81
Coinheritance (DNA), 66

Colitis
  initial therapy for life-threatening, *629t*
  neutropenic. *See* Typhlitis
  recommended therapy for life-threatening, *624t*
Colloids, 139
  clinical implications between crystalloid and, 139–140, *139t*
  implications on intracranial pressure, 140
  physiology and pharmacology, 139
Colonic diverticulosis
  diagnosis, 492
  hemorrhage in the critically ill, 492
  pathogenesis, 492
  treatment, 492
Coma
  anatomy of consciousness, 245–246, *246f, 247f*
  apnea in, *249t*
  barbiturates and, 239
  coma dépassé, 275
  death by brain criteria, 250
  definition, 244–245
  diagnosis and management in the intensive care unit, 244–252
  evaluation guidelines, 250–252, *251t*
  examination of patients with altered consciousness, 246–247, *248t, 249t*
  herniation syndromes, 247–249
    central, 247–248
    cerebellar tonsillar, 249
    lateral mass, 248–249
    subfalcine, 248–249
    upward transtentorial, 249
  key points, 252
  "Ondine's curse," *249t*
  persistent vegetative state, 249–250
  psychogenic unresponsiveness, 250
Coma cocktail. *See* Thiamine
Coma dépassé, 275
Committee on Medical Research of the Association of Medical Colleges, 73
Community-acquired pneumonia (CAP), 385–387
  complications, 387
  diagnosis, 385–386, *386t*
  epidemiologic associations for organisms causing, *386t*
  treatment, 386–387
Community hospitals
  acute care medicine in, 29–44
  admitting diagnoses, 43, *43t*
  critical care, 33–38, *35f, 36t, 37t, 38t, 39f, 40f, 41t*
  hospital organization involvement, 38
  intraoperative care, 33
  key points, 43–44
  philosophical and practical approach to acute care medicine, 38, 42
  postoperative care, 33
  practice framework, 29–38
  preoperative evaluation clinic, 32–33, 33t, *34f*
  recruiting and training of anesthesiologists, 38, 42

role of hospitalist teams in acute care services, 42–43, *43t*
  surgical clinical pathways, 33
Compensatory antiinflammatory response syndrome (CARS), care of the patient with multiple trauma and, 794
Complete blood count (CBC)
  for control of infection in burn patients, 806
  in heart transplantation, 701
Compound heterozygosity, 64
Computed tomography (CT)
  abdominal imaging in the intensive care unit, 849–854
  for aortic transections, 845, *845f*
  for blunt thoracic trauma, 844–845
  for chest wall trauma, 846
  comatose patients and, 245, *246f*
  for cytomegalovirus, 844
  for diagnosis of infection, 620
  for diagnosis of shock, 194
  for diagnosis of subarachnoid hemorrhage, 265–266
  for diaphragmatic rupture, 845
  for evaluation of the central nervous system, 854–855
  for fungal infections, 844, *844f*
  for invasive pulmonary aspergillosis, 844, *844f*
  for left lower-quadrant conditions, 853–854
  for left upper-quadrant conditions, 852–853, *852f*
  for lower-quadrant conditions, 853, *853f*
  for *Mycobacterium* infection, 843–844
  for perioperative evaluation of pulmonary disease, 380
  for *Pneumocystis carinii,* 843
  for pulmonary embolism, 846–847, *847f*
  for right upper-quadrant conditions, 851–852, *851f*
  for searching for a source of infection, sepsis, or fever, 843
  for septic emboli, 843, *844f*
  for thoracic spine injury, 845–846
  for thoracic valvular disease, 846
  for tracheobronchial tears, 845
  xenon-enhanced, 278
Computerized Intensity Intervention Score (CIIS), 24
Confidentiality, 46
Conflict of interest, in critical care medicine, 76–77
Congenital heart disease, 780–783, *781t*
  development issues, 781
  initial postoperative assessment and critical care management, 781
  perioperative metabolism, 783
  perioperative nutrition, 783
  perioperative pain, 783
  perioperative sedation, 783
  physiology, 781
  postoperative issues in common cardiac lesions, 781, *782t*

pulmonary dysfunction after cardiothoracic surgery, 783
  treatment of postoperative cardiovascular failure, 781–783
Congestive heart failure (CHF)
  effect on drug disposition, 188–189
  mechanical ventilation and, 466
  postural drainage and, 434
  preoperative assessment of patient, 8–9
  tracheal intubation and, 89
  treatment of ischemia and, 311
Consciousness
  anatomy, 245–246, *246f, 247f*
  brainstem activity and, 259
  decreased level after neurosurgery, 259–260
  definition, 244
  examination of patients with altered, 246–247, *248t, 249t*
  testing of clinical syndromes, *251t*
Constipation, tube feeding problems and, *180t*
Contact-activation pathway, 549, *550f*
Continuous arteriovenous hemodiafiltration (CAVHDF)
  for acute renal failure, 793
  for poisoning, 829
  for renal replacement therapy, 526
Continuous arteriovenous hemodialysis (CAVHD), for renal replacement therapy, 526
Continuous arteriovenous hemofiltration (CAVH), for renal replacement therapy, 526
Continuous cardiac output (CCO), 111
Continuous positive airway pressure (CPAP)
  death by brain criteria and, 250
  for inhalation injury, 812
Continuous renal replacement therapy (CRRT), 181
  for acute renal failure, 793
  for renal replacement therapy, 525, *526t*
Continuous venovenous hemodiafiltration (CVVHDF)
  for poisoning, 829
  for renal replacement therapy, 526
Continuous venovenous hemodialysis (CVVHD), for renal replacement therapy, 526
Continuous venovenous hemofiltration (CVVH), for renal replacement therapy, 525–526
Contractility, 289
Controlled clinical trials, 57
Contusions, computed tomography for detection of, 846
Cook Critical Care catheter, 98
COPD. *See* Chronic obstructive pulmonary disease
Copper, daily requirements in total parenteral nutrition, *182t*
COR. *See* Cervicoocular reflex
Cornelia de Lange syndrome, *779t*
Coronary artery bypass graft (CABG), 3. *See also* Minimally invasive direct coronary artery bypass

direct, 355
myocardial ischemia and, 305
off-pump, 355–356
perioperative epinephrine and, *316f*
Coronary artery disease (CAD)
cardiac function and, 287
pathophysiology, 303–305, *304f*
patients at risk for, 5, 305–306, *305t*
pharmacologic stress for detection, 6–8
Coronary artery surgery study (CASS), 5
Coronary perfusion pressure (CPP),
cardiogenic shock and, 290
Corticosteroids, *441t*
for asthma, 379
for diffuse alveolar hemorrhage, 743
for fever, 578
for intraoperative management of heart
transplantation, 703–704
long-term therapy, 639
for myasthenia gravis, 420
in orthotopic heart transplantation, 709
perioperative coverage, 9, *10t*
for septic shock, 639
in transplantation, 693–694, *694t*
Corynebacterium jeikeium, 655, 656
Corynebacterium spp., as complication of
hematopoietic stem cell
transplantation, 746, *746t*
Cosegregation (DNA), 66
Cost–benefit analysis
of accelerated surgical recovery, 355
of decision support systems, 84
in the intensive care unit, 24–25
of research, 76
technology and therapy research in the
intensive care unit, 71
Coxiella burnetii (Q fever), 636, 680
CPAP. *See* Continuous positive airway
pressure
CPB. *See* Cardiopulmonary bypass
CPDA-1. *See* Citrate phosphate dextrose
adenine
CPP. *See* Cerebral perfusion pressure;
Coronary perfusion pressure
CPR. *See* Cardiopulmonary resuscitation
CPS. *See* Cardiopulmonary status
Cranial vault contents, 237
Craniofacial dysostosis, *779t*
Craniotomy, postoperative care, 254–255
Creatine clearance, renal dysfunction and,
510–511, *510f, 510t*
CREST (calcinosis, Raynaud syndrome,
esophageal dysmotility,
scleroderma, and telangiectasia)
syndrome, 491
Creutzfeld–Jakob disease (CJD), blood
transfusions and, 567
CRH. *See* Central reflex hyperpnea
CRI. *See* Goldman Cardiac Risk Index
Critical care medicine (CCM)
cardiopulmonary status, 533
care of the critically ill obstetric patient,
765–775
care of the poisoned patient, 818–840
comatose patient diagnosis and
management, 244–252

in community hospitals, 29–44
conflict of interest in, 76–77
erythropoietin in critically ill patients, 575
fluid management in critically ill patients,
137–146
genomics in perioperative, 63–69
management of acute renal failure in the
critically ill patient, 521–532
nurses, 17–18
nutrition support, 176–185
perioperative management of infants and
children, 776–790
pharmacokinetic and pharmacodynamic
principles in, 186–191
philosophical and practical approach to,
38, 42
practice guidelines, 21–22
prognosis of patients with hematopoietic
stem cell transplantation, 749
research in, 70–79
rounds, 33–34
staffing, 17–19
standards of practice in medicine, 20–21
venous thromboembolism/pulmonary
embolism, 533–548
Critical illness polyneuropathy (CIP), *163t*
Crohn disease
evaluation with computed tomography in
the intensive care unit, 853–854
nutrition and, 179
Cromolyn sodium, *441t*
for asthma, 379
CRRT. *See* Continuous renal replacement
therapy
Cryoprecipitate, 572–573
Cryptococcus neoformans, 617, 649, 651, 684
evaluation with computed tomography in
the intensive care unit, 844
recommended therapy for life-threatening,
625t
Cryptococcus spp.
following kidney transplantation, 734
following liver transplantation, 730, 731
in postoperative management of heart
transplantation, 709
Cryptogenic sepsis, without identified local
infection, 627, 630
Cryptosporidium, 476, 654, 677
Crystalloids, 139
clinical implications between colloid and,
139–140, *139t*
implications on intracranial pressure, 140
physiology and pharmacology, 139
CSP. *See* Cyclosporine
CT. *See* Computed tomography
Curare (tubocurarine), for intensive care unit
use, *155t*
Cushing syndrome
perioperative management of infants and
children, 779
preoperative assessment of patient, 9
CVP. *See* Central venous pressure catheter
CVVH. *See* Continuous venovenous
hemofiltration
CVVHD. *See* Continuous venovenous
hemodialysis

CVVHDF. *See* Continuous venovenous
hemodiafiltration
CY. *See* Cyclophosphamide
Cyclic adenosine monophosphate (cAMP)
cardiogenic shock and, 292
shock and, 201
Cyclic antidepressants (CAs)
antidotes for overdose, *830t*
evaluation and management for
intoxication of, 834–836
toxic syndromes, *820t*
Cyclophosphamide (CY)
as complication of hematopoietic stem cell
transplantation, 745
in transplantation, *694t*
Cyclosporine A
acute tubular necrosis and, 505–506
as cause of qualitative platelet disorders,
555t
Cyclosporine (CSP, Rapamycin, Rapamune)
causing hypertension, 339
drug interactions, *696t, 708t*
following kidney transplantation, 734, *735t*
following liver transplantation, 732, *732t*
for intraoperative management of heart
transplantation, 703–704
for liver disease, 724
in pediatric transplantation, 783, *784t*
for postoperative management of heart
transplantation, 707
for renal failure, 745
in transplantation, *694t*, 695, *696t*
Cystic fibrosis (CF), perioperative evaluation,
377–378, *378t*
Cytokines
in acute lung injury/acute respiratory
distress syndrome (ALI/ARDS),
410–411
care of the patient with multiple trauma
and, 794
during catabolic phase of response to
injury, 176
continuous removal in the systemic
inflammatory response syndrome
(SIRS), 529–530
levels after trauma, 794
multiple organ dysfunction syndrome and,
592–593
role in transplantation rejection and graft
injury, 691–692
Cytomegalovirus (CMV), 491, 616, 651
blood transfusions and, 567
computed tomography for detection of,
844
following kidney transplantation, 734
following liver transplantation, 730–731
with hematopoietic stem cell
transplantation, 747–748, *748f,*
748t
in HIV-positive patients, 666
in immunocompromised patients, 661
in postoperative management of heart
transplantation, 709
recommended therapy for life-threatening,
627t
treatment, 662

Cytovene (ganciclovir)
  adverse effects, 686
  as antiviral prophylaxis, 640
  distribution and elimination, 686
  dosing, *622t*
  for Epstein-Barr infection, 626
  in immunocompromised patients, *652t*
  nephrotoxic effects, *745t*
  for viral infections, 626

D

Daclizumab (Zenapax), following kidney
    transplantation, 734, *735t*
DAD. *See* Diffuse alveolar damage
DAH. *See* Diffuse alveolar hemorrhage
Danazol, for autoimmune thrombocytopenia
    purpura, 562–563
DARE. *See* Database of Abstracts of Reviews
    of Effectiveness
DAT. *See* Positive direct antiglobulin test
Database of Abstracts of Reviews of
    Effectiveness (DARE), 57
Databases, 84
Data collection, 81–82
  measurement and interpretation of
    hemodynamic assessment, 123
Data mining, 84
DDAVP. *See* 1-Deamino-8-D-arginine
    vasopressin
D-dimer, 550
1-Deamino-8-D-arginine vasopressin
    (DDAVP), 555
Death, 46
  airway management and, 99
  by brain criteria, 250
  brain death determination and diagnosis,
    276–277, *276t*
  cerebral, 277
  from cyclic antidepressants, 836
  definition, 275
  diagnosis and management of brain-dead
    and nonheart-beating organ
    donors, 275–286
  during dialysis for acute renal failure, 527
  hematolic manifestations of fetal, 772–773
  irreversible, 277
  sudden, 527
  testing for brain death, 277–278, *277t*
Death and Dignity Act, 51
Debridement, in multiple organ dysfunction
    syndrome, 595
Decerebrate rigidity, 247
Decision making
  for the incapacitated patient, 46–47
  shared, 51
  surrogate, 47
Decontamination techniques, for care of the
    poisoned patient, 822–831
Decorticate rigidity, 247
Deep-breathing, postoperative, 401
Deep sternal wound infection (DSWI), in the
    cardiac surgical patient, 352
Deferoxamine, as neuroprotectant, 232
Defibrillation
  in cardiopulmonary resuscitation, 367–368
  defibrillators, 367–368

duration and electric pattern, 367
  energy requirements and adverse effects,
    368
Defibrillators, in cardiopulmonary
    resuscitation, 367–368
Defibrotide, for hepatic venoocclusive disease,
    744
Delirium, definition, 245
Demeclocycline, for syndrome of
    inappropriate antidiuretic
    hormone, 214
Dental injuries, airway management and, 99
Department of Health Services, 23
Desmopressin
  for diabetes insipidus, 753
  for hypernatremia, 215
  side effects, 753
Dexamethasone, perioperative management
    of infants and children, 780
Dexamethasone sodium phosphate, *441t*
Dexmedetomidine
  as antihypertensive drug, 342
  comparison with other intensive care unit
    sedative drugs, *150t*
  in the intensive care unit, 149
  as neuroprotectant, 234
  for perioperative myocardial ischemia, 315
  as a sedative in the intensive care unit,
    151t
Dextran
  as cause of fever, *585t*
  as cause of qualitative platelet disorders,
    555t
Dextrose
  for fluid replacement therapy, 141
  for poisoning, 822
D fragment, 550
Diabetes insipidus
  emergency treatment, 752–753
  pediatric, 779
  treatment, 215
Diabetes mellitus. *See also* Diabetes insipidus;
    Insulin
  as an emergency, 760–762, *761t*, *762t*
  in critically ill obstetric patients, 772
  gestational, 766
  heart transplantation and, 701
  in immunocompromised patients,
    668–669
  otitis and, 669
  pancreas transplantation and, 736, *736t*
  preoperative assessment, 9
  rhinocerebral mucormycosis and, 669
  risk for coronary artery disease, 5
Diabetic ketoacidosis (DKA), 761–762,
    761t
  clinical features, 761
  in critically ill obstetric patients, 766
  diagnosis, 761
  electrolyte alterations during, *761t*
  laboratory features, 761
  treatment, 761–762
Diagnosis-related group (DRG) coding, 81
*Diagnostic and Statistical Manual of Mental
    Disorders, Fourth Edition
    (DSM-IV)*, 245

Diagnostic bronchoalveolar lavage (BAL), for
    diagnosis of complications of
    hematopoietic stem cell
    transplantation, 743–744
Dialysis
  for acute renal failure, 793
  complications in acute renal failure,
    527–528
  fever during, 527–528
  first-use syndrome, 527
  hemorrhage during, 528
  hopotension during, 527
  hypoxemia during, 527
  liver, for fulminant hepatic failure, 500
  principles of water and solute removal by,
    524–525
  sudden death during, 527
  techniques of renal replacement therapy,
    525–527
Dialysis disequilibrium syndrome, 527
  prevention, 527
Dialyzer membrane biocompatibility, during
    renal replacement therapy, 529
Diaphragmatic rupture, computed
    tomography for detection of, 845
Diarrhea
  in the perioperative intensive care unit
    patient, 475–476
  tube feeding problems and, *180t*
Diazepam
  in the intensive care unit, 147–148
  as a sedative in the intensive care unit,
    151t
  for seizures, 836
Diazoxide, as antihypertensive drug, 340
DIC. *See* Disseminated intravascular
    coagulopathy
DICOM, 82
Diffuse alveolar damage (DAD), as
    complication of hematopoietic
    stem cell transplantation, 742
Diffuse alveolar hemorrhage (DAH), as
    complication of hematopoietic
    stem cell transplantation, 742–743,
    743f
Diflucan (fluconazole), 626, *683t*
  adverse effects, 685
  distribution and elimination, 685
  dosing, *622t*
  in immunocompromised patients, *652t*
DiGeorge syndrome, 782
Digibind, for digoxin toxicity, 831
Digitalis
  for cardiac insufficiency as complication of
    hematopoietic stem cell
    transplantation, 745
  for shock, 201, *201t*
  toxic syndromes, *820t*
Digitalis glycosides, antidotes for overdose,
    830t
Digital subtraction angiography (DSA), for
    determination of brain death, 278
Digoxin
  abnormal cardioactive response in the
    denervated heart, 706–707, *706t*
  for atrial fibrillation, 323

dosage adjustments in the intensive care unit, *523t*

evaluation and management for intoxication of, 831

for overdose of digitalis glycosides, *830t*

as prophylaxis against atrial fibrillation, 351

for rate control in atrial flutter or atrial fibrillation, 322–323

for supraventricular tachyarrhythmias, 322

Digoxin-Specific Antibody Fragments (Digibind), for digoxin toxicity, 831

Diltiazem hydrochloride

for acute myocardial ischemia, 311, *312t*

as antihypertensive drug, 342–343, *342t*

for multifocal atrial tachycardia, 324

for pheochromocytoma, 760

for rate control in atrial flutter or atrial fibrillation, 322–323

Dimethyl sulfoxide, as neuroprotectant, 232

Dipyridamole, pharmacologic stress for detection of coronary artery disease, 7

Dipyridamole thallium scintigraphy (DTS), for myocardial ischemia, 307

Dipyridimole, as cause of qualitative platelet disorders, *555t*

Direct coronary artery bypass, 355

Disclosure, 46

Diseases, research pathophysiology, 71–72

Dismutase, as neuroprotectant, 232

Disopyramide, acquired prolonged repolarization syndromes and, *329t*

Disorientation, 211, *211t*

Disputes, mediating, 49–50

Disseminated intravascular coagulopathy (DIC)

airway management and, 95

blood transfusions and, 568

perioperative hemostasis and coagulopathy, 555–558, *556t*

Distributive justice, 45

Diuretics

for cardiac insufficiency as complication of hematopoietic stem cell transplantation, 745

for hypertension in the intensive care unit, 339–340

loop, 511–512

in acute renal failure, 523

for prevention and treatment of renal injury, 511–513

as renal protective agents, 353

resistance, *512t*

Dizocilpine, as neuroprotectant, 232

DKA. *See* Diabetic ketoacidosis

DLT. *See* Double-lung transplant

DNA

coinheritance, 66

cosegregation, 66

linkage dysequilibrium, 65

testing, 64

DNR. *See* Do-not-resuscitate orders

Dobutamine

in the cardiac surgical patient, 347, *348t*

for pediatric treatment of postoperative cardiac failure, 782

pharmacologic stress for detection of coronary artery disease, 7

for shock, 201, *201t*, 202

Dobutamine stress echocardiography, for preoperative care in liver transplantation, 726

Donors. *See* Organ donors

Do-not-resuscitate (DNR) orders, 47, 48

Dopamine

for acute renal failure, 793

in acute renal failure, 522–523

in animal studies for acute renal failure, *522t*

for bradyarrhythmias, 320

in the cardiac surgical patient, 347, *348t*

for cardiogenic shock, 292

for fulminant hepatic failure, 499

in management of organ donors, 280, *281f*, 282

for pediatric treatment of postoperative cardiac failure, 782

for prevention and treatment of renal injury, 513–514

for shock, *201t*, 202, *202f*

Dopaminergic agonists, for prevention and treatment of renal injury, 513–514

Dopexamine

for prevention and treatment of renal injury, 514

for shock, 201, *201t*

Doppler ultrasonography

to determine cardiac output in hemodynamic assessment, 130

transcranial, 254

Dorsalis pedis artery, in arterial cannulation, 104

Double burst stimulation, 159

Double-lung transplant (DLT), 711

Down syndrome, *779t*

Doxacurium (nuromax), for intensive care unit use, *155t*, 157, 164

Doxycycline

dosing, *622t*

for malaria, 636

for rickettsial infections, 636

DPI. *See* Dry-powder inhaler

Drains, following surgery, 172

DRG. *See* Diagnosis-related group coding

Droperidol, antiemetic therapy perioperative management of infants and children, 780

Drug fever, 585, *585t*

infections and, 617–618

Drug therapy. *See also* individual drug names

abnormal cardioactive drug responses in the denervated heart, 706–707, *706t*

aerosolized, 439–440

agents for clinical transportation in transplantation, 693–694, *694t*

antibacterial, 624–625

antibiotics for intraoperative management of heart transplantation, 703–704

antifungal, 625–626, *625t*

antihypertensive drugs in pregnancy, *337t*

antiinfective therapy, 620–627, *628t–629t*, *637f*, *638t*

antimicrobial therapy in immunocompromised patients, *652t*

antiviral, 626–627, *627t*

dosing, *622t*

beta-lactams, 620–621, *622t–623t*, *624t*

in cardiopulmonary resuscitation, 368–370, *368t*

clearance, 187

drug disposition after single intravenous dose, 186, *187f*

effect on coagulation, 313–314, *314t*

elimination by first-order process, 186

first-order and dose-dependent kinetics, 186–188

drug accumulation and loading dose, 187–188

volume of distribution and clearance, 186–187

following kidney transplantation, 734

following liver transplantation, 730

for hypertension in the intensive care unit, 339–343

inhalation agents, *441t*

interactions with neuromuscular blocking drugs, *156t*

key points, 190

medications causing hypertension, 339

minimum inhibitory concentration, 620

for multiresistant gram-positive cocci, 623

for myocardial ischemia, 311, *312t*

neuroresuscitative agents, 242

non–first-order drug kinetics, 188–189, *189t*

drug disposition in elderly patients, 189

drug interactions, 189, *189t*

effect of changes in plasma protein binding on drug disposition, 189

effect of heart failure on drug disposition, 188–189

effect of liver failure on drug disposition, 188

effect of renal failure on drug disposition, 188

pharmacokinetic and pharmacodynamic principles, 186–191

pharmacologic immunosuppression, 693–698, *694t*

pharmacologic neuroprotectants, 231–234

practical use of plasma drug concentration, 189–190, *190f*

pulse-steroid therapy, 694

recommended therapy for life-threatening infections, *624t*

routes of administration, 370

toxicity in pediatric multiorgan failure, 788

Dry-powder inhaler (DPI), 442

DSA. *See* Digital subtraction angiography

DSWI. *See* Deep sternal wound infection

DTS. *See* Dipyridamole thallium scintigraphy

D-tubocurarine, for intensive care unit use, 157

Dubowitz syndrome, *779t*

Duraclon (clonidine)
  as antihypertensive drug, 342
  for preoperative antihypertensive
      medication, 338–339
  toxic syndromes, *820t*
Dyspnea, tube feeding problems and, *180t*
Dysrhythmias
  in the cardiac surgical patient, 351–352
  long-term management, 352
  in postoperative care of thoracic surgical
      patients, 420

E
EAE. *See* Effective arterial elastance
Eaton–Lambert syndrome, *163t*, 419
EBM. *See* Evidence-based medicine
ECG. *See* Electrocardiogram
Echinocandin, 626
Echocardiography
  for detection of coronary artery disease, 7–8
  for diagnostic evaluation of pulmonary
      embolism, 541–542, *542t*
  hemodynamic information acquired, *132t*
ECMO. *See* Extracorporeal membrane
      oxygenation
Edema
  in the cardiac surgical patient, 354
  as complication of subarachnoid
      hemorrhage, 270
  effect of renal failure on drug disposition,
      188
  pulmonary, following lung transplantation,
      717
  thermal damage to the lungs and, 811–812
EDPVR. *See* End-diastolic pressure volume
      relationship
Education, of the preoperative patient, 397
Effective arterial elastance (EAE), shock and,
      195
E fragment, 550
Ehlers-Danlos syndrome, predisposition to
      subarachnoid hemorrhage, 264
Eisenmenger syndrome
  in critically ill obstetric patients, 769
  as indication for heart-lung transplant, 720
Elderly. *See also* Age
  drug disposition in, 189
  mechanical ventilation and, 467–468, *468f*
  mechanical ventilation in, 467–468, *468f*
Electrical injury, 812–813
Electrocardiogram (ECG)
  changes in the cardiac surgical patient,
      350–351
  for preoperative testing, 32–33
Electrolytes
  abnormalities in the pediatric intensive care
      unit, 779
  in acute renal failure, 524
  alterations during diabetic ketoacidosis,
      761t
  in the critically ill patient, 182, *182t*
  deficiency, *163t*
  diagnosis and management of
      abnormalities, 206–224
  effect on organ donors, 281–282
  toxicity, *163t*

Electronic mail (e-mail), 84–85
Electronic medical record (EMR), 80–82
Electrophysiology, for consciousness testing,
      251t
Elimination, for care of the poisoned patient,
      828–830, *830t*
E-mail. *See* Electronic mail
Embolectomy, for mesenteric ischemia, 480
Embolism, in critically ill obstetric patients,
      772
Emergency medicine
  after pediatric neurologic surgery, 780
  endocrine emergencies, 752–764
  hyperglycemic emergencies, 760–762,
      761t, *762t*
  poisoning, 821–822, *821t*
  stabilization and supportive care of the
      poisoned patient, 821–822, *821t*
Emesis. *See* Vomiting
EMMT. *See* European Multicenter Milrinone
      Trial
Emphysema
  centrilobular, 377
  panacinar, 377
  perioperative evaluation, 376–377, *377t*
  preoperative assessment of patient, 8
EMR. *See* Electronic medical record
Enalapril, acute tubular necrosis and, 505
Encephalitis, recommended therapy for
      life-threatening, *627t*
Encephalopathy, hypertensive, 335
Encryption, medical informatics, 85–86
End-diastolic pressure volume relationship
      (EDPVR) shock and, 195
Endocarditis
  acute infective, 630–631
  initial therapy for life-threatening, *628t*
  recommended therapy for life-threatening,
      624t
Endocrine diseases
  adrenal insufficiency, 757–759, *757t*
  carcinoid syndrome, 760
  diabetes insipidus, 752–753
  diabetes mellitus, 760–762, *761t*, *762t*
  emergencies, 752–764
  hyperglycemic emergencies, 760–762,
      761t, *762t*
  key points, 762–763
  parathyroid disease, 753–754, *754t*
  pheochromocytoma, 759–760
  preoperative assessment, 9
  thyroid disease, 754–757
      hyperthyroidism, 756–757, *756t*
      hypothyroidism (myxedema), 755–756,
          755t
Endocrine system, effect on organ donors,
      280–281, *280f*, *281f*
End-of-life issues, 45–54
Endoscopic retrograde
      cholangiopancreatography (ERCP),
      479
Endotracheal intubation, mechanical
      ventilation and, 403
Endotracheal tube
  changing, 97–98
  mechanical ventilation and, 403

End-systolic pressure volume relationship
      (ESPVR), shock and, 195
Energy balance, nutrition support in the
      critically ill patient, 179
Engraftment, with hematopoietic stem cell
      transplantation, 741
Enteral nutrition
  benefits, 180–181
  care of the patient with multiple trauma
      and, 794, 796
  in the critically ill patient, 180–181, *180t*
  following liver transplantation, 731
  for fulminant hepatic failure, 499
  jejunostomy and, 172
  pediatric perioperative management, 778
Enteric infections, 634
Enterobacteriaceae, recommended therapy,
      624t
Enterobacter spp., 621
  fever and, 584
Enterococcus
  as complication of hematopoietic stem cell
      transplantation, 746, *746t*
  recommended therapy, *624t*
Enterococcus faecalis, 623, 680–681
Enterocutaneous fistulas, 172–173
Environment, protected, in the intensive care
      unit, 640
Ephedrine, abnormal cardioactive response in
      the denervated heart, 706–707,
      706t
Epidemic typhus (*Rickettsia prowazekii*), 636
Epidural analgesia, 425–426
Epinephrine, *441t*
  in the cardiac surgical patient, 347, *348t*
  in cardiopulmonary resuscitation, 368–369
  in management of organ donors, 280,
      281f
  for pediatric treatment of postoperative
      cardiac failure, 782
  for perioperative myocardial ischemia, 315,
      315f
  for shock, *201t*, 202, *202f*
Epoprostenol, for pulmonary hypertension in
      critically ill obstetric patients, 769
Epstein-Barr virus
  as complication of hematopoietic stem cell
      transplantation, 747–748, *748t*
  following liver transplantation, 730
Eptifibatide
  for acute coronary syndromes, *314t*
  effect on coagulation, 313
ERCP. *See* Endoscopic retrograde
      cholangiopancreatography
Erhlichia chaffeensis (erhlichiosis), 636
Erhlichia phagocytophilia (erhlichiosis), 636
Erhlichiosis (*Erhlichia chaffeensis, Erhlichia
      phagocytophilia*), 636
Erysipelas, following surgery in the intensive
      care unit, 170
Erythromycin, 621, 677
  adverse reactions, 677
  antibiotic management of renal and hepatic
      dysfunction in the intensive care
      unit, *675t*
  dosing, *622t*

drug interactions in critically ill patients, *189t*

Erythropoietin
causing hypertension, 339
in critically ill patients, 575

Escharotomy incisions, 802, *803f*

Escherichia coli, 633, 634, 674
fluid management and, 140
sepsis and, 606
with thrombocytopenia, 563

Esmolol
for acute myocardial ischemia, 311, *312t*
as antihypertensive drug, 341, *341t*
for aortic dissection, 336
for Marfan syndrome in critically ill obstetric patients, 769
for paroxysmal supraventricular tachycardia, 322
for rate control in atrial flutter or atrial fibrillation, 322–323

Esophageal tracheal Combitube (ETC), in cardiopulmonary resuscitation, 365

Esophagitis, 491. See also Mucosal erosive disease

ESPVR. See End-systolic pressure volume relationship

Estradiol, as neuroprotectant, 232

Estrogen, as neuroprotectant, 232

ETC. See Esophageal tracheal Combitube

Ethanol, poisoning and, 829–830, *830t*

Ethical issues, 45–54
advance directives, 47–48
allocation of medical resources, 52
in caring for patients, 45
do-not-resuscitate orders, 47, 48
in genomics in perioperative critical care, 67
health care system reform, 52–53
hospital ethics committees, 53
key points, 54
legal problems and, 53
managed care, 53
mediating disputes, 49–50
versus moral issues, 45
pediatric, 50–51
physician-assisted suicide and active euthanasia, 51–52, *51t*, *52t*
physicians' obligations, 45–47
withdrawal of basic life support, 49
withdrawal of life-sustaining treatment, 48–49, *49f*

Ethylene glycol
antidotes for overdose, *830t*
poisoning and, 829–830
toxic syndromes, *820t*

Etomidate
in the intensive care unit, 149
as neuroprotectant, 233–234, *233t*, 234
for tracheal intubation, 92

ETT. See Existing endotracheal tube

European Multicenter Milrinone Trial (EMMT), 299

Euthanasia, 51–52, *51t*, *52t*
definitions, *51t*

Eutonyl (pargyline), for hypertension, 337

Evidence-based medicine (EBM), 55–62

definition, 56–57
information websites, *60t*
key points, 61
literature review, 57
need for, 55, *56t*
search strategy, 56–68
skill sets required, 55–61
base clinical set, 57
critical appraisal process, 55–56
levels of evidence, 56
primary evidence, 56
randomized controlled trial (RCT), 56
secondary evidence, 56
web sites, 57

Evidence-Based Medicine Working Group, 56

Evidence-based standards, 21

Excision, of burn wounds, 808

Excitatory amino acid receptor antagonists, as neuroprotectants, 232

Excitotoxicity, cerebral injury and, 229

Exercise
decreased activity, *180t*
importance of tolerance, 5–6, *6t*

Exercise testing, in perioperative management of pulmonary diseases, 399

Existing endotracheal tube (ETT), 97–98

External jugular venous cannulation, in the intensive care unit, 107, *107f*

Extracellular fluid volume, regulation, 138–139

Extracorporeal membrane oxygenation (ECMO), for pediatric treatment of postoperative cardiac failure, 782–783

Extubation. See also Reintubations
in the cardiac surgical patient, 349
unplanned, 469–470, *470t*
versus weaning failure, 470

F

Fascial disruption, following surgery, 170

Fasciitis
initial therapy for life-threatening, *629t*
necrotizing, 634

Fat, for nutrition support in the critically ill patient, 181

FDA. See U.S. Food and Drug Administration

FDPs. See Fibrinogen-degradation products

Febrile nonhemolytic transfusion reaction (FNHTR), 568

Febrile response, to fever in the intensive care unit, 577–578

Fecal elimination, for care of the poisoned patient, 828–829

Feeding. See also Nutrition
nutrition support in the critically ill patient, 180–181, *180t*

Femoral artery, in arterial cannulation, 104

Femoral venous catheterization, in the intensive care unit, 108

Fenoldapam
in acute renal failure, 522–523
in animal studies for acute renal failure, *522t*
as antihypertensive drug, 342
for fulminant hepatic failure, 499

for hypertensive encephalopathy, 335
for prevention and treatment of renal injury, 514

Fentanyl
in the intensive care unit, 151–152
for tracheal intubation, 92

Fetal heart rate monitoring (FHRM), in critically ill obstetric patients, 767, *768f*

Fetus
beat-to-beat variability in critically ill obstetric patients, 767
hematologic manifestations of death, 772–773
maternal–fetal interactions during pregnancy, 766–767, *767f*
viability, 765

Fever. See also Temperature
clinical evaluation, 579
computed tomography for detection of, 843
during dialysis for acute renal failure, 527–528
evaluation, 578–579, *579f*, *580f*
in the intensive care unit, 577–587
febrile response, 577–578
beneficial and adverse effects, 578
pathophysiology, 577–578, *578f*
treatment, 578
in immunocompromised patients, 668
infection and, 617
infectious sources of, 579–584
abdominal infection, 582–583, *583f*
catheter-related infection, 580–582, *581f*, *582f*, *582t*
nosocomial pneumonia, 583–584
sinusitis, 584
urinary tract infection, 584
ventilator-associated pneumonia (VAP), 583–584, *584f*
initial empiric antibiotic therapy in patients with neutropenia and, *658t*
key points, 586
noninfectious causes in immunocompromised patients, 655
noninfectious causes of, 584–585
drug fever, 585, *585t*
malignant hyperthermia, 585
neuroleptic malignant syndrome, 585
transfusion reactions, 585
postoperative, 169–170, 585–586
in transplant patients without a defined source, 661

FEVT. See Forced expired volume timed

FHF. See Fulminant hepatic failure

FHRM. See Fetal heart rate monitoring

Fiberoptic intubation, 95–96, *95f*

Fibrinogen-degradation products (FDPs), 550

Fibrinogenolysis, definition, 550

Fibrinolysis
definition, 550
laboratory testing, 552
for vasospasm, 256

Fibrinopeptides, 550

Fibromuscular dysplasia, predisposition to subarachnoid hemorrhage, 264

Fibrosing alveolitis, acute lung injury/acute respiratory distress syndrome (ALI/ARDS) and, 411

FIRDA. *See* Frontally predominant rhythmic delta activity

First-degree burns, 801

First-use syndrome, in dialysis, 527

Fisoneb, 439

Fistulas
    aortoenteric, 491
    enterocutaneous, 172–173

FK506. *See* Tacrolimus

Flagyl, for *Clostridium difficile* colitis, 476

Flow (cardiac output), definition, 534

Flow volume loops, perioperative evaluation, 381–382

Fluconazole (Diflucan), 626, *683t*
    adverse effects, 685
    distribution and elimination, 685
    dosing, *622t*
    in immunocompromised patients, *652t*

Flucytosine (Ancobon), 626, *683t*
    adverse effects, 684–685
    distribution and elimination, 684
    dosing, *622t*

Fludrocortisone, for septic shock, 639

Fluid management in critically ill patients, 137–146
    in acute care of burns, 804, *804t*
    in acute lung injury/acute respiratory distress syndrome (ALI/ARDS), 413
    in acute renal failure, 524
    after kidney transplantation, 733–734, *734t*
    after pediatric neurologic surgery, 780
    clinical experience with hypertonic fluid management, 143
    clinical implications of choices between crystalloid and colloid, 139–140, *139t*
    colloids, crystalloids, and hypertonic solutions, 139
    effect on organ donors, 281–282
    fluid replacement therapy, 140–143, *141t, 142f, 143t*
        clinical implications of hypertonic fluid administration, 142–143, *143t*
        dextrose, 141
        maintenance requirements for water, sodium, and potassium, 140–141
        management, 141
        surgical fluid requirements, 141–142, *141t, 142f*
    fluid status, assessment, and monitoring, 143–145, *145t*
        of hypovolemia and tissue hypoperfusion, 143–145, *145t*
    following kidney transplantation, 733–734, *734t*
    implications of crystalloid and colloid infusions on intracranial pressure, 140
    intracranial hypertension, 236–239

key points, 145

in management of organ donors, 281

as nutritional support, 182

for pancreatitis, 479

pediatric calculations, *778t*

perioperative management in infants and children, 778, *778t*

pheochromocytoma, 760

physiologic principles of volume homeostasis, 137–139, *138f*
    body fluid compartments, 137, *138f*
    distribution of infused fluids, 137
    prediction of plasma volume expansion using kinetic analysis, 137–138
    regulation of extracellular fluid volume, 138–139

in postoperative care of thoracic surgical patients, 420

sepsis and, 610–612

shock and, 197, 200

testing for consciousness, *251t*

Flumadine (rimantadine)
    as antiviral prophylaxis, 640
    for viral infections, 626

Flumazenil
    for fulminant hepatic failure, 499
    for overdose of benzodiazepines, *830t*
    for poisoning, 822

Flunisolide, *441t*

Fluorides, antidotes for overdose, *830t*

Fluoroquinolones
    dosing, *623t*
    for infections, 623–624
    for pancreatitis, 480

Fluticasone propionate, *441t*

FNHTR. *See* Febrile nonhemolytic transfusion reaction

Folate, 177

Folinic acid, in immunocompromised patients, *652t*

Forced expired volume timed (FEVT), 375, *376f*

Forced vital capacity (FVC), 375

Fortaz (ceftazidime), 620

Foscarnet (Foscavir)
    dosing, *622t*
    nephrotoxic effects, *745t*
    for viral infections, 626

Foscavir (Foscarnet)
    dosing, *622t*
    nephrotoxic effects, *745t*
    for viral infections, 626

Fractures
    computed tomography for detection of, 846
    stabilization in multiple organ dysfunction syndrome, 595

Frank, Otto, 195

Frank-Starling relation, 288, *288f*

"Fraud squad," 25

FRC. *See* Functional residual capacity

Free radical scavengers, in animal studies for acute renal failure, *522t*

Frontally predominant rhythmic delta activity (FIRDA), 251

FTE. *See* Full-time equivalent resident

Full-time equivalent (FTE) resident, 81

Fulminant hepatic failure (FHF), 495–502
    cardiovascular complications, 496–497
    clinical presentation, 495–496
    coagulation complications, 497, *497f, 498f*
    definition, 495
    etiology, 495
    gastrointestinal complications, 498
    infectious complications, 497–498
    key points, 501
    liver support devices, 500
    liver transplantation, 500
    malnutrition and, 498
    mediator therapy, 499–500
    metabolic disorders and, 498
    neurologic complications, 496, *496t*
    pulmonary complications, 497
    renal dysfunction and failure, 498–499
    treatment, 499

Functional residual capacity (FRC), in airway management, 92

Fungal infections
    computed tomography for detection of, 844, *844f*
    with hematopoietic stem cell transplantation, 747, *747f*
    recommended therapy for life-threatening, *625t*

Fungizone (amphotericin B deoxycholate), 625

Furosemide
    as antihypertensive drug, 339–340
    as cause of qualitative platelet disorders, *555t*
    in management of organ donors, 282
    for prevention and treatment of renal injury, 511–512

Fusarium, 625, 656
    recommended regimens for treatment of multiresistant, *638t*
    recommended therapy for life-threatening, *625t*

FVC. *See* Forced vital capacity

G

GABA. *See* Gamma-aminobutyric acid

Gamma-aminobutyric acid (GABA), benzodiazepines and, 147–148

Ganciclovir (Cytovene)
    adverse effects, 686
    as antiviral prophylaxis, 640
    distribution and elimination, 686
    dosing, *622t*
    for Epstein-Barr infection, 626
    in immunocompromised patients, *652t*
    nephrotoxic effects, *745t*
    for viral infections, 626

Gangliosides, for cerebral ischemia, 260

Gangrene, synergistic, 634

Gas transport
    in cardiopulmonary resuscitation, 365
    in critically ill obstetric patients, 766

Gastric emptying
    factors that cumulatively increase the appropriateness of, 823, *824t*
    for poisoning, 823

Gastrointestinal hemorrhage (GIH)
in the critically ill patient, 485–494
fulminant hepatic failure and, 498
key points, 493
lower gastrointestinal bleeding, 492, *492t*
colonic diverticulosis, 492
vascular anomalies, 492
in orthotopic heart transplantation, 709
resuscitation protocol, 486, 488, *488t*
upper gastrointestinal bleeding, 485–492, *486t*
aortoenteric fistulas, 491
initial triage, 485–486, *487f*, *488t*
Mallory-Weiss syndrome, 490–491
mucosal erosive disease, 491
peptic ulcer disease, 486, 488–489, *488t*, *489t*
portal hypertension, 489–490, *489t*
stress-related erosive syndrome (SRES), 490
tumors, 492
vascular anomalies, 491–492
Gastrointestinal motility, poisoning and, 823
Gastrointestinal obstruction, evaluation with computed tomography in the intensive care unit, 853
Gastrointestinal perforation, evaluation with computed tomography in the intensive care unit, 853
Gastrointestinal system, fulminant hepatic failure and, 498
Gastrointestinal tract
evaluation with computed tomography in the intensive care unit, 852–853
infections associated with, *618t*
in liver transplantation, 731
sepsis and, 609
Gatifloxacin (Tequin), 624
dosing, *623t*
GCS. *See* Glasgow Coma Scale
"Gene chips." *See* Oligonucleotide microarrays
Genes, map of the human leukocyte antigen, 692, *692f*
Genetic association, 65
polymorphism and predisposition to acute renal failure, 506, *507t*
Genomics, 63–69
analytical validity, 64–65
categories of critical care genotypes, 63–65
circumstantial evidence for genomic causation, 66
clinical utility, 67
clinical validity, 65
definition, 63
ethical, legal, and social issues, 67
experimental evidence for biologic causation, 66–67
Human Genome Project, 53–54
key points, 68
phenotype issues in genomic causation, 67
profiling, 64
shortcomings in perioperative critical care, 68
statistical evidence for genomic causation, 65–66

family-based segregation analysis, 66
population-based Genomic Association studies, 65–66
Genotypes
categories of critical care, 63–65
definition, 63
Gentamicin, 621
for control of infection in burn patients, 806
dosage adjustments in the intensive care unit, *523t*
dosing, *623t*
effect of renal failure on drug disposition, 188
Gentamicin sulfate, 676
Gestation
diabetes mellitus and, 766
preterm, 765
GFR. *See* Glomerular filtration rate
Giant aneurysms, operative management, 269–270
Giardia, 654, 679
GIH. *See* Gastrointestinal hemorrhage
Glasgow Coma Scale (GCS), 10, *10t*
comatose patients, 245, *245t*
decreased level of consciousness, 259
fever and, 579
in the head-injured patient, 796
in postoperative management of aneurysms, 272
traumatic brain injuries and, 236, *237t*
Glomerular filtration rate (GFR), 138
in the cardiac surgical patient, 353
potassium abnormalities and, 215
Glomerulonephritis, hypertension and, 336
Glucagon
during catabolic phase of response to injury, 176
for overdose of beta-blockers, *830t*
Glucocorticoids
for acute lung injury/acute respiratory distress syndrome (ALI/ARDS), *413t*
in acute lung injury/acute respiratory distress syndrome (ALI/ARDS), 414
during catabolic phase of response to injury, 176
perioperative coverage, *10t*
for subarachnoid hemorrhage, 270
Glucose
intolerance as adverse reaction to β-blockers, 341
for nutrition support in the critically ill patient, 181
Glutamate receptors, 229
Glycopeptides, 677–678
adverse effects, 678
distribution and elimination, 678
resistance, 681–682, *682t*
Glycopyrrolate, for tracheal intubation, 91–92
Goldenhar syndrome, *779t*
Goldman Cardiac Risk Index (CRI), 2–3, 394
Government agencies, mandatory practice standards, 23

Grafts
engraftment with hematopoietic stem cell transplantation, 741
failure in pediatric transplantation, 785
in liver transplantation, 724, 729–730
pancreatitis following pancreas transplantation, 737
Graft-versus-host disease (GVHD), with hematopoietic stem cell transplantation, 740
Granulocytopenia
infections associated with, *618t*
initial therapy for life-threatening, *628t*, *629t*
Grateful Med, 58–59
Growth hormones
in animal studies for acute renal failure, *522t*
in immune-enhancing diets, 182
Guanethidine sulphate, for preoperative antihypertensive medication, 339
Guanine nucleoside analogs
adverse effects, 686
distribution and elimination, 686
in the intensive care unit, 686
"Guidelines 2000 for Cardiopulmonary Resuscitation and Emergency Cardiovascular Care," 320, 322, *323f*, 328, *329f*
Guillain-Barré, *163t*
GVHD. *See* Graft-versus-host disease
Gynecologic infections, 634

H

HAART. *See* Highly active antiretroviral treatment
HACEK *(Haemophilus aphrophilus, Actinobacillus actinomycetemcomitans, Cardiobacterium hominus, Eikenella corrodens,* and *Kingella)*, 630–631
Haemophilus influenzae, 385, 626, 630
fever and, 584
in postoperative management of lung transplantation, 719
recommended therapy, *624t*
Halothane, as neuroprotectant, 233
Hantaan virus (Korean), recommended therapy for life-threatening, *627t*
Hantavirus, 626, 632
recommended therapy for life-threatening, *627t*
Haplotype, 66
HCFA. *See* Health Care Financing Administration
HCV. *See* Hepatitis C virus
Head trauma
care of the patient with, 796–797
management in the intensive care unit, 236–243
mechanical ventilation with closed-head trauma, 466–467, *467f*
neuromuscular blocking agents and, 164
Health, assessment, 394
Health Care Financing Administration (HCFA), 23, 25

Health care system, reform, 52–53
Health Insurance Portability and
  Accountability Act (HIPAA), 25
Health maintenance organizations (HMOs),
  346
Heart. *See also* Cardiogenic shock
  cardiac function, 287–289
  care of the patient with blunt cardiac
    injury, 797
  heart-lung transplantation, 720–721
  heterotopic transplant, 710–711
  orthotopic transplant, 351, 699–710
  pediatric transplantation, 786
Heart failure. *See* Congestive heart failure
Heart–lung transplantation
  adult, 720–721
  pediatric, 786
Heart rate (HR)
  in asymptomatic patients with
    bradyarrhythmias, 320
  in cardiogenic shock, 287
Helicobacter pylori, 486, 489
HELLP. *See* Hemolysis, elevated liver
    transaminases, low platelets
    syndrome
Hematemesis, 211, *211t*
Hematologic diseases
  management in lung transplantation, 718
  preoperative assessment, 10
Hematomas, computed tomography for
    detection of, 846
Hematopoietic stem cell transplantation
    (HSCT), 740–751. *See also* Bone
    marrow transplant
  allogeneic transplantation, 740–741
  autologous transplantation, 740
  bacterial infections and, 746, *746t*
  cardiac insufficiency, 745–746
  common viral infections as complication of
    hematopoietic stem cell
    transplantation, 747–748, *748t*
  cytomegalovirus, 747–748, *748f, 748t*
  diagnosis of pulmonary complications
    743–744, *743f*
  engraftment, 741
  four-year survival rates, 741–742, *742t*
  fungal infections, 747, *747f*
  hepatic venoocclusive disease and, 744
  indications, 741, *741t*
  infections in recipients, 746–748, *746f*
  key points, 750
  outcomes, 741–742, *742t*
  preparative regimens, 741
  prognosis of critically ill recipients, 749
  pulmonary complications, 742–743,
    743f
  renal failure and, 744–745, *745t*
  thrombotic microangiopathy, 748–749
Hemihypertrophy, *779t*
Hemodialysis
  for fulminant hepatic failure, 499
  for hyperkalemia, 217
  intermittent, for renal replacement therapy,
    525
  for poisoning, 829
  for removal of salicylates, 833

for syndrome of inappropriate antidiuretic
    hormone, 214
Hemodilution in Stroke Study Group,
    260
Hemodynamic assessment
  arterial pressure wave to determine cardiac
    output, 130
  catheter passage, 126–127
  catheter presence in the pulmonary artery,
    127
  central venous cannulation, 126
  clinical application of pulmonary artery
    monitoring, 131–132, *131f*
  continuous cardiac output catheter, 130
  in critically ill obstetric patients, 765,
    766t
  in the critically ill patient, 122–136
  data measurement and interpretation, 123
  Doppler ultrasonography to determine
    cardiac output, 130
  hemodynamic pressure monitoring, 123,
    123f
  key points, 135
  lithium dilution to determine cardiac
    output, 130
  mixed-venous oxygen-saturation catheters,
    128–129, *128f, 129f*
  partial CO_2 rebreathing to determine
    cardiac output, 130–131
  pediatric perioperative management,
    777–778, *777t*
  perioperative interventions and
    pathophysiology, 124–126, *125f,
    125t*
  physical complications of pulmonary artery
    catheter monitoring, 126, *126t*
  Poiseuilles law and, 534, *534f*
  principles of thermodilution cardiac output
    measurement, 127–128
  pulmonary artery catheter, 122–123
    efficacy, 132
  right ventricular ejection fraction catheter,
    129–130
  special purpose pulmonary artery catheters,
    128
  thoracic impedance cardiography to
    determine cardiac output, 130
  transesophageal echocardiography,
    132–134, *132t, 133t*
Hemodynamic monitoring
  in acute lung injury/acute respiratory
    distress syndrome (ALI/ARDS),
    413
  in the intensive care unit, 102
  in liver transplantation, 728
Hemolysis, elevated liver transaminases, low
    platelets (HELLP) syndrome
  in critically ill obstetric patients, 771
  with microangiopathic hemolysis, 563
  with perioperative hemostasis and
    coagulopathy, 554
Hemolytic transfusion reaction (HTR),
    568–569
Hemolytic uremic syndrome (HUS), with
    perioperative hemostasis and
    coagulopathy, 554

Hemoperfusion
  for poisoning, 829, 830
  for removal of salicylates, 833
Hemorrhage. *See also* Gastrointestinal
    hemorrhage
  as cause of hypovolemic shock, 197
  causes of perioperative bleeding, 553, *553t*
  causes of prolonged bleeding time, 551,
    551t
  during dialysis, 528
  interpleural in postoperative care of
    thoracic surgical patients, 423
  intrapulmonary in postoperative care of
    thoracic surgical patients, 422–423
Hemorrhagic fever virus, recommended
    therapy for life-threatening, *627t*
Hemorrhagic shock
  in critically ill obstetric patients, 773
  perioperative management in infants and
    children, 786–788
  children at risk for postoperative
    hemorrhage, 786–787
  early recognition and treatment of
    hemorrhage, 787
  late recognition and treatment, 787
  multiple organ failure syndrome during
    the perioperative period, 787–788
Hemostasis and blood coagulopathy, 549–565
  bedside assessment, 553, *553t*
  disseminated intravascular coagulation,
    555–558, *556t*
  heparin-induced thrombocytopenia, 562
  hypothermia and, 559
  idiopathic thrombocytopenic purpura
    (ITP) and, 562–563
  key points, 564
  laboratory assessment, 553–555
    coagulation studies, 553–554
    platelet count, 554–555, *554t*
      aspirin and, 555
      hereditary thrombocytopathies, 555,
        556f
      qualitative platelet disorders,
        554–555, *555t*
  laboratory methods, 550–553
    activated clotting time (ACT), 552
    fibrinolysis testing, 552
    primary hemostasis testing, 550–551,
      551t
    secondary hemostasis testing, 551–552
    Sonoclot, 552–553
    thromboelastograph (TEG), 552–553,
      553f
  liver disease and, 558
  massive transfusion and, 561
  normal hemostasis, 549–550, *550f*
  in orthotopic heart transplantation, 707
  post-cardiopulmonary bypass, 560–561
  posttransfusion purpura, 563
  secondary, 549
  thrombocytopenia and, 561–562
  thrombocytopenia with microangiopathic
    hemolysis, 563–564
  vitamin K deficiency and, 558–559, *559f*
Hemothorax, computed tomography for
    detection of, 846

Heparin
  for acute coronary syndromes, *314t*
  effect on coagulation, 313
  in management of organ donors, 282
  outcome versus thrombolysis in clinical
    trials for pulmonary embolism,
    543–544, *544t*
  for pulmonary embolism, 540
  for pulmonary hypertension in critically ill
    obstetric patients, 769
Heparin-induced thrombocytopenia and
  thrombosis syndrome (HITTS),
  562
Heparin-induced thrombocytopenia (HIT),
  562
Hepatic disease
  with hematopoietic stem cell
    transplantation, 744
  in liver transplantation, 729–730
  preoperative assessment, 9
Hepatic dysfunction
  antibiotic management in the intensive care
    unit, *675t*
  sepsis and, 609
Hepatic encephalopathy, 496, *496t*
Hepatic failure
  effect on drug disposition, 188
  fulminant hepatic failure, 495–502
  in immunocompromised patients, 669
  nutrition support in the critically ill
    patient, 183
Hepatic surgery, perioperative renal
  protection, 508
Hepatitis, preoperative assessment, 10
Hepatitis A
  blood transfusions and, 567
  as cause of fulminant hepatic failure,
    495
Hepatitis B, as cause of fulminant hepatic
    failure, 495
Hepatitis C
  blood transfusions and, 566–567
  as cause of fulminant hepatic failure, 495
  virus epidemiology, 725
Hepatitis C virus (HCV), following liver
    transplantation, 731
Hepatitis D, as cause of fulminant hepatic
    failure, 495
Hepatitis E, as cause of fulminant hepatic
    failure, 495
Hepatobiliary stone disease, 479
Hepatorenal syndrome (HRS), 498–499
  acute tubular necrosis and, 505
  as complication of hematopoietic stem cell
    transplantation, 744–745
  following liver transplantation, 731
Hereditary thrombocytopathies, laboratory
    assessment, 555, *556t*
Herniation syndromes, 247–249
  central, 247–248
  cerebellar tonsillar, 249
  lateral mass, 248–249
  subfalcine, 248–249
  upward transtentorial, 249
Heroics, with intracranial hypertension,
    239

Herpes simplex virus (HSV), 491, 616, 651
  as complication of hematopoietic stem cell
    transplantation, 747–748, *748t*
  following kidney transplantation, 734
  recommended therapy for life-threatening,
    627t
Heterotopic heart transplantation, 710–711
Heterotopic ossification. *See* Myositis
    ossificans
Heterozygosity, 64
^{99m}Tc-hexa-methylpropylene amine oxime
    (^{99m} Tc-HMPAO), 278
HFV. *See* High-frequency ventilation
HHNS. *See* Hyperglycemic hyperosmolar
    nonketotic syndrome
Hibernating myocardium, 303
High-anion gap metabolic acidosis, 838
High-frequency ventilation (HFV), 453
Highly active antiretroviral treatment
    (HAART), 688
HIPAA. *See* Health Insurance Portability and
    Accountability Act
Hirudin, for acute coronary syndromes, *314t*
Histoplasma, in postoperative management of
    heart transplantation, 709
Histoplasma capsulatum, 617, 654, 660
  evaluation with computed tomography in
    the intensive care unit, 844
  recommended therapy for life-threatening,
    625t
HIT. *See* Heparin-induced thrombocytopenia
HITTS. *See* Heparin-induced
    thrombocytopenia and thrombosis
    syndrome
HIV. *See* Human immunodeficiency virus
HL-7, 82
HLA. *See* Human leukocyte antigen
HMOs. *See* Health maintenance
    organizations
Homozygosity, 64
Hormones
  for cardiogenic shock, 293
  in management of organ donors, 280
  as neuroprotectants, 232
Hospital-acquired pneumonia (HAP),
    387–389
  definitions, 387, *387t*
  diagnosis, 388, *388t*
  in the intensive care unit, 583–584
  prevention, 388
  treatment, 388–389
Hospitalist, role of teams in acute care
    services, 42–43, *43t*
Hospitals. *See also* Community hospitals
  acute care medicine in community, 29–44
  admission for cardiac surgery, 346–347,
    347t
  critical care medicine in community, 29–44
  ethics committees, 53
  organization involvement, 38
Host defenses, to infection, 649, 651
HR. *See* Heart rate
HRS. *See* Hepatorenal syndrome
HSCT. *See* Hematopoietic stem cell
    transplantation; Human leukocyte
    antigen

HSV. *See* Herpes simplex virus
HTR. *See* Hemolytic transfusion reaction
Human Genome Project, 53–54. *See also*
    Genomics
Human herpesvirus-6, as complication of
    hematopoietic stem cell
    transplantation, 747–748, *748t*
Human immunodeficiency virus (HIV)
    infection
  adrenal insufficiency and, 757–758
  blood transfusions and, 566
  in the intensive care unit, 632
  preoperative assessment, 10
Human leukocyte antigen (HLA), 692, *692f*,
    740. *See also* Hematopoietic stem
    cell transplantation
  pediatric transplantation and, 783
Humidification
  for airway management, 433–434
  for inhalation injury, 812
Humoral immune defects, infection and,
    667–668
Hunt-Hess scale, comparison of neurologic
    surgeons' grading scales, 266, *266t*
Hurler syndrome, *779t*
HUS. *See* Hemolytic uremic syndrome
Hydralazine
  as antihypertensive drug, 340
  as cause of fever, *585t*
  infection and, 618
Hydrazide, infection and, 618
Hydrocephalus, as complication of
    subarachnoid hemorrhage, 270
Hydrocortisone
  for adrenal insufficiency, 759
  as cause of qualitative platelet disorders,
    555t
  for hypercalcemia, 219
  perioperative coverage, *10t*
  for septic shock, 639
Hydrofluoric acid, 813
Hydroxyethyl starch, 140
  as cause of qualitative platelet disorders,
    555t
Hyperacute rejection, 691
Hypercalcemia, 753, *754t*
  diagnosis and management, 219
Hyperchloremic acidosis, 141
Hypercholesterolemia, risk for coronary artery
    disease, 5
Hyperdynamic shock, 195–196, *195f*, *196f*
  interrelationship with cardiogenic and
    hypovolemic shock, 192–193,
    192f
Hyperemia, subarachnoid hemorrhage and,
    271–272
Hyperglycemia
  as an emergency, 760–762, *761t*, *762t*
  in liver transplantation, 730
  preoperative assessment of patient, 9
Hyperglycemic hyperosmolar nonketotic
    syndrome (HHNS), 761–762
  clinical features, 761
  diagnosis, 761
  laboratory features, 761
  treatment, 761–762

Hyperkalemia, *330f*
  diagnosis and management, 216–217,
      217f, 217t
  treatment, 216, *217t*
Hypermagnesemia, diagnosis and
      management, 221
Hypernatremia
  acute treatment, *214t*
  diagnosis and management, 214–215,
      214f, 214t, 215f
  perioperative management of infants and
      children, 780
Hyperparathyroidism, 753
Hyperphosphatemia
  diagnosis and management, 222
  treatment, *219t*
Hypertension
  airway management and, 99
  aortic dissection and, 335–336, 336
      clinical features, 336
      management, 336
      pathophysiology, 336
  care of the patient in the intensive care
      unit, 333–345
  causes of intraabdominal, 171, *171t*
  classification, 333, *334t*
  definition, 333
  excess catecholamines and, 337
  hypertensive emergencies and urgencies,
      334, *334t*
  hypertensive encephalopathy, 335
      clinical features, 335
      management, 335
      pathology, 335
  identifiable/secondary causes, *334t*
  intraoperative, 339
      induction, 339
      maintenance, 339
      measurement, 339
      stress response and pathophysiology, 339
  key points, 344
  kidney and, 336
      pathophysiology, 336
      renal failure, 336
  left ventricular failure and, 335
      management, 335
      pathophysiology, 335
  malignant, 334–335
      clinical findings, 334–335
      management, 335
      outcome, 335
      pathogenesis/pathology, 334
  myocardial ischemia and, 335
  neurologic syndromes and, 336–337
  parenteral pharmacologic antihypertensive
      therapy, 339–343
      adrenergic agents, 340–342, *341t*
      angiotensin-converting enzyme
          inhibitors, 343
      calcium channel blockers, 342–343,
          342t
      diuretics, 339–340
      peripheral vasodilators, 340
  pathophysiology, 333–334
      cardiac output, 333–334
      hemodynamics of blood pressure, 333

  systemic vascular resistance, 334
  perioperative, 337–339
      history and definitions, 337, *338f*
      medications causing hypertension, 339
      preoperative antihypertensive
          medication, 338–339
      preoperative assessment, 338
  perioperative renal protection and,
      508–509
  in pregnancy, 336, *337t*
  risk for coronary artery disease, 5
  treatment algorithm of perioperative, *338f*
Hypertensive encephalopathy, 335
  clinical features, 335
  management, 335
  pathology, 335
Hypertensive hypervolemic therapy, 258
Hyperthermia, as source of fever, 585
Hyperthyroidism
  as an emergency, 756–757, *756t*
  diagnosis, 756
  etiologies, 756, *756t*
  preoperative assessment of patient, 9
  treatment, 756
Hypertonic fluids
  clinical implications of administration,
      142–143, *143t*
  management, 143
  for poisoning, 822
  resuscitation advantages and disadvantages,
      143t
Hypertonic solutions, 139
  physiology and pharmacology, 139
Hyperventilation, 209, *209t*
  for cerebroprotective intervention,
      230–231
  traumatic brain injury and, 238
Hypnotics, toxic syndromes, *820t*
Hypocalcemia, 753, *754t*
  acquired prolonged repolarization
      syndromes and, *329t*
  diagnosis and management, 218, *219t*
  treatment, 218, *219t*
Hypogammaglobulinemia, infections
      associated with, *618t*
Hypoglycemia, preoperative assessment of
      patient, 9
Hypokalemia
  acquired prolonged repolarization
      syndromes and, *329t*
  in the critically ill patient, 182
  diagnosis and management, 215–216
Hypomagnesemia
  acquired prolonged repolarization
      syndromes and, *329t*
  diagnosis and management, 220–221, *221t*
  therapy of magnesium depletion, *221t*
  treatment, 220
Hyponatremia
  in the critically ill patient, 182
  diagnosis and management, *13f*, 211–214,
      212f
  perioperative management of infants and
      children, 780
  treatment, 213, *213f*
Hypoparathyroidism, 753

Hypophosphatemia
  in the critically ill patient, 182
  diagnosis and management, 221–222
Hypoproteinemia, 177
  in critically ill patients, 140
Hypotension
  in the cardiac surgical patient, 349–350
  during dialysis for acute renal failure,
      527
  etiology of acute, 115, *116t*
  in management of organ donors, 280
Hypothermia
  care of the patient with multiple trauma
      and, 793–794
  for cerebroprotective intervention, 231
  pediatric perioperative management,
      778
  perioperative hemostasis and coagulopathy,
      559
  postoperative, 316
  for traumatic brain injury, 239
Hypothyroidism (myxedema)
  as an emergency, 755–756, *755t*
  treatment, 755–756
Hypovolemia. *See also* Oliguria
  diagnosis and management, 212
  fluid status, assessment, and monitoring,
      143–145, *145t*
Hypovolemic shock, 197–198, *198f*
  definition, 197
  interrelationship with cardiogenic and
      hyperdynamic shock, 192–193,
      192f
Hypoxemia
  definition, 428
  during dialysis for acute renal failure, 527
  fulminant hepatic failure and, 497
  shock and, 193
Hypoxia, definition, 428

I

IABP. *See* Intraaortic balloon pump
IAC-CPR. *See* Interposed abdominal
      compression-CPR
IAIMS. *See* Integrated Advanced Information
      Management Systems
Ibuprofen
  acute tubular necrosis and, 505
  for fever, 578
Ibutilide, for atrial flutter or atrial fibrillation,
      323–324, *324f*
ICDs. *See* Implantable cardioverter
      defibrillators
ICP. *See* Intracranial pressure
ICU. *See* Intensive care unit
Idiopathic acute fatty liver of pregnancy
      (AFLP), in critically ill obstetric
      patients, 773–774
Idiopathic pneumonia syndrome, as
      complication of hematopoietic
      stem cell transplantation, 743–744
Idiopathic thrombocytopenic purpura (ITP)
  plate concentrates and, 573
Idiopathic thrombocytopenic purpura (ITP),
      with perioperative hemostasis and
      coagulopathy, 562–563

IEEE. *See* Institute of Electric and Electronic Engineering
IEEE 1073 Standard for Medical Device Communications, 82
Ifosfamide, for renal failure, 744
Ileus, *476t*
　in the perioperative intensive care unit patient, 476–477
iLGF. *See* Insulin-like growth factor
Imaging. *See also* Computed tomography; Magnetic resonance imaging; Thoracic computed tomography
　abdominal imaging in the intensive care unit, 849–854
　chest applications, 843–847
　evaluating complex pleural disease in the intensive care unit patient, 847–849
　　central venous catheter complications, 849
　　drainage in refractory pleural effusions or pneumothoraces, 849
　　lung abscess versus empyema, 848
　　malignant pleural effusion, 848–849
　　pleural space infection, 848, *848f*
　　thoracic interventional procedures, 849, *850f*
　in immunocompromised patients, 654–655
　in the intensive care unit, 841–858
　perioperative evaluation, 380
　for pheochromocytoma, 759
Imidazole derivatives. *See* Azoles
Imipenem, 675
　for bacteria in the intensive care unit, *673t*
　dosage adjustments in the intensive care unit, *523t*
　for pancreatitis, 480
　for pneumonia, 389
Imipenem-cilastatin (Primaxin), 621
　dosing, *622t*
Imipramine, acquired prolonged repolarization syndromes and, *329t*
Immune defects. *See* Host defenses
Immune dysfunction, care of the patient with multiple trauma and, 794
Immune serum globulin (ISG)
　in the intensive care unit, 640
　for prevention of toxic shock syndrome, 635
Immune system, immune-enhancing diets, 182–183
Immunobiology, 691–693
　graft injury, 691–692
　rejection
　　mediated by antibody, 691
　　mediated by T-lymphocytes, 691
　　role of cytokines in, 691–692
　　role of major histocompatibility complex in, 692–693, *692f, 693f*
Immunologic testing, nutrition support in the critically ill patient, 178
Immunomodulation
　in blood transfusion, 569
　therapies for care of the patient with multiple trauma and, 794

Immunosuppression
　acute tubular necrosis and, 505–506
　common causes and major infections in immunocompromised patients, 649, *650t*
　diagnostic approach, 653, *654f*
　drug interactions, 707–708, *708t*
　in kidney transplantation, 734, *735t*
　in liver transplantation, 732, *732t*
　in lung transplantation, 718
　in orthotopic heart transplantation, 707–708, *708t*, 710
　pediatric, 783, *784t*
Impedance (resistive element), definition, 534
Implantable cardioverter defibrillators (ICDs), 701
Imuran. *See* Azathioprine
Incentive spirometry, for airway management, 434
Indirect antigen presentation, 692, *693f*
Indomethacin
　acute tubular necrosis and, 505
　for fever, 578
Infants. *See* Pediatric care
Infarction, in postoperative care of thoracic surgical patients, 423
Infections
　abdominal, 582–583, *583f*
　　in the perioperative intensive care unit patient, 481–482
　in acquired immune deficiency syndrome, 663–667, *664t, 665f, 667f*
　　in the intensive care unit, 636–637
　acute infective endocarditis, 630–631
　aminoglycosides, 621
　of antibacterials, 624–625
　antiinfective therapy, 620–627, *625t*
　　for infectious disease syndromes, 627–637, *628t–629t, 637f, 638t*
　antiviral drugs, 626–627, *627t*
　babesiosis, 636
　bacterial in liver transplantation, 730–731
　beta-lactams, 620–621, *622t–623t, 624t*
　in bone marrow transplant recipients, 662–663, *662f*
　in the cardiac surgical patient, 352
　care of the patient with multiple trauma and, 793
　catheter-related infection, 580–582, *581f, 582f, 582t*
　as cause of mucosal erosive disease, 491
　causes in immunocompromised patients, 649, *650t*
　clinical approach to the infected, immunocompromised patient, 653–655, *654f*
　computed tomography for detection of, 843, 844, *844f*
　continuous patient assessment, 620
　cryptogenic sepsis without identified local infection, 627, 630
　cystic fibrosis and, 378
　deep sternal wound infection, 352
　diagnosis, 616–620
　diagnostic studies, 618–620
　diarrhea and, 475–476

　drugs for multiresistant gram-positive cocci, 623
　enteric, 634
　evaluating pleural space infection with computed tomography, 848, *848f*
　evaluating with computed tomography in the intensive care unit, 855
　fever as source of, 579–584
　fluoroquinolones, 623–624
　focused antiinfective therapy, 637
　following kidney transplantation, 734
　fulminant hepatic failure and, 497–498
　geographic, recommended therapy for life-threatening, *625t*
　gynecologic, 634
　with hematopoietic stem cell transplantation, 746, *746t*
　host defenses to, 649, 651
　in the immunocompromised patient, 649–671
　intraabdominal, 633–634
　　acalculous cholecystitis, 633
　　cholangitis, 633
　　secondary peritonitis/intraabdominal abscess, 633
　　spontaneous bacterial peritonitis, 633
　　typhlitis, 633–634
　key points, 641
　line sepsis, 631–632
　in liver transplantation, 730–731
　lung diagnosis, 438, *438t*
　in lung transplantation, 719
　macrolides, 621
　malaria, 636
　management of life-threatening in the intensive care unit, 616–648. *See also* individual drug names
　meningitis, 632–633
　metastatic, *624t*
　in the neutropenic patient, 655–657, *658t*
　noninfectious syndromes mimicking infection, 617–618
　nonspecific immunodeficiency states and, 668–669
　in orthotopic heart transplantation, 709, 710
　pathogens at site of, *618t*
　in patients with humoral immune defects, asplenia, or complement deficiency, 667–668
　patterns of, 617, *618t, 619f*
　pediatric posttransplant, 784–785
　pneumococcal, 668
　pneumonia, 632
　in postoperative care of thoracic surgical patients, 424
　posttransplantation, 660
　prevention, 616–617
　　in the intensive care unit, 640
　　　antiviral prophylaxis, 640
　　　basic infection control practices, 640
　　　immune serum globulin, 640
　　　protected environments, 640
　　　technologic innovations, 640

Infections (*contd.*)
principles in assessment of, 651–653, *652t*
pulmonary function complications, 455–456
reactivation of latent, *618t*
in recipients with hematopoietic stem cell transplantation, 746–748, *746f*
recommended therapy for life-threatening, *624t*
in the renal transplant patient, 659–660, *659f*
rickettsial, 636
sinusitis, 632
skin, 634
soft-tissue, 634
in solid-organ transplant recipients, 657–662, *659f*
source control, 620
supportive therapy, 637–640
adjunctive therapies, 638–639
circulatory support, 638
toxic shock syndrome (TSS), 635–636
treatment of antimicrobial-resistant, 637, *637f, 638t*
urosepsis, 634
vancomycin, 621, 623
viral
meningoencephalitis, 633
recommended therapy for life-threatening, *627t*
in wound management in acute care of burns, 806–807
Infectious diseases. *See also* Human immunodeficiency virus
following surgery in the intensive care unit, 169–170
initial therapy for life-threatening, *628t–629t*
preoperative assessment, 10
transmission in blood transfusions, 566–567, *568t*
Infectious Diseases Society, 387
Inflammation, cerebral injury and, 230
Inflammatory mediators, in multiple organ dysfunction syndrome, 590–592
Influenza virus
as complication of hematopoietic stem cell transplantation, 747–748, *748t*
recommended therapy for life-threatening, *627t*
Information systems, as quality management tool, 24
Informed consent, 46
research and, 76, 77
Inhalation agents, 440–442, *441t*
as neuroprotectant, 233–234, *233t*
Inhalation injury, 808–812
characteristics of sites of, 810, *810t*
incidence and mortality related to age and presence of, 809, *809t*
incidence and mortality related to total body surface area burn and presence of, 809, *809t*
treatment, 812
Injuries. *See also* Burns; Trauma; Traumatic brain injury

acute tubular necrosis and, 504–506
computed tomography for detection of thoracic spine injury, 845–846
electrical, 812–813
inhalation, 808–812
in the intensive care unit, 168
lung, 569
metabolic response to, 176, *177f*
neutrophil-dependent lung, 410
oxidant, 229–230
pathophysiology of cerebral, 228–230
prevention and treatment of renal injury, 511–517, *511f, 511t, 512t*
renal injury and failure, 503–504
spinal cord syndromes, 240–242
ventilator-induced lung injury, 410
Inotropic agents
for cardiac surgical patients, 347, *348t*
shock and, 201
Insecticides, acquired prolonged repolarization syndromes and, *329t*
Institute of Electric and Electronic Engineering (IEEE), 82
Institutional Review Board (IRB), role in research, 76
Insulin. *See also* Diabetes insipidus; Diabetes mellitus
during catabolic phase of response to injury, 176
characteristics, 762, *762t*
following pancreas transplantation, 736, *736t*
for hyperkalemia, 217
regular infusion protocol, *37t*
Insulin-like growth factor (iLGF)
for acute renal failure, 793
in immune-enhancing diets, 182
Integrated Advanced Information Management Systems (IAIMS), 80
Integrity, professional, 45–46
Intensive care unit (ICU)
abdominal imaging, 849–854
acquired immunodeficiency syndrome in, 636–637
acute abdominal conditions in the perioperative patient, 474–484
administrative structure, 15–16
advanced imaging in, 841–858
analgesic drugs in, 147
antibiotic selection, 672–673, *673t*
arterial cannulation in, 102–105, *103f, 104f, 105f, 105t*
care of the hypertensive patient in, 333–345
care of the patient with multiple trauma, 791–800
care of the poisoned patient, 818–840
central venous catheterization in, 105–106, *106t*
complications, 108–109
clinical protocol, *36t*
"closed" unit model, 17
comatose patient diagnosis and management, 244–252
continuous patient assessment, 620
detection of renal dysfunction in, 509–511

tubular function tests and evaluation of oliguria, 509–511, *509t*
urine flow rate and oliguria, 509
dosage adjustments for medications, *523t*
ensuring quality of care, 19–22
critical care clinical practice guidelines, 21–22
evidence-based standards, 21
morbidity and mortality review, 20
performance improvement, 21
quality assurance programs, 20
quality management techniques, 19–20
standards of practice in critical care medicine, 20–21
evaluation of fever in, 577–587
external jugular venous cannulation technique in, 107, *107f*
extubating patients in, 98–99
complications, 99
reintubating patients for whom extubation fails, 98–99
femoral venous catheterization technique in, 108
gastrointestinal hemorrhage in the critically ill, 485–494
head and spinal cord injury management, 236–243
hemodynamic monitoring in, 102
initiation and adequacy of renal replacement therapy in, 529
integrative or translational research in, 72–73
internal jugular vein catheterization techniques in, 106–107
key points, 26, 120
management, 15–19
of brain-dead and nonheart-beating organ donors, 278
of life-threatening infection in, 616–648. *See also* individual drug names
mandatory practice standards, 22–25
clinical information systems as quality management tool, 24
cost-benefit analysis, 24–25
government agencies, 23
Health Care Financing Administration (HCFA), 25
Health Insurance Portability and Accountability Act (HIPAA), 25
Joint Commission on Accreditation of Healthcare Organizations (JCAHO), 22
Medicare, 25
patient acuity systems as quality assessment tools, 23–24
payor-mandated assessment of quality of care, 23
medical informatics in, 80–88
models of care, 16–17
neuromuscular blocking agents in, 152–165
"open" unit model, 16–17
percutaneous dilational tracheostomy (PcT) in, 118–119, *118f, 118t, 119f*

perioperative management of infants and children, 776–790
peripherally inserted central venous (PICC lines) catheters in, 107–108
postoperative management
of aneurysms, 272
of arteriovenous malformations, 272–273
in liver transplantation, 726–728
of subarachnoid hemorrhage, 272–273
preoperative management, in liver transplantation, 726
prevalence of infection in, 616, *617f*
prevention of infection in, 640
procedures, 102–121
pulmonary artery catheterization in, 109–110, *109t, 110f, 110t, 111f*
pulmonary artery catheter variants, 111
research problems in, 77
risk indices for mortality and utilization, 11–12
sedatives in, 157
staffing, 17–19
critical care nurses, 17–18
nutritionist, 18
pharmacists, 18
physician, 17
respiratory therapists, 18
social worker, 18
subclavian venous catheterization technique in, 108
surgical, 346
surgical considerations in, 168–175
transesophageal echocardiography (TEE) in, 111–112, *112t*
transpulmonary thermodilution, 111, *112f*
triage for upper gastrointestinal bleeding, 486, *487f*
two-dimensional examination in, 112–116, *113f, 114f, 115f, 116f, 116t, 117f*
left-ventricular filling or volume status, 113–114
left ventricular performance, 114–115, *114f, 115f, 116t, 117f*
use of antimicrobials in, 672–689
Intercostal analgesia, 425
Interferon-alpha (Roferon-A), for viral infections, 626
Interleukin-1, during catabolic phase of response to injury, 176
Interleukin-6, during catabolic phase of response to injury, 176
Intermittent hemodialysis, for renal replacement therapy, 525
Intermittent positive pressure breathing (IPPB), 400
for airway management, 435–436
Internal jugular vein catheterization, in the intensive care unit, 106–107
Internet, 84–85
Interpleural analgesia, 425
Interpleural hemorrhage, in postoperative care of thoracic surgical patients, 423
Interposed abdominal compression-CPR (IAC-CPR), 366, *366f*

Intraabdominal hypertension, perioperative renal protection and, 508–509
Intraabdominal infections, 633–634
recommended therapy for life-threatening, *624t*
Intraaortic balloon pump (IABP), 701
for cardiogenic shock, 291–292
for myocardial ischemia, 311
Intracerebral hemorrhage
evaluation with computed tomography in the intensive care unit, 854
postoperative care, 261–262
Intracranial compliance, 237, *237f*
Intracranial hemorrhage, acquired prolonged repolarization syndromes and, *329t*
Intracranial hypertension, 236–239
fluid therapy, 239
heroics, 239
management, 238–239
pathophysiology and treatment rationale, 236–238
pediatric perioperative management, 779
postoperative care, 260–261
Intracranial pressure (ICP)
in the head-injured patient, 796
implications of crystalloid and colloid infusions on, 140
measurement, 238
postural drainage and, 434
in traumatic brain injury, 236–237, *237f*
Intrapulmonary hemorrhage, in postoperative care of thoracic surgical patients, 422–423
Intrinsic pathway, 549, *550f*
Intrinsic sympathomimetic activity (ISA), hypertension and, 339
Intubation
fiberoptic, 95–96, *95f*
laryngeal mask airway, 96, *96f*
nasotracheal, 94–95
orotracheal, with rigid laryngoscope, 94, *94f*
tracheal, 90–101
Invasive pulmonary aspergillosis (IPA)
computed tomography for detection of, 844, *844f*
evaluation with computed tomography in the intensive care unit, 844, *844f*
Iodine, contraindications, 757
ION. *See* Ischemic optic neuropathy
IPA. *See* Invasive pulmonary aspergillosis
IPPB. *See* Intermittent positive pressure breathing
Ipratroprium bromide, *441t*
IRB. *See* Institutional Review Board
Iron
daily requirements in total parenteral nutrition, *182t*
for poisoning, 823
ISA. *See* Intrinsic sympathommetic activity
Ischemia, in the perioperative intensive care unit patient, 480
Ischemia cascade, *304f*
Ischemic bowel disease, evaluation with computed tomography in the intensive care unit, 853–854

Ischemic optic neuropathy (ION), 575
ISHLT. *See* Registry of the International Society for Heart and Lung Transplantation
Isocarboxazid (Marplan), for hypertension, 337
Isoetharine hydrochloride, *441t*
Isoflurane, as neuroprotectant, 233
Isolator blood culture system, 619
Isoniazid
antidotes for overdose, *830t*
as cause of fulminant hepatic failure, 495
toxic syndromes, *820t*
Isonicotinic acid, infection and, 618
Isoproterenol, *441t*
for bradyarrhythmias, 320
in management of organ donors, 280
for shock, 201, *201t*
ITP. *See* Idiopathic thrombocytopenic purpura
Itraconazole (Sporanox), 626, *683t*
adverse effects, 685
distribution and elimination, 685
dosing, *622t*
in immunocompromised patients, *652t*

J

Japanese B encephalitis virus, 633
JCAHO. *See* Joint Commission on Accreditation of Healthcare Organizations
Jehovah's Witness, refusal of blood transfusion, 46
Jejunostomy, for enteral nutrition, 172
JK *Corynebacterium,* 621, 630, 631
JNC. *See* Joint National Committee on Detection, Evaluation, and Treatment of High Blood Pressure
Joint Commission on Accreditation of Healthcare Organizations (JCAHO), 22
Joint National Committee (JNC) on Detection, Evaluation, and Treatment of High Blood Pressure, 333, *334t*, 337
Jugular venous cannulation
external, in the intensive care unit, 107, *107f*
internal, in the intensive care unit, 106–107

K

Kallikrein-kinen system, multiple organ dysfunction syndrome and, 591, *591f*
Kanamycin sulfate, 676
Kayexalate (sodium polystyrene sulfonate resin), for hyperkalemia, 217
Kernohan notch, 248
Ketamine
in the intensive care unit, 149
as neuroprotectant, *233t*
for tracheal intubation, 92
Ketoconazole (Nizoral), 626, *683t*, 685
for acute lung injury/acute respiratory distress syndrome (ALI/ARDS), *413t*

Ketoconazole (Nizoral) (*contd.*)
  drug interactions in critically ill patients, *189t*
Key points
  acid-base abnormalities, 222–223
  acute abdominal conditions in the perioperative intensive care unit patient, 483
  acute care medicine in community hospitals, 43–44
  acute care of burns, 813
  acute lung injury/acute respiratory distress syndrome (ALI/ARDS), 415
  acute therapy in patients with cardiac arrhythmias, 332
  advanced imaging in the intensive care unit, 856
  airway management and tracheal intubation, 100
  analgesic drugs, 165
  antimicrobial therapy in the intensive care unit, 688–689
  application of pharmacokinetic and pharmacodynamic principles in critically ill patients, 190
  biology of transplantation, 698
  cardiogenic shock, 300
  cardiopulmonary resuscitation, 370
  cardiopulmonary transplantation, 721
  care of critically ill obstetric patients, 774
  care of the patient with endocrine emergencies, 762–763
  care of the patient with multiple trauma, 798
  care of the poisoned patient, 838
  cerebroprotection, 234
  diagnosis and management of comatose patients, 252
  electrolyte abnormalities, 222–223
  ethical and end-of-life issues, 54
  evaluation of fever in the intensive care unit, 586
  evidence-based medicine (EBM), 61
  fluid management in critically ill patients, 145
  fulminant hepatic failure, 501
  gastrointestinal hemorrhage in the critically ill, 493
  genomics in perioperative critical care, 68
  hematopoietic stem cell transplantation, 750
  hemodynamic assessment in the critically ill patient, 135
  hypertensive patient in the intensive care unit, 344
  infections in the immunocompromised patient, 670
  intensive care unit, 26
  kidney transplantation, 737–738
  liver transplantation, 737–738
  management of acute renal failure in the critically ill patient, 530
  management of life-threatening infection in the intensive care unit, 641

  mechanical ventilation, 458, 471
  medical informatics in the intensive care unit, 86
  multiple organ dysfunction syndrome, 597
  myocardial ischemia, 317
  neuromuscular blocking drugs, 165
  nonheart-beating organ donors, 284
  nutrition support in the critically ill patient, 184
  pancreas transplantation, 737–738
  patient with sepsis or systemic inflammatory response syndrome, 612
  perioperative evaluation of pulmonary diseases and function, 383
  perioperative hemostasis and coagulopathy, 564
  perioperative management
    of the cardiac surgical patient, 358–359
    of infants and children, 788
    of obstructive and restrictive pulmonary diseases, 405
    of thoracic surgical patients, 426
  perioperative renal protection, 517
  pneumonia, 391–392
  postoperative care of the neurosurgical patient, 262
  preoperative assessment, 12
  procedures in the intensive care unit, 120
  renal replacement therapy, 530
  research in critical care medicine, 78
  respiratory care, 444
  sedatives, 165
  shock, etiology and pathyphysiology, 203–204
  spinal cord injuries, 242
  subarachnoid hemorrhage and cerebrovascular accident, 273
  surgical considerations in the intensive care unit, 174
  transfusion medicine for the intensivist, 575
  transplantation, 284
  traumatic brain injury, 242
Kidneys
  hypertension and, 336
  pediatric transplantation, 785–786
Kidney transplantation, 733–735
  contraindications, 733
  postoperative care, 733–735
    fluid management, 733–734, *734t*
    immunosuppression, 734, *735t*
    rejection, 734–735
  preoperative care, 733
Kidney Transplant Registry of the United Network for Organ Sharing (UNOS), 283
Kjeldahl method, 179
Klebsiella pneumonia, 634, 674
  blood transfusions and, 567–568
Klebsiella spp., in postoperative management of lung transplantation, 719
Klippel–Feil syndrome, *779t*
Korean Hantaan virus, recommended therapy for life-threatening, *627t*

K-receptor agents, as neuroprotectants, 234
Kwashiorkor, 177

L
Labetalol
  as antihypertensive drug, 341, *341t*
  for aortic dissection, 336
  for cerebral ischemia, 260
  for pheochromocytoma, 760
Labetalol hydrochloride, for acute myocardial ischemia, 311, *312t*
Lacerations, computed tomography for detection of, 846
β-Lactam antibiotics, 673
  resistance, 681–682, *682t*
β-Lactamase inhibitors, 674
  antibiotic selection in the intensive care unit, *673t*
β-Lactam/beta-lactamase inhibitors
  for infections, 620–621, *622t–623t,* *624t*
  for pneumonia, 389
Large bowel obstruction, 477
Laryngeal mask airway (LMA), 92
  in cardiopulmonary resuscitation, 365
  intubation, 96, *96f*
Laryngoscopy, difficult rigid, 89, *90t*
Laser bronchoscopy, 417
Lassa fever virus, recommended therapy for life-threatening, *627t*
Lead, toxic syndromes, *820t*
Left ventricular assist devices (LVAD), 701
Left ventricular compliance, factors that decrease, 124–125, *125t*
Left ventricular end-diastolic pressure (LVEDP), in myocardial ischemia, 303–304
Left ventricular failure
  hypertension and, 335
  management, 335
  pathophysiology, 335
Left ventricular preload (LVEDV), in cardiogenic shock, 291
Legal issues
  ethical issues and, 53
  in genomics in perioperative critical care, 67
Legionella pneumophila, 620, 677
Legionella spp., 385, 391, 621, 653, 654, 655, 660
  following liver transplantation, 730
  in postoperative management of heart transplantation, 709
  recommended therapy, *624t*
Legislation
  "Baby Doe" case, 50–51
  Patient Self-Determination Act, 47
  physician-assisted suicide, 51–52
  for surrogate decision making, 47
  Uniform Anatomical Gift Act, 76
  Uniform Determination of Death Act, 275
Leptospira spp., 674
Leuconostoc, 655–656
Leukemia
  adult T-cell blood transfusions and, 567
  in immunocompromised patients, 668
Leukocyte-depleted blood products, 573

Leukotrienes, multiple organ dysfunction syndrome and, 591–592
Levalbuterol, *441t*
Levaquin (levofloxacin), 624
  dosing, *623t*
Levofloxacin (Levaquin), 624
  dosing, *623t*
Lidocaine
  bronchoscopy and, 439
  in cardiopulmonary resuscitation, 369–370
  for radial artery cannulation, 102, *103f*
  for tracheal intubation, 92, 95
  for treatment of tachyarrhythmias, 330–331
Life support, withdrawal, 49
Life-sustaining treatment
  sedatives and analgesics administration during, 48–49
  withdrawal, 48–49, *49f*
Lincosamides
  adverse reactions, 677
  distribution and elimination, 677
Line sepsis, 631–632
Linezolid (Zyvox)
  adverse effects, 680
  antibiotic management of renal and hepatic dysfunction in the intensive care unit, *675t*
  distribution and elimination, 680
  dosing, *623t*
  for multiresistant gram-positive cocci, 623
Linkage dysequilibrium, 65
Lipids, in the critically ill patient, 181
Lipolysis, sepsis and, 610
Liposomal amphotericin, in the intensive care unit, 684
Lisinopril, acute tubular necrosis and, 505
Lisofylline, for acute lung injury/acute respiratory distress syndrome (ALI/ARDS), *413t*
Listeria monocytogenes, 651
  recommended therapy, *624t*
Listeria spp.
  following kidney transplantation, 734
  following liver transplantation, 730
Lithium
  dilution to determine cardiac output, 130
  evaluation and management for intoxication of, 831–832
  poisoning and, 829–830
  for syndrome of inappropriate antidiuretic hormone, 214
  toxic syndromes, *820t*
Liver
  acute fatty liver in critically ill obstetric patients, 773–774
  dialysis, for fulminant hepatic failure, 500
  evaluation with computed tomography in the intensive care unit, 851
  transplantation
    adult, 500, 724–732, 834
    pediatric, 785
  venoocclusive disease, 744

Liver disease
  Child's classification, 489, *489t*
  end-stage, 724
  fulminant hepatic failure, 495–502
  with perioperative hemostasis and coagulopathy, 558
  support devices, 500
  transplantation, 500
Liver failure
  acute tubular necrosis and, 505
  effect on drug disposition, 188
Liver transplantation, 500, 724–732
  candidacy, 724
  complications, 728–732
    coagulation, 728, *728f,* 730
    graft function, 729–730
    hemodynamic, 728
    immunosuppression, 732, *732t*
    infection, 730–731
    neurologic, 729
    nutrition/gastrointestinal function, 731
    pulmonary, 728–729
    rejection, 731–732
    renal function, 731
  contraindications, 725, *725t*
  epidemiology, 725
  postoperative care, 726–728, *728f*
  preoperative care, 726, *727f*
  registrations, 725, *725f*
LMA. *See* Laryngeal mask airway
LMWH. *See* Low-molecular-weight heparin
Locked-in-syndrome, definition, 244
Loop diuretics
  in acute renal failure, 523
  in animal studies for acute renal failure, *522t*
  for prevention and treatment of renal injury, 511–512
Lorazepam
  comparison with other intensive care unit sedative drugs, *150t*
  in the intensive care unit, 147–148
  as a sedative in the intensive care unit, *151t*
  for seizures, 836
Losartan, acute tubular necrosis and, 505
Lower gastrointestinal bleeding, 492, *492t*
Low-molecular-weight heparin (LMWH)
  with perioperative hemostasis and coagulopathy, 552
  for pulmonary embolism, 540
Lung
  computed tomography for detection of parenchymal injury, 846
  diagnosis of infections in, 437, *438t*
  evaluation lung abscess versus empyema with computed tomography, 848
  heart-lung transplantation, 720–721
  in immunocompromised patients, 654–655
  infections, 378
  lesions from thermal damage, 811
  pediatric transplantation, 786
  postoperative care of thoracic surgical patients, 424
Lung injury
  neutrophil-dependent, 410

from positive pressure ventilation, 452–453
  from smoke inhalation, 809–810
  transfusion-related, 569
  ventilator-induced, 411
Lung sounds, interpretation in perioperative evaluation, *380t*
Lung transplantation, 424, 711–720, *711f*
  acute postoperative management, 717–720
    airway complications, 717–718
    cardiovascular management, 718
    hematologic management, 718
    hyperacute and acute rejection, 718–719
    immunosuppression, 718
    infectious complications, 719
    long-term complications, 719–720, *719t*
    respiratory management, 717
  bilateral sequential single-lung transplant (BSSLT), 711
  choice of lung transplant procedure, 712–713
  "clam shell" incision, 716, *716f*
  contraindications to, 712
  distribution by indication, 711–712, *711t*
  donor lung procurement, 714
  donor lung selection, 713–714
  double-lung transplant (DLT), 711
  indications and selection criteria for, 711–712, *711t*
  intraoperative management, 714–717, *716f*
  left lung transplant anatomy, 715, *716f*
  outcome following, 720
  preoperative preparation, 714
  single-lung transplant (SLP), 711
Lung-volume reduction surgery (LVRS), 419
Lupogenic drugs, infection and, 618
LVAD. *See* Left ventricular assist devices
LVEDP. *See* Left ventricular end-diastolic pressure
LVEDV. *See* Left ventricular preload
LVRS. *See* Lung-volume reduction surgery
Lymphocytic choriomeningitis virus, 633

M
MAC. *See* Minimal anesthetic concentration or monitored anesthetic care
Macroglossia, *779t*
Macrolides
  adverse reactions, 677
  for bacteria in the intensive care unit, *673t*
  distribution and elimination, 677
  infection and, 621
Mafenide acetate, for control of infection in burn patients, 806
Magnesium
  daily requirements in total parenteral nutrition, *182t*
  diagnosis and management of abnormalities, 219–221
  monitoring in the critically ill patient, 182
  replacement protocol, *36t*
Magnetic resonance imaging (MRI)
  comatose patients and, 245, *247f*
  for diagnosis of subarachnoid hemorrhage, 265–266

Magnetic resonance imaging (MRI) (*contd.*)
for perioperative evaluation of pulmonary disease, 380
Major histocompatibility complex (MHC), 692–693, *692f, 693f*
Malaria, 621
initial therapy for life-threatening, *629t*
recommended therapy for life-threatening, *627t*
Malignant hypertension (MHT), 334–335
clinical findings, 334–335
management, 335
outcome, 335
pathogenesis/pathology, 334
Malignant hyperthermia, as source of fever, 585
Mallory-Weiss syndrome
diagnosis, 491
hemorrhage in the critically ill, 490–491
pathogenesis, 490
treatment, 491
Malnutrition
in the critically ill patient, 177, *178t*
fulminant hepatic failure and, 498
Managed care, 53
Management Strategy and Prognosis of Pulmonary Embolism Registry (MAPPET), 537–538
Manganese, daily requirements in total parenteral nutrition, *182t*
Mannitol
for acute renal failure, 793
in animal studies for acute renal failure, *522t*
for brain parenchyma reduction, 238
for care of the head-injured patient, 796
in management of organ donors, 282
as neuroprotectant, 231, 232
for prevention and treatment of renal injury, 512–513
prophylactic use, 512–513
MAOIs. *See* Monoamine oxidase inhibitors
MAP. *See* Mean arterial pressure
MAPPET. *See* Management Strategy and Prognosis of Pulmonary Embolism Registry
Marasmus, 177
Marburg virus, recommended therapy for life-threatening, *627t*
Marfan syndrome
in critically ill obstetric patients, 769
predisposition to subarachnoid hemorrhage, 264
Marplan (isocarboxazid), for hypertension, 337
Mask
aerosol and T-piece, 432–433
non-rebreathing, *431f*, 432
partial rebreathing, 431, *431f*
Venturi, 431–432, *432f*
Massive transfusion, 561, 573–574
coagulopathy, 573–574, *574t*
metabolic complications, 574
Mass median aerodynamic diameter (MMAD), 439
MAT. *See* Multifocal atrial tachycardia
Maxipime (cefepime), 620, 621, 674

antibiotic management of renal and hepatic dysfunction in the intensive care unit, *675t*
dosing, *622t*
MDF. *See* Myocardial depressant factor
MDI. *See* Metered-dose inhaler
Mean arterial pressure (MAP), 225
in the cardiac surgical patient, 349
in management of organ donors, 280
Mechanical obstruction, in the abdomen of the perioperative intensive care unit patient, 477–478
Mechanical ventilation, 447–459
in acute lung injury/acute respiratory distress syndrome (ALI/ARDS), 412–413
alveolar recruitment and gas exchange, 450–452
inspiratory flow pattern and inspiratory–expiratory time manipulations, 451–452
positive end-expiratory pressure, 450–451, *452f*
chronic obstructive pulmonary disease and, 465–466, *466f, 466t*
clinical practice guidelines—evidence-based weaning recommendations, 471
closed head trauma and, 466–467, *467f*
congestive heart failure and, 466
controlling delivery of sedatives to reduce time on the ventilator, 465
in critically ill obstetric patients, 770
design principles, 447–448, *448f, 449t, 450t*
duration, 460, *461f*
key points, 458, 471
lung injury from positive pressure ventilation, 452–453
modes of ventilatory support, *450t*
modified ventilatory support protocol used by the National Institutes of Health ARDS Network, 452, 456–458
assessment for tolerance, 457–458
full-support ventilation orders, 456
full vent support, 456
inspiration:expiration ratio goals, 457
oxygenation goals, 457
pH goals, 456
plateau pressure goals, 456–457
weaning, 457
in multiple organ dysfunction syndrome, 595
myocardial infarction and, 466
neurosurgery patients, 466–467, *467f*
non–pressure-related complications of mechanical ventilation, 455–456
oxygen toxicity, 455
patient ventilator interface complications, 455
pulmonary infectious complications, 455–456
ventilator management protocols, 456
in older patients, 467–468, *468f*
for patients requiring endotracheal intubation, 403

patient subgroups, 465–468
patient–ventilator interactions, 453–455
breath cycling, 455
ventilator breath triggering, 453
ventilator-derived flow pattern, 453–455, *455f*
pneumonia in, *438t*
positive-pressure ventilation and cardiac function, 455
in postoperative care of thoracic surgical patients, 421
prolonged and failure to wean, 468–469, *469t*
protocol for routine ventilator management, *41t*
reintubations, 469–470
extubation versus weaning failure, 470
rates, 469
unplanned extubation, 469–470, *470t*
ventilation and respiratory system mechanics, 448–450
distribution of ventilation, 449–450, *451f*
equation of motion, 448–449
intrinsic positive end-expiratory pressure and the ventilatory pattern, 449
pressure targeted versus flow/volume targeted breaths, 449
weaning, 354, 457, 460–473, *464t*
randomized controlled trials, 460–465
withdrawal algorithm, 49, *49f*
Mediastinal shift, in perioperative care of thoracic surgical patients, 420
Mediator therapy, for fulminant hepatic failure, 499–500
Medicaid, 23
Medical Device Communications Industry Group, 82
Medical informatics. *See also* Technology
clinical management databases, 84
benchmarking, 84
data mining, 84
decision support systems, 83–84
cost reduction, 84
expert systems, 83
methods, 83
support technology, 83–84
electronic medical record, 80–82
adopting an electronic medical record system, 82
advantages, 80–81
data collection, 81–82
encryption, 85–86
information-seeking behavior, 86
in the intensive care unit, 80–88
the Internet, 84–85
audio, video, and teleconferencing, 85
electronic mail, 84–85
key points, 86
security, 85–86
wireless technology, 85
Medical information bus (MIB), 82
Medical records
electronic, 80–82
paper, 80–81
Medical resources, allocation, 52

Medical Subject Headings (MeSH) browser, 56–57, 59

Medicare, 23, 25
  diagnosis-related group coding, 81

MEDLINE, 56–57, 58–59

Meningitis, 632–633
  recommended therapy for life-threatening, *624t*

Meningoencephalitis, viral, 633

Menstruation, toxic shock syndrome and, 636

Mental status, perioperative management of infants and children, 780

Meperidine, in the intensive care unit, 152

Meprobamate, for poisoning, 823

Meropenem (Merren), 621, 675
  dosing, *622t*

Merren (meropenem), 621, 675
  dosing, *622t*

Mesenteric ischemia, in the perioperative intensive care unit patient, 480

MeSH. *See* Medical Subject Headings Browser

Metabolic acidosis
  diagnosis and management, 207–208, *208t, 209t*
  high-anion gap, 838

Metabolic alkalosis, diagnosis and management, 207, *207f, 207t, 208t*

Metabolic disorders, fulminant hepatic failure and, 498

Metabolic equivalents (METS), in cardiac assessment, 306, *308f*

Metabolism
  alterations in critically ill obstetric patients, 766
  altered aerobic with sepsis, 608–609
  as cause of qualitative platelet disorders, *555t*
  perioperative management in infants and children, 778, 783
  peripheral, 610
  response to injury, 176, *177f*
  spinal cord injuries and, 242
  support of the hypermetabolic response to thermal injury, 804–806

Metaproterenol, *441t*

Metastatic infection, recommended therapy for life-threatening, *624t*

Metered-dose inhaler (MDI), 440

Methanol
  antidotes for overdose, *830t*
  poisoning and, 829–830
  toxic syndromes, *820t*

Methicillin
  resistance in *Staphylococcus aureus,* 64
  resistance to coagulase-negative *Staphylococcus epidermidis* (MRCNS), 616
  vancomycin and, 621

Methotrexate, for renal failure, 744

Methyldopa
  infection and, 618

α-methyldopa, for preoperative antihypertensive medication, 339

Methylprednisolone
  as cause of qualitative platelet disorders, *555t*

for diffuse alveolar hemorrhage, 743

following kidney transplantation, 734, *735t*

following liver transplantation, 732, *732t*

for intraoperative management of heart transplantation, 704

in management of organ donors, 280

in pediatric transplantation, *784t*

for postoperative management of heart transplantation, 707

for spinal cord injuries, 242

4-Methylpyrazole (pomepizole), for poisoning, *830t*

Methylxanthines, as cause of qualitative platelet disorders, *555t*

Metocurine, for intensive care unit use, 157

Metoprolol
  for acute myocardial ischemia, 311, *312t*
  as antihypertensive drug, 341, *341t*

Metoprolol in Acute Myocardial Infarction (MIAMI), 312

Metronidazole
  adverse effects, 680
  antibiotic management of renal and hepatic dysfunction in the intensive care unit, *675t*
  for bacteria in the intensive care unit, *673t*
  for *Clostridium difficile* colitis, 476
  for colitis, 634
  distribution and elimination, 679–680
  dosage adjustments in the intensive care unit, *523t*
  dosing, *623t*
  for enteric infections, 634

METS. *See* Metabolic equivalents

Mezlin (mezlocillin), 620
  dosing, *622t*

Mezlocillin (Mezlin), 620
  dosing, *622t*

MG. *See* Myasthenia gravis

MHC. *See* Major histocompatibility complex

MHT. *See* Malignant hypertension

MIAMI. *See* Metoprolol in Acute Myocardial Infarction

MIB. *See* Medical information bus

MIC. *See* Minimum inhibitory concentration

Microangiopathy, with hematopoietic stem cell transplantation, 748–749

Micrognathia, *779t*

Midazolam
  comparison with other intensive care unit sedative drugs, *150t*
  in the intensive care unit, 147–148
  as a sedative in the intensive care unit, *151t*
  for tracheal intubation, 92

MIDCAB. *See* Minimally invasive direct coronary artery bypass

Miller–Dieker syndrome, *779t*

Milrinone
  in the cardiac surgical patient, 347, *348t*
  for cardiogenic shock, 292, 293
  clinical trials, 299
  for pediatric treatment of postoperative cardiac failure, 782
  for shock, 201, *201t*

Mineralocorticoid deficiency, 216, *217t*

Minerals, 182

Minimal anesthetic concentration (MAC) anesthesia, 32–33

Minimally invasive direct coronary artery bypass (MIDCAB), 355–357, *356t. See also* Coronary artery bypass graft
  comparison of surgical techniques, *356t*
  direct coronary artery bypass, 355
  off-pump coronary artery bypass, 355–356
  port-access surgery, 355
  transmyocardial laser revascularization, 356–357

Minimum inhibitory concentration (MIC), 620

Mini-sequencing, 65

Misoprostol, for mucosal erosive disease, 491

Mitral regurgitation, cardiogenic shock and, 294

Mitral stenosis (MS), in critically ill obstetric patients, 768–769

Mivacron (mivacurium), for intensive care unit use, *155t,* 156–157

Mivacurium (mivacron), for intensive care unit use, *155t,* 156–157

Mivazerol
  as antihypertensive drug, 342
  for perioperative myocardial ischemia, 315

Mixed pressor agents, shock and, 202, *202f*

MMAD. *See* Mass median aerodynamic diameter

MMF. *See* Mycophenolate mofetil

Moclobemide, for hypertension, 337

MODS. *See* Multiorgan dysfunction syndrome; Multiple organ dysfunction syndrome

Molecular beacons, 65

Molecular mechanisms, of cerebral injury, 228–229

Molybdenum, daily requirements in total parenteral nutrition, *182t*

Monoamine oxidase inhibitors (MAOIs), for hypertension, 337

Monobactams, 675–676
  adverse reactions, 675–676, *676t*
  distribution and elimination, 675, *675t*

Monoclonal antibodies, in animal studies for acute renal failure, *522t*

Moral issues, versus ethical issues, 45

Moraxella catarrhalis, 385, 677
  fever and, 584

Morbidity and mortality review, 20

Morphine
  effect of renal failure on drug disposition, 188
  in the intensive care unit, 151–152, *151t*

MRCNS. *See* Methicillin, resistance to coagulase-negative *Staphylococcus epidermidis*

MRI. *See* Magnetic resonance imaging

MS. *See* Mitral stenosis

Mucocutaneous infection, in immunocompromised patients, 649, *650t*

Mucor spp., 656
  following kidney transplantation, 734
  following liver transplantation, 731

Mucosal erosive disease
diagnosis, 491
hemorrhage in the critically ill, 491
pathogenesis, 491
treatment, 491
Mucoviscidosis. *See* Cystic fibrosis
Multicenter trials, 57
research, 74, *74t*
Multifocal atrial tachycardia (MAT), 321,
324, *325f*
Multiple myeloma, in immunocompromised
patients, 668
Multiple organ dysfunction syndrome
(MODS), 588–600
fever and, 578–579
fulminant hepatic failure and, 496
key points, 597
pathophysiology, 588–595, *589t*
apoptosis, 594, *594f*
complex nonlinear systems, 594–595
cytokines, 592–593
derangements in oxygen delivery and
consumption, 588–590, *589f*
derangements in the barrier function of
the intestinal mucosa, 593–594
nitric oxide, 592–593, *593f*
role of inflammatory and vasoactive
mediators, 590–592
coagulation system, 591
complement, neutrophils, and reactive
oxygen metabolites, 590–591, *590t*
kallikrein-kinin system, 591, *591f*
prostaglandins, leukotrienes, and
platelet-activating factor, 591–592
during the perioperative period in infants
and children, 787–788
peritonitis and, 171
prevention and treatment, 595–597
debridement of dead tissue and fracture
stabilization, 595
infection, 595–596
catheter-related sepsis, 596
intraabdominal sepsis, 596
pulmonary sepsis, 596
sepsis, 596
mechanical ventilation, 595
nutrition support, 596–597
resuscitation, 595
research, 70
sepsis and, 604–610
shock and, 193, 203
supportive therapy, 637–638
transition from sepsis, 603
Multiple trauma, 791–800
Mumps, 178
Mupirocin, in the intensive care unit, 681
Murine typhus *(Rickettsia typhi)*, 636
Muromonab-CD3 (OKT3), in pediatric
transplantation, *784t*
Muscular dystrophies, *163t*
Myasthenia gravis (MG), *163t*
in perioperative care of thoracic surgical
patients, 419–420
in postoperative care of thoracic surgical
patients, 424
Mycobacterium avium, 677

Mycobacterium spp., computed tomography
for detection of, 843–844
Mycobacterium tuberculosis, 438t, 617
bland-aerosol therapy and, 439
genomic identification, 64
Mycophenolate mofetil (MMF)
clinical trials, 695
following kidney transplantation, 734, *735t*
following liver transplantation, 732, *732t*
in pediatric transplantation, 783, *784t*
for postoperative management of heart
transplantation, 707
in transplantation, *694t,* 695
Mycoplasma pneumoniae, 677
Mycoplasma spp., 385, 680
Myocardial depressant factor (MDF), shock
and, 195
Myocardial depression
sepsis and, 605–608, *606f, 607f*
Myocardial infarction (MI)
acquired prolonged repolarization
syndromes and, *329t*
cardiogenic shock and, 289–290, *291t*
clinical evaluation in patients undergoing
noncardiac surgery, 3–4
clinical presentation, 290, *291t*
in critically ill obstetric patients, 769
evolution of pump failure, 290
mechanical ventilation and, 466
pathophysiology of acute, 289–290
shock and, 194
Myocardial ischemia
acquired prolonged repolarization
syndromes and, *329t*
airway management and, 99
anesthetic management, 314–316
intraoperative period, 314–315, *315f,
316f*
postoperative period, 315–316
cardiac risk assessment and preoperative
evaluation, 306–308, *308t, 309t*
clinical and perioperative presentation,
305–306, *305t, 306f, 307f*
hypertension and, 335
key points, 317
monitoring, 309–311, *310f*
pathophysiology, 303–305, *304f*
perioperative, 303–319
prevention, 309, *310f*
treatment, 311–314
β-adrenergic receptor blockers, 312–313
angiotensin-converting enzyme
inhibitors, 314
calcium-channel blockers, 313
drugs that affect coagulation, 313–314,
314t
organic nitrates, 311–312
pharmacologic, 311, *312t*
Myositis ossificans (heterotopic ossification),
neuromuscular blocking agents
and, 165
Myxedema. *See* Hypothyroidism

N
NAC. *See* N-acetylcysteine
N-acetylcysteine (NAC)

for acetaminophen toxicity, 834
for overdose of acetaminophen, *830t*
Nafcillin
antibiotic management of renal and hepatic
dysfunction in the intensive care
unit, *675t*
dosing, *623t*
for toxic shock syndrome, 635
Naloxone
for overdose of opiates, *830t*
for poisoning, 822
for spinal cord injuries, 242
Naproxen, for fever, 578
Naproxysyn, acute tubular necrosis and, 505
Nardil (phenelzine), for hypertension, 337
Nasal cannula, 431
Nasal trumpet, for airway management, 95
Nasotracheal intubation, 94–95
contraindications, 90
National Acute Spinal Cord Injury Study,
242
National Center for Biotechnology
Information (NCBI), 59
National Diabetes Data Group, 772
National Health Service (NHS) Centre for
Reviews and Dissemination, 57
National Heart, Lung and Blood Institute
(NHLBI), 72
National Institute of Drug Abuse, 837
National Institutes of Health (NIH), 73
modified ventilatory support protocol, 452,
456–458
National Library of Medicine (NLM) of the
United States, 58–59
National Marrow Donor Program, 740–741
National Nosocomial Infections Surveillance
system, 603
Natriuretic peptides, in animal studies for
acute renal failure, *522t*
NCBI. *See* National Center for Biotechnology
Information
Nebulizers
small-volume, 440
ultrasonic, 439
Necrotizing fasciitis, 634
initial therapy for life-threatening, *629t*
Necrotizing pancreatitis, following surgery,
173
Neisseria meningitidis, 630, 651, 674, 680
Neomycin sulfate, 676
Neonates. *See* Pediatric care
Nephrotoxicity, in acute renal failure, 523,
523t
Nephrotoxic vasomotor nephropathy,
505–506
Nephrotoxins, acute renal failure and, 506,
506t
Nerve stimulators, 157–158, *158f*
Netilmicin sulfate, 676
Neuraminidase inhibitors
adverse effects, 686
distribution and elimination, 686
in the intensive care unit, 686
Neurocognitive deficits, in the cardiac surgical
patient, 353–354, *353t*
Neurogenic shock, 198

Neuroimaging, for consciousness testing, *251t*

Neuroleptic malignant syndrome, as source of fever, 585

Neurologic disease
fulminant hepatic failure and, 496, *496t*
hypertension and, 336–337
in liver transplantation, 729
management of infants and children after surgery, 778–780
in orthotopic heart transplantation, 709
preoperative assessment, 10

Neurology
comparison of neurologic surgeons' grading scales, 266, *266t*
neurologic examination in spinal cord injuries, 239–240, *240t, 241f*

Neuromuscular blocking agents (NMBAs)
adverse effects, *156t*
central nervous system effects, 164
considerations for perioperative pulmonary complications, 396–397
depolarizing neuromuscular block, 156
drug action, 155–156
drug interactions with, *156t*
head trauma and, 164
indications and interactions in the intensive care unit, 152–165, 154, *154t, 155t, 156t*
intermediate-acting, 157
key points, 165
long-acting, 157
monitoring, 157–158, *158f*
limitations, 159, *160f*
myositis ossificans (heterotopic ossification) and, 165
nondepolarizing (competitive) neuromuscular block, 156
patterns of stimulation, 158–159, *159f, 160t*
physiology of the neuromuscular junction, 152–154, *152f, 153f, 154f*
recording responses of neuromuscular junction, 159
reversal of neuromuscular blockade, 164–165
short-acting, 156–157
side effects in the intensive care unit, 159–162, *161t*
pharmacologic, 161–162
physiologic, 162
toxic, 162
structure–activity relationship, 155, *156f*
toxic neuromyopathies in intensive care unit patients, 162–165, *163f, 163t*
recommendations to avoid prolonged weakness during use, 164
selected, prospective studies, 164
tracheal intubation and, 92

Neuromuscular junction
physiology, 152–154, *152f, 153f, 154f*
recording responses, 159
accelerography, 159
visual and tactile, 159

Neuromyopathies, in intensive care unit patients, 162–165, *163f, 163t*

Neuroprotectants
nonpharmacologic, 230–231
pharmacologic, 231–234

Neuroresuscitative agents, 242

Neurosurgery
acute intracerebral hemorrhage, 261–262
acute intracranial hypertension, 260–261
arteriovenous malformation (AVM), 259
carotid endarterectomy, 253–254
cerebral ischemia, 260
cerebral vascular lesions, 255–258
aneurysm, 255–256, *255t*
vasospasm after subarachnoid hemorrhage, 256–258, *257f, 258f, 258t*
craniotomy, 254–255
critical care and initial resuscitation in traumatic brain injury, 236, *237t*
decreased level of consciousness and, 259–260
key points, 262
management issues, 259–262
mechanical ventilation and, 466–467, *467f*
postoperative care of the neurosurgical patient, 253–263

Neutropenia
infections and, 655–657, *658t*
initial empiric antibiotic therapy in patients with fever, *658t*

Neutropenic colitis. *See* Typhlitis

Neutrophil-dependent lung injury, 410

New York Carnegie Foundation for the Advancement of Teaching, 73

New York Heart Association (NYHA), 699

NHBD. *See* Nonheart-beating donor organs

NHLBI. *See* National Heart, Lung and Blood Institute

NHS. *See* National Health Service Centre for Reviews and Dissemination

Nicardipine
as antihypertensive drug, 342–343, *342t*
for hypertensive encephalopathy, 335
for ischemia, 313
for pheochromocytoma, 760
for vasospasm, 257

Nicardipine hydrochloride, for acute myocardial ischemia, 311, *312t*

Nicotinic acetylcholine receptors, schematic drawing, *154f*

Nifedipine
as antihypertensive drug, 342–343, *342t*
for malignant hypertension, 335

NIH. *See* National Institutes of Health

Nimbex (cisatracurium), for intensive care unit use, *155t*, 157, 164

Nimodipine
for cerebral ischemia, 260
for vasospasm, 257

Nitrates, for acute myocardial ischemia, 311, *312t*

Nitric oxide (NO)
for acute lung injury/acute respiratory distress syndrome (ALI/ARDS), *413t*
in acute lung injury/acute respiratory distress syndrome (ALI/ARDS), 414
for acute respiratory distress syndrome, 298
for cardiogenic shock, 297
clinical applications of inhaled, *298t*
donors, 515
in multiple organ dysfunction syndrome, 592–593, *593f*
for prevention and treatment of renal injury, 515
synthase inhibitors as neuroprotectants, 232
toxicity, 229–230

Nitrofurantoin, as cause of qualitative platelet disorders, *555t*

Nitrofurazone, for control of infection in burn patients, 806

Nitrogen, balance in nutrition support in the critically ill patient, 178–179

Nitroglycerin
for acute myocardial ischemia, 311, *312t*
as antihypertensive drug, 340
for cardiogenic shock, 297
for reducing pulmonary vascular resistance, *298t*
for shock, 203

Nitrous oxide, with phenylephrine for right ventricular dysfunction, 298

Nitrovasodilators, for pediatric treatment of postoperative cardiac failure, 782

Nizoral (ketoconazole), 626, *683t*, 685
for acute lung injury/acute respiratory distress syndrome (ALI/ARDS), *413t*
for acute lung injury/acute respiratory distress syndrome (ALI/ARDS), *413t*
drug interactions in critically ill patients, *189t*

NLM. *See* National Library of Medicine of the United States

NMBAs. *See* Neuromuscular blocking agents

NMDA. *See* N-methyl-d-aspartate

N-methyl-d-aspartate (NMDA), 229

NNRTIs. *See* Nonnucleoside analogue reverse transcriptase inhibitors

NO. *See* Nitric oxide

Nocardia asteroides, 651, 653, 660
recommended therapy, *624t*

Nocardia spp.
following kidney transplantation, 734
following liver transplantation, 730

Nonheart-beating donor (NHBD) organs, 283

Noninvasive positive pressure ventilation (NPPV), postoperative management, 402–403, *402t*

Nonmaleficence, 45

Nonnucleoside analogue reverse transcriptase inhibitors (NNRTIs), 687–688, *687t*

Nonspecific interstitial pneumonia (NSIP), as complication of hematopoietic stem cell transplantation, 742

Nonsteroidal antiinflammatory drugs
(NSAIDS)
acute tubular necrosis and, 505
as cause of fulminant hepatic failure, 495
as cause of qualitative platelet disorders,
555t
causing hypertension, 339
for fever, 578
in the intensive care unit, 150–151
for peptic ulcer disease, 486
for postthoracotomy analgesia, 425
preoperative assessment, 10
Noonan's syndrome, *779t*
Norcuron (vecuronium), for intensive care
unit use, *155t,* 157, 164
Norepinephrine
in the cardiac surgical patient, 347, *348t*
in management of organ donors, *281f*
for perioperative myocardial ischemia, 315,
315f
for prevention and treatment of renal
injury, 516
for shock, 201, *201t*
Norepinephrine bitartrate, abnormal
cardioactive response in the
denervated heart, 706–707, *706t*
Normeperidine, in the intensive care unit, 152
Nortriptyline, acquired prolonged
repolarization syndromes and, *329t*
Nosocomial pneumonia. *See*
Hospital-acquired pneumonia
NRTIs. *See* Nucleoside analog reverse
transcriptase inhibitors
NSAIDS. *See* Nonsteroidal antiinflammatory
drugs
NSIP. *See* Nonspecific interstitial pneumonia
N-tert-butyl-(2-sulfophenyl)-nitrone
(S-PBN), as neuroprotectant, 232
Nucleoside analog reverse transcriptase
inhibitors (NRTIs), 687–688, *687t*
Nuromax (doxacurium), for intensive care
unit use, *155t,* 157, 164
Nurse practitioner, 19
Nutrients, in the critically ill patient, 181
Nutrition
assessment of nutrition status, 176–177,
178t
in burn patients, 805
care of the patient with multiple trauma
and, 794–796
assessment of nutritional requirements,
795–796
early enteral nutrition, 796
stress versus starvation, 795
chronic caloric deficiency, 177
daily requirements of trace elements, *182t*
electrolytes, 182, *182t*
enteral, 172
in the critically ill patient, 180–181,
180t
fluids, 182
hepatic failure and, 183
history of, 177
how to feed, 180–181, *180t*
immune-enhancing diets, 182–183
in immunocompromised patients, 668

key points, 184
kwashiorkor, 177
laboratory evaluation, 178–179
biochemical parameters, 178
energy balance, 179
immunologic tests, 178
laboratory-based nutritional assessment,
179
nitrogen balance, 178–179
lipids and, 181
in liver transplantation, 731
in lung-transplant recipients, 424
malnutrition and, 177, *178t*
in fulminant hepatic failure, 498
marasmus, 177
metabolic response to injury, 176, *177f*
nutrients, 181
glucose and fat, 181
protein, 181
perioperative management in infants and
children, 778, 783
physical examination of the patient, 177
renal failure and, 183
respiratory failure and, 183
specialty formulas, 597
subjective global assessment, 177–178
support in acute renal failure, 524
support in multiple organ dysfunction
syndrome, 596–597
support in the critically ill patient, 176–185
techniques for tube placement, 181
total parenteral, 181
vitamins, 182
when to feed, 180
Nutritionist, 18
NYHA. *See* New York Heart Association
Nystatin
for control of infection in burn patients,
806
in pediatric transplantation, 785

O

Obesity
preoperative assessment of patient, 8
as risk factor for perioperative pulmonary
complications, 395–396
Obstetrics. *See also* Pregnancy
care of the critically ill patient, 765–775
perioperative renal protection in
complicated, 508
peripartum hemorrhagic shock, 773
Obstruction
in the abdomen of the perioperative
intensive care unit patient,
477–478
airway, 418–419, 421
gastrointestinal, 853
large bowel, 477
mechanical, 477–478
small bowel, 476–477
Obstructive lung disease
perioperative evaluation, 375
as risk factor for perioperative pulmonary
complications, 395
Obstructive ventilatory defects (OVDs), 375
Obtundation, definition, 245

Off-pump coronary artery bypass (OPCAB),
355–356
Ofloxacin, 679
Ogilvie syndrome, 477
OHT. *See* Orthotopic heart transplant
OKT-3
following kidney transplantation, 735
in pediatric transplantation, *784t*
in transplantation, 697
OKTD, in transplantation, 697
Oligonucleotide microarrays ("gene chips"),
65
Oliguria, 143. *See also* Hypovolemia
in the cardiac surgical patient, 352–353,
353t
tubular function tests and, 509–511, *509t*
urine flow rate and, 509
OLT. *See* Liver transplantation
Omega-3 fatty acids
for care of the patient with multiple trauma
and, 796
in immune-enhancing diets, 182
Omega-6 polyunsaturated fatty acids, for care
of the patient with multiple trauma
and, 796
Ondansetron, antiemetic therapy in
perioperative management of
infants and children, 780
"Ondine's curse," in comatose patients, *249t*
OPCAB. *See* Off-pump coronary artery
bypass
Operating room (OR), DNR and foregoing
treatment orders in, 48
Opiates
antidotes for overdose, *830t*
as neuroprotectants, *233t*
Opioids
in the intensive care unit, 151–152, *151t*
intrathecal in postoperative care of thoracic
surgical patients, 425
toxic syndromes, *820t*
OR. *See* Operating room
Organ donors. *See also* Transplantation
anesthetic management, 282
cardiovascular effects and interactions,
278–280, *279f*
determination and diagnosis of brain
death, 276–277, *276t*
diagnosis and management of brain-dead
and nonheart-beating, 275–286
donor heart procurement, 702–703
donor lung procurement, 714
donor lung selection, 713–714
donor-recipient matching in orthotopic
heart transplantation, 702
endocrine effects, 280–281, *280f, 281f*
exclusions, 278
fluids and electrolytes, 281–282
for hematopoietic stem cell transplantation,
740–741
key points, 284
management of brain-dead and
nonheart-beating, 278
nonheart-beating, 282–283, 283
priority status level, 702
procurement procedure, 282

registrations, 725, *725f*
respiratory management, 280
selection in heart transplantation, 702
shortage, 713
temperature regulation and coagulation, 282
testing for brain death, 277–278, *277t*
Organ failure, definition, *589t*
Organic nitrates, for myocardial ischemia, 311–312
Organophosphate insecticides
acquired prolonged repolarization syndromes and, *329t*
antidotes for overdose, *830t*
Organ transplantation. *See* Transplantation
Orogastric lavage
clinical trials, 825
complications, 825
contraindications, 826
for poisoning, 825–826
Orotracheal intubation, with rigid laryngoscope, 94, *94f*
Orthotopic heart transplant (OHT), 351, 699–710, *700f*
acute postoperative management, 705–709
cardiovascular support, 705–707, *706t*
corticosteroid use, 709
gastrointestinal bleeding, 709
hemostasis and blood coagulation, 707
immunosuppression, 707–708, *708t*
infectious complications, 709
neurologic complications, 709
rejection complications, 708, *708t*
respiratory support, 707
contraindications to, 701, *701t*
donor heart procurement, 702–703
donor-recipient matching, 702
donor selection, 702
indications for, 699–701, *700f, 701f*
intraoperative management, 703–705, *704f, 705f*
long-term complications
cardiovascular complications, 709–710
immunosuppressive therapy, 710
outcome following transplant, 710
priority status level, 702
recipient preoperative management, 703
recipient selection, 701
treatment of right ventricular dysfunction following, 705–706, *706t*
Orthotopic liver transplantation (OLT). *See* Liver transplantation
Oseltamivir (Tamiflu)
adverse effects, 686
as antiviral prophylaxis, 640
distribution and elimination, 686
for viral infections, 626
Osler-Weber-Rendu syndrome, 491
Osmotherapy, as neuroprotectant, 231
Osteogenesis imperfecta, *779t*
Otitis, in diabetic patients, 669
Ovassapian airway, 95, *95f*
OVDs. *See* Obstructive ventilatory defects
Oxacillin, dosing, *623t*
Oxazolidinediones

adverse effects, 680
distribution and elimination, 680
Oxidant injury, 229–230
Oxizolidinones
for bacteria in the intensive care unit, *673t*
for multiresistant gram-positive cocci, 623
Oxygenation
shock and, 199–200
supply–demand paradigm, 504–505
Oxygen delivery
in cardiogenic shock, 291
for cerebroprotective intervention, 230
derangements in, 588–590, *589f*
in multiple organ dysfunction syndrome, 588–590
Oxygen supplementation, for perioperative pulmonary management for risk reduction, 401
Oxygen supply, utilization of cerebral, *227t*
Oxygen therapy, 428–433
aerosol mask and T-piece, 432–433
complications, 433
disorders of oxygenation, 428–429, *429f*
high-flow systems, 431
low-flow systems, 430–431, *430t*
nasal cannula, 431
non-rebreathing mask, 431f, 432
oxygen absorption atelectasis, 433, *433f*
oxygen administration, 429
oxygen content, 429–430
oxygen delivery systems, 430, *430t*
oxygen toxicity, 433
partial-rebreathing mask, 431, *431f*
simple face mask, 431
suppression of respiratory drive, 433
tracheostomy collars, 431
Venturi mask, 431–432, *432f*
Oxygen toxicity, mechanical ventilation and, 455

P
Pacing
for bradyarrhythmias, 320
in the cardiac surgical patient, 349
for pediatric treatment of postoperative cardiac failure, 782
"Packed cells." *See* Red blood cells
PACU. *See* Postanesthesia care unit
Pain
analgesic drugs and, 150
assessment algorithm, *39f*
destroyed by burn injury, 801
nonsurgical etiologies of abdominal, 478, *479t*
perioperative management in infants and children, 783
Pancreas, evaluation with computed tomography in the intensive care unit, 851–852, *851t*
Pancreas transplantation, 735–737
candidacy, 735–736
isolated, 735
postoperative care, 736–737, *736t*
preoperative care, 736
simultaneous pancreas kidney (SPK), 735–736

Pancreatitis
following pancreas transplantation, 737
fulminant hepatic failure and, 498
necrotizing, 173
in the perioperative intensive care unit patient, 479–480
Pancuronium bromide, abnormal cardioactive response in the denervated heart, 706–707, *706t*
Pancuronium (pavulon), for intensive care unit use, *155t*, 157, 164
PAOP. *See* Pulmonary arterial occlusion pressure
PAP. *See* Pulmonary artery pressure
Parainfluenza virus, as complication of hematopoietic stem cell transplantation, 747–748, *748t*
Paralytics, for airway management, 92
Parasites, 651
Parathyroid disease, 753–754, *754t*
Parathyroid hormone (PTH), calcium abnormalities and, 218
Paravertebral blockade, in postoperative care of thoracic surgical patients, 426
Parenteral nutrition, for fulminant hepatic failure, 499
Pargyline (Eutonyl), for hypertension, 337
Parnate (tranylcypromine)
for hypertension, 337
Paroxysmal supraventricular tachycardia (PSVT), cause, 321–322
Parsonnet Index, 3
Partial thromboplastin time (PTT)
airway management and, 95
with perioperative hemostasis and coagulopathy, 551
PAS. *See* Physician-assisted suicide
Pasteurella mutocida, 674
Patient care
acute care of burns, 801–817
bedside assessment of perioperative hemostasis and coagulopathy, 553, *553t*
with blunt cardiac injury, 797
clinical approach to the infected, immunocompromised patient, 653–655, *654f*
continuous assessment in the intensive care unit, 620
of the critically ill obstetric patient, 765–775
endocrine emergencies and, 752–764
ethical issues, 45. See also Ethical issues
of the head-injured patient, 796–797
identification of high-risk, 506
with increased abdominal pressure, 797
infections in the immunocompromised patient, 649–671
initial empiric antibiotic therapy in patients with neutropenia and fever, *658t*
management of acute renal failure in the critically ill patient, 521–532
patient–ventilator interactions, 453–455
patient with multiple trauma, 791–800
position in pulmonary function, 374

Patient care (*contd.*)
  postoperative care of the neurosurgical
      patient, 253–263
  preoperative education and training, 397
  prognosis with hematopoietic stem cell
      transplantation, 749
  protocol standardization, 34
Patient Outcomes Research Team (PORT),
      385, *386t*
Patients
  assessment before tracheal intubation,
      89–91, *90t*
  autonomy, 45
  death and dying, 46
  decision making for the incapacitated,
      46–47
  drug disposition in elderly, 189
  end-of-life issues, 45–54
  ethical issues, 45–54
  evaluation with pulmonary disease, 8–9, *8t*
  fluid management in the critically ill,
      137–146
  hemodynamic assessment in the critically
      ill, 122–136
  history of nutrition, 177
  laboratory evaluation of, 178–179
  nutrition support in the critically ill,
      176–185
  pharmacokinetic and pharmacodynamic
      principles in critically ill, 186–191
  physical examination of, 177
  physicians' obligations to, 45–47
  preparation for tracheal intubation, 91–92
  privacy and confidentiality, 46
  privacy and security in an intensive care
      unit, 25
  refusal of treatment, 46
  surgical approach to, 6–8, *7f*
  symptoms of suffering, 49, *50f*
Patient Self-Determination Act (PSDA), 47
PAV. *See* Proportional assist ventilation
Pavulon (pancuronium), for intensive care
      unit use, *155t*, 157, 164
PBN. *See* α-phenyl-n-tert-butyl-nitrone
PCD. *See* Programmed cell death
PCP. *See* Phencyclidine
PCR. *See* Polymerase chain reaction
PcT. *See* Percutaneous dilational tracheostomy
PDE. *See* Phosphodiesterase fraction III
      inhibitors
PE. *See* Pulmonary embolism
Peak expiratory flow rate (PEFR), 395
Pediatric care
  airway management, 776–777
  breathing, 777
  circulation, 777–778, *777t*
  congenital heart disease, 780–783, *781t*
    developmental issues, 781
    initial postoperative assessment and
        critical care management, 781
    perioperative care
      metabolism, 783
      nutrition, 783
      pain, 783
      perioperative sedation, 783
      physiology, 781

  postoperative issues in common cardiac
      lesions, 781, *782t*
  pulmonary dysfunction after
      cardiothoracic surgery, 783
  treatment of postoperative cardiovascular
      failure, 781–783
ethical and end-of-life issues, 50–51
fluid management, 778, *778t*
hemorrhagic shock and multiorgan failure,
      786–788
  children at risk for postoperative
      hemorrhage, 786–787
  early recognition and treatment of
      hemorrhage, 787
  late recognition and treatment, 787
  multiple organ failure syndrome during
      the perioperative period, 787–788
key points, 788
management after neurologic surgery,
      778–780
  diagnoses, 778–779, *779t*
  emergency procedures, 780
  fluid management, 780
  medications, 780
  monitoring, 779
  physical examination, 779–780
metabolic acidosis in, 208
metabolism, 778
nutrition, 778
perioperative care, 776–790
poisoning, 818. *See also* Poisoning
syrup of ipecac for poisoning and,
      823–825, *825t*
transplantation, 783–786
  heart, 786
  immunosuppressive medications, 783,
      784t
  kidney, 785–786
  liver, 785
  lung, 786
  multivisceral abdominal organ, 786
  posttransplant infection, 784–785
  posttransplant rejection, 783–784
  preoperative management, 783
Pediatric intensive care unit (PICU),
      perioperative management of
      infants and children, 776–790
PEFR. *See* Peak expiratory flow rate
PEG. *See* Percutaneous endoscopic
      gastrotomy
Penicillin G
  for bacteria in the intensive care unit, *673t*
  dosing, *623t*
  for toxic shock syndrome, 635
Penicillins, 620
  antibiotic management of renal and hepatic
      dysfunction in the intensive care
      unit, *675t*
  antipseudomonal, 674
  for bacteria in the intensive care unit, *673t*
  as cause of fever, *585t*
  as cause of qualitative platelet disorders,
      555t
  dosing, *622t*
  for gram-positive organisms, 674
  in immunocompromised patients, *652t*

  for infection following surgery, 170
  in the intensive care unit, 673–674
  for pneumonia, 389
Pentamidine
  acquired prolonged repolarization
      syndromes and, *329t*
  dosing, *622t*
  in immunocompromised patients, *652t*
Pentamidine isethionate, for
      bronchoconstriction, 439
Pentoxifylline, for cerebral ischemia, 260
Peptic ulcer disease
  diagnosis, 486
  hemorrhage in the critically ill, 486,
      488–489, *488t*, *489t*
  pathogenesis, 486
  treatment, 486, 488–489, *488t*, *489t*
Percussion, for airway management, 435
Percutaneous dilational tracheostomy (PcT)
  complications, *118t*
  equipment, *119t*
  in the intensive care unit, 118–119, *118f*,
      118t, *119f*
  placement, *118f*, *119f*
Percutaneous endoscopic gastrotomy (PEG),
      181
Percutaneous transluminal coronary
      angioplasty (PTCA), 346
Performance improvement, 21
Perioperative medicine
  acute abdominal conditions in the
      perioperative intensive care unit
      patient, 474–484
  care of thoracic surgical patients, 417–427
  causes of perioperative bleeding, 553, *553t*
  definition, 32, *32t*
  evaluation of pulmonary diseases and
      function, 374–384
  fulminant hepatic failure, 495–502
  genomics in critical care, 63–69
  interventional and pathophysiology of
      hemodynamic assessment,
      124–126, *125f*, *125t*
  management
    of the cardiac surgical patient, 346–362
    of infants and children, 776–790
    of obstructive and restrictive pulmonary
        diseases, 393–407
  myocardial ischemia, 303–319
  perioperative hemostasis and coagulopathy,
      549–565
  renal protection, 503–520
  stabilization in the cardiac surgical patient,
      347–348, *348t*
Perioperative risk
  cardiac evaluation decision analysis form,
      29, *30f–31f*
  multifactorial influences on, 1, *2t*
Peripherally inserted central venous (PICC
      lines) catheters, 181
  in the intensive care unit, 107–108
Peripheral vasodilators, for hypertension in
      the intensive care unit, 340
Peritonitis
  following surgery, 171
  initial therapy for life-threatening, *629t*

recommended therapy for life-threatening, *624t*

secondary/intraabdominal abscess, 633

spontaneous bacterial, 633

Permissive diagnosis, 250

Permissive hypercapnia, 452–453

PFT. *See* Pulmonary function, testing

PGP. *See* Pretty Good Privacy encryption

Pharmacist, 18

Pharmacodynamic principles

in critically ill patients, 186–191

definition, 186

Pharmacokinetic principles

in critically ill patients, 186–191

definition, 186

Pharmacology

abnormal cardioactive drug responses in the denervated heart, 706–707, *706t*

for acute lung injury/acute respiratory distress syndrome, *413t*

agents for clinical transportation in transplantation, 693–694, *694t*

antibacterial, 624–625

antibiotics for intraoperative management of heart transplantation, 703–704

antifungal drugs, 625–626, *625t*

antihypertensive drugs in pregnancy, *337t*

antimicrobial therapy in immunocompromised patients, *652t*

antiviral drugs, 626–627, *627t*

dosing, *622t*

beta lactams, 620–621, *622t–623t, 624t*

as cause of qualitative platelet disorders, *555t*

drugs for multiresistant gram-positive cocci, 623

following kidney transplantation, 734

following liver transplantation, 730

for hypertension in the intensive care unit, 339–343

immunosuppression, 693–698, *694t*

intervention during withdrawal of life-sustaining treatment, 48–49, *49f*

medications causing hypertension, 339

minimum inhibitory concentration, 620

for prevention and treatment of renal injury, 511–516

pulse-steroid therapy, 694

recommended therapy for life-threatening infections, *624t*

toxicity in pediatric multiorgan failure, 788

Phencyclidine (PCP), 149

toxic syndromes, *820t*

Phenelzine (Nardil), for hypertension, 337

Phenobarbital, for poisoning, 823

Phenobarbitone, drug interactions in critically ill patients, *189t*

Phenothiazines

acquired prolonged repolarization syndromes and, *329t*

as cause of qualitative platelet disorders, *555t*

in the intensive care unit, 149–150

toxic syndromes, *820t*

Phenotypes

definition, 63

issues in genomic causation, 67

Phenoxybenzamine, for pheochromocytoma, 759–760

Phentolamine, for left ventricular failure, 335

Phenylephrine

with nitrous oxide for right ventricular dysfunction, 298

for shock, 201, *201t*

for tracheal intubation, 95

α-phenyl-n-tert-butyl-nitrone (PBN), as neuroprotectant, 232

Phenytoin

as cause of fever, *585t*

dosage adjustments in the intensive care unit, *523t*

drug interactions in critically ill patients, *189t*

infection and, 618

perioperative management of infants and children, 780

Pheochromocytoma, 759–760

diagnosis, 759

symptoms, 759

treatment, 759–760

Phosphate, diagnosis and management of abnormalities, 221–222

Phosphodiesterase (PDE) fraction III inhibitors

for cardiogenic shock, 292

as cause of qualitative platelet disorders, *555t*

Phosphorus, daily requirements in total parenteral nutrition, *182t*

Phototoxicity, with tetracyclines, 680

Physician, 17

basic obligations, 45–47

autonomy, 45

beneficence or nonmaleficence, 45

death and dying, 46

decision making for the incapacitated patient, 46–47

disclosure and informed consent, 46

distributive justice, 45

patient refusal of treatment, 46

privacy and confidentiality, 46

professional integrity, 45–46

ethical and end-of-life issues, 45–54

obligations to patient, 45–47

Physician assistant, 19

Physician-assisted suicide (PAS), 51–52, *51t, 52t*

definitions, *51t*

guidelines for justifiable, *52t*

legislation, 51–52

Physician extender, 19

Physiological and Operative Severity Score for Enumeration of Mortality and Morbidity (POSSUM), 11, *11t*

Physiology, response to surgery, 168–172, *171t, 172t*

Physostigmine, for overdose of anticholinergic agents, *830t*

PI. *See* Principal investigator

PICC lines. *See* Peripherally inserted central venous catheters

PiCCO. *See* Pulse contour cardiac output monitor

Picis CareSuite, 82

PICU. *See* Pediatric intensive care unit

Pierre–Robin sequence, *779t*

Pigskin, for burn patients, 807

PIOPED. *See* Prospective Investigation of Pulmonary Embolism Diagnosis

Pipecuronium (arduan), for intensive care unit use, *155t*

Piperacillin

antibiotic management of renal and hepatic dysfunction in the intensive care unit, *675t*

dosage adjustments in the intensive care unit, *523t*

dosing, *622t*

Piperacillin (Pipracil), 620

Piperacillin-tazobactam (Tazocin, Zosyn), 620–621

dosing, *622t*

Pipercuronium, for intensive care unit use, 157

Pipracil (piperacillin), 620

Pirbuterol, *441t*

PIs. *See* Protease inhibitors

PKE. *See* Public key encryption

Placenta, function in critically ill obstetric patients, 767, *767f, 768f*

Plasma, fresh frozen, 572–573

Plasma drug concentrations, practical use of, 189–190, *190f*

Plasma exchange, for myasthenia gravis, 420

Plasma protein binding, effect of changes in drug disposition, 189

Plasma volume expansion, prediction, using kinetic analysis, 137–138

Plasmodium falciparum, 636

recommended therapy for life-threatening, *627t*

Plasmodium spp., 636

Platelet, concentrates, 573

Platelet-activating factor, multiple organ dysfunction syndrome and, 591–592

Platelet count, laboratory assessment, 554–555, *554t*

Platelet disorders

causes, *555t*

laboratory assessment in qualitative, 554–555, *555t*

Platelet inhibitors

for acute coronary syndromes, *314t*

in animal studies for acute renal failure, *522t*

Pleural effusion

drainage, 849

evaluation with computed tomography, 848, *848f*

malignant, 848–849

in postoperative care of thoracic surgical patients, 423

Pneumatoceles, computed tomography for detection of, 846

Pneumocystis aeruginosa, 617, *619f*
Pneumocystis carinii, *438t*, 617, 649
  computed tomography for detection of, 843
  following liver transplantation, 730
  in pediatric transplantation, 784–785
  in postoperative management of heart transplantation, 709
Pneumonia, 385–392, 632
  acquired in the intensive care unit, 583–584
  community-acquired, 385–387
    complications, 387
    diagnosis, 385–386, *386t*
    epidemiologic associations for organisms causing, *386t*
    treatment, 386–387
  as complication of hematopoietic stem cell transplantation, 742
  in HIV-positive patients, 666
  hospital-acquired, 387–389
    definitions, 387, *387t*
    diagnosis, 388, *388t*
    prevention, 388
    treatment, 388–389
  in immunocompetent patients, *438t*
  in immunocompromised patients, 649, *650t*
  key points, 391–392
  nosocomial. See Hospital-acquired pneumonia
  recommended therapy for life-threatening, *624t*, *627t*
  ventilator-associated, 389–391
    autopsy studies, 390
    diagnosis, 390–391
    mechanisms, 389, *389f*
    prevention, 391
    treatment, 391
Pneumonitis, as complication of hematopoietic stem cell transplantation, 748, *748f*
Pneumothorax
  as complication of venous cannulation, 126
  computed tomography for detection of, 843, 846
  in postoperative care of thoracic surgical patients, 422
Poiseuille's law, 534, *534f*
Poisondex, 819
Poisoning, 818–840
  antidotes for overdose, 830–831, *830t*
  in children, 818
  decontamination techniques, 822–831
    adsorption of unabsorbed toxin, 826–828
    antidotes, 830–831, *830t*
    enhanced fecal elimination, 828–829
    enhanced renal elimination, 829–830, *830t*
    evacuation of unabsorbed toxin, 822–826, *824t*, *825t*
  diagnosis, 818–821
    drugs, toxins, and toxic syndromes, 819, *820t*
    toxic syndromes, 819, *819t*

emergency stabilization and supportive care, 821–822, *821t*
  epidemiology, 818
  evaluation and management of specific intoxications, 831–838
    acetaminophen, 833–834, *835f*
    cocaine, 837–838
    cyclic antidepressants, 834–836
    digoxin, 831
    lithium, 831–832
    salicylates, 832–833
    theophylline, 836–837
    -induced high-anion gap metabolic acidosis, 838
  key points, 838
  management, 821–822, *821t*
  nontoxic household items, *821t*
Polyclonal antisera, for postoperative management of heart transplantation, 707
Polycystic kidney disease
  hypertension and, 336
  predisposition to subarachnoid hemorrhage, 264
Polymerase chain reaction (PCR), 64–65
  in immunocompromised patients, 653
Polymorphic ventricular tachycardia (PVT), 328, *328f*
Polymorphism, predisposition to acute renal failure, 506, *507t*
Polyuria, in pediatric transplantation, 785–786
Polyvinyl chloride (PVC), thermal damage to the lungs, 811
Pomepizole (4-methylpyrazole), for poisoning, *830t*
PORT. *See* Patient Outcomes Research Team
Port-access surgery, 355
Portal hypertension
  diagnosis, 489
  hemorrhage in the critically ill, 489–490, *489t*
  pathogenesis, 489
  treatment, 489–490
Positive direct antiglobulin (DAT) test, 568
Positive end-expiratory pressure (PEEP)
  definition, 450–451
  extubating patients in the intensive care unit, 98
  in management of organ donors, 280
  shock and, 194
  during withdrawal of life-sustaining treatment, 49, *49f*
POSSUM. *See* Physiological and Operative Severity Score for Enumeration of Mortality and Morbidity
Postanesthesia care unit (PACU), 253
Postcardiotomy vasodilatory shock, 293
Posterior cord syndrome, 240
Posterior tibial artery, in arterial cannulation, 104
Posthyperventilation apnea, in comatose patients, *249t*
Postoperative care, 33
Posttransfusion purpura, with perioperative hemostasis and coagulopathy, 563

Posttransplant lymphoproliferative disorder (PTLD), 661
Postural drainage, for airway management, 434, *434f*
Potassium
  diagnosis and management of abnormalities, 215–217
  maintenance requirements for fluid replacement therapy, 140–141
  monitoring in the critically ill patient, 182
  replacement protocol, *38t*
Povidone iodine, for control of infection in burn patients, 806
Practice standards. *See also* Health Care Financing Administration; Health Insurance Portability and Accountability Act; Joint Commission on Accreditation of Healthcare Organizations; Medicare
  clinical information systems as quality management tool, 24
  cost-benefit analysis, 24–25
  government agencies and, 23
  patient acuity systems as quality assessment tools, 23–24
  payor-mandated assessment of quality of care, 23
Prednisone
  perioperative coverage, *10t*
  for typhoid fever, 639
Preeclampsia
  in critically ill obstetric patients, 771–772, *771t*
  definition, 771
  signs and symptoms, *771t*
Pregnancy. *See also* Obstetrics
  antihypertensive drugs in, *337t*
  complicated obstetrics and perioperative renal protection, 508
  hypertension in, 336, *337t*
  key points, 774
  maternal–fetal interactions during, 766–767, *767f*
  nonobstetric diseases in critically ill obstetric patients, 767–771
    cardiac disease, 768–769
    cardiopulmonary resuscitation, 770–771, *770f*
    pulmonary disease, 769–770
  normal and abnormal, 765
  obstetric diseases in critically ill obstetric patients, 771–774
    acute fatty liver, 773–774
    amniotic fluid embolism (AFE), 772
    diabetes mellitus in, 772
    hematologic manifestations of fetal death, 772–773
    obstetric peripartum hemorrhagic shock, 773
    severe preeclampsia, 771–772, *771t*
  physiologic changes secondary to, 765–766
    blood volume, 765
    gas exchange and acid-base changes, 766
    hemodynamics, 765, *766t*
    metabolic alterations, 766

placental function, 767, *767f, 768f*
preterm gestation, 765
Preload, 287–288, *288f*
Preoperative assessment, 1–14
  in cardiac disease, 2–8
  components of evaluation, 1, *2t*
  in endocrine diseases, 9
  evaluation clinic, 32–33, *33t, 34f*
  in hematologic and infectious issues, 10
  in hepatic disease, 9
  key points, 12
  in neurologic disease, 10
  for noncardiac surgery, 29–30, *30f–31f*
  perioperative corticosteroid coverage, *10t*
  perioperative risk, 1, *2t*
  in renal disease, 9–10
  in respiratory disease, 8–9
  risk indices for intensive care unit mortality
    and utilization, 11–12
President's Commission for the Study of
    Ethical Problems, 48, 275–276,
    284
Pressure support ventilation (PSV), 354
Pretty Good Privacy (PGP) encryption,
    85–86
Primary hemostasis, laboratory testing,
    550–551, *551t*
Primaxin (imipenem-cilastatin), 621
  dosing, *622t*
Principal investigator (PI), role in research, 75
Privacy, 46
Probucol, acquired prolonged repolarization
    syndromes and, *329t*
Procainamide
  acquired prolonged repolarization
    syndromes and, *329t*
  for atrial flutter or atrial fibrillation,
    323–324, *324f*
  as cause of fever, *585t*
  infection and, 618
  for supraventricular tachyarrhythmias,
    322
Procarbazine, as cause of fever, *585t*
Procysteine, for acute lung injury/acute
    respiratory distress syndrome
    (ALI/ARDS), *413t*
Professional Standards Review Organization,
    23
Programmed cell death (PCD), cerebral
    injury and, 230
Prolonged repolarization syndromes, 328,
    329t
Propofol
  comparison with other intensive care unit
    sedative drugs, *150t*
  in the intensive care unit, 148–149
  as neuroprotectant, *233t*, 234
  as a sedative in the intensive care unit, *151t*
  for tracheal intubation, 92
Proportional assist ventilation (PAV), 455
Propranolol hydrochloride
  for acute myocardial ischemia, 311, *312t*
  as antihypertensive drug, 340–341, *341t*
Prospective Investigation of Pulmonary
    Embolism Diagnosis (PIOPED),
    539

Prostaglandin E₁, for acute lung injury/acute
    respiratory distress syndrome
    (ALI/ARDS), *413t*
Prostaglandins, multiple organ dysfunction
    syndrome and, 591–592
Prostate, transurethral resection of, 2
Protease inhibitors (PIs), 687–788,
    687t
Protected environment, in the intensive care
    unit, 640
Protein
  chronic deficiency, 177
  for nutrition support in the critically ill
    patient, 181
Proteus mirabilis, 674
Proteus spp., 634
Prothrombin time (PT), airway management
    and, 95
PSDA. *See* Patient Self-Determination Act
Pseudallescheria boydii, 625, 683
  recommended regimens for treatment of
    multiresistant, *638t*
  recommended therapy for life-threatening,
    625t
Pseudohyponatremia, diagnosis and
    management, 211
Pseudomonas aeruginosa, 389, 391, 616, 621,
    653
  antibiotic selection in the intensive care
    unit, *673t*
  in cystic fibrosis, 378
  fever and, 584
  following liver transplantation,
    730
  in postoperative management of heart
    transplantation, 709
  recommended regimens for treatment of
    multiresistant, *638t*
  recommended therapy, *624t*
Pseudomonas fluorescens, 681
Pseudomonas spp.
  in burn patients, 810
  evaluation with computed tomography in
    the intensive care unit, 855
  in inhalation injury, 812
Pseudoobstruction, 477
PSV. *See* Pressure support ventilation
PSVT. *See* Paroxysmal supraventricular
    tachycardia
Psychiatric medications, as cause of qualitative
    platelet disorders, *555t*
Psychogenic unresponsiveness, 250
PT. *See* Prothrombin time
PTA. *See* Pancreas transplantation, isolated
PTCA. *See* Percutaneous transluminal
    coronary angioplasty
PTH. *See* Parathyroid hormone
PTLD. *See* Posttransplant lymphoproliferative
    disorder
PTT. *See* Partial thromboplastin time
Public key encryption (PKE), 85–86
PubMed, 58–59
Pulmonary arterial occlusion pressure
    (PAOP), 140
  following surgery in the intensive care unit,
    169

Pulmonary artery
  anatomic position, *123f*
  monitoring, 131–132, *131f*
    complications, 126, *126t*
  physical complications of monitoring, 126,
    126t
Pulmonary artery catheterization
  efficacy, 132
  hemodynamic assessment, 122–123
  insertion in the intensive care unit, 111
  in the intensive care unit, 109–111, *109t,
    110f, 110t, 111f*
Pulmonary artery pressure (PAP), cardiogenic
    shock and, 297
Pulmonary diseases
  anesthetic factors, 382–383
  assessment of perioperative pulmonary risk,
    397–399
    exercise testing, 399
    preoperative pulmonary function tests,
      397–398, *398t*
    recommendations for preoperative
      pulmonary function tests,
      398–399
  atelectasis, 383
  clinical risk factors for perioperative
    pulmonary complications,
    394–396, *394t*
    age, 394
    general health and cardiovascular status,
      394
    obesity, 395–396
    obstructive lung disease, 395
    smoking, 395
  common chronic respiratory diseases,
    376–379
    asthma, 378–379, *378t*
    bronchiectasis, 377, *377t*
    chronic bronchitis, 376, *376t*
    cystic fibrosis (mucoviscidosis),
      377–378, *378t*
    emphysema, 376–377, *377t*
  in critically ill obstetric patients,
    769–770
  evaluation of the patient with, 8–9,
    8t
  evaluation of the patient with respiratory
    disease and, 379–382
    arterial blood gas studies, 380–381
    flow volume loops, 381–382
    imaging, 380
    interpretation of lung sounds, *380t*
    pulmonary function testing, 381, *381f,
      382f*
  fulminant hepatic failure and, 497
  with hematopoietic stem cell
    transplantation, 742–743, *743f*
  infections associated with, *618t*
  key points, 383, 405
  in liver transplantation, 728–729
  mechanical ventilation for patients
    requiring endotracheal intubation,
    403
  noninvasive positive pressure ventilation in
    postoperative patients, 403
  obstructive lung disease, 375

Pulmonary diseases (*contd.*)
perioperative considerations for restrictive, 403–404
perioperative ventilatory support, 404
risk factor assessment, 403–404
perioperative evaluation, 374–384
perioperative management of obstructive and restrictive, 393–407
perioperative pulmonary management for risk reduction, 399–402
anesthesia choice, 400
noninvasive ventilatory assistance, 402–403
optimal preoperative medical therapy for obstructive lung diseases, 400
oxygen supplementation, 401
postoperative deep-breathing maneuvers, 401
pulmonary rehabilitation and incentive spirometry training, 400
smoking cessation, 399–400
surgical techniques, 401
venous thromboembolism prophylaxis, 401–402, *401t*
perioperative risk management strategy, *404t*
postoperative management of respiratory decompensation, 402–403, *402t*
prediction tools for estimation of postoperative pulmonary outcome, 399
pulmonary pathology, 375
respiratory physiology, 374
reversible versus irreversible disease, 375–376, *376f*
surgical and anesthetic considerations for perioperative pulmonary complications, 396–397
operative anesthetic techniques, 396
perioperative neuromuscular blockade, 396–397
preoperative patient education and training, 397
surgical anatomic site, technique, and duration, 396, *396t*, *397t*
Pulmonary dysfunction, after cardiothoracic surgery in infants and children, 783
Pulmonary edema
in the cardiac surgical patient, 354
following lung transplantation, 717
Pulmonary embolism (PE). *See also* Venous thromboembolism
cardiac arrest and, 544–545
clinical manifestations, 535–536
computed tomography for detection of, 846–847, *847f*
in critically ill obstetric patients, 769–770
in the critically ill patient, 533–548
diagnostic approach, 540–542, *540t*, *541f*, *541t*, *542t*
diagnostic findings, 539–540, *539t*
diagnostic-therapeutic approach to, *541f*
echocardiography in diagnostic evaluation, 541–542, *542t*
key points, 545
outcome, 533, *534f*

of thrombolysis versus heparin in clinical trials for, 543–544, *544t*
pathophysiologic model, 534–535, *537f*
relationship between shock, embolism size, and outcome, 540–541, *540t*
relationship between shock and outcome, *541t*
shock model and physiology, 534–536, *534f*, *535f*, *535t*, *536f*, *537f*
therapeutic approach, 542–544, *543t*, *544t*
thrombolytic therapy for, 543, *543f*
in transit, 544–545
Pulmonary function
infectious complications, 455–456
pathology, 375
recommendations for preoperative testing, 398–399
testing in perioperative evaluation, 381, *381f*, *382f*
testing in perioperative management of pulmonary diseases, 397–398, *398t*
Pulmonary hypertension
in critically ill obstetric patients, 769
impact on right ventricular function, *297t*
Pulmonary insufficiency, from smoke inhalation, 810
Pulmonary resection, 417
Pulmonary sepsis, in multiple organ dysfunction syndrome, 596
Pulse contour cardiac output monitor (PiCCO), 111
Pulse-steroid therapy, 694
Pulse therapy, 806
Purine nucleoside analog
adverse effects, 687
distribution and elimination, 687
in the intensive care unit, 687
Purpura
autoimmune thrombocytopenia. *See* Idiopathic thrombocytopenic purpura
posttransfusion, 563
thrombotic thrombocytopenic, 553
PVC. *See* Polyvinyl chloride
PVT. *See* Polymorphic ventricular tachycardia
Pyelonephritis, hypertension and, 336
Pyrethamine, in immunocompromised patients, *652t*
Pyridoxine, for overdose of isoniazid, *830t*

Q
Q fever *(Coxiella burnetii)*, 636, 680
Qualitative platelet disorders, laboratory assessment, 554–555, *555t*
Quality assurance programs, 20
in research, 74
Quality management techniques, 10–20
Quality of care
certification process, 21
critical care clinical practice guidelines, 21–22
ensuring, 19–22
evidence-based standards, 21
models of care, 16–17
morbidity and mortality review, 20
payor-mandated assessment of, 23

performance improvement, 21
quality assurance programs, 20
quality management techniques, 19–20
standard of care definition, 21
standards of practice in critical care medicine, 20–21
Quinidine
acquired prolonged repolarization syndromes and, *329t*
as cause of fever, *585t*
as cause of qualitative platelet disorders, *555t*
infection and, 618
Quinidine gluconate, dosing, *622t*
Quinine
for babesiosis, 636
dosing, *622t*
for malaria, 636
Quinolones
adverse effects, 679
antibiotic management of renal and hepatic dysfunction in the intensive care unit, *675t*
distribution and elimination, 679
in immunocompromised patients, *652t*
in the intensive care unit, 678–679, *678t*
resistance, 681–682, 682, *682t*
Quinupristin/dalfopristin, antibiotic management of renal and hepatic dysfunction in the intensive care unit, *675t*
Quinupristin-dalfopristin (Synercid)
adverse effects, 681
distribution and elimination, 681
dosing, *623t*
in the intensive care unit, 680–681
for multiresistant gram-positive cocci, 623

R
Radial artery cannulation
direct cannulation, 102–103, *103f*, *104f*
in the intensive care unit, 102–104, *105f*, *106f*
transfixation cannulation technique, 103–104, *104f*
Radiation therapy, as complication of hematopoietic stem cell transplantation, 745
Radical scavengers, as neuroprotectants, 232
Radionuclide angiography (RNA), compared with two-dimensional transesophageal echocardiography, 134
Ramsay sedation scale, 147, *148t*, 245, *245t*
Randomized clinical trials (RCTs), 57
Randomized controlled trial (RCT), 132
Rapacuronium (raplon)
for airway management, 92
for intensive care unit use, *155t*
Rapamune Global Study Group, 696
Rapamycin (Sirolimus), in transplantation, *694t*, 696
Raplon (rapacuronium), for intensive care unit use, *155t*
RBCs. *See* Red blood cells
RBF. *See* Renal blood flow

RCT. *See* Randomized clinical trials; Randomized controlled trial
Red blood cells (RBCs), 570–572
"Red-man syndrome," 621, 623
Registry of the International Society for Heart and Lung Transplantation (ISHLT), 699
Rehabilitation
  of the cardiac surgical patient, 349
  pulmonary, 400
Reintubations, 469–470. *See also* Extubation
  extubation versus weaning failure, 470
  rates, 469
  unplanned extubation, 469–470, *470t*
Relenza (zanamavir), for viral infections, 626
Renal blood flow (RBF), regulation, 138
Renal critical care
  antibiotic management in the intensive care unit, *675t*
  perioperative renal protection, 503–520
Renal disease
  dysfunction and failure, 498–499
  end-stage, 733
  preoperative assessment, 9–10
Renal dysfunction
  care of the patient with multiple trauma and, 792–793
  evaluation with computed tomography in the intensive care unit, 852, *852f*
Renal elimination, for care of the poisoned patient, 829–830, *830t*
Renal failure, 503–520
  continuous renal replacement therapy, 181
  detection of renal dysfunction in the intensive care unit, 509–511
    tubular function tests and evaluation of oliguria, 509–511, *509t*
      creatinine clearance, 510–511, 510f, *510t*
      sodium conservation, 509–510
      tubular concentrating ability, 509
      urine flow rate and oliguria, 509
  effect on drug disposition, 188
  etiology of acute, 503, *504t*
  evaluation with computed tomography in the intensive care unit, 852
  following liver transplantation, 731
  genetic polymorphism and predisposition to acute renal failure, 506, *507t*
  with hematopoietic stem cell transplantation, 744–745, *745t*
  high-risk procedures and events, 506–509
    biliary tract and hepatic surgery, 508
    cardiac surgery, 506–507
    complicated obstetrics, 508
    intraabdominal hypertension, 508–509
    rhabdomyolysis, 508–509
    trauma, 508–509
    urogenital surgery, 508
    vascular surgery, 507–508
  hypertension and, 336
  identification of the high-risk patient, 506
  in immunocompromised patients, 669
  key points, 517
  natural history of perioperative acute renal failure, 506, *506t, 507f*

nutrition support in the critically ill patient, 183
pathogenesis of acute, 503–506
  renal injury and failure, 503–504
  tubular necrosis, 504–506
patterns of postoperative, *507f*
preexisting renal insufficiency, 506
prevention and treatment of renal injury, 511–517, *511f, 511t, 512t*
  pharmacologic interventions, 511–516
    angiotensin-converting enzyme inhibitors, 515
    atrial natriuretic peptide, 515–516
    calcium channel blockers, 514–515
    diuretics, 511–513
    dopaminergic agonists, 513–514
    nitric oxide donors, 515
    renal ischemic preconditioning and adenosine, 516
    vasopressor therapy in vasodilated shock, 516–517
      arginine vasopressin, 516–517
      norepinephrine, 516
Renal function, in liver transplantation, 731
Renal insufficiency
  preoperative assessment of patient, 9
  sepsis and, 609–610
Renal perfusion pressure, in acute renal failure, 522
Renal replacement therapy
  continuous, 525–527, *526t*
  controversies, 528–530
  in the critically ill patient, 528–530
  indications for, 524, *524t*
  mode of, 528
  techniques, 525–527
RES. *See* Reticuloendothelial system
Rescue breathing, 364
Research
  advances, 72–75, *75f*
  on brain-dead organ donors, 283–284
  for cardiogenic shock, 297
  clinical trials, 73–74
  conflict of interest in critical care, 76–77
  cost estimates, 76
  in critical care medicine, 70–79
  in endovascular technology, 273
  funding sources, 76
  history in critical care medicine, 70
  integrative or translational in the intensive care unit, 72–73
  intensive care unit technology and therapy, 71
  key points, 78
  multicenter trials, 74, *74t*
  natural history, risk, and outcomes analysis, 71
  optimal personnel and resources utilization, 71
  organizational structure within the institution, 75–76
  pathophysiology of diseases, 71–72
  problems in the intensive care unit, 77
  quality assurance, 74
  respiratory care, 444
  role of the institutional review board, 76
  role of the principal investigator, 75

role of the study coordinator, 76
  on shock, 203
Resection, *476t*
Reserpine, for preoperative antihypertensive medication, 339
Resident, full-time equivalent, 81
Resistive element (impedance), definition, 534
Respiratory abnormalities
  in comatose patients, *249t*
  in lung transplantation, 717
  in orthotopic heart transplantation, 707
Respiratory acidosis
  diagnosis and management, 209–210
  treatment, 210
Respiratory alkalosis, diagnosis and management, 209, *209t*
Respiratory care, 428–446
  aerosol therapy, 439–443
  airway clearance techniques, 433–439
  complications of oxygen therapy, 433
  department organization, 443–444, *444f*
  future, 444
  key points, 444
  oxygen therapy, 428–433
Respiratory decompensation, postoperative management, 402–403, *402t*
Respiratory disease
  evaluation of the patient with pulmonary disease, 8–9, *8t*
  perioperative evaluation, 376–379
  preoperative assessment, 8–9
Respiratory failure
  in HIV-positive patients, 665–666
  nutrition support in the critically ill patient, 183
  in spinal cord injuries, 240–241
Respiratory function, physiology, 374
Respiratory syncytial virus (RSV)
  in children, 440
  as complication of hematopoietic stem cell transplantation, 747–748, *748t*
Respiratory system, effect on organ donors, 280
Respiratory therapist, 18
Respirgard II, 439
Resting metabolic rate (RMR), nutrition and, 179
Restriction fragment length polymorphism (RFLP), 64
Restrictive lung disease, preoperative assessment of patient, 8
Restrictive ventilatory defects (RVDs), 375
Resuscitation
  care of the patient with multiple trauma and, 791–792
  in multiple organ dysfunction syndrome, 595
  protocol for upper gastrointestinal bleeding, 486, 488, *488t*
  in spinal cord injuries, 239
  in traumatic brain injury, 236, *237t*
Reticular formation (RF), 244
Reticuloendothelial system (RES), idiopathic thrombocytopenic purpura and, 562–563

Return of spontaneous circulation (ROSC), in cardiopulmonary resuscitation, 369
Revascularization, transmyocardial laser, 356–357
RFLP. *See* Restriction fragment length polymorphism
Rhabdomyolysis, perioperative renal protection and, 508–509
Rhinocerebral mucormycosis, in diabetic patients, 669
Rhinovirus, as complication of hematopoietic stem cell transplantation, 747–748, *748t*
Ribavirin
    adverse effects, 687
    distribution and elimination, 687
    dosing, *622t*
    for respiratory syncytial virus in children, 440
Ribavirin (Virazole), for viral infections, 626
Rib fractures, computed tomography for detection of, 846
Rickets, 177
Rickettsia akari (Rickettsialpox), 636
Rickettsial infections, 636
    initial therapy for life-threatening, *629t*
Rickettsialpox *(Rickettsia akari),* 636
Rickettsia rickettsii (Rocky Mountain Spotted Fever), 636, 680
Rickettsia spp., 680
Rickettsia typhi (murine typhus), 636
Rickettsia typhus (epidemic typhus), 636
Right ventricular ejection fraction (RVEF) catheter, 111
    hemodynamic assessment, 129–130
Right ventricular failure, 296–298, *297f, 297t, 298t*
Right ventricular function, impact of pulmonary hypertension on, *297t*
Rigid bronchoscopy, 417
Riker Sedation-Agitation scale (SAS), 147, *148t*
Rimantadine (Flumadine)
    as antiviral prophylaxis, 640
    for viral infections, 626
Rimfampicin, drug interactions in critically ill patients, *189t*
Ringer solution, 141
Risk indices
    cardiac risk stratification for noncardiac surgical procedures, *5t*
    cardiac surgery specific, 3, *4t*
    for mortality and utilization in the intensive care unit, 11–12, *11t*
    in myocardial ischemia, 306–308, *308t, 309t*
    noncardiac, 2–3
    for perioperative cardiac surgery, 358
    for perioperative pulmonary complications, 394–396
    perioperative strategy, *404t*
    for restrictive pulmonary diseases, 403–404
    value of, 11–12
RMR. *See* Resting metabolic rate
RNA. *See* Radionuclide angiography
Rocephin (ceftriaxone), 620

Rockall Severity Score, 486, *488t*
Rocky Mountain Spotted Fever *(Rickettsia rickettsii),* 636, 680
Rocuronium (zemuron), for intensive care unit use, *155t,* 157, 164
Roferon-A (interferon-alpha) for viral infections, 626
ROSC. *See* Return of spontaneous circulation
RSV. *See* Respiratory syncytial virus
Rupture, cardiogenic shock and, 294–295
Russell–Silver syndrome, *779t*
RVDs. *See* Restrictive ventilatory defects
RVEF. *See* Right ventricular ejection fraction catheter

S
SAH. *See* Subarachnoid hemorrhage
Salbutamol, for hyperkalemia, 217
Salicylates
    evaluation and management for intoxication of, 832–833
    poisoning and, 829–830
    toxic syndromes, *820t*
Saline, for hypovolemia, 214
Salmeterol, *441t*
    for asthma, 378–379
Salmonella spp., 476, 634
SAPS. *See* Simplified Acute Physiology Score
SAS. *See* Sedation Agitation scale
SCA. *See* Society of Cardiovascular Anesthesiologists
SCCM. *See* Society of Critical Care Medicine
SCUF. *See* Slow continuous ultrafiltration
Scurvy, 177
Seckel syndrome, *779t*
Secondary hemostasis
    definition, 549
    laboratory testing, 551–552
Second-degree burns, 801
Security, in medical informatics, 85–86
Sedation-Agitation scale (SAS), 147, *148t*
Sedatives, 147–150, *148t, 150t, 151t*
    administration during life-sustaining treatment, 48–49
    for cardiac surgical patients, 346
    comparison of intensive care unit drugs, *150t*
    controlling delivery to reduce time on the ventilator, 465
    perioperative management in infants and children, 783
    pharmacokinetic variables, *151t*
    toxic syndromes, *820t*
    for tracheal intubation, 92
Seizures
    after a craniotomy, 254
    as complication of subarachnoid hemorrhage, 270–271
    poisoning and, 836
Selective estrogen receptor modulator (SERM), as neuroprotectant, 232
Selegiline, for hypertension, 337
Selenium, daily requirements in total parenteral nutrition, *182t*
Sepsis, 601–615. *See also* Systemic inflammatory response syndrome

acute-phase response, 601–602
acute respiratory distress syndrome, 604–605, *604t*
altered aerobic metabolism, 608–609
altered physiologic responses and current therapy, 603–604
biliary, 173
catechol-resistant vasodilation, 608
catheter-related, 596
computed tomography for detection of, 843
cryptogenic without identified local infection, 627, 630
definitions, *589t,* 601, *602t*
fluid and vasopressor administration, 610–612
gastrointestinal tract and, 609
hepatic dysfunction, 609
initial therapy for life-threatening, *628t*
intraabdominal, 596
key points, 612
line, 631–632
in lung-transplant recipients, 424
in multiple organ dysfunction syndrome, 596
myocardial depression, 605–608, *606f, 607f*
nervous system and, 610
normal response to, 601–604
organ dysfunction, 604–610
peripheral metabolism and, 610
pulmonary, 596
renal insufficiency, 609–610
septic response, 602–603, *602t*
shock and, 195
transition to multiple organ dysfunction syndrome, 603
Septic emboli, computed tomography for detection of, 843, *844f*
Septicemia, 409, *410f*
    in immunocompromised patients, 668
Septic encephalopathy, 610
Septic reactions, to blood transfusions, 567–568, *568t*
Septic shock
    acute tubular necrosis and, 505
    in immunocompromised patients, 649, *650t*
    treatment, 759
Sequential single-lung transplantation (SSLT), 419
SERM. *See* Selective estrogen receptor modulator
Serratia, 621, 634
    recommended regimens for treatment of multiresistant, *638t*
Shigella dysenteriae, with thrombocytopenia, 563
Shigella spp., 476, 634
Shock, 192–205
    in acute pulmonary embolism, 540
    blood transfusions and, 568
    cardiogenic, 196–197, *197f*
    classification, 193–198, *194t*
    in critically ill obstetric patients, 773
    definition, 198

hyperdynamic, 195–196, *195f, 196f*
hypovolemic, 197–198, *198f*
interrelationships of hyperdynamic, hypovolemic, and cardiogenic shock states, 192–193, *192f*
key points, 203–204
monitoring and therapy, 198–203, *199f*
  fluids, 200
  inotropic or chronotropic agents, 201
  mixed pressor agents, 202, *202f*
  oxygenation and acid-base balance, 199–200
  steroids, 203
  vasoconstrictor agents, 201–202
  vasodilator agents, 202–203
  vasopressor agents, 200, *201t*
mortality, 192
neurogenic, 198
obstructive mechanisms of, 193–195
postcardiotomy vasodilatory, 293
relationship between outcome and, *541t*
relationship between shock, embolism size, and outcome, 540–541, *540t*
research on, 203
septic. *See* Septic shock
spinal, 240
vasodilator, 516–517
"Shock lung." *See* Acute respiratory distress syndrome
Shunting
  anatomic, 428–429
  true, 429
SIADH. *See* Syndrome of inappropriate antidiuretic hormone
SICU. *See* Surgical intensive care unit
SID. *See* Strong ion difference
Silver nitrate, for control of infection in burn patients, 806
Silver sulfadiazine, for control of infection in burn patients, 806
Simplified Acute Physiology Score (SAPS), 11, *11t*, 24
Simultaneous pancreas kidney (SPK) transplantation, 735–736
SIMV. *See* Synchronized intermittent mandatory ventilation
Single-lung transplant (SLP), 711
Single nucleotide polymorphisms (SNPs), 65
Single twitch, 158–159
Sinusitis
  in the intensive care unit, 632
  as source of fever, 584
Sirolimus (rapamycin)
  in pediatric transplantation, *784t*
  in transplantation, *694t*, 696–697
SIRS. *See* Systemic inflammatory response syndrome
Skin infections, 634
  initial therapy for life-threatening, *629t*
SLED. *See* Sustained low-efficiency daily dialysis
Sleep apnea, as surgical risk factor, 395–396
Slow continuous ultrafiltration (SCUF), for renal replacement therapy, 526
SLP. *See* Single-lung transplant
Small bowel obstruction, 476–477, *476t*

Small-particle aerosol generator (SPAG), for respiratory syncytial virus in children, 440
Small-volume nebulizers (SVN), 440
Smith–Lemli–Opitz syndrome, *779t*
Smoking. *See also* Tobacco use
  cessation, 399–400
  hypertension and, 338
  respiratory disease and, 379
  as risk factor for perioperative pulmonary complications, 395
SNOMED. *See* Standard Nomenclature of Medicine
SNP. *See* Sodium nitroprusside
SNPs. *See* Single nucleotide polymorphisms
Social issues, in genomics in perioperative critical care, 67
Social worker, 18
Society of Cardiovascular Anesthesiologists (SCA), 133, 306
Society of Critical Care Medicine (SCCM), 21–22, 35, 38, 71, 463
  Consensus Statement on the Triage of Critically Ill Patients, 52
Sodium
  diagnosis and management of abnormalities, 211–215
  maintenance requirements for fluid replacement therapy, 140–141
  monitoring in the critically ill patient, 182
  renal dysfunction and, 509–510
Sodium bicarbonate, in cardiopulmonary resuscitation, 370
Sodium nitroprusside (SNP)
  as antihypertensive drug, 340
  for aortic dissection, 336
  for cardiogenic shock, 297
  as cause of qualitative platelet disorders, *555t*
  for hypertensive encephalopathy, 335
  for malignant hypertension, 335
  for reducing pulmonary vascular resistance, *298t*
  for shock, 203
Sodium polystyrene sulfonate resin (Kayexalate), for hyperkalemia, 217
Soft-tissue infections, 634
  initial therapy for life-threatening, *629t*
  recommended therapy for life-threatening, *624t*
Soft-tissue injuries, airway management and, 99
Solutes, principles of removal by dialysis, 524–525
Sonoclot, in perioperative hemostasis and coagulopathy, 552–553
Sotalol
  acquired prolonged repolarization syndromes and, *329t*
  for atrial fibrillation, 323
SPAG. *See* Small-particle aerosol generator
S-PBN. *See* α-phenyl-tert-butyl-(2-sulfophenyl)-nitrone
Spetzler-Martin grading scale, 266, *267t*
Spinal cord injuries, *163t*
  Brown-Séquard syndrome, 240
  central cord syndrome, 240

complete cord lesion, 240
computed tomography for detection of, 845–846
cord injury syndromes, 240–242
initial resuscitation, 239
key points, 242
management in the intensive care unit, 236–243
metabolic effects, 242
neurologic examination, 239–240, *240t, 241f*
neuroresuscitative agents, 242
pathophysiology, 239
posterior cord syndrome, 240
shock and, 198
spinal shock, 240
systemic effects, 240–242
  autonomic hyperreflexia, 242
  cardiovascular, 241–242
  respiratory, 240–241
Spinal shock, 240
Spirometry training, for pulmonary rehabilitation, 400
SPK. *See* Simuntaneous pancreas kidney transplantation
Spleen, in T-cell-dependent immune responses, 651
Splenectomy, infections associated with, *618t*
Spontaneous bacterial peritonitis, 633
Sporanox (itraconazole), 626, *683t*
  adverse effects, 685
  distribution and elimination, 685
  dosing, *622t*
  in immunocompromised patients, *652t*
Sporothrix spp., recommended therapy for life-threatening, *625t*
SRES. *See* Stress-related erosive syndrome
SSLT. *See* Sequential single-lung transplantation
Standard Nomenclature of Medicine (SNOMED), 84
Standard of care, definition, 21
Staphylococcus aureus, 389, 630, 631, 635
  blood transfusions and, 567–568
  as complication of hematopoietic stem cell transplantation, 746, *746t*
  fever and, 581, 582
  following liver transplantation, 730
  fulminant hepatic failure and, 498
  in inhalation injury, 812
  in the intensive care unit, 616
    antibiotic selection, *673t*
    evaluation with computed tomography, 855
  methicillin-resistant, 64
  in postoperative management of heart transplantation, 709
  recommended regimens for treatment of multiresistant, *638t*
  recommended therapy, *624t*
  secondary to sepsis, 603
Staphylococcus epidermidis
  blood transfusions and, 567–568
  fulminant hepatic failure and, 498
  methicillin-resistant coagulase-negative, 616

Staphylococcus pneumoniae, 385, 387, 617, 620, 630
  recommended regimens for treatment of multiresistant, *638t*
Staphylococcus spp.
  in burn patients, 807, 810
  as complication of hematopoietic stem cell transplantation, 746, *746t*
Starvation, care of the patient with multiple trauma and, 795
Stasis, Virchow triad, 536, *537t*
Statistics
  evidence for genomic causation, 65–66
  family-based genomic segregation analysis, 66
  population-based Genomic Association studies, 65–66
Stenotrophomonas maltophilia, 391, 655, 674
  recommended therapy, *624t*
Steroid myopathy, *163t*
Steroids
  for brain edema, 238–239
  in management of organ donors, 280
  perioperative management of infants and children, 780
  pulse-steroid therapy, 694
  shock and, 203
  side effects, 694, *694t*
  for spinal cord injuries, 242
Stomas, surgery and, 170–171
Stomatitis, recommended therapy for life-threatening, *627t*
Streptococcus pneumonia, 651, 674
  fever and, 584
  in the intensive care unit
    antibiotic selection, *673t*
    evaluation with computed tomography, 855
  penicillin-resistant, 616
  recommended therapy, *624t*
Streptococcus pyogenes, 630
Streptococcus viridans
  as complication of hematopoietic stem cell transplantation, 746, *746t*
Streptogramins, for bacteria in the intensive care unit, *673t*
Streptokinase, for pulmonary embolism, 537–538
Streptomyces venezuelae, 680
Streptomycin sulfate, 676
Stress, effect on asthma, 378
Stress echocardiography, for detection of coronary artery disease, 7–8
Stress-related erosive syndrome (SRES)
  diagnosis, 490
  hemorrhage in the critically ill, 490
  pathogenesis, 490
  treatment, 490
Stroke. *See* Cerebral ischemia
Strong ion difference (SID), 206
Strongyloides, 660
Strongyloides stercoralis, 660–661
Study coordinator, role in research, 76
Stupor, definition, 245
Sturge–Weber syndrome, *779t*
Subarachnoid hemorrhage (SAH)

and cerebrovascular accident, 264–274
classification systems, 266–267, *266t*, *267t*
complications, 270–271
diagnosis, 265–266
epidemiology, 264–265
evaluation with computed tomography in the intensive care unit, 854, *855f*
future developments, 273
grades of, *255t*
hyperemia and normal perfusion pressure breakthrough, 271–272
key points, 273
operative management, 268–270
outcome, 273
pathophysiology, 265
postoperative care, 256–258, *257f*, *258f*, *258t*
postoperative management in the intensive care unit, 272–273
preoperative management, 267–268
surgical alternatives, 270
Subclavian venous catheterization, in the intensive care unit, 108
Succinylcholine
  for airway management, 92
  for intensive care unit use, 155–156
Suctioning, for airway management, 436
Sudden death, during dialysis for acute renal failure, 527
Suffering, 49–50, *50f*
Suicide, physician-assisted, 51–52, *51t*, *52t*
Sulbactam sodium, 674
Sulfadiazine, in immunocompromised patients, *652t*
Sulfonamides
  adverse effects, 679
  as cause of fever, *585t*
  distribution and elimination, 679
  in the intensive care unit, 679
Supraventricular tachyarrhythmias
  acute therapy in patients with, 321–327, *323f*, *324f*, *325f*, *326f*, *327f*
  in patients with accessory pathways, 325–327, *326f*, *327f*
Surfactant therapy, for acute lung injury/acute respiratory distress syndrome (ALI/ARDS), 413–414
Surgery. *See also* Lung transplantation
  abdominal compartment syndrome (ACS) and, 171–172, *171t*, *172t*
  anatomic site, technique, and duration, 396, *396t*, *397t*
  antifibrinolytic therapy for postoperative bleeding, 357
  approach to the patient, 6–8, *7f*
  for bleeding ulcer, 488–489, *489t*
  cardiac, 29, *30f–31f*, 346–362, 506–507, 781, *782t*
  cardiac risk stratification for noncardiac surgical procedures, *5t*
  cardiac surgery specific risk indices, 3, *4t*
  clinical evaluation in patients undergoing noncardiac surgery, 3–8, *4t*, *5t*, *6t*, *7f*
  considerations for perioperative pulmonary complications, 396–397

cost reduction of accelerated recovery, 355
fascial disruption and, 170
fluid requirements for, 141–142, *141t*, *142f*
guidelines for replacement of fluid shifts during, 142
importance of exercise tolerance, 5–6, *6t*
importance of surgical procedure, 5, *5t*
in the intensive care unit, 168–175, 346
intraoperative care, 33
management of infants and children after neurologic, 778–780
management of the open abdomen, 172–173
  biliary sepsis, 173
  enterocutaneous fistulas, 172–173
  necrotizing pancreatitis, 173
  tubes and drains, 172
perioperative
  renal protection, 506–509
perioperative management
  of the cardiac surgical patient, 346–362
  in infants and children, 781, *782t*
  of thoracic surgical patients, 417–427
peritonitis following, 171
physiologic response to surgical insult, 168–172, *171t*, *172t*
port-access, 355
postoperative care, 33
  deep-breathing maneuvers, 401
  fever, 169–170, 585–586
  hyponatremia, 212
  in kidney transplantation, 733–735
  in liver transplantation, 726–728, *728f*
  of the neurosurgical patient, 253–263
  of respiratory decompensation, 402–403, *402t*
  of the surgical patient, 174
during pregnancy, 508
preoperative care
  evaluation clinic, 32–33, *33t*, *34f*
  in kidney transplantation, 733
  in liver transplantation, 726, *727f*
  of the patient with endocrine disease, 9
risk of ischemic events after major vascular operation, 307, *309t*
stomas and, 170–171
surgical clinical pathways, 33
sustained systemic inflammatory response (SIRS) and, 169
timing, in subarachnoid hemorrhage, 268
tubes and drains following, 172
urogenital, 508
vascular, 507–508
video-assisted thoracoscopic, 419
Surgical intensive care unit (SICU), 346
  sepsis and, 601–615
  systemic inflammatory response syndrome and, 601–615
Sustained low-efficiency daily dialysis (SLED), for renal replacement therapy, 526
Sustained systemic inflammatory response, 169
SVN. *See* Small-volume nebulizers
SVR. *See* Systemic vascular resistance
Symadine (amantadine)
  adverse effects, 686

as antiviral prophylaxis, 640
distribution and elimination, 686
dosing, *622t*
for viral infections, 626
Symmetrel (amantadine)
adverse effects, 686
as antiviral prophylaxis, 640
distribution and elimination, 686
dosing, *622t*
for viral infections, 626
Sympathoadrenal stimulation, for cardiogenic
shock, 291
Sympathomimetic drugs. *See also* individual
drug names
for asthma, 378–379
for cardiogenic shock, 292
hypertension and, 337
interaction, 337
Synchronized intermittent mandatory
ventilation (SIMV), 354
Synchrony, definition, 454
Syndrome of inappropriate antidiuretic
hormone (SIADH), 212–213
pediatric, 779
Synercid (quinupristin-dalfopristin)
adverse effects, 681
distribution and elimination, 681
dosing, *623t*
in the intensive care unit, 680–681
for multiresistant gram-positive cocci, 623
Synergistic gangrene, 634
Synergy, 681
Syrup of ipecac
availability, 824
clinical studies, 824
complications, 824
contraindications, 824
dose, 824
for poisoning, 823–825, *825t*
Systemic analgesia, 425–426
Systemic inflammatory response syndrome
(SIRS), 601–615. *See also* Sepsis
care of the patient with multiple trauma
and, 794
continuous removal of cytokines in,
529–530
definitions, *602t*
fever and, 578–579
following surgery, 169
in the intensive care unit, 617
risk factors for developing, 602, *602t*
shock and, 192
treatment in the intensive care unit, 639
Systemic vascular resistance (SVR)
hypertension and, 334
in management of organ donors, 279
shock and, 193

T
Tachyarrhythmias, acute therapy in patients
with, 321–331
Tachycardia, airway management and, 99
Tacrolimus (FK506, Prograf)
agents potentially altering metabolism and
blood levels following liver
transplantation, 732, *732t*

following kidney transplantation, 734, *735t*
following liver transplantation, 732, *732t*
for intraoperative management of heart
transplantation, 703–704
for liver disease, 724
in pediatric transplantation, *784t*
for postoperative management of heart
transplantation, 707
in transplantation, *694t*, 695–696
Tamiflu (oseltamivir)
adverse effects, 686
as antiviral prophylaxis, 640
distribution and elimination, 686
for viral infections, 626
Task Force on Research in Cardiopulmonary
Dysfunction in Critical Care
Medicine, 72
Tazicef (ceftazidime), 620
Tazidime (ceftazidime), 620
Tazobactam, 674
Tazocin (piperacillin-tazobactam), 620
dosing, *622t*
TBI. *See* Traumatic brain injury
TBSA. *See* Total body surface area
TCD. *See* Transcranial Doppler
ultrasonography
T cells, 691. *See also* T-lymphocytes
⁹⁹ᵐ Tc-HMPAO. *See*
99mTc-hexa-methylpropylene
amine oxime
Technology. *See also* Medical informatics
research, 71
support for medical informatics, 83–84
wireless, 85
TEE. *See* Transesophageal echocardiography
TEG. *See* Thromboelastograph
Teicoplanin, 678
nephrotoxic effects, *745t*
Teleconferencing, 85
Temperature. *See also* Fever
control in perioperative management of
infants and children, 779
environmental heating in burn patients,
805
regulation in organ donors, 282
Tequin (gatifloxacin), 624
dosing, *623t*
Terbutaline, *441t*
TESS. *See* Toxic Exposure Surveillance System
Testing
for brain death, 277–278, *277t*
exercise, 399
fibrinolysis, 552
the immunocompromised patient,
653–655, *654f*
immunologic, in the critically ill patient,
178
positive direct antiglobulin (DAT), 568
preoperative pulmonary function tests,
397–398, 398–399, *398t*
primary hemostasis, 550–551, *551t*
pulmonary function in perioperative
evaluation, 381, *381f, 382f*
for renal dysfunction in the intensive care
unit, 509–511, *509t*
secondary hemostasis, 551–552

Tetanus, 159
Tetracyclines
adverse effects, 680
for bacteria in the intensive care unit, *673t*
distribution and elimination, 680
in the intensive care unit, 680
Tetralogy of Fallot, pediatric treatment,
781–782
THA. *See* Total hip arthroplasty
THAM. *See* Tris
(hydroxymethyl)-aminomethane
Theophylline
dosage adjustments in the intensive care
unit, *523t*
effect of heart failure on drug disposition,
188–189
evaluation and management for
intoxication of, 836–837
poisoning and, 829–830
toxic syndromes, *820t*
Therapeutic Intervention Scoring System
(TISS), 23–24
Therapy, research, 71
Thermodilution, principles of cardiac output
measurement, 127–128
Thiamine, 182
for poisoning, 822
Thiopental, for tracheal intubation, 92
Thioridazine, acquired prolonged
repolarization syndromes and, *329t*
Third-degree burns, 801
Thoracic computed tomography, 842–843
Thoracic impedance cardiography (TIC), to
determine cardiac output, 130
Thoracic spine injury, computed tomography
for detection of, 845–846
Thoracic surgery, perioperative care, 417–427
assessment, indications, and intraoperative
considerations, 417–420
bronchoscopy, 417–418
myasthenia gravis and thymoma,
419–420
operations for major airway obstruction,
418–419
key points, 426
postoperative care and complications,
420–424
air leakage, 421–422
airway obstruction, 421
atelectasis and mediastinal shift, 420
bronchopleural fistula, 422
bronchoscopy, 421
cardiac herniation, 423
dysrhythmias, 420
fluid management, 420
interpleural hemorrhage, 423
intrapulmonary hemorrhage, 422–423
lung transplantation, 424
mechanical ventilation, 421
myasthenia gravis, 424
pleural effusion, 423
pneumothorax, 422
postoperative infections, 424
postthoracotomy analgesia, 424
torsion or infarction, 423
T-tube insertion and changes, 421

Thoracic surgery, perioperative care (*contd.*)
  systemic analgesia, 425–426
    epidural analgesia, 425–426
    intercostal analgesia, 425
    interpleural analgesia, 425
    intrathecal opioids, 425
    paravertebral blockade, 426
    transcutaneous electric nerve stimulation
      (TENS), 426
Thoracic valvular disease, computed
    tomography for detection of, 846
Thoracoscopic surgery, video-assisted, 419
Thoracotomy, analgesia in postoperative care
    of thoracic surgical patients, 424
Thrombectomy, for mesenteric ischemia, 480
Thrombin inhibitors, for acute coronary
    syndromes, *314t*
Thrombin time (TT), with perioperative
    hemostasis and coagulopathy, 552
Thrombocytopenia
  causes, 554, *554t*
  heparin-induced, 562
  hereditary, 555, *556t*
  with microangiopathic hemolysis, 563–564
  with perioperative hemostasis and
    coagulopathy, 561–562
Thromboelastogram, *497f, 498f*
Thromboelastograph (TEG), for
    perioperative hemostasis and
    coagulopathy, 552–553, *553f*
Thrombolysis, outcome versus heparin in
    clinical trials for pulmonary
    embolism, 543–544, *544t*
Thrombolytic agents
  for cerebral ischemia, 260
  effect on coagulation, 313–314
  for pulmonary embolism, 543, *543t*
Thrombosis, *476t*
Thrombotic microangiopathy (TM), with
    hematopoietic stem cell
    transplantation, 748–749
Thrombotic thrombocytopenic purpura
    (TTP), with perioperative
    hemostasis and coagulopathy, 553
Thromboxane, in animal studies for acute
    renal failure, *522t*
Thymectomy, for myasthenia gravis, 420
Thymoma, in perioperative care of thoracic
    surgical patients, 419–420
Thyroid disease
  as an emergency, 754–757
  diagnosis, 755, *755t*
  preoperative assessment, 9
  thyroid storm, 756–757
Thyroid hormone, for cardiogenic shock, 293
Thyroxine, in animal studies for acute renal
    failure, *522t*
TIC. *See* Thoracic impedance cardiography
Ticarcillin-clavulanate (Timentin), 620
Ticarcillin (Ticar), 620
  dosing, *622t*
Ticarillin-clavulanate (Timentin)
  dosing, *622t*
Ticar (ticarcillin), 620
  dosing, *622t*
Ticlopidine, effect on coagulation, 313

Timentin (ticarcillin-clavulanate), 620
  dosing, *622t*
TIPS. *See* Transjugular intrahepatic
    portosystemic stent-shunt
Tirofiban
  for acute coronary syndromes, *314t*
  effect on coagulation, 313
TISS. *See* Therapeutic Intervention Scoring
    System
Tissue analysis, for consciousness testing,
    251t
Tissue-factor pathway, 549, *550f*
Tissue hypoperfusion, fluid status, assessment,
    and monitoring, 143–145, *145t*
Tissue plasminogen activator (TPA), for
    cerebral ischemia, 260
Title 22, California Administrative Code, 23
TLC. *See* Total lung capacity
T-lymphocytes. *See also* T cells
  in transplantation, 691
TM. *See* Thrombotic microangiopathy
TMLR. *See* Transmyocardial laser
    revascularization
TMP. *See* Trimethoprim-sulfamethoxazole
TMP-SMX. *See*
    Trimethoprim-sulfamethoxazole
TNF. *See* Tumor necrosis factor
Tobacco use. *See also* Smoking
  preoperative assessment of patient, 8
  risk for coronary artery disease, 5
Tobramycin
  dosage adjustments in the intensive care
    unit, *523t*
  dosing, *623t*
Tobramycin sulfate, 676
Toddlers. *See* Pediatric care
TOF. *See* Train-of-four ratio
Tolypocladium inflatum gams, 695
Torsades de pointes, 328, *329t*
Torsion, in postoperative care of thoracic
    surgical patients, 423
Torulopsis glabrata, 656
Total body surface area (TBSA)
  calculating percentage burned, 802, *803t*
  incidence and mortality related to burns,
    809, *809t*
  influence of age on, 802, *802f*
Total body water (TBW), 137, *138f*
Total hip arthroplasty (THA), 569–570
Total lung capacity (TLC), 375
Total parenteral nutrition (TPN)
  in the critically ill patient, 181
  daily requirements of trace elements in,
    182t
  for mechanical obstruction, 477
Toxic Exposure Surveillance System (TESS),
    818
Toxicity
  of amphotericin B, 625
  diarrhea and, 476
  nitric oxide, 229–230
  oxygen, 433
    mechanical ventilation and, 455
  in pediatric multiorgan failure, 788
Toxicology screens, 820–821
Toxic shock syndrome (TSS), 635–636

  initial therapy for life-threatening, *629t*
  menstruation and, 636
Toxic syndromes, 819, *819t*
Toxins
  as cause of fulminant hepatic failure, 495
  evacuation of unabsorbed, 822–826, *824t,*
    825t
  shock and, 195
Toxoplasma gondii, 617, 649, 653, 677
  following liver transplantation, 730
  in postoperative management of heart
    transplantation, 709
Toxoplasma spp., following kidney
    transplantation, 734
TPA. *See* Tissue plasminogen activator
TPN. *See* Total parenteral nutrition
Trace elements, administration in the
    critically ill patient, 182, *182t*
Tracheal intubation, 89–101
  changing the endotracheal tube, 97–98
  difficult airway, 96–97, *97f*
  equipment, 91, *91f*
  extubating patients in the intensive care
    unit, 98–99
    complications, 99
    reintubating patients for whom
      extubation fails, 98–99
  indications for, 89, *90t*
  key points, 100
  medical evaluation, 89, *90t*
  neuromuscular blocking agents and, 92
  patient assessment before, 89–91, *90t*
  patient preparation, 91–92
  procedures for, 92–96, *93f, 94f, 95f, 96f*
    fiberoptic intubation, 95–96, *95f*
    intubating laryngeal mask airway, 96,
      96f
    nasotracheal intubation, 94–95
    orotracheal intubation with rigid
      laryngoscope, 94, *94f*
Tracheal resection, 419
Tracheobronchial tears, computed
    tomography for detection of, 845
Tracheostomy, percutaneous dilational,
    118–119, *118f, 118t, 119f*
Tracheostomy collars, 431
Tracrium (atracurium), for intensive care unit
    use, *155t,* 157, 164
Training, for the preoperative patient, 397
Train-of-four (TOF) ratio, 98, 159, *160f,*
    160t
TRALI. *See* Transfusion-related acute lung
    injury
Transcranial Doppler (TCD) ultrasonography
  to identify cerebral hyperperfusion
    syndrome, 254
  to identify vasospasm after subarachnoid
    hemorrhage, 256
Transcutaneous electric nerve stimulation
    (TENS), in postoperative care of
    thoracic surgical patients, 426
Transesophageal echocardiography (TEE)
  for cardiac surgical patients, 346
  compared with radionuclide angiography,
    134
  complete examination, *113f*

hemodynamic assessment and, 132–134, *132t, 133t*
  in the intensive care unit, 111–112
    indications for, *112t*
  perioperative practice guidelines, *133t*
Transfusion. *See* Blood transfusion
Transfusion-related acute lung injury (TRALI), 569
Transjugular intrahepatic portosystemic stent-shunt (TIPS), for portal hypertension, 490
Transmyocardial laser revascularization (TMLR), 356–357
Transplantation. *See also* Organ donors
  anesthetic management, 282
  biology of, 690–698
  cardiopulmonary, 699–723
  cardiovascular effects and interactions, 278–280, *279f*
  clonal anergy, 690
  diagnosis and management of brain-dead and nonheart-beating organ donors, 275–286
  endocrine effects, 280–281, *280f, 281f*
  fluids and electrolytes, 281–282
  heart, perioperative management in infants and children, 786
  heart–lung, 378
  hematopoietic stem cell, 740–751
  history, 275–276
  immunobiology, 691–693
    rejection
      mediated by antibody, 691
      mediated by T-lymphocytes, 691
      role of cytokines in rejection and graft injury, 691–692
      role of major histocompatibility complex in rejection, 692–693, *692f, 693f*
  immunosuppressive medications in pediatric, 783, *784t*
  induction of immunologic tolerance, 690–691
  infections
    in bone marrow transplant recipients, 662–663, *662f*
    in the renal transplant patient, 659–660, *659f*
    in transplant recipients, 657–662, *659f*
  key points, 284, 698
  kidney, 733–735
    perioperative management in infants and children, 785–786
  liver, 500, 724–732, 834
    perioperative management in infants and children, 785
  lung, perioperative management in infants and children, 786
  multivisceral abdominal organ, perioperative management in infants and children, 786
  nonheart-beating organ donors, 282–283
  organ donor procurement procedure, 282
  orthotopic heart transplant, 351
  pancreas, 735–737
  of the pancreas, 281
  pediatric, *784t*
  perioperative management in infants and children, 783–786
  pharmacologic immunosuppression, 693–698, *694t*
    anti-IL-2 receptor-α (CD25), 697–698
    antilymphocyte globulin, 697
    azathioprine, 694
    corticosteroids, 693–694, *694t*
    cyclosporine, 695, *696t*
    mycophenolate mofetil (MMF), 695
    OKT3, 697
    sirolimus, 696–697
    tacrolimus, 695–696
  posttransplantation infections, 660
    perioperative management in infants and children, 784–785
  posttransplant rejection, perioperative management in infants and children, 7830784
  preoperative management in infants and children, 783
  respiratory management, 280
  temperature regulation and coagulation, 282
Transpulmonary thermodilution, in the intensive care unit, 111, *112f*
Transthoracic echocardiography (TTE), in the intensive care unit, 116, *117f*
Transurethral resection of the prostate (TURP), 2
Tranylcypromine (Parnate), for hypertension, 337
Trauma, *476t. See also* Injuries
  care of the head-injured patient, 796–797
  care of the patient with blunt cardiac injury, 797
  care of the patient with increased abdominal pressure, 797
  care of the patient with multiple trauma, 791–800
  chest wall, computed tomography for detection of, 846
  coagulopathy and, 793–794
  evaluation with computed tomography in the intensive care unit, 855
  head, neuromuscular blocking agents and, 164
  hypothermia and, 793–794
  immune dysfunction and, 794
    cytokine levels after trauma, 794
    immunomodulatory therapies, 794
  in the intensive care unit, 168
  key points, 798
  multiple, 791–800
  nutritional support and, 794–796
    assessment of nutritional requirements, 795–796
    early enteral nutrition, 796
    stress versus starvation, 795
  outcome of oxygen delivery to, 145, *145t*
  perioperative renal protection and, 508–509
  renal dysfunction in, 792–793
  resuscitation of the patient with, 791–792
  ventilatory support and, 792
Trauma Injury Severity Score (TRISS), 11

Traumatic brain injury (TBI), 228, 236–239
  intracranial hypertension, 236–239
    fluid therapy, 239
    heroics, 239
    management, 238–239
    pathophysiology and treatment rationale, 236–238
  key points, 242
  principles of neurosurgical critical care and initial resuscitation, 236, *237t*
Treacher Collins syndrome, *779t*
Treatment
  foregoing policies, 47
  patient refusal of, 46
  withdrawal of life-sustaining, 48–49, *49f*
Trendelenburg position, for subclavian venous catheterization, 108
Treponema pallidum, 674
Triamcinalone acetonide, *441t*
Triazoles, *683t*
Trichomonas spp., 679
Trichosporon, 625, 656
  following liver transplantation, 731
  recommended regimens for treatment of multiresistant, *638t*
  recommended therapy for life-threatening, *625t*
Tricyclic amines
  adverse effects, 686
  distribution and elimination, 686
  in the intensive care unit, 686
Tricyclic antidepressants
  acquired prolonged repolarization syndromes and, *329t*
  as cause of fulminant hepatic failure, 495
  as cause of qualitative platelet disorders, *555t*
Trifluoperazine, acquired prolonged repolarization syndromes and, *329t*
Trimethoprim-sulfamethoxazole (TMP-SMX)
  antibiotic management of renal and hepatic dysfunction in the intensive care unit, *675t*
  for bacteria in the intensive care unit, *673t*
  dosing, *622t, 623t*
  in immunocompromised patients, *652t*
Tris (hydroxymethyl)-aminomethane (THAM), 792
TRISS. *See* Trauma Injury Severity Score
True shunting, 429
TSS. *See* Toxic shock syndrome
TT. *See* Thrombin time
TTE. *See* Transthoracic echocardiography
TTP. *See* Thrombotic thrombocytopenic purpura
T-tube insertion, 419
Tubes. *See also* Extubation; Reintubations
  computed tomography for detection of malpositioned chest, 846
  feeding problems and their causes, 180, *180t*
  following surgery, 172
  techniques for placement in the critically ill patient, 181
  T-tube insertion in postoperative care of thoracic surgical patients, 421

Tubocurarine (curare), for intensive care unit use, *155t*

Tubular function tests
creatine clearance, 510–511, *510f, 510t*
and evaluation of oliguria, 509–511, *509t*
sodium conservation, 509–510
tubular concentrating ability, 509

Tubular necrosis, perioperative renal protection and, 504–506

Tumor lysis syndrome, 744

Tumor necrosis factor (TNF)
blood transfusions and, 568
during catabolic phase of response to injury, 176

Tumors
carcinoid syndrome, 760
hemorrhage in the critically ill, 492
infections associated with, *618t*
pheochromocytoma, 759–760

Turner syndrome, *779t*

TURP. *See* Transurethral resection of the prostate

Two-dimensional examination, in the intensive care unit, 112–116, *113f, 114f, 115f, 116f, 116t, 117f*

Typhlitis, 633–634
evaluation with computed tomography in the intensive care unit, 853

Typhus, 680

Tyrosine
for shock, 202, *202f*

U

UGIB. *See* Upper gastrointestinal bleeding

Unasyn (ampicillin-sulbactam), 620
dosing, *622t*

Uniform Anatomical Gift Act, 76

Uniform Determination of Death Act, 275

United Network for Organ Sharing (UNOS), 283, 726
for heart transplantation, 702
for liver transplantation, 500

UNOS. *See* United Network for Organ Sharing

UPET. *See* Urokinase Pulmonary Embolism Trial

Upper gastrointestinal bleeding (UGIB), 485–492, *486t*
causes, *486t*

UpToDate, 58

Urinary tract infection, as source of fever, 584

Urine
flow rate and oliguria, 509
nutrition and, 179
output in the cardiac surgical patient, 348

Urogenital surgery, perioperative renal protection, 508

Urokinase, for pulmonary embolism, 537–538

Urokinase Pulmonary Embolism Trial (UPET), 537–538

Urokinase-Streptokinase Pulmonary Embolism Trials (USPET), 537–538

Urosepsis, 634
initial therapy for life-threatening, *629t*
recommended therapy for life-threatening, *624t*

U.S. Food and Drug Administration (FDA), 342, 440
drug alerts, 81
role of the principal investigator and, 75

U.S. Renal Data System (USRDS), 695

The User's Guides to the Medical Literature, 56

USPET. *See* Urokinase-Streptokinase Pulmonary Embolism Trials

USRDS. *See* U.S. Renal Data System

V

Vancomycin, 677–678
adverse effects, 678
antibiotic management of renal and hepatic dysfunction in the intensive care unit, *675t*
for bacteria in the intensive care unit, *673t*
distribution and elimination, 678
dosage adjustments in the intensive care unit, *523t*
dosing, *623t*
for infections, 621, 623
for methicillin-resistant *Staphylococcus aureus* (MRSA), 621
nephrotoxic effects, *745t*
for pneumonia, 389
resistance, 682–683
side effects, 621, 623
for toxic shock syndrome, 635

Vancomycin hydrochloride, in immunocompromised patients, *652t*

VAP. *See* Ventilator-associated pneumonia

Varicella-zoster virus (VZV), 616, 651
as complication of hematopoietic stem cell transplantation, 747–748, *748t*
recommended therapy for life-threatening, *627t*

VAS. *See* Visual analog scale

Vascular anastomosis, *476t*

Vascular anomalies
diagnosis, 491
lower gastrointestinal bleeding and, 492
pathogenesis, 491
treatment, 492
upper gastrointestinal bleeding and, 491–492

Vascular surgery, perioperative renal protection, 507–508

Vasoactive mediators, in multiple organ dysfunction syndrome, 590–592

Vasoconstrictor agents
for cardiogenic shock, 296
shock and, 201–202

Vasodilation, catechol-resistant, 608

Vasodilators
abnormal cardioactive response in the denervated heart, 706–707, *706t*
in acute lung injury/acute respiratory distress syndrome (ALI/ARDS), 414

for cardiac insufficiency as complication of hematopoietic stem cell transplantation, 745
for hypertension in the intensive care unit, 340
for pediatric treatment of postoperative cardiac failure, 782
pharmacologic stress for detection of coronary artery disease, 7
shock and, 202–203
side effects, 340

Vasomotor nephropathy, 505

Vasopressin
for cardiogenic shock, 293–294, *293t*
in cardiopulmonary resuscitation, 369
for hypernatremia, 215
for portal hypertension, 489–490
for shock, 201–202

Vasopressor agents
in cardiopulmonary resuscitation, 368–369
for prevention and treatment of renal injury, 516–517
sepsis and, 610–612
shock and, 200, *201t*

Vasospasm
after subarachnoid hemorrhage, 256–258, *257f, 258f, 258t*
complications, 271

VATS. *See* Video-assisted thoracoscopic surgery

Vecuronium (norcuron), for intensive care unit use, *155t*, 157, 164

VEDP. *See* Ventricular end-diastolic pressure

VEDV. *See* Ventricular end-diastolic volume

Vegetative state, persistent, 249–250

Venoocclusive disease (VOD), with hematopoietic stem cell transplantation, 744

Venous thromboembolism (VTE). *See also* Pulmonary embolism
in the critically ill patient, 533–548
diagnostic findings, 538–540, *539t*
incidence and presentation, 536–538, *537t, 538t*
key points, 545
prophylaxis, 401–402, *401t*, 537, *538t*
risk factors for, *537t*

Ventilation
in cardiopulmonary resuscitation, 364
care of the patient with multiple trauma and, 792
clinical practice guidelines—evidence-based weaning recommendations, 471
high-frequency, 453
management protocols, 456
mechanical, in acute lung injury/acute respiratory distress syndrome (ALI/ARDS), 412–413
modes of ventilatory support, *450t*
in multiple organ dysfunction syndrome, 595
noninvasive assistance, 402–403
noninvasive positive pressure in postoperative patients, 403
patient interface complications, 455

perioperative support, 404
positive-pressure and cardiac function, 455
pressure support, 354
proportional assist, 455
respiratory system mechanics, 448–450
  distribution of ventilation, 449–450,
    451f
  equation of motion, 448–449
  intrinsic positive end-expiratory pressure
    and the ventilatory pattern, 449
  pressure targeted versus flow/volume
    targeted breaths, 449
synchronized intermittent mandatory, 354
ventilator-derived flow pattern, 453–455,
  455f
weaning, 354, 457, 460–473
  in the cardiac surgical patient, 354
  duration, 460, *461f*
  randomized controlled trials, 460–465
Ventilation-perfusion (V/Q) lung scanning,
  shock and, 194
Ventilator-associated pneumonia (VAP),
  389–391
autopsy studies, 390
diagnosis, 390–391
mechanisms, 389, *389f*
prevention, 391
as source of fever, 583–584, *584f*
tracheal intubation and, 91
treatment, 391
Ventilator-induced lung injury, 410
Ventricular dysrhythmias, in the cardiac
  surgical patient, 352
Ventricular end-diastolic pressure (VEDP),
  shock and, 195
Ventricular end-diastolic volume (VEDV),
  shock and, 195
Ventricular septal rupture, cardiogenic shock
  and, 294–295
Ventricular tachyarrhythmias, acute therapy
  in patients with, 327–328, *327f,
  328f, 329f, 329t, 330t*
Ventricular tachycardia
  diagnosis, 327, *328f*
  hyperkalemic, 329, *330f*
Venturi mask, 431–432, *432f*
Verapamil
  for acute myocardial ischemia, 313
  as antihypertensive drug, 342–343,
    342t
  for multifocal atrial tachycardia, 324
  for rate control in atrial flutter or atrial
    fibrillation, 322–323
Vestibuloocular reflex (VOR), 247–248
Vibration, for airway management, 435
Video-assisted thoracoscopic surgery (VATS),
  419
Vinblastine sulfate, as cause of qualitative
  platelet disorders, *555t*
Vinca alkaloids, for autoimmune
  thrombocytopenia purpura,
  562–563
Vincristine sulfate, as cause of qualitative
  platelet disorders, *555t*
Viral infections, recommended therapy for
  life-threatening, *627t*

Viral meningoencephalitis, 633
Virazole (ribavirin), 626
  for viral infections, 626
Virchow triad of stasis, 536, *537t*
Vistide (cidofovir)
  dosing, *622t*
  for viral infections, 626
Visual analog scale (VAS), 150
VisualCare, 82
Vitamin A, 182
Vitamin B$_6$, for overdose of isoniazid, *830t*
Vitamin B$_{12}$, 177
Vitamin C, 177, 182
Vitamin D, 177
  in parathyroid disease, 753
Vitamin E, 177, 182
Vitamin K, 182
  deficiency with perioperative hemostasis
    and coagulopathy, 558–559, *559f*
  for fulminant hepatic failure, 499
  for nutritional support with acute renal
    failure, 524
Vitamins
  antioxidant, 182
  for nutrition support in the critically ill
    patient, 182
VOD. *See* Venoocclusive disease
Volatile anesthetics, as cause of fulminant
  hepatic failure, 495
Volume homeostasis
  body fluid compartments, 137, *138f*
  distribution of infused fluids, 137
  physiological principles, 137–139,
    138f
  prediction of plasma volume expansion
    using kinetic analysis, 137–138
  regulation of extracellular fluid volume,
    138–139
Volume of distribution (V$_d$), 190
Volume reservoir (capacitance), definition,
  534
Volume resuscitation, in management of
  organ donors, 281
Vomiting
  poisoning and, 823
  tube feeding problems and, *180t*
von Willibrand factor (vWF), in normal
  hemostasis, 549
VOR. *See* Vestibuloocular reflex
Voriconazole, 685
V/Q. *See* Ventilation-perfusion lung scanning
VTE. *See* Venous thromboembolism
VZV. *See* Varicella-zoster virus

W
Water
  maintenance requirements for fluid
    replacement therapy, 140–141
  principles of removal by dialysis, 524–525
WBC. *See* White blood cell count
Wernicke encephalopathy, 822
West Nile encephalitis virus, 633
White blood cell (WBC) count, in
  immunocompromised patients,
  653
Whole-bowel irrigation, for poisoning, 829

Wide-complex tachyarrhythmias, acute
  therapy in patients with, 328–330,
  330f, 331f
William syndrome, *779t*
Wolff-Parkinson-White syndrome, 321,
  325–326, *326f, 327f*
Wounds
  biological dressings as alternatives to topical
    antimicrobial agents, 807-808
  burn-wound pathology, 801
  complications in the intensive care unit,
    170
  control of infection by conservative
    methods, 806–807
  debridement, 807–808
  excision of burn wounds, 808
  management of acute burns, 806–808
  use of cadaver allograft, 808, *808t*

X
Xenografting, for fulminant hepatic failure,
  500
Xenon-enhanced computed tomography, for
  determination of brain death, 278
X fragment, 550

Y
Yersinia enterocolitica, blood transfusions and,
  567–568
Yersinia spp., 476
Y fragment, 550

Z
Zafirlukast (Accolate), for asthma, 379
Zanamivir (Relenza), for viral infections, 626
Zemuron (rocuronium), for intensive care
  unit use, *155t*, 157, 164
Zenapax (daclizumab), following kidney
  transplantation, 734, *735t*
Ziehl-Nielson stain, 653
Zinc, daily requirements in total parenteral
  nutrition, *182t*
Zithromax (azithromycin), 621
  for babesiosis, 636
  dosing, *622t*
Zoster, recommended therapy for
  life-threatening, *627t*
Zosyn (piperacillin-tazobactam), 620–621
Zovirax (acyclovir)
  adverse effects, 686
  as antiviral prophylaxis, 640
  distribution and elimination, 686
  dosing, *622t*
  in immunocompromised patients, *652t*
  nephrotoxic effects, *745t*
  for viral infections, 626
Zygomycetes, recommended therapy for
  life-threatening, *625t*
Zyvox (linezolid)
  adverse effects, 680
  antibiotic management of renal and hepatic
    dysfunction in the intensive care
    unit, *675t*
  distribution and elimination, 680
  dosing, *623t*
  for multiresistant gram-positive cocci, 623

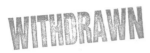